D1311292

Diseases OF THE Nervous System Clinical Neurobiology

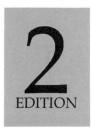

2 EDITION

Diseases OF THE Nervous System Clinical Neurobiology Volume I

Edited by

Arthur K. Asbury, M.D.

Van Meter Professor of Neurology
Vice Dean for Research
University of Pennsylvania School of Medicine
Philadelphia, Pennsylvania

Guy M. McKhann, M.D.

Professor of Neurology
Director
The Zanvyl Krieger Mind/Brain Institute
Johns Hopkins University
Baltimore, Maryland

W. Ian McDonald, Ph.D., F.R.C.P.

Professor of Clinical Neurology
Institute of Neurology
Honorary Consultant Physician
National Hospital for Neurology and Neurosurgery
Queen Square and
Moorfield's Eye Hospital
London

with 150 contributors

W.B. SAUNDERS COMPANY

Harcourt Brace Jovanovich, Inc.

Philadelphia   London   Toronto   Montreal   Sydney   Tokyo

W. B. SAUNDERS COMPANY
Harcourt Brace Jovanovich, Inc.

The Curtis Center
Independence Square West
Philadelphia, Pennsylvania 19106

Library of Congress Cataloging-in-Publication Data

Diseases of the nervous system : clinical neurobiology / [edited by] Arthur K. Asbury, Guy M. McKhann, W. Ian McDonald.—2nd ed.

p. cm

ISBN 0–7216–3208–4

1. Nervous system—Diseases.   2. Neurobiology.
   I. Asbury, Arthur K.   II. McKhann, Guy M.
   III. McDonald, W. Ian.

[DNLM: 1. Nervous System Diseases. WL 100 D611]

RC346.D56 1992

616.8—dc20

DNLM/DLC   91-43058

Editor: Linda Mills
Developmental Editor: Kathleen McCarthy
Designer: Nina McDaid Ikeda
Cover Designer: Michelle Maloney
Production Manager: Bill Preston
Manuscript Editors: Judith Gandy, Mary Prescott, and Terry Russell
Illustration Specialist: Peg Shaw
Indexer: Katherine Garcia

Diseases of the Nervous System: Clinical Neurobiology   ISBN 0–7216–3209–2 Volume I
                                                                     0–7216–3211–4 Volume II
                                                                     0–7216–3208–4 set

Copyright © 1992, 1986, by W. B. Saunders Company

All rights reserved. No part of this publication may be reproduced or transmitted in any form or by any means, electronic or mechanical, including photocopy, recording, or any information storage and retrieval system, without permission in writing from the publisher.

Printed in United States of America.

Last digit is the print number: 9   8   7   6   5   4   3   2   1

*This monograph is dedicated
to our many friends and colleagues
who wrote the chapters,
for their diligence, for their intellectual rigor,
and for their belief in the vision of
scientific and clinical excellence
on which these volumes are predicated.*

Contributors

Marilyn S. Albert, Ph.D.
Associate Professor of Psychiatry and Neurology, Harvard Medical School; Attending Physician, Massachusetts General Hospital, Boston, Massachusetts
The Effects of Age: Normal Variation and Its Relation to Disease

Garrett E. Alexander, M.D., Ph.D.
Professor of Neurology, Department of Neurology, Emory University School of Medicine; Active Staff, Emory University Hospital, Atlanta, Georgia
Central Mechanisms of Initiation and Control of Movement

Michael J. Aminoff, M.D., F.R.C.P.
Professor of Neurology, Department of Neurology, School of Medicine, University of California, San Francisco; Attending Physician, University of California Medical Center, San Francisco, California
Aneurysms and Vascular Malformations

Barry G.W. Arnason, M.D.
Professor, Pritzker School of Medicine, University of Chicago; Attending Physician, Chief of Neurology Service, Bernard Mitchell Hospital, University of Chicago, Chicago, Illinois
Cell-Mediated Immunity and Neurologic Disease

Arthur K. Asbury, M.D.
Ruth Wagner Van Meter and J. Ray Van Meter Professor of Neurology and Vice Dean for Research, University of Pennsylvania School of Medicine, Philadelphia, Pennsylvania
Pathophysiology of Nervous System Diseases; Disorders of Peripheral Nerve

Michael Baraitser, F.R.C.P.
Consultant Clinical Geneticist at the Hospital for Sick Children, London, United Kingdom
Neurocutaneous Disorders

Robert L. Barchi, M.D., Ph.D.
David Mahoney Professor of Neuroscience, University of Pennsylvania School of Medicine, Philadelphia, Pennsylvania
Pathophysiology of Myotonia and Periodic Paralysis

J. Richard Baringer, M.D.
Professor and Chairman, Department of Neurology, University of Utah School of Medicine; Chief, Neurology Service, University Hospital; Staff Neurologist, Veterans Administration Medical Center, Salt Lake City, Utah
Viral Infections

David Barnes, M.D.
Senior Registrar, Institute of Neurology; Senior Registrar in Neurology, Guys Hospital, London, United Kingdom
Diseases of the Optic Nerve

Günter Baumgartner, M.D.
Late Professor of Neurology, Faculty of Medicine, University of Zürich; Director, Department of Neurology, University Hospital, Zürich, Switzerland
Psychophysics and Central Processing

Christopher D. Betts, M.B.Ch.B., F.R.C.S. Ed.
Research Registrar, National Hospital for Neurology and Neurosurgery; Urology Registrar, Royal London Hospital, London, United Kingdom
Sexual Dysfunction in Neurologic Disease; Bladder Dysfunction in Neurologic Disease

A. Lorris Betz, M.D., Ph.D.
Professor, Departments of Pediatrics and Neurosurgery, University of Michigan School of Medicine; Attending Physician, University of Michigan Hospitals, Ann Arbor, Michigan
Blood Vessels and the Blood-Brain Barrier

Shawn J. Bird, M.D., Ph.D.
Assistant Professor of Neurology, University of Pennsylvania; Staff Neurologist, Hospital of the University of Pennsylvania, Philadelphia, Pennsylvania
Disorders of Peripheral Nerve

Peter M. Black, M.D., Ph.D.
Frank D. Ingram Professor of Neurosurgery, Harvard Medical School; Neurosurgeon in Chief, Brigham and Women's Hospital and Children's Hospital, Boston, Massachusetts
Chronic Increased Intracranial Pressure

Charles F. Bolton, M.D., C.M., F.R.C.P.C.
Professor of Neurology, Department of Clinical Neurological Sciences, Faculty of Medicine, The University of Western Ontario; Professor of Neurology and Director, EMG Laboratory, Victoria Hospital, London, Ontario, Canada
Neurologic Manifestations of Renal Diseases

Thomas Brandt, M.D.
Professor and Chairman of Neurology, University of Munich; Director of Neurology, Klinikum Grosshadern, University of Munich, Munich, Germany
Vertigo and Dizziness

Richard P. Bunge, M.D.
Professor of Neurological Surgery and Cell Biology and Anatomy, University of Miami School of Medicine, Miami, Florida
The Cell of Schwann

David Burke, M.D., D.Sc., F.R.A.C.P.
Professor of Clinical Neurophysiology, University of New South Wales School of Medicine; Neurologist, The Prince Henry and Prince of Wales Hospitals, Sydney, Australia
The Myotatic Unit and Its Disorders

John J. Caronna, M.D.
Professor of Clinical Neurology, Cornell University Medical College; Attending Neurologist, The New York Hospital, New York, New York
Neurologic Manifestations of Cardiac Diseases

Paul E. Cooper, M.D., F.R.C.P.C.
Associate Professor, Department of Clinical Neurological Sciences and Department of Medicine, The University of Western Ontario; Chief of Clinical Neurological Sciences, St. Joseph's Health Centre, London, Ontario, Canada
Hypothalamic-Pituitary Function and Dysfunction

James J. Corbett, M.D.
Professor and Chairman of Neurology and Professor of Ophthalmology, Department of Neurology, University of Mississippi Medical Center; Attending Physician, University of Mississippi Medical Center, Methodist Rehabilitation Hospital, Jackson, Mississippi
Pupillary Function and Dysfunction

W. Maxwell Cowan, B.M.B.Ch., D.Phil., F.R.S.
Vice-President and Chief Scientific Officer; Howard Hughes Medical Institute, Bethesda, Maryland
Development of the Nervous System

Thomas O. Crawford, M.D.
Assistant Professor of Neurology, Johns Hopkins University; Attending Physician, Active Full-Time Staff, Johns Hopkins Hospital, Baltimore, Maryland
Pathophysiology of Neuronal and Axonal Degenerations; Motor Neuron Diseases

Antonio R. Damasio, M.D., Ph.D.
Professor of Neurology, University of Iowa College of Medicine; Professor and Head, Department of Neurology, University of Iowa Hospitals and Clinics, Iowa City, Iowa
The Agnosias

Larry E. Davis, M.D., F.A.C.P.
Professor of Neurology and Microbiology, University of New Mexico School of Medicine; Chief, Neurology Service, Veterans Administration Medical Center, Albuquerque, New Mexico
Spirochetal Disease

David M. Dawson, M.D.
Associate Professor of Neurology, Harvard Medical School; Chief, Neurology Service, Brockton/West Roxbury Veterans Administration Hospital, Boston, Massachusetts
Antineoplastic Drugs

Mahlon R. DeLong, M.D.
Professor and Chairman, Department of Neurology, Emory University School of Medicine; Active Staff, Emory University Hospital, Atlanta, Georgia
Central Mechanisms of Initiation and Control of Movement

Martha Bridge Denckla, M.D.
Professor of Neurology and Pediatrics, Johns Hopkins University School of Medicine; Director, Developmental Neurobehavior Clinic, The Kennedy Institute, Baltimore, Maryland
Developmental Dyslexia

J. Raymond DePaulo
Associate Professor, Johns Hopkins University School of Medicine; Director, Affective Disorders Clinic, Johns Hopkins Hospital, Baltimore, Maryland
Neurologic Complications of Psychotropic Drugs

Ivan Diamond, M.D., Ph.D.
Professor and Vice-Chair, Department of Neurology, and Professor of Pediatrics and Pharmacology, University of California, San Francisco; Director, Ernest Gallo Clinic and Research Center, University of California, San Francisco; Attending and Consulting Physician, Neurology, University of California, San Francisco, San Francisco General Hospital, and Veterans Administration Hospital, San Francisco, California
Alcohol Neurotoxicity

Mark A. Dichter, M.D., Ph.D.
Professor of Neurology, University of Pennsylvania; Director, Comprehensive Epilepsy Center, Graduate Hospital, Philadelphia, Pennsylvania
Cellular Pathophysiology and Pharmacology of Epilepsy

Salvatore DiMauro, M.D.
Professor of Neurology, Columbia-Presbyterian Medical Center, New York, New York
Pathophysiology of Metabolic Myopathies

James O. Donaldson III, M.D.
Professor of Neurology, University of Connecticut, School of Medicine, Farmington, Connecticut
Neurologic Complications of Pregnancy

Richard L. Doty, Ph.D.
Associate Professor of Psychology in Otorhinolaryngology–Head and Neck Surgery, University of Pennsylvania School of Medicine; Director, Smell and Taste Center, Hospital of the University of Pennsylvania, Philadelphia, Pennsylvania
Smell and Taste and Their Disorders

Daniel B. Drachman, M.D.
Professor of Neurology and Neurosciences, Johns Hopkins University; Director, Neuromuscular Unit, Attending Physician, Active Full-Time Staff, Johns Hopkins Hospital, Baltimore, Maryland
Motor Neuron Diseases

Paul Eslinger, Ph.D.
Associate Professor, Department of Neurology, Penn State University College of Medicine and Milton F. Hershey Medical Center, Hershey, Pennsylvania
The Agnosias

Stanley Fahn, M.D.
H. Houston Merritt Professor of Neurology, Columbia University College of Physicians and Surgeons; Attending Neurologist, Neurological Institute of New York, Presbyterian Hospital, New York, New York
Parkinson's Disease and Other Basal Ganglion Disorders

Kenneth H. Fischbeck, M.D.
Associate Professor of Neurology, University of Pennsylvania School of Medicine; Physician, Hospital of the University of Pennsylvania, Philadelphia, Pennsylvania
Structure and Function of Striated Muscle

David R. Fish, M.A., M.R.C.P., M.D.
Senior Lecturer in Clinical Neurophysiology, Institute of Neurology and National Hospitals for Neurology and Neurosurgery; Honorary Consultant in Clinical Neurophysiology, National Hospital for Neurology and Neurosurgery, London, United Kingdom
Disorders of Sleep

Robert A. Fishman, M.D.
Professor and Chairman, Department of Neurology, University of California, San Francisco; Chief, Neurology Service, University of California, San Francisco; Consultant in Neurology, San Francisco General Hospital and Veterans Administration Hospital, San Francisco, California
Neurologic Manifestations of Electrolyte Disorders

Christopher G. Fowler, M.R.C.P., F.R.C.S. Urol.
Senior Lecturer in Urology, The London Hospital Medical College, University of London; Consultant Urological Surgeon, The Royal London Hospital and Community Trust and Newham Health Authority; Honorary Consultant Urological Surgeon, The National Hospital for Neurology and Neurosurgery, London, United Kingdom
Sexual Dysfunction in Neurologic Disease; Bladder Dysfunction in Neurologic Disease

Clare J. Fowler, M.Sc., M.R.C.P.
Honorary Senior Lecturer at Institute of Urology; Honorary Senior Clinical Lecturer, Department of Medicine, University College; Consultant in Uro-Neurology, National Hospital for Neurology and Neurosurgery; Consultant Clinical Neurophysiologist, Middlesex and University College Hospitals, London, United Kingdom
Sexual Dysfunction in Neurologic Disease; Bladder Dysfunction in Neurologic Disease

Hans-Joachim Freund, M.D.
Professor of Neurology, University of Düsseldorf; Chairman, Department of Neurology, Neurologische Klinik der Universität Düsseldorf, Düsseldorf, Germany
The Apraxias

H. Harris Funkenstein, M.D.
Late Associate Professor of Neurology, Harvard Medical School, Boston, Massachusetts
The Effects of Age: Normal Variation and Its Relation to Disease

Roy E. Furman, M.D., Ph.D.
Media, Pennsylvania
Pathophysiology of Myotonia and Periodic Paralysis

Roger W. Gilliatt, D.M., F.R.C.P.
Late Professor Emeritus, University of London; Former Chairman, University Department of Clinical Neurology, Institute of Neurology, London, United Kingdom; Visiting Scientist, National Institutes of Health, Bethesda, Maryland
Syncope and Nonepileptic Seizures

Sid Gilman, M.D.
Professor and Chairman, Department of Neurology, University of Michigan Medical School; Chief, Neurology Service, University of Michigan Hospitals, Ann Arbor, Michigan
Cerebellum and Motor Dysfunction

Myron D. Ginsberg, M.D.
Professor and Vice-Chairman, Department of Neurology, Professor of Radiology, and Director, Cerebral Vascular Disease Research Center, University of Miami School of Medicine; Attending Neurologist, Jackson Memorial Hospital, Miami, Florida
Cerebral Circulation: Its Regulation, Pharmacology, and Pathophysiology

Michael J. Glantz, M.D.
Assistant Professor of Neurology, University of Minnesota, Minneapolis, Minnesota
Harmful Effects of Radiation on the Nervous System

Gary W. Goldstein, M.D.
Professor, Departments of Neurology and Pediatrics, Johns Hopkins School of Medicine and Johns Hopkins Hospital; President, Kennedy Institute, Baltimore, Maryland
Blood Vessels and the Blood-Brain Barrier

Barry Gordon, M.D., Ph.D.
Associate Professor of Neurology and Psychology, Johns Hopkins University School of Medicine; Director, Cognitive Neurology, and Member, Mind/Brain Institute, Johns Hopkins Hospital, Baltimore, Maryland
Memory Systems and Their Disorders

Scott T. Grafton, M.D.
Clinical Instructor, School of Medicine, University of California, Los Angeles; Attending Physician, University of California, Los Angeles, Medical Center, Los Angeles, California
Cerebral Pathophysiology Evaluated with Positron Emission Tomography

Jack A. Grebb, M.D.
Assistant Professor of Psychiatry, New York University School of Medicine; Research Scientist, The Nathan S. Kline Institute for Psychiatric Research; Guest Investigator, Laboratory of Molecular and Cellular Neuroscience, The Rockefeller University; Associate Attending Psychiatrist, Bellevue Hospital, New York, New York
Schizophrenia

Diane E. Griffin, M.D., Ph.D.
Professor of Medicine and Professor of Neurology, Johns Hopkins University School of Medicine; Active Staff, Department of Medicine, Johns Hopkins Hospital, Baltimore, Maryland
Host Responses to Infection of the Nervous System

John W. Griffin, M.D.
Professor and Associate Director, Department of Neurology, and Professor of Neuroscience, Johns Hopkins University School of Medicine and Johns Hopkins Hospital, Baltimore, Maryland
The Cell of Schwann; Pathophysiology of Neuronal and Axonal Degenerations

Robert C. Griggs, M.D.
Professor and Chair, Department of Neurology, University of Rochester School of Medicine and Dentistry; Chief of Neurology, Strong Memorial Hospital, Rochester, New York
Neurologic Manifestations of Respiratory Diseases

A.E. Harding, M.D., F.R.C.P.
Professor of Clinical Neurology, Institute of Neurology, University of London; Consultant Neurologist, National Hospitals for Neurology and Neurosurgery and West Middlesex University Hospital, London, United Kingdom
Molecular Genetic Techniques and Their Applications to Clinical Neurology; Hereditary Ataxias and Related Disorders

Hans-Peter Hartung, M.D.
Professor of Neurology, Department of Neurology, Neurologische Klinik, Universität Wuerzburg, Germany
Circulating Immune Factors

David Healy, M.D., M.R.C. Psych.
Senior Lecturer, Department of Psychological Medicine, Cardiff; Senior Lecturer, Academic Subdepartment of Psychological Medicine, North Wales Hospital, Denbigh, Clwyd, United Kingdom
Neurochemistry of Mood Disorders

Kenneth M. Heilman, M.D.
The James E. Rooks Jr. Professor of Neurology, Director, Center for Neuropsychology Studies, and Professor of Clinical Psychology, University of Florida; University of Florida Teaching Hospital (Shands) and Veterans Administration Medical Center, Gainesville, Florida
Neglect

Michael G. Hennerici, M.D.
Professor of Neurology and Chairman, University of Heidelberg, Mannheim Hospital, Germany
Atherosclerotic and Hypertensive Vascular Disease

Paul N. Hoffman, M.D., Ph.D.
Assistant Professor, Department of Ophthalmology and Neurology, Johns Hopkins University School of Medicine; Neuro/Ophthalmology Unit, Wilmer Ophthalmological Institute, Johns Hopkins Hospital, Baltimore, Maryland
Pathophysiology of Neuronal and Axonal Degenerations

Orest Hurko, M.D.
Associate Professor of Neurology and Medicine, Center for Medical Genetics, Johns Hopkins University School of Medicine, Baltimore, Maryland
Heritable Disorders of The Nervous System

Peter R. Huttenlocher, M.D.
Professor of Pediatrics and Neurology, Committee on Neurobiology, University of Chicago; Attending Physician, Wyler Childrens Hospital, Chicago, Illinois
Neural Plasticity

Bryan Jennett, M.D., F.R.C.S.
Professor of Neurosurgery, University of Glasgow; Consultant Neurosurgeon, Institute of Neurological Sciences, Southern General Hospital, Glasgow, Scotland
Head Trauma

Ralph H. Johnson, D.M., D.Sc., D.Phil., F.R.C.P.G., F.R.A.C.P., F.R.S.E.
Director, Postgraduate Medical Education, Oxford University, and Professional Fellow of Wadham College, Oxford; Honorary Consultant Physician and Neurologist, John Radcliffe Hospital, Oxford, United Kingdom
Autonomic Function and Dysfunction

Richard T. Johnson, M.D.
Director and Professor, Department of Neurology, Professor of Molecular Biology and Genetics, and Professor of Neuroscience, Johns Hopkins University School of Medicine; Neurologist-in-Chief, Johns Hopkins Hospital, Baltimore, Maryland
Host Responses to Infection of the Nervous System; Parasitic Infections

S.J. Jones, Ph.D.
Honorary Lecturer, Institute of Neurology; Senior Scientist, The Medical Research Council, National Hospital for Neurology and Neurosurgery, London, United Kingdom
Evoked Potentials: Their Contribution to the Diagnosis and Understanding of Neurologic Disease

Robert J. Joynt, M.D., Ph.D.
Professor of Neurology and Neurobiology/Anatomy, University of Rochester School of Medicine; Vice President and Vice Provost for Health Affairs, University of Rochester, Rochester, New York
Ependyma

Christopher Kennard, Ph.D., F.R.C.P.
Professor of Clinical Neurology, Charing Cross and Westminster Medical School, University of London; Honorary Consultant Neurologist, Charing Cross Hospital, London, United Kingdom
Pathophysiology of Vision

Charles P. Kimmelman, M.D., F.A.C.S.
Professor and Acting Chairman, Department of Otolaryngology, New York Medical College; Chairman, Department of Otolaryngology–Head and Neck Surgery, New York Eye and Ear Infirmary, New York, New York
Smell and Taste and Their Disorders

Roman S. Kocen, M.D.
Honorary Senior Lecturer in Neurology, Institute of Neurology, University of London; Consultant Neurologist, National Hospital for Neurology and Neurosurgery, and Civil Consultant in Neurology, Royal Air Force, London, United Kingdom
Tuberculosis of the Nervous System

Ralph W. Kuncl, M.D., Ph.D.
Associate Professor of Neurology, Johns Hopkins University; Co-Director, Neuro-muscular Clinical Laboratory, and Attending Physician, Active Full-Time Staff, Johns Hopkins Hospital, Baltimore, Maryland
Motor Neuron Diseases

David G. Lambie, B.Sc., Ph.D., B.B.S.
Departmental Manager, Department of Health, Wellington, New Zealand
Autonomic Function and Dysfunction

James W. Lance, M.D., F.R.C.P.(Lond.), F.R.A.C.P., F.A.A.
Professor of Neurology, School of Medicine, University of New South Wales; Chairman, Department of Neurology, and Director, Institute of Neurological Sci-ences, The Prince Henry and Prince of Wales Hospitals, Sydney, Australia
The Myotatic Unit and Its Disorders; Headache and Migraine

Robert B. Layzer, M.D.
Professor of Neurology, University of California, San Francisco, Medical School; Director of Muscle Clinic, University of California, San Francisco, Medical Center; Attending Physician, Moffitt-Long Hospitals, San Francisco, California
Pathophysiology of Metabolic Myopathies; Neurologic Manifestations of Endocrine Diseases

R. John Leigh, M.D.
Professor of Neurology, Case Western Reserve University; Consultant, Cleveland Department of Veterans Affairs Medical Center, Cleveland, Ohio
Oculomotor Control: Normal and Abnormal

Pamela M. Le Quesne, D.M., F.R.C.P.
Honorary Senior Lecturer, University College and Middlesex School of Medicine, Medical Research Council Toxicology Unit; Honorary Consultant Neurologist, The Middlesex Hospital, London, United Kingdom
Metal Neurotoxicity

Ronald P. Lesser, M.D.
Associate Professor of Neurology and Neurosurgery, Johns Hopkins University School of Medicine; Director, Johns Hopkins Epilepsy Center, Johns Hopkins Hospital, Baltimore, Maryland
Smell and Taste and Their Disorders

David E. Levy, M.D.
Clinical Associate Professor of Neurology, Cornell University Medical College; Associate Attending Neurologist, New York Hospital, New York, New York; Central Nervous System Research Director, Knoll Pharmaceutical, Whippany, New Jersey
Neurologic Manifestations of Cardiac Diseases

Ulf Lindblom, M.D., D.M.Sc.
Professor, Karolinska Institute; Chairman, Department of Neurology, Karolinska Hospital, Stockholm, Sweden
Somatosensory Function and Dysfunction

Phillip A. Low, M.D.
Professor of Neurology, Mayo Medical School; Consultant in Neurology, St. Mary's Hospital and Rochester Methodist Hospital, Rochester, Minnesota
Sudomotor Function and Dysfunction

Linda M. Luxon, B.Sc., F.R.C.P.
Consultant Physician in Neuro-otology, National Hospital for Neurology and Neurosurgery, London, United Kingdom
Disorders of Hearing

William W. Lytton, M.D.
Senior Research Associate, Computational Neurobiology Laboratory, Salk Institute, La Jolla; Assistant Clinical Professor, Department of Neuroscience, University of California, San Diego; Attending Medical Staff, University of California, San Diego, Medical Center, San Diego, California
Computational Neuroscience

Raymond Maciewicz, M.D.
Associate Professor, Institute of Health Professions, Massachusetts General Hospital; Associate Professor of Neurology in Neuroscience, Harvard Medical School; Active Staff Neurology/Psychiatry, and Director, Spaulding Pain Rehabilitation Program; Associate Neurologist, Massachusetts General Hospital, Boston, Massachusetts
Organization of Pain Pathways

Joseph A. Madsen, M.D.
Staff Physician, Brigham and Women's Hospital and Children's Hospital, Boston, Massachusetts
Chronic Increased Intracranial Pressure

William R. Markesbery, M.D.
Professor of Neurology and Pathology; Director, Sanders-Brown Center on Aging; Commonwealth Chair in Aging, University of Kentucky College of Medicine; Associate Neurologist and Associate Pathologist, University Hospital; Consultant in Neurology and Neuropathology, Veterans Administration, Lexington, Kentucky
Alzheimer's Disease

C. David Marsden, F.R.C.P., F.R.S.
Professor and Chairman, University Department of Neurology, Institute of Neurology, National Hospital for Neurology and Neurosurgery, London, United Kingdom
Motor Dysfunction and Movement Disorders

Joseph B. Martin, M.D., Ph.D.
Professor of Neurology and Dean, School of Medicine, University of California, San Francisco; Attending Physician, Moffitt/Long Hospitals and San Francisco General Hospital, San Francisco, California
Hypothalamic-Pituitary Function and Dysfunction

W. Bryan Matthews, B.M., F.R.C.P.
Emeritus Professor of Clinical Neurology, University of Oxford, Oxford, United Kingdom
Neurologic Manifestations of Sarcoidosis

John C. Mazziotta, M.D., Ph.D.
Professor of Neurology and Radiological Sciences, School of Medicine, University of California, Los Angeles; Attending Physician, University of California, Los Angeles, Medical Center, Los Angeles, California
Cerebral Pathophysiology Evaluated with Positron Emission Tomography

Justin C. McArthur, M.B.B.S., M.P.H.
Associate Professor of Neurology, Johns Hopkins School of Medicine and Johns Hopkins Hospital, Baltimore, Maryland
Neurologic Manifestations of Human Immunodeficiency Virus Infection; Neurologic Manifestations of Infection with Human T Cell Lymphotropic Virus Type I

Rosaleen A. McCarthy, M.D.
University of Cambridge, Cambridge, United Kingdom
Disorders of Memory

W. Ian McDonald, Ph.D., F.R.C.P.
Professor of Clinical Neurology, Institute of Neurology; Honorary Consultant Physician, National Hospital for Neurology and Neurosurgery, Queen Square, and Moorfield's Eye Hospital, London, United Kingdom
Pathophysiology of Nervous System Diseases; Diseases of the Optic Nerve, Multiple Sclerosis and Its Pathophysiology

Paul R. McHugh, M.D.
Director, Department of Psychiatry, and Henry Phipps Professor of Psychiatry, Johns Hopkins University School of Medicine; Psychiatrist-in-Chief, Johns Hopkins Hospital, Baltimore, Maryland
Food Intake and Its Disorders

Guy M. McKhann, M.D.
Professor of Neurology and Director, The Zanvyl Krieger Mind/Brain Institute, Johns Hopkins University, Baltimore, Maryland
Pathophysiology of Nervous System Diseases

James G. McLeod, M.B.B.S., B.Sc. Med., D.Phil.(Oxon.), F.R.A.C.P., F.R.C.P.(Lond.)
Bushell Professor of Neurology, University of Sydney; Chairman, Institute of Clinical Neurosciences, Royal Prince Alfred Hospital, Sydney, Australia
Vasomotor Function and Dysfunction

Thomas H. McNeill, Ph.D.
Associate Professor of Gerontology and Neurobiology, University of Southern California, Los Angeles, California
Ependyma

David H. Miller, M.R.Ch.B., M.D., F.R.A.C.P.
Senior Lecturer in Clinical Neurology, Institute of Neurology; Honorary Consultant Neurologist, National Hospital for Neurology and Neurosurgery, London, United Kingdom
Neurologic Manifestations of Collagen-Vascular Diseases

J.P. Mohr, M.D.
Sciarra Professor of Clinical Neurology, College of Physicians and Surgeons, Columbia University, New York, New York
Acquired Language Disorders

John A. Morgan-Hughes, M.D., F.R.C.P.
Consultant Physician, Institute of Neurology, National Hospital for Neurology and Neurosurgery, London, United Kingdom
Diseases of Striated Muscle

Hugo W. Moser, M.D.
University Professor of Neurology and Pediatrics, Johns Hopkins University; Director of Neurogenetics, Kennedy Institute, Baltimore, Maryland
Genetic and Metabolic Diseases: Mechanisms and Potential for Therapy

Dwight E. Moulin, M.D.
Assistant Professor, Department of Clinical Neurological Sciences, University of Western Ontario; Attending Physician, Victoria Hospital, London, Ontario, Canada
Neuropharmacology of Pain

John Newsom-Davis, M.D.
Professor of Clinical Neurology, University of Oxford; Honorary Consultant, Radcliffe Infirmary, Oxford, United Kingdom
Diseases of the Neuromuscular Junction

Charles P. O'Brien, M.D., Ph.D.
Professor and Vice-Chairman of Psychiatry, University of Pennsylvania School of Medicine; Chief of Psychiatry, Philadelphia Veterans Affairs Medical Center, Philadelphia, Pennsylvania
Neurologic Consequences of Drug Abuse

José Ochoa, D.Sc., M.D., Ph.D.
Professor of Neurology and Neurosurgery, Oregon Health Sciences University; Director, Neuromuscular Unit, Good Samaritan Hospital and Medical Center, Portland, Oregon
Somatosensory Function and Dysfunction

Mitsuhiro Osame, M.D.
Professor and Chairman, The Third Department of Internal Medicine, Faculty of Medicine, Kagoshima University; Director, World Health Organization, Collaborating Centre for Human Retroviral Infections Associated with Neurological Disorders, Kagoshima, Japan
Neurologic Manifestations of Infection with Human T Cell Lymphotropic Virus Type I

Gavril W. Pasternak, M.D., Ph.D.
Professor of Neurology and Neuroscience and Professor of Pharmacology, Cornell University Medical College; Member, Memorial Sloan-Kettering Cancer Center; Attending Neurologist, Memorial Hospital, New York, New York
Neuropharmacology of Pain

Eugene S. Paykel, M.D., F.R.C.P., F.R.C. Psych.
Professor of Psychiatry, University of Cambridge Clinical School; Head, Department of Psychiatry, Addenbrooke's Hospital, Cambridge, United Kingdom
Neurochemistry of Mood Disorders

John B. Penney, Jr., M.D.
Professor of Neurology, Harvard Medical School; Neurology Service, Massachusetts General Hospital, Boston, Massachusetts
Pharmacologic Aspects of Motor Dysfunction

David Pleasure, M.D.
Professor of Neurology and Pediatrics, University of Pennsylvania School of Medicine; Director, Neurology Research, Children's Hospital of Philadelphia, Philadelphia, Pennsylvania
Third Messengers That Regulate Neural Gene Transcription

Fred Plum, M.D.
Titzell Professor and Chairman, Department of Neurology and Neuroscience, Cornell University Medical College; Neurologist in Chief, New York Hospital, New York, New York
Cerebral Metabolism and Hypoxic-Ischemic Brain Injury

Roger J. Porter, M.D.
Deputy Director, National Institute of Neurological and Communicative Disorders and Stroke, Bethesda, Maryland
Management of Epilepsy

Jerome B. Posner, M.D.
Professor of Neurology and Neurosciences, Cornell University Medical College; Chairman, Department of Neurology, Memorial Sloan-Kettering Cancer Center, New York, New York
Secondary Neoplastic Disease; Paraneoplastic Syndromes

Michael Powell, M.A.(Oxon.), M.B.B.S.(Lond.), F.R.C.S. Eng.
Consultant Neurosurgeon, The National Hospital for Neurology and Neurosurgery, London, United Kingdom
Neurologic Manifestations of Vertebral Column Disorders

Arthur L. Prensky, M.D.
Allen P. and Josephine B. Green, Professor of Pediatric Neurology, Washington University; Pediatrician and Neurologist, St. Louis Children's Hospital and Barnes Hospital, St. Louis, Missouri
Mental Retardation

James W. Prichard, M.D.
Professor of Neurology, Yale University; Attending Physician, Yale–New Haven Medical Center, New Haven, Connecticut
Magnetic Resonance Spectroscopy of Cerebral Metabolism in Vivo

William A. Pulsinelli, M.D., Ph.D.
Professor of Neurology and Neuroscience, Cornell University Medical College; Attending Neurologist, The New York Hospital, New York, New York
Cerebral Metabolism and Hypoxic-Ischemic Brain Injury

Marcus E. Raichle, M.D.
Professor of Neurology and Radiology, Washington University School of Medicine; Attending Physician, Barnes Hospital, St. Louis, Missouri
Cortical Information Processing in the Normal Human Brain

Isabelle Rapin, M.D.
Professor of Neurology and Pediatrics (Neurology), Albert Einstein College of Medicine; Attending Neurologist and Child Neurologist, Einstein Affiliated Hospitals, Bronx, New York
The Normal and Abnormal Acquisition of Language

Anthony T. Reder, M.D.
Assistant Professor of Neurology, University of Chicago; Attending Physician, University of Chicago Hospitals and Clinics, Chicago, and Oak Forest Hospital, Oak Forest, Illinois
Cell-Mediated Immunity and Neurologic Disease

Trevor J. Resnick, M.D.
Assistant Professor of Pediatrics and Neurology, University of Miami; Director of Developmental Neurology and Attending Neurologist, Miami Children's Hospital, Miami, Florida
The Normal and Abnormal Acquisition of Language

E. Osmund R. Reynolds, M.D., F.R.C.P., F.R.C.O.G
Professor of Neonatal Paediatrics and Head of Department of Paediatrics, University College and Middlesex School of Medicine; Consultant Neonatal Paediatrician, University College Hospital, London, United Kingdom
Perinatal Brain Injury

Alan Richens, M.B.B.S., B.Sc., Ph.D., F.R.C.P.
Professor of Pharmacology and Therapeutics, University of Wales College of Medicine; Consultant Physician, University Hospital of Wales and Llandough Hospital, Cardiff, United Kingdom
Anticonvulsant Pharmacokinetics

Richard C. Roberts, M.A., D.Phil., B.M.B.Ch., M.R.C.P.(U.K.)
Senior Lecturer, Neurology, Department of Medicine, University of Dundee; Consultant Neurologist, Royal Infirmary, Dundee, Scotland
Syncope and Nonepileptic Seizures

Martin K. Robinson, M.B.B.S., F.R.A.C.P.
Lecturer in Clinical Pharmacology, Department of Pharmacology and Therapeutics, University of Wales College of Medicine, Cardiff, United Kingdom; Neurologist (Visiting), Queen Elizabeth Hospital, Adelaide, South Australia
Anticonvulsant Pharmacokinetics

Maria A. Ron, M.Phil., Ph.D., F.R.C. Psych.
Reader in Neuropsychiatry, Institute of Neurology; Consultant Psychiatrist, National Hospital for Neurology and Neurosurgery, London, United Kingdom
Neurologic Aspects of Functional Disorders

Allan H. Ropper, M.D.
Professor of Neurology, Tufts University School of Medicine; Chief of Neurology, St. Elizabeth's Hospital, Boston, Massachusetts
Coma and Acutely Raised Intracranial Pressure

M. Rossor, M.D., F.R.C.P.
Senior Lecturer, Institute of Neurology; Consultant Neurologist, National Hospital for Neurology and Neurosurgery and St. Mary's Hospital, London, United Kingdom
Dementia

Jeffrey D. Rothstein, M.D., Ph.D.
Assistant Professor of Neurology, Johns Hopkins University School of Medicine; Attending Physician, Active Full-Time Staff, Johns Hopkins Hospital, Baltimore Maryland
Motor Neuron Diseases; Neurologic Manifestations of Hepatic and Gastrointestinal Diseases

David A. Rottenberg, M.D.
Professor of Neurology, University of Minnesota School of Medicine; Chief, Neurology Service, and Chief, PET Imaging Service, Minneapolis Veterans Administration Medical Center, Minneapolis, Minnesota
Harmful Effects of Radiation on the Nervous System

Lewis P. Rowland, M.D.
Henry and Lucy Moses Professor and Chairman, Department of Neurology, Columbia University College of Physicians and Surgeons; Director, Neurology Service, Presbyterian Hospital, New York, New York
Pathophysiology of Metabolic Myopathies

K.H. Ruddock, B.Sc., A.R.C.S., Ph.D., D.I.C
Professor of Biophysics, Imperial College of Science, Technology and Medicine, University of London, London, United Kingdom
Pathophysiology of Vision

Judith M. Rumsey, Ph.D.
Research Psychologist, Child Psychiatry, National Institute of Mental Health, Bethesda, Maryland
Development Dyslexia

R.W. Ross Russell, D.M., F.R.C.P.
Physician, National Hospital for Neurology and Neurosurgery, St. Thomas Hospital, and Moorfield's Eye Hospital, London, United Kingdom
Miscellaneous Cerebrovascular Diseases

Gérard Said
Professor of Neurology, Université Paris-XI; Chef du Service de Neurologie, Hôpital de Bicêtre, Bicêtre, France
Pathophysiology of Nerve and Root Disorders

Martin A. Samuels, M.D.
Associate Professor of Neurology, Harvard Medical School; Chief of Neurology, Brigham and Women's Hospital, Boston, Massachusetts
Neurologic Manifestations of Hematologic Diseases

John W. Scadding, M.D., F.R.C.P.
Senior Lecturer, Institute of Neurology; Consultant Neurologist, National Hospital for Neurology and Neurosurgery, London, United Kingdom
Neuropathic Pain

Herbert H. Schaumburg, M.D.
Professor and Chairman, Department of Neurology, Albert Einstein College of Medicine/Montefiore Medical Center; Director of Neurology, Montefiore Medical Center, Bronx, New York
Chemical Neurotoxicity

W. Michael Scheld, M.D.
Professor of Internal Medicine and Neurosurgery and Associate Chair for Residency Programs, University of Virginia Health Sciences Center, Charlottesville, Virginia
Bacterial Infections in Adults

Geoffrey D. Schott, M.D., F.R.C.P.
Consultant Neurologist, National Hospital for Neurology and Neurosurgery, and Royal National Orthopedic Hospital, London, and Warford General Hospital, Warford, United Kingdom
Neurologic Manifestations of Bone and Joint Diseases

Terrence J. Sejnowski, Ph.D.
Investigator, Howard Hughes Medical Institute; Professor, Computational Neurobiology Laboratory, Salk Institute; Professor, Departments of Biology and Physics, University of California, San Diego, La Jolla, California
Computational Neuroscience

Michael E. Selzer, M.D., Ph.D.
Professor of Neurology, University of Pennsylvania School of Medicine; Director, Center for Neurologic Rehabilitation and Attending Neurologist, Hospital of the University of Pennsylvania, Philadelphia, Pennsylvania
Cellular Pathophysiology and Pharmacology of Epilepsy

Joan R. Shapiro, Ph.D.
Director, Neuro-Oncology Research, Barrow Neurological Institute, St. Joseph's Hospital and Medical Center, Phoenix, Arizona
Primary Brain Tumors

William R. Shapiro, M.D.
Chairman, Division of Neurology, Barrow Neurological Institute, St. Joseph's Hospital and Medical Center, Phoenix, Arizona
Primary Brain Tumors

Simon D. Shorvon, M.A.B.Ch., M.D., F.R.C.P.
Senior Lecturer in Neurology, Institute of Neurology; Consultant Neurologist, National Hospital for Neurology and Neurosurgery; Medical Director, Chalfont Centre for Epilepsy, London, United Kingdom
Epidemiology and Etiology of Epilepsy; Classification and Clinical Characteristics of Epilepsy

Ira Shoulson, M.D.
Louis C. Lasagna Professor of Experimental Therapeutics and Professor of Neurology, Pharmacology and Medicine, University of Rochester School of Medicine and Dentistry; Neurologist and Physician, Strong Memorial Hospital, Rochester, New York
Huntington's Disease

Roger P. Simon, M.D.
Professor of Neurology, University of California, San Francisco; Chief of Neurology, San Francisco General Hospital, San Francisco, California
Pathophysiology of Respiratory Dysfunction

R.K. Small, B.A., Ph.D.
Lecturer, Institute of Neurology, London, United Kingdom
Glial Cell Lineages in Development and Disease

Solomon H. Snyder, M.D.
Distinguished Service Professor of Neuroscience, Pharmacology and Psychiatry and Director, Department of Neuroscience, Johns Hopkins University School of Medicine; Psychiatrist, Active Staff, Johns Hopkins Hospital, Baltimore, Maryland
Neurotransmitters

Lawrence Steinman, M.D.
Professor of Neurology and Neurological Sciences, Pediatrics and Genetics, Stanford University; Neurologist, Stanford University Hospital; Pediatric Neurologist, Lucille Packard Childrens Hospital at Stanford, Stanford, California
Immunosuppressive Therapy of Neurologic Disease

John R. Sutton, M.D.
Head, Department of Biological Sciences, Cumberland College of Health Sciences, The University of Sydney, Sydney, Australia
Neurologic Manifestations of Respiratory Diseases

P.K. Thomas, D.Sc., M.D.
Professor of Neurology, Royal Free Hospital School of Medicine and Institute of Neurology; Consultant Neurologist, Royal Free Hospital and National Hospital for Neurology and Neurosurgery, London, United Kingdom
Pathophysiology of Nerve and Root Disorders

A.J. Thompson, M.D., M.R.C.P.I.
Honorary Senior Lecturer, Department of Clinical Neurology, Institute of Neurology; Consultant Neurologist, National Hospital for Neurology and Neurosurgery and The Whittington Hospital, London, United Kingdom
Multiple Sclerosis and Its Pathophysiology

H. Stanley Thompson, M.D.
Professor of Ophthalmology, Department of Ophthalmology, University of Iowa College of Medicine and University of Iowa Hospitals and Clinics, Iowa City, Iowa
Pupillary Function and Dysfunction

Klaus V. Toyka, M.D.
Professor and Chairman, Department of Neurology, Neurologische Klinik, Universität Wuerzburg, F.R. Germany
Circulating Immune Factors

Daniel Tranel, Ph.D.
Associate Professor, Department of Neurology, University of Iowa College of Medicine and University of Iowa Hospitals and Clinics, Iowa City, Iowa
The Agnosias

Roger R. Tuck, M.B.B.S., B.Sc., Ph.D., F.R.A.C.P.
Staff Neurologist, Royal Prince Alfred Hospital, Sydney, Australia
Vasomotor Function and Dysfunction

Larry E. Tune, M.D.
Associate Professor of Psychiatry, Johns Hopkins University School of Medicine, Baltimore, Maryland
Neurologic Complications of Psychotropic Drugs

Allan R. Tunkel, M.D., Ph.D.
Assistant Professor of Internal Medicine, Medical College of Pennsylvania, Philadelphia, Pennsylvania
Bacterial Infections in Adults

Harold C. Urschel III, M.D.
Associate Medical Director and Director of Chemical Dependency Treatment, Southwestern Psychiatric Services, Dallas, Texas
Neurologic Consequences of Drug Abuse

Edward Valenstein, M.D.
Professor, Department of Neurology, University of Florida College of Medicine; Attending Neurologist, University of Florida Clinic, Shands Hospital, Gainesville, Florida
Neglect

Maurice Victor, M.D.
Professor of Medicine and Neurology, Dartmouth Medical School, Hanover, New Hampshire; Distinguished Physician of the Veterans Administration, White River Junction, Vermont
Neurologic Manifestations of Hepatic and Gastrointestinal Diseases

Kenneth S. Warren, M.D.
Professor of Medicine, New York University Medical Center; Adjunct Professor of Medicine, Rockefeller University; Director for Science, Maxwell Communication Corporation, New York, New York
Parasitic Infections

Elizabeth K. Warrington, D.Sc.
Professor of Clinical Neuropsychology, Institute of Neurology; Head of Psychology Department, National Hospital for Neurology and Neurosurgery, London, United Kingdom
Disorders of Memory

Robert T. Watson, M.D.
Professor of Neurology and Senior Associate Dean for Educational Affairs, University of Florida College of Medicine; Member, Board of Directors, University of Florida Teaching Hospital (Shands), Gainesville, Florida
Neglect

Stephen G. Waxman, M.D., Ph.D.
Professor and Chairman, Department of Neurology, Yale University Medical School; Neurologist-in-Chief, Yale–New Haven Hospital, New Haven; Director, Neuroscience Research Center, Veterans Administration Hospital, West Haven, Connecticut
Molecular Organization and Pathophysiology of Axons

Daniel R. Weinberger, M.D.
Associate Professor of Neurology and Psychiatry, George Washington University School of Medicine; Chief, Clinical Brain Disorders Branch, Intramural Research Program, National Institute of Mental Health, Neurosciences Center at Saint Elizabeth's, Washington, D.C.
Schizophrenia

John S. Wyatt, M.B.B.S., M.R.C.P.
Senior Lecturer in Neonatal Paediatrics, University College and Middlesex School of Medicine; Consultant Paediatrician, University College Hospital, London, United Kingdom
Perinatal Brain Injury

Richard Jed Wyatt, M.D.
Consulting Professor of Psychiatry, Duke University School of Medicine, Durham, North Carolina; Adjunct Professor of Psychiatry, Uniformed Services University School of Medicine, Bethesda, Maryland; Visiting Professor of Psychiatry, Columbia University, New York, New York; Chief, Neuropsychiatry Branch, Intramural Research Program, National Institute of Mental Health, Neurosciences Center at Saint Elizabeth's, Washington, D.C.
Schizophrenia

Anne B. Young, M.D., Ph.D.
Julieanne Dorn Professor of Neurology, Harvard Medical School; Chief, Neurology Service, Massachusetts General Hospital, Boston, Massachusetts
Pharmacologic Aspects of Motor Dysfunction

G. Bryan Young, M.D., F.R.C.P.C.
Associate Professor, Department of Clinical Neurological Sciences, University of Western Ontario; Director, EEG Laboratory, Victoria Hospital, London, Ontario, Canada
Neurologic Manifestations of Renal Diseases

Robert R. Young, M.D.
Professor of Neurology, Harvard Medical School; Chief, Spinal Cord Injury Service, Brockton/West Roxbury Veterans Administration Medical Center, Boston, Massachusetts
Tremor

David S. Zee, M.D.
Professor of Neurology, Johns Hopkins University School of Medicine and Department of Neurology, Johns Hopkins Hospital, Baltimore, Maryland
Oculomotor Control: Normal and Abnormal

Preface

When we were preparing the first edition of this textbook, and then revising the second, the question would occasionally arise, "Why another textbook of neurology?" We, as editors, view these volumes as more than a textbook of neurology. Rather, we place emphasis on the subtitle, *Clinical Neurobiology*. With that subtitle we imply, and hope that we have implemented, a bridging of the gap between the basic neuroscience and clinical neurology. In doing so we attempted to supplement the necessary description of the characteristics and management of neurologic disease with discussions of the mechanisms of disease, newer approaches to understanding disease, and the potential for new effective therapies. These were the premises on which the first edition was based, and they remain so for the second edition.

We did not feel held to the table of contents for the first edition. For disorders for which there have been relatively few advances through research, we did not feel the need to repeat the information already presented in the first edition. In other areas, we asked authors to approach a subject considered in the first edition from a different point of view. For example, in the area of neurotransmitters and receptors, we focus more on intercellular responses (Chapter 4) and intracellular responses (Chapter 5) than we did in the first edition. Similarly, in organizing the section on brain and motor control, we combined the chapters on supraspinal motor systems, cortical control of movement, and organization of basal ganglia into a single overview chapter (Chapter 21).

Another goal we had was to gradually change authors from one edition to the next. We did not do this because of any dissatisfaction with the first contributors. Rather, we thought that for certain areas, approaching a problem from a different point of view than the previous one would be worthwhile.

Finally, some areas have grown in importance since the first edition was planned 6 or 7 years ago, either because of clinical interest or because of advances in research. Such is the case for Lyme disease, hereditary spastic paresis, diseases associated with prions, and AIDS, to name a few.

We would be remiss not to acknowledge the support of two editors previously with W. B. Saunders Company: Mr. Albert E. Meier was our guiding mentor for the first edition, and his basic strategies helped to shape the second edition. The implementation of this edition was initially carried out with the able assistance of Mr. Martin Wonsiewicz. Finally, Ms. Linda Mills stepped in at a crucial moment and carried this edition through to completion.

A special word of thanks goes to the many authors who participated in producing these two volumes. As in the first edition, our busy colleagues enthusiastically contributed their expertise, were remarkably cooperative when we suggested changes in direction or emphasis, and most important, delivered on time. Any success that these volumes have is due to them.

If we were honest, the editors would have their names in small print and those of our secretaries in capital letters. We gratefully acknowledge the efforts of Ms. Anne Kruger, Ms. Charlotte Card, Ms. Jenifer Lewis, and Ms. Maria Porretti.

ARTHUR K. ASBURY, M.D.
GUY M. McKHANN, M.D.
W. IAN McDONALD, PH.D., F.R.C.P.

Preface to the
First Edition

The premise on which these volumes are based states that physicians dealing with diseases of the nervous system need to know what scientific investigation has disclosed about these diseases. It is axiomatic that our ability to control, treat, or prevent a given neurological disorder depends upon the depth of our knowledge and understanding of it. In recent decades, study of nervous system disease by a host of techniques, many of them growing out of basic neuroscientific research, has surged forward. As a result, the complexity of clinical neurology has multiplied and development of special areas of knowledge within neurology has proceeded rapidly. Witness the emergence of such areas as neurobehavior, neurooncology, neuroophthalmology, clinical neurophysiology, neuromuscular disorders, epileptology, neuroepidemiology, clinical neuropharmacology, and the subspecialty of cerebral circulation and stroke. While this Balkanization of neurology has resulted in geometric growth of knowledge, it has also made it difficult to keep abreast.

The overall purposes of this monographic effort are two-fold: (1) to examine and bring together what scientific inquiry has taught us about the phenomena of neurologic dysfunction and the causes of neurological diseases, and (2) to present in summary fashion an up-to-date account of the major groups of neurological disorders, their pathogeneses, and their management. Our justification for yet another reference book in the field of neurology is the perceived need to summarize and synthesize what research has taught us about the mechanisms of neurological disease.

How the information is set forth will be evident upon inspection of the table of contents. The first several sections deal with the organization and function of particular cellular components and systems of the brain and its extensions, and the later sections deal with groups of disorders clustered either by anatomic system or cause. The final three chapters deal with the application of three major new methodologies to the study of neurological disorders, including evoked potentials, positron emission tomography, and magnetic resonance techniques. For those wishing to read in more depth on any of the subjects discussed, key references are indicated which leave a bibliographic trail for the interested to pursue.

The readership for whom these pages are intended includes neuroscientists of any persuasion or background, students pursuing doctoral degrees, physicians trained in disciplines other than neurology, and of course, neurologists, neurosurgeons and psychiatrists and those training in these fields. No attempt has been made to describe the fundamentals of the neurological examination or the standard diagnostic techniques used in clinical neurology. These are fully described in other texts. Nevertheless, readers with only passing familiarity with clinical neurology should experience no difficulty grasping the subject matter presented within these covers.

Many disorders and phenomena are considered in several chapters, generally from different points of view and at varying depth. As a policy, we encouraged this apparent duplication on the basis that it avoided artificial demarcations between topics, and that it added a richness to the texture of the book. To guide the reader, cross-referencing is used generously.

Development of this publishing project and of the principles which guided it took place over several years. Initial planning involved exchanges of ideas between the editors and also with Mr. Albert E. Meier, Editor and Publisher of Ardmore Medical Books at W. B. Saunders Company. Drs. Robert A. Fishman and Jerome B. Posner also lent their considerable talents to this early planning phase. From these discussions emerged a number of principles. These included: first, that the major emphasis would be on the pathophysiology of nervous diseases; second, that basic neuroscience would be presented but mainly to the extent that it was necessary to illuminate a particular phenomenon or disease; we felt it was beyond the scope of these volumes to attempt a comprehensive account of all of fundamental neuroscience; third, that each chapter topic would be shaped in such a way that it could be summarized in 4000 to 8000 words (there are a couple of exceptions); fourth, that where possible chapter authors should be clinicians experienced in the disorders of the human nervous system as well as recognized authorities on the neuroscientific basis of understanding in their own particular area of interest; fifth, that the depth at which each chapter covered its topic was to be uniform throughout. We trust the volumes reflect an adherence to these principles.

A project of this magnitude requires many hands. We extend our thanks and gratitude to each and every one who helped. We especially wish to recognize our long suffering secretaries Ms. Sharon Brubaker, Ms. Jane Cook, Ms. Kerry Pearce, and Ms. Judy DiStefano. Mr. Albert E. Meier of W. B. Saunders Company and Mr. Richard Barling of William Heinemann Medical Books Ltd. were steadfast in their support and unerring guidance. But it is to the chapter authors themselves to whom we owe the greatest debt of gratitude. They produced the substance of this book, and they deserve the credit. Any errors are our own.

A.K. ASBURY, M.D.
G.M. MCKHANN, M.D.
W.I. MCDONALD, PH.D., F.R.C.P.

Contents

Muscle and the Neuromuscular Junction

Peripheral Nerve, Root, and Spinal Cord

The Brain and Motor Control

24

Pharmacologic Aspects of Motor Dysfunction,   342

Anne B. Young
John B. Penney, Jr.

25

Tremor,   353

Robert R. Young

26

Oculomotor Control: Normal and Abnormal,   368

R. John Leigh
David S. Zee

Cranial Nerves and Their Disorders

27

Smell and Taste and Their Disorders,   390

Richard L. Doty
Charles P. Kimmelman
Ronald P. Lesser

28

Pathophysiology of Vision,   404

Christopher Kennard
K.H. Ruddock

29

Diseases of the Optic Nerve,   421

W. Ian McDonald
David Barnes

30

Disorders of Hearing,   434

Linda M. Luxon

31

Vertigo and Dizziness,   451

Thomas Brandt

Bodily Functions

32

Vasomotor Function and Dysfunction,   469

Roger R. Tuck
James G. McLeod

Disorders of Development

Disorders of Psychic Function

Intracranial Pressure

Vascular Diseases

Infection

Neuroimmunology

Neurologic Manifestations of Systemic Diseases

Approaches to the Study of Neurologic Pathophysiology

Introduction

1

Pathophysiology of Nervous System Diseases

Guy M. McKhann
W. Ian McDonald
Arthur K. Asbury

Pathophysiology "attempts to explain the biological basis of disease, making use of what ever scientific disciplines may be pertinent" (Smith and Thier, 1981). In the case of diseases of the nervous system, a wide array of scientific disciplines and approaches has been brought to bear. In this book we intend to emphasize the pathophysiology of neurologic disease. We use this term, *pathophysiology*, in its broadest sense, to mean the interface between basic biologic and physical mechanisms and clinical problems. The purpose of this introduction is to place contemporary efforts to elucidate neurologic pathophysiology into historical and clinical perspective. Each succeeding chapter has as its subject a particular topic within the field of neurology, but in this chapter we treat the specialty as a whole.

Since the first edition there have been remarkable new challenges and advances. In the introductory chapter to the first edition we concluded by saying: "The challenge for the clinician scholar and for the basic investigator interested in the diseases of the human nervous system is to persist in looking for the opportunities where rapid advances in the basic neurosciences and other areas can be applied to diseases of the nervous system. Fortuitous clinical events can also lead to new approaches to basic questions. This is an exciting time for the neurosciences and for clinical neurology. Neurology no longer should be viewed as a descriptive field, because the key questions can now be asked in virtually all neurological conditions: what is the pathophysiology and what can be done to restore function toward normal?" Can understanding the pathophysiology lead to approaches to therapy? Can we achieve a restoration of function?

NEW CHALLENGES

We should explore further a sentence from the previous paragraph: "Fortuitous clinical events can also lead to new approaches to basic questions." Nowhere is this statement more true than in the challenges offered by the interaction of three infectious agents with the nervous system. At the time of the first edition, infection with human immunodeficiency virus (HIV) was just being recognized and its neurologic manifestations characterized. It is now clear that there is a distinctive HIV encephalopathy and that this encephalopathy does not appear to be related to direct involvement of neural cells by HIV. Various indirect mechanisms have been proposed and are being evaluated. This devastating disease not only bridges the interface between neuroimmunology and neurovirology, but also emphasizes that understanding the pathophysiology of the encephalopathy may well depend on first understanding the interaction among HIV, its products, and neurobiologic processes.

The search for viral mechanisms for chronic neurologic disease has a long and varied history. The establishment of the association of the viral agent

1

human T cell lymphotrophic virus type I (HTLV-I) with chronic progressive spastic paraparesis opens a new chapter in this area of research. As with HIV, however, the question remains, by what mechanisms does this virus damage specific neuronal systems?

In addition, our understanding of the mechanisms of slowly progressive transmissible diseases, the spongiform encephalopathies, is becoming clearer. A relatively small protein (a prion) is associated with infectivity in the disease in animals (scrapie). A similar protein, cellular prion protein (PrP^c), is normally present in healthy animals. By some unknown mechanism, this normal protein is converted into the scrapie prion protein (PrP^{Sc}) by a post-translational change. Furthermore, it has been suggested that the scrapie prion enhances its own replication by a feedback mechanism. In the human spongiform encephalopathies—kuru, Creutzfeldt-Jakob disease, and the rare familial form, Gerstmann-Straussler syndrome—it has been suggested that alterations of prions underlie the pathophysiology. This hypothesis has been strengthened by the establishment of a strain of transgenic mice carrying the genetic abnormality of the Gerstmann-Straussler syndrome and expressing the characteristic pathologic changes (Hsiao, 1990). This novel mechanism of disease, a self-replicating protein, remains controversial and will clearly continue to be the focus of attention in coming years.

In the previous edition we cited observations that the meperidine analogue MPTP (1-methyl-4-phenyl-1,2,3,6-tetrahydropyridine) can produce in humans and in experimental animals a disease remarkably similar to naturally occurring Parkinson's disease. This fortuitous clinical observation has led to a new area of research in which MPTP is the model for the study of the role of nigrostriatal pathways in the control of movement; the evaluation of newer therapies for Parkinson's disease, including transplant of adrenal or fetal brain tissue; and the study of the role of susceptibility to a brain toxin in the neurobiology of aging. In addition, knowledge of the mechanisms of action of MPTP has raised the question of whether a similar agent in the environment may play a role in naturally occurring Parkinson's disease. Also, studies with this model have suggested newer approaches to therapy, including the use of selegiline (Deprenyl) (Langston, 1990).

The list of challenges continues, but perhaps the greatest challenge has been the use of new technologies, both to pose questions and to attempt to obtain answers about normal and abnormal neural functions.

THE NEW TECHNOLOGIES

There are many advances from which to choose, but certainly the most outstanding, the ones that border on science fiction, are the advances in molecular biology as they are applied to understanding cellular functions. These approaches have been useful for establishing genetic markers for a number of diseases of the nervous system, and the number grows almost weekly. In addition, the techniques of reverse genetics have been used to identify previously unknown gene products. A striking example is the identification of dystrophin in the Duchenne form of muscular dystrophy (Hoffman et al., 1987). Important as these advances are for diagnosis and understanding the genetic mechanisms of the disease, molecular biology has led to other striking developments. The ability to introduce DNA components into host cells has allowed in vitro production of large amounts of proteins that previously were barely detectable. Thus, the field of growth factors has exploded, and the role of trophic factors in disease mechanisms and as putative therapeutic agents is being studied. The development of transgenic animals in which normal and abnormal genes can be introduced and expressed has provided unique models of disease.

One could argue that molecular biology has led to a reductionist approach to the nervous system, in which specific subtypes of receptors and channels, rather than only cells, are examined. At the other extreme are the newer techniques of imaging that allow questions to be asked about how the human brain processes information as it performs higher cognitive functions. The advances in positron emission tomography, the use of intradural electrodes to stimulate and record from the cerebral cortex, and the evaluation of event-related potentials all provide approaches to mapping human brain functions. These techniques alone and in combination allow questions about not only the location of cortical processes, but also the temporal sequencing of information processing. On the horizon loom other imaging methodologies, including magnetic resonance imaging and magnetoencephalography, which may also add to the ability to evaluate neural processing in awake functioning humans.

NEWER CONCEPTS OF NEUROLOGIC DISEASE

A crucial question is whether the recognition of new challenges and the use of new technologies allow development of new concepts of pathophysiology of neurologic disease. The answer is unequivocally yes. The concept of neural damage from a number of types of insults, such as anoxia, ischemia, and trauma, has changed. The initial damage is followed by secondary effects that produce tissue damage only after a latency of hours or even days. Recognition of these delayed effects offers a therapeutic window during which intervention may be possible. For example, excitatory amino acids, glutamate, aspartate, and related compounds, have been proposed as agents responsible for delayed neuronal damage in ischemia, anoxia, some forms of trauma, and seizures. Study of the interactions of these excitatory amino acids with specific receptors and of the blocking of these interactions is an extraordinarily active area of research. This new concept of neurologic disease will likely result in clinical trials of agents that can prevent damage to the brain. A closely related question is whether endogenous excitatory compounds play a role in chronic progressive degenerative diseases of the nervous system, such as Huntington's disease. Animal models suggest that this hypothesis is possible.

Perhaps the greatest change, however, has not been a difference in concepts of neurologic disease, but in attitudes toward neurologic disease. Clinician scholars are no longer satisfied to accept an explanation that a particular disease is a viral disease of the nervous system, is immunologically mediated, or is a degenerative disease of the nervous system. They are now asking why and by what mechanism. The study of the interrelationship between the nervous system and the immune system is a striking example of this change. Neural function clearly influences immunologic function and vice versa. In addition, the immune system is no longer considered to be simply antibodies and antigens; cytokines and other soluble factors are now included as intermediaries in damage to the nervous system.

In asking why, scholars are conceptualizing about the brain as a series of systems—interrelated, interdependent systems. We have seen the advent of computational approaches to the evaluation of neural processing of information. These computational techniques, which model both normal and abnormal brain function, provide a valuable adjunct to the usual biologic methods of studying the nervous system.

THE DECADE OF THE BRAIN

In January 1990 President George Bush of the United States signed a proclamation declaring the 1990s as the Decade of the Brain. This recognition underscores the remarkable progress made in approaching brain functions and emphasizes the challenges and opportunities before us. A committee appointed by the Council of the Neurology Institute of the National Institutes of Health, on which two of us (Guy McKhann and Arthur Asbury) served, selected areas in which it was thought that there are unique opportunities for both understanding and altering disease processes (Table 1–1). We should add one other category: the overlap between brain and behavior. This area, traditionally the province of psychiatrists, has become more biologically oriented as genetic markers of psychiatric disease are proposed, abnormalities in transmitter metabolism are identified, and responses to therapeutic agents are

Table 1–1. AREAS WITH OPPORTUNITIES FOR UNDERSTANDING AND ALTERING DISEASE PROCESSES

The Developing Brain
  Developmental disorders
  Epilepsy
  Huntington's disease and other inherited diseases
The Injured Brain
  Head injury
  Spinal cord injury
  Cerebrovascular accident (stroke) and cerebrovascular disease
  Brain tumors
The Failing Brain
  The dementias, including Alzheimer's disease
  Multiple sclerosis
  Nerve and muscle disorders, including diabetic neuropathy and amyotrophic lateral sclerosis (Lou Gehrig's disease)
  Acquired immunodeficiency syndrome (AIDS) and other infections of the brain
  Parkinson's disease and motor system disorders
The Feeling Brain
  Effect of drugs on the brain
  Pain
Training for the Future

characterized. We include more discussions of behavior in this book than in the traditional neurology textbook because we believe that there is a great overlap of these fields. Understanding brain functions and abnormalities may yield great progress in both explaining and modifying behavior.

Identifying the 1990s as the Decade of the Brain implies a promise of significant advances. The reader can make his or her own speculations and predictions. Some are obvious, but the unexpected provides the excitement. Part of this excitement also comes from the increasing blurring of the margins of traditional approaches to the nervous system. Partly driven by the new technologies, anatomy and physiology converge around identification, localization, and characterization of receptor subtypes. Previously categorized by binding of pharmacologic agents, structure-function correlations based on molecular biologic identification are beginning to provide explanations of how a single neurotransmitter, such as dopamine or acetylcholine, can be involved in diverse neurologic functions. These new methods of studying neurotransmission may have implications for the treatment of seizures, abnormalities of motor control, pain, behavior disorders, and ischemic-anoxic brain injury.

The basis for the technical advances that we have discussed has not come from the neurosciences. Rather, molecular biologists, physicists, and chemists, among others, have provided this underpinning. That trend should continue and should be encouraged. The theoretic basis for understanding how the brain works and can become abnormal is not a natural approach for many biologically based clinician scholars, but it is for physicists and mathematicians. It is quite likely that in this decade those who model brain functions on the basis of real data will provide new insights into the pathophysiology of disease (Mesulam, 1990).

The final common pathway, however, remains the clinician scholar. We are the ones who know the vagaries of the human nervous system, we are the ones who provide our colleagues with meaningful characterizations of neurologic disease, and we are the ones who devise and evaluate the clinical trials of new therapies. We have an ever-expanding intellectual base from which to grow. Effective use of that new information to understand and alter diseases of the nervous system remains the goal of the Decade of the Brain.

References

Hsiao K.K., Scott M., Foster D., et al. Spontaneous neurodegeneration in transgenic mice with mutant prion protein. *Science* 250:1587–1590, 1990.

Hoffman E.P., Brown R.H., Kunkel L.M. Dystrophin: the protein product of the Duchenne muscular dystrophy locus. *Cell* 51:919–928, 1987.

Langston J.W. Selegiline as neuroprotective therapy in Parkinson's disease: concepts and controversies. *Neurology* 5:143–147, 1990.

Mesulam M.M. Large-scale neurocognitive networks and distributed processing for attention, language and memory. *Ann. Neurol.* 28:597–613, 1990.

Smith L.H. Jr., Thier S.O., eds. Preface. In *Pathophysiology: The Biological Principles of Disease*. Philadelphia, Saunders, 1981.

Organization of the Nervous System Neurons

2

Development of the Nervous System

W. Maxwell Cowan

Any consideration of the development of the nervous system must address a number of related, if formally separable, issues: How and when does neural tissue arise? How and where do neuronal precursors proliferate? How do their progeny reach their definitive locations? How do neurons acquire their distinctive morphologic, physiologic, and biochemical properties? Most important, how do they come to form connections with other nerve cells or innervate such effector tissues as striated muscle and glands? Developmental neurobiologists have been attempting to answer these and other questions for almost a century (Patterson and Purves, 1982), but it is still not possible to give a completely satisfying account of the development of any single region of either the central or the peripheral nervous system, let alone of the entire nervous system. This chapter summarizes some of the more general aspects of the development of the vertebrate nervous system in general and the human nervous system in particular and then gives a brief account of each of the major events in neurogenesis and their later modification and refinement. It is hardly necessary to emphasize that a sound grasp of these features of neuronal development is essential for an understanding of not only many of the problems encountered in pediatric neurology and neuropathology but also many of the more serious conditions encountered in clinical neurology. This chapter incorporates several more recent findings, especially those bearing on some of the molecular events associated with neural induction, the analysis of neuronal lineages, the genetic specification of nerve cells, and the mechanisms involved in axonal pathfinding.

THE ORIGIN OF NEURAL TISSUE AND THE GENERAL DEVELOPMENT OF THE NERVOUS SYSTEM

Neural Induction

The development of the nervous system may be said to begin when, under the influence of the invaginating *chorda mesoderm*, the ectoderm along the dorsal midline becomes irrevocably transformed into the *neuroepithelium* of the *medullary* or *neural plate*. Coincident with this, the ectoderm surrounding the neural plate, in what is sometimes referred to as the *neurosomatic junctional region*, becomes committed to form the future *neural crest*. Both these transformations appear to be brought about by the *inductive* influence of the underlying chorda mesoderm. As the developing *notochord* extends forward from the region of the *Hensen node* (corresponding to the dorsal lip of the blastopore in lower vertebrates), it seems to determine sequentially, within the neural plate, the major regions of the future central nervous system (CNS): the forebrain, midbrain, and hindbrain rostrally and the spinal cord caudally.

The nature of the inductive influence of the chorda mesoderm on the overlying ectoderm has not yet been established, but in the past 2–3 years, much has been learned about the transformation of the cells that come to form the invaginating mesoderm. Experiments in amphibian embryos (in which *primary induction* was first discovered by Spemann and Mangold [1924]) suggest that mesodermal induction is brought about by one or more growth factors, most probably members of the transforming growth factor family (transforming growth factor β and the related activins), but the fibroblast growth factors (fibroblast growth factors α and β) may also be implicated (see Thomsen et al., 1990). The corresponding inducing agent that transforms the overlying ectoderm into neural tissue remains to be isolated. However, it is widely believed that it exerts its influence on the ectoderm in a graded fashion so that the last region of the ectoderm to come under its influence (and hence, the region influenced for the shortest time) becomes the forebrain; the tissue first exposed to the inducing factor (and hence, exposed for the longest period or at the highest concentration) later forms the spinal cord.

Formation of the Neural Tube

When it is first recognizable, about the middle of the third week after conception, the human neural plate is roughly paddle shaped and is marked by only a slight increase in the height of its columnar epithelial cells. However, shortly thereafter, a longitudinal furrow appears in the midline, and as this deepens, the initially flat neural plate becomes converted into a distinct *neural groove* flanked by the elevated *neural folds*. The accumulation of contractile filaments around the perimeter of the apical or free poles of the epithelial cells that form the neural plate changes them from their initial cylindric form to truncated cones. As this process proceeds, the neural groove appears to sink down and the lateral walls of the plate become progressively elevated until the neural folds on either side approach each other and begin to fuse along the dorsal midline; because the adjoining somatic ectoderm fuses in the same way, the neural tube comes to lie deep to the overlying ectoderm that later forms the epidermis.

In humans, the fusion of the neural folds begins toward the end of the third or early in the fourth week of gestation at what will later be the cervical region and extends zipper-like both rostrally and caudally, turning the original neural plate into the *neural tube* (Fig. 2–1). For a short time, the neural tube is open to the amniotic cavity at its rostral and caudal ends, but by the end of the fourth week, it becomes sealed off, with the closure of the anterior

and posterior *neuropores*. With the closure of the neural tube, the ectoderm that formed the lips of the neural folds separates from the tube to form a fairly distinct crest of tissue that extends initially along the length of the neural tube. This is the *neural crest*, a pleomorphic tissue that gives rise to several components of the peripheral nervous system (PNS) as well as a number of non-neural tissues (see later).

Almost immediately after the closure of the neural tube, its lateral walls begin to thicken, while its dorsal and ventral surfaces become much reduced to form the future *roof* and *floor plates*, respectively. The actual origin of the floor plate (which has come to assume a new significance since the demonstration of its important role in both the induction of the motor columns of the spinal cord and the guidance of commissural axons that cross the midline of the cord) has been clarified. It appears to be derived not from the neural plate as was commonly believed but from cells in and around the Hensen node, which may account for its inductive and polarizing properties. The thickening of the lateral wall of the neural tube has been attributed to the inductive influence of the somatic mesoderm on either side of it, but the evidence for this has been called in question and the nature of the inductive influence (if it exists) is unknown. The progressive thickening of the lateral walls of the neural tube results in an apparent crowding of the cells together so that their nuclei come to lie at several levels, giving the tube a stratified appearance. However, near its superficial or apical surface, each cell retains its attachment to its neighbors through specialized membrane contacts known as junctional complexes, and because each cell has a peripheral process that reaches to the *basal lamina* that surrounds the entire neural tube, the neuroepithelium is regarded as a *pseudostratified columnar epithelium*. As we shall see, this has important implications for the way cells proliferate in the neural tube and its various derivatives.

The Neural Crest

Concurrently with the changes in the neural tube, the cells of the neural crest begin to disperse by migrating along well-defined pathways: one population of cells migrates dorsolaterally to join the developing epidermis; it gives rise, in time, to most of the pigment cells of the body. A second group migrates ventrally through the somatic mesoderm alongside the neural tube. During its migration, this group of cells is apparently influenced by both the neural tube and the somatic mesoderm, and when its cells have completed their migration, they form the *prevertebral* and *paravertebral ganglia* of the sympathetic nervous system. A third group migrates ventrolaterally but becomes arrested alongside the neural tube; its cells form the *dorsal root* or *sensory ganglia*. Still other components of the neural crest, which are not discussed here, migrate into the ventral

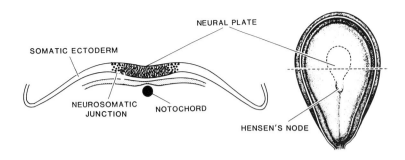

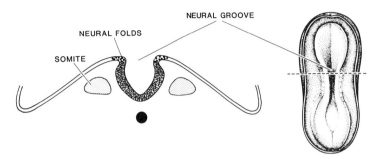

Figure 2–1. The appearance of the neural plate as seen from the dorsal aspect *(upper right)*, and in transverse section *(upper left)*, the neural groove, and the early neural tube shortly after the fusion of the neural folds *(lower)*. (Redrawn from Cowan W.M. The development of the brain. *Sci. Am.* 241[3]:113–133, 1979. Copyright © by Scientific American, Inc. All rights reserved.)

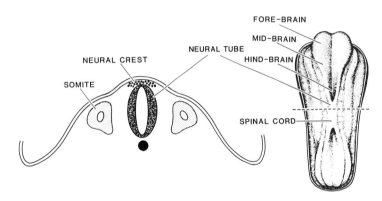

mesentery to form the medulla of the adrenal gland, migrate rostrally into the head region and form parts of the visceral skeleton, or give rise to various components of the so-called APUD system (whose cells are characterized by their amine precursor uptake and decarboxylation) and to parts of certain endocrine glands (e.g., the calcitonin-secreting cells of the thyroid gland).

The migratory patterns of the neural crest cells are remarkably consistent, and it is now evident from a variety of different types of experimentation that the characteristic phenotype of each class of cell is determined in part by the migratory route its cells take but largely by the final location they come to occupy (for review, see Le Douarin, 1982). For example, a substantial portion of the neural crest from the trunk region gives rise to the adrenal medulla and to sympathetic ganglion cells, which synthesize and release *norepinephrine*. If, at early stages, this tissue is excised and transplanted to the head region of a donor embryo (most of this work has been done in chick embryos), the same crest cells migrate into the gut, where they give rise to *cholinergic* neurons. Similarly, in vitro studies have established that this

type of change is not due to the clonal selection of cells from an initially mixed population but rather that individual neurons can switch their transmitter phenotype from one type to another.

The Ectodermal Placodes

There is one other source of neural tissue: the so-called ectodermal placodes. As the neural tube expands and grows, at a number of sites it secondarily induces the overlying ectoderm to form the precursors of certain sensory epithelia and components of cranial nerve ganglia. Such ectodermal placodes include the olfactory placode, which gives rise to the olfactory epithelium; the trigeminal placode, which after invaginating joins with a neural crest component to form the trigeminal ganglion; the auditory or acousticovestibular placode, which gives rise to the spiral and vestibular ganglia; and the facial, vagal, and glossopharyngeal placodes, which form the sensory ganglia of the related cranial nerves. The further fate of these placodal derivatives is not discussed, except to say that they give rise to both neuronal and supportive (glial) elements in the respective ganglia and that in almost every respect, other than their origin, they resemble neural crest derivatives.

Changes in Gross Morphology of the Developing Central Nervous System

Shortly after the closure of the neural tube, a series of three vesicle-like swellings appears at its rostral end. These are the three primary brain vesicles usually referred to as the *prosencephalic,* or forebrain, vesicle; the *mesencephalic,* or midbrain, vesicle; and the *rhombencephalic,* or hindbrain, vesicle. The presumptive spinal cord extends caudally from the hindbrain vesicle as a structure of essentially uniform diameter (see Fig. 2–1). As the result of differential growth of the three brain vesicles and a number of complex foldings or flexures, the original elongated and rather unremarkable neural tube becomes converted quite rapidly into the generally recognized parts of the CNS. It is unnecessary to describe these changes in detail here; they are well described in most textbooks of embryology and their major features are shown diagrammatically in Figure 2–2. It need only be stated that the forebrain vesicle ultimately gives rise to the *telencephalon* (including the greatly expanded *cerebral hemispheres* and the *diencephalon*); the midbrain vesicle changes the least and forms the definitive *midbrain;* and from the ventral

part of the hindbrain vesicle, the *pons* and *medulla* develop fairly early, and at a somewhat later stage, the major part of the *cerebellum* develops from the dorsal region of the hindbrain.

THE PRIMARY PROCESSES OF NEURONAL DEVELOPMENT

The transformation of each region of the developing brain and spinal cord into the various components that compose its adult structure is brought about by a series of cytogenetic and morphogenetic events that may be referred to collectively as the *primary processes of neurogenesis* (Cowan, 1978). These events are both *progressive* (or additive) and *regressive.* More or less in the order in which they occur, the progressive events are *cell proliferation, neuronal migration, selective cell aggregation, cytodifferentiation, axonal outgrowth,* and *synapse formation.* The first regressive event occurs at about the time when the neurons in each population begin to form connections within their respective projection fields: this phase in development is marked by the *selective death* of a substantial proportion (generally about 50%) of the initial population of cells. Later, many of the connections that were initially formed are eliminated as certain axon terminals are withdrawn and, in some cases, extensive early-formed axon collaterals are removed. Thus, the definitive form of each region of the

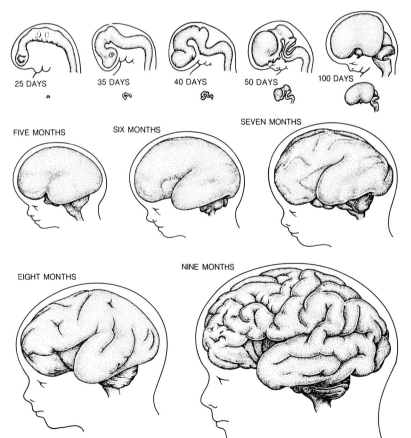

Figure 2–2. The appearance of the developing human brain at each of several stages from the fourth week of gestation to term. The drawings in the upper row are magnified; those just beneath them are drawn to the same scale as the figures in the lower two rows. (Redrawn from Cowan W.M. The development of the brain. *Sci. Am.* 241[3]:113–133, 1979. Copyright © by Scientific American, Inc. All rights reserved.)

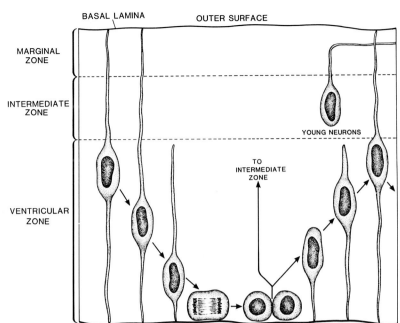

Figure 2–3. The to-and-fro movements of the nuclei of the cells in the neuroepithelium and the rounding up of the ventricular cells before division. After cytokinesis, the cells may either repeat the cycle or move out of the ventricular zone into the developing intermediate zone. The marginal zone is formed predominantly by the basal processes of ventricular cells and the axons of young neurons in the intermediate zone.

Cell Proliferation

The wall of the neural tube is formed initially by a pseudostratified columnar epithelium that rests on an external basement membrane (or basal lamina): each cell extends a peripheral process to the basal lamina and a central process to the luminal surface of the tube, where it is joined to the central processes of neighboring cells by typical junctional complexes. The nuclei of the cells lie at different levels within the neuroepithelium, except for those in the later stages of mitosis (i.e., metaphase, anaphase, and telophase), which are consistently found along the luminal aspect of the epithelium. This appearance

nervous system is fashioned by the addition of new cellular elements and the establishment of new cell-to-cell relationships and is later refashioned by the selective removal of some fraction of the initial group of cellular elements and the controlled elimination of some of the earlier-established intercellular relationships (Cowan et al., 1985). In the following discussion, each of these several events is described in some detail and certain of the underlying descriptive and experimental evidence is briefly summarized. The account given refers principally to the development of the vertebrate CNS; for the most part, the same series of events occurs in the development of the PNS, but there are some significant differences (see later). The development of the nervous system in invertebrates is, in its overall form, quite different, but in a number of important details, neurogenesis in vertebrates and invertebrates is strikingly similar; much of our knowledge of the molecular and genetic mechanisms involved derives from studies of certain invertebrates, especially the fruit fly *Drosophila* and the nematode worm *Caenorhabditis elegans*.

led the great German embryologist Wilhelm His (whose careful reconstructions of early embryonic brains are the basis for Fig. 2–2) to suggest that the neuroepithelium consists of two cell types: *germinal cells*, which, he thought, gave rise to neurons, and *spongioblasts*, which were said to form all the glial elements of the CNS. This interpretation of the structure of the neuroepithelium was challenged by Schaper (1897) shortly after it was propounded, and it is now known to be incorrect—although, curiously, the term spongioblast has lingered in the neuropathologic literature as the cellular basis of certain ill-defined CNS tumors. As Schaper first recognized, and as subsequent work has confirmed, the cells that form the neuroepithelium initially compose a single more or less uniform population, and the distribution of their nuclei simply reflects the various stages in the mitotic cycle through which the proliferating cells pass. Feulgen spectrophotometry (which is used to measure the DNA content of individual nuclei) and [³H]thymidine autoradiography have established that the resting or interphase nuclei are located in the basal and middle regions of the neuroepithelium, and it is here that DNA synthesis begins. Subsequently, as the cells enter prophase, their nuclei begin to move superficially toward the luminal surface of the epithelium. By the time they enter metaphase, they withdraw their peripheral processes and appear to round up before telophase. After cytokinesis (which usually occurs in a plane orthogonal to the luminal surface [Fig. 2–3]), the resulting daughter cells again extend a peripheral process toward the basal lamina, and the nucleus once more migrates away from the lumen toward the midlevel of the epithelium, where it remains until the next round of DNA synthesis.

This characteristic to-and-fro movement of the nuclei of the neuroepithelial cells is termed *interkinetic nuclear migration*, and it is typical of cell proliferation in all pseudostratified epithelia (Sauer, 1935). It is not known why nuclei move toward the surface of the epithelium before dividing, but it is known that the process of nuclear migration is dependent on the integrity of microfilaments in the luminal part of the cell; if these are disrupted (by treatment with the drug cytochalasin B), the nuclei do not move toward the lumen, and division is arrested. Experimental treatment of the neuroepithelium with colchicine (which disrupts microtubules, including those that form the mitotic spindle) also causes mitotic arrest and results in a massive pile-up of metaphase figures at and immediately deep to the luminal surface (for review, see Cowan, 1981).

Continued cell proliferation leads at first to a general expansion of the surface area of the neuroepithelium in parallel with the rapid growth of the brain and spinal cord. However, this early phase of more or less exponential growth in the numbers of neuroepithelial cells soon gives way to the differential production of neurons and glia of specific types or lineages. This phase of early neuronal and glial differentiation is marked by the withdrawal of cells from the neuroepithelium (or as it is now termed, the *ventricular zone*) and their movement basally into a newly emerging *intermediate zone* (formerly called the mantle zone).

Although it is not known why cells of particular lineages begin to withdraw from the proliferative pool when they do, the technique of [³H]thymidine autoradiography has made it possible to determine the time of generation (or the birth dates) of specific types of neurons in many regions of the nervous system and in a variety of vertebrates. From this work (Cowan, 1981), the following generalizations can be drawn:

1. Each population of neurons is generated during a distinct period in embryonic or fetal life. With a few notable exceptions, such as the granule cells of the cerebellar cortex and of the dentate gyrus (a part of the hippocampal formation), this period is usually quite short, lasting as a rule just a few days to a week or two at most.

2. The sequence in which cells withdraw from the proliferative pool is well defined, so that it is possible to speak of distinct *gradients* in cell production in most regions. The actual sequence—or the direction of the gradient—varies from region to region. Thus, in the retina, the ganglion cells (which in the mature state are farthest removed from the original ventricular zone) are generated first, followed in turn by the cells in the inner nuclear layer and finally the photoreceptors (i.e., the cells are generated in an outside-in gradient). In the cerebral cortex, the sequence is the exact reverse of this: the deepest cells (i.e., those that later come to occupy layer VI and are topographically closest to the ventricular zone) are generated first, whereas those that occupy successively more superficial layers withdraw from the cell cycle in an orderly inside-out sequence.

3. In most regions, there is also evidence of (a) a general ventral-to-dorsal gradient, which ensures that motor systems tend to be generated earlier than the related sensory systems, and (b) either a rostrocaudal or center-to-periphery sequence of cell generation and overall maturation. Thus, in the spinal cord, cells in the basal plate are generated, on average, some days before the cells in the alar plate, and the cells of any given class tend to be generated earlier at cervical than at lumbosacral levels. This pattern is common also in the brain stem but, significantly, not in the forebrain. Similarly, in the retina, there is a general center-to-periphery sequence in the development of all classes of neurons. Several other variants of this gradient theme could be cited, but these examples should serve to make the general point that neurogenesis is highly programmed in both space and time.

4. The characteristic segmental arrangement of neurons in the spinal cord appears not to be due to an underlying segmental pattern of cell proliferation but rather to the later segmental grouping of neurons into discrete pools, or laminae. However, because the segmental arrangement of the sensory (or dorsal root) ganglia is due to the inductive influence of the neighboring mesodermal somites, it remains possible that there is a similar, but covert, action of somatic mesoderm on the cord itself.

   A special case can be made for the segmental proliferation of cells in the hindbrain, where a number of distinct swellings (or *neuromeres*) can be recognized at an early stage in development. Although the significance (and even the existence) of neuromeres has been debated for almost half a century, there is now fairly compelling evidence that they are a distinctive feature of rhombencephalic development in all vertebrates and that they reflect regions of relatively high cell proliferation separated by narrow zones where proliferation proceeds at a low rate. That certain homologues of the homoeotic or segment-determining genes found in *Drosophila* are selectively expressed in some of the neuromeres is further evidence not only that these transient structures are important but also that the hindbrain is segmentally organized (Lumsden, 1990; Stern and Keynes, 1988).

5. Neurons were once thought to be generated before the glial cells in the same region; this is now known to be incorrect. In all regions of the developing nervous system that have been carefully studied, neuronal and glial cell precursors (identifiable on the basis of immunocytochemical staining with appropriate markers) have been found to coexist side by side within the proliferative zone (Levitt et al., 1981), and the existence of a population of glial cells with radially directed processes plays an important role in the early outward migration of young neurons (see later). However, what does seem to be true is that, even

though glial cells are evident as early as the first neurons, glial proliferation may continue for some time after all the neurons in the region have been generated. Furthermore, in some cases, there appears to be a close correlation between the number of certain glial cells generated and the number of neurons or neuronal processes in the region; the rapid proliferation of oligodendrocytes at the time of myelination of axons is perhaps the best example of this phenomenon (see later).

6. In nearly every region, the larger neurons tend to be generated earlier than the smaller neurons of the same general type. This has sometimes mistakenly been taken to mean that projection neurons are always generated before local circuit neurons, or interneurons. In most regions this is true, but in the cerebral cortex, for example, the small stellate cells in layer IV are nearly all generated before the larger pyramidal neurons (which give rise to corticocortical connections) in layers II and III.

Although in most regions of the CNS cell proliferation is limited to the ventricular zone, in some regions there is an early outward migration of cells into a subjacent zone where the proliferation of both neuronal and glial precursors continues, often for considerable periods of time. These subjacent or specialized proliferative regions are variously termed *subependymal* or *subventricular zones* or are often named for the specific region in which they occur (e.g., the rhombic lip and the external granular layer of the cerebellum). In most respects, cell proliferation in these areas is similar to that in the ventricular zone, except that there is no indication of any form of interkinetic nuclear migration. The most prominent subventricular zones in the human brain are found in the striatum (in the angle between the corpus callosum and the head of the caudate nucleus), in the hilar region of the dentate gyrus (from which most of the dentate granule cells arise), in the rhombic lip (from which certain of the pontine and olivary nuclei are derived), and in the external granular layer of the cerebellum (which gives rise to the various interneurons found in the cerebellar cortex and to the enormous number of cerebellar granular cells).

The birth date of a neuron or of a population of neurons is an important landmark in its developmental history for several reasons. It appears to be the trigger for the outward migration of the cells from the ventricular zone. In addition, the *phenotype* of the cell is often determined at this time, as is the locus to which the cells migrate. Perhaps most important of all, it seems as though at this time neurons acquire a set of rather fixed instructions regarding the site or sites to which their axons later project (Cowan, 1979a).

The lineages of the different neuronal and glial cell types has been a vexing question for several years mainly because there were few, if any, reliable cytochemical markers for specific classes of cells and

no easy way to trace the fates of individual progenitor cells. Fortunately, as a result of a number of technical developments, this issue has been greatly clarified (see Stent, 1985), and it is now known that many long-held views (for example, that each neuroepithelial cell can give rise to cells of only one class) are erroneous.

The development of cell class–specific antibodies that could be used immunocytochemically to identify both immature and mature cells was the first useful approach to this issue. It has been used particularly well to clarify the lineages and the relationships between the major classes of central glial cells. There are three major classes of glial cells in the CNS: *oligodendrocytes* and two types of *astrocytes* (referred to as type 1 and type 2); there are now good cytochemical markers for each class. From a careful study of the development of the rat optic nerve (which, developmentally, is a central fiber pathway), Raff and colleagues established that type 1 astrocytes arise at an early stage from a distinctive precursor, whereas type 2 astrocytes and oligodendrocytes arise later from a common precursor. Type 1 astrocytes seem to produce a growth factor (probably platelet derived growth factor) that in vitro causes the oligodendrocyte/type 2 astrocyte progenitor cells to keep dividing. A second signal—thought to be the protein known as ciliary neurotrophic factor—causes these progenitor cells to stop producing oligodendrocytes and to begin producing type 2 astrocytes (see Raff, 1989). The early appearance, in vitro, of type 1 astrocytes followed some days later, at approximately the day of birth, by oligodendrocytes and about a week later by the type 2 astrocytes is in keeping with these findings. Raff's studies also provided evidence that the type 1 astrocytes are involved in the initial formation of the optic stalk and that the oligodendrocyte/type 2 astrocyte progenitor cells secondarily invade the developing optic nerve from the basal forebrain.

A second approach to the analysis of cell lineages involved the selective marking of individual progenitor cells in the neuroepithelium either by the *intracellular injection* of a long-lasting marker (such as the enzyme horseradish peroxidase, for which there is an effective cytochemical procedure that gives rise to a distinctive reaction product) or by *genetically* using an engineered retrovirus into which a suitable reporter gene (such as the *Escherichia coli lacZ* gene, which encodes a β-galactosidase) has been inserted (Sanes, 1989). Horseradish peroxidase labeling was first used to study cell lineages in the amphibian neural retina, which, as a direct derivative of the forebrain, has proved to be an excellent model for studies of CNS development. The most significant findings from this work are that a single neuroepithelial cell can give rise to both retinal neurons and supporting cells (the so-called Müller cells of the retina) and furthermore that its progeny can include any of the different classes of retinal neurons— photoreceptors, bipolar cells, amacrine cells, and ganglion cells (Holt et al., 1988). The use of retroviral vectors confirmed these findings in the mammalian retina and demonstrated essentially the same type of lineage relationships for many of the different classes of neurons in the cerebral cortex (Turner and Cepko, 1987; Walsh and Cepko, 1988).

A related but less direct genetic approach that has been used to follow certain cell lineages in the mammalian nervous system involves the use of chimeric mice generated by fusing blastomeres from two genetically distinct strains (e.g., wild-type and *lurcher* mutants) and subsequently examining the distribution of cells from each parental line in the adult CNS (for a critique of this approach, see Herrup, 1988; Jennings, 1988).

The most complete analysis of neural cell lineages has been carried out in the nematode worm *C. elegans* by Horvitz and colleagues (for reviews, see Ambros and Horvitz, 1987; Horvitz, 1987, 1990). Because the nematode is essentially translucent and contains fewer than 1000 cells in all, it has been possible, using Nomarski optics, to observe directly the fate of every cell, including the 300 or so neurons. By generating large numbers of mutants, many of which affect the lineages of specific neurons, it has been possible to identify a number of genes that specify the fate of individual precursor cells. So far, the complexity of the mammalian nervous system has precluded any comparable genetic analysis of neuronal cell lineages, but there is every reason to believe that homologous or functionally related genes exist in mammals and will in time be identified.

Neuronal Migration

In the PNS, neural crest and placodal precursor cells migrate along predetermined, but as yet molecularly undefined, pathways to their various loci in the cranial, spinal, or autonomic ganglia, and it is only on reaching their definitive locations that they undergo their major phase of proliferation. However, in the CNS, the situation is quite different. Because essentially all proliferation occurs in either the *ventricular* or the *subventricular zone*, all neurons have to undergo at least one phase of migration during which they are translocated from the region in which they are generated to their definitive locations in the brain or the spinal cord. Although much remains to be learned about neuronal migration, several general features of this important phase in neurogenesis are quite well understood (Sidman and Rakic, 1974) and can be briefly summarized as follows:

1. The initial impetus for migration of a young neuron appears to be its withdrawal from the cell cycle, although the nature of the actual stimulus to migrate is not known. However, there is circumstantial evidence that suggests quite strongly that the cells have acquired a distinct "address" by the time they begin to migrate out of the ventricular or subventricular zone.

2. The process of neuronal migration is ameboid,

with the cells extending leading processes into which the nucleus is actively drawn and then gradually retracting their trailing processes. The forward propulsion of the cells appears to be brought about by the adhesion of the leading edge of the cell to an underlying substrate through some form of receptor-ligand interaction and a consequent signal to motile elements within the cytoskeleton.

3. All such cellular movements require the presence of an appropriate substratum along which the cells can move; one obvious substratum that exists in all regions of the CNS is the system of radial glial processes. These are the processes of a special type of astrocyte-like progenitor cell that have their cell bodies in the ventricular zone and extend lengthy processes to the lumen of the neural tube and to the basal lamina surrounding the developing brain and spinal cord. As such, they can be thought of as persisting columnar cells from the original neuroepithelium that, at an early stage, acquire some of the properties of astrocytes (e.g., they contain the glial fibrillary acidic protein). In most regions of the human brain and spinal cord, these radial glia subsequently disappear, but in many lower vertebrates, they may persist into adult life. It is generally assumed that, when they disappear, they become transformed into typical astrocytes, but there is no direct evidence for this. Electron micrographs of developing neural tissue during the period of cell migration often show several young neurons closely applied to the surface of a single radial glial process (Fig. 2–4).

4. That the relationship between migrating neurons and radial glial processes is not merely fortuitous is suggested by the finding that in at least one type of mouse neurologic mutant in which the granule cells of the cerebellum are arrested in their migration from the external to the internal granular layers, there is an early breakdown of the relevant radial glial processes (Rakic and Sidman, 1973).

5. The molecular basis of the cell interactions that are such an essential feature of neuronal migration remain to be determined but there is now good evidence for the involvement of a number of cell surface adhesion molecules such as the neural-glial cell adhesion molecule NG-CAM, N-cadherin, cytotactin, and astrotactin (see Hatten, 1990; Jessell, 1988). It is likely also that members of the *integrin* family that are known to be involved in process outgrowth are also implicated in neuronal migration through interactions with extracellular matrix molecules such as laminin and fibronectin (Tomaselli et al., 1988).

6. It is important to note that not all neuronal migrations in the CNS are in a predominantly radial direction and also that, in some cases, the cells migrate well beyond the limits of the related radial glial processes. The substrates along which such migrations occur are not known at present, nor is it known how migrating cells identify the sites at

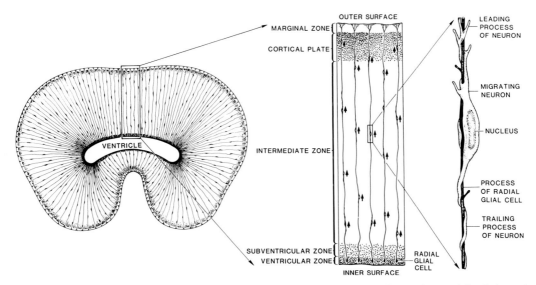

Figure 2–4. Young neurons generally migrate outward from the ventricular zone along the surfaces of a specialized class of glial cell (the so-called radial glial). The drawing on the left shows the disposition of the radial glial in a section through the developing cerebral hemisphere, and the inset drawings to the right show how they span the entire thickness of the wall of the hemisphere and provide a substrate for the migrating neurons as they move out to form the cortical plate. (Redrawn from Cowan W.M. The development of the brain. *Sci. Am.* 241[3]:113–133, 1979. Copyright © by Scientific American, Inc. All rights reserved. Based originally on observations by Dr. Pasko Rakic.)

which they should detach themselves from the substratum and begin to aggregate with other cells of like kind to form the anlagen or precursors of particular nuclear groups or cortical layers.

There are several reports in the neuropathologic literature of what are called *neuronal ectopias,* which are best thought of as errors in the migratory process—the cells migrating too far, not far enough, or occasionally in an inappropriate direction. The cause of such ectopias is unknown, but it is probably significant that they are often associated with other disturbances in brain development such as *lissencephaly.* These grossly abnormal neuronal migrations are to be distinguished from the not infrequent displacement of occasional cells that are found to lie outside the boundaries of the relevant nuclear group or cortical layer as a whole. Many such cells seem to be able to receive and form the appropriate connections and to function as integral components of their respective populations (O'Leary and Cowan, 1982). It is also worth mentioning that, contrary to an earlier opinion, the essential phenotype of central (as opposed to peripheral) neurons is not determined by the locus they come to occupy. This has been clearly demonstrated in yet another neurologic mutant (the *reeler* mouse) in which, even though most types of cortical neurons end up in the wrong places, they succeed in making the right types of connections and have the appropriate functional properties (Lemmon and Pearlman, 1981).

As mentioned earlier, neuronal migrations in the PNS also seem to follow predetermined pathways, but as yet no morphologically identifiable cellular substrates comparable to the radial glia in the CNS have been recognized. It is generally assumed that subtle and covert differences in the distribution of

extracellular matrix molecules form the basis of these predetermined pathways, and for some migrating neural crest derivatives, there is growing evidence that this is so. In addition, there is a good deal of evidence that the neuronal phenotype of most neural crest cells is largely determined by the regions through which they migrate and the definitive loci in which they come to reside. In part, at least, this is because, in the PNS, the majority of the migrating cells are *precursors* or *stem cells* rather than differentiated young neurons, and they undergo their major phase of proliferation after, rather than before, migrating (see earlier).

Selective Cell Aggregation

The cessation of migration and the selective aggregation of cells of like kind to form the anlagen of the various nuclear groups and cortical laminae have been among the first of the primary events in neurogenesis to begin to be understood at the molecular level. Using the experimental paradigm suggested by Holtfreter (1939) (who originally demonstrated that dissociated embryonic cells can reaggregate in vitro in cell type–specific ways—ectodermal cells with other ectodermal cells, mesodermal with mesodermal, and so on), several workers examined the selective adhesivity of brain cells and established the following major points (for reviews, see Edelman, 1984; Gottlieb and Glaser, 1980):

1. All neural cells have a tendency to adhere to other neural cells from the same region and, in some cases, to cells from other regions with which they are synaptically linked.
2. The patterns of adhesivity vary from region to region and, within any region, from tissue to

tissue at different stages during normal development (i.e., the adhesivity is temporally modulated).

3. The adhesion of cells to each other can be selectively inhibited by neuronal membrane fragments and by antibodies directed against certain cell surface components.

Edelman and colleagues used an ingenious immunologic approach to isolate a number of cell adhesion molecules (CAMs) from the brain and other tissues. One of the former (designated N-CAM because in adult animals it is largely limited to neurons) is of special interest in neural development. This is a large sialoglycoprotein that exists in several forms, each encoded by a distinct mRNA generated by alternative splicing from a single large gene. N-CAM is found on the surfaces of all neurons (and, to a lesser extent, muscle cells) and undergoes a characteristic change from an embryonic form to the mature, or adult, form by the selective elimination of several sialic acid residues. Antibodies against N-CAM not only block cell reaggregation in vitro but also disrupt normal cell aggregation in vivo and prevent the selective fasciculation of nerve fibers. N-CAM is present at an early stage in development (at the blastoderm stage), in the region that fate-mapping studies have identified as presumptive neural tissue (Edelman, 1984). It subsequently appears at specific times in the development of all neural centers and undergoes conversion from the embryonic to the adult form at certain well-defined times in each region. Although in adults N-CAM is essentially confined to neural tissue, it appears transiently during the induction of several organs and tissues such as the lens of the eye and the mesonephros. Interestingly, in the PNS, it is said to be present in the neural crest but disappears during the migration of the cells to their several locations, only to reappear again as the cells aggregate to form neuronal ganglia. It is normally absent from the neuromuscular junction but reappears after transection of the motor axons.

The ubiquitous distribution of N-CAM marks it as a molecule of unusual importance in both neural development and the maintenance of the established nervous system. However, it is clearly only one of a number of neuron- and/or glial cell–related adhesion molecules. A second molecule, called NG-CAM by Edelman and colleagues (1985), has been identified and partially characterized. Unlike N-CAM, which is homophilic in its interactions (i.e., it binds to N-CAM on other nerve cells), NG-CAM is heterophilic and may play a key role in the association between neurons and the surrounding glia, for example, during neuronal migration. More recently, a number of other cell adhesion and cell substrate molecules have been identified, some of which (including the *cadherins*) are calcium dependent, whereas others, such as N-CAM, are calcium independent. Although on the surface it may seem difficult to account for the assemblage of so many different cellular aggregates

in the CNS on the basis of just a few key molecules, as Edelman (1984) pointed out, the spatial and temporal modulation of a molecule such as N-CAM confers on it enormous potential for selectivity. It remains to be determined just which of these various CAMs participate in the assembly of particular neuronal aggregates in the CNS or PNS and what changes in cell adhesivity occur as the anlagen of the different nuclear groups and ganglia are remodeled to accommodate the ingrowth of axons, dendrite formation, and the establishment of synapses.

Neuronal Cytodifferentiation

Although it is clear that the cells that migrate out of the ventricular or subventricular zones in the developing CNS are already differentiated (in the sense that they are distinguishable morphologically and cytochemically as either young neurons or glial precursors), it is only after completing the phases of migration and association with other cells in a presumptive nuclear group or cortical sheet that most central neurons undergo their major phase of cytodifferentiation. Included under this term are three related classes of events:

1. The development of a number of processes—usually a single axon and one or more dendrites.
2. The acquisition of a distinctive set of membrane properties and, antecedent to this, the synthesis of the necessary ion channels and their insertion into the cell membrane.
3. A commitment to a particular mode of cell-to-cell transmission. In most mammalian neurons, this involves the appearance of the appropriate transmitter-synthesizing and -degrading enzymes, and the related transmitter receptors, but in some, it involves the appearance of the necessary molecular mechanisms for the formation of gap junctions for electrical transmission.

For simplicity, these three classes of events may be referred to as morphologic, physiologic, and molecular differentiation, respectively.

Morphologic Differentiation

Some neurons begin to "spin out" an axon even while migrating, but the majority do so only after coming to reside in their definitive locations. Although at a later stage the distinction between axons and dendrites is usually quite clear, initially all the outgrowing processes are rather similar and contain the same complement of organelles, including ribosomes. For this reason, they are conveniently referred to by the noncommittal term *neurite*. It is not known what determines the emergence of a neurite from a particular point along the cell's perimeter, but it often appears as though the cell has acquired some form of polarity at an early stage in its development. Exactly what polarity in this context means in molecular terms is still not clear, nor is it known what antecedent changes occur within growing neurons such as the redistribution of microtubules and other cytoskeletal elements (Dotti et al., 1988). However, it has been known for about 80 years that all neuronal processes are extensions of the cell body or of other processes and are not formed (as was at one time believed) by glial or other cells. Almost from the beginning, most new processes are distinguished at their growing tips by expanded swellings—the *growth cones.* These are regions of rapid membrane movement and are characterized by the presence of large numbers of motile, finger-like processes called *microspikes,* or *filopodia,* separated by veil-like membranous sheets, or *lamellipodia.* The interior of the growth cone is filled with membranous sacs and tubules, whereas the filopodia are packed with actin filaments. Microtubules and neurofilaments, which are such a prominent feature of the axon itself, are absent from the growth cone (see Bunge, 1973) (Fig. 2–5).

Neural processes grow by the continuous addition of new cytoplasmic and membrane components that are delivered to the growth cones by the process of rapid *anterograde axonal transport* with a velocity in excess of 200 mm/day. As the axon becomes elongated, there is a progressive addition of neurofilaments and microtubules, which are transported at a much slower rate (~1 mm/day) near the distal end of the growing processes. Many of these components continue to be supplied to the axon throughout its life to replace those lost by turnover or those returned

to the cell soma by the process of *retrograde axonal transport.* However, a few transported proteins have been identified that seem to be specifically involved in axonal growth. The genes for these growth-associated proteins (GAPs) appear to be turned off when the neurons establish connections in their projection field and thereafter are either not expressed or are expressed at only low levels in most central neurons. However, where axonal regeneration is possible (in the peripheral nervous system of mammals or in most central pathways in fish and amphibians), the genes that encode the GAPs may continue to be expressed at low levels throughout life and are apparently capable of being expressed at substantially higher levels during the process of regeneration (Skene, 1984). One GAP, GAP-43, has been studied especially intensively and the gene that encodes it has been cloned (Karns et al., 1987). GAP-43 is an axonally transported phosphoprotein, enriched in growth cones, and although it is not an integral membrane protein, it is known to be closely associated with the axolemma. When transfected into non-neuronal cells, GAP-43 can cause the cells to form growth cone–like extensions and to assume neuron-like morphologic features. The cellular distribution and the developmental regeneration of GAP-43 strongly suggest that it plays a key role in axonal elongation, but its precise function in the economy of growing and regenerating neurons remains to be determined.

The vigorous extension and retraction of filopodia that one observes in growing neurites in vitro strongly suggest that they actively "sample" the various substrata that they contact, selectively adhering to some, while totally ignoring others. This form of growth cone–substrate interaction seems to be critical in axonal pathfinding and has been the subject of intensive study (see later).

In many neurons, the axon is the first process to be formed and its development often precedes that of the dendrites by several hours or even some days. The appearance of the axon as a morphologically distinct entity is marked by the initial neurite's becoming more uniform in diameter, losing its early content of ribosomes, and at somewhat later stages, taking on all the characteristics of a mature axon, including, in many instances, the acquisition of a myelin sheath. The growth rate of neurites is somewhat variable, but in mammals, axons usually grow at a rate of about 1–5 mm/day. Less is known about the growth of dendrites, but it is now clear that they too have growth cones at their ends, and some evidence suggests that dendritic growth and reorganization may continue throughout life. Because neurons are usually classified morphologically according to the number, arrangement, and disposition of their dendrites, a good deal of attention has been paid to the factors that determine the form of dendritic arbors. In many cases, the general form of the neuron's dendritic tree appears to be intrinsically determined, because it can be effectively reproduced in vitro when the cells are cultured in relative isolation

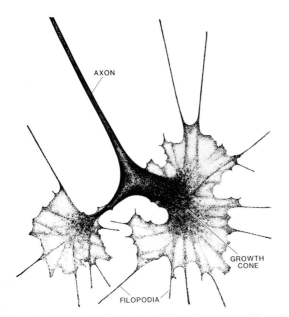

Figure 2–5. Axons grow by the deposition of new materials at their growing tips or growth cones. This drawing (which is based on an original electron micrograph of the growth cone of a cultured sympathetic neuron by Dr. Mary B. Bunge) shows the appearance of a typical growth cone with its expanded lamellipodia and finger-like filopodia, which are extended and retracted as the growth cone senses its way along the substratum.

(Banker and Cowan, 1979; Kriegstein and Dichter, 1983). However, in at least one other case (the granule cells of the dentate gyrus), the in vitro form of the dendrites bears little relationship to their normal in vivo arrangement but, interestingly, is strikingly similar to the appearance of the displaced granule cells found in the mutant reeler mouse (Boss et al., 1983). This suggests, and there is considerable evidence to support the idea, that the detailed three-dimensional arrangement of most dendritic trees is shaped largely by extrinsic factors, such as the presence of various mechanical barriers, the ingrowth of specific afferent pathways, and even competition for available growth factors by surrounding dendrites (Cowan, 1979a). There is also some evidence that retrogradely transported signals from the region of the cell's axon may be involved, but the nature of the signals and how they act are quite unknown.

Physiologic Differentiation

The characteristic membrane properties of neurons do not all appear fully formed ab initio; rather, they appear to emerge in characteristic sequences of which the following seems to be one of the more common. At the earliest stages of development, the cells can be shown to be electrically coupled to each other through gap junctions. Subsequently, as the cells become electrically uncoupled (this usually occurs as they withdraw from the cell cycle), they display long-lasting (10–100 ms) action potentials that are due to transitory changes in Ca^{2+} influx. Later, there is a phase during which much shorter-lasting (1–2 ms) Na^+ action potentials are superimposed on the Ca^{2+} fluxes. Finally, in most instances, the Ca^{2+} action potentials disappear entirely, leaving only the Na^+ action potentials typical of most mature neurons (Spitzer, 1981). It is not known why such a developmental sequence should be obligatory for many (if not all) classes of neurons, but it clearly reflects the temporally programmed expression of the genes involved in the synthesis of the various ion-specific membrane channels. The analysis of neuronal gene expression at this level has only just begun, but now that the genes for most of the major classes of ion channels have been cloned, one can expect substantial progress along these lines within the next several years.

Molecular Differentiation

Although each of the above-mentioned events requires the expression of specific genes and the synthesis of the appropriate macromolecules, there are, in addition, a number of changes in each class of nerve cell that collectively determine its phenotype and its mode of synaptic transmission. For most cells, this includes

1. The synthesis of at least one group of transmitter-synthesizing enzymes, and commonly the synthe-

sis of one or more neuropeptides and their post-translational modification
2. The synthesis of one or, commonly, several types of transmitter receptor molecules as well as receptors for various growth factors (see later) and their insertion into the appropriate postsynaptic sites on the cell membrane
3. In all cases, the continued synthesis of the large number of polypeptides and lipids (and their subsequent modifications) that are required for the continuous maintenance of the cell and all its processes

A detailed consideration of these events is beyond the scope of this chapter; some aspects are dealt with elsewhere in this volume and, for a general review, see the volumes edited by Black (1984) and Edelman et al. (1985).

Formation of Connections

It is generally acknowledged that the central issue in developmental neurobiology is how the enormously intricate patterns of connections that characterize the adult nervous system come to be established. Given the complexity of the problem, it is perhaps not surprising that many workers who first addressed the issue favored the view that connections are initially formed in an entirely random and fortuitous manner and that function and experience serve to select those pathways and connections that prove to be adaptive. However, from the beginning, there were strong objections to this functionalist point of view, and since the pioneering studies of Roger Sperry in the 1940s and 1950s, no one has seriously championed it (see Sperry, 1965). Indeed, all the available evidence indicates that each class of neuron is specified to form connections with certain subsets of cells in one or more target fields and that, under normal circumstances, the axons of each class of cell grow along clearly definable pathways to reach their target regions. It is impossible in a short overview to summarize adequately all this evidence, and the following simply considers some of the principles involved and the types of experimental analysis that have been brought to bear on them.

It is important to note at the outset that the formation of connections involves at least three distinct sets of issues. The first concerns how each nerve cell or small population of cells becomes topographically distinguishable from other neurons within the same general region. To cite a specific example from the system that has been most intensively studied from this point of view, it is important to know how ganglion cells in the inferior nasal quadrant of the retina are distinguished from those in the superior temporal quadrant, because this type of distinction must antecede and finally determine that the axons from the two regions terminate in different parts of their terminal projection fields (in this case, the lateral geniculate nucleus and the superior colliculus). The key question, in other words, is how do nerve cells acquire the *positional information* that establishes their local addresses? The second set of issues concerns the outgrowth of axons and the pathways they take to reach their appropriate destinations: how do axons find their way? The third set of issues is rather more complex. It concerns how axons find their appropriate targets, selecting the appropriate target region (e.g., a specific nucleus or a particular cortical area in the brain and a particular muscle or part of the skin in the periphery), homing in on the appropriate subregion within those target structures, and within that subregion, synapsing with the proper subset of target cells, whether they be neurons, muscle fibers, or sensory receptors.

Acquisition of Positional Information by Neurons

There is a good deal of evidence that all nerve cells have position-dependent properties that determine the ordered patterns of connections they can form. Yet little is known about the nature of the positional information they acquire, how this information is encoded in the cells, and how it is later expressed in the outgrowth of their axons and in the recognition of their target sites. Studies of the developing retina and certain other regions of the nervous system indicate that some cells at least acquire this information at an early stage in development, perhaps as early as the initial regional determination of the neural plate. However, it also is clear that the information acquired at this stage is not "fixed" irrevocably. Under some circumstances, it can be overridden if the normal topographic relationships of the region are altered. For example, if the eye rudiment of a frog is rotated 180° at an early stage (e.g., when the optic vesicle first appears), the retina later projects in a completely normal manner on the contralateral optic tectum. However, if the rotation is done a short while later (at early optic cup stages), the retinotectal projection is reversed along the nasotemporal axis but not in the dorsoventral dimension. If the eye rotation is done some 5–10 hours later, the entire retinotectal projection is reversed, indicating that by this time the polarity of the developing eye is fixed in some way. Interestingly, at this stage, only a small fraction of the total number of retinal ganglion cells has been generated, and none of the cells have sent an axon into the optic nerve (see Cowan and Hunt, 1985).

Because essentially the same results can be obtained if the eye is transplanted to the flank and later returned to the orbit, it appears that the retina (and presumably other parts of the nervous system) is under the influence of some general polarity-determining influence that operates throughout the body to assign positional addresses to the developing nerve cells. Although these initial assignments may for a period be reversible, after a certain critical stage the addresses of the first-formed cells in the population become fixed, and the cells that are subsequently generated acquire, in orderly fashion, a set of similarly fixed addresses. In the case of a two-dimensional sheet of cells, as in the retina, these addresses may be considered as being defined either by a set of Cartesian coordinates in which the position of each cell (or more probably, each small group of cells) is defined by a specific x and y value or by an angular and a radial coordinate value (Hunt, 1975). Although these notions have a certain heuristic value, they leave unresolved the *cellular basis* of the addressing mechanism. For this, there is no better suggestion than Sperry's original hypothesis that, during development, these positional addresses become encoded on the surfaces of the cells in the form of a set of cytochemically distinct labels and that these labels enable the axons of the cells to identify their preferred pathways and to recognize their appropriate targets. Cells in the target area are considered to bear a matching or complementary set of position-dependent labels that mediate the requisite axon-cell recognition. This, in essence, is the *chemoaffinity hypothesis* (Hunt and Cowan, 1990; Sperry, 1963) (see later).

Axonal Pathfinding

In normal individuals, the paths taken by axons from their sites of origin to their target destinations are rather constant and reproducible from individual to individual. This suggests that, during development, axonal outgrowth is fairly rigidly controlled and highly constrained. However, experimental studies clearly show that axons can, if necessary, pursue a number of highly irregular courses and yet still reach their preferred target region. There are reports of retinal axons in amphibians that have fortuitously regenerated back to the optic tectum along the course of the oculomotor nerve, and even when parts of the optic nerves have been experimentally misrouted and made to approach the tectum through a quite abnormal route, they can still regrow back to the appropriate sectors of the tectum. This indicates that axons can home in and sense when they have reached their predetermined targets, regardless of the route they follow. Despite this, during *normal* development, most axons follow rather stereotyped pathways, and to do this they seem to be able to adopt a number of different strategies. Among the more important known strategies are the following:

Selective Axonal Fasciculation. Axons of neighboring neurons often grow together over considerable distances and use some form of fiber-fiber interaction as an important cuing mechanism. In many situations, a small number of pioneering fibers grow to their appropriate target using some of the guiding cues discussed later. Later-formed axons follow these pioneering fibers, apparently using axoaxonal interactions, or selective fasciculation, as their primary guiding mechanism. Among the molecules involved in this type of axon fasciculation, N-CAM and some of its homologues in invertebrates (e.g., the fasciculins in *Drosophila* [see Grenningloh et al., 1991]) seem to be especially important. Thus, antibodies to N-CAM can be shown to disrupt the normally ordered growth of optic nerve fibers into the chick optic tectum and to disrupt the normal process of target recognition.

Axon-Substrate Interactions. Most axons seem to show a strong preference for certain substrates instead of others, one important feature in the substrate being its adhesivity (Letourneau, 1979). The existence on neurites of a variety of cell surface molecules, such as the various integrins that function as receptors for molecular determinants in the underlying substrata (including, for example, fibronectin or laminin) seems to be particularly important. That such substrata seem to promote process formation and elongation has been taken as further evidence that selective axonal outgrowth commonly follows pre-existing pathways laid down in the form of selective substrate distributions.

Axonal Tropisms. In at least one case, a specific protein (nerve growth factor [NGF] [see later]) has been shown to exert a strong tropic influence on growing sympathetic axons, the fibers apparently being attracted by a high local concentration of NGF, which may even cause them to change direction and to grow for some distance along the applied concentration gradient (Gundersen and Barrett, 1979). Until recently, it was not known how general this phenomenon might be, although as Ramón y Cajal first pointed out near the turn of the century, chemotropic mechanisms of this kind could account for the selective growth of most axonal pathways (see Ramón y Cajal, 1960). Several studies carried out both in vivo and in vitro provided rather compelling evidence that certain tissues can release and set up gradients of soluble factors that direct axonal growth along defined pathways. One of the most striking examples of this comes from studies of the earliest-formed axons in the chick spinal cord. These commissural axons grow initially toward the midline, where they cross to the opposite side. They appear to be drawn toward the midline by a factor produced by the cells in the floor plate (Tessier-Lavigne et al., 1988). Heffner et al. (1990) similarly showed that pontine tissue grown in vitro can cause corticospinal axons to give off collaterals that grow toward the explanted pontine tissue in a manner that is reminiscent of the cortico-pontine collateral projection seen in vivo.

Other Gradient Effects. Several types of experiment suggest that growing axons may be strongly influenced by other gradients that operate along the rostrocaudal or mediolateral dimension of the entire neuraxis. For example, in the case of the giant Mauthner cells in amphibian larvae, it has been found that their large axons always grow first from lateral to medial across the midline and then from rostral to caudal down the spinal cord regardless of the initial position or orientation of the parent cell, as if they sequentially come under the influence of a general

lateral-to-medial and then rostral-to-caudal gradient mechanism. The nature of these gradients is not known but is likely to be the subject of intense study during the next few years.

In any given situation, it seems likely that the growth cones of at least the initial population of axons respond to one or more of these mechanisms. Later axons may be guided to their targets by following these first-formed axons. However, it is recognized that, even in fiber systems that show a fairly high degree of topographic order throughout their course, such as the visual pathways, individual axons often diverge markedly from their neighbors, even though they may ultimately terminate in the same region and even on the same cells.

Target Recognition

That growing axons are able to identify correctly the region in which they should terminate, even though they are misdirected along a quite aberrant pathway, clearly implies that they are endowed with a powerful discriminatory capacity. This capacity enables them to identify not only the appropriate target region but also the appropriate topographic sector within that region and the appropriate class of neurons within the target field. Several hypotheses have been put forward to account for this. Among these, the most enduring have been the following:

Mechanical Guidance, or Morphogenetics. According to this view, the axons of neighboring neurons in the projecting population tend to remain closely associated with each other throughout their course so that when they enter their designated projection field, they maintain their appropriate topographic relationships. Selective axonal fasciculation is important in the development of many pathways (see earlier) and, together with the known topographic order found in many central pathways such as the dorsal columns and the optic nerve, provides the strongest evidence for the morphogenetic hypothesis. However, despite its resilience (for review, see Horder and Martin, 1978), this hypothesis has been difficult to sustain, given the evidence that axons of neighboring neurons often diverge from one another during normal development. Also, perhaps even more seriously damaging to this hypothesis is the finding that regenerating axons can sort themselves out after having been intentionally scrambled. That under these circumstances axons can successfully track down and innervate an appropriate target region, when this has been experimentally dislocated and even rotated through 90–180°, makes it clear that, at best, the simplistic notion of mechanical guidance can be relevant in only a few special situations such as seem to obtain in certain invertebrate neural pathways. Certainly it cannot by itself account for target recognition in the vertebrate nervous system.

Temporal Sequencing. According to the temporal sequencing hypothesis, the patterns of connections that are formed simply reflect the temporal order in which the axons innervate the target field. The most telling evidence against this idea comes from experiments in amphibians in which the normal temporal sequence of innervation of the optic tectum by retinal axons is reversed yet the retinotectal map that is formed is quite normal. Similarly, it has been shown in chick embryos that, if the portion of the projecting neuronal population that normally innervates the first region of the target to be invaded is removed (either before the outgrowth of the first axons or before the regeneration of the entire fiber system), axons from the remaining part of the projecting population usually by-pass, and leave uninnervated, the first region of the target field that they encounter and continue to grow until they reach the appropriate sector of the target. Although experiments of this type argue strongly against the sequence of innervation as the key factor in setting up the initial topographic pattern of connections, it is worth noting that the distribution of synaptic sites *within* the appropriate part of the target field is often determined on a first come, first served principle (Gottlieb and Cowan, 1972).

Functional Selection. One of the earliest suggestions, and one vigorously advocated by the distinguished developmental biologist Paul Weiss (1936), is that the initial pattern of connections in most systems is essentially random and that from this random connectivity the connections that prove to be functionally adaptive come to be selected, and in some way validated and maintained. There is a phase during development when connections do become stabilized, and the stabilization process is in some way activity dependent (see later); nevertheless, the overwhelming weight of evidence argues against the notion of randomness in the initial patterns of connections either during development or after regeneration. Whenever the pattern of connections is intentionally disrupted (e.g., by eye rotation in amphibians and by peripheral nerve crosses in mammals), the ensuing behavior is always maladaptive and does not improve with experience (Sperry, 1965).

Chemoaffinity Mechanisms. Almost a century ago, Langley pointed out that the selective reinnervation of the superior cervical ganglion after interruption of the preganglionic chain could be accounted for only by postulating that the incoming preganglionic fibers and the neurons in the ganglion were chemically distinguished in some way (Langley, 1898). Yet it was not until the 1950s that Sperry was able to generalize this notion by advancing what has come to be known as the chemoaffinity hypothesis (Sperry, 1963). According to this hypothesis, each developing neuron (or more probably, each small group of neurons) acquires a distinct chemical label or set of labels that defines both its functional class and its three-dimensional position within the population of which it is a part; the presence of these labels on the growth cones of their axons enables them to identify and form connections with their appropriate target cells, presumably because the target cells bear on their surfaces a matching or complementary set of chemical labels. Although no specific chemical labels that might be involved in this process have been identified, the chemoaffinity hypothesis has withstood a broad range of experimental tests and, to date, has not been controverted by any experimental finding. The one conceptual challenge that has been leveled at the hypothesis is that it presupposes such a multitude of different cytochemical markers that they could not all be encoded by the limited number of genes in the genome (about 10^5 in humans). However, as Sperry (1965) first pointed out, if the molecules in question were graded in their distribution or systematically modulated in their structure, it would be possible, at least theoretically, to encode the position of every neuron in a two-dimensional sheet, such as the retina, with only two molecules or the position of all neurons in a three-dimensional complex, such as a nuclear group in the brain, with just three basic molecules.

More recently, work on CAMs suggested that much of the connectivity in the nervous system could (again, in principle) be determined by a relatively small number of CAMs whose molecular structure, like that of N-CAM, is temporally modulated (Edelman, 1984). The finding that there are cell surface molecules in the retina and optic tectum that show a striking gradient in their distribution across either their dorsoventral or rostrocaudal dimensions (see, for example, Constantine-Paton et al., 1986; Trisler et al., 1981) not only is consonant with Sperry's view but also suggests that the search for the postulated molecular labels may soon prove fruitful.

The search for the molecular mechanisms that underlie the remarkably specific patterns of connections in both the CNS and the PNS is currently one of the most active in the field, but so far, progress has been slow and the problems continue to be rather intractable. Moreover, it is now evident that, at least in the CNS, neurons may bear several distinct specificities. Collectively, these determine that inhibitory afferents nearly always terminate on cell somas, the proximal parts of dendrites, or the initial segments of axons, whereas most excitatory inputs end either on the intermediate or distal dendritic segments and often on dendritic spines, and that most, but not all, inputs are topographically segregated on the recipient neurons. The factors that determine specificity at this level are completely unknown, although it remains possible that the receptors for different types of neurotransmitters and/or the receptors for selected growth factors may be implicated.

Synaptogenesis

The actual process of synaptogenesis is poorly understood. Descriptive morphologic studies indicate that after coming into fairly close apposition with some region of the postsynaptic cell surface, the growth cone or the terminal part of an axonal branch accumulates vesicles, which initially are rather variable in size, but later become more uniform (approximately 45–55 nm). Approximately concurrently with this, the characteristic specializations appear on the apposed presynaptic and postsynaptic membranes. However, in some cases in which it has been possible to study the appearance of synaptic transmission physiologically, it appears that these morphologic developments are relatively late features of synaptogenesis and that functional transmission can occur long before the emergence of any morphologic specializations. This is especially clear at the neuromuscular junction, whose development can be readily studied in vitro. From such studies, it is clear that functional transmission (associated with acetylcholine release, the binding of the transmitter to receptor molecules on the surface of a muscle cell, and the opening of the relevant ion channels) usually occurs within just a few minutes after the initial contact of the axon and the muscle fiber (Kiddokoro and Yeh, 1982). Subsequently, there is a dramatic aggregation of receptor molecules at the site of the developing neuromuscular junction (partly as the result of the diffusion of receptors from neighboring regions of the muscle and partly by de novo synthesis), which seems to be induced by one or more factors released by the axon terminal (Harris et al., 1988; Magill et al., 1987; New and Mudge, 1986). Again, as in the case of the early emergence of the membrane properties of neurons, there is a progressive evolution in certain of the biophysical features of the junctional region. Thus, the mean quantal size, which is initially quite variable, becomes progressively more uniform, and the mean opening time of the acetylcholine channel becomes appreciably shorter.

One factor released by motor neuron axons that promotes the aggregation of acetylcholine receptors and the degradative enzyme acetylcholinesterase has been extensively studied by McMahon and colleagues (Magill et al., 1987). This is the protein *agrin*. Agrin has been cloned from several species and appears to be enriched in the basal lamina at the neuromuscular junction. It remains to be seen whether other synaptic sites, and especially those in the CNS, undergo similar developmental changes. However, one feature that seems to be generally true is that initially many more axons form synapses on the target cells than survive into maturity and that, over a period of some days or weeks, there is a progressive loss of many of the first-formed contacts, even though at the same time the surviving axons may continue to make new synapses on the postsynaptic cells.

Validation and Refinement of Connections

Although it is generally agreed that the initial pattern of connections that is established during development is both orderly and specific, it is evident that the early wiring of the nervous system is neither precise nor free from errors and, indeed, is subject to appreciable modification at later stages. The definitive circuitry of the nervous system is sculpted from an earlier, less precise pattern by two major regressive phenomena, namely, cell death and selective process elimination.

Cell Death During Normal Neural Development

That degenerating cells can be seen in the developing nervous system was first reported near the turn of the century, but it was not until the late 1940s that it came to be widely appreciated that most neuronal populations undergo a phase of substantial cell death during their development. Since that time, considerable evidence has been presented that in all but a few neural systems about 50% of the cells that initially assemble to form the precursors of the various nuclear groups, cortical layers, or peripheral ganglia degenerate, usually when the population as a whole begins to form connections within its projection field (Cowan, 1973; Hamburger and Oppenheim, 1982). Moreover, if part or all of the projection field is experimentally ablated (before the outgrowth of axons from the projecting population), there is a corresponding and proportional increase in the number of cells that die. That the additional cell death occurring under these circumstances takes place during the same time frame as the naturally occurring or spontaneous neuronal death suggests that the critical factor responsible for the latter is found in the target field rather than within the neurons themselves. This idea has been strengthened by the finding that in some cases the numbers of surviving neurons can be substantially increased by providing the cells with an expanded target area (e.g., by transplanting supernumerary eyes or limbs).

The critical factor appears to be the availability of certain trophic, or growth, factors within the target field that can be taken up by active axons but are available in only limited amounts. Because of the limited availability of these materials, only a proportion of the neurons can survive. At present, the only such factor that has been chemically isolated and adequately characterized is NGF, which is essential for the survival and growth of sympathetic and dorsal root ganglion cells (see Levi-Montalcini, 1982). Administering exogenous NGF to developing limb buds in chick embryos effectively eliminates the degeneration of 40–50% of the related dorsal root ganglion cells that normally die, as the NGF is taken up by the sensory fibers and is retrogradely transported to their somas in the dorsal root ganglia. By analogy, it is assumed that most target regions normally produce a limited amount of a trophic factor that is specific for the survival of the innervating neurons and that the axons of the cells compete among themselves for this trophic material: those that are successful survive, whereas those that are unsuccessful die.

Considerable effort is currently being directed toward the isolation and characterization of other neurotrophic factors. A number, including the so-called brain-derived neurotrophic factor and a ciliary neurotrophic factor have been identified and cloned, and their distribution within the developing nervous system is being mapped. It has become evident that many of the growth factors that have been extensively studied in non-neural tissues, such as fibroblast growth factor, epidermal growth factor, the insulin-like growth factors, and platelet-derived growth factor, are present in the nervous system and, at least in vitro, are capable of maintaining dissociated neurons from many different regions of the brain and spinal cord (see, for example, Baskin et al., 1988; Walicke et al., 1986). The widespread distribution and general growth-supporting characteristics of these trophic factors led to the view that most central and peripheral neurons depend for their survival on both general and specific growth factors, although, to date, few neuron-type specific growth factors have been identified.

Although it may seem surprising that there should be an initial overproduction of neurons and the later elimination of a significant proportion of the cells, it is now clear from a variety of experimental studies that cell deaths of this kind match the size of each neuronal population to the size or the functional needs of the region or regions it innervates and, at the same time, eliminate many cells whose axons have grown to an inappropriate target or to an inappropriate region within their target field (see Cowan et al., 1985).

This phenomenon of target-related naturally occurring neuronal degeneration is to be distinguished from the earlier elimination of certain neurons that occurs at, or immediately after, this last division. In the nematode C. elegans, programmed cell deaths of this kind occur quite commonly and consistently eliminate one of the daughter cells in certain neuronal lineages. In these cases, the death of the cells occurs before they have extended axons toward their putative target fields and is clearly genetically programmed. The evidence for this derives from the isolation of a number of cell death mutants affecting several genes. In the absence of the normally programmed cell death in these mutants, certain cell lineages are extended beyond their normal limits and result in abnormal cell numbers. The identification of the relevant cell death genes has been an important step in the analysis of the control of neuronal numbers in this organism and has led to the active search for homologous genes in vertebrates and especially in mammals (Horvitz, 1990).

Process and Synapse Elimination

Not only is there an initial overproduction of neurons, but also most neurons seem to make many more connections than they can (or need to) maintain. As a result, in most neural systems, there is a second regressive phase during which a proportion of the initial connections formed are selectively elim-

inated. This phenomenon was first identified at the neuromuscular junction. Whereas most mature muscle fibers in mammals are usually innervated by only a single axon, early in development they are commonly innervated by up to six or seven separate axons and only much later are the supernumerary axons removed. Essentially the same findings have now been made in autonomic ganglia and in several regions in the CNS, so that it may now be regarded as a rather general feature of early neuronal development (Purves, 1988; Purves and Lichtman, 1980). It is not yet known why certain axon terminals persist while others are selectively eliminated, but it is interesting that, even as certain axon terminals are being eliminated, the axons that persist continue to make additional synapses on their target cells. It seems therefore unlikely that, in these situations, process elimination can be ascribed simply to a limitation in the number of synapses that the postsynaptic cells can support.

It is now clear also that process and synapse elimination of this kind is not confined to axon terminals, nor is it purely a local phenomenon that serves to fine tune the initial neuronal circuitry; in some cases, it can lead to the elimination of entire neural pathways. The first evidence of this came from studies of the callosal connections linking the visual cortex of the two sides. In mature animals, such connections are limited to the region of representation of the vertical meridian, along the border between areas 17 and 18. However, in young animals, callosally projecting cells are found throughout the entire visual cortex, and in kittens (in which this issue has been most carefully studied), it is not until the third or fourth postnatal week that the projection becomes restricted to its characteristic adult distribution (Innocenti, 1981). Similar observations have been made in other cortical areas and for other cortical projection systems, but what is perhaps of greatest interest has been the finding that the limitation of these pathways is brought about not by the death of the relevant neurons, but by the selective elimination of specific axon collaterals, with the parent neuron and its other axonal branches apparently being unaffected (for review, see Cowan et al., 1985). Just how widespread this phenomenon of long axon collateral elimination may be is not known, nor are the developmental factors responsible for it known. It is noteworthy, however, that, in animals in which an experimental strabismus has been induced, the callosal collaterals are no longer limited to the border between areas 17 and 18 but persist over a considerable part of both areas, suggesting that functional factors play an important role in selecting which axons die and which survive.

The finding of selective axon collateral elimination during the development of the cerebral cortex has helped to clarify one of the more puzzling features of cortical ontogeny, namely, how the many different cortical fields come to be distinguished in terms of the connections they form. In an elegant series of experimental studies involving the excision of pieces of cortex from one area (e.g., the primary visual cortex) and their heterotopic transplantation to another region (e.g., the sensorimotor cortex), O'Leary and Stanfield (1989) showed that initially all cortical areas are equivalent in the sense that they all form essentially the same initial patterns of connections. Only later, apparently as the result of the ingrowth into each cortical field of its specific afferents from the thalamus, do the efferent connections become specific for each field. This connectional specificity is again brought about by the selective elimination of certain early-formed collateral projections. Thus, pyramidal cells in layer V of all cortical fields initially send a projection into the corticospinal tract; in the case of the visual cortex, this spinal projection is later eliminated (without the death of the parent cells), whereas in the motor cortex, it is maintained throughout life (see O'Leary and Stanfield, 1989).

By analogy with what is known of the effects of NGF, it has been postulated that not only the death of certain cells but also the elimination of particular axon branches may be attributable to the limited availability of trophic materials. When NGF-dependent sympathetic neurons are grown in specially designed three-chambered culture dishes (in which it is possible to selectively withdraw NGF from one or more chambers), it has been found that all neurites that do not have direct access to NGF die back, even though the parent cell persists. As long as one or more neurites have access to NGF, the cell and the relevant neurite are maintained (Campenot, 1977). A single mechanism of this kind would provide a parsimonious explanation of both cell death and selective process elimination during development. However, until the other postulated trophic factors have been identified and characterized, and until it can be shown in what way functional activity mediates cell survival and the preferential persistence of axonal branches, this notion remains entirely speculative. Nevertheless, it is becoming increasingly clear that cell death and collateral elimination are extremely important in normal development and that together they determine the final form of the mature nervous system. At the same time, the early existence of an excessive number of cells and the rich exuberance of early connections may provide the essential substratum for many aspects of developmental plasticity in the immature CNS. Certainly many of the morphologic findings that have been reported after early CNS injury seem now to be attributable to the persistence of preformed connections rather than to the de novo generation of new and unusual patterns of connections.

Neuronal Plasticity

The potential modifiability of the connections that are initially formed provides the basis for what has come to be known as *neuromorphologic plasticity*. This term actually refers to a number of different phenomena, including the ability of axons to sprout and form new connections in the adult brain, the reinnervation of regions that have been partially denervated, and the expansion or reduction of axonal projection fields during development. Only the latter is applicable here: for a review of the whole range of phenomena associated with plasticity, see Lund (1978) and Cotman (1978).

One of the best documented examples of developmental plasticity is that seen during the development of eye dominance columns, or stripes, in layer IV of the visual cortex of primates. In mature monkeys, the inputs to layer IV from each eye (relayed, of course, through the lateral geniculate nucleus) are rather sharply segregated into a complex series of stripes (confusingly referred to as eye dominance columns), each about 400 μm wide. However, when the afferents from the lateral geniculate first reach layer IV, they tend to overlap extensively, and neither anatomically nor physiologically is there any indication of the characteristic alternating left eye and right eye columns. These columns appear only gradually during the first month or so postnatally, apparently as the result of some form of competitive interactions between the inputs from the two eyes. Thus, if at birth the eyelids of one eye are sutured closed, the eye dominance stripes associated with that eye are found some 2–3 months later to be considerably reduced in width, whereas those connected to the nondeprived eye are correspondingly enlarged (Hubel et al., 1977). The expansion of the axon terminals associated with the nondeprived eye is apparently reversible, at least for some time, because, if the sutured eyelids are reopened and the eyelids of the opposite eye closed, the formerly shrunken eye dominance stripes expand while those that had expanded become progressively reduced in width.

That the emergence of the eye dominance columns is dependent on the activity of the retinal ganglion cells has been clearly documented in kittens by injecting the sodium channel blocking agent tetrodotoxin into both eyes throughout the critical period for deprivation effects. Under these circumstances, the inputs to layer IV from the two eyes do not segregate and eye dominance columns are not formed (Stryker, 1981). This finding is but one of many similar observations that collectively suggest that neuronal activity is involved in some way in the refinement of most neural circuits. Indeed, as a general principle, the formation of connections involves two quite separate mechanisms: (1) a mechanism that depends on the presence of distinctive cytochemical labels, which establishes the initial connectional patterns, and (2) one that is mediated by electrical activity, which is critical for the refinement and maintenance of the connections.

CONCLUSION

Although much has been learned about neuronal development in the past few decades, it is evident from even this brief survey of the field that much remains to be discovered. This is especially true of the mechanisms responsible for neural induction, for the control of cell proliferation in the CNS, and for the molecular and functional mechanisms involved in the formation of connections. Fortunately, advances in other areas of cellular and molecular biology have greatly improved the prospects that at least some of these issues will be amenable to more critical investigation. The emergence in the past few years of a number of new methods, such as those involved in the identification, isolation, cloning, and sequencing of genes and their products, the hybridoma method for producing monoclonal antibodies, techniques for isolating molecules that are present in only minute amounts, improved methods for tracing connections in the developing nervous system, and in situ hybridization techniques for identifying where specific genes are being expressed, should greatly facilitate the analysis of these and other developmental problems. It can be confidently anticipated that, by the imaginative application of these methods and those that will undoubtedly be developed in the near future, a much more satisfying account of each aspect of normal neuronal development and new insights into the causation and prevention of many of the disorders to which the developing nervous system seems to be heir will be possible.

References

(Key references are designated with an asterisk.)

Ambros V., Horvitz H.R. The *lin 14* locus of *Caenorhabditis elegans* controls the time of expression of specific postembryonic developmental events. *Genes Dev.* 1:398–414, 1987.

Banker G.A., Cowan W.M. Further observations on hippocampal neurons in dispersed cell culture. *J. Comp. Neurol.* 187:469–494, 1979.

Baskin D.G., Wilcox B.J., Figlewicz D.P., et al. Insulin and insulin-like growth factors in the CNS. *Trends Neurosci.* 3:107–111, 1988.

Black I.B., ed. *Cellular and Molecular Biology of Neuronal Development.* New York, Plenum Publishing, 1984.

Boss B.D., Condon T.P., Lanz E., et al. Dispersed cell cultures from the dentate gyrus of neonatal rats. *Soc. Neurosci. Abstr.* 9:240, 1983.

Bunge M.B. Fine structure of nerve fibers and growth cones of isolated sympathetic neurons in culture. *J. Cell Biol.* 56:713–735, 1973.

Campenot R.B. Local control of neurite development by nerve growth factor. *Proc. Natl. Acad. Sci. U.S.A.* 74:4516–4519, 1977.

Constantine-Paton M., Blum A.S., Mendez-Otero R., et al. A cell surface molecule distributed in a dorsoventral gradient in the perinatal rat retina. *Nature* 324:459–462, 1986.

Cotman C.W., ed. *Neuronal Plasticity.* New York, Raven Press, 1978.

Cowan W.M. Neuronal death as a regulative mechanism in the control of cell number in the nervous system. In Rockstein M., ed. *Development and Aging in the Nervous System.* New York, Academic Press, pp. 19–41, 1973.

*Cowan W.M. Aspects of neural development. In Porter, R., ed. *International Review of Physiology III.* Baltimore, University Park Press, pp. 149–191, 1978.

Cowan W.M. Selection and control in neurogenesis. In Schmitt F.O., Worden F.C., eds. *Fourth Study Program.* Cambridge, MA, M.I.T. Press, pp. 59–79, 1979a.

*Cowan W.M. The development of the brain. *Sci. Am.* 241(3):113–133, 1979b.

Cowan W.M. The development of the vertebrate central nervous system: an overview. In Garrod D.R., Feldman J.D. eds. *Development in the Nervous System.* New York, Cambridge University Press, pp. 3–33, 1981.

Cowan W.M., Hunt R.K. The development of the retino-tectal projection: an overview. In Edelman G.M., Gall E., Cowan W.M., eds. *Molecular Bases of Neural Development.* New York, Wiley, pp. 389–428, 1985.

*Cowan W.M., Fawcett, J.W., O'Leary D.D.M., et al. Regressive phenomena in the development of the vertebrate nervous system. *Science* 225:1258–1265, 1985.

Dotti C.G., Sullivan C.A., Banker G.A. The establishment of polarity by hippocampal neurons in culture. *J. Neurosci.* 8:1454–1468, 1988.

*Edelman G.M. Modulation of cell adhesion during induction, histogenesis, and perinatal development of the nervous system. *Annu. Rev. Neurosci.* 7:339–375, 1984.

Edelman G.M., Gall E., Cowan W.M., eds. *Molecular Bases of Neural Development.* New York, Wiley, 1985.

Gottlieb D.I., Cowan W.M. Evidence for a temporal factor in the occupation of available synaptic sites during the development of the dentate gyrus. *Brain Res.* 41:452–456, 1972.

Gottlieb D.I., Glaser L. Cellular recognition during neural development. *Annu. Rev. Neurosci.* 3:303–318, 1980.

Grenningloh G., Bieber A., Rehm J., et al. Molecular genetics of neuronal regulation in *Drosophila*: evolution and function of immunoglobulin superfamiliar adhesion molecules. *Cold Spring Harbor Symp. Quant. Biol.* (in press).

Gundersen R.W., Barrett J.N. Neuronal chemotaxis. Chick dorsal root axons turn toward high concentration of nerve growth factor. *Science* 206:1079–1080, 1979.

Hamburger V., Oppenheim R.W. Naturally occurring neuronal death in vertebrates. *Neurosci. Commentaries* 1:39–55, 1982.

Harris D.A., Falls D.L., Dill Revor R.M., et al. Acetylcholine receptor-inducing factor from chicken brain increases the level of mRNA encoding the receptor alpha subunit. *Proc. Natl. Acad. Sci. U.S.A.* 85:1983–1987, 1988.

*Hatten M.E. Riding the glial monorail: a common mechanism for glial-guided neuronal migration in different regions of the mammalian brain. *Trends Neurosci.* 13:179–184, 1990.

Heffner C.D., Lumsden A.G.F., O'Leary D.D.M. Target control of collateral extension and directional axon growth in the mammalian brain. *Science* 247:217–220, 1990.

Herrup K. What do genetic mosaics tell us about cell lineages in the mammalian CNS? A reply. *Trends Neurosci.* 11:49–50, 1988.

Holt C., Bertsch T.W., Ellis H.M., et al. Cellular determination in the *Xenopus* retina is independent of lineage and birthdate. *Neuron* 1:15–26, 1988.

Holtfreter J. Gewebeaffinität, ein Mittel der embryonalen Form bildung. *Arch. Exp. Zellforsch.* 23:169–209, 1939.

Horder T.J., Martin K.A.C. Morphogenetics as an alternative to chemospecificity in the formation of nerve connections. *Symp. Soc. Exp. Biol.* 32:275–358, 1978.

Horvitz H.R. Genetics of cell lineage. In Wood W.B., ed. *The Nematode Caenorhabditis elegans Cell Lineages.* Cold Spring Harbor, NY, Cold Spring Harbor Laboratory, pp. 157–190, 1987.

*Horvitz H.R. Genetic control of *Caenorhabditis elegans* cell lineages. *Harvey Lect.* 84:65–77, 1990.

Hubel D.H., Wiesel T.N., LeVay S. Plasticity of ocular dominance columns in monkey striate cortex. *Philos. Trans. R. Soc. Lond.* [*Biol.*] 278:377–404, 1977.

Hunt R.K. Developmental programming for retinotectal patterns. *Ciba Found. Symp.* 29:131–159, 1975.

Hunt R.K., Cowan W.M. The chemoaffinity hypothesis: an appreciation of Roger W. Sperry's contributions to developmental biology. In Trevarthen C., ed. *Brain Circuits and Functions of the Mind. Essays in Honor of Roger W. Sperry.* New York, Cambridge University Press, pp. 19–74, 1990.

Innocenti G.M. Growth and reshaping of axons in the establishment of visual callosal connections. *Science* 212:824–827, 1981.

Jennings C.G.B. What do chimaeras tell us about cell lineages in the mammalian CNS. *Trends Neurosci.* 11:46–49, 1988.

*Jessell T.M. Adhesion molecules and the hierarchy of neural development. *Neuron* 1:3–13, 1988.

Karns L.R., Shi-Chung N., Freeman J.A., et al. Cloning of complementary DNA for GAP-43, a neuronal growth related protein. *Science* 236:597–600, 1987.

Kiddokoro Y., Yeh E. Initial synaptic transmission at the growth cone in *Xenopus* nerve-muscle cultures. *Proc. Natl. Acad. Sci. U.S.A.* 79:6727–6731, 1982.

Kreigstein A.R., Dichter M.A. Morphological classification of rat cortical neurons in cell culture. *J. Neurosci.* 3:1634–1647, 1983.

Langley J.N. On the regeneration of preganglionic and of post-ganglionic visceral nerve fibers. *J. Physiol. (Lond.)* 22:215–230, 1898.

*Le Douarin N.M. *The Neural Crest.* New York, Cambridge University Press, 1982.

Lemmon V., Pearlman A.L. Does laminar position determine the receptive field properties of cortical neurons? A study of cortico-tectal cells in area 17 of the normal mouse and the reeler mutant. *J. Neurosci.* 1:83–93, 1981.

Letourneau P.C. Cell-substratum adhesion of neurite growth cones, and its role in neurite elongation. *Exp. Cell Res.* 124:127–138, 1979.

*Levi-Montalcini R. Developmental neurobiology and the natural history of nerve growth factor. *Annu. Rev. Neurosci.* 5:341–362, 1982.

Levitt P., Cooper M.L., Rakic P. Co-existence of neuronal and glial precursor cells in the cerebral ventricular zone of the fetal monkey: an ultrastructural immunoperoxidase analysis. *J. Neurosci.* 1:27–39, 1981.

Lumsden A. The cellular basis of segmentation in the developing hindbrain. *Trends Neurosci.* 13:329–335, 1990.

Lund R.D. *Development and Plasticity of the Brain.* New York, Oxford University Press, 1978.

Magill C., Reist N.E., Fallon J.R., et al. Agrin. *Prog. Brain Res.* 71:391–396, 1987.

New H.V., Mudge A.W. Calcitonin gene–related peptide regulates muscle acetylcholine receptor synthesis. *Nature* 323:809–811, 1986.

O'Leary D.D.M., Cowan W.M. Further studies on the development of the isthmo-optic nucleus with special reference to the occurrence and fate of ectopic and ipsilaterally projecting neurons. *J. Comp. Neurol.* 212:399–416, 1982.

O'Leary D.D.M., Stanfield B.B. Selective elimination of axons extended by developing cortical neurons is dependent on regional locale. Experiments utilizing fetal cortical transplants. *J. Neurosci.* 9:2230–2246, 1989.

*Patterson P., Purves D. *Readings in Developmental Neurobiology.* Cold Spring Harbor, NY, Cold Spring Harbor Laboratory, 1982.

Purves D. *Body and Brain: A Trophic Theory of Neural Connections.* Cambridge, MA, Harvard University Press, 1988.

Purves D., Lichtman J.W. Elimination of synapses in the developing nervous system. *Science* 210:153–157, 1980.

Raff M.C. Glial cell diversification in the optic nerve. *Science* 243:1450–1455, 1989.

Rakic P., Sidman R.L. Sequence of developmental abnormalities leading to granule cell deficit in cerebellar cortex of weaver mutant mice. *J. Comp. Neurol.* 152:103–132, 1973.

*Ramón y Cajal S. *Studies on Vertebrate Neurogenesis* (translated by L. Guth). Springfield, IL, Thomas, 1960.

Rupp F., Payan D.G., Magill-Sole C., et al. Structure and expression of a rat agrin. *Neuron* 6:811–823, 1991.

Sanes J. Analysing cell lineage with a recombinant retrovirus. *Trends Neurosci.* 12:21–28, 1989.

Sauer F.C. The cellular structure of the neural tube. *J. Comp. Neurol.* 63:13–23, 1935.

Schaper A. Die fruhesten Differenzierungsvorgange in Central-nervensystem. *Arch. Entwicklungsmech. Org.* 5:8–132, 1897.

Sidman R.L., Rakic P. Neuronal migration in human brain development. In Berenberg S.R., Masse N.P., eds. *Pre and Post-Natal Development of the Human Brain.* Vol. 13. *Modern Problems in Pediatrics.* Basel, Karger, pp. 13–43, 1974.

Skene J.H.P. Growth associated proteins and the curious dichotomies of nerve regeneration. *Cell* 37:697–700, 1984.

Spemann H., Mangold H. Uber Induktion von Embryonalanlagen durch Implantation artfremder Organisatoren. *Arch. Mikrosk. Anat. Entwicklungsmech.* 100:599–638, 1924.

*Sperry R.W. Chemoaffinity in the orderly growth of nerve fiber patterns and connections. *Proc. Natl. Acad. Sci. U.S.A.* 50:703–710, 1963.

Sperry R.W. Embryogenesis of behavioral nerve nets. In DeHaan R.L., Ursprung H., eds. *Organogenesis.* Philadelphia, Saunders, pp. 161–186, 1965.

*Spitzer N. Development of membrane properties in vertebrates. *Trends Neurosci.* 4:169–172, 1981.

Stent G.D. The role of cell lineage in development. *Philos. Trans. R. Soc. Lond. [Biol.]* 312:3–19, 1985.

Stern C.D., Keynes R.J. Spatial patterns of homeobox gene expression in the developing mammalian CNS. *Trends Neurosci.* 5:190–192, 1988.

Stryker M.P. Late segregation of geniculate afferents to the cat's visual cortex after recovery from binocular impulse blockade. *Soc. Neurosci. Abstr.* 7:842, 1981.

Tessier-Lavigne M., Placzek M., Lunsden A.G.S., et al. Chemotropic guidance of developing axons in the mammalian central nervous system. *Nature* 336:775–778, 1988.

*Thomsen G., Woolf T., Whitman M., et al. Activins are expressed early in *Xenopus* embryogenesis and can induce axial mesoderm and anterior structures. *Cell* 63:485–493, 1990.

Tomaselli J.J., Neugebauer K.M., Bixby J., et al. Cadherin and integrins: two receptor systems that mediate neuronal process outgrowth on astrocytes. *Neuron* 1:33–43, 1988.

Trisler G.D., Schneider M.D., Nirenberg M. A topographic gradient of molecules in retina can be used to identify neuron position. *Proc. Natl. Acad. Sci. U.S.A.* 78:2145–2149, 1981.

Turner D.L., Cepko C.L. A common progenitor for neurons and glia persists in rat retina late in development. *Nature* 328:131–136, 1987.

Walicke P., Cowan W.M., Ueno N., et al. Fibroblast growth factor promotes the survival of dissociated hippocampal neurons and enhances neurite extension. *Proc. Natl. Acad. Sci. U.S.A.* 83:3012–3016, 1986.

Walsh C., Cepko C.L. Clonally related cortical cells show several migration patterns. *Science* 241:1342–1345, 1988.

Weiss P. Selectivity controlling the central-peripheral relations in the nervous system. *Biol. Rev.* 11:494–531, 1936.

*Whitman M., Melton D.A. Growth factors in early embryogenesis. *Annu. Rev. Cell Biol.* 5:93–117, 1989.

3

Molecular Organization and Pathophysiology of Axons

Stephen G. Waxman

The axon, interposed between the initial segment (at the somadendritic pole of the neuron) and its presynaptic terminals, plays a crucial role in neuronal function. Possibly reflecting its adaption to this role, the axon exhibits a complex functional organization. This functional motif applies especially to the mammalian myelinated fiber, which is characterized by a differentiation of the myelin-forming cell, the myelin sheath, and the axon membrane itself. This chapter will examine the conduction properties and molecular organization of normal and pathologic mammalian axons; it will also examine the substrates for abnormal axonal function in disease of the peripheral nervous system (PNS) and central nervous system (CNS).

THE MYELINATED AXON

Because myelinated fibers are commonly affected by pathologic processes, attention will be focused on this group of axons and their associated myelin sheaths. The myelin sheath originates from the elaborated membrane of the Schwann cell in the PNS (Geren, 1954; Robertson, 1955) and the oligodendrocyte in the CNS (Bunge et al., 1962; Peters, 1960). The periodic radial structure of myelin reflects its origin as a relatively compact spiral of Schwann cell (PNS) or oligodendroglial (CNS) membranes (Fig. 3–1). A thin extension of the extracellular space (about 10 Å wide) is maintained between adjacent lamellae (Hirano et al., 1969); however, tight junctions par-

tially isolate the intramyelinic extracellular compartment from the generalized extracellular space (Schnapp and Mugnaini, 1978). As a result of this anatomic arrangement, the myelin sheath exhibits a high transverse resistance and a low capacitance. These characteristics permit the myelin to function as an electrical insulator.

The peripheral myelin sheath is surrounded by the Schwann cell from which it is derived (Fig. 3–2). In contrast, the oligodendroglial cell body is located at some distance from the myelin sheath; only a thin cytoplasmic bridge with it is maintained in adult white matter (Fig. 3–3). It has been estimated that 30–50 myelinated segments are supported by a single oligodendrocyte in rat optic nerve (Peters and Proskauer, 1969). The relatively tenuous cytoplasmic connection between the oligodendroglial cell body and its myelin sheaths, together with the fact that numerous myelin sheaths are supported by a single glial cell, may be reflected in the relative paucity of remyelination after damage to CNS myelin. Nevertheless, evidence suggests that oligodendroglia can divide after injury (Aranella and Herndon, 1984), and it is now clear that remyelination can be mediated by oligodendrocytes under some circumstances (Ludwin, 1988).

As viewed along the length of the axon, the myelin is organized into segments with a length corresponding to that of the myelin-forming cells or processes. These myelin segments are separated by nodes of Ranvier. In normal PNS and CNS fibers, each node extends for only a short distance (less than 1 μm) along the fiber axis. On either side of the node, the myelin terminates in an ordered fashion, innermost layers terminating farthest from the node. Pockets of paranodal Schwann cell or oligodendroglial cytoplasm are present at the terminal loop of each myelin

Work in the author's laboratory has been supported in part by grants from the National Institutes of Health and the National Multiple Sclerosis Society, by the Medical Research Service of the Veterans Administration, and by support from the Daniel Heumann Fund and the Allen Charitable Trust.

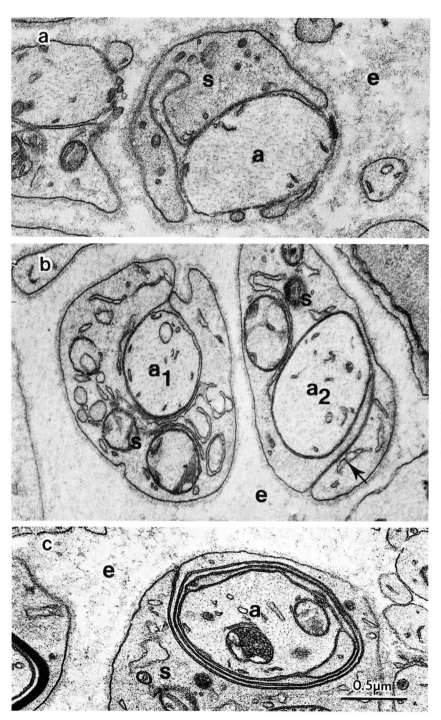

Figure 3–1. Myelination in baby mouse sciatic nerve shown in transverse section electron micrographs. $KMnO_4$ fixation. *(a)* A Schwann cell(s) has established a one-to-one relationship with an axon (a). *(b)* Axons a_1 and a_2 at early stages of myelination. A Schwann cell (s) has surrounded axon a_1 but has not yet formed a spiral wrapping in this plane of section. The Schwann cell associated with axon a_2 has begun to form a spiral wrap *(arrow)*. *(c)* Axon (a) surrounded by myelinating Schwann cell (s), which has formed two loops around the axon. An inner tongue of Schwann cell cytoplasm extends within the forming sheath. e = extracellular space. × 36,000.

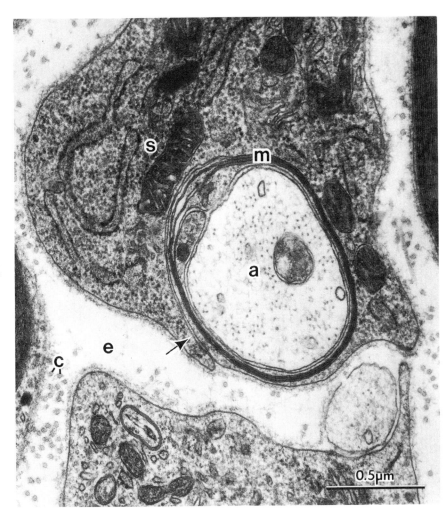

Figure 3–2. Compact myelin sheath (m) surrounding an axon (a) from baby mouse sciatic nerve. A mesaxon *(arrow)* connects the myelin sheath to the plasma membrane of the Schwann cell. e = extracellular space; c = collagen within sciatic nerve. × 53,700.

layer and in most cases are closely apposed to the axon surface, with which they form a specialized paranodal axoglial junction (Hirano and Dembitzer, 1978) that exhibits a paracrystalline structure in freeze-fracture replicas (Schnapp and Mugnaini, 1978; Wiley and Ellisman, 1980). Electron microscopic studies with extracellular tracers demonstrate that under some experimental conditions, the paranodal space between axon and terminating myelin loops can be penetrated by markers such as lanthanum and microperoxidase. Nevertheless, it is likely that the paranodal axoglial junctions partially isolate the internodal axon from the general extracellular space. Hirano and Dembitzer (1978) pointed out that even subtle pathologic alterations of the paranodal junction may expose the internodal axon to the general extracellular space, thereby shunting the entire internode, even if the integrity of the myelin per se is maintained. This view is supported by biophysical data (Funch and Faber, 1984).

In the PNS, a network of finger-like processes extends from the paranodal Schwann cell cytoplasm to form a network surrounding the nodal axon within the paranodal space (Elfvin, 1961; Robertson, 1959). These microvillous processes bear an indistinct ex-

tracellular coating and can approach the axolemma to within 20–50 Å (Rydmark and Berthold, 1983). The regularity of this structure is so striking that it has been considered as part of a paranodal apparatus, which has been suggested to play a role in nodal function (Landon, 1981). A similar network of paranodal astrocytic processes contacts CNS nodes of Ranvier (Fig. 3–4); these paranodal astrocytic processes were first described by Hildebrand (1971a,b) and their presence has been amply confirmed since then (Raine, 1984; Waxman and Black, 1984). Because these astrocytic processes are present at developing nodes (Hildebrand and Waxman, 1984), even in tissue that has been experimentally rendered glial cell deficient and where random axoglial interactions are minimized (Sims et al., 1985), there is probably a developmental interaction between the perinodal astrocyte and the node of Ranvier (Fig. 3–5). There is evidence for regional specialization of the astrocyte membrane (Landis, 1981; Newman, 1984; Waxman and Black, 1984), which is consistent with a role of the perinodal astrocyte in maintaining extracellular ionic homeostasis at the node of Ranvier. As noted later, there is also evidence for the presence of sodium channels in perinodal astrocytes (Black et al.,

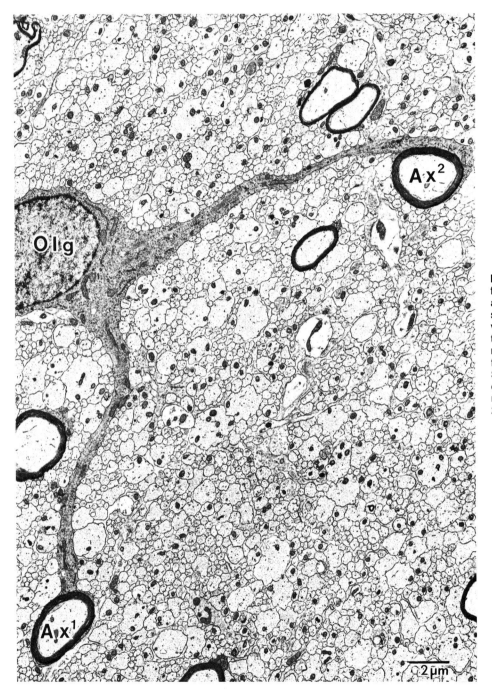

Figure 3–3. Oligodendrocyte (Olg) forming myelin sheaths around two axons (Ax[1], Ax[2]) in developing spinal cord. Note the connections, via thin cytoplasmic processes, between the oligodendrocyte and the myelin sheaths. × 6300. (Modified from Waxman S.G., Sims T.J. Specificity in central myelination: evidence for local regulation of myelin thickness. *Brain Res.* 292:179–185, 1984.)

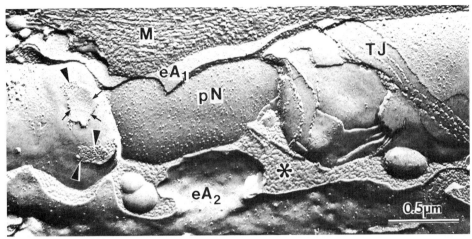

Figure 3–4. Freeze-fracture electron micrograph showing a node of Ranvier from an optic nerve. Terminating myelin lamellae are seen on both sides of the node, where the axon P face is visualized (pN). Note the tight junctions (TJ) within the myelin sheath to the right, and the gap junction *(arrowheads)* formed between the terminating oligodendrocyte to the left and an adjacent cell. * = perinodal extracellular space. Two astrocytic membranes (eA₁, eA₂) approach the node. M = myelin sheath of a neighboring fiber. × 39,000. (Modified from Waxman S.G., Black J.A. Freeze-fracture structure of the perinodal astrocyte and associated glial junctions. *Brain Res.* 308:77–87, 1984.)

1989) and in Schwann cell processes adjacent to the node of Ranvier (Ritchie et al., 1990), which suggests a physiologic role for these crucially located glial cell processes. This raises the possibility that gliosis per se may alter nodal function, even in otherwise structurally intact axons.

SPECIFICITY AND MOLECULAR CONTROL OF MYELINATION

There is a high degree of specificity in the interaction between the myelin-forming cell and the axon during myelination. For example, myelin thickness and internode distance are matched to fiber size and type; for a review, see Waxman and Foster (1980a). This specificity extends to the level of the single axon. Thus, in the case of central tracts in which numerous axons of different sizes are myelinated by a single oligodendrocyte, myelin thicknesses for fibers of different diameters are matched to diameter (despite origin from a common oligodendrocyte). Regulation of myelin thickness is therefore distributed within the oligodendroglial processes and is subject to local modulation by the axon (Waxman and Sims, 1984). In this regard, it is interesting that there is evidence, during myelination, for increased membrane turnover in distal oligodendrocyte proc-

Figure 3–5. Astrocytes are related to nodes of Ranvier in a highly specific manner. This electron micrograph shows a developing node of Ranvier from spinal cord rendered glial cell deficient by x-irradiation at the time of gliogenesis. A thin astrocytic process *(arrowheads)* extends from a perinodal astrocyte (AP) and contacts the nodal axon. Another process *(arrows)* extends to a nearby axon (a). PN = paranodal oligodendroglial loop; NA = nodal axon. × 45,000. (Modified from Sims T.J., Waxman S.G., Black J.A., et al. Perinodal astrocytic processes at nodes of Ranvier in developing normal and glial cell deficient rat spinal cord. *Brain Res.* 337:321–333, 1985.)

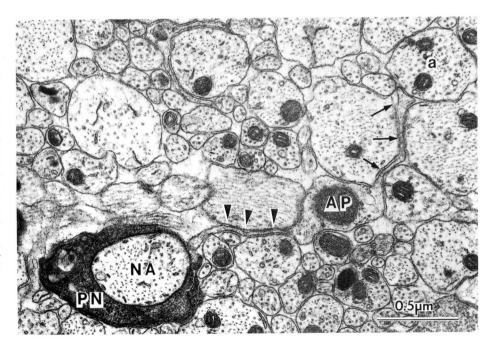

esses, that is, in the part of the oligodendrocyte that is located closest to the forming myelin sheaths (Waxman et al., 1988). This result suggests that myelin biosynthesis may occur, at least in part, within the oligodendroglial processes close to the axons.

On the basis of cross-union experiments, it is now well known that the axon determines whether myelination will occur (Aguayo et al., 1976; Weinberg and Spencer, 1976). Spencer and Weinberg (1978) and Waxman and Foster (1980a) suggested that myelination is, at least in part, regulated by cell surface–related signals. Several research groups have demonstrated structural changes in the axon surface that delineate nodal from internodal membrane regions in premyelinated fibers before formation of myelin or mature paranodal junctions and that may serve as membrane markers (Waxman and Foster, 1980; Wiley-Livingston and Ellisman, 1980). Moreover, there are distinct differences in the macromolecular structure of the axon membrane of myelinated, compared with nonmyelinated, nerve fibers (Waxman and Black, 1988).

Black et al. (1982) demonstrated, by freeze-fracture techniques, distinct changes in the ultrastructure of the P face of the axon membrane that occur at about the time of contact of premyelinated axons by glial cells (Fig. 3–6a and b). Examining axons that developed in a glial cell–deficient environment, Black et al. (1985) showed that these changes in axon membrane structure do not depend on glial contact but, on the contrary, occur even in axons deprived of ensheathment by myelin-forming cells (Fig. 3–6c). It has been suggested that this reorganization of the axon membrane reflects incorporation of a cell sur-

face–mediated signal for myelination (Waxman, 1987). The glial cell surface probably contains a template of complementary molecules, and development of myelinated fibers probably involves a complex sequence of axoglial interactions (Waxman, 1987). Studies of remyelinating axons have shown increased metabolic activity related to high-molecular-weight proteins (possibly related to recognition functions between axons and myelin-forming cells) in the period before remyelination (M.E. Smith et al., 1984).

MODES OF IMPULSE CONDUCTION

The axon membrane of most nonmyelinated axons exhibits a relatively uniform molecular structure (Black et al., 1981), in accord with the generally held view that conduction in these fibers occurs continuously. Conduction velocity in nonmyelinated fibers is proportional to the square root of the diameter. As a result of high longitudinal core resistance, together with the capacitance of the axon membrane, nonmyelinated fibers require a large diameter if they are to conduct impulses at high velocities.

The conduction velocity–diameter relationship for myelinated fibers is approximately linear (Fig. 3–7). At a diameter larger than about 0.2 μm, myelinated fibers conduct more rapidly than nonmyelinated axons of the same size (Waxman and Bennett, 1972). Tasaki and Takeuchi (1942) and Huxley and Stampfli (1949) demonstrated saltatory conduction in peripheral myelinated fibers and showed that excitability of these fibers was localized to the region of nodes of Ranvier, with the internode acting as a set of resistances and capacitances in parallel. Mechanisms of

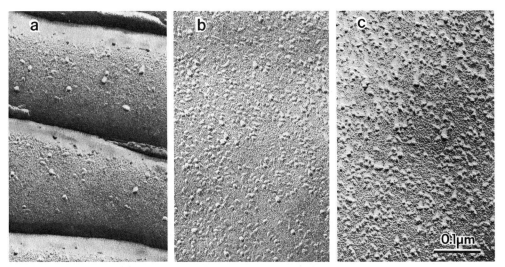

Figure 3–6. The axon membrane expresses a new population of membrane protein molecules (seen as intramembranous particles) at the time when it becomes competent to trigger myelin formation by nearby glial cells. These freeze-fracture electron micrographs show the protoplasmic membrane leaflet of developing dorsal column axons. *(a)* Axon membrane structure in 3-day-old premyelinated axons. *(b)* Axon membrane of a 19-day-old myelinated axon. Note the incorporation of an increased density of particles into the axon membrane. *(c)* Axon membrane of a 19-day-old axon deprived of glial contact by x-irradiation at the time of gliogenesis. Despite absence of glial ensheathment, axon membrane structure has changed as in *b.* × 125,000. (Modified from Black J.D., Sims T.J., Waxman S.G., et al. Membrane ultrastructure of developing axons in glial deficient rat spinal cord. *J. Neurocytol.* 14:79–104, 1985. Published by Chapman & Hall.)

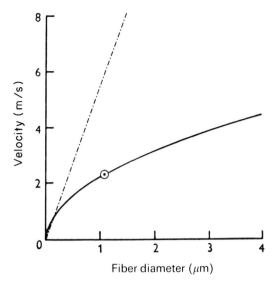

Figure 3–7. Relationship between conduction velocity and diameter for nonmyelinated fibers (solid line) and myelinated fibers (dashed line). The two relationships intersect at a point corresponding to a diameter of 0.2 μm, which indicates that at a larger diameter, myelinated fibers exhibit higher conduction velocities than nonmyelinated fibers of the same size. (Modified from Waxman S.G., Bennett M.V.L. Relative conduction velocities of small myelinated and non-myelinated fibres in the central nervous system. Reprinted by permission from *Nature* [*New Biol.*] vol. 238 p. 217. Copyright © 1972 Macmillan Magazines Ltd.)

conduction in CNS myelinated fibers are less clearly understood. The available results suggest that saltatory conduction occurs in at least some central myelinated axons (Bement and Ranck, 1969; Funch and Faber, 1982; Kocsis and Waxman, 1981).

SAFETY FACTOR

The safety factor of myelinated fibers (operationally defined as current available to stimulate a given node/current required to stimulate node) is higher in myelinated than in nonmyelinated fibers. The available evidence suggests a safety factor of 5–7 in normal myelinated fibers (Brill et al., 1977; Tasaki, 1953). Because the safety factor is inversely related to temperature (Rasminsky, 1973; Westerfield et al., 1978), this consideration may be especially important in the mammalian nervous system. In addition, the refractory period is shorter in myelinated than in nonmyelinated fibers, so that the former can sustain high-frequency impulse trains for longer periods (Paintal, 1978; Swadlow and Waxman, 1976).

AXON MEMBRANE ORGANIZATION

The demonstration of saltatory conduction in myelinated fibers raises important questions about organization of the axon membrane. For conduction to occur in a saltatory manner, the axon membrane at the node must exhibit electrical excitability. However,

the demonstration of saltatory conduction does not indicate whether the internodal axon membrane, which is normally covered by the myelin sheath, is excitable. The internodal axon membrane could, in principle, contain voltage-sensitive sodium channels that are not normally activated, because the transmembrane potential is attenuated by the overlying myelin. Alternatively, the internodal membrane could be inexcitable as a result of a low density of sodium channels. The latter possibility would not necessarily lead to conduction block in normal fibers, because the majority of action current is shunted via the myelinated internode, from one node of Ranvier to the next. The low density of sodium channels in the internodal axon membrane would be expected to interfere with conduction in demyelinated axons in which action current is shunted through the demyelinated (former internodal) membrane. Although conduction block is observed in some demyelinated fibers, this does not allow axon membrane properties in the internode to be predicted with certainty, because conduction failure may also occur in the presence of excitable internodal membrane, as a result of impedance mismatch (related largely to capacitative current loss) in the demyelinated region (Waxman and Brill, 1978).

In an important study, Rasminsky and Sears (1972) used longitudinal current analysis to study conduction in single ventral root axons in situ after demyelination with diphtheria toxin. The spatial resolution of the technique in these early experiments was not sufficient to determine whether the internode exhibited excitability. Nevertheless, this early study was important, because it focused attention on the question of membrane properties of the internodal axon.

SODIUM CHANNELS

The axon membrane in myelinated fibers is a highly ordered structure, in which the voltage-sensitive sodium channels are clustered in high density at the node of Ranvier, and the fast potassium channels (which tend to hold the membrane near resting potential) exhibit a complementary localization within the internodal axon membrane. The differentiation of the axon membrane has been studied by several experimental techniques.

Morphologic differentiation between nodal and internodal axon membrane is revealed by cytochemical studies with ferric ion–ferrocyanide staining after fixation in cacodylate-buffered aldehydes (Quick and Waxman, 1977). The cytoplasmic surface of the axon membrane at the node is specifically stained by this method, but the internodal membrane is not stained. The nodal membrane exhibits a cytochemical structure similar to that of the initial segment membrane, which is a site of high sodium channel density (Dodge and Cooley, 1973). Comparative studies in systems in which only some nodes exhibit impulse electrogenesis demonstrate the specific cytochemical differentiation of the axolemma at the excitable nodes (Quick and Waxman, 1977). The cytochemical findings suggest that the nodal membrane is a site of high sodium channel density and provide a useful method for the study of membrane differentiation at normal and pathologic nodes of Ranvier. Cytochemical studies also demonstrate that the axolemma undergoes structural reorganization during normal development (Waxman and Foster, 1980b) and that the internodal membrane may exhibit structural reorganization after demyelination (Coria et al., 1984; Foster et al., 1980).

In axons examined by freeze-fracture methods, the external (E face) membrane leaflet at the node of Ranvier differs from that of most other biologic membranes (Kristol et al., 1978; Rosenbluth, 1976, 1981). A high density (about $1300/\mu m^2$) of intramembranous particles, which represent integral membrane proteins, is present in the E face of the nodal axon membrane (Fig. 3–8). In contrast, the internodal/paranodal membrane contains, in most regions, a much lower density ($100–200/\mu m^2$) of E face particles. Rosenbluth (1976) suggested that the large E face particles at the node may be related to sodium channels.

The axolemma of nonmyelinated fibers contains, in most cases, E face particles that are distributed in a homogeneous manner at a density of about $150–300/\mu m^2$ (Black et al., 1981). This density is only twofold higher than that of the internodal axolemma. Because the available physiologic evidence suggests that the internodal membrane is inexcitable under usual circumstances (see later), the absence of a more dramatic difference between these two types of membrane suggests several possibilities:

1. E face membrane particles may not represent sodium channels in a one-to-one manner; rather, a subset of particles may be related (possibly in a one-to-many or many-to-one manner) to some ionic channels.

2. If internodal E face particles represent functional sodium channels, then (assuming that the internodal membrane is inexcitable) either the sodium channel density in nonmyelinated membrane is just above the density required to support impulse conduction or the internodal channel density is close to the value necessary for electrical excitability. This possibility is consistent with the suggestion that minor changes in membrane structure could lead to continuous conduction in some demyelinated fibers. As noted later, there is evidence that relatively low densities of sodium channels ($<5/\mu m^2$) can support conduction in some fibers with high input impedance (Waxman et al., 1988), so that, alternatively, increases in input impedance may permit a small number of internodal sodium channels to mediate conduction after demyelination.

3. Channel precursors or channels that have been altered so as to be inoperative may be present in the internodal axolemma; this suggestion, if correct, would have important implications for the development of continuous conduction in demyelinated fibers.

The precise identification of the various classes of intramembranous particles remains to be accomplished. Even in the absence of such identification, however, the freeze-fracture method provides a morphologic marker for nodal membrane and demon-

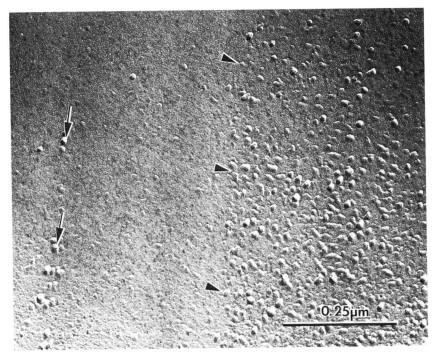

Figure 3–8. Freeze-fracture electron micrograph showing structural specialization of the axon membrane at the node of Ranvier. Note the increased density of E face membrane particles in the nodal axon membrane (to the right of the arrowheads). These intramembranous particles may be related to sodium channels, which are clustered at the node. The paranode is located to the left of the arrowheads. Shallow ridges indent the axon between terminating myelin loops, and a few particles *(arrows)* are located in these ridges. × 125,000.

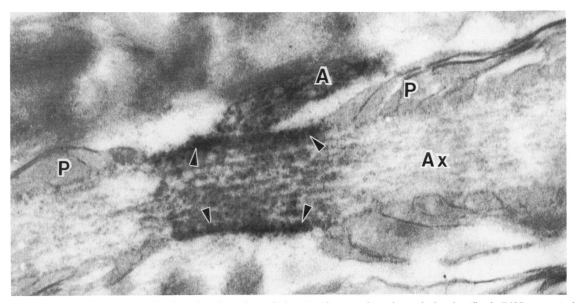

Figure 3–9. Ultrastructural immunolocalization of sodium channels in rat optic nerve by using polyclonal antibody 7493 generated against purified sodium channel α subunits. A myelinated axon (Ax) is shown at a node of Ranvier. Nodal parts of the axon membrane are densely immunoreactive *(arrowheads)*, whereas the axon membrane below the paranodal oligodendroglial loops (P) is not immunoreactive. Note that sodium channel immunoreactivity is also present in perinodal astrocyte processes (A) that contact the node, which suggests a possible role of astrocytes in development or maintenance of the nodal axon membrane. × 55,000. (Modified from Black J.A., Friedman B., Waxman S.G., et al. Immuno-ultrastructural localization of sodium channels at nodes of Ranvier and perinodal astrocytes in rat optic nerve. *Proc. R. Soc. Lond. [Biol.]* 238:39–51, 1989.)

strates the structural differentiation of nodal membrane from other biologic membranes, including the internodal/paranodal axolemma.

Sodium channels have been localized to the nodal membrane in mammalian white matter by using ultrastructural immunocytochemical methods (Black et al., 1989). These immunolocalization studies have used polyclonal antibodies generated against purified α subunits of mammalian sodium channels (Elmer et al., 1990). These studies demonstrated the specific localization of immunoreactivity in the axon membrane of the node of Ranvier, but not in the internodal axon membrane (Fig. 3–9). It is interesting that perinodal astrocyte processes also show sodium channel immunoreactivity, which suggests a role of astrocytes in development and/or maintenance of the axon membrane at the node of Ranvier (Black et al., 1989). Patch-clamp studies also demonstrate sodium channels in mammalian astrocytes, although the density of these channels is too low to support electrogenesis (Southeimer et al., 1990). It may be possible, in the future, to definitively identify specific intramembranous particles as sodium channels by using fracture-label methods.

Saxitoxin-binding studies (which use a ligand that binds specifically to sodium channels), pioneered by Ritchie and colleagues, have provided important information about localization and density of sodium channels in myelinated fibers. These studies suggest a sodium channel density of about $10^4/\mu m^2$ in the axon membrane at the node of Ranvier and a sodium channel density of less than $25/\mu m^2$ in the internodal axon membrane under the myelin sheath in normal myelinated fibers. This estimate of internodal sodium channel density falls below the value necessary for electrical excitability under most circumstances (Ritchie and Rogart, 1977). In mammalian nonmyelinated axons (C fibers), saxitoxin-binding studies suggest (if uniform channel distribution is assumed) a sodium channel density of $100–200/\mu m^2$ (Ritchie et al., 1976); this value is close to that predicted by computer simulations (Hodgkin, 1975) to maximize conduction velocity in nonmyelinated axons. In some premyelinated axons, action potential conduction is supported by low densities of sodium channels (as low as $2/\mu m^2$); conduction in these fibers is facilitated by a high input impedance (Waxman et al., 1989). A similar mechanism may support conduction in some demyelinated axons.

Nodal and internodal membranes also exhibit different properties when studied by voltage clamp, with inward sodium currents being limited to the former site (Chiu and Ritchie, 1981). A maximum of 82,000 sodium channels per node (corresponding to a density of about $1500/\mu m^2$) is suggested by gating current measurements at rabbit PNS nodes (Chiu, 1980). Current fluctuation analysis demonstrates a mean of 21,000 sodium channels at nodes in rat sciatic nerve (Neumcke and Stampfli, 1982). Although there is some variation between these and other estimates, it is clear that sodium channel density in the nodal membrane is at least $10^3/\mu m^2$. The electrophysiologic data are thus consistent with the cytochemical and freeze-fracture results in demonstrating a heterogeneous distribution of sodium channels in myelinated fibers. Voltage-sensitive sodium channels are present in high density at the node of Ranvier (where they are required for saltatory conduction), and in low density (probably too low to support impulse conduction under usual circumstances) in the internodal axon membrane under the myelin sheath.

The mechanisms by which sodium channels are clustered at the nodal region have been studied. One hypothesis suggests that the paranodal axoglial junction serves as a barrier to diffusion of channels within the membrane (Rosenbluth, 1976). Alternatively, it has been suggested that the axon exhibits a capability for the development, independent of myelin formation, of nodal domains. Ionic channels at the node may be cross-linked to one another, to other membrane structures, or to nonmembranous elements (either in a submembranous cytoskeleton or outside the membrane) (Ellisman, 1979; Waxman and Quick, 1978).

Patches of nodal membrane develop at the sites of immature nodes before the formation of paranodal axoglial junctions (Tao-Cheng and Rosenbluth, 1982; Waxman and Foster, 1980b; Wiley-Livingston and Ellisman, 1980). Membrane patches with increased E face particle density (presumably corresponding to "hot spots" of increased sodium channel density) have also been observed along nonmyelinated fibers in the retinal nerve fiber layer (Black et al., 1984). Similar node-like membrane patches, with a high density of large E face particles, develop in axons that are experimentally deprived of glial ensheathment (Black et al., 1985). There is also ultrastructural evidence for the presence of foci of node-like membrane in some dysmyelinated (Bray et al., 1979; Rosenbluth, 1979) and demyelinated (Blakemore and Smith, 1983) fibers. The development of φ nodes (which are thought to represent clusters of sodium channels) in PNS fibers demyelinated with lysophosphatidyl choline has been observed physiologically at the sites of developing nodes before formation of new myelin (Bostock et al., 1980; K.J. Smith et al., 1982).

Thus, circumferential ensheathment by myelin-forming cells is not a prerequisite for the development of patches of nodal membrane. There is, however, a close spatial relationship between these foci of node-type membrane and specifically located, radially oriented astrocytic or Schwann cell processes (Blakemore and Smith, 1983; Hildebrand and Waxman, 1983; Rosenbluth, 1979). The nature of the interaction between axons and astrocytes at these sites is not clear, although it is known that axon-astrocyte contact is present early in development (see Fig. 3–5) and that axoglial junctions of the paranodal type are not present in these regions (Black et al., 1985; Sims et al., 1985). Sodium channel–related immunoreactivity has been observed in perinodal astrocyte processes (see Fig. 3–9), which suggests that sodium channels, channel precursors, and/or channel breakdown products may be present in these processes (Black et al., 1989). It has been suggested (Bevan et al., 1985; Gray and Ritchie, 1985) that glial

cells may function as extraneuronal sites of ion channels, which are subsequently transported to the axon. Type 2 astrocytes in the optic nerve, which are thought to give rise to perinodal astrocyte processes that contact the node, express sodium channels with steady-state inactivation properties and kinetics similar to those of neurons (Southeimer et al., 1991). The presence of sodium channels provides additional evidence for a role of astrocytes in the development and/or maintenance of the axon membrane at the node of Ranvier.

It is possible that mammalian myelinated axons contain several types of sodium channels. The presence of a population of slowly inactivating sodium channels in sensory axons is suggested by sustained bursting after blockade of potassium conductance (Kocsis and Waxman, 1987) and is further supported by observations of sodium influx into depolarized axons in anoxic optic nerve (Stys et al., 1991). In this regard, it is interesting that sensory and motor axons exhibit different responses to potassium channel blockade (Bowe et al., 1985), which suggests that different types of nerve fibers may express different populations of sodium channels.

POTASSIUM CHANNELS

Voltage-sensitive potassium channels in the axolemma of myelinated fibers have distributions different from those of sodium channels. There is now evidence for at least two classes of potassium channels in mammalian myelinated fibers: "fast" and "slow" channels. Notably, the available evidence indicates that the classic model of action potential electrogenesis (in which repolarization of the action potential depends on the activation of voltage-sensitive potassium channels) may not pertain to mammalian myelinated fibers. Thus, although voltage-sensitive potassium conductance mediates repolarization of the action potential in mammalian nonmyelinated fibers (Bostock et al., 1978; Kocsis et al., 1981; Preston et al., 1983), repolarization of the action potential at the node of Ranvier appears to depend on rapid sodium inactivation, large leakage currents, or both (Brismar, 1980; Chiu et al., 1979). Voltage-clamp studies of the node of Ranvier in mammalian peripheral nerve suggest a paucity of potassium channels (Brismar, 1980; Chiu et al., 1979). Potassium channel organization in central myelinated fibers has been studied by using intra-axonal and current-clamp techniques (Gordon et al., 1988; Kocsis and Waxman, 1980, 1981). Pharmacologic agents, which specifically block various types of potassium channels, have provided probes that are useful for determining the distribution of these channels in myelinated fibers. These probes include 4-aminopyridine (4-AP), which specifically blocks the rapidly activating (or fast) potassium channel (g_{Kf}), and tetraethylammonium (TEA), which blocks the delayed rectifying (or slow) potassium channel (g_{Ks}). Intra-axonal recordings (Fig. 3–10) in myelinated axons in situ in mammalian CNS

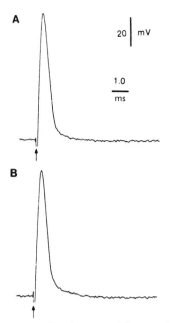

Figure 3–10. Intra-axonal action potentials recorded from myelinated fiber in rat dorsal columns, before *(A)* and after *(B)* injection with the potassium channel–blocking agent tetraethylammonium. Note that blockade of potassium channels does not lead to a delay in repolarization (which would be expected to produce broadening of the action potential as in Fig. 3–11); in normal mammalian myelinated fibers, voltage-sensitive potassium channels are not required for action potential repolarization. (Modified from Kocsis J.D., Waxman S.G. Action potential electrogenesis in mammalian central axons. In Waxman S.G., Ritchie J.M., eds. *Demyelinating Disease: Basic and Clinical Electrophysiology.* New York, Raven Press, pp. 299–372, 1981.)

show that repolarization in these fibers is not mediated by TEA-sensitive potassium channels (Kocsis and Waxman, 1980). Similarly, duration of the action potential in mammalian myelinated fibers is not prolonged by externally applied 4-AP.

4-AP–sensitive (fast) potassium channels, although rare in the nodal membrane, appear to be present in paranodal and internodal axon membrane under the myelin sheath. Developmental studies (Waxman and Foster, 1980a), carried out with optic nerve, show that before myelination both sodium and 4-AP–sensitive potassium channels contribute to action potential waveform; however, after myelination the contribution of 4-AP–sensitive potassium conductance to action potential waveform is attenuated. Voltage-clamp experiments with sciatic nerve have demonstrated the appearance of potassium conductance in mammalian nerve fibers after acute disruption of the myelin (Chiu and Ritchie, 1980). Kocsis et al. (1982b) demonstrated that in regenerating mammalian sciatic nerve fibers before myelin formation pharmacologic blockade of potassium channels with 4-AP leads to delayed action potential repolarization and consequent spike broadening (Fig. 3–11). Voltage-clamp (Brismar, 1981) and longitudinal current analysis data (Bostock et al., 1981) for demyelinated PNS fibers also indicate the presence of outward currents related to fast potassium channels in the internodal axon

membrane, which is normally covered by the myelin sheath. It has been suggested that these internodal fast potassium channels have a role in stabilizing the axon so as to prevent abnormal repetitive firing in response to single stimuli (Kocsis et al., 1983; Ritchie and Chiu, 1981). The possibility that internodal potassium channels contribute to the resting potential of the myelinated fiber has also been proposed (Chiu and Ritchie, 1984).

More recent studies (Baker et al., 1987; Kocsis et al., 1986, 1987) demonstrated that slow potassium channels are also present in the axon membrane in some mammalian myelinated fibers. These channels, which are blocked by TEA, are activated by pro-

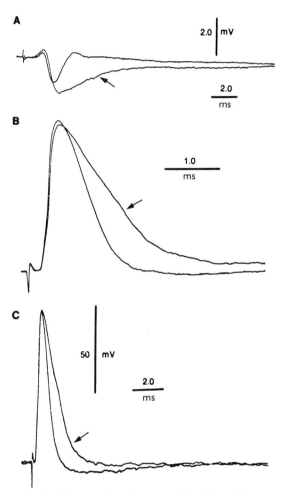

Figure 3–11. Compound action potentials *(A)* and intra-axonal action potentials *(B, C)* recorded from premyelinated regenerating rat sciatic nerve, before and after blockade of potassium channels with 4-AP (0.5 mmol/L). *(A)* Note prolongation of compound action potential after blockade of potassium conductance *(arrow)*. *(B)* Prolongation of the action potential *(arrow)* recorded intra-axonally from a single premyelinated axon, after blockade of potassium channels. *(C)* Attenuation of after-hyperpolarizing potential after blockage of potassium channels with 4-AP *(arrow)*. These results demonstrate the participation of voltage-sensitive potassium channels in action potential electrogenesis in premyelinated fibers. (Modified from Kocsis J.D., Waxman S.G., Hildebrand C., et al. Regenerating mammalian nerve fibres: changes in action potential waveform and firing characteristics following blockage of potassium conductance. *Proc. R. Soc. Lond.* [Biol.] 217:77–87,1982.)

A

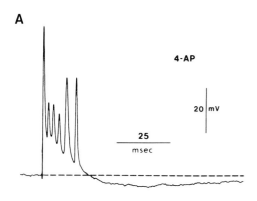

4-AP

20 | mV

25
——
msec

B

60
——
msec

4-AP + TEA

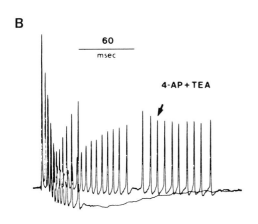

C

7.5 | mV

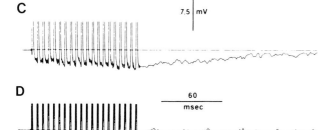

D

60
——
msec

Figure 3–12. Slow potassium channels modulate repetitive firing in myelinated axons. *(A, B)* Modulation of repetitive firing in rat sensory axon after blockade of slow potassium channels with TEA. An after-hyperpolarizing potential (below resting potential, indicated by the dashed line in *A*) terminates action potential burst activity. This potential is attenuated *(B)* by TEA. Note the increased burst behavior after attenuation of the after-hyperpolarization by blockade of slow potassium channels, which suggests that the after-hyperpolarizing potential modulates burst activity. *(C, D)* Recordings from motor axon in rat sciatic nerve. Note that an after-hyperpolarizing potential is present after repetitive activity *(C)* and is attenuated by blockade of slow potassium channels with TEA *(D)*. (Modified from Kocsis J.D., Eng D.L., Gordon T.R., et al. Functional differences between 4-aminopyridine and tetraethylammonium-sensitive potassium channels in myelinated axons. *Neurosci. Lett.* 75:193–198, 1987.)

longed depolarization. These channels do not mediate repolarization of single action potentials but are activated during high-frequency discharge. Activation of slow potassium channels mediates an after-hyperpolarization (Fig. 3–12), which appears to par-

ticipate in the modulation of repetitive firing (Baker et al., 1987; Kocsis et al., 1986, 1987). These slow potassium channels appear to play a role in determining adaptive properties in sensory axons (Bowe et al., 1985). They have a pharmacologic signature similar to that of delayed rectifier channels (Gordon et al., 1988, 1989). The available evidence suggests a nodal, and possibly also an internodal, location for these slow potassium channels.

There is also evidence for a fourth type of ion channel, the inward rectifier (g_{IR}), in the axon membrane of mammalian myelinated fibers (Baker et al., 1987; Eng et al., 1990). These channels activate in response to hyperpolarization of the axon membrane. It appears likely that both sodium and potassium ions permeate these channels. Because the inward rectifier channels limit the degree of hyperpolarization that the axon can sustain, these channels appear to play a role in modulating the excitability of the membrane and/or in modulating the degree to which the membrane can be hyperpolarized by other channels or pumps.

Figure 3–13 presents a simplified working model that summarizes current understanding of ion channel organization of the myelinated fiber (Black et al., 1990b). According to this working model, myelinated fiber organization is characterized by a relative segregation of voltage-sensitive sodium and fast potassium channels into nodal and paranodal/internodal domains of the axolemma, respectively. With respect to pathophysiology, the membrane differentiation at the node provides several mechanisms by which conduction may be altered after demyelination. Given the low sodium channel density that characterizes the normal internodal axon membrane, it is clear that after acute demyelination of a sufficient area of the internode, excitability will be reduced and even lost (Ritchie and Rogart, 1977; Waxman, 1977). This result, in addition to the capacitative loading imposed by paranodal or segmental demyelination

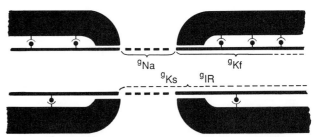

Figure 3–13. Schematic model of ion channel organization in mammalian myelinated fibers. Sodium channels are present in high density in the axon membrane at the node of Ranvier but are present in low densities (too low to sustain impulse conduction under usual circumstances) in the internodal axon membrane. 4-AP–sensitive potassium channels have a complementary distribution and are present in the internodal axon membrane where they are masked by the overlying myelin. The focal distribution of these two channels has important implications for axonal pathophysiology. g_{Na} = sodium channels; g_{Kf} = fast (4-AP–sensitive) potassium channels; g_{Ks} = slow (TEA-sensitive) potassium channels; g_{IR} = inward rectifier channels.

(Rasminsky and Sears, 1972), will tend to produce conduction block. In addition, demyelination should unmask the internodal (fast) potassium conductance, which would be expected to hold the membrane close to the potassium equilibrium potential E_K (i.e., close to resting potential) (Ritchie and Chiu, 1981; Sherratt et al., 1980). This latter consideration provides a rationale for examining the effect of potassium channel blockade on conduction in demyelinated fibers (Davis and Schauf, 1981; Sears and Bostock, 1981; Waxman et al., 1985).

ABNORMAL MODES OF IMPULSE CONDUCTION

Injured and demyelinated nerve fibers exhibit a number of abnormalities of impulse conduction (Fig. 3–14) that can be broadly categorized as negative in the jacksonian sense, with reduction in conduction velocity or block of conduction, or positive, with de novo production of abnormal impulses or pathologic amplification or transduction of signals.

Decreased conduction velocity was one of the first abnormalities to be observed in demyelinated fibers (McDonald, 1963; McDonald and Sears, 1970). Longitudinal current analysis demonstrates that internodal conduction time can be increased to over 500 μs after demyelination, compared with about 20 μs in normal fibers (Rasminsky and Sears, 1972). The increased internodal conduction time reflects, in part, the increased time necessary for charging of the exposed (formerly internodal) capacity (Koles and Rasminsky, 1972).

McDonald (1977) has presented measurements of the extent (3–30 mm, mean 10.5 mm) of demyelinated plaques in the optic nerve of patients with multiple sclerosis. Assuming that (before demyelination) the fiber diameter was less than 3 μm and that the internode distance was about 200 μm, there should be about 50 internodal lengths in a plaque 1 cm long. Using a value of 500 ms for internodal conduction time in the demyelinated fibers, McDonald estimated that a conduction delay of about 25 ms is interposed by a 1-cm plaque. This prediction corresponds, to at least a first approximation, to the delay measured in the visual evoked response in patients with multiple sclerosis. As noted by McDonald, this estimate is based on the assumption that data derived from large myelinated fibers can be extrapolated to small myelinated fibers; this assumption remains to be tested. In addition, abnormalities of synaptic summation (possibly reflecting temporal dispersion) are not taken into account in this argument. Moreover, continuous conduction can occur along some demyelinated axons (see later) with a greatly reduced conduction velocity (Bostock and Sears, 1976, 1978). Nevertheless, it is likely that slowed conduction, possibly in a saltatory mode, occurs in demyelinated fibers.

Decreased conduction velocity need not necessarily lead to clinical deficits in all cases. It is well known that the visual evoked response exhibits prolonged latency in some patients with multiple sclerosis after clinical recovery from optic neuritis (Halliday and McDonald, 1977). It is interesting that asymptomatic slowing of conduction is more common along visual than along somatosensory pathways in patients with

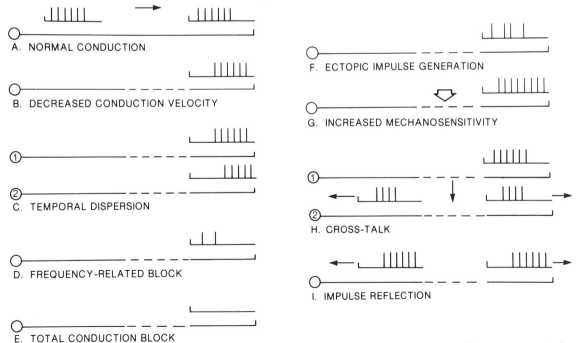

Figure 3–14. Abnormal nodes of impulse conduction in demyelinated and injured axons. Negative abnormalities are represented on the left *(B to E)*, and positive abnormalities are represented on the right *(F to I)*.

multiple sclerosis, despite the longer conduction distance along somatosensory tracts (Hume and Waxman, 1988.)

Studies of the effect of temperature on demyelinated fibers indicate that, although increased temperature leads to increased conduction velocity (Swadlow et al., 1981), it also produces clinical worsening related to conduction block (Davis and Jacobson, 1971; Namerow, 1968; Rasminsky, 1973). The important conclusion is that, for some pathways, decreased conduction velocity may be less important than conduction block in producing clinical deficits. Nevertheless, decreased conduction velocity (or temporal dispersion) can lead to significant clinical abnormalities in some systems. It has been shown, for example, that some specialized motor fibers function as precisely timed delay lines (Waxman, 1975). Moreover, some postsynaptic cells are quite sensitive to small changes (less than 1 ms) in the timing of incoming impulses (Yasargil and Diamond, 1968), so that any alteration in conduction velocity in the incoming fibers leads to distortion of the synaptic message.

Temporal dispersion, or the loss of synchrony of action potentials carried in fibers demyelinated to different degrees, occurs as a corollary of decreased conduction velocity. This dispersion is often observed in clinical electrophysiologic studies. This abnormality has been cited as a mechanism underlying the loss of deep tendon reflexes and vibration sensibility in patients with early diabetic neuropathy, in which there are only moderate reductions in maximal conduction velocity (Gilliatt and Willison, 1962).

There is also evidence for *conduction block* in demyelinated fibers (Denny-Brown and Brenner, 1944; McDonald, 1963; McDonald and Sears, 1970; Rasminsky and Sears, 1972). Conduction block can be frequency related, with low-frequency impulse trains conducting relatively reliably and high-frequency impulse trains failing to propagate; or conduction failure can be complete, with no transmission of impulses across the lesion site (Waxman, 1988b). Conduction block may reflect inexcitability of the exposed demyelinated axon membrane, with a consequent decrease in current density through excitable membrane (Ritchie and Rogart, 1977; Waxman, 1977). Alternatively, conduction block can occur as a result of the impedance mismatch imposed by myelin thinning and/or pathologic exposure of excitable axon membrane in demyelinated regions; in this case, capacitative loading will result in decreased current density and a consequent failure to reach threshold (Waxman, 1977). In addition, the exposed (former internodal) potassium channels will tend to hold the demyelinated membrane close to the potassium equilibrium potential (Waxman, 1982). Pump-mediated hyperpolarization (Bostock and Grafe, 1985) will also decrease the safety factor and interfere with conduction of bursts of impulses.

In addition to the above-mentioned abnormalities, there are a number of positive (in the jacksonian sense) conduction abnormalities in demyelinated fibers, as outlined in Figure 3–14. *Ectopic impulse generation* has been observed, for example, in chronically demyelinated axons in cat dorsal columns (K.J. Smith and McDonald, 1980). *Impulse reflection,* which is predicted on the basis of abrupt changes in input impedance (Goldstein and Rall, 1974; Ramon et al., 1975), has also been demonstrated in demyelinated fibers (Burchiel, 1980).

There is also evidence for *abnormal cross-talk* (ephaptic interaction) between abnormally myelinated axons. Subthreshold ephaptic interactions have been documented even in normal neighboring axons (Kocsis et al., 1982a). However, suprathreshold effects of ephaptic transmission have been described in acutely (Wall et al., 1974) and chronically injured axons. Studies of single fibers have demonstrated cross-talk, with abnormal impulse generation, in abnormally myelinated fibers in the dystrophic mouse (Rasminsky, 1980) and in fibers ending in neuromas (Kocsis et al., 1984), although it has not been observed in axons demyelinated with lysophosphatidyl choline (Targ and Kocsis, 1985).

Some studies also suggest *increased mechanosensitivity* in demyelinated fibers (Howe et al., 1977; K.J. Smith and McDonald, 1980). This abnormality probably accounts for Lhermitte's sign in the case of cervical spinal cord lesions (K.J. Smith and McDonald, 1980), Tinel's sign in the case of peripheral nerve lesions, and radiculopathic paresthesias in the case of straight leg raising or straight arm raising in patients with spinal root or plexus pathology (Waxman, 1979). The mechanism remains unexplained, although even normal axons exhibit a degree of mechanosensitivity.

Demyelinated fibers are highly sensitive to temperature, with the safety factor for transmission falling as the temperature increases (Rasminsky, 1973; Schauf and Davis, 1974). This sensitivity causes conduction block to develop as temperature increases. This thermal sensitivity is due to the decreased time integral of inward current at higher temperatures and may explain the worsening of clinical symptoms in some patients with multiple sclerosis as body temperature is raised (Guthrie, 1951). It is interesting that a similar thermosensitivity is not clinically apparent in most patients with peripheral neuropathies. In addition, changes in metabolic status and in the composition of the extracellular milieu can alter excitability and conduction velocity of demyelinated (Davis et al., 1977; Schauf and Davis, 1974) as well as normal nonmyelinated (Malenka et al., 1981) fibers. Thus, structure-function relationships in excitable tissues are dynamic, reflecting, for example, temperature and metabolic status. In this regard, changes in the exogenous milieu, as well as alterations in axonal structure, can play a role in determining clinical symptoms related to demyelinated fibers.

STRUCTURAL AND FUNCTIONAL PLASTICITY OF THE AXON

The available evidence suggests that, in some fibers, remyelination can restore conduction after loss of myelin (K.J. Smith et al., 1979). However, the well-established clinical observation of asymptomatic plaques in multiple sclerosis (Ghatak et al., 1974; Mackay and Hirano, 1967) suggests that remyelination may not be a necessary prerequisite for recovery of function (conversely, clinical worsening in patients with multiple sclerosis need not imply de novo demyelination in all cases). Moreover, the time course of recovery of vision in some patients with optic neuritis is more rapid than could be accounted for by remyelination (Halliday and McDonald, 1977).

Clinicopathologic relationships in demyelinating diseases are complex and suggest a variety of pathophysiologic mechanisms. In some cases, the asymptomatic demyelinated plaque may be explained on the basis of redundant conduction pathways and/or the utilization of alternative conduction pathways. Another set of mechanisms may include the presence of normal nonmyelinated fibers carrying biologically important information along the affected pathway. In other cases, recovery may be attributed to resolution of cerebral edema or to central adaptive mechanisms (e.g., sprouting). Although these mechanisms may contribute to functional recovery in some instances, the available evidence indicates that demyelinated fibers per se may conduct biologically useful information in some cases. Clinical observations provide strong evidence for this conclusion: for example, Wisniewski et al. (1976) described a patient with preserved vision despite total demyelination, observed at postmortem examination, extending for more than 2 cm along the optic nerves. In such cases, conduction at biologically relevant frequencies along the demyelinated axons can be inferred.

There have now been several direct demonstrations of the conduction of action potentials along demyelinated axon regions. Bostock and Sears (1976, 1978) have demonstrated, in rat ventral roots demyelinated with diphtheria toxin, continuous conduction along demyelinated regions. These observations imply the development of electrical excitability in the demyelinated (former internodal) membrane. Cytochemical studies have demonstrated the spread of nodal membrane characteristics through demyelinated axon regions, thus providing a morphologic demonstration of plasticity of the demyelinated axon region (Coria et al., 1984; Foster et al., 1980). More recently, immunoelectron microscopic studies with antibodies directed against mammalian CNS sodium channels have demonstrated reorganization of sodium channels in demyelinated axons (Black et al., 1991).

In some small-diameter fibers that do not have myelin, a low density of sodium channels ($<5/\mu m^2$) can support impulse conduction (Waxman et al., 1989). For example, in premyelinated axons in neonatal rat optic nerve, which are not yet myelinated or ensheathed by glial cells, action potential conduction is supported by a sodium channel density of approximately $2/\mu m^2$. This result is due to the fact that input resistance, for cylindric axons, is proportional to $(diameter)^{-3/2}$. As a result of the high input resistance of small-diameter axons, activation of a small number of sodium channels can depolarize the fiber to threshold. Waxman et al. (1989) have suggested that, in some small demyelinated fibers, a similar mechanism may contribute to restoration of conduction. Although the density of sodium channels in the internodal axon membrane is much lower than that at the node (see earlier), the available results suggest that some sodium channels are present in the internodal axon membrane (Ritchie and Rogart, 1977; Waxman and Quick, 1978). In this regard, it is important to recall that axon diameter is often reduced in demyelinated regions (Prineas and Connell, 1978, 1979). Moreover, it is possible that the diameter is reduced in demyelinated axon regions without a loss of sodium channels. These factors may permit restoration of conduction, on the basis of preexisting sodium channels (at a density too low to support conduction without a decrease in diameter), without imposing the need for additional sodium channel incorporation into the demyelinated axon membrane.

Conduction in demyelinated regions may not always occur in a continuous manner. A nonuniform mode of conduction, involving φ nodes, which probably represent aggregations of sodium channels at the site of developing nodes of Ranvier, has been described several days before remyelination in ventral root axons demyelinated with lysophosphatidyl choline (Bostock et al., 1980; K.J. Smith et al., 1982). Impulse conduction of this type appears to have a low safety factor and is highly temperature sensitive. The important point, however, is that there is evidence for membrane plasticity in the demyelinated axon, with the development of distributed or clustered sodium channels along the previously inexcitable internode. It has not yet been determined, in these cases of conduction through demyelinated fibers, whether the acquisition of excitability in demyelinated regions reflects redistribution of pre-existing sodium channels or the production of new channels and their insertion into the membrane, or both.

As noted by Rasminsky (1978), the fact that remyelinated fibers conduct at velocities close to normal, despite their reduced internode distances, suggests the development of near-normal properties at newly formed nodes after remyelination. Electron microscopic studies indicate that nodes formed along remyelinated fibers in spinal cord recapitulate normal cytochemical properties (Weiner et al., 1980). In remyelinated peripheral nerve, there is an increase in saxitoxin binding that is proportional to the increase in the nodal area imposed by the shorter spacing between nodes (Ritchie et al., 1981); this finding suggests that newly formed (remyelinated) nodes exhibit a relatively normal density of sodium channels, presumably reflecting channel biosynthesis after demyelination. The role of the cell body in the response to demyelination is under investigation.

IMPEDANCE MISMATCH AFTER DEMYELINATION

Waxman (1978) and Sears et al. (1978) have called attention to the fact that increased threshold, or impedance mismatch as a result of inadequate current density at the junction between normally myelinated and demyelinated axon regions, may constitute a physiologic barrier with respect to invasion of action potentials into demyelinated axon regions.

Impedance matching could be mediated by reduction in diameter of the demyelinated region (Bostock and Sears, 1978; Prineas and Connell, 1978), by the interposition of short internodes proximal to the demyelinated region (Waxman and Brill, 1978), or by the development of larger than normal nodes or higher than normal sodium channel densities at nodes proximal to the demyelinated zone (Fig. 3–15).

Alternatively, minor changes in axon membrane properties at the transition region between a myelinated zone and the region without myelin may promote impulse invasion (Fig. 3–16). In particular, increasing sodium conductance or decreasing potassium conductance promotes invasion (Waxman and Wood, 1984). As a result of the nonlinear behavior of excitable membranes, the spatial distribution of the ionic channels at a demyelinated region, as well

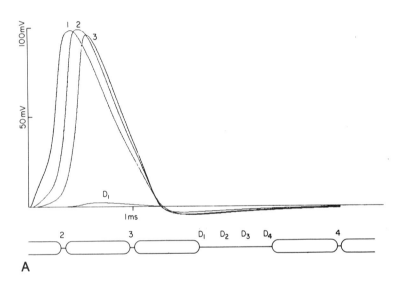

A

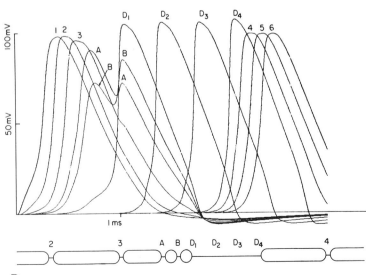

B

Figure 3–15. Conduction block can occur in demyelinated fibers as a result of impedance mismatch. *(A)* Computed action potentials for a fiber focally demyelinated in the region between D_1 and D_4 under the assumption that the demyelinated axon membrane had developed a high density of sodium channels (similar to that of normal nodal membrane). Despite the assumption of excitability in the demyelinated zone, there is failure of invasion of the action potential from the normal region into the demyelinated region. This conduction block is a result of inadequate current density at the transition region between myelinated and demyelinated zones, primarily because of capacitative current loss. *(B)* Computed action potentials for a demyelinated fiber similar to that in *A* showing the effect of interposing several short internodes (A–B; B–D_1) proximal to the demyelinated zone. Nodes A and B are assumed to have normal nodal properties. Under these conditions, the action potential invades and passes through the demyelinated region. (From Waxman S.G., Brill M.H. Conduction through demyelinated plaques in multiple sclerosis: computer simulation of facilitation by short internodes. *J. Neurol. Neurosurg. Psychiatry* 41:408–417, 1978.)

Figure 3–16. Computed action potentials showing effect of altered ionic channel distribution on invasion of demyelinated zone. *Inset* shows action potentials at subsequent nodes at 2-mm distances along a fiber with demyelination beginning at 2.0 cm; conduction block occurs at the beginning of the demyelinated region (D). When a transition zone, 50 μm long and with a sodium channel density 50% higher than normal, is located at the beginning of the demyelinated region, the action potential invades the demyelinated axon and propagates at a slower conduction velocity. Decreased potassium conductance in the transition zone (not shown) similarly promotes invasion. (Modified from Waxman S.G., Wood S.L. Impulse conduction in inhomogeneous axons: effects of variation in voltage-sensitive ionic conductances on invasion of demyelinated axon segments and preterminal fibers. *Brain Res.* 294:111–123, 1984.)

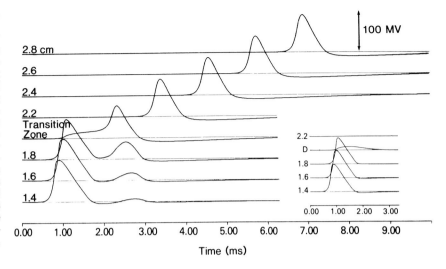

as their number, is predicted to have significant effects on impulse invasion properties. Thus, relatively minor degrees of membrane reorganization (possibly involving redistribution of channels via lateral diffusion within the membrane) may lead to functional changes with respect to impulse invasion of demyelinated regions (Waxman and Wood, 1984). If the prerequisites for the invasion of demyelinated axon regions are met, a density of sodium channels in the demyelinated zone, which is considerably lower than that at normal nodes, can sustain continuous conduction (Waxman and Brill, 1978).

STRUCTURE-FUNCTION RELATIONSHIPS

Conduction velocity and fiber diameter in normal myelinated fibers are related via an approximately linear relationship, with an increase in conduction velocity of 5.5 m/s for each 1 μm in diameter (Waxman and Bennett, 1972). Myelin thickness also plays a role in determining conduction velocity. For any given axon diameter (measured within the myelin sheath), conduction velocity increases with increasing sheath thickness (R.S. Smith and Koles, 1970). For a fixed fiber diameter (axon plus myelin sheath), an optimal value of myelin thickness tends to maximize conduction velocity; the optimal value of the ratio (axon diameter/fiber diameter) is independent of diameter and falls between 0.6 and 0.7 (Moore et al., 1978; Rushton, 1951). Observed values for this ratio fall in this range for many classes of PNS and CNS axons (Friede and Samorajski, 1967; Waxman and Bennett, 1972).

Internode distance also plays a role in determining conduction velocity. Huxley and Stampfli (1949) suggested that, at any given diameter, conduction velocity should exhibit a maximum at a particular internode distance. These workers also suggested that the curve relating conduction velocity to internode distance should have a relatively flat maximum. Brill et al. (1977) quantitatively studied the internode

distance–conduction velocity relationship. If axon diameter and myelin thickness are fixed, the conduction velocity is maximized when the ratio between internode distance and axon diameter falls between 100 and 200; this value for this ratio is observed in most normal peripheral myelinated fibers. There is only a moderate decrease in conduction velocity for moderately decreased internode distances. For significant reductions in internode distance, as are observed both in normal preterminal axons and in some remyelinated fibers, there can be substantial decreases in conduction velocities (Fig. 3–17). In terms of conduction in remyelinated fibers, these relationships are based on the assumption that relatively normal nodal properties are re-established after remyelination (Rasminsky, 1978).

The pattern of myelination departs from the general (main trunk) pattern in certain specialized axon regions, where it is altered to meet particular requirements. For example, internode distances are reduced (compared with those of most normal fibers) so as to

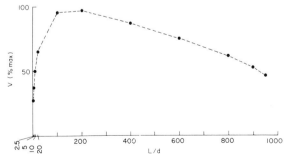

Figure 3–17. Relationship between conduction velocity (expressed as a percentage of the maximal conduction velocity V at any given diameter) and internode length (expressed as the ratio L/d between internode length and diameter). Note that conduction velocity is maximized when L/d falls between 100 and 200, as occurs in normal myelinated fibers. (Modified from Brill M.H., Waxman S.G., Moore J.W., et al. Conduction velocity and spike configuration in myelinated fibres: computed dependence on internode distance. *J. Neurol. Neurosurg. Psychiatry* 40:769–774, 1977.)

permit "delay line" operation in some electromotor systems that require a high degree of synchrony of neuronal discharge in cells separated by widely varying distances (Meszler et al., 1974; Waxman, 1972). In these systems, internode distances are matched to specific timing requirements. Reduction in internode distance is also observed proximal to regions where changes in fiber architecture might otherwise impose impedance mismatch, for example, near the bifurcation leading to the crus commune of dorsal root ganglion cells (Ito and Takahashi, 1960), in the preterminal axon just proximal to nonmyelinated terminals of peripheral (Zenker, 1964) and central (Waxman, 1972) axons, and close to receptor potential generation zones in sensory fibers (Quick et al., 1979). At these sites, reduction in internode distance results in an increase in the current density at sites of capacitive (and, to a lesser degree, resistive) loading and thus facilitates impulse invasion (Revenko et al., 1973). As noted earlier, the matching of internode distances to specific functional requirements requires local mechanisms for the control of myelin sheath characteristics. It is likely that the axon provides molecular cues that specify the length and thickness of the myelin sheaths that are produced by Schwann cells and oligodendrocytes (Waxman, 1987).

Structure-function relationships are not static but vary with external conditions and the history of prior impulse transmission along the fiber. Conduction velocity depends, for example, on temperature; the biophysical basis for this temperature dependence is discussed by Moore et al. (1978). Experimental data for mammalian axons suggest a Q_{10} of about 1.6 for conduction velocity in the temperature range 27–37°C (Paintal, 1978). A Q_{10} of 1.51 has been found both for motor and for sensory human PNS fibers (DeJesus et al., 1973). Similarly, there is a dependence of conduction velocity on temperature in mammalian CNS axons, which show an increase in conduction velocity of approximately 2.5%/°C (Swadlow et al., 1981). Together with the dependence of conduction properties on extracellular ionic concentrations (Malenka et al., 1981; Schauf and Davis, 1974) and on prior impulse activity (Swadlow and Waxman, 1976), this temperature dependence emphasizes that conduction velocity should not be viewed as an invariant characteristic of the axon but rather as a dynamic property. The safety factor, too, varies with external conditions and the history of impulse conduction in the fiber in question; these alterations in excitability can be significant with respect to invasion of axonal arbors in the neuropil (Chung et al., 1970; Swadlow et al., 1980).

Because the safety factor is normally high along the trunk of myelinated axons, conduction usually occurs with high reliability in white matter. After demyelination, however, the safety factor may fall so that activity-dependent changes in excitability will lead to significant alterations in conduction. In this regard, it is interesting that Kaji and Sumner (1989) demonstrated reversal in high-frequency conduction

block in demyelinated fibers after treatment with cardiac glycosides, as predicted from pump-mediated hyperpolarization, which has been observed in mammalian PNS (Bostock and Grafe, 1985) and CNS (Gordon et al., 1990) axons as a result of high-frequency activity.

The above-discussed considerations suggest that several strategies should be explored in attempting to develop symptomatic therapies to increase conduction in demyelinated fibers. These strategies include the development of pharmacologic agents that will predictably alter ion channel properties so as to increase the flow of net inward current and thereby improve the safety factor in demyelinated axons, and the development of pharmacologic agents that will permit the therapeutic alteration of pump-mediated changes in excitability. Also, as noted earlier, the safety factor is inversely related to temperature in demyelinated fibers. Therefore, the development of pharmacologic agents that lower core body temperature without causing clinically unacceptable side effects is also an attractive strategy in the search for symptomatic therapies for use in demyelinating disorders.

References

(Key references are designated with an asterisk.)

Aguayo A., Epps J., Charron L., et al. Multipotentiality of Schwann cells in cross-anastomosed and grafted myelinated and unmyelinated nerves: quantitative microscopy and radioautography. *Brain Res.* 104:1–20, 1976.

Aranella L.S., Herndon R.M. Mature oligodendrocytes: division following experimental demyelination in adult animals. *Arch. Neurol.* 41:1162–1165, 1984.

Baker M., Bostock H., Grafe P., et al. Function and distribution of three types of rectifying channel in rat spinal root myelinated axons. *J. Physiol. (Lond.)* 383:45–67, 1987.

Bement S., Ranck J.B. A quantitative study of electrical stimulation of central myelinated fibers. *Exp. Neurol.* 24:147–170, 1969.

Bevan S., Chiu S.Y., Gray P.T.A., et al. The presence of voltage-gated sodium, potassium and chloride channels in rat cultured astrocytes. *Proc. R. Soc. Lond. [Biol.]* 225:299–313, 1985.

Black J.A., Foster R.E., Waxman S.G. Freeze-fracture ultrastructure of rat CNS and PNS nonmyelinated axolemma. *J. Neurocytol.* 19:981–993, 1981.

Black J.A., Foster R.E., Waxman S.G. Rat optic nerve: freeze-fracture studies during development of myelinated axons. *Brain Res.* 250:1–10, 1982.

Black J.A., Waxman S.G., Hildebrand C. Membrane specialization and axo-glial association in the rat retinal nerve fiber layer: freeze-fracture observations. *J. Neurocytol.* 13:417–430, 1984.

Black J.A., Sims T.J., Waxman S.G., et al. Membrane ultrastructure of developing axons in glial deficient rat spinal cord. *J. Neurocytol.* 14:79–104, 1985.

Black J.A., Friedman B., Waxman S.G., et al. Immuno-ultrastructural localization of sodium channels at nodes of Ranvier and perinodal astrocytes in rat optic nerve. *Proc. R. Soc. Lond. [Biol.]* 238:39–51, 1989.

Black J.A., Friedman B., Elmer L.W., et al. Sodium channel immuno-localization in astrocytes and Schwann cells in vitro and in vivo. In Jeserich G., Althaus H.H., Waehneldt T.V., eds. *Cellular and Molecular Biology of Myelination.* New York Springer-Verlag, pp. 81–98, 1990a.

*Black J.A., Kocsis J.D., Waxman S.G. Ion channel organization of the myelinated fiber. *Trends Neurosci.* 13:42–54, 1990b.

Black J.A., Felts P., Smith K.J., et al. Distribution of sodium channels in chronically demyelinated axons: immuno-ultrastructural localization and electrophysiological observations. *Brain Res.* 544:59–70, 1991.

Blakemore W.F., Smith K.J. Node-like axonal specializations along demyelinated central nerve fibers: ultrastructural observations. *Acta Neuropathol. (Berl.)* 60:291–296, 1983.

Bostock H., Grafe P. Activity-dependent excitability changes in normal and demyelinated spinal root axons. *J. Physiol. (Lond.)* 365:239–257, 1985.

Bostock H., Sears T.A. Continuous conduction in demyelinated mammalian nerve fibers. *Nature* 263:786–787, 1976.

Bostock H., Sears T.A. The internodal axon membrane: electrical excitability and continuous conduction in segmental demyelination. *J. Physiol. (Lond.)* 280:273–301, 1978.

Bostock H., Sherratt M., Sears T.A. Overcoming conduction block in demyelinated fibres by prolonging action potentials. *Nature* 274:385–387, 1978.

Bostock H., Hall S.M., Smith K.J. Demyelinated axons can form "nodes" prior to remyelination. *J. Physiol. (Lond.)* 308:21P–23P, 1980.

Bostock H., Sears T.A., Sherratt R.M. The effects of 4-aminopyridine and tetraethylammonium ions on normal and demyelinated mammalian nerve fibers. *J. Physiol. (Lond.)* 313:301–315, 1981.

Bowe C.M., Kocsis J.D., Waxman S.G. Differences between mammalian ventral and dorsal spinal roots in response to blockade of potassium channels during maturation. *Proc. R. Soc. Lond. [Biol.]* 224:355–366, 1985.

Bray G.M., Cullen M.J., Aguayo A.J., et al. Node-like areas of intermembranous particles in the unensheathed axons of dystrophic mice. *Neurosci. Lett.* 13:203–207, 1979.

Brill M.H., Waxman S.G., Moore J.W., et al. Conduction velocity and spike configuration in myelinated fibers: computed dependence on internode distance. *J. Neurol. Neurosurg. Psychiatry* 40:769–774, 1977.

Brismar T. Potential clamp analysis of membrane currents in rat myelinated nerve fibers. *J. Physiol. (Lond.)* 298:171–184, 1980.

Brismar T. Specific permeability properties of demyelinated rat nerve fibers. *Acta Physiol. Scand.* 113:167–176, 1981.

Bunge M.B., Bunge R.P., Pappas G.D. Electron microscopic demonstration of connections between glia and myelin sheaths in the developing mammalian central nervous system. *J. Cell Biol.* 12:448–453, 1962.

Burchiel K.J. Abnormal impulse generation in focally demyelinated trigeminal roots. *J. Neurosurg.* 53:674–683, 1980.

Chiu S.Y. Asymmetry currents in the mammalian myelinated nerve. *J. Physiol. (Lond.)* 309:449–514, 1980.

Chiu S.Y., Ritchie J.M. Potassium channels in nodal and internodal axonal membrane in mammalian myelinated fibers. *Nature* 284:170–171, 1980.

Chiu S.Y., Ritchie J.M. Evidence for the presence of potassium channels in the internodal region of acutely demyelinated mammalian single nerve fibers. *J. Physiol. (Lond.)* 313:415–437, 1981.

Chiu S.Y., Ritchie J.M. On the physiological role of internodal potassium channels and the security of conduction in myelinated nerves. *Proc. R. Soc. Lond. [Biol.]* 220:415–422, 1984.

Chiu S.Y., Ritchie J.M., Rogart R.B., et al. A quantitative description of membrane currents in rabbit myelinate nerve. *J. Physiol. (Lond.)* 292:149–166, 1979.

Chung S.H., Raymond S.A., Lettvin J.Y. Multiple meaning in single visual units. *Brain Behav. Evol.* 3:72–101, 1970.

Coria F., Berciano M.T., Berciano J., et al. Axon membrane remodeling in lead-induced demyelinating neuropathy in the rat. *Brain Res.* 291:369–372, 1984.

Davis F.A., Jacobson S. Altered thermal sensitivity in injured and demyelinated nerve. *J. Neurol. Neurosurg. Psychiatry* 34:551–561, 1971.

Davis F.A., Schauf C.L. Approaches to the development of pharmacological interventions in multiple sclerosis. In Waxman S.G., Ritchie J.M., eds. *Demyelinating Diseases: Basic and Clinical Electrophysiology.* New York, Raven Press, pp. 505–510, 1981.

Davis F.A., Becker F.O., Michael J.A., et al. Effect of intravenous sodium bicarbonate, disodium edetate (Na_2EDTA), and hyperventilation on visual and oculomotor signs in multiple sclerosis. *J. Neurol. Neurosurg. Psychiatry* 33:723–732, 1977.

DeJesus P.V., Hausmanowa-Petrusewicz I., Barchi R.L. The effect

of cold on nerve conduction in human slow and fast nerve fibers. *Neurology (Minneap.)* 23:1182–1188, 1973.

Denny-Brown D., Brenner C. Paralysis of nerve induced by direct pressure and by tourniquet. *Arch. Neurol. Psychiatry* 51:1–26, 1944.

Dodge F.A. Jr., Cooley J.W. Action potential of the motoneuron. *IBM J. Res. Dev.* 17:219–229, 1973.

Elfvin L.-G. The ultrastructure of the nodes of Ranvier in cat sympathetic nerve fibers. *J. Ultrastruct. Res.* 5:374–387, 1961.

Ellisman M. Molecular specializations of the axon membrane at nodes of Ranvier are not dependent upon myelination. *J. Neurocytol.* 8:719–735, 1979.

Elmer L.W., Black J.A., Waxman S.G., et al. The voltage-dependent sodium channel in mammalian PNS and CNS: antibody characterization and immunocytochemical localization. *Brain Res.* 532:222–231, 1990.

Eng D.L., Gordon T.R., Kocsis J.D., et al. Current clamp analysis of time-dependent rectification in rat optic nerve axons. *J. Physiol. (Lond.)* 421:185–202, 1990.

Foster R.E., Whalen C.C., Waxman S.G. Reorganization of the axonal membrane of demyelinated nerve fibers: morphological evidence. *Science* 210:661–663, 1980.

Friede R.L., Samorajski T. Relation between the number of myelin lamellae and axon circumference in fibers of vagus and sciatic nerves of mice. *J. Comp. Neurol.* 130:223–232, 1967.

Funch P.G., Faber D.S. Action-potential propagation and orthodromic impulse initiation in the Mauthner axon. *J. Neurophysiol.* 47:1214–1231, 1982.

Funch P.G., Faber D.S. Measurement of myelin sheath resistances: implications for axonal conduction and pathophysiology. *Science* 225:538–540, 1984.

Geren B.B. The formation from the Schwann cell surface of myelin in peripheral nerves of chick embryos. *Exp. Cell Res.* 7:558–562, 1954.

Ghatak N.R., Hirano A., Listmaer M., et al. Asymptomatic demyelinated plaque in the spinal cord. *Arch. Neurol.* 30:484–486, 1974.

Gilliatt R.W., Willison R.G. Peripheral nerve conduction in diabetic neuropathy. *J. Neurol. Neurosurg. Psychiatry* 25:11–18, 1962.

Goldstein S.S., Rall W. Changes of action potential shape and velocity for changing core conductor geometry. *Biophys. J.* 14:731–757, 1974.

Gordon T.R., Kocsis J.D., Waxman S.G. Evidence for the presence of two types of potassium channels in rat optic nerve. *Brain Res.* 447:1–10, 1988.

Gordon T.R., Kocsis J.D., Waxman S.G. Pharmacological sensitivities of two afterhyperpolarizations in rat optic nerve. *Brain Res.* 502:252–258, 1989.

Gordon T.R., Kocsis J.D., Waxman S.G. Electrogenic pump activity in rat optic nerve. *Neuroscience* 37:829–837, 1990.

*Gray P.T.A., Ritchie J.M. Ion channels in Schwann and glial cells. *Trends Neurosci.* 8:411–415, 1985.

Guthrie T.C. Visual and motor changes in patients with multiple sclerosis. *Arch. Neurol. Psychiatry* 65:437–440, 1951.

*Halliday A.M., McDonald W.I. Pathophysiology of demyelinating disease. *Br. Med. Bull.* 33:21–27, 1977.

Hildebrand C. Ultrastructural and light-microscopic studies of the nodal region in large myelinated fibers of the adult feline spinal cord white matter. *Acta Physiol. Scand. Suppl.* 364:43–80, 1971a.

Hildebrand C. Ultrastructural and light-microscopic studies of the developing feline spinal cord white matter. I. The nodes of Ranvier. *Acta Physiol. Scand. Suppl.* 364:81–101, 1971b.

Hildebrand C., Waxman S.G. Regional node-like membrane specializations in non-myelinated axons of rat retinal nerve fiber layer. *Brain Res.* 258:23–32, 1983.

Hildebrand C., Waxman S.G. Postnatal differentiation of rat optic nerve fibers: electron microscopic observations on the development of nodes of Ranvier and axo-glial relations. *J. Comp. Neurol.* 224:25–38, 1984.

Hirano A., Becker M.H., Zimmerman H.M. Isolation of the periaxonal space of central myelinated fibers with regard to diffusion of peroxidase. *J. Histochem. Cytochem.* 17:512–516, 1969.

Hirano A., Dembitzer H.M. Morphology of normal central myelinated axons. In Waxman S.G., ed. *Physiology and Pathobiology of Axons.* New York, Raven Press, pp. 65–82, 1978.

*Hodgkin A.L. *The Conduction of the Nervous Impulse.* Springfield, IL, Thomas, 1964.

Hodgkin A.L. The optimum density of sodium channels in the unmyelinated nerve. *Philos. Trans. R. Soc. Lond. [Biol.]* 270:297–300, 1975.

Howe J.F., Loeser J.D., Calvin W.H. Mechanosensitivity of dorsal root ganglia and chronically injured axons: a physiological basis for the radicular pain of nerve root compression. *Pain* 3:25–41, 1977.

Hume A.L., Waxman S.G. Evoked potentials in suspected multiple sclerosis: diagnostic value and prediction of clinical course. *J. Neurol. Sci.* 83:191–210, 1988.

Huxley A.F., Stampfli R. Evidence for saltatory conduction in peripheral myelinated nerve fibres. *J. Physiol. (Lond.)* 108:315–339, 1949.

Ito M., Takahashi I. Impulse transmission through spinal ganglion. In Katsuki Y., ed. *Electrical Activity of Single Cells.* Tokyo, Igaku-Shoin Medical Publishers, pp. 159–179, 1960.

Kaji R., Sumner A.J. Effect of digitalis on central demyelinative conduction block in vivo. *Ann. Neurol.* 25:159–195, 1989.

Kocsis J.D., Waxman S.G. Absence of potassium conductance in central myelinated axons. *Nature* 287:348–349, 1980.

Kocsis J.D., Waxman S.G. Action potential electrogenesis in mammalian central axons. In Waxman S.G., Ritchie J.M., eds. *Demyelinating Diseases: Basic and Clinical Electrophysiology.* New York, Raven Press, pp. 299–312, 1981.

Kocsis J.D., Waxman S.G. Ion channel organization of normal and regenerating mammalian axons. *Prog. Brain Res.* 71:89–102, 1987.

Kocsis J.D., Malenka R.C., Waxman S.G. Enhanced parallel fiber frequency-following after reduction of postsynaptic activity. *Brain Res.* 207:321–331, 1981.

Kocsis J.D., Ruiz J.A., Cummins K. Modulation of axonal excitability mediated by surround electrical activity: an intra-axonal study. *Exp. Brain Res.* 47:151–153, 1982a.

Kocsis J.D., Waxman S.G., Hildebrand C., et al. Regenerating mammalian nerve fibres: changes in action potential waveform and firing characteristics following blockage of potassium conductance. *Proc. R. Soc. Lond. [Biol.]* 217:277–287, 1982b.

Kocsis J.D., Ruiz J.A., Waxman S.G. Maturation of mammalian myelinated fibers: changes in action potential characteristics following 4-aminopyridine application. *J. Neurophysiol.* 50:449–463, 1983.

Kocsis J.D., Preston R.J., Targ E.F. Retrograde impulse activity and horseradish peroxidase tracing of nerve fibers entering neuroma studied in vitro. *Exp. Neurol.* 85:400–412, 1984.

Kocsis J.D., Gordon T.R., Waxman S.G. Mammalian optic nerve fibers display two pharmacologically distinct potassium channels. *Brain Res.* 393:357–361, 1986.

Kocsis J.D., Eng D.L., Gordon T.R., et al. Functional differences between 4-aminopyridine and tetraethylammonium-sensitive potassium channels in myelinated axons. *Neurosci. Lett.* 75:193–198, 1987.

Koles Z.J., Rasminsky M. A computer simulation of conduction in demyelinated nerve fibres. *J. Physiol. (Lond.)* 227:351–364, 1972.

Kristol C., Sandri C., Akert K. Intramembranous particles at nodes of Ranvier of the cat spinal cord: a morphometric study. *Brain Res.* 142:391–400, 1978.

Landis D.M.D. Membrane structure in mammalian astrocytes. *J. Exp. Biol.* 95:35–48, 1981.

Landon D.N. Structure of normal peripheral myelinated nerve fibres. In Waxman S.G., Ritchie J.M., eds. *Demyelinating Diseases: Basic and Clinical Electrophysiology.* New York, Raven Press, pp. 25–49, 1981.

*Ludwin S.K. Remyelination in the central nervous system and the peripheral nervous system. In Waxman S.G., ed. *Functional Recovery in Neurological Disease.* New York, Raven Press, pp. 215–253, 1988.

McDonald W.I. The effects of experimental demyelination in conduction in peripheral nerve: a histological and electrophysiological study: II. Electrophysiological observations. *Brain* 86:501–524, 1963.

McDonald W.I. Pathophysiology of conduction in central nerve fibres. In Desmedt J.E., ed. *Visual Evoked Potentials in Man: New Developments.* Oxford, Clarendon Press, pp. 427–437, 1977.

McDonald W.I., Sears T.A. The effects of experimental demyelination on conduction in the central nervous system. *Brain* 93:583–598, 1970.

Mackay R.P., Hirano A. Forms of benign multiple sclerosis: report of two "clinically silent" cases discovered at autopsy. *Arch. Neurol.* 17:588–600, 1967.

Malenka R.C., Kocsis J.D., Ransom B.R., et al. Modulation of parallel fiber excitability by postsynaptically mediated changes in extracellular potassium. *Science* 214:339–341, 1981.

Meszler R.M., Pappas G.D., Bennett M.V.L. Morphology of the electromotor system in the spinal cord of the electric eel, *Electrophorus electricus.* *J. Neurocytol.* 3:251–261, 1974.

Moore J.W., Joyner R.W., Brill M.H., et al. Simulation of conduction in uniform myelinated fibers: relative sensitivity to changes in nodal and internodal parameters. *Biophys. J.* 21:147–160, 1978.

*Morrell P., ed. *Myelin.* 2nd ed. New York, Plenum Publishing, 1984.

Namerow N.S. Circadian temperature rhythm and vision in multiple sclerosis. *Neurology* 18:417–422, 1968.

Neumcke B., Stampfli R. Sodium currents and sodium-current fluctuations in rat myelinated nerve fibers. *J. Physiol. (Lond.)* 329:163–184, 1982.

Newman E.A. Regional specialization of retinal glial cell membrane. *Nature* 309:155–157, 1984.

Paintal A.S. Conduction properties of normal peripheral mammalian axons. In Waxman S.G., ed. *Physiology and Pathobiology of Axons.* New York, Raven Press, pp. 131–144, 1978.

Peters A. The structure of myelin sheaths in the central nervous system of *Xenopus laevis* (Daudin). *J. Biophys. Biochem. Cytol.* 7:121–126, 1960.

Peters A., Proskauer C.C. The ratio between myelin segments and oligodendrocytes in the optic nerve of the adult rat. *Anat. Rec.* 163:243, 1969.

Preston R.J., Waxman S.G., Kocsis J.D. Effects of 4-aminopyridine on rapidly- and slowly-conducting fibers of rat corpus callosum. *Exp. Neurol.* 79:808–820, 1983.

Prineas J.W., Connell F. The fine structure of chronically active multiple sclerosis plaques. *Neurology* 28(Part 2):68–75, 1978.

Prineas J., Connell F. Remyelination in multiple sclerosis. *Ann. Neurol.* 5:22–31, 1979.

Quick D.C., Waxman S.G. Specific staining of the axon membrane at nodes of Ranvier with ferric ion and ferrocyanide. *J. Neurol. Sci.* 31:1–11, 1977.

Quick D.C., Kennedy W.R., Donaldson L. Dimensions of myelinated nerve fibers near the motor and sensory terminals in cat tenuissimus muscles. *Neuroscience* 4:1089–1096, 1979.

Raine C.S. On the association between perinodal astrocytic processes and the nodes of Ranvier in the CNS. *J. Neurocytol.* 13:21–27, 1984.

Ramon F., Joyner R.W., Moore J.W. Propagation of action potentials in inhomogeneous axon regions. *Fed. Proc.* 38:1357–1363, 1975.

Rasminsky M. The effects of temperature on conduction in demyelinated single nerve fibers. *Arch. Neurol.* 28:287–292, 1973.

Rasminsky M. Physiology of conduction in demyelinated axons. In Waxman S.G., ed. *Physiology and Pathobiology of Axons.* New York, Raven Press, pp. 361–376, 1978.

Rasminsky M. Ephaptic transmission between single nerve fibers in spinal nerve roots of dystrophic mice. *J. Physiol. (Lond.)* 305:151–169, 1980.

Rasminsky M., Sears T.A. Internodal conduction in undissected demyelinated nerve fibers. *J. Physiol. (Lond.)* 227:323–350, 1972.

Revenko S.-V., Timin Y.N., Khodorov B.I. Special features of the conduction of nerve impulses from the myelinized part of the axon into the nonmyelinated terminal. *Biophysics* 18:1140–1145, 1973.

*Ritchie J.M., Chiu S.Y. Distribution of sodium and potassium channels in mammalian myelinated nerve. In Waxman S.G., Ritchie J.M., eds. *Demyelinating Diseases: Basic and Clinical Electrophysiology.* New York, Raven Press, pp. 329–342, 1981.

Ritchie J.M., Rogart R.B. The density of sodium channels in mammalian myelinated nerve fibers and the nature of the axonal membrane under the myelin sheath. *Proc. Natl. Acad. Sci. U.S.A.* 74:211–215, 1977.

Ritchie J.M., Rogart R.B., Strichartz G. A new method for labelling saxitoxin and its binding to nonmyelinated fibres of the rabbit vagus, lobster walking leg, and garfish olfactory nerve. *J. Physiol. (Lond.)* 261:477–494, 1976.

Ritchie J.M., Rang H.P., Pellegrino R. Sodium and potassium channels in demyelinated and remyelinated mammalian nerve. *Nature* 294:257–259, 1981.

Ritchie J.M., Black J.A., Waxman S.G., et al. Sodium channels in the cytoplasm of Schwann cells. *Proc. Natl. Acad. Sci. U.S.A.* 87:9290–9294, 1990.

Robertson J.D. The ultrastructure of adult vertebrate peripheral myelinated fibers in relation to myelinogenesis. *J. Biophys. Cytol.* 1:271–278, 1955.

Robertson J.D. Preliminary observations on the node of Ranvier. *Z. Zellforsch.* 50:553–560, 1959.

Rosenbluth J. Intramembranous particle distribution at the node of Ranvier and adjacent axolemma in myelinated axons of the frog brain. *J. Neurocytol.* 5:731–745, 1976.

Rosenbluth J. Aberrant axon-Schwann cell junctions in dystrophic mouse nerves. *J. Neurocytol.* 8:655–672, 1979.

Rosenbluth J. Freeze-fracture approaches to ionophore localization in normal and myelin-deficient nerves. In Waxman S.G., Ritchie J.M., eds. *Demyelinating Diseases: Basic and Clinical Electrophysiology.* New York, Raven Press, pp. 391–418, 1981.

Rushton W.A.H. A theory of the effects of fibre size in medullated nerve. *J. Physiol. (Lond.)* 115:102–122, 1951.

Rydmark M., Berthold C. Electron microscopic serial section analysis of nodes of Ranvier in lumbar spinal roots of the cat. *J. Neurocytol.* 12:537–565, 1983.

Schauf C.L., Davis F.A. Impulse conduction in multiple sclerosis: a theoretical basis for modification by temperature and pharmacological agents. *J. Neurol. Neurosurg. Psychiatry* 37:152–161, 1974.

Schnapp B., Mugnaini E. Membrane architecture of myelinated fibers as seen by freeze-fracture. In Waxman S.G., ed. *Physiology and Pathobiology of Axons.* New York, Raven Press, pp. 83–123, 1978.

*Sears T.A., Bostock H. Conduction failure in demyelination: is it inevitable? In Waxman S.G., Ritchie J.M., eds. *Demyelinating Diseases: Basic and Clinical Electrophysiology.* New York, Raven Press, pp. 357–375, 1981.

Sears T.A., Bostock H., Sheratt M. The pathophysiology of demyelination and its implications for the symptomatic treatment of multiple sclerosis. *Neurology* 28(Part 2):21–26, 1978.

Sherratt R.M., Bostock H., Sears T.A. Effects of 4-aminopyridine on normal and demyelinated mammalian nerve fibers. *Nature* 283:570–572, 1980.

Sims T.J., Waxman S.G., Black J.A., Gilmore S.A. Perinodal astrocytic processes at nodes of Ranvier in developing normal and glial cell deficient rat spinal cord. *Brain Res.* 337:321–333, 1985.

Smith R.S., Koles Z.J. Myelinated nerve fibers: computed effect of myelin thickness on conduction velocity. *Am. J. Physiol.* 219:1256–1258, 1970.

Smith K.J., McDonald W.I. Spontaneous and mechanically evoked activity due to a central demyelinating lesion. *Nature* 286:154–155, 1980.

Smith K.J., Blakemore W.F., McDonald W.I. Central remyelination restores secure conduction. *Nature* 280:395–396, 1979.

Smith K.J., Bostock H., Hall S.M. Saltatory conduction precedes remyelination in axons demyelinated with lysophosphatidyl choline. *J. Neurol. Sci.* 54:13–31, 1982.

Smith M.E., Kocsis J.D., Waxman S.G. Myelin protein metabolism in demyelination and myelination in the sciatic nerve. *Brain Res.* 270:37–44, 1984.

Southeimer H., Ransom B.R., Cornell-Bell A., et al. Na⁺ current expression in rat hippocampal astrocytes in vitro: alterations during development. *J. Neurophysiol.* 65:3–19, 1990.

Southeimer H., Minturn J.F., Black J.A., et al.: Two types of Na⁺ currents in cultured rat optic nerve astrocytes. *J. Neurosci. Res.* (in press).

Spencer P.S., Weinberg H.J. Axonal specification of Schwann cell expression and myelination. In Waxman S.G., ed. *Physiology and Pathobiology of Axons.* New York, Raven Press, pp. 389–404, 1978.

Stys P.K., Waxman S.G., Ransom B.R. Na⁺-Ca²⁺ exchanger mediates Ca²⁺ influx during anoxia in mammalian CNS white matter. *Ann. Neurol.* (in press).

Swadlow H.A., Waxman S.G. Variations in conduction velocity and excitability following single and multiple impulses of visual callosal axons in the rabbit. *Exp. Neurol.* 53:128–150, 1976.

Swadlow H.A., Kocsis J.D., Waxman S.G. Modulation of impulse conduction along the axonal tree. *Annu. Rev. Biophys. Biomed. Eng.* 9:143–179, 1980.

Swadlow H.A., Waxman S.G., Weyand T.G. Effects of variations in temperature on impulse conduction along nonmyelinated axons in the mammalian brain. *Exp. Neurol.* 71:383–389, 1981.

Targ E.F., Kocsis J.D. 4-Aminopyridine leads to restoration of conduction in demyelinated rat sciatic nerve. *Brain Res.* 328:358–361, 1985.

Tao-Cheng J.H., Rosenbluth R. Development of nodal and paranodal membrane specializations in amphibian peripheral nerves. *Dev. Brain Res.* 3:577–594, 1982.

Tasaki I. *Nervous Transmission.* Springfield, IL, Thomas, 1953.

Tasaki I., Takeuchi T. Weitere Studien ueber den Aktions-strom der markhaltigen Nervenfaser und ueber die elektrosaltatorische Uebertragung des Nervenimpulses. *Pfluegers Arch. Gesamte Physiol. Menschen Tiere* 245:764–782, 1942.

Wall P.D., Waxman S.G., Basbaum A.I. Ongoing activity in peripheral nerve: injury discharge. *Exp. Neurol.* 45:576–589, 1974.

Waxman S.G. Regional differentiation of the axon: a review with special reference to the concept of the multiplex neuron. *Brain Res.* 47:269–288, 1972.

Waxman S.G. Integrative properties and design principles of axons. *Int. Rev. Neurobiol.* 18:1–40, 1975.

Waxman S.G. Conduction in myelinated, unmyelinated, and demyelinated fibers. *Arch. Neurol.* 34:585–590, 1977.

Waxman S.G., ed. *Physiology and Pathobiology of Axons.* New York, Raven Press, 1978.

Waxman S.G. The flexion-adduction sign in neuralgic amyotrophy. *Neurology* 29:1301–1304, 1979.

Waxman S.G. Membranes, myelin, and the pathophysiology of multiple sclerosis. *N. Engl. J. Med.* 306:1529–1533, 1982.

Waxman S.G. Rules governing membrane reorganization and axoglial interactions during the development of myelinated fibers. *Prog. Brain Res.* 71:121–142, 1987.

*Waxman S.G. Biophysical mechanisms of impulse conduction in demyelinated axons. In Waxman S.G., ed. *Functional Recovery in Neurological Disease.* New York, Raven Press, pp. 185–214, 1988a.

*Waxman S.G. Clinical course and electrophysiology of multiple sclerosis. In Waxman S.G., ed. *Functional Recovery in Neurological Disease.* New York, Raven Press, pp. 175–184, 1988b.

Waxman S.G., Bennett M.V.L. Relative conduction velocities of small myelinated and non-myelinated fibres in the central nervous system. *Nature (New Biol.)* 238:217–219, 1972.

Waxman S.G., Black J.A. Freeze-fracture structure of the perinodal astrocyte and associated glial junctions. *Brain Res.* 308:77–87, 1984.

Waxman S.G., Black J.A. Unmyelinated and myelinated axon membrane from rat corpus callosum: differences in macromolecular structure. *Brain Res.* 453:337–343, 1988.

Waxman S.G., Brill M.H. Conduction through demyelinated plaques in multiple sclerosis: computer simulations of facilitation by short internodes. *J. Neurol. Neurosurg. Psychiatry* 41:408–417, 1978.

Waxman S.G., Foster R.E. Ionic channel distribution and heterogeneity of the axon membrane in myelinated fibers. *Brain Res. Rev.* 2:205–240, 1980a.

Waxman S.G., Foster R.E. Development of the axon membrane during differentiation of myelinated fibers in spinal nerve roots. *Proc. R. Soc. Lond. [Biol.]* 209:441–446, 1980b.

Waxman S.G., Quick D.C. Intra-axonal ferric ion-ferrocyanide staining of nodes of Ranvier and initial segments in central myelinated fibers. *Brain Res.* 144:1–10, 1978.

*Waxman S.G., Ritchie J.M., eds. *Demyelinating Diseases: Basic and Clinical Electrophysiology.* New York, Raven Press, 1981.

Waxman S.G., Sims T.J. Specificity in central myelination: evidence for local regulation of myelin thickness. *Brain Res.* 292:179–185, 1984.

Waxman S.G., Wood S.L. Impulse conduction in inhomogeneous axons: effects of variation in voltage-sensitive ionic conductances on invasion of demyelinated axon segments and preterminal fibers. *Brain Res.* 294:111–123, 1984.

Waxman S.G., Kocsis J.D., Eng D.L. Ligature-induced injury in peripheral nerve: electrophysiological observations on changes in action potential characteristics following blockade of potassium conductance. *Muscle Nerve* 8:85–92, 1985.

Waxman S.G., Sims T.J. Gilmore S.A. Cytoplasmic membrane elaborations in oliodendrocytes during myelination of spinal motoneuron axons. *Glia* 1:286–292, 1988.

Waxman S.G., Black J.A., Kocsis J.D., et al. Low density of sodium channels supports action potential conduction in axons of neonatal optic nerve. *Proc. Natl. Acad. Sci. U.S.A.* 86:1406–1410, 1989.

Weinberg H.J., Spencer P.S. Studies on the control of myelinogenesis. II. Evidence for neuronal regulation of myelin production. *Brain Res.* 113:363–378, 1976.

Weiner L.P., Waxman S.G., Stohlman S.A., et al. Remyelination following virus-induced demyelination: ferric ion-ferrocyanide staining of nodes of Ranvier within the CNS. *Ann. Neurol.* 8:580–583, 1980.

Westerfield M., Joyner R.W., Moore J.W. Temperature-sensitive conduction failure at axonal branch points. *J. Neurophysiol.* 41:1–8, 1978.

Wiley-Livingston C.A., Ellisman M.H. Development of axonal membrane specializations defines nodes of Ranvier and precedes Schwann cell myelination. *Dev. Biol.* 79:334–355, 1980.

Wiley C.A., Ellisman M.H. Rows of dimeric particles within the axolemma and juxtaposed particles within glia, incorporated into a new model for the paranodal axo-glial junction. *J. Cell Biol.* 84:261–280, 1980.

Wisniewski H.M., Oppenheimer D., McDonald W.I. Relation between myelination and function in EAE and MS. *J. Neuropathol. Exp. Neurol.* 35:327, 1976.

Yasargil G.M., Diamond J. Startle-response in teleost fish: elementary circuit for neural discrimination. *Nature* 230:241–243, 1968.

*Zagoren J.D., Federoff S., eds. *The Node of Ranvier.* New York, Academic Press, 1984.

Zenker W. Internodienlängen und Faserkaliber der terminalen Verlaufsstrecke motorische Fasern der äusseren Augenmuskeln und des M. thyreoarytaenoideus des Rhesusaffen. *Z. Zellforsch.* 62:531–545, 1964.

4

Neurotransmitters

Solomon H. Snyder

With few exceptions communication among the billions of neurons in the brain occurs at synapses via specific neurotransmitters. Thus, neurotransmitters are fundamental to all central nervous system information processing. Essentially all drugs used in neurology and psychiatry act via one or another neurotransmitter system. Accordingly, it is not surprising that the virtual explosion of molecular neuroscience beginning in the 1970s has resulted in large part from advances in our understanding of neurotransmitters.

One of the most striking features of neurotransmitters lies in their diversity. Until the mid 1960s the only known neurotransmitters were the handful of biogenic amines. In the late 1960s the role of amino acids, such as γ-aminobutyric acid (GABA), glycine, and glutamate, as neurotransmitters became apparent. The decade of the 1970s witnessed the appreciation of peptides as neurotransmitters, sparked in large part by the widespread attention devoted to the enkephalins as the endogenous ligands for opiate receptors. Peptides represent the most diverse group of transmitters, with between 50 and 100 discrete peptides currently implicated in neurotransmission. However, in terms of the numbers of synapses involved, peptides have a low abundance; no known peptide accounts for more than 1% of synapses in the brain. By contrast, amino acids are the most abundant neurotransmitters. GABA, the major inhibitory neurotransmitter, accounts for 25–40% of synapses, depending on the brain region under consideration. Biogenic amines account for relatively small proportions of synapses, usually between 1 and 3% in a given brain region. However, in the caudate nucleus, dopamine terminals are 10% or more of all synapses.

ACETYLCHOLINE

Acetylcholine is the first of the major neurotransmitters to have been definitively identified. This identification dates to the 1920s and the classic studies of Otto Loewi. Despite its acceptance for many years as the neurotransmitter of parasympathetic nerves, only in the 1960s did it become clear that acetylcholine is a neurotransmitter in specific neuronal pathways in the brain (Kuhar, 1978). Histochemical localization of cholinesterase demonstrated a major cholinergic pathway with cell bodies in the basal nucleus of Meynert and axons ascending to terminate in various areas of the cerebral cortex. A closely related pathway was also observed with cell bodies in the lateral septum and axons proceeding via the fimbria to terminate in the hippocampus. Subsequent studies localizing the acetylcholine-synthesizing enzyme choline acetyltransferase have confirmed the cholinergic nature of these systems (Kasa, 1986; Rossier, 1979). Both of them appear to degenerate in Alzheimer's disease, findings that have prompted numerous attempts to treat Alzheimer's disease by "correcting" the acetylcholine deficiency (Collerton, 1986) (Table 4–1). A review of acetylcholine metabolism and receptor action provides insights into possible therapeutic strategies.

Biosynthesis

Acetylcholine is formed by the action of choline acetyltransferase, which links choline to acetyl coenzyme A. Choline acetyltransferase occurs in the cytoplasm of nerve terminals, so that the acetylcholine formed must be accumulated in synaptic vesicles by an ATP-dependent uptake and binding process.

Often a biosynthetic enzyme represents the major regulatory step in the formation of a neurotransmitter. This is not the case for acetylcholine. Variations

Supported by U.S. Public Health Service grants MH-18501 and DA-00266 and Research Scientist Award DA-00074.

Table 4–1. CENTRAL NERVOUS SYSTEM DRUG ACTIONS AND DISEASES INVOLVING NEUROTRANSMITTERS

Drug Action or Disease	Molecular Mechanism
Acetylcholine	
Alzheimer's disease	Degeneration of cholinergic neuronal input to the hippocampus and the cerebral cortex
Myasthenia gravis	Acetylcholine potentiated by acetylcholinesterase inhibitors, which compensates for autoimmune loss of skeletal muscle receptors
Norepinephrine and Serotonin	
Tricyclic antidepressants	Inhibit reuptake mechanism, which potentiates synaptic activity
Monoamine oxidase inhibitors	Elevate intraterminal levels of amine, which spill out into synapse
Dopamine	
Neuroleptics	Block D_2 receptors to relieve schizophrenic symptoms
L-Dihydroxyphenylalanine	Converted by dopa decarboxylase to dopamine to relieve dopamine deficiency in Parkinson's disease
Central nervous system–selective agonists (e.g., bromocriptine, pergolide)	Directly stimulate dopamine D_2 receptors to relieve parkinsonian symptoms
GABA	
Benzodiazepines, barbiturates	Facilitate synaptic effects of GABA by acting at sites allosteric to the GABA recognition site on $GABA_A$ receptors

in choline acetyltransferase activity are not the major determinant of acetylcholine formation. Instead, the accumulation of choline in cholinergic nerve terminals is the principal regulatory event (Jope, 1979). Uptake systems occur for choline in all cells of the body, because choline is required for the formation of membrane phospholipids. In addition to possessing the low-affinity general choline uptake mechanism, cholinergic neurons have a high-affinity uptake system for choline that has an absolute requirement for sodium and energy. The velocity of this choline uptake system varies in close conjunction with increases or decreases in the rate of firing of cholinergic neurons (Kuhar, 1978). Inhibitors of the choline uptake system block acetylcholine formation.

Catabolism

Acetylcholine is degraded by acetylcholinesterase, which hydrolyzes the transmitter to choline and acetate (Massoulie and Bon, 1982). The acetate enters general metabolic pathways, and choline is recycled as a precursor for new transmitter synthesis. Acetylcholinesterase acts rapidly and accounts for the inactivation of synaptically released acetylcholine. At the neuromuscular junction, acetylcholinesterase is highly concentrated in the postsynaptic membrane near the acetylcholine receptors. In the brain, besides postsynaptic localizations, acetylcholinesterase occurs throughout the membrane of cholinergic neurons for which it can serve as a marker, although cholinesterase activity occurs also in noncholinergic neurons and in non-neuronal cells.

Cholinergic synaptic activity is potentiated by cholinesterase-inhibiting drugs. Clinically these are effective in the therapy of myasthenia gravis (see Table 4–1). Organophosphate cholinesterase inhibitors have been used both as insecticides and in chemical warfare.

Receptors

The two major subdivisions of cholinergic receptors are nicotinic and muscarinic. The nicotinic receptor of skeletal muscle involves a protein different from that of nicotinic receptors of ganglia and the brain (Changeux et al., 1984). Drug specificity differs so that the snake toxin α-bungarotoxin, a potent agent in skeletal muscle, does not influence nicotinic receptors of ganglia and the brain.

Muscarinic sites represent the major acetylcholine receptors in the brain and the autonomic nervous system. Recent molecular cloning has distinguished at least four and possibly five distinct muscarinic receptor subtypes (Bonner et al., 1988; Dohlman et al., 1989; Peralta et al., 1987). These subtypes differ in their localization throughout the brain, in the second messengers with which they interact, and in their drug specificity. Some of these receptor subtypes act by stimulating phosphoinositide turnover; others act by inhibiting adenylate cyclase (Nathanson, 1987). Differences in drug specificity of these receptors can have therapeutic importance, particularly in the parasympathetic nervous system. For instance, muscarinic receptors mediate cholinergic slowing of the heart and enhanced gastric acid formation. Nonspecific muscarinic antagonists, such as atropine and related agents, have been used to treat the hyperacidity of peptic ulcers, but they accelerate the heart rate. Drugs such as pirenzepine, which are selective for the M_1 receptor of the stomach but not the M_2 receptor of the heart, can decrease gastric acid secretion without affecting cardiac activity (Hammer et al., 1980). Receptor subtype–selective agents in the brain may similarly exhibit therapeutic selectivity. Developing such selective cholinergic agonists is a particular goal for treatment of Alzheimer's disease.

CATECHOLAMINES

Norepinephrine is the major neurotransmitter of sympathetic neurons, whereas both norepinephrine and epinephrine are secreted from the adrenal medulla. Dopamine is the metabolic precursor of norepinephrine. However, in certain brain regions dopamine occurs in specific neuronal systems in the

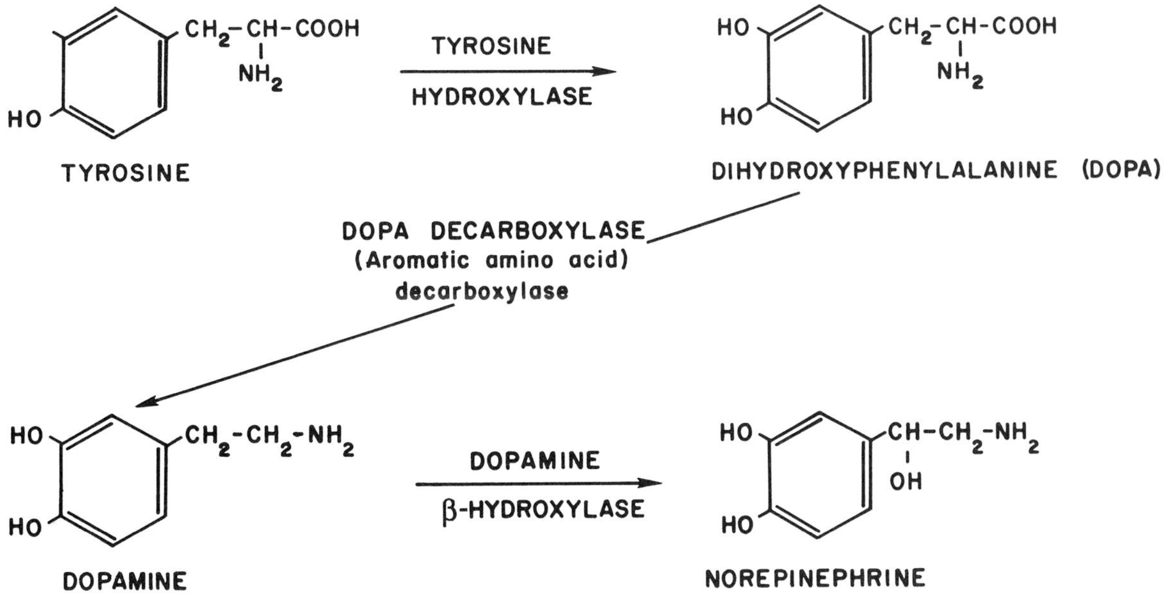

Figure 4–1. Pathway of catecholamine biosynthesis.

absence of norepinephrine and thus is itself a transmitter.

The development of histochemical techniques based on fluorescent derivatives of the catecholamines permitted the localization of catecholamine neuronal pathways in the early 1960s, a major step forward in our understanding of these neurotransmitters (Lindvall and Bjorklund, 1978; Moore and Bloom, 1979). The catecholamines were the first neurotransmitters whose localizations were mapped throughout the brain. The localization of neurotransmitters has proved to be one of the most powerful tools in understanding their function.

The major dopamine pathway in the brain has cell bodies in the substantia nigra with axons ascending in the medial forebrain bundle to terminate in the caudate nucleus and putamen, a localization that implies a role in extrapyramidal motor function. Lesions of this nigrostriatal pathway produce motor abnormalities in animals, and idiopathic Parkinson's disease in humans is associated with a degeneration of the nigrostriatal pathway.

A role of dopamine in emotional function is implied by the disposition of the mesolimbic pathway (Hokfelt et al., 1984). Cell bodies occur in the ventral tegmental nuclei of the brain stem, with terminals in the nucleus accumbens, central nucleus of the amygdala, and phylogenetically older parts of the cerebral cortex associated with the limbic system. It is thought that the therapeutic antischizophrenic actions of neuroleptic drugs derive from blockade of dopamine D_2 receptors in this part of the brain, whereas receptor blockade in the caudate nucleus and putamen gives rise to parkinsonian extrapyramidal side effects (Snyder, 1984).

A neuroendocrine role is associated with the dopamine pathway whose cell bodies are in the arcuate nucleus of the hypothalamus with terminals in the median eminence in association with the portal capillary system to the pituitary. Dopamine released into these capillaries acts at receptors in the pituitary to inhibit the release of prolactin. Thus, neuroleptic drugs increase plasma levels of prolactin and thereby cause amenorrhea.

The great majority of norepinephrine-containing neurons in the brain have their cell bodies in the small locus ceruleus in the midbrain with axons ascending or descending to innervate almost all parts of the central nervous system. The exact functions of norepinephrine pathways are not well established, but they seem to involve emotional behavior. Stimuli that accelerate the firing of neurons in the locus ceruleus are associated with anxiety.

Biosynthesis

The dietary precursor of the catecholamines is the amino acid tyrosine. Tyrosine is hydroxylated to L-dihydroxyphenylalanine (dopa) by the enzyme tyrosine hydroxylase, which requires molecular oxygen and a pteridine cofactor tetrahydrobiopterin (Fig. 4–1). Because the K_m for tyrosine hydroxylase is in the micromolar range, the enzyme is saturated by physiologic levels of tyrosine. Thus, one cannot alter tissue levels of catecholamines even with relatively high doses of tyrosine (Molinoff and Axelrod, 1971).

Dopa is decarboxylated by dopa decarboxylase (aromatic-L-amino-acid decarboxylase), a pyridoxal phosphate–requiring enzyme. The enzyme protein is identical with the serotonin-forming enzyme 5-hydroxytryptophan decarboxylase, which has a broad substrate specificity and so is also formally designated aromatic-L-amino-acid decarboxylase.

Dopa decarboxylase has a relatively high K_m and V_{max}. Physiologic levels of dopa are extremely low, so that exogenous dopa is rapidly converted to dopamine, which accounts for the efficacy of levodopa as a therapeutic agent in Parkinson's disease.

Dopamine β-hydroxylase, like tyrosine hydroxylase, is a mixed function oxidase that uses molecular oxygen. Ascorbic acid provides the source of electrons, and copper is involved in the electron transfer reaction. Thus, copper chelators, such as disulfiram, which are used in the treatment of alcoholism, inhibit this enzyme and can prevent the formation of norepinephrine. Dopamine β-hydroxylase is partially particulate, associated with the membranes of norepinephrine storage vesicles, and some of it is contained in the cytoplasm of the vesicles and is released on exocytotic liberation of norepinephrine (Weinshilboum et al., 1971).

In the adrenal medulla, phenylethanolamine *N*-methyltransferase transfers the methyl group of *S*-adenosylmethionine to the nitrogen of norepinephrine to form epinephrine. Epinephrine occurs in low concentrations in the brain in association with a discrete system of epinephrine-containing neurons in the brain stem, which play a role in blood pressure regulation.

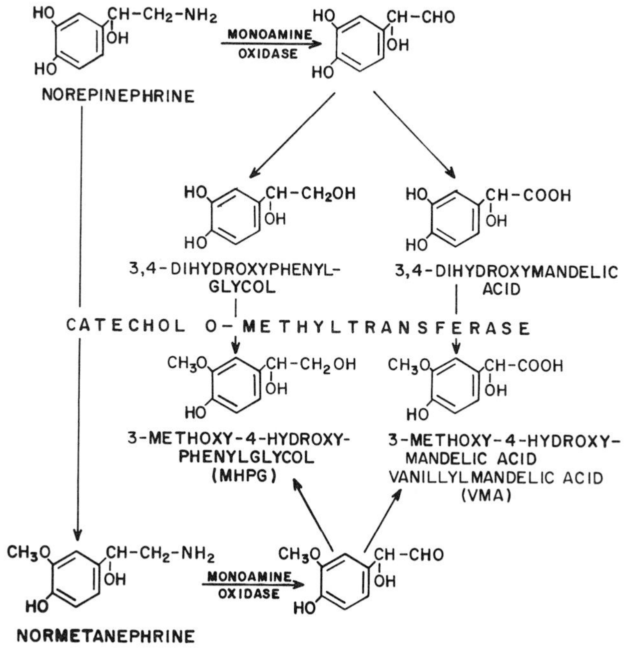

Storage

Catecholamines are stored in vesicles together with ATP and acidic proteins, which in the adrenal are referred to as chromogranins (Stjarne, 1975). This storage process can be disrupted by reserpine, which depletes catecholamines and serotonin by inhibiting the pump-like mechanism that concentrates the amines within the vesicles. When reserpine releases catecholamines or serotonin from the vesicles, the amines are degraded by monoamine oxidase (MAO) in nearby mitochondria so that only metabolites escape the neuron and the pharmacologic effects of reserpine are equivalent to those of amine depletion rather than synaptic release of amines. Accordingly, the behavioral depression in humans that is associated with reserpine treatment is presumably due to a deficiency of the biogenic amines, whose levels are reduced by such treatment to virtually negligible values.

Metabolism

Catecholamines are degraded primarily by two enzymes, MAO and catechol *O*-methyltransferase (COMT) (Fig. 4–2). MAO occurs in the outer membrane of mitochondria in cells throughout the body (Costa and Sandler, 1972). Because nerve terminals possess extremely high densities of mitochondria, MAO, which acts on catecholamines and serotonin, is localized within amine-storing nerve terminals. MAO rarely if ever acts on synaptically released

Figure 4–2. Catecholamine catabolism.

amine transmitters. COMT occurs in the cytoplasm of neural and non-neural tissues and primarily acts on extracellular catecholamines.

The names of these enzymes indicate their substrate specificity. MAO can act on any monoamine including serotonin and histamine. COMT can act on any catechol, including acid metabolites of the catecholamines. The substrate preferences of these enzymes account for the complex pattern of metabolic degradation of catecholamines, which can proceed via initial actions of either MAO or COMT followed by the action of the other enzyme. MAO converts the amines into their corresponding aldehydes, which can then be either reduced to the corresponding alcoholic glycol or oxidized to an acid. In the brain the reductive pathway predominates, whereas in the periphery oxidation plays the major role. Accordingly, in the brain the major final product of catecholamine metabolism is 3-methoxy-4-hydroxyphenylglycol, whereas in the periphery the final product is 3-methoxy-4-hydroxymandelic acid, also referred to as vanillylmandelic acid. Because of these differences in central and peripheral metabolism of catecholamines, much research has dealt with the possibility that urinary levels of 3-methoxy-4-hydroxyphenylglycol reflect the brain disposition of catecholamines. However, it now appears that more than half of 3-methoxy-4-hydroxyphenylglycol in the urine derives from the metabolism of catecholamines coming from sympathetic nerves or the adrenal. Inhibitors of MAO cause a build-up of amines in nerve terminal cytoplasm, and substantial amounts then leak out into the synaptic cleft. Administration of MAO inhibitors increases brain levels of biogenic amines. MAO inhibitors were the first widely used antidepressant drugs and provided a basis for theo-

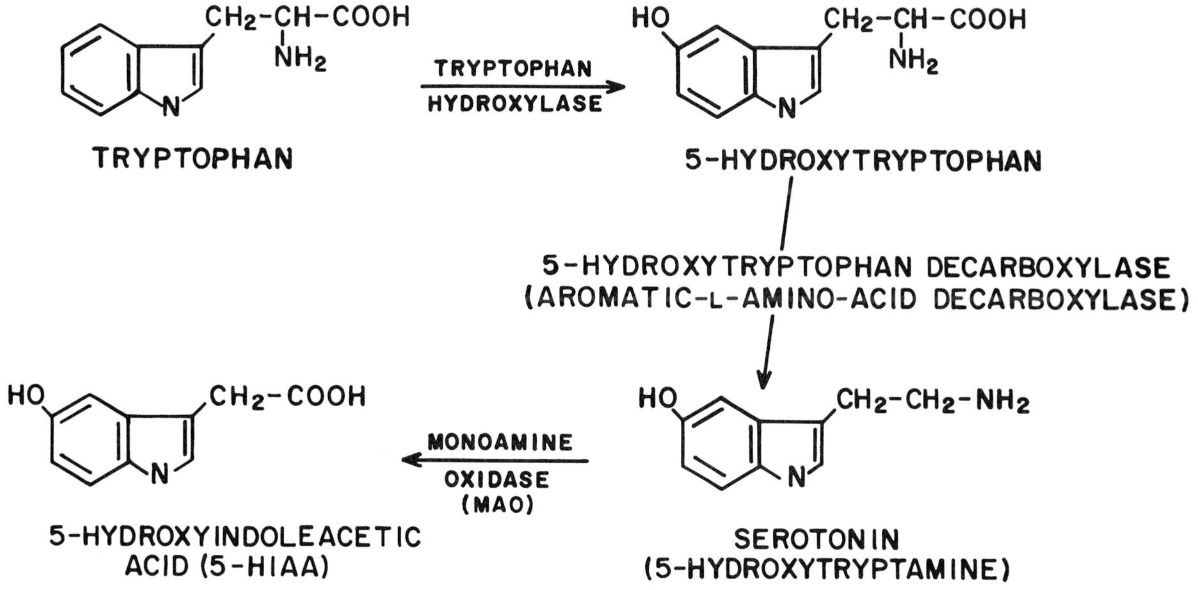

Figure 4–3. Serotonin metabolism.

ries linking biogenic amines and mood regulation (see Table 4–1).

Reuptake

Neither MAO nor COMT accounts for synaptic inactivation of catecholamines. Thus, synaptic activity of sympathetic nerves is not potentiated by inhibitors of MAO or COMT. Instead, a reuptake pump plays the major role.

The reuptake inactivation of catecholamines was discovered and characterized by Julius Axelrod in the late 1950s and early 1960s, when he showed that peripherally administered radiolabeled catecholamines were highly concentrated into sympathetically innervated organs in the nerve terminals (Axelrod, 1971). Drugs that blocked this uptake process potentiated the effects of sympathetic nerve stimulation. This reuptake system has now been well characterized in isolated nerve terminal preparations, and the uptake recognition site, or uptake receptor, has been molecularly characterized by the binding of radiolabeled forms of potent uptake-inhibiting drugs (Javitch et al., 1985; Snyder, 1986a,b). The uptake recognition sites for dopamine and norepinephrine differ so that drugs can be designed to selectively inhibit the uptake of one or the other catecholamine. However, the general features of the uptake systems are quite similar, requiring energy and having an absolute requirement for sodium, thus resembling the choline "precursor" uptake system. Uptake systems now appear to represent the major mode for neurotransmitter inactivation and account for the inactivation of serotonin as well as the amino acid transmitters, but not for neuropeptides.

SEROTONIN

Serotonin-containing neurons have their cell bodies in a group of midline nuclei located in the medulla oblongata and midbrain, referred to as the raphe nuclei. From the raphe magnus serotonin cells in the medulla, axons descend to the spinal cord. The dorsal and median raphe nuclei in the midbrain project axons that ascend through the medial forebrain bundle to terminate predominantly in the hypothalamus and limbic system but also in numerous areas of the brain, including most of the cerebral cortex. Because of their discrete localization it is possible to lesion the raphe nuclei and examine behavioral alterations. Lesions of the midbrain raphe nuclei are associated with sleep disturbances. Electrical stimulation of the raphe magnus causes analgesia, which is presumably related to the terminations of this pathway in association with enkephalin-containing neurons in the spinal cord. Actions of tricyclic antidepressant drugs on serotonin also imply a role for these neurons in mood regulation (see Table 4–1).

Metabolism

The dietary precursor of serotonin is the amino acid tryptophan. Tryptophan is hydroxylated to 5-hydroxytyptophan by a mixed function oxygenase that requires molecular oxygen and tetrahydrobiopterin (Snyder, 1988) (Fig. 4–3). In many ways tryptophan hydroxylase resembles tyrosine hydroxylase. However, its K_m is relatively high, higher than the physiologic levels of tryptophan in the brain. Thus, administration of tryptophan augments brain levels of serotonin. Orally administered tryptophan in humans facilitates sleep, which is thought to be associated with increased brain levels and synaptic release of serotonin. 5-Hydroxytryptophan is decarboxylated by aromatic-L-amino-acid decarboxylase, the same enzyme protein that accounts for dopa decarboxylase activity.

Serotonin is metabolized by MAO, which is located primarily in the mitochondria of serotonin-containing nerve terminals, again analogous to the interaction of catecholamines and MAO. The aldehyde formed by the actions of MAO on serotonin is almost completely converted to the acid 5-hydroxyindoleacetic acid. Accordingly, levels of 5-hydroxyindoleacetic acid, the only end product of serotonin metabolism, provide the most efficient means of assessing serotonin turnover. Monitoring this metabolite in human cerebrospinal fluid has clarified serotonin disposition in humans.

Reuptake

Like the catecholamines, serotonin is inactivated by an energy- and sodium-requiring uptake system. Tricyclic antidepressants at therapeutic concentrations inhibit this uptake pump. Some of the older, widely used antidepressants, such as imipramine and amitriptyline, have similar potencies in inhibiting uptake of norepinephrine and serotonin, so that one cannot readily distinguish whether potentiation of one or the other is primarily responsible for the therapeutic effect of these drugs. Desmethylimipramine is 1000 times more potent in inhibiting norepinephrine uptake than serotonin or dopamine uptake, which indicates that potentiation of norepinephrine alone can have antidepressant actions. Highly selective inhibitors of serotonin uptake, such as fluoxetine, have been used clinically and appear to be highly effective agents, so that facilitating synaptic activities of serotonin alone can have therapeutic actions in depression. Most antidepressants are weak inhibitors of dopamine uptake, and this amine does not appear to have a role in mood regulation.

AMINO ACIDS

γ-Aminobutyric Acid

GABA is the major inhibitory neurotransmitter in the brain. Although GABA was identified in 1951 as a brain-selective amino acid (Roberts and Frankel, 1951), its role as an inhibitory neurotransmitter was definitively established only in the mid 1960s (Gottlieb, 1988). GABA occurs both in long neuronal pathways and in small interneurons in all areas of the central nervous system. Its highest concentration is in the substantia nigra, where it is localized to the nerve terminals of the descending striatonigral pathway. This tract reciprocally regulates the ascending dopamine-containing nigrostriatal system.

Metabolism

GABA is formed from the amino acid glutamic acid by glutamate decarboxylase, a pyridoxal phosphate–requiring enzyme. It is degraded by GABA transaminase, which also uses pyridoxal phosphate as a cofactor. In the transaminase reaction, GABA is converted to succinic semialdehyde, and α-ketoglutarate is reciprocally converted to glutamate. In this way catabolism of GABA is associated with the formation of its precursor glutamate. The succinic semialdehyde is oxidized to succinic acid.

GABA is inactivated by a high-affinity, sodium- and energy-requiring uptake system. Although this uptake is most enriched in GABA-containing nerve terminals, it also occurs in glia. Astrocytic glia ensheath synapses and may play a major role in synaptic inactivation of released GABA. Glial uptake either does not exist or is minor for biogenic amines. Its greater role in amino acid inactivation may relate to the much higher levels of released amino acid neurotransmitters, which may require a combination of nerve terminals and glia to provide an adequate uptake system for inactivation.

Receptor Actions

GABA inhibits neurons by hyperpolarizing them (Bormann, 1988), which is accomplished by increasing chloride ion conductance. Molecular cloning has revealed that the $GABA_A$ receptor mediating these effects contains within the same molecule both the recognition site for GABA and the chloride ion channel (Barnard et al., 1987). Convulsant drugs, such as bicuculline and picrotoxin, act by blocking GABA receptors. Bicuculline competes with GABA at its recognition site, whereas picrotoxin acts at a site more closely linked to the chloride ion channel. Benzodiazepines, such as diazepam and clonazepam, facilitate the synaptic effects of GABA, which accounts for their anticonvulsant, sedative, and antianxiety influences. The benzodiazepines act at a site separate from the GABA recognition site, which allosterically increases the affinity of GABA for its binding site (see Table 4–1).

Glycine

Glycine is an inhibitory neurotransmitter primarily in the spinal cord and brain stem, where it acts at up to 25% of synapses. In higher brain regions, glycine does not appear to play a role as a neurotransmitter itself but may act synergistically with glutamate at certain receptors (see later). In the spinal cord and brain stem, glycine occurs exclusively in small interneurons. In the spinal cord these neurons make synaptic contact with ventral horn motor neurons.

A neurotransmitter role for glycine was first suspected in the mid 1960s when the effects of physiologic inhibition in the spinal cord were shown to involve enhanced chloride ion conductance and to be blocked selectively by strychine (Johnston, 1975). Both GABA and glycine increase chloride conductance. However, strychnine blocks the effects of glycine but not of GABA. Molecular cloning reveals that the glycine receptor incorporates both the glycine-binding site and the chloride ion channel (Grenningloh et al., 1987). Moreover, there are substantial homologies in the amino acid sequences of glycine, $GABA_A$, and nicotinic cholinergic receptors.

Like the effects of GABA and the biogenic amines, the synaptic effects of glycine are terminated by a high-affinity, sodium- and energy-requiring uptake system (Snyder et al., 1973).

Because glycine is incorporated into proteins and participates in general intermediary metabolism, it has been difficult to distinguish the neurotransmitter pool of glycine from the more general metabolic pools. Concentrations of glycine are several-fold higher in the spinal cord and lower brain stem than in the cerebral cortex. Thus, it is thought that in these lower centers most endogenous glycine is contained in the transmitter pool. One can label the transmitter pool of glycine selectively via the high-affinity uptake system with radiolabeled glycine.

Glycine clearly plays a role in the physiologic regulation of skeletal muscle tone. Genetic diseases of mice and cows have been identified in which muscle spasticity is associated with a profound decrease in numbers of glycine receptors. The neuroleptic mutant mouse *spastic* displays pronounced myoclonus, associated with a profound depletion in numbers of glycine receptor–binding sites labeled with [³H]strychnine (Becker, 1990). Knowledge of the molecular genetics of the glycine receptor coupled with transgenic mouse technology may permit elucidation of the molecular abnormality and its correction. Poll Hereford cattle, which are myoclonic, also display a marked loss of glycine receptors, which can account for the pathophysiology of the disease (Gundlach, 1990; Gundlach et al., 1988).

Glutamate

Glutamate appears to be the major excitatory neurotransmitter in the brain. Although definitive estimates are difficult, glutamate is probably a transmitter at 35–40% of all synapses in the brain (McGeer and McGeer, 1989). Because of difficulties in discriminating transmitter and nontransmitter pools of glutamate, researchers have been unable to image glutamatergic neurons selectively. However, glutamate is likely contained in both long neuronal pathways and small interneurons. It is unclear whether any unique metabolic pathway exists for neurotransmitter pools of glutamate.

Glutamate acts at a variety of receptor subtypes (Lodge, 1987). The NMDA subtypes are so designated because N-methyl-D-aspartate is selectively po-

tent, whereas quisqualate and kainate subtypes are selectively activated by these rigid glutamate derivatives. At NMDA and kainate receptors, glutamate acts by opening ion channels. The NMDA receptor also has a recognition site for glycine that is clearly distinct from the glycine receptor associated with synaptic inhibition in the spinal cord and brain stem (Ascher and Nowak, 1987). At the NMDA receptor, glycine, at physiologic concentrations, facilitates the actions of glutamate. This effect of glycine is not influenced by strychnine. Glycine appears to be absolutely required for the normal functioning of glutamate at the NMDA receptor, which thus is a unique receptor whose activity depends on the simultaneous presence of two amino acids.

Two quisqualate-selective receptors exist, one of which involves ion channels, whereas the other involves stimulation of the phosphoinositide second-messenger system. The ionotropic quisqualate, kainate, and NMDA receptors are associated with channels permitting the conductance of sodium, but the NMDA receptor also admits calcium ions and is blocked by magnesium. With normal physiologic activity, the NMDA channel is inactive, being blocked by magnesium. High-frequency stimulation relieves the block and permits the entry of calcium. The high rates of firing of excitatory neurons consequent to cerebral ischemia maximally activate NMDA receptors, with an attendant influx of large amounts of calcium. By activating calcium-dependent proteases, this calcium may be responsible for neurotoxicity. With cerebral ischemia, neuronal damage often extends far beyond zones directly infarcted by the initial insult. This secondary loss of neural tissue likely occurs consequent to hyperexcitation via NMDA receptors. Thus, NMDA antagonist drugs may be therapeutic in stroke. In gerbils with a ligated cerebral artery, hippocampal neuronal death can be prevented by treatment with NMDA antagonists up to 2 hours after artery ligation (Choi, 1988).

PEPTIDES

Numerous peptides have been identified as neurotransmitters in the brain (Snyder, 1980). Some, such as the enkephalins, were first identified as neurotransmitters. Others, such as cholecystokinin, were well known intestinal hormones that were subsequently shown to occur in the brain. Pituitary peptides and hypothalamic releasing factor peptides also occur in neuronal pathways throughout the brain. Peripherally circulating peptides, such as bradykinin and angiotensin, are also neurotransmitters in the brain. One of the major challenges of molecular neuroscience is to ascertain why nature has provided so many different neuropeptide systems. A partial compilation of these peptides is contained in Table 4–2. In the interest of brevity, the focus here is on substance P and the enkephalins.

Peptide neurotransmitters are formed by proteo-

Table 4–2. PEPTIDE NEUROTRANSMITTER
CANDIDATES

Gut-Brain Peptides
Vasoactive intestinal polypeptide
Cholecystokinin octapeptide
Substance P
Neurotensin
Met-enkephalin
Leu-enkephalin
Neuropeptide Y

Hypothalamic-Releasing Hormones
Thyrotropin-releasing hormone
Luteinizing hormone–releasing hormone
Somatostatin (growth hormone release–inhibiting factor)

Pituitary Peptides
Adrenocorticotropin
β-Endorphin
α-Melanocyte-stimulating hormone
Vasopressin
Oxytocin

Others
Angiotensin II
Bradykinin
Carnosine
Bombesin
Calcitonin gene–related peptide
Galanin

lytic cleavage from large protein precursors in which the peptides are flanked on both sides by pairs of basic amino acids (Lynch and Snyder, 1987). The peptides are liberated from their precursors by the sequential actions of trypsin-like and carboxypeptidase B–like enzymes (Martin et al., 1987). Similar processing is involved in the biosynthesis of hormonal peptides such as insulin. It is yet unclear whether highly selective processing enzymes exist for each neuropeptide. The neuropeptides are degraded by peptidases. Some peptidases may be selective; others are more general. Most of the peptidase activities for neuropeptides are as yet unidentified.

Substance P

Substance P was identified in the 1930s in powdered (hence substance P) extracts of the hypothalamus as a substance that caused contraction in certain smooth muscle systems. Its structure was finally elucidated almost 40 years later (Leeman and Mroz, 1975). Immunohistochemical localization of substance P has suggested specific neurotransmitter functions (Pernow, 1983). It is localized in thin, unmyelinated, sensory C fibers, which are involved in pain perception (Jessell, 1983). Stimulation of these nerves releases substance P in the dorsal spinal cord, where it excites spinal neurons. Substance P occurs in numerous neuronal systems in the brain. The most prominent one has cell bodies in the caudate nucleus and axons that descend to terminate in the substantia nigra.

Enkephalins

The enkephalins were isolated from brain extracts as substances that mimic the effects of morphine at opiate receptor–binding sites in the brain and in peripheral smooth muscle. There are two enkephalins that differ only in their COOH-terminal amino acid, which is leucine for leu-enkephalin and methionine for met-enkephalin (Miller, 1983).

Met-enkephalin and leu-enkephalin are derived from different precursors coded for by different genes (Costa et al., 1987). Thus, it is not surprising that met-enkephalin and leu-enkephalin are predominantly stored in different neuronal systems. It is yet unclear whether the leu-enkephalin and met-enkephalin systems have different functions.

The localization of enkephalin-containing neurons throughout the brain and spinal cord closely parallels the localization of opiate receptors (Lynch and Snyder, 1986). This observation establishes definitively that the enkephalins are the physiologic neurotransmitters for opiate receptors.

Besides the enkephalins, other, larger peptides, containing within them the met-enkephalin sequence, have been identified and are referred to generically as endorphins, a term that also designates any opiate-like peptide, including the enkephalins (Akil and Watson, 1983; Bloom, 1988). Because their localization in the brain largely differs from that of opiate receptors, the nonenkephalin endorphins are probably not major neurotransmitters at opiate receptors. The most abundant one, β-endorphin, occurs in much higher concentrations in the anterior pituitary than in the brain. It is formed from the same precursor as adrenocorticotropin and is coreleased with adrenocorticotropin from the pituitary. Thus, the major function of β-endorphin is likely to be as a pituitary hormone acting on some peripheral target, which has not yet been definitively identified.

References

(Key references are designated with an asterisk.)
Akil H., Watson S.J. Beta endorphin and biosynthetically related peptides in the central nervous system. In Iversen L.L., Iversen S.D., Snyder S.H., eds. *Handbook of Psychopharmacology.* Vol. 16. New York, Plenum Publishing, pp. 209–254, 1983.
*Ascher P., Nowak L. Electrophysiological studies of NMDA receptors. *Trends Neurosci.* 10:248–288, 1987.
Axelrod J. Noradrenaline: fate and control of its biosynthesis. *Science* 173:598–606, 1971.
*Barnard E.A., Darlison M.G., Seeburg P. Molecular biology of the GABA-A receptor: the receptor channel superfamily. *Trends Neurosci.* 10:502–509, 1987.
Becker C.M. Disorders of the inhibitory glycine receptor—the spastic mouse. *FASEB J.* 4:2767–2774, 1990.
Bloom F.E. Neurotransmitters: part, present and future directions. *FASEB J.* 2:32–41, 1988.
Bonner T.A., Young A.C., Brann M.R., et al. Cloning and expression of the human and rat M₅ muscarinic acetylcholine receptor genes. *Neuron* 1:403–410, 1988.
Bormann J. Electrophysiology of GABA-A and GABA-B receptor subtypes. *Trends Neurosci.* 11:112–116, 1988.

Changeux J.-P., Devillers-Thiery A., Chemouilli P. Acetylcholine receptor: an allosteric protein. *Science* 25:1335–1345, 1984.

*Choi D.W. Glutamate neurotoxicity and diseases of the nervous system. *Neuron* 1:623–634, 1988.

Collerton D. Cholinergic function and intellectual decline in Alzheimer's disease. *Neuroscience* 19:1–28, 1986.

Costa E., Sandler M., eds. *Monoamine Oxidase: New Vistas.* New York, Raven Press, 1972.

Costa E., Mocchetti I., Supattapone S., et al. Opioid peptide biosynthesis: enzymatic selectivity and regulatory mechanisms. *FASEB J.* 1:16–21, 1987.

Dohlman H.G., Caron M.G., Lefkowitz R.J. A family of receptors coupled to guanine nucleotide regulatory proteins. *Biochemistry* 26:2657–2664, 1989.

Gottlieb D.I. GABAergic neurons. *Sci. Am.* 258(2):38–45, 1988.

Grenningloh G., Rienitz A., Schmitt B., et al. The strychnine-binding subunit of the glycine receptor shows homology with nicotinic acetylcholine receptors. *Nature* 328:215–220, 1987.

Gundlach A. Disorder of the inhibitory glycine receptor: inherited myoclonus in Poll Hereford calves. *FASEB J.* 4:2761–2766, 1990.

Gundlach A.L., Dodd P.R., Grabara S.C.G., et al. Deficit of glycine/strychnine receptors in inherited myoclonus of Poll Hereford calves. *Science* 241:1807–1810, 1988.

Hammer R., Berrie C.P., Birdsall N.M.J., et al. Pirenzipine distinguishes between subclasses of muscarinic receptors. *Nature* 283:90–92, 1980.

Hokfelt T., Johannson O., Goldstein M. Chemical anatomy of the brain. *Science* 225:1326–1334, 1984.

Javitch J.A., Strittmatter S.M., Snyder S.H. Differential visualization of dopamine and norepinephrine uptake sites in rat brain using [^{3}H]mazindol autoradiography. *J. Neurosci.* 5:1513–1521, 1985.

Jessell T.M. Substance P in the nervous system. In Iversen L.L., Iversen S.D., Snyder S.H., eds. *Handbook of Psychopharmacology.* Vol. 16. New York, Plenum Publishing, pp. 1–106, 1983.

Johnston G.A.R. Biochemistry of glycine, taurine, glutamate and aspartate. In Iversen L.L., Iversen S.D., Snyder S.H. eds. *Handbook of Psychopharmacology.* Vol. 4. New York, Plenum Publishing, pp. 59–82, 1975.

Jope R. High affinity choline uptake and acetylcholine production in brain. Role in regulation of ACh synthesis. *Brain Res. Rev.* 1:313–344, 1979.

Kasa P. The cholinergic systems in brain and spinal cord. *Prog. Neurobiol.* 26:211–272, 1986.

Kuhar M.J. Central cholinergic pathways: physiologic and pharmacologic aspects. In Lipton M.A., Dismascio A., Killam K.F., eds. *Psychopharmacology, a Generation of Progress.* New York, Raven Press, pp. 199–204, 1978.

Leeman S.E., Mroz E.A. Substance P. *Life Sci.* 15:2033–2044, 1975.

Lindvall O., Bjorklund A. Organization of catecholamine neurons in the rat central nervous system. In Iversen L.L., Iversen S.D., Snyder S.H., eds. *Handbook of Psychopharmacology.* Vol. 9. New York, Plenum Publishing, pp. 139–231, 1978.

*Lodge D. Modulating glutamate pharmacology. *Trends Pharmacol. Sci.* 10:263–301, 1987.

Lynch D.R., Snyder S.H. Neuropeptides: multiple molecular forms, metabolic pathways, and receptors. *Annu. Rev. Biochem.* 55:773–799, 1986.

Lynch D.R., Snyder S.H. Enkephalins: focus on biosynthesis. In Martin J., Brownstein M., Krieger D., eds. *Brain Peptides Update.* Vol. 1. New York, Wiley, pp. 164–173, 1987.

Martin J.B., Brownstein M.J., Krieger D.T., eds. *Brain Peptides Update.* New York, Wiley, 1987.

Massoulie J., Bon S. The molecular forms of acetylcholinesterase and cholinesterase in vertebrates. *Annu. Rev. Neurosci.* 5:57–106, 1982.

McGeer P.L., McGeer E.G. Amino acid neurotransmitters. In Siegel G., Agranoff B., Albers R.W., et al., eds. *Basic Neurochemistry.* 4th ed. New York, Raven Press, pp. 312–332, 1989.

Miller R.J. The enkephalins. In Iversen L.L., Iversen S.D., Snyder S.H., eds. *Handbook of Psychopharmacology.* Vol. 16. New York, Plenum Publishing, pp. 107–208, 1983.

Molinoff P.B., Axelrod J. Biochemistry of catecholamines. *Annu. Rev. Biochem.* 40:465–500, 1971.

Moore R.Y., Bloom F.E. Central catecholamine neuron systems. *Annu. Rev. Neurosci.* 2:113–168, 1979.

*Nathanson N. Molecular properties of the muscarinic acetylcholine receptor. *Annu. Rev. Neurosci.* 10:195–236, 1987.

*Peralta E.G., Ashkenazi A., Winslow J.W., et al. Distinct primary structures, ligand binding properties and tissue-specific expression of four human muscarinic acetylcholine receptors. *EMBO J.* 6:3923–3929, 1987.

Pernow B. Substance P. *Pharmacol. Rev.* 35:85–141, 1983.

Roberts E., Frankel S. Glutamic acid decarboxylase in brain. *J. Biol. Chem.* 188:789–795, 1951.

Rossier J. Choline acetyltransferase: a review with special reference to its cellular and subcellular localization. *Int. Rev. Neurobiol.* 20:283–337, 1979.

Snyder S.H. Brain peptides as neurotransmitters. *Science* 209:976–983, 1980.

Snyder S.H. Drug and neurotransmitter receptors in the brain. *Science* 224:22–31, 1984.

Snyder S.H. Brain receptors: the emergence of a new pharmacology. *Trends Neurosci.* 9:455–459, 1986a.

Snyder S.H. Neuronal receptors. *Annu. Rev. Physiol.* 48:461–471, 1986b.

*Snyder S.H. *Drugs and the Brain.* New York, Freeman, 1988.

Snyder S.H., Young A.B., Bennett J.P., et al. Synaptic biochemistry of amino acids. *Fed. Proc.* 32:2039–2047, 1973.

Stjarne L. Basic mechanisms and local feedback control of secretion of adrenergic and cholinergic neurotransmitters. In Iversen L.L., Iversen S.D., Snyder S.H., eds. *Handbook of Psychopharmacology.* Vol. 6. New York, Plenum Publishing, pp. 179–233, 1975.

Weinshilboum R.M., Thoa N.B., Johnson D.G., et al. Proportional release of norepinephrine and dopamine-β-hydroxylase from sympathetic nerves. *Science* 174:1349–1351, 1971.

5

Third Messengers That Regulate Neural Gene Transcription

David Pleasure

The changes in structure of the nervous system that occur during development, learning, aging, and disease are governed by signals from the environment (e.g., hormones, cytokines, neuropeptides, and neurotransmitters) that modulate the transcriptional activity of neural cell–specific genes. This chapter considers the mechanisms that permit this coupling between the extracellular milieu and the nucleus and focuses on a group of nuclear third-messenger proteins that influence phenotype by activating or repressing the transcription of neural genes.

REGULATION OF NEURAL PHENOTYPE AND FUNCTION: ROLE OF DIFFERENTIATION-SPECIFIC PROTEINS AND EFFECTS OF EXTRACELLULAR STIMULI

Phenotype and function of neural cells are dictated by the proteins they express. For example, a neuron forms dendrites and axons because it is rich in tubulin and microtubule-associated proteins (Black and Baas, 1989; Mitchisen and Kirschner, 1988), maintains an excitable plasma membrane because it has gated plasma membrane ion channels (Hess, 1990; Unwin, 1989), and communicates with other neurons by virtue of neurotransmitter-synthetic enzymes. An oligodendrocyte forms myelin because it can synthesize cell-cell adhesion proteins (e.g., myelin-associated glycoprotein) that are necessary for adhesion to axons, structural proteins (e.g., proteolipid) that stabilize repetitive wraps of myelin (Lemke, 1988), and enzymes (e.g., ceramide galactosyltransferase) that catalyze production of myelin lipids.

The proteins that a cell expresses are in large part determined by the genes accessible for transcription in that cell. This gene repertoire is governed by the lineage of the cell and its stage of commitment within that lineage (Vandenbergh et al., 1989). Most lineages have one or more branch points, and the choice of a particular course of commitment and differentiation is influenced by the environment (Anderson, 1989; Lillien and Raff, 1990).

Two examples of the regulation of neural phenotype by environmental factors serve to illuminate these points, as follows.

1. Oligodendroglial precursor cells are stimulated to proliferate and then differentiate into myelin-forming oligodendroglia by platelet-derived growth factor, a paracrine growth factor synthesized within the brain by type 1 astrocytes, microglia, and endothelial cells. Another protein synthesized in brain, basic fibroblast growth factor, also stimulates proliferation of oligodendroglial precursor cells, but, in the presence of platelet-derived growth factor, prevents their differentiation (Bogler et al., 1990; McKinnon and Dubois-Dalcq, 1990). Yet a third protein, ciliary neurotrophic growth factor, induces oligodendroglial precursor cells to differentiate into type 2 astrocytes rather than oligodendrocytes. The numbers of precursor cells, oligodendroglia, and type 2 astroglia are regulated, then, by the relative concentrations of these three growth factors in the milieu (Grinspan et al., 1990; Lillien and Raff, 1990). These growth factor effects must be communicated from the plasma membrane, where specific receptors for these growth factors reside (Courty et al., 1988; Heldin and Westermark, 1989; Ruta et al., 1989), to the nucleus, where entry into the cell cycle or tran-

scription of proteins characteristic of differentiated oligodendroglia (e.g., myelin basic protein) or type 2 astroglia (e.g., glial fibrillary acidic protein) takes place.

2. Neural crest neuroepithelial cells are stimulated by glucocorticoids to become adrenal chromaffin cells. Alternatively, they are induced by nerve growth factor (NGF) to differentiate into process-bearing, postmitotic autonomic neurons (Anderson, 1989; Naujoks et al., 1982). Transduction of the signal delivered by NGF to the plasma membrane of the neuroepithelial cells is initiated by binding of this growth factor to high-affinity trans–plasma membrane NGF receptors (Johnson et al., 1986). Expression of NGF receptors by the neuroepithelial cells requires prior exposure to fibroblast growth factor (Birren and Anderson, 1990). Fibroblast growth factor can, as well, duplicate some of the neuron-differentiating effects of NGF (Rydel and Greene, 1987). The autonomic neurons generated from the neuroepithelial cells by the action of NGF are then directed by ciliary neurotrophic growth factor and other trophic proteins toward various neurotransmitter-specific phenotypes (Ernsberger et al., 1989; Nawa and Patterson, 1990; Yamamori et al., 1989).

These two examples pertain to the developing nervous system. However, terminally differentiated neurons and glia are also subject to modulation of phenotype in response to environmental stimuli. For example, in adult hippocampal neurons, transcription of proenkephalin is augmented and neurite sprouting is initiated by seizures (Sonnenberg et al., 1989c), and, in *Aplysia,* neuronal synthesis of a group of proteins that participate in learning is initiated by neurotransmitter-mediated long-term facilitation (Barzilai et al., 1989).

How do these various extracellular signals modulate the expression of the proteins that govern neural phenotype?

AMPLIFICATION OF ENVIRONMENTAL SIGNALS AND DISSEMINATION OF THEM THROUGHOUT THE CELL BY SECOND MESSENGERS

Some extracellular signals are communicated directly to the cell interior. For example, steroid hormones are sufficiently hydrophobic to pass through the plasma membrane lipid bilayer. They then bind to intracellular steroid receptors, thereby enhancing the capacity of these receptors to interact with specific DNA target sequences (Evans and Arriza, 1989). Other signals, for example, extracellular Ca^{2+}, gain entry via specific channels (Hess, 1990).

Protein hormones and growth factors, peptide neuromodulators, and neurotransmitters must act indirectly, by inducing modifications in the structure of plasma membrane receptors that, in turn, alter the configuration of transmembrane ion channels (Lester and Jahr, 1989) or the activity of enzyme systems on the inner aspect of the plasma membrane (Gilman,

1987; Huang, 1989). These alterations then lead to changes in intracellular ion concentrations or to the generation of such second messengers as cyclic AMP, diacylglycerol, and inositol triphosphate, which serve to amplify the original signal and propagate it through the cytosol and to the nucleus (Berridge and Irvine, 1989; Huang, 1989; Nishizuka, 1988). Disorders in this transduction process, caused, for example, by mutations affecting plasma membrane-associated G proteins that couple receptors and adenylate cyclase, can grossly perturb cell function (Lyons et al., 1990).

The number of known second messengers is still relatively small. Response specificity is achieved by temporally and spatially graded rises in second-messenger levels (Berridge and Irvine, 1989), by recruitment of various combinations of second messengers after a single stimulus (Nishizuka, 1988), and by regional variations in the intracellular targets on which the second messengers act (Huang, 1989; Nishizuka, 1988; Tobimatsu and Fujisawa, 1989).

Second messengers influence phenotype by a variety of mechanisms. For example, cyclic AMP enhances cytoplasmic protein kinase activity and stimulates phosphorylation of various cytosolic proteins (e.g., intermediate filament peptides and glycogenolytic enzymes), thereby changing their structural and catalytic properties (Rothermel et al., 1984). Cyclic AMP also enhances phosphorylation of a nuclear cyclic AMP response element–binding protein (Berkowitz and Gilman, 1990; Montminy et al., 1990), thus stimulating transcription of genes (e.g., tyrosine hydroxylase, somatostatin) that contain the consensus cyclic AMP response element 5'-TGACGTCA-3' (Goodman, 1990; Jones and Jones, 1989; Maekawa et al., 1989; Montminy and Bilezikjian, 1987; Montminy et al., 1990).

Because prolonged action of the second messengers can lead to cell transformation or death, a network of regulatory mechanisms is in place to ensure that they are degraded or sequestered within milliseconds to seconds (Boekhoff et al., 1990). Signaling via the second messengers, therefore, is a good way to elicit rapid activation or repression of cellular events, but they are unsuitable as long-term modulators (Sheng and Greenberg, 1990). Another feature of the second messengers is that they are relatively small molecules; hence, the number of functional domains they express that could contribute to specificity of binding to proteins or DNA is small. These characteristics of the second messengers have made a nuclear third-messenger system necessary for extracellular-nuclear coupling to occur over time and with a degree of binding specificity appropriate for precise and effective modulation of protein transcription.

COUPLING OF EXTRACELLULAR SIGNALS WITH NUCLEAR PROTEIN TRANSCRIPTION BY THIRD MESSENGERS

The third messengers are a group of nuclear proteins, normally expressed at extremely low levels,

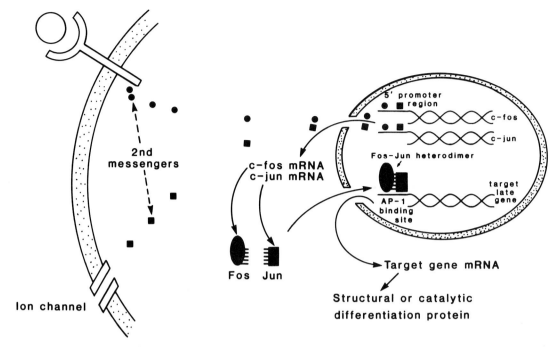

Figure 5–1. Signals conveyed by second messengers reach the nucleus. Although the diagram suggests that the second messengers penetrate the nuclear membrane and then bind to promoter or enhancer regions of immediate early genes, this description may be an oversimplification. After activation by the second messengers of immediate early gene transcription, translation of immediate early gene mRNA takes place in cytosol. The resulting third-messenger proteins enter the nucleus and bind to regulatory sequences of the target genes that they activate (e.g., tyrosine hydroxylase and proenkephalin). In the case of Fos and Jun, the protein species bound is a heterodimer complex (AP-1), which interacts with a consensus DNA sequence 5′-TGACGTCA-3′ in the regulatory region of the target gene. The induction of these target genes, because it depends on translation of the immediate early genes, is blocked by inhibitors of protein synthesis.

that are induced by a variety of extracellular signals and that bind to specific nucleotide sequences in the promoter and enhancer regions of genes (Mitchell and Tjian, 1989). There, in concert with other transcriptional factors, they exert powerful excitatory or inhibitory effects on the initiation of RNA synthesis. The third messengers are encoded by immediate early genes, also referred to as primary response genes or competence genes.

Many immediate early genes were initially recognized because they are the normal nuclear homologues of transforming retroviral oncogenes (e.g., v-*fos*); others were cloned from human cancers (e.g., N-*myc*) (Bishop, 1985, 1987). Additional immediate early genes were identified because they are rapidly induced during entry into the cell cycle (Lau and Nathans, 1985) or within minutes after treatment of cells with agents (e.g., NGF) that eventually cause differentiation (e.g., NGF1-A) (Milbrandt, 1987; Tirone and Shooter, 1989). Most recently, immediate early genes have been cloned from expression or genomic libraries by virtue of sequence homology to known immediate early genes, because they code for proteins with structural features characteristic of DNA-binding proteins (e.g., "zinc fingers" and "leucine zippers") or because they bind with high affinity

to known promoter or enhancer motifs (Maekawa et al., 1989). By now, almost 100 immediate early genes and corresponding proteins have been recognized, which has engendered a bewildering alphabet soup of abbreviations, particularly because many immediate early genes were independently discovered in several contexts and continue to be referred to by several names. Figure 5–1 illustrates the general features of the system relating immediate early gene and third messengers.

The most fully studied of the immediate early genes is c-*fos*. Changes in the tertiary structure of the c-*fos* gene are detectable within a minute after a cell is stimulated, first appearing in regulatory regions of the gene and then propagating into coding regions (Feng and Villeponteau, 1990). Transcription of c-*fos* increases within a few minutes, and the steady-state level of c-*fos* mRNA peaks by 30 minutes. Decay of the c-*fos* response is only slightly less rapid, because transcription of c-*fos* falls abruptly and its half-life in cytosol is short (Herrlich and Ponta, 1989). Degradation of Fos protein is also rapid. Hence, the total time during which the level of Fos is elevated in response to environmental signals is brief in comparison to the half-life of most other structural and catalytic proteins, although it is several orders of magnitude longer than that of the second messengers induced by such signals.

Fos binds to DNA as a component of a heterodimer complex with Jun or other members of the Jun family. Both Fos and Jun contain α-helical domains in which a leucine is present as each seventh amino acid on one face of the helix. These leucine zipper regions of Fos and Jun interdigitate during dimer formation (Gentz et al., 1989), and this interdigitation is stabilized when the dimer binds to DNA (Shuman et al., 1990). Adjacent basic amino acid–rich regions of the two proteins then bind to AP-1 sequences in the regulatory regions of genes that are susceptible to transcriptional regulation by this complex (Abate et al., 1990; Bohmann et al., 1987; Rauscher et al., 1988). The coordinate "scissors grip" binding to the major groove of DNA by the two proteins of the complex stabilizes the protein-DNA interaction (O'Neil et al., 1990; Shuman et al., 1990; Talanian et al., 1990).

Binding of Fos-Jun complexes to AP-1 sites increases the rate of transcription of such target genes as tyrosine hydroxylase, proenkephalin, and neurotensin/neuromedin N (Gizang-Ginsberg and Ziff, 1990; Kislauskis and Dobner, 1990; Sonnenberg et al., 1989c). Inhibitors of protein synthesis, such as cycloheximide, block activation of the late response genes by the immediate early genes because they prevent the production of Fos, Jun, and other third messengers.

Some other genes are repressed by Fos. For example, the Fos protein itself, in the absence of Jun, can inhibit transcription of c-*fos* (Gius et al., 1990). This inhibition results in a feedback-inhibitory loop by which accumulation of Fos in the nucleus down-regulates synthesis of c-*fos* mRNA and of Fos. As would be predicted, the combination of an appropriate environmental stimulus and an inhibitor of protein synthesis, which blocks this feedback loop, causes the superinduction of c-*fos* (Lau and Nathans, 1985).

Fine-tuning of the effects of the third messengers on gene transcription is accomplished by a complex network of controls. Several molecules of a given third messenger may interact in a nonlinear fashion with other transcriptional factors at gene transcription regulatory regions (Mitchell and Tjian, 1989; Pettersson and Schaffner, 1990; Ptashne and Gann, 1990; Visvader et al., 1988). Post-translational modifications of third messengers, particularly phosphorylation, influence these interactions. The composition of third-messenger complexes also varies as a function of time after activation. For example, members of the Fos family other than Fos itself (Fos-related antigens, or Fra) are also induced by extracellular signals, but with a longer latency and half-life than Jun itself. As the Fos response decays with time, levels of Fra in the AP-1 protein complexes increase. This increase may serve to diminish the efficacy with which DNA-binding activity recognizing AP-1 sites modulates transcription of target genes, thus leading to a period during which the cell may be relatively refractory to extracellular stimuli

(Gizang-Ginsberg and Ziff, 1990; Morgan and Curran, 1989; Sonnenberg et al., 1989a).

Specificity of the transcriptional responses to various extracellular stimuli is achieved in some instances by variations in the pattern of immediate early gene activation (Iwaki et al., 1990). For example, immediate early genes expressed by cells of the rat pheochromocytoma line PC12 are activated by either potassium-induced plasma membrane depolarization or binding of NGF to high-affinity NGF receptors. However, the steroid receptor–related gene nur/77 (NGF1-B) (Watson and Milbrandt, 1989) is more markedly induced by membrane depolarization than by NGF, whereas the zinc finger motif gene zif/268 (NGF1-A) is induced to a much greater extent by NGF than by potassium. In some instances, however, such a differential third-messenger response is less evident. For example, PC12 cells express high-affinity receptors for epidermal growth factor as well as for NGF, and both growth factors elicit apparently identical patterns of immediate early gene activation, yet epidermal growth factor, unlike NGF, fails to elicit PC12 cell differentiation or growth arrest (Bartel et al., 1989; Greenberg et al., 1985). This result suggests that immediate early genes other than those currently recognized are involved in the differential response to these two stimuli or, alternatively, that response specificity is achieved by some other mechanism, perhaps a signal-specific variation in post-translational processing of third messengers.

THIRD MESSENGERS AND NEUROLOGIC DISEASE

A role for the third messengers in the pathogenesis of neurologic disease has been best established with respect to neuroectodermal tumors. Genomic amplification of N-*myc* occurs in a sizable proportion of human neuroblastomas and is correlated with poor prognosis (Amler and Schwab, 1989; Brodeur et al., 1984). Overexpression of c-*myc*, either because of genomic amplification or translocation, is present in some primary human medulloblastomas and in the majority of medulloblastoma cell lines (Bigner et al., 1990; MacGregor and Ziff, 1990; Wasson et al., 1990). These nuclear proteins are down-regulated during normal neural development (Caubet, 1989; Pfeifer-Ohlsson et al., 1985). Although the functions of the *myc* family are not known, it has been established that permanent transfection of various primary cell cultures with a cDNA coding for members of this family causes immortalization and contributes to transformation (Birren and Anderson, 1990; Haltmeier and Rohrer, 1990; Schwab and Bishop, 1988). It is likely, therefore, that persistent overexpression of N- or c-*myc* contributes to the failure of the neuroectodermal cells that make up these tumors to terminally differentiate and exit from the cell cycle in the presence of factors and receptors that would normally elicit such a transition (Baker et al., 1989;

Pleasure et al., 1990). Experimentally induced over-expression of other third messengers may also interfere with neuronal differentiation in response to appropriate environmental stimuli (lto et al., 1991) or may render cells abnormally susceptible to tumorigenic influences in the environment (Schuh et al., 1990).

The third-messenger system is also involved in the pathogenesis of retinoblastoma, a neuroectodermal malignancy caused by inactivation in the immature retina of both copies of the tumor suppressor gene *RB-1*. In sporadic cases of retinoblastoma, the tumor arises as a consequence of separate somatic mutations that inactivate each copy of *RB-1*, whereas in the familial form a germline mutation has inactivated one copy of *RB-1*, and tumors arise after a somatic mutation of the second copy of the gene (Dunn et al., 1988; Knudson, 1985). In each instance, clonal expansion of the affected cell is due to the absence of Rb, the protein encoded by *RB-1*. It has been shown that Rb represses transcription of c-*fos* and that the lack of Rb causes overexpression of c-*fos* and results in greater than normal expression of genes activated by the AP-1 complex (Robbins et al., 1990).

A role for the third messengers is also likely in human gliomas and meningiomas in which there is tumor cell overexpression of a member of the fibroblast growth factor family or a platelet-derived growth factor isoform (Libermann et al., 1987; Takahashi et al., 1990). Here, the third messengers merely serve to link an excessive autocrine growth factor signal to the nucleus.

Immediate early genes and the third messenger system also play a role in the pathophysiology of epilepsy (Sheng and Greenberg, 1990; Shin et al., 1990; Sonnenberg et al., 1989a,c). Immunohistologic and in situ hybridization studies demonstrate that c-*fos*, *egr*-1, and Fra genes are activated in mesial temporal structures during generalized seizures induced by pentylenetetrazole and that Fos immunoreactivity accumulates in regions of cerebral cortex kindled during temporal lobe seizures (Drugunow and Robertson, 1987; Sonnenberg et al., 1989a). Qualitative and quantitative alterations in AP-1 complexes persist for hours after relatively brief seizures (Sonnenberg et al., 1989a). These third-messenger perturbations, which are blocked by anticonvulsants, link the seizures to the alterations in late response neurotransmitter synthetic and neuromodulator synthetic genes (e.g., proenkephalin) caused by the seizures (Sonnenberg et al., 1989c).

A role for the third messengers in other neurologic diseases is more speculative. Fos is induced in tactile and visual pathways by appropriate sensory inputs (Kornhauser et al., 1990; Sager and Sharp, 1990; Wisden et al., 1990), and perturbations of third-messenger metabolism may cause long-term aberrations in polysynaptic interaction within such pathways (e.g., in reflex sympathetic dystrophy and disorders of circadian rhythms). It is clear that immediate early genes are activated and third messengers synthesized during the excitation-transcription coupling that occurs in the early stages of long-term potentiation and long-term facilitation (Barzilai et al., 1989; Cole et al., 1989; Goelet et al., 1986), and it is possible that third-messenger effects may contribute in some circumstances to impaired memory consolidation. Immediate early gene mutations, if not lethal, may influence commitment of stem cells to the various neural lineages and result in abnormal patterns of differentiation of neurons or glia (Caubet, 1989; Jimenez and Campos-Ortega, 1990).

CONCLUSIONS

Third messengers encoded by immediate early genes are a necessary link in the coupling of extracellular stimuli to gene transcription. Data already in hand convincingly prove a central role for these nuclear proteins in normal neural development and plasticity and strongly support their participation in the pathogenesis of neural tumors and the pathophysiology of epilepsy. But "the devil is in the details"—much further work will be necessary to understand the mechanisms by which the requisite specificity of third-messenger responses is achieved and to learn how to modify these responses in interesting and desirable ways.

References

Abate C., Luk D., Gentz R., et al. Expression and purification of the leucine zipper and DNA-binding domains of Fos and Jun: both Fos and Jun contact DNA directly. *Proc. Natl. Acad. Sci. U.S.A.* 87:1032–1036, 1990.

Amler L.C., Schwab M. Amplified N-*myc* in human neuroblastoma cells is often arranged in clustered tandem repeats of differently recombined DNA. *Mol. Cell. Biol.* 9:4903–4913, 1989.

Anderson D.J. The neural crest lineage problem: neuropoeisis? *Neuron* 3:1–12, 1989.

Baker D.L., Reddy U.R., Pleasure D., et al. Analysis of nerve growth factor receptor expression in human neuroblastoma and neuroepithelioma cell lines. *Cancer Res.* 40:4142–4146, 1989.

Bartel D.P., Sheng M., Lau L.F., et al. Growth factors and membrane depolarization activate distinct programs of early response gene expression: dissociation of *fos* and *jun* activation. *Genes Dev.* 3:304–313, 1989.

Barzilai A., Kennedy T.E., Sweatt J.D., et al. 5-HT modulates protein synthesis and the expression of specific proteins during long-term facilitation in *Aplysia* sensory neurons. *Neuron* 2:1577–1586, 1989.

Berkowitz L.A., Gillman M.J. Two distinct forms of active transcription factor CREB (cAMP response element binding protein). *Proc. Natl. Acad. Sci. U.S.A.* 87:5258–5262, 1990.

Berridge M.J., Irvine R.F. Inositol phosphates and cell signalling. *Nature* 341:197–205, 1989.

Bigner S.H., Friedman H.S., Vogelstein B., et al. Amplification of the c-*myc* gene in human medulloblastoma cell lines and xenografts. *Cancer Res.* 50:2347–2350, 1990.

Birren S.J., Anderson D.J. A v-*myc*–immortalized sympathoadrenal progenitor cell line in which neuronal differentiation is initiated by FGF but not NGF. *Neuron* 4:189–201, 1990.

Bishop J.M. Viral oncogenes. *Cell* 42:23–38, 1985.

Bishop J.M. The molecular genetics of cancer. *Science* 235:305–311, 1987.

Black M.M., Baas P.W. The basis of polarity in neurons. *Trends Neurosci.* 12:211–214, 1989.

Boekhoff I., Tareilus E., Strotmann J., et al. Rapid activation of alternative second messenger pathways in olfactory cilia from rats by different odorants. *EMBO J.* 9:2453–2458, 1990.

Bogler O., Wren D., Barnett S.C., et al. Cooperation between two growth factors promotes extended self-renewal and inhibits differentiation of oligodendrocyte-type-2 astrocyte (O-2A) progenitor cells. *Proc. Natl. Acad. Sci. U.S.A.* 87:6368–6372, 1990.

Bohmann D., Bos T.J., Admon A., et al. Human proto-oncogene c-*jun* encodes a DNA binding protein with structural and functional properties of transcription factor AP-1. *Science* 238:1386–1392, 1987.

Brodeur G.M., Seeger R.C., Schwab M., et al. Amplification of N-*myc* in untreated human neuroblastomas correlates with advanced disease stage. *Science* 224:1121–1124, 1984.

Caubet J.-F. c-*fos* proto-oncogene expression in the nervous system during mouse development. *Mol. Cell. Biol.* 9:2269–2272, 1989.

Cole A.J., Saffen D.W., Baraban J.M., et al. Rapid increase of an immediate early gene messenger RNA in hippocampal neurons by synaptic NMDA receptor activation. *Nature* 340:474–476, 1989.

Courty J., Dauchel M.C., Mereau A., et al. Presence of basic fibroblast growth factor receptors in bovine brain membranes. *J. Biol. Chem.* 263:11217–11220, 1988.

Drugunow M., Robertson H.A. Kindling stimulation induces c-*fos* protein(s) in granule cells of the rat dentate gyrus. *Nature* 329:441–442, 1987.

Dunn J.M., Phillips R.A., Becker A.J., et al. Identification of germline and somatic mutations affecting the retinoblastoma gene. *Science* 241:1797–1800, 1988.

Ernsberger U., Sendtner M., Rohrer H. Proliferation and differentiation of embryonic chick sympathetic neurons: effects of ciliary neurotrophic factor. *Neuron* 2:1275–1284, 1989.

Evans R.M., Arriza J.L. A molecular framework for the actions of glucocorticoid hormones in the nervous system. *Neuron* 2:1105–1112, 1989.

Feng J., Villeponteau B. Serum stimulation of the c-*fos* enhancer induces reversible changes in c-*fos* chromatin structure. *Mol. Cell. Biol.* 10:1126–1133, 1990.

Gentz R., Rauscher F.J. III, Abate C., et al. Parallel association of Fos and Jun leucine zippers juxtaposes DNA binding domains. *Science* 246:1622–1625, 1989.

Gilman A.G. G proteins: transducers of receptor-generated signals. *Annu. Rev. Biochem.* 56:615–649, 1987.

Gius D., Cao X., Rauscher F.J. III, et al. Transcriptional activation and repression by Fos are independent functions: the C-terminus represses immediate-early gene expression via CArG elements. *Mol. Cell. Biol.* 10:4243–4255, 1990.

Gizang-Ginsberg E., Ziff E.B. Nerve growth factor regulates tyrosine hydroxylase gene transcription through a nucleoprotein complex that contains c-*fos*. *Genes Dev.* 4:447–491, 1990.

Goelet P., Castellucci V.F., Schacher S., et al. The long and the short of long-term memory—a molecular framework. *Nature* 322:419–422, 1986.

Goodman R.H. Regulation of neuropeptide gene expression. *Annu. Rev. Neurosci.* 13:111–127, 1990.

Greenberg M.E., Greene L.A., Ziff E.B. Nerve growth factor and epidermal growth factor induce rapid transient changes in proto-oncogene transcription in PC12 cells. *J. Biol. Chem.* 260:14101–14110, 1985.

Grinspan J., Stern J., Pustilnik S., et al. Cerebral white matter contains PDGF-responsive precursors to O2A cells. *J. Neurosci.* 10:1866–1873, 1990.

Haltmeier H., Rohrer H. Distinct and different effects of the oncogenes v-*myc* and v-*src* on avian sympathetic neurons: retroviral transfer of v-*myc* stimulates neuronal proliferation whereas v-*src* transfer enhances neuronal differentiation. *J. Cell Biol.* 110:2087–2098, 1990.

Heldin C.-H., Westermark B. Platelet-derived growth factor: three isoforms and two receptor types. *Trends Genet.* 5:108–111, 1989.

Herrlich P., Ponta H. Nuclear oncogenes convert extracellular stimuli into changes in the genetic program. *Trends Genet.* 5:112–116, 1989.

Hess P. Calcium channels in vertebrate cells. *Annu. Rev. Neurosci.* 13:337–356, 1990.

Huang K.-P. The mechanism of protein kinase C activation. *Trends Neurosci.* 12:425–432, 1989.

Ito E., Sweterlitsch L.A., Tran P.B.-V., et al. Inhibition of PC-12 cell differentiation by the immediate early gene FRA-1. *Oncogene* (in press).

Iwaki K., Sukhatme V.P., Shubeita H.E., et al. Alpha- and beta-adrenergic stimulation induces distinct patterns of immediate early gene expression in neonatal rat myocardial cells. *J. Biol. Chem.* 265:13809–13817, 1990.

Jimenez F., Campos-Ortega J.A. Defective neuroblast commitment in mutants of the achaete-scute complex and adjacent genes of *D. melanogaster*. *Neuron* 5:81–89, 1990.

Johnson D., Lanahan A., Buck C.R., et al. Expression and structure of the human NGF receptor. *Cell* 47:545–554, 1986.

Jones R.H., Jones N.C. Mammalian cAMP-responsive element can activate transcription in yeast and binds a yeast factor(s) that resembles the mammalian transcription factor ATF. *Proc. Natl. Acad. Sci. U.S.A.* 86:2176–2180, 1989.

Kislauskis E., Dobner P.R. Mutually dependent response elements in the cis-regulatory region of the neurotensin/neuromedin N gene integrate environmental stimuli in PC12 cells. *Neuron* 4:783–795, 1990.

Knudson A.G. Jr. Hereditary cancer, oncogenes, and antioncogenes. *Cancer Res.* 45:1437–1443, 1985.

Kornhauser J.M., Nelson D.E., Mayo K.E., et al. Photic and circadian regulation of c-*fos* gene expression in the hamster suprachiasmatic nucleus. *Neuron* 5:127–134, 1990.

Lau L.F., Nathans D. Identification of a set of genes expressed during the G_0/G_1 transition of cultured mouse cells. *EMBO J.* 4:3145–3151, 1985.

Lemke G. Unwrapping the genes of myelin. *Neuron* 1:535–543, 1988.

Lester R.A.J., Jahr C.E. Quisqualate receptor–mediated depression of calcium currents in hippocampal neurons. *Neuron* 4:741–749, 1990.

Libermann T.A., Friesel R., Jaye M., et al. An angiogenic growth factor is expressed in human glioma cells. *EMBO J.* 6:1627–1632, 1987.

Lillien L.E., Raff M.C. Differentiation signals in the CNS: type-2 astrocyte development in vitro as a model system. *Neuron* 5:111–119, 1990.

Lyons J., Landis C.A., Harsh G., et al. Two G protein oncogenes in human endocrine tumors. *Science* 249:655–659, 1990.

MacGregor D.N., Ziff E.B. Elevated c-*myc* expression in childhood medulloblastomas. *Pediatr. Res.* 28:63–68, 1990.

Maekawa T., Sakura H., Kanei-Ishii C., et al. Leucine zipper structure of the protein CRE-BP1 binding to the cyclic AMP response element in brain. *EMBO J.* 8:2023–2028, 1989.

McKinnon R.D., Dubois-Dalcq M. Fibroblast growth factor blocks myelin basic protein gene expression in differentiating O-2A glial progenitor cells. *Ann. N. Y. Acad. Sci.* 605:358–359, 1990.

Milbrandt J. A nerve growth factor–induced gene encodes a possible transcriptional regulatory factor. *Science* 238:797–799, 1987.

Mitchell P.J., Tjian R. Transcriptional regulation in mammalian cells by sequence-specific DNA binding proteins. *Science* 245:371–378, 1989.

Mitchisen T., Kirschner M. Cytoskeletal dynamics and nerve growth. *Neuron* 1:761–772, 1988.

Montminy M.R., Bilezikjian L.M. Binding of a nuclear protein to the cyclic-AMP response element of the somatostatin gene. *Nature* 328:175–178, 1987.

Montminy M.R., Gonzalez G.A., Yamamoto K.K. Regulation of cAMP-inducible genes by CREB. *Trends Neurosci.* 13:184–188, 1990.

Morgan J.I., Curran T. Stimulus-transcription coupling in neurons: role of cellular immediate-early genes. *Trends Neurosci.* 12:459–462, 1989.

Naujoks K.W., Korsching S., Rohrer H., et al. Nerve growth factor–mediated induction of tyrosine hydroxylase and of neurite outgrowth in cultures of bovine adrenal chromaffin cells: dependence on developmental stage. *Dev. Biol.* 92:365–379, 1982.

Nawa H., Patterson P.H. Separation and partial characterization of neuropeptide-induced factors in heart cell conditioned medium. *Neuron* 2:269–277, 1990.

Nishizuka Y. The molecular heterogeneity of protein kinase C and its implications for cellular recognition. *Nature* 334:661–665, 1988.

O'Neil K.T., Hoess R.H., DeGrado W.F. Design of DNA-binding peptides based on the leucine zipper motif. *Science* 249:774–778, 1990.

Pettersson M., Schaffner W. Synergistic activation of transcription by multiple binding sites for NF-kB even in absence of co-operative factor binding to DNA. *J. Mol. Biol.* 214:373–380, 1990.

Pfeifer-Ohlsson S., Rydnert J., Goustin A.S., et al. Cell-type–specific pattern of *myc* protooncogene expression in developing human embryos. *Proc. Natl. Acad. Sci. U.S.A.* 82:5050–5054, 1985.

Pleasure S., Reddy U.R., Venkatakrishnan G., et al. Introduction of nerve growth factor (NGF) receptors (NGFRs) into a medulloblastoma cell line results in expression of high and low affinity NGFRs but not NGF-mediated differentiation. *Proc. Natl. Acad. Sci.* 87:8496–8500, 1990.

Ptashne M., Gann A.A.F. Activators and targets. *Nature* 346:329–331, 1990.

Rauscher F.J. III, Sambucetti L.C., Curran T., et al. Common DNA binding site for Fos protein complexes and transcription factor AP-1. *Cell* 52:471–480, 1988.

Robbins P.D., Horowitz J.M., Mulligan R.C. Negative regulation of human c-*fos* expression by the retinoblastoma gene product. *Nature* 346:668–671, 1990.

Rothermel J.D., Perillo N.L., Marks J.S., et al. Effects of the specific cAMP antagonist, (R$_p$)-adenosine cyclic 3′,5′-phosphorothoate, on the cAMP-dependent protein kinase–induced activity of hepatic glycogen phosphorylase and glycogen synthase. *J. Biol. Chem.* 259:15294–15300, 1984.

Ruta M., Burgess W., Givol D., et al. Receptor for acidic fibroblast growth factor is related to the tyrosine kinase encoded by the FMS-like gene (FLG). *Proc. Natl. Acad. Sci. U.S.A.* 86:8722–8726, 1989.

Rydel R.E., Greene L.A. Acidic and basic fibroblast growth factors promote stable neurite outgrowth and neuronal differentiation in cultures of PC12 cells. *J. Neurosci.* 7:3639–3652, 1987.

Sager S.M., Sharp F.R. Light induces a Fos-like nuclear antigen in retinal neurons. *Mol. Brain Res.* 7:17–21, 1990.

Schuh A.C., Keating S.J., Monteclaro F.S., et al. Obligatory wounding requirement for tumorigenesis in v-*jun* transgenic mice. *Nature* 346:756–760, 1990.

Schwab M., Bishop J.M. Sustained expression of the human protooncogene MYCN rescues rat embryo cells from senescence. *Proc. Natl. Acad. Sci. U.S.A.* 85:9585–9589, 1988.

Sheng M., Greenberg M.E. The regulation and function of c-*fos* and other immediate early genes in the nervous system. *Neuron* 4:447–485, 1990.

Shin C., McNamara J.O., Morgan J.I., et al. Induction of c-*fos*

mRNA expression by afterdischarge in the hippocampus of naive and kindled rats. *J. Neurochem.* 55:1050–1055, 1990.

Shuman J.D., Vinson C.R., McKnight S.L. Evidence of changes in protease sensitivity and subunit exchange rate on DNA binding by C/*ERB*. *Science* 249:771–774, 1990.

Sonnenberg J.L., Macgregor-Leon P.F., Curran T., et al. Dynamic alterations occur in the levels and composition of transcription factor AP-1 complexes after seizure. *Neuron* 3:359–365, 1989a.

Sonnenberg J.L., Mitchelmore C., Macgregor-Leon P.F., et al. Glutamate receptor agonists increase the expression of Fos, Fra, and AP-1 binding activity in the mammalian brain. *J. Neurosci. Res.* 24:72–80, 1989b.

Sonnenberg J.L., Rauscher P.J. III, Morgan J.I., et al. Regulation of proenkephalin by Fos and Jun. *Science* 246:1622–1625, 1989c.

Takahashi J.A., Mori H., Fukumoto M., et al. Gene expression of fibroblast growth factors in human gliomas and meningiomas: demonstration of cellular source of basic fibroblast growth factor mRNA and peptide in tumor tissues. *Proc. Natl. Acad. Sci. U.S.A.* 87:5710–5714, 1990.

Talanian R.V., McKnight C.J., Kim P.S. Sequence-specific DNA binding by a short peptide dimer. *Science* 249:769–771, 1990.

Tirone F., Shooter E.M. Early gene regulation by nerve growth factor in PC12 cells: induction of an interferon-related gene. *Proc. Natl. Acad. Sci. U.S.A.* 86:2088–2092, 1989.

Tobimatsu T., Fujisawa H. Tissue-specific expression of four types of rat calmodulin-dependent protein kinase II mRNAs. *J. Biol. Chem.* 264:17907–17912, 1989.

Unwin N. The structure of ion channels in membranes of excitable cells. *Neuron* 3:665–676, 1989.

Vandenbergh D.J., Wuenschell C.W., Mori N., et al. Chromatin structure as a molecular marker of cell lineage and developmental potential in neural crest-derived chromaffin cells. *Neuron* 3:507–518, 1989.

Visvader J., Sassone-Corsi P., Verma I.M. Two adjacent promoter elements mediate nerve growth factor activation of the c-*fos* gene and bind distinct nuclear complexes. *Proc. Natl. Acad. Sci. U.S.A.* 85:9474–9478, 1988.

Wasson J.C., Saylors R.L. III, Zeltzer P., et al. Oncogene amplification in pediatric brain tumors. *Cancer Res.* 50:2987–2990, 1990.

Watson M.A., Milbrandt J. The NGFI-B gene, a transcriptionally inducible member of the steroid receptor gene superfamily: genomic structure and expression in rat brain after seizure induction. *Mol. Cell. Biol.* 9:4213–4219, 1989.

Wisden W., Errington M.L., Williams S., et al. Differential expression of immediate early genes in the hippocampus and spinal cord. *Neuron* 4:603–614, 1990.

Yamamori T., Fukada K., Aebersold R., et al. The cholinergic neuronal differentiation factor from heart cells is identical to leukemia inhibitory factor. *Science* 246:1412–1416, 1989.

6

Neural Plasticity

Peter R. Huttenlocher

Plasticity refers to adjustments of the nervous system to changes in its internal or external milieu (Jacobson, 1978). It is a property that is especially prominent in the developing nervous system, but it persists to some extent throughout the life span. Although it is often adaptive and may play a role in the recovery from brain injury, examples of plasticity that are maladaptive also exist (Finger and Almli, 1985). Plasticity may be expressed as structural rearrangements involving changes in neuron number as well as in number and direction of outgrowth of axons, in dendritic development, or in synaptic contacts (Purves and Lichtman, 1985). Such structural rearrangements may be associated with changes in function (functional plasticity). Key examples of plasticity, both structural and functional, are presented in this chapter, with emphasis on examples that have relevance to clinical situations.

PLASTICITY IN SENSORY SYSTEMS

Visual System

Studies of Animals

Effects of changes in the external milieu on structure and function of the developing nervous system tend to be prominent in sensory systems. Such effects have been clearly delineated in the classic work of Wiesel and Hubel on the developing visual system (Wiesel, 1982; Wiesel and Hubel 1963, 1965). Effects of visual input on structure and function of the visual cortex have been found to occur during a well-defined vulnerable or sensitive period, during which normal visual input is critical for development. In the kitten, the sensitive period, during which aberrant visual input affects the organization of the visual cortex, extends from about age 3 weeks to about age 3 months (Hubel and Wiesel, 1970). Effects on neuronal activity and on synaptic connectivity are more

marked when there is asymmetric rather than bilateral deprivation of vision, which indicates important influences based on bilateral interaction and competition. Monocular deprivation of formed visual images (pattern vision) during the sensitive period leads to an increase in the number of neurons in the visual cortex that respond to stimulation of the unaffected eye and to a marked reduction in response from the deprived eye, as well as to a decrease in the number of binocularly driven cells. Behaviorally, decreased visual responsiveness occurs in the deprived eye. These changes in function are accompanied by structural changes indicative of major rearrangements of synaptic connections. In the normal adult, alternating vertical columns of cells in layer 4c of the calcarine cortex receive predominant input from one or the other eye (ocular dominance columns). In the kitten, these columns develop during the postnatal period (LeVay et al., 1978), whereas in the monkey their development begins prenatally (Rakic, 1981). Development of ocular dominance columns is markedly changed in response to monocular visual deprivation during the sensitive period, with enlargement in the width of the columns related to the seeing eye and contraction of columns related to the deprived eye (Hubel et al., 1977).

The effects of changes in visual input that have been described up to now have primarily negative consequences as far as function is concerned. Positive effects are observed also. In animals with monocular deprivation early in the sensitive period, both the induced anatomic changes in the visual cortex and functional impairments can be reversed if pattern vision to the deprived eye is restored before the end of the sensitive period.

Changes in visual input that are more subtle than complete deprivation of pattern vision also have powerful effects on the development of visual functions. Induction of artificial squint or strabismus in kittens by unilateral section of an eye muscle such as the lateral rectus leads to a decrease in binocularly driven neurons and a decrease in the number of neurons driven by stimuli presented to the squinting eye (Hubel and Wiesel, 1965). Fitting kittens with goggles that allow viewing of only vertical or horizontal lines increases the number of cortical neurons that respond selectively to lines oriented in the direction of prior experience (Leventhal and Hirsch, 1975).

Observations of Human Infants

Counterparts to the findings in animals occur in human infants. Although little is known of structural changes related to aberrant visual input during infancy, that such changes occur can be inferred from effects on visual function that are striking and are remarkably similar to those observed in kittens and subhuman primates. Observations in human infants indicate the existence of a sensitive period similar to that found experimentally but extending over a much longer age span, from infancy to age 6 or 7 years, in keeping with the slower development of the human central nervous system (Von Noorden and Crawford, 1979). In infants with congenital cataracts, removal of the cataracts must be carried out before age 4 to 6 months to avoid permanent visual impairment (Gelbart et al., 1982; Lewis et al., 1986). The sensitive period appears to begin some time between birth and this 4- to 6-month limit. More subtle alterations in visual input during the sensitive period produce changes that may become irreversible also. Strabismus that has its onset before about age 6 years often leads to visual loss (amblyopia) in the squinting eye (Jacobsen et al., 1981). Conversely, patching of the good eye, thus forcing the child to use the squinting eye, is effective in preventing and even reversing amblyopia if it is carried out before age 6 or 7 years (Assaf, 1982). The effects in adults are quite different. Squint or loss of binocularity related to eye muscle paralysis does not cause amblyopia but rather leads to permanent diplopia.

Mechanism of Adaptation

What is the mechanism by which the developing visual cortex adapts to visual inputs? Available evidence indicates that there is a close linkage of plasticity to the process of synapse formation, or synaptogenesis. In the visual cortex, there is an early period during which there is rapid synaptogenesis. In humans, this period occurs between ages 3 and 4 months (Huttenlocher and DeCourten, 1987; Huttenlocher et al., 1982), a time during which visual responsiveness also increases rapidly and during which the visual functions that depend on cortical processing first appear (Wilson, 1988). In kittens and monkeys, rapid synaptogenesis occurs at corresponding developmental stages, also in the postnatal period (Cragg, 1975; O'Kusky and Colonnier, 1982; Rakic et al., 1986). This early period is one of exuberant synaptogenesis, during which the total num-

ber of synaptic contacts that are formed greatly exceeds the number that remain in the adult. It has been suggested that only the general outlines of neural connectivity are genetically determined and that formation of synaptic contacts, although constrained by a general developmental scheme, also has a random aspect. Many of these early synaptic contacts are thought to be redundant (Changeux and Danchin, 1976). Some of the early synaptic contacts become incorporated into functional systems, either by becoming linked to afferent inputs or by being involved in intrinsic neural circuits, a process referred to as *functional validation*. Synaptic contacts that are incorporated into functional units tend to persist, whereas others are resorbed. Synapse elimination has indeed been confirmed to exist in many neural systems, both simple ones such as the neuromuscular junction and complex ones such as the cerebral cortex. In the visual cortex of humans, synapse elimination begins at about age 6 months and is complete by age 6 or 7 years (Fig. 6–1). By late childhood the total number of synaptic contacts in human visual cortex is little more than half that found in infancy. As pointed out earlier, the period between 6 months and 7 years is also the sensitive period during which plasticity of the system can be demonstrated. It appears likely that the availability of redundant synapses during this time contributes to the observed increase in functional plasticity. This does not imply that synaptic connections become totally fixed after age 7 years. As a matter of fact, adjustments of the central nervous system to changes in afferent input continue to be demonstrable at maturity. Although the total synapse number stays constant in the adult, there is likely to be continued elimination of synaptic contacts, balanced by formation of new synaptic connections.

The schema presented in Figure 6–2 illustrates the process of synaptogenesis and synapse elimination in layer 4c of the human visual cortex and the way in which this process may be modified by amblyopia in infancy and by patching of the eye that is preferred for fixation. Approximately 50% of the synapses formed by age 6 months are eliminated between the ages of 6 months and 7 years. This process is normally symmetric and results in alternate areas of predominant input from each eye, the ocular dominance columns. In strabismus, synapse elimination is asymmetric, and by maturity there are not sufficient connections from the squinting eye for normal visual function. However, up to the end of the sensitive period, sufficient redundant synapses are available to achieve a normal number of connections related to the squinting eye, provided that input to the visual cortex via the squinting eye is modified by patching of the eye that is preferred for fixation. Not all aspects of these processes are clearly understood. For example, it is not known how the great regularity of ocular dominance columns is achieved in normal persons, each column having the same width as the next. A subtle periodic variation in the density of afferent fibers may be produced by a genetically

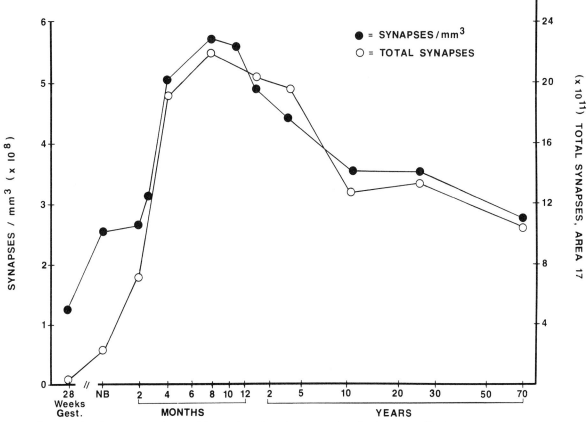

Figure 6-1. Synaptic density and an estimate of the total number of synapses in calcarine cortex (Brodmann area 17) in humans. (Reprinted with permission from Neuropsychologia, vol. 28, Huttenlocher P.R., Morphometric study of human cerebral cortex development, Copyright 1990, Pergamon Press PLC.)

determined developmental program. This difference may then become magnified by competition between the two eyes, with progressive strengthening of the input that is stronger from the start, and weakening of the input from the opposite eye (Hubel et al., 1977).

Bilateral deprivation of input from the retina during the sensitive period has effects that differ markedly from those of asymmetric input. The early physiologic observations of Wiesel and Hubel (1965) showed much less effect of bilateral than of unilateral visual deprivation on the function of neurons in visual cortex. More recent studies have further characterized the effects of bilateral deprivation. Total blockade of retinal impulses in the cat during the sensitive period by injection of tetrodotoxin into the eyes results in persistence of diffuse retinal inputs from both eyes to layer 4c of the visual cortex and prevents formation of the ocular dominance columns (Stryker and Harris, 1986). Apparently, the competition between inputs from the two eyes that normally results in formation of the ocular dominance columns depends on afferent activity. A similar effect may occur in the developing human visual system. Evidence for this comes from measurements of the regional metabolic rate of the cerebral cortex by positron emission tomography. The resting metabolic rate of the cerebral cortex is thought to be closely

linked to synaptic density (Chugani et al., 1987). It has been shown that congenitally blind adults have high rates of metabolism in the calcarine cortex (Veraart et al., 1990). This effect is not seen in blindness acquired later in life, when metabolic activity is low in the visual cortex, similar to the level found in normal subjects who have eyes closed. These observations in the human suggest that synapse elimination in the visual cortex may fail to occur normally when the system is deprived of visual input from an early age. Persistence of redundant synaptic circuits may have negative effects on the function of the cerebral cortex and may provide the basis for the frequent occurrence of epileptiform discharges in the visual cortex in congenitally blind persons.

Somatosensory System

Information concerning plasticity in sensory systems other than the visual system is more limited. However, interesting effects have been observed in the somatosensory system. In rodents, the most important somatosensory system is related to the vibrissae, which have a distinct cortical representation in the so-called barrel fields of the sensory cortex. Each vibrissa is represented in the cerebral cortex by a single, well-demarcated cortical region (barrel). It has been found that developing sensory cortex forms the exact number of barrels needed for the number

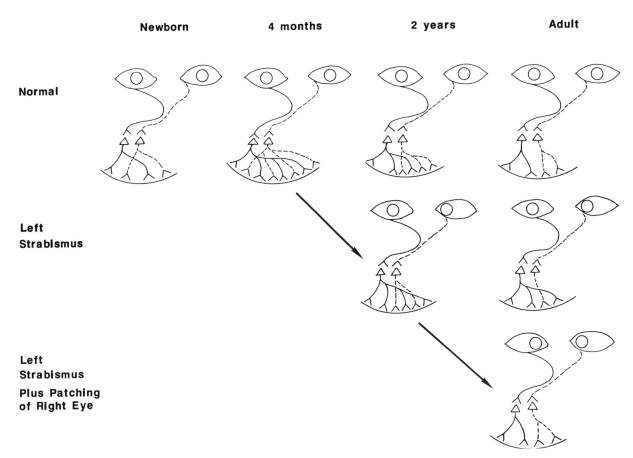

Figure 6–2. Schema illustrating the postulated effects of strabismus on input to the visual cortex from the two eyes (see text). *(Top Row)* Normal synaptogenesis and synapse elimination. *(Middle Row)* Effect of strabismus. *(Bottom Row)* Effect of patching the eye that is preferred for fixation before the end of the sensitive period.

of vibrissae. Removal of vibrissae during the sensitive period of development results in a decrease in the number of cortical barrels (Van der Loos and Doerfl, 1978; Van der Loos and Welker, 1985). Here again, sensory input to cortex during the sensitive period determines the development of cortical structure.

In the somatosensory system, plasticity has been demonstrated to persist to a considerable extent in the adult. In primates, section of the median nerve or amputation of a digit results in a rearrangement of the cortical map in the somatosensory cortex, so that neighboring regions of skin enlarge their cortical representations into the region formerly specified for the median nerve (Merzenich et al., 1983). A new, precise cortical map is created within a few weeks after the injury. This rearrangement almost certainly involves the disappearance of prior cortical connections, axonal sprouting, and creation of new synaptic contacts in adult brain.

Auditory System

We know little about plasticity in the developing auditory system. However, it is quite likely that aberrant input during critical periods of development has effects on the functioning of this system as well.

Evidence comes from the study of children with transient hearing impairments during infancy. Even partial transient hearing loss in the infant, which is a common occurrence related to otitis media, has long-lasting effects on the emergence of language functions (Hubbard et al., 1985; Teele et al., 1984). It is likely that a sensitive period exists in this system during which normal auditory input is important for its normal development, but the limits of this sensitive period are as yet unknown.

PLASTICITY IN SYSTEMS SUBSERVING HIGHER CORTICAL FUNCTIONS

Language Functions

Remarkable recovery of language functions occurs when the normal language areas are destroyed during the fetal, infancy, or early childhood periods. For the large majority of humans, language functions are localized to the left cerebral hemisphere. Anatomic evidence suggests that this lateralization is determined before birth. In most newborn infants, the region in the left hemisphere that subserves language functions, especially the left posterior temporal area, is significantly larger than the corresponding area in the right hemisphere. (Galaburda et al., 1987; Geschwind and Levitsky, 1968). Yet, early destruction of the language cortex on the left does not lead to aphasia. After extensive unilateral cortical lesions in the infant, and even after surgical hemidecortication, language development proceeds in a nearly normal fashion, although subtle effects on syntactic comprehension have been reported (Dennis and Kohn, 1975; Woods and Carey, 1979). In the child who has already acquired language functions, similar lesions produce a transient expressive aphasia. However, language functions recover within a few days of the cortical injury. Recovery after destruction of language areas in the left cerebral hemisphere becomes less after about age 8 years (Woods and Teuber, 1978a).

Several possible explanations have been advanced concerning the recovery of language functions in young children. The most cogent hypothesis holds that language is initially represented bilaterally. However, there is competition for language processing between the two hemispheres, and the left usually becomes predominant. Loss of function in circuits related to language processing in the right hemisphere leads to gradual disappearance of these circuits—another possible example of selective, normally occurring synapse elimination during cortical development. In the normal adult state, the right hemisphere has only limited residual language functions, mainly related to prosody, or the melody of language (Ross, 1981; Weintraub et al., 1981).

Association Cortex

In cortical regions concerned with higher-level processing, as in primary sensory areas, there is evidence that input to the system during early development affects the system's eventual organization. Evidence in humans comes from electrophysiologic studies of persons with congenital deafness. Neville and associates (1983) have found that visual evoked responses in areas remote from the occipital cortex, including the temporal and frontal areas, are larger in subjects with congenital deafness than in those with normal hearing. Apparently, circuits that would have been specified for the processing of auditory information have been recruited for visual processing. Such changes may underlie the remarkable ability of persons who have lost one sensory modality to utilize others, such as, for example, a deaf person's ability to perform lip reading.

Intellectual Functions

Undoubtedly, systems subserving cognitive functions partake in the plasticity that is a property of other cortical regions. In animal studies, numerous attempts have been made to enhance cortical structure and function by early environmental enrichment. Effects of enriched environments on the de-

velopment of the cerebral cortex have been reported in rodents. These effects include an increase in the width of the cortical mantle (Diamond, 1967), an increase in the number of synapses per neuron, a decrease in neuronal density, and an increase in capillary growth (Sirevaag and Greenough, 1988; Turner and Greenough, 1985).

In humans, there is evidence that early environmental stimulation, in the preschool years, improves learning and that such effects carry over into later childhood years. A benefit of early intervention has been shown both in normal children (McCartney, 1984; McCartney et al., 1985; Ramey et al., 1984; The Infant Health and Development Program, 1990) and in those with developmental disabilities (Francis-Williams and Davies, 1974; Wetherby et al., 1989), including Down's syndrome (Carr, 1970).

Also, interesting data suggest the persistence of plasticity during normal aging in centers that are important for cognitive processes, such as the frontal lobes. In aging human cerebral cortex, surviving neurons appear to compensate for neuronal loss by sprouting and consequent enlargement of their dendritic trees (Buell and Coleman, 1979, 1981). Similar enlargement of cortical dendritic trees has not been observed in the cerebral cortex from patients with senile dementia. It has been suggested that the compensatory dendritic growth that occurs normally may be important for maintenance of normal higher cortical functions during aging.

Unfortunately, the plasticity of cerebral cortex may also have major negative consequences relative to the development of cognitive functions. Developing cerebral cortex is particularly vulnerable to damage, especially during the period of dendritic development, synaptogenesis, and myelination that spans the first year of life. A number of metabolic disturbances and endocrine deficiencies have profound effects on brain structure and function when they occur during the vulnerable period of development. These disorders include inborn metabolic errors such as phenylketonuria and galactosemia, nutritional deficiencies, and deficiency of thyroid hormone. Structural changes in the cerebral cortex, including impaired growth of dendrites and impaired myelination of the subcortical white matter, have been described in these disorders. Functionally, the major effect is impairment of intellectual abilities. These effects are largely irreversible, even when the metabolic disturbances are corrected at a later date. This fact has given rise to neonatal screening programs to identify affected infants before the appearance of central nervous system damage and in time for therapeutic intervention.

PLASTICITY IN MOTOR SYSTEMS

Peripheral Motor System

Structural plasticity in the peripheral motor system has been demonstrated both at neuromuscular junctions and in spinal motor neurons. The processes of overproduction of synapses and subsequent synapse elimination have been well documented at the developing neuromuscular junction. In the embryo, each myocyte receives innervation from several motor neurons. However, in the mature mammal, innervation from only a single motor neuron persists. The other contacts are withdrawn, around the time of birth in rodents and probably during the fetal period in humans (Dennis et al., 1981).

Regressive changes occur in motor neurons in the spinal cord at a somewhat earlier age than does synapse elimination at the neuromuscular junction. About half of the initially formed motor neurons degenerate in most species studied, in what has been called programmed cell death (Cowan et al., 1984). Normally occurring cell death has been studied most intensively in the chick embryo (Hamburger, 1975). Cell death in the chick spinal motor neuron pool can be influenced by manipulation of the size of the target. Decreasing target size by amputation of a limb in the embryo increases cell death of motor neurons. Of more interest, programmed cell death is diminished by transplantation of an extra limb in the embryo, which thereby increases the target available for innervation (Hollyday and Hamburger, 1976). It has been proposed that persistence of embryonic neurons depends on target finding: neurons that find a target for innervation persist, whereas neurons that fail to find targets degenerate. This may not be the only mechanism, however. Spinal motor neurons that will eventually undergo normal cell death appear to make neuromuscular synapses before degeneration. Functional activity appears to be a factor in neuronal death in this system. Neuromuscular blockade at the critical time for neuronal death prevents it (Pittman and Oppenheim, 1979), and excessive stimulation of developing muscle enhances it (Oppenheim and Nunez, 1982). Programmed cell death has been observed to occur in many developing systems, including several brain stem nuclei (Rogers and Cowan, 1973) and the mammalian retina (Rakic and Riley, 1983). However, it appears not to be universal. For example, it appears to play a minor role in the development of mammalian cerebral cortex, with only a 15% loss of neurons in the visual cortex of monkeys between birth and maturity (O'Kusky and Colonnier, 1982), and with no loss of neurons demonstrated during late fetal and postnatal development of human visual cortex (Huttenlocher, 1990). This difference in the importance of cell death may be related to the availability of numerous targets in a system of great complexity, such as cerebral cortex, compared, for example, with retinal ganglion cells, which have only a limited and specific target for innervation. Programmed cell death occurs prenatally in most systems. Its importance to pathologic processes is therefore limited to prenatal developmental disorders. It is likely that excessive cell death during embryogenesis plays a role in some types of fetal malformation. For example, it has been observed to occur in a genetic cerebellar malformation in the

mouse, the weaver mutation, in which there is excessive death of granule cells (Sotelo and Changeux, 1974).

Central Motor Systems

Plasticity in central motor pathways has been studied extensively in the developing pyramidal motor system in rodents. In the rat, the pyramidal tract is normally an almost entirely crossed system. Ablation of motor cortex on one side before about 10 days postnatal age results in the formation of an uncrossed corticospinal tract in addition to the normal crossed projection, both originating from the remaining normal cerebral hemisphere (D'Amato and Hicks, 1978; Hicks, 1975; Hicks and D'Amato, 1977). This change is accomplished by enlargement of the cortical areas in which pyramidal tract cells occur—an example of modification of cortical representation secondary to focal brain damage (Huttenlocher and Raichelson, 1989) (Fig. 6–3). Formation of the aberrant uncrossed tract appears to depend in part on the availability of a pool of transient corticospinal axons that are normally present in the postnatal rat. These transient fibers grow into the upper spinal cord, but in the normal situation they apparently fail to find targets for innervation (Joosten et al., 1987). They are withdrawn after postnatal day 10, at about the time when development of the brain in rodents approximates that of the human neonate. Ingrowth of fibers into the ipsilateral spinal cord never occurs normally. The formation of an uncrossed corticospinal tract after neonatal motor cortex ablation therefore appears to be an example of de novo formation of connections

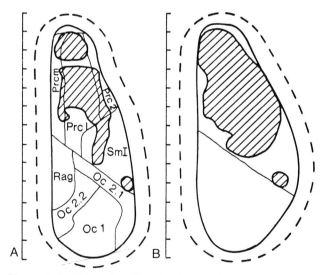

Figure 6–3. Maps of regions in the cerebral cortex in which pyramidal motor neurons are found. *(A)* Normal map, with the motor cortex shaded and outlines of cortical regions according to Zilles et al. (1980). Prc = precentral; Sm = sensorimotor; Rag = area retrosplenialis agranularis; Oc = occipital areas. *(B)* Map of the motor cortex region in the remaining cerebral hemisphere after postnatal hemispherectomy. (Modified from Huttenlocher P.R., Raichelson R.M. Effects of neonatal hemispherectomy on location and number of corticospinal neurons in the rat. *Dev. Brain Res.* 47:59–69, 1989.)

in response to injury in the central nervous system. It differs from regeneration in that it is not a regrowth of a pathway that has been severed, but rather a redirection of growing fibers that as yet have not found a target. Regeneration in the sense of regrowth of severed connections has been observed to occur to a limited extent in the mammalian central nervous system. It can be enhanced by insertion of splints made of peripheral nerve segments into transected central fiber tracts (Aguayo et al., 1982a,b). It has been postulated that regeneration of axons requires surfaces that contain adhesion molecules such as laminin, which are absent in the central nervous system after the embryonic period but which are provided by peripheral nerve sheaths.

The growth of an uncrossed corticospinal tract after neonatal unilateral cortical injury in the rat appears to be of functional significance. Animals with neonatal lesions have better motor function than those with later ablations (Kolb and Whishaw, 1989). Similar observations in monkeys, made many years ago by Kennard (Kennard, 1942), were not confirmed in a later study (Passingham et al., 1983); however, lesions may have been made past the period for maximal plasticity in monkeys. In the human, clinical observations provide evidence for limited functional plasticity in motor systems. Prenatal or early postnatal destruction of the motor cortex on one side causes significant, permanent motor deficits, especially of the upper limb, where hand and finger movements are severely impaired. Gait is less affected, and even patients with total hemidecortication early in childhood walk remarkably well (Ueki, 1966). In part, this finding may be related to normal bilateral representation of gait. More direct evidence of plasticity in motor systems comes from the occurrence of mirror movements, which are especially prominent in persons with early unilateral central motor lesions. Mirror movements occur on voluntary movement of both the normal side and the paretic side, which suggests that the same system, presumably in the remaining intact hemisphere, subserves volitional movements on both sides (Woods and Teuber, 1978b).

MECHANISMS

Plasticity in the immature brain, which may underlie both enhanced recovery from injury and certain forms of developmental error (for example, strabismic amblyopia), is almost certainly, at least in part, related to overproduction of neural elements, which occurs as a normal developmental event. Overproduction may involve neurons, axonal and dendritic processes, and synapses. Plasticity appears to be mediated by the persistence of structures that are normally transient. Several examples of persistence of transient structures were described earlier in this chapter, especially in the discussion of plasticity in motor systems. Factors that lead to persistence of

normally transient structures include enlargement of targets that are available for innervation and changes in afferent input during critical developmental periods. A general schema of mechanisms of plasticity is provided in Table 6–1.

Plasticity persists to a lesser extent in the adult brain. The observed effects, such as those described for the somatosensory cortex (Calford and Tweedale, 1990; Merzenich et al., 1983) and for motor systems (Sanes et al., 1990), may be related in part to the unmasking of connections by removal of inhibitory influences. For example, in any given region of somatosensory cortex, there is an overlap of synaptic input from adjacent regions of skin. Elimination of the major input by local anesthesia or by sensory nerve section removes inhibitory influences normally exerted by the major innervation and thereby reveals weaker connections from adjacent areas. This effect has been shown to exist by the study of cortical sensory maps immediately after nerve block (Calford and Tweedale, 1990). Limited degrees of axonal sprouting and the formation of new synapses may also be factors. Regrowth of severed axons does not occur in the mammalian central nervous system, but mature axons do have the capacity to adjust to damage in such a way as to affect function, a property that is discussed in Chapter 3.

CONCLUSION

Available evidence suggests considerable functional plasticity for several years after birth in humans, especially in cortical systems. At the same time, it is clear that many developmental events, especially those in subcortical structures, follow relatively fixed sequences that take place during specific and immutable developmental periods. Also, plasticity is associated with increased vulnerability, with sensitive periods during which abnormal influences may lead to developmental errors that may be irreversible. This problem is well illustrated by the effects of asymmetric visual input on development of the

Table 6–1. SCHEMA ILLUSTRATING MAJOR MECHANISMS OF PLASTICITY IN THE DEVELOPING NERVOUS SYSTEM

Period	Mechanism
Early development (relatively fixed genetic program)	Overproduction of neurons Exuberant growth of axons Exuberant dendritic sprouting Overproduction of synapses
Late development (modifiable by environment)	Programmed neuronal death Axon withdrawal Pruning of dendrites Synapse elimination
Factors that modify late development	Change in target size Neuronal activity Other (growth factors, metabolic and endocrine changes)

visual cortex and by the special vulnerability of developing cerebral cortex to damage by metabolic disturbances.

Positive effects of plasticity on function occur mainly after certain types of unilateral brain damage. The outstanding example in humans is the recovery of language functions after early dominant hemisphere injury. Plasticity may also play an important role in early learning. Enrichment programs designed for both normal children and those at risk for developmental disabilities appear to be most effective when applied during the preschool years, that is, during the period when plasticity of the human cerebral cortex is known to be high. However, solid data regarding the optimal ages for such effects, their limits, and their mechanisms are still lacking.

References

(Key references are designated with an asterisk.)

Aguayo A.J., David S., Richardson P., et al. Axonal elongation in peripheral and central nervous system transplants. *Adv. Cell Neurobiol.* 3:215–234, 1982a.

Aguayo A.J., Richardson P.M., Benrey M. Transplantation of neurons and sheath cells—a tool for the study of regeneration. In Nicholls J.G., ed. *Repair and Regeneration of the Nervous System.* Life Sciences Research Report 24. Berlin, Springer-Verlag, pp. 91–106, 1982b.

Assaf A.A. The sensitive period: transfer of fixation after occlusion for strabismic amblyopia. *Br. J. Ophthalmol.* 66:64–70, 1982.

Buell S.J., Coleman P.D. Dendritic growth in the aged human brain and failure of growth in senile dementia. *Science* 206:854–856, 1979.

Buell S.J., Coleman P.D. Quantitative evidence for selective dendritic growth in normal human aging but not in senile dementia. *Brain Res.* 214:23–41, 1981.

Calford M.B., Tweedale R. Interhemispheric transfer of plasticity in the cerebral cortex. *Science* 244:805–807, 1990.

Carr J. Mental and motor development of young mongol children. *J. Ment. Defic. Res.* 14:205–220, 1970.

*Changeux J.-P., Danchin A. Selective stabilization of developing synapses as a mechanism for the specification of neuronal networks. *Nature* 264:705–712, 1976.

*Chugani H.T., Phelps M.E., Mazziotta J.C. Positron emission tomography of human brain functional development. *Ann. Neurol.* 22:487–497, 1987.

*Cowan W.M., Fawcett J.W., O'Leary D.D.M., et al. Regressive events in neurogenesis. *Science* 225:1258–1265, 1984.

Cragg B.G. The development of synapses in the visual system of the cat. *J. Comp. Neurol.* 160:147–166, 1975.

D'Amato C.J., Hicks S.P. Normal development and posttraumatic plasticity of corticospinal neurons in rats. *Exp. Neurol.* 60:557–569, 1978.

Dennis M., Kohn B. Comprehension of syntax in infantile hemiplegias after cerebral hemidecortication: left hemisphere superiority. *Brain Lang.* 2:472–482, 1975.

Dennis M.J., Ziskind-Conhaim L., Harris A.J. Development of neuromuscular junctions in rat embryos. *Dev. Biol.* 81:266–279, 1981.

Diamond M.C. Extensive cortical depth measurements and neuron size increases in the cortex of environmentally enriched rats. *J. Comp. Neurol.* 131:357–364, 1967.

Finger S., Almli C.R. Brain damage and neuroplasticity: mechanisms of recovery or development? *Brain Res. Rev.* 10:177–186, 1985.

Francis-Williams J., Davies P.A. Very low birth weight and intelligence. *Dev. Med. Child Neurol.* 16:709–728, 1974.

Galaburda A.M., Corsiglia J., Rosen G.D., et al. Planum temporale asymmetry: reappraisal since Geschwind and Levitsky. *Neuropsychologia* 25:853–868, 1987.

Gelbart S.S., Hoyt C.S., Jastrebski G., et al. Long-term visual results in bilateral congenital cataracts. *Am. J. Ophthalmol.* 93:615–621, 1982.

Geschwind M., Levitsky W. Human brain: left-right asymmetrics in temporal speech region. *Science* 161:186–187, 1968.

Hamburger V. Cell death in the development of the lateral motor column of the chick embryo. *J. Comp. Neurol.* 160:535–546, 1975.

Hicks S.P. Functional adaptation after brain injury and malformation in early life in rats. In Ellis, N. ed. *Aberrant Development in Infancy.* Hillsdale, NJ, Erlbaum, pp. 27–47, 1975.

Hicks S.P., D'Amato J.C. Locating corticospinal neurons by retrograde axonal transport of horseradish peroxidase. *Exp. Neurol.* 56:410–420, 1977.

Hollyday M., Hamburger V. Reduction of the naturally occurring motor neuron loss by enlargement of the periphery. *J. Comp. Neurol.* 170:311–320, 1976.

Hubbard T.W., Paradise J.L., McWilliams B.J., et al. Consequences of unremitting middle-ear disease in early life: otologic, audiologic and developmental findings in children with cleft palate. *N. Engl. J. Med.* 312:1529–1534, 1985.

Hubel D.H., Wiesel T.N. Binocular interaction in striate cortex of kittens reared with artificial squint. *J. Neurophysiol.* 26:994–1059, 1965.

Hubel D.H., Wiesel T.N. The period of susceptibility to the physiological effects of unilateral eye closure in kittens. *J. Physiol. (Lond.)* 206:419–436, 1970.

Hubel D.H., Wiesel T.N., LeVay S. Plasticity of ocular dominance columns in the monkey striate cortex. *Philos. Trans. R. Soc. Lond.* [*Biol.*] 278:377–409, 1977.

Huttenlocher P.R. Morphometric study of human cerebral cortex development. *Neuropsychologia* 28:517–527, 1990.

Huttenlocher P.R., deCourten C. The development of synapses in striate cortex of man. *Hum. Neurobiol.* 6:1–9, 1987.

Huttenlocher P.R., Raichelson R.M. Effects of neonatal hemispherectomy on location and number of corticospinal neurons in the rat. *Dev. Brain Res.* 47:59–69, 1989.

Huttenlocher P.R., deCourten C., Garey L.G., et al. Synaptogenesis in human visual cortex—evidence for synapse elimination during normal development. *Neurosci. Lett.* 33:247–252, 1982.

Jacobsen S.G., Mohindra I., Held R. Age of onset of amblyopia in infants with esotropia. In Maffei L., ed. *Documents in Ophthalmology Proceedings Series.* Vol. 30. The Hague, Junk Publishers, pp. 210–216, 1981.

Jacobson M. *Developmental Neurobiology.* 2nd ed. New York, Plenum Publishing, 1978.

Joosten E.A.J., Gribnau A.A.M., Dederen P.J.W.C. An anterograde tracer study of the developing corticospinal tract in the rat: three components. *Dev. Brain Res.* 36:121–130, 1987.

Kennard M.A. Cortical reorganization of motor function: studies on a series of monkeys of various ages from infancy to maturity. *A.M.A. Arch. Neurol.* 48:227–240, 1942.

Kolb B., Whishaw I.Q. Plasticity in the neocortex: mechanisms underlying recovery from early brain damage. *Prog. Neurobiol.* 32:235–276, 1989.

LeVay S., Stryker M.P., Shatz C.J. Ocular dominance columns and their development in layer IV of the cat's visual cortex: a quantitative study. *J. Comp. Neurol.* 179:223–244, 1978.

Leventhal A.G., Hirsch V.V.B. Cortical effects of early selective exposure to diagonal lines. *Science* 190:902–904, 1975.

Lewis T.L., Maurer D., Brent H.P. Effect on perceptual development of visual deprivation during infancy. *Br. J. Ophthalmol.* 70:214–220, 1986.

McCartney K. Effects of quality of day care environment on children's language development. *Dev. Psychol.* 20:244–260, 1984.

McCartney K., Scarr S., Phillips D. Day care as intervention: comparisons of varying quality programs. *J. Appl. Dev. Psychol.* 6:247–260, 1985.

Merzenich M.M., Kaas J.H., Wall J.T., et al. Progression of change following median nerve section in the cortical representation of the hand in areas 3b and 1 in adult owl and squirrel monkeys. *Neuroscience* 10:639–665, 1983.

Neville H.H., Schmidt A., Kutas M. Altered visual-evoked potentials in congenitally deaf adults. *Brain Res.* 266:127–132, 1983.

O'Kusky J., Colonnier M. Postnatal changes in the number of neurons and synapses in the visual cortex (A17) of the macaque monkey. *J. Comp. Neurol.* 210:291–306, 1982.

Oppenheim R.W., Nunez R. Electrical stimulation of hindlimb increases neuronal cell death in chick embryo. *Nature* 295:57–59, 1982.

Passingham R.E., Perry V.H., Wilkinson F. The long-term effects of removal of sensorimotor cortex in infant and adult rhesus monkeys. *Brain* 106:675–705, 1983.

Pittman R., Oppenheim R.W. Cell death of motoneurons in the chick embryo spinal cord. IV. Evidence that a functional neuromuscular interaction is involved in the regulation of naturally occurring cell death and the stabilization of synapses. *J. Comp. Neurol.* 187:425–446, 1979.

*Purves D., Lichtman J.W. *Principles of Neural Development.* Sunderland, MA, Sinauer Associates, 1985.

Rakic P. Development of visual centers in the primate brain depends on binocular competition before birth. *Science* 214:928–931, 1981.

Rakic P., Riley K.P. Overproduction and elimination of retinal axons in fetal rhesus monkey. *Science* 219:1441–1444, 1983.

Rakic P., Bourgeois J.-P., Eckenhoff M.F., et al. Concurrent overproduction of synapses in diverse regions of primate cerebral cortex. *Science* 232:232–234, 1986.

Ramey C.T., Yeates K.O., Short E.J. The plasticity of intellectual development: insights from preventive intervention. *Child Dev.* 55:1913–1925, 1984.

Rogers L.A., Cowan W.M. The development of the mesencephalic nucleus of the trigeminal nerve in the chick. *J. Comp. Neurol.* 147:291–320, 1973.

Ross E.D. The aprosodias: functional anatomic organization of the affective components of language in right hemisphere. *Arch. Neurol.* 38:561–569, 1981.

Sanes J.N., Suner S., Donoghue J.P. Dynamic organization of primary motor cortex output to target muscles in adult rats. *Exp. Brain Res.* 79:479–491, 1990.

Sirevaag A.M., Greenough W.T. A multivariate statistical summary of synaptic plasticity measures in rats exposed to complex, social and individual environments. *Brain Res.* 441:386–392, 1988.

Sotelo C., Changeux J.-P. Bergmann fibers and granular cell migration in the cerebellum of homozygous weaver mutant mouse. *Brain Res.* 77:484–491, 1974.

Stryker M.P., Harris W.A. Binocular impulse blockade prevents the formation of ocular dominance columns in cat visual cortex. *J. Neurosci.* 6:2117–2133, 1986.

Teele D.W., Klein J.O., Rosner B.A. Otitis media with effusion during the first three years of life and development of speech and language. *Pediatrics* 74:282–287, 1984.

The Infant Health and Development Program. Enhancing the outcomes of low-birth-weight, premature infants. A multisite, randomized trial. *J.A.M.A.* 263:3035–3042, 1990.

Turner A.M., Greenough W.T. Differential rearing effects on rat visual cortex synapses. I. Synaptic and neuronal density and synapses per neuron. *Brain Res.* 329:195–203, 1985.

Ueki K. Hemispherectomy in the human with special reference to the preservation of function. *Prog. Brain Res.* 21:285–338, 1966.

Van der Loos H., Doerfl J. Does the skin tell the somatosensory cortex how to construct a map of the periphery? *Neurosci. Lett.* 7:23–30, 1978.

Van der Loos H., Welker E. Development and plasticity of somatosensory brain maps. In *Development, Organization, and Processing in Somatosensory Pathways.* New York, Liss, pp. 53–67, 1985.

Veraart C., De Volder A.G., Wanet-Defalque M.C., et al. Glucose utilization in human visual cortex is abnormally elevated in blindness of early onset but decreased in blindness of late onset. *Brain Res.* 510:115–121, 1990.

*Von Noorden G.K., Crawford M.L.J. The sensitive period. *Trans. Ophthalmol. Soc. U.K.* 99:442–446, 1979.

Weintraub S., Mesulam M.-M., Kramer L. Disturbances in prosody: a right hemisphere contribution to language. *Arch. Neurol.* 38:742–744, 1981.

Wetherby A., Yonclas D., Bryan A. Communicative profiles of 289 preschool children with handicaps: implications for early intervention. *J. Speech Hear. Disord.* 54:148–158, 1989.

*Wiesel T.N. Postnatal development of the visual cortex and the influence of environment. *Nature* 299:583–591, 1982.

Wiesel T.N., Hubel D.H. Single cell responses in striate cortex of kittens deprived of vision in one eye. *J. Neurophysiol.* 26:1003–1017, 1963.

Wiesel T.N., Hubel D.H. Comparison of the effects of unilateral and bilateral eye closure on cortical unit responses in kittens. *J. Neurophysiol.* 28:1029–1040, 1965.

Wilson H.R. Development of spatiotemporal mechanisms in infant vision. *Vision Res.* 28:611–628, 1988.

Woods B.T., Carey S. Language deficits after apparent clinical recovery from childhood aphasia. *Ann. Neurol.* 6:405–409, 1979.

Woods B.T., Teuber H.L. Changing patterns of childhood aphasia. *Ann. Neurol.* 3:273–280, 1978a.

Woods B.T., Teuber H.L. Mirror movements after childhood hemiparesis. *Neurology* 28:1152–1158, 1978b.

Zilles K., Zilles B., Schleicher A. A quantitative approach to cytoarchitectonics. IV. The areal pattern of the cortex of the albino rat. *Anat. Embryol.* 159:335–360, 1980.

7

Glial Cell Lineages in Development and Disease

R.K. Small

Glial precursor cells in the central nervous system (CNS) are generated in the germinal matrix of the subventricular zone and then migrate to target regions where differentiation occurs. This sequence, composed of proliferation and migration followed by differentiation, is a general scheme that can be broadly applied to both the neurons and the glial cells of the CNS. Glial cells retain the capacity for proliferation long after they have migrated from the ventricular layers, whereas migrating neurons are postmitotic cells. Neural cell populations are generated in successive but overlapping waves, and as each population undergoes its sequence of development, the embryonic neural tube is gradually transformed from a single-layered epithelial sheet into the complex structure of the adult brain. The orderly manner in which mammalian development proceeds suggests that regulatory mechanisms operate on many levels to ensure the proper timing of proliferation, guidance of migration, and induction of differentiation.

A necessary first step to untangling cellular interactions of this complexity has been to unambiguously identify the key participants. The use of cell type–specific antibodies has provided a basis for distinguishing the various neural cell types and for isolating and purifying glial cells for in vitro studies of function. These advances have highlighted the central role played by glial cells in early events of CNS development. In addition, antibodies directed against specific cellular and substrate components have, in several instances, permitted an identification of candidate molecules that mediate early cellular interactions.

TYPES AND FUNCTIONS OF CNS GLIA

Radial Glia

The earliest glia found in the embryonic CNS are radial glia, a class of cells with radial processes that span the entire thickness of the developing CNS. In the primate brain, radial glia can be detected as early as the sixth week of gestation (Levitt and Rakic, 1980). Radial glia are thought to provide positional information for young neurons migrating from the ventricular surface into the developing cortical plate. Neuroblasts in embryonic brain and spinal cord have been shown by electron microscopy to adhere closely to glial processes, and it is thought that these radial fibers provide guidance pathways that direct neurons to their final positions in the developing gray matter (Rakic, 1971; Sidman and Rakic, 1973.) Trajectories of radial glia vary throughout the CNS, perhaps creating regionally unique migratory pathways that contribute to the architectonic distinctions observed in the CNS (Rakic, 1981).

There is considerable variation in the intermediate filament subunits expressed by radial glia. The occasional presence of subunits of glial fibrillary acidic protein (GFAP) in radial glia of some species, as well as ultrastructural features that are characteristic of astrocytes (e.g., puncta adhaerentia), has been taken as evidence that radial glia give rise to astrocytes. Transitional cell types showing features intermediate to radial glia and astrocytes have been described in the cortex (Schmechel and Rakic, 1979). Studies of the embryonic spinal cord, however, suggest that radial glia may serve as common precursors for both

72

astrocytes and oligodendrocytes (Hirano and Goldman, 1988). The exact relationship of the embryonic radial glia to cell types occurring later in development requires further study.

Most radial glia do not persist in the mature CNS. Two notable exceptions are the Bergmann glia of the cerebellum and the Müller cells of the retina. Both of these unique classes of glia maintain a radial orientation in the mature brain but differ from embryonic radial glia by positioning the cell bodies midway along their radial processes rather than in the ventricular layers (Fig. 7–1). They also retain intermediate filament characteristics that are associated with immature glia. In mature astrocytes, intermediate filaments are heteropolymers composed primarily of GFAP and, to a lesser extent, vimentin subunits; in immature cells, intermediate filaments consist largely of vimentin subunits. Müller cells of most species and Bergmann glia of avian species express the immature vimentin-type filaments. It is interesting that Müller cells can express GFAP and do so in response to retinal injury or pathologic changes (Bignami and Dahl, 1979). Techniques for obtaining purified cultures of retinal Müller cells (e.g., Scherer and Schnitzer, 1989; Small et al., 1991) may prove useful for examining the functions and interactions of radial types of glia and may reveal factors that trigger their expression of GFAP.

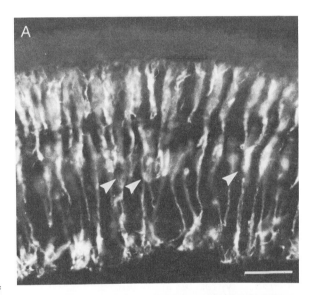

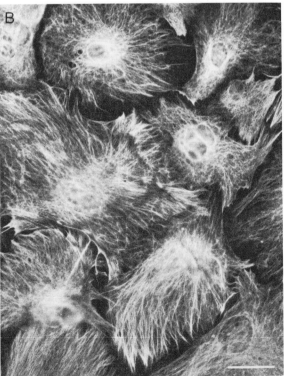

Figure 7–1. Müller cells of the retina (shown here) and Bergmann glia of the cerebellum are unique classes of glia that retain a radial orientation of the mature CNS. They differ from embryonic radial glia by positioning their cell bodies midway along their radial processes *(arrowheads* in *A)* rather than in the ventricular layers. *(A)* Müller cells are the only class of glial cells present in the guinea pig retina. Their intermediate filaments can be immunolabeled with monoclonal antibodies to vimentin but not with antibodies to GFAP. *(B)* When Müller cells from guinea pig retina are maintained in cell culture, they continue to express vimentin but not GFAP in their intermediate filaments. Scale bar for *A* = 20 μm, for *B* = 50 μm.

The molecular basis of neuronal migration on glial fibers is not yet understood, but coculture studies indicate that this interaction involves a mechanism common to neurons and glia in general. Neurons display a similar rate (10–60 μm/hour) and mode of locomotion while migrating on glia derived from diverse brain regions (Hatten, 1990). Membrane-mediated interactions between cultured neurons and glia have been shown to inhibit glial cell proliferation and to cause an alteration in glial cell shape by inducing extension of cell processes (Hatten, 1985). These effects may well be involved in the formation and maintenance of radial pathways during the period of neuronal migration.

Astrocytes

Astrocytes are the most numerous cell type in the CNS. Their name derives from the star-shaped or stellate morphology that is commonly observed. Although astrocytes can assume a variety of forms in different CNS regions, they are readily identified in vivo by immunolabeling with antibodies to the intermediate filament protein GFAP. Astrocytes in cell culture express receptors for most of the known CNS neurotransmitters, which suggests that they are highly responsive to their neurochemical milieu. The most frequent receptor class found on astrocytes is the β-adrenergic receptor. Although the function of intermediate filaments in glial cells is not known, activation of the β-adrenergic receptor has been shown to induce phosphorylation of the intermediate filament proteins GFAP and vimentin (McCarthy et al., 1985). Astrocytes are heterogeneous with respect to the class of adrenergic receptor expressed by individual cells (Lerea and McCarthy, 1989), and such differences may provide a basis for subdividing the astrocyte population in future studies.

Astroctyes account for approximately 70% of the glial cells in the rat optic nerve at birth; they thus represent the major glial cell type present during the peak period of axonal outgrowth. It is widely recognized that astrocytes promote the survival of neurons in culture and that they provide a preferred surface for neurite outgrowth (Fallon, 1985; Noble et al., 1984). When neurons are cultured on nonglial cell monolayers, there is a marked tendency for neuronal cell bodies to show aggregation and for neurites to form large fascicles. Neurons grown on astrocyte monolayers remain dispersed as single cells, and their neurites are less fasciculated. Astrocytes in culture produce extracellular matrix proteins such as laminin and fibronectin (Liesi et al., 1983; Price and Hynes, 1985). The bulk of the neurite-promoting activity present in medium conditioned by astrocyte monolayers can be assigned to fractions containing a highly sulfated laminin complex and, to a lesser extent, to free fibronectin (Matthiessen et al., 1989).

The end feet of astrocyte processes form a continuous boundary at junctions of neuroectodermal and mesenchymal tissues such as the glia limitans at the pial surface and the perivascular membrane surrounding CNS blood vessels. The formation of perivascular membranes is correlated developmentally with the appearance of a permeability barrier in the CNS, and evidence suggests that astrocytes may induce endothelial cells to express tight permeability features. When astrocytes are transplanted to peripheral locations such as the chick chorioallantoic membrane, the blood vessels that invade the cell aggregate show a permeability barrier to vascular tracers that resembles the blood-brain barrier of the CNS (Janzer and Raff, 1987).

Oligodendrocytes

Oligodendrocytes are the myelin-forming cells of the CNS. Galactocerebroside (GalC), a major glycolipid of myelin, is a specific marker for oligodendrocytes in the CNS. Myelination of CNS tracts can be regarded as the last stage in the development of the CNS. It is a protracted process that is initiated at postnatal ages and continues well into the first decade of human life. The myelin sheaths, or internodes, produced by oligodendrocytes are essential for the rapid and efficient conduction of nerve impulses along axons. Each oligodendrocyte of the CNS gives rise to 20 or more internodes on different axons, in contrast to the peripheral nervous system in which each Schwann cell is responsible for a single internode.

Mature oligodendrocytes have recently been shown to provide a nonpermissive substrate for neuronal adhesion and neurite outgrowth (Schwab and Caroni, 1988). Two membrane proteins have been identified in myelin fractions that mediate these nonpermissive effects. Absorption of oligodendrocytes or myelin fractions with antibodies generated against these proteins markedly improves or neutralizes their inhibitory substrate properties (Caroni and Schwab, 1988). These inhibitory proteins are absent in myelin isolated from peripheral nerves or in cultured Schwann cells, which may explain why axons of the CNS can show regenerative growth into transplanted peripheral nerves but show little or no growth within the adult CNS (e.g., Benfey and Aguayo, 1982). In many CNS tracts, myelin formation has been shown to begin well after the period of axonal growth (e.g., Looney and Elberger, 1986), so that elongating axons and their growth cones would not normally encounter mature oligodendrocytes. The different regenerative capacity observed in neonatal versus adult CNS tracts (e.g., Small and Leonard, 1983), as well as the existence of critical periods for successful regrowth in the neonate, may in part be based on the schedule of oligodendrocyte maturation in particular fiber tracts.

Studies of glial cells in the developing optic nerve have yielded some of our most accurate information on the time of appearance of different classes of glia as well as the identity of factors that coordinate the proliferation and differentiation of glial populations. Moreover, an analysis of glial lineage relationships in the optic nerve has led to new ideas about the sequence of events leading to the formation of myelinated tracts in the CNS.

TWO DISTINCT GLIAL LINEAGES IN THE OPTIC NERVE

The optic nerve provides a simple model system that is uniquely suited to examining questions of gliogenesis in the mammalian CNS. Embryonically, the nerve is derived from the optic stalk, which is an extension of the neural tube composed of germinal neuroepithelium. The neural cell population of the mature nerve is composed exclusively of glial cells, which provide the functional and structural support for axons projecting from the ganglion cells of the retina to the brain. The nerve contains no intrinsic neuronal cell bodies and this greatly simplifies its cellular profile. Two types of glial cells occur in the nerve: astrocytes and oligodendrocytes. (Cells of non-neuroectodermal origin are also present in the nerve, such as meningeal cells and small numbers of endothelial cells, pericytes, and macrophages.) The simplicity of the nerve's neural cell composition has made it a valuable preparation for establishing criteria for distinguishing glial cell types, for analyzing their lineage relationships, and for determining the origins of precursors for the different glial populations of the nerve.

By using antibodies specific for cell types, Raff et al. (see 1989 for review) have identified two distinct glial precursor cells in the developing rat optic nerve. One is a type 1 astrocyte precursor that gives rise to astrocytes, the first mature glial cells found in the developing nerve. Astrocytes can be detected in the nerve as early as embryonic day 16 (E16) by their expression of GFAP, the intermediate filament protein. Type 1 astrocytes are the only mature glial cells present in the nerve at ages when growing neurites of retinal ganglion cells enter the nerve to reach targets in the brain. Five days later, on the day of birth (E21), the first immature oligodendrocytes are detected in the nerve, and their numbers continue to increase during the following weeks (Skoff et al., 1976a,b). Oligodendrocytes are derived from a second type of precursor cell, which can be identified by antibodies to cell surface gangliosides (A_2B_5) and glycoproteins (e.g., NSP-4). The oligodendrocyte precursor is a small cell with a perikaryon of approximately 7 μm from which long bipolar processes extend (Fig. 7–2). The cell processes terminate in a structure resembling the axonal growth cone, a membranous expansion with many fine filopodial projections (see Fig. 7–2C).

In vitro experiments suggest that oligodendrocyte precursors are biopotential cells (Raff et al., 1983): when cultured in chemically defined medium, these precursors differentiate into oligodendrocytes, but when cultured in medium containing 10% fetal calf serum, they fail to express oligodendrocyte differentiation markers and instead express GFAP, the astrocyte marker (Fig. 7–3). Oligodendrocyte precursors have thus been called oligodendrocyte–type 2 astrocyte, or O-2A, progenitor cells on the basis of their bipotential behavior in vitro. Type 2 astrocytes are multipolar cells that express A_2B_5 and NSP-4 on their surface. In contrast, type 1 astrocytes are non–process-bearing, or epithelioid, cells that lack these markers (Table 7–1). Type 2 astrocytes have proved to be difficult to identify unambiguously in vivo (compare Skoff, 1990 and Miller et al., 1985), and current research is focused on identifying and defining this cell's role in the CNS. The formation of myelinated tracts during CNS development requires the presence of a pool of oligodendrocyte precursors in developing tracts at ages when axons become myelin competent. Each O-2A precursor cell can generate an oligodendrocyte clone of variable size when the precursor is cultured in the presence of appropriate growth factors (Temple and Raff, 1986).

Glial cell cultures derived from human fetal optic nerves display many properties similar to those observed in cultures of rat optic nerve glia (Kennedy and Fok-Seang, 1986). Oligodendrocytes appear to be derived from A_2B_5-positive precursor cells, and two populations of GFAP-positive astrocytes can be distinguished on the basis of A_2B_5 labeling. When human optic nerve suspensions are treated with A_2B_5 antibody and complement, oligodendrocytes fail to develop in culture. However, unlike rat optic nerve cultures, A_2B_5-positive astrocytes as well as A_2B_5-positive cells that are negative for both GalC and GFAP are still present in human optic nerve cultures after complement treatment. Because of these results, it has not been possible to determine if human A_2B_5-positive precursors are bipotential cells capable of giving rise to both oligodendrocytes and astrocytes. A possible cause for the differences in rat and human optic nerve cultures is that the gestational age of the human cultures (16–18 weeks) is likely to represent an earlier stage of development than the perinatal rat cultures. Bipotential O-2A precursor cells resembling those of the rat optic nerve have been demonstrated in a variety of regions of rodent brain including the cerebrum (Behar et al., 1988; Williams et al. 1985) and the cerebellum (Levi et al., 1986).

SEPARATE ORIGINS FOR THE TWO GLIAL LINEAGES OF THE OPTIC NERVE

The identification of two cell lineages within the optic nerve, based on the time of appearance of each lineage and the phenotypic differences of the precursor cells, has been reinforced by in vivo developmental studies that indicate that precursors of these two lineages are generated from separate germinal sources in the CNS (Small, 1986; Small et al.,

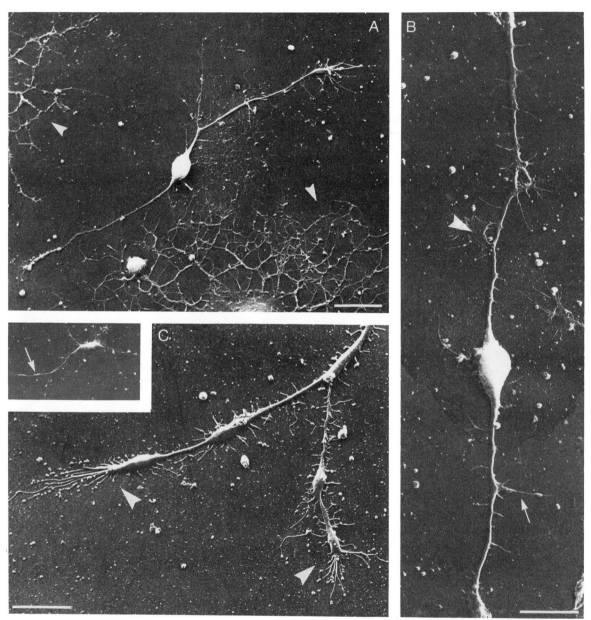

Figure 7–2. *(A)* Precursors of the myelin-forming oligodendrocytes of the CNS are small motile cells with long bipolar cell processes. These precursors differentiate in vitro into multipolar oligodendrocytes *(arrowheads)* when cultured in chemically defined medium. *(B)* Fine filopodial branches *(arrow)*, as well as lamellipodia *(arrowhead)*, are seen along the processes of the cell. *(C)* The cell processes terminate in small growth cone–like structures with long filopodial extensions *(arrowheads)*. Time-lapse microcinematography of precursors in vitro reveals that these growth cones are highly motile structures that expand and retract as they probe the substrate. The directional movement of the oligodendrocyte precursor is ultimately determined by the behavior of the growth cone. Scale bars for *A* and *B* = 10 μm, for *C* = 5 μm.

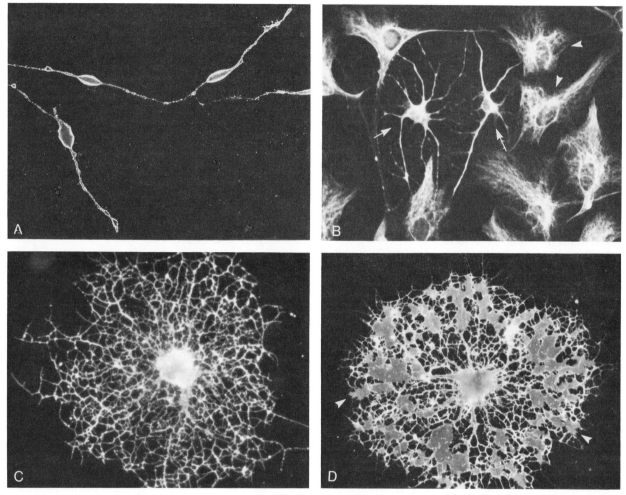

Figure 7–3. Glial cells cultured from the neonatal rat optic nerve are distinguished in vitro on the basis of both morphologic and antigenic features. *(A)* Oligodendrocyte precursors are small cells with long bipolar processes. Precursors are shown labeled with the A$_2$B$_5$ antibody, which is directed against cell surface gangliosides. *(B)* When optic nerve cells are cultured in 10% fetal calf serum, oligodendrocyte precursors fail to express myelin-specific markers and instead express GFAP. These type 2 astrocytes *(arrows)* are stellate cells that label with the A$_2$B$_5$ antibody (not shown). In contrast, the early type 1 astrocytes of the nerve *(arrowheads)* are epithelioid cells that do not label with the A$_2$B$_5$ antibody. *(C)* When cultured in the absence of serum, oligodendrocyte precursors stop dividing and differentiate into multipolar oligodendrocytes. GalC, the myelin-specific glycolipid, is expressed on the membrane of the cell body and processes. *(D)* Within 7 days in culture, anastomosing sheets of flattened membrane *(arrowheads)* appear along the cell processes as oligodendrocytes begin to synthesize myelin proteins. *A, B* × 1100; *C, D* × 2000.

Table 7–1. ANTIGENIC PHENOTYPE OF OPTIC NERVE GLIA

Cell Type (Morphology in Culture)	Immunolabeling Characteristics
O-2A precursor cells	
Neonatal (bipolar)	$A_2B_5^+$, $O4^-$, vimentin$^+$, NSP-4$^+$, GalC$^-$, GFAP$^-$
Adult (unipolar)	$A_2B_5^+$, $O4^+$, vimentin$^-$, NSP-4$^+$, GalC$^-$, GFAP$^-$
Oligodendrocytes (multipolar)	GalC$^+$, $O4^+$, $A_2B_5^{+/-}$,* vimentin$^-$, GFAP$^-$
Type 2 astrocytes (multipolar)	$A_2B_5^+$, NSP-4$^+$, vimentin$^+$, GFAP$^+$, GalC$^-$
Type 1 astrocytes (epithelioid)	GFAP$^+$, $A_2B_5^-$, NSP-4$^-$, vimentin$^+$, $O4^-$, GalC$^-$

*Oligodendrocytes lose A_2B_5 expression during maturation.

1987). Type 1 astrocyte precursors appear to be derived at early ages from the *intrinsic* neuroepithelial cells of the optic stalk, and these precursors are present in the nerve at the youngest ages examined. In contrast, O-2A precursors are highly motile cells that arise from a source (or sources) *extrinsic* to the nerve; O-2A precursor cells are not present in the nerve until late stages of development, after growing neurites have reached targets in the brain. These precursors then gradually populate the developing nerve in a progressive wave that spreads from the optic chiasm into the nerve (Small et al., 1987).

The separate origins of the optic nerve's two glial lineages highlight an organizational feature of the CNS germinal matrix that has only recently become apparent: Regions of the germinal neuroepithelium appear to be restricted in their potential to generate the different neural cell types. Thus, the optic nerve's germinal neuroepithelium is committed to generating astrocytes but not neurons or oligodendrocytes. The retinal germinal neuroepithelium displays a similar restriction in potential. Clonal analysis based on retroviral marking techniques reveals that retinal clones are composed of mixtures of various neuronal cell types and Müller (glial) cells but that no labeling is detected in the astrocytes of the retina (Turner and Cepko, 1987). Instead, retinal astrocytes appear to be derived from migratory cells that enter the retina from the region of the optic nerve head shortly before birth in the rat (Watanabe and Raff, 1988).

The optic nerve is an ideal CNS region for tracking movements of migratory precursor cells because the nerve presents a discrete linear pathway of sufficient length to permit local analyses of cell populations. Immunolabeling of the cells present in different regions of the nerve reveals that the first O-2A precursor cells detected in the nerve are localized exclusively in the region closest to the optic chiasm (Table 7–2). With increasing age, the size of the nerve's O-2A precursor population increases, and these precursors gradually spread toward the retinal pole of the nerve. Just before birth, small numbers of precursors have reached the segment of nerve closest to the retina, but the distribution of O-2A precursors remains steeply graded along the axis of the nerve. It is not until the end of the first postnatal week that a gradient is no longer detected and approximately equal numbers of precursors are present throughout the nerve. The first appearance of O-2A precursors in the optic nerve coincides with the arrival of axons from retinal ganglion cells at targets in the brain. This temporal juxtaposition raises the possibility that axons destined for myelination may have an active role in recruiting myelin-forming precursor cells into target regions and perhaps serve as a guidance pathway.

Motility of O-2A Precursors

O-2A precursor cells are highly motile in culture. Time-lapse microcinematography shows that when they are cultured in the presence of medium containing astrocyte-derived factors, precursors translocate over long distances; they move at an average rate of 21 μm/hour and can achieve maximal rates of 100 μm/hour for short periods (Small et al., 1987). When O-2A precursor cells divide, the two daughter cells migrate in opposite directions, each pursuing a path that is orientated along the original processes of the parent cell. The specialized structure seen at the tip of the precursor's bipolar processes in Figure 7–2C resembles a neuritic growth cone, suggesting that it may have motile and chemotactic properties (Small, 1985). Time-lapse cinematography provides strong support for this suggestion. This terminal structure can be seen expanding and retracting as it probes the substrate and ultimately, the path selected by this growth cone determines the direction of move-

Table 7–2. DISTRIBUTION OF O-2A PROGENITOR CELLS IN PERINATAL RAT OPTIC NERVES*

Age	Number of Progenitor Cells per Nerve Segment			Total Number of O-2A Progenitors per Nerve
	Retinal	*Middle*	*Chiasmal*	
Embryonic day 16	0	17 ± 5	89 ± 18	106
Embryonic day 17	9 ± 6	73 ± 12	236 ± 31	318
Birth	417 ± 82	728 ± 102	1,194 ± 84	2,339
Postnatal day 5	2,787 ± 106	2,846 ± 91	3,884 ± 129	9,517
Postnatal day 9	4,001 ± 463	5,380 ± 634	5,438 ± 609	14,819

*Optic nerves were divided into three equal segments termed retinal, middle, and chiasmal. Cells from each segment were dissociated and plated for 3–4 h before immunolabeling. O-2A progenitor cells were defined as $A_2B_5^+$, NSP-4$^+$, GalC$^-$, and GFAP$^-$.

Data from Small R.K., Riddle P., Noble M. Evidence for migration of oligodendrocyte-type 2 astrocyte progenitor cells into the developing rat optic nerve. *Nature* 328:155–157, 1987.

ment of the precursor cell. The motility of the O-2A precursor cell is in sharp contrast to the relative absence of movement observed after O-2A precursor cells assume a multipolar morphology and differentiate along either the oligodendrocyte or the type 2 astrocyte pathway. Multipolar cells in these cultures show minimal movement, and this is usually associated with growth of the cell's processes. In culture, O-2A precursor cells exhibit an absence of directional movement, often reversing and migrating back along their original paths. This finding is in contrast to the situation in vivo, in which developmental studies indicate that recruitment of the O-2A lineage into the optic nerve may be highly directional. The optic tract, the CNS continuation of the optic nerve beyond the optic chiasm, remains largely devoid of glia at perinatal ages when the nerve becomes filled with glia, which suggests a spatially and/or temporally discrete origin for glia of the optic tract.

Considerable evidence from a variety of experimental approaches supports the view that oligodendrocytes, their precursors, or both are capable of long-distance migration in vivo. For example, transplantation of bits of normal neonatal brain into shiverer mice, a mutant whose myelin lacks myelin basic protein (MBP), results in pockets of MBP-containing myelin located at long distances from the graft site (Lachapelle et al., 1984). Similarly, irradiation of the neonatal spinal cord is followed by a cephalocaudal infiltration of oligodendrocytes, leading to limited myelination of the rostral portion of the irradiated area (Beal and Hall, 1974; Blakemore and Patterson, 1975).

Chick-quail chimeric embryos have been used to directly visualize the process of O-2A precursor cell migration during the development of the optic nerve (Balaban and Small, 1989). When transplants of CNS tissue are exchanged at early embyonic ages between these two closely related avian species, grafts are readily integrated into the host CNS with little or no scarring (Le Douarin, 1973). The nucleus of quail cells is distinguished from that of the chick by the presence of one or more prominent clusters of heterochromatin. Any quail cells that have migrated after transplantation into the surrounding chick tissue are thus easily detected. Chimeras were constructed by unilaterally transplanting the embryonic chick optic stalk isotopically into a quail host at the 11–15 somite stage. At later ages, a population of GalC-positive oligodendrocytes derived from the quail host brain (i.e., bearing the quail nuclear marker) was present in the transplanted chick optic nerve (Fig. 7–4). Progressive infiltration of the transplant by quail-derived cells was observed when chimeras were examined at various ages after transplantation. Quail-derived cells showed a centrifugal spread along the nerve, as well as a radial spread from central to more peripheral locations in the nerve.

REGULATION OF MIGRATION OF GLIAL PRECURSOR CELLS BY DISTINCT MOLECULES

How specific are the molecules guiding the movements of glial precursor cells within the developing brain? Cell migration is a feature shared by all cells of the brain, and the striking differences in cellular distribution suggests that each cell type responds to different chemotactic cues or adhesion molecules. Young neurons appear to be guided by processes of radial glial cells as they migrate from the ventricular surface into the developing cortical plate. Astrocytes have been shown to migrate into the developing retina in close association with retinal blood vessels (Watanabe and Raff, 1988), and astrocytes transplanted into the adult CNS have been found preferentially localized along the basement membrane delimiting the perivascular space of blood vessels (Emmett et al., 1988; Goldberg and Bernstein, 1988). These observations suggest that molecules associated with blood vessels, such as laminin or other extracellular matrix molecules, may serve as specific signals that guide astrocyte migration.

In vitro studies indicate that the migratory behavior of different types of glial cells is stimulated by specific attractant molecules (Armstrong et al., 1990). Chemotaxis, or directed movement, of glia has been assayed in vitro by introducing cells into a chamber separated by a filter from a second compartment containing candidate molecules, and then counting cells that migrate through the pores of the filter. Oligodendrocyte precursors selectively migrate toward platelet-derived growth factor (PDGF) but not toward laminin or C5a (a 12-kd cleavage product of complement activation), both of which serve as attractants for astrocytes. Type 1 astrocytes synthesize the A chain of PDGF in culture (Richardson et al., 1988), and O-2A precursor cells express the PDGF α receptor (McKinnon et al., 1990). The fact that type 1 astrocytes are present throughout the optic nerve well before O-2A precursor cells have colonized the nerve raises the attractive possibility that astrocytes may provide a gradient of PDGF that guides O-2A precursor cells into the nerve and that may even contribute to the timing of migration.

A COMPARISON OF OLIGODENDROCYTE DEVELOPMENT IN VIVO AND IN VITRO

The ability to identify and isolate O-2A precursor cells with similar characteristics from the optic nerve, cerebrum, and cerebellum has provided an opportunity to study factors that regulate the proliferation and differentiation of oligodendrocyte precursor cells under defined culture conditions.

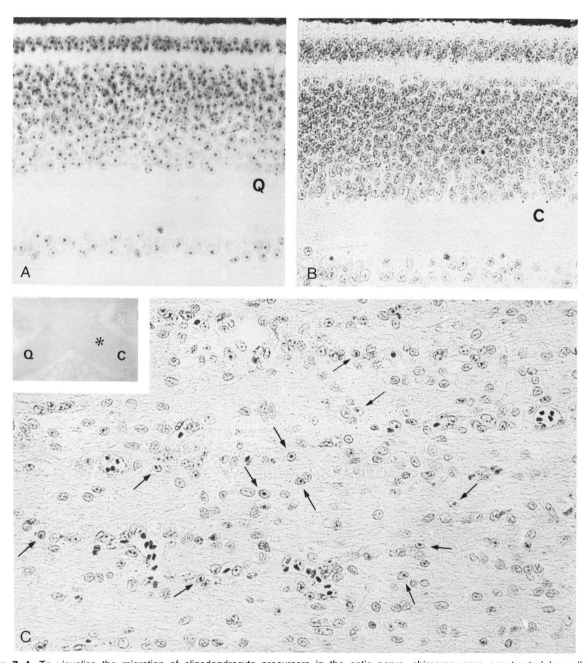

Figure 7–4. To visualize the migration of oligodendrocyte precursors in the optic nerve, chimeras were constructed by unilaterally transplanting a chick optic vesicle into a quail host at the 11–15 somite stage (i.e., 30–35 hours of incubation). The 13-day chimeric embryo contains a retina and optic nerve derived from the quail (Q) host *(A)* whose cells are readily distinguished by the prominent nuclear marker from cells derived from the chick (C) graft on the contralateral side *(B). (Inset)* The grafted chick optic nerve forms a normal decussation at the optic chiasm with no apparent scarring. The region of chick nerve at the asterisk is shown at higher magnification in *C*. A population of quail-derived cells *(arrows* in *C)* has migrated into the chick optic nerve, and many of these cells are found to express GalC, the oligodendrocyte-specific marker (Balaban and Small, 1989).

In Vivo Development

Oligodendrocyte maturation in vivo progresses through an orderly sequence in which first the lipid components of myelin and then the major proteins of myelin are expressed. This sequence is completed within each CNS tract shortly before the initiation of myelination. In the rat optic nerve, the O4 antigen (Sommer and Schnachner, 1981) is first detected the day before birth (E20) on a small number of NSP-4-positive , GalC-negative precursor cells located at the chiasmal end of the nerve. The O4 antibody recognizes an antigen complex consisting of sulfatide, seminolipid, and an unidentified antigen (Bansal et al., 1989; Sommer and Schnachner, 1981). GalC labeling can be detected a day later, at birth, on a subpopulation of O4-positive cells that again are restricted to the chiasmal end of the nerve (Small, 1988). Myelin proteins appear almost synchronously toward the end of the first postnatal week before axonal ensheathment is observed. Myelin gene products include MBP, a cytoplasmic protein associated with the major dense line of myelin; myelin-associated glycoprotein, a cell adhesion molecule thought to mediate contact between oligodendrocyte and axon membranes; proteolipid protein, a hydrophobic acylated transmembrane protein involved in myelin compaction; and 2′,3′-cyclic-nucleotide phosphohydrolase, whose function is unknown. Each of the myelin proteins occurs in several isoforms that are generated by alternative splicing of mRNA derived from single-copy genes. In situ hybridization has revealed that one of the isoforms of MBP, the exon 2–containing transcript, is present only during the initial stages of myelination both during development and in remyelination subsequent to experimentally induced demyelination (Jordon et al., 1989a,b; 1990) A similar sequence of oligodendrocyte development has been demonstrated in a variety of CNS white matter tracts, including the optic nerve and the cerebellum (Reynolds and Wilkin, 1988).

In Vitro Development

The development of oligodendrocyte precursors cultured in defined medium follows a similar sequence of appearance of differentiation markers to that observed in vivo. This sequence appears to be independent of neuronal control because it is observed when oligodendrocyte precursors are cultured in the absence of neurons. Oligodendrocyte precursors are initially bipolar cells that express cell surface gangliosides (A_2B_5) and glycoproteins (NSP-4) and contain vimentin-positive intermediate filaments. As the cells mature, they become tripolar and multipolar (see Fig. 7–3) and can be labeled with the O4 antibody (Sommer and Schachner, 1981; 1984). Cells positive for O4 can differentiate into either oligodendrocytes or astrocytes (Trotter and Schachner, 1989). The glycolipid GalC is observed soon after the ap-

pearance of O4, at a stage when the cells have become more multipolar and branched (Sommer and Schachner, 1982). Myelin proteins such as MBP, myelin-associated glycoprotein, and proteolipid protein emerge in sequence 5–7 days after the appearance of GalC (Dubois-Dalcq et al., 1986). Each of these proteins is initially confined to the cell body region and then spreads to the cell processes, with myelin-associated glycoprotein appearing first followed by MBP and proteolipid protein. As shown in Figure 7–3D, extensive flattened sheets of myelin-containing membrane appear at multiple sites along the processes of oligodendrocytes after about a week in culture (Knapp et al., 1987). During the course of differentiation, A_2B_5 expression is lost and intermediate filaments of vimentin or other known classes can no longer be detected in mature oligodendrocytes (see Table 7–2). These in vitro studies clearly indicate that oligodendrocyte differentiation through stages of myelin gene expression is regulated independent of neuronal influence.

Oligodendrocytes and their precursors express the neural cell adhesion molecule (N-CAM) on their surface. N-CAM encompasses a group of related molecules that appear to mediate intercellular adhesion through homophilic binding between cells expressing N-CAM (reviewed in Edelman, 1986). Structural diversity in the N-CAM molecule is generated by extensive transcriptional and post-translational modification of a single-copy gene. Stage-specific variation in the N-CAM molecule may underlie the diversity of developmental roles assigned to this molecule, which include cell migration, axon fasciculation, and stabilization of cell assemblies. The form of N-CAM expressed on the oligodendrocyte lineage has been shown to vary with the stage of differentiation. Bipolar A_2B_5-positive precursor cells have the highly sialylated, embryonic form of N-CAM on their surface, whereas more mature oligodendrocytes express only the adult 120-kd and 140-kd forms of the N-CAM molecule (Trotter et al., 1989). The transition from the embryonic to the adult form of the molecule is correlated with the expression of the O4 antigen on O-2A precursor cells. Embryonic N-CAM has been found to be less adhesive than the adult form of N-CAM (Sadoul et al., 1983) and it may thus facilitate the motility of migratory precursor cells. Similarly, the shift to the adult form of N-CAM may be associated with the reduction in motility that is observed in vitro as oligodendrocytes begin to mature (Small et al., 1987).

Factors Regulating Differentiation of O-2A Precursor Cells in Vitro

When cells are dissociated from neonatal rat optic nerves and cultured in defined medium, most O-2A precursor cells rapidly stop dividing and differentiate into oligodendrocytes within 48 hours (Raff et al., 1983). This differentiation is premature because in vivo the division of O-2A precursor cells extends for several weeks, during which time oligodendrocytes are continuously produced (Skoff et al., 1976a,b). The correct timing of oligodendrocyte differentiation can be restored in vitro by culturing O-2A precursor cells in the presence of type 1 astrocytes or factors secreted by type 1 astrocytes (Noble and Murray, 1984). One factor produced by type 1 astrocytes that stimulates O-2A precursor cell division has been identified as the A chain of PDGF (Richardson et al., 1988), the same molecule that acts as a chemoattractant for O-2A precursor cells. In the presence of PDGF, O-2A precursor cells continue to divide, but when PDGF is withdrawn, these cells differentiate prematurely. However, even in the continued presence of PDGF, O-2A precursor cells eventually stop dividing and differentiate into oligodendrocytes. This loss of responsiveness to PDGF occurs after a number of divisions so that a timely generation of oligodendrocytes is observed in vitro that resembles the extended period of oligodendrocyte production seen in vivo (Raff et al., 1985).

The development of oligodendrocytes in vitro is influenced by several polypeptide growth factors in addition to PDGF. Insulin-like growth factor I also acts as a mitogen for O-2A precursor cells, and, in addition, it promotes expression of the differentiation antigen GalC (McMorris and Dubois-Dalcq, 1988). Basic fibroblast growth factor (bFGF) affects the differentiation of oligodendrocytes and can induce division in cells expressing GalC (Eccleston and Silberberg, 1985; Saneto and de Vellis, 1985). bFGF is an even more potent mitogen for O-2A precursor cells than is PDGF (McKinnon et al., 1990). Moreover, bFGF may play a critical role in controlling the timing of myelination of specific fiber tracts by an action that modulates the interaction of PDGF with O-2A precursor cells: bFGF has recently been shown to induce a high level of expression of PDGF α receptors in precursor cells and thus to increase their sensitivity to PDGF (McKinnon et al. 1990). Dividing O-2A precursor cells initially express high levels of the PDGF α receptor, but differentiation along the oligodendrocyte pathway is marked by a significant reduction in receptor level (Hart et al., 1989). FGF is known to promote the outgrowth of neurites (reviewed in Barde, 1989) and to be localized within developing fiber tracts of the CNS (Gonzalez et al., 1990). Because myelination of the various CNS fiber tracts is initiated at different developmental ages, bFGF may serve a critical role in coordinating the expansion of the O-2A population to meet the needs of particular axon populations through its induction of PDGF receptors on precursor cells.

These studies indicate that the differentiation of O-2A precursor cells is influenced by a variety of growth factors that are present during early development. It is clear that several of these factors have complex actions, which include modulation of responsiveness to other known factors. Current research is focused on examining how growth factors interact to regulate the timing of division, migration, and differentiation of O-2A precursor cells.

MIGRATORY OLIGODENDROCYTE PRECURSORS IN THE ADULT OPTIC NERVE

Cells migrating out of explants of both neonatal and adult rat optic nerves have been shown to myelinate cerebellar explants previously depleted of myelin-forming cells (Wolf et al., 1986). This demonstration suggests that the adult optic nerve contains a population of migratory oligodendrocyte precursors. Indeed, a small population of dividing, bipotential O-2A precursor cells has been identified in the optic nerve of adult rats (ffrench-Constant and Raff, 1986; Wolswijk and Noble, 1989).

O-2A precursor cells in the adult optic nerve are distinguished from their neonatal counterparts on the basis of antigenic phenotype and function (see Table 7–1). Adult O-2A precursor cells, in common with neonatal precursors, are labeled with the A_2B_5 and NSP-4 monoclonal antibodies and do not express GalC. However, unlike O-2A precursors in the neonate, most adult precursor cells express the O4 surface antigen and lack intermediate filaments, features that are also observed in mature oligodendrocytes (Wolswijk and Noble, 1989). In comparison to O-2A precursors from neonates, the adult O-2A precursors migrate significantly more slowly (4 versus 21 μm/hour), have a longer cell cycle (65 versus 18 hours), and require twice the time to express differentiation antigens in cell culture (5 versus 2 days) (Wolswijk and Noble, 1989). It is apparent that the functional differences observed in O-2A precursor cells of neonates and adults are well suited to the respective requirements of a developing and a mature CNS. The rapidly dividing precursor cells of the young animal can generate large colonies of highly motile O-2A lineage cells that are capable of rapid migration to specific targets and differentiation into myelin-forming cells at the initial stages of myelination. In the adult, limited numbers of slowly dividing precursor cells can generate only small colonies of myelin-forming cells, which show minimal motility and which may serve as a localized source for replacing oligodendrocytes lost during normal cell turnover. The predominant phenotype of the O-2A precursor population in the rat optic nerve shows a gradual transition from neonatal to adult during the first 4 weeks postnatally, with a few cells expressing an adult phenotype as early as postnatal day 7 and a few cells still expressing a neonatal phenotype at 1 month after birth (Wolswijk et al., 1990). Myelination of the CNS tracts is a progressive process that continues well into late postnatal ages and for which the presence of small numbers of O-2A precursor cells with a neonatal phenotype would be required.

The differences between neonatal and adult precursor cells are consistent with the observations of

Wolf et al. (1986) showing that although myelin-forming cells migrate out of both adult and neonatal optic nerves, cells from adult nerves migrate shorter distances into the explants and take longer to myelinate the explants. The different functional properties of neonatal and adult O-2A precursor cells may also be related to clinical observations (Kriss et al., 1988; McDonald, 1983) showing that children recover more readily from optic neuritis, a demyelinating disease of the optic nerve, than do adults. The characteristics of adult precursor cells suggest that these cells are not well suited to repair large-scale losses of oligodendrocytes that are associated with demyelinating diseases such as multiple sclerosis.

GUIDANCE AND RESTRICTION IN THE REGULATION OF MIGRATION

Studies of the optic pathway suggest that strong factors may restrict the migration of oligodendrocyte precursors into unmyelinated regions of the CNS such as the retina. One of the sharpest transitions between myelinated white matter and unmyelinated gray matter occurs at the lamina cribrosa, the retrobulbar zone where the optic nerve emerges from the eye. The intraretinal portions of ganglion cell axons are unmyelinated within the retinas of most mammals and remain unmyelinated until after passing through the heavily vascularized lamina cribrosa. Beyond the lamina cribrosa, the vast majority of optic axons become myelinated within a transitional zone of 100 μm. What prevents the highly motile O-2A precursor cells from migrating through the lamina cribrosa to reach the retina? Berliner (1931) suggested that the lamina cribrosa may serve as a barrier to the migration of oligodendrocytes based on his observation that the rabbit lacks a lamina cribrosa and that unlike most mammals, its retina contains a central myelinated zone known as medullary streak.

Experimental evidence supports the view that factors associated with the lamina cribrosa may normally prevent oligodendrocyte precursors from reaching the retina (Perry and Lund, 1990). When fetal retinas are transplanted to the midbrain, they differentiate to form a well-laminated retina containing an optic fiber layer. These fibers project from the transplant and form functional connections with the host brain (Klassen and Lund, 1987). Because a lamina cribrosa is not present in the axon fascicles that emerge from the transplants, migratory oligodendrocyte precursors from the surrounding host tissue can invade the transplant and myelinate the intraretinal portion of axons contained within the optic fiber layer. Thus, ganglion cell axons within the retina appear to be myelin competent but are not normally myelinated because O-2A precursors are prevented from entering the retina. This restriction on O-2A migration is in contrast to the ability of astrocytes to traverse this region of nerve at slightly younger ages (Watanabe and Raff, 1988) and may reflect developmental

changes in the microenvironment of the lamina cribrosa as well as the different dependencies of these two cell types on molecules that guide and restrict their movement.

The specific features of the lamina cribrosa that prevent oligodendrocyte precursor cells from reaching the retina are not known. However, as noted by Perry and Lund (1990), the lamina cribrosa, in common with the subfornical region and the pituitary stalk, has a leaky blood-brain barrier (Tso et al., 1975), and such regions contain little or no myelin. These authors suggested that exposure to plasma proteins may restrict the migration of O-2A precursor cells and/or their differentiation. Indeed, the in vitro studies of Raff (1989) clearly show that when O-2A precursor cells are exposed to fetal calf serum, they fail to develop into oligodendrocytes.

Inhibition of oligodendrocyte development by serum proteins may have clinical significance in cases of demyelinating diseases of the CNS such as multiple sclerosis. Breakdown of the blood-brain barrier is a consistent early feature of clinical relapse in multiple sclerosis (reviewed in McDonald and Barnes, 1989). The specific sensitivity of the oligodendrocyte lineage to molecules present in serum may contribute to both the formation of demyelinating lesions (see Chapter 90) and the extremely restricted capacity for remyelination seen in adults, in spite of the presence of a population of O-2A precursor cells in the adult CNS (Wolswijk and Noble, 1989).

It has been demonstrated that oligodendrocytes as well as O-2A precursor cells present in the adult rat CNS are uniquely susceptible to lysis by the complement present in normal serum (Scolding et al., 1989b; Wren and Noble, 1989). In the absence of antibodies, these cells bind and activate complement, which leads to cell lysis or reversible injury, depending on the complement concentration (Scolding et al., 1989a). Susceptibility to complement is not a characteristic of other neural cells such as myelin-forming Schwann cells of the peripheral nervous system, meningeal cells, astrocytes, or O-2A precursor cells with a neonatal phenotype. It is interesting to note that small numbers of O-2A precursor cells with an adult phenotype are detected for the first time in the rat optic nerve at the end of the first postnatal week (Wolswijk et al., 1990), the age at which increasing numbers of precursors have migrated into the retinal pole of the optic nerve (see Table 7–1). It is interesting to speculate on whether precursors that have migrated the length of the nerve to reach the lamina cribrosa might represent the complement-sensitive subpopulation of precursor cells. Exposure to normal serum in regions of blood-brain barrier disruption in patients with multiple sclerosis may lead to the destruction of both myelin-competent oligodendrocytes and complement-sensitive precursors, the potential cellular source for myelin repair. The gradual transition of O-2A cells from a population composed predominantly of cells with a neonatal phenotype to one composed of cells with the adult vulnerability to complement may also be relevant to the greater capacity for myelin repair that is observed in childhood (Kriss et al., 1988).

RESPONSES OF GLIAL CELLS IN THE ADULT CENTRAL NERVOUS SYSTEM

Both astrocytes and oligodendrocytes in the adult CNS retain a capacity for division that can be enhanced under pathologic and experimental conditions. Although little division of astrocytes is observed in the normal adult brain, the response of astrocytes to injury includes proliferation, migration to sites of injury, and marked hypertrophy of cell processes that are enriched in intermediate filaments. Gliotic scars persist throughout life and consist mainly of GFAP filaments. Reactive astrocytes initially express high levels of glutamine synthetase, the enzyme that catalyzes the conversion of the neurotransmitters γ-aminobutyric acid and glutamate to glutamine. It has been suggested that reactive astrocytes may re-express properties seen in astrocytes during early development, which may promote repair mechanisms. Reactive astrocytes in vivo produce laminin (Liesi et al., 1984), an extracellular matrix component that promotes neurite outgrowth and that is present in the basal lamina of the glia limitans as well as in the perivascular membrane surrounding blood vessels. In culture, astrocytes produce a number of growth factors including nerve growth factor, PDGF, and insulin-like growth factor, in addition to matrix components such as laminin and fibronectin.

Evidence suggests that astrocytes may participate in immune reactions in the CNS. Cultured astrocytes produce interleukin-1, a molecule released by activated macrophages that promotes T cell proliferation and secretion of interleukin-2 (Fontana et al., 1982). Cultured astrocytes can also be induced to express class I and class II molecules of the major histocompatibility complex, and such activated astrocytes can act as antigen-presenting cells for antigens such as MBP (Fontana et al., 1984). The differential capacity of astrocytes from different rat strains to express class II molecules has been correlated with the susceptibility of strains to experimental autoimmune encephalomyelitis, a laboratory model of multiple sclerosis.

In vivo studies indicate that undifferentiated O-2A precursor cells may not be the only source of new oligodendrocytes in the adult CNS. GalC-positive oligodendrocytes in the optic nerve can be labeled 1 hour after an injection of [³H]thymidine, in contrast to in vitro studies that indicate that GalC-positive oligodendrocytes are postmitotic (Skoff et al., 1989). Proliferation can be induced in GalC-positive oligodendrocytes in vitro but requires the presence of growth factors such as bFGF (Eccleston and Silberberg, 1985). Morphologic studies have also provided

evidence that mature oligodendrocytes that have established myelin sheaths are capable of division in vivo (Sturrock and McRae, 1980). Differences observed in the behavior of oligodendrocytes in vitro and in vivo underscore the importance of understanding the responses of oligodendrocytes to growth factors that may be present during development and disease. Successful remyelination is seen after induction of demyelination with virus or agents such as cuprizone or lysolecithin. The generation of new oligodendrocytes in response to demyelinating agents has been demonstrated by using [³H]thymidine autoradiography (e.g., Arenella and Herndon, 1984; Herndon et al., 1977; Ludwin, 1981; Ludwin and Bakker, 1988). These studies clearly show that the adult CNS has the capacity for myelin repair, and further studies are required to clarify the relative contributions of existing oligodendrocytes and adult O-2A precursor cells to remyelination. Delineating the factors that can enhance the proliferation of oligodendrocytes and/or their precursors in vivo, as well as the factors that selectively damage oligodendrocytes (e.g., susceptibility to complement), is crucial for understanding the relative failure of remyelination seen in demyelinating diseases of the adult CNS such as multiple sclerosis.

References

Arenella L.S., Herndon R.M. Mature oligodendrocytes. Division following experimental demyelination in adult animals. *Arch. Neurol.* 41:1162–1165, 1984.

Armstrong R.C., Harvath L., Dubois-Dalcq M.E. Type-1 astrocytes and oligodendrocyte-type 2 astrocyte glial progenitors migrate toward distinct molecules. *J. Neurosci. Res.* 27:400–407, 1990.

Balaban E., Small R. The use of avian chimaeras to study the origin of myelin-forming cells in the optic nerve. *J. Cell Biol.* 109:58a, 1989.

Bansal R., Warrington A.E., Gard A.L., et al. Multiple and novel specificities of monoclonal antibodies O1, O4, and R-mAb used in the analysis of oligodendrocyte development. *J. Neurosci. Res.* 24:548–557, 1989.

Barde, Y.-A. Trophic factors and neuronal survival. *Neuron* 2:1525–1534, 1989.

Beal J.A., Hall J.L. A light microscopic study of the effects of X-irradiation on the spinal cord of neonatal rats. *J. Neuropathol. Exp. Neurol.* 33:128–143, 1974.

Behar T., McMorris F.A., Novotny E.A., et al. Growth and differentiation properties of O-2A progenitors purified from rat cerebral hemispheres. *J. Neurosci. Res.* 21:168–180, 1988.

Benfey M., Aguayo A.J. Extensive elongation of axons from rat brain into peripheral nerve grafts. *Nature* 296:150–152, 1982.

Berliner M.L. Cytologic studies on the retina: I. Normal coexistence of oligodendroglia and myelinated nerve fibers. *Arch. Ophthalmol.* 6:740–751, 1931.

Bignami, A., Dahl, D. The radial glia of Müller in the rat retina and their response to injury. An immunofluorescence study with antibodies to the glial fibrillary acidic (GFA) protein. *Exp. Eye Res.* 28:63–69, 1979.

Blakemore W.F., Patterson R.C. Observations on the interactions of Schwann cells and astrocytes following X-irradiation of neonatal rat spinal cord. *J. Neurocytol.* 4:573–585, 1975.

Caroni P., Schwab M.E. Antibody against myelin-associated inhibitor of neurite growth neutralizes nonpermissive substrate properties of CNS white matter. *Neuron* 1:85–96, 1988.

Dubois-Dalcq M., Behar R., Hudson L., et al. Emergence of three myelin proteins in oligodendrocytes cultured without neurons. *J. Cell Biol.* 102:284–392, 1986.

Eccleston P.A., Silberberg D.H. Fibroblast growth factor is a mitogen for oligodendrocytes in vitro. *Dev. Brain Res.* 21:315–318, 1985.

Edelman G.M. Cell adhesion molecules in the regulation of animal form and tissue pattern. *Annu. Rev. Cell Biol.* 2:81–116, 1986.

Emmett C.J., Lawrence J.M., Seeley P.J. Visualization of migration of transplanted astrocytes using polystyrene microspheres. *Brain Res.* 447:223–233, 1988.

Fallon J.R. Preferential outgrowth of central nervous system neurites on astrocytes and Schwann cells as compared with nonglial cells in vitro. *J. Cell Biol.* 100;198–207, 1985.

Fontana A., Kristensen F., Dubs R., et al. Production of prostaglandin E and interleukin-1 like factors by cultured astrocytes an C-6 glioma cells. *J. Immunol.* 129:2413–2419, 1982.

Fontana A., Fierz W., Weberle H. Astrocytes present myelin basic protein to encephalitogenic T cell lines. *Nature* 307:273–276, 1984.

ffrench-Constant C., Raff M.C. Proliferating bipotential glial progenitor cells in adult rat optic nerve. *Nature* 319:499–502, 1986.

Goldberg W.J., Bernstein J.J. Fetal cortical astrocytes migrate from cortical homografts throughout the host brain and over the glial limitans. *J. Neurosci. Res.* 20:38–45, 1988.

Gonzalez A.-M., Buscaglia M., Ong M., et al. Distribution of basic fibroblast growth factor in the 18-day rat fetus: localization in the basement membranes of diverse tissues. *J. Cell Biol.* 110:753–765, 1990.

Hart I.K., Richardson W.D., Heldin C.-H., et al. PDGF receptors on cells of the oligodendrocyte–type 2 astrocyte (O-2A) cell lineage. *Development* 105:595–603.

Hatten M.E. Neuronal regulation of astroglial morphology and proliferation in vitro. *J. Cell Biol.* 100:384–396, 1985.

Hatten M.E. Riding the glial monorail: a common mechanism for glial-guided neuronal migration in different regions of the developing mammalian brain. *Trends Neurosci.* 13:179–184, 1990.

Herndon R.M., Price D.L., Weiner L.P. Regeneration of oligodendroglia during recovery from demyelinating disease. *Science* 195:693–694, 1977.

Hirano M., Goldman J.E., Gliogenesis in rat spinal cord: evidence for origin of astrocytes and oligodendrocytes from radial precursors. *J. Neurosci. Res.* 21:155–167, 1988.

Janzer R.C., Raff M.C. Astrocytes induce blood-brain barrier properties in endothelial cells. *Nature* 325:253–257, 1987.

Jordan C.A., Friedrich V.L. Jr., de Ferra F., et al. Differential exon expression in myelin basic protein transcripts during central nervous system (CNS) remyelination. *Cell. Mol. Neurobiol.* 10:3–18, 1990.

Jordan C.A., Friedrich V. Jr., Dubois-Dalcq M. In situ hybridization analysis of myelin gene transcripts in developing mouse spinal cord. *J. Neurosci.* 9:248–257, 1989a.

Jordan C.A., Friedrich V. Jr., Godfraind C., et al. Expression of viral and myelin gene transcripts in a murine CNS demyelinating disease caused by a coronavirus. *GLIA* 2:318–329, 1989b.

Kennedy P.G.E., Fok-Seang J. Studies on the development, antigenic phenotype and function of human glial cells in tissue culture. *Brain* 109:1261–1277, 1986.

Klassen H.J., Lund R.D. Retinal transplants can drive a pupillary reflex in host rat brains. *Proc. Natl. Acad. Sci. U.S.A.* 84:6958–6960, 1987.

Knapp P.E., Bartlett W.P., Skoff R.P. Cultured oligodendrocytes mimic in vivo phenotypic characteristics: cell shape, expression of myelin-specific antigens, and membrane production. *Dev. Biol.* 120:356–365, 1987.

Kriss A., Francis D.A., Cuendet F., et al. Recovery after optic neuritis in childhood. *J. Neurol. Neurosurg. Psychiatry* 51:1253–1258, 1988.

Lachapelle F., Gumpel M., Baulac M., et al. Transplantation of CNS fragments into the brain of shiverer mutant mice: extensive myelination by implanted oligodendrocytes. I. Immunohistochemical studies. *Dev. Neurosci.* 6:325–334, 1984.

Le Douarin N.M. A biological cell labelling technique and its use in experimental embryology. *Dev. Biol.* 30:217–222, 1973.

Lerea L.S., McCarthy K.D. Astroglial cells in vitro are heterogeneous with respect to expression of the α_1-adrenergic receptor. *GLIA* 2:135–147, 1989.

Levi G., Gallo V., Viotti M.T. Bipotential precursors of putative fibrous astrocytes and oligodendroctyes in rat cerebellar cultures express distinct surface features and "neuron-like" γ-aminobutyric acid transport. *Proc. Natl. Acad. Sci. U.S.A.* 83:1504–1508, 1986.

Levitt P., Rakic P. Immunoperoxidase localization of glial fibrillary acidic protein in radial glial cells and astroctyes of the developing rhesus monkey brain. *J. Comp. Neurol.* 193:417–448, 1980.

Liesi P., Dahl D., Vaheri A. Laminin is produced by early rat astrocytes in primary culture. *J. Cell Biol.* 96:920–924, 1983.

Liesi P., Kaakkola S., Dahl D. Laminin is induced in astrocytes of adult brian by injury. *EMBO J.* 3:683–686, 1984.

Looney G.A., Elberger A.J. Myelination of the corpus callosum in the cat: time course, topography, and functional implications. *J. Comp. Neurol.* 248:336–347, 1986.

Ludwig S.K. Pathology of demyelination and remyelination. *Adv. Neurol.* 31: 123–168, 1981.

Ludwin S.K., Bakker D.A. Can oligodendrocytes attached to myelin proliferate? *J. Neurosci.* 8:1239–1244, 1988.

Matthiessen H.P., Schmalenbach C., Müller H.W. Astroglia-released neurite growth-inducing activity for embryonic hippocampal neurons is associated with laminin bound in a sulfated complex and free fibronectin. *GLIA* 2:117–188, 1989.

McCarthy K.D., Prime J., Harmon T., et al. Receptor-mediated phosphorylation of astroglial intermediate filament proteins in cultured astroglia. *J. Neurochem.* 44:723–730, 1985.

McDonald W.I. Doyne lecture: The significance of optic neuritis. *Trans. Ophthalmol. Soc. U.K,* 103:230–246, 1983.

McDonald W.I., Barnes D. Lessons from magnetic resonance imaging in multiple sclerosis. *Trend Neurosci.* 12:376–379, 1989.

McKinnon R.D., Matsui T., Dubois-Dalcq M., et al. FGF modulates the PDGF-driven pathway of oligodendrocyte development. *Neuron* 5:603–614, 1990.

McMorris F.A, Dubois-Dalcq, M. Insulin-like growth factor 1 promotes cell proliferation and oligodendroglial commitment in rat glial progenitor cells developing in vitro. *J. Neurosci. Res.* 21:199–209, 1988.

Miller R.H., David S., Patel R., et al. A quantitative immunohistochemical study of macroglial cell development in the rat optic nerve: in vivo evidence for two distinct astrocyte lineages. *Dev. Biol.* 111:35–41, 1985.

Noble M., Murray, K. Purified astroctyes promote the in vitro division of a bipotential glial progenitor cell. *EMBO J.* 3:2243–2247, 1984.

Noble M., Fok-Seang J., Cohen J. Glia are a unique substrate for the in vitro growth of CNS neurons. *J. Neurosci.* 4:1892–1903, 1984.

Perry V.H., Lund R.D. Evidence that the lamina cribrosa prevents intraretinal myelination of retinal ganglion cell axons. *J. Neurocytol.* 19:265–272, 1990.

Price J., Hynes R.O. Astrocytes in culture synthesize and secrete a variant form of fibronectin. *J. Neurosci.* 5:2205–2211, 1985.

Raff M.C. Glial cell diversification in the rat optic nerve. *Science* 243:1450–1455, 1989.

Raff M.C., Miller R.H. Noble M. A glial progenitor cell that develops in vitro into an astrocyte or an oligodendrocyte depending on culture medium. *Nature* 303:390–396, 1983.

Raff M.C., Abney E.R., Fok-Seang, J. Reconstitution of a developmental clock in vitro: a critical role for astrocytes in the timing of oligodendrocyte differentiation. *Cell* 42:61–69, 1985.

Rakic P. Neuron-glial relationships during granule cell migration in developing cerebellar cortex. *J. Comp. Neurol.* 141:282–312, 1971.

Rakic P. Neuron-glial interaction during brain development. *Trends Neurosci.* 4:184–187, 1981.

Reynolds R., Wilkin G.P. Development of macroglial cells in rat cerebellum: II. An in situ immunohistochemical study of oligodendroglial lineage from precursor to mature myelinating cell. *Development* 102:409–425, 1990.

Richardson W.D., Pringle N., Mosley M.J., et al. A role for platelet-derived growth factor in normal gliogenesis in the central nervous system. *Cell* 53:309–319, 1988.

Sadoul R., Hirn M., Deagostini-Brazin H., et al. Adult and embryonic mouse neural cell adhesion molecules have different binding properties. *Nature* 304:347–379, 1983.

Saneto R.P., de Vellis J. Characterization of cultured rat oligodendrocytes proliferating in a serum-free, chemically defined medium. *Proc. Natl. Acad. Sci. U.S.A.* 82:3509–3513, 1985.

Scherer J., Schnitzer J. The rabbit retina: a suitable mammalian tissue for obtaining astroglia-free Müller cell cultures. *Neurosci. Lett.* 97:51–56, 1989.

Schmechel D.E., Rakic P. A Golgi study of radial glial cells in developing monkey telencephalon: morphogenesis and transformation into astrocytes. *Anat. Embryol. (Berl.)* 156:115–152, 1979.

Schwab M.E., Caroni P. Oligodendrocytes and CNS myelin are nonpermissive substrates for neurite growth and fibroblast spreading in vitro. *J. Neurosci.* 8:2381–2393, 1988.

Scolding N.J., Houston W.A.J., Morgan B.P., et al. Reversible injury to cultured rat oligodendroctyes by complement. *Immunology* 67:441–446, 1989a.

Scolding N.J., Morgan B.P., Houston W.A.J., et al. Normal rat serum cytotoxicity against syngeneic oligodendrocytes: complement activation and attack in the absence of anti-myelin antibodies. *J. Neurol. Sci.* 89:289–300, 1989b.

Sidman, R.L., Rakic, P. Neuronal migration with special reference to the developing human: a review. *Brain Res.* 62:1–35, 1973.

Skoff R.P. Gliogenesis in rat optic nerve: astrocytes are generated in a single wave before oligodendrocytes. *Dev. Biol.* 139:149–168, 1990.

Skoff R., Price D., Stocks A. Electron microscopic autoradiographic studies of gliogenesis in rat optic nerve. I. Cell proliferation. *J. Comp. Neurol.* 169:291–312, 1976a.

Skoff R., Price D., Stocks A. Electron microscopic autoradiographic studies of gliogenesis in rat optic nerve. II. Time of origin. *J. Comp. Neurol.* 169:313–333, 1976b.

Skoff R., Knapp P.E., Bartlett W.P. Astrocyte diversity in the optic nerve: a cytoarchitectural study. In Federoff S., Vernadakis A. eds. *Astrocytes.* Vol. I. New York: Academic Press, pp. 269–291, 1986.

Skoff R.P., Knapp P.E., Ghandour S. Neuroglial cell lineage: in vivo and in vitro differences. *Soc. Neurosci. Abstr.* 15:14, 1989.

Small R.K. Membrane specializations of neuritic growth cones in vivo: a quantitative IMP analysis. *J. Neurosci. Res.* 13:39–53, 1985.

Small R.K. Migration of oligodendrocyte-type 2 astrocyte progenitor cells in the developing rat optic nerve. *Soc. Neurosci. Abstr.* 12:183, 1986.

Small R.K. Differentiation of a migratory bipotential glial progenitor cell in the developing rat optic nerve. In Gorio A., et al. eds. *Neural Development and Regeneration.* Berlin: Springer-Verlag. NATO ASI Series 22:677–680, 1988.

Small R.K., Leonard C.M. Rapid fiber reorganization after olfactory tract section and bulbectomy in the golden hamster. *J. Comp. Neurol.* 214:353–369, 1983.

Small R.K., Patel P., Watkins B.A.. The response of Müller cells to growth factors alters with time in culture. *GLIA* (in press).

Small R.K., Riddle P., Noble M. Evidence for migration of oligodendrocyte-type 2 astrocyte progenitor cells into the developing rat optic nerve. *Nature* 328:155–157, 1987.

Sommer I., Schachner M. Monoclonal antibodies (O1 to O4) to oligodendrocyte cell surfaces: an immunocytological study in the central nervous system. *Dev. Biol.* 83:311–327, 1981.

Sommer I., Schachner, M. Cells that are O4 antigen–positive and O1 antigen–negative differentiate into O1 antigen–positive oligodendrocytes. *Neurosci. Lett.* 29:183–188, 1982.

Sommer I., Schachner M. Stage-specific antigens on oligodendrocyte cell surfaces. In Duprat A.M., Kato A.C., Weber M., eds. *The Role of Cell Interactions in Early Neurogenesis.* New York, Plenum Publishing. NATO ASI Series 77:201–205, 1984.

Sturrock R.R., McRae D.A. Mitotic division of oligodendrocytes which have begun myelination. *J. Anat.* 131:577–582, 1980.

Temple S., Raff M.C. Clonal analysis of oligodendrocyte development in culture: evidence for a developmental clock that counts cell divisions. *Cell* 44:773–779, 1986.

Trotter J., Schachner M. Cells positive for the O4 surface antigen isolated by cell sorting are able to differentiate into astrocytes or oligodendrocytes. *Dev. Brain Res.* 46:115–122, 1989.

Trotter J., Bitter-Suermanm D., Schachner M. Differentiation-regulated loss of the polysialylated embryonic form and expression of the different polypeptides of the neural cell adhesion molecule by cultured oligodendrocytes and myelin. *J. Neurosci. Res.* 22:369–383, 1989.

Tso M.O.M., Shih C.-Y., McLean M.I.W. Is there a blood-brain barrier at the optic nerve head? *Arch. Ophthalmol.* 93:815–825, 1975.

Turner D.L., Cepko C.L. A common progenitor for neurons and glia persists in rat retina late in development. *Nature* 328:131–136, 1987.

Watanabe T., Raff M.C. Retinal astrocytes are immigrants from the optic nerve. *Nature* 332:834–836, 1988.

Williams B.P., Abney E.R., Raff M.C. Macroglial cell development in embryonic rat brain: studies using monoclonal antibodies, fluorescence activated cell sorting, and cell culture. *Dev. Biol.* 112:126–134, 1985.

Wolf M.K., Brandenberg M.C., Billings-Gagliardi S.J. Migration and myelination by adult glial cells: reconstructive analysis of tissue culture experiments. *J. Neurosci.* 6:3731–3738, 1986.

Wolswijk G., Noble M. Identification of an adult-specific glial progenitor cell. *Development* 105:387–400, 1989.

Wolswijk G., Riddle P.N., Noble M. Coexistence of perinatal and adult forms of a glial progenitor cell during development of the rat optic nerve. *Development* 109:691–698; 1990.

Wren D.R., Noble M. Oligodendrocytes and oligodendrocyte/type-2 astrocyte progenitor cells of adult rats are specifically susceptible to the lytic effects of complement in absence of antibody. *Proc. Natl. Acad. Sci. U.S.A.* 86:9025–9029, 1989.

8

The Cell of Schwann

Richard P. Bunge
John W. Griffin

The function of Schwann cells is to house axons and to provide for these axons a hollow tubular channel of extracellular matrix (ECM) within the connective tissues of peripheral nerve; these channels provide physical strength and are useful for guiding nerve fibers regenerating within the peripheral nerve trunk. In addition, Schwann cells provide myelin segments for larger nerve fibers. The insulating qualities of these myelin segments and the partitioning of the axolemmal function that they engender allow saltatory conduction of the nerve impulse, which increases the velocity of nerve conduction as much as 100 times. The large number of Schwann cells present in essentially all parts of the peripheral nervous system facilitates the processes of remyelination and nerve fiber regeneration after injury; these processes occur more satisfactorily in peripheral than in central neural tissues.

SOURCES OF CELLULAR AND CONNECTIVE TISSUE COMPONENTS IN PERIPHERAL NERVE TRUNKS

It is generally accepted that Schwann cells derive, along with sensory and autonomic neurons, from neural crest (and placodes of the head region) during embryogenesis (LeDouarin, 1982). Crest cells migrate before they express overt differentiation; thus the exact point at which the Schwann cell lineage diverges from neuronal precursors is not clear. Schwann cells appear early among the developing nerve cells of cranial and peripheral ganglia (Tennyson, 1965) and subsequently migrate outward along axonal fasciculi as the peripheral nerve trunks form. During and subsequent to this migration, their numbers increase (Aguayo et al., 1976b; Asbury, 1967). This developmental scenario explains the ubiquity of the Schwann cell populations in peripheral nerve trunks, save for the ventral nerve roots; ventral roots derive their Schwann cells from neural crest cells migrating ventrally along the lateral aspect of the neural tube.

Harrison (1924) tested this point by removing neural crest cells in early embryos before ventral migration of crest cells had begun. In these regions the ventral root axons grew out from the spinal cord to form plexuses and provide muscle innervation as expected, but in their early development these axons were entirely devoid of ensheathing cells. This compelling evidence for the crest origin of Schwann cells has now been supported by studies in chick-quail chimeras (LeDouarin, 1982).

When the Schwann cell numbers are initially low, they position themselves between bundles of axons and the surrounding mesenchyme, from which they are separated by an intervening basal lamina. The cells then migrate interiorly into the axonal bundles and partition these bundles into groups, or families (for review see Webster and Favilla, 1984). As the Schwann cells isolate smaller and smaller bundles of axons, each cell begins to acquire its own basal lamina. Increasing cell numbers now provide sufficient Schwann cells to sequester large axons (for individual ensheathment and myelination) or to provide several unmyelinated axons a form of "harbor" within furrows in the Schwann cell surface. Groups of axon–Schwann cell units are interspersed with fibroblasts and become surrounded with a complex sleeve of flattened cells forming the perineurium (P.K. Thomas and Olsson, 1984). The cellular and extracellular components within this perineurial sleeve compose the endoneurium.

Work in the laboratory of R.P. Bunge is supported by grants NS 19923 and NS 09923 from the National Institutes of Health and funds from the Miami Project to Cure Paralysis. Work in the laboratory of J.W. Griffin is supported by grants NS 14784 and PO1 22849 from the National Institutes of Health.

In addition to including cellular components, peripheral nerve trunks contain substantial amounts of connective tissue (for review, see M.B. Bunge et al., 1983). This connective tissue gives peripheral nerves their characteristic cord-like consistency (in contrast to central nervous system tissue). About one-third of the protein in peripheral nerve trunks is collagen. Electron microscopic, biochemical, and immunocytochemical studies have established that the ECM components of peripheral nerve include types I, III, IV, and V collagen. Electron micrographs show collagen fibrils disposed linearly between the axon–Schwann cell units of peripheral nerve trunks. The other major ECM component is the basal lamina, which surrounds each axon–Schwann cell unit over its entire external circumference. This basal lamina is known to be composed of type IV collagen, laminin, heparan sulfate proteoglycan, and fibronectin; these are universal components of basal lamina throughout the body (Cornbrooks et al., 1983; Eldridge et al., 1986; Laurie et al., 1983). Laminin, which functions generally in binding epithelial cells to basal laminae, is disposed around each axon–Schwann cell unit and delineates the position of the basal lamina; fibronectin is more generally disposed throughout the extracellular spaces of the endoneurium. There are also major collagen components in the surrounding perineurium and epineurium. (For a complete review of the connective tissue components of peripheral nerve, see P.K. Thomas and Olsson, 1984.)

In addition to Schwann cells and axons, fibroblasts, endothelial cells of capillaries, and other cells occupy the endoneurium; thus the cellular source of the ECM components in nerve trunks has been uncertain. Tissue culture studies undertaken after separation of specific cell populations from peripheral nerve tissues have clarified this issue. Pure cultures are available of sensory neuron, Schwann cell, and fibroblast populations; which can be cocultured in various combinations (for review, see M.B. Bunge, 1991; McGarvey et al., 1984) (Figs. 8–1 to 8–3). When Schwann cells are cocultured with neurons in a fibroblast-free system, the function of the Schwann cell can (under suitable culture conditions) progress to axonal ensheathment and myelination (see Fig. 8–2). Concomitantly, basal lamina is formed around each axon–Schwann cell unit and collagenous fibrils are deposited in adjacent regions (see Fig. 8–3). The amount of fibrous collagen is considerably augmented if fibroblasts are added to the culture. If the neurons are removed from a culture of Schwann cells and neurons after a substantial basal lamina is deposited, this basal lamina is retained. But if this basal lamina is removed by trypsin digestion, the orphaned Schwann cell will not form a new basal lamina. If neurons are added back, basal lamina will again be formed (M.B. Bunge et al., 1982). These tissue culture observations correlate with observations in vivo, which indicate that Schwann cells free of axonal contact during migratory phases are not surrounded by basal lamina (Billings-Gagliardi et al., 1974). Thus it appears that axon contact induces basal lamina formation by Schwann cells, that Schwann cells can form basal lamina components without the aid of fibroblasts and that fibroblasts and Schwann cells cooperate in the formation of fibrous collagen of the endoneurium.

Biochemical analysis of these same types of culture preparation supports and adds to these morphologic observations (for review see M.B. Bunge et al., 1983). When radiolabeled peptides released into culture medium by Schwann cells are analyzed after separation on gels, it is evident that these cells have substantial secretory activity. Among the secreted products are types I, III, IV, and V collagen as well as laminin, entactin (like laminin, a component of basal lamina), proteoglycans, and a small amount of fibronectin. Type IV collagen and laminin, which are two major components of basal lamina, are particularly prominent products of Schwann cells. When Schwann cells that are driven by neuronal contact are compared with Schwann cells that are separated from axonal influence, axonal contact specifically influences (increases) type IV collagen production;

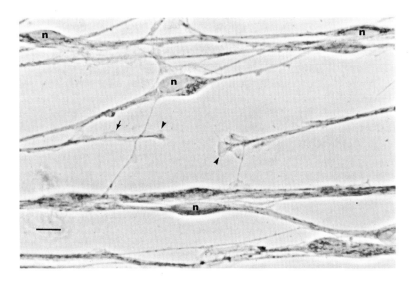

Figure 8–1. A pure population of Schwann cells in culture. The nuclei of several of the Schwann cells are marked with an n. Cytoplasmic organelles are concentrated in the perinuclear region. Despite their isolation from axonal contact, these Schwann cells maintain a characteristic linear configuration. The extended ends of the Schwann cell processes show lamellipodial extensions *(arrowheads)*. These lamellipodia can also be seen along the shafts of the Schwann cell processes *(arrow)*. Under these conditions (free of axonal contact), the cells do not organize a basal lamina. Sudan black stain of a Schwann cell preparation, photographed with phase microscopy. Bar = 10 μm. (Prepared by P. Wood.)

Figure 8–2. Myelinating and unmyelinating Schwann cells are shown in this culture preparation stained with Sudan black to emphasize the tubular myelin sheaths. The cell nuclei related to the myelin segments are marked ms; those related to unmyelinated axons are marked us. A bundle of axons related to unmyelinated Schwann cells is bracketed by the arrowheads. A node of Ranvier between two adjacent myelin segments is marked n. The Schwann cell cytoplasm (c) on the external aspect of one of the myelin segments is visible in this phase micrograph. Under these conditions each axon–Schwann cell unit, both myelinated and un-myelinated, is surrounded by a basal lamina. A collagen substratum required for this degree of differentiation of Schwann cell in tissue culture forms the fibrous background. An electron micrograph of this preparation is shown in Figure 8–3. Bar = 5 μm. (From a preparation by Charles Eldridge.)

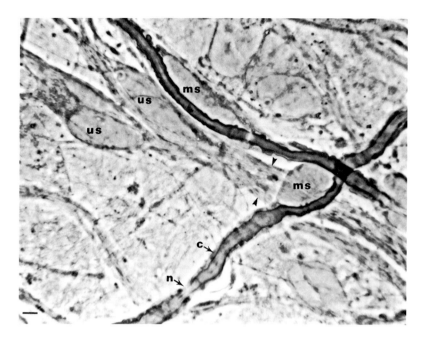

laminin production proceeds in the presence or absence of neurons (Carey et. al., 1983; Cornbrooks et al., 1983). Immunocytochemical studies have confirmed these biochemical observations. Of particular note is the observation that Schwann cells in all situations studied (whether in contact with neurons or not) express laminin on their surface. Thus, axonal contact seems to specifically influence type IV collagen release, which in turn allows basal lamina organization.

Tissue culture experiments have also helped to clarify the long-standing uncertainty of whether Schwann cells or fibroblasts (or both) are responsible for forming the cellular barrier surrounding each nerve fascicle, the perineurium. M.B. Bunge et al. (1989) introduced genetic markers into purified populations of cultured fibroblasts and Schwann cells and then added these in various combinations to purified sensory neurons in a culture system capable of supporting histiotypic development, including

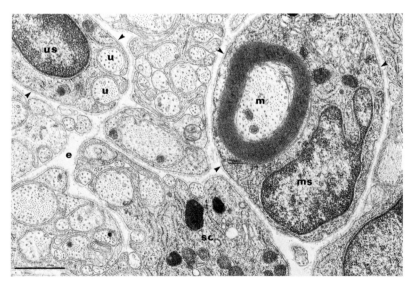

Figure 8–3. An electron micrograph showing myelinated (m) and unmyelinated (u) axons with characteristic Schwann cell ensheathment. The myelinating Schwann cell (nucleus marked ms) has provided a spiral extension of its plasmalemma, which, on compaction, forms the myelin sheath. The unmyelinating Schwann cell (nucleus marked us) harbors unmyelinated axons within troughs characteristic of the ensheathment provided throughout the peripheral nervous system for smaller axons. Both myelinated and unmyelinated axons are characterized by the circular profiles of microtubules, interspersed with neurofilaments. The basal lamina surrounding both types of cell is marked with arrowheads. Characteristic Schwann cell cytoplasm is seen in a third cell (sc). This cytoplasm includes granular endoplasmic reticulum, mitochondria, elements of the Golgi apparatus, and dense inclusions belonging to the lysosomal system. The extracellular space of the endoneurium (e) in this preparation contains few collagenous fibrils because this electron micrograph is of a culture of neurons and Schwann cells but no fibroblasts. In the normal peripheral nerve (and in cultures to which fibroblasts have been added), this space would contain bundles of fibrillar collagen. Bar = 1 μm. (From material prepared by P. Wood, P. Bates, and B. Tiffany.)

myelination and perineurium formation. Only cells of fibroblast lineage were found to contribute to the perineurial sheaths formed in these cultures.

THE CYTOLOGY OF THE SCHWANN CELL

The following description of Schwann cell cytology derives largely from electron microscopic observations (for a complete description see Peters et al., 1976; P.K. Thomas and Ochoa, 1984) and from the more recent characterization of the Schwann cell molecular components revealed by immunocytochemistry.

The cytologic characteristics of the cell of Schwann (see Figs. 8–2 and 8–3) and those of the satellite cells of peripheral neuronal somas are similar. The ovoid nucleus contains a substantial amount of condensed chromatin, often clumped both in the nuclear periphery and near the center of the nucleus (where one or more nucleoli are seen). The cytoplasm is dense, containing both free and membrane-associated ribosomes. Many rounded mitochondria and the Golgi apparatus are concentrated in the perinuclear zone. The cytoplasm contains lysosomes and multivesicular bodies; peroxisomes approximately 0.2 μm in diameter are common. Schwann cells also contain microtubules of standard dimension and intermediate filaments. Occasionally, single cilia of unknown function project from Schwann cells. Schwann cells related to unmyelinated nerve fibers provide ensheathment via indentations of the surface of the Schwann cells where individual axons reside in separate troughs (see Fig. 8–3). Frequently 5–20 axons are ensheathed by a single Schwann cell.

This basic pattern of ensheathment of unmyelinated nerve fibers is modified in several body parts. In the olfactory nerve, Schwann cells provide common ensheathment for several dozen small-diameter axons within each trough. In autonomic nerve plexuses, it is also common for small groups of axons to be enclosed within each trough of Schwann cell cytoplasm.

Electrophysiologic studies of peripheral neurons grown in culture without Schwann cells show that these isolated neurons may generate standard nerve impulses (Higgins and Burton, 1982). Thus, ensheathment of unmyelinated axons in the peripheral nervous system is not necessary for action potential conduction. It has been noted that certain unmyelinated Schwann cells in the peripheral nervous system express intermediate filaments marked by the same antibody as are the intermediate filaments of central astrocytes (Yen and Fields, 1981).

Substantially modified ensheathing cells are also found in the myenteric plexus of the gut wall (Jessen and Mirsky, 1983). Here the non-neuronal cells provide communal ensheathment both for nerve cell bodies and for nerve processes without separation of these neural elements by intervening cytoplasmic extensions. These cells surround the miniature ganglia and connectives of the gut plexuses in a manner reminiscent of the glia limitans provided by astrocytes on the surface of the central nervous system. It is interesting that they also contain an intermediate filament that appears to be similar to that found in astrocytes.

The cytoplasm of the myelin-related Schwann cell (see Fig. 8–3) is not manifestly different from that described for unmyelinating Schwann cells. Pioneering electron microscopic analysis in the 1950s established that the myelin sheath was formed by the spiral deposition of the plasma membrane of the cell of Schwann (Robertson, 1962). The cell cytoplasm is retained inside and outside of the compacted myelin lamellae (see Figs. 8–2 and 8–3), with the cell nucleus located midway between the nodes of Ranvier. Retention of the Schwann cell cytoplasm leads to the distinctive paranodal region and to the interruption of myelin compaction in the clefts of Schmidt-Lanterman. Special junctions are formed between the paranodal loops of the Schwann cell cytoplasm and the axolemma in the paranodal region (for details see Schnapp and Mugnaini, 1975; P.K. Thomas and Ochoa, 1984). The compaction of membrane in the myelin sheath is a unique cellular mechanism and derives from unusually close apposition between both the cytoplasmic and the external surfaces of the spiraled Schwann cell plasma membrane. The manner in which the known molecular constituents of myelin membrane may be organized to facilitate compaction was discussed by Braun et al. (1980).

The development of antibodies to Schwann cell components has aided in delineating subtypes of the Schwann cell family. Mirsky and Jessen (1984) reviewed the differences that can be observed among myelinating and unmyelinating Schwann cells, satellite cells, and enteric glia by using a battery of antibodies to certain surface components (Ran-1, Ran-2, A5E3) and to the intermediate filaments, glial fibrillary acidic protein and vimentin.

INTERACTIONS OF AXONS AND SCHWANN CELLS

The regulation of basal lamina production by axonal contact is but one of at least four ways in which axons influence the function of the Schwann cell. The other known influences include regulation of Schwann cell numbers, effects on axon diameter, and induction of myelination.

The influence of axon numbers on Schwann cell populations during embryogenesis has been documented by Aguayo et al. (1976b). In tissue culture preparations in which nerve cells and Schwann cells are separated and recombined, it is possible to demonstrate directly that axons influence Schwann cell proliferation (McCarthy and Partlow, 1976; Wood and Bunge, 1975) and, moreover, that direct contact between the axon and the Schwann cell is required. Later work (Salzer and Bunge, 1980; Salzer et al.,

1980) indicated that the mitogenic agent is a component of the axon surface. Axolemmal preparations derived from central white matter are also mitogenic (DeVries et al., 1982; Sobue et al., 1983). The initial assumption was that the mitogenic moiety was a glycoprotein; later evidence indicated that the mitogenic activity expressed on rat cultured sensory neurons is associated with a membrane-related proteoglycan (Ratner et al., 1985).

The method of Brockes et al. (1979), which permits preparation of large populations of pure Schwann cells, has allowed a general analysis of agents capable of inducing Schwann cell proliferation (for review see Ratner et al., 1986). Brockes and co-workers (1980) obtained a potent mitogen from bovine pituitary gland (a peptide termed *glial growth factor*), which has now been obtained in highly purified form. Davis and Stroobant (1990) tested a wide variety of growth factors on Schwann cells in vitro and established that transforming growth factor (β_1 and β_2) is mitogenic for these cells, as are also acidic and basic fibroblast growth factor and several forms of platelet-derived growth factor (when used in combination with agents that raise intracellular cyclic AMP levels). Characteristics of the substratum on which Schwann cells are grown have also been shown to influence Schwann cell proliferation (Dubois-Dalcq et al., 1981, among others).

Interactions between axons and Schwann cells influence both Schwann cell size and axon size. A review of the evidence that maturation of axons to full diameter depends not only on neuronal factors but also on the presence of normal Schwann cells and myelin sheaths is available (Aguayo et al., 1979). Axon diameter is decreased in demyelinating neuropathies, in trembler mice (in which Schwann cell myelination is defective), and in the naked axons in the spinal roots of dystrophic mice. Remyelination increases axon diameters of demyelinated axons; ensheathment increases axonal diameter in dystrophic mice; and transplants of normal Schwann cells increase the abnormally small diameter of axons of the trembler mouse. Tissue culture experiments provided direct demonstration that axon diameters are increased in areas of a culture containing Schwann cell (or glial) ensheathment when compared with adjacent regions where axons remained naked (Windebank et al., 1985).

Axons manifestly influence Schwann cell size, inasmuch as the length and the thickness of myelin segments are proportional to axon diameter (Friede and Samorajski, 1967). Thus, the longitudinal and radial extension of Schwann cells is greater when these are related to large-diameter fibers.

It has been accepted for several decades that axons instruct Schwann cells to deposit myelin (for review see Aguayo et al., 1976a; Weinberg and Spencer, 1975). Several types of experiments have shown that Schwann cells from a segment of nerve that is normally unmyelinated will provide myelin sheaths if axons from a nerve containing myelinated fibers are allowed to grow into this Schwann cell population. Because it can be observed that unmyelinated axons in dorsal roots become myelinated by oligodendrocytes as they course through the region of the glia limitans of the root entry zone, some differences in signaling for myelination must exist between central and peripheral neural tissues (Berthold et al., 1984).

New information is available on the mechanisms by which myelin segments are constructed. The role of myelin-specific Schwann cell components has been reviewed (Lemke, 1988). One of the earliest expressed of the myelin-specific components, myelin-associated glycoprotein, is believed to be involved in the early interactions of axons and Schwann cells, in the segregation of axons destined to be myelinated (Owens and Bunge, 1990), and in the maintenance of the inner cytoplasmic collar of Schwann cell cytoplasm (Trapp et al., 1981). Galactocerebroside is implicated in the initiation of the myelin spiral (Ranscht et al., 1987). The components P_0 and myelin basic protein are believed to be involved in the compaction of the forming sheaths (Lemke, 1988). The lengthening of the membranous spiral of the forming myelin sheath is thought to occur by the progression of the inner lip of the Schwann cell over the surface of the axon (R.P. Bunge et al., 1989).

ROLE OF THE SCHWANN CELL IN REGENERATION

Regeneration in the Peripheral Nervous System

When the fibers of a peripheral nerve trunk are interrupted, the distal segment of the nerve undergoes a process termed *wallerian degeneration*, in which the axons and the myelin sheaths distal to the injury undergo degeneration (for review see Fawcett and Keynes, 1990). In the distal segment the Schwann cells and their attendant basal lamina, as well as the collagen components of the endoneurium, persist for many weeks. In the first week after injury the Schwann cells in this distal segment begin to multiply, and thus a substantial population of cells is retained in the longitudinal spaces provided by the retained basal lamina. Spencer et al. (1981) presented evidence that this Schwann cell proliferation occurs both during the degenerative phase of wallerian degeneration and in response to the regenerating axons. These linear cellular arrays are called *bands of Büngner*. The regenerating axons grow from the intact proximal stump and elongate through the columns of Schwann cells contained within the basal lamina. The regenerated axons are eventually ensheathed by Schwann cells, after which the axonal caliber gradually increases.

The type of injury influences the quality of regeneration; restoration of structure and function is greatest after a crush injury, presumably because the tough basal lamina tubes (unlike the delicate axons) are not directly interrupted and retain continuity to direct axonal growth toward peripheral targets. If the nerve is physically interrupted, axons can grow across considerable distances (1–2 cm) to reach the peripheral stump, but in this case functional recovery tends to be incomplete because of disruption of the guiding basal lamina tubes at the site of injury. It has generally been thought that Schwann cells within these distal bands are instrumental in providing trophic support for the regrowing axons. Several lines of evidence show that isolated peripheral nerve segments can attract the growth of axons regenerating from intact proximal nerve trunks (for review see Kuffler, 1989). It is, however, not clear which cell types in the peripheral nerve stumps may be the source of tropic agents.

The facilitation of axonal growth in peripheral nerve regeneration is also influenced by the presence of the basal lamina retained in the bands of Büngner. In one study, Ide and collaborators (1983) used freezing and thawing to kill the cellular elements in the peripheral nerve stump but to retain the ECM materials. They observed prompt nerve fiber growth into these distal stumps and observed the growth cones and nerve fibers directly applied to the internal aspect of the basal lamina of the bands of Büngner. In this case the axons grew into these basal lamina tubes ahead of a Schwann cell front, which subsequently migrated into the frozen nerve, which indicates the importance of ECM components in promoting regeneration within peripheral nerve.

Regeneration in the Central Nervous System

During the past decade, it was established that many of the central neurons of higher vertebrates (which were generally thought to lack the capacity to regenerate several axons) would exhibit regenerative capacity if the damaged axon was provided with access to peripheral nerve tissue (for review see Carter et al., 1989). In these experiments, a segment of peripheral nerve was inserted into the parenchyma of the central nervous system and time was allowed for nerve fibers derived from central neurons to enter this stump and to elongate. After several weeks the distal part of the peripheral nerve stump was treated with horseradish peroxidase. The central nervous system parenchyma in the region in which the nerve entered the central nervous system was then examined to determine whether nerve cell bodies there had been marked by retrograde transport of horseradish peroxidase from the distal site. In a variety of experiments of this type these and other workers showed that central nervous system neurons extend axons into the environment of the peripheral nerve stump, sometimes for a distance of several centimeters. Axons from a variety of central nervous system neurons from cortical, thalamic, brain stem, and basal

ganglia tissues will sponsor axon growth into grafted peripheral nerve segments. These observations indicate that components of peripheral nerve trunks promote and facilitate the growth of the central axons. It remains to be determined whether the neurons that have the capability of extending axons into these peripheral nerve stumps constitute special populations or whether such responses are typical of central neurons.

These remarkable observations raise the question of which components of the peripheral nerve are critical for engendering the regenerative response. Regenerating axons within peripheral nerves are known to grow in the space between the basal lamina left behind by the former axon–Schwann cell unit and the orphaned Schwann cells still resident within these basal lamina tubes; they do not grow in the endoneurial spaces (Scherer and Easter, 1984). Both basal lamina components and Schwann cell surfaces are known to promote axon growth (for review see R.P. Bunge and Hopkins, 1991). When peripheral nerves to be used as grafts are treated to remove their cellular content, leaving only the framework of ECM, axon regeneration will progress, at least for short distances, into these acellular constructs.

In experiments with the peripheral nervous system, the growth of regenerating axons has been compared after placing either cellular or acellular (frozen and thawed) grafts into defects within the peripheral nerve trunk. Both promote regeneration, but the cellular graft is superior (for discussion, see Sketelj et al., 1989). Related experiments have been undertaken in tissue culture by Ard et al. (1987). Schwann cells can be grown under culture conditions in which they may or may not produce a basal lamina; basal lamina deposited by Schwann cells can be prepared and the Schwann cells subsequently removed. Testing neurite growth on these preparations indicated that both Schwann cell surfaces and Schwann cell–derived basal lamina were effective in promoting neurite growth.

Results were different, however, when growth of certain central neurons was examined by using similar cellular versus noncellular substrates. Both embryonic (Kleitman et al., 1988) and adult (R.P. Bunge and Hopkins, 1991) retinal ganglion cells will extend axons onto the surfaces of cocultured Schwann cells (Fig. 8–4) but not onto Schwann cell–derived basal lamina material. Similarly, tests in two systems in vivo indicate that certain types of central neurites will regenerate axons only when provided with implants containing living Schwann cells. Retinal ganglion cells will not extend axons into acellular grafts of peripheral nerve (Berry et al., 1988), nor will neurons of the forebrain septal region regenerate on transplants of ECM devoid of Schwann cells, whereas growth is noted when these transplants retain their Schwann cell population (Kromer and Cornbrooks, 1985).

These data point to the importance of the living

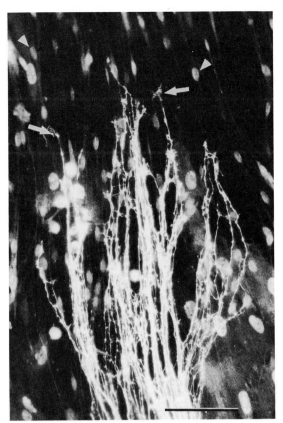

Figure 8–4. Regenerating axons from retinal ganglion neurons extending on the surface of Schwann cells. An underlying bed of Schwann cells purified from neonatal rat sciatic nerve (Brockes et al., 1979) was first established at high density on a collagen substrate, which alone does not support retinal ganglion neuron growth. An explant of retina taken from a 15-day rat embryo was placed on the Schwann cell bed and allowed to grow for 5 days. The neurite growth cones *(arrows)* are growing along the surfaces of the fusiform Schwann cells. Schwann cell nuclei are indicated by the arrowheads. The cell adhesion molecule L1 is implicated in mediating this promotion of neurite growth (see text). The neurites are marked with an antibody specific for neurofilaments, stained with a secondary fluorescent antibody, and photographed in a fluorescence microscope. Bar = 50 μm. (Preparation and photograph by N. Kleitman.)

Schwann cell in providing surface components capable of engendering a regenerative response in central neurons. Cell surface components responsible for prompting neurite growth are rapidly being identified (for review see Bixby and Harris, 1991). The generation of antibodies that block neurite growth on cell surfaces has allowed identification of the major proteins that promote neuronal process growth on Schwann cells (Bixby et al., 1988). These developments suggest that the Schwann cell may be instrumental in fostering central regeneration because its surface is unusually well endowed with proteins capable of interacting with growing neurites to promote regenerative growth. Schwann cells are also known to be sources of trophic factors, such as nerve growth factor, which are instrumental in maintaining neuronal health (for review see Taniuchi et al., 1988).

Role of Schwann Cells in Limb Regeneration in Amphibians

Regeneration of appendages (in vertebrates with this capability) is known, in several instances, to be influenced by the state of innervation of the regenerating member; this applies to fin regeneration in fish and to limb regeneration in amphibians (for a general review, see Brockes, 1984). This nerve dependence was extensively studied in urodeles. After limb amputation in adult urodeles, a growth zone (the blastema) forms, which is enlarged as blastemal cells proliferate; later these cells undergo differentiation and morphogenesis to replace specific tissues of the missing part. The proliferation of blastemal cells goes through a nerve-dependent stage that is generally believed to result from the release of growth factors from axons regenerating into the blastema tissue. Work by Brockes (1984) established that a growth factor (glial growth factor described earlier) is present in the newt blastema during regeneration and that its activity is decreased on denervation. Brockes developed monoclonal antibodies to newt blastema cells that have allowed demonstration that certain of the blastema progenitor cells are of muscle and others are of Schwann cell origin. This work suggests that the nerve may contribute growth factors as well as cell stock to the developing blastema population; the fact that direct contact between axon and blastema cells may influence their proliferation must also be considered.

SCHWANN CELL BEHAVIORS IN DISEASE

The foregoing sections have discussed Schwann cell behavior and axon–Schwann cell interactions in normal nerves, while drawing on lessons from nerve development, cell culture, and axonal regeneration. In considering Schwann cells in the setting of nervous system disease, it is useful to focus on two aspects of their behavior: their phenotypic characteristics, including participation or abstention from myelin formation, and their entry and exit from the cell cycle. The changes in these behaviors in a wide variety of diseases have recurrent themes. For example, nervous system injury or disease prompts a reversion to a dedifferentiated phenotype. Schwann cells of myelinated fibers cease or reduce synthesis of myelin-related constituents and begin synthesis of new molecules, including nerve growth factor (NGF) and its receptor. In addition, in most diseases Schwann cells re-enter the cell cycle. In normal nerves after early development, Schwann cell division is rare. Schwann cells of myelinated fibers usually do not divide for the life of the organism, and those of unmyelinated fibers proliferate at an extremely low level. In disease, they proliferate vigorously. In particular, the Schwann cells of unmyelinated fibers provide a reservoir of cells especially responsive to neural injury, even if the unmyelinated nerve fibers themselves are not directly affected by the disease process.

From a pathogenetic standpoint, nervous system diseases are conveniently classified into those that affect primarily the neuron or its axon, thus producing axon loss, and those that result in demyelination, related to injury either to myelin specifically or to the Schwann cell more generally. The behaviors of Schwann cells in diseased nerves, which are best illustrated by the process of wallerian degeneration after nerve transection, are briefly summarized and then compared with other types of axonal degeneration and with the responses in demyelination.

Wallerian Degeneration

Aspects of the Schwann cell responses to loss of the axon were cited earlier; this section summarizes the sequence of cellular events in wallerian degeneration, as a basis for comparison with other types of injury. Transection of an axon in the mammalian peripheral nervous system is followed by prompt breakdown of the axon itself. The time course of this degeneration is similar in both myelinated and unmyelinated fibers. For example, in peripheral nerves of most laboratory rodents, the axoplasm of the distal stump is converted to granular debris in most fibers within 24–48 hours, and in all fibers within 72–96 hours. The responses of the Schwann cells and of hematogenous macrophages, summarized in Figure 8–5, is a sequence common to all species. The specific timing described here applies to the young rat. At 24 hours, a time when the axoplasm has been degraded and the axolemma has disappeared in most fibers, the myelin sheath remains continuous longitudinally and roughly circular in cross-section. However, by 48 hours the myelin sheath has begun to undergo periodic interruptions, which results in formation of a series of closed chambers, oval or elliptical in longitudinal section, termed *ovoids*. The myelin of these ovoids becomes collapsed and folded, and ultimately the myelin debris is removed from the Schwann cells by the phagocytic activity of hematogenous macrophages (Beuche and Friede, 1984, 1986; Scheidt and Friede, 1987; Stoll et al., 1990).

Schwann cells enter the cell cycle early in the course of wallerian degeneration (Clemence et al., 1989; Pellegrino et al., 1986). For example, in the rat the Schwann cell division peaks on days 3 and 4 (D.R. Archer and J.W. Griffin, unpublished; Clemence et al., 1989). Proliferation at a lower level continues at least for the first 3 weeks after injury, with Schwann cells of both unmyelinated and myelinated fibers dividing. The total number of divisions has been correlated with the original distance between adjacent Schwann cells; Schwann cells with close Schwann cell–Schwann cell spacing divide only a few times, whereas those with much longer spacing (for example, Schwann cells of myelinated fibers with

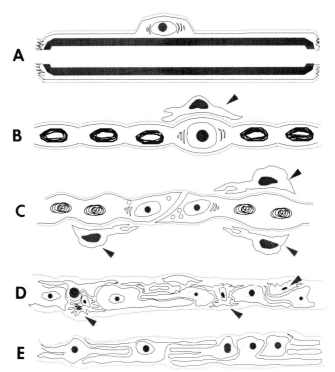

Figure 8–5. Schematic diagrams illustrating the sequential stages of wallerian degeneration and the Schwann cell responses as seen in laboratory rodents. *(A)* At 24 hours after nerve transection. At this stage, the myelin sheath and the Schwann cell appear to be relatively normal. However, in such fibers the axoplasm has already been reduced to granular and amorphous debris. *(B)* At 48 hours after nerve transection. By this stage, the Schwann cell perikaryon has "hypertrophied" to occupy the full cross-sectional area of the nerve fiber; macrophages *(arrow)* have entered to lie next to some of the degenerating fibers; and the myelin has begun segmentation into early ovoids. *(C)* By 4 days, the Schwann cell has undergone its first longitudinal division, the process of ovoid formation is more advanced, and macrophages *(arrows)* are much more numerous. *(D)* By 14 days, myelin has been completely removed from many of the degenerating nerve fibers, and Schwann cell proliferation has resulted in numerous Schwann cells with interdigitating processes. In addition, macrophages within the Schwann cell tube are abundant *(arrows)*. *(E)* By 30 days, the Schwann cell tube (band of Büngner) contains only Schwann cells with their interdigitated processes and overlying basal lamina. Note that from day 4 onward, NGF production by the Schwann cells of the distal stump is abundant, and NGF receptor has been inserted into the plasmalemma of the Schwann cells.

long internodes) divide many more times (G.A. Thomas, 1948). These observations suggest that division continues until a relatively short Schwann cell–Schwann cell spacing is achieved, a process requiring many more divisions in fibers with long internodes than with short ones.

The precise signal that stimulates Schwann cell proliferation associated with axon loss is unknown, but indirect evidence suggests that the mitogen or mitogens may be diffusible. At the same time that the Schwann cells of degenerating fibers enter the cell cycle, the nearby endoneurial fibroblasts, endothelial cells, and perineurial cells also enter the cell cycle. In a model in which only the lumbar ventral roots were transected, so that only the myelinated motor fibers in the sciatic nerve degenerated, the Schwann cells of nearby, structurally normal unmyelinated fibers (not undergoing any axonal degeneration) also proliferated. Indeed, the Schwann cells of unmyelinated fibers were the most numerous cell type dividing on days 3 and 4 after initiation of the lesion (D.R. Archer and J.W. Griffin, unpublished). These results suggest the action of a diffusible factor released into the endoneurial space by degeneration of axons (Griffin et al., 1987). The source of this factor or factors is undetermined, but candidates include soluble fragments of the degenerating axon itself (Chen and DeVries, 1991), the Schwann cells of degenerating fibers (Eccleston et al., 1990), and the hematogenous macrophages recruited into the lesion.

At early times after axotomy, the Schwann cell changes its synthetic program, with a marked reduction in synthesis of myelin constituents, including lipids (White et al., 1989) and proteins (Trapp et al., 1988). In the Schwann cells of myelinating fibers from young rats, a fall in content of mRNAs for myelin proteins is easily detected within 2 days, and the levels have fallen to 5% of the preaxotomy levels by 5 days (Trapp et al., 1988). In general, maintenance of the myelin sheath requires integrity of the axon. However, an exception of particular interest is the model of double myelination, in which a second myelin sheath is maintained around a myelinated fiber. This type of myelination occurs in the sympathetic nervous system of older rats. In this setting, the outer myelin sheath has no axonal contact (Kidd and Heath, 1988). Surprisingly, when the axon undergoes degeneration, these outer myelin sheaths remain intact (G.J. Kidd, J.W. Heath, and B.D. Trapp, personal communication). In this specific setting, the maintenance of myelin by Schwann cells has lost its axonal dependence.

Early in wallerian degeneration, the Schwann cell loses other phenotypic markers associated with the myelin-maintaining Schwann cell, and re-expresses those associated with premyelinated or unmyelinated fibers (Jessen and Mirsky, 1984; Jessen et al., 1987). In addition, within 2–3 days of axonal injury, Schwann cells begin synthesis of NGF and NGF receptor. The sequence leading to the synthesis of NGF, which is a trophic factor that supports axonal outgrowth in specific susceptible neurons, has proved to be particularly instructive. Sustained production of NGF by denervated Schwann cells requires the presence of the cytokine interleukin-1 (Lindholm et al., 1987). Interleukin-1 is produced by the macrophages that invade the distal stump (Lindholm et al., 1988). Macrophages are increasingly recognized to have critical roles in influencing the behavior of the non-neural cells in peripheral nervous system disease.

The daughter Schwann cells thus produce NGF and retain some NGF on their plasmalemma by means of the NGF receptor. They remain within the basal lamina of the Schwann cell band. The final product of this process of wallerian degeneration is thus a longitudinal band of Schwann cells, which provides an attractive pathway for regenerating axons (Johnson et al., 1988).

Demyelination

Acquired Disorders. Demyelination of individual internodes occurs in a variety of acquired disorders. In some, there is an attack on the myelin sheath, whereas in others there is a dysfunction of the whole Schwann cell. An example of an immune-mediated attack on myelin is the Guillain-Barré syndrome. A closely related, but not identical, experimental model is allergic neuritis resulting from immunization of animals with whole myelin or specific constituents of peripheral myelin. A few toxic and metabolic disorders result in demyelination, including intoxication with lead (in experimental animals), tellurium, hexachlorophene, diphtheria toxin, and buckthorn toxin. In all of these acquired disorders, the responses of the Schwann cells have several shared features. As the process of demyelination is initiated, the Schwann cells down-regulate synthesis of myelin constituents. In addition, they begin to synthesize and express NGF receptor on their surface (Fig. 8–6) (G. Stoll and J.W. Griffin, unpublished).

Schwann cells also proliferate, much as they do in wallerian degeneration. As in wallerian degeneration, the Schwann cells of nearby unmyelinated fibers, apparently unaffected by the demyelination, can also proliferate (Griffin et al., 1990). Schwann cells begin dividing on day 3 after demyelination (Hall and Gregson, 1974) and continue at lower levels during the first 14 days (Griffin et al., 1990). In demyelinating fibers, the initial division is accompanied by the perikaryal region of the Schwann cell separating from the remainder of the Schwann cell and the damaged myelin sheath forming a smaller cell. The Schwann cells of damaged internodes divide several times. After these divisions, some of the daughter cells remain within the basal lamina of the nerve fiber, but others appear outside the basal lamina and form a ring of supernumerary Schwann cells. A small number of these supernumerary Schwann cells are found in most demyelinating neuropathies, and if remyelination supervenes they disappear, presumably as a result of involution and death.

A few neuropathies are characterized by numerous redundant Schwann cells' forming large and apparently stable structures termed *onion bulbs*. These structures are typically seen in some of the heritable disorders described here, but they can, as shown in Figure 8–7, be prominent in acquired neuropathies as well. It is widely suggested that repeated demyelination is the stimulus for formation of these structures, but why they stabilize and persist in some settings and not in others is not understood.

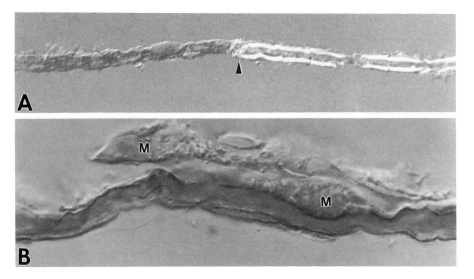

Figure 8–6. Teased nerve fibers undergoing segmental demyelination related to experimental allergic neuritis. In *A*, the internode to the left of the arrowhead has been demyelinated and stains darkly with antibodies against NGF receptor; the internode to the right has intact myelin (bright in this optical system) and does not express NGF receptor. In *B*, the remyelinating nerve fiber is positive for NGF receptor, but the nearby macrophages (M) are negative.

Genetic Disorders. In a few heritable disorders in humans, enzymatic defects result in abnormal Schwann cells. These disorders include some of the recessively inherited lysosomal storage diseases. For example, in metachromatic leukodystrophy, a defect in arylsulfatase A results in accumulation of sulfatides within Schwann cells, defective myelination, and high turnover of Schwann cells. Similarly, in globoid cell (Krabbe's) leukodystrophy, a defect in β-galactosidase results in accumulations of galactocerebroside within macrophages and Schwann cells, again with recurrent demyelination.

Several mouse mutants express inherited disorders of Schwann cell function, some of which have proved to be particularly instructive (for reviews see Aguayo and Bray, 1984; Aguayo et al., 1979; Baumann, 1980). For example, the *twitcher* mouse provides a murine counterpart to human globoid cell leukodystrophy. Recurrent demyelination and endoneurial edema result in the accumulation of macrophages containing massive inclusions of the stored lipid. This disorder has been exploited to examine the extent to which such inherited disorders are correctable by providing a population of macrophages and other bone marrow–derived cells from normal animals (Scaravilli and Jacobs, 1981). Bone marrow transplantation has been shown to result in substantially longer life and milder peripheral nerve disease.

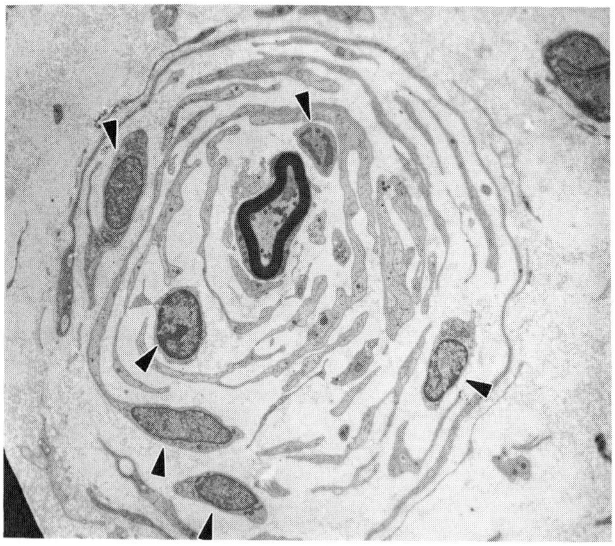

The *trembler* mutation, transmitted by dominant inheritance, is a disorder in which peripheral myelin is abnormally thin, poorly compacted, or absent. Abnormal persistence of Schwann cell multiplication leads to a several-fold increase in Schwann cell numbers within myelinated nerves. It is interesting that the unmyelinating Schwann cells in this model have no abnormalities and do not undergo excessive proliferation. This model has been exploited to ask whether the primary defect is within the Schwann cell or within the axon that "signals" the Schwann cell responses. When segments of trembler nerve were grafted into normal nerves and normal axons were allowed to regenerate through the grafts, the defective myelination typical of the trembler model was seen within the graft (Aguayo et al., 1977, 1979). Conversely, when normal nerve segments were grafted into trembler hosts, the trembler axons regenerating through the normal grafts were normally myelinated. These studies definitively demonstrated that the trembler Schwann cell is both necessary and sufficient for the trait.

The *dystrophic* mouse mutation affects both muscular and peripheral nerve tissues. Minor abnormalities of axonal ensheathment are present throughout the peripheral nervous system, but in certain spinal roots (both dorsal and ventral) axonal segments are

Figure 8–7. Major onion bulbs, composed of concentric layers of supernumerary Schwann cells organized around individual nerve fibers, from a patient with chronic inflammatory demyelinating neuropathy. The demyelination in this disorder is presumed to be immunologically mediated. Similar onion bulbs are characteristic of some of the heritable demyelinating neuropathies. The nuclei of the Schwann cells of the onion bulb are indicated by arrowheads.

completely devoid of Schwann cell ensheathment (including myelin). In these regions, naked axonal segments lie in direct contact with one another. It has been suggested that abnormal impulse conduction and initiation in these regions, rather than a genetic abnormality in muscle, may explain the prominent muscle lesions that develop as these animals grow older. Tissue culture studies have established that the Schwann cell abnormality is intrinsic to the Schwann cell and does not result from faulty axonal signaling. The fact that Schwann cell ensheathment failure can be substantially corrected if axon–Schwann cell units are provided with surrounding tissues from normal mice is a particularly intriguing aspect of this disorder (R.P. Bunge et al., 1981; Peterson and Bray, 1984).

The *shiverer* mouse and the *myelin-deficient* mouse are both recessively inherited disorders with an essential absence of a specific myelin component—the myelin basic protein. The myelin in the central nervous system is decreased in abundance, and the myelin that is present is poorly compacted and lacks major dense lines. In both of these models the myelin of the peripheral nervous system, also lacking myelin basic protein, is little affected. These observations indicate that myelin basic protein plays a less critical role in the peripheral nervous system than in the central nervous system. The shiverer mouse mutant has provided a particularly instructive example of the potential for correction of gene defects by molecular genetic techniques. Shiverer animals have been made phenotypically normal by introducing myelin basic protein transgene in ovo that corrects the abnormal shiverer gene (Readhead et al., 1987).

A final mutant, the C57BL/6/Ola mouse, is proving instructive because its nervous system survives and functions too well in disease, rather than because of inherent defects that lead to disease. When nerve fibers are severed in this substrain, the distal stumps undergo wallerian degeneration in slow motion, at a rate that is about 10-fold slower than in normal C57BL/6 mice. For example, fibers of the sciatic nerves remain relatively normal structurally for 2 weeks, and many fibers survive for 4 weeks after transection (as described earlier, axons in normal mice are reduced to granular debris within 24–48 hours) (Glass and Griffin, 1991; Lunn et al., 1989; Perry et al., 1990a,b). This capacity for prolonged survival of the distal stump is an autosomal dominant trait (Perry et al., 1990b). The "defect" lies within the nerve rather than the macrophage system, as demonstrated by bone marrow chimeras (Perry et al., 1990a). This model is being used to examine the fate of axoplasm that no longer has continuity with the cell body (see Chapter 17) (Glass and Griffin, 1991) and to examine the Schwann cell responses. For example, the down-regulation of myelin mRNA content after nerve transection is markedly delayed in the C57BL/6/Ola mouse (Thomson et al., 1991), which reflects the fact that the Schwann cell is responding to the axon.

In humans, several heritable disorders of peripheral nerves reflect abnormalities of Schwann cell myelination (for review see Ouvrier et al., 1990). Both the pathologic abnormalities and the clinical consequences range from relatively subtle to extremely severe. Perhaps the most severe disorder is *congenital absence of peripheral nerve myelin*. This rare abnormality, probably inherited at least in some forms as an autosomal recessive trait, can produce complete paralysis beginning with earliest development in utero. Such a defect results in fixed joint contractures (the joints have never moved normally) and is usually incompatible with survival beyond infancy. In one such case, studied to determine at what stage the sequence leading to myelination was arrested, the Schwann cells were found to have segregated individual nerve fibers and to have begun elongation of the mesaxon (Charnas et al., 1988) (Fig. 8–8). However, they failed to elongate the mesaxon to produce a spiral wrapping (noncompact myelin) in most fibers, and in all fibers compact myelin was absent. In addition, the cells failed to grow normally longitudinally, so that the Schwann cell–Schwann cell spacing along the nerve was abnormally short. Such a defect may reflect problems in both longitudinal and radial growth of the Schwann cell.

Another rare disorder is Dejerine-Sottas disease, an autosomal recessive neuropathy in which all peripheral myelin sheaths are abnormally thin, internodes are relatively short, and there are numerous supernumerary Schwann cells arranged in large on-

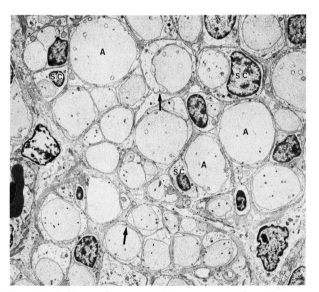

Figure 8–8. Transverse section of a nerve from a patient with congenital absence of peripheral nerve myelin. Note the complete absence of myelin. There is normal segregation of most of the large axons (examples are indicated by A) into a 1:1 relationship with the Schwann cell (examples of the Schwann cell nuclei are indicated by SC). Examples of external mesaxons are shown by arrows. All of these mesaxons extend less than one turn around the axon, and no compact myelin is formed. (From Charnas L., Trapp B.D., Griffin J.W. Congenital absence of peripheral myelin. *Neurology* 38:966–974, 1988.)

ion bulbs around the nerve fibers. Children with this disorder are neurologically abnormal in infancy and often have relatively severe neurologic disabilities. The nature of the cellular and molecular defects is unknown.

A somewhat similar but much milder disorder, transmitted by dominant inheritance, is a demyelinating neuropathy termed *Charcot-Marie-Tooth disease type I*, or hereditary motor sensory neuropathy type I. The early manifestations of this disorder may be restricted to high arched feet and poor athletic performance. Neurologic presentation may not occur until the third or fourth decade of life (or later), usually with footdrop and weakness in the ankles as the predominant features. The pathologic characteristics of this disorder are in many ways similar to those of Dejerine-Sottas disease, but milder. Again, large onion bulbs surround most myelinated fibers, similar to those in Figure 8–7. Because they take up so much space within the nerve, the nerves become visibly and palpably enlarged, which produces a "hypertrophic" neuropathy. At the present time, chromosomal linkage studies have indicated at least two different disorders, with different linkage, within this group of patients. It remains a matter of controversy as to whether the primary defect is within the Schwann cell or within the axon (Dyck, 1984), and the molecular defect is not known.

References

(Key references are designated with an asterisk.)

Aguayo A.J., Bray G.M. Cell interactions studied in the peripheral nerves of experimental animals. In Dyck P.J., Thomas P.K., Lambert E.H., et al., eds. *Peripheral Neuropathy*. Vol. I. 2nd ed. Philadelphia, Saunders, pp. 360–377, 1984.

Aguayo A.J., Epps J., Charron L., et al. Multipotentiality of Schwann cells in cross anastomosed and grafted myelinated and unmyelinated nerves—quantitative microscopy and radioautography. *Brain Res.* 104:1–20, 1976a.

Aguayo A.J., Peyronnard J.M., Terry L.C., et al. Neonatal neuronal loss in rat superior cervical ganglia: retrograde effects on developing preganglionic axons and Schwann cells. *J. Neurocytol.* 5:137–155, 1976b.

Aguayo A.J., Kasarjian J., Samene E., et al. Myelination of mouse axons by Schwann cells transplanted from normal and abnormal human nerves. *Nature* 268:753–755, 1977.

Aguayo A.J., Bray G.M., Perkins C.S. Axon–Schwann cell relationships in neuropathies of mutant mice. *Ann. N. Y. Acad. Sci.* 317:512–531, 1979.

Ard M.D., Bunge R.P., Bunge M.B. Comparison of the Schwann cell surface and Schwann cell extracellular matrix as promoters of neurite growth. *J. Neurocytol.* 16:539–555, 1987.

Asbury A.K. Schwann cell proliferation in developing mouse sciatic nerve. *J. Cell Biol.* 34:735–743, 1967.

Baumann N. *Neurological Mutations Affecting Myelination*. INSERM Symposium No. 14. Amsterdam, Elsevier North Holland Biomedical Press, 1980.

Berry M., Hall S., Follows R., et al. Response of axons and glia at the site of anastomosis between the optic nerve and cellular or acellular sciatic nerve grafts. *J. Neurocytol.* 17:727–744, 1988.

Berthold C.-H., Carlstedt T., Corneliuson O. Anatomy of the nerve root at the central-peripheral transitional region. In Dyck P.J., Thomas P.K., Lambert E.H., et al., eds. *Peripheral Neuropathy*. Vol. I. 2nd ed. Philadelphia, Saunders, pp. 156–170, 1984.

Beuche W., Friede R.L. The role of non-resident cells in wallerian degeneration. *J. Neurocytol.* 13:767–796, 1984.

Beuche W., Friede R.L. Myelin phagocytosis in wallerian degeneration depends on silica-sensitive, bg/bg-negative and Fc-positive monocytes. *Brain Res.* 378:97–106, 1986.

Billings-Gagliardi S., Webster H. deF., O'Connell M.F. In vivo and electron microscopic observations on Schwann cells in developing tadpole nerve fibers. *Am. J. Anat.* 141:375–392, 1974.

Bixby J.L., Harris W.A. Molecular mechanisms of axon growth and guidance. *Annu. Rev. Cell Biol.* (in press).

Bixby J.L., Lilien J., Reichardt L.F. Identification of the major proteins that promote neuronal process outgrowth on Schwann cells in vitro. *J. Cell Biol.* 107:353–361, 1988.

*Brockes J.P. Mitogenic growth factors and nerve dependence of limb regeneration. *Science* 225:1280–1287, 1984.

Brockes J.P., Fields K.L., Raff M.C. Studies on cultured rat Schwann cells. I. Establishment of purified populations from cultures of peripheral nerve. *Brain Res.* 165:105–118, 1979.

Brockes J.P., Lemke G.E., Balzer D.R. Jr. Purification and preliminary characterization of a glial growth factor from bovine pituitary. *J. Biol. Chem.* 255:8374–8377, 1980.

Bunge M.B. Schwann cell regulation of extracellular matrix biosynthesis and assembly. In Dyck P.J., Thomas P.K., Griffin J., et al., eds. *Peripheral Neuropathy*. 3rd ed. Philadelphia, Saunders, in press.

Bunge M.B., Williams A.K., Wood P.M. Neuron–Schwann cell interaction in basal lamina formation. *Dev. Biol.* 92:449–460, 1982.

*Bunge M.B., Bunge R.P., Carey D.J., et al. Axonal and nonaxonal influences on Schwann cell development. In Coates P.W., Markwald R.R., Kenny A.D., eds. *Developing and Regenerating Vertebrate Nervous Systems*. New York, Liss, pp. 71–105, 1983.

Bunge M.B., Wood P.M., Tynan L.B., et al. Perineurium originates from fibroblasts: demonstration in vitro with a retroviral marker. *Science* 243:229–231, 1989.

Bunge R.P., Hopkins J.M. The role of peripheral and central neuroglia in neural regeneration in vertebrates. *Semin. Neurosci.* 2:509–518, 1991.

Bunge R.P., Bunge M.B., Williams A.K., et al. Does the dystrophic mouse nerve lesion result from an extracellular matrix abnormality? In Shotland D., ed. *Disorders of the Motor Unit*. New York, Wiley, pp. 23–35, 1981.

Bunge R.P., Bunge M.B., Bates M. Movements of the Schwann cell nucleus implicate progression of the inner (axon-related) Schwann cell process during myelination. *J. Cell Biol.* 109:273–284, 1989.

Carey D.J., Eldridge C.F., Cornbrooks C.J., et al. Biosynthesis of type IV collagen by cultured rat Schwann cells. *J. Cell Biol.* 97:473–479, 1983.

Carter D.A., Bray G.M., Aguayo A.J. Regenerated retinal ganglion cell axons can form well-differentiated synapses in the superior colliculus of adult hamsters. *J. Neurosci.* 9:4042–4050, 1989.

Charnas L., Trapp B.D., Griffin J.W. Congenital absence of peripheral myelin. *Neurology* 38:966–974, 1988.

Chen S.-J., DeVries G.H. Alpha-FGF is an axonal mitogen for cultured oligodendrocytes. *Trans. Am. Soc. Neurochem.* (in press).

Clemence A., Mirsky R., Jessen K.R. Non–myelin-forming Schwann cells proliferate rapidly during wallerian degeneration in the rat sciatic nerve. *J. Neurocytol.* 18:185–192, 1989.

Cornbrooks C.J., Carey D.J., McDonald J.A., et al. In vivo and in vitro observations on laminin production by Schwann cells. *Proc. Natl. Acad. Sci. U.S.A.* 80:3850–3854, 1983.

Davis J.B., Stroobant P. Platelet-derived growth factors and fibroblast growth factors are mitogens for rat Schwann cells. *J. Cell Biol.* 110:1353–1360, 1990.

DeVries G.H., Salzer J.L., Bunge R.P. Axolemma-enriched fractions isolated from PNS and CNS are mitogenic for cultured Schwann cells. *Brain Res.* 255:295–299, 1982.

Dubois-Dalcq M., Rentier B., Baron-Van Evercooren A., et al. Structure and behavior of rat primary and secondary Schwann cells in vitro. *Exp. Cell Res.* 131:283–297, 1981.

Dyck P.J. Inherited neuronal degeneration and atrophy affecting peripheral motor, sensory, and autonomic nerves. In Dyck P.J., Thomas P.K., Lambert E.H., et al., eds. *Peripheral Neuropathy*. Vol. I. 2nd ed. Philadelphia, Saunders, pp. 1600–1655, 1984.

Eccleston P.A., Collarini E.J., Jessen K.R., et al. Schwann cells secrete a PDGF-like factor: evidence for an autocrine growth mechanism involving PDGF. *Eur. J. Neurosci.* 2:985–992, 1990.

Eldridge C.F., Sanes J.R., Chiu A.Y., et al. Basal lamina–associated heparan sulfate proteoglycan in the rat PNS: characterization and localization using monoclonal antibodies. *J. Neurocytol.* 15:37–51, 1986.

Fawcett J.W., Keynes R.J. Peripheral nerve regeneration. *Annu. Rev. Neurosci.* 13:43–60, 1990.

Friede R., Samorajski T. Relation between the number of myelin lamellae and axon circumference in fibers of vagus and sciatic nerves of mice. *J. Comp. Neurol.* 130:223–231, 1967.

Glass J.D., Griffin J.W. Neurofilament redistribution in transected nerves: evidence for bidirectional transport of neurofilaments. *J. Neurosci.* (in press).

Griffin J.W., Drucker N., Gold B.G., et al. Schwann cell proliferation and migration during paranodal demyelination. *J. Neurosci.* 7:682–699, 1987.

Griffin J.W., Stocks E.A., Fahnestock K., et al. Schwann cell proliferation following lysolecithin-induced demyelination. *J. Neurocytol.* 19:367–384, 1990.

Hall S.M., Gregson N.A. The effects of mytomycin C on remyelination in the peripheral nervous system. *Nature* 252:303–305, 1974.

Harrison R.G. Neuroblast versus sheath cell in the development of peripheral nerves. *J. Comp. Neurol.* 37:123–205, 1924.

Higgins D., Burton H. Electrotonic synapses are formed by fetal rat sympathetic neurons maintained in a chemically-defined culture medium. *Neuroscience* 7:2241–2253, 1982.

Ide C., Tohyama K., Yokota R., et al. Schwann cell basal lamina and nerve regeneration. *Brain Res.* 288:61–75, 1983.

Jessen K.R., Mirsky R. Astrocyte-like glia in the peripheral nervous system: an immunohistochemical study of enteric glia. *J. Neurosci.* 3:2206–2218, 1983.

Jessen K.R., Mirsky R. Nonmyelin-forming Schwann cells coexpress surface proteins and intermediate filaments not found in myelin-forming cells: a study of Ran-2, A5E3 and glial fibrillary acidic protein. *J. Neurocytol.* 12:923–934, 1984.

Jessen K.R., Mirsky R., Morgan L. Axonal signals regulate the differentiation of non–myelin-forming Schwann cells: an immunohistochemical study of galactocerebroside in transected and regenerating nerves. *J. Neurosci.* 7:3362–3369, 1987.

Johnson E.M. Jr., Taniuchi M., DiStefano P.S. Expression and possible function of nerve growth factor receptors on Schwann cells. *Trends Neurosci.* 11:299–304, 1988.

Kidd G.J., Heath J.W. Double myelination of axons in the sympathetic nervous system of the mouse. II. Mechanisms of formation. *J. Neurocytol.* 17:263–276, 1988.

Kleitman N., Wood P., Johnson M.I., et al. Schwann cell surfaces but not extracellular matrix organized by Schwann cells support neurite outgrowth from embryonic rat retina. *J. Neurosci.* 8:653–663, 1988.

Kromer L.F., Cornbrooks C.J. Transplants of Schwann cell cultures promote axonal regeneration in the adult mammalian brain. *Proc. Natl. Acad. Sci. U.S.A.* 82:6330–6334, 1985.

Kuffler D.P. Regeneration of muscle axons in the frog is directed by diffusible factors from denervated muscle and nerve tubes. *J. Comp. Neurol.* 281:416–425, 1989.

Laurie G.W., Leblond C.P., Martin G.R. Light microscopic immunolocalization of type IV collagen, laminin, heparan sulfate proteoglycan and fibronectin in the basement membranes of a variety of rat organs. *Am. J. Anat.* 167:71–82, 1983.

LeDouarin N. *The Neural Crest.* New York, Cambridge University Press, 1982.

Lemke G. Unwrapping the genes of myelin. *Neuron* 1:535–543, 1988.

Lindholm D., Heumann R., Meyer M., et al. Interleukin-1 regulates synthesis of nerve growth factor in non-neuronal cells of rat sciatic nerve. *Nature* 330:658–659, 1987.

Lindholm D., Heumann R., Hengerer B., et al. Interleukin-1 increases stability and transcription of mRNA encoding nerve growth factor in cultured rat fibroblasts. *J. Biol. Chem.* 263:16348–16351, 1988.

Lunn E.R., Perry V.H., Brown M.C., et al. Absence of wallerian degeneration does not hinder regeneration in peripheral nerve. *Eur. J. Neurosci.* 1:27–33, 1989.

McCarthy K., Partlow L. Neuronal stimulation of [³H]thymidine incorporation by primary cultures of highly purified non-neuronal cells. *Brain Res.* 114:415–426, 1976.

McGarvey M.L., Baron-Van Evercooren A., Kleinman H.K., et al. Synthesis and effects of basement membrane components in cultured rat Schwann cells. *Dev. Biol.* 105:18–28, 1984.

Mirsky R., Jessen K.R. Molecular heterogeneity in peripheral glia. In Duprat A.M., Kato A.C., Weber M., eds. *The Role of Cell Interactions in Early Neurogenesis.* New York, Plenum Publishing, pp. 181–190, 1984.

Ouvrier R.A., McLeod J.G., Pollard J.D. *Peripheral Neuropathy in Childhood.* New York, Raven Press, 1990.

Owens G., Bunge R.P. Schwann cells expressing myelin-associated glycoprotein but not galactocerebroside initiate but cannot continue the process of myelination. *GLIA* 3:113–124, 1990.

Pellegrino R.G., Politis M.J., Ritchie J.M., et al. Events in degenerating cat peripheral nerve: induction of Schwann cell S phase and its relation to nerve fibre degeneration. *J. Neurocytol.* 15:17–28, 1986.

Perry V.H., Brown M.C., Lunn E.R., et al. Evidence that very slow wallerian degeneration in C57BL/Ola mice is an intrinsic property of the peripheral nerve. *Eur. J. Neurosci.* 2:802–808, 1990a.

Perry V.H., Lunn E.R., Brown M.C., et al. Evidence that the rate of wallerian degeneration is controlled by a single autosomal dominant gene. *Eur. J. Neurosci.* 2:408–413, 1990b.

Peters A., Paley S.L., Webster H.DeF. *The Fine Structure of the Nervous System: The Neurons and Supporting Cells.* Philadelphia, Saunders, 1976.

Peterson A.C., Bray G.M. Normal basal laminas are realized on dystrophic Schwann cells in dystrophic shiver chimera nerves. *J. Cell Biol.* 99:1831–1837, 1984.

Ranscht B., Wood P.M., Bunge R.P. Inhibition of in vitro peripheral myelin formation by monoclonal anti-galactocerebroside. *J. Neurosci.* 7:2936–2947, 1987.

Ratner N., Bunge R.P., Glaser L.A neuronal cell surface heparan sulfate proteoglycan is required for dorsal root ganglion neuron stimulation of Schwann cell proliferation. *J. Cell Biol.* 101:741–754, 1985.

Ratner N., Bunge R.P., Glaser L. Schwann cell proliferation in vitro. An overview. *Ann. N.Y. Acad. Sci.* 486:170–181, 1986.

Readhead C., Popko B., Takahashi N., et al. Expression of a myelin basic protein gene in transgenic shiverer mice: correction of the dysmyelinating phenotype. *Cell* 48:703–712, 1987.

Robertson J.D. The unit membrane of cells and mechanisms of myelin formation. In Korey S.R., Pope A., Robins E., eds. *Ultrastructure and Metabolism of the Nervous System. Proceedings of the Association of Research on Nervous and Mental Diseases.* Vol. 40. Baltimore, Williams & Wilkins, 1962.

Salzer J.L., Bunge R.P. Studies of Schwann cell proliferation. I. An analysis in tissue culture of proliferation during development, wallerian degeneration and direct injury. *J. Cell Biol.* 84:739–752, 1980.

Salzer J.L., Bunge R.P., Glaser L. Studies of Schwann cell proliferation. III. Evidence for the surface localization of the neurite mitogen. *J. Cell Biol.* 84:767–778, 1980.

Scaravilli F., Jacobs J.M. Peripheral nerve grafts in hereditary leukodystrophic mutant mice (twitcher). *Nature* 290:56–58, 1981.

Scheidt P., Friede R.L. Myelin phagocytosis in wallerian degeneration. Properties of Millipore diffusion chambers and immunohistochemical identification of cell populations. *Acta Neuropathol.* 75:77–84, 1987.

Scherer S.S., Easter S.S. Degenerative and regenerative changes in the trochlear nerve of the goldfish. *J. Neurocytol.* 13:519–565, 1984.

Schnapp B., Mugnaini E. The myelin sheath: electron microscopic studies with thin sections and freeze-fracture. In Santini M., ed. *Golgi Centennial Symposium Proceedings.* New York, Raven Press, p. 209, 1975.

Sketelj J., Bresjanac M., Popovic M. Rapid growth of regenerating axons across the segments of sciatic nerve devoid of Schwann cells. *J. Neurosci. Res.* 24:153–162, 1989.

Sobue G., Krieder B., Asbury A.K., et al. Specific and potent mitogenic effect of axolemmal fraction or Schwann cells from sciatic nerves in serum-containing and defined media. *Brain Res.* 280:263–275, 1983.

*Spencer P.S., Politis M.J., Pellegrino R.G., et al. Control of Schwann cell behavior during nerve degeneration and regeneration. In Gorio A., Millesi H., Mingrino S., eds. *Symposium *on Post-Traumatic Peripheral Nerve Regeneration*. New York, Raven Press, pp. 411–426, 1981.

Stoll G., Griffin J.W., Li C.Y., et al. Wallerian degeneration in the peripheral nervous system: participation of both Schwann cells and macrophages in myelin degradation. *J. Neurocytol.* 18:671–683, 1990.

Taniuchi M., Clark H.B., Schweitzer J.B., et al. Expression of nerve growth factor receptors by Schwann cells of axotomized peripheral nerves: ultrastructural location, suppression by axonal contact, and binding properties. *J. Neurosci.* 8:664–681, 1988.

Tennyson V.M. Electron microscopic study of the developing neuroblast of the dorsal root ganglion of the rabbit embryo. *J. Comp. Neurol.* 124:267–282, 1965.

Thomas G.A. Quantitative histology of wallerian degeneration. II. Nuclear population in two nerves of different fibre spectrum. *J. Anat.* 82:135–145, 1948.

*Thomas P.K., Ochoa J. Microscopic anatomy of peripheral nerve fibers. In Dyck P.J., Thomas P.K., Lambert E.H., et al., eds. *Peripheral Neuropathy*. Vol. I. 2nd ed. Philadelphia, Saunders, pp. 39–96, 1984.

*Thomas P.K., Olsson Y. Microscopic anatomy and function of the connective tissue components of peripheral nerve. In Dyck P.J., Thomas P.K., Lambert E.H., et al., eds. *Peripheral Neuropathy*. Vol. I. 2nd ed. Philadelphia, Saunders, pp. 121–155, 1984.

Thomson C.E., Mitchell L.S., Griffiths I.R., et al. Retarded wallerian degeneration following peripheral nerve transection in C57BL/6/Ola mice is associated with delayed down-regulation of the P_0 gene. *Brain Res.* 538:157–160, 1991.

Trapp B.D., Itoyama Y., Sternberger N.H., et al. Immunocytochemical localization of P_0 protein in Golgi complex membranes and myelin of developing rat Schwann cells. *J. Cell Biol.* 90:1–6, 1981.

Trapp B.D., Hauer P., Lemke G. Axonal regulation of myelin protein mRNA levels in actively myelinating Schwann cells. *J. Neurosci.* 8:3515–3521, 1988.

*Webster H.DeF., Favilla J.T. Development of peripheral nerve fibers. In Dyck P.J., Thomas P.K., Lambert E.H., et al., eds. *Peripheral Neuropathy*. Vol. I. 2nd ed. Philadelphia, Saunders, pp. 329–359, 1984.

Weinberg H.J., Spencer P.S. Studies on the control of myelinogenesis. I. Myelination of regenerating axons after entry into a foreign unmyelinated nerve. *J. Neurocytol.* 4:395–418, 1975.

White F.V., Toews A.D., Goodrum J.F., et al. Lipid metabolism during early stages of wallerian degeneration in the rat sciatic nerve. *J. Neurochem.* 52:1085–1092, 1989.

Windebank A.J., Wood P., Bunge R.P., et al. Myelination determines the caliber of dorsal root ganglion neurons in culture. *J. Neurosci.* 5:1563–1569, 1985.

Wood P.M., Bunge R.P. Evidence that sensory axons are mitogenic for Schwann cells. *Nature* 256:662–664, 1975.

Yen S.-H., Fields K.L. Antibodies to neurofilament, glial filament and fibroblast intermediate filament proteins bind to different cell types of the nervous system. *J. Cell Biol.* 88:115–126, 1981.

9

Ependyma

Thomas H. McNeill
Robert J. Joynt

The ependyma is a layer of epithelial cells that line the ventricular cavities of the cerebrum, brain stem, and central canal of the spinal cord. Ependymal cells originate in a single layer of undifferentiated proliferative epithelium termed the *ventricular zone* (Boulder Committee, 1970) derived from the developing ectoderm of the neural plate (Jacobson, 1978). As the plate develops, undifferentiated ventricular cells proliferate and develop into two differentiated cell lines that ultimately form all cellular components of the central nervous system (CNS). At the time of embryonic differentiation, cells destined to form the ependyma, as well as other neuroglial cells, continue to be referred to as ventricular cells, or in some cases as spongioblasts, whereas the predecessors of neurons are termed *neuroblasts*. According to this nomenclature, ventricular cells are considered to be the predecessors of all neurons, macroglia, and ependymal cells in the CNS.

As development progresses, the original single layer of undifferentiated ventricular cells rapidly proliferates and forms a pseudostratified layer of columnar epithelium (Angevine, 1970). As premitotic ventricular cells initiate DNA replication (S phase), their nuclei migrate to the ventricular surface from deeper layers of stratum. When the nuclei are at the surface, they divide (mitosis). After division, the daughter cells move away from the surface as the cell elongates to take on its original columnar form and the cycle recurs. As the neural tube develops, ventricular cells continue to divide to form two fundamental zones around the central canal (Angevine, 1970). The innermost zone is the ventricular zone with cells abutting directly on the inner limiting membrane of the neurocanal. The ventricular zone is composed of a homogeneous population of proliferative ventricular cells and is confined to the area in which both mitotic division and intermitotic migration of ventricular cells takes place. The outer or marginal zone contains few

cells and forms the future white matter of the CNS across which nerve processes will extend. At the time of neural tube closure, cells of the ventricular zone still form a pool of undifferentiated daughter cells. Later, however, ventricular cells will divide to form both undifferentiated ventricular cells and embryonic neuroblasts.

By the end of the development, ventricular cells destined to become ependymal cells stop dividing and begin to differentiate into their characteristic cell morphology (Fujita, 1963). Although junctional complexes are not present at this time, the lateral cell borders of the developing ependyma do have cytoplasmic interdigitations of plasma membrane with prominent thickening that are thought to facilitate cellular communication. Ultrastructural features of embryonic ependyma include free polyribosomes, mitochondria, a well-defined Golgi complex, granular endoplasmic reticulum, and microvilli on the ventricular surface (Lyser, 1964). Cilia are thought to develop just before birth, with the final stages of ependyma development taking place shortly thereafter. At that time, neonatal ependymal cells resemble those of the adult and form a single layer of mostly ciliated cuboidal cells lining the cavities of the brain and the spinal cord.

CILIATED EPENDYMAL CELLS

Although squamous and columnar cell types line some regions of the ventricular surface, the most common type of ependymal cell is the ciliated cuboidal epithelium (Fig. 9–1). In toluidine blue–stained plastic-embedded sections, ependymal cells have prominent and centrally located nuclei, a nucleoplasm of even density, and a homogeneously stained cytoplasm with few distinguishing features (Millhouse, 1975). Because of the basophobic nature of

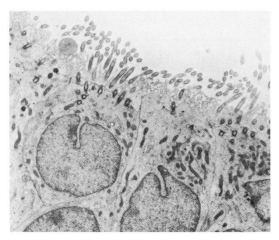

Figure 9–1. Transmission electron micrograph of ciliated ependymal cells lining the thalamic wall of the third ventricle of the monkey *Macaca fascicularis*. Ciliated ependymal cells have a characteristic round, centrally located nucleus, a relatively homogeneous cytoplasm with mitochondria, and Golgi cisternae concentrated on the luminal border. × 4850.

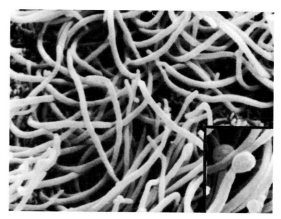

Figure 9–2. Scanning electron micrograph of the ventricular surface of the thalamic wall of the duck *Anas platyrhynchos*. Cilia are distributed over much of the ventricular surface with an even density. Individual cilia have spherical, knob-like configurations at their tips (*inset*). × 10,125.

the cytoplasm, ependymal cells are easily distinguished from the more darkly staining adjacent neuropil. In light microscopic preparations, ependymal cells have numerous cilia on their ventricular surfaces, as well as many underlying microvilli that extend into the ventricular lumen. Owing to the heavy density of cilia (Fig. 9–2), the ventricular surface takes on a heterogeneous topography with distinguishing regional differences, as seen with the scanning electron microscope (Scott and Paull, 1983; Weindl and Joynt, 1972).

Studies have shown that the architectural organization of the ventricular surface is relatively consistent across most mammalian and nonmammalian species, with only a few exceptions (Bruni et al., 1972; Scott and Paull, 1983; Weindl and Joynt, 1972). In general, the surfaces of the cerebral ventricles and the spinal canal are covered by a densely packed layer of cilia, which gradually decreases in density across a zone of transition adjacent to the circumventricular organs (CVOs) (Hofer, 1958). In the third ventricle, the dorsal two-thirds of the ventricular wall is lined by ependymal cells with long cilia that extend into the lumen of the ventricle. This type of surface topography extends from the lamina terminalis, rostrally, to the cerebral aqueduct, caudally. Along the ventral one-third of the ventricle, ependymal cells form a transition zone that blends into a sparsely ciliated ependymal surface on the floor of the infundibular recess. Based on the species examined, there may be an abrupt or gradual transition between ciliated and nonciliated cell surfaces.

Ultrastructurally, ependymal cells are characterized by numerous long cilia; a round, centrally located nucleus; and a relatively homogeneous cytoplasm (see Fig. 9–1). In addition, ciliated ependymal cells have relatively few cytoplasmic projections into the ventricular lumen. Polyribosomes are distributed throughout the cytoplasm, with mitochondria and

the Golgi cisternae concentrated along the luminal border. Cilia may be distributed over the ventricle surface with either an even density or clusters of small patches or isolated islands (see Fig. 9–2). Although all cilia have the characteristic in 9 + 2 configuration of microtubules, individual cilia show marked variations in size and shape depending on the species examined.

The presence of cilia over a large area of the ventricular surface has suggested that cilia are used in influencing the kinetics of local cerebrospinal fluid (CSF) flow. Scanning electron microscope studies have shown that cilia are distributed in wave-like patterns along the ventricular surface, which suggests that cilia are able to move CSF through coordinated beating (Scott et al., 1974a). Studies with fresh tissue showed that cilia of ependymal cells beat rapidly and can direct CSF flow toward the foramina of Luschka and Magendie of the fourth ventricle (Cathcart and Worthington, 1964). In addition, cilia can remove small masses of cellular debris from

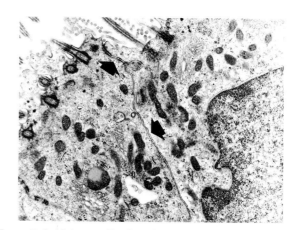

Figure 9–3. High-magnification electron micrograph of a junction (*arrow*) between two ciliated ependymal cells. Most ciliated ependymal cells are joined either by gap junctions or by zonulae adherens. × 11,250.

ependymal surfaces and inhibit the collection of small fragments of tissue debris in blind recesses of the ventricular system. Previous studies revealed that when there is damage to cilia because of increased ventricular pressure such as in hydrocephalus, a stagnation may occur in CSF flow at the infundibular recess, thus forming a frequent implantation site for metastases from CNS tumors. Thus, not only do cilia provide a mechanism to facilitate local CSF flow, but they do so by removing cellular debris and metastatic cells before they have a chance to initiate a new site of disease.

Neighboring ependymal cells throughout most of the ventricular surface are joined by specialized junctional complexes termed *gap junctions* or *zonulae adherens* along the lateral cell borders (Brightman and Palay, 1963; Brightman and Reese, 1969). Previous studies reported that these junctions do not form a complete seal around the cell and therefore provide for the free movement of large molecules and proteins from the CSF into the neuropil (Fig. 9–3). Because gap junctions form a discontinuous barrier to the movement of large molecules, it has been suggested that they may serve more of a purpose in intercellular communication (Revel and Karnovsky, 1967). Previous studies showed that when horseradish peroxidase is injected into the CSF of the third ventricle, it can traverse the gap junctions and migrate between ependymal cells into the underlying neuropil. Conversely, cellular metabolites from the subadjacent neuropil may move freely into the CSF, a sampling of which has been used as a tool in the study of cell metabolism in neurodegenerative diseases of the CNS.

NONCILIATED EPENDYMAL CELLS

Regions along the cerebral ventricles where the morphologic characteristic of the ependymal cells

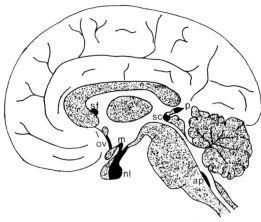

Figure 9–4. Schematic diagram of a midsagittal section through the human brain showing the ventricular system and the circumventricular organs: the median eminence (m), the subcommissural organ (sc), the organum vasculosum of the lamina terminalis (ov), subfornical organ (sf), the area postrema (ap), the neural lobe (nl), and pineal gland (p).

deviates from the common ciliated cuboidal cell type occur along the ventricular surfaces of the CVOs (Hofer, 1958). Figure 9–4 is a schematic diagram of a midsagittal section through the human brain showing the ventricular system and the CVOs. These organs include the median eminence, the subcommissural organ, the organum vasculosum of the lamina terminalis, the subfornical organ, the area postrema, the neural lobe, and the pineal gland. Another structure that is not normally considered to be a CVO but that has many features similar to those of the CVOs is the paraventricular organ (Kappers, 1920–1921; Mikami, 1975), which forms a bilateral groove in the wall of the third ventricle and is most pronounced in submammalian species (Fig. 9–5).

Except for the area postrema, all of the CVOs including the paraventricular organ are located along

Figure 9–5. Low-magnification micrograph of a subependymal cell of the paraventricular organ, whose cells have ventricular processes that extend into the ventricular lumen. (*Inset*) Scanning electron micrograph showing the surface appearance of the ventricular protrusions. × 4920.

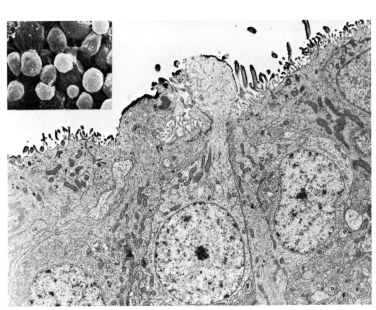

the walls of the third ventricle and share many morphologic similarities with respect to their vascular, neuronal, and ependymal organization (Weindl and Joynt, 1972). These regions of the brain are covered by nonciliated ependymal cells with many microvilli on the ventricular surface. In addition, some cells show cytoplasmic extensions or protrusions at the surface of the cell (Fig. 9–6) that extend into the lumen of the ventricle. Most notable are the intraventricular cytoplasmic swellings of the paraventricular organ (Vigh and Vigh-Teichmann, 1973; Vigh-Teichmann et al., 1969). These bulb-shaped swellings have been shown to contain well-developed mitochondria and numerous dense core vesicles. In addition, fluorescence histochemical and immunocytochemical studies of these processes have shown them to be an extension of subependymal serotoninergic or dopaminergic neurons, which extend into the ventricular lumen (Baumgarten and Braak, 1967; Sano et al., 1983; Sharp and Follett, 1986).

In general, nonciliated ependymal cells have irregular shapes, an indented or lobulated nucleus, and numerous microvilli (Figs. 9–7 and 9–8). Microtubules, endoplasmic reticulum, polyribosomes, and Golgi cisternae are also present within the cytoplasm (Peters et al., 1976). In contrast to ciliated cells, neighboring nonciliated ependymal cells of the CVOs are joined by tight junctions (or zonulae occludens) (Brightman et al., 1975) (Fig. 9–9), which form a complete seal around the cell and an impermeable barrier for the movement of most molecules between the CSF and the adjacent neuropil (Feder et al., 1969; Reese and Karnovsky, 1967). Previous studies showed that when horseradish peroxidase is injected intravenously, it rapidly crosses the fenestrated endothelium of the blood vessels of the CVOs and diffuses into the excellular tissue space (Brightman, 1968). However, passage of the enzyme into the CSF is blocked by the tight junctions between ependymal cells. Conversely, an intraventricular infusion of

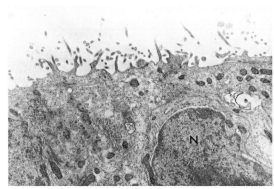

Figure 9–7. Electron micrograph of nonciliated ependymal cells in the median eminence of the monkey *M. fascicularis.* Nonciliated ependymal cells have numerous microvilli on their surface and a lobulated or indented nucleus (N). × 8700.

horseradish peroxidase rapidly diffuses between ciliated ependymal cells in the dorsal regions of the ventricle but does not cross between ependymal cells of the CVOs. Thus, the tight junction adjoining ependymal cells of the CVOs prevents the infusion of molecules that can cross the fenestrated capillaries of the CVOs into the CSF. However, although large molecules such as proteins are restricted from crossing the ependyma, small ions and water can pass with little restriction. Thus, the ependymas of CVOs are not impermeable to all substances.

The ventricular surfaces of nonciliated ependymal cells are covered by numerous microvilli as well as large apical processes that protrude into the CSF (Millhouse, 1975; Scott and Paull, 1983). Classically, microvilli have been shown to increase the cell surface of existing cells to allow for increased absorptive or secretory activity; a similar role has been suggested for ependymal cells of the CVOs (Knowles, 1972). In addition, the large variability in the presence and size of the apical processes (see Fig. 9–6) of the ventricular surfaces from animal to animal and spe-

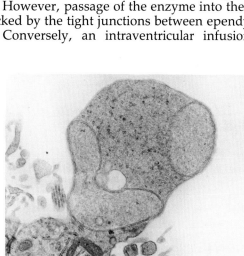

Figure 9–6. High-magnification electron micrograph of an apical process of a nonciliated ependymal cell in the median eminence of the mouse. × 11,125.

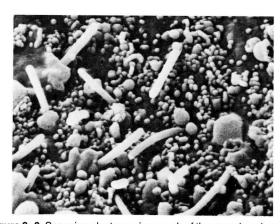

Figure 9–8. Scanning electron micrograph of the ependymal surface of the organum vasculosum of the lamina terminalis of the duck *A. platyrhynchos.* Most notable is the lack of cilia on the surface of the ependyma. × 8100.

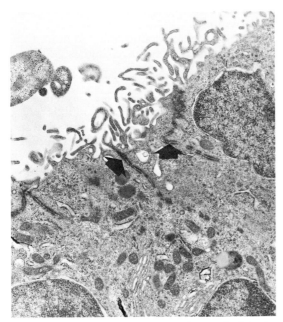

Figure 9–9. High-magnification electron micrograph of the junction between two ependymal cells of the median eminence of the monkey. Nonciliated ependymal cells of most CVOs are joined by tight junctions *(arrows)* or by zonulae occludens to form a complete seal around the cell. × 13,500.

cies to species has suggested that these variations may reflect changes in the neuroendocrine dynamics or in the metabolic states of ependymal cell function (Knowles, 1972; Knowles and Anand-Kumar, 1967). However, previous studies have shown that although ependymal cells are capable of both absorbing and transporting many biologically active substances, they also transplant many substances with little biologic significance such as microperoxidase and nonmetabolized amino acids (Scott et al., 1973, 1974b; Silverman et al., 1972). Thus, it has been argued that the ability of nonciliated cells to transport molecules between the CSF and the adjacent tissue may be a general cellular phenomenon that is not necessarily linked to a specific neuroendocrine event.

Unlike ciliated ependymal cells, which have flattened or ovoid bases, ependymal cells of the CVOs have a long, radially oriented process that reaches deep into the neuropil. Specialized nonciliated ependymal cells, whose basal processes stretch to the outer surface of the brain, are called tanycytes or stretch cells and were first described by Horstmann in 1954. In mammals, tanycyte ependymal cells are found along the CVOs of the third ventricle. In most cases tanycyte end feet terminate on subependymal capillaries of the neuropil or on the fenestrated blood vessels of the median eminence and organum vasculosum (Millhouse, 1972). Similar to the case for astrocytes, tanycytic end feet are separated from the blood vessel endothelium by a basal lamina (Peters et al., 1976). Studies of the median eminence have shown that tanycyte processes are interposed between peptide-containing axon terminals ending on

the fenestrated portal capillaries (Monroe et al., 1972; Scott et al., 1972). This arrangement has led some to speculate that the end feet of tanycytes may perform a neuroregulatory mechanism by governing the amount of surface area of fenestrated capillary at the neurohemal contact zone available for diffusion of neurosecretory hormones (Lichtensteiger and Richards, 1975; Lichtensteiger et al., 1978).

Studies by Lichtensteiger et al. (1978) have shown that injections of nicotine, which produce pronounced reductions in growth hormone and prolactin levels, are paralleled by a reduction in the surface area covered by the non-neuronal profiles along the contact zone of the median eminence. In addition, the inhibition of both the reduction of prolactin levels and the degree to which non-neuronal profiles cover pericapillaries of the median eminence can be reversed by pretreatment with the dopamine receptor blocker pimozide. However, whether there is a true functional link between the neuroendocrine parameters and ultrastructural changes in non-neuronal elements in the median eminence remains to be proved.

SUPRAEPENDYMAL CELLS

Two types of supraependymal cells have been found on the surface of the ventricular cavities (Clementi and Marini, 1972; Coats, 1973a,b,c; Paull et al., 1977; Scott and Paull, 1983; Scott et al., 1974a, 1977). The majority of these cells, in most mammalian species, are considered to be quiescent histiocytes with long filopodia interconnecting adjacent cells. Their cell cytoplasm contains numerous lysosomes and is thought to be active only during an inflammatory reaction or in response to some type of pathophysiologic change. The second type of supraependymal cell is the so-called CSF-contacting neuron (Vigh-Teichman and Vigh, 1974) (Fig. 9–10). These cells show ultrastructural characteristics similar to those of neurons of the CNS and have numerous processes that course over the ventricular surface

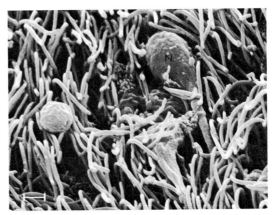

Figure 9–10. Scanning electron micrograph of CSF-contacting neuron (N) in the dorsal wall of third ventricle. Scale bar = 2 μm.

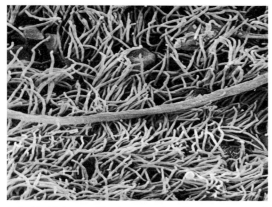

Figure 9–11. High-magnification scanning electron micrograph of a supraependymal cell process traversing the ciliated ependymal surface of the dorsal thalamic wall. Scale bar = 2 μm.

(Fig. 9–11). In some species cells are bound into a small cluster resembling a large ganglion on the floor of the infundibular recess (Card and Mitchell, 1978). It has been speculated that supraependymal neurons may act as a type of receptor cell to monitor the chemical composition of the CSF (McKenna and Rosenbluth, 1974) In this way they may serve to integrate functionally various specialized regions of the brain (Scott and Paull, 1983). However, the contribution of supraependymal neurons to the overall regulation of neuroendocrine homeostasis is not yet fully understood.

ROLE OF EPENDYMINS IN LEARNING AND MEMORY

Ependymins are a unique family of brain extracellular glycoproteins first described in goldfish (Shashoua, 1976). Two forms of ependymin have been isolated (i.e., β and γ), and their amino acid compositions (R. Schmidt and Shashoua, 1983) and DNA sequences (Konigstorfer et al., 1989a,b) have been determined. Radioimmunoassay studies of the regional and subcellular distribution of ependymins have demonstrated that they are specific to the nervous system (R. Schmidt and Lapp, 1987) and are highly concentrated in fluid extracts of brain extracellular matrix and CSF (R. Schmidt and Lapp, 1987). These data are consistent with previous immunocytochemical studies that have found that ependymins are synthesized in specialized cells in the periventricular gray of the ependymal zone surrounding the ventricular cavities of the brain as well as in neurons of the optic tectum and vagal lobes of various species of fish (Benowitz and Shashoua, 1977; R. Schmidt, 1985; R. Schmidt et al., 1986). Ependymins have also been found in reactive astrocytes associated with gliosis after brain injury (J.T. Schmidt and Shashoua, 1988) and in embryonic pyramidal neurons of the rat hippocampus (R. Schmidt et al., 1986). However, ependymin-like proteins have not been detected in

adult rats by immunocytochemistry with antisera to fish ependymin.

Although the role of ependymins in brain function remains unclear, studies have suggested that they participate in the formation of new synaptic circuits associated with long-term memory consolidation. This hypothesis is based on a substantial literature that has documented that the consolidation of long-term memory involves the synthesis of new protein (Agranoff, 1981; Dunn, 1980) and that the release of proteins into the extracellular space may be an essential component of the intercellular communication that is required to facilitate neuronal differentiation, growth, and regeneration (Banker, 1980; Caroni et al., 1988; Cotman and Anderson, 1988; Gage et al., 1988). Studies with double-labeling techniques reported that the steady-state concentrations of ependymins increase in the brain of fish after a new pattern of swimming behavior is learned (R. Schmidt, 1987; Shashoua, 1976, 1979) and that the injection of antiependymin into the fourth ventricle up to 20 hours after training is initiated can impair long-term memory of the new behavior without influencing short-term memory of the physical ability to perform the new task (Shashoua and Moore, 1978). In addition, the ability of antiependymin to inhibit long-term memory consolidation is not task specific but has been shown to inhibit active avoidance learning as well as classical conditioning in goldfish (Piront and Schmidt, 1988; Shashoua and Hesse, 1989). Studies have also reported that the infusion of antiependymin into the ventricles of the optic tectum can block the sharping of the retinotectal maps of regenerating optic nerve fibers after an optic nerve crush (J.T. Schmidt and Shashoua, 1988).

How ependymins regulate synaptogenesis is currently unclear. However, previous studies (R. Schmidt and Shashoua, 1983) have suggested that based on their protein sequences, the N-linked carbohydrate chains of both ependymin β and γ share a common eptitope with calcium-dependent cell adhesion molecules such as neural cell adhesion molecule and myelin-associated glycoprotein. In addition, biochemical studies have reported that in the presence of low calcium levels, ependymins form insoluble fibrous aggregates that cannot be redissolved in most protein solvents (Shashoua, 1985). On the basis of these biochemical characteristics (Kruse et al., 1984; Shashoua, 1985), it is hypothesized that the synthesis of ependymin is carefully regulated in the brain and that when ependymins are secreted into the extracellular matrix they polymerize in response to the lowering of local calcium concentrations in the extracellular matrix after sustained synaptic activity (Krnjevic et al., 1982; Marciani et al., 1982). Thus, similar to what has been postulated for the role of the extracellular matrix in the growth of immature synapses in the developing nervous system (Sanes, 1983), the formation of fibrous extracellular template formed by the polymerized ependymins at the site of potentiated synapses provides a physical substrate on which the growth of new synapses or the elongation of existing synapses can be directed (Shashoua, 1985; Shashoua and Hesse, 1989). However, whether this model of ependymin function can be applied to higher animals, including humans, remains to be determined because it is unclear whether a mammalian homologue of fish ependymin exists in the adult brain of either laboratory rodents or primates.

THE EPENDYMA AND DISEASE

Although ependymal cells form an important interface that separates the CSF and the surrounding brain tissue, mature ependymal cells react little to disease processes and have little ability to proliferate or to regenerate in adults. The most common pathologic change of ependymal cells is a consequence of a generalized inflammatory reaction or irritation termed *granular ependymitis* (Duchen, 1984). This reaction is characteristically seen along the floor of the fourth ventricle and in severe cases in the anterior horns of the lateral ventricles. Inflammation of the ependymal surface follows many types of viral and bacterial infections and is best known as a characteristic of neurosyphilis (Sahs and Joynt, 1984). In hematoxylin-eosin–stained paraffin sections, small granulations appear as a collection of neurological cells that may be partly or entirely covered by an ependyma, with possible necrosis of the ependymal lining of the ventricular wall. In most cases, granular ependymitis is accompanied by a moderate ventricular dilation related to the obstruction of CSF flow out of the fourth ventricle. Microscopically, the ventricular cavity can be filled with numerous inflammatory cells such as polymorphonuclear leukocytes and large mononuclear phagocytes (Figs. 9–12 and 9–13). In severe cases, the ventricular wall is disrupted, with the spaces filled with inflammatory cells, most of which are polymorphonuclear leuko-

cytes. In such cases the ventricular cavity serves as a bacterial reservoir for the spread of infection.

Ependymal cells are also especially vulnerable to mumps virus, and infection with this virus may be accompanied by a loss of ependymal cells (Johnson, 1974, 1980). On the basis of experiments with animals, virus replication in the CNS is limited initially to meningeal and ependymal cells, with undifferentiated cells being the most susceptible to infections. Viral infections of ependymas may also produce a blockage of CSF flow, which results in hydrocephalus. Virus-induced aqueductal stenosis accompanied by hydrocephalus has been reported in newborn hampsters after an infection with mumps virus (Johnson, 1968), as well as from an obstruction of the CSF flow by inflammatory cells or neoplastic transformed meningeal cells. In humans, electron microscopic evidence of virus-induced hydrocephalus resulting from ependymitis has been described by Herndon et al. (1974). They reported that ependymal cells infected with viral nucleocapsid-like material was found in the CSF of six patients with mumps meningitis and provided morphologic support for the conclusion that mumps virus can cause a granular ependymitis and an ependymal cell loss in adult human brain.

Neoplastic ependymomas are the most common cellular pathologic condition of ependymal cells. As a group, tumors of ependymal cells present a wide spectrum of cellular subtypes, with many types of tumors being correlated with specific clinical and pathologic parameters. With regard to location, the histologic identification of various cellular subtypes within a tumor should be approached with caution because previous studies have reported that the number of cell types found in a tumor specimen may be substantially influenced by the amount of tissue obtained at the biopsy (Shuman et al., 1975). Neoplastic ependymomas are most frequently found in a posterior intracranial fossa, with the next most common site being the cauda equina. In general, neoplastic ependymal cells form rosettes of either

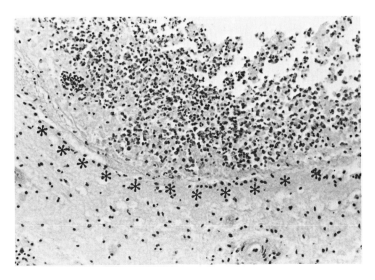

Figure 9–12. Low-magnification micrograph of the ependymal surface (*) of the fourth ventricle showing a case of granular ependymitis. The ventricular cavity is filled with numerous inflammatory cells. × 144.

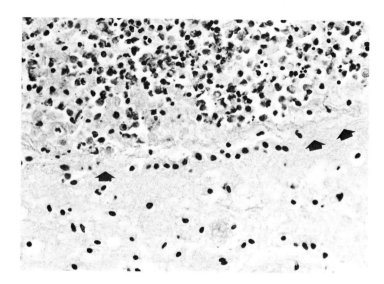

Figure 9–13. High-magnification micrograph of the ependymal surface showing disruption of the ependymal lining *(arrows)* and loss of ependymal cells. × 288.

cuboidal or columnal epithelium around a central lumen. At times, the lumen may be lined by a limiting membrane.

Although the rosette formation is quite variable, the ependymal cells tend to arrange in groups or cords with few mitotic figures and are easily recognized with hematoxylin-eosin stain (Lantos, 1983). At high magnification, phosphotungstic acid–hematoxylin stains will stain small, rod-shaped structures at the base of the cilia to enable the identification of the apical surface. Neoplastic cells of ependymomas also stain with glial fibrillary acidic protein, a water-soluble protein isolated from plaques rich in fibrillary astrocytes that are found in patients with multiple sclerosis. As a diagnostic tool, glial fibrillary acidic protein staining is most useful for identifying the glial origin of a neoplasm with few apparent neurofibrils present. In general, neoplastic cells of ependymomas show considerable variations in glial fibrillary acidic protein staining intensity, with the stain most intense in the perivascular and rosette-forming cells. This pattern suggests that filaments in neoplastic ependymal cells may share a common immunologic origin with other neuroglia.

Clinicopathologic studies of ependymomas (Ilgren et al., 1984a,b) have correlated a number of clinical and pathologic parameters including age, sex, duration of preoperative symptoms, and tumor histology. These findings suggest that both patient age and site of tumor were correlated with the duration of preoperative symptoms, as well as tumor cell number and histology. In addition, patients with ependymomas in the posterior fossa were found to live for a shorter time after treatment than those with tumors of the cauda equina. Also, younger patients apparently do not survive as long as older patients with posterior fossa tumors. In contrast, patient age did not correlate with survival of patients with cauda equina tumors. Although it is not fully understood why differences exist, ependymomas of the cauda equina clearly have a different set of clinical and pathologic characteristics from ependymomas of the brain, and these differences are of special importance when considering the clinical management of patients with these tumors.

References

(Key references are designated with an asterisk.)

Agranoff B.W. Learning and memory: biochemical approaches. In Siegel, G.J., Albers R.W., Agranoff, B.W., et al., eds. *Basic Neurochemistry.* 3rd ed. Boston, Little Brown, pp. 801–820, 1981.

Angevine J.B. Critical cellular events in the shaping of neural centers. In Schmitt F.O., ed. *The Neurosciences Second Study Program.* New York, Rockefeller University Press, pp. 62–72, 1970.

Banker G.A. Trophic interactions between astroglial cells and hippocampal neurons in culture. *Science* 209:809–819, 1980.

Baumgarten H.G., Braak H. Catecholamine in Hypothalamus vom Goldfisch (*Crassius auratus*). *Z. Zellforsch.* 80:246–263, 1967.

Benowitz L.I., Shashoua V.E. Localization of a brain protein metabolically linked with behavioral plasticity in the goldfish. *Brain Res.* 136:227–242, 1977.

Boulder Committee. Embryonic vertebrate central nervous system: revised terminology. *Anat. Rec.* 166:257–261, 1970.

Brightman M.W. The intracerebral movement of proteins injected into blood and cerebrospinal fluid of mice. *Prog. Brain Res.* 29:29–37, 1968.

Brightman M.W., Palay S.L. The fine stucture of ependyma in the brain of the rat. *J. Cell Biol.* 19:415–439, 1963.

Brightman M.W., Reese T.S. Junctions between intimately apposed cell membranes in the vertebrate brain. *J. Cell Biol.* 40:648–677, 1969.

*Brightman M.W., Prescott L., Reese T.S. Intercellular junctions of special ependyma. In Knigge K.M., Scott D.E., Kobayashi H., et al., eds. *Brain-Endocrine Interaction II. The Ventricular System. 2nd International Symposium, Shizuoka, 1974.* Basel, Karger, pp. 146–165, 1975.

Bruni J.E. Montemurro D.G., Clattenburg R.E., et al. A scanning electron microscopic study of the ependymal surface of the third ventricle of the rabbit, rat, mouse and human brain. *Anat. Rec.* 174:407–420, 1972.

Card J.P., Mitchell J.A. Electron microscopic demonstration of a supraependymal cluster of neuronal cells and processes in the hamster third ventricle. *J. Comp. Neurol.* 180:43–58, 1978.

Caroni P., Szvio T., Schwab M.E. Central nervous system regeneration: oligodendrocytes and myelin as non-permissive substrates for neurite growth. *Prog. Brain Res.* 78:363–370, 1988.

Cathcart R.S., Worthington W.C. Ciliary movement in the rat cerebral ventricles: clearing action and direction of current. *J. Neuropathol. Exp. Neurol.* 23:609–618, 1964.

Clementi F., Marini D. The surface fine structure of wall of the cerebral ventricles and of the choroid plexus in cat. *Z. Zellforsch.* 123:82–95, 1972.

Coates P.W. Supraependymal cells and surface specializations on the floor of the monkey third ventricle. Scanning microscopic study. *Anat. Rec.* 1975:294A, 1973a.

Coates P.W. Supraependymal cells in the recesses of the monkey third ventricle. *Am. J. Anat.* 136:533–539, 1973b.

Coates P.W. Supraependymal cells: light and transmission electron microscopy extends scanning electron microscopic demonstration. *Brain Res.* 57:502–507, 1973c.

Cotman C.W., Anderson K.J. Synaptic plasticity and functional stabilization in the hippocampal formation: possible role in Alzheimer's disease. In Waxman S., ed. *Physiological Basis for Functional Recovery in Neurological Disease.* New York, Raven Press, pp. 313–336, 1988.

Duchen L.W. General pathology of neurons and neuroglia. In Adams J.H., Corsellis J.A.N., Duchen L.W., eds. *Greenfield's Neuropathology.* New York, Wiley–Medical Publications, pp. 1–52, 1984.

Dunn A.J. Neurochemistry of learning and memory: an evaluation of recent data. *Annu. Rev. Psychol.* 31:343–390, 1980.

Feder N. Reese T.S., Brightman M.W. Microperoxidase, a new tracer of low molecular weight. A study of the interstitial compartments of the mouse brain. *Abstr. J. Cell Biol.* 43:24A–26A, 1969.

Fujita S. The matrix cell and cytogenesis in the developing central nervous system. *J. Comp. Neurol.* 120:37–42, 1963.

Gage F.H., Olejniczak P., Armstrong D.M. Astrocytes are important for sprouting in the septohippocampal circuit. *Exp. Neurol.* 102:2–13, 1988.

*Herndon R.M., Johnson R.T., Davis L.E., et al. Ependymitis in mumps virus meningitis. Electron microscopical studies of cerebrospinal fluid. *Arch. Neurol.* 30:475–479, 1974.

Hofer H. Zur Morphologie der circumventrikularen Organe der Saugetiere. *Verh. Dtsch. Zool. Ges.* 202–251, 1958.

Horstmann E. Die Faserglia des Selachiergehirns. *Z. Zellforsch. Mikrosk. Anat.* 39:588–617, 1954.

*Ilgren E.B., Stiller C.A., Hughes J.T., et al. Ependymoas: a clinical and pathological study. Part I—biologic features. *Clin. Neuropathol.* 3:113–121, 1984a.

Ilgren E.B., Stiller C.A., Hughes J.T., et al. Ependymoas: a clinical and pathological study. Part II—survival features. *Clin. Neuropathol.* 3:122–127, 1984b.

Jacobson M., ed. *Developmental Neurobiology.* 2nd ed. New York, Plenum Publishing, 1978.

Johnson R.T. Mumps virus encephalitis in the hamster. Studies of the inflammatory response and noncytopathic infection of neurons. *J. Neuropathol. Exp. Neurol.* 27:80–95, 1968.

Johnson R.T. Pathophysiology and epidemiology of acute viral infections of the nervous system. *Adv. Neurol.* 6:27–40, 1974.

Johnson R.T. Selective vulnerability of neural cells to viral infections. *Brain* 103:447–472, 1980.

Kappers C.U.A. *Die vergleichende Anatomie des Nervensystems der Wirbeltiere und des Menschen.* Bd. I, II and III. Bohn, Haarlem, 1920–1921.

Knowles F. Ependyma of the third ventricle in relation to pituitary function. *Prog. Brain Res.* 38:550–570, 1972.

Knowles F., Anand-Kumar, T.C. Structural changes, related to reproduction, in the hypothalamus and in the pars tuberalis of the rhesus monkey. Part I. The hypothalamus. Part II. The pars tuberalis. *Philos. Trans. R. Soc. London Ser. B* 256:357–375, 1967.

Königstorfer A., Sterrer S., Eckerskorn C., et al. Molecular characterization of an ependymin precursor from goldfish brain. *J. Neurochem.* 52:310–312, 1989a.

Königstorfer A., Sterrer S., Hoffmann W. Biosynthesis of ependymins from goldfish brain. *J. Biol. Chem.* 264:13689–13692, 1989b.

Krnjevic K., Morris M.E., Reiffenstein R.J. Stimulation evoked changes in extracellular K^+ and Ca^{2+} in pyramidal layers of the rat's hippocampus. *Can. J. Physiol. Pharmacol.* 60:1643–1657, 1982.

Kruse J., Mailhammer R., Wernecke H., et al. Neural cell adhesion molecules and myelin-associated glycoprotein share a common carbohydrate moiety recognized by monoclonal antibodies. *Nature* 311:153–155, 1984.

Lantos P.L. Histochemistry of the tumours of the nervous system. In Filipe M.I., Lake B.D., eds. *Histochemistry in Pathology.* New York, Churchill Livingstone, pp. 70–81, 1983.

Lichtensteiger W., Richards J.G. Tuberal DA neurons tanycytes: response to electrical stimulation and nicotine (abstract). *Experientia* 31:742, 1975.

Lichtensteiger W., Richards J.G., Kopp H.G. Possible participation of non-neuronal elements of median eminence in neuroendocrine effects of dopaminergic and cholinergic systems. In Scott D.E., Kozlowski E.P., Weindl A., eds. *Brain-Endocrine Interaction III. Neural Hormones and Reproduction. 3rd International Symposium, Wurzburg, 1977.* Basel, Karger, pp. 251–262, 1978.

Lyser K.M. Early differentiation of motor neuroblasts in the chick embryo as studied by electron microscopy. I. General aspects. *Dev. Biol.* 10:433–466, 1964.

Marciani M.G., Louvel J., Heinemann U. Aspartate induced changes in extracellular free calcium in "in vitro" hippocampal slices of rats. *Brain Res.* 238:272–277, 1982.

McKenna O., Rosenbluth J. Cytological evidence for catecholamine containing sensory cells bordering the ventricle of the toad hypothalamus. *J. Comp. Neurol.* 54:133–148, 1974.

Mikami S.-I. A correlative ultrastructural analysis of the ependymal cells of the third ventricle of Japanese quail. (*Coturnix coturnix japonica*). In Knigge K.M., Scott D.E., Kobayashi H., et al., eds. *Brain-Endocrine Interaction II. The Ventricular System. 2nd International Symposium, Shizuoka, 1974.* Basel, Karger, pp. 80–93, 1975.

Millhouse O.E. Light and electron microscopic studies of the ventricular wall. *Z. Zellforsch.* 127:149–174, 1972.

*Millhouse O.E. Lining of the third ventricle in the rat. In Knigge K.M., Scott D.E., Kobayashi H., et al., eds. *Brain-Endocrine Interaction II. The Ventricular System. 2nd International Symposium, Shizuoka, 1974.* Basel, Karger, pp. 3–18, 1975.

Monroe B.G., Newman B.L., Schapiro S. Ultrastructure of the median eminence of neonatal and adult rats. In Knigge K.M., Scott D.E., Weindl A., eds. *Brain-Endocrine Interaction. Median Eminence: Structure and Function. International Symposium, Munich, 1971.* Basel, Karger, pp. 7–26, 1972.

Paull W.K., Martin H., Scott D.E. Scanning electron microscopy of the third ventricular floor of the rat. *J. Comp. Neurol.* 175:301–310, 1977.

Peters A., Palay S.L., Webster H. deF. *The Fine Structure of the Nervous System: The Neurons and Supporting Cells.* Philadelphia, Saunders, 1976.

Piront M.-L., Schmidt R. Inhibition of long-term memory formation by antiependymin antisera after active shock-avoidance learning in goldfish. *Brain Res.* 442:53–62, 1988.

Reese T.S., Karnovsky M.J. Fine structural localization of a blood-brain barrier to exogenous peroxidase. *J. Cell Biol.* 34:207–217, 1967.

Revel J.P., Karnovsky M.J. Hexagonal array of subunits in intercellular junctions of the mouse heart and liver. *J. Cell Biol.* 33:C7–C12, 1967.

Sahs A.L., Joynt R.J. Bacterial meningitis. In Baker A.B., Baker L.H., eds. *Clinical Neurology.* Vol. 2. Philadelphia, Harper & Row, 1984.

Sanes J.R. Roles of extracellular matrix in neural development. *Annu. Rev. Physiol.* 45:581–600, 1983.

*Sano Y., Ueda S., Yamada H., et al. Immunohistochemical demonstration of serotonin-containing CSF-contacting neurons in the submammalian paraventricular organ. *Histochemistry* 77:423–430, 1983.

Schmidt J.T., Shashoua V.E. Antibodies to ependymin block the sharpening of the regenerating retinotectal projection in goldfish. *Brain Res.* 446:269–284, 1988.

Schmidt R. Involvement and function of specific goldfish brain glycoproteins (ependymins) in two different learning paradigms (abstract). *J. Neurochem.* 44:S21, 1985.

Schmidt R. Changes in subcellular distribution of ependymins in goldfish brain induced by learning. *J. Neurochem.* 48:1870–1878, 1987.

Schmidt R., Lapp H. Regional distribution of ependymins in goldfish brain measured by radioimmunoassay. *Neurochem. Int.* 10:383–390, 1987.

Schmidt R., Shashoua V.E. Structural and metabolic relationships between goldfish brain glycoproteins participating in functional plasticity of the central nervous system. *J. Neurochem.* 40:652–660, 1983.

Schmidt R., Löffler F., Müller H.W., et al. Immunological cross-reactivity of cultured rat hippocampal neurons with goldfish brain proteins synthesized during memory consolidation. *Brain Res.* 386:245–257, 1986.

*Scott D.E., Paull W.K. Scanning electron microscopy of the mammalian cerebral-ventricular system. *Micron* 14:165–186, 1983.

Scott D.E., Krobisch G., Dudley G.K., et al. The mammalian median eminence: a comparative and experimental model. In Knigge K.M., Scott D.E., Weindl A., eds. *Brain-Endocrine Interaction. Median Eminence: Structure and Function. International Symposium, Munich, 1971.* Basel, Karger, pp. 35–49, 1972.

Scott D.E., Kozlowski G.P., Paull W.K., et al. Scanning electron microscopy of the human cerebral ventricular system. II. The fourth ventricle. *Z. Zellforsch. Mikrosk. Anat.* 139:61–68, 1973.

Scott D.E., Kozlowski G.P., Sheridan M.N. Scanning electron microscopy in the ultrastructural analysis of the mammalian cerebral ventricular system. *Int. Rev. Cytol.* 37:349–388, 1974a.

Scott D.E., Krobisch-Dudley G., Knigge K.M. The ventricular system in neuroendocrine mechanisms. II. In vivo monamine transport by ependyma of the median eminence. *Cell Tissue Res.* 154:1–16, 1974b.

Scott D.E., Krobisch-Dudley G., Paull W.K., et al. The ventricular system in neuroendocrine mechanisms. III. Supraependymal neuronal networks in the primate brain. *Cell Tissue Res.* 179:235–254, 1977.

Sharp P.J., Follett B.K. The distribution of monoamines in the hypothalamus of the Japanese quail, *Coturnix coturnix japonica. Z. Zelforsch.* 90:245–262, 1968.

Shashoua V.E. Brain metabolism and the acquisition of new behaviors. I. Evidence for specific changes in the pattern of protein synthesis. *Brain Res.* 111:347–364, 1976.

Shashoua V.E. Brain metabolism and the acquisition of new behaviors. III. Evidence for secretion of two proteins into the brain extracellular fluid after training. *Brain Res.* 166:349–358, 1979.

Shashoua V.E. The role of brain extracellular proteins in neuro-plasticity and learning. *Cell. Mol. Neurobiol.* 5:183–207, 1985.

Shashoua V.E., Hesse G.W. Classical conditioning leads to changes in extracellular concentrations of ependymin in goldfish brain. *Brain Res.* 484:333–339, 1989.

Shashoua V.E., Moore M.E. Effect of antisera to β and γ goldfish brain proteins on the retention of a newly acquired behavior. *Brain Res.* 148:441–449, 1978.

Shashoua V.E., Moore M.E. Role of brain extracellular proteins in the mechanism of long term potentiation in rat brain hippocampus. *Soc. Neurosci. Abstr.* 11:782, 1985.

Shuman R.M., Alvord E.C., Leech R.W. The biology of childhood ependymomas. *Arch. Neurol.* 32:731–739, 1975.

Silverman A.J., Knigge K.M., Peck W.A. Median eminence: in vitro transport of amino acids, thyroxin and thyrotropin releasing hormone (TRF) (abstract). *Anat. Rec.* 169:429, 1972.

Vigh B., Vigh-Teichmann I. Comparative ultrastructure of the cerebrospinal fluid–contacting neurons. *Int. Rev. Cytol.* 35:189–251, 1973.

Vigh-Teichmann I., Vigh B. The infundibular cerebrospinal fluid contacting neurons. *Adv. Anat. Embryol. Cell Biol.* 50:7–89, 1974.

Vigh-Teichmann I., Vigh B., Aros B. Phylogeny and ontogeny of the paraventricular organ. In Sterba G., ed. *Zirkumventriculare Organ und Liquor.* Jena, Fischer, 1969.

*Weindl A., Joynt R.J. Ultrastructure of the ventricular walls. Three-dimensional study of regional specialization. *Arch. Neurol.* 26:420–427, 1972.

10

Blood Vessels and the Blood-Brain Barrier

Gary W. Goldstein
A. Lorris Betz

The brain capillary is the structure responsible for the formation of the blood-brain barrier (BBB). In addition to limiting the exchange of substances between the blood and the brain, the capillaries have metabolic and transport properties that are important in brain function and in the pathophysiology of some metabolic encephalopathies. Furthermore, injury to the capillaries can produce leakage of plasma proteins and vasogenic brain edema. This reaction is particularly prominent in brain tumors, acute lead encephalopathy, cerebritis, and head injury. In some of these disorders the damage may be so severe as to cause complete loss of capillary integrity and frank hemorrhage. Ironically, the opening of the barrier that occurs in disease may enhance the delivery of chemotherapeutics to the brain. Methods are also now available to safely open the normal BBB for short times, and these procedures may provide the means for delivery of therapeutic agents normally excluded from the brain.

In this chapter we review the structure and physiology of the brain capillary and we attempt, when possible, to relate capillary function to disease processes and therapeutic interventions. Several review articles (Betz and Goldstein, 1984; Betz et al., 1989a; Goldstein and Betz, 1983, 1986; Pardridge, 1983) and three monographs (Bradbury, 1979; Neuwelt, 1989; Rapoport, 1976) cover some of these subjects in more detail.

STRUCTURE

Capillaries are microvessels with diameters generally between 3 and 7 μm. The capillary wall does not contain smooth muscle cells, which are found in arterioles and some venules. In addition to the absence of muscle and elastic fibers, capillaries can be distinguished from these other microvessels by their smaller size. Surrounding the capillary endothelial cell is a basement membrane within which another cell, the pericyte, may be embedded (Fig. 10–1). In brain capillaries there is an additional close association with astrocytes. Each of these components is considered separately.

Endothelial Cell

The brain capillary endothelial cell forms a continuous, nonfenestrated endothelium that restricts the movement of many polar solutes between the blood and the brain. The classic studies of Reese and Karnovsky (1967) and Brightman and Reese (1969) clearly demonstrated two unusual properties of endothelial cells in brain capillaries that explain the formation of a BBB (Fig. 10–2). The first is the presence in brain capillaries of continuous tight junctions, which prevent the transcapillary movement of protein tracers. The second major difference is the smaller number of plasmalemma vesicles in brain capillary endothelium. In other tissues, these vesicles appear to transfer protein across the capillary via the sequential steps of endocytosis on one side of the cell and exocytosis on the other side (Simionescu et al., 1978). The low density of these plasmalemma vesicles in brain capillaries is consistent with the low permeability of the BBB to proteins. Vesicular transport of proteins across the BBB may occur, however, after a variety of insults such as hypertension and ischemia with reperfusion (Westergaard, 1977). An additional morphologic feature of brain capillary endothelial cells is their high density of mitochondria.

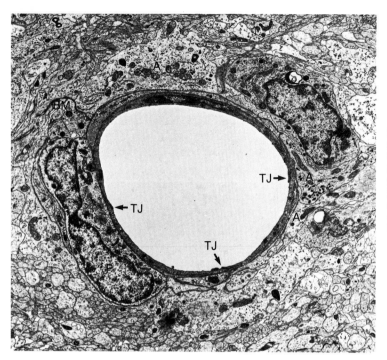

Figure 10–1. Ultrastructure of a normal brain capillary. A mouse brain capillary is shown with the endothelial cell, the pericyte (P), the basement membrane (BM), and astrocytic foot processes (A). Note the tight junctions (TJ) and low number of intraendothelial vesicles. (From Wolinsky J.S., Johnson R.T. Viruses in chronic neurological diseases. In Fraenkel-Conrat H., Wagner, R.R., eds. *Comprehensive Virology*. Vol. 16. New York, Plenum Publishing, p. 261, 1980.)

Oldendorf et al. (1977) calculated that the percentage of capillary endothelial cell volume occupied by mitochondria is four to five times greater than that in systemic capillaries. This increased mitochondrial density may reflect a higher metabolic activity related to the barrier function of these capillaries.

Not all areas of the brain contain capillaries that produce a barrier. In these nonbarrier regions, the morphologic features of the capillaries are similar to those of systemic microvascular beds (see Fig. 10–2). Thus, the tight junctions are discontinuous, there are more plasmalemma vesicles and fewer mitochondria, and some endothelial cells even exhibit fenestrations (Brightman, 1977). Table 10–1 lists brain regions that contain capillaries of this type. The absence of a BBB in many of these regions may relate to a feedback role in regulation of hormone release. In the case of the choroid plexus, the capillaries are freely permeable, but a blood–cerebrospinal fluid (CSF) barrier is produced by the choroid plexus epithelial cells, which secrete CSF.

The microvasculature of brain tumors is frequently more permeable than that of normal brain tissue. This enhanced permeability is noted clinically by the increased uptake of contrast agents and radionuclides during imaging by computed tomography or nuclear brain scanning. Figure 10–3 demonstrates the enhanced entry of radioactive rubidium, a potassium analogue, into a brain tumor imaged by positron emission tomography (Brooks et al., 1984). The morphologic basis for this altered permeability is related to a change in the structure of the capillary endothelial cells in or near the tumor (Brightman, 1977; Long, 1970; Stewart et al., 1985).

As shown in Figure 10–4, the endothelial cells in a brain tumor capillary contain open intercellular clefts and fenestrations, and the normal glial foot processes are absent. In addition, endothelial hyperplasia and extensive vesicle formation may be present. These latter changes could be the result of the rapid capillary growth induced by the tumor. Similar features may result in the enhanced capillary permeability that is seen in the new blood vessels found around an area of infarction or abscess. In both of these pathologic states, vasogenic brain edema is prominent. The underlying mechanism of this type of edema appears to be the passage of plasma proteins across the abnormal endothelial cells (Betz et al., 1989b; Fishman, 1975). The efficacy of steroid therapy is most convincingly demonstrated in the setting of brain tumor edema; however, the mechanism for improvement is not known.

Basement Membrane and Pericyte

The *basement membrane* of brain capillaries is a thin extracellular matrix of collagen, other proteins, and proteoglycans located between the antiluminal membrane of the endothelial cell and the foot process of the astrocyte (see Fig. 10–1). The functions most

Table 10–1. AREAS OF BRAIN WITHOUT A BLOOD-BRAIN BARRIER

Pituitary gland
Median eminence
Area postrema
Preoptic recess
Paraphysis
Pineal gland
Endothelium of the choroid plexus

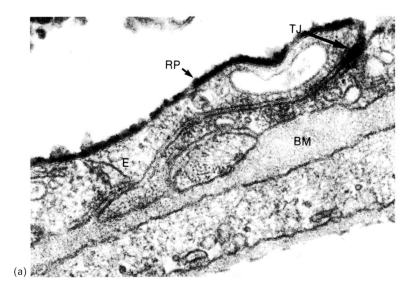

(a)

Figure 10–2. Comparison of endothelial permeability in the cerebrum and the choroid plexus. The protein tracer horseradish peroxidase (approximately 40 kd) was administered intravenously and allowed to circulate for 45 minutes. The tissues were then sampled and developed for ultrastructural localization of the peroxidase reaction product (RP). (*a*) The tight junction (TJ) of a normal cerebral endothelial cell (E) prevents the movement of tracer from the vessel lumen into the basement membrane (BM). (*b*) The choroid plexus endothelium (E) has open intercellular junctions and fenestrations (F) that allow the protein tracer to enter the space between the choroid plexus epithelial cells (CP). (*a* from Westergaard E., Brightman W.W. Transport of protein across cerebral arterioles. *J. Comp. Neurol.* 152:17–44, 1973. *b* courtesy of M.W. Brightman, National Institutes of Health.)

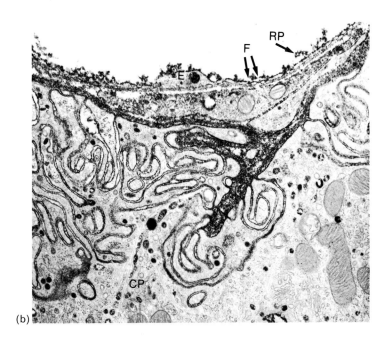

(b)

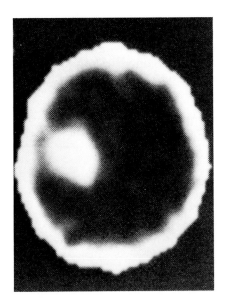

Figure 10–3. Uptake of rubidium by a brain tumor. This positron emission tomograph illustrates the extremely low permeability of the BBB to the potassium ion analogue ^{82}Rb. In contrast, the isotope accumulates within the tumor, which lacks normal brain capillaries. (From Brooks D.J., Beaney R.P., Lammertsma A.A., et al. Quantitative measurement of blood-brain barrier permeability using rubidium-82 and positron emission tomography. *J. Cereb. Blood Flow Metab.* 4:535–545, 1984.)

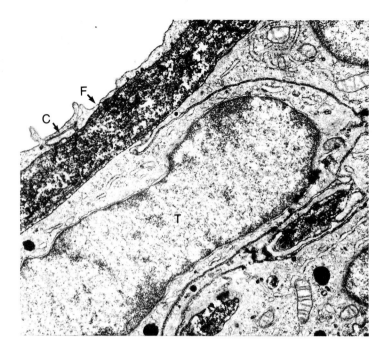

Figure 10–4. Ultrastructure of a capillary in a brain tumor. An experimental brain tumor was obtained by direct injection of a simian virus 40–induced choroid plexus papilloma into the cerebral cortex of a newborn hamster. Microvascular permeability was examined 6 months later by using horseradish peroxidase. The tracer readily penetrated the large perivascular space because of the endothelial fenestrations (F) and open interendothelial cleft (C). Tumor cells (T) are seen immediately adjacent to the perivascular space. (Courtesy of L. Prescott and M.W. Brightman, National Institutes of Health.)

frequently ascribed to the basement membrane are supporting cellular structures, acting as a semipermeable filter, and providing a framework for cell migration and differentiation during development (Betz and Goldstein, 1984). Because of the tensile properties of basement membrane, we believe that it provides an important physical support to maintain capillary integrity and to prevent microvascular hemorrhage. The capillary basement membrane thickens in hypertension, diabetes mellitus, and aging, and this abnormality may be related to an accumulation of collagen fibrils.

Pericytes are found within the basement membrane of brain capillaries. Because of their periendothelial location, proposed roles for these cells include synthesis of basement membrane, phagocytosis of exogenous protein, support and protection of endothelial cells, and regulation of endothelial cell growth. They may also control the diameter of the capillary wall and thus regulate blood flow at the level of the individual capillary.

Glial–Endothelial Cell Relationship

A special relationship exits between capillaries and astrocytes of the brain. With few exceptions, cerebral capillaries are almost completely ensheathed by astrocytic processes (see Fig. 10–1). In fact, early investigators thought that the glial cells were the anatomic site of the BBB. However, ultrastructural studies demonstrated that proteins can freely permeate the space between astrocytic foot processes and enter the basement membrane up to but not past the tight junctions connecting the endothelial cells (Brightman and Reese, 1969). The close contact between astrocytes and endothelial cells suggests a functional interaction (Goldstein, 1988). This possibility is supported by the fact that foot processes of the same astrocyte contact neurons or ependymal cells. Potential interactions include transfer of substances, regulation of capillary activity, and induction of specialized endothelial properties. Support for the importance of glial cells for the function of brain capillaries is found in brain tumors in which a loss of the normal glial–endothelial cell relationship is associated with the absence of a BBB.

FUNCTION

As shown in Figure 10–1, the brain capillary endothelial cell presents a continuous barrier formed by its plasma membrane and tight junctions. The rate at which a molecule crosses this barrier is determined by a number of factors (Table 10–2). Most molecules move down a concentration gradient as they traverse the barrier, and their rate of uptake by the brain increases as their concentration in blood is raised. In addition, different types of molecules vary

Table 10–2. DETERMINANTS OF SOLUTE FLUX ACROSS THE BLOOD-BRAIN BARRIER

Concentration gradient
Permeability
    Capillary integrity
    Lipid solubility
    Transport
Surface area
    Capillary density
    Capillary recruitment
Capillary metabolism
    Active pumps
    Intracellular modification

in their ability to cross a barrier with normal integrity. Lipid-soluble compounds can penetrate this barrier by virtue of their ability to enter cell membranes, but most polar solutes are excluded. However, the entry of essential polar molecules such as D-glucose and large neutral amino acids is facilitated by specific transport carriers. The number of capillaries that are perfused in a given brain region can change, which alters the surface area available for solute transport. Also, some solutes are enzymatically modified as they pass through the endothelial cell cytoplasm, the capillary thus functioning as a metabolic barrier.

Nonspecific Permeability

One factor that determines the ability of a substance to cross the BBB is its lipid solubility. Respiratory gases, for example, are highly lipid soluble and are readily exchanged between the blood and the brain. Substances of therapeutic interest vary greatly in their ability to cross the barrier; in large part, this variability is related to lipid solubility. Figure 10–5 demonstrates this relationship for the selected examples discussed here.

Most antibiotics, including penicillin, do not enter the brain well because of their poor lipid solubility (Norrby, 1978). Chloramphenicol is an exception. It is quite lipid soluble and readily achieves therapeutic concentrations in the central nervous system (CNS). One way to overcome low permeability of a drug is to raise its serum concentration because the amount that enters the brain is proportional to the product

of its permeability and its concentration. The penicillins remain useful antibiotics for susceptible organisms despite their low BBB permeability because they are well tolerated and can be administered in high doses. For most drugs, however, side effects limit this approach. Thus, methotrexate is an effective drug for CNS neoplasms, but low permeability and high toxicity limit its usefulness when administered systemically.

Several of the most lipid-soluble drugs with the highest BBB permeability are the ones most subject to abuse. They include heroin, nicotine, ethanol, and diazepam (see Fig. 10–5). These substances are almost entirely extracted by the brain in a single pass through the cerebral vasculature. This rapid entry of psychoactive agents may encourage their abuse because of the close association between administration and effect. For example, the cerebral effect of nicotine is noted 3–4 seconds after tobacco smoke is inhaled (Oldendorf, 1983). This interval corresponds to the circulation time from the pulmonary bed through the left ventricle and into the brain circulation. The high capillary extraction thus accounts for the rapid onset of the effect.

In a similar manner, high lipid solubility and high brain capillary extraction underlie the rapid onset of diazepam's anticonvulsant activity after intravenous administration. Phenytoin and phenobarbital, on the other hand, are slower to act in status epilepticus. This delayed onset of activity is explained by lower capillary extraction, which is in part the result of binding to plasma proteins (Cornford et al., 1983).

Water itself readily crosses the BBB (see Fig. 10–

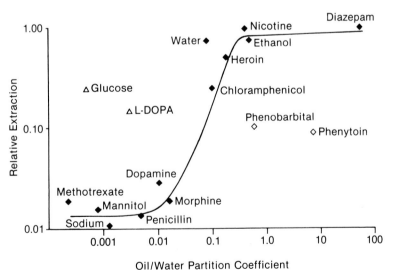

Figure 10–5. Relationship between lipid solubility and brain uptake of selected compounds. The distribution into olive oil relative to water for each test substance serves as a measure of its lipid solubility. Brain uptake is determined by comparing the extraction of each test substance relative to a highly permeable tracer during a single passage through the cerebral circulation. In general, compounds with higher oil-to-water partition coefficients show increased entry into the brain (♦). The uptake of the two anticonvulsants phenobarbital and phenytoin is lower than that predicted from their lipid solubility partly because of their binding to plasma proteins (◇). This result explains the slower onset of anticonvulsant activity of these agents compared with diazepam. The uptake of glucose and L-dopa is greater than that predicted by their lipid solubility because specific carriers facilitate their transport across the brain capillary (△). Data for diazepam and chloramphenicol are estimates. (Data, except those for diazepam and chloramphenicol, from Oldendorf W.H. The blood-brain barrier. *Exp. Eye Res.* 25:177–190, 1977; and Oldendorf W.H. The blood-brain barrier and its relevance to modern nuclear medicine. In Magistretti P.L., ed. *Functional Radionuclide Imaging of the Brain.* New York, Raven Press, pp. 1–10, 1983.)

5). At any given time, therefore, the brain is in osmotic equilibrium with the blood in its capillaries. For this reason, administration of an osmotically active compound with low BBB permeability such as mannitol causes a net movement of water from the brain into the bloodstream. The nearly 100-fold difference in BBB permeability between water and mannitol provides the basis of a method for dehydrating brain tissue as a therapeutic intervention for the control of increased intracranial pressure.

Specific Transport Systems

Not all molecules with low lipid solubility are restricted in their passage across the BBB. Although glucose and mannitol are similar in size and structure, the brain extraction of glucose is 20- to 30-fold greater than that of mannitol (see Fig. 10–5). This apparently anomalous relationship is also observed for other metabolically essential compounds (Table 10–3). The high permeability of these polar compounds is mediated by specific transport carriers in the plasma membrane of the endothelial cells. Such carriers are similar to enzymes except that they move solutes across a cell membrane. Like enzymes, their transport activity is regulated by the amount of carrier present in the membrane and by the affinity of the receptor site for the molecule being transported. The receptor sites are subject to competition for occupancy by structurally related compounds. Thus, the presence of specific transport carriers not only enhances the movement of essential substrates across the BBB but also provides a mechanism for regulating barrier permeability.

Glucose is the primary energy substrate of the brain; its metabolism accounts for nearly all of the brain's oxygen consumption. Because entry of glucose into the brain is critical, mechanisms for glucose transport across the BBB are particularly well studied (Kalaria et al., 1988; Lund-Andersen, 1979; Pardridge, 1983). Highly specific carriers are present in brain capillary endothelial cells and mediate the passage of this polar substrate through the BBB. Ordinarily, the activity of these carriers is more than sufficient to meet the metabolic needs of the brain. Under

some circumstances, however, transport of glucose across the BBB may limit brain metabolism. For example, in extreme hypoglycemia, the concentration of glucose in the blood may fall to a level so low that an inadequate amount is transported into the brain. In another situation, when the metabolic demand of the brain increases, such as during hypoxia and seizures, the number of carriers may be inadequate to sustain function even in the presence of a normal concentration of glucose in the blood.

Patients with diabetes mellitus present a special problem for glucose entry into the brain (Fig. 10–6). When the blood glucose concentration is chronically elevated, a compensatory decrease may occur in the number of glucose carriers in the brain capillary (Gjedde and Crone, 1981; McCall et al., 1982). The reduced number of carriers is adequate for glucose entry because of the elevated glucose concentration. Difficulty arises, however, when the blood glucose level is rapidly brought to normal. Because the number of carriers remains low for several hours after return to a normal blood concentration, glucose transfer across the BBB may be too slow and, paradoxically, symptoms of hypoglycemia may develop. This clinical example illustrates that the number of transport carriers in the BBB is important and that this number is subject to regulation by metabolic factors.

Another way to alter carrier-mediated transport systems present in the BBB is by competition at receptor sites. This competition becomes clinically important when several substrates interact with the same carrier and each is present in the blood at concentrations near their affinity for the receptor. This situation exists for the essential large neutral amino acids (Pardridge, 1983; Smith et al., 1987) (Fig. 10–7). In phenylketonuria, the plasma level of phenylalanine is markedly elevated, and an excess of this amino acid is transported into the brain. Other amino acids that share the same carrier must compete for transport with phenylalanine, and even though their blood concentration may be normal, their uptake into the brain is greatly reduced (Oldendorf, 1973). The resulting deficiency of essential amino acids may contribute to the brain injury that occurs in untreated phenylketonuric patients.

Table 10–3. BLOOD-BRAIN BARRIER TRANSPORT SYSTEMS

Transport System	Representative Substrate	Affinity (mmol/L)	Maximal Rate (nmol/g/min)
Hexose	Glucose	9.0	1600
Monocarboxylic acid	Lactate	1.9	120
Large neutral amino acid	Phenylalanine	0.12	30
Basic amino acid	Lysine	0.10	6
Acidic amino acid	Glutamate	0.04	0.4
Amine	Choline	0.44	10
Purine	Adenine	0.027	1
Nucleoside	Adenosine	0.018	0.7

Modified from Pardridge W.M. Neuropeptides and the blood-brain barrier. *Annu. Rev. Physiol.* 45:73–82, 1983. Reproduced, with permission, from the Annual Review of Physiology, Vol. 45, © 1983 by Annual Reviews Inc.

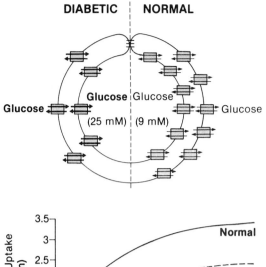

Figure 10–6. Effect of diabetes on glucose transport from the blood to the brain. Under normal circumstances, glucose moves across the brain capillary endothelium by successive transport steps from the blood to the endothelial cell to the brain. The maximal rate of transport is directly related to the number of transport carriers present in the endothelial cell membrane. In experimentally induced chronic hyperglycemia, the maximal rate of brain glucose uptake decreases. This change is best explained by a down-regulation of the number of glucose carriers. However, even though the maximal rate is lower, the actual rate of brain glucose uptake is unchanged because of the higher plasma glucose concentration. Kinetic constants for the graph were obtained from Gjedde and Crone (1981).

endothelial cells in the brain-to-blood direction (Betz et al., 1980). The affinity of capillary Na^+,K^+-ATPase is half-saturated at a potassium concentration of 2.8 mmol/L. Therefore, it should respond to physiologic deviations in the concentration of potassium in the brain's interstitial fluid (Goldstein, 1979). Return of potassium to the blood may be mediated by a cation channel in the luminal membrane (Vigne et al., 1989). Thus, these ion-transporting systems in the endothelial cell may assist the astrocytes in maintaining a stable concentration of potassium in sites around neuronal activity (Kimelberg and Norenberg, 1989) and may allow for the long-term maintenance of a concentration gradient for potassium between the blood and the brain.

The antiluminal location of Na^+,K^+-ATPase in brain capillary endothelial cells is similar to the cellular polarity of many fluid-transporting epithelial cells. In such tissues, transepithelial movement of water is driven by the transcellular transport of sodium and chloride. The major energy-requiring step is the active extrusion of sodium across the antiluminal membrane mediated by Na^+,K^+-ATPase. When this movement is coupled to a passive entry of sodium on the luminal membrane, the net result is active transport of sodium across the cell from lumen to interstitial space. Simultaneous transfer of chloride maintains electroneutrality, and water follows to offset osmolar gradients. Production of CSF by the choroid plexus involves this same general scheme (Spector and Johanson, 1989). Because brain capillaries also appear to contribute to CSF production (Milhorat et al., 1971), it is not surprising to find that they have a similar transport polarity for ions.

At least two separate sodium transport systems are present in the luminal membrane of brain capillary endothelial cells (Betz, 1983). One is inhibited by low concentrations of the diuretic amiloride and

Ion and Fluid Homeostasis

Even molecules as small as ions are restricted in their passage across the BBB (see Figs. 10–3 and 10–5). This limited permeability provides the opportunity for strict regulation of the ionic composition of the brain's interstitial fluid. For example, the concentration of potassium in the CSF and the interstitial fluid of the brain is 2.8 mmol/L, which is significantly lower than its concentration in blood (3–5 mmol/L). Furthermore, changes in the blood concentration of potassium do not result in changes in the interstitial fluid concentration of potassium (Davson, 1976).

Two cellular mechanisms in the capillary appear to be important in this homeostasis. The luminal (blood surface) plasma membrane and tight junction of the capillary wall have a low permeability to potassium (Hansen et al., 1977), whereas, as shown in Figure 10–8, the antiluminal (brain surface) plasma membrane contains Na^+,K^+-ATPase, which can pump potassium from the interstitial fluid into the

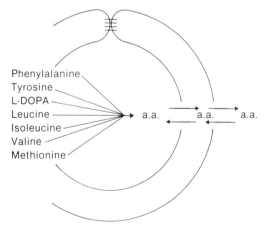

Figure 10–7. Transport of large neutral amino acids across the brain capillary. A single type of transport carrier mediates the transcapillary movement of structurally related amino acids (a.a.). As a result, these compounds must compete with each other for entry into brain, and an elevation in the plasma level of one may inhibit entry of others. This schematic shows some of the amino acids whose uptake would be reduced under these circumstances.

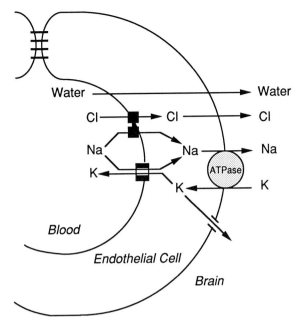

Figure 10–8. Transport of sodium and water across the brain capillary. Sodium has a central role in the transport functions of the brain capillary. The luminal membrane of the endothelial cell has two transport systems for sodium entry, which are distinguished by their sensitivity to diuretics (Betz, 1983). The cotransport carrier of sodium and chloride can be inhibited by furosemide and the cation channel by amiloride. These entry systems, when coupled with the active extrusion of sodium across the antiluminal membrane by Na^+,K^+-ATPase (Betz et al., 1980), are responsible for transendothelial movement of sodium and water. Na^+,K^+-ATPase may also contribute to the regulation of the potassium concentration in the interstitial fluid. After potassium is inside the endothelial cell, it could either move into the blood through the cation channel (Vigne et al., 1989) or return to the brain through a channel in the antiluminal membrane, depending on whether or not the physiologic state required conservation of potassium by the brain.

is therefore similar to a sodium pore found in some tight epithelia. This system may be the same cation channel that allows potassium to leave the endothelial cell (Vigne et al., 1989). The other luminal sodium transport system is inhibited by furosemide and is probably a sodium-chloride cotransport system. Thus, transport of sodium and water from the blood to the brain across the capillary involves entry of sodium into the endothelial cell across the luminal membrane via either of two transport systems, followed by active pumping of sodium from the endothelial cell to brain interstitial fluid across the antiluminal membrane by Na^+,K^+-ATPase (see Fig. 10–8). The fact that ions move across the BBB by means of biologic transport systems rather than simple diffusion opens the way for manipulation of brain volume by specific drugs, including diuretics, ion channel blockers, hormones, and inhibitors of critical enzymes such as carbonic anhydrase and Na^+,K^+-ATPase.

Metabolism

Active transport systems such as Na^+,K^+-ATPase are large consumers of metabolic energy. The greater

number of mitochondria in brain capillary endothelial cells compared with the number in other vascular endothelia (Oldendorf et al., 1977) is undoubtedly related to this increased metabolic demand. In contrast to other brain cells, cerebral capillaries can use a variety of substrates for energy production. Isolated brain microvessels readily oxidize glucose, fatty acids, β-hydroxybutyrate, and pyruvate to carbon dioxide (Betz and Goldstein, 1984). Fatty acid metabolism may be particularly important to brain capillaries, because maximal ion transport into isolated cerebral microvessels can be achieved only if palmitate is present in addition to glucose (Goldstein, 1979).

Other metabolic processes in the brain capillary are important to BBB function. Most neurotransmitters present in the blood do not enter the brain because of their low lipid solubility and lack of specific transport carriers in the luminal membrane of the capillary endothelial cell. This case is illustrated for dopamine in Figure 10–5. In contrast, L-dopa, the precursor of dopamine, has affinity for the large neutral amino acid transport system (see Fig. 10–7) and more easily enters the brain from the blood than would be predicted by its lipid solubility. This is why patients with Parkinson's disease are treated with L-dopa rather than with dopamine. However, the entry of L-dopa into the brain is limited by the presence of the enzymes aromatic-L-amino-acid decarboxylase and monoamine oxidase within the capillary endothelial cell (Fig. 10–9) (Hardebo and Owman, 1979).

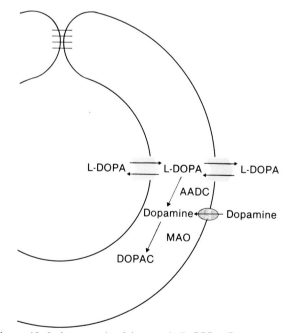

Figure 10–9. An example of the metabolic BBB. L-Dopa enters and exits the endothelial cell by means of the large neutral amino acid transport system. Inside the endothelial cell, it is subject to enzymatic conversion to dopamine and dihydroxyphenylacetic acid (DOPAC) by aromatic-L-amino-acid decarboxylase (AADC) and monoamine oxidase (MAO). These conversions decrease the amount of L-dopa available for transport into the brain. In addition, dopamine can enter the endothelial cell across the antiluminal membrane and be converted to dihydroxyphenylacetic acid. This mechanism may remove active neurotransmitters from the interstitial fluid.

This enzymatic BBB limits transendothelial passage of L-dopa into the brain and explains the need for large doses of this agent in the treatment of Parkinson's disease. Therapy is currently enhanced by concurrent treatment with an inhibitor of peripheral aromatic-L-amino-acid decarboxylase.

Intracapillary monoamine oxidase may also play a role in the inactivation of neurotransmitters released by neuronal activity, because monoamines are actively accumulated and metabolized by isolated brain capillaries (Hardebo and Owman, 1979). The fact that monoamines show extremely little uptake when presented from the luminal side suggests that the uptake systems are present only on the antiluminal membrane of the brain capillary endothelial cell (see Fig. 10–9).

Capillary Perfusion

In addition to depending on barrier permeability, the amount of solute entering the brain depends on the capillary surface area that is available for exchange (see Table 10–2). It appears that capillary surface area does not remain constant because not all capillaries in the brain are being perfused at any given time (Weiss et al., 1982). Instead, there may be intermittent opening and closing of capillaries in response to the local needs of the tissue. This process not only changes the microregional blood flow but also alters the capillary surface area (Hertz and Paulson, 1982; Phelps et al., 1981) (Fig. 10–10). Over long periods the total number of capillaries in a region can change and thereby alter the capillary density. The best example of this situation is the increase in capillary density seen during development (Bär,

Table 10–4. RECEPTORS ASSOCIATED WITH BRAIN MICROVESSELS*

α_2-Adrenergic receptor
β-Adrenergic receptor
Dopamine
Histamine
Adenosine
Prostaglandins
Insulin
Vasoactive intestinal polypeptide
Parathyroid hormone
Arginine vasopressin
Angiotensin II
Atrial natriuretic factor

*The presence of neurotransmitter or hormonal receptors was assayed either by measuring increases in cyclic AMP activity or by quantitating the binding of radioactive ligands.
Data from Betz and Goldstein (1986), Chabrier et al. (1987), Harik (1984), Huang and Rorstad (1984), Pearlmutter et al. (1988), Speth and Harik (1985).

1980). Growth of new capillaries also occurs around a tumor or an area of infarction. The enhanced entry of radiographic tracers observed with these lesions may reflect an increase in density as well as permeability of the new blood vessels.

The close matching of regional blood flow with metabolic demand implicates regulatory processes in the control of microvascular perfusion. These processes may include innervation of the capillaries (Rennels et al., 1977), as well as direct responses to local chemical mediators (Berne et al., 1981). Such regulators would serve to fine tune the response of larger-resistance vessels to the needs of specific microregions of brain. Table 10–4 gives receptors present in brain capillaries that may be used in the control of either capillary perfusion or permeability.

BY-PASSING THE BLOOD-BRAIN BARRIER

A number of agents of potential therapeutic importance do not readily enter the brain because they have low lipid solubility and are not transported by the specific carriers present in the BBB. Consequently, there is considerable interest in devising ways to enhance drug entry into the CNS, and a number of schemes have been developed (Table 10–5).

The most obvious method of circumventing the BBB is to inject the agents directly into the CSF.

Brain Uptake = P×S×C

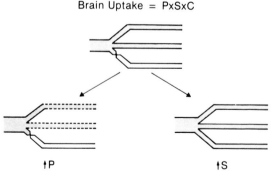

Figure 10–10. Determinants of solute uptake by brain. The amount of a substance entering the brain depends on the product of the permeability of the capillary wall (P), the surface area of the capillary to which the substance has access (S), and the concentration of substance in the blood (C). The permeability of the capillary can be enhanced by increasing the number of transport carriers, increasing the lipid solubility of the substance, or damaging the integrity of the endothelial cell (↑ P). Because capillaries are not continuously perfused, it is possible to increase the accessible surface area available for transport by opening the capillary bed or by increasing the capillary density in the brain (↑ S). Brain uptake can also be enhanced by increasing the concentration of the substance in the blood.

Table 10–5. METHODS FOR BY-PASSING THE BLOOD-BRAIN BARRIER

Intrathecal administration
Intracarotid infusion
Inhibition of capillary enzymes
Enhancement of capillary permeability
Drug modification
Increase lipid solubility
Transport by carriers

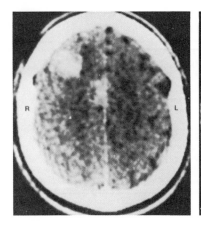 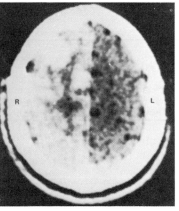

Figure 10–11. Osmotic opening of the BBB. The computed tomographic scan on the left shows two contrast-enhancing metastatic tumors. Infusion of a hypertonic mannitol solution into the right carotid artery increased capillary permeability throughout the cerebral hemisphere, as documented by markedly increased uptake of contrast agent (*right*). (Reproduced, with permission, from Neuwelt E.A., Diehl J.T., Vu L.H., et al., Monitoring of methotrexate delivery in patients with malignant brain tumors after osmotic blood-brain barrier disruption. *Ann. Intern. Med.* 1981; 94:449–454.)

Although ventricular or cisternal access sites may be used, intrathecal administration of antineoplastic agents is usually accomplished by intralumbar injection. Drug clearance and the need for repeated administration are drawbacks to this approach. A more complete discussion of the limitations of the intrathecal route is presented elsewhere (Riccardi et al., 1983). Alternatively, a reservoir may be used for repeated access to the ventricular fluid. The reservoir offers the advantages of maintaining therapeutic levels of drug in the CSF and avoiding the initially high and potentially toxic concentrations that follow a single intralumbar injection. Because of limited drug penetration into brain substance, these routes are most often used in patients with chronic meningitis and leukemia.

Enhanced delivery of a drug into the brain can be accomplished by raising its concentration in the blood, but this approach is often limited by the occurrence of systemic side effects. Similar high drug concentrations in the brain vasculature may be achieved by infusing the drug directly into the carotid artery (Eckman et al., 1974; Greenberg et al., 1984). In this way the same total systemic dose produces a much higher concentration gradient across the BBB and leads to a greater brain uptake.

Another way to enhance delivery is to increase the permeability of the BBB. The disease itself may produce this effect, which is why the rate of penicillin passage into brain is highest early in the course of meningitis. However, if the capillaries are intact, some intervention is necessary to open the barrier. The infusion of hyperosmolar solutions into the carotid circulation has been extensively studied as a method of altering BBB permeability in experimental animals (Rapoport et al., 1980). This work has been extended to patients with brain tumors (Neuwelt et al., 1981). Figure 10–11 shows the effect of such an infusion on the uptake of a radiographic contrast agent in a cerebral hemisphere containing a brain tumor. This change in permeability appears to be caused by separation of the tight junctions, which normally seal together the endothelial cells in brain capillaries (Brightman, 1977; Dorovini-Zis et al., 1983, 1984). Although the increase in BBB permeability is

reversible and apparently well tolerated, its effectiveness for chemotherapy of brain tumors remains to be shown. In addition, as shown in Figure 10–11, the effect of the hypertonic solution is greatest on the BBB of normal brain (Warnke et al., 1987). This effect could lead to undesirable toxic reactions.

Designing drugs with high BBB permeability is a more selective way to improve their delivery into the brain. In fact, most neuroactive drugs are effective because they are lipid soluble and enter the brain easily. A good example of the importance of chemical structure and lipid solubility is provided by comparison of the brain uptake of heroin and morphine (Oldendorf et al., 1972) (Fig. 10–12). These compounds are similar in structure except for the two acetyl groups of heroin, which make it more lipid soluble (see Fig. 10–5). This greater lipid solubility explains its more rapid onset of action. After heroin

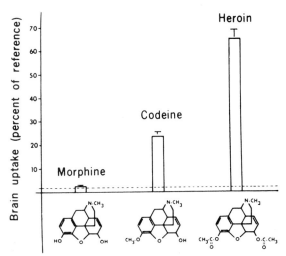

Figure 10–12. Uptake of morphine, codeine, and heroin by the brain. The greater uptake of heroin is due to blocking of the polar hydroxyl groups of morphine by less polar acetyl groups. After heroin is in the brain, the acetyl groups are removed to form morphine, which is trapped. Application of this principle could lead to enhanced uptake of other drugs by the brain. (From Oldendorf W.H., Hyman S., Braun L., et al. Blood-brain barrier: penetration of morphine, codeine, heroin, and methadone after carotid injection. *Science* 178:984–986, 1972. Copyright 1972 by the American Association for the Advancement of Science.)

is within the brain, its acetyl groups are removed to produce morphine, which leaves the brain only slowly. This process would seem to provide the basis for developing new drugs that readily enter but then are trapped within the CNS.

CONCLUSION

The BBB was once considered to be an impermeable wall of unclear structure. We now know that the barrier is produced by the endothelial cells in brain capillaries and that many of the transport properties of these cells are controlled by specific carriers, channels, and enzymes. Furthermore, the density of capillaries and the amount of microvascular perfusion also appear to be carefully regulated. A better understanding of these processes may lead to the development of new ways to manipulate BBB function and improve therapy of CNS diseases. At times it would be desirable to increase BBB permeability to enhance brain uptake of drugs and substrates, whereas in other cases it would be advantageous to decrease permeability and limit the formation of brain edema. Current research concerning the biology of the brain endothelium is directed at these goals.

References

(Key references are designated with an asterisk.)

Bär T. The vascular system of the cerebral cortex. In Brodal A., van Limborgh J., Ortmann R., et al., eds. *Advances in Anatomy, Embryology and Cell Biology.* Berlin, Springer-Verlag, pp. 1–62, 1980.

Berne R.M., Winn H.R., Rubio R. The local regulation of cerebral blood flow. *Prog. Cardiovasc. Dis.* 24:243–260, 1981.

Betz A.L. Sodium transport from blood to brain: inhibition by furosemide and amiloride. *J. Neurochem.* 41:1158–1164, 1983.

*Betz A.L., Goldstein G.W. Brain capillaries. Structure and function. In Lajtha A., ed. *Handbook of Neurochemistry.* New York, Plenum Publishing, pp. 465–484, 1984.

Betz A.L., Goldstein G.W. Specialized properties and solute transport in brain capillaries. *Annu. Rev. Physiol.* 48:241–250, 1986.

Betz A.L., Firth J.A., Goldstein G.W. Polarity of the blood-brain barrier: distribution of enzymes between the luminal and antiluminal membranes of brain capillary endothelial cells. *Brain Res.* 192:17–28, 1980.

Betz A.L., Goldstein G.W., Katzman R. Blood-brain–cerebrospinal fluid barriers. In Siegel G.J., Agranoff B., Albers R.W., et al., eds. *Basic Neurochemistry: Molecular, Cellular, and Medical Aspects.* New York, Raven Press, pp. 591–606, 1989a.

Betz A.L., Iannotti F., Hoff J.T. Brain edema: a classification based on blood-brain barrier integrity. *Cerebrovasc. Brain Metab. Rev.* 1:133–154, 1989b.

*Bradbury M. *The Concept of a Blood-Brain Barrier.* Chichester, Wiley, 1979.

*Brightman M.W. Morphology of blood-brain interfaces. *Exp. Eye Res.* 25:1–25, 1977.

Brightman M.W., Reese T.S. Junctions between intimately apposed cell membranes in the vertebrate brain. *J. Cell Biol.* 40:648–677, 1969.

Brooks D.J., Beaney R.P., Lammertsma A.A., et al. Quantitative measurement of blood-brain barrier permeability using rubidium-82 and positron emission tomography. *J. Cereb. Blood Flow Metab.* 4:535–545, 1984.

Chabrier P.E., Roubert P., Braquet P. Specific binding of atrial natriuretic factor in brain microvessels. *Proc. Natl. Acad. Sci. U.S.A.* 84:2078–2081, 1987.

Cornford E.M., Pardridge W.M., Braun L.D., et al. Increased blood-brain barrier transport of protein-bound anticonvulsant drugs in the newborn. *J. Cereb. Blood Flow Metab.* 3:280–286, 1983.

Davson H. The blood-brain barrier. *J. Physiol.* (Lond.) 255:1–28, 1976.

Dorovini-Zis K., Bowman P.D., Betz A.L., et al. Hyperosmotic arabinose solutions open the tight junctions between brain capillary endothelial cells in tissue culture. *Brain Res.* 302:383–386, 1984.

Dorovini-Zis K., Sato M., Goping G., et al. Ionic lanthanum passage across cerebral endothelium exposed to hyperosmotic arabinose. *Acta Neuropathol.* 60:49–60, 1983.

Eckman W.W., Patlak C.S., Fenstermacher J.D. A critical evaluation of the principles governing the advantages of intra-aterial infusions. *J. Pharmacokinet. Biopharm.* 2:257–285, 1974.

*Fishman R.A. Brain edema. *N. Engl. J. Med.* 293:706–711, 1975.

Gjedde A., Crone C. Blood-brain glucose transfer: repression in chronic hyperglycemia. *Science* 214:456–457, 1981.

Goldstein G.W. Relation of potassium transport to oxidative metabolism in isolated brain capillaries. *J. Physiol.* (Lond.) 286:185–195, 1979.

Goldstein G.W. Endothelial cell–astrocyte interactions. A cellular model of the blood-brain barrier. *Ann. N. Y. Acad. Sci.* 529:31–39, 1988.

Goldstein G.W., Betz A.L. Recent advances in understanding brain capillary function. *Ann. Neurol.* 14:389–395, 1983.

*Goldstein G.W., Betz A.L. The blood-brain barrier. *Sci. Am.* 254(3):74–83, 1986.

Greenberg H.S., Ensminger W.D., Chandler W.F., et al. Intra-arterial BCNU chemotherapy for treatment of malignant gliomas of the central nervous system. *J. Neurosurg.* 61:423–429, 1984.

Hansen A.J., Lund-Andersen H., Crone C. K$^+$-permeability of the blood-brain barrier, investigated by aid of a K$^+$-sensitive microelectrode. *Acta Physiol. Scand.* 101:438–445, 1977.

*Hardebo J.E., Owman C. Barrier mechanisms for neurotransmitter monoamines and their precursors at the blood-brain barrier. *Ann. Neurol.* 8:1–11, 1979.

Harik S.I. Neurotransmitter receptors in cerebral microvessels. In MacKenzie E.T., Seylaz J., Bes A., eds. *Neurotransmitters and the Cerebral Circulation.* New York, Raven Press, pp. 1–9, 1984.

Hertz M.M., Paulson O.B. Transfer across the human blood-brain barrier: evidence for capillary recruitment and for a paradox glucose permeability increase in hypocapnia. *Microvasc. Res.* 24:364–376, 1982.

Huang M., Rorstad O.P. Cerebral vascular adenylate cyclase: evidence for coupling to receptors for vasoactive intestinal peptide and parathyroid hormone. *J. Neurochem.* 43:849–856, 1984.

Kalaria R.N., Gravina S.A., Schmidley J.W., et al. The glucose transporter of the human brain and blood-brain barrier. *Ann. Neurol.* 24:757–764, 1988.

*Kimelberg H.K., Norenberg M.D. Astrocytes. *Sci. Am.* 260(4):66–76, 1989.

Long D.M. Capillary ultrastructure and the blood-brain barrier in human malignant brain tumors. *J. Neurosurg.* 32:127–144, 1970.

Lund-Andersen H. Transport of glucose from blood to brain. *Physiol. Rev.* 59:305–352, 1979.

McCall A.L., Millington W.R., Wurtman R.J. Metabolic fuel and amino acid transport to the brain in experimental diabetes mellitus. *Proc. Natl. Acad. Sci. U.S.A.* 79:5406–5410, 1982.

Milhorat T.H., Hammock M.K., Rall D.P., et al. Cerebrospinal fluid production by the choroid plexus and brain. *Science* 173:330–332, 1971.

Neuwelt, E.A. *Implications of the Blood-Brain Barrier and Its Manipulation.* New York, Plenum Publishing, 1989.

Neuwelt E.A., Diehl J.T., Vu L.H., et al. Monitoring of methotrexate delivery in patients with malignant brain tumors after osmotic blood-brain barrier disruption. *Ann. Intern. Med.* 94:449–454, 1981.

Norrby R. A review of the penetration of antibiotics into CSF and its clinical significance. *Scand. J. Infect. Dis.* 14:296–309, 1978.

Oldendorf W.H. Saturation of blood-brain barrier transport of amino acids in phenylketonuria. *Arch. Neurol.* 28:45–48, 1973.

Oldendorf W.H. The blood-brain barrier. *Exp. Eye Res.* 25:177–190, 1977.

Oldendorf W.H. The blood-brain barrier and its relevance to modern nuclear medicine. In Magistretti P.L., ed. *Functional Radionuclide Imaging of the Brain.* New York, Raven Press, pp. 1–10, 1983.

Oldendorf W.H., Hyman S., Braun L., et al. Blood-brain barrier: penetration of morphine, codeine, heroin, and methadone after carotid injection. *Science* 178:984–986, 1972.

Oldendorf W.H., Cornford M.E., Brown W.J. The large apparent work capacity of the blood-brain barrier: a study of the mitochondrial content of capillary endothelial cells in brain and other tissues of the rat. *Ann. Neurol.* 1:409–417, 1977.

*Pardridge W.M. Brain metabolism: a perspective from the blood-brain barrier. *Physiol. Rev.* 63:1481–1535, 1983.

Pearlmutter A.F., Szkrybala M., Kim Y., et al. Arginine vasopressin receptors in pig cerebral microvessels, cerebral cortex and hippocampus. *Neurosci. Lett.* 87:121–126, 1988.

Phelps M.E., Huang S.-C., Hoffman E.J., et al. Cerebral extraction of N-13 ammonia: its dependence on cerebral blood flow and capillary permeability–surface area product. *Stroke* 12:607–619, 1981.

Rapoport S.I. *Blood-Brain Barrier in Physiology and Medicine.* New York, Raven Press, 1976.

Rapoport S.I., Fredericks W.R., Ohno K., et al. Quantitative aspects of reversible osmotic opening of the blood-brain barrier. *Am. J. Physiol.* 238:R421–R431, 1980.

Reese T.S., Karnovsky M.J. Fine structural localization of a blood-brain barrier to exogenous peroxidase. *J. Cell Biol.* 34:207–217, 1967.

Rennels M.L., Forbes M.S., Anders J.J., et al. Innervation of the microcirculation in the central nervous system and other tissues. In Owman C., Edvinsson L., eds. *Neurogenic Control of the Brain Circulation.* Oxford, Pergamon Press, pp. 91–104, 1977.

*Riccardi R., Bleyer W.A., Poplack D.G. Enhancement of delivery of antineoplastic drugs into cerebrospinal fluid. In Wood J.H., ed. *Neurobiology of Cerebrospinal Fluid.* New York, Plenum Publishing, pp. 453–466, 1983.

Simionescu N., Simionescu M., Palade G.E. Structural basis of permeability in sequential segments of the microvasculature. II. Pathways followed by microperoxidase across the endothelium. *Microvasc. Res.* 15:17–36, 1978.

Smith Q.R., Momma S., Aoyagi M., et al. Kinetics of neutral amino acid transport across the blood-brain barrier. *J. Neurochem.* 49:1651–1658, 1987.

*Spector R., Johanson C.E. The mammalian choroid plexus. *Sci. Am.* 261(5):68–74, 1989.

Speth R.C., Harik S.I. Angiotensin II receptor binding sites in brain microvessels. *Proc. Natl. Acad. Sci. U.S.A.* 82:6340–6343, 1985.

Stewart P.A., Hayakawa K., Hayakawa E., et al. A quantitative study of blood-brain barrier permeability ultrastructure in a new rat glioma model. *Acta Neuropathol. (Berl.)* 67:96–102, 1985.

Vigne P., Champigny G., Marsault R., et al. A new type of amiloride-sensitive cationic channel in endothelial cells of brain microvessels. *J. Biol. Chem.* 264:7663–7668, 1989.

Warnke P.C., Blasberg R.G., Groothius D.R. The effect of hyperosmotic blood-brain barrier disruption on blood-to-tissue transport in ENU-induced gliomas. *Ann. Neurol.* 22:300–305, 1987.

Weiss H.R., Buchweitz E., Murtha T.J., et al. Quantitative regional determination of morphometric indices of the total and perfused capillary network in the rat brain. *Circ. Res.* 51:494–503, 1982.

Westergaard E. The blood-brain barrier to horseradish peroxidase under normal and experimental conditions. *Acta Neuropathol.* 39:181–187, 1977.

Wolinsky J.S., Johnson R.T. Viruses in chronic neurological diseases. In Fraenkel-Conrat H., Wagner R.R., eds. *Comprehensive Virology.* New York, Plenum Publishing, pp. 257–296, 1980.

Muscle and the Neuromuscular Junction

11

Structure and Function of Striated Muscle

Kenneth H. Fischbeck

Understanding the structure and function of normal human muscle is the key to determining the cause of muscle disease. The underlying gene defects are now being identified in a number of hereditary neuromuscular disorders. Whether we can apply this information to understanding the pathogenesis of these diseases and formulating a reasoned approach to treatment will depend on how much we know of the basic cell biology of muscle.

MUSCLE EMBRYOGENESIS AND DEVELOPMENT (Table 11–1)

Myoblasts, the cells that give rise to muscle, develop from the same embryonic mesenchymal cells that give rise to bone, cartilage, and connective tissue. Several regulatory factors, *MyoD, myf5,* and *myogenin,* initiate myogenesis by inducing the expression of muscle-specific genes (Braun et al., 1990; Davis et al., 1990; Wright et al., 1989). Muscle colony-forming cells may be cultured from human embryos as early as the fifth week of development, soon after the limb buds form (Hauschka, 1974). These cells increase in density six- to sevenfold and spread distally in the growing limb between 5 and 14 weeks of development. In the seventh week the myogenic cells become recognizable for the first time as they become more compact and elongated and assume a parallel alignment. These myoblasts then begin to fuse and form multinucleated *myotubes.*

The process of *myoblast fusion* has been well studied in animal and human cells in tissue culture. Before the cells fuse they become committed to differentiation, probably as a result of the influence of growth factors and hormones (Hauschka et al., 1982; Turo and Florini, 1982). The process of myoblast fusion is dependent on calcium and appears to be mediated by prostaglandin E_1 and protein kinase C (David et al., 1990). Monoclonal antibodies have been used to identify surface antigens specific to myoblasts and lost during subsequent development (Gower et al., 1989; Kaufman et al., 1985). Human muscle cells grown in culture can form mature myotubes (Fig.

Table 11–1. MILESTONES IN HUMAN MUSCLE DEVELOPMENT

Developmental Age	Event
5 wk	First muscle colony-forming cells can be cultured from early limb buds
7 wk	First identifiable myoblasts and myotubes (cell fusion begins)
9–10 wk	First neuromuscular contacts
18–19 wk	First muscle fiber type differentiation
20–30 wk	Cell fusion ends
Birth	Fiber type differentiation nearly complete

The author is supported by grants from the National Institutes of Health (NS 08075), the March of Dimes Birth Defects Foundation, and the Muscular Dystrophy Association.

123

11–1), with striations and occasionally spontaneous contractions, but further biochemical and morphological maturation does not occur, whether the muscle is grown by itself or cocultured with spinal cord neurons (Blau and Webster, 1981; Iannaccone et al., 1982; Witkowski and Dubowitz, 1975).

Primary myotubes in the embryo are found in clusters, with gap junctions between cells that probably allow electrical and metabolic coupling (Kelly, 1983). As the muscle matures, the primary cells separate into independent units each surrounded by its own basal lamina. Adherent myoblasts continue to replicate and fuse with the maturing primary myotubes; others fuse with each other to form *secondary myotubes*. Cell fusion is particularly active at 10–12 weeks of development and continues until 20–30 weeks (Fidziańska, 1980; Hauschka, 1974). A number of mononuclear myogenic cells remain within the basal lamina as *satellite cells,* adherent but not fused with the mature muscle fibers.

Intramuscular nerves are present at 8 weeks of development, and neuromuscular contacts begin to form at 9–10 weeks (Juntunen and Teräväinen, 1972). Innervation has been shown in animal embryos to stimulate muscle proliferation (Bonner, 1980; Harris, 1981) as well as muscle fiber type differentiation. In human muscle, fiber types can be distinguished after 18–19 weeks of gestation (Carpenter and Karpati, 1984). Thereafter the proportion of undifferentiated fetal muscle fibers (histochemical type 2C) declines as fibers with mature histochemical staining characteristics appear. The process of fiber type differentiation has been well studied in rat, which is much less mature at birth; it appears that primary myotubes develop into slow-twitch (type 1) muscle fibers and secondary myotubes into fast-twitch (type 2) fibers, probably as a result of the sequence and pattern of innervation (Kelly, 1983).

After birth and through childhood until adolescence, human muscle fibers gradually increase in length and diameter. The increase in fiber size is due to addition of the myofibrils that make up the contractile apparatus. The nuclei and organelles involved in protein synthesis and cellular "housekeeping"

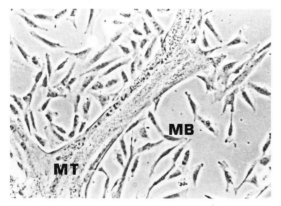

Figure 11–1. Human muscle cells in tissue culture. MB = myoblasts; MT = myotube.

functions remain small and peripherally placed. Throughout adulthood muscle fibers remain capable of regeneration; cells that have been damaged in situ or removed and grown in culture retain the remarkable ability to revert to myoblasts and recapitulate the process of myogenesis.

TISSUE ORGANIZATION OF MATURE MUSCLE

Cellular Interactions

Satellite cells are small, flat cells with scant cytoplasm scattered in shallow troughs along the length of muscle fibers (Campion, 1984). They are closely adherent to the underlying muscle fiber, although no specialized connection appears to exist. They are contained within the muscle fiber's basal lamina sheath and, in human muscle, account for about 4% of the nuclei found within the sheath (Schmalbruch and Hellhammer, 1976). When muscle is injured and undergoes necrosis, the satellite cells become stimulated to form myoblasts, which fuse to regenerate the damaged fibers.

The *motor end plate* is the site of interaction between nerve and muscle. At the end plate the terminal axons of the nerve lose their myelin coats and branch over the surface of the muscle fiber in a patch approximately 200–300 μm² in area. The axon terminal is capped by a Schwann cell. The nerve terminal itself contains mitochondria, neurofilaments, and synaptic vesicles, which are frequently clustered adjacent to the muscle surface. Freeze-fracture electron microscopy shows assembly of intramembranous particles in clusters and short rows of "active zones" in the presynaptic membrane. The muscle fiber is highly specialized in the end-plate region, with prominent infolding of the plasma membrane. Mitochondria, muscle fiber nuclei, and other noncontractile cytoplasmic organelles such as endoplasmic reticulum are commonly found near the end plate. The basal lamina separates nerve from muscle at the end plate and penetrates each infolding in the synaptic cleft. Contained in the basal lamina are the proteins *s-laminin* and *agrin*, which can serve as guides for reinnervation and re-formation of the end-plate structure after damage to the nerve or the muscle (Hunter et al., 1989; Magill-Solc and Mc-Mahan, 1988).

The *myotendinous junction* is the site of coupling between the contractile apparatus of the muscle fiber and the collagen of the tendon. Here the muscle fiber and tendon are interdigitated, with large, irregular invaginations and evaginations of the muscle plasma membrane. The force of contraction is carried by a set of fine filaments connected to the actin of the myofibrils in the muscle fiber interior and traversing the plasma membrane to the extracellular space (Trotter et al., 1983). This mechanical connection is maintained when the plasma membrane is solubilized with detergent. In chick muscle, this connection between muscle and tendon appears to be mediated at least in part by the protein *integrin* (Bozyczko et al., 1989).

The *vascular supply* of muscle is provided by arteries that run in the connective tissue between fascicles and give rise to arterioles that penetrate among the muscle fibers to the central portion of each fascicle. The arterioles branch into a rich network of capillaries that course longitudinally along the muscle fibers with frequent transverse anastomoses like rungs on a ladder. The number of capillaries varies with age, exercise, and fiber type.

The *muscle spindle* is a specialized structure with several muscle fibers surrounded by a connective tissue capsule. The fibers within the spindle, termed *intrafusal muscle fibers,* are of two general types: *nuclear chain fibers,* which are narrow (10–15 μm in diameter) and short, and *nuclear bag fibers,* which are larger (up to 50 μm in diameter). The nuclear bag fibers can be further subdivided according to twitch characteristics and histochemical staining (Banks et al., 1977; Carpenter and Karpati, 1984). The intrafusal muscle fibers have specialized motor innervation (the γ efferents) and at least two types of sensory nerve endings. The spindles provide sensory feedback from muscle contraction and thereby facilitate muscle coordination and maintain proper tone.

Muscle Fiber Histochemistry

Muscle fibers are separable into distinct categories on the basis of physiology, structure, and biochemistry. Fibers can be differentiated by speed of contraction and resistance to fatigue. Slow-twitch fibers tend to be fatigue resistant; they have abundant mitochondria and lipid granules and make greater use of the Krebs cycle and oxidative metabolism. Fast-twitch fibers tend to have higher glycogen content and derive much of their metabolic energy from the glycolytic pathway. Muscle histochemistry allows identification of fiber types in frozen sections of human muscle using a variety of specific stains. Histochemical staining procedures have been reviewed by Dubowitz (1985) and Brumback and Leech (1984). Most reliable for differentiating fiber types is the myosin ATPase stain, and, although the correlation with fiber type differentiation by other characteristics is not always exact, this stain is generally accepted as the standard for identification of fiber types in human muscle.

The fiber types defined by ATPase stain are based on the pH dependence of myosin ATPase activity, which relates closely to antigenic differences in myosin between fast- and slow-twitch muscles (Table 11–2). *Type 1 fibers,* which are slow twitch and have oxidative metabolism, show little ATPase activity at "standard" incubating conditions (pH 9.4) but good activity (dark staining) after preincubation at pH 4.3–4.6. *Type 2A fibers* are fast twitch but relatively fatigue

Table 11–2. MUSCLE FIBER TYPES

Histochemical Classification	Description	ATPase Stain		
		pH 9.4	*pH 4.6*	*pH 4.3*
Type 1	Slow twitch, oxidative	Light	Dark	Dark
Type 2A	Fast twitch, oxidative/glycolytic	Dark	Light	Light
Type 2B	Fast twitch, glycolytic	Dark	Dark	Light
Type 2C	Fetal	Dark	Dark	Dark

resistant, with both oxidative and glycolytic metabolism; they are reactive for ATPase stain at pH 9.4 but not pH 4.6 or 4.3. *Type 2B fibers* are fast twitch, rapidly fatiguing, and dependent on glycolysis as a primary energy source; they have ATPase activity at pH 9.4 and 4.6 but not 4.3. *Type 2C fibers* are common in fetal muscle; they show ATPase activity with both alkaline (pH 9.4) and acid (pH 4.3 and 4.6) preincubation.

There is strong evidence from animal experiments that fiber type is determined by innervation. Cross-innervation of a predominantly fast-twitch muscle with a slow-twitch nerve will cause conversion of the muscle fibers from fast to slow and vice versa. All of the muscle fibers within each motor unit, that is, all of the fibers innervated by a single motor neuron, have the same fiber type. Because motor units are normally intermingled, fibers of each type are not clustered in normal muscle but dispersed in a checkerboard pattern. Although some variation from one muscle to another might be expected, the usual ratio of type 1 to type 2 fibers in human muscles available for biopsy is 1:2. About half of the type 2 fibers are 2A and half 2B; type 2C fibers are rarely seen in normal mature muscle.

CELLULAR ORGANIZATION OF MUSCLE

By electron microscopy, muscle fibers are seen to be nearly filled with *myofibrils*, which contain the filamentous proteins, actin and myosin, responsible for generating the force of muscle contraction. Other structures found within muscle fibers or associated with their surface serve to maintain the integrity of the cells, to propagate the signal to contract to the vicinity of the contractile apparatus, to couple excitation with contraction, and to provide energy for contraction to occur (Fig. 11–2).

The *basal lamina* lies on the external surface of the muscle fiber. Under experimental and pathologic conditions it is shown to be a durable sheath, which can maintain its cylindric shape even when the underlying fiber is destroyed. External to the basal lamina is a loosely woven network of collagen fibrils, referred to as the reticular lamina. The basal lamina itself is granular and amorphous, about 30 nm thick, and separated from the plasma membrane by a thin electron-lucid gap that is occasionally traversed by

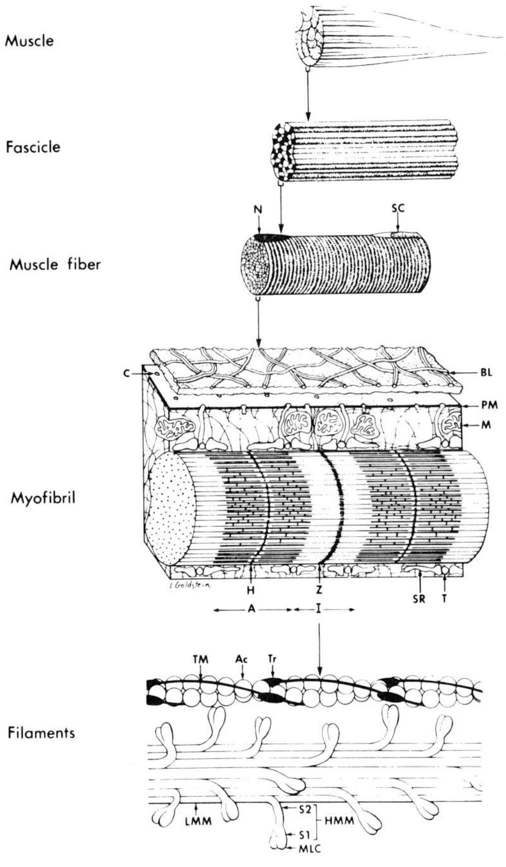

Figure 11–2. Human muscle structure. Muscle fiber: N = nucleus; SC = satellite cell. Myofibril (with adjacent plasma membrane and cell surface): BL = basal lamina; PM = plasma membrane; C = caveola; M = mitochondria; H = H zone; Z = Z line; A = A band; I = I band; SR = sarcoplasmic reticulum; T = T tubule. Muscle filaments: Ac = actin; TM = tropomyosin; Tr = troponin. Myosin: LMM = light meromyosin (rod); HMM = heavy meromyosin with S1 and S2 subfragments; MLC = myosin light chains.

trabeculae (Bonilla, 1983). The composition of the basal lamina has been studied with immunohistochemical technique in rat muscle (Sanes, 1982); the identified proteins include laminin, fibronectin, and collagen.

The *muscle plasma membrane* has flask-shaped invaginations called *caveolae*. The functional role of caveolae is not clear; they appear to be fixed structures rather than pinocytotic vesicles, in that they flatten with supraphysiologic stretch and fill with extracellular markers (Dulhunty and Franzini-Armstrong, 1975). A minority of caveolae are connected to T tubules. In human muscle caveolae may vary in density with the underlying sarcomere structure; the overall density is about $18/\mu m^2$ (Bonilla et al., 1981).

A *cytoskeleton* of filamentous proteins underlies the plasma membrane in muscle, as in other cells. These proteins form an intricate array that preserves the structural integrity of the muscle fiber during contraction and relaxation (Wang, 1983). Thin filaments underlying the muscle plasma membrane are composed primarily of *cytoplasmic actin,* which is antigenically distinct from actin found in the myofibrils (Lubit and Schwartz, 1980). In chick muscle, these cytoplasmic actin filaments interact with circumferential bands of *spectrin* and *vinculin,* which are closely adherent to the internal surface of the plasma membrane. Spectrin and vinculin show a regular repeating pattern coincident with the sarcomere structure in the contractile apparatus, indicating that they serve

as a link between membrane and myofibril, perhaps helping to keep the two in register during contraction (Pardo et al., 1983; Repasky et al., 1982).

Dystrophin is a large (427-kd) protein that was identified by its involvement in Duchenne's muscular dystrophy (Hoffman et al., 1987, 1988). Sequence analysis indicates that it has a long, rod-shaped configuration (Koenig et al., 1988). There is sequence homology to the actin-binding domain of α-actinin at the NH_2-terminal end, so it is likely that dystrophin binds to actin in the sarcolemmal cytoskeleton. Immunocytochemical studies localize dystrophin to the muscle plasma membrane, where it seems to provide structural support as the muscle contracts and relaxes (Bonilla et al., 1988; Watkins et al., 1988; Zubrzycka-Gaarn et al., 1988).

Intermediate filaments run through the interior of the muscle fiber within and between sarcomeres in the myofibrils, forming a scaffolding for the contractile proteins. The filaments are deployed longitudinally, ensheathing each myofibril, and transversely, connecting myofibrils at the Z and M lines. The principal components of intermediate filaments in mature muscle are *desmin* (skeletin) and *synemin.* Another intermediate filament protein, *vimentin,* is found in developing muscle (Thornell et al., 1983).

The *sarcoplasmic reticulum and T tubules* constitute a membranous system that runs through the interior of the muscle fiber, around each myofibril, and mediates excitation-contraction coupling. The *T sys-*

tem is a network of narrow tubules that course transversely into the muscle fiber interior around each myofibril at the level of the A-I junction (this feature distinguishes mammalian skeletal muscle from cardiac muscle and muscles in fish and amphibians, in which the T system is at the level of the Z lines). The T tubule is formed by invagination of the plasma membrane and resembles it biochemically. In mature muscle the T system remains continuous with the muscle plasma membrane, connecting via caveolae at the fiber surface, and the interior of the T tubules is continuous with the extracellular space, allowing the tubules to carry action potentials from the surface into the central portions of the muscle fiber.

The *sarcoplasmic reticulum* (SR) is a vesicular network that surrounds each myofibril. Dilated sacs of SR called terminal cisternae abut the T tubules on either side of the A-I junction, forming SR-T-SR *triads*. At the point of contact between SR and T tubule there are bridging structures; these are composed of the *ryanodine receptor* and *dihydropyridine receptor* (Block et al., 1988), the proteins that mediate excitation-contraction coupling, as discussed later. Near the fiber surface, the SR may come in contact with the plasma membrane in a manner analogous to the SR-T junction; such contacts are called *peripheral couplings*. The terminal cisternae of SR contain dense material that is largely the calcium-binding protein calsequestrin. The major protein constituent of the SR membrane is Ca^{2+}-ATPase. The function of SR is to release calcium in response to depolarization of the plasma membrane and T system, thereby triggering actin-myosin interaction and muscle contraction, then subsequently to reaccumulate calcium actively to allow relaxation.

Mitochondria are arrayed through the muscle fiber interior in a pattern that appears to allow delivery of ATP to the sites where it is most needed in energy-requiring processes such as contraction and ion transport. Mitochondria may be numerous in the endplate region and near the fiber surface beneath the plasma membrane. In the muscle fiber interior mitochondria are clustered around the myofibrils near the A-I junction. Mitochondria are more sparse in type 2B fibers than in type 1 or 2A fibers.

Myofibrils are the structural units that actually mediate contraction of the muscle fiber (Fig. 11–3). They are densely packed in the cell, accounting for more than three-fourths of the volume. The myofibrils are about 1 μm in diameter and can run the length of the muscle fiber (up to several centimeters). They have a characteristic regularly repeating transverse band pattern: dark, anisotropic, or *A bands* containing longitudinal thick filaments alternate with lighter, isotropic or *I bands* containing thin filaments. At the center of the A band is the dark transverse *M line* surrounded by a somewhat lighter region, the *H zone*. At the center of the I band runs the dense *Z line* (or disc). The repeating unit from one Z line to the next is called a *sarcomere*. All the myofibrils in the fiber are held in register, presumably by inter-

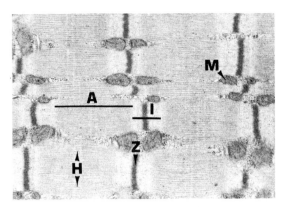

Figure 11–3. Thin-section electron micrograph of muscle contractile apparatus. Labeling as in Figure 11–2.

mediate filaments that connect adjacent Z lines. This gives the fiber as a whole its striated appearance. The sarcomere length varies from about 2 to 3 μm, depending on the degree of contraction. The lengths of the thick filaments (about 1.5 μm) and thin filaments (1.0–1.25 μm) do not vary as the sarcomere shortens, but the region of overlap does, hence the *sliding filament model* for muscle contraction, in which the force of contraction is generated by thick and thin filaments sliding past each other in the sarcomere.

The thick filaments in the myofibrils are composed primarily of myosin and the thin filaments of actin with the regulatory proteins troponin and tropomyosin. Fine cross-bridges between thick and thin filaments sometimes seen in the area of overlap by electron microscopy have been identified as the double-head portion of the myosin molecule (see later). The thick filaments are cross-linked in a hexagonal lattice at the level of the M line; proteins identified with this structure include myomesin, M protein, and the MM form of creatine kinase (Grove et al., 1984). The thin filaments are held in place by the dense meshwork of the Z line, which has been found to contain α-actinin, as well as a rim of desmin, which connects to the scaffolding of intermediate filaments running around and between the myofibrils.

The long, filamentous proteins *titin* and *nebulin* also run longitudinally within the myofibrils, apparently providing structural support for the cell (Horowits et al., 1986). Titin is the largest polypeptide yet described, with molecular mass of about 3000 kd. Partial sequence analysis indicates a regular repeat pattern similar to that of other muscle proteins (Labeit et al., 1990).

The major known structural proteins of vertebrate skeletal muscle are listed in Table 11–3.

MOLECULAR ORGANIZATION OF MUSCLE

Muscle fibers convert a signal of acetylcholine released by the nerve terminal at the neuromuscular

Table 11–3. MAJOR STRUCTURAL PROTEINS IN VERTEBRATE MUSCLE

Location	Protein
Basal lamina	Laminin
	Fibronectin
	Collagen (IV and V)
Cytoskeleton	Cytoplasmic actin
	Spectrin
	Vinculin
	Dystrophin
Intermediate filaments	Desmin (skeletin)
	Synemin
	Vimentin
Myofibrils	Titin
	Nebulin
Z lines	Desmin
	α-Actin
M lines	Myomesin
	M protein
	Creatine kinase (MM)
Thick filaments	Myosin
	C protein
Thin filaments	α-Actin
	Tropomyosin
	Troponin

junction to mechanical force generated by the coordinated contraction of thousands of sarcomere units. Necessary to this process are (1) excitation of the muscle plasma membrane and T system, (2) coupling of excitation to contraction by the SR, and (3) contraction by interaction of actin and myosin in the myofibrils. The structure and function of key proteins in each of these steps have been subjects of extensive research, both in muscle and in other tissues where they occur. Some of this work is summarized in the following. Molecular aspects of muscle energy supply are discussed by Rowland et al. in Chapter 12.

Muscle Fiber Excitation

Across the muscle plasma membrane is a potential of about 90 mV, inside negative. As in nerve cells, this *resting potential* results from an unequal distribution of ions across the membrane and selective permeability of the membrane to these ions. Na^+ and Cl^- have a higher concentration outside the cell and K^+ a higher concentration inside. The membrane has a greater permeability to Cl^- and K^+; thus the resting potential is close to the equilibrium potential of these ions. Acetylcholine causes depolarization of the plasma membrane at the neuromuscular junction by inducing an increase in membrane permeability to both Na^+ and K^+ at the acetylcholine receptor. Depolarization beyond a threshold point leads to a regenerative *action potential,* which propagates the length of the fiber by successive voltage- and time-dependent increases in conductance of the membrane first to Na^+ (causing depolarization) and subsequently to K^+ (causing repolarization). Accounts of the mechanisms of generation of the resting potential, neuromuscular transmission, and propagation of the action potential are given by Kuffler et al. (1984) and elsewhere in this book (see Chapters 3 and 13). A brief discussion of the major proteins involved in these processes follows (Table 11–4).

The unequal distribution of Na^+ and K^+ across the muscle membrane that gives rise to the resting potential is maintained by the membrane protein Na^+,K^+-*ATPase,* which actively transports Na^+ out of the cell and K^+ in. This protein has been isolated from mammalian kidney, purified, reconstituted into artificial liposomes in active form, cloned, and sequenced (Jørgensen, 1982; Shull et al., 1985). It is composed of two subunits; the larger α subunit (about 110 kd) binds ATP and mediates ion transfer;

Table 11–4. PROTEINS INVOLVED IN MUSCLE EXCITATION AND EXCITATION-CONTRACTION COUPLING

Protein	Major Location in Muscle	Ligand	Source for Isolation or Identification	Subunits, Molecular Mass (kd)	References
Acetylcholine receptor	Plasma membrane (end plate)	Bungarotoxin	Electric organ, muscle	$α_2$, 50 β, 54 γ, 56 δ, 58	Changeux et al., 1984
Acetylcholinesterase	Basal lamina (end plate)		Electric organ, muscle	80 (up to 12-mers ± collagen tail)	Brimijoin, 1983; Skau, 1986
Na^+,K^+-ATPase	Plasma membrane	Ouabain	Kidney	α, 110 β, 35	Jørgensen, 1982 Shull et al., 1985
Na^+ channel	Plasma membrane	Tetrodotoxin, saxitoxin	Electric organ, brain, muscle	260 (33–38)	Catterall, 1986, 1988; Barchi, 1988
K^+ channel	Plasma membrane		*Drosophila,* muscle	~70	Koren et al., 1990
Ca^{2+} channel	T tubules, plasma membrane	Dihydropyridine	Muscle	170	Tanabe et al., 1987
Ca^{2+} release protein	Sarcoplasmic reticulum	Ryanodine	Muscle	560	Zorzato et al., 1990
Ca^{2+}-ATPase	Sarcoplasmic reticulum		Muscle	110	MacLennan et al., 1985 Inesi, 1985

the smaller β subunit is a glycoprotein of about 35 kd. In frog muscle plasma membrane, Na^+,K^+-ATPase density has been estimated by ouabain binding to be about 2500 molecules/μm^2 (Venosa and Horowicz, 1981).

Acetylcholine receptor is the protein that, when binding acetylcholine at the neuromuscular junction, allows ion flow across the plasma membrane to produce depolarization. A major advance in understanding of this protein came with the isolation of cDNA for each of the receptor subunits; this made available the complete amino acid sequence of the protein (see review by Changeux et al., 1984). The receptor is composed of two identical α subunits and three nonidentical subunits, β, γ, and δ. The α subunits bind acetylcholine and α-bungarotoxin, the ligand used to purify the protein. The five subunits are arranged in a ring about a central ion channel. There is 10–60% homology in amino acid sequence among the subunits; each has at least four hydrophobic membrane-spanning domains. Receptor proteins may form dimers by disulfide linkage between the δ subunits and also appear to be anchored via a 43-kd protein to cytoplasmic actin in the submembranous cytoskeleton. The acetylcholine receptor gene initially isolated from *Torpedo* electric organ has been used to find the genes for the receptors in calf and human muscle. There is considerable homology (about 80%) between *Torpedo* and the mammals in the amino acid sequences for the α subunit, less for the γ chain. The receptor can be synthesized by oocytes injected with subunit-specific mRNAs; in this system each of the subunits is necessary for normal activity of the receptor protein.

Acetylcholinesterase is the enzyme responsible for degrading acetylcholine at the neuromuscular junction, thereby terminating the signal to contract. This enzyme exists in a variety of forms in various tissues (reviewed by Brimijoin, 1983; Skau, 1986). The different forms are multimers of a subunit of 80 kd; the largest consists of 12 of these subunits attached to a collagen tail. In muscle, acetylcholinesterase is most highly concentrated at the neuromuscular junction, where it is secreted by the muscle fiber under neural influence and is fixed to the basal lamina. A study with monoclonal antibodies showed much homology between acetylcholinesterase at the human neuromuscular junction and the enzyme present in human red blood cells (Fambrough et al., 1982), suggesting that these two forms may be coded by the same, or very similar, genes.

The *sodium channel protein* initiates and propagates action potentials in muscle plasma membrane by mediating transient voltage-dependent increases in Na^+ conductance. The density of channels in muscle membrane has been estimated to be 200–400/μm^2. The protein has been isolated and purified from electric organ, rat brain, and rat muscle by virtue of its binding to the highly selective ligands tetrodotoxin and saxitoxin (reviewed by Barchi, 1988; Catterall, 1986, 1988). Antibodies to isolated rat sodium channel cross-react with human muscle plasma membrane

(Haimovich et al., 1984). The purified channel protein has been reconstituted into artificial liposomes, where it shows toxin-binding and ion flux–mediating properties similar to those in the plasma membrane. The sodium channel has a large glycosylated subunit (about 260 kd). In mammalian preparations additional subunits of 33–38 kd have been reported. These smaller subunits do not appear to be necessary to channel function, because functional sodium channels can be expressed in oocytes injected with mRNA for the major subunit alone (Noda et al., 1986). As with acetylcholine receptor, isolation of the sodium channel gene (Noda et al., 1984) was a major advance in appreciating the correlation of structure with function in this protein. Subsequently, two separate sodium channel genes that correspond to the tetrodotoxin-sensitive and -insensitive forms of the protein were cloned from mammalian skeletal muscle mRNA (Kallen et al., 1990; Trimmer et al., 1989; see also Chapter 13).

Potassium, calcium, and chloride channels are also present in muscle plasma membrane and the T system. Potassium channels mediate the time- and voltage-dependent increase in K^+ conductance that allows repolarization of the membrane after an action potential. Calcium channels allow Ca^{2+} influx with membrane depolarization and in some preparations allow the propagation of action potentials when sodium channels are blocked with tetrodotoxin. Chloride channels allow a fixed, relatively high membrane permeability to Cl^-, which stabilizes the membrane and prevents repetitive firing. Sequence analysis of the cloned sodium, potassium, and calcium channels indicates that they are all members of the same gene family (Catterall, 1988). The voltage-activated potassium channel, first cloned in *Drosophila*, has been cloned from rat muscle as well (Koren et al., 1990); it is smaller than the sodium and calcium channels and probably exists in the plasma membrane in multimeric form. The calcium channel that mediates long-lasting Ca^{2+} currents has been isolated and cloned by virtue of its ability to bind dihydropyridines such as nifedipine (Tanabe et al., 1987). This dihydropyridine-binding calcium channel is particularly concentrated in the T system, in which it has been shown to play an important role in excitation-contraction coupling.

Excitation-Contraction Coupling

Spread of depolarization from the muscle plasma membrane through the T system leads to the release of Ca^{2+} from the SR that surrounds each myofibril. The transfer of signal from the T system to the SR is facilitated by the close juxtaposition of the dihydropyridine receptor (calcium channel) protein in the T system membrane and a large protein, the ryanodine receptor, that bridges the gap between SR and T system and mediates calcium release from the SR (Block et al., 1988). The ryanodine receptor gene has

Table 11–5. MUSCLE CONTRACTILE PROTEINS

Protein	Location	Subunits, Molecular Mass (kd)	References
α-Actin	Thin filaments	G-actin, 42	Holmes et al., 1990
Myosin	Thick filaments	2 heavy chains, 200 4 light chains, 15–27	Warrick and Spudich, 1987
Tropomyosin	Thin filaments	α, 33.5 β, 37	Zot and Potter, 1987 Ohtsuki et al., 1986
Troponin	Thin filaments	Troponin C, troponin T, troponin I, 75 total	Ohtsuki et al., 1986; Zot and Potter, 1987

been cloned; it encodes a 560-kd protein with over 5000 amino acids (Zorzato et al., 1990). The Ca^{2+} concentration, which is normally quite low in the intracellular space (about 0.1 μmol/L, $\frac{1}{1000}$ the extracellular concentration), rapidly increases in the vicinity of the contractile apparatus, allowing actin-myosin interaction and contraction to occur. The fiber relaxes when Ca^{2+} is actively pumped back into the SR, and low intracellular Ca^{2+} concentration is restored. Apparent from this sequence of events is the need to maintain intracellular Ca^{2+} at a low resting level. This is accomplished by Na^+-Ca^{2+} exchange and active Ca^{2+} transport at the plasma membrane and, most important, reuptake of Ca^{2+} into SR by Ca^{2+}-ATPase.

Ca^{2+},Mg^{2+}-activated ATPase (Ca^{2+}-ATPase) is the principal protein in the SR membrane. Two separate Ca^{2+}-ATPase genes, representing fast-twitch and slow-twitch isoforms, have been cloned from mammalian muscle mRNA (Brandl et al., 1986). The protein consists of a single peptide (about 110 kd), which most likely is present in the SR in dimeric or multimeric form (Inesi, 1985). The bulk of each subunit is on the external (cytoplasmic) surface of the SR membrane, where it can be visualized with negative staining and is subject to tryptic cleavage. The protein is anchored in the lipid bilayer by hydrophobic domains. Ca^{2+}-ATPase shares many features with the α subunit of Na^+,K^+-ATPase, described earlier. Both couple ATPase activity to ion transport, and they are similar in molecular weight, amino acid sequence at the active (phosphorylation) site, proteolytic fragment pattern, and sensitivity to inhibition by vanadate (Hiatt et al., 1984).

Ca^{2+}-ATPase is stimulated in the presence of cytoplasmic Ca^{2+} by *calmodulin*, a small (16.5 kd) protein that binds four Ca^{2+} ions and interacts with a broad variety of Ca^{2+}-activated enzymes (reviewed by Tomlinson et al., 1984). Calmodulin is widespread in eukaryotic organisms; its 148-amino-acid sequence is well conserved, reflecting the crucial role that it and Ca^{2+} play in the regulation of cell functions.

Muscle Contraction

Muscle contraction results from interaction between actin and myosin subfragment S1. ATP is hydrolyzed by the myosin, and a conformational change shifts the actin and myosin filaments relative to each other a distance of 10 nm. In the resting state, actin-myosin interaction is blocked by tropomyosin. Contraction is initiated when Ca^{2+} released by the SR is bound by troponin, which shifts tropomyosin and allows actin-myosin interaction to occur. The mechanism of muscle contraction has been reviewed by Hibberd and Trentham (1986), Cooke (1986), Goldman (1987), and Zot and Potter (1987). A description of the major proteins and molecular aspects of their interactions is given next and in Table 11–5.

Actin, although originally discovered in muscle, probably exists in some form in every eukaryotic cell. It consists of globular subunits (G-actin) of 42 kd that polymerize to form a long, double-helical filament (F-actin). Six different mammalian actins have been identified, four muscle (skeletal α, cardiac α, and smooth α and γ) and two cytoplasmic (β and γ), on the basis of variations in amino acid sequence. Several of the human actin genes have been isolated (J.N. Engel et al., 1981; Gunning et al., 1983). There may be as many as 20–30 human actin genes in all, scattered throughout the genome (Soriano et al., 1982). Cross-linking studies have suggested that the portion of actin that binds to myosin is near the NH_2-terminal end (Sutoh, 1982). The detailed structure of the F-actin filament has been determined by x-ray diffraction studies (Holmes et al., 1990).

Myosin is the principal component of the thick filaments in myofibrils. It is a large protein of about 470 kd, is about 160 nm long, and is composed of two heavy chains (200 kd each) and four light chains (15–27 kd). The heavy chains consist of globular heads of about 117 kd (S1) connected by filamentous necks (S2) to long, narrow rods. The two heavy chains that make up the bulk of each myosin protein are paired so that their tails are intertwined. Proteolytic treatment produces the characteristic fragments light meromyosin, which constitutes the paired heavy chain tails, and heavy meromyosin, made up of the S1 and S2 subfragments. Two light chains are associated with each S1 segment. The S1 segments have ATPase and actin-binding capability. In muscle the myosin molecules are stacked in parallel, roughly 300 per thick filament, with the paired S1 head groups protruding as cross-bridges every 14.3 nm. Under appropriate conditions, myosin can self-associate to form thick filament–like structures in vitro (Pepe, 1983). A number of myosin heavy chain genes have been cloned and sequenced (see review by

Warrick and Spudich, 1987). Sequence comparison shows relatively high homology in portions of the head region, consistent with the importance of this portion of the protein in actin interactions. The rod sequence is highly repetitive, with about 40 cycles of a 28-amino-acid repeat. This rod sequence has been used to predict that parallel myosin molecules interact optimally when staggered by 98 residues, corresponding to a distance of 14.6 nm, close to the known separation between myosin heads in thick filaments (Karn et al., 1982). As with actin, multiple myosin heavy chain genes are represented in the vertebrate genome. It has been suggested that there are 13 separate heavy chain genes in the rat. Leinwand et al. (1983) have identified four distinct human myosin heavy chain genes, located in a cluster on chromosome 17.

The nature of the interaction between myosin and actin that gives rise to muscle tension has been studied with a variety of biochemical and biophysical techniques, but the exact mechanism remains elusive (see reviews by Cooke, 1986; Goldman, 1987; Hibberd and Trentham, 1986). There is contact between actin and myosin subfragment S1, which also contains the ATPase site. It is unlikely that major conformational changes occur in either actin or myosin subfragment S2, to which S1 is attached; it appears instead that the S1 cross-bridge origin on the thick filament remains fixed with contraction and that the structural changes are either at the site of actin-myosin contact or nearby within S1 itself. Movement of the thick filament relative to the thin filament is the result of a cycle of repeated actin-myosin interactions.

Actin-myosin interaction is controlled by the thin filament proteins tropomyosin and troponin (el-Saleh et al., 1986; Ohtsuki et al., 1986; Zot and Potter, 1987). *Tropomyosin* is a long, narrow protein that lies along the actin double helix in the thin filament. Two subunits of tropomyosin have been identified in muscle, α (33.5 kd) and β (37 kd). Tropomyosin is also found in nonmuscle tissues, where it has a lower molecular mass. The protein is about 38 nm long; in the thin filament each tropomyosin molecule interacts with seven actin subunits. In the resting state, this interaction between tropomyosin and actin prevents the actin from binding myosin. X-ray diffraction studies show a change in configuration of tropomyosin preceding cross-bridge movement and the generation of tension.

The change in tropomyosin that allows contraction to occur is triggered by *troponin*, a 75-kd protein found in pairs at 38-nm intervals along the thin filaments, one for every tropomyosin molecule (see Fig. 11–2). Troponin consists of three subunits: troponin C, which binds Ca^{2+}; troponin T, which binds tropomyosin; and troponin I, which mediates the inhibition of contraction in the absence of Ca^{2+}. Troponin C is closely related to calmodulin (discussed earlier). Binding of Ca^{2+} to troponin C induces conformational changes in troponin and tropomyosin that allow actin to interact with myosin and contraction to take place. As with most contractile proteins, troponin varies from one muscle to another, depending on fiber type and stage of muscle development.

HEREDITARY DEFECTS IN MUSCLE PROTEINS

Hereditary diseases that cause muscle dysfunction are generally the result of mutations in genes that code for proteins important to muscle structure and function. Over the past several years, the identification of genetic defects in a number of muscle diseases has led to increased understanding not only of the pathogenesis of these diseases but also of the nature of the proteins that are altered. These disorders are covered in more detail elsewhere in this text. A brief summary is given in Table 11–6 and in the following discussion.

As mentioned earlier, the protein dystrophin was first identified as the normal product of the gene that is altered in Duchenne's and Becker's muscular dystrophies (Hoffman et al., 1987, 1988). Subsequent studies have shown that the distribution of mutations in the dystrophin gene is not uniform and that the severity of the disease varies with type and location

Table 11–6. HEREDITARY DEFECTS IN MUSCLE PROTEINS

Protein	Disease	Evidence	References
Dystrophin	Duchenne's and Becker's muscular dystrophies	Gene defects, protein abnormalities	Hoffman et al., 1987, 1988; Koenig et al., 1989
Acetylcholine receptor, acetylcholinesterase	Congenital myasthenia	Protein abnormality	A.G. Engel, 1984
Na^+ channel	Periodic paralysis	Genetic linkage	Fontaine et al., 1990
Ca^{2+} channel (dihydropyridine receptor)	Muscular dysgenesis (mice)	Protein abnormality	Knudson et al., 1989; Tanabe et al., 1988
Ca^{2+} release protein (ryanodine receptor)	Malignant hyperthermia	Genetic linkage	MacLellan et al., 1990; McCarthy et al., 1990
Myosin heavy chain (cardiac)	Familial hypertrophic cardiomyopathy	Gene defect	Geisterfer-Lowrance et al., 1990; Tanigawa et al., 1990

of the mutation (Koenig et al., 1989). These studies indicate that a cysteine-rich domain near the COOH terminus is particularly important to the stability of the protein, because patients with mutations affecting the translation of this domain invariably have severe disease. Other patients with mutations limited to the central rod domain may have unusually mild disease, indicating that this portion of the protein is less critical to its function (Gospe et al., 1989).

Different forms of congenital myasthenia have been found to be associated with either a deficiency or abnormality of acetylcholine receptor or a deficiency of acetylcholinesterase at the neuromuscular junction (reviewed by A.G. Engel, 1984). Specific mutations have not yet been identified in the genes for these proteins, but it is likely that they exist.

The genes for two channel proteins, the voltage-dependent sodium channel and the SR calcium release protein (or ryanodine receptor), have been implicated by genetic linkage analysis and physiologic studies as candidate genes in hyperkalemic periodic paralysis and malignant hyperthermia, respectively (Fontaine et al., 1990; MacLennan et al., 1990; McCarthy et al., 1990). Another channel protein, the T system calcium channel (dihydropyridine receptor) has been found to be deficient in mice with muscular dysgenesis, and replacement with cDNA for this protein restores excitation-contraction coupling, which is defective in these animals (Knudson et al., 1989; Tanabe et al., 1988). Specific genetic defects have been identified in the cardiac isoforms of myosin heavy chain in familial hypertrophic cardiomyopathy (Geisterfer-Lowrance et al., 1990; Tanigawa et al., 1990).

It is likely that the list of known hereditary defects in muscle proteins will expand greatly as more genes responsible for hereditary muscle diseases are identified and we come to recognize the roles of the protein products of these genes in normal muscle structure and function.

References

(Key references are designated with an asterisk.)

Banks R.W., Harker D.W., Stacey M.J. A study of mammalian intrafusal muscle fibers using a combined histochemical and ultrastructural technique. *J. Anat.* 123:783–796, 1977.

Barchi R.L. Probing the molecular structure of the voltage-dependent sodium channel. *Annu. Rev. Neurosci.* 11:455–495, 1988.

Blau H.M., Webster C. Isolation and characterization of human muscle cells. *Proc. Natl. Acad. Sci. U.S.A.* 78:5623–5627, 1981.

Block B.A., Imagawa T., Campbell K.P., et al.: Structural evidence for direct interaction between the molecular components of the transverse tubule/sarcoplasmic reticulum junction in skeletal muscle. *J. Cell Biol.* 107:2587–2600, 1988.

Bonilla E. Ultrastructural study of the muscle cell surface. *J. Ultrastruct. Res.* 82:341–345, 1983.

Bonilla E., Fischbeck K., Schotland D.L. Freeze-fracture studies of muscle caveolae in human muscular dystrophy. *Am. J. Pathol.* 104:167–173, 1981.

Bonilla E., Samitt C.E., Miranda A.F., et al. Duchenne muscular dystrophy: deficiency of dystrophin at the muscle cell surface. *Cell* 54:447–452, 1988.

Bonner P.H. Differentiation of chick embryo myoblasts is tran-

siently sensitive to functional denervation. *Dev. Biol.* 76:79–86, 1980.

Bozyczko D., Decker C., Muschler J., et al. Integrin on developing and adult skeletal muscle. *Exp. Cell Res.* 183:72–91, 1989.

Brandl C.J., Green N.M., Korczak B., et al. Two Ca^{2+} ATPase genes: homologies and mechanistic implications of deduced amino acid sequences. *Cell* 44:597–607, 1986.

Braun T., Winter B., Bober E., et al. Transcriptional activation domain of the muscle-specific gene-regulatory protein myf5. *Nature* 346:663–665, 1990.

Brimijoin S. Molecular forms of acetylcholinesterase in brain, nerve and muscle: nature, localization and dynamics. *Prog. Neurobiol.* 21:291–322, 1983.

Brumback R.A., Leech R.W. *Color Atlas of Muscle Histochemistry.* Littleton, MA, PSG Publishing, 1984.

Campion D.R. The muscle satellite cell: a review. *Int. Rev. Cytol.* 87:225–251, 1984.

*Carpenter S., Karpati G. *Pathology of Skeletal Muscle.* New York, Churchill Livingstone, 1984.

Catterall W.A. Molecular properties of voltage-sensitive sodium channels. *Annu. Rev. Biochem.* 55:953–985, 1986.

*Catterall W.A. Structure and function of voltage-sensitive ion channels. *Science* 242:50–61, 1988.

Changeux J.P., Devillers-Thiery A., Chemouilli P. Acetylcholine receptor: an allosteric protein. *Science* 225:1335–1345, 1984.

Cooke R. The mechanism of muscle contraction. *Crit. Rev. Biochem.* 21:53–118, 1986.

David J.D., Faser C.R., Perrot G.P. Role of protein kinase C in chick embryo skeletal myoblast fusion. *Dev. Biol.* 139:89–99, 1990.

Davis R.L., Cheng P.F., Lassar A.B., et al. The MyoD DNA binding domain contains a recognition code for muscle-specific gene activation. *Cell* 60:733–748, 1990.

Dubowitz V. *Muscle Biopsy: A Practical Approach.* 2nd ed. London, Bailliere Tindall, 1985.

Dulhunty A.F., Franzini-Armstrong C. The relative contributions of the folds and caveolae to surface membrane of frog skeletal muscle fibers at different sarcomere lengths. *J. Physiol. (Lond.)* 250:513–539, 1975.

el-Saleh S.C., Warber K.D., Potter J.D. The role of tropomyosin-troponin in the regulation of skeletal muscle contraction. *J. Muscle Res. Cell Motil.* 7:387–404, 1986.

Engel A.G. Myasthenia gravis and myasthenic syndromes. *Ann. Neurol.* 16:519–534, 1984.

*Engel A.G., Banker B.Q., eds. *Myology.* New York, McGraw-Hill, 1986.

Engel J.N., Gunning P.W., Kedes L. Isolation and characterization of human actin genes. *Proc. Natl. Acad. Sci. U.S.A.* 78:4674–4678, 1981.

Fambrough D.M., Engel A.G., Rosenberry T.L. Acetylcholinesterase of human erythrocytes and neuromuscular junctions: homologies revealed by monoclonal antibodies. *Proc. Natl. Acad. Sci. U.S.A.* 79:1078–1082, 1982.

Fidziańska A. Human ontogenesis. I. Ultrastructural characteristics of developing human muscle. *J. Neuropathol. Exp. Neurol.* 39:476–486, 1980.

Fontaine B., Khurana T.S., Hoffman E.P., et al. Hyperkalemic periodic paralysis and the adult muscle sodium channel α-subunit gene. *Science* 250:1000–1002, 1990.

Geisterfer-Lowrance A.A.T., Kass S., Tanigawa G., et al. A molecular basis for familial hypertrophic cardiomyopathy: a β cardiac myosin heavy chain missense mutation. *Cell* 62:999–1006, 1990.

Goldman Y.E., ed. Special topic: molecular mechanism of muscle contraction. *Annu. Rev. Physiol.* 49:629–709, 1987.

Gospe S.M., Lazaro R.P., Lava N.S. et al. Familial X-linked myalgia and cramps: a nonprogressive myopathy associated with a deletion in the dystrophin gene. *Neurology* 39:1277–1280, 1989.

Gower H.J., Moore S.E., Dickson G., et al. Cloning and characterization of a myoblast cell surface antigen defined by 24.1D5 monoclonal antibody. *Development* 105:723–731, 1989.

Grove B.K., Kurer V., Lehner C., et al. A new 185,000-dalton skeletal muscle protein detected by monoclonal antibodies. *J. Cell Biol.* 98:518–524, 1984.

Gunning P., Ponte P., Okayama H., et al. Isolation and characterization of full-length cDNA clones for human α-, β-, and γ-actin mRNAs: skeletal but not cytoplasmic actins have an amino-terminal cysteine that is subsequently removed. *Mol. Cell. Biol.* 3:787–795, 1983.

Haimovich B., Bonilla E., Casadei J., Barchi R. Immunocytochemical localization of the mammalian voltage-dependent sodium channel using polyclonal antibodies against the purified protein. *J. Neurosci.* 4:2259–2268, 1984.

Harris A.J. Embryonic growth and innervation of rat skeletal muscles. I. Neural regulation of muscle fiber numbers. *Philos. Trans. R. Soc. Lond. [Biol.]* 293:258–277, 1981.

Hauschka S.D. Clonal analysis of vertebrate myogenesis. III. Developmental changes in the muscle-colony-forming cells of the human fetal limb. *Dev. Biol.* 37:345–368, 1974.

Hauschka S.D., Rutz R., Linkhart T.A., et al. Skeletal muscle development. In Schotland D.L., ed. *Disorders of the Motor Unit.* New York, Wiley, pp. 903–923, 1982.

Hiatt A., McDonough A.A., Edelman I.S. Assembly of the (Na$^+$ + K$^+$)-adenosine triphosphatase. Post-translational membrane integration of the α subunit. *J. Biol. Chem.* 259:2629–2685, 1984.

Hibberd M.G., Trentham D.R. Relationships between chemical and mechanical events during muscle contraction. *Annu. Rev. Biophys. Biophys. Chem.* 15:119–161, 1986.

Hoffman E.P., Brown R.H., Kunkel L.M. Dystrophin: the protein product of the Duchenne muscular dystrophy locus. *Cell* 51:919–928, 1987.

Hoffman E.P., Fischbeck K.H., Brown R.H., et al. Characterization of dystrophin in muscle-biopsy specimens from patients with Duchenne's or Becker's muscular dystrophy. *N. Engl. J. Med.* 318:1363–1368, 1988.

Holmes K.C., Popp D., Gebhard W., et al. Atomic model of the actin filament. *Nature* 347:44–49, 1990.

Horowits R., Kempner E.S., Bisher M.E., et al. A physiological role for titin and nebulin in skeletal muscle. *Nature* 323:160–164, 1986.

Hunter D.D., Shah V., Merlie J.P., et al. A laminin-like adhesive protein concentrated in the synaptic cleft of the neuromuscular junction. *Nature* 338:229–234, 1989.

Iannaccone S.T., Nagy B., Samaha F.J. Partial biochemical maturation of aneurally cultured human skeletal muscle. *Neurology (N. Y.)* 32:846–851, 1982.

Inesi G. Mechanism of calcium transport. *Annu. Rev. Physiol.* 47:573–601, 1985.

*Ishikawa H. Fine structure of skeletal muscle. In Dowben R.M., Shay J.W., eds. *Cell and Muscle Motility.* Vol. 4. New York, Plenum Publishing, 1983.

Jørgensen P.L. Mechanism of the Na$^+$,K$^+$ pump. Protein structure and conformations of the pure (Na$^+$ + K$^+$)-ATPase. *Biochim. Biophys. Acta* 694:27–68, 1982.

Juntunen J., Teräväinen H. Structural development of myoneural junctions in the human embryo. *Histochemie* 32:107–112, 1972.

Kallen R.G., Sheng Z.H., Yang J., et al. Primary structure and expression of a sodium channel characteristic of denervated and immature rat skeletal muscle. *Neuron* 4:233–242, 1990.

Karn J., McLachlin A.D., Barnett, L. Heavy-chain gene of *Caenorhabditis elegans*: genetics, sequence, structure. In Pearson M.C., Epstein H.F., eds. *Muscle Development: Molecular and Cellular Control.* Cold Spring Harbor, NY, Cold Spring Harbor Laboratory, 1982.

Kaufman S.J., Foster R.F., Haye K.R., et al. Expression of a developmentally regulated antigen on the surface of skeletal and cardiac muscle cells. *J. Cell Biol.* 100:1977–1987, 1985.

Kelly A.M. Emergence of specialization in skeletal muscle. In Peachey L.D., Adrian R.H., Geiger S.R., eds. *Handbook of Physiology.* Section 10. *Skeletal Muscle.* Bethesda, American Physiological Society, pp. 507–537, 1983.

Knudson C.M., Chaudhari N., Sharp A.H., et al. Specific absence of the α$_1$ subunit of the dihydropyridine receptor in mice with muscular dysgenesis. *J. Biol. Chem.* 264:1345–1348, 1989.

Koenig M., Monaco A.P., Kunkel L.M. The complete sequence of dystrophin predicts a rod-shaped cytoskeletal protein. *Cell* 53:219–228, 1988.

Koenig M., Beggs A.H., Moyer M., et al. The molecular basis for

Duchenne versus Becker muscular dystrophy: correlation of severity with type of deletion. *Am. J. Hum. Genet.* 45:498–506, 1989.

Koren G., Liman E.R., Logothetis D.E., et al. Gating mechanism of a cloned potassium channel expressed in frog oocytes and mammalian cells. *Neuron* 2:39–51, 1990.

Kuffler S.W., Nicholls J.G., Martin A.R. *From Neuron to Brain.* 2nd ed. Sunderland, MA, Sinauer Associates, 1984.

Labeit S., Barlow B.P., Gantel M., et al. A regular pattern of two types of 100-residue motif in the sequence of titin. *Nature* 345:273–276, 1990.

Leinwand L.A., Saez L., McNally E., Nadal-Ginard B. Isolation and characterization of human myosin heavy chain genes. *Proc. Natl. Acad. Sci. U.S.A.* 80:3716–3720, 1983.

Lubit B.W., Schwartz J.H. An antiactin antibody that distinguishes between cytoplasmic and skeletal muscle actins. *J. Cell Biol.* 86:891–897, 1980.

MacLennan D.H., Brandl C.J., Korczak B., et al. Amino-acid sequence of a Ca^{2+} + Mg^{2+}-dependent ATPase from rabbit muscle sarcoplasmic reticulum, deduced from its complementary DNA sequence. *Nature* 316:696–700, 1985.

MacLennan D.H., Duff C., Zorzato F., et al. Ryanodine receptor gene is a candidate for predisposition to malignant hyperthermia. *Nature* 343:559–561, 1990.

Magill-Solc C., McMahan U.J. Motor neurons contain agrin-like molecules. *J. Cell Biol.* 107:1825–1833, 1988.

McCarthy T.V., Healy J.M.S., Heffron J.J.A., et al. Localization of the malignant hyperthermia susceptibility locus to human chromosome 19q12-13.2. *Nature* 343:562–564, 1990.

Noda M., Shimizu S., Tanabe T., et al. Primary structure of *Electrophorns electricus* sodium channel deduced from cDNA sequence. *Nature* 312:121–127, 1984.

Noda M., Ikeda T., Suzuki H., et al. Expression of functional sodium channels from cloned cDNA. *Nature* 322:826–828, 1986.

Ohtsuki I., Maruyama K., Ebashi S. Regulatory and cytoskeletal proteins of vertebrate skeletal muscle. *Adv. Protein Chem.* 38:1–67, 1986.

Pardo J.V., Siliciano J.D'A., Craig S.W. A vinculin-containing cortical lattice in skeletal muscle: transverse lattice elements ("costameres") mark sites of attachment between myofibrils and sarcolemma. *Proc. Natl. Acad. Sci. U.S.A.* 80:1008–1012, 1983.

Pepe F.A. Macromolecular assembly of myosin. In Stracher A., ed. *Muscle and Nonmuscle Motility.* Vol. 1. New York, Academic Press, 1983.

Repasky E.A., Granger B.L., Lazarides E. Wide-spread occurrences of avian spectrin in non-erythroid cells. *Cell* 29:821–833, 1982.

Sanes J.R. Laminin, fibronectin, and collagen in synaptic and extrasynaptic portions of muscle fiber basement membrane. *J. Cell Biol.* 93:442–451, 1982.

Schmalbruch H., Hellhammer U. The number of satellite cells in normal human muscle. *Anat. Rec.* 185:279–288, 1976.

Shull G.E., Schwartz A., Lingrel J.B. Amino-acid sequence of the catalytic subunit of the (Na$^+$ + K$^+$) ATPase deduced from a complementary DNA. *Nature* 316:691–695, 1985.

Skau K.A. Mammalian acetylcholinesterase molecular forms. *Comp. Biochem. Physiol.* 83C:225–227, 1986.

Soriano P., Szabo P., Bernardi G. The scattered distribution of actin genes in the mouse and human genomes. *EMBO J.* 1:579–583, 1982.

Sutoh K. Identification of myosin-binding sites on the actin sequence. *Biochemistry* 21:3654–3661, 1982.

Tanabe T., Takeshima H., Mikami A., et al. Primary structure of the receptor for calcium channel blockers from skeletal muscle. *Nature* 328:313–318, 1987.

Tanabe T., Beam K.G., Powell J.A., et al. Restoration of excitation-contraction coupling and slow calcium current in dysgenic muscle by dihydropyridine receptor complementary DNA. *Nature* 336:134–139, 1988.

Tanigawa, G., Jarcho J.A., Kass S., et al. A molecular basis for familial hypertrophic cardiomyopathy: an α/β cardiac myosin heavy chain hybrid gene. *Cell* 62:991–998, 1990.

Thornell L.E., Eriksson A., Edstrom L. Intermediate filaments in human myopathies. In Dowben R.M., Shay J.W., eds. *Cell and Muscle Motility.* Vol. 4. New York, Plenum Publishing, 1983.

Tomlinson S., MacNeil S., Walker S.W., et al. Calmodulin and cell function. *Clin. Sci.* 66:497–508, 1984.

Trimmer J.A., Cooperman S.S., Tomiko S.A., et al. Primary structure and functional expression of a mammalian skeletal muscle sodium channel. *Neuron* 3:33–49, 1989.

Trotter J.A., Eberhard S., Samora A. Structural domains of the muscle-tendon junction. I. The internal lamina and the connecting domain. *Anat. Rec.* 207:573–591, 1983.

Turo K.A., Florini J.R. Hormonal stimulation of myoblast differentiation in the absence of DNA synthesis. *Am. J. Physiol.* 243:C278–C284, 1982.

Venosa R.A., Horowicz P. Density and apparent location of the sodium pump in frog sartorius muscle. *J. Membr. Biol.* 59:225–232, 1981.

Wang K. Membrane skeleton of skeletal muscle. *Nature* 304:485–486, 1983.

*Warrick H.M., Spudich J.A. Myosin structure and function in cell motility. *Annu. Rev. Cell Biol.* 3:379–421, 1987.

Watkins S.C., Hoffman E.P., Slayter H.S., et al. Immunoelectron microscopic localization of dystrophin in myofibers. *Nature* 333:863–866, 1988.

Witkowski J.A., Dubowitz V. Growth of diseased human muscle in combined cultures with normal mouse embryonic spinal cord. *J. Neurol. Sci.* 26:203–220, 1975.

Wright W.E., Sassoon D.A., Lin V.K. Myogenin, a factor regulating myogenesis, has a domain homologous to MyoD. *Cell* 56:607–617, 1989.

Zorzato F., Fujii J., Otsu K., et al. Molecular cloning of cDNA encoding human and rabbit forms of the Ca^{2+} release channel (ryanodine receptor) of skeletal muscle sarcoplasmic reticulum. *J. Biol. Chem.* 265:2244–2256, 1990.

Zot A.S., Potter J.D. Structural aspects of troponin-tropomyosin regulation of skeletal muscle contraction. *Annu. Rev. Biophys. Chem.* 16:535–559, 1987.

Zubrzycka-Gaarn E.E., Bulman D.E., Karpati G., et al. The Duchenne muscular dystrophy gene product is localized in sarcolemma of human skeletal muscle. *Nature* 333:466–469, 1988.

12

Pathophysiology of Metabolic Myopathies

Lewis P. Rowland
Robert B. Layzer
Salvatore DiMauro

INTRODUCTION

The term *metabolic myopathy* is used to designate conditions in which there is a recognized disorder of energy metabolism in skeletal muscle. These conditions include the glycogen storage diseases, lipid storage myopathies, lack of muscle carnitine palmitoyltransferase (CPT), mitochondrial myopathies, and AMP deaminase (adenylic acid deaminase) deficiency (Table 12–1).

The most common symptom in all of these diseases is weakness of limb muscles. In some mitochondrial diseases, ocular muscles are most severely affected and there is progressive limitation of eye movements or progressive external ophthalmoplegia. Other symptoms in these diseases are myalgia, cramps (actually contractures as they occur in disorders of glycolysis), myoglobinuria, and exercise intolerance. Our task is to relate these symptoms to abnormalities of muscle metabolism.

Definitions: Fatigue, Exercise Intolerance, and Weakness

The major symptoms of metabolic myopathies merge with one another: weakness, fatigue, and exercise intolerance (Hainaut and Duchateau, 1989). Each term can be considered separately but the features overlap. Weakness and fatigue, moreover, each have two meanings, one physiologic and the other clinical.

Muscle Fatigue

Edwards (1979, 1984) has defined *weakness* as failure to generate force. *Fatigue*, in contrast, is failure to sustain force or power output in a prolonged or repetitive contraction. However, in a state of fatigue, muscle typically fails to generate normal initial force (Bigland-Ritchie and Woods, 1984), so that weakness and fatigue occur together, even in normal individuals.

Edwards (1984) has tried to dissect the molecular basis of fatigue and weakness, focusing on three fundamental properties of muscle: electromechanical activation, fuel supply, and contractile machinery (Fig. 12–1).

Fatigue in normal muscle has been studied physiologically in mammalian preparations and in humans. In fatigued muscle, abnormalities have been identified at several different anatomic sites: transmission at the neuromuscular junction, excitation of the muscle surface membrane, excitation-contraction coupling, and activation of the contractile elements.

In a normal person, the kind of fatigue that occurs during intense exercise seems to be of metabolic origin, directly related to changes in intracellular concentration of intermediates of energy metabolism. During exercise, the muscle concentration of creatine phosphate (CP) declines and the concentrations of inorganic phosphate (P_i) and hydrogen ions increase. Metabolic fatigue correlates most closely with increased levels of hydrogen ions and diprotonated P_i, as determined by nuclear magnetic resonance (NMR) spectroscopy (Boska et al., 1990; Miller et al., 1987, 1988; Wilson et al., 1988); both of these substances inhibit the interaction of actin with myosin. Recovery

135

Table 12–1. METABOLIC MYOPATHIES

Metabolic Defect	Manifestations
Ammonia metabolism	
AMP deaminase	Myalgia, fatigue (debated)
Glycogen metabolism	
Phosphorylase	Recurrent myoglobinuria; cramps
Phosphorylase kinase	(contracture) almost universal;
Phosphofructokinase	fixed weakness uncommon,
Phosphoglycerate kinase	may occur alone
Phosphoglycerate mutase	
Lactate dehydrogenase	
Brancher, debrancher;	Fixed limb or respiratory
α-glucosidase	weakness; no cramps or
	myoglobinuria
Lipid metabolism	
Carnitine	Recurrent myoglobinuria; no
palmitoyltransferase	weakness
Muscle carnitine deficiency	Fixed limb or respiratory
	weakness; myoglobinuria
	exceptional
Systemic carnitine	Encephalopathy, cardiopathy,
deficiency	limb weakness, myoglobinuria
β oxidation	Encephalopathy, cardiopathy,
	limb weakness, myoglobinuria
Mitochondrial myopathies	
Substrate utilization	Infantile encephalomyopathy;
(pyruvate	lactic acidosis
dehydrogenase)	
Krebs' cycle (fumarase)	Infantile encephalomyopathy
Energy transduction	Euthyroid hypermetabolism
(Luft's disease)	
Respiratory chain: NADH–	Encephalomyopathy MELAS;*
CoQ reductase (complex	Leber's optic atrophy; exercise
I)	intolerance; lactic acidosis
Succinate–CoQ reductase	Weakness, myoglobinuria
(complex II); coenzyme	
Q_{10}	
Reduced CoQ–cytochrome	Encephalomyopathy, exercise
c reductase (complex III)	intolerance, lactic acidosis
Cytochrome c oxidase	Fatal or benign infantile
(complex IV)	myopathy, encephalomyopathy
	(Leigh's)
Multiple complexes	Encephalomyopathy (Kearns-
(mitochondrial DNA	Sayre syndrome) or ocular
deletions)	myopathy with ragged red
	fibers

*MELAS = mitochondrial encephalopathy, lactic acidosis, and stroke.

from metabolic fatigue occurs fairly rapidly, usually within an hour. In contrast, low-intensity exercise produces a nonmetabolic fatigue that lasts for several hours. Intracellular energy metabolites are present in normal concentration, but excitation-contraction coupling is altered, as deduced from observations that the tension of a single muscle twitch is depressed much more than the tension of a maximal voluntary contraction or tetanus (Moussavi et al., 1989). The mechanism of nonmetabolic fatigue is not known.

As long suspected by clinicians, muscle weakened by any neurogenic or myopathic disorder is probably also more susceptible to fatigue than is normal muscle. Even chronic disuse or lack of muscle activity can increase the fatigability of muscle. However, the precise nature of fatigue in neuromuscular disorders

is largely unknown, because the patients have not been studied by techniques that could correlate metabolic and physiologic changes. Nevertheless, Lenman et al. (1989) studied patients with different neurologic diseases, all characterized by signs of upper motor neuron lesions with spastic paraparesis or paraplegia. Maximal tensions were measured after voluntary contraction or contractions induced by repetitive electrical stimulation in trains lasting 3 minutes. The fatigability of the patients' muscles uniformly exceeded that of control subjects' muscles, and some of the features suggested that calcium uptake mechanisms were less effective than in controls. Hainaut and Duchateau (1989) also noted that exercise training helped both strength and endurance, not one or the other alone.

Similarly, in patients with primary myopathies, Milner-Brown and Miller (1988) found reduced values for maximum force and also for what they called a *fatigue index* in patients with different kinds of muscle disease. Measures of both strength and fatigue improved with training exercises. Miller et al. (1990) found that muscles weakened by neurogenic disorders were also more susceptible to fatigue.

Clinically, patients with myopathies of any kind do not complain of fatigue. Symptoms are almost always due to weakness or exercise intolerance. However, there is no disease in which the patient starts out with normal strength and then becomes profoundly weak after exercise. In myasthenia gravis, abnormal fatigability (inability to sustain the height of the evoked end plate potential in a train of stimuli) is actually a defining *physiologic* characteristic of the disease. Even in myasthenia gravis, however, the patients do not complain of inability to sustain activity. Rather, they note specific symptoms that are due to weakness—dysarthria, dysphagia, ptosis, or weak limbs—and that may or may not become worse with repetition.

Physiologically and clinically, therefore, it is not necessary to consider fatigue as a primary symptom. Nor is the fatigability of a perpetually weak muscle a defining characteristic in any disease. In glycogen diseases, however, for several complicated reasons, patients may not be able to sustain activity under circumstances that would not bother a normal person. These reasons will be considered later.

Muscle Weakness

In the terms proposed by Edwards (1984) (see Fig. 12–1), only a few diseases can be assigned a proper explanation. Myasthenia and other disorders can be considered aberrations of neuromuscular transmission. The myotonias, periodic paralysis, and, perhaps, Duchenne's dystrophy can be considered diseases of muscle surface membranes and therefore indicative of disorders of electromechanical activation, but that is not certain.

In almost all myopathies that are characterized by permanent or progressive limb weakness, the disor-

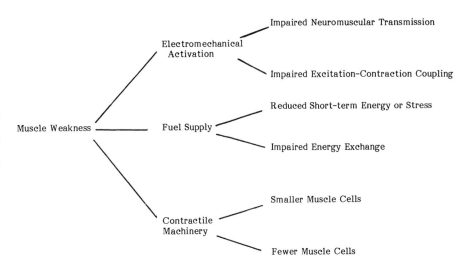

Figure 12–1. The pathophysiology of muscle weakness. (Modified from Edwards R.H.T. Physiological analysis of skeletal muscle weakness and fatigue. *Clin. Sci. Mol. Med.* 54:463–470, 1978.)

der has been ascribed to the last category proposed by Edwards (see Fig. 12–1)—"muscle cells too few." The conventional explanation is based on morphology, even in metabolic myopathies in which there is fixed weakness rather than exercise intolerance. That is, muscle fibers are lost because the rate of degeneration of fibers exceeds the rate of regeneration. With fewer functioning fibers, the muscle cannot exert full force. The results of electromyography reinforce this impression; the "myopathic" pattern includes motor unit potentials that are small in amplitude and shorter in duration than normal because there are fewer fibers in each motor unit.

The same argument—loss of functional fibers—has been advanced to explain the fixed limb weakness of the glycogen storage diseases. However, the conditions characterized by lack of phosphorylase or phosphofructokinase (PFK) provide evidence against the view that physical disruption of muscle fibers is the major cause of weakness. In these diseases, myoglobinuria and myalgia are the common early symptoms and there may be no weakness at all. Yet the muscles are stuffed with glycogen, disrupting the normal architecture; there is also evidence of degeneration and regeneration. Some patients with these diseases do show clinical weakness, but it has not been demonstrated that there is more degeneration of muscle fibers in symptomatically weak patients than there is in patients with only recurrent myoglobinuria (and no limb weakness between attacks).

In metabolic myopathies, it is logical to ascribe symptoms to failure of energy production, and that, in turn, could lead to a failure of electromechanical activation or a disorder of the contractile machinery. In the past decade, many studies with NMR spectroscopy have contributed to this interpretation, as we shall see when we consider individual diseases. Nevertheless, there are some inconsistencies:

1. In some mitochondrial myopathies, the major symptom is fixed limb weakness; in other disorders, there is exercise intolerance without limb weakness (DiMauro et al., 1987; Zeviani et al., 1989).

2. In some mitochondrial myopathies, the histochemical appearance of "ragged red fibers" implies that there is an abnormally increased number, size, or structure of muscle mitochondria. However, particularly in syndromes of progressive external ophthalmoplegia, there may be no weakness in the same limb muscles for which biopsy specimens have shown the ragged red fibers.

3. If one mitochondrial enzyme is missing (CPT), the clinical syndrome is recurrent myoglobinuria. However, if the substrate for the same enzyme system (carnitine) is limited in amount, the reverse is true; there is fixed limb weakness and no myoglobinuria.

4. In some glycogen storage myopathies, there is fixed weakness but no myoglobinuria (as in debrancher deficiency). In others, the reverse is true, and there is myoglobinuria without fixed weakness in conditions caused by any one of the several enzymes involved in glycogen degradation.

5. An attack of myoglobinuria can be regarded as the ultimate energy crisis in muscle, but diseases of electron transport are not ordinarily associated with myoglobinuria. However, myoglobinuria has been associated with two defects of the respiratory chain: coenzyme Q_{10} deficiency (Ogasahara et al., 1989) and complex II deficiency (Haller et al., 1990).

6. There is debate about the relation of AMP deaminase deficiency to clinical symptoms; the enzyme may be missing in asymptomatic people.

Therefore, clinical syndromes of permanent limb weakness are difficult to analyze in molecular terms. Even in metabolic myopathies, fixed weakness may be due to morphologic loss of functional muscle fibers, and the disordered metabolism may be the basis of other symptoms: exercise intolerance, myoglobinuria, and cramps or contracture.

Exercise Intolerance

Inability to sustain normal patterns of work or exercise has emerged as a major symptom of the mitochondrial myopathies, but the term *exercise intolerance* is difficult to define and, therefore, the syndrome is difficult to diagnose. In the broadest terms, a person may find it impossible to carry out normal physical activities. Physicians may analyze the problem and finally ascribe the disorder to either impaired cardiovascular adjustments or impaired muscle metabolism. Sometimes, there is a gross systemic disorder with lactic acidosis and congestive heart failure; sometimes, there is only lactic acidosis. Sometimes, there is only exertional dyspnea. Another factor may be related to brain stem control of respiration because ventilatory drive responses are depressed in some patients (Barohn et al., 1990).

Sometimes, there is no cardiopulmonary problem, only failure of limb functions in patients who show no abnormality when they are examined at rest; there is no weakness in manual muscle testing, and there is no functional abnormality of routine limb functions. However, the patients rapidly fail in attempts to sustain or repeat effort. There may be an aching sense of tiredness in the legs. In glycogen storage diseases this failure to continue work is accompanied by forced flexion of the affected joint and by painful swelling of the shortened muscle (contracture).

One precondition for the occurrence of exercise-induced myoglobinuria is that the patient must be strong enough to perform sufficiently rigorous exercise. This may be the reason why metabolic defects that are severe enough to cause fixed weakness may also "protect" the patient from attacks of myoglobinuria. Examples abound. In glycogen metabolism, deficiency of phosphoglycerate kinase (PGK) causes myoglobinuria only in the milder "muscle" form of the condition, not the severe form in which there is fixed limb weakness. In lipid metabolism, CPT deficiency causes myoglobinuria without weakness, whereas carnitine deficiency is accompanied by weakness but not pigmenturia. Moreover, in conditions caused by defects of the respiratory chain, only the milder ones seem to be accompanied by myoglobinuria; in the others, hypotonia and paresis of the limbs of affected infants are a common (protective?) feature. In the dystrophies, exercise-induced myoglobinuria is not common but seems to be more frequent in patients with the less severe Becker's dystrophy; in the severe form, Duchenne's dystrophy, myoglobinuria has been induced by general anesthesia but exercise-induced attacks have not been recorded. All of these examples indicate that exercise-induced myoglobinuria requires a high level of activity.

Chronic Fatigue Syndrome

The major problem in differential diagnosis of fatigue syndromes is fatigue itself as a symptom. It is worth reiterating that patients with metabolic my-opathies, any other kind of myopathy, or myasthenia gravis—patients with disordered physiology—do not complain of fatigue. When patients do complain of fatigue (in contrast to the specific symptoms of limb or cranial muscle weakness), they usually describe inability to get started in the morning, a sense of overwhelming exhaustion in doing housework or routine tasks, an unrelenting sense of tiredness, a constant need to rest and to lie down, or a need to pace the day's work if there is to be some social or physical activity in the evening. Myalgia and tenderness of the skin or muscles are frequent concomitants of this disorder, usually with no true symptoms of limb weakness or evidence of overt weakness on manual muscle testing and no abnormality of serum enzymes, muscle biopsy, or electromyography. This disorder, in our minds, is usually psychogenic, often a manifestation of depression.

Yet many physicians seem unwilling to consider fatigue a psychogenic disorder, and there has been a parade of chronic fatigue syndromes, with other names as well: chronic infectious mononucleosis, chronic Epstein-Barr viral infection, chronic Lyme disease, epidemic neuromyalgia, or Iceland disease. Although it is conceivable that chronic viral infection or some long-lasting effects of viral infection in muscle might alter the metabolism of skeletal muscle, Yonge (1988) found no NMR spectroscopic evidence of impaired energy metabolism in patients with "postviral" syndromes, and mitochondrial studies have also been unrewarding (Byrne and Trounce, 1987).

Another version of this syndrome is the "fading athlete syndrome" of skilled competitive athletes as they reach age 30 or thereabout. They find that they cannot compete as effectively as they did in youth; rather than admit the inexorable effects of age, they insist that something must be wrong with their muscles. If an athlete suffers a true myopathy, the symptoms affect the activities of daily living, not professional weightlifting or marathon running. Sometimes, a high-school athlete is deemed an Olympic talent by his or her parents (themselves former athletes) or a coach, but the young person simply does not live up to expectations. Rather than recognize human limits or unrealistic goals, the parents or coach attributes the subchampionship performance to a muscle disease. These seem to be psychogenic disorders, but the symptoms merge with the exercise intolerance of mitochondrial disorders.

Relation of Metabolic Abnormality to Clinical Manifestations: Fuels for Exercise

The type of fuel for muscle exercise has been a subject of study in the last 20 years, especially since the introduction of needle biopsies (Edwards et al., 1980) and NMR spectroscopy (Arnold et al., 1988), techniques that permit repeated study of the same muscle. The following conclusions have been discussed in several reviews (Edwards et al., 1980; Felig and Wahren 1975; Havel, 1971, 1972; Karlsson et al., 1981; Poehlman, 1989):

1. At rest, muscle uses predominantly lipid for energy.
2. The immediate source of energy for muscle contraction is ATP, which is rapidly replenished at the expense of CP through phosphorylation of ADP by creatine kinase.
3. In exercise of high-intensity, near-maximal aerobic power, additional ATP is generated through anaerobic glycogen breakdown and glycolysis.
4. During exercise of moderate intensity, the type of fuel used depends on the duration of work. At the beginning of exercise, glycogen is the main source of energy, but after 5 or 10 minutes glucose in blood becomes the more important carbohydrate fuel. As work continues, fatty acid utilization increases and, after about 4 hours, lipid is the principal fuel, although oxidation of branched chain amino acids also contributes substantially in prolonged exercise (Felig and Wahren, 1975).
5. Intense exercise is performed in essentially anaerobic conditions; mild or moderate exercise is accompanied by increased blood flow to exercising muscles, facilitating provision of substrates and favoring aerobic metabolism (Coleman et al., 1986).

These formulations are oversimplified because they do not take into account other important variables that influence fuel utilization, such as training, nutritional status, and muscle fiber type composition. In the following discussion, it will be seen that abnormalities of energy supply can account for exercise intolerance, myalgia, contracture, and myoglobinuria. The cause of weakness remains uncertain.

WEAKNESS AND EXERCISE INTOLERANCE IN SPECIFIC METABOLIC DISORDERS

Disorders of Carbohydrate Metabolism

Nine well-defined hereditary enzyme defects of glycogen metabolism or glycolysis affect muscle (Fig. 12–2; see also Chapter 14) (DiMauro, 1979; Servidei and DiMauro, 1989; Servidei et al., 1988).

Of these, one (branching enzyme deficiency) affects glycogen synthesis and another (acid maltase deficiency) affects a lysosomal enzyme of glycogen degradation. Presumably, neither of these two pathways is directly involved in energy provision during exercise. A third enzyme defect (phosphorylase *b* kinase deficiency) has been documented in muscle in only a few patients, and the clinical picture remains to be defined.

Of the remaining six, two (phosphorylase deficiency and debrancher deficiency) affect glycogen

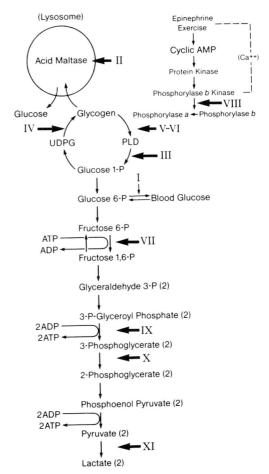

Figure 12–2. Scheme of glycogen metabolism. Roman numerals and arrows indicate sites of enzyme defects that affect muscle. See text for discussion. (From DiMauro S., Bresolin N., Papadimitriou A. Fuels for exercise: clues from disorders of glycogen and lipid metabolism. In Serratrice G., Cros P., Desnuelle C., et al., eds. *Neuromuscular Diseases.* New York, Raven Press, pp. 45–50, 1984.)

breakdown and four (PFK, PGK, phosphoglycerate mutase [PGAM], and lactate dehydrogenase deficiencies) affect glycolysis.

Impaired energy production from carbohydrate is the common consequence of these enzyme defects and should result in similar exercise-related symptoms and signs. Except for debrancher deficiency, this is true. Most patients with phosphorylase, PFK, PGK, PGAM, and lactate dehydrogenase deficiencies are not weak but have exercise intolerance, cramps, and pigmenturia when they engage in strenuous activities, particularly isometric exercise such as lifting heavy weights or wrestling (DiMauro and Bresolin, 1985; DiMauro et al., 1984). Moderate exercise typically causes premature myalgia, but these symptoms are usually overcome by a brief rest or slowing of pace, after which patients find that they can resume or continue exercise without problems. This "second wind" phenomenon has been attributed to both early mobilization of fatty acids and increased blood flow to exercising muscles (Havel, 1972). In patients with phosphorylase deficiency who exercise at a constant workload, second wind can also be induced by administration of glucose or fructose (Lewis et al., 1985; Pernow et al., 1967; Porte et al., 1966), substrates that enter the glycolytic pathway below the metabolic block.

Braakhekke et al. (1986) found evidence of two phases in patients with McArdle's disease. For the first 15 minutes there was an adaptation phase, in which there was progressive fatigue and weakness, followed by rapid and complete recovery. Then the second wind phase commenced. In the first phase, the patients could not use glycogen as fuel, as evidenced by the appearance of excessive amounts of ammonia in venous blood. There was a reduction of 40–75% in the force generation of individual motor units. To compensate, there was an increase in cardiac output, which could have served to increase muscle blood flow and deliver free fatty acids and glucose as alternative fuels. Lewis and Haller (1986) named this adjustment a *hyperkinetic circulatory response*. There was also evidence that metabolic pathways had shifted in the first few moments because there was slight lactate production, which was attributed to the appearance of hexose phosphates in muscle. Also, blood levels of glucose decreased more in patients than in controls, implying greater peripheral utilization.

Braakhekke et al. (1986) found that as exercise continued there was evidence of change in the respiratory exchange ratio, indicating a switch to fatty acids, earlier than in controls. Electromyographic activity increased, presumably a measure of the recruitment of more motor units to compensate for the failure of force generation. During the second wind period itself, there was no difference between patients and controls in circulatory factors or measures of metabolism.

In the four defects of glycolytic enzymes—PFK, PGK, PGAM, and lactate dehydrogenase—blood glucose cannot be used as a source of energy. Even so, symptoms are not more severe than in phosphorylase deficiency, suggesting that impaired glycogen utilization is indeed the fundamental problem in McArdle's disease.

Application of these findings in therapeutic trials has been largely unsuccessful, but glucagon administration (to promote hepatic glycogenolysis and raise blood glucose levels) was effective in improving the exercise tolerance of at least one patient with phosphorylase deficiency (Kono et al., 1984). In another patient, muscle endurance (tested by bicycle ergometry and by performance in recreational activities) improved after both short-term and long-term ingestion of protein (Slonim and Goans, 1985). Increased provision of branched chain amino acids may simply favor a compensatory phenomenon that occurs spontaneously in patients with McArdle's disease; in these patients isoleucine, leucine, and alanine are taken up rather than released by muscle during exercise.

In the glycogen storage diseases, there must be a common final pathway that leads to the similar symptoms. Because energy from anaerobic glycolysis is not available, high-energy phosphate (phosphagen) is depleted by intense exercise and cannot be promptly replenished; this sequence can cause a severe and prolonged energy crisis, presumably with depletion of ATP, but that has never been proved (Argov et al., 1987).

Edwards and colleagues (Edwards et al., 1982a,b; Wiles et al., 1981) have explored the phenomenon of fatigue (failure to maintain sustained force), which occurs more rapidly in patients with myophosphorylase deficiency than in controls after repetitive nerve stimulation under ischemic conditions. The rapid decline of force was accompanied by a concomitant decline in the amplitude of evoked potentials; unlike the pattern in normal subjects, action potentials in patients did not recover as long as ischemia was maintained (Edwards et al., 1982a,b; Wiles et al., 1981). These findings suggested that a metabolic event was responsible for the premature fatigue, but muscle concentration of ATP at fatigue was normal by chemical measurement in needle biopsies (Edwards et al., 1980) or ^{31}P NMR spectroscopy (Ross et al., 1981). Fatigue was attributed to failure of muscle excitation, most likely a failure in maintenance of the electrical properties of the sarcolemma (Edwards et al., 1982a,b; Wiles et al., 1981). Premature failure of muscle excitation might have a protective effect, preventing muscle from going into rigor through depletion of ATP, as discussed later.

The clinical similarities of phosphorylase, PFK, PGAM, and PGK deficiencies suggest the same pathophysiologic basis. It is therefore difficult to explain why symptoms differ in debrancher deficiency. Patients with debrancher deficiency have hepatomegaly and fasting hypoglycemia in childhood, but these problems usually disappear around puberty and most patients lead normal adult lives. In a few patients, a progressive myopathy becomes manifest in the third or fourth decade, with proximal limb weakness and, sometimes, distal wasting but no cramps or myoglobinuria. It is not clear why an enzyme defect that affects the same pathway as phosphorylase deficiency should have such different clinical consequences. Not only is the lack of cramps and myoglobinuria difficult to explain, but also the mechanism of weakness is obscure; why some but not all patients are affected is still another question.

There are other theories about the origin of muscle symptoms in phosphorylase-deficient muscle. R.G. Cooper et al. (1989) found evidence that myofibrillar activation failed more than excitation failed and that there was abnormal slowing of relaxation mechanisms. They attributed these abnormalities to accumulation of metabolites. Although there is little decline in ATP levels (Argov et al., 1987), there is an accumulation in muscle of P_i and ADP (Lewis et al., 1985), metabolites that may inhibit several ATPase activities including myofibrillar, Ca^{2+}-activated, and Na^+,K^+-ATPases (Lewis and Haller, 1986). Moreover, the alterations in adenine phosphates changethe muscle phosphorylation potential, a secondary abnormality of oxidative metabolism.

Therefore, abnormal glycogen metabolism may account for the weakness and exercise intolerance of these diseases, but some questions remain to be resolved.

Disorders of Lipid Metabolism

CPT deficiency causes symptoms and signs that are usually but not always related to exercise. Myalgia, a subjective feeling of muscle stiffness (without observable contractures), and myoglobinuria may follow prolonged exercise that need not be of high intensity. Fasting, alone or with exercise, is another important precipitating factor (DiMauro and Papadimitriou, 1985). In a normal person, after a few hours of uninterrupted exercise of moderate intensity, fatty acids provide the main source of energy for muscle. Fasting increases the dependence of normal muscle on fatty acid oxidation by reducing the concentration of muscle glycogen and the availability of blood glucose. The circumstances in which myalgia and myoglobinuria occur in CPT deficiency correspond to those in which oxidation of fatty acids prevails in normal muscle. This confirms the conclusions drawn from studies of normal individuals and suggests that impairment of energy production is the common cause of exercise intolerance and myoglobinuria in different metabolic myopathies (see Table 12–1).

The excessive dependence of CPT-deficient patients on carbohydrate metabolism is manifested by higher than normal respiratory quotients at rest and during exercise and also by abnormal release of creatine kinase after either prolonged exercise or prolonged fasting (DiMauro and Papadimitriou, 1985). This critical need for carbohydrate fuel was also shown in one patient by unusually severe intolerance for exercise after his muscle glycogen had been depleted by combined exercise and ketogenic diet (Layzer et al., 1980). These experimental conditions could be used in other patients to determine the concentrations of ATP and CP in muscle at the time of exhaustion, either by needle biopsies and chemical analysis or by NMR. Exercise after fasting or ketogenic diet should be approached cautiously, however, because of the risk of massive myoglobinuria. The lack of cramps in patients with CPT deficiency is puzzling if the common final pathway to myoglobinuria involves a critical drop of ATP concentration. The main difference between CPT deficiency and the glycogenoses with myoglobinuria is that type 1 rather than type 2 fibers are affected by the metabolic block of CPT deficiency. Selective decrease of ATP concentration in type 1 fibers could cause necrosis (and myoglobinuria) without contracture, but that remains to be demonstrated.

Mitochondrial Myopathies

Exercise intolerance, without cramps or pigmenturia, has been prominent in some patients with blocks of the respiratory chain affecting complex I or complex III (DiMauro et al., 1985, 1987; Lombes et al., 1989; Morgan-Hughes, 1982; Petty et al., 1986; Zeviani et al., 1989). Most were normal in infancy and early childhood, but around age 10 they had to rest after walking increasingly shorter distances and even mild exercise caused shortness of breath, myalgia, dyspnea, and sometimes vomiting. In a few patients, weakness at rest was specifically excluded at first but became apparent later. All patients had lactic acidosis at rest and an abnormal increase of venous lactic acid concentration with exercise.

In one patient with complex III deficiency, ^{31}P NMR studies at age 17 showed a markedly reduced ratio of CP to P_i concentration at rest (approximately 1.5 compared with normal values of about 10) (Eleff et al., 1984). It is not clear why severe block of complex III should cause relatively mild symptoms for many years, in contrast to the severe generalized weakness of patients with complex IV (cytochrome c oxidase) deficiency, which is usually fatal in infancy. The block of the respiratory chain in patients with complex I deficiency is incomplete, affecting oxidation of NAD-dependent but not of flavoprotein-dependent substrates, and this may explain the milder symptoms. A related question is why these patients do not have myoglobinuria; lactic acidosis is exacerbated by physical activity and may be a protecting factor by causing general malaise that keeps the patient from exercising excessively.

In experimental animals, Byrne and Morgan-Hughes (1989) found that administration of dinitrophenol, an uncoupler of oxidative metabolism in mitochondria, led to progressive failure of contractility, followed by failure of the muscle action potential and then an electrically silent contracture. This sequence was accelerated by external work but the same changes occurred at rest, unlike the situation in human mitochondrial diseases. Another mitochondrial poison is diphenylene iodonium, which inhibits site I. Administration of this compound also led to failure of twitch tension and action potential, but contracture occurred less consistently than with dinitrophenol (J.M. Cooper et al., 1988). If the preparation was allowed to rest, there was recovery of twitch responses; then restimulation led to a state of pathologic fatigability similar to that seen in human patients. Heller et al. (1988) have used dinitrophenol to reproduce the effects of exercise in stress studies of human muscle biopsy specimens.

It has been difficult to assess the lactic acidosis of patients with mitochondrial diseases, although this systemic disorder presumably plays a role in limiting capacity for exercise and could also be important in distinguishing between metabolic and psychogenic exercise intolerance. However, as pointed out by Nashel and Lane (1989), analysis of the studies has been impeded because "exercise regimens have ranged from minutes to several hours in duration, and from 'light work' to 'exercise to exhaustion' and have not been standardized with regard to age, weight and sex of subjects."

Nashel and Lane (1989) therefore devised a physiologic exercise test, based on the calculation of an "anaerobic threshold" in terms of oxygen consumption measured during exercise and measured ventilatory variables and blood lactate levels. They found abnormal results in six patients with mitochondrial myopathies (four with ragged red fibers, one with normal biopsy, and one with nonspecific histologic changes) and a false-positive rate of 7% in normal controls.

Argov et al. (1987) used NMR spectroscopy to study 12 adults with different mitochondrial myopathies. All had abnormalities at rest, and 11 had abnormal patterns of recovery from exercise. During exercise there were abnormalities in the five patients who could exercise adequately, and exercise-induced acidosis was less than normal in nine patients. They discerned two major groups: those with primary abnormalities of energy metabolism and those with what seemed to be less specific secondary NMR abnormalities.

The increasing attention to mitochondrial myopathies may lead to better understanding of exercise intolerance and weakness.

AMP Deaminase Deficiency

Exercise intolerance, with cramps or myalgia, is the most common complaint of patients with AMP deaminase deficiency. Increased serum creatine kinase activity at rest or after exercise has been found in some patients, but pigmenturia has been reported only in rare and exceptional patients with apparently isolated AMP deaminase deficiency (Hyser et al., 1989; Tonin et al., 1990). The paucity of attacks of myoglobinuria and the asymptomatic state of many (if not most) people with this enzymatic disorder have raised doubt about the clinical significance of the biochemical anomaly (Rowland, 1984a,b). Sinkeler et al. (1988) studied a family in which there was clear evidence of autosomal recessive inheritance. However, only two of the eight individuals with the biochemical abnormality had myalgic symptoms; the other six affected members of the family were asymptomatic.

Nevertheless, there is evidence that the enzymatic deficit causes metabolic abnormality. In formal exercise tests, four patients with AMP deaminase deficiency produced less work than normal controls or patients with myalgia but without AMP deaminase deficiency (Sabina et al., 1984). The decrease of total phosphagen (creatine phosphate + ATP) level for a unit of work was greater in patients than in asymptomatic or symptomatic controls. The disruption of the purine nucleotide cycle caused by AMP deami-

nase deficiency could impair energy production and limit exercise tolerance by at least three different mechanisms:

1. Loss of the anaplerotic role of fumarate in the Krebs cycle.
2. Reduction of the adenylate energy charge with accumulation of AMP, ADP, and adenosine during muscle contractions.
3. Loss of the buffering role of NH_3 (normally generated in the AMP deaminase reaction) for the hydrogen ions produced during ATP hydrolysis and inhibition of myosin ATPase.

OTHER SYMPTOMS

Pain, Cramps, and Contracture

Muscle pain and cramps are characteristic of some metabolic myopathies (Layzer, 1984, 1985a,b; Rowland, 1985). In McArdle's disease and other disorders of the energy-yielding glycolytic pathway, pain and cramps tend to occur early during moderate or intense exercise; residual muscle soreness may persist for several days. In CPT deficiency, muscle pain tends to occur after prolonged exercise but also occurs at rest, especially when carbohydrate intake is restricted. In AMP deaminase deficiency, muscle pain does not have a consistent pattern but may occur mainly during intense exercise. True muscle cramps are not a feature of either CPT or AMP deaminase deficiency, and neither pain nor cramps are typical of acid maltase deficiency, carnitine deficiency, or disorders of the mitochondrial electron transport system.

Although the physiology of muscle pain is incompletely understood, it seems likely that several mechanisms are involved (Edwards, 1986; Mense and Schmidt, 1977; Mills et al., 1982). The pain of muscle cramps is caused mainly by excitation of pain nerves that are sensitive to mechanical stimulation. But the exertional pain experienced by patients with metabolic muscle disease may also be related to the pain that occurs in patients with intermittent claudication, which is not associated with muscle spasm. In normal persons, continuous exercise eventually engenders a deep, aching muscle pain that increases rapidly, forcing them to stop exercising. With rest, the pain subsides in a few seconds. When the same exercise is conducted after circulation has been occluded by a tourniquet, pain develops much more quickly and does not go away until the circulation is restored. The rapidity of onset of this ischemic or metabolic pain is roughly proportional to the intensity of the exercise (Mills et al., 1982; Rodbard, 1975).

Several authors have hypothesized that some pain-producing chemical substance diffuses out of muscle cells into the interstitial fluid during contraction, but the putative metabolite has never been identified. Originally, lactic acid was proposed for this role, but then it was discovered that patients with McArdle's disease have severe exertional pain, yet do not generate lactate or hydrogen ions. Of course, the mechanical effects of a severe contracture could account for pain in McArdle's disease. A more convincing objection to the lactate-induced pain theory is the lack of severe exertional pain in patients with mitochondrial myopathies who generate excessive amounts of lactic acid. Although ammonium ions are normally produced during intense or ischemic exercise, they probably do not mediate ischemic pain, because patients with AMP deaminase deficiency do not generate ammonia in muscle. Other unsupported candidates for the pain substance include potassium ions, creatine, and the adenine nucleotides.

A third type of pain is that associated with muscle damage. This pain is most noticeable a day or two after the injury and is accompanied by muscle swelling and tenderness, features that suggest an inflammatory basis for the pain (Armstrong, 1984). Experiments with animals have shown that muscle pain afferents are excited by chemical mediators of inflammation such as bradykinin, prostaglandins, serotonin, and histamine, chemicals that accumulate slowly in injured tissues (Mense and Schmidt, 1977). Inflammatory pain is probably responsible for the delayed and long-lasting muscle soreness that occurs after exercise in patients with McArdle's disease and AMP deaminase deficiency and either during rest or after exercise in patients with CPT deficiency.

The cramps of McArdle's disease and related disorders differ from ordinary muscle cramps in several ways. Unlike those of McArdle's disease, ordinary cramps tend to occur at rest, during sleep, or after trivial effort; often start and end with muscle twitching; have an explosive onset; may wax and wane for several minutes; and can usually be terminated by passive stretching of the affected muscle (Layzer, 1985a). In contrast, the cramps of McArdle's disease occur only during exercise, and the severity of the cramping is related to the intensity of the exercise. Furthermore, electromyographic recordings of the muscle spasm show profuse electrical discharges in an ordinary cramp (Denny-Brown, 1953) and electrical silence in the McArdle cramp (Brandt et al., 1977). Ordinary cramps are attributed to spontaneous discharges of motor nerves; the painful shortening of muscle in McArdle's disease is a physiologic *contracture* or rigor.

Contracture has several possible mechanisms. The inappropriate shortening may be triggered by an elevated intracellular concentration of free calcium ions, either because the calcium stored in the sarcoplasmic reticulum is released without preceding electrical stimulation or because calcium released by electrical stimulation fails to be reaccumulated by the sarcoplasmic reticulum. Another possibility is an abnormal interaction between actin and myosin in the presence of normal calcium concentrations. Which of these occurs in McArdle's disease has not been determined. However, in an experimental analogue of McArdle's disease, frog muscle poisoned by 1-fluoro-2,4-dinitrobenzene (FDNB), which inhib-

its the enzyme creatine kinase, showed a sudden increase of calcium efflux at the same time that contracture developed, presumably reflecting an increase of intracellular calcium concentration (Nauss and Davies, 1966).

What is the biochemical basis of the contracture in McArdle's disease and related glycolytic disorders? In vivo ^{31}P NMR spectroscopy of muscle in patients with McArdle's disease (Ross et al., 1981) and PFK deficiency (Argov et al., 1987) showed, as expected, that ordinary exercise causes CP levels to fall and P_i levels to rise much more rapidly than normal. However, cramping occurred before the CP stores were exhausted, at a time when ATP levels were unchanged (Ross et al., 1981). Biopsy studies had given similar results (Edwards et al., 1980; Rowland et al., 1965). These findings seem to imply that a low ATP concentration in whole muscle is not the cause of the contracture.

Experiments with animal models have given contradictory results. In frog muscle, rigor develops after treatment with either FDNB (Murphy, 1966), which prevents the conversion of ADP to ATP, or iodoacetic acid (Sahlin et al., 1981), which interrupts glycolysis by inhibiting the enzyme glyceraldehyde-3-phosphate dehydrogenase. After repeated stimulation of muscle, both ATP concentration and muscle tension gradually decline; rigor appears when both tension and ATP concentration have fallen to about half of the original values. But studies of rats poisoned with iodoacetic acid (Ruff and Weissman, 1989) showed that ATP concentrations in muscle did not decline until after the onset of contracture, which seemed to correlate best with elevated levels of ADP (determined by calculation). Preliminary studies indicated that elevated levels of ADP may promote contracture by increasing the interaction of actin with myosin. Also, intracellular acidosis normally protects against contracture by inhibiting actin-myosin interaction, but in McArdle's disease acidosis does not occur. This may explain why contracture occurs in the glycolytic disorders of muscle and not in the other disorders of muscle energy metabolism.

Recurrent Myoglobinuria

Grossly visible myoglobinuria implies destruction of at least 200 g of muscle. In an individual case, the cause may be only one of more than 50 different known disorders, or there may be combinations of etiologies (Rowland, 1984a,b; Tonin et al., 1990). These diverse causes, however, can be grouped under a few headings: direct muscle damage (by muscle exertion, crush, or ischemia); metabolic depression (after drug overdose or severe distortion of salt and water homeostasis, especially hypokalemia); exposure to drugs or toxins, especially those that affect muscle surface membranes; and extremes of body temperature (hypothermia or hyperthermia). The metabolic myopathies are probably analogous to the agents that cause metabolic depression or ischemia.

The logic used to explain myoglobinuria is similar to that used to explain contracture. That is, the integrity of muscle surface membranes undoubtedly requires adequate supplies of ATP. During ischemic work or prolonged isotonic contraction (in which there is relative ischemia of the vigorously contracted muscle), normal individuals use stored glycogen to replenish the ATP and CP that have been consumed for the contraction. Individuals who lack phosphorylase, PFK, PGK, or PGAM, however, cannot call on glycogen, and ATP levels may fall below some critical level, leading to contracture first and then disrupting the muscle surface membrane.

The theory is logical, and no alternative theory has been forthcoming in 20 years. However, as explained earlier, it has not been possible to demonstrate the presumed fall in ATP levels. Alternative theories have been too difficult to test, but there could be a fall in a local intracellular compartment (such as sarcoplasmic reticulum) or in some but not all muscle fibers; focal changes of either kind would not be evident in measurements of ATP content of the whole muscle.

If this explanation is correct, defective energy metabolism in the mitochondrial myopathies might also lead to clinical myoglobinuria, but that has not yet been seen. Another conundrum has to be explained.

OVERALL VIEW

Metabolic myopathies are rare diseases. They have been intensively studied for two reasons: the tissues are available for investigation, and the studies provide important information about normal muscle as well as the diseases under scrutiny. Ingenious electrophysiologic methods have been developed to study normal and abnormal muscle contraction in humans, separating the effects of neuromuscular transmission, membrane activation, excitation-contraction coupling, and activation of myofibrils. Underlying all of this complex physiology is energy metabolism, which has been studied by direct biochemical analysis of muscle biopsy specimens or by isolating mitochondria for functional assessment (two separate technologies) and, in the past decade, by magnetic resonance spectroscopy. Nevertheless, there are still unanswered questions and therapy of these diseases remains largely unsatisfactory. There is still work to be done.

References

(Key references are designated with an asterisk.)

Argov Z., Bank W.J., Maris J., et al. Muscle energy metabolism in McArdle's syndrome by in vivo phosphorus magnetic resonance spectroscopy. *Neurology* 37:1720–1724, 1987.

Armstrong R.B. Mechanisms of exercise-induced delayed onset muscular soreness: a brief review. *Med. Sci. Sports Exerc.* 16:529–538, 1984.

Arnold D.L., Taylor D.J., Radda G.K. Investigation of human mitochondrial myopathies by phosphorus magnetic resonance spectroscopy. *Ann. Neurol.* 18:189–196, 1988.

Barohn R.J., Clanton T., Sahenk Z., et al. Recurrent respiratory insufficiency and depressed ventilatory drive complicating mitochondrial myopathies. *Neurology* 40:103–106, 1990.

Bigland-Ritchie B., Woods J.J. Changes in muscle contractile properties and neural control during human muscle fatigue. *Muscle Nerve* 7:691–699, 1984.

Boska M.D., Moussavi R.S., Carson P.J., et al. The metabolic basis of recovery after fatiguing exercise of human muscle. *Neurology* 40:240–244, 1990.

Braakhekke J.P., DeBuin M.I., Stegeman D.F., et al. The second wind phenomenon in McArdle's disease. *Brain* 109:1087–1101, 1986.

Brandt N.J., Buchthal F., Ebbesen F., et al. Post-tetanic mechanical tension and evoked action potentials in McArdle's disease. *J. Neurol. Neurosurg. Psychiatry* 40:920–925, 1977.

Byrne E., Morgan-Hughes J.A. Prolonged aerobic exercise; physiological studies in rat gastrocnemius with additional observations on the effects of acute mitochondrial blockade. *J. Neurol. Sci.* 92:215–227, 1989.

Byrne E., Trounce I. Chronic fatigue and myalgia syndrome; mitochondrial and glycolytic studies in skeletal muscle. *J. Neurol. Neurosurg. Psychiatry* 50:743–746, 1987.

Coleman R.A., Stajich J.M., Pact V.W., et al. The ischaemic exercise test in normal adults and in patients with weakness and cramps. *Muscle Nerve* 9:216–221, 1986.

Cooper J.M., Petty R.K.H., Hayes D.J., et al. An animal model of mitochondrial myopathy: a biochemical and physiological investigation of rats treated in vivo with NADH-CoQ reductase inhibitor, diphenyleneiodonium. *J. Neurol. Sci.* 83:335–347, 1988.

Cooper R.G., Stokes M.J., Edwards R.H.T. Myofibrillar activation failure in McArdle's disease. *J. Neurol. Sci.* 93:1–10, 1989.

Denny-Brown D. Clinical problems in neuromuscular physiology. *Am. J. Med.* 15:368–390, 1953.

DiMauro S. Metabolic myopathies. *Handb. Clin. Neurol.* 41:175–234, 1979.

DiMauro S., Bresolin N. Phosphorylase deficiency. In Engel A.G., Banker B.Q., eds. *Myology.* New York, McGraw-Hill, pp. 1585–1601, 1985.

DiMauro S., Eastwood A.B. Disorders of glycogen and lipid metabolism. *Adv. Neurol.* 17:123–142, 1977.

DiMauro S., Papadimitriou A. Carnitine palmitoyltransferase (CPT) deficiency. In Engel A.G., Banker B.Q., eds. *Myology.* New York, McGraw-Hill, pp. 1697–1708, 1985.

*DiMauro S., Bresolin N., Hays A.P. Disorders of glycogen metabolism of muscle. *CRC Crit. Rev. Clin. Neurobiol.* 1:83–116, 1984.

*DiMauro S., Bonilla E., Zeviani M., et al. Mitochondrial myopathies. *Ann. Neurol.* 17:521–538, 1985.

DiMauro S., Bonilla E., Zeviani M., et al. Mitochondrial myopathies. *J. Inherited Metab. Dis.* 10(Suppl. 1):113–128, 1987.

Edwards R.H.T. Physiological and metabolic studies of the contractile machinery of human muscle in health and disease. *Phys. Med. Biol.* 24:237–249, 1979.

*Edwards R.H.T. New techniques for studying human muscle function, metabolism, and fatigue. *Muscle Nerve* 7:599–609, 1984.

Edwards R.H.T. Muscle fatigue and pain. *Acta Med. Scand.* [Suppl.] 711:179–188, 1986.

Edwards R.H.T., Wiles C.M. Energy exchange in human skeletal muscle during isometric contraction. *Circ. Res.* 48(Suppl. 1):11–17, 1981.

Edwards R.H.T., Young A., Wiles M. Needle biopsy of skeletal muscle in the diagnosis of myopathy and the clinical study of muscle function and repair. *N. Engl. J. Med.* 302:261–271, 1980.

Edwards R.H.T., Dawson M.J., Wilkie D.R., et al. Clinical use of NMR in the investigation of myopathy. *Lancet* 1:725–731, 1982a.

Edwards R.H.T., Wiles C.M., Gohil K., et al. Energy metabolism in human myopathy. In Schotland D.L., ed. *Disorders of the Motor Unit.* New York, Raven Press, pp. 715–728, 1982b.

Eleff S., Kennaway N.G., Buist N.R.M., et al. ^{31}P-NMR study of improvement in oxidative phosphorylation by vitamins K3 and

C in a patient with a defect in electron transport at complex III in skeletal muscle. *Proc. Natl. Acad. Sci. U.S.A.* 81:3529–3533, 1984.

Felig P., Wahren J. Fuel homeostasis in exercise. *N. Engl. J. Med.* 293:1078–1084, 1975.

Hainaut K., Duchateau J. Muscle fatigue, effects of training and disuse. *Muscle Nerve* 12:660–669, 1989.

Haller R.G., Henriksson K.G., Jorfeldt L., et al. Muscle succinate dehydrogenase deficiency: exercise pathophysiology of a novel mitochondrial myopathy. *Neurology* 40(Suppl. 1):413, 1990.

Havel R.J. Influence of intensity and duration of exercise on supply and use of fuels. *Adv. Exp. Med. Biol.* 11:315–325, 1971.

Havel R.J. Caloric homeostasis and disorders of fuel transport. *N. Engl. J. Med.* 287:1186–1192, 1972.

Heller S.L., Brooke M.H., Kaiser K.K., et al. 2,4-Dinitrophenol, muscle biopsy, and McArdle's disease. *Neurology* 38:15–19, 1988.

Hyser C.L., Clarke P.R.H., DiMauro S., et al. Myoadenylate deaminase deficiency and exertional myoglobinuria. *Neurology* 39(Suppl. 1):335, 1989.

Karlsson J., Sjodin B., Jacobs I., et al. Relevance of muscle fiber type of fatigue in short intense and prolonged exercise in man. In *Ciba Found. Symp.* 82:59–74, 1981.

Kono N., Mineo I., Sim Sumi S., et al. Metabolic basis of improved exercise tolerance: muscle phosphorylase deficiency after glucagon administration. *Neurology* 34:1471–1476, 1984.

*Layzer R.B. *Neuromuscular Manifestations of Systemic Disease*. Philadelphia, Davis, 1984.

*Layzer R.B. Muscle pain, cramps and fatigue. In Engel A.G., Banker B.Q., eds. *Myology*. New York, McGraw-Hill, 1985a.

Layzer R.B. McArdle's disease in the 80's. *N. Engl. J. Med.* 312:370–371, 1985b.

Layzer R.B., Havel R.J., McIlroy M.B. Partial deficiency of carnitine palmityltransferase. *Neurology* 30:627–633, 1980.

Lenman A.J.R., Tulley F.M., Vrbova G., et al. Muscle fatigue in some neurological disorders. *Muscle Nerve* 12:938–942, 1989.

Lewis S.F., Haller R.G. The pathophysiology of McArdle's disease; clues to regulation of exercise and fatigue. *J. Appl. Physiol.* 61:391–401, 1986.

Lewis S.F., Haller R.G., Cook J.D., et al. Muscle fatigue in McArdle's disease studied by ^{31}P-NMR; effect of glucose infusion. *J. Appl. Physiol.* 59:1991–1994, 1985.

Lombes A., Bonilla E., DiMauro S. Mitochondrial encephalomyopathies. *Rev. Neurol. (Paris)* 145:671–689, 1989.

Mense S., Schmidt R.F. Muscle pain: which receptors are responsible for the transmission of noxious stimuli? In Rose F.C., ed. *Physiological Aspects of Clinical Neurology*. Oxford, Blackwell Scientific Publications, pp. 265–278, 1977.

Miller R.G., Gianinni D., Layzer R.B., et al. Effects of fatiguing exercise on high-energy phosphates, force and EMG; evidence for 3 phases of recovery. *Muscle Nerve* 10:810–821, 1987.

Miller R.G., Boska M.D., Moussavi R.S., et al. ^{31}P nuclear magnetic resonance studies of high energy phosphates and pH in human muscle fatigue. Comparison of anaerobic and aerobic exercise. *J. Clin. Invest.* 81:1190–1196, 1988.

Miller R.G., Green A.T., Moussavi R.S. Excessive muscular fatigue in patients with spastic paraparesis. *Neurology* 40:1271–1274, 1990.

Mills K.R., Newham D.J., Edwards R.H.T. Force, contraction frequency and energy metabolism as determinants of ischemic muscle pain. *Pain* 14:149–154, 1982.

Milner-Brown H.S., Miller R.G. Muscle strengthening through high-resistance weight training in patients with neuromuscular disorders. *Arch. Phys. Med. Rehabil.* 69:14–19, 1988.

*Morgan-Hughes J.A. Defects of the energy pathways of skeletal muscle. *Adv. Clin. Neurol.* 3:1–46, 1982.

Moussavi R.S., Carson P.J., Boska M.D., et al. Nonmetabolic fatigue in exercising human muscle. *Neurology* 39:1222–1226, 1989.

Murphy R.A. Correlations of ATP content with mechanical properties of metabolically inhibited muscle. *Am. J. Physiol.* 211:1082–1088, 1966.

Nashel L., Lane R.J.M. Screening for mitochondrial cytopathies: the subanaerobic threshold exercise test (SATET). *J. Neurol. Neurosurg. Psychiatry* 52:1090–1094, 1989.

Nauss K.M., Davies R.E. Changes in phosphate compounds during the development and maintenance of rigor mortis. *J. Biol. Chem.* 24:2818–2922, 1966.

Ogasahara S., Engel A.G., Frens D., et al. Muscle coenzyme Q deficiency in familial mitochondrial encephalomyopathy. *Proc. Natl. Acad. Sci. U.S.A.* 86:2379–2382, 1989.

Pernow B.B., Havel R.J., Jennings D.B. The second wind phenomenon in McArdle's syndrome. *Acta Med. Scand. [Suppl.]* 472:294–307, 1967.

Petty R.K.H., Harding A.E., Morgan-Hughes J.A. The clinical features of mitochondrial myopathy. *Brain* 109:915–938, 1986.

Poehlman E.T. A review: exercise and its influence on resting energy metabolism in man. *Med. Sci. Sports Exerc.* 21:515–525, 1989.

Porte D., Crawford D.W., Jennings D.B., et al. Cardiovascular and metabolic response to exercise in a patient with McArdle's syndrome. *N. Engl. J. Med.* 275:406–412, 1966.

Rodbard S. Pain in contracting muscle. In Crue B.L. Jr., ed. *Pain: Research and Treatment*. New York, Academic Press, pp. 183–196, 1975.

Ross B.D., Radda G.K., Gadian D.G., et al. Examination of a case of suspected McArdle's syndrome by ^{31}P nuclear magnetic resonance. *N. Engl. J. Med.* 304:1338–1342, 1981.

Rowland L.P. Myoglobinuria. *Can. J. Neurol. Sci.* 11:1–13, 1984a.

Rowland L.P. The membrane theory of Duchenne dystrophy: where is it? *Ital. J. Neurol. Sci.* 5(Suppl. 3):13–28, 1984b.

*Rowland L.P. Muscle cramps, spasms and stiffness. *Rev. Neurol. (Paris)* 4:261–273, 1985.

Rowland L.P., Araki S., Carmel P. Contracture in McArdle's disease. *Arch. Neurol.* 13:541–544, 1965.

Ruff R.L., Weissman J. Possible role of ADP in contracture of muscle with impaired myoglycolysis (abstract). *Neurology* 39(Suppl. 1):360, 1989.

Sabina R.L., Swain J.L., Olanow C.W., et al. Myoadenylate deaminase deficiency. Functional and metabolic abnormalities associated with disruption of the purine nucleotide cycle. *J. Clin. Invest.* 73:720–730, 1984.

Sahlin K., Eldstrom L., Sjoholm H., et al. Effects of lactic acid accumulation and ATP decrease on muscle tension and relaxation. *Am. J. Physiol.* 240:C121–C126, 1981.

Servidei S., DiMauro S. Disorders of glycogen metabolism of muscle. *Neurol. Clin.* 7:159–178, 1989.

Servidei S., Shanske S., Zeviani M., et al. McArdle's disease: biochemical and molecular genetic studies. *Ann. Neurol.* 24:774–781, 1988.

Sinkeler S.P.T., Joosten E.M.G., Wevers R.A., et al. Myoadenylate deaminase deficiency: a clinical, genetic, and biochemical study in nine families. *Muscle Nerve* 11:312–317, 1988.

Slonim A.E., Goans P.J. Myopathy in McArdle's syndrome. Improvement with high-protein diet. *N. Engl. J. Med.* 312:355–359, 1985.

Tonin P., Lewis P., Servidei S., et al. Metabolic causes of myoglobinuria. *Ann. Neurol.* 27:181–185, 1990.

Wiles C.M., Jones D.A., Edwards R.H.T. Fatigue in human metabolic myopathy. *Ciba Found. Symp.* 82:1–18, 1981.

Wilson J.R., McCully K.K., Mancini D.M., et al. Relationship of muscular fatigue to pH and diprotonated P_i in humans: a ^{31}P-NMR study. *J. Appl. Physiol.* 64:2333–2339, 1988.

Yonge R.P. Magnetic resonance muscle studies: implications for psychiatry. *J. R. Soc. Med.* 81:322–326, 1988.

Zeviani M., Bonilla E., De Vivo D.C., et al. Mitochondrial diseases. *Neurol. Clin.* 7:123–156, 1989.

13

Pathophysiology of Myotonia and Periodic Paralysis

Robert L. Barchi
Roy E. Furman

Since the work of Adrian and colleagues in the early 1970s (Adrian et al., 1970), neurobiologists have recognized that the spreading wave of excitation in muscle that follows the appearance of a signal at the neuromuscular junction is produced by a carefully choreographed sequence of membrane conductance changes to sodium and potassium ions. During the past 10 years, researchers have made remarkable progress in understanding the processes that control this excitation in skeletal muscle and its ultimate coupling to contraction. Progress has been especially dramatic in the area of membrane ion channels and the events that underlie the generation of an action potential. As with many such advances in the basic sciences, the impact of this information is rapidly being seen in clinical neurobiology.

Membrane channels controlling the movement of sodium ions, potassium ions, calcium ions, and chloride ions have been examined at the level of a single channel using patch-clamp and planar bilayer technology. Work with muscle acetylcholine receptors and with sodium and calcium channels has progressed to include the complete sequencing of their mRNAs, the unraveling of their primary amino acid sequences, and the generation of reasonable models of their three-dimensional structure (for reviews, see Barchi, 1988; Barrantes, 1988; Hosey and Lazdunski, 1988). The relationship among gating events observed at the level of single channels, the membrane currents associated with synaptic events, and the structure of the membrane proteins is the focus of active research.

From this rapidly growing base of information, a clearer picture of the pathophysiology of muscle disorders that are characterized by abnormalities of membrane excitability is beginning to emerge. In some cases, these disorders can be discussed in terms of specific membrane defects and channel abnormalities, and these defects can be related with reasonable certainty to the clinical expression of the disease.

This chapter reviews two groups of diseases that are associated with abnormalities of membrane excitability. The myotonic syndromes are characterized by an abnormal increase in membrane excitability, with persistent runs of action potentials appearing in the surface membrane. The periodic paralyses, on the other hand, are characterized by episodic failure of membrane excitability that leads to functional paralysis of the muscle. In both disease types, significant progress has been made toward defining some of the factors involved in their pathogenesis at the molecular level. This progress, as well as its integration into a more general pathophysiologic construct, is the primary subject of this chapter.

THE MYOTONIC SYNDROMES

The myotonic syndromes are easily identified among the disorders of the neuromuscular system by their characteristic mechanical and electrical features. Clinically, myotonia is seen as the delayed relaxation of skeletal muscle after a voluntary contraction or contraction induced by electrical or mechanical stimuli. Myotonia is a hallmark of a number of diseases that vary widely in their inheritance, pathologic features, and prognosis; these diseases include myotonia congenita, myotonic dystrophy, paramyotonia congenita, chondrodystrophic myotonia, and forms of hyperkalemic periodic paralysis. Myotonia indistinguishable from that found in these naturally occurring disorders is also seen as a reaction

Table 13–1. DISEASES AND DRUGS ASSOCIATED WITH MYOTONIA

Genetic Diseases

Human
  Dominant myotonia congenita
  Recessive generalized myotonia
  Myotonic dystrophy
  Paramyotonia congenita
  Hyperkalemic periodic paralysis
  Chondrodystrophic myotonia

Goat
  Congenital myotonia

Dog
  Congenital myotonia
  Cushingoid myotonia

Horse
  Congenital myotonia

Drugs and Chemicals

Aromatic carboxylic acids
  2,4-Dichlorophenoxyacetic acid
  Anthracene-9-carboxylic acid
  Diuretics
Inhibitors of sterol synthesis
  20,25-Diazacholesterol
  Hypocholesterolemic drugs—clofibrate (Atromid-S), triparanol
Halides
  Iodine
Steroids in dogs

Other

Hypochloremia
Propranolol (unmasked latent MyMD*)
Vincristine (unmasked latent MyMD)
Sulfhydryl-inhibiting *para*-substituted mercuribenzoates

*MyMD = myotonic muscular dystrophy.

to several classes of drugs and chemicals and can be reproduced in laboratory animals (Table 13–1).

The clinical features of myotonia are remarkably constant, despite the widely varying presentations of the diseases in which it occurs. Patients typically have painless muscular stiffness on initiation of movement that slowly resolves during 5–15 seconds. The first efforts to use a muscle after a period of rest are the most severely affected by the delayed relaxation. Repeated use of the muscle generally leads to increased mobility, but another rest period often permits muscular stiffness to return. Minimal muscular contractions are often not impaired, whereas forceful contractions can cause the muscles to lock briefly in a contracted state. Other factors that can

aggravate myotonia include muscle cooling, fasting, menstruation, potassium ingestion, and sudden emotional arousal. Any muscle of the body can be affected, including those of the trunk and the face, and the degree of involvement can vary widely in different muscle groups.

When patients with myotonia are examined by concentric needle electromyography, they exhibit a common picture of increased insertional activity and prolonged, repetitive discharges of motor unit potentials that wax and wane in frequency and amplitude (Fig. 13–1). These discharges may persist for many seconds after needle movement, muscle percussion, or voluntary contraction. This spontaneous repetitive electrical activity correlates with the mechanical delay

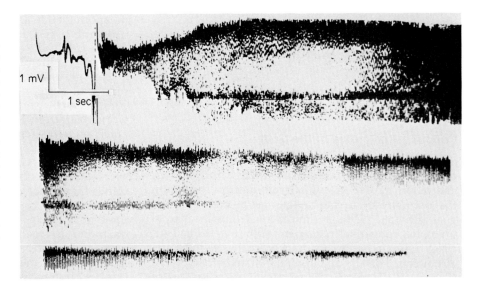

Figure 13–1. An electromyographic recording from the tibialis anterior muscle illustrating the waxing-and-waning repetitive electrical discharges found in the myotonic syndromes. Although typical of the recordings made in human diseases, this particular example is from the 20,25-diazacholesterol model of myotonia in the rat. A similar syndrome was first discovered in humans undergoing hypocholesterolemic therapy with 20,25-diazacholesterol (Winer et al., 1965). (From Furman R.E., Barchi, R.L. 20,25-Diazacholesterol myotonia: an electrophysiological study. Reprinted with permission from *Annals of Neurology,* volume 10, pages 251–260, 1981.)

1 mV

1 sec

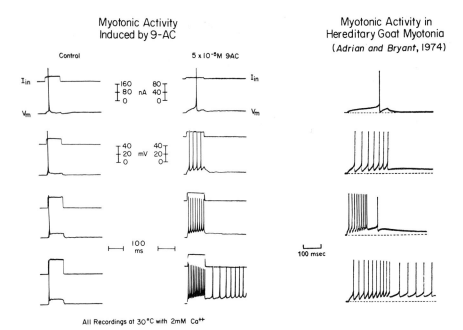

Figure 13–2. The similarities between the naturally occurring myotonia congenita in the goat *(right)* and the myotonic syndrome produced in normal rat muscle by a specific inhibitor of sarcolemmal chloride conductance, anthracene-9-carboxylic acid (9-AC) *(left)*. In the myotonic syndromes, threshold depolarizing currents produce action potentials with long latencies, whereas in controls, action potentials begin shortly after the onset of the stimulus. Successively increasing the depolarizing current in myotonic muscle generates multiple action potentials during the stimulus until the afterdepolarization after the stimulus reaches threshold and initiates the spontaneous, repetitive myotonic discharge. I_{in} = stimulus current delivered via an intracellular microelectrode; V_m = intracellularly recorded membrane potential. Records were obtained from the diaphragm in the rat (Furman and Barchi, 1978) and the external intercostal muscle in the goat (Adrian and Bryant, 1974).

in muscular relaxation and is thought to account for the abnormality of contraction. The waxing-and-waning frequency of these discharges produces the crescendo-decrescendo sound patterns on an audio monitor that led to the term *dive bomber potentials*, which is common in the older literature.

The remarkable similarity of the clinical and electrical appearance of myotonia in a variety of disorders initially led investigators to seek a common underlying pathogenetic mechanism that would explain this phenomenon at the membrane level in all diseases. However, research during the past 20 years has shown that this is not the case. Although members of one major group of myotonic disorders do share a common mechanism, myotonia appears to be a common expression for a number of otherwise unrelated defects that affect the behavior of membrane ion channels (for review, see Rudel and Lehmann-Horn, 1985). In the following discussion, the various myotonic disorders are reviewed briefly and some of the common themes relating to the appearance of repetitive electrical discharges are considered.

Myotonia Caused by Abnormal Chloride Conductance

Congenital Myotonia of the Goat

Much of the knowledge of the pathophysiology of myotonia is based on the detailed electrophysiologic and biophysical studies by Bryant and colleagues on the naturally occurring congenital myotonia of the goat (Bryant, 1979), a clinical syndrome similar to myotonia congenita in humans (White and Plaskett, 1904). Early experiments quickly established the sarcolemma as the site of pathologic change in myotonia (Brown and Harvey, 1939). Later in vitro studies of

single muscle fibers from external intercostal biopsies of myotonic goats displayed the typical features of abnormal excitability (Adrian and Bryant, 1974). These myotonic bursts persisted in spite of motor nerve section or neuromuscular blockade.

When intercostal muscle fibers from myotonic goats were impaled with microelectrodes and depolarized with long constant currents just above threshold, a repetitive series of driven action potentials were seen, followed by a long, depolarizing afterpotential that continued after the stimulus was terminated (Adrian and Bryant, 1974) (Fig. 13–2). The amplitude of this depolarizing afterpotential was proportional to the number of preceding driven action potentials. If the afterpotential became large enough, long trains of self-sustaining, spontaneous action potentials were triggered. Normal goat fibers, on the other hand, showed only a few driven action potentials, much smaller after-depolarizations, and no spontaneous activity.

Bryant (1962) first proposed that these myotonic discharges in the goat could be explained by a lowered muscle membrane permeability to chloride, but it was not until 1971 that the presence of a marked reduction in chloride conductance (88%) was actually confirmed (Bryant and Morales-Aguilera). Further work characterizing the permeability and conductance sequences of the chloride channel in normal and myotonic goat fibers (Bryant and Owenburg, 1980) led to the conclusion that the myotonic membrane had a reduced density of chloride channels rather than a normal number of channels with modified conductance properties. Voltage clamp of myotonic goat fibers (Valle and Bryant, 1980) also demonstrated a small but significant increase in the potassium conductance of the delayed rectifier and an increased time constant for potassium inactivation. Although the marked reduction in chloride conductance is the primary abnormality in goat myotonia, these other membrane defects raise the possibility of a more widespread process.

The delayed relaxation of myotonic muscle fibers is believed to be the consequence of repetitive membrane firing, which in turn triggers normal contractile activation. Unfortunately, there have been few direct measurements of excitation-contraction coupling in myotonic goats. In one study, changes in voltage-dependent contractile activation (Bryant, 1979) were interpreted as indicating enhanced calcium reuptake by the sarcoplasmic reticulum, and other findings (Swift et al., 1979) on purified sarcoplasmic reticulum fragments also suggested an excitation-contraction abnormality. A thorough study of sarcoplasmic reticulum function in chemically skinned single fibers from myotonic goat (Wood et al., 1980), however, found that contractures in response to caffeine and other release and reuptake variables were normal.

Human Recessive Myotonia Congenita

Myotonia congenita in humans is an inherited disorder that occurs in autosomal dominant and autosomal recessive forms. Although similar in appearance, the two forms are pathophysiologically distinct. The dominant form (Thomsen's disease) is not associated with abnormal chloride conductance and will be discussed further later. Recessive generalized myotonia (RGM) is characterized by a marked reduction in membrane chloride conductance and seems in many ways the human counterpart of goat myotonia.

In RGM, myotonia appears later in the first or second decade of life. Myotonia is prominent and generalized; it usually represents the major clinical symptom. There is a 3:1 male predominance. Although patients with RGM have particularly well-developed musculature, mild myopathic features often develop progressively with age, along with a curious thinning of the forearm musculature. Other organ systems are not involved.

The experimental data on human myotonia congenita are not extensive, but studies of the recessive form (RGM) are consistent with the concept of a primary defect in muscle membrane chloride conductance. Electrophysiologic measurements were made on external intercostal muscle biopsy specimens from six patients with myotonia congenita (Lipicky et al., 1971). These myotonic fibers had a greatly increased resting membrane resistance and a lowered internal resistivity compared with controls, whereas other membrane characteristics were unchanged. The principal defect was attributed to decreased chloride conductance on the basis of the increased specific membrane resistance and the clinical similarity of the disease to congenital myotonia of the goat. Subsequently, a specific reduction in sarcolemmal chloride conductance of greater than 90% was confirmed in four intercostal muscle biopsy specimens using cable analysis techniques (Lipicky

and Bryant, 1973). Studies using intracellular recording with isolated resealed muscle fiber segments from patients with RGM also support the concept of a reduced membrane chloride conductance, although the degree of reduction varied considerably among the seven patients studied (Franke et al., 1991).

Although the major channel defect identified in the recessive form of myotonia congenita involves the chloride channel, there is some evidence of minor changes in the properties of other channels as well. Measurements of sodium currents in myoballs prepared from muscle biopsies (Rudel et al., 1989) revealed small changes in the time constants for sodium channel activation and inactivation in patients with the recessive form of myotonia congenita. The remainder of the sodium channel properties were normal. A subsequent study using patch-clamp techniques with isolated, resealed muscle fiber segments from patients with RGM revealed abnormal single-channel behavior for the sodium channel, with frequent reopenings of the channel during prolonged depolarization that are not observed in controls (Franke et al., 1991). It is possible that the abnormal repetitive membrane electrical activity seen in RGM is due to a combination of a reduced chloride conductance and abnormal sodium channel kinetics. Alternatively, the sodium channel changes could be the result of secondary effects on, or modification of, the channel protein produced by a primary defect in chloride conductance. The specific molecular defect producing RGM remains to be defined.

Myotonia in Periodic Paralysis

Myotonia is also seen in several of the inherited forms of periodic paralysis. It is a prominent feature of paramyotonia congenita, in which generalized myotonia can appear with cold exposure, or localized myotonia can occur with focal cooling of a limb. Myotonia is also seen as an associated feature in hyperkalemic periodic paralysis. In the latter disorder, the genetic defect has been linked to a defect in the gene encoding the skeletal muscle tetrodotoxin-sensitive sodium channel on chromosome 17 (Fontaine et al., 1990), confirming electrophysiologic studies pointing to abnormalities in sodium channel function. These disorders are discussed in more detail in the section on the periodic paralyses.

Myotonia Induced by Aromatic Carboxylic Acids

Carboxylic acids have long been known to induce myotonia (Pohl, 1917). The plant herbicide 2,4-dichlorophenoxyacetic acid produces a myotonic syndrome in humans after accidental ingestion (Bucher, 1946). This toxic myotonia was subsequently studied in rats (Eyzaguirre et al., 1948); twitch, tetanic, and percussion myotonia was found after the injection of 2,4-dichlorophenoxyacetic acid. A group of 33 hydrocarbon- and halogen-substituted benzoic acids produced myotonic symptoms after intraperitoneal injection in mice, rats, dogs, cats, chickens, rabbits, and rhesus monkeys (Tang et al., 1968).

In a comparative study of normal and myotonic goats, Bryant and Morales-Aguilera (1971) concluded that these carboxylic acids produced myotonia by specific block of chloride conductance pathways. Further support for this idea came from a study of 25 monocarboxylic aromatic acids (Palade and Barchi, 1977b). Nineteen of the tested compounds reduced membrane chloride conductance in vitro in a dose-dependent manner. The inhibitory constant for chloride channel block correlated directly with the drugs' physicochemical properties.

These compounds partition into the membrane lipid phase and bind at a single class of intramembranous sites. Conductance and permeability sequence measurements suggested that the compounds altered channel selectivity rather than sterically blocking the channel pore (Palade and Barchi, 1977b). Most of these compounds had no effect on potassium conductance. Subsequently, nine of the compounds were tested for their ability to induce myotonia in isolated rat muscle (Furman and Barchi, 1978). The concentration of each compound that produced myotonia closely correlated with the concentration that blocked chloride conductance, and intracellular recordings demonstrated the same changes observed by Adrian and Bryant (1974) in myotonic goat fibers (see Fig. 13–2).

Theoretic Models of Myotonia

Early computer models of space-clamped muscle fibers (Barchi, 1975; Bretag, 1973) confirmed that myotonic discharges could result from reducing membrane chloride conductance. These model discharges were also sensitive to a number of other membrane variables. For example, increasing the potassium equilibrium potential or slightly reducing the sodium conductance led to suppression of myotonic activity, even in the presence of an extremely low chloride conductance. In a more elaborate computer model that included propagated action potentials, a T tubule system, and luminal potassium accumulation, Adrian and Marshall (1976) found that small variations in the rate constants for sodium activation and inactivation also strongly modulated this myotonic activity.

These observations were experimentally verified in aromatic carboxylic acid–induced myotonia by altering temperature and external cations or by using drugs in ways known to effect changes in sodium or potassium channel kinetics under conditions of controlled reduction in chloride conductance (Furman and Barchi, 1978). In both theoretic and experimental models, chloride conductance must be reduced to between 10 and 20% of normal before myotonic activity appears under otherwise normal circumstances.

Physiologic Basis of Myotonia with Reduced Chloride Conductance

The repetitive electrical discharges seen in each of the myotonic disorders discussed earlier can be explained on the basis of the marked reduction in membrane chloride conductance that they share. At the resting potential, muscle membranes are three to five times more permeable to chloride ions than to potassium ions, whereas sodium permeability accounts for less than 1% of the total membrane permeability (Palade and Barchi, 1977a). In response to a depolarizing stimulus, the sodium and potassium ion permeabilities undergo time- and voltage-dependent changes that result in the generation of an action potential (Fig. 13–3). The upstroke of the action potential is produced by a rapid increase in membrane sodium permeability (activation) that causes the membrane potential to shift in a positive direction toward the sodium equilibrium potential. This increase in sodium conductance is transient, however, and its inactivation quickly restores membrane permeability for sodium to its resting value. Concurrently, but with a slower time course, potassium permeability increases. These two processes repolarize the membrane and are responsible for the slower downstroke of the action potential. Chloride permeability remains high and constant during the action potential, and chloride ion fluxes passively follow cation movements.

During normal muscle activity, action potentials are propagated both longitudinally along the surface sarcolemma and radially into the fiber interior along elements of the T tubule system. With each action potential, small quantities of potassium ions move out of the cell, while small amounts of sodium and chloride ions move inward. The potassium ions released into the large volume of the extracellular space have little impact, but the same amounts released into the restricted space of the T tubule system can raise the luminal potassium ion concentration significantly. Calculations show that a single action potential can increase luminal potassium concentration by 0.3 mM; this change can depolarize the T tubule membrane by as much as 1.7 mV (Adrian and Bryant, 1974). Normally, this depolarization is not reflected in the surface membrane potential because of the large stabilizing chloride conductance present in the sarcolemma. In the absence of this chloride shunt, however, the potassium accumulation in the T tubule lumen produced by a series of action potentials can locally depolarize the surface membrane sufficiently to initiate self-sustaining action potentials. The observed increase in the afterpotential of 1 mV/impulse seen in myotonic fibers is compatible with this mechanism. A study (Almers, 1972) showing that potassium diffuses from the T tubule with a time constant of 0.4 second compares favorably with the afterpotential decay time of 0.5 second observed in intact muscle fibers (Adrian and Bryant, 1974).

The behavior of myotonic fibers can be reproduced in normal skeletal muscle fibers by blocking chloride

Membrane Ion Channels and The Action Potential

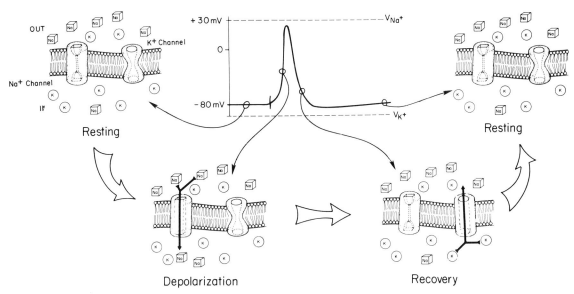

Figure 13-3. The time- and voltage-dependent changes of the sodium and potassium channels in the membrane during the generation of an action potential. The resting potential is determined by the equilibrium potential of the predominant resting permeability to potassium ions. A time- and voltage-dependent increase in the sodium permeability leads to a rapid influx of sodium ions and the rapid, depolarizing upstroke of the action potential. Repolarization and recovery to the resting potential are governed by the increase in potassium permeability and the decrease in sodium permeability. During the short duration of the action potential, chloride permeability remains constant and helps return the membrane potential to the resting state. The dotted, horizontal lines represent the potential the membrane would assume if it were permeable to either sodium (+55 mV) or potassium (-70 mV) alone.

conductance through substitution of an impermeant anion for chloride (Bretag, 1971; Bryant and Morales-Aguilera, 1971; Rudel and Senges, 1972) or by specific channel-blocking compounds (Furman and Barchi, 1978). Disconnecting the T tubule system from the surface membrane by glycerol shock, however, abolishes the long-lasting, depolarizing afterpotential and sustained spontaneous activity, confirming the role of the T tubule system in their generation (Adrian and Bryant, 1974). Figure 13-4 summarizes several

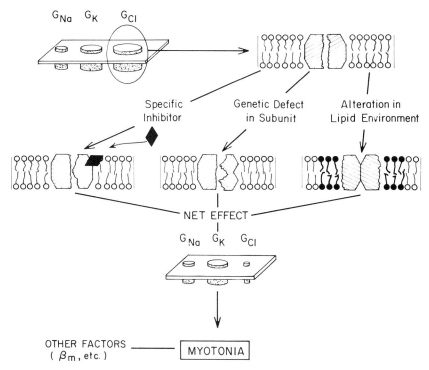

Figure 13-4. A reduction in the intrinsic chloride conductance (G_{Cl}) by any of several mechanisms produces a myotonic syndrome. Hypochloremia or specific drug blockers of the channel have been used to produce animal models of myotonia. Hereditary defects reducing the numbers or functionality of chloride channels have been hypothesized for myotonia congenita. Reduction of chloride conductance produced by abnormal lipid-protein interactions has also been suggested. Extrinsic factors such as temperature, extracellular ionic concentrations, or changes in sodium kinetics can modulate the extent and severity of myotonia produced by low sarcolemmal chloride conductance. (From Barchi R.L. Muscle membrane chloride conductance and the myotonic syndromes. *Electroencephalogr. Clin. Neurophysiol. [Suppl.]* 34:559–570, 1978.)

mechanisms that might lead to the reduced chloride conductance observed in these myotonic diseases.

Although a reduction in sarcolemmal chloride conductance may be the principal factor underlying repetitive firing in these disorders, small changes in the kinetics of sodium channel activation or inactivation can markedly influence the prominence of myotonic activity in the presence of a low but constant chloride conductance (Adrian and Marshall, 1976; Furman and Barchi, 1978). Several investigators reported small but potentially significant changes in sodium channel kinetics in goat myotonia and in recessively inherited generalized myotonia in humans (Rudel et al., 1989). The cause of these changes remains to be defined.

The dive bomber discharges of myotonia heard during audio monitoring of the electromyographic signal show signs of adaptation: the firing frequency may increase and then decrease with time, while the amplitude decreases. The actual mechanisms responsible for the termination of the repetitive activity are not known, but several hypotheses used to explain slow adaptation in neural membranes may apply (Jack et al., 1975). For example, slow, temporal changes in the maximal conductance or gating kinetics of potassium and/or sodium channels could decrease the frequency and the amplitude of repetitive firing. Alternatively, repetitive activity can stimulate electrogenic ion pumps, such as the Na^+,K^+-ATPase, to generate hyperpolarizing currents, which also decrease membrane excitability. The inward shift of potassium ions can block myotonia by increasing the potassium equilibrium potential.

More work remains to be done to clarify the mechanisms underlying percussion myotonia, the warm-up phenomenon, the putative hyperosmolarity of myotonic goat muscle (Lipicky and Bryant, 1966), the abolition of myotonia by water deprivation, and the negative Q_{10} of chloride conductance (Lipicky and Bryant, 1972), as well as mechanisms underlying the control of chloride conductance in the membrane.

Myotonia Not Caused by Low Chloride Conductance

Human Myotonic Dystrophy

Although first described by Steinert in 1909, myotonic muscular dystrophy (MyMD) was cited in the literature even before that time. MyMD is a multisystem disease affecting a variety of tissues in addition to skeletal muscle. The disease is inherited in an autosomal dominant pattern with variable expressivity, with a higher prevalence (between 2.4 and 4.9 cases per 100,000 persons) than that of myotonia congenita. Although symptoms can occur in infancy, patients usually first experience myotonia and weakness of the distal musculature in the early adult years. The course is marked by steady progression of weakness affecting facial, oropharyngeal, truncal,

and limb musculature. Death usually occurs in the fifth or sixth decade from cardiac arrhythmia, respiratory failure, or intercurrent infection. Associated abnormalities include early frontal baldness, subcapsular cataracts, hyperostosis cranii, small sella turcica, enlarged paranasal sinuses, high-arched palate, mental deficiency, cardiac conduction defects, elevation of one or both hemidiaphragms, smooth muscle dysfunction, testicular atrophy, low basal metabolic rate, and reduced serum immunoglobulin G level. Electromyography shows the classic high-frequency discharges, as well as myopathic changes resulting from the dystrophic process affecting skeletal muscle. Extensive clinical, biochemical, and morphologic studies have documented a spectrum of defects related to cell membrane function (for review, see Roses et al., 1979), but the fundamental pathophysiology of this disorder is still unknown.

The primary electrophysiologic defect producing abnormal electrical activity in MyMD is not known, but numerous abnormalities have been reported. In vivo resting potentials are normal or reduced. Intracellular sodium concentration is increased (Hofmann and DeNardo, 1968; Lipicky, 1977), but membrane resistance is either normal or only minimally reduced (Lipicky, 1977). Chloride conductance is slightly lower than normal and is certainly not reduced sufficiently to be the cause of the myotonic activity. Dystrophic fibers have an enhanced mechanical sensitivity to microelectrode impalement (Lipicky, 1977). Wood et al. (1980) found a large reduction in the caffeine concentration required to release calcium from the sarcoplasmic reticulum in chemically skinned fibers but no change in contractile protein function.

One study using primary muscle tissue cultures of human MyMD muscle suggested that the myotubules have a decreased membrane potential, increased hyperexcitability, and decreased after-hyperpolarizations (Merickel et al., 1981). Voltage-clamp studies showed slower activation of outward current, but the steady-state current was only slightly decreased. These intriguing observations could not be duplicated in a subsequent study in another laboratory, however (Tahmoush et al., 1983). More recent biophysical measurements with patch-clamp recording in myoballs derived from MyMD muscle biopsy specimens indicated small increases in the time constants for sodium channel activation and inactivation but no alteration in the voltage dependence of these key channel properties (Rudel et al., 1989).

Abnormalities in chemical and physical properties of MyMD erythrocyte membranes have been reported, including increased Na^+,K^+-ATPase activity (Mishra et al., 1980), decreased membrane-bound protein kinase level, altered stoichiometry of the sodium pump, and increased stomatocyte formation (Appel and Roses, 1977).

The multisystem nature of MyMD and the multiple membrane defects reported in this disorder led researchers to postulate an abnormality of the lipid membrane as the basic pathogenetic element in this disease. Early reports using physical probes of membrane structure suggested a generalized increase in membrane fluidity (Butterfield et al., 1976), but subsequent reports using both electron spin resonance probes (Gaffney et al., 1980) and fluorescence polarization techniques (Chalikian and Barchi, 1980b) failed to confirm this finding. The fundamental defect in this disorder remains to be defined.

Dominant Myotonia Congenita

Dominantly inherited myotonia congenita (DMC) is best exemplified by a single extended kinship that can be traced to a mutation affecting the family of Dr. Asmus Thomsen (Leyden, 1874; Thomsen, 1876). The natural history and clinical presentation of the disease have been studied extensively by Becker (1977). DMC affects both sexes with a low prevalence (between 0.3 and 0.6 cases per 100,000 persons). The onset of myotonia is usually noted in early childhood, sometimes being recognized by astute family members at birth. In DMC, the myotonic symptoms are typically generalized but not progressive. Myotonia in DMC is usually not aggravated by cold exposure and improves with repeated use of a muscle, giving rise to the clinically described warm-up phenomenon.

Although early reports suggested that DMC was characterized by markedly reduced sarcolemmal G_{Cl} (Lipicky et al., 1971), it now appears that this conclusion may reflect insufficient distinction between the dominant and recessive forms of congenital myotonia. In more recent studies on isolated resealed muscle fibers from eight patients with DMC, seven of eight had normal G_{Cl} and the eighth showed only a modest reduction in this membrane conductance (Iaizzo et al., 1991). However, patch-clamp studies showed that sodium channels in all eight patients exhibited persistent abnormal reopenings during depolarization, a finding seen only rarely in normal muscle. An abnormality of sodium channel kinetics may produce the hyperexcitability characteristic of this disorder.

Myotonia Induced by 20,25-Diazacholesterol

The most interesting experimental myotonia, from the viewpoint of generalized lipid membrane defects, is that produced by the drug azacosterol (20,25-diazacholesterol [20,25-D]). 20,25-D is an inhibitor of the enzyme Δ^{24}-reductase, which converts desmosterol to cholesterol in vivo. Winer et al. (1965) reported that hypercholesterolemic patients receiving 20,25-D developed a myotonic syndrome, which subsided several weeks after the drug administration was discontinued. Plasma, erythrocytes, and whole muscle in these patients showed an increase in desmosterol levels. The apparent correlation of the severity of the myotonic syndrome with the amount of desmosterol present triggered renewed interest in

the possibility that disorders of membrane lipid metabolism could be responsible for the abnormalities seen in some of the human myotonic disorders.

Rats treated with 20,25-D exhibit numerous biochemical abnormalities in their cell surface membranes reminiscent of those found in MyMD. These defects include increased erythrocyte Na^+,K^+-ATPase (Chalikian and Barchi, 1980a; Peter et al., 1973), increased ouabain binding (Seiler et al., 1974), decreased Ca^{2+}-ATPase activity, and increased membrane fluidity (Butterfield and Watson, 1977; Chalikian and Barchi, 1980b). Thus, 20,25-D–induced myotonia is a potentially important model for the study of lipid-protein interactions leading to altered membrane function, even though not all the findings are seen in human diseases.

Electrophysiologic studies of 20,25-D–induced myotonia have demonstrated that low membrane chloride conductance is not the primary abnormality in this disorder (Furman and Barchi, 1981). Membrane chloride conductance decreases transiently shortly after initiation of 20,25-D treatment but rises again with continued exposure at a time when myotonia is still prominent (D'Alonzo and McArdle, 1982). In some studies, the electromyographic evidence of myotonia and the delayed relaxation appeared to be independent phenomena (Furman and Barchi, 1981). Moreover, intracellular recordings do not show spontaneous activity unless electrode penetration of the membrane produces a current leak. Studies with skinned muscle fibers and measurements of sarcoplasmic reticulum regulation of calcium failed to demonstrate any abnormality in the intracellular handling of this divalent cation (Furman et al., 1982). The pathogenesis of the membrane hyperexcitability in this disorder has not been discovered, but alterations in the kinetics of sodium or potassium channels are the most likely abnormalities.

Other Mechanisms for Myotonia

No single explanation exists for mechanisms of repetitive electrical activity in the myotonic disorders that are not associated with low chloride conductance. Oscillatory electrical activity is not unusual in nerve and muscle, and other mechanisms that would produce myotonia can easily be imagined. Experimental evidence of such mechanisms, however, is scant. Repetitive action potentials could arise from changes in sodium or potassium channel kinetics. More rapid activation of sodium permeability would decrease the electrical threshold for firing and promote hyperexcitability. Failure of a small fraction of abnormal sodium channels to inactivate could produce a net inward current of sufficient magnitude to drive repetitive action potentials while still being too small to induce inactivation of normal channels and consequent muscular paralysis. An increased rate of recovery from sodium inactivation would reprime the sodium channel more quickly for initiation of the next action potential. Faster recovery of potassium permeability to the resting value would permit more rapid firing and hyperexcitability. These factors alone, or in combination with reduced chloride conductance, could under appropriate physiologic conditions generate repetitive firing.

Other Myotonic Syndromes

Myotonia also occurs naturally in mice, dogs, horses, chickens, and probably other species. Sufficient electrophysiologic data do not yet exist to classify these syndromes. The myotonia in the rare disease chondrodystrophic myotonia, which is characterized by progressive myopathy, dwarfism, bone disease, and abnormal facies, may reside at the neuromuscular junction (Fowler et al., 1974). The myotonia in some forms of hyperkalemic periodic paralysis and paramyotonia congenita is discussed later.

THE PERIODIC PARALYSES

The periodic paralyses are primary disorders of skeletal muscle characterized by transient attacks of muscle weakness, which are often associated with alterations of serum potassium concentration. Other organ systems, including cardiac and smooth muscle, are not affected in these disorders. In most cases, these rare syndromes are familial with autosomal dominant inheritance, but there are clinically indistinguishable sporadic cases. Striking alterations in serum potassium concentration often correlate with the onset of paralysis and have led to classification of the periodic paralyses into hypokalemic and hyperkalemic forms. The clinical features of the most common forms are presented in Table 13–2. Additionally, there are acquired forms associated with chronic potassium depletion or thyrotoxicosis, which resemble hypokalemic periodic paralysis.

Periodic Paralyses Associated with Reduced Serum Potassium Levels

Hypokalemic Periodic Paralysis

The distinguishing clinical features of hypokalemic periodic paralysis include episodes of weakness or flaccid paralysis with electrically unexcitable skeletal muscles, sensitivity to carbohydrates and insulin, absence of electromyographic signs of myotonia, and marked hypokalemia during an attack. Between attacks of paralysis, the resting membrane potential in skeletal muscle fibers is reduced, but the contractile apparatus responds normally to directly applied calcium (Engel and Lambert, 1969) (Fig. 13–5). During the onset of a paralytic episode, muscle strength declines in direct proportion to the loss of muscle electrical excitability. During paralysis, muscle fibers cannot be excited by a depolarizing pulse but remain capable of generating action potentials after a hyperpolarizing conditioning pulse.

Shifts in electrolytes occur during the attack, recovery, and interictal phases of hypokalemic paralysis. Attacks are attended by movement of potassium from the small extracellular pool into skeletal muscle, reducing the serum potassium level to as low as 1.5 mEq/L. Spontaneous or induced recovery is accompanied by a prompt shift of the excessive intracellular potassium back into the serum. Between attacks, total-body potassium stores and serum potassium concentration are slightly reduced; intracellular potassium concentration is lower, and sodium concentration slightly higher, than normal. In vitro muscle fibers show a paradoxical depolarization with either insulin administration or decrease of the external potassium concentration.

Voltage-clamp studies (Rudel et al., 1984) of external intercostal muscles from three patients with familial hypokalemic periodic paralysis provided the best documentation of the membrane defects in this disease. Membrane potentials in normal external potassium ion concentration at 37°C were found to be slightly depolarized compared with those in controls. Marked depolarization occurred either with lowering external potassium ion concentrations to 1 mM or with cooling to 27°C. Increasing extracellular potassium ion concentrations or rewarming caused only slight repolarization, but membrane potentials could be restored by brief perfusion with low-chloride solutions before returning to normal potassium ion concentrations.

All diseased fibers showed reduced membrane excitability, even when hyperpolarized. During induced depolarization, fibers were unexcitable with

Table 13–2. CLINICAL FEATURES OF THE PERIODIC PARALYSES

Parameter	Hypokalemic Periodic Paralysis	Hyperkalemic Periodic Paralysis	Paramyotonia Congenita
Age at onset	First or second decade	>10 y	Infancy
Ictal serum K^+	1.5–3	5.0–8.0	Normal
Attack severity	+ + +	+ (often only mild weakness)	+ +
Attack duration	Often prolonged (1–12 h)	Frequently brief (<1 h)	Variable
Predisposing factors	Carbohydrate load	Low carbohydrate or fasting	Cold
	Stress	Rest after exercise	Rest after exercise
	Rest after exercise	Cold	
Myotonia	–	+ (in some forms)	+ + + (paradoxical)
Inheritance	Autosomal dominant (occasional sporadic)	Autosomal dominant	Autosomal dominant
Provocative test	Glucose plus insulin	Oral potassium chloride after exercise	Limb cooling

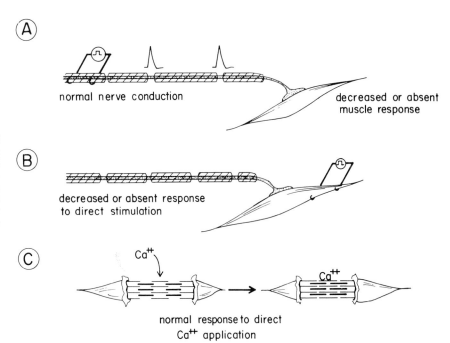

Figure 13–5. Muscles during an attack of hypokalemic periodic paralysis are electrically unexcitable to indirect *(A)* or direct *(B)* stimulation, but the contractile proteins respond normally to externally applied calcium in a skinned muscle fiber *(C)*. This evidence points to the sarcolemma as the site of major pathogenesis in hypokalemic periodic paralysis.

direct electrical stimulation. Repolarization of the fibers, however, restored baseline excitability.

When specific membrane conductance pathways were examined, potassium and chloride conductances were found to be normal under all conditions. The abnormal membrane depolarization was ascribed to a TTX-insensitive increase in resting sodium conductance in the diseased fibers. Other evidence of increased steady-state sodium permeability of the muscle surface membrane includes the increased intracellular sodium concentration and the hyperpolarization produced by decreasing the extracellular sodium concentration (Hofmann and Smith, 1970).

Thyrotoxic Periodic Paralysis

A sporadic form of periodic paralysis is occasionally seen in conjunction with hyperthyroidism (Layzer and Goldfield, 1974; Okinaka et al., 1957). Thyrotoxic periodic paralysis is clinically similar to the familial hypokalemic form, but 90% of the cases occur among male Asians. In a review of 10 cases, Kelley et al. (1989) reported that all developed paralytic attacks nearly coincident with the onset of hyperthyroidism, and in each case, the paralytic episodes resolved when a euthyroid state was attained. In this series, attacks were most often precipitated by rest after exercise and less frequently by ingestion of a large carbohydrate load. Little information is available on the pathophysiology of this disorder. Insulin levels have been reported as elevated during spontaneous attacks, and the symptoms are abolished by β-adrenergic blockade (Conway et al., 1974).

Thyroid hormone increases both the activity and the number of Na^+,K^+-ATPase sites in muscle membranes (Edelman, 1979). It is possible that attacks

may result from increased internal sodium concentration in genetically susceptible individuals.

Experimental Models of Hypokalemic Periodic Paralysis

There are no known naturally occurring animal models of periodic paralysis, but two experimental models mimic many of the features of hypokalemic periodic paralysis: barium poisoning and chronic potassium depletion.

Barium Poisoning. In humans, intoxication with barium induces reversible muscle weakness (Pa-Ping disease) (Allen, 1969) associated with serum hypokalemia and vacuolar myopathic changes comparable with those seen in hypokalemic periodic paralysis. A similar syndrome can be produced experimentally in laboratory animals (Schott and McArdle, 1974). Barium, an alkaline earth divalent cation, is a voltage- and use-dependent blocker of potassium channels (Armstrong et al., 1982; Donaldson and Bean, 1982) and is also highly permeant through calcium channels. In vitro experiments with mammalian muscle have shown that barium reversibly depolarizes the muscle cells, prolongs the action potential duration, and transiently potentiates contractility before inhibiting it (Gallant, 1983). These effects are antagonized by increased external potassium concentration but are not influenced by calcium channel blockers.

These observations are consistent with the hypothesis that barium selectively blocks the inwardly rectifying potassium channels of skeletal muscle membranes. Reduced potassium permeability shifts the membrane potential in the depolarizing direction toward the sodium equilibrium potential, as well as significantly retarding the leakage of intracellular potassium. This shift in membrane potential may be opposed for a time by the electrogenic pumping of the Na^+,K^+-ATPase, but the coupled Na^+-K^+ fluxes, in the face of reduced potassium permeability, ultimately lead to a shift of extracellular potassium into the cell and intracellular sodium out. In this model, reduced potassium permeability is the primary defect; hypokalemia is the consequence and not the cause of the depolarization.

Chronic Potassium Deficiency. Chronic potassium deficiency is a second model of hypokalemic paralysis in which the defects can be explained by a reduced membrane potassium conductance. Mammals receiving a potassium-free diet soon experience chronic hypokalemia, decreased intracellular potassium and increased sodium concentrations, and skeletal muscle depolarization (Bilbrey et al., 1973; Kao and Gordon, 1975). Dogs, but apparently not rats, are subject to transient episodes of weakness with further decreases in plasma potassium concentration, either spontaneously or after epinephrine administration. Both species show an unusual response to insulin. After insulin exposure, normal muscles hyperpolarize and increase membrane resistance, whereas potassium-deficient muscles with low extracellular potassium concentration show marked depolarization with secondary flaccid paralysis and further hypokalemia.

The mechanism of chronic potassium deficiency is speculative. Proffered explanations have suggested increased sodium permeability and/or decreased potassium permeability. Insulin-induced decreases in potassium permeability lead to depolarization and hypokalemia analogous to the situation in barium poisoning. Alternatively, increased basal sodium permeability depolarizes the resting potential toward the sodium equilibrium potential, whereas insulin stimulation of Na^+,K^+-ATPase leads to potassium accumulation by the muscle and further membrane depolarization.

Periodic Paralysis Associated with Elevated Serum Potassium Levels

The nosological classification of hyperkalemic periodic paralysis on clinical grounds has historically generated debate. Two forms of hyperkalemic periodic paralysis, the adynamia episodica of Gamstorp (1956) and paramyotonia congenita of Eulenburg (1886), were considered by most investigators to be separate entities, but other workers argued for their identity (Drager et al., 1958; Layzer et al., 1967). Adynamia episodica is characterized by periodic paralysis and hyperkalemia, whereas the salient features of paramyotonia congenita are myotonia that appears with cold exposure and worsens with exercise (paradoxical myotonia) and cold-induced paresis. Some investigators have suggested further subdivision of adynamia episodica into additional syndromes when the paresis is associated with true

myotonia or with paradoxical myotonia (Lehmann-Horn et al., 1983).

Paramyotonia Congenita (Eulenburg)

The myotonia seen in patients with hyperkalemic paralysis may be clinically indistinguishable from that in myotonia congenita, but more often the former is paradoxical—continued exercise of an affected part exacerbates rather than diminishes the myotonia. It is also believed to be more susceptible to cold than is classic myotonia (Ricker et al., 1977). Cold exposure often leads to a stiffness or to passive resistance to stretch, preceding the onset of paralysis. This stiffness differs from the delayed relaxation of myotonia and is often associated with decreased rather than increased electrical activity.

Lehmann-Horn et al. (1981) reported an extensive in vitro voltage-clamp study of external intercostal muscle from three male patients with paramyotonia congenita (see also companion clinical study by Haass et al., 1981) and three normal control subjects. At 37°C, the membrane potential in the muscle from paramyotonic patients was normal, but cooling to 27°C produced a slow depolarization of membrane potential. Several minutes of spontaneous electrical and mechanical activity occurred before the depolarization stabilized at -40 mV, with failure of both membrane action potentials and contraction. Rewarming did not restore the membrane potential. All these effects, however, could be prevented by pretreatment with TTX, a specific blocker of the voltage-sensitive sodium channel.

Cooling produced a marked increase in sodium conductance in all diseased fibers, whereas potassium and chloride conductance remained normal (Lehmann-Horn et al., 1987b). Exposure of muscle fibers in vitro to 7 mM potassium chloride did not induce excessive depolarization, loss of electrical excitability, or paralysis. Clinical improvement in paralysis has been noted with tocainide, an orally administrable derivative of lidocaine, that affects the sodium channel, but not with other antiarrhythmic agents, such as procainamide or phenytoin, which are also known to affect sodium conductance (Ricker et al., 1980).

These data are consistent with a temperature-dependent abnormality of the sarcolemmal sodium channel. The defect may be in the channel protein itself or could represent an abnormality of the lipid milieu, producing abnormal lipid-protein interactions in the ion channels. The myotonic patients may have an additional defect of chloride conductance at physiologic temperatures. The nosological and physiologic implications of these findings await further experimentation.

Adynamia Episodica (Gamstorp)

Adynamia episodica was described first by Hellweg-Larsen et al. (1955) and subsequently in a detailed report by Gamstorp (1956), whose name is often associated with the disease. Like the more common hypokalemic form of periodic paralysis, the disease is characterized by intermittent episodes of weakness or paresis but, in this case, is associated with elevation in serum potassium concentration. Weakness is more common than paralysis; both can be brought on by fasting, rest after exercise, or artificial elevation of the serum potassium concentration. The disease is usually inherited as an autosomal dominant trait.

Intracellular recordings have been made from a number of patients with adynamia episodica with or without myotonic features (Lehmann-Horn et al., 1983, 1987a; Ricker et al., 1989). In all cases, fibers exhibited a normal resting membrane potential at 37°C in 3.5 mM potassium chloride and did not depolarize when cooled. Increasing extracellular potassium concentration to 9 mM resulted in prompt depolarization and electrical unexcitability associated with the appearance of an abnormal, noninactivating sodium current. This current, along with the potassium chloride–induced depolarization, could be reversibly blocked by TTX. Electrical excitability at high potassium chloride concentrations could be restored by lowering the pH without affecting the membrane potential; pH altered the abnormal slow inactivation properties of the channel.

Steady-state potassium and chloride conductances in the presence of TTX were normal. Without TTX, total membrane conductance was normal in the hyperpolarizing direction, but with depolarization, an inward sodium current was seen that was more pronounced in high external potassium concentration. The contractile properties were normal in low-sodium solutions or with sodium channels blocked with TTX.

The presumed defect in this disease is, again, an abnormal sodium channel that has both increased conductance and altered kinetics, leading to hyperexcitability and depolarization induced by hyperkalemia. The cloning and sequencing of two sodium channel isoforms from rat skeletal muscle (Kallen et al., 1990; Trimmer et al., 1989) have opened the way for direct testing of this hypothesis. Probes generated to the rat TTX-sensitive skeletal muscle sodium channel were used to clone the human TTX-sensitive skeletal muscle channel (A. George, R.L. Barchi, and R.G. Kallen, in preparation). A clone including unique sequence in the 3'-untranslated region of this human channel was then used to localize the gene; it was encoded to the long arm of chromosome 17 between q23.1 and q25.3 (George et al., 1991). Fontaine et al. (1990), taking advantage of the high degree of homology between similar sodium channel isoforms in rat and human muscle, used the polymerase chain reaction to clone a fragment of the human muscle channel encoding the region between the third and fourth homologous repeat domains (see section on sodium channels). By using a restriction fragment length polymorphism within the genomic DNA encoding this region, they screened a

family with hyperkalemic periodic paralysis for linkage between the expression of the disease phenotype and the sodium channel gene locus. Tight linkage was found with an LOD score of 4.0 at 0.0 recombinant frequency.

In a subsequent electrophysiologic study, Cannon et al. (1991) carried out single-channel measurements on sodium channels in cultured myotubes grown from biopsy samples from the same family with hyperkalemic periodic paralysis that was used for linkage studies and from normal control subjects. In this elegant study, a clear potassium-sensitive abnormality in sodium channel kinetics was demonstrated. Control muscle sodium channels opened briefly and then inactivated normally after depolarization, whether exposed to normal or elevated extracellular potassium ion concentration. Sodium channels from diseased muscle showed normal kinetic behavior at the normal potassium ion concentration of 3.5 mM; when this concentration was increased to 10 mM, however, a fraction of the channels intermittently shifted between the normal kinetic mode and an alternate kinetic state characterized by failure of inactivation during a depolarizing current pulse. The resulting persistent channel openings, even in a small fraction of the total channel population, generated a small but significant noninactivating sodium current. This current can lead to further membrane depolarization and subsequent inactivation of normal sodium channels in the surrounding membrane. Thus the abnormal inactivation properties of a small percentage of channels can ultimately produce inactivation of all sodium channels, failure of membrane excitation, and paralysis (Barchi, 1991). Work is now under way in a number of laboratories to clone the defective gene from families with this disorder and to identify the specific deletion or mutation responsible for the potassium ion concentration–sensitive kinetic abnormality.

Membrane Potential and Excitability in Periodic Paralysis

For normal muscle contraction, electrical impulses originating in motor neurons must be chemically transmitted across the neuromuscular junction to the muscle membrane, where action potentials once more take over to spread the excitation signal along the muscle surface and into the fiber interior via the T tubule system. Depolarization of the T tubule system triggers calcium release from the sarcoplasmic reticulum, activation of the actomyosin system, and muscle contraction. In the periodic paralyses, muscle weakness is due to the failure of the normal excitation process responsible for the spread of action potentials along the muscle surface membrane. Paradoxically, this refractory state is due to persistent depolarization of the surface membrane. A brief review of the physiology of the membrane action potential clarifies this point.

In skeletal muscle, the action potential is largely the result of a transient increase in membrane permeability to sodium ions that is mediated by a voltage-dependent sodium ion channel. The classic studies of Hodgkin and Huxley (1952) described three possible states for this sodium channel: resting, activated, and inactivated. The equilibrium distribution of all membrane sodium channels among these states is dependent on the membrane potential. Resting sodium channels convert to the activated state with rapid membrane depolarization, increasing membrane sodium conductance to produce an action potential. The lifetime of the activated state is brief, however, and the channels quickly convert to the nonconducting, inactivated state with maintained depolarization. Inactivated channels cannot be reopened; they return to the resting state only when the membrane is repolarized. This repolarization normally occurs at the end of an action potential in parallel with the opening of a membrane potassium channel.

Prolonged depolarization progressively reduces the number of sodium channels that are available for activation at a given time. The percentage of membrane sodium channels that is available for activation in the resting state at a particular voltage is described by the steep sigmoid curve in Figure 13–6. Because an action potential can be generated only when the net inward sodium current is greater than all other outward currents across the cell membrane, the number of sodium channels that can be opened is critical. At normal resting potentials, when more than 70% of the sodium channels are available, this condition is easily met and the membrane exhibits normal excitability. With persistent depolarization of more than 10–20 mV, however, the number of available channels is sharply reduced and the membrane becomes incapable of producing an action potential, even though the channels themselves may be normal in function.

Shifts of the voltage dependence of sodium acti-

vation kinetics in a depolarizion direction, or inactivation kinetics in a hyperpolarization direction, could also reduce membrane excitability. For example, the reduced excitability of fibers in hypokalemic paralysis despite experimentally induced hyperpolarization, which was observed by Rudel et al. (1984), may reflect additional, more complicated abnormalities of sodium channel kinetics in this disease.

To understand the episodic depolarizations that trigger the periodic paralyses, the origin of the muscle resting membrane potential should be considered. Ions at equilibrium across a membrane adjust their concentration gradients to satisfy the Nernst equation. When several permeant ions are present, some of whose concentrations are fixed by energy-requiring ion pumps, the membrane potential is in a steady state: passive diffusion of an ion down its electrochemical gradient is counterbalanced by active pumping of that ion against the gradient. The membrane potential in this condition is described by the more complex Goldman equation (Fig. 13–7). In muscle, the principal permeant ions are sodium, potassium, and chloride. Because chloride is passively distributed across muscle membranes, any change in membrane potential causes chloride to redistribute itself so as eventually to approach equilibrium. In contrast, the steady-state membrane potential can be altered by changing the concentrations of sodium or potassium ions across the membrane. An important outcome of the relationship expressed in the Goldman equation is that the same effect on membrane potential can be produced merely by altering the relative permeabilities of the membrane to these ions. The membrane potential can vary between the limits set by the sodium ($+55$ mV) and potassium equilibrium potentials (-75 mV) without requiring any change in the actual concentration of these ions.

The membrane potential may also be altered by ion pumps independently of permeability or concentration changes if pumping creates a net movement

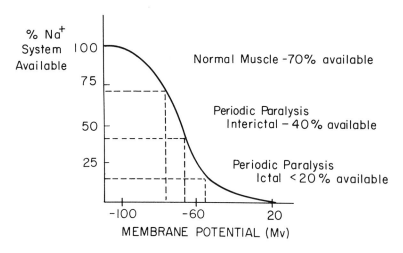

Figure 13–6. The number of sodium channels able to respond with a permeability increase to a depolarizing stimulus decreases sigmoidally as the membrane is depolarized. In the steady state, sodium channels are distributed between resting and inactivated states. The curve represents the number of sodium channels in a resting state during a maintained membrane potential (h_∞ curve in Hodgkin-Huxley terminology). A 10-mV depolarization from the resting potential of -77 mV reduces the sodium channels available to generate an action potential to 40%. An additional 10-mV depolarization during a periodic paralysis attack inactivates most sodium channels, so that the requirements for action potential generation are no longer fulfilled.

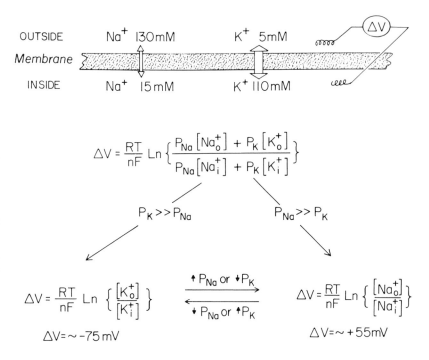

Figure 13–7. The concentrations of sodium and potassium ions across a membrane as well as the permeability of the membrane to those ions determine the electrical potential (ΔV) measured across the membrane. The potential can be calculated knowing the ion concentrations ([Na], [K]), membrane permeabilities (P_{Na}, P_K), and absolute temperature (T) from the Goldman equation. If one ionic permeability is much greater than the other, the Goldman equation reduces to the Nernst equation for the equilibrium potential across the membrane. By altering the relative ion permeabilities, the membrane potential can shift from a potassium equilibrium potential of -75 mV to a sodium equilibrium potential of $+55$ mV. R, F, and n are constants representing the gas constant, the Faraday constant, and the ionic valence, respectively.

of charge across the membrane. In skeletal muscle, the Na^+,K^+-ATPase is electrogenic, exchanging three internal sodium ions for every two external potassium ions. Increased pump activity hyperpolarizes the membrane slightly by extruding intracellular sodium, whereas decreased pumping depolarizes the membrane. The potential generated by this mechanism is equal to the net charge extruded per square centimeter of membrane divided by the membrane capacitance and may amount to 5–10 mV under normal conditions.

The Goldman equation predicts that the depolarization seen in periodic paralysis could occur as the result of any of the following changes: lowering internal sodium or potassium concentration, increasing external sodium or potassium concentration, increasing sodium permeability, or decreasing potassium permeability. Decreasing electrogenic ion pumping also depolarizes the membrane (Fig. 13–8). In the periodic paralyses, the depolarization seems to be due largely to an abnormal increase in membrane sodium conductance. External factors, such as

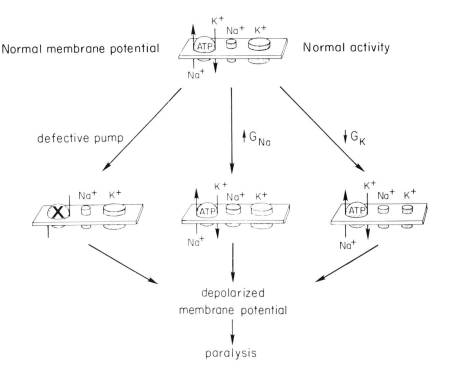

Figure 13–8. The electrogenic effect of the Na^+,K^+-ATPase as well as the membrane ion permeabilities determines the membrane potential. Alterations in any of these factors in the periodic paralyses can lead to membrane depolarization and attacks of paralysis. G = conductance.

cooling, that lead to further transient increases in sodium conductance tip the delicately balanced membrane to a more depolarized state, resulting in inactivation of the voltage-sensitive sodium channel, failure of activation, and paralysis.

The details of the interplay among serum potassium concentration, membrane potential, and paralysis in the individual disorders remain to be clarified, but shifts in serum potassium ion concentration probably reflect coupling to sodium movements through the Na^+,K^+-ATPase pump system. This coupling can result in either hypokalemia or hyperkalemia, depending on the functional state of the Na^+,K^+-ATPase itself. The increased inward sodium ion movement that is associated with an increase in membrane sodium conductance is a potent stimulus for pump activity. A sudden increase in sodium conductance from any further triggering event additionally stimulates this pump. Because the Na^+,K^+-ATPase exchanges extracellular potassium ions for intracellular sodium ions, this pumping activity can rapidly reduce the potassium ion concentration in the limited volume of the extracellular space and produce hypokalemia. It is essentially this sort of coupling that produces net potassium ion movement into the cells of normal individuals after the administration of glucose and insulin. Conversely, if the Na^+,K^+-ATPase cannot increase its rate sufficiently to keep pace with an increased sodium ion leakage, the necessary result is a compensatory outward movement of potassium ions and secondary hyperkalemia. It is important to realize that either hyperkalemia or hypokalemia can result from the same fundamental defect in membrane sodium conductance, depending on the capacity of the Na^+,K^+-ATPase to respond to the additional sodium load.

A muscle membrane in delicate balance as the result of an increased inward sodium ion leak just compensated by a maximally activated pump could also be thrown out of balance by the selective slowing of pump activity. This could easily occur with a reduction of temperature, for example, because the temperature dependence of energy-dependent pumping is nearly threefold greater than that for ion movement through an aqueous membrane channel.

Molecular Characterization of Muscle Sodium Channels

During the past few years, the primary sequence for both the principal TTX-sensitive sodium channel of adult rat skeletal muscle and the TTX-insensitive sodium channel found in denervated muscle has been determined through the cloning of their respective cDNAs (Kallen et al., 1990; Trimmer et al., 1989). These channels join a larger group, including those from eel electroplax, rat brain, and *Drosophila*, whose primary structures are known. All these sodium channels share a number of common features. Each consists primarily of a single, large 260,000-polypeptide chain that contains all the necessary components

needed to form a functional sodium channel. Each is heavily glycosylated. One or more smaller subunits are present in the mammalian channels, but they are not necessary for basic channel function (for review, see Barchi, 1988).

The sequences of all known sodium channels show a remarkable degree of homology. All contain four large regions of internal homology, encompassing 200–300 amino acids each, which are clearly derived from the same primordial gene element. Within each domain are six putative transmembrane helixes, including one, S4, with a remarkably constant positively charged amino acid (arginine or lysine) at every

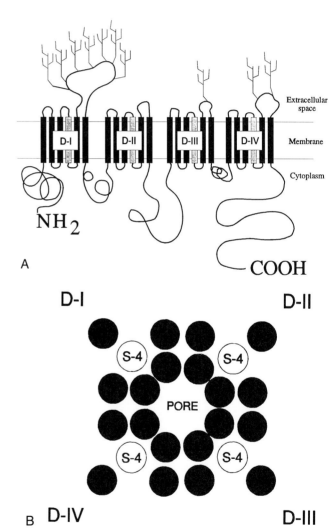

Figure 13–9. The voltage-dependent sodium channel in muscle consists of a large 260-kd α subunit and two smaller β subunits of 30–40 kd. *(A)* The α subunit contains all the functional elements of the channel. This α subunit includes about 2000 amino acids organized into four internal repeat domains, each of which has six putative transmembrane helixes. *(B)* In the membrane, the repeat domains probably organize themselves in a pseudosymmetric fashion around a central ion pore. The walls of the pore are formed from one or two amphipathic helixes contributed from each of the repeat domains. The fourth helix in each domain contains a positive charge at every third residue; these helixes may be the voltage-sensitive elements controlling channel activation.

Table 13–3. MEMBRANE ABNORMALITIES IN THE PERIODIC PARALYSES

Parameter	Hypokalemic Periodic Paralysis	Adynamia Episodica	Paramyotonia Congenita
Membrane potential			
Interictal	Normal or slightly decreased	Normal	Normal
Ictal	Depolarized	Depolarized	Depolarized
Provoking factors in vitro	$\downarrow [K^+]_{out}$	$\uparrow [K^+]_{out}$	Cooling to 27°C
TTX block	No	Yes	Yes
Membrane conductance during paralysis			
G_{Na}	Increased	Increased	Increased
G_K	Normal	Normal	Normal
G_{Cl}	Normal	Normal	Normal or reduced

third position. These S4 helixes are thought to play a central role in the voltage gating of the channel.

Current models of channel tertiary structure envision the internal repeat domains organized in a pseudosymmetric fashion about a central pore, much like the staves of a barrel. The pore, or ion channel, is formed by the hydrophilic surfaces of one or two amphipathic helixes contributed by each of the repeat domains (Fig. 13–9). The regions of protein linking the repeat domains, as well as the NH_2 and COOH termini, are located on the cytoplasmic surface of the membrane (Noda et al., 1986).

The human homologues of the two rat skeletal muscle sodium channels have also been cloned (Gellens et al., 1991; George et al., 1990). These channels share a high degree of sequence identity with their rodent counterparts. The TTX-sensitive channel in human muscle, for example, is much more closely related to the rat TTX-sensitive channel than it is to the TTX-insensitive channel in human muscle. Both the human channels have now been localized to specific chromosomes; the muscle TTX-sensitive sodium channel maps to the long arm of chromosome 17 (George et al., 1991), whereas the TTX-insensitive channel found in denervated skeletal muscle and in heart is located on chromosome 3.

With evidence linking a defect in the gene encoding the human skeletal muscle TTX-sensitive sodium channel to the pathophysiology of the periodic paralyses, an opportunity exists to explore issues related to the structure and function of this channel in vivo. These disorders are natural mutagenic experiments in which the channel alterations can be precisely defined and their functional consequences documented. Undoubtedly, the details of this story will be evolving rapidly during the next few years.

Summary

Table 13–3 summarizes the electrophysiologic defects in periodic paralysis. Each disease appears to be clinically and physiologically different, but each has in common a possible defect in a sarcolemmal membrane sodium channel. It is interesting to speculate that these may all be different abnormalities of the voltage-dependent sodium channel protein. In hypokalemic paralysis, the pathologic feature may

be a TTX-insensitive, leaky sodium channel with decreased excitability. In some patients with hyperkalemic paralysis, sodium channels may inactivate inappropriately near the resting potential. The genetic sodium channel defect in paramyotonia congenita may prove to induce a conformation that is stable at normal temperatures but, owing to entropic effects, becomes unstable when temperature is lowered, leading to persistent channel activation and depolarization. Are these diseases the ion channel analogues of the hemoglobinopathies in which critical amino acid substitutions alter the functionality of the protein? Rapidly accelerating advances in the study of molecular biology and genetics of ion channels will someday provide the answer.

References

(Key references are designated with an asterisk.)

*Adrian R.H., Bryant S.H. On the repetitive discharge in myotonic muscle fibers. *J. Physiol. (Lond.)* 240:505–515, 1974.

Adrian R.H., Marshall M.W. Action potentials reconstructed in normal and myotonic muscle fibers. *J. Physiol. (Lond.)* 258:125–143, 1976.

Adrian R.H., Chandler W.K., Hodgkin A.L. Voltage-clamp experiments in skeletal muscle fibers. *J. Physiol. (Lond.)* 208:607–644, 1970.

Allen A.S. Pa Ping, or Kiating paralysis. *Clin. Med. J.* 51:296–301, 1969.

Almers W. Potassium conductance changes in skeletal muscle and the potassium concentration in the transverse tubules. *J. Physiol. (Lond.)* 225:33–56, 1972.

Appel S.H., Roses A.D. Membranes and myotonia. In Rowland L.P., ed. *Pathogenesis of Human Muscular Dystrophies.* Amsterdam, Excerpta Medica, pp. 747–758, 1977.

Armstrong C.M., Swenson R.P. Jr., Taylor S.R. Block of squid axon K channels by internally and externally applied barium ions. *J. Gen. Physiol.* 80:663–682, 1982.

Barchi R.L. Myotonia: an evaluation of the chloride hypothesis. *Arch. Neurol.* 32:175–180, 1975.

*Barchi R.L. Probing the molecular structure of the voltage-dependent sodium channel. *Annu. Rev. Neurosci.* 11:455–495, 1988.

Barchi R. Bad channel genes and weak muscles. *Curr. Biol.* (in press).

Barrantes F.J. Muscle endplate cholinoreceptors. *Pharmacol. Ther.* 38:331–385, 1988.

Becker P.E. Myopathies. In Becker P.E., ed. *Humangenetik.* Vol. 3/1. Stuttgart, Thieme, 1964.

Becker P.E. *Myotonia Congenita and Syndromes Associated with Myotonia.* Stuttgart, Thieme, 1977.

Bilbrey G.L., Herbin L., Carter N.W., et al. Skeletal muscle resting membrane potential in potassium deficiency. *J. Clin. Invest.* 52:3011–3018, 1973.

Bretag A.H. Further modelling of the myotonic phenomenon. *Proc. Austr. Physiol. Pharmacol. Soc.* 2:22, 1971.

Bretag A.H. Mathematical modelling of the myotonic action potential. In Desmedt J.E., ed. *New Developments in Electromyography and Clinical Neurophysiology.* Vol. 1. Basel, Karger, pp. 464–482, 1973.

Brown G.L., Harvey A.M. Congenital myotonia in the goat. *Brain* 62:341–363, 1939.

Bryant S.H. Muscle membrane of normal and myotonic goats in normal and low external chloride. *Fed. Proc.* 21:312–315, 1962.

Bryant S.H. Myotonia in the goat. *Ann. N.Y. Acad. Sci.* 317:314–324, 1979.

*Bryant S.H., Morales-Aguilera A. Chloride conductance in normal and myotonic muscle fibres and the action of monocarboxylic aromatic acids. *J. Physiol. (Lond.)* 219:367–383, 1971.

Bryant S.H., Owenburg K. Characteristics of the chloride channel in skeletal-muscle fibers from myotonic and normal goats. *Fed. Proc.* 39:579–583, 1980.

Bucher N.L. Effects of 2,4-dichlorophenoxyacetic acid on experimental animals. *Proc. Soc. Exp. Biol. Med.* 63:204–205, 1946.

Butterfield D.A., Watson W.E. Electron spin resonance studies of an animal model of human congenital myotonia: increased erythrocyte membrane fluidity in rats with 20,25-diazacholesterol–induced myotonia. *J. Membr. Biol.* 32:165–176, 1977.

Butterfield D.A., Roses A.D., Appel S.H., et al. Electron spin resonance studies of membrane proteins in erythrocytes in myotonic muscular dystrophy. *Arch. Biochem. Biophys.* 177:226–234, 1976.

Cannon S.C., Brown R.H., Corey D.P. A sodium channel defect in hyperkalemic periodic paralysis: potassium-induced failure of inactivation. *Neuron* 6:619–626, 1991.

Chalikian D.M., Barchi R.L. 20,25-Diazacholesterol myotonia—biochemical characteristics of the sarcolemma. *Neurology (N.Y.)* 30:423–424, 1980a.

Chalikian D.M., Barchi R.L. Fluorescent-probe analysis of erythrocyte-membranes in myotonic-dystrophy. *Neurology (N.Y.)* 30:277–285, 1980b.

Conway M.J., Seibel J.A., Eaton R.P. Thyrotoxicosis and periodic paralysis: improvement with beta blockade. *Ann. Intern. Med.* 81:332–336, 1974.

D'Alonzo A.J., McArdle J.J. An evaluation of fast- and slow-twitch muscle from rats treated with 20,25-diazacholesterol. *Exp. Neurol.* 78:46–66, 1982.

Donaldson P.L., Bean K.G. Calcium currents in mammalian skeletal muscle. *Biophys. J.* 37:340a, 1982.

Drager G.A., Hammill J.F., Shy G.M. Paramyotonia congenita. *A.M.A. Arch. Neurol. Psychiatry* 80:1–9, 1958.

Edelman I.S. Effect of thyroid hormones on biochemical processes. *Prog. Clin. Biol. Res.* 31:685–689, 1979.

Engel A.G., Lambert E.H. Calcium activation of electrically inexcitable muscle fibers in primary hypokalemic periodic paralysis. *Neurology (Minneap.)* 19:851–858, 1969.

Eulenburg A. Uber eine familiare, durch 6 Generationen verfolgbare Form congenitaler Paramyotonie. *Neurol. Zbl.* 12, 1886.

Eyzaguirre C., Folk B.P., Zierler K.L., et al. Experimental myotonia and repetitive phenomena: the veratrinic effect of 2,4-dichlorophenoxyacetate (2,4-D) in the rat. *Am. J. Physiol.* 155:69–77, 1948.

Fontaine B., Khurana T.S., Hoffman E.P., et al. Hyperkalemic periodic paralysis and the adult muscle sodium channel alpha-subunit gene. *Science* 250:1000–1002, 1990.

Fowler W.M. Jr., Layzer R.B., Taylor T.D., et al. The Schwartz-Jampel syndrome: its clinical, physiological and histological expressions. *J. Neurol. Sci.* 22:127, 1974.

Franke C., Iaizzo P.A., Hatt H., et al. Altered Na$^+$ channel activity and reduced Cl$^-$ conductance cause hyperexcitability in recessive generalized myotonia. *Muscle Nerve* (in press).

Furman R.E., Barchi R.L. The pathophysiology of myotonia produced by aromatic carboxylic acids. *Ann. Neurol.* 4:357–365, 1978.

Furman R.E., Barchi R.L. 20,25-Diazacholesterol myotonia: an electrophysiological study. *Ann. Neurol.* 10:251–260, 1981.

Furman R.E., Mollman J.E., Wood D., et al. Transmembrane Ca^{++} movement in 20,25-diazacholesterol myotonia. *Neurology (N.Y.)* 32:A145, 1982.

Gaffney B.J., Drachman D.B., Lin D.C., et al. Spin-label studies of erythrocytes in myotonic dystrophy: no increase in membrane fluidity. *Neurology (N.Y.)* 30:272–276, 1980.

Gallant E.M. Barium-treated mammalian skeletal muscle: similarities to hypokalaemic periodic paralysis. *J. Physiol. (Lond.)* 335:577–590, 1983.

Gamstorp I. Adynamia episodica hereditaria. *Acta Paediatr.* 45(Suppl. 108):1–126, 1956.

Gellens M.E., George A.L., Chen I., et al. Primary structure of a human cardiac muscle sodium channel. *Biophys. J.* 59:69A, 1991.

George A.L., Kallen R.G., Barchi R.L. Isolation of a human skeletal muscle sodium channel cDNA clone. *Biophys. J.* 57:108A, 1990.

George A.L., Ledbetter D.H., Kallen R.G., et al. Assignment of a human skeletal muscle sodium channel gene (SCN4A) to 17q23.1-25.3. *Genomics* 9:555–556, 1991.

Haass A., Ricker K., Rudel R., et al. Clinical study of paramyotonia congenita with and without myotonia in a warm environment. *Muscle Nerve* 4:388–395, 1981.

Hellweg-Larsen A.H., Hauge M., Sagild U. Hereditary transient muscular paralysis in Denmark: genetic aspects of family periodic paralysis and family periodic adynamica. *Acta Genet. Stat. Med.* 5:263–281, 1955.

Hodgkin A.L., Huxley A.F. A quantitative description of membrane current and its application to conduction and excitation in nerve. *J. Physiol. (Lond.)* 117:500–544, 1952.

Hofmann W.W., Smith R.A. Hypokalemic periodic paralysis studied in vitro. *Brain* 93:445–474, 1970.

Hofmann W.W., DeNardo G.L. Sodium flux in myotonic muscular dystrophy. *Am. J. Physiol.* 214:330–336, 1968.

Hosey M.M., Lazdunski M. Calcium channels: molecular pharmacology, structure, and regulation. *J. Membr. Biol.* 104:81–105, 1988.

Iaizzo P.A., Franke C., Hatt H., et al. Altered sodium channel behavior causes myotonia in dominantly inherited myotonia congenita. *Neuromuscular Dis.* (in press).

Jack J.J.B., Noble D., Tsien R.W. *Repetitive Activity in Excitable Cells in Electric Current Flow in Excitable Cells.* Oxford, Clarendon Press, 1975.

Kallen R.G., Sheng Z., Yang J., et al. Primary structure and expression of a sodium channel characteristic of denervated and immature rat skeletal muscle. *Neuron* 4:233–242, 1990.

Kao I., Gordon A.M. Mechanism of insulin produced paralysis of muscle from potassium-depleted rats. *Science* 188:740–741, 1975.

Kelley D., Gharib H., Kennedy F., et al. Thyrotoxic periodic paralysis: report of 10 cases and review of the electromyographical findings. *Arch. Intern. Med.* 149:2597–2600, 1989.

Layzer R.B., Goldfield E. Periodic paralysis caused by abuse of thyroid hormone. *Neurology (Minneap.)* 24:949–952, 1974.

Layzer R.B., Lovelace R.E., Rowland L.P. Hyperkalemic periodic paralysis. *Arch. Neurol.* 16:455–472, 1967.

Lehmann-Horn F., Rudel R., Dengler R., et al. Membrane defects in paramyotonia congenita with and without myotonia in a warm environment. *Muscle Nerve* 4:396–406, 1981.

Lehmann-Horn F., Rudel R., Ricker K., et al. Two cases of adynamia episodica hereditaria: in vitro investigation of muscle cell membrane and contraction parameters. *Muscle Nerve* 6:113–121, 1983.

Lehmann-Horn F., Kuther G., Ricker K., et al. Adynamia episodica hereditaria with myotonia: a non-inactivating sodium current and the effect of extracellular pH. *Muscle Nerve* 10:363–374, 1987a.

*Lehmann-Horn F., Rudel R., Ricker K. Membrane defects in paramyotonia congenita. *Muscle Nerve* 10:633–641, 1987b.

Lewis E.D., Griggs R.C., Moxley R.T. III. Regulation of plasma potassium in hyperkalemic periodic paralysis. *Neurology (Minneap.)* 29:1131–1137, 1979.

Leyden E. *Klin. Rukenmarkskrankheiten* 1:128, 1874.

Lipicky R.J. Studies in human myotonic dystrophy. In Rowland L.P., ed. *Pathogenesis of Human Muscular Dystrophies.* Amsterdam, Excerpta Medica, pp. 729–738, 1977.

Lipicky R.J., Bryant S.H. Sodium, potassium and chloride fluxes in intercostal muscle from normal goats and goats with hereditary myotonia. *J. Gen. Physiol.* 50:89–111, 1966.

Lipicky R.J., Bryant S.H. Temperature effects on cable parameters and K efflux in normal and myotonic goat muscle. *Am. J. Physiol.* 222:213–215, 1972.

*Lipicky R.J., Bryant S.H. A biophysical study of human myotonias. In Desmedt J.E., ed. *New Developments in Electromyography and Clinical Neurophysiology*. Vol. 1. Basel, Karger, pp. 451–463, 1973.

Lipicky R.J., Bryant S.H., Salmon J.H. Cable parameters, sodium, potassium, chloride and water content, and potassium efflux in isolated external intercostal muscles of normal volunteers and patients with myotonia congenita. *J. Clin. Invest*. 50:2091–2103, 1971.

Merickel M., Gray R., Chauvin P., et al. Cultured muscle from myotonic muscular dystrophy patients: altered membrane electrical properties. *Proc. Natl. Acad. Sci. U.S.A*. 78:648–652, 1981.

Mishra S.K., Hobson M., Desaiah D. Erythrocyte membrane abnormalities in human myotonic dystrophy. *J. Neurol. Sci*. 46:333–340, 1980.

Noda M., Ikeda T., Kayano T., et al. Existence of distinct sodium channel mRNAs in rat brain. *Nature* 320:188–192, 1986.

Okinaka S., Shizume K., Wantanabe A., et al. The association of periodic paralysis and hyperthyroidism in Japan. *J. Clin. Endocrinol*. 17:1454–1459, 1957.

Palade P.T., Barchi R.L. Characteristics of the chloride conductance in muscle fibers of the rat diaphragm. *J. Gen. Physiol*. 69:325–342, 1977a.

Palade P.T., Barchi R.L. On the inhibition of muscle membrane chloride conductances by aromatic carboxylic acids. *J. Gen. Physiol*. 69:875–896, 1977b.

Peter J.B., Andiman R.M., Bowman R.L., et al. Myotonia induced by diazacholesterol: increased (Na + K)-ATPase activity of erythrocyte ghosts and development of cataracts. *Exp. Neurol*. 41:738–744, 1973.

Pohl J. Physiologische Wirkung des tetrahydroatophans. *Z. Exp. Path. Ther*. 19:198, 1917.

Ricker K., Hertel G., Langscheid K., et al. Myotonia not aggravated by cooling. *J. Neurol*. 216:9–20, 1977.

Ricker K., Haass A., Rüdel R., et al. Successful treatment of paramyotonia congenita (Eulenburg): muscle stiffness and weakness prevented by tocainide. *J. Neurol. Neurosurg. Psychiatry* 43:268–271, 1980.

Ricker K., Camacho L., Grafe P., et al. Adynamia episodica hereditaria: what causes the weakness? *Muscle Nerve* 12:883–891, 1989.

Riecker G., Bolte, H.D. Membranpotentiale einzelner Skeletmuskelzellen bei hypokalamischer periodischer Muskelparalyse. *Klin. Wochenschr*. 44:804–807, 1966.

Roses A.D., Harper P.S., Bossin E.H. Myotonic muscular dystrophy. In Vinken P.J., Bruyn G.W., Ringel S.P., eds. Diseases of Muscle. Part 2. *Handbook of Clinical Neurology*. Vol. 41. New York, Elsevier North Holland Biomedical Press, 1979.

*Rudel R., Lehmann-Horn F. Membrane changes in cells from myotonic patients. *Physiol. Rev*. 65:310–356, 1985.

Rudel R., Senges J. Experimental myotonia in mammalian skeletal muscle. Changes in membrane properties. *Pfluegers Arch*. 331:324–334, 1972.

*Rudel R., Lehmann-Horn F., Ricker K., et al. Hypokalemic periodic paralysis: in vitro investigation of muscle fiber membrane parameters. *Muscle Nerve* 7:110–120, 1984.

Rudel R., Ruppersberg J.P., Spittelmeister W. Abnormalities of the fast sodium current in myotonic dystrophy, recessive generalized myotonia, and adynamia episodica. *Muscle Nerve* 12:281–287, 1989.

Ruff R.L., Simoncini L., Stuhmer W. Slow sodium channel inactivation in mammalian muscle: a possible role in regulating excitability. *Muscle Nerve* 11:502–510, 1988.

Schott G.D., McArdle B. Barium-induced skeletal muscle paralysis in the rat, and its relationship to human familial periodic paralysis. *J. Neurol. Neurosurg. Psychiatry* 37:32–39, 1974.

Seiler D., Fiehn W., Kuhn E. Disturbances in cholesterol biosynthesis as a cause of experimental myotonia. In Bradley W.D., ed. *Recent Advances in Myology*. Amsterdam, North Holland, pp. 429–433, 1974.

Steinert H. Myopathologische Beitrage: Uber das klinische und anatomische Bild des Muskelschwunds der Myotoniker. *Dtsch. Z. Nervenheilkd*. 37:58–104, 1909.

Swift L.L., Atkinson J.B., Lequire V.S. Composition and calcium-transport activity of the sarcoplasmic-reticulum from goats with and without heritable myotonia. *Lab. Invest*. 40:384–390, 1979.

Tahmoush A.J., Askanas V., Nelson P.G., et al. Electrophysiologic properties of aneurally cultured muscle from patients with myotonic muscular-atrophy. *Neurology (N.Y.)* 33:311–316, 1983.

Tang A.H., Schroeder L.A., Keasling H.H. U-23,223 (3-chloro-2,5,6-trimethylbenzoic acid), a veratrinic agent selective for the skeletal muscles. *Arch. Int. Pharmacodyn. Ther*. 175:319–329, 1968.

Thomsen J. Tonische Krämpfe in willkurlich beweglichen Muskeln in Folge von ererbter psychischer Disposition. *Arch. Psychiatr*. 6:702–718, 1876.

*Trimmer J.S., Cooperman S., Tomiko S., et al. Primary structure and functional expression of a mammalian skeletal muscle sodium channel. *Neuron* 3:33–49, 1989.

Valle R., Bryant S.H. Potassium conductance in myotonic and normal mammalian skeletal-muscle fibers. *Fed. Proc*. 39:2073, 1980.

White G.R., Plaskett J. "Nervous," "stiff-legged," or "fainting" goats. *Am. Vet. Rev*. 28:556–560, 1904.

Winer N., Martt J.M., Somers J.E., et al. Induced myotonia in man and goat. *J. Lab. Clin. Med*. 66:758–769, 1965.

Wood D.S., Lipicky R.J., Bryant S.H. Myotonic dystrophy: in vitro physiologic analysis of intact and skinned fibers. *Neurology (N.Y.)* 30:423, 1980.

14

Diseases of Striated Muscle

John A. Morgan-Hughes

Many human diseases alter the structure and function of skeletal muscle. In some, myopathy is but a minor facet of the overall clinical picture, whereas in others it is the major or exclusive presenting manifestation. This chapter is concerned largely with the latter group.

GENETIC MYOPATHIES

The Muscular Dystrophies

Muscular dystrophies are a heterogeneous group of genetically determined diseases that cause primary degeneration of skeletal muscle. The slow and selective decline in muscle strength so characteristic of these disorders is due to a gradual reduction in muscle cell mass, largely brought about through repeated episodes of segmental muscle fiber necrosis (Cullen and Mastaglia, 1980). Despite repair and regeneration, the necrotic process eventually leads to the virtual disappearance of muscle fibers and their replacement by fat cells embedded in a network of fibrous connective tissue. The altered or missing gene products primarily responsible for these changes remained elusive until 1987 when, through the use of reverse genetics, the Duchenne muscular dystrophy (DMD) gene and its encoded protein, dystrophin, were isolated and characterized (Hoffman et al., 1987; Koenig et al., 1987). Since then it has become evident that DMD and its allelic form, Becker's muscular dystrophy (BMD), as well as several newly recognized dystrophy phenotypes, are caused by genetic abnormalities of dystrophin, a large (427 kd) cytoskeletal protein located on the cytoplasmic face of the sarcolemmal membrane (Arahata et al., 1989; Koenig et al., 1988). Although

similar molecular genetic strategies are actively being applied to other muscular dystrophies and myotonic disorders and are narrowing the search for the abnormal genes (Wijmenga et al., 1990; Yamaoka et al., 1990), the biochemical defects underlying these disorders remain to be identified. Until this information becomes available, it is convenient to classify these diseases according to mode of inheritance (Table 14–1), age at onset, rate of progression, and pattern of muscle involvement.

X-Linked Dystrophies

Defects of Dystrophin

Duchenne's Muscular Dystrophy

This dystrophy is the most common X-linked recessive dystrophy, with an incidence of about 1 per 3500 live male births (Moser, 1984). It is caused by mutations in the dystrophin gene on the short arm of the X chromosome at p21 (Koenig et al., 1987, 1989). Most mutations resulting in DMD are dele-

Table 14–1. TYPES OF MUSCULAR DYSTROPHIES

X-linked recessive	Autosomal dominant
Defects of dystrophin	Facioscapulohumeral
DMD	Limb-girdle
BMD	Scapuloperoneal
Congenital	Distal
Quadriceps	Oculopharyngeal
Myalgia and cramps	
Defects unknown	
Emery-Dreifuss	
Scapuloperoneal	
Autosomal recessive	
Limb-girdle	
Scapulohumeral	
Pelvifemoral	
Childhood	
Congenital	

The author is grateful to the Muscular Dystrophy group of Great Britain, the Brain Research Trust, and the Wellcome Foundation for financial support.

tions, with breakpoints that in more than 90% of cases disrupt the translational reading frame of the encoded protein dystrophin (Gillard et al., 1989; Koenig et al., 1989). The presence of a frameshift deletion should lead to the synthesis of a truncated gene product, which being functionally incompetent, would be rapidly degraded. This scenario is consistent with the complete absence of dystrophin in DMD muscle when visualized by immunocytochemistry or immunoblotting, as demonstrated in Figure 14–1 (Arahata et al., 1989; Nicholson et al., 1990).

DMD is virtually confined to boys but is occasionally expressed in girls with the Turner syndrome or the Turner mosaic syndrome, a structural aberration of the X chromosome or a balanced X autosomal translocation (see Worton and Thompson, 1988). In all translocation cases, the breakpoint on the X chromosome has occurred within the DMD locus at Xp21. In these patients the normal X chromosome is preferentially inactivated, presumably because expression of the autosomal genes attached to the broken X is essential for survival. Preferential inactivation of the normal X chromosome also accounts for clinically manifesting female carriers who are heterozygous for the DMD mutation (Bonilla et al., 1990; Richards et al., 1990). The mutation rate for DMD, which is of the order of 1 per 10,000 per gene per generation, is higher than that in any other X-linked recessive disease and is currently thought to be equal in the male and female germ cells (Moser, 1984). The high mutation frequency, which accounts for about one-third of all cases, may reflect the enormous size of the dystrophin gene, which contains more than 70 exons and spans more than 2000 kilobase pairs of genomic DNA (Den Dunen et al., 1989; Koenig et al., 1987, 1988).

Although the earliest pathologic changes are evident in muscle taken at or before the 20th week of gestation (Fidziańska et al., 1984), the disease usually goes unnoticed until early childhood. Delayed motor development is common, and approximately half the patients are still unable to walk by the age of 18 months. Early features that are due to selective involvement of the pelvic girdle musculature include a waddling, lordotic gait; difficulties with running and with climbing stairs; and a tendency to fall frequently. When attempting to get up, the child initially has to push with a hand on one knee, but as the weakness progresses the child turns ·to the prone position and climbs up the legs, by using the Gowers maneuver. Weakness begins in the gluteal, iliopsoas, and quadriceps muscles of the lower limbs and the latissimus dorsi, deltoid, biceps, triceps, brachioradial, and pectoral muscles of the arms. As the disease advances, the weakness spreads to involve most muscle groups in the limbs and trunk, but calf, forearm, and hand muscles remain relatively spared (Emery, 1988; Hyser and Mendell, 1988). Weakness of the neck flexor muscles, with an inability to lift the head against gravity, occurs in almost all cases and may be one of the earliest features of the disease. Calf hypertrophy is almost invariable

(Fig. 14–2), and other muscles, such as the deltoid, the quadriceps of the thigh, the masseter, and the tongue, may also be enlarged. The limb reflexes are depressed or absent, except for the ankle jerks, which are the last to disappear.

Patients with DMD become wheelchair bound between the ages of 8 and 12 years. The later stages of the disease are characterized by the development of muscular contractures, progressive kyphoscoliosis, and increasing obesity or cachexia. Death occurs in the late teens or early 20s from respiratory insufficiency, cardiac failure, or both.

The mean IQ of patients with DMD is 15–20 points lower than that of the normal population, and about one-third of all patients have a significant but nonprogressive mental handicap (Hyser and Mendell, 1988). Cardiomyopathy occurs in all cases but rarely causes symptoms except in the terminal stages of the disease, when arrhythmias and congestive heart failure may occur. The electrocardiogram (ECG) shows tall R waves from the right-sided chest leads and deep Q waves from the limb and left-sided chest leads. The smooth muscle of the gastrointestinal tract may be affected in some cases and may cause bouts of abdominal pain and distention or, rarely, may lead to gastric dilatation (Hyser and Mendell, 1988). The serum creatine kinase (CK) activity is increased at birth and rises to extremely high values (up to 100 times normal) during the ambulant phase, but it later falls. The electromyogram (EMG) shows myopathy, and muscle biopsy shows hypercontracted fibers and groups of fibers undergoing segmental necrosis and phagocytosis. Striking proliferation of the endomysial connective tissue occurs in the later stages. Although the above-mentioned investigations, together with the clinical features and family history, are sufficient to establish the diagnosis in most cases, new diagnostic tests based on the molecular definition of DMD (see Fig. 14–1) are rapidly becoming incorporated into routine clinical use. These tests are briefly reviewed in a later section and are fully discussed by Beggs and Kunkel (1990).

Becker's Muscular Dystrophy

BMD is similar to DMD and is caused by mutations in the same dystrophin gene (Hoffman et al., 1989). As in DMD, most mutations are deletions, but unlike DMD the deletion breakpoints usually bring together exons that maintain the translational reading frame of the encoded protein (Koenig et al., 1989; Monaco et al., 1988). The presence of an in-frame deletion results in the synthesis of a partially functional dystrophin protein that is reduced in size, abundance, or both (Hoffman et al., 1987, 1989) (see Fig. 14–1*D*). In a few cases, duplications of the dystrophin gene result in the synthesis of a larger dystrophin protein.

BMD is less common than DMD, with an incidence of about 1 per 30,000 males, begins somewhat later in life, and runs a more benign clinical course (Hyser and Mendell, 1988; Walton and Gardner-Medwin,

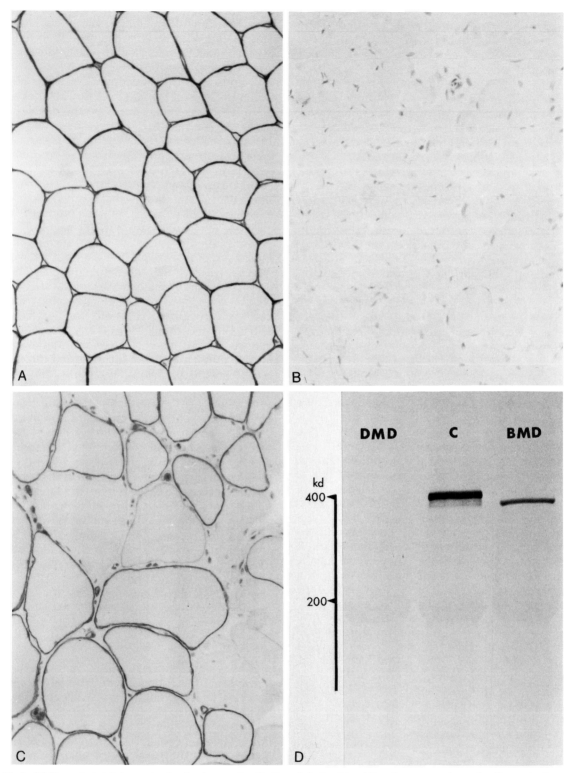

Figure 14–1. *(A)* Normal skeletal muscle showing immunolocalization of dystrophin at the plasma membrane in all muscle fibers. Indirect peroxidase technique, with a monoclonal antibody to dystrophin, followed by peroxidase-labeled rabbit antimouse immunoglobulins. × 250. *(B)* Skeletal muscle fibers in a patient with DMD show no labeling for dystrophin. Indirect peroxidase technique; a hematoxylin counterstain was used to show cell nuclei. × 250. *(C)* Manifesting carrier of DMD: a mosaic of dystrophin-positive and dystrophin-negative fibers is present. Indirect peroxidase technique. × 250. *(D)* Western blot of skeletal muscle from a normal control (C), a patient with DMD, and a patient with BMD. A monoclonal antibody to the COOH terminus of dystrophin was used. Normal control muscle shows a strong positive band at around 400 kd. No dystrophin is detectable in the muscle from the DMD patient. In the muscle from the BMD patient, a protein of reduced size and decreased abundance is present. (Courtesy of Louise Nicholson, M.D., and Margaret Johnson, M.D., Muscular Dystrophy Research Laboratories, Newcastle General Hospital, Newcastle-upon-Tyne, England.)

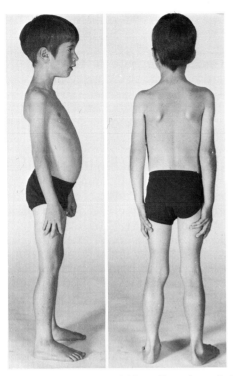

Figure 14–2. DMD in a 6-year-old boy. Note the typical lordotic posture, enlargement of the calves, and early winging of the scapulae.

1988). Most patients present between the ages of 5 and 20 years with pelvic girdle weakness associated with a waddling, lordotic gait and difficulties with running and with climbing stairs. As the disease progresses, the shoulder girdle muscles, biceps, triceps, brachioradial muscle, and neck flexors become involved. Calf hypertrophy is invariable and may antedate the onset of overt weakness (Fig. 14–3). As in DMD, other muscles may also be enlarged. Exertional myalgia and muscle cramps, sometimes associated with myoglobinuria, may be early features in some cases (Hoffman et al., 1989). Most patients remain ambulatory until the third or fourth decade of life, but a few become wheelchair bound in the middle teens and others retain the ability to walk until the sixth decade of life (England et al., 1990; Hoffman et al., 1989). Contractures, scoliosis, and respiratory insufficiency are less common than in DMD, and nonprogressive mental retardation occurs in only a minority of cases. Cardiomyopathy is also thought to be less common than in DMD, but arrhythmias, congestive heart failure, and significant ECG changes have been described (Hoffman et al., 1989; Hyser and Mendell, 1988).

As in DMD, the serum CK activity is markedly raised during the ambulant phase (20–50 higher than normal), the EMG shows myopathy, and the muscle biopsy specimen typically shows hypercontracted fibers, segmental myonecrosis with phagocytosis, and endomysial connective tissue proliferation in the later stages of the disease.

Atypical Duchenne's and Becker's Phenotypes

An absence of muscle dystrophin was demonstrated in three patients with a congenital muscular dystrophy of the Fukuyama type (Arahata et al., 1989; Arikawa et al., 1990). All three patients initially had weakness and evidence of cerebral disease in infancy and had delayed developmental milestones. Dystrophin was normal, however, in a number of other reported cases with Fukuyama congenital muscular dystrophy (Arahata et al., 1988c, 1989).

Gospe et al. (1989) described a family with an X-linked recessive myopathy that was characterized by myalgia, muscle cramps, and calf hypertrophy without muscular weakness. There were nine affected male members from two generations, with ages ranging from 4 to 33 years. Symptoms began in childhood but did not worsen. Cramping occurred at rest as well as during exertion, and one patient was said to have had an episode of pigmenturia. All affected members had a high resting serum CK value, and EMG studies performed for four patients showed normal results in two and myopathic results in two. Muscle biopsy samples for three patients showed nonspecific myopathic changes, but necrotic fibers were not observed. DNA analysis identified a deletion in the first third of the dystrophin gene, and immunoblots of muscle showed a normal amount of abnormally small dystrophin protein.

Dystrophin abnormalities of the BMD type have also been described in four unrelated men who presented with quadriceps myopathy, which in three

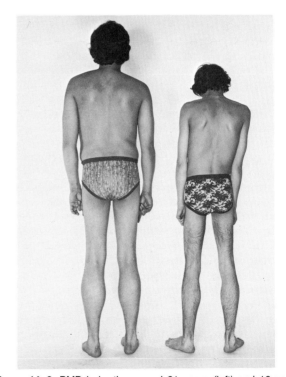

Figure 14–3. BMD in brothers aged 21 years *(left)* and 16 years *(right)*. Note the enlarged calves and early winging of the scapulae.

patients was associated with enlargement of the calves. Two of these patients had cardiomyopathy (dilated heart). All four patients had deletions in the dystrophin gene and reduced amounts of an abnormally small dystrophin protein.

Molecular Genetics and Pathogenesis

Dystrophin is 3685 amino acids long and has a predicted molecular size of 427 kd (Koenig et al., 1988). The NH_2- and COOH-terminal domains are bridged by a large rod domain containing 24 repeat segments, followed by a 280-amino-acid cysteine-rich segment (Koenig et al., 1988, 1990). Dystrophin is most abundant in skeletal and cardiac muscle, but it constitutes only a minute amount (less than 0.01%) of the total muscle protein. It is also a normal component of all myogenic cells and is present in other tissues, including the brain (Hoffman et al., 1987). The brain dystrophin isoform, however, is transcribed from a specific promoter that is different from the one used in muscle (Chelly et al., 1990).

Of patients with DMD or BMD, 65% have deletions, or less commonly, insertions, which can be detected by Southern blotting and by multiplex polymerase chain reaction amplification of candidate exon subsets (Beggs and Kunkel, 1990). Most cases (92%) conform to the reading frame rule, that is, frameshift deletions or duplications result in DMD and in-frame deletions (or duplications) result in BMD. Exceptions to this rule have been described, particularly in cases with deletions involving exons 3 to 7 (Baumbach et al., 1989; Gillard et al., 1989; Malhotra et al., 1988). Various mechanisms have been proposed to explain the occurrence of the milder Becker's phenotype in some patients with frameshift deletions (Gillard et al., 1989; Koenig et al., 1989; Malhotra et al., 1988). They include (1) creation of an in-frame message by splicing out exons flanking the deletion; (2) inclusion of intron sequences; (3) the presence of dual promoters; (4) creation of a new in-frame translational start site; and (5) partial compensation for the defect by dystrophin-related proteins, such as the one encoded on chromosome 6 (Love et al., 1989).

The relative importance of the different dystrophin domains with respect to disease phenotype has also been examined in a large series of patients (Koenig et al., 1989). On the basis of the assumption that dystrophin is synthesized as predicted by the reading frame rule, deletions within the NH_2-terminal domain or within the first 13 or last 8 repeats of the rod domain usually result in BMD. Deletions involving the cysteine-rich segment and the first half of the COOH-terminal domain usually result in DMD. The presence of a specific brain-type promoter that is different from the one used in muscle raises the interesting possibility that certain mutations of the dystrophin gene may affect IQ more than do other mutations. So far, however, no clear correlations between IQ and deletion type have emerged (Gillard et al., 1989).

The mechanism of segmental myonecrosis in dystrophies caused by mutations of the dystrophin gene remains to be determined. Structural similarities to α-actinin and spectrin suggest that dystrophin functions as a component of the membrane cytoskeleton (Koenig et al., 1988). This proposal is consistent with its localization to the cytoplasmic face of the sarcolemmal membrane in normal skeletal muscle. The observations that dystrophin forms tight complexes with several sarcolemmal glycoproteins and that at least one of these is markedly deficient in DMD muscle suggest that dystrophin may play a crucial role in anchoring the myofiber membrane to the underlying components of the cytoskeleton (Ervasti et al., 1990). The absence of dystrophin, as in DMD, or the presence of a functionally abnormal dystrophin protein, as in BMD, could render the sarcolemmal membrane more susceptible to contraction-induced damage. This damage could lead to myonecrosis through an influx of ionic calcium and an activation of calcium-dependent endogenous proteases. Such a mechanism would be consistent with an already large body of evidence pointing to a primary abnormality of the muscle fiber membrane in DMD and BMD (see Engel, 1986b).

Prevention

Carrier detection and prenatal diagnosis are currently the only means of preventing DMD and BMD, but this situation may change as a result of myoblast transplantation or gene therapy. Traditional methods of carrier detection and prenatal diagnosis have been superseded by DNA analysis and dystrophin screening. The merits and limitations of these new molecular tests are fully discussed elsewhere (Beggs and Kunkel, 1990) and are mentioned only briefly here.

In patients with detectable deletions (65% of cases), the diagnosis can be established by Southern blotting and multiplex polymerase chain reaction analysis. These techniques can also be applied to carrier detection and to prenatal diagnosis by using amniotic fluid cells or chorionic villus biopsy. The accuracy of DNA analysis for carrier detection is limited by the gene dosage effect (carriers have one normal copy of the dystrophin gene) and by the fact that 35% of cases harbor mutations that are not detectable by current assays. Because of the high mutation rate, prenatal diagnosis should be performed for mothers who are not detectable carriers to exclude germline mosaicism (Baker et al., 1989). In families without a detectable mutation, carrier detection must rely on linkage studies that utilize Southern blotting and polymerase chain reaction–based assays with probes that recognize restriction fragment length polymorphisms within and flanking the dystrophin gene.

Dystrophin screening is assuming greater importance in carrier detection. Biopsied muscle from a manifesting or nonmanifesting carrier may show a mosaic of dystrophin-positive and dystrophin-negative fibers depending on whether the normal or abnormal X chromosome is inactivated. The sensitivity of dystrophin screening for carrier detection can be enhanced by examining cloned myoblast cultures (Hurko et al., 1989).

Defects Unknown

Benign X-Linked Dystrophy with Early Contractures (the Emery-Dreifuss Dystrophy)

This rare form of X-linked dystrophy begins before the age of 10 years and runs a benign clinical course compatible with survival well into middle age (Emery, 1982; Rowland et al., 1979). It is characterized by slowly progressive proximal weakness beginning in the pelvic girdle musculature, cardiac abnormalities, and the presence of early flexion contractures at the elbows and shortening of the heel cords. Lower facial weakness is common, and cardiac involvement with arrhythmias and sudden death have been reported. The early contractures, facial weakness, and absence of muscular hypertrophy distinguish this disorder from BMD. The serum CK activity is moderately elevated, and myopathic changes have been demonstrated by EMG and muscle biopsy examination. The serum CK activity is elevated in about 50% of female carriers. The gene for the X-linked form has been mapped to the distal part of the long arm of chromosome X at Xq28 (Hodgson et al., 1986). An autosomal recessive variant of the Emery-Dreifuss muscular dystrophy has also been described (Takamoto et al., 1984).

X-Linked Scapuloperoneal Muscular Dystrophy

This disorder is similar to if not identical with the Emery-Dreifuss dystrophy (Thomas et al., 1972). In this disorder, however, the wasting and weakness typically involve the proximal muscles of the upper limbs and the anterior tibial and peroneal groups in the legs. The disease begins during the first decade of life, runs a slowly progressive course, and is associated with early contractures of the posterior cervical muscles, the elbow flexors, and the calves. Cardiac abnormalities including arrhythmias and sudden death have been reported. Serum CK activity is moderately elevated, the EMG has myopathic changes, and the muscle biopsy sample shows variation in muscle fiber size and occasional necrotic fibers.

Autosomal Recessive Muscular Dystrophies

Limb-Girdle Dystrophy

Limb-girdle dystrophy is a term that probably encompasses a number of different recessively inherited myopathies that manifest with slowly progressive proximal weakness, usually in the second to the fourth decades of life (Walton and Gardner-Medwin, 1981). In the scapulohumeral form, weakness and wasting may remain confined to the scapular and upper arm muscles for many years before eventually spreading to involve the proximal muscles of the lower limbs. Winging of the scapulae and difficulty in raising the arms above the head are early features related to selective involvement of the upper trapezius, rhomboids, and anterior serratus. The neck flexors, biceps, triceps, and brachioradial muscle are also affected early, but the deltoid and forearm muscles are relatively spared and may appear to be enlarged because of atrophy of adjacent muscles.

The pelvifemoral form presents with difficulties in climbing stairs and getting out of a low chair, related to early weakness of the iliopsoas, glutei, and quadriceps femoris. Most patients develop weakness of the scapulohumeral muscles. Both forms of the disease run a slowly progressive course that usually leads to severe disability between the fourth and sixth decades of life. Apart from sternomastoid weakness, the cranial muscles are spared, intellect is normal, and the heart is usually unaffected. The limb reflexes may be obtainable until quite late.

The serum CK activity is moderately elevated, the EMG indicates myopathy, and the muscle biopsy sample shows nonspecific dystrophic changes with hypertrophied fibers, internal nucleation, connective tissue proliferation, and occasional myonecrosis. The differential diagnosis includes spinal muscular atrophy, acid maltase deficiency, chronic polymyositis, nemaline myopathy, and clinically manifesting carriers of the dystrophin gene.

Childhood Muscular Dystrophy

This disorder closely resembles DMD but affects both sexes and runs a somewhat more benign clinical course. The disease usually is first seen in early childhood, and most patients become wheelchair bound during the second or third decades of life. Mild facial weakness is common, and there may be hypertrophy of the calves and other muscles. The serum CK activity is markedly elevated, and the EMG and muscle biopsy findings are similar to those seen in DMD.

The Congenital Muscular Dystrophies

This heterogeneous group of myopathies begins in the neonatal period with generalized hypotonic weakness often associated with widespread muscular contractures (Fukuyama and Osawa, 1982; McMenamin et al., 1982). There is often a history of reduced fetal movements, and major feeding and breathing difficulties may become apparent soon after birth. Facial weakness is common, but mental development is usually normal and cardiac abnormalities are rare. The clinical course is highly variable and sometimes leads to death from ventilatory insufficiency in infancy or early childhood. The majority of patients survive infancy, but some remain severely disabled and unable to walk or stand without support. Others, however, eventually become ambulant and may lead a relatively independent existence. The serum CK activity is raised, particularly in the early stages, the EMG has myopathic alterations, and the muscle biopsy changes resemble those seen in progressive muscular dystrophy. The frequent occurrence of congenital muscular dystrophy in siblings indicates autosomal recessive inheritance.

Several clinical variants have been described, including the Fukuyama type of congenital muscular dystrophy, which is rare outside Japan and is associated with severe mental retardation, seizures, diffuse muscle wasting, weakness, and widespread muscular contractures (Fukuyama and Osawa, 1982). Although improvement may occur in early childhood, most patients die during the first decade of life. Histologic studies show dystrophic changes in muscle and diffuse micropolygyria of the cerebral cortex, hypoplasia of the cerebellar vermis, ventricular dilatation, and thickening of the leptomeninges (Fukuyama et al., 1981).

A further clinical subgroup of patients with congenital muscular dystrophy is the so-called muscle, eye, and brain disease described by Santavuori et al. in 1978. In addition to having mental retardation and hypotonic weakness, these patients show prominent ocular changes, including extreme myopia, glaucoma, hypoplasia of the retina and optic nerve, and mature cataracts (Korinthenberg et al., 1984). Fukuyama's congenital muscular dystrophy and muscle, eye, and brain disease are inherited as autosomal recessive traits.

Autosomal Dominant Muscular Dystrophies

Facioscapulohumeral Dystrophy

Facioscapulohumeral (FSH) dystrophy is the most common dominantly inherited dystrophy, with an incidence of 0.5–5.0 per 100,000. Penetrance is virtually complete, but phenotypic expression is highly variable, even in the same pedigree, and sometimes the disease goes unnoticed throughout life (Walton and Gardner-Medwin, 1981). Onset in infancy or early childhood heralds a poor prognosis and usually leads to severe disability by the second or third decade. Most cases present in the late teens or early 20s, but there may have been a lifelong inability to whistle or blow up a balloon and a tendency to sleep with the eyes half open. Profound facial weakness is an early feature of the disease and causes pouting of the lips and a transverse smile. The pattern of limb muscle involvement is similar to that of the scapulohumeral form of limb-girdle dystrophy, but as the disease progresses weakness spreads to the pelvic girdle musculature and to the anterior tibial and

peroneal groups. Winging of the scapulae is an early feature and is associated with difficulty in lifting the arms above the head. The deltoid muscles are relatively spared, and when the patient attempts to abduct the arms, the scapulae typically ride up the posterior chest wall to become visible from the front (Fig. 14–4). The calves, deltoids, and levator scapulae may be enlarged. Progression of disease is associated with increasing lumbar lordosis and bilateral footdrop, which gives rise to a waddling, high-stepping gait. The long forearm extensor muscles are commonly affected in the later stages. Except for early-onset cases, FSH dystrophy rarely leads to severe disability before the fourth or fifth decades of life and is compatible with a relatively normal life span.

Early-onset FSH dystrophy has occasionally been reported in association with sensorineural deafness (Korf et al., 1985), with or without retinal vascular changes resembling Coats' syndrome (Taylor et al., 1982). The vascular changes include retinal telangiectasis and exudation, sometimes leading to retinal detachment and visual loss. A fluorescein study of a large group of unselected patients with FSH dystrophy indicates, however, that telangiectasis and retinal exudation are more common than has been previously supposed (Fitzsimons et al., 1987). Fifty-six of 75 patients with FSH dystrophy showed telangiectasis, sometimes accompanied by retinal exudation (Fig. 14–5), but only 2 had significant visual loss.

The serum CK activity may be normal or only slightly elevated, the EMG is normal or shows my-

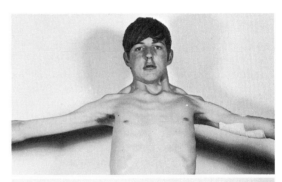

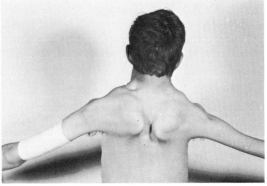

Figure 14–4. FSH dystrophy in a 16-year-old boy. Note the myopathic facies and elevation of the scapulae on abduction of the arms.

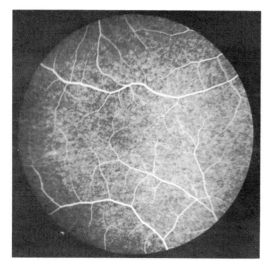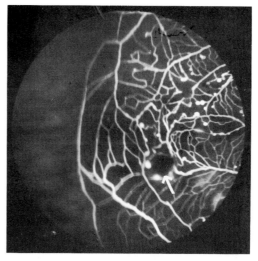

Figure 14–5. Fluorescein angiograms of the temporal periphery of the right retina from a control subject *(left)* and from a patient with FSH dystrophy *(right)*. The patient's angiogram shows capillary closure on the left of the picture and telangiectasis and fluorescein leakage on the right. A small hemorrhage *(arrow)* obscures the underlying choroidal circulation. (Courtesy of Dr. R. Fitzsimons, Institute of Neurology, Queen Square, London.)

opathy, and muscle biopsy gives evidence of mild dystrophic changes typically associated with atrophic angulated muscle fibers. A marked inflammatory exudate resembling that seen in polymyositis occurs in some cases. The differential diagnosis includes FSH forms of spinal muscular atrophy, centronuclear myopathy, congenital myasthenic syndromes, mitochondrial myopathy, and inclusion body myositis. The gene for FSH dystrophy has been mapped to chromosome 4 (Wijmenga et al., 1990).

Late-Onset Autosomal Dominant Limb-Girdle Dystrophy

A few families with a dominantly inherited limb-girdle dystrophy have been described (Chukow et al., 1986; Gilchrist et al., 1988). The weakness typically begins in the proximal muscles of the lower limbs but slowly spreads to involve the deltoids, biceps, and triceps in the upper limbs. Mild distal weakness may also occur. Onset is usually in the third or fourth decade of life. The absence of facial weakness and winging of the scapulae distinguishes this disorder from FSH dystrophy. The serum CK activity may be moderately increased, the EMG demonstrates myopathy, and muscle biopsy results show nonspecific myopathic changes, sometimes associated with vacuoles and lobulated ("moth-eaten") fibers. The disorder is slowly progressive and may lead to loss of ambulation in later life.

Autosomal Dominant Scapuloperoneal Myopathy

This rare disorder typically begins in adult life with footdrop related to early involvement of the anterior tibial and peroneal groups (Thomas et al., 1975). The short extensor muscle of the toes is characteristically

spared and may be hypertrophied, a feature that distinguishes this condition from neurogenic forms of scapuloperoneal weakness. The weakness in the upper limbs usually begins in the scapular muscles and may spread to involve the deltoids, biceps, and triceps. The disease runs a benign course and is rarely associated with severe disability. Mild facial and sternomastoid weakness occurs in some cases. The serum CK activity is usually elevated, the EMG presents myopathy, and muscle biopsy results show nonspecific myopathic changes.

Distal Myopathy of Welander

This myopathy is rare outside Sweden and is seen initially either in childhood or in adult life with slowly progressive, predominantly distal wasting and weakness (Markesbery et al., 1977). The serum CK activity may be normal or mildly elevated, and the EMG indicates myopathy with spontaneous discharges. A variety of changes as seen on muscle biopsy samples evidence primary muscle disease. Necrotic fibers have been described in some cases, and in others the fibers have contained rimmed vacuoles (Markesbery and Griggs, 1986).

Oculopharyngeal Muscular Dystrophy

This dominantly inherited disorder typically begins in adult life with ptosis and extraocular weakness, usually without significant diplopia (Victor et al., 1962). Dysphagia is a prominent symptom in some cases. The face and sternomastoid muscles are frequently affected, and most patients develop weakness in the limbs. The serum CK activity is usually elevated, the EMG indicates myopathy, and the muscle biopsy sample shows rimmed vacuoles in a proportion of the muscle fibers.

Myotonic Disorders

Myotonic Dystrophy

Myotonic dystrophy (MyD) is a dominantly inherited multisystem disease with an incidence of 4–5 per 100,000. The genetic locus for MyD is on the long arm of chromosome 19 at q13.2-q13.3 (Yamaoka et al., 1990). Penetrance is virtually complete, but expression is highly variable and sometimes the disease remains asymptomatic throughout life (Harper, 1979). Occasionally, MyD presents in the neonatal period with ptosis, facial weakness, profound generalized hypotonia, feeding and breathing difficulties, and mental retardation. Myotonia is absent clinically but can usually be detected on the EMG. Patients with early-onset disease who survive infancy tend to improve during childhood and adolescence but later follow the typical downhill clinical course. In congenital cases, the mother is almost invariably the affected parent, which suggests that some unknown maternal factor may determine the early onset of the disease (Harper, 1979).

MyD more commonly is first noted in adult life with vague symptoms that may be more related to mental apathy and personality change than to muscular weakness. Most patients admit to weakness of grip, with difficulty in letting go, and some complain of a tendency to fall. Other presenting symptoms include poor vision related to ptosis or cataracts, impotence caused by testicular atrophy, loss of libido, dysphagia, syncopal episodes sometimes related to cardiac arrhythmias, and excessive sweating. The disease is easily recognized in the outpatient clinic. Patients are often of below-average intelligence; are apathetic; and have a haggard appearance because of the combination of frontal baldness, ptosis, facial weakness, and striking atrophy of the temporal, masseter, and sternomastoid muscles (Fig. 14–6). The lower jaw tends to sag, and the speech is slurred because of weakness and myotonia of the tongue. Weakness and wasting in the limbs are predominantly distal in distribution and mainly affect the muscles of the forearms, hands, calves, and anterior tibial and peroneal groups. Myotonia can be demonstrated by percussion of the tongue or thenar muscles or by asking the patient to open and close the fist. The disease is slowly progressive, most patients becoming severely disabled and unable to walk by the fourth or fifth decade of life. Death occurs before the expected normal age from cardiac failure, a fatal arrhythmia, or pulmonary hypoventilation caused by severe weakness of the diaphragm and intercostal muscles.

Virtually all patients develop posterior subcapsular cataracts that may require extraction. Cardiac conduction defects occur in 70% of patients and may lead to syncope or sudden death. Characteristic endocrine abnormalities include testicular atrophy with unresponsiveness to follicle-stimulating hormone, failure of adrenal androgenic function, and insulin

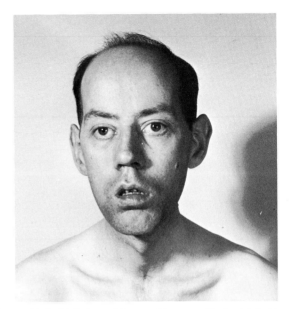

Figure 14–6. MyD in a 32-year-old man with frontal baldness, sagging of the jaw, and atrophy of the temporal, masseter, and sternomastoid muscles.

resistance with hyperinsulinemia in response to a glucose load (Moxley et al., 1984). Approximately one-third of patients have a low IQ and an abnormal personality (Bird et al., 1983).

The serum CK activity is normal or only slightly increased, the EMG shows myopathy with myotonic discharges, and the muscle biopsy sample typically shows chains of central nuclei, ring fibers, and selective atrophy of the type 1 muscle fibers. Plasma immunoglobulin G levels are low because of hypercatabolism of this immunoglobulin. MyD is thought to be due to a generalized membrane abnormality, but the product of the defective gene has not been identified. The myotonia may be related to a disturbance of the membrane potassium ion conductance system (Merickel et al., 1981) (also see Chapter 13).

Autosomal Dominant Myotonia Congenita (Thomsen's Disease)

Thomsen's disease typically begins in infancy or early childhood with widespread myotonia and diffuse muscular hypertrophy without significant weakness. The myotonia is generalized, is accentuated by rest and cold, and tends to wear off during muscular activity. Affected children need to warm up before participating in vigorous exercise or they may fall. Muscular hypertrophy persists throughout life, but myotonia tends to diminish with age. Physiologic studies suggest that the myotonia in Thomsen's disease may be due to decreased membrane conductance to chloride ions (Barchi, 1975, 1982).

Autosomal Recessive Myotonia Congenita (Becker's Type)

This disorder is somewhat similar to Thomsen's disease but is seen rather later in childhood and is often associated with distal weakness that is usually nonprogressive.

Paramyotonia Congenita of Eulenburg

This dominantly inherited disease is characterized by generalized myotonia that is induced or exacerbated by exposure to cold. Some patients also develop episodes of focal or generalized flaccid weakness similar to those seen in hyperkalemic periodic paralysis, although in these patients the serum potassium level remains normal. Physiologic studies suggest that the myotonia and the weakness in this condition may be due to a temperature-dependent abnormality of the sodium conductance pathway in the muscle membrane (Lehmann-Horn et al., 1981). Lowering the temperature of the muscle causes an increase in sodium ion permeability and progressive membrane depolarization. As depolarization proceeds, hyperexcitability and myotonia give way to paralysis. (See Chapter 13.)

Specific Congenital Myopathies

These disorders typically begin with hypotonic weakness in infancy or early childhood, but late-onset cases have been described (Fardeau, 1982). There may be a history of reduced fetal movements, and motor milestones are often somewhat delayed, but walking is usually achieved between the ages of 2 and 4 years. The weakness may improve during childhood and adolescence but may later worsen. Muscle bulk is reduced but focal wasting is unusual. Minor skeletal deformities and congenital hip dislocation are common. The diagnosis depends on the muscle biopsy appearances.

Central Core Disease

This disease was first described by Shy and Magee (1956) and is characterized by the presence of one or more cores that run axially along the length of the muscle fibers (Fig. 14–7). The cores lack mitochondria and contain tightly packed myofilaments that show varying degrees of disorganization. Cores are confined to the histochemical type 1 fibers, which are the predominant and sometimes the only fiber type present in the biopsied sample. Severe disability is exceptional and the disease is usually compatible with a normal ambulant life. Minor skeletal deformities and congenital hip dislocation are relatively common. Malignant hyperthermia that follows general anesthesia has been reported in several cases (Frank et al., 1980). Eleven of 13 patients described by Shuaib et al. (1987) were considered to be at risk for malignant hyperthermia on the basis of the in vitro contracture test.

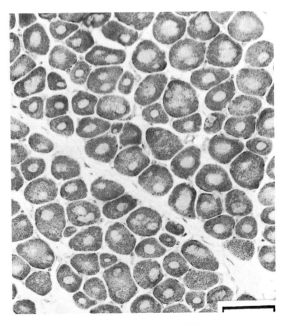

Figure 14–7. Transverse section of the left biceps from an 8-year-old girl with central core disease. The succinate dehydrogenase reaction shows the presence of one or more cores in the majority of fibers. Scale = 100 μm.

Multicore Disease

Multicore disease is thought to be a distinct nosological entity characterized by small focal areas of myofibrillar disorganization on muscle biopsy. The clinical features are somewhat similar to those of central core disease, but the mode of inheritance is different. Unlike central core disease, the extraocular muscles are sometimes involved.

Nemaline Myopathy

Nemaline myopathy is characterized by the presence of peripheral collections of rod-shaped bodies in a variable proportion of the muscle fibers (Fig. 14–8). The rods are best seen in sections stained with the modified Gomori's trichrome stain. At an ultrastructural level, the rods show a periodicity similar to that of the Z bands from which they are thought to be derived (see Fig. 14–8).

Three main types of nemaline myopathy have been described (Banker, 1986; Martinez and Lake, 1987). The severe neonatal form is characterized by dysmorphic features, profound generalized hypotonic weakness, and a fatal outcome, usually before the age of 2 years. Inheritance is thought to be autosomal recessive. In the more benign early-onset form, which is often associated with dysmorphic features, the weakness may remain static during childhood or adolescence but may later progress to cause respiratory insufficiency in the third or fourth decade of life. Inheritance is uncertain but may be autosomal dominant in some cases. In the adult-onset form, which is almost always sporadic and is not associated with dysmorphic features, the weakness is usually

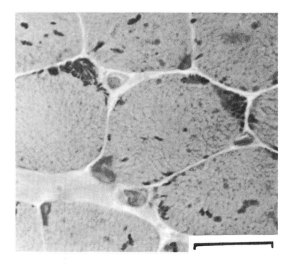

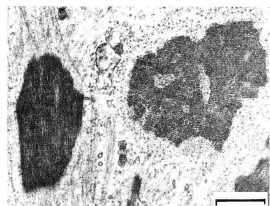

Figure 14–8. Nemaline myopathy in an 8-year-old boy. *(Top)* Modified Gomori's trichrome stain to show collections of rods at the periphery of the muscle fibers. Scale = 25 μm. *(Bottom)* Electron micrograph showing longitudinal *(left)* and transverse *(right)* views of the rods. Note the lattice-like appearance of the rods in transverse section. Scale = 0.5 μm. (Courtesy of Dr. D.N. Landon, Institute of Neurology, Queen Square, London.)

progressive and may lead to severe disability. Facial and sternomastoid weakness is common, and cardiomyopathy may also occur.

Centronuclear Myopathy

This disorder also exists in several different forms. Early-onset cases typically begin in the neonatal period with ptosis, limitation of eye movements, facial weakness, and generalized hypotonia. Motor milestones are delayed, and the weakness may progress in childhood or early adolescence and lead to severe disability in the second or third decade of life. A severe X-linked form of centronuclear myopathy, with a high mortality during the neonatal period, especially in affected males, has also been described (Barth et al., 1975). These cases also show ptosis, limitation of eye movements, and contractures. Patients who survive infancy may show some improvement during childhood and adolescence.

Late-onset centronuclear myopathy manifests with

proximal limb girdle weakness, usually without ptosis or extraocular involvement. The weakness is usually progressive and may lead to severe disability in the fourth or fifth decade. Muscle biopsy samples in all forms of centronuclear myopathy show chains of central nuclei that are typically surrounded by a clear zone that is devoid of myofibrillar ATPase activity. These appearances resemble myotubes. In some cases the type 1 fibers are small and the type 2 fibers are either normal or enlarged.

Congenital Fiber Type Disproportion

This relatively benign congenital myopathy is associated with abnormally small type 1 muscle fibers. The condition manifests with hypotonic weakness in the neonatal period, often associated with contractures and mild skeletal abnormalities, including congenital hip dislocation. Motor milestones are delayed, but the weakness may improve during childhood and adolescence. A severe form of the disorder, with death from respiratory insufficiency, has also been described (Fardeau, 1982). Other congenital myopathies with specific morphologic features have been

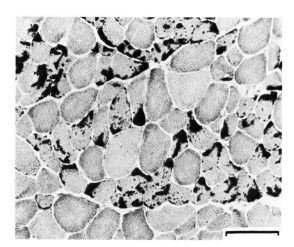

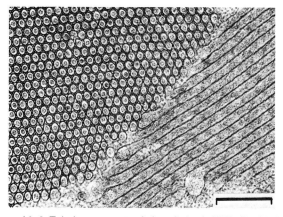

Figure 14–9. Tubular aggregates in hypokalemic FPP. *(Top)* NADH-tetrazolium reductase preparation showing densely staining areas, mainly at the periphery of the type 2 fibers. Scale = 100 μm. *(Bottom)* Electron micrograph showing component tubules in longitudinal *(right)* and transverse *(left)* section. Scale = 1 μm. (Courtesy of Dr. D.N. Landon, Institute of Neurology, Queen Square, London.)

described in isolated cases. They include fingerprint body myopathy, reducing body myopathy, zebra body myopathy, and sarcotubular myopathy. These disorders have been extensively reviewed by Fardeau (1982) and Banker (1986).

The Familial Periodic Paralyses

The familial periodic paralyses (FPPs) are dominantly inherited diseases that manifest with recurrent episodes of flaccid, areflexic weakness caused by partial depolarization and loss of excitability of the muscle plasma membrane (Layzer, 1984). They are classified as hypokalemic, normokalemic, and hyperkalemic on the basis of the serum potassium level at the time of an attack. Although the molecular events leading to membrane depolarization and inexcitability are probably different in the three forms, they share many common features (Table 14–2) (see also Chapter 13).

Muscle biopsy in all three types of FPP may show vacuolar changes and tubular aggregates (Fig. 14–9).

Hypokalemic Form

Hypokalemic FPP is more common in males and usually presents in the first or second decade of life. The attacks of adynamia vary both in frequency and in severity and may disappear in later life. The weakness typically comes on during sleep after unaccustomed physical activity, a large meal, or both. It begins in the trunk and proximal muscles and then spreads distally. The cranial and respiratory muscles are rarely affected. Tendon reflexes are depressed or absent at the height of the attack, and paralyzed

muscles are electrically inexcitable. Studies suggest that loss of excitability of the muscle membrane may be due to an increased sodium conductance (Rudel et al., 1984). Strength usually returns within a few hours, but slight residual weakness may persist for several days. Mild attacks can sometimes be aborted by gentle exercise. Fixed proximal weakness may develop later in life.

During an attack there is a shift of potassium, sodium, and chloride ions into the muscle and a lowering of the serum potassium level. The urinary excretion of these ions and water also falls. The ECG may show changes of hypokalemia with U waves, reduced or flattened T waves, and ST depression.

Provocative tests should be carefully monitored and avoided in the presence of weakness or hypokalemia. They include oral glucose (50–100 g) or sodium chloride (2–4 g) loading followed by vigorous exercise for 15–20 minutes. Soluble insulin (10–20 IU subcutaneously) with an oral glucose load increases the chances of provoking an attack. The weakness usually responds to 2–4 g potassium chloride given orally. Prophylaxis includes a low-sodium diet containing less than 60 mEq/day and avoidance of large meals, cold, and emotional stress. Acetazolamide, 250 mg three times daily, or chlorothiazide, 500 mg daily, may help to prevent attacks in patients unable to adhere to a low-sodium diet.

Hyperkalemic Form

This disorder occurs with equal frequency in both sexes and usually appears before the age of 10 years. Attacks are precipitated by rest after exercise, exposure to cold, emotional stress, or missing a meal. Gentle exercise or a light carbohydrate meal may

Table 14–2. FAMILIAL PERIODIC PARALYSES

Parameter	Hypokalemic Form	Hyperkalemic Form	Normokalemic Form
Inheritance	Autosomal dominant	Autosomal dominant	Autosomal dominant
Male/female ratio	2:1	1:1	1:1
Age at onset	First or second decade	First decade	First decade
Type of paralysis	Usually generalized	Focal or generalized	Usually generalized
Onset	During sleep	Variable	During sleep
Muscles affected	Limbs and trunk	Limbs and trunk	Limbs and trunk
Duration	Hours or days	Minutes or hours	Usually days
Tendon reflexes	Diminished or absent	Diminished or absent	Diminished or absent
Precipitating factors	Rest after exercise, a high carbohydrate or sodium intake, alcohol, cold, emotional stress	Rest after exercise, fasting, high potassium intake, cold, emotional stress	Rest after exercise, alcohol, cold, emotional stress
Provocative tests	Glucose ± insulin, sodium chloride, glucocorticoids, epinephrine	Potassium chloride	Potassium chloride
Response to electrical stimulation	Diminished or absent	Diminished or absent	Diminished or absent
Treatment of attacks	Salt restriction, potassium chloride	Calcium gluconate	Sodium chloride
Prophylaxis	Salt restriction, acetazolamide or chlorothiazide	Acetazolamide or chlorothiazide	Acetazolamide
Myopathology	Vacuolated fibers, tubular aggregates	Vacuolated fibers, tubular aggregates	Vacuolated fibers, tubular aggregates

stave off an attack. As in hypokalemic FPP, the tendon reflexes are diminished or absent and paralyzed muscles are electrically inexcitable because of partial depolarization of the muscle fiber membrane (Lehmann-Horn et al., 1981). The attacks of paralysis are usually briefer than those in the hypokalemic form and often less severe. Myotonia of the eyelids, face, tongue, and thenar and other muscles, which is exacerbated by the cold, can be elicited both during and between attacks of paralysis in some, but not all, cases. The myotonic form of hyperkalemic periodic paralysis is similar to if not identical with paramyotonia congenita. As in other forms of FPP, mild fixed weakness may develop later in life. During an attack, potassium moves out of the muscle cells, and the serum potassium level rises but not necessarily to abnormal values. The renal excretion of potassium, sodium, and water increases. The ECG may show increased T wave amplitude in the precordial leads.

Weakness may be provoked by orally administered potassium chloride given in a dose of 2 g and repeated every 2 hours for up to four doses. The patient should be carefully observed with continuous ECG monitoring and repeated serum electrolyte estimations. The tests should not be undertaken in the presence of weakness, hyperkalemia, or impaired renal function. Prophylaxis includes avoidance of precipitating factors and if necessary acetazolamide or chlorothiazide by mouth.

Normokalemic FPP

This form is rare, and its existence as a distinct nosologic entity remains in some doubt. In most respects, reported cases have been similar to the hyperkalemic type, except that the serum potassium level remains normal during an attack (Poskanzer and Kerr, 1961). As in the hyperkalemic variety, attacks of weakness can be provoked by rest after exercise, exposure to cold, and potassium loading.

Other Causes of Periodic Paralysis

Thyrotoxic Hypokalemic Periodic Paralysis

This sporadic disorder is largely but not exclusively confined to Asian males who appear to be genetically predisposed to this complication of thyroid overactivity (Yeo et al., 1978). The attacks of paralysis are virtually indistinguishable from those occurring in hypokalemic FPP, except that they rarely occur before the third or fourth decade of life. As in the familial form, paralyzed muscles are electrically inexcitable, possibly because of increased activity of the sodium-potassium pump (Layzer, 1984). Attacks of paralysis are abolished by treatment of the thyrotoxicosis but may recur unless the euthyroid state is maintained.

Secondary Hypokalemic Periodic Paralysis

This condition may occur in a variety of situations, including primary hyperaldosteronism, excessive thiazide therapy, renal tubular acidosis, and disorders that cause a loss of potassium from the gastrointestinal tract (see Engel, 1981). Secondary hyperkalemic periodic paralysis occurs in chronic renal or adrenal insufficiency (Engel, 1981).

METABOLIC MYOPATHIES

Except for acid maltase deficiency, defects of muscle metabolism that have been identified biochemically involve key reactions in the pathways of muscle energy production (Morgan-Hughes, 1982). They can be divided into two groups, according to whether the biochemical error is cytosolic or involves the processes of oxidative metabolism, which take place exclusively within the mitochondrial inner membrane and matrix space (see also Chapter 12).

Cytosolic (and Lysosomal) Deficiencies

These disorders are given in Table 14–3 and are illustrated schematically in Figure 14–10.

Acid Maltase Deficiency (Glycogenosis Type II)

Acid maltase is a lysosomal enzyme with α-1,4- and α-1,6-glucosidase activity. It hydrolyzes glycogen, maltose, and other linear oligosaccharides to

Table 14–3. METABOLIC MYOPATHIES: LYSOSOMAL AND CYTOSOLIC ENZYME DEFICIENCIES

Disorder	Basis of Deficiency
Acid maltase deficiency	Absent enzyme protein Catalytically inactive enzyme protein Low level of normal enzyme
Debrancher deficiency	Defect of transferase activity Defect of α-1,6-glucosidase activity Combined deficiency
Myophosphorylase deficiency	Absent enzyme protein Catalytically inactive enzyme protein
Phosphorylase *b* kinase deficiency	
Phosphofructokinase deficiency	Absent enzyme protein Catalytically inactive enzyme protein
Phosphoglycerate kinase deficiency	Mutant enzyme with low catalytic activity
Phosphoglycerate mutase deficiency	Absence of muscle isoenzyme
Lactate dehydrogenase deficiency	Absence of muscle isoenzyme
Myoadenylate (AMP) deaminase deficiency	Absence of muscle isoenzyme

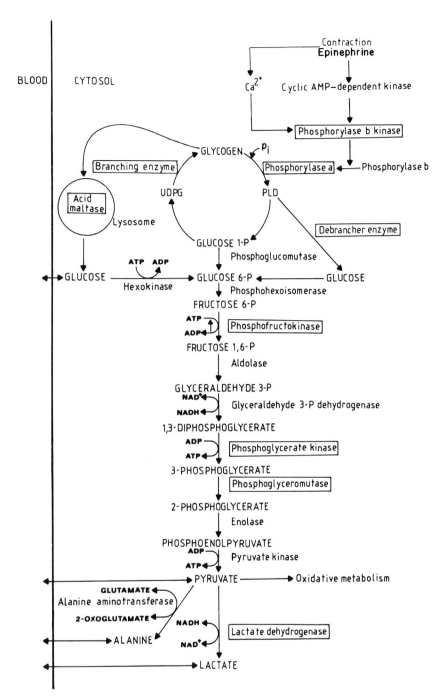

Figure 14–10. Scheme of carbohydrate metabolism in muscle. Defects that have been identified in humans involve the enzymes enclosed in boxes.

yield free glucose (Huijing, 1975). The acid maltase gene has been mapped to chromosome 17, and the nucleotide sequence of the complete coding region has been determined (Martiniuk et al., 1990). Three clinically distinct forms of acid maltase deficiency have been described (DiMauro et al., 1984).

The Fatal Infantile Form

This variety is noted first in the neonatal period with rapidly progressive generalized flaccid weakness, feeding and breathing difficulties, massive cardiomegaly, and variable enlargement of the liver and tongue (DiMauro et al., 1984). Cardiorespiratory failure invariably causes death before the age of 2 years. The serum CK value is increased, and the ECG shows a shortened PR interval with giant QRS complexes in all leads. The EMG indicates myopathy with increased insertional activity, fibrillation, high-frequency discharges, and pseudomyotonia. Glycogen, both free and membrane bound (lysosomal), is deposited in massive amounts in muscle, liver, and heart and to a lesser extent in all tissues including neurons of the cerebral cortex, brain stem and spinal cord, glial cells, Schwann cells, blood lymphocytes, smooth muscle, and kidney. Glycogen also accumulates in fibroblast and muscle cultures. The muscle fibers contain multiple vacuoles packed with periodic acid–Schiff–positive material that stains intensely for the lysosomal marker enzyme acid phosphatase. Acid maltase activity is undetectable in all tissues except kidney, which contains a genetically distinct α-1,4-glucosidase with a broad pH optimum (Dreyfus and Poenaru, 1980). Most patients with the infantile-onset form lack the mature enzyme protein, but a catalytically inactive mutant protein was demonstrated in a few cases. Studies of fibroblast cultures derived from patients with the infantile form provide evidence for considerable molecular heterogeneity (Martiniuk et al., 1990; Reuser et al., 1987). The findings in these and other studies suggest that loss of enzyme activity may be caused by abnormalities of precursor synthesis, post-translational processing, or maturation of α-glucosidase into its catalytically active form within the lysosomal system. Northern blot analysis of 10 infantile-onset cases provided evidence for at least three different mutations: (1) absence of both mRNA and enzyme protein; (2) presence of both mRNA and enzyme protein; and (3) presence of mRNA but absence of enzyme protein (Martiniuk et al., 1990).

The Childhood Form

This form is largely restricted to skeletal muscle and runs a more benign clinical course (Servidei and DiMauro, 1989). Motor milestones may be delayed owing to weakness of the limb girdle muscles and trunk. Involvement of the respiratory muscles, including the diaphragm, may lead to recurrent pneumonia and ventilatory insufficiency. There may be hypertrophy of the calves and a nasal speech because of palatal weakness. Unlike the situation in infantile form, the heart and liver are rarely enlarged. The weakness is slowly progressive and usually leads to death from pneumonia and respiratory failure in the second or third decade of life.

The serum CK value is moderately elevated but the ECG is usually normal. EMG changes are similar to but less marked than in the infantile form. Muscle glycogen deposition is also less marked and may not affect all fibers. Glycogen accumulates in blood lymphocytes and in fibroblast and muscle cultures, but excessive glycogen in other organs, such as heart, liver, or central nervous system (CNS), may be minimal or absent. Childhood cases show some residual acid maltase activity in muscle and in cultured fibroblasts. The residual enzyme shows normal kinetic and electrophoretic characteristics, which suggests that the childhood form may be due to decreased synthesis of enzyme protein (Servidei and DiMauro, 1989). Studies suggest that the childhood form is also heterogeneous at a molecular genetic level (Reuser et al., 1987).

The Adult Form

This variety begins between the second and fourth decade as a slowly progressive proximal myopathy

mimicking limb-girdle dystrophy or chronic polymyositis (Engel et al., 1973). Chronic ventilatory insufficiency related to selective involvement of the diaphragm may be a common early manifestation and its presence is a major clue to diagnosis (Trend et al., 1985). Diaphragmatic paralysis can be detected by measuring the vital capacity in the supine and the upright positions or by recording transdiaphragmatic pressures. In such cases, ventilatory support, particularly during sleep with a rocking-bed or cuirass ventilator, may delay clinical deterioration and allow patients to live a more active life (Trend et al., 1985). Respiratory failure is the eventual cause of death in most cases, the heart and liver being unaffected. In the adult form, glycogen deposition is restricted to skeletal muscle and peripheral blood lymphocytes (DiMauro et al., 1984). It also occurs in fibroblast and muscle cultures. Muscle histologic appearance is variable and may be normal, particularly if the biopsy sample is taken from a strong muscle. In a typical sample, however, the appearances of the vacuolated fibers are indistinguishable from those in other forms of the disease (Fig. 14–11). The serum CK activity is moderately increased, and the EMG shows myopathy, but spontaneous discharges are often minimal or absent. In adult-onset cases, residual acid maltase activity is usually significantly higher than that in the other forms, but exceptions have been described (Martiniuk et al., 1990; Reuser et al., 1987). On the basis of mRNA and enzyme activity, three different mutations have been identified: (1) normal mRNA and 25% enzyme activity, (2) small mRNA and 2% enzyme activity, and (3) normal-sized mRNA with almost undetectable enzyme activity (Martiniuk et al., 1990).

Autosomal recessive inheritance has been demonstrated in all three forms of the disease (Rowland and DiMauro, 1983). Complementation experiments suggest that the infantile and late-onset forms may be allelic, a finding that would explain the single occurrence of both types of disease in the same

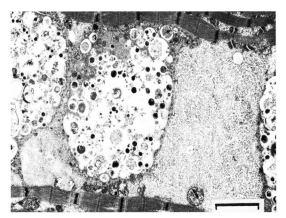

Figure 14–11. Adult acid maltase deficiency. Electron micrograph showing excess glycogen and massive secondary lysosomes containing granular and membranous cellular debris. Scale = 2 μm. (Courtesy of Dr. D.N. Landon, Institute of Neurology, Queen Square, London.)

pedigree (Loonen et al., 1981). Absence of acid maltase activity in cultured amniotic fluid cells affords a reliable method for prenatal diagnosis.

Treatment is directed at maintaining adequate ventilatory support, particularly during sleep, and combating intercurrent infection. Attempts at enzyme replacement have proved unsuccessful. The beneficial effects of a high-protein diet, rich in branched chain amino acids, warrant further study (Slonim et al., 1983).

Debrancher Deficiency (Glycogenosis Type III)

Debranching enzyme catalyzes the two-stage removal of the last four glucose residues from the glycogen side chains. The transferase and α-1,6-glucosidase activities reside on a single enzyme protein. This deficiency typically manifests in infancy or early childhood with hepatomegaly, ketonuria, fasting hypoglycemia, seizures, and growth retardation with normal intellectual development. In most cases, the symptoms and signs resolve spontaneously during adolescence despite persistence of the enzyme deficiency.

Myopathy has been the major presenting feature in 22 patients with this deficiency (Cornelio et al., 1984; DiMauro et al., 1984). Of these patients, seven showed symptoms in childhood when the hepatic features of the disease were still evident. Five showed diffuse muscle weakness, and in two patients, one of whom had additional hepatic glucose-6-phosphatase deficiency, the clinical picture was dominated by exercise-induced myalgia, weakness, and muscle cramps without myoglobinuria (Cornelio et al., 1984). The remaining 15 patients had slowly progressive weakness, usually in the third or fourth decade of life, although there was often a history of hepatomegaly, growth retardation, or hypoglycemia in early childhood. Mild exercise intolerance without muscle pain or cramp preceded the onset of overt weakness in six patients. In debrancher deficiency myopathy, the muscle wasting and weakness are often more marked distally, which may initially suggest either anterior horn cell disease or a peripheral motor neuropathy (Cornelio et al., 1984).

The serum CK value increased in all patients with myopathy; and EMG studies show myopathic features combined with increased insertional activity, fibrillations, positive sharp waves, and pseudomyotonia. Mild slowing of peripheral nerve conduction was also reported. The forearm ischemic exercise lactate test is usually flat but may show a small rise possibly because of the action of myophosphorylase on the glycogen side chains. The ECG shows left ventricular or biventricular hypertrophy in most cases, but cardiac symptoms are rare. Mild glucose intolerance is common, but the normal hyperglycaemic response to epinephrine or glucagon is lacking in all cases. Unlike patients with hepatic glucose-6-phosphatase deficiency, these patients show a normal hyperglycemic response to galactose. Muscle biopsy shows a vacuolar myopathy related to the deposition of glycogen with abnormally short side chains. Muscle histologic features are similar in childhood and adult cases, regardless of whether myopathy is present. Because of the absence of tissue-specific isoenzymes, debrancher deficiency is expressed in all tissues, including brain, liver, muscle, heart, erythrocytes, and leukocytes and in fibroblast and muscle cultures (DiMauro et al., 1984). A high-protein diet has proved beneficial in the hepatic form but failed to improve muscle strength in one patient with myopathy (Cornelio et al., 1984).

Myophosphorylase Deficiency (Glycogenosis Type V)

This disorder was identified biochemically by Mommaerts et al. and Schmid and Mahler in 1959, but the typically clinical features were first recognized by McArdle in 1951. Most patients present in childhood or early adolescence with recurrent episodes of painful muscle stiffness and weakness, induced by strenuous exercise and relieved by rest. During vigorous exercise muscles develop intensely painful cramp-like contractures that are electrically silent. In a severe attack, muscle symptoms may persist for hours and may be associated with myoglobinuria and renal insufficiency. The level of exercise needed to induce symptoms varies from case to case, but leisurely activity is rarely curtailed. Patients typically experience the so-called second wind if they reduce the level of exercise when symptoms first appear. This is due to a greatly increased muscle blood flow and to enhanced utilization of blood-borne energy substrates, particularly glucose, free fatty acids, and possibly alanine (Morgan-Hughes, 1982). In its typical form, the disease runs a benign course and becomes less troublesome with age as the level of activity decreases. Most patients are normal between attacks, but mild nonprogressive proximal weakness of the upper limbs occurs in about 20% of cases.

Rare clinical variants of myophosphorylase deficiency have been reported. They include a fatal infantile form that begins with rapidly progressive generalized weakness in the neonatal period and leads to death from respiratory failure in early infancy (Miranda et al., 1979). Myopathic forms starting with progressive proximal weakness, without muscle pain or cramp, in infancy or adult life have also been described (Cornelio et al., 1983; Pournand et al., 1983).

The serum CK level is raised at rest and may rise to extremely high levels during an attack of myoglobinuria. As in other muscle glycogenoses, the venous lactate level fails to rise during ischemic exercise (DiMauro et al., 1984). Muscle biopsy results show multiple subsarcolemmal vacuoles that are positive for periodic acid–Schiff and contain glycogen lying free within the peripheral sarcoplasm. Absence of the enzyme can be demonstrated by histochemical methods or by direct biochemical assay. A muscle sample taken after an attack of myoglobinuria shows myonecrosis and regenerating fibers that paradoxically exhibit normal myophosphorylase activity (Mitsumoto, 1979). The reappearance of phosphorylase in regenerating muscle fibers and in myophosphorylase-deficient muscle grown in tissue culture is due to the presence of a genetically distinct fetal isoenzyme (DiMauro et al., 1984). In most cases, tissues other than voluntary muscle are not clinically affected. Although mental retardation, seizures, and ECG changes have occasionally been described, they are not thought to be directly related to the biochemical error as the muscle phosphorylase isoenzyme makes only a relatively small contribution to the total phosphorylase activity in these organs (Miranda et al., 1979). Normal adult voluntary muscle contains a single phosphorylase isoenzyme that in myophosphorylase deficiency either is undetectable by immunologic and electrophoretic methods or is present but catalytically inactive (DiMauro et al., 1984).

There appears to be no correlation between clinical expression and the presence or absence of the enzyme protein. In a study of 48 patients with McArdle's disease, myophosphorylase protein was undetectable in 41 patients and was present in markedly reduced amounts in 6 (Servidei et al., 1988). Only one patient, an alcoholic, with otherwise typical symptoms had a normal amount of cross-reacting material. Patients lacking the enzyme protein included two with benign congenital weakness, two with late-onset progressive weakness, and three with a mild, virtually subclinical form of the disease. Northern blot analysis for four of these patients showed normal mRNA in two patients, one with absent enzyme protein and the other with reduced enzyme protein, and an abnormally short mRNA in a third, also with no detectable enzyme protein. mRNA was not detected in the fourth patient, but the enzyme protein was not examined. These combined results were consistent with at least five different mutations in the myophosphorylase gene or its flanking regulatory regions, but there were no obvious correlations with clinical phenotype.

Despite a 3:1 preponderance of affected males, the disorder is transmitted as an autosomal recessive trait (Rowland and DiMauro, 1983). The myophosphorylase gene has been mapped to the long arm of chromosome 11 and has been cloned and sequenced (Burke et al., 1987). Therapeutic attempts to by-pass the metabolic block by giving glucose or fructose have been unsuccessful, but improvement in exercise intolerance has been reported after the administration of glucagon (Kono et al., 1984) or after a high-protein diet (Slonim and Goans, 1985).

Phosphorylase b Kinase Deficiency

Phosphorylase b (inactive form) predominates in resting muscle. It is converted into the a (active) form by phosphorylase b kinase (PHK), which itself is activated by calcium ions released from the sarcoplasmic reticulum during muscular contraction. PHK may be phosphorylated to a more active form that functions at lower calcium ion concentrations by cyclic AMP–dependent protein kinase (Krebs and Beavo, 1979). PHK is composed of four different polypeptides and has a subunit composition of $\alpha_4\beta_4\gamma_4\delta_4$ (van den Berg and Berger, 1990). The α and β subunits confer regulation of catalytic activity by phosphorylation (catalyzed by cyclic AMP–dependent protein kinase). The δ subunit, which is a member of the calmodulin family, confers calcium ion sensitivity, and the γ subunit carries the catalytic site (Kilimann, 1990). The genes encoding the α, β, and γ subunits have been mapped to Xq12-13, 16q12-13, and chromosome 7, respectively (Francke et al., 1989; Kilimann, 1990). These subunits exist as multiple tissue-specific isoforms (Bender and Emerson, 1987; Francke et al., 1989), and the α and β isoforms are generated by differential mRNA splicing (Francke et al., 1989).

Deficiency of the human enzyme is clinically heterogeneous probably because of genetic mutations affecting the different tissue-specific subunits. Four clinical variants have been identified (Table 14–4).

PHK deficiency confined to skeletal muscle manifests with progressive weakness or exercise intolerance and muscle cramps in childhood (Iwamasa et al., 1983; Ohtani et al., 1982) or adult life (Abarbanel et al., 1986; Clemens et al., 1990; Servidei et al., 1987). Exercise-induced myoglobinuria and electrically silent muscle contractures have been described (Abarbanel et al., 1986; Servidei et al., 1987). Lactate production during ischemic exercise may be normal, mildly impaired, or absent. In both muscle variants, the EMG usually exhibits myopathy, and muscle biopsy results show the changes of a glycogen storage myopathy with or without myofibrillar degeneration and myonecrosis (Clemens et al., 1990).

PHK deficiency involving muscle and liver is dominated by hepatic disease (Bashan et al., 1981). PHK deficiency confined to the heart has been described in two unrelated infants who died of cardiac arrest (Eishi et al., 1985; Mizuta et al., 1984; Servidei et al., 1988a).

Muscle Phosphofructokinase Deficiency (Glycogenosis Type VII)

Except for erythrocytosis and a mild hemolytic tendency related to partial deficiency of red blood

Table 14–4. CLINICAL PHENOTYPES OF PHOSPHORYLASE b KINASE DEFICIENCY

Tissues Affected	Inheritance
Liver	X-linked recessive, autosomal recessive
Liver and muscle	Autosomal recessive
Muscle	Unknown
Heart	Unknown

cell phosphofructokinase (PFK), the typical clinical features are indistinguishable from those of myophosphorylase deficiency (DiMauro et al., 1984). Episodes of exercise-induced myalgia and muscle cramp usually begin in childhood, but pigmenturia and renal insufficiency are less common than in McArdle's disease. Inheritance is autosomal recessive, but 14 of the 19 reported cases have been male. Rare clinical variants have been described, including a fatal infantile form and a late-onset myopathic form (DiMauro et al., 1984).

The serum CK level is usually elevated at rest and may reach extremely high levels during an attack of myoglobinuria. Venous lactate levels fail to rise during ischemic exercise, and the EMG displays myopathy. The muscle biopsy appearances are similar to those in myophosphorylase deficiency except that a small proportion of the muscle fibers in some, but not all, cases may contain filamentus polysaccharide deposits that are partially resistant to α-amylase (Hays et al., 1981).

Human PFK is a tetrameric enzyme composed of muscle-specific (M), liver-specific (L), and platelet-specific subunits (Vora, 1982). Normal adult muscle expresses only the M subunit and contains a single M_4 tetramer that is either absent or present but catalytically inactive in PFK-deficient muscle (Miranda et al., 1982). Normal erythrocytes express both M and L subunits and contain two homotetramers (M_4 and L_4) and three hybrid forms. In PFK deficiency, red blood cells lack the M subunit so that only the L_4 tetramer remains to give approximately 50% of normal PFK activity (Vora, 1982). Partial deficiency of red blood cell PFK may account for the hemolytic tendency, but a reduced concentration of 2,3-diphosphoglycerate has also been implicated. Expression of all three PFK subunits in immature muscle accounts for the presence of PFK activity in cultured PFK-deficient muscle (Davidson et al., 1983). During development, the isoenzyme pattern changes and leaves only the M_4 tetramer in adult muscle. Other tissues, such as heart and brain, also express all three PFK subunits and probably show a partial enzyme deficiency, but cardiac and cerebral symptoms have not been reported in a typical case. As in McArdle's disease, immunologic studies have shown that PFK deficiency is genetically heterogeneous in that some patients lack the enzyme protein, whereas others show a catalytically inactive mutant protein (Miranda et al., 1982).

Phosphoglycerate Kinase Deficiency

Phosphoglycerate kinase deficiency, an X-linked disease that normally manifests with hemolytic anemia, was identified as a cause of exercise-induced myalgia, myoglobinuria, and renal insufficiency in a 15-year-old boy with symptoms dating back to early childhood (DiMauro et al., 1983). Erythrocyte phosphoglycerate kinase activity, which measured 5% of the normal mean, was shown to be due to the

presence of a mutant enzyme with increased substrate affinity. A forearm ischemic exercise test resulted in a severe and sustained contracture, but there was no rise in venous lactate. Muscle biopsy results showed a slight excess of lipid without glycogen storage.

Phosphoglycerate Mutase Deficiency

DiMauro et al. (1984) also documented a deficiency of muscle phosphoglycerate mutase in a 17-year-old girl and two unrelated adult males with recurrent attacks of exercise-induced muscle pain and myoglobinuria since adolescence. Clinical examination was normal between attacks. In each case, there was a small rise in venous lactate during ischemic exercise, and the muscle biopsy results showed a slight excess of glycogen. Muscle phosphoglycerate mutase activity, which was reduced to about 5% of normal, was due to the presence of the brain-specific BB isoenzyme, the muscle-specific (MM) and hybrid (MB) forms being undetectable. Phosphoglycerate mutase activity was normal in muscle cultures prepared from all three cases because of the presence of the BB homodimer, the sole isoenzyme in immature muscle (DiMauro et al., 1984). Reduced phosphoglycerate mutase activity in muscle from the parents of one patient was consistent with autosomal recessive transmission.

Lactate Dehydrogenase Deficiency

Muscle lactate dehydrogenase deficiency, caused by the absence of the muscle-specific subunit, was reported in a Japanese family with exercise-related symptoms and recurrent pigmenturia (Kanno et al., 1980). A forearm ischemic exercise test on the prepositus showed a marked rise in venous pyruvate but little or no rise in lactate concentration. Residual muscle lactate dehydrogenase activity, which measured 5% of the normal mean, was attributed to the presence of the heart-specific (H_4) tetramer. Studies of other affected members in this family indicated autosomal recessive inheritance consistent with the assignment of the lactate dehydrogenase muscle-specific subunit to chromosome 11.

Myoadenylate (AMP) Deaminase Deficiency

Myoadenylate deaminase (MADA) is a major enzyme of the purine nucleotide cycle that plays an important supportive role in muscle bioenergetics through: (1) the removal of AMP, (2) the regulation of glycolysis through the production of IMP and NH_3, (3) its anaplerotic effect through the production of fumarate, and (4) the production of purine nucleotides, which may be used to replenish ATP after exercise (Fig. 14–12).

MADA deficiency, first described by Fishbein et al. (1978), is the most common of known muscle

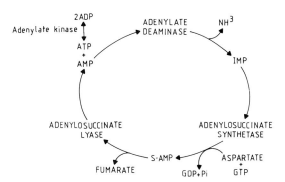

Figure 14–12. Scheme of the purine nucleotide cycle.

enzyme deficiencies, with an incidence in most muscle biopsy series of about 2% (Fishbein et al., 1984). Two-thirds of reported cases manifest in childhood or early adult life with exercise-related symptoms consisting of easy fatigability, myalgia, and postexercise cramp. Clinical examination is usually normal, but mild proximal weakness has been reported. The serum CK activity is usually raised, especially after exercise, but the EMG result may be normal. Venous ammonia and hypoxanthine levels fail to rise during ischemic exercise, but lactate production is normal. Muscle biopsy results are normal or mildly myopathic. The enzyme defect can be demonstrated by histochemical or biochemical assay. The defect is inherited as an autosomal recessive trait and is associated with the absence of an immunologically detectable muscle enzyme protein (Fishbein et al., 1984). Enzyme activity in other tissues and in cultured MADA-deficient muscle is normal, the latter owing to the presence of a genetically distinct fetal isoenzyme (DiMauro et al., 1980a).

In addition to its occurrence in patients with exercise-related symptoms, MADA deficiency has been reported as a coincidental finding in patients with other well-defined neuromuscular diseases, including hypokalemic periodic paralysis, motor neuron disease, muscular dystrophy, mitochondrial myopathy, myasthenia gravis, and benign congenital hypotonia (Sabina et al., 1984). Although absence of the muscle enzyme in such diverse conditions has cast doubt on the significance of the defect in patients with exercise-induced muscle pain, the incidence is much higher in the latter group (Kelemen et al., 1982). Biochemical studies of patients with MADA deficiency suggest that these patients have a reduced capacity for muscle energy production when compared with age-matched control subjects (Sabina et al., 1984).

Defects of Mitochondrial Metabolism

These defects are a newly recognized group of inborn metabolic errors that impinge directly on the pathways of aerobic energy production in the mitochondrial inner membrane and matrix space (Di-

Mauro et al., 1990; Morgan-Hughes, 1986). The spectrum of reported biochemical abnormalities includes defects that impair the entry of high-energy substrates into the mitochondria or the capacity to generate reducing potential from these substrates, as well as those that block the oxidative phosphorylation pathway itself (Table 14–5). For reviews see DiMauro et al. (1990), Lombes et al. (1989), and Zeviani et al. (1989).

Defects of Substrate Transport

Muscle Carnitine Deficiency

This disorder manifests with progressive weakness in infancy, childhood, or adult life (Engel and Rebouche, 1984). The weakness tends to fluctuate in severity and may be exacerbated by exercise, pregnancy, or a prolonged fast. Muscle biopsy results show an excess of neutral lipid droplets, particularly in type 1 and type 2A muscle fibers (Fig. 14–13). Total muscle carnitine levels are reduced to about 20% of normal in skeletal muscle but are usually normal in serum and in other tissues. Some patients respond to oral DL-carnitine (3–6 g daily), prednisone, or both, but muscle carnitine levels usually show little change. The disease, which appears to be transmitted as an autosomal recessive trait, is thought to be due to defective transport of carnitine into muscle (Rebouche and Engel, 1984).

Systemic Carnitine Deficiency

Primary systemic carnitine deficiency is an autosomal recessive disorder that may manifest with hypoketotic hypoglycemic coma in infancy or with progressive hypertrophic cardiomyopathy and skeletal muscle weakness in childhood (Stanley et al., 1990; Tein et al., 1990). Total carnitine levels are markedly reduced in plasma, liver, and muscle, and

Table 14–5. DEFECTS OF MITOCHONDRIAL METABOLISM

Type of Defect	Disorder
Substrate transport	Carnitine deficiency, myopathic
	Carnitine deficiency, systemic
	Carnitine palmitoyl transferase deficiency
Substrate utilization	Deficiencies of pyruvate dehydrogenase complex
	Defects of β oxidation
Krebs' cycle	Fumarase deficiency
	Dehydrolipoyl dehydrogenase deficiency
Respiratory chain	Complex I deficiency
	Complex II deficiency
	Coenzyme Q_{10} deficiency
	Complex III deficiency
	Complex IV deficiency
	Multiple defects
Energy conservation and transduction	Luft's disease
	H^+-ATPase deficiency

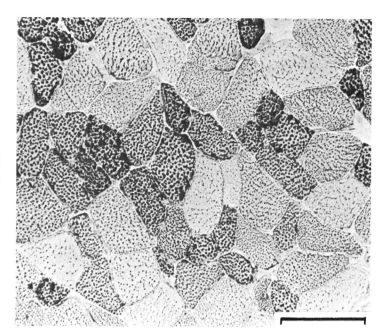

Figure 14–13. Transverse section of the quadriceps muscle of the thigh from a patient with carnitine deficiency. Sudan black B fat stain shows excess of neutral lipid droplets in the type 1 and type 2A muscle fibers. Scale = 100 μm.

the renal conservation of carnitine is severely impaired. The disorder is thought to be due to a defect of the carrier-mediated carnitine uptake mechanism in kidney and probably also in skeletal muscle. The carnitine transport defect is expressed and can be identified in cultured fibroblasts. Muscle biopsy results show a lipid storage myopathy. Treatment with oral carnitine (3–6 g daily) has proved beneficial, particularly in patients with cardiomyopathy.

Severe carnitine deficiency also occurs as a secondary phenomenon in association with a number of inborn metabolic errors, some of which are accompanied by episodes of hypoketotic hypoglycemia (Engel, 1986a). They include organic acidurias, defects of β oxidation, and deficiencies involving the mitochondrial respiratory chain and oxidative phosphorylation system. The mechanism of secondary carnitine deficiency in these disorders may relate to carnitine's role in converting acyl coenzyme A derivatives, which accumulate in the mitochondrial matrix (as a result of the metabolic block) into innocuous acylcarnitines, thereby freeing coenzyme A for other metabolic reactions. The acylcarnitines are then transported out of the mitochondria and are excreted virtually unchanged in the urine. This mechanism imposes a considerable drain on carnitine stores and may eventually lead to secondary carnitine depletion.

Carnitine Palmitoyl Transferase Deficiency

This disease is autosomal recessive and manifests with recurrent bouts of muscle pain, weakness, myoglobinuria, and renal insufficiency, which are typically precipitated by prolonged vigorous exercise, especially in the cold, after fasting, or after a high-fat, low-carbohydrate diet (DiMauro et al., 1980b). A muscle biopsy sample taken between attacks is usually normal, but samples obtained immediately after an episode of myoglobinuria typically show an excess of neutral lipid droplets, particularly in the type 1 muscle fibers. The enzyme defect appears to be generalized and has been demonstrated in liver, leukocytes, platelets, and cultured fibroblasts. Exercise tolerance may be improved by a high-carbohydrate diet.

A rare hepatic form of carnitine palmitoyl transferase deficiency was described as manifesting with hypoketotic hypoglycemic coma in early infancy (Demaugre et al., 1990). The defect, which is thought to involve the CPT1 isoform, is expressed in liver and cultured fibroblasts but not in skeletal muscle. This finding would suggest the presence of these isoforms.

Defects of Substrate Utilization

Deficiencies of the Pyruvate Dehydrogenase Complex

These disorders may manifest with (1) severe and rapidly fatal congenital lactic acidosis, (2) progressive encephalopathy with neuropathologic features of Leigh's disease, which leads to death or severe disability in early childhood, or (3) a mild disease characterized by intermittent ataxia often precipitated by a high-carbohydrate intake, intercurrent infection, or emotional stress (Robinson et al., 1989). The defect in many patients with the severe disorder has involved the α subunit of the first catalytic enzyme pyruvate dehydrogenase, which is encoded on the X chromosome (Brown et al., 1989).

Defects of β Oxidation

This group of disorders includes (1) deficiencies of long chain, medium chain, and short chain fatty acyl-

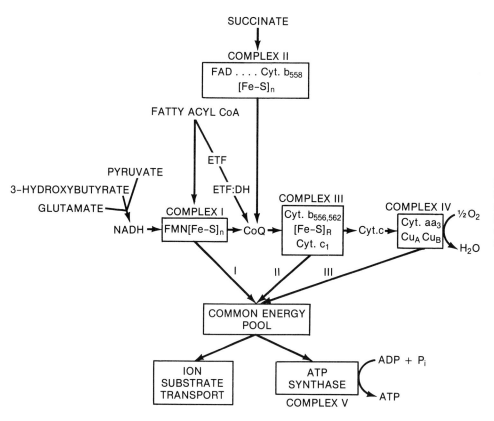

Figure 14–14. Scheme of the mitochondrial respiratory chain and oxidative phosphorylation system to show the respiratory enzyme complexes (I–V) and the three coupling sites.

CoA dehydrogenases, (2) deficiencies of the electron transfer flavoprotein, and (3) deficiencies of electron transfer flavoprotein–ubiquinone oxidoreductase (Vianey-Liaud et al., 1987). These disorders usually manifest with episodes of hypoketotic hypoglycemic coma in infancy or early childhood. The attacks are precipitated by fasting or intercurrent infection and are characterized by urinary organic acid and acylcarnitine excretion profiles that reflect the site of the metabolic block. Some patients with defects of this type may develop muscle weakness, carnitine deficiency, and a lipid storage myopathy.

Defects of the Krebs Cycle

Specific deficiencies of two Krebs' cycle enzymes have been described.

Fumarase deficiency causes a progressive encephalopathy in early infancy associated with increasing lethargy, psychomotor retardation, generalized hypotonia, and microcephaly (Gellera et al., 1990). Urinary organic acid analysis shows increased levels of fumarase and succinate. The enzyme defect has been demonstrated in various tissues including brain, liver, kidney, and heart, as well as in cultured fibroblasts. Both cytosolic and mitochondrial forms of fumarase are deficient in most cases. The two isoforms are encoded by a single gene on human chromosome 1. Dihydrolipoamide dehydrogenase deficiency causes a severe lactic acidosis and progressive encephalopathy in early infancy (Robinson et al., 1989). Autopsy studies showed loss of myelin

with cystic lesions in the basal ganglia, thalamus, and brain stem, consistent with Leigh's syndrome. All cases have shown a combined deficiency in the activities of the pyruvate dehydrogenase, α-ketoglutarate dehydrogenase, and branched chain keto acid dehydrogenase complexes, with elevated levels of lactate, pyruvate, α-ketoglutarate, and branched chain amino acids in the blood.

Defects Involving Different Respiratory Enzyme Complexes

These disorders (Fig. 14–14; see Table 14–5) exhibit a wide range of clinical presentations that vary according to the distribution and severity of the metabolic block (DiMauro et al., 1985, 1990; Morgan-Hughes, 1986; Morgan-Hughes et al., 1985; Petty et al., 1986). Various organs may be affected, either singly or in different combinations. They include the CNS, peripheral nervous system, retina, liver, kidneys, skeletal muscle, and heart. Reported cases fall into two main categories according to whether the disease predominantly affects the brain or skeletal muscle. Cases with major CNS involvement manifest with a fluctuating encephalopathy, which may begin at any age from infancy to late adult life. Patients with the early-onset disorder develop a varied combination of clinical features that include vomiting, somnolence, mental regression, focal or generalized seizures, ataxia, visual failure, generalized hypotonic weakness, and respiratory insufficiency. Cardiomyopathy and hepatopathy have been the major presenting features in some cases. Early onset usually heralds a poor prognosis, most patients dying of cardiorespiratory insufficiency and a severe metabolic acidosis in infancy or early childhood.

Patients with the late-onset disorder typically show varying degrees of dementia and cerebellar ataxia, often accompanied by myoclonic jerks, choreoathetoid movements, or dystonia. The illness may be punctuated by recurrent stroke-like episodes associated with headache, somnolence, visual failure, and focal seizures. Other features appearing in some, but not all, cases include sensorineural deafness, pigmentary retinal degeneration, growth retardation, peripheral neuropathy, and cardiopathy. Myopathy, which may affect the extraocular muscles as well as muscles of the limbs and trunk, may be only a minor feature of the overall clinical picture and in some cases may be clinically undetectable. In both early-onset and late-onset cases, the illness tends to fluctuate in severity and may be exacerbated by intercurrent infection, fasting, or other types of environmental stress. Respiratory chain deficiencies with major CNS involvement usually result in severe disability and may lead to coma and sudden death (Petty et al., 1986). Laboratory investigations show EEG and ECG changes, raised lactate and pyruvate levels with an increased lactate/pyruvate ratio in the blood and in the cerebrospinal fluid, an elevated cerebrospinal fluid protein value, and various abnormalities on the computed tomographic brain scan, including cerebral and cerebellar atrophy, low-density areas in the hemispheres, and calcification of the basal ganglia (Fig. 14–15).

Patients without major CNS disease usually begin with muscle weakness, exercise intolerance, and a fluctuating lactic acidemia in early childhood, although late-onset illness has been described (Di-

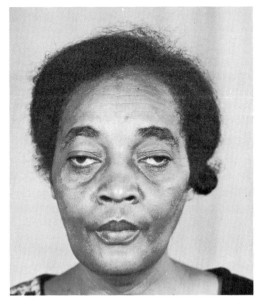

Figure 14–16. A 46-year-old woman with a mitochondrial myopathy resulting in ptosis, external ophthalmoplegia, and fatigable weakness of the limbs. Studies of isolated muscle mitochondria showed a deficiency of complex III with normal cytochromes.

Mauro et al., 1985; Morgan-Hughes et al., 1985). The extraocular and bulbar muscles (Fig. 14–16), as well as muscles of the limbs and trunk, may be affected in some cases, and other tissues such as retina, heart, liver, and peripheral nervous system may also be involved.

In the past few years, mutations of the mitochondrial genome have been identified in a number of mitochondrial myopathies with defects of the respiratory chain. These mutations are given in Table 14–6. Large deletions affecting a variable proportion of mitochondrial DNAs (mtDNAs) were demonstrated

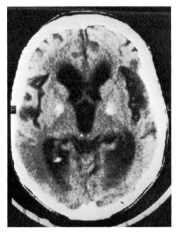

Figure 14–15. Computed tomographic brain scan of a 41-year-old woman with a mitochondrial encephalomyopathy who initially had drop attacks in her late 20s and then developed fatigable weakness, dementia, cerebellar ataxia, sensorineural deafness, pigmentary retinopathy, seizures, and left hemiparesis. Studies of isolated muscle mitochondria showed a deficiency of complex I. Note extensive cerebral and cortical atrophy with calcification in the region of the basal ganglia.

Table 14–6. MITOCHONDRIAL MYOPATHIES: DISEASE-ASSOCIATED MUTATIONS OF MITOCHONDRIAL DNA

Mutation	Phenotype*
Deletions (and Duplications)	
Large single deletions (heteroplasmic)	PEO + limb weakness
	PEO + retinopathy and/or deafness
	Kearns-Sayre syndrome
	Pearson's bone marrow–pancreas syndrome
Large multiple deletions (heteroplasmic)	Autosomal dominant PEO
Tandem duplication (heteroplasmic)	Kearns-Sayre syndrome
Point Mutations	
A-G at base pair 8344 in the TψC loop of tRNA^{Lys}	MERRF
A-G at base pair 3243 in the dihydrouridine loop of tRNA$^{Leu\ (UUR)}$	MELAS PEO

*PEO = progressive external ophthalmoplegia; MERRF = myoclonic epilepsy and ragged red fibers; MELAS = mitochondrial encephalopathy, lactic acidosis, and stroke.

in about 30% of cases (Harding et al., 1990; Mita et al., 1990). All patients harboring large-scale deletions initially had progressive external ophthalmoplegia, and many showed additional features such as heart block, pigmentary retinopathy, and/or CNS disease consistent with the Kearns-Sayre phenotype. The deletions eliminated structural genes for two or more respiratory chain polypeptides as well as the intervening tRNA genes but did not extend to the origins of replication or transcription of the heavy or light strands of mtDNA. Analyses of the breakpoint regions of the deleted mtDNAs identified short nucleotide sequences ranging from 5 to 13 base pairs, which occur in the normal genome as direct repeats flanking the deleted region. The association with direct repeats has led to the slip replication theory of origin (Mita et al., 1990). The absence of detectable deletions in the mothers of affected patients suggests that deletions arise during oogenesis or embryonic development.

Although at least 17 different deletions have been characterized at a nucleotide level (Mita et al., 1990), their precise role in the pathogenesis of these diseases remains unclear. Large deletions invariably eliminate one or more tRNA genes, so that protein-coding sequences not encompassed by the deletion would not be translated unless complementation occurred. Complementation would require the presence of normal as well as deleted genomes within the same organelle.

Two studies addressed this question, one by applying the techniques of in situ hybridization (Mita et al., 1989) and the other by examining mtDNA transcription and translation in cloned fibroblast cultures containing 60% of deleted genomes (Nakase et al., 1990). Taken together, these studies show that deleted mtDNAs are transcribed probably at a normal rate but that mitochondria containing deleted genomes lack the capacity to translate these transcripts into proteins. The failure to translate genes not encompassed by the deletion implies that complementation does not occur and suggests that the normal and deleted genomes may be segregated in different organelles. These studies also show that mitochondria containing deleted mtDNAs are virtually confined to cytochrome oxidase–negative ragged red fibers (Mita et al., 1989).

Multiple deletions of muscle mtDNA have been identified in affected members of a large pedigree with an autosomal dominant mitochondrial myopathy, characterized by progressive external ophthalmoplegia, limb weakness, cataract, and premature death (Zeviani et al., 1989). The deletion breakpoints were different in the individual members, indicating that the heteroplasmic mtDNAs were not transmitted from one generation to the next and must have arisen de novo by some common mechanism. The findings in this family could be explained by a mutation of a nuclear gene encoding a protein involved in mtDNA replication.

A heteroplasmic point mutation in the TψC loop of mitochondrial tRNA^{Lys} has been identified in several pedigrees with a maternally inherited mitochondrial encephalomyopathy associated with myoclonic epilepsy and/or cerebellar ataxia (Shoffner et al., 1990; Zeviani et al., 1991). This mutation is associated with a combined deficiency of complexes I and IV and was shown to be associated with reduced synthesis of the larger mtDNA translation products. A similar transitional mutation involving the dihydrouridine loop of mitochondrial tRNA$^{Leu(UUR)}$ has been identified in 26 of 31 unrelated patients with a mitochondrial encephalopathy associated with stroke-like episodes and lactic acidosis (MELAS) and in one patient with progressive external ophthalmoplegia (Goto et al., 1990).

Defects of the Phosphorylation System

These disorders include Luft's euthyroid hypermetabolism and mitochondrial ATPase deficiency (DiMauro et al., 1985). Only two patients with Luft's disease have been described, and both initially had severe heat intolerance, hyperthermia, excessive sweating, polyphagia, polydypsia, and mild generalized fatigable weakness in early childhood. The basal metabolic rate was grossly elevated in each case, but tests of thyroid function were consistently normal. Biochemical studies showed abnormally high mitochondrial respiratory activity, even in the absence of ADP, which may have been related to an inability of the mitochondria to retain calcium ions (DiMauro et al., 1985). Two cases of mitochondrial ATP synthase deficiency have also been described, one manifesting a nonprogressive mitochondrial myopathy and the other predominantly CNS disease associated with a carnitine-deficient lipid storage myopathy (Clark et al., 1984).

The morphologic hallmark of defects localized to the mitochondrial respiratory chain and phosphorylation system is the so-called ragged red muscle fiber, which owes its appearance, in frozen sections stained with the modified Gomori's trichrome method, to large peripheral collections of structurally abnormal mitochondria (Morgan-Hughes and Landon, 1983). Ragged red fibers show an intense cytochemical reaction for the exclusively intramitochondrial enzyme succinate dehydrogenase; at an ultrastructural level, the fibers are packed with structurally abnormal mitochondria, often containing paracrystalline inclusions (Fig. 14–17). There is also an excess of glycogen and neutral lipid, the latter being particularly prominent in patients with secondary carnitine deficiency. Similar changes in mitochondrial morphologic characteristics have also been described in neurons, Schwann cells, hepatocytes, and cardiac muscle.

Metabolic Myopathies of Uncertain Pathogenesis

Malignant Hyperthermia

This dominantly inherited trait has variable penetrance and in the majority of cases becomes clinically

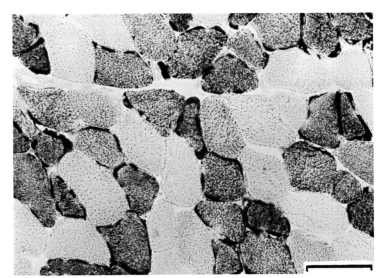

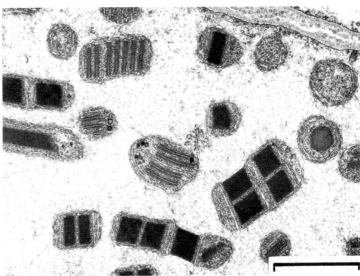

Figure 14–17. Mitochondrial myopathy. *(Top)* Transverse section of the quadriceps muscle of the thigh from a 20-year-old girl with mitochondrial myopathy and a deficiency of cytochromes *b* and *c*. The succinate dehydrogenase reaction illustrates subsarcolemmal staining in a high proportion of the fibers. Scale = 100 μm. *(Bottom)* Electron micrograph of the periphery of a muscle fiber showing excess glycogen and structurally abnormal mitochondria containing type 1 and type 2 paracrystals. Scale = 1 μm. (Courtesy of Dr. D.N. Landon, Institute of Neurology, Queen Square, London.)

manifest only under general anesthesia (Gronert, 1980). Agents that precipitate an attack include halothane, ether, cyclopropane, chloroform, methoxyflurane, enflurane, ketamine, and suxamethonium. During anesthesia, there is a rapid rise in body temperature, generalized muscular rigidity, tachycardia, tachypnea, cyanosis, metabolic acidosis, lactic acidemia, hyperkalemia, myoglobinemia, and myoglobinuria. Until the introduction of dantrolene, mortality was about 70%. Treatment consists of stopping the anesthetic, vigorous cooling, correction of the acidosis with sodium bicarbonate, and intravenous dantrolene, 1–2 mg/kg given in repeated doses every 10–15 minutes up to a total of 10 mg/kg (Gronert, 1980). Patients thought to be at risk of developing malignant hyperthermia should be carefully screened by measuring the serum CK level and by examining muscle biopsy tissue for evidence of a subclinical myopathy and an abnormal contraction response on exposure to halothane, caffeine, or both (Harriman, 1982).

Most experimental findings in human and porcine

malignant hyperthermia point to defective regulation of intracellular free ionic calcium in skeletal muscle, although the mechanism is unknown (Heffron, 1984). A rise in intracellular free ionic calcium would activate PHK and myosin ATPase and so lead to accelerated glycogen breakdown and abnormal contraction. Overloading of the muscle mitochondria with calcium ions may also lead to uncoupling of oxidative phosphorylation and excessive heat production. One study showed close linkage between malignant hyperthermia and the ryanodine receptor gene mapped to the q13.1 region of human chromosome 19, which encodes the calcium release channel of the sarcoplasmic reticulum (MacLennan et al., 1990).

Malignant hyperthermia has also been reported in occasional patients with myotonic dystrophy, myotonia congenita, and central core disease.

Idiopathic Paroxysmal Myoglobinuria

This disorder presents with acute attacks of muscle pain, weakness, and myoglobinuria, sometimes leading to renal insufficiency. The serum CK value is grossly elevated during an attack, and muscle biopsy samples show extensive myonecrosis and regenerative activity. Although there are a number of known exogenous and endogenous causes for this type of syndrome, such as viruses, drugs, alcohol, toxins, and inherited metabolic defects, in a substantial number of patients the etiology remains unknown. In some cases the attacks tend to be precipitated by vigorous exercise but in others they may be related to intercurrent infection. Treatment is symptomatic, but renal dialysis may be indicated.

ACQUIRED MYOPATHIES

The Inflammatory Diseases

The inflammatory diseases of muscle comprise a large and heterogeneous group of acquired myopathies that fall into three broad categories: infective, drug induced, and idiopathic (Table 14–7). Myositides, caused by known infective agents such as viruses, bacteria, and parasites, have been extensively reviewed and are not considered further here (Kagen, 1984; Mastaglia and Ojeda, 1985a,b).

The Idiopathic Inflammatory Myopathies

Polymyositis (PM) and dermatomyositis (DM) are a complex group of autoimmune diseases that affect all age groups but show peaks in late childhood and in the fourth and fifth decades of life (Whitaker, 1982). The reported annual incidence ranges from two to five cases per million of the population, with a 2:1 preponderance of affected females, especially in the younger age groups and in black patients.

The clinical features and natural history of these diseases are remarkably pleomorphic (Mastaglia and Ojeda, 1985a,b; Whitaker, 1982). Rarely, the onset is

---

Table 14–7. INFLAMMATORY MYOPATHIES

Infective
  Viral: influenza virus A and B, parainfluenza virus,
    coxsackievirus, echovirus, adenovirus
  Bacterial: *Staphylococcus aureus, Streptococcus pyogenes*
  Parasitic: toxoplasmosis, cysticercosis, trichinosis

Drug Induced
  D-Penicillamine
  Cimetidine
  Procainamide

Idiopathic
  Dermatomyositis
    Childhood
    Adult
  Polymyositis
  Overlap myositis
  Paraneoplastic myositis
  Inclusion body myositis
  Granulomatous myositis
  Eosinophilic myositis
  Focal myositis

---

acute with fever, malaise, myalgia, and rapidly evolving weakness of the limb girdle and trunk muscles, sometimes associated with bulbar involvement and ventilatory insufficiency (Venables et al., 1982). There may be extensive edema of the skin and subcutaneous tissues, particularly in the periorbital regions and in areas overlying weak and tender muscles. In acute cases, the rapid and widespread destruction of muscle fibers may lead to myoglobinuria and renal insufficiency. Muscle biopsy examination is necessary to exclude other forms of rhabdomyolysis, such as those caused by viruses (Kagen, 1984), drugs, toxins, and inborn metabolic errors (Morgan-Hughes, 1982).

More commonly, PM and DM begin insidiously, with slowly progressive weakness of the limb girdle, trunk, and neck flexor muscles that develops over the course of weeks, months, or even years. In subacute and chronic cases, particularly those without major skin involvement, the clinical features may resemble those seen in muscular dystrophy and late-onset forms of acid maltase deficiency or nemaline myopathy. In PM, however, the weakness is typically more diffuse, the muscle wasting is less pronounced, and the reflexes are characteristically preserved or even hyperactive. Other distinguishing features that may be present in different combinations include dysphagia, Raynaud's phenomenon, muscle pain, flitting arthralgia, and symptoms referable to myocardial involvement (Askari, 1984) or interstitial lung disease (Salmeron et al., 1981).

The typical skin changes of DM consist of edema and heliotropic discoloration of the eyelids and a raised scaly erythematous rash involving the face (butterfly rash), the shoulders, and the upper parts of the chest and back, and the extensor surfaces of the limbs overlying the knuckles, wrists, elbows, and knees. Periungual erythema and telangiectasis are common, particularly in childhood DM, and in both childhood and adult forms, small ulcerated vasculitic skin lesions may develop over the bony prominences of the digits, wrists, elbows, knees, and ankles. Soft tissue calcification over pressure areas is also common in childhood DM but rare in adult cases (Pachman and Maryjowski, 1984).

Atypical presentations of PM include patients in whom the weakness is localized to one limb or is predominantly distal or facioscapulohumeral in distribution and a chronic adult form with selected involvement of the long forearm flexor, brachioradialis, and quadriceps femoris (Mastaglia and Ojeda, 1985a,b). As the name implies, localized nodular myositis typically manifests as a painful muscle mass that initially may mimic a muscle abscess, hematoma, or even a malignant tumor (Heffner and Barron, 1981). Such cases, however, usually develop a much more symmetric and typical clinical picture.

Overlap Polymyositis

Overlap polymyositis is a term applied to an inflammatory myopathy within the context of a connective tissue disease, such as systemic lupus erythematosus, rheumatoid arthritis, mixed connective tissue disease, or systemic sclerosis (Isenberg, 1984). The incidence of PM in these disorders may have been overestimated in the past, partly because myalgia and disuse atrophy are relatively common and partly because the strict diagnostic criteria for PM laid down by Bohan and Peter (1975a,b) have not always been applied. Despite these shortcomings, PM probably occurs in most patients with mixed connective tissue disease (Sharp, 1981) and in 5–15% of patients with systemic lupus erythematosus, rheumatoid arthritis, systemic sclerosis, and Sjögren's syndrome (Isenberg, 1984). The clinical and histologic features of overlap myositis are similar to those of isolated PM except that vasculitic lesions are often more pronounced. In systemic lupus erythematosus and in polyarteritis nodosa, involvement of small and medium-sized intramuscular blood vessels may lead to focal areas of muscle infarction. Estimation of the serum CK activity, EMG studies, and muscle biopsy examination are essential to establish the presence of an overlap myositis and to ensure that muscle weakness and wasting are not due to disuse, denervation, or drug treatment. In addition to the above-named disorders, PM has also been reported in association with myasthenia gravis, autoimmune thyroiditis, graft-versus-host disease, and monoclonal gammopathy (Mastaglia and Ojeda, 1985a,b).

Paraneoplastic Myositis

This disorder accounts for about 10% of all cases of PM and DM. The association with malignant disease is rare in childhood DM, isolated PM, and overlap syndromes, but it rises to more than 20% in older patients with DM, particularly those with prominent vasculitic skin lesions (Callen, 1984). The most frequent associations are with carcinoma of the breast, ovary, lung, and gastrointestinal tract. The neoplasm may present before or after the onset of muscle symptoms or may occur concurrently.

The Diagnosis of PM and DM

Diagnosis depends on the following criteria, as laid down by Bohan and Peter (1975a,b) and Bohan et al. (1977), on the basis of a computer-assisted analysis of more than 150 cases:

1. The presence of progressive, symmetric weakness of the limb girdle and neck flexor muscles, with or without dysphagia
2. Muscle biopsy evidence of segmental myonecrosis, regeneration, and interstitial or perivascular inflammatory exudates consisting predominantly of mononuclear cells or perifascicular atrophy with or without adjacent inflammatory change

3. Increased serum levels of muscle enzymes, particularly CK
4. EMG changes of myopathy, with increased insertional activity and fibrillation potentials

Ideally, all four criteria should be fulfilled, but most authorities agree that in practice three are sufficient to institute treatment.

Pathogenesis

Humoral and cell-mediated immune mechanisms appear to be central to the pathogenesis of PM and DM, but the factors that trigger these responses remain unknown (Denman, 1984; Mastaglia and Ojeda, 1985a,b; Plotz et al., 1989). Most patients have one or more circulating antibodies directed against antigens that are normally present in the cell nucleus or in the cytoplasm (Reichlin and Arnett, 1984; Targoff, 1989). Although no single antibody is exclusive to any one clinical subset, some show relative disease specificity. For example, antibody to the Jo-1 antigen, which itself has been identified as the protein component of histidyl-tRNA synthetase (Mathews and Bernstein, 1983), occurs in about 20% of patients with isolated PM and in up to 70% of patients with PM and interstitial lung disease but appears to be less common in DM and overlap syndromes (Mathews et al., 1984). Antibodies to four other aminoacyl-tRNA synthetases (threonyl, alanyl, isoleucyl, and glycyl) and to another as-yet unidentified component of the translational machinery (anti-KJ) have also been described in association with PM and interstitial lung disease (Targoff, 1989). Other myositis antibodies with relative disease specificities include anti–Mi-2 in DM, anti–PM-Scl in DM and systemic sclerosis, and antinuclear ribonucleoprotein in overlap syndromes of PM with systemic lupus erythematosus.

Additional evidence for humoral immunity is provided by the presence of circulating immune complexes; the deposition of immunoglobulins and complement components in the walls of intramuscular blood vessels, particularly in DM (Emslie-Smith and Engel, 1990); and the observation that PM serum and immunoglobulin G accelerate the degradation of acetylcholine receptors in cultured rat muscle (Mastaglia and Ojeda, 1985a,b; Pestronk and Drachman, 1985). Although the factors that initiate these immune responses have so far remained elusive, the identification of antigens recognized by some of these circulating autoantibodies has led to the hypothesis of a viral origin (Bernstein and Mathews, 1984). Several of the target antigens are components of the translational machinery that could theoretically be rendered immunogenic by interacting with viral RNA.

The role of cell-mediated immunity has been extensively evaluated by using monoclonal antibodies directed against cell surface antigens to identify lymphocyte subsets in muscle biopsy material (Arahata and Engel, 1984, 1988a,b; Engel and Arahata, 1984). The findings from these studies are consistent with antigen-specific, major histocompatibility complex–restricted, T cell–mediated muscle fiber damage in isolated PM and inclusion body myositis but not in DM or systemic sclerosis. In the former conditions, there is a preponderance of CD8$^+$ cytotoxic T cells, which were observed invading and destroying non-necrotic muscle fibers. Enhanced expression of major histocompatibility complex class I antigens on regenerating muscle fibers and on noninvaded as well as T cell–invaded fibers suggests that other factors are required for T cell–mediated myotoxicity. In systemic sclerosis, the findings suggested a T cell–mediated response directed against connective tissue and vascular elements rather than the muscle fibers themselves. In DM, the results were more in keeping with a humoral immune response in that B cells and CD4$^+$ predominated and invasion of non-necrotic muscle fibers by mononuclear cells was rarely seen. These findings are consistent with the view that small and medium-sized blood vessels are the primary target of the immune response in DM. The observation that intramuscular capillary density is significantly reduced in the early stages of DM before major structural alterations occur provides further confirmatory evidence (Emslie-Smith and Engel, 1990).

Studies of HLA antigens in PM and DM suggest that as in other autoimmune diseases, genetic factors may influence host susceptibility and determine the pattern of the immunologic response. An increased incidence of HLA-B8 and HLA-DR3 has been reported in adult PM and childhood DM, and there appears to be a strong association between the Jo-1 antibody in adult PM and HLA-DR3 or HLA-DRw6 (Garlepp and Dawkins, 1984; Plotz et al., 1989).

Treatment of PM and DM

Therapy is directed toward immunosuppression. It is generally agreed that prednisone is the drug of choice, commencing with a single daily dose of between 40 and 80 mg. High doses need to be maintained until there has been a significant clinical response and the serum CK value has fallen to normal or near-normal levels. Thereafter, the prednisone can be tapered slowly by 2.5–5 mg/week, but most patients require a maintenance dose of 10–30 mg/day for several months. In such cases, potassium and calcium supplements may be required. Alternate-day therapy, which reduces the incidence of steroid side effects, may be instituted after a satisfactory remission has been obtained. Azathioprine (2.5–3.0 mg/kg body weight/day) may be used concurrently with prednisone or reserved for patients who are resistant to steroid treatment. Patients who fail to respond to prednisone alone may be treated with maximal doses of azathioprine, methotrexate, or cyclophosphamide. Other regimens, such as plasmapheresis, low-dose total-body or nodal irradiation,

and thymectomy, have not been clearly evaluated but can be considered as last lines of treatment in patients with refractory and life-threatening disease (Mastaglia and Ojeda, 1985a,b). The prognosis in inflammatory myopathies depends on the underlying disease process. In isolated PM or DM and in overlap syndromes, 60–70% of patients show a favorable response, but treatment may have to be continued for several months or even years.

OTHER INFLAMMATORY MYOPATHIES

Inclusion Body Myositis

This myopathy is thought to be a distinct variety of inflammatory myopathy on the basis of the clinical and myopathologic features and resistance to immunosuppressive treatment (Carpenter and Karpati, 1981; Lotz et al., 1989). It is more common in the older age groups, runs a benign and protracted clinical course, and is not usually associated with malignancy, skin changes, or connective tissue disease. The weakness is often more marked in the lower limbs and not uncommonly affects distal as well as proximal muscle groups. Facial weakness and dysphagia have also been reported. The serum CK value is usually normal, and the EMG typically shows neurogenic as well as myopathic changes. In addition to mononuclear inflammatory cell infiltration, myonecrosis, and regenerative activity, the muscle biopsy sample typically shows fibers containing rimmed or membrane-bound sarcoplasmic vacuoles and occasional eosinophilic inclusions. Electron microscopy shows distinctive cytoplasmic and intranuclear masses of randomly oriented filaments or filamentous microtubules 10–20 nm in diameter and 1–3 μm in length. Doubts have been expressed concerning the nosology of inclusion body myositis, because similar morphologic changes have been observed in a patient with Sjögren's syndrome and in a patient with otherwise typical DM who showed a favorable response to steroid therapy (Lane et al., 1985).

Granulomatous Myositis

This myositis is a rare manifestation of sarcoidosis, although asymptomatic muscle granulomas are not uncommon in this disorder. Occasionally, however, patients with or without evidence of sarcoidosis in other organs may develop slowly progressive proximal weakness, sometimes associated with skin changes resembling DM (Itoh et al., 1980). The serum CK value may be normal, but the muscle biopsy sample shows circumscribed granulomatous lesions consisting of histiocytes, epithelioid cells, and Langhans giant cells. Response to steroids is variable and is usually less favorable in chronic cases. Granulomatous myositis may also occur in Crohn's disease, Wegener's granulomatosis, and a rare syndrome consisting of myositis, giant cell myocarditis, myasthenia gravis, and autoimmune thyroiditis sometimes associated with thymoma (Namba et al., 1974).

Eosinophilic Polymyositis

This disorder occasionally occurs as part of the hypereosinophilic syndrome and may be associated with hypergammaglobulinemia, rash, pulmonary and cardiac involvement, peripheral neuropathy, and anemia (Stark, 1979). The serum CK activity is usually increased, and a muscle biopsy sample shows myonecrosis, regeneration, and perivascular and interstitial inflammatory exudates consisting largely of eosinophils. The response to immunosuppressive treatment is variable.

Eosinophilic Fasciitis

This benign disorder may mimic DM in the early stages. It presents with induration and swelling of the skin over the forearms and upper trunk, associated with pain, stiffness, and limitation of movement. Muscle biopsy results are usually normal but may show eosinophilic infiltration. Most cases show a rapid response to corticosteroid treatment (Simon et al., 1982).

ENDOCRINE MYOPATHIES

Hyperthyroidism

Hyperthyroidism may be associated with a myopathy, exophthalmic ophthalmoplegia, hypokalemic periodic paralysis, or myasthenia gravis (Kendall-Taylor and Turnbull, 1983). Myopathy with proximal or sometimes diffuse muscle weakness occurs in 80% of untreated cases but is rarely the major presenting complaint. Clinical symptoms include difficulty in climbing stairs or getting up from a seated or squatting position. Bulbar and respiratory muscle involvement is rare. The weakness is often out of proportion to the degree of muscle atrophy, and the limb reflexes are normal or hyperactive. The EMG indicates myopathy, the serum CK activity is normal, and muscle biopsy results may show an increased proportion of histochemical type 2 muscle fibers. Thyrotoxic myopathy is probably due to several factors including an abnormally low resting muscle membrane potential, reduced membrane excitability, and increased relaxation rate. Treatment of the hyperthyroidism results in complete recovery.

Graves' ophthalmopathy is thought to be an organ-specific autoimmune disease associated with inflammatory infiltration and edema of the orbital contents, including the extraocular muscles, lacrimal glands,

and connective tissue elements. The two main symptoms are exophthalmos, which may be painful, and diplopia related especially to weakness of upward and lateral gaze. The proptosis that results from increased retro-orbital pressure may be severe and may lead to chemosis, corneal ulceration, papilledema, optic atrophy, and visual loss. The condition may be unilateral or bilateral and is independent of thyroid status. It is associated with the presence of circulating autoantibody to a soluble eye muscle antigen (Kodama et al., 1982). Tarsorrhaphy may be necessary to protect the cornea, and orbital decompression, together with high doses of corticosteroids, is indicated when vision is threatened.

Thyrotoxic hypokalemic paralysis and myasthenia gravis are discussed elsewhere (Chapters 13, 15, and 117).

Hypothyroidism

Hypothyroidism is commonly associated with myalgia, cramps, and muscle stiffness, sometimes accompanied by mild proximal weakness. Occasionally, there is striking muscle hypertrophy (Hoffmann's syndrome). The tendon reflex relaxation time is delayed, and the muscles may show percussion myoedema. The EMG displays myopathy, the serum CK activity is elevated, and muscle biopsy results may show a reduced proportion of histochemical type 2 muscle fibers, which are sometimes atrophic. Muscle function is restored to normal by replacement therapy.

Cushing's Syndrome

This disorder is almost always associated with a proximal myopathy, which is typically confined to the lower limbs and is associated with depressed or absent reflexes. The serum CK value is usually normal, the EMG indicates myopathy, and muscle biopsy sample shows selective atrophy of the histochemical type 2B fibers and an excess of neutral lipid droplets in the type 1 fibers. The condition is indistinguishable from steroid-induced myopathy and responds to treatment of Cushing's syndrome. The weakness in both conditions may be due to a decrease in the synthesis of muscle proteins, an increase in the breakdown of muscle proteins, or the effects of corticosteroids on the function of the muscle fiber membrane or sarcoplasmic reticulum (Kendall-Taylor and Turnbull, 1983).

Addison's Disease

Addison's disease is also associated with weakness and fatigue, which is probably related to changes in body water and electrolyte content. The symptoms respond promptly to steroid replacement therapy.

Table 14–8. TOXIC AND DRUG-INDUCED MYOPATHIES

Acute Rhabdomyolysis	**Inflammatory Myopathy**
Alcohol	D-Penicillamine
Heroin	Cimetidine
Amphetamine	Procainamide
Methadone	
Barbiturates	**Painless Proximal Myopathy**
Diazepam	Corticosteroids
Amphotericin B	Chloroquine
Carbenoxolone	Perhexiline
Phencyclidine	
	Myalgia, Cramps, and
Subacute Necrotizing	**Myokymia**
Myopathy	Clofibrate
Alcohol	Lithium
Clofibrate	Salbutamol
ε-Aminocaproic acid	Cimetidine
Emetine	Isoetharine
Heroin	
	Myotonia
Hypokalemic Myopathy	20,25-Diazocholesterol
Diuretics	
Purgatives	
Licorice	
Carbenoxolone	
Amphotericin B	

Acromegaly

Acromegaly is initially associated with increased muscle bulk and strength but later may cause mild proximal weakness with an elevated serum CK level, myopathic changes on the EMG, and muscle fiber degeneration as seen on muscle biopsy examination.

Hyperparathyroidism

Hyperparathyroidism, either primary or secondary, may be associated with a proximal myopathy characterized by a waddling gait, easy fatigability, and pain on movement. Muscle wasting is usually minimal, strength is variable because of pain, and reflexes are typically hyperactive. The serum CK level is normal, the EMG shows myopathy, and muscle biopsy results may show selective atrophy of the type 2B muscle fibers. The serum calcium value is elevated in primary hyperparathyroidism but may be normal in osteomalacia, although the alkaline phosphatase level is invariably increased. The diagnosis of a myopathy related to hyperparathyroidism or osteomalacia depends on careful clinical, radiologic, and biochemical assessment, which may include measurement of blood parathyroid hormone and vitamin D levels, bone biopsy, and estimation of urinary calcium and phosphorus excretion. Osteomalacic myopathy occurs in vitamin D deficiency, malabsorption syndromes, renal tubular acidosis, chronic renal failure, and long-standing anticonvulsant intoxication. The myopathy of primary hyperparathyroidism responds to removal of the adenoma; osteomalacic myopathy usually responds to treatment with vitamin D.

TOXIC AND DRUG-INDUCED MYOPATHIES

A wide range of drugs and toxic agents, including alcohol, can produce an acute or subacute necrotizing myopathy with muscle pain, tenderness, and weakness, sometimes associated with myoglobinuria and renal insufficiency (Argov and Mastaglia, 1988). The more important ones are given in Table 14–8. The serum CK value may be grossly elevated, the EMG indicates myopathy, and the muscle biopsy sample may show extensive myonecrosis with profuse regenerative activity. The mechanism of most drug-induced myopathies is not known, but some are thought to act by causing profound hypokalemia (see Table 14–8). Drug-induced myopathies are usually dose dependent and are reversible provided the drug is withdrawn promptly. Some drugs cause a syndrome of myalgia, muscle cramps, and myokymia, whereas others, particularly corticosteroids, cause a progressive proximal myopathy that is painless.

References

(Key references are designated with an asterisk.)

Abarbanel J.M., Bashan N., Potashnik R., et al. Adult muscle phosphorylase "B" kinase deficiency. *Neurology* 36:560–562, 1986.

Ahtani Y., Matsuda I., Iwomasa T., et al. Infantile glycogen storage myopathy in a girl with phosphorylase kinase deficiency. *Neurology* 32:833–838, 1982.

*Arahata K., Engel A.G. Monoclonal antibody analysis of mononuclear cells in myopathies. I. Quantitation of subsets according to diagnosis and sites of accumulation and demonstration and counts of muscle fibres invaded by T cells. *Ann. Neurol.* 16:193–208, 1984.

Arahata K., Engel A.G. Monoclonal antibody analysis of mononuclear cells in myopathies. IV. Cell-mediated cytotoxicity and muscle fibre necrosis. *Ann. Neurol.* 23:168–173, 1988a.

Arahata K., Engel A.G. Monoclonal antibody analysis of mononuclear cells in myopathies. V. Identification and quantitation of T8⁺ cytotoxic and T8⁺ suppressor cells. *Ann. Neurol.* 23:493–499, 1988b.

Arahata K., Ishiura S., Ishiguro T., et al. Immunostaining of skeletal and cardiac muscle surface membrane with antibody against Duchenne muscular dystrophy peptide. *Nature* 333:861–863, 1988c.

Arahata K., Hoffman V.P., Kunkel L.M., et al. Dystrophin diagnosis: comparison of dystrophin abnormalities by immunofluorescence and immunoblot analysis. *Proc. Natl. Acad. Sci. U.S.A.* 86:7154–7158, 1989.

Argov Z., Mastaglia F.L. Drug-induced neuromuscular disorders in man. In Walton J.A., ed. *Disorders of Voluntary Muscle.* 5th ed. London, Churchill Livingstone, pp. 981–1014, 1988.

Arikawa E., Arahata K., Nonaka I., et al. Dystrophin analysis in congenital muscular dystrophy (abstract). *Neurology* 40(Suppl. 1):206, 1990.

Askari A.D. Cardiac abnormalities. *Clin. Rheum. Dis.* 10:131–149, 1984.

Bakker E., Veenema H., Den Dunnen J.T., et al. Germinal mosaicism increases the recurrence risk for "new" Duchenne muscular dystrophy mutations. *J. Med. Genet.* 26:553–558, 1989.

Banker B.Q. The congenital myopathies. In Engel A.G., Banker B.Q., eds. *Myology.* New York, McGraw-Hill, pp. 1527–1579, 1986.

Barchi R.L. Myotonia. An evaluation of the chloride hypothesis. *Arch. Neurol.* 32:175–180, 1975.

Barchi R.L. A mechanistic approach to the myotonic syndromes. *Muscle Nerve* 5:560–563, 1982.

Barth P.G., van Wijngaarden G.K., Bethlem J. X-linked myotubular myopathy with fatal neonatal asphyxia. *Neurology* 25:531–536, 1975.

Bashan N., Iancu T.C., Lermer A., et al. Glycogenesis due to liver and muscle phosphorylase kinase deficiency. *Pediatr. Res.* 15:299–303, 1981.

Baumbach L.L., Chamberlain J.S., Ward P.A., et al. Molecular and clinical correlations of deletions leading to Duchenne and Becker muscular dystrophies. *Neurology* 39:465–474, 1989.

Beggs A.H., Kunkel L.M. Improved diagnosis of Duchenne/Becker muscular dystrophy. *J. Clin. Invest.* 85:613–619, 1990.

Bender P.K., Emerson C.P. Jr. Skeletal muscle phosphorylase kinase catalytic subunit mRNAs are expressed in heart tissue but not in liver. *J. Biol. Chem.* 262:8799–8805, 1987.

Bernstein R.M., Mathews M.B. From virus infection to autoantibody production. *Lancet* 1:42, 1984.

Bird T.B., Follett C., Griep E. Cognitive and personality function in myotonic muscular dystrophy. *J. Neurol. Neurosurg. Psychiatry* 46:971–980, 1983.

Bohan A., Peter J.B. Polymyositis and dermatomyositis. Part one. *N. Engl. J. Med.* 292:344–347, 1975a.

Bohan A., Peter J.B. Polymyositis and dermatomyositis. Part two. *N. Engl. J. Med.* 292:403–407, 1975b.

Bohan A., Peter J.B., Bowman R.L., et al. A computer assisted analysis of 153 patients with polymyositis and dermatomyositis. *Medicine* 56:255–286, 1977.

Bonilla E., Younger D.S., Chang H.W., et al. Partial dystrophin deficiency in monozygous twin carriers of the Duchenne gene discordant for clinical myopathy. *Neurology* 40:1267–1270, 1990.

Bradley W.G., Jones M.Z., Mussini J.M., et al. Becker-type muscular dystrophy. *Muscle Nerve* 1:111–132, 1978.

Brown R.M., Dahl H-H.M., Brown G.K. X chromosome localization of the functional gene for the E1α subunit of the human pyruvate dehydrogenase complex. *Genomics* 4:174–181, 1989.

Burke J., Hwang P., Anderson L., et al. Intron/exon structure of the human gene for the muscle isozyme of glycogen phosphorylase. *Proteins* 2:177–187, 1987.

Callen J.P. Myositis and malignancy. *Clin. Rheum. Dis.* 10:117–130, 1984.

*Carpenter S., Karpati G. The major inflammatory myopathies of unknown cause. *Pathol. Annu.* 16:205–237, 1981.

Chelly J., Hamard G., Koulakoff A., et al. Dystrophin gene transcribed from different promoters in neuronal and glial cells. *Nature* 344:64–65, 1990.

Chutkow J.G., Heffner R.R., Cramer A.A., et al. Adult-onset autosomal dominant limb-girdle muscular dystrophy. *Ann. Neurol.* 20:240–248, 1986.

Clark J.B., Hayes D.J., Morgan-Hughes J.A., et al. Mitochondrial myopathies: disorders of the respiratory chain and oxidative phosphorylation. *J. Inherited Metab. Dis.* 7:62–68, 1984.

Clemens P.R., Yamamoto M., Engel A.G. Adult phosphorylase *b* kinase deficiency. *Ann. Neurol.* 28:529–538, 1990.

Cornelio F., Bresolin N., DiMauro S., et al. Congenital myopathy due to phosphorylase deficiency. *Neurology (N.Y.)* 33:1383–1385, 1983.

*Cornelio F., Bresolin N., Singer P.A., et al. Clinical varieties of neuromuscular disease in debrancher deficiency. *Arch. Neurol.* 41:1027–1032, 1984.

Cullen M.J., Mastaglia F.L. Morphological changes in dystrophic muscle. *Br. Med. Bull.* 36:145–152, 1980.

Davidson M., Miranda A.F., Bender A.N., et al. Muscle phosphofructokinase (PFK) deficiency: immunological and biochemical studies of PFK isozymes in muscle culture. *J. Clin. Invest.* 72:545–550, 1983.

Demaugre F., Bonnefont J.P., Cepance C., et al. Immuno quantitative analysis of human carnitine palmitoyltransferase I, II defects. *Pediatr. Res.* 27:497–500, 1990.

Den Dunen J.T., Grootscholten P.M., Bakker E., et al. Topography of the Duchenne muscular dystrophy (DMD) gene: FIGE and cDNA analysis of 194 cases reveals 115 deletions and 13 duplications. *Am. J. Hum. Genet.* 45:835–847, 1989.

Denman A.M. Inflammatory disorders of muscle. Aetiology. *Clin. Rheum. Dis.* 10:9–33, 1984.

DiMauro S., Miranda A.F., Hays A.P., et al. Myoadenylate deaminase deficiency. Muscle biopsy and muscle culture in a patient with gout. *J. Neurol. Sci.* 47:191–202, 1980a.

*DiMauro S., Trevisan C., Hays A. Disorders of lipid metabolism in muscle. *Muscle Nerve* 3:369–388, 1980b.

DiMauro S., Dalakas M., Miranda A.F. Phosphoglycerate kinase (PGK) deficiency: another cause of recurrent myoglobinuria. *Ann. Neurol.* 13:11–19, 1983.

*DiMauro S., Bresolin E., Hays A.P. Disorders of glycogen metabolism of muscle. *Crit. Rev. Clin. Neurobiol.* 1:83–116, 1984.

*DiMauro S., Bonilla E., Zeviani M., et al. Mitochondrial myopathies. *Ann. Neurol.* 11:521–538, 1985.

DiMauro S., Bonilla E., Lombes A., et al. Mitochondrial encephalomyopathies. *Neurol. Clin.* 8:483–505, 1990.

Dreyfus J.C., Poenaru L. White blood cells and a diagnosis of alpha-glucosidase deficiency. *Pediatr. Res.* 14:342–344, 1980.

Eishi Y., Takemura T., Sone R. Glycogen storage disease confined to the heart with deficient activity of cardiac phosphorylase kinase: a new type of glycogen storage disease. *Hum. Pathol.* 16:193–197, 1985.

Emery A.E.H. Muscular dystrophy, benign X-linked with contractures. In Vinken P.J., Bruyn G.W., eds. *Handbook of Clinical Neurology.* Vol. 43. Part II. Amsterdam, North Holland, pp. 38–89, 1982.

Emery A.E.H. *Duchenne Muscular Dystrophy.* Revised ed. *Oxford Monographs on Medical Genetics.* Vol. 15. New York, Oxford University Press, 1988.

Emslie-Smith A.M., Engel A.G. Microvascular changes in early and advanced dermatomyositis: a quantitative study. *Ann. Neurol.* 27:343–356, 1990.

Engel A.G. Metabolic and endocrine myopathies. In Walton J.N., ed. *Disorders of Voluntary Muscle.* 4th ed. Edinburgh, Churchill Livingstone, pp. 664–711, 1981.

Engel A.G. Carnitine deficiency syndromes and lipid storage myopathies. In Engel A.G., Banker B.Q., eds. *Myology.* New York, McGraw-Hill, pp. 1663–1696, 1986a.

Engel A.G. Duchenne dystrophy. In Engel A.G., Banker B.Q., eds. *Myology.* New York, McGraw-Hill, pp. 1185–1240, 1986b.

*Engel A.G., Arahata K. Monoclonal antibody analysis of mononuclear cells in myopathies. II. Phenotypes of autoinvasive cells in polymyositis and inclusion body myositis. *Ann. Neurol.* 16:209–215, 1984.

*Engel A.G., Rebouche C.J. Carnitine metabolism and inborn errors. *J. Inherited Metab. Dis.* 7:38–43, 1984.

Engel A.G., Gomez M.R., Seybold M.E., et al. The spectrum and diagnosis of acid maltase deficiency. *Neurology (Minneap.)* 23:95–106, 1973.

England S.B., Nicholson I.V.B., Johnson M.A., et al. Very mild muscular dystrophy associated with the deletion of 46% of dystrophin. *Nature* 343:180–182, 1990.

Ervasti J.M., Ohlendieck K., Kahl S.D., et al. Deficiency of a glycoprotein component of the dystrophin complex in dystrophic muscle. *Nature* 344:315–319, 1990.

*Fardeau M. Congenital myopathies. In Mastaglia F.L., Walton J., eds. *Skeletal Muscle Pathology.* Edinburgh, Churchill Livingstone, pp. 161–203, 1982.

Fidziańska A., Goebel H.H., Kosswig R., et al. "Killer" cells in Duchenne disease: ultrastructural study. *Neurology (N.Y.)* 34:295–303, 1984.

Fishbein W.N., Armbrustmacher V.W., Griffin J.L. Myoadenylate deaminase deficiency: a new disease of muscle. *Science* 299:545–548, 1978.

Fishbein W.N., Armbrustmacher V.W., Griffin J.L., et al. Levels of adenylate deaminase, adenylate kinase, and creatine kinase in frozen human muscle biopsy specimens relative to type 1/type 2 fiber distribution: evidence for a carrier state of myoadenylate deaminase deficiency. *Ann. Neurol.* 15:271–277, 1984.

Fitzsimons R.B., Gurwin E.B., Bird A.C. Retinal vascular abnormalities in facioscapulohumeral muscular dystrophy. *Brain* 110:631–648, 1987.

Francke U., Darras B.T., Zander N.F., et al. Assignment of human genes for phosphorylase kinase subunits α (PHKA) to Xq12-q13 and β (PHKB) to 16q12-q13. *Am. J. Hum. Genet.* 45:276–282, 1989.

Frank J.B., Harati Y., Butler I.J., et al. Central core disease and malignant hyperthermia syndrome. *Ann. Neurol.* 7:11–17, 1980.

Fukuyama Y., Osawa M. Congenital muscular dystrophy: clinico-nosological aspects. In Ebashi S., ed. *Muscular Dystrophy*. Tokyo, University of Tokyo Press, pp. 399–424, 1982.

Fukuyama Y., Osawa M., Suzuki H. Congenital progressive muscular dystrophy of the Fukuyama-type. Clinical, genetic and pathological considerations. *Brain Dev.* 3:1–29, 1981.

Garlepp M.J., Dawkins R.L. Immunological aspects. *Clin. Rheum. Dis.* 10:35–51, 1984.

Gellera C., Uziel D., Rimoldi M., et al. Fumarase deficiency is an autosomal recessive encephalopathy affecting both the mitochondrial and the cytosolic enzymes. *Neurology* 40:494–499, 1990.

Gilchrist J.M., Periac-Vance M., Silverman L., et al. Clinical and genetic investigation in autosomal dominant limb girdle muscular dystrophy. *Neurology* 38:5–9, 1988.

Gillard E.F., Chamberlain J.S., Murphy E.G., et al. Molecular and phenotypic analysis of patients with deletions within the deletion-rich region of the Duchenne muscular dystrophy (DMD) gene. *Am. J. Hum. Genet.* 45:507–520, 1989.

Gospe S.M., Lazaro R.P., Lava N.S., et al. Familial X-linked myalgia and cramps: a non-progressive myopathy associated with a deletion in the dystrophin gene. *Neurology* 39:1277–1280, 1989.

Goto Y., Nonaka I., Horai S. A mutation in the tRNA^Leu (UUR) gene associated with the MELAS subgroup of mitochondrial encephalomyopathies. *Nature* 348:651–653, 1990.

Gronert G.A. Malignant hyperthermia. *Anesthesiology* 53:395–423, 1980.

Harding A.E., Hold I.J., Cooper J.M., et al. Mitochondrial myopathies: genetic defects. *Biochem. Soc. Trans.* 18:519–522, 1990.

*Harper P.S. *Myotonic Dystrophy. Major Problems in Neurology.* Vol. 9. Philadelphia, Saunders, 1979.

Harriman D.G.F. The pathology of malignant hyperthermia. In Mastaglia F., Walton J., eds. *Skeletal Muscle Pathology.* Edinburgh, Churchill Livingstone, pp. 575–591, 1982.

Hays A.P., Hallett M., Delfs J., et al. Muscle phosphofructokinase deficiency: abnormal polysaccharide in a case of late-onset myopathy. *Neurology (N.Y.)* 31:1077–1086, 1981.

Heffner R.R., Barron S.A. Polymyositis beginning as a focal process. *Arch. Neurol.* 38:439–442, 1981.

Heffron J.J.A. Mitochondrial and plasma membrane changes in skeletal muscle in the malignant hyperthermia syndrome. *Biochem. Soc. Trans.* 12:360–362, 1984.

Hodgson S., Boswinkel E., Cole C., et al. A linkage study of Emery-Dreifuss muscular dystropy. *Hum. Genet.* 74:409–411, 1986.

Hoffman E.P., Brown R.H., Kunkel L.M. Dystrophin: the protein product of the Duchenne muscular dystrophy locus. *Cell* 51:919–928, 1987.

Hoffman E.P., Kunkel L.M., Angelini C., et al. Improved diagnosis of Becker muscular dystrophy by dystrophin testing. *Neurology* 39:1011–1017, 1989.

Huijing F. Glycogen metabolism and glycogen storage disease. *Physiol. Rev.* 55:609–658, 1975.

Hurko O., Hoffman E.P., McKee L., et al. Dystrophin analysis in clonal myoblast derived from a Duchenne muscular dystrophy carrier. *Am. J. Hum. Genet.* 44:820–826, 1989.

Hyser C.L., Mendell J.R. Recent advances in Duchenne and Becker muscular dystrophy. *Neurol. Clin.* 6:429–453, 1988.

*Isenberg D. Myositis in other connective tissue disorders. *Clin. Rheum. Dis.* 10:151–174, 1984.

Itoh J., Akiguchi I., Midorikawa R., et al. Sarcoid myopathy with typical rash of dermatomyositis. *Neurology (N.Y.)* 30:1118–1121, 1980.

Iwamasa T., Fukuda S., Tokumitsu S. Myopathy due to glycogen storage disease: pathological and biochemical studies in relation to glycogenosome formation. *Exp. Mol. Pathol.* 38:405–420, 1983.

*Kagen L.J. Less common causes of myositis. *Clin. Rheum. Dis.* 10:175–187, 1984.

Kanno T., Sudo K., Takeuchi I., et al. Hereditary deficiency of lactate dehydrogenase M-subunit. *Clin. Chim. Acta* 108:267–276, 1980.

Kelemen J., Rice D.R., Bradley W.G., et al. Familial myoadenylate deaminase deficiency and exertional myalgia. *Neurology (N.Y.)* 32:857–863, 1982.

Kendall-Taylor, Turnbull D.M. Endocrine myopathies. *Br. Med. J.* 287:705–708, 1983.

Kilimann M.W. Molecular genetics of phosphorylase kinase: cDNA cloning, chromosomal mapping and isoform structure. *J. Inherited Metab. Dis.* 13:435–441, 1990.

Kodama K., Sikorska H., Bandy-Dafoe P., et al. Demonstration of a circulating auto-antibody against a soluble I-muscle antigen in Graves' ophthalmopathy. *Lancet* 2:1353–1356, 1982.

Koenig M., Kunkel L.M. Detailed analysis of the repeat domain of dystrophin reveals four potential segments that may confer flexibility. *J. Biol. Chem.* 265:4560–4566, 1990.

Koenig M., Hoffman E.P., Bertelson C.J., et al. Complete cloning of the Duchenne muscular dystrophy (DMD) cDNA and preliminary genomic organization of the DMD gene in normal and affected individuals. *Cell* 50:509–517, 1987.

Koenig M., Monago A.P., Kunkel L.M. The complete sequence of dystrophin predicts a rod-shaped cytoskeletal protein. *Cell* 53:219–228, 1988.

Koenig M., Beggs A.H., Moyer M., et al. The molecular basis for Duchenne versus Becker muscular dystrophy: correlation of severity with type of deletion. *Am. J. Hum. Genet.* 45:498–506, 1989.

Kono N., Mineo I., Sumi S., et al. Metabolic basis of improved exercise tolerance: muscle phosphorylase deficiency after glucagon administration. *Neurology* 34:1471–1476, 1984.

Korf B.R., Bresnan M.J., Schapiro F., et al. Facioscapulohumeral dystrophy presenting in infancy with facial diplegia and sensorineural deafness. *Ann. Neurol.* 17:513–516, 1985.

Korinthenberg R., Palm D., Schlake W., et al. Congenital muscular dystrophy, brain malformation and ocular problems (muscle, eye and brain disease) in 2 German families. *Eur. J. Pediatr.* 142:64–68, 1984.

Krebs E.G., Beavo J.A. Phosphorylation-dephosphorylation of enzymes. *Annu. Rev. Biochem.* 48:923–959, 1979.

Lane R.J.M., Fulthorpe J.J., Hudgson P. Inclusion body myositis: a case with associated collagen vascular disease responding to treatment. *J. Neurol. Neurosurg. Psychiatry* 48:270–273, 1985.

Layzer R.B. Pathophysiology of the periodic paralyses: overview and theoretical aspects. In Serratrice G., Cros D., Desnuelle C., et al., eds. *Neuromuscular Diseases.* New York, Raven Press, pp. 173–177, 1984.

Lehmann-Horn F., Rudel R., Dengler R., et al. Membrane defects in paramyotonia congenita with and without myotonia in a warm environment. *Muscle Nerve* 4:396–406, 1981.

Lombes A., Bonilla E., DiMauro S. Mitochondrial encephalomyopathies. *Rev. Neurol.* 145:671–689, 1989.

Loonen M.C.B., Busch H.S.M., Koster J.F., et al. A family with different clinical forms of acid maltase deficiency (glycogenosis type II): biochemical and genetic studies. *Neurology (N.Y.)* 31:1209–1216, 1981.

Lotz B.P., Engel A.G., Nishino H., et al. Inclusion body myositis. Observations in 40 patients. *Brain* 112:727–747, 1989.

Love D.R., Hill D.F., Dickson G., et al. An autosomal transcript in skeletal muscle with homology to dystrophin. *Nature* 339:55–58, 1989.

MacLennan D.H., Duff C., Zorzato F., et al. Ryanodine receptor gene is a candidate for predisposition to malignant hyperthermia. *Nature* 343:559–561, 1990.

Malhotra S.B., Hart K.A., Klamut H.J., et al. Frame-shift deletions in patients with Duchenne and Becker muscular dystrophy. *Science* 242:755–758, 1988.

Markesbery W.R., Griggs R.C. Distal myopathies. In Engel A.G., Baker B.Q., eds. *Myology.* New York, McGraw-Hill, pp. 1313–1325, 1986.

Markesbery W.R., Griggs R.C., Herr B. Distal myopathy: electron microscopic and histochemical studies. *Neurology (Minneap.)* 27:727–735, 1977.

Martinez B.A., Lake B.D. Childhood nemaline myopathy—a review of clinical presentation in relation to prognosis. *Dev. Med. Child Neurol.* 29:815–820, 1987.

Martiniuk F., Meyler M., Tzall S., et al. Extensive genetic heterogeneity in patients with acid alpha glucosidase deficiency as detected by abnormalities of DNA and mRNA. *Am. J. Hum. Genet.* 47:73–78, 1990.

*Mastaglia F.L., Ojeda V.J. Inflammatory myopathies. Part one. *Ann. Neurol.* 17:215–227, 1985a.

*Mastaglia F.L., Ojeda V.J. Inflammatory myopathies. Part two. *Ann. Neurol.* 17:317–323, 1985b.

Mathews M.B., Bernstein R.M. Myositis autoantibody inhibits histidyl-tRNA synthetase: a model for autoimmunity. *Nature* 304:177–179, 1983.

Mathews M.B., Reichlen M., Hughes G.R.V., et al. Anti-threonyl-tRNA synthetase. A second myositis-related autoantibody. *J. Exp. Med.* 160:420–434, 1984.

McArdle B. Myopathy due to a defect in muscle glycogen breakdown. *Clin. Sci.* 10:13–33, 1951.

McMenamin J.B., Becker L.E., Murphy E.G. Congenital muscular dystrophy: a clinico-pathological report of 24 cases. *J. Paediatr.* 100:692–697, 1982.

Merickel M., Gray R., Shauvin P., et al. Cultured muscle from myotonic muscular dystrophy patients: altered membrane electrical properties. *Proc. Natl. Acad. Sci. U.S.A.* 78:648–652, 1981.

Miranda A.F., Nette E.G., Hartlage P.L., et al. Phosphorylase isoenzymes in normal and myophosphorylase-deficient human heart. *Neurology* 29:1538–1541, 1979.

Miranda A.F., Schanske S., DiMaur S. Developmentally regulated isozyme transitions in normal and diseased human muscle. In Pearson M.L., Epstein H.F., eds. *Muscle Development: Molecular and Cellular Control.* Cold Spring Harbor, NY, Cold Spring Harbor Laboratory, pp. 515–552, 1982.

Mita S., Schmidt B., Schon E.A., et al. Detection of "deleted" mitochondrial genomes in cytochrome-*c*–oxidase-deficient muscle fibers of a patient with Kearns-Sayre syndrome. *Proc. Natl. Acad. Sci. U.S.A.* 86:9509–9513, 1989.

Mita S., Rizzuto R., Moraes C.T., et al. Recombination via flanking direct repeats is a major cause of large-scale deletions of human mitochondrial DNA. *Nucleic Acids Res.* 18:561–567, 1990.

Mitsumoto H. McArdle's disease: phosphorylase activity in regenerating muscle fibres. *Neurology* 29:258–262, 1979.

Mizuta K., Hashimoto E., Tsutou A. A new type of glycogen storage disease caused by deficiency of cardiac phosphorylase kinase. *Biochem. Biophys. Res. Commun.* 119:582–587, 1984.

Mommaerts W.F.H.M., Illingworth B., Pearson C.M., et al. A functional disorder of muscle associated with absence of phosphorylase. *Proc. Natl. Acad. Sci. U.S.A.* 45:791–797, 1959.

Monaco A.P., Bertelson C.J., Leichti-Gallati S., et al. An explanation for the phenotypic differences between patients bearing partial deletions of the DMD locus. *Genomics* 2:90–95, 1988.

Morgan-Hughes J.A. Defects of the energy pathways of skeletal muscle. In Matthews W.B., Glaser G.H. (eds) *Recent Advances in Clinical Neurology.* Vol. 3. Edinburgh, Churchill Livingstone, pp. 1–46, 1982.

Morgan-Hughes J.A. Mitochondrial myopathies. In Engel A.G., Banker B.Q., eds. *Myology.* New York, McGraw-Hill, pp. 1709–1743, 1986.

Morgan-Hughes J.A., Landon D.N. Mitochondrial respiratory chain deficiencies in man. Some histochemical and fine-structural observations. In Scarlato G., Cerri G., eds. *Mitochondrial Pathology in Muscle Disease.* Padua, Piccin Medical Books, pp. 21–37, 1983.

Morgan-Hughes J.A., Hayes D.J., Cooper M., et al. Mitochondrial myopathies: deficiencies localized to complex I and complex III of the mitochondrial respiratory chain. *Biochem. Soc. Trans.* 13:648–630, 1985.

Morgan-Hughes J.A., Schapira A.H.V., Cooper J.M., et al. Molecular defects of NADH-ubiquinone oxidoreductase (complex I) in mitochondrial diseases. *J. Bioenerg. Biomembr.* 20:365–382, 1988.

Morgan-Hughes J.A., Cooper J.M., Holt I.J., et al. Mitochondrial myopathies: clinical defects. *Biochem. Soc. Trans.* 18:523–525, 1990.

Moser H. Duchenne muscular dystrophy. Pathogenetic aspects and genetic prevention. *Hum. Genet.* 66:17–40, 1984.

Moxley R.T., Corbett A.J., Minaker K.L., et al. Whole body insulin resistence in myotonic cystrophy. *Ann. Neurol.* 15:157–162, 1984.

Nakase H., Moraes C.T., Rizzuto R., et al. Transcription and translation of deleted mitochondrial genomes in Kearns-Sayre syndrome: implications for pathogenesis. *Am. J. Hum. Genet.* 46:418–427, 1990.

Namba T., Brunner M.G., Grob N. Idiopathic giant cell polymyositis. Report of a case and review of the syndrome. *Arch. Neurol.* 31:27–30, 1974.

Nicholson L.V.B., Johnson M.A., Gardner-Medwin D., et al.

Heterogeneity of dystrophin expression in patients with Duchenne and Becker dystrophies. *Acta Neuropathol.* 80:239–250, 1990.

Ohtani Y., Matsuda I., Iwamasa T., et al. Infantile glycogen storage myopathy in a girl with phosphorylase kinase deficiency. *Neurology (N.Y.)* 32:833–838, 1982.

*Pachman L.M., Maryjowski M.C. Juvenile dermatomyositis and polymyositis. *Clin. Rheum. Dis.* 10:95–115, 1984.

Pestronk A., Drachman D. Polymyositis: reduction of acetylcholine receptors in skeletal muscle. *Muscle Nerve* 8:233–239, 1985.

Petty R.K.H., Harding A.E., Morgan-Hughes J.A. The clinical features of mitochondrial myopathy. *Brain* 109:915–938, 1986.

Plotz P.H., Dalakas M., Leff R.L., et al. Current concepts in the idiopathic inflammatory myopathies: polymyositis, dermatomyositis and related disorders. *Ann. Intern. Med.* 111:143–157, 1989.

Poskanzer D.C., Kerr D.M.S. A third type of periodic paralysis with normokalemia and favourable response to sodium chloride. *Am. J. Med.* 31:328–342, 1961.

Pournand R., Sanders D.B., Corwin M.H. Late-onset McArdle's disease with unusual electromyographic findings. *Arch. Neurol.* 40:374–378, 1983.

Rebouche C.J., Engel A.G. Kinetic compartmental analysis of carnitine metabolism in the human carnitine deficiency syndromes: evidence for alterations in tissue carnitine transport. *J. Clin. Invest.* 73:857–867, 1984.

Reichlin M., Arnett F.C. Multiplicity of antibodies of myositis sera. *Arthritis Rheum.* 27:1150–1156, 1984.

Reuser A.J.J., Kroos M., Willemsen R., et al. Clinical diversity in glycogenosis type II. *J. Clin. Invest.* 79:1689–1699, 1987.

Richards C.S., Watkins S.C., Hoffman E.P., et al. Skewed X inactivation in female MZ twins results in Duchenne muscular dystrophy. *Am. J. Hum. Genet.* 46:672–681, 1990.

Robinson B.H., Chun K., Mackay N., et al. Isolated and combined deficiencies of the α-keto acid dehydrogenase complexes. *Ann. N. Y. Acad. Sci.* 573:337–346, 1989.

Rosing H.S., Hopkins L.C., Wallace D.C., et al. Maternally inherited mitochondrial myopathy and myoclonic epilepsy. *Ann. Neurol.* 17:228–237, 1985.

*Rowland L.P., DiMauro S. Glycogen-storage diseases of muscle: genetic problems. In Kety S.S., Rowland L.P., Sidman R.L., et al., eds. *Genetics of Neurological and Psychiatric Disorders.* New York, Raven Press, pp. 239–253, 1983.

Rowland L.P., Fetell M., Olarte M., et al. Emery-Dreifuss muscular dystrophy. *Ann. Neurol.* 5:111–117, 1979.

Rudel R., Lehmann-Horn F., Ricker K., et al. Hypokalemic periodic paralysis: in vitro investigation of muscle fiber membrane parameters. *Muscle Nerve* 7:110–120, 1984.

*Sabina R.L., Swain J.L., Olanow C.W., et al. Myoadenylate deaminase deficiency. Functional and metabolic abnormalities associated with disruption of the purine nucleotide cycle. *J. Clin. Invest.* 73:720–730, 1984.

Salmeron G., Greenberg D., Lidski M.D. Polymyositis and diffuse interstitial lung disease. A review of the pulmonary histopathologic findings. *Arch. Intern. Med.* 141:1005–1010, 1981.

Santavuori T., Leisti J., Kruus S., et al. Muscle, eye and brain disease: a new syndrome. *Doc. Ophthalmol. Proc. Ser.* 17:393–396, 1978.

Schmid R., Mahler R. Chronic progressive myopathy with myoglobinuria: demonstration of a glycogenolytic defect in muscle. *J. Clin. Invest.* 38:2044–2058, 1959.

Servidei S., DiMauro S. Disorders of glycogen metabolism of muscle. *Neurol. Clin.* 7:159–178, 1989.

Servidei S., Metlay L.A., Booth F.A., et al. Clinical and biochemical heterogeneity of phosphorylase kinase deficiency (abstract). *Neurology* 37(Suppl. 1):139, 1987.

Servidei S., Metlay L.A., Chodosh J., et al. Fatal infantile cardiopathy caused by phosphorylase *b* kinase deficiency. *J. Pediatr.* 113:82–85, 1988a.

Servidei S., Shanske S., Zeviani M., et al. McArdle's disease: biochemical and molecular genetic studies. *Ann. Neurol.* 24:774–778, 1988b.

Sharp G.C. Mixed connective tissue disease and overlap syndromes. In Kelly W.N., Harris E.D., Ruddy S., eds. *Textbook of Rheumatology.* Philadelphia, Saunders, pp. 1151–1161, 1981.

Shoffner J.M., Lott M.T., Lezza A.M.S., et al. Myoclonic epilepsy and ragged-red fiber disease (MERRF) is associated with a mitochondrial DNA tRNA^{Lys} mutation. *Cell* 61:931–937, 1990.

Shuaib A., Paasuke R.T., Brownell K.W. Central cord disease: clinical features in 13 patients. *Medicine* 66:389–396, 1987.

Shy G.M., Magee K.R. A new congenital non-progressive myopathy. *Brain* 79:610–621, 1956.

Simon D.B., Ringel S.P., Sufit R.L. Clinical spectrum of fascial inflammation. *Muscle Nerve* 5:525–537, 1982.

Slonim A.E., Goans P.J. Myopathy in McArdle's syndrome. Improvement with a high-protein diet. *N. Engl. J. Med.* 312:355–359, 1985.

Slonim A.E., Coleman R.A., McElligot M.A., et al. Improvement of muscle function in acid maltase deficiency by high-protein therapy. *Neurology (N.Y.)* 33:34–39, 1983.

Stanley C.A., Treem W.R., Hale D.E., et al. A genetic defect in carnitine transport causing primary carnitine deficiency. In Tanaka K., Coates P.M., eds. *Fatty Acid Oxidation. Clinical Biochemical and Molecular Aspects.* New York, Liss, pp. 457–464, 1990.

Stark R.J. Eosinophilic polymyositis. *Arch. Neurol.* 36:71–72, 1979.

Sunohara N., Arahata K., Hoffman E.P., et al. Quadriceps myopathy: forme fruste of Becker muscular dystrophy. *Ann. Neurol.* 28:634–639, 1990.

Takamoto K., Hirose K., Uono M., et al. A genetic variant of Emery-Dreifuss disease. *Arch. Neurol.* 41:1292–1293, 1984.

Targoff I.N. Immunologic aspects of myositis. *Curr. Opin. Rheumatol.* 1:432–442, 1989.

Taylor D.A., Carroll J.E., Smith M.E., et al. Facioscapulohumeral dystrophy associated with hearing loss and Coats syndrome. *Ann. Neurol.* 12:395–398, 1982.

Tein I., DeVivo D.C., Bierman S., et al. Impaired skin fibroblast carnitine uptake in primary systemic carnitine deficiency manifested by childhood carnitine-responsive cardiomyopathy. *Pediatr. Res.* 28:247–255, 1990.

Thomas P.K., Calne D.B., Elliot C.F. X-linked scapuloperoneal syndrome. *J. Neurol. Neurosurg. Psychiatry* 35:208–215, 1972.

Thomas P.K., Schott G.D., Morgan-Hughes J.A. Adult onset scapuloperoneal myopathy. *J. Neurol. Neurosurg. Psychiatry* 38:1008–1015, 1975.

Trend P. St J., Wiles C.M., Spencer G.T., et al. Acid maltase deficiency in adults: diagnosis and management in 5 cases. *Brain* 108:845–860, 1985.

van den Berg I.E.T., Berger R. Phosphorylase B kinase deficiency in man: a review. *J. Inherited Metab. Dis.* 13:442–451, 1990.

Venables G.S., Bates D., Carllidge N.E.F., et al. Acute polymyositis with subcutaneous oedema. *J. Neurol. Sci.* 55:161–164, 1982.

Vianey-Liaud C., Divry P., Gregersen N., et al. The inborn errors of mitochondrial fatty acid oxidation. *J. Inherited Metab. Dis.* 10(Suppl. 1):159–198, 1987.

Victor M., Hayes R., Adams R.D. Oculopharyngeal muscular dystrophy. A familial disease of late life characterized by dysphagia and progressive ptosis of the eyelids. *N. Engl. J. Med.* 267:1267–1272, 1962.

Vora S. Isozymes of phosphofructokinase. *Curr. Top. Biol. Med. Res.* 6:119–167, 1982.

Walton J.A., Gardner-Medwin D. Progressive muscular dystrophy and the myotonic disorders. In Walton J.A., ed. *Disorders of Voluntary Muscle.* 4th ed. Edinburgh, Churchill Livingstone, pp. 481–524, 1981.

Walton J.A., Gardner-Medwin D. The muscular dystrophies. In Walton J.A., ed. *Disorders of Voluntary Muscle.* 5th ed. London, Churchill Livingstone, pp. 519–568, 1988.

Whitaker J.N. Inflammatory myopathy: a review of etiologic and pathogenetic factors. *Muscle Nerve* 5:573–592, 1982.

Wijmenga C., Frants R.R., Brouwer O.F., et al. Location of facioscapulohumeral muscular dystrophy gene on chromosome IV. *Lancet* 1:651–653, 1990.

Worton R.G., Thompson M.W. Genetics of Duchenne muscular dystrophy. *Annu. Rev. Genet.* 22:601–629, 1988.

Yamaoka L.H., Pericak-Vance M.A., Speer M.C., et al. Tight linkage of creatine kinase (CKMM) to myotonic dystrophy chromosome 19. *Neurology* 40:222–226, 1990.

Yeo P.P.B., Chan S.H., Lui K.F., et al. HLA and thyrotoxic periodic paralysis. *Br. Med. J.* 2:930, 1978.

Zeviani M., Bonilla E., DeVivo D.C., et al. Mitochondrial disease. *Neurol. Clin.* 7:123–155, 1989.

Zeviani M., Amati P., Bresolin N., et al. Rapid detection of the A-G$^{(8344)}$ mutation of mtDNA in Italian families with myoclonus epilepsy and ragged-red fibers (MERRF). *Am. J. Hum. Genet.* 48:203–211, 1991.

15

Diseases of the Neuromuscular Junction

John Newsom-Davis

Improvement in prognosis for the principal disorders of the neuromuscular junction reflects the increased understanding of their causes and the expanded knowledge of the basic biology of the neuromuscular junction, particularly at the molecular level. These advances have been dependent on the application of many new investigative techniques. Foremost among them has been the use of specific ligands for the acetylcholine receptor (AChR) such as α-bungarotoxin (α-Bgt), which enabled the receptors to be quantified and was crucial in establishing the autoimmune nature of myasthenia gravis (MG).

THE NORMAL NEUROMUSCULAR JUNCTION

Development

The mechanism by which innervation of muscle leads to the clustering of AChRs at the nerve-muscle junction is not fully understood. According to one hypothesis, trophic factors released by the motor neuron cause the local accumulation of AChRs, whereas another theory argues that cell contact alone is sufficient to induce AChR clustering (Bloch and Pumplin, 1988).

Morphology

Although one motor nerve cell may supply as many as 1500 muscle fibers, each adult muscle fiber is supplied by only a *single* axonal branch and has only one neuromuscular junction. With appropriate staining, neuromuscular junctions are readily seen by light microscopy. Both the presynaptic nerve

terminals and the postsynaptic membrane can be visualized simultaneously by the use of a combined silver-cholinesterase staining method (Pestronk and Drachman, 1978) (Fig. 15–1A). The junction is roughly elliptic, with a branched pattern of nerve terminals within the cholinesterase-stained area. Pharmacologic denervation causes elongation and increased branching of the nerve terminals (Fig. 15–1B).

At the ultrastructural level (Fig. 15–2), the nerve terminal membrane is closely applied to the postsynaptic muscle membrane, with a space of about 50 nm separating the two. The basement membrane, or

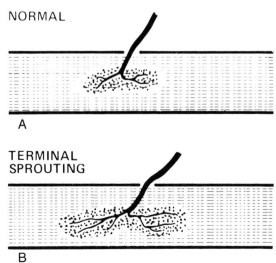

Figure 15–1. Mammalian neuromuscular junctions (combined silver-cholinesterase stain). *(A)* Normal junction. Note nerve terminal branches extending throughout elliptic cholinesterase-stained area. *(B)* Effect of pharmacologic denervation produced by treatment with botulinum toxin. Note elongation and increased branching of the nerve terminals and enlargement of the end-plate area.

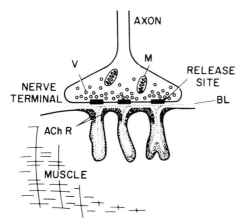

Figure 15–2. A normal neuromuscular junction. V = synaptic vesicle; M = mitochondrion; AChR = acetylcholine receptors; BL = basal lamina.

basal lamina, an amorphous-appearing but functionally important layer, intervenes between nerve and muscle membranes in the junctional region. The nerve terminal contains an abundance of synaptic vesicles, some of which tend to cluster around slight thickenings in the nerve terminal membrane, the release sites or active zones. The large membrane particles found at the active zones are thought to represent voltage-gated calcium channels (VGCCs) (Pumplin et al., 1981). In humans, the particles are about 10 nm in mean diameter and are arranged as an orderly array of double parallel rows, with 3–15 particles per row (Fukunaga et al., 1982). The muscle membrane underlying the nerve terminals is thrown into a series of complex folds, which increase its surface area. AChRs are concentrated at the peaks of these folds, directly opposite the nerve terminal's release sites, thus minimizing the distance that the transmitter must travel to reach the receptor sites. Acetylcholinesterase (AChE) at the neuromuscular junction is synthesized chiefly, if not exclusively, by the muscle cell and is bound to the basal lamina within the synaptic folds.

Neuromuscular Transmission

The major function of acetylcholine (ACh) transmission at the neuromuscular junction is to trigger contractions of skeletal muscle. In addition, there is compelling evidence that ACh transmission plays an important role in the nerve's trophic regulation and maintenance of skeletal muscle.

Presynaptic Mechanisms

ACh is synthesized in the nerve terminal through the catalytic action of the enzyme choline acetyltransferase and is stored in vesicles for subsequent release. It has been estimated that each vesicle, or quantum, contains 5000–10,000 ACh molecules. Quanta of ACh

are released by a calcium-dependent process of *exocytosis* that occurs both *spontaneously* and *in response to impulses*. In addition, *spontaneous nonquantal* ACh release occurs at motor nerve terminals.

Quantal release begins with fusion of the ACh-containing vesicles to the nerve membrane at the preferred release sites. The fused vesicles then open outward, liberating their contents into the synaptic clefts. High-resolution electron microscopy reveals the vesicles in the act of transmitter release; they can be seen as Ω-shaped profiles. After emptying, the vesicles are recycled within the nerve terminals, presumably in preparation to release ACh again. The released ACh crosses the synaptic space and combines with the AChR, causing a transient increase of permeability to sodium and potassium, with resultant electrical depolarization (see later).

Spontaneous Quantal Acetylcholine Release. The spontaneous release of individual quanta of ACh gives rise to local end-plate depolarizations of small amplitude, termed *miniature end-plate potentials* (MEPPs), that are readily detected with intracellular microelectrodes. MEPPs have been recorded from muscles in humans and a wide variety of other vertebrates; they typically occur with a frequency of 1–5/second and an amplitude of about 1 mV. They do not lead to propagated action potentials or muscle contractions.

Impulse-Dependent Acetylcholine Release. When an electrical nerve impulse invades the motor nerve terminal, it causes VGCCs in the nerve terminal to open, allowing calcium to enter. This triggers the release of approximately 50–100 quanta of ACh (in humans). The process of synaptic vesicle fusion with the nerve terminal membrane is calcium dependent and is believed to involve synapsin I, a phosphoprotein that normally links synaptic vesicles to the cytoskeleton (Sudhof et al., 1989). The local influx of Ca^{2+} leads to phosphorylation of synapsin I, causing the synaptic vesicles to be released and allowing their fusion with the postsynaptic membrane and subsequent exocytosis. The resulting near-synchronous release of many quanta produces a large depolarization, the *end-plate potential* (EPP). The amplitude of the EPP is normally sufficient to initiate an action potential that is propagated along the muscle membrane and leads to muscle contraction.

Spontaneous Nonquantal Release. In addition to its quantal release, ACh is liberated from motor nerve terminals by a nonquantal mechanism of continuous leakage. Nonquantal release is believed to be responsible for a much larger proportion of the ACh liberated spontaneously from motor nerve terminals than is quantal release. Release may be mediated by an ACh transport system (Edwards et al., 1985). Its functional role is uncertain, because the released ACh may not be able to penetrate the barrier of AChE in the synaptic cleft.

Postsynaptic Mechanisms

When ACh is released from the motor nerve terminal, it crosses the synaptic cleft and binds to the

AChR. This induces a rapid increase in permeability to sodium and potassium, as well as the divalent cations Ca^{2+} and Mg^{2+}. Noise analysis and patch clamping permit detailed analysis of the events that occur at single AChR channels. At rest, the channel is in the closed state. When it is activated by binding of ACh, the AChR channel opens abruptly, remaining open on the order of 1 ms (Neher and Sakman, 1976). Each open channel permits the flux of ions at a rate of 1–10 million/second (Changeux et al., 1984).

The amplitude of the depolarization resulting from a neurotransmission event depends on the number of interactions between ACh molecules and receptor molecules. After a nerve impulse, the amplitude of the EPP is normally more than necessary to trigger a muscle action potential. The excess is termed the *safety margin* of neuromuscular transmission. Any change that reduces the probability of interaction—and thus the safety margin—increases the risk of failure of neuromuscular transmission. This principle is basic to an understanding of the pathophysiology of disorders of the neuromuscular junction.

The entire process of neuromuscular transmission is rapid, on the order of milliseconds. It is terminated by the removal of ACh, in part by diffusion away from the AChRs and in part by the action of AChE, which rapidly hydrolyzes ACh. If the action of ACh is *not* rapidly terminated, the AChR may undergo a change that has been termed *desensitization*. It becomes unresponsive to further application of ACh, although the muscle cell does not remain depolarized. Desensitization of AChRs can be produced by agents that prolong or mimic the agonist action of ACh. Thus, the application of ACh itself or the use of stable ACh analogues or anti-AChE agents can induce receptor desensitization.

The Acetylcholine Receptor

A great deal is now known about the nicotinic AChR, the first ion channel for which the genes were cloned and sequenced. This progress was initiated by the discovery of specific toxins from the venoms of elapid snakes such as cobras and kraits. α-Bgt purified from the venom of the many-banded krait and toxins from several species of cobras bind specifically to the active sites of AChRs and have served as probes for the identification, purification, and quantitative measurement of AChRs. Another factor that spurred research in this field was the availability of extremely rich sources of AChR in the electric organs of certain eels and rays. These organs consist of great numbers of neuromuscular junction–like structures. When triggered by ACh transmission, they generate large electrical discharges, used to stun their prey. AChR purified from these sources has been extensively characterized.

The AChR is composed of five subunits (α_2, β, γ/ε, δ) arranged around a central ion channel. The ACh- and α-Bgt–binding sites are on the two α subunits (amino acid residues 186–198). The γ subunit present in fetal (and denervated) muscle is replaced by an ε in innervated muscle. The genes coding for the different subunits have been cloned and sequenced in several species, including (in humans) those for α (Beeson et al., 1990b; Noda et al., 1983), β (Beeson et al., 1989), γ (Shibahara et al., 1985), and δ (Luther et al., 1989) subunits. The sequences of the different subunits show considerable homology within and between species, indicating that the molecules have been highly conserved through evolution. Each subunit has a relatively large extracellular NH_2-terminal domain and probably four transmembrane segments, with a short extracellular COOH-terminal domain. The subunits have been localized in humans to chromosome 2 in the case of γ (Cohen-Haguenauer et al., 1987), α, and δ subunits (Beeson et al., 1990a) and to chromosome 17 in the case of β (Beeson et al., 1990a). Evidence in humans indicates that there are two isoforms of the α subunit, alternative splicing leading to either the inclusion or the exclusion of an exon (3A) coding for 25 amino acids (Beeson et al., 1990b). It is not yet known whether membrane expression of the 3A isoform occurs.

Evidence that the subunit arrangement outlined earlier is functional comes from studies in which either injection of *Xenopus* oocytes with mRNAs (Mishina et al., 1984) or transfection of mouse fibroblasts with cDNAs (Claudio et al., 1987) coding for the different subunits leads to a fully functional receptor. The first three transmembrane regions of the δ subunits are thought to play a key role in AChR gating.

Acetylcholine Receptor Turnover. AChRs in muscle cells undergo active turnover (Pumplin and Fambrough, 1982). In normally innervated muscles, AChRs are present nearly exclusively at neuromuscular junctions, and their turnover rate is relatively slow (i.e., average half-life = 10 days in the rat). After denervation in vivo, there is a marked increase of synthesis of extrajunctional AChRs, which turn over more than 10 times as fast as the more stable junctional receptors. An increase in the turnover rate of junctional AChRs induced by antibodies is believed to play an important role in the pathogenesis of MG (see later).

Acetylcholinesterase

AChE (Massoulie and Bon, 1982) is a glycoprotein enzyme that is concentrated at the postsynaptic membrane of the neuromuscular junction, although lesser amounts are detectable throughout the entire muscle fiber. AChE is synthesized within the muscle cell and is secreted and bound to the basal lamina within the synaptic cleft. AChE exists in various molecular forms that differ in the *number of catalytic subunits* per molecule (1–12) and the presence or absence of a *collagen tail*. One particular molecular form of AChE (12 subunits plus collagen tail) predominates at most mammalian neuromuscular junctions and is regulated by a trophic influence of the

Table 15–1. CLASSIFICATION OF MAIN DISORDERS OF NEUROMUSCULAR TRANSMISSION

Disorder	Age at Presentation	Pathophysiology	Disease Mechanism
Myasthenia gravis	>1 y	Loss of functional AChRs	IgG* anti-AChR antibody
Juvenile MG	1–16 y	As for MG	As for MG
Neonatal MG	Birth	Transient loss of functional AChRs	Placental transfer of maternal IgG anti-AChR antibody
Congenital myasthenia	<2 y; some later	Heterogeneous (presynaptic or postsynaptic; see Table 15–4)	Inherited, heterogeneous
Lambert-Eaton myasthenic syndrome	>1 y	Reduced nerve-evoked quantal release of acetylcholine	IgG antibody to nerve terminal VGCCs; associated small cell carcinoma in two-thirds of cases
Botulism	Any	Reduced nerve-evoked and spontaneous quantal release of acetylcholine	Toxin acting within nerve terminal

*IgG = immunoglobulin G.

motor nerve. The chief function of AChE at the neuromuscular junction is to hydrolyze ACh rapidly, which (1) terminates the synaptic event, (2) permits repetitive activation of muscle fibers, and (3) prevents receptor desensitization.

DISORDERS OF NEUROMUSCULAR TRANSMISSION

A classification of disorders of neuromuscular transmission is given in Table 15–1. The two major forms are autoimmune. In MG, anti-AChR antibodies lead to loss of postsynaptic AChRs; in the Lambert-Eaton myasthenic syndrome (LEMS), immunoglobulin G (IgG) antibodies cause loss of functional VGCCs at the motor nerve terminals. LEMS is paraneoplastic in about 60% of cases, associating specifically with small cell lung carcinoma (SCLC). Congenital (hereditary) myasthenia describes a heterogeneous group of disorders in which the immune system is not implicated. Botulism is due to the actions of a toxin that gains access to motor nerve terminals and interferes with ACh release.

Myasthenia Gravis

MG may occur from early childhood to old age. Its prevalence is variably estimated at 5–9 per 100,000. In MG, there is evidence of heterogeneity of disease

expression (Table 15–2), which may reflect differences in etiologic mechanisms (Compston et al., 1980). Some cases without detectable serum anti-AChR antibody may prove to have an immunologically distinct form of MG (see Table 15–2, group E).

Immunopathogenesis

Anti–Acetylcholine Receptor Antibody

Anti-AChR antibody is an IgG antibody in which all four subclasses may be represented; it may be of κ or λ light chain. Human anti-AChR is normally measured by a radioimmununoassay using solubilized human receptor extracted from calf muscle of patients undergoing leg amputation and labeled with ^{125}I-labeled α-Bgt. After incubation with serum, any AChR bound by antibody is precipitated with an anti–(human) IgG; the radioactivity in the pellet provides a measure of the anti-AChR present.

Anti-AChR appears to be highly specific for MG in whites (Vincent and Newsom-Davis, 1985) (Table 15–3). It is not detectable in healthy individuals, including the elderly, or in neurologic controls. A low incidence (7%) was found, however, in an elderly group (older than 65 years) selected for an autoimmune predisposition by the presence of a markedly raised antithyroid antibody titer. By contrast, elderly Japanese individuals have an anti-AChR incidence of 18%, indicating an influence of racial and/or environmental factors. Raised titers without clinical evidence

Table 15–2. CLINICAL HETEROGENEITY IN MYASTHENIA GRAVIS

Group	Clinical Features	Onset Age (y)	Thymus Pathology*	Anti-AChR Titer†	HLA Association‡
A	Generalized	<40	Hyperplasia	+ + +	A1, B8, DR3
B	Generalized	>40	Involution	+	A3, B7, DR2
C	Generalized	Any	Thymoma	+ +	? None
D	Ocular only	Any	NA	+, ±, or 0	NA
E	Generalized	Any	? Involution	0	NA

*Typical features.
†Average titer for the group: + + + = high; + + = intermediate; + = low; ± = very low; 0 = absent.
‡In whites. NA = not available.

Table 15–3. DIAGNOSTIC TESTS IN DISORDERS OF NEUROMUSCULAR TRANSMISSION*

Test	Myasthenia Gravis	Congenital Myasthenia	Lambert-Eaton Syndrome	Botulism	Principal False-Positive Conditions
Anti-AChR antibody†	85–90%	0%	0%	0%	Penicillamine myasthenia, tardive dyskinesia, elderly with autoimmune predisposition
Edrophonium responsiveness	+	±‡	±	±	Anterior horn cell disease, peripheral neuropathy
Electrophysiology CMAP (initial amplitude)	Normal	Normal	Reduced	Normal or reduced	Anterior horn cell disease, peripheral neuropathy, primary muscle disease
Decrement at 3 Hz > 10%	±	±‡	±	±	Anterior horn cell disease
Post-tetanic potentiation > 25%§	−	−	+	±	
SFEMG jitter	+	+	+	+	Anterior horn cell disease, peripheral neuropathy, primary muscle disease

*+ = positive; ± = variable; − = absent; CMAP = compound muscle action potential; SFEMG = single-fiber electromyography.
†Proportion of cases in whom anti-AChR antibody is detectable in serum.
‡See Table 15–4.
§Increment in amplitude in the compound muscle action potential immediately after 15 s of maximal voluntary contraction.

of MG also occur occasionally in patients with tardive dyskinesia, in those with nonmyasthenic thymoma, in the unaffected identical twin of patients with MG, and more rarely, in other relatives of those with MG. In addition, anti-AChR is usually detectable in patients with MG who are in clinical remission.

Anti-AChR is detectable in serum in 85–90% of patients with generalized MG and in about 70% of those with ocular MG. Titers correlate poorly with muscle weakness between individuals, probably reflecting the heterogeneity of the antibody. Thus, the *absolute* antibody titer is not a measure of disease severity. By contrast, serial measurements show a good correlation between antibody titer and muscle weakness in individual patients (e.g., Oosterhuis et al., 1983), especially if functional aspects of the antibody are considered (Drachman et al., 1982); several studies have shown that remission after thymectomy, for example, is associated with a progressive decline in anti-AChR titer. Thus the *relative* rather than the *absolute* titer provides an index of disease severity.

Anti-AChR antibody is heterogeneous; differences in specificities have been demonstrated by several means, including antibody reactivity with different receptor preparations and competition studies using monoclonal antibodies raised against the receptor. Many of the antibodies are directed against determinants in the main immunogenic region (residues 60–75) of the α subunit of the receptor (Lindstrom, 1983), but some are directed elsewhere, including to the γ subunit (Whiting et al., 1986). A relatively small proportion of the antibody is directed against the α-Bgt–binding sites (of which there are two for each AChR). Studies using polyclonal anti-idiotype sera raised in rabbits suggested that there is also heterogeneity of anti-AChR idiotypes (Lang et al., 1985).

Seronegative Myasthenia Gravis

Those patients in whom anti-AChR is not detectable in the standard radioimmunoassay (seronegative

MG) appear by other criteria to have typical MG. In some cases with a short history, anti-AChR may initially be undetectable because it is all bound to receptor. Others may remain persistently anti-AChR negative. These latter patients may respond to plasma exchange, pointing to a humoral factor. Passive transfer studies to mice using Ig prepared from the patients' plasma confirmed the presence of a humoral factor, presumably antibody, that can interfere with neuromuscular transmission (Mossman et al., 1986). Some of these patients have antibodies against other end-plate determinants (e.g., vinculin [Yamamoto et al., 1987]) but the functional role of these is unknown. Studies indicate the presence in some of these patients of IgM anti-AChR antibodies, and perhaps also in patients with seropositive MG, that may exert a blocking action (Yamamoto et al., 1991).

Other Autoantibodies

Anti–striated muscle antibody is heterogeneous and is detectable by immunofluorescence in about 30% of all cases of MG but much more frequently (about 90%) in those with thymoma. Anti–cross-striational antibody can be distinguished from that staining the surface of skeletal muscle cells, which probably recognizes sarcolemmal antigens. The former antibody is itself heterogeneous, binding with the A band and/or the I band and also stains thymic muscle-like (myoid) cells. Antibodies against the muscle cell surface appear closely related to an antibody to citric acid extract of skeletal muscle, which is highly specific for thymoma cases. This antibody can thus serve as a serum marker for this tumor. Studies using polyclonal antisera to the citric acid extract have demonstrated that epithelial thymoma cells and skeletal muscle share common antigens (Gilhus et al., 1984/1985).

Other organ-specific and non–organ-specific auto-antibodies are also present at increased frequency.

End-Plate Morphology

Striking changes are seen at the end plate in severe cases of MG (Fig. 15–3). There is simplification of the postsynaptic folds and widening of the postsynaptic cleft, which may also contain degradative products of the postsynaptic membrane. α-Bgt labeling demonstrates loss of AChR (Fambrough et al., 1973). End plates are typically elongated, suggesting remodeling as a response to immunologically mediated damage. Light microscopic and electron microscopic immunohistologic studies show both IgG and the third component of complement (C3) largely confined to the postsynaptic membrane, but in severe cases they can be located on fragments in the synaptic cleft (A.G. Engel, 1980). C9, the terminal lytic component of the complement cascade, has also been located on short segments of the postsynaptic membrane and, more intensively than IgG or C3, on the fragments shed into the synaptic cleft. In further confirmation, the membrane attack complex (C5b–9) has been visualized by immunofluorescence at the end plate in MG but not in control muscle and was sometimes observed in the absence of detectable α-Bgt binding, implying C′-mediated destruction of the receptors (A.G. Engel and Arahata, 1987).

Lymphocytic collections (lymphorrhages) have been recognized in MG muscle but are not located at the end plate. They are seen more frequently in thymoma cases in which anti–striated muscle antibody is usually detectable (see earlier).

Immunogenetics

The well-recognized association of MG with particular human leukocyte antigens (HLAs) relates to the

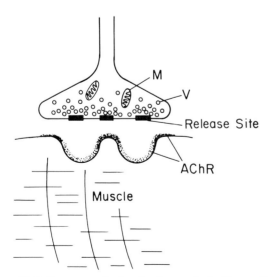

Figure 15–3. Neuromuscular junction from patient with myasthenia gravis. Compare with Figure 15–2. Note the reduced numbers of acetylcholine receptors (AChRs) *(stippling)*; sparse, shallow postsynaptic folds; widened synaptic space; and normal nerve terminal. M = mitochondrion; V = synaptic vesicle.

type of disease and to the race of the patient. Table 15–2 gives the associations in whites. In Japanese patients with early-onset MG (<3 years), HLA-DR9 associates (Matsuki et al., 1990), as in Chinese patients (Chin et al., 1987); no association with B8, DR3 was observed.

Particular IgG heavy chain markers (δ) associate with MG in Japanese (Gm1, 2, 21), especially in thymoma cases (Nakao et al., 1980). Restriction fragment length polymorphism typing in white patients with a probe for the C_μ switch region shows a clear association of the 2.6-kb homozygous phenotype with late-onset MG, contrasting with that in the early-onset form (Demaine et al., 1987) and providing further evidence of disease phenotype heterogeneity. Association with particular T cell receptor V_α and C_α alleles was also found in a series of 17 patients with MG (Oksenberg et al., 1989).

Thymus Histology

The thymus is a lymphoepithelial structure that reaches its full size at birth. From puberty onward, involution occurs with fatty replacement. Its cellular constitution has been elucidated by immunohistologic techniques. The thymus contains myoid cells, and these can express AChR in culture (Kao and Drachman, 1977). AChR has been demonstrated in human thymic myoid cells in situ, both in healthy controls and in patients with MG, by using double-staining immunofluorescence with a panel of monoclonal anti–human AChR antibodies and antisera for muscle proteins (Schluep et al., 1987).

Abnormalities of the thymus are common in MG. Nine percent of patients have a *thymoma*. Thymomas are epithelial tumors. Immunohistologic studies (N. Willcox et al., 1987) using several different cell markers show that they exhibit unusual phenotypes, often expressing the two sets of markers that normally distinguish subcapsular or medullary thymic epithelium from cortical. They may arise from rare cortical epithelial cells that are keratin positive and express markers not only for cortical epithelium but also for subcapsular or medullary epithelium. About 30% of thymomas show local invasion.

The majority of those with early-onset (younger than 40 years) MG show *hyperplasia* of the thymic medulla, characterized by relative attenuation of the thymic cortex, by the presence in the medulla of many germinal centers and their surrounding T cell areas, and by hypertrophy of the medullary epithelium. Germinal centers are rare in non-MG thymus. The germinal centers contain Ig-positive material, plasma cells, B cells, helper T cells, and probably also follicular dendritic (antigen-presenting) cells. The appearances of these germinal centers are similar to those in other lymphoid tissue. The T cell zones that surround the germinal centers have heavy fibronectin deposits, together with helper T cells, interdigitating cells, and occasional CD8-positive T cells. In advanced cases, the laminin bands separating epithelial cell areas from the peripheral lymph node–like areas are fenestrated, thus apparently allowing communication among the medullary epithelium, the T cell zones, and germinal centers (Bofill et al., 1985). Myoid cells are found mainly in the medullary epithelium, T cell areas, and septal regions. They have not been identified in germinal centers. They are HLA-DR negative, and there is uncertainty about whether they are a focus of immunologic attack (Kirchner et al., 1988; Schluep et al., 1987).

Immunosuppression with corticosteroids in patients with early-onset MG appears to lead rapidly to an involuted thymus in patients who otherwise would be expected to show hyperplasia. Cell loss is most striking from the cortex.

Production of Anti–Acetylcholine Receptor Antibody

Anti-AChR antibody can be synthesized in vitro by cells from thymus, peripheral blood, lymph node, and bone marrow only in patients with MG. Cultured thymic cells produce anti-AChR spontaneously, but in the case of the others, mitogen stimulation is usually required. Highest levels of spontaneous production are shown by thymic cells from patients with medullary hyperplasia (Scadding et al., 1981). Amounts from atrophic or thymomatous thymus are low or absent. Spontaneous production of specific antibody is probably more dependent on plasma cells than on B cells. The rate of anti-AChR antibody synthesis in culture by thymic cells correlates strongly with the serum anti-AChR titer (Newsom-Davis et al., 1987). Furthermore, the fine specificities of the antibodies in the culture supernatants, defined by competition studies, closely match those in the patients' serum (Heidenreich et al., 1988). Neither total IgG nor other specific antibodies show similar spontaneous synthesis; this suggests that thymic cells have been selectively preactivated by thymic AChR. Thymic antigen (AChR)–presenting cells may underlie the selective enhancement of anti-AChR production by peripheral blood lymphocytes when they are cocultured with autologous thymic cells (Newsom-Davis et al., 1981).

Helper T cells are almost certainly required for anti-AChR antibody production, as is the case for most antibodies including anti-AChR antibodies in experimental autoimmune MG. In addition, production of anti-AChR antibodies by peripheral blood lymphocytes cocultured with autologous irradiated thymic cells is abrogated if all T cells are depleted (H.N. Willcox et al., 1984). Several groups have reported reactivity of peripheral blood or thymic T cells, or lines and clones derived from them, to native or recombinant *Torpedo* AChR and human AChR and to synthetic peptide sequences of the α subunit (Harcourt et al., 1988; Hohlfeld et al., 1984, 1985, 1987, 1988; Melms et al., 1989; Newsom-Davis et al., 1989). The α subunit has been studied in greatest detail so far, and a number of different epitopes on

the extracellular and cytoplasmic domains have been identified, both in MG and non-MG individuals, and their HLA class II restriction has been defined. It has not yet been shown convincingly that these AChR-specific T cell clones can provide cognate help for specific antibody production.

The proportion of cytotoxic suppressor T cells in peripheral blood may be slightly decreased in MG, particularly in patients with early-onset disease (Berrih et al., 1981). Some functional decrease in suppression is also shown by the concanavalin A suppression assay. Specific suppression of anti-AChR production by suppressor T cells has not been demonstrated (Lisak et al., 1984).

Etiologic Factors

Is a single etiologic factor likely to underlie MG? Evidence suggests not. First, the heterogeneity of the disorder argues against this (see Table 15–2). One interpretation of these differences is diversity of triggering factors and of the mechanisms by which tolerance to AChR is lost (Compston et al., 1980). Second, anti-AChR specificities between these subgroups are not identical: competition studies using monoclonal anti–human AChR antibodies show differences between thymoma and nonthymoma anti-AChR (Whiting et al., 1985). There are also striking differences in the ratio of reactivity with denervated and with normal (i.e., junctional) AChR between those with high titers (in whom the ratio tends to be high) and those with low titers (0.1–2 nmol/L) in whom the ratio is low. This suggests that the autoimmune response in this latter group is primarily against junctional AChR, whereas that in the high-titer group is against extrajunctional (non–end-plate) AChR, which is present on developing muscle, denervated muscle, and presumably also thymus myoid cells.

Penicillamine-induced MG provides a direct example of an independent triggering factor in MG. This drug may induce myasthenia that is otherwise clinically indistinguishable from spontaneously acquired MG and that typically subsides when penicillamine administration is stopped. Serum anti-AChR is detectable in these patients and shows the same characteristics as in other recent-onset cases (Vincent and Newsom-Davis, 1982). The HLA association, however, is with Bw35 and DR1, and the frequencies of B8 and DR3 are reduced compared with those in idiopathic MG (Garlepp et al., 1983).

Attempts to implicate viruses as possible agents in precipitating autoimmunity in MG have been unsuccessful. Antibody titers against a number of common viruses do not differ from those in matched controls (Klavinskis et al., 1985), and virus could not be cultured from MG thymus tissue in recent-onset cases (Aoki et al., 1985). Stefansson et al. (1985) reported sharing of antigenic determinants between (*Torpedo*) AChR and proteins from some bacteria (*Escherichia coli*, *Proteus vulgaris*, and *Klebsiella pneu-*

moniae), raising the possibility that mutations might render these determinants immunogenic, perhaps only in those of a particular immunogenetic type. Reactivity with MG sera could not, however, be detected.

Clinical Features

MG is characterized by weakness of skeletal muscle that increases with muscle activity (fatigability). The distribution of weakness is highly variable and often asymmetric. Eye muscles are the first to be affected in about 60% of cases and are affected at some stage in the illness in about 90%.

Examination often confirms fatigability. Facial weakness has a characteristic snarling appearance and, together with ptosis, may be seen to increase as the patient describes his or her symptoms. The fluctuation in muscle strength that is sometimes observed when power is being assessed should not necessarily be interpreted as fluctuation in effort, although in other ways it may appear indistinguishable. Tendon reflexes are typically brisk for the degree of weakness.

Progress of the disease is variable. In a small proportion of cases, symptoms remain confined to eye muscles (ocular myasthenia), and the probability of this is high when symptoms have remained confined to eye muscles for 2 years or longer. At the other extreme, weakness may be rapidly progressive, leading to respiratory muscle paralysis within a few weeks. Factors such as stress, pregnancy, and infection may initiate symptoms and also cause exacerbation in established disease.

The natural history of the disease is rarely observable because of the use of immunologic treatments. Earlier accounts described an initial labile phase that lasts for up to 7 years. In this period, most spontaneous remissions and deaths were seen (particularly in the first year), and thymectomy was most effective. In stage 2, slow progression usually occurred, but deaths were less frequent, and thymectomy became less effective. Beyond 15 years (stage 3), the response to anticholinesterase drugs became refractory and muscle wasting occurred. The impact of long-term anticholinesterase treatment on these latter changes is uncertain.

Pregnancy. In pregnancy, myasthenic symptoms may be unstable, particularly during the puerperium (Plauché, 1979).

Neonatal Myasthenia Gravis. Neonatal MG is a transient disorder affecting one in eight babies born to MG mothers. Anti-AChR antibody can be detected both in unaffected and in affected infants but persists longer in the latter, possibly because of transient synthesis of the antibody by the infant (Lefvert and Österman, 1983).

Diagnosis

Table 15–3 sets out the principal diagnostic procedures. By far the most specific finding is the presence of anti-AChR antibody (Vincent and Newsom-Davis, 1985), which, in whites, is virtually confined to MG patients (see earlier).

The edrophonium (Tensilon) test is less specific, but the strongest response is seen in MG and congenital myasthenia. A test dose of 2 mg intravenously should first be given, followed at 1 minute by a larger dose (4–8 mg); 4 mg is often adequate and is less likely to cause side effects. The response occurs in 30–60 seconds and subsides within 4–5 minutes. Adverse reactions occasionally occur, including syncope, and appropriate precautions should therefore be taken.

The maximal decrement in the compound muscle action potential evoked by a train of five shocks at 3 Hz is less than 10% in normal persons, when the fifth is compared with the first. In MG and congenital myasthenia, decrement may be increased. This is present in about 50% of those with mild disease and in 80% of those with moderate-to-severe weakness. Postactivation exhaustion can be demonstrated by repeating the above procedure at 30-second intervals for 5 minutes after a 15-second period of maximal voluntary contraction. Cooling the limb improves the response.

Single-fiber electromyography allows selective recording from two or more muscle fibers of the same motor unit (i.e., innervated by the same motor neuron). Impairment of transmission leads to jitter in their timing relationship and sometimes demonstrates block. Jitter can be quantified and the normal range defined (Sanders, 1983). When a range of muscles is studied, including frontalis, abnormal transmission may be detected in 95% of those with generalized weakness and in 84% of those with restricted ocular MG. As Table 15–3 indicates, this test is by no means specific for MG.

Several other diagnostic tests are available but are not in general use. These include the regional curare test, stapedial reflex fatigue, and several tests of ocular muscle function. Special techniques applied to biopsied muscle (usually intercostal muscle) can be used in the investigation of intractable diagnostic problems. These methods allow the number of receptors to be quantified (by ^{125}I-labeled α-Bgt binding), electrophysiologic variables to be measured (e.g., MEPP amplitudes and quantal content), and the presence of postsynaptic IgG and complement to be identified by immunohistologic techniques.

Management

The outline of an approach to management is indicated in Figure 15–4. Management decisions, of course, have to take into account other factors not included in the diagram—for example, the patient's acceptance of the side effects associated with therapy.

Removal of a *thymoma* is normal practice because of risks of local infiltration. If operative removal is incomplete, radiotherapy or chemotherapy is indicated. Myasthenic symptoms in thymoma cases usu-

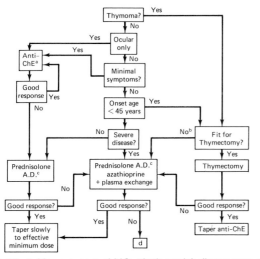

Figure 15–4. Management of MG. [a]Antiacetylcholinesterase drugs (pyridostigmine, prostigmine). [b]Thymectomy can be reconsidered when response to plasma exchange and/or immunosuppressive drugs has developed. [c]Alternate days. [d]Consider other immunosuppressive drugs or lymphoid irradiation (see text).

ally fail to respond to surgery; immunosuppressive drug treatment should then be considered.

Anticholinesterase preparations (prostigmine, pyridostigmine) are of greatest value for the treatment of mild symptoms. Dosage should be every 3–4 hours, usually excluding night doses, and high dosage should be avoided. Cholinergic toxicity can cause a clinical crisis. Chronic high dosage may lead to AChR loss, as has been demonstrated in animals, thus exacerbating the effects of anti-AChR antibody. In patients responding well to immunologic treatment, anticholinesterase treatment can be tapered and withdrawn.

Ocular myasthenia may respond to anticholinesterase medication, but the response is typically incomplete. Alternate-day prednisolone treatment should be considered in these cases. The dose can be increased by 5 mg weekly from a low initial dose (5 mg) until symptoms resolve or the maximal acceptable dose is reached. When remission occurs, the dosage can be tapered to define the effective minimal dosage. Remission can be expected in about 65% of cases, the majority of these being controlled by a prednisolone dosage of 20 mg or less on alternate days. Improvement occurs in most of the remainder, and total lack of response is an indication to review the diagnosis.

Most clinical studies have indicated that *thymectomy* is of greatest value in the younger-onset patient (younger than 45 years). A retrospective computer-matched comparison of thymectomy versus medical (nonimmunologic) treatment clearly demonstrated the benefits of surgery (Buckingham et al., 1976). Pooled results from several large series suggest a remission rate of about 25%, worthwhile improvement in 45%, and a neutral effect in the remainder. Remission is associated with a fall in anti-AChR. There is no convincing evidence of a deleterious

effect of thymectomy on the individual's immune responsiveness. Juvenile MG also responds to thymectomy. Increased remission rates were evident, particularly in those without ocular signs, with a short history, and with onset after the age of 12 years (Rodriguez et al., 1983). Evidence that older-onset (older than 45 years) patients benefit from thymectomy is less convincing; the thymus removed from such cases is typically atrophic.

The transcervical approach to thymectomy has been advocated because it is better tolerated by patients. Unfortunately, studies indicate that this is often an incomplete procedure (Masaoka et al., 1981; Matell et al., 1981), and that has been the author's own experience in two cases operated on elsewhere.

Prednisolone has been used increasingly in MG, and its effectiveness has been demonstrated by studies using historical controls. It has replaced adrenocorticotropin as a therapeutic agent. Alternate-day treatment appears to reduce side effects and lessens the risk of exacerbation of symptoms during treatment induction. Patients can be managed satisfactorily with dosage given only in this way. Alternate days of symptom fluctuation may initially be pronounced, but this diminishes as overall improvement develops. In severe cases, alternate-day dosage up to 100–120 mg may be given. Because exacerbation of symptoms may occur during induction of treatment, patients with appreciable weakness may require hospitalization. Increasing the dose in 10-mg steps from a low initial value (e.g., 10 mg) reduces the risk of initial deterioration. Plasma exchange may be useful in controlling symptoms at this time.

Improvement can be expected in more than 70% of patients. Remission of symptoms or substantial improvement allows a reduction in steroid dosage with the aim of defining the effective minimal dose. A slow reduction rate (e.g., 5 mg/month) reduces the risk of a rapid and uncontrollable relapse. When symptoms recur, the dose should be increased until control is reestablished.

The value of *azathioprine* in the treatment of MG is now becoming increasingly clear. A dose of 2.5 mg/kg is usually optimal. The drug is slow in its action; the $t_{1/2}$ for anti-AChR decline exceeds 6 months. A few individuals are acutely intolerant of the drug. Mild but stable abnormalities of liver function are not necessarily grounds for withdrawing the drug unless there are associated symptoms. Patients require full blood count and liver function tests weekly for 8 weeks and monthly thereafter. When remission is achieved, dose reduction should be instituted slowly (e.g., 25 mg/3 months). Teratogenic effects and risk of infection or inducing malignancy have to be kept in mind. In severe cases, prednisolone combined with azathioprine is probably the most effective regimen, but this has not yet been established in controlled trials.

A course of *plasma exchange* (55 ml/kg of body weight daily for 5 days) typically produces a short-term improvement, reaching its peak 2–5 days after the last exchange and lasting for 2–4 weeks. It is therefore useful for controlling acute relapse or in preparing patients for thymectomy and in controlling symptoms by repeated use in severe cases while the beneficial effects of thymectomy or of immunosuppressive drugs develop. Many reports of plasma exchange in MG are available, but there is no convincing evidence of a positive interaction (i.e., synergy) of plasma exchange with immunosuppressive drug treatment. In severely affected patients resistant to, or intolerant of, the treatment outlined earlier, lymphoid or total-body irradiation (W.K. Engel et al., 1981) and the use of other cytotoxic agents (e.g., cyclophosphamide) should be considered.

Neonatal MG requires treatment by anticholinesterase medication until spontaneous recovery occurs; occasionally, assisted ventilation may be needed. Remission after exchange transfusion has been observed.

Lambert-Eaton Myasthenic Syndrome

LEMS is caused by IgG autoantibodies that interfere with ACh release at motor nerve terminals and probably also at parasympathetic postganglionic terminals. It is associated with small (oat) cell carcinoma of the lung in about 60% of cases (O'Neill et al., 1988), typically preceding radiologic evidence of tumor, sometimes by up to 5 years. The incidence of the disorder in cases of small cell carcinoma is about 3% (Elrington et al., 1991; Hawley et al., 1980).

Immunopathogenesis

Autoimmune Mechanism

In LEMS, there is a decrease in the nerve-evoked quantal release of ACh, as shown by physiologic and pharmacologic studies (Lambert and Elmqvist, 1971; Molenaar et al., 1982). The molecular leakage of ACh is also decreased. MEPP frequency, by contrast, is normal at the resting (polarized) membrane potential. The abnormality does not appear to be due to a deficiency in storage or synthesis of ACh because ACh content and choline acetyltransferase activity are normal in LEMS muscle (Molenaar et al., 1982). Freeze-fracture electron microscopic studies indicate that the pathologic process affects the active zones and active zone particles because these are reduced and disorganized at the LEMS nerve terminal (Fukunaga et al., 1982). Postsynaptic function is normal.

The evidence that the physiologic defect in LEMS is due to IgG antibodies comes from clinical and experimental studies. Plasma exchange in both the carcinomatous and noncarcinomatous forms of the disease produced a statistically significant improvement in the amplitude of the compound muscle action potential (Newsom-Davis and Murray, 1984). This reached its peak at 10–15 days after the course of exchange and was associated with clinical improvement.

IgG prepared from LEMS plasma and injected repeatedly into mice transfers the main physiologic abnormalities (Lang et al., 1981). There is a highly significant decrease in the quantal content of the EPP compared with that in animals receiving control human IgG, and plasma is no more effective in inducing this than is IgG, indicating that the latter contains the active factor (Lang et al., 1983). The effects of LEMS IgG do not seem dependent on later components in the complement cascade, because C5-deficient animals are as susceptible to LEMS IgG as animals with normal levels of C5.

A likely target for the antibody is the VGCC at the motor nerve terminal. First, the observed defects in transmitter release are Ca^{2+} dependent. Second, active zone particles (which are believed to represent VGCCs) are reduced in number and disorganized in mice receiving LEMS IgG (Fukunaga et al., 1983), as in the human disease. Third, in these mice, the slope of the relationship between log quantal content and external log Ca^{2+} concentration is similar to that in control mice but is shifted to the right, consistent with the loss of function of about 40% of VGCCs (Lang et al., 1987). Loss of functional VGCCs appears to result from their cross-linking by IgG antibodies and consequent down-regulation (Nagel et al., 1988). In freeze-fracture electron microscopic studies of the nerve terminal, the earliest change in LEMS IgG–injected mice was a reduced distance between active zone particles in the outside pairs of rows. Later changes were clustering of active zone particles and finally a reduction in their numbers. Adjacent active zone particles are close enough to be cross-linked by divalent anti-VGCC antibodies. These effects were not observed with monovalent Fab.

Anti–Voltage-Gated Calcium Channel Antibodies

At least three types of neuronal VGCCs (T, L, and N) have been identified by electrophysiologic means (Nowycky et al., 1985). Studies in which whole-cell voltage-clamp techniques were used have shown that LEMS IgG contains antibodies that interfere with L-type channels in adrenal chromaffin cells (Kim and Neher, 1988) and in a murine hybrid neuroblastoma cell line NG108 (Peers et al., 1990). However, ACh release is believed to depend on N-type channels, suggesting that the anti–L-type activity may not be responsible for the muscle weakness but may represent either cross-reactivity or a different antibody specificity. Interference with N-type VGCCs has not yet been shown in single-cell studies.

The marine snail toxin ω-conotoxin binds N-type VGCCs and blocks ACh release at the neuromuscular junction in the frog but not in mice. Radiolabeled toxin has formed the basis for an assay for anti-VGCC antibodies (Lennon and Lambert, 1989; Leys et al., 1989, 1991; Sher et al., 1989). Antibodies are detected at clearly raised titers in 45–65% of patients with LEMS in assays that use either SCLC or neuroblastoma cell lines as the source of antigen. As in MG, the serum titer of specific antibody does not correlate with disease severity among patients. In preliminary longitudinal studies, however, it appears that in individual patients antibody titer correlates with disease severity (Leys et al., 1991). This assay may prove useful in diagnosis, although it remains to be determined whether the antibodies detected in this assay are those that interfere with nerve terminal VGCC function.

Associated Autoimmune Disease

Autoimmune disease is associated with LEMS at an apparently increased frequency, particularly in the noncarcinomatous form of the disease. There is also an increased frequency of organ-specific autoantibodies. Lennon et al. (1982) found one or more organ-specific autoantibodies in 52% of 46 patients with noncarcinomatous disease and in 28% of 18 patients with tumor. In an age-matched group of patients with miscellaneous neurologic disease, 17% had one or more specific autoantibodies.

Immunogenetics

A highly significant increase in HLA-B8 was observed in LEMS ($P < .001$), which was stronger in non–SCLC-associated LEMS than in LEMS with SCLC ($P < .001$ and $P = .02$, respectively) (N. Willcox et al., 1985). The frequencies of HLA-DR3 and -A1 were slightly increased in the nontumor group but did not reach significance levels. There was also a significant increase for all cases in the frequency of the IgG heavy chain marker Glm(2) (N. Willcox et al., 1985). No increase was found in small cell carcinoma cases without LEMS. The biologic significance of the Gm association is not clear, but one possibility is that the V_H genes coding for antibodies that can recognize the restricted antigenic determinants that may be shared by the carcinoma cells and the motor nerve terminal are in linkage disequilibrium with those coding for Glm(2).

Role of Associated Carcinoma

SCLC is by far the most common tumor associated with this syndrome (O'Neill et al., 1988). Other reported tumors (single cases) include malignant thymoma, leukemia, and gastric and renal carcinoma. An early suggestion that small cell carcinoma, known to be a neurosecretory tumor, might be releasing a biologically active peptide that interferes with neuromuscular transmission has not been confirmed. Moreover, Lambert and Lennon (1982) transplanted metastatic small (oat) cell carcinoma from LEMS into athymic nude mice and observed no change in neuromuscular transmission in mice subsequently bearing large tumors.

SCLC cells can generate Ca^{2+} spikes and cultured SCLC cell lines show K^+-stimulated (voltage-gated)

Ca^{2+} flux (Roberts et al., 1985), indicating that these tumors express VGCCs. This is not unexpected in view of their presumed neuroectodermal origin. Experimental evidence of the potential role of SCLC cells in LEMS with SCLC was the finding that LEMS IgG (from either SCLC or noncancer cases) significantly inhibited K^+-stimulated Ca^{2+} flux into cultured SCLC cell lines (Roberts et al., 1985). Moreover, the degree of inhibition correlated significantly with the compound muscle action potential amplitude, an electromyographic index of disease severity (Lang et al., 1989). Thus SCLC-associated LEMS may be triggered by tumor VGCC determinants. Cross-reaction of the autoantibodies with similar determinants at motor nerve terminals, and perhaps also at cholinergic terminals in the parasympathetic system, leads to the neurologic syndrome. In strong support of this hypothesis is the finding that resection or irradiation of SCLC in LEMS cases is often followed by improvement in or recovery from the neurologic disorder (Chalk et al., 1990).

Clinical Features

Patients typically have fatigability and weakness, particularly affecting walking (O'Neill et al., 1988). There may be mild bilateral ptosis. Bulbar muscles are unaffected, and only in occasional cases does weakness significantly affect respiratory muscles. Autonomic features are nearly always present, notably a dry mouth, sexual impotence, and occasionally sphincter disorders. Examination of mild cases often reveals little abnormality in strength when formally tested, but the gait may be abnormal with a slow and waddling characteristic. In advanced cases, weakness may be generalized but especially severe proximally. Augmentation of strength often occurs during the first few seconds of a maximal effort. Reflexes are depressed or absent but can be transiently restored by a short period (e.g., 15 seconds) of maximal voluntary contraction (post-tetanic potentiation).

Diagnosis

Response to edrophonium may be present but is typically less than that in MG (see Table 15–3). The amplitude of the compound muscle action potential in resting muscle on supramaximal nerve stimulation is reduced (Lambert et al., 1961). After maximal voluntary contraction for 15 seconds, an increase in amplitude greater than 25% is highly suggestive of LEMS (Newsom-Davis and Murray, 1984), and values greater than 100% are diagnostic. Increased jitter is often evident on single-fiber electromyography. Nerve conduction velocities are normal. Measurement of serum anti-VGCC antibodies may prove useful in some cases (see earlier).

Management

An approach to management is indicated in Figure 15–5 (see also Newsom-Davis, 1985). When a tumor

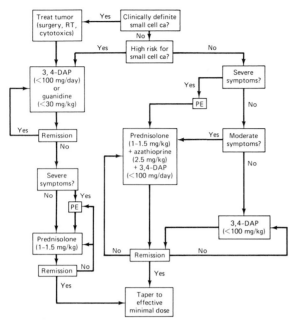

Figure 15–5. Management of LEMS. RT = radiotherapy; 3,4-DAP = 3,4-diaminopyridine; ca = carcinoma; PE = plasma exchange.

has been demonstrated, its treatment by surgery (only rarely possible), by deep radiotherapy, or by cytotoxic drugs may well improve the neurologic syndrome. Drugs that increase ACh release should be the first line of drug treatment in these cases and in those in whom the risk of carcinoma is high (e.g., smokers). 3,4-Diaminopyridine (10–20 mg four or five times daily) is effective and relatively nontoxic (Lundh et al., 1984; McEvoy et al., 1989). Perioral and sometimes more widespread paresthesias usually occur about 1 hour after ingestion. Guanidine (30 mg/kg of body weight) is also effective but much more toxic. If the response to these drugs is poor, prednisolone (up to 1–1.5 mg/kg of body weight on alternate days) coupled with plasma exchange should be considered.

In patients with non–SCLC-associated LEMS with mild symptoms, 3,4-diaminopyridine is the drug of choice. In the remainder, immunosuppressive treatment is indicated. The combination of prednisolone (dosage as earlier) and azathioprine (2.5 mg/kg of body weight) given together appears to be the most effective regimen, but response is slow and improve-

ment may not be evident for at least 6 months. Plasma exchange may provide a useful boost to the response and, in mild cases, may be sufficient to bring the compound muscle action potential into the normal range. When remission has been obtained, the dosage of prednisolone should be reduced slowly (5 mg/month) to define the effective minimal dose. It is unlikely that immunosuppressive drugs can be completely withdrawn without a return of symptoms. Thus, patients should be told of the probable need for long-term treatment with these drugs.

Congenital Myasthenia

Congenital myasthenia constitutes a heterogeneous set of inherited disorders of neuromuscular transmission in which immunologic mechanisms are not implicated.

Classification

Table 15–4 summarizes the main features of the several forms of congenital myasthenia that are defined by electrophysiologic, biochemical, morphologic, and other studies of biopsied muscle (see also A.G. Engel, 1984). The further application of these techniques is likely to increase the range of defined disorders.

Familial Infantile Myasthenia

Fluctuating ophthalmoplegia and ptosis, feeding difficulties, and episodic apnea occur in infancy (Mora et al., 1987). Inheritance is autosomal recessive. Symptoms may improve with age and respond to anticholinesterase drugs. A decremental electromyographic response to 2-Hz stimulation is observed either in rested muscle or sometimes only after exercise. Similarly, MEPP and EPP amplitudes are often normal in rested muscle but diminish after nerve stimulation at 10 Hz. Ultrastructure of the junction is normal, and there is no AChR loss. Morphometric studies have shown that the synaptic vesicles are abnormally small in rested muscle, although vesicle size did not correlate with MEPP amplitude (Mora et al., 1987).

Vincent et al. (1981) described a patient who had

Table 15–4. CLASSIFICATION AND MAIN DIAGNOSTIC FEATURES OF CONGENITAL MYASTHENIA

Disorder	Inheritance	Typical Age at Onset	Edrophonium/ Anticholinesterase Response*	Electrophysiologic Responses	
				Single Shock	*Train*
Familial infantile myasthenia	Recessive	Infancy	+ or −	Normal	Decrement
AChE deficiency	Recessive	Infancy	−	Repetitive	Decrement
Prolonged AChR open time	Dominant	Infancy to adulthood	−	Repetitive	Decrement
Deficiency of AChRs	Recessive	<2 y	+	Normal	Decrement

*+ = positive; − = absent.

weakness at birth that affected limb, truncal, and bulbar muscles but spared ocular muscles. Weakness responded to edrophonium, anticholinesterase preparations, and 4-aminopyridine (a drug that increases transmitter release). A decremental response was present. MEPP amplitudes in rested muscle were decreased but α-Bgt binding was normal. Acetylcholine content was also normal. The findings were consistent with a decrease in the number of ACh molecules in each quantum.

Acetylcholinesterase Deficiency

A.G. Engel et al. (1977) reported a 16-year-old Hindu boy whose weakness was evident soon after birth and who was unresponsive to anticholinesterase preparations. There was a decremental response to repetitive nerve stimulation and a repetitive response to a single shock.

Electrophysiologic studies showed prolonged MEPPs and EPPs and a decrease in quantal content. MEPP frequency was reduced. Nerve terminal size was also decreased and the postsynaptic folds showed focal degeneration. ACh receptors appeared normal. The principal abnormality was absence of AChE at the end plate. This disorder appeared to be due to a congenital defect in molecular assembly of AChE or in its attachment to the postsynaptic membrane.

Prolonged Open Time of the Acetylcholine Receptor

Prolonged AChR open time was first described by A.G. Engel et al. (1982); other cases have since been reported (Oosterhuis et al., 1987). Onset was in adult life or infancy and varied, even within the same family. Inheritance was autosomal dominant. There was relatively selective involvement of scapular muscles and finger extensors, with associated wasting, and variable weakness of facial, masticatory, and cervical muscles. Electrophysiologic studies on biopsied muscle specimens showed a prolonged time course for the MEPP and for the miniature end-plate current; MEPP amplitudes were slightly reduced and quantal content was normal. Morphologic studies revealed atrophic fibers, and tubular aggregates together with vacuoles occurred close to the end plates. Focal degeneration of the postsynaptic folds was seen, and there was associated loss of AChR; MEPP amplitudes were decreased where these morphologic changes were prominent. Calcium accumulation was observed at the end plate in one case. This syndrome can be accounted for by a prolonged open time of the ACh-induced ion channel.

Deficiency of Acetylcholine Receptors

In several families and in sporadic cases, the principal abnormality has been decreased binding of ^{125}I-labeled α-Bgt associated with a decrease in MEPP amplitude but no prolongation of its time course (thus excluding the slow channel syndrome). Vincent et al. (1981) described four cases with onset in infancy or early childhood, of whom two were brothers and one was the son of a cousin marriage. The inheritance appears to be autosomal recessive. The end plate was elongated, and in one case, α-Bgt binding was slowly reversible, suggesting possible abnormality of the AChR affecting the α-Bgt–binding site. Morgan-Hughes et al. (1981) reported a patient in whom α-Bgt binding was decreased. Onset in this man was in adulthood; his parents were first cousins. Weakness affected ocular, bulbar, and limb muscles. A decreased response to repetitive stimulation was present and jitter was increased. Affinity was normal for α-Bgt and increased for tubocurarine. The meaning of this finding is not clear. Tubular aggregates were present.

Treatment

Anti-AChE treatment is effective in some but not all types of congenital myasthenia (see Table 15–4). Pyridostigmine is the most useful drug, and the dose should be given four or five times daily. The dosage in infants is 5–10 mg orally, and in older children, 10–30 mg, depending on age and response. In adults, the initial dose is 30–60 mg, and this can be increased if required to 120 mg. Higher dosage should be avoided because of the evidence that this down-regulates AChRs. There appear to be no special advantages in combining pyridostigmine with prostigmine.

3,4-Diaminopyridine, which increases transmitter release from the nerve terminal, is effective in some forms of congenital myasthenia and can be used with pyridostigmine (Palace et al., 1991).

Botulism

The paralysis in botulism is caused by the toxin released by the bacillus *Clostridium botulinum*. The toxin is approximately 900 kd and is among the most potent of human poisons.

Pathophysiology

The toxin interferes with transmitter release at motor nerve terminals and at presynaptic cholinergic terminals. MEPP frequencies and EPP amplitudes are greatly reduced but not abolished. It acts within the nerve terminal, possibly by reducing sensitivity to Ca^{2+}, and it does not affect ACh synthesis. Its effects, therefore, although presynaptic, differ from those present in LEMS.

Clinical Features

Botulism may arise from ingestion of infected material, by wound infection, and by production of toxin within the gut in infants. The incubation period typically ranges from 6 to 36 hours. Autonomic features occur early and include dry mouth, constipation, and urinary retention. Difficulty in focusing may be an initial symptom, and ocular symptoms can predominate, especially sixth nerve palsy (Terranova et al., 1979). Other symptoms include weakness of facial, bulbar, cervical, limb, and respiratory muscles. Tendon reflexes may be normal, decreased, or absent (Hughes et al., 1981). Recovery may take many weeks. *Infant botulism* may present with constipation, floppiness, ophthalmoplegia, ptosis, bulbar weakness, and respiratory arrest (Turner et al., 1978) and may be a cause of sudden infant death (Arnon et al., 1978).

Diagnosis

There may be a response to intravenous edrophonium, but this is often not striking (see Table 15–3). The amplitude of the compound muscle action potential may be reduced; post-tetanic potentiation occurs less prominently than in LEMS (Gutmann and Pratt, 1976). Increased jitter can be expected. *C. botulinum* can sometimes be cultured from the stool and gastric contents, and circulating toxin can be detected by the mouse neutralization test.

Treatment

Assisted ventilation may be required. Botulinum antitoxin should be given. Guanidine has been used to treat botulinum poisoning, but 3,4-diaminopyridine may prove to be as effective and appears to be less toxic.

References

(Key references are designated with an asterisk.)

Aoki T., Drachman D.B., Asher D.M., et al. Attempts to implicate viruses in myasthenia gravis. *Neurology* 35:185–192, 1985.

Arnon S.S., Midura T.F., Damus K., et al. Intestinal infection and toxin production by *Clostridium botulinum* as one cause of sudden infant death syndrome. *Lancet* 1:1272–1277, 1978.

Beeson D., Brydson M., Newsom-Davis J. Nucleotide sequence of human muscle acetylcholine receptor beta-subunit. *Nucleic Acids Res.* 17:4391, 1989.

Beeson D., Jeremiah S., West L.F., et al. Assignment of the human nicotinic acetylcholine receptor genes: the alpha and delta subunit genes to chromosome 2 and the beta subunit gene to chromosome 17. *Ann. Hum. Genet.* 54:199–228, 1990a.

Beeson D., Morris A., Vincent A., et al. The human muscle nicotinic acetylcholine receptor α-subunit exists as two isoforms: a novel exon. *EMBO J.* 9:2101–2106, 1990b.

Berrih S., Gaud C., Bach M-A., et al. Evaluation of T cell subsets in myasthenia gravis using anti-T cell monoclonal antibodies. *Clin. Exp. Immunol.* 45:1–8, 1981.

Bloch R.J., Pumplin D.W. Molecular events in synaptogenesis: nerve-muscle adhesion and postsynaptic differentiation. *Am. J. Physiol.* 254:C345–C364, 1988.

*Bofill M., Janossy G., Willcox N., et al. Microenvironments in the normal and myasthenia gravis thymus. *Am. J. Pathol.* 119:462–473, 1985.

Buckingham J.M., Howard F.M., Bernatz P.E., et al. The value of thymectomy in myasthenia gravis. *Ann. Surg.* 184:453–458, 1976.

Chalk C.H., Murray N.M.F., Newsom-Davis J., et al. Response of the Lambert-Eaton myasthenic syndrome to treatment of associated small cell lung carcinoma. *Neurology* 40:1552–1556, 1990.

Changeux J.-P., Devilliers-Thiery A., Chemouilli P. Acetylcholine receptor: an allosteric protein. *Science* 115:1335–1345, 1984.

Chiu H.-C., Hsieh R.-P., Hsieh K.-H., et al. Association of HLA-DRw9 with myasthenia gravis in Chinese. *J. Immunogenet.* 14:203–207, 1987.

Claudio T., Green W.N., Hartman D.S., et al. Genetic reconstitution of functional acetylcholine receptor channels in mouse fibroblasts. *Science* 238:1688–1694, 1987.

Cohen-Haguenauer O., Barton P.J.R., Merlie J., et al. Localisation of the human acetylcholine receptor gamma subunit gene to 2q32 – qter. *Cytogenet. Cell Genet.* 46:595, 1987.

Compston D.A.S., Vincent A., Newsom-Davis J., et al. Clinical, pathological, HLA antigen and immunological evidence for disease heterogeneity in myasthenia gravis. *Brain* 103:579–601, 1980.

Demaine A.G., Welsh K.I., Willcox N., et al. Genetic susceptibility to myasthenia gravis studies by DNA hybridization. *Ann. N. Y. Acad. Sci.* 505:800–802, 1987.

*Drachman D.B., Adams R.N., Stanley E.F., et al. Mechanisms of acetylcholine receptor loss in myasthenia gravis. *J. Neurol. Neurosurg. Psychiatry* 43:601–610, 1980.

Drachman D.B., Adams R.N., Josifek L.F., et al. Functional activities of autoantibodies to acetylcholine receptors and the clinical severity of myasthenia gravis. *N. Engl. J. Med.* 307:769–775, 1982.

Edwards C., Dolezal V., Tucek S., et al. Is an acetylcholine transport system responsible for nonquantal release of acetylcholine at the rodent myoneural junction? *Proc. Natl. Acad. Sci. U.S.A.* 82:3514–3518, 1985.

Elmqvist D., Hofmann W.M., Kugelberg J., et al. An electrophysiological investigation of neuromuscular transmission in myasthenia gravis. *J. Physiol. (Lond.)* 174:417–434, 1964.

Elrington G.M., Murray N.M.F., Spiro S.G., et al. Neurological paraneoplastic syndromes in patients with small cell lung cancer: a prospective survey of 150 patients. *J. Neurol. Neurosurg. Psychiatry* (in press).

Engel A.G. Morphologic and immunopathologic findings in myasthenia gravis and in congenital myasthenic syndromes. *J. Neurol. Neurosurg. Psychiatry* 43:577–589, 1980.

*Engel A.G. Myasthenia gravis and myasthenic syndromes. *Ann. Neurol.* 16:519–534, 1984.

Engel A.G., Arahata K. The membrane attack complex of complement at the endplate in myasthenia gravis. *Ann. N. Y. Acad. Sci.* 505:326–332, 1987.

Engel A.G., Lambert E.H., Gomez M.R. A new myasthenia syndrome with end-plate acetylcholinesterase (AChE) deficiency, small nerve terminals, and reduced acetylcholine release. *Ann. Neurol.* 1:315–330, 1977.

Engel A.G., Lambert E.H., Mulder D.M., et al. A newly recognized congenital myasthenic syndrome attributed to a prolonged open time of the acetycholine-induced ion channel. *Ann. Neurol.* 11:553–569, 1982.

Engel W.K., Lichter A.S., Dalakas M.C. Splenic and total-body irradiation treatment of myasthenia gravis. *Ann. N. Y. Acad. Sci.* 377:744–754, 1981.

Fambrough D., Drachman D.B., Satyamurti S. Neuromuscular junction in myasthenia gravis. Decreased acetylcholine receptors. *Science* 182:293–295, 1973.

Fukunaga H., Engel A.G., Osame M., et al. Paucity and disorganization of presynaptic membrane active zones in the Lambert-Eaton myasthenic syndrome. *Muscle Nerve* 5:686–697, 1982.

Fukunaga H., Engel A.G., Lang B., et al. Passive transfer of Lambert-Eaton myasthenic syndrome with IgG from man to mouse depletes the presynaptic membrane active zones. *Proc. Natl. Acad. Sci. U.S.A.* 80:7636–7640, 1983.

Garlepp M.J., Dawkins R.L., Christiansen F.T. HLA antigens and acetylcholine receptor antibodies in penicillamine induced myasthenia gravis. *Br. Med. J.* 286:340, 1983.

Gilhus N.E., Aarli J.A., Christensson B., et al. Rabbit antiserum to a citric acid extract of human skeletal muscle staining thymomas from myasthenia gravis patients. *J. Neuroimmunol.* 7:55–64, 1984/1985.

Guttmann L., Pratt L. Pathophysiologic aspects of human botulism. *Arch. Neurol.* 33:175–179, 1976.

Harcourt G.C., Sommer N., Rothbard J., et al. A juxta-membrane epitope on the human acetylcholine receptor recognized by T cells in myasthenia gravis. *J. Clin. Invest.* 82:1295–1300, 1988.

Hawley R.J., Cohen M.H., Saini N., et al. The carcinomatous neuromyopathy of oat cell lung cancer. *Ann. Neurol.* 7:65–72, 1980.

Heidenreich F., Vincent A., Willcox N., et al. Anti–acetylcholine receptor antibody specificities in serum and in thymic cell culture supernatants from myasthenia gravis patients. *Neurology* 38:1784–1788, 1988.

Hohlfeld R., Toyka K.V., Heininger K., et al. Autoimmune human T lymphocytes specific for acetylcholine receptor. *Nature* 310:244–246, 1984.

Hohlfeld R., Conti-Tronconi B., Kalies I., et al. Genetic restriction of autoreactive acetylcholine receptor–specific T lymphocytes in myasthenia gravis. *J. Immunol.* 135:2392–2399, 1985.

Hohlfeld R., Toyka K.V., Tzartos S.J., et al. Human T helper lymphocytes in myasthenia gravis recognize the nicotinic receptor α-subunit. *Proc. Natl. Acad. Sci. U.S.A.* 84:5379–5383, 1987.

Hohlfeld R., Toyka K., Miner L., et al. Amphipathic segment of the nicotinic receptor alpha subunit contains epitopes recognized by T lymphocytes in myasthenia gravis. *J. Clin. Invest.* 81:657–660, 1988.

Hokkanen E. Epidemiology of myasthenia gravis in Finland. *J. Neurol. Sci.* 9:463–478, 1969.

*Hughes J.M., Blumenthal J.R., Merson M.H., et al. Clinical features of types A and B food-borne botulism. *Ann. Intern. Med.* 95:442–445, 1981.

Kao I., Drachman D.B. Thymic muscle cells bear acetylcholine receptors: possible relation to myasthenia gravis. *Science* 195:74–75, 1977.

Kim Y.I., Neher E. IgG from patients with Lambert-Eaton syndrome blocks voltage-dependent calcium channels. *Science* 239:405–408, 1988.

Kirchner T., Hoppe F., Schalke B., et al. Microenvironment of thymic myoid cells in myasthenia gravis. *Virchows Arch. [B]* 54:295–302, 1988.

Klavinskis L.S., Willcox N., Oxford J.S., et al. Antivirus antibodies in myasthenia gravis. *Neurology* 35:1381–1384, 1985.

Lambert E.H., Elmqvist D. Quantal components of end-plate potentials in the myasthenic syndrome. *Ann. N. Y. Acad. Sci.* 183:183–199, 1971.

Lambert E.H., Lennon V.A. Neuromuscular transmission in nude mice bearing oat cell tumours from Lambert-Eaton myasthenic syndrome. *Muscle Nerve* 5:S39–S45, 1982.

Lambert E.H., Rooke E.D., Eaton L.M., et al. Myasthenic syndrome occasionally associated with bronchial neoplasm: neurophysiologic studies. In Viets H.R., ed. *Myasthenia Gravis.* Springfield, IL, Thomas, pp. 362–410, 1961.

*Lang B., Newsom-Davis J., Wray D., et al. Autoimmune aetiology for myasthenic (Eaton-Lambert) syndrome. *Lancet* 2:224–226, 1981.

Lang B., Newsom-Davis J., Prior D., et al. Antibodies to motor nerve terminals: an electrophysiological study of a human myasthenic syndrome transferred to mouse. *J. Physiol. (Lond.)* 344:335–345, 1983.

Lang B., Roberts A.J., Vincent A., et al. Anti–acetylcholine receptor idiotypes in myasthenia gravis analysed by rabbit anti-sera. *Clin. Exp. Immunol.* 60:637–644, 1985.

Lang B., Newsom-Davis J., Peers C., et al. The effect of myasthenic syndrome antibody on presynaptic calcium channels in the mouse. *J. Physiol. (Lond.)* 390:257–270, 1987.

Lang B., Vincent A., Murray N.M.F., et al. Lambert-Eaton myasthenic syndrome: immunoglobulin G inhibition of Ca^{2+} flux in tumour cells correlates with disease severity. *Ann. Neurol.* 25:265–271, 1989.

Lefvert A.K., Osterman P.O. Newborn infants to myasthenic mothers: a clinical study and an investigation of acetylcholine receptor antibodies in 17 children. *Neurology (N.Y.)* 33:133–138, 1983.

Lennon V.A., Lambert E.H. Autoantibodies bind solubilized calcium channel–ω–conotoxin complexes from small cell lung carcinoma: a diagnostic aid for Lambert-Eaton myasthenic syndrome. *Mayo Clin. Proc.* 64:1498–1504, 1989.

Lennon V.A., Lambert E.H., Whittingham S., et al. Autoimmunity in the Lambert-Eaton myasthenic syndrome. *Muscle Nerve* 5:S21–S25, 1982.

Leys K., Lang B., Vincent A., et al. Calcium channel autoantibodies in Lambert-Eaton myasthenic syndrome (letter). *Lancet* 2:1107, 1989.

*Leys K., Lang B., Johnston I., et al. Calcium channel autoantibodies in the Lambert-Eaton myasthenic syndrome. *Ann. Neurol.* 29:307–314, 1991.

Lindstrom J. Using monoclonal antibodies to study acetylcholine receptors and myasthenia gravis. *Neurosci. Commentaries* 1:139–156, 1983.

Lisak R.P., Laramore C., Levinson A.I., et al. In vitro synthesis of antibodies to acetylcholine receptor by peripheral blood cells: Role of suppressor T cells in normal subjects. *Neurology (N.Y.)* 34:802–805, 1984.

Lundh H., Nilsson O., Rosen I. Treatment of Lambert-Eaton syndrome: 3,4-diaminopyridine and pyridostigmine. *Neurology (N.Y.)* 34:1324–1330, 1984.

Luther M.A., Schoepfer R., Whiting P., et al. A muscle acetylcholine receptor is expressed in the human cerebellar medulloblastoma cell line TE671. *J. Neurosci.* 9:1082–1096, 1989.

Masaoka A., Monden Y., Seike Y., et al. Reoperation after transcervical thymectomy for myasthenia gravis. *Neurology (N.Y.)* 32:83–85, 1982.

Massoulie J., Bon S. The molecular forms of cholinesterase and acetylcholinesterase in vertebrates. *Annu. Rev. Neurosci.* 5:57–106, 1982.

Matell G., Lebram G., Osterman P.O., et al. Follow-up comparison of suprasternal VS transsternal method of thymectomy in myasthenia gravis. *Ann N. Y. Acad. Sci.* 377:844–845, 1981.

Matsuki K., Juji T., Tokunaga K., et al. HLA antigens in Japanese patients with myasthenia gravis. *J. Clin Invest.* 86:392–399, 1990.

McEvoy K.M., Windebank A.J., Daube J.R., et al. 3,4-Diaminopyridine in the treatment of Lambert-Eaton myasthenic syndrome. *N. Engl. J. Med.* 321:1567–1571, 1989.

Melms A., Chrestel S., Schalke B.C.G., et al. Autoimmune T lymphocytes in myasthenia gravis. Determination of target epitopes using T cell lines and recombinant products of the mouse nicotinic acetylcholine receptor gene. *J. Clin. Invest.* 83:785–790, 1989.

Mishina M., Kurosaki T., Tobimatsu T., et al. Expression of functional acetylcholine receptor from cloned cDNAs. *Nature* 307:604–608, 1984.

Molenaar P.C., Polak R.L., Miledi R., et al. Acetylcholine in intercostal muscle from myasthenia gravis patients and in rat diaphragm after blockade of acetylcholine receptors. *Prog. Brain Res.* 49:449–492, 1979.

Molenaar P.C., Newsom-Davis J., Polak R.L., et al. Eaton-Lambert syndrome: acetylcholine and choline acetyltransferase in skeletal muscle. *Neurology (N.Y.)* 32:1061–1065, 1982.

*Mora M., Lambert E.H., Engel A.G. Synaptic vesicle abnormality in familial infantile myasthenia. *Neurology* 37:206–214, 1987.

Morgan-Hughes J.A., Lecky B.R.F., Landon D.N., et al. Alteration in the number and affinity of junctional acetylcholine receptors in a myopathy with tubular aggregates: a newly recognized receptor defect. *Brain* 104:279–295, 1981.

Mossman S., Vincent A., Newsom-Davis J. Myasthenia gravis without acetylcholine-receptor antibody: a distinct disease entity. *Lancet* 1:116–118, 1986.

Nagel A., Engel A.G., Lang B., et al. Lambert-Eaton myasthenic syndrome IgG depletes presynaptic membrane active zone particles by antigenic modulation. *Ann. Neurol.* 24:552–558, 1988.

Nakao Y., Miyazaki T., Ota K., et al. Gm allotypes in myasthenia gravis. *Lancet* 1:677–680, 1980.

Neher G., Sakman B. Single channel currents recorded from membrane of denervated muscle fibers. *Nature* 260:799–802, 1976.

*Newsom-Davis J. The Lambert-Eaton myasthenic syndrome. In Johnson R.T., ed. *Current Therapy in Neurologic Disease.* Toronto, Decker, pp. 371–375, 1985.

Newsom-Davis J., Murray N.M.F. Plasma exchange and immunosuppressive drug treatment in the Lambert-Eaton myasthenic syndrome. *Neurology (N.Y.)* 34:480–485, 1984.

Newsom-Davis J., Willcox H.N.A., Calder L. Thymus cells in myasthenia gravis selectively enhance production of anti–acetylcholine receptor antibody by autologous blood lymphocytes. *N. Engl. J. Med.* 305:1313–1318, 1981.

Newsom-Davis J., Willcox N., Schluep M., et al. Immunological heterogeneity and cellular mechanisms in myasthenia gravis. *Ann. N. Y. Acad. Sci.* 505:12–26, 1987.

Newsom-Davis J., Harcourt G., Sommer N., et al. T-cell reactivity in myasthenia gravis. *Autoimmunity* 2:101–108, 1989.

Noda M., Furutani Y., Takahashi H., et al. Cloning and sequence analysis of calf cDNA and human genomic DNA encoding α-subunit precursor of muscle acetylcholine receptor. *Nature* 305:818–823, 1983.

Nowycky M.C., Fox A.P., Tsien R.W. Three types of neuronal calcium channel with different calcium agonist sensitivity. *Nature* 316:440–443, 1985.

Oksenberg J.R., Sherritt M., Becogich A.B., et al. T-cell receptor V_α and C_α alleles associated with multiple sclerosis and myasthenia gravis. *Proc. Natl. Acad. Sci. U.S.A.* 86:988–992, 1989.

*O'Neill J.H., Murray N.M.F., Newsom-Davis J. The Lambert-Eaton myasthenic syndrome: a review of 50 cases. *Brain* 111:577–596, 1988.

*Oosterhuis H.J.G.H. *Myasthenia Gravis.* Edinburgh, Churchill Livingstone, 1984.

Oosterhuis H.J.G.H., Limburg P.C., Hummel-Tappel E. Antiacetylcholine receptor antibodies in myasthenia gravis. Part 2. Clinical and serological follow-up of individual patients. *J. Neurol. Sci.* 58:371–385, 1983.

Oosterhuis H.J.G.H., Newsom-Davis J., Wokke J.H.J., et al. The slow channel syndrome: two new cases. *Brain* 110:1061–1079, 1987.

Palace J., Wiles C.M., Newsom-Davis J. 3,4–Diaminopyridine in the treatment of congenital (hereditary) myasthenia. *J. Neurol. Neurosurg Psychiatry* (in press).

Peers C., Lang B., Newsom-Davis J., et al. Selective action of myasthenic syndrome antibodies on calcium channels in a rodent neuroblastoma × glioma cell line. *J. Physiol. (Lond.)* 421:293–308, 1990.

Pestronk A., Drachman D.B. A new stain for quantitative measurement of sprouting at neuromuscular junctions. *Muscle Nerve* 1:70–74, 1978.

Plauché W.C. Myasthenia gravis in pregnancy: an update. *Am. J. Obstet. Gynecol.* 135:691–697, 1979.

Pumplin D.W., Fambrough D.M. Turnover of acetylcholine receptors in skeletal muscle. *Annu. Rev. Physiol.* 44:319–335, 1982.

Pumplin D.W., Reese T.S., Llinas R. Are the synaptic membrane particles the calcium channels? *Proc. Natl. Acad. Sci. U.S.A.* 78:7210–7213, 1981.

Roberts A., Perera S., Lang B., et al. Paraneoplastic myasthenic syndrome IgG inhibits $^{45}Ca^{2+}$ flux in a human small cell carcinoma line. *Nature* 317:737–739, 1985.

Rodriguez M., Gomez M.R., Howard F.M., et al. Myasthenia gravis in children: long term follow-up. *Ann. Neurol.* 13:504–510, 1983.

Sanders D.B. Electrodiagnosis of myasthenia gravis: recent techniques. In Albuquerque E.X., Elderfrawi A.T. eds. *Myasthenia Gravis.* London, Chapman & Hall, pp. 275–295, 1983.

Scadding G.K., Vincent A., Newsom-Davis J., et al. Acetylcholine receptor antibody synthesis by thymic lymphocytes: correlation with thymic histology. *Neurology (N.Y.)* 31:935–943, 1981.

Schluep M., Willcox N., Vincent A., et al. Acetylcholine receptors in human myoid cells in situ: an immunohistological study. *Ann. Neurol.* 22:212–222, 1987.

Sher E., Gotti C., Canal N., et al. Specificity of calcim channel autoantibodies in Lambert-Eaton myasthenic syndrome. *Lancet* 2:640–643, 1989.

Shibahara S., Kubo T., Perski H.J., et al. Cloning and sequence analysis of human genomic DNA encoding γ subunit precursor of muscle acetylcholine receptor. *Eur. J. Biochem.* 146:15–22, 1985.

Stefansson K., Dieperink M.E., Richman D.P., et al. Sharing of antigenic determinants between the nicotinic acetylcholine receptor and proteins in *Escherichia coli*, *Proteus vulgaris* and *Klebsiella*. *N. Engl. J. Med.* 312:221–225, 1985.

Sudhof T.C., Czernik A.J., Kao H.T., et al. Synapsins: mosaics of shared and individual domains in a family of synaptic vesicle phosphoproteins. *Science* 245:1474–1480, 1989.

Terranova W., Palumbo J.N., Breman J.G. Ocular findings in botulism type B. *J.A.M.A.* 241:475–477, 1979.

Turner H.D., Brett E.M., Gilbert R.J., et al. Infant botulism in England. *Lancet* 1:1277–1278, 1978.

Vincent A., Newsom-Davis J. Acetylcholine receptor antibody characteristics in myasthenia gravis. II. Patients with penicillamine-induced myasthenia or idiopathic myasthenia of recent onset. *Clin. Exp. Immunol.* 49:266–272, 1982.

*Vincent A., Newsom-Davis J. Acetylcholine receptor antibody as a diagnostic test for myasthenia gravis: results in 153 validated cases and 2967 diagnostic assays. *J. Neurol. Neurosurg. Psychiatry* 48:1246–1252, 1985.

Vincent A., Cull-Candy S.G., Newsom-Davis J., et al. Congenital myasthenia, endplate acetylcholine receptors and electrophysiology in five cases. *Muscle Nerve* 4:306–318, 1981.

Vincent A., Newsom-Davis J., Newton P., et al. Acetylcholine receptor antibody and clinical response to thymectomy in myasthenia gravis. *Neurology (N.Y.)* 33:1276–1282, 1983.

Whiting P., Vincent A., Newsom-Davis J. Monoclonal antibodies to the human acetylcholine receptor. *Biochem. Soc. Trans.* 13:116–117, 1985.

Whiting P.J., Vincent A., Newsom-Davis J. Myasthenia gravis: monoclonal antihuman acetylcholine receptor antibodies used to analyse antibody specificities and responses to treatment. *Neurology* 36:612–617, 1986.

Willcox H.N.A., Newsom-Davis J., Calder L.R. Cell types required for anti–acetylcholine receptor antibody synthesis by cultured thymocytes and blood lymphocytes in myasthenia gravis. *Clin. Exp. Immunol.* 58:97–106, 1984.

Willcox N., Demaine A.G., Newsom-Davis J., et al. Increased frequency of IgG heavy chain marker Glm(2) and of HLA-B8 in Lambert-Eaton myasthenic syndrome with and without associated lung carcinoma. *Hum. Immunol.* 14:29–36, 1985.

Willcox N., Schluep M., Ritter M.A., et al. Myasthenic and nonmyasthenic thymoma: an expansion of a minor cortical epithelial subset? *Am. J. Pathol.* 127:447–460, 1987.

Yamamoto T., Sato T., Sugita H. Antifilamin, antivinculin and antitropomyosin antibodies in myasthenia gravis. *Neurology* 37:1329–1333, 1987.

Yamamoto T., Vincent A., Ciulla T.A., et al. Seronegative myasthenia gravis: a plasma factor inhibiting agonist induced acetylcholine receptor function co-purifies with IgM. *Ann. Neurol.* (in press).

Peripheral Nerve, Root, and Spinal Cord

16

Somatosensory Function and Dysfunction

Ulf Lindblom

José Ochoa

The best service to the reader interested in sensation in the context of neurologic disease is to recommend Chapter VIII in *Introduction to Clinical Neurology* (Holmes, 1946), which considers the classic neurology of sensation. The following offers a brief version that includes advances in basic and applied knowledge, with emphasis on pathophysiologic aspects of somatosensory dysfunction.

It need not be emphasized that sensation, a subjective function, requires by definition a conscious and cooperative subject for its expression. Although the neurologic examination of sensory signs is a psychophysical exercise that relies on subjective estimation, signs of sensory deficit become validated pari passu with their anatomic or physiologic consistency and can thus be regarded as objective "signs." Eliciting reflexes and recording evoked nerve or brain potentials test preserved conduction of afferent pathways objectively, but the cerebral functions of sensory decoding can be explored only by psychophysical testing of conscious cooperative subjects.

Disorders of somatic sensation fall into two major categories: negative and positive phenomena.

Negative Phenomena. Hypoesthesia and hypoalgesia reflect failure at any level along sensory channels. The patient may or may not be aware of the deficit, and a routine sensory examination may or may not disclose it. For sensory deficit to be demonstrable by conventional sensory testing, a significant percentage of afferent channels may need to be out

of action (Buchthal and Rosenfalck, 1966). Altogether, negative sensory symptoms are relatively late indicators of afferent dysfunction, but subclinical deficit may be unmasked by quantitative sensory testing (Dyck et al., 1984; Lindblom and Tegnér, 1989) and by electrodiagnostic testing: recording of sensory nerve action potentials (Gilliatt, 1978) and somatosensory cerebral evoked potentials (Desmedt, 1980; Halliday, 1982; Treede and Bromm, 1988).

Positive Phenomena. Positive manifestations also reflect dysfunction at any level in the sensory pathways, but are expressed clinically mostly as symptoms only, without signs. They are largely due to abnormal generation of impulses in sensory channels. A commonplace example is ectopic cortical discharge, traditionally documented by electroencephalograms, in sensory epilepsy. Ectopic discharges generated in primary sensory units underlie spontaneous paresthesias (and pain) of peripheral nerve origin (Ochoa and Torebjörk, 1980) and abnormal sensations provoked by mechanical pressure on pathologic sensory pathways, as in the signs of Tinel, Lasègue, Spurling, and Lhermitte. These discharges can be documented, with difficulty, through microneurography (Nordin et al., 1984; Ochoa et al., 1982, 1987) (see Figs. 16–7 and 16–8).

A significant category of positive sensory phenomena involves inadequate subjective response to natural stimulation of receptors. Examples are pain in response to non-noxious stimuli (allodynia) or excessive pain response to noxious stimuli (hyperalgesia) (for definitions of pain terms, see Merskey, 1986 and Linblom, 1985). Mechanisms behind these abnormalities may include sensitization of pain receptors (Cline et al., 1989), abnormal patterns of discharge on transmission through neuromas (Tegnér and Borg, 1988), and derangement of central neuronal processing (Fruhstorfer and Lindblom, 1984; Lindblom and Verrillo, 1979; Wahrén et al., 1989; Yarnitsky and Ochoa, 1990).

Activity in a few sensory channels, especially if at higher frequency, can definitely evoke perceptible and even disturbing subjective symptoms (Ochoa and Torebjörk, 1983, 1989). Obviously, positive sensory manifestations are subtle indicators of afferent dysfunction, and the paucity of accompanying physical signs should not be misconstrued as evidence of a primarily psychologic origin.

The idea that some spontaneous positive sensory symptoms may be due to release of normally inhibited neural activity remains viable (Noordenbos, 1959; Wahrén et al., 1989; Yarnitsky and Ochoa, 1990).

SOMATOSENSORY PSYCHOPHYSICAL FUNCTIONS

When given a punctate mechanical stimulus somewhere on the skin, one can correctly recognize a touch, a prick or tickle sensation of a certain strength, felt in a precise point. Although such everyday experience is taken for granted, it must be recognized that physical attributes of a locally acting stimulus have been captured (encoded) by a range of primary sensory units, transmitted up, and decoded by the brain as subjective attributes of a natural sensation. Thus, a simple touch somewhere on the body surface must involve coding and decoding of rate, depth, and duration of skin displacement, which is perceived as a specific sensory quality, of a certain magnitude, somatotopically localized.

Intensity Coding

When Adrian and Zotterman discovered that trains of unitary messages spelled by sensory nerve fibers are a frequency code that reflects *intensity* of the natural stimulus, they logically proposed that afferent impulse frequency is decoded by the brain only as the magnitude of a sensation.

It started on a gloomy November morning in 1925 in Cambridge when Adrian and I recorded the electrical response of a single sensory nerve fibre to various grades of stimulation of the muscle spindle. That very day we conceived that the nerve fibre transmits information according to the principle of impulse frequency modulation. Consequently, the simple code transmitted by the nerve fibre can only inform us about the strength and duration of the stimulus, and the process of adaptation in the receptor (Zotterman, 1973).

In other words, *temporal summation* of afferent impulses is a key determinant of the subjective magnitude of a sensation. However, increasing intensity of a natural stimulus results not only in increased firing frequency of discharge but also in recruitment of more and more sensory units (*spatial summation*), and there are reasons to believe that either mechanism of summation might contribute to determine subjective magnitude. Classic psychophysical measurements, in which subjective magnitude of a sensation is plotted as a function of the intensity of a natural stimulus, suggested initially that such relationship is logarithmic (i.e., equal stimulus ratios produce *equal sensation differences* [Fechner's law, 1860]). Later, the prevailing relationship was shown to be described by a power function (i.e., equal stimulus ratios produce *equal sensation ratios* [Stevens' law, 1957]), with different slopes (exponents) on a logarithmic plot for the different somatosensory submodalities. Eventually, Mountcastle's group related both the intensity of a natural stimulus and the magnitude of its sensation with the frequency of the afferent impulses in single sensory units, in parallel experiments in monkeys and humans (Mountcastle, 1967). The correlation has also been achieved in strictly human experiments comparing neural and psychophysical thresholds during microneurographic recordings (Knibestöl and Vallbo, 1980). These studies showed that stimulus intensity is related both to impulse frequency of the unitary response and to psychophysical magnitude by a power function, but the shapes of the curves and the existence of linearity are disputed. These studies are based on natural stimulation, through which temporal and spatial summation may take place concurrently. When temporal summation is assessed separately from spatial summation, the frequency content of an afferent message per se carries information decodable as subjective magnitude (Torebjörk and Ochoa, 1980).

Localization Function (Topognosia, Locognosia)

If one accepts that the ability to localize a stimulus on the body surface is a function of the cortex, the existence of a somatotopic homunculus in the postcentral gyrus satisfies the intuitive requirement that there should be a cortical representation of the body map. Amazingly, the columnar modular organization of the somatosensory cortex is not only somatotopic but also submodality specific (Mountcastle, 1957). In other words, modular loci of the cortex are exclusively concerned with particular kinds of sensory units projecting from particular parts of the body. Because cutaneous localization in humans is precise for input from different kinds of sensory units (Schady et al., 1983a,b), the additional requirement emerges that there should exist multiple, submodality-specific, somatotopically arranged homunculi in the cortex. This has been demonstrated in animals

(Dykes, 1983; Kaas et al., 1979). It is also remarkable that a train of impulses initiated in a single low-threshold mechanoreceptor unit is sufficient to provide fairly good localization. Indeed, when felt, just a single impulse from a single microstimulated rapidly adapting unit may be enough for localization. Thus, the conscious human brain may resolve the body map at the single-channel level. Said colloquially, the brain knows the address of individual cutaneous receptors, at least in fingers (Ochoa and Torebjörk, 1983, 1989).

Quality of Somatosensory Submodalities

Because impulse frequency is the only variable within the messages spelled by single afferent units (and frequency is decoded as subjective magnitude of sensation), the subjective quality must be determined by some other measure. Zotterman (1971) was convinced that sensory qualities ("touch, tickle and pain") are determined not by the contents of the afferent message but by the nature of the messenger channel and its specific central processing, as von Frey had also advocated in the *specificity theory* to explain the quality of cutaneous submodalities (for a brief, excellent review in English, see von Frey, 1906).

In the 1950s, the Oxford group challenged the specificity (or pathway) theory of sensory quality by proposing the pattern theory, which was based heavily on the fact that in the cornea only naked endings can be seen under the microscope, although several qualities might be aroused by stimulation. The particular energy of the stimulus casts a particular code of nerve impulses along otherwise uncommitted receptors and pathways, and characteristic patterns of impulses evoke particular sensations (Weddell, 1955). "One and the same type of ending can mediate different forms of sensation, according to the physical conditions to which it is exposed" (Sinclair, 1955).

In addition to the bulk of electrophysiologic evidence in favor of the specificity theory, obtained at all levels from peripheral receptors to the cerebral cortex and referred to elsewhere in this chapter, various clinical lesions, affecting different sensory nerve fibers or tracts, produce profiles of sensory impairment that cannot be explained on the basis of a pattern theory. This holds also for blocking experiments in healthy human subjects, which repeatedly have demonstrated a specific relation between type of nerve fiber and sensory submodality. Intraneural microstimulation of identified primary sensory units of awake subjects (Ochoa and Torebjörk, 1983, 1989; Torebjörk and Ochoa, 1980) provides further documentation of specificity for submodality within the somatic afferent system. By permitting the administration of various patterned trains of impulses to identified sensory units, this method also provides evidence against the pattern theory (Ochoa and Torebjörk, 1980; Ochoa et al., 1984).

ANATOMY AND PHYSIOLOGY OF THE PERIPHERAL SENSORY SYSTEM: ORDER AND DISORDER

Structure and Stimulus-Response Characteristics of Primary Sensory Units

The "apparatus that intervenes between stimulus and sensation" (Adrian, 1931) is exposed to natural energies at end organs of primary sensory neurons. A peripheral sensory unit is composed of a single afferent nerve fiber together with its endings, cell body, and central processes; "it could be considered as the sensory equivalent of the neuromotor unit" (Tower, 1940).

The range of morphologically identifiable sensory end organs in the human skin is shown in Figure 16–1. Some are encapsulated, whereas others are simple naked nerve endings. *Nociceptors* and *thermoreceptors* have unmyelinated or thinly myelinated slowly conducting nerve fibers and naked endings. The encapsulated endings are connected to neurons with large myelinated fibers and are low-threshold mechanoreceptors: some mechanoreceptors are superficial (and have German names), others are deep (and have Italian names).

The area from which impulse activity can be excited in any sensory unit is called a unitary *receptive field.* Any discrete point of skin contains sensory receptors from a variety of units. In human finger pulps, there are about 240 low-threshold mechanoreceptor units represented per square centimeter (Johansson and Vallbo, 1979). This ensures considerable overlap of receptive fields of different units in any point of richly innervated skin and thus both uniform and multimodality sensitivity.

Although sensory units may sometimes be activated by different types of energy, they are usually particularly sensitive to one energy; such is the *adequate stimulus.* Sensory receptors are variously responsive to an adequate stimulus, requiring relatively more or less energy to be activated (i.e., they have a high or low threshold). To reach the axon of a sensory ending, the stimulus must pass through intervening tissues: *stimulus accession.* Next, the stimulus energy is transformed into electrical energy: *transduction.* This stage is incompletely understood, but involves depolarization of the axon terminal in proportion to the amount of energy applied. Thus, the *generator potential* is a graded response, unlike the all-or-nothing *action potentials* propagated up along nerve fibers. Trains of such action potentials are triggered by suprathreshold generator potentials at the pacemaker region adjacent to the axon terminal (for review, see Loewenstein, 1971). The amplitude of the generator potential determines the frequency at which action potentials are initiated, but intrinsic properties of the sensory receptors determine how sustained the impulse activity is. Thus, in the presence of a sustained adequate stimulus, receptors may respond with fairly sustained firing, or their response

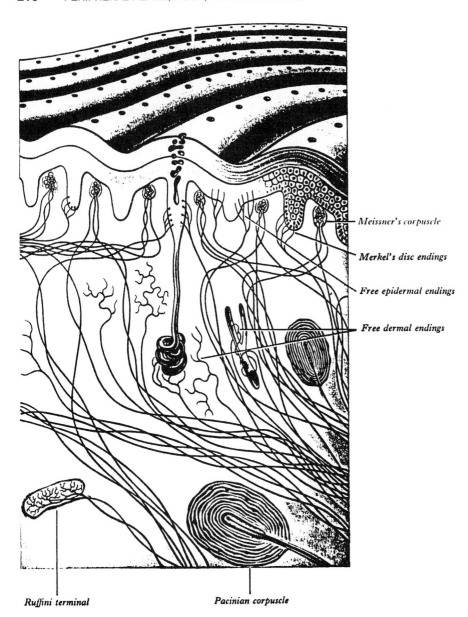

Figure 16–1. Schematic illustration of some of the principal sensory endings of thick (hairless) skin and associated structures, including various types of encapsulated and "free" endings, of the epidermis, the dermis, and subcutaneous connective tissue. (From Williams P.L., Warwick R., eds. *Gray's Anatomy*. 36th ed. Edinburgh, Churchill Livingstone, 1980.)

Meissner's corpuscle

Merkel's disc endings

Free epidermal endings

Free dermal endings

Ruffini terminal

Pacinian corpuscle

may quickly die out (i.e., they are *slowly or rapidly adapting*).

Human sensory units can be usefully classified according to nature of the *adequate stimulus, threshold, adaptation rate,* and *conduction velocity.* Because the histologic end organs of animal sensory units expressing stimulus-response characteristics comparable with those of the human are known (see Iggo, 1973), an integrated morphophysiologic classification of human sensory units is offered in Table 16–1.

Cutaneous Receptor Dysfunction

Receptors wither away with aging, in dying-back neuropathies, and in all situations in which axons degenerate. Local skin trauma or disease may cause receptor decay. Otherwise normal receptors may change their response characteristics from intense or prolonged usage. For example, *fatigue* of the receptor response to reiterated activation is a common feature of nociceptors with C fibers. Mechanical or thermal stimuli repeated at short intervals excite fewer and fewer impulses from such receptors, and a pause of several minutes may be needed to restore excitability.

Under special conditions, nociceptors may become sensitized. A superficial burn lowers their threshold for mechanical and thermal excitation, and their responses to suprathreshold stimuli become excessive. Such sensitization of nociceptors leads to hyperalgesia (La Motte et al., 1982), as in sunburn. C nociceptors become sensitized as part of the phenomenon of neurogenic inflammation, typically induced by neurotoxins such as capsaicin (Culp et al., 1989; Szolcsanyi, 1977). Nociceptor sensitization may also occur as a consequence of disease in humans (Cline et al., 1989). This type of sensitization has been suggested in the pathogenesis of vascular headaches

Table 16–1. HISTOLOGIC TYPES OF NERVE TERMINALS IN HUMAN GLABROUS SKIN, FUNCTIONAL RECEPTOR CHARACTERISTICS, NERVE FIBER TYPES, AND SUBJECTIVE SENSORY CORRELATES

| Histology | Receptor Characteristics | | | Electrophysiologic Symbol | Nerve Fiber Type | Sensory Quality |
	Adequate Stimuli	Field Organization	Adaptation			
Meissner corpuscles	Weak contact as single or oscillatory event	Multiple spots (12–17) within distinct border	Rapidly adapting; on-off discharge _stimulus duration_	RA	Large myelinated	Discrete taps Flutter (texture recognition)
Pacini corpuscles	Light contact, single or oscillating	Single spot within indistinct border	Comparable to RA-Meissner but even more dynamic	PC	Myelinated	Vibration Tickle
Merkel discs	Sustained orthogonal pressure	Multiple spots (4–7) within distinct border	Slowly adapting	SA-I	Large myelinated	Continuous pressure
Ruffini organs	Sustained orthogonal pressure; shearing skin	Single spot within indistinct border	Slowly adapting, often spontaneously active	SA-II	Large myelinated	No sensation when activated in isolation Possibly proprioception
Naked endings	Noxious mechanical stimuli	One or two spots within distinct border	Slowly adapting	Nociceptors with A δ fibers	Small myelinated	Sharp stinging, "fast" pain
Naked endings	Noxious stimuli: 1. mechanical 2. thermal—above 43°C and below 14°C 3. various chemicals	Multiple spots (2–7) within distinct border	Intermediate rate of adaptation Afterdischarges common	Polymodal or multisensitive nociceptors with C fibers	Unmyelinated	Dull or burning, "slow" pain Itch
Naked endings	Thermal 34–50°C	Single spot	Rapidly and slowly adapting	Warm receptors	Unmyelinated	Warmth
Naked endings	Thermal	Unknown in humans	Unknown in humans	Cold receptors	Small myelinated	Cold

Presented in 1981 to the American Academy of Neurology, Annual Course in Neurophysiology. Reproduced by courtesy of J. Ochoa and H. E. Torebjörk.

(Moskowitz et al., 1986) and might be a component of neuropathic pain and even arthritis (Guilbaud, 1988; Levine et al., 1985).

Sensory Nerve Fibers

Practically all somatic nerves have a contingent of sensory fibers. Cutaneous nerves in humans contain a single-size population of unmyelinated fibers, three or four times more abundant than the summated populations of large and small myelinated fibers (Ochoa and Mair, 1969), as seen in Figure 16–2. Of course, nerves connected with skin contain mostly afferent fibers and a proportion of efferent postganglionic sympathetic fibers to sweat glands and to smooth muscle for piloerection and cutaneous vasomotility. Deep nerves connected with muscle and deep tissues contain a sizable proportion of proprioceptive afferent myelinated fibers from muscle spindles and Golgi tendon organs, in addition to thin afferent fibers from nociceptors (supplying musculoskeletal tissues, including joints) and sympathetic efferents.

That the nerve conduction velocity is a function of axon diameter and degree of myelination is expressed in the compound nerve action potential. When a nerve trunk is stimulated electrically, the compound nature of the propagated wave can be displayed by recording at a suitable conduction distance: each elevation reflects more or less synchronous conduction in nerve fibers of a particular population (Erlanger and Gasser, 1924, 1930) (Fig. 16–3). The accepted composition of the sensory nerve action potential includes A α (72–30 m/second), A δ (30–4 m/second), and C (2–0.4 m/second) elements (Burgess and Perl, 1973).

Sensory Nerve Fiber Dysfunction

Both negative and positive manifestations may result from nerve fiber dysfunction. Although personal experience of transient positive and negative nerve symptoms is commonplace, a simple experiment, to remind the clinician of both, should at some stage be self-administered by every neurologist.

Negative Manifestations

Experiment Part A. Inflate a sphygmomanometer cuff around the upper arm, above systolic pressure.

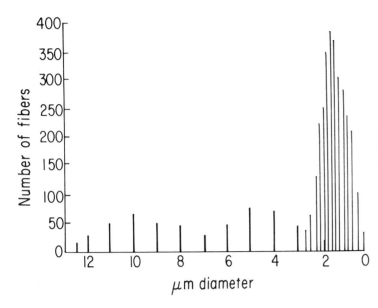

Figure 16–2. Compound size frequency histogram from two sural nerve fascicles of a young man. It shows a trimodal distribution of large myelinated, small myelinated, and unmyelinated axons. (Modified in reverse from Ochoa J., Mair W.G.P. The normal sural nerve in man. I. Ultrastructure and numbers of fibres and cells. *Acta Neuropathol.* 13:197–216, 1969.)

Leave in place for longer than 30 minutes. Avoid movement: it elicits muscle pain. Transitory ischemic paresthesia appears within a few minutes and progressive centripetal numbness thereafter. Routine sensory examination of fingertips reveals a dissociated deficit: light touch, vibration, and cold are lost first, followed by pricking pain, whereas warmth and dull pain persist longer. This is because compression-ischemia blocks conduction as a function of fiber diameter (Lewis et al., 1931). If at this stage the numb skin is stimulated electrically and the conducted signals are picked up further proximally with an intraneural electrode, only the late C components representing afferent unmyelinated fibers are found to be present (Torebjörk and Hallin, 1973) (Fig. 16–4). This simple experiment illustrates the segregation of sensation as a function of submodality and also how it feels to have no feeling—and to feel pure C pain.

Clinical Expression. Clinically, loss of sensation is largely described by the patient as numbness and is witnessed on examination as an elevated perception threshold or a reduced suprathreshold magnitude of sensation. Most daily life stimuli and also clinical bedside tests are suprathreshold, and altered suprathreshold magnitude is thus detected before

threshold changes. It is not well recognized in clinical thinking that both functions can be assessed and that they may be intrinsically linked to each other, as illustrated in Figure 16–5. The thick solid line in Figure 16–5A represents the most common sensory disturbance, characterized by increased perception threshold and subnormal intensity of sensation at all suprathreshold stimulus levels. Hypoesthesia is primarily considered a sign of reduced number of conducting elements, but peripheral lesions that do not prevent conduction of action potentials may disperse or impoverish the afferent barrages. This is most critical for sensory submodalities that depend heavily on spatial and temporal resolution (e.g., tactile discrimination and vibration sense) or on summation (e.g., warm sensation).

The discovery of central mechanisms of modulation of sensory transmission provided a basis for understanding functional alterations of somatic sensation (Towe, 1973). Dynamic alterations might be superimposed on structural abnormalities or may occur in isolation. A clinical expression of the later mechanism is the spectacular hysterical anesthesia or analgesia that occurs as a reversible suppression of perception of somatic stimulation. The condition is not reversed by naloxone (U. Lindblom, unpublished observation), which suggests that modulatory systems other than the endorphin system are responsible. Functional sensory loss occurs in other clinical conditions (e.g., in chronic pain, recovery of sensibility was documented after pain-relieving measures [Lindblom, 1985]).

Evaluation. Important levels of discrepancy in the evaluation of sensory disturbances call for clarification. In the first, patients may complain of numbness while no sensory loss is found on examination, even when perception thresholds for multiple submodalities are carefully tested. This presumably occurs because the feeling of numbness, contrary to first-hand belief, is not always the awareness of loss of

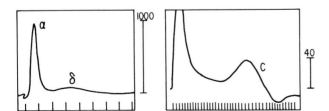

Figure 16–3. Compound action potentials recorded from the sural nerve of the cat. Three main elevations are seen, today labeled A α, A δ, and C deflections. (Modified from Gasser H.S. Conduction in nerves in relation to fiber types. *Proc. Assoc. Res. Nerv. Ment. Dis.* 15:35–59, 1934.)

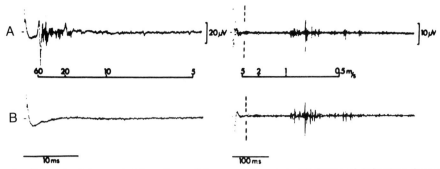

Figure 16–4. Compound action potential recorded from the radial nerve in humans. *(A)* Series of deflections from myelinated fibers *(left)* and unmyelinated fibers *(right)*. *(B)* After nerve compression for 40 minutes, impulse transmission was blocked in myelinated fibers *(left)* but not in unmyelinated fibers *(right)*. With only C fibers conducting, sensations of warmth, heat, itch, and delayed pain can still be perceived. (Modified from Torebjörk H.E., Hallin R.G. Perceptual changes accompanying controlled preferential blocking of A and C fibre response in intact human skin nerves. *Exp. Brain Res.* 16:321–332, 1973.)

conducting sensory elements, but a mild positive symptom that may, or may not, be associated with loss of sensation. Typically, spinal cord injury patients with extensive sensory loss seldom complain of numbness. An alternative explanation may be that the demonstration of normal thresholds is not sufficient to exclude a sensory dysfunction that might be confined to the suprathreshold stimulus range, as illustrated by the thin solid line in Figure 16–5*A*. Therefore, a wider use of discriminative tests is recommended, such as figure writing (graphesthesia), which is a simple and sensitive test of spatiotemporal and magnitude discrimination (Bender et al., 1982).

The second discrepancy between symptoms and signs is of the opposite character: sensory impairment is revealed by testing in the absence of subjective complaints. Not surprisingly, impairment of vibration sense (and lack of myotatic reflexes) is not noted by the patients because the sensory inflow via the pacinian system (or from muscle spindles) is not a part of conscious experience in the daily perceptual world. What is more surprising is that significant defects of cutaneous sensation often escape subjective recognition when they are protracted and unaccompanied by positive phenomena that attract attention. This applies to thermal, tactile, and nociceptive

sensibility, and not only to loss of sensation but also to some extent to its abnormal exaggeration. Toxic and metabolic neuropathies are common examples of this discrepancy that necessitate quantitative sensory testing even when the patient denies sensory symptoms.

Positive Manifestations

Experiment Part B. After 20 minutes or more, release the cuff. Usually, within seconds, the cold pale hand becomes red and feels hot. Then a stereotyped sequence of *paresthesias* follows: they peak by 1½ minutes and slowly wane thereafter. As long suspected, this nerve equivalent of sensory epilepsy reflects the generation of spontaneous paroxysmal discharges from within afferent nerve fibers (Ochoa and Torebjörk, 1980; Torebjörk et al., 1979) (Fig. 16–6). Diabetics and elderly people are *less* prone to postischemic paresthesias (for a discussion of the ionic phenomena, see Culp et al., 1982). In addition to familiarizing the clinician with an assortment of abnormal sensations, such as tingling, buzzing, pricking, and pseudocramp, this simple experiment emphasizes the role of ectopic impulse generators as

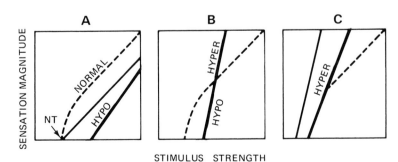

Figure 16–5. Diagrammatic illustration of principal quantitative abnormalities of common sensation as can be assessed separately for each modality by means of selective mechanical, thermal, or painful stimulation. Stimulus strength *(abscissa)* is plotted against subjective magnitude of sensation quantified by magnitude estimation or similar psychophysical techniques. Normal intensity functions *(hatched lines)* are typically power functions (Stevens' law). NT on abscissa indicates normal threshold. Thick solid lines in *A, B,* and *C* indicate observed functions of hypoesthesia, hypo-hyperesthesia, and hyperesthesia, respectively. Thin solid lines represent hypothetic functions of hypoesthesia with retained threshold in *A,* and hyperesthesia with lowered threshold in *C.*

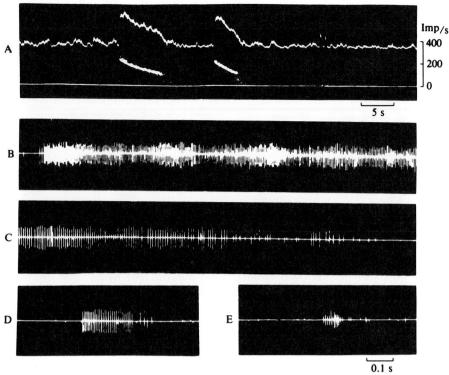

Figure 16–6. Prolonged high-frequency discharges in a single unit recorded from the median nerve at elbow level. Unitary bursts appeared during the second minute after release of cuff compression around the forearm, maintained for 25 minutes. *(A)* Integrated neurogram *(upper trace)* shows four abrupt deflections, representing single-unit discharges, also displayed in *B* through *E*. Instantaneous frequency plot *(lower trace)* shows initial frequency of about 220 Hz with exponential fall to about 150 Hz and subsequent breakdown. Duration of consecutive bursts diminished from an initial maximum of 7 seconds. *B* displays the beginning and *C*, the end of first unitary burst shown in *A*. Note regular firing frequency at the beginning, and missing beats toward the end. Last two bursts in *A* are displayed in *D* and *E*. (From Ochoa J., Torebjörk H.E. Paresthesiae from ectopic impulse generation in human sensory nerves. *Brain* 103:835–852, 1980, by permission of Oxford University Press.)

symptom determinants in the peripheral nervous system. Spontaneous discharges, originating ectopically in pathologic nerve fibers, have been reported in symptomatic patients (Nordin et al., 1984; Ochoa et al., 1982, 1987).

Provocation Tests. In the realm of positive sensory phenomena, a third, rather common, discrepancy between symptoms and signs arises when the patient reports paresthesias or pains and the examiner fails to document dysfunction by conventional clinical or electrodiagnostic testing or even by quantitative sensory testing of patients relaxed in the physician's office. Provocation tests may be helpful in this situation, for example, the classic maneuvers of Tinel, Lasègue, Lhermitte, Phalen, and Spurling (Figs. 16–7 and 16–8). For several of these tests, microneurography has confirmed that abnormal discharges are actually produced in the sensory pathway, as suspected from the patient's report (Nordin et al., 1984; Ochoa et al., 1987). Provocation may also induce a transitory conduction block and a measurable increase in sensory threshold, which reveal the site of a suspected lesion (Borg and Lindblom, 1986).

Neuropathic Pain. That spontaneously ongoing chronic pain, after injury to nerves or nerve roots, may reflect release of the input from pain fibers caused by lack of inhibition from damaged large-

diameter afferents (fiber dissociation theory) was strongly advocated by Noordenbos (1959). However, a dropout of large-diameter afferents is not a consistent finding in painful local nerve lesions (Ochoa and Noordenbos, 1979). Spontaneous impulse generation from pathologic fibers within the pain pathways is a serious alternative, originally put forward by Wall and Gutnick (1974). Spontaneous afferent discharges remain to be demonstrated in humans with chronic neuropathic pain, although excessive numbers of immature sprouts, a pathologic substrate reputed as potentially capable of spontaneous impulse generation, have been consistently found trapped at the site of neuroma and Tinel's sign in surgical specimens from such patients (Ochoa, 1982; Ochoa and Noordenbos, 1979).

Ephaptic cross-talk, known to follow acute nerve injury, has been recurrently entertained as a possible basis for chronic neuralgic pain (see Chapter 3). Because cross-talk was categorically shown as viable in naturally occurring pathologic animal nerves (Rasminsky, 1978, 1980), interest in ephapses revived, and in the pain context, Seltzer and Devor (1979) made a case for cross-talk in rat amputation neuromas. Ephapses involving C fibers have been claimed (Blumberg and Jänig, 1981), and the anatomic proximity of C afferent and sympathetic fibers in nerve

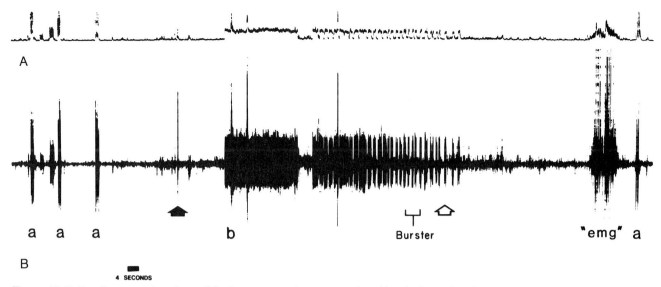

Figure 16–7. Bursting nerve impulse activity in sensory unit, propagated antidromically to site of intraneural recording from cutaneous fascicle in ulnar nerve at wrist level. Patient had a C-8 radiculopathy and consistently experienced pain and paresthesias on extension and left lateral flexion of the neck. The recording captures the sequence of ectopic discharge provoked by positioning the neck. *(A)* Integrated neurogram. *(B)* Simultaneous discriminated neurogram. a = stimulation of receptive field of a low-threshold mechanoreceptor unit in little finger; solid arrow = neck flexed to left and extended; b = onset of abnormal unitary bursting, temporally correlating with verbalized report of paresthesias reaching the hand; open arrow = head returned to neutral position; "emg" = voluntary muscle artifact; a = original receptive field reconfirmed. (From Ochoa J., Cline M., Dotson R., et al. Pain and paresthesias provoked mechanically in human cervical root entrapment [sign of Spurling]. Single sensory unit antidromic recording of ectopic, bursting, propagated nerve impulse activity. In Pubols L.M., Sessle B.J., eds. *Effects of Injury on Trigeminal and Spinal Somatosensory Systems.* New York, Liss, pp. 389–397, 1987.)

trunks (see Ochoa, 1984) might be taken as a basis for sympathetic dependent pain (causalgia). Whether or not ephaptic cross-talk may be implicated in spontaneous ongoing pain, this aberration remains conceivable in recurrent pain triggered by non-noxious stimuli, as in some paroxysmal neuralgias and in some forms of pain abnormally evoked by non-noxious stimulation of sensory receptors (Lindblom, 1985). Certain clinical phenomena of (1) altered quality, (2) excessive spatial distribution, and (3) overlasting duration of stimulus-evoked sensations might be explained, respectively, by (1) abnormal transfer of afferent information to the wrong type of channel, (2) disinhibited central spread of discharges, and (3) after discharge at either peripheral or central levels. (See also Chapter 65.)

CENTRAL CONNECTIONS

The first sensory station for most afferent fibers is the *dorsal horn*. Here the primary sensory neurons relay on an intricate but orderly laminated system of small secondary neurons. Fibers that form the spinothalamic tracts emerge from the dorsal horn and cross anterior to the ependyma to the opposite half of the cord (see Chapter 64). Accurate mapping by means of retrograde transport of a marker (Trevino and Carstens, 1975) made it possible to establish with certainty the location of the cells of origin of the spinothalamic tracts in laminae I, VII, and VIII in the monkey. Segregation of afferent fiber systems in the

cord explains selective loss of sensory modalities after strategic lesions.

Descending tracts have been discovered in the spinal cord, with cells of origin in the periaqueductal gray in the brain stem, which cause *inhibition of spinothalamic neurons*. Some of these inhibitory neurons have receptors that are specifically activated by opiates. Thus, morphine abolishes pain by indirectly inhibiting spinothalamic discharges (Fields and Basebaum, 1979). Other descending inhibitory influences are well known; for example, the corticospinal tracts, in addition to activating the motor neurons for voluntary muscle contraction, inhibit the excitation exerted by spindle afferents on motor neurons.

Spinal Cord and Brain Stem Dysfunction

Negative Manifestations. Traditional sensory syndromes (Holmes, 1946) resulting from spinal cord lesions are well known and are beyond the scope of this chapter. Dissociation of sensory submodality deficit in focal spinal cord lesions is another expression of specificity, because submodality-specific afferent systems are segregated in the cord. Thus, tactile discrimination and "deep" sensation (joint position and vibration sense) are affected in posterior column disease, whereas pain and temperature sensibility are affected in spinothalamic lesions. Current understanding calls for qualification of this simple concept: correlating negative sensory phenomena with focal anatomic lesions, although certainly revealing of the functions that concern a particular pathway, is partly misleading. Indeed, it is fallacious

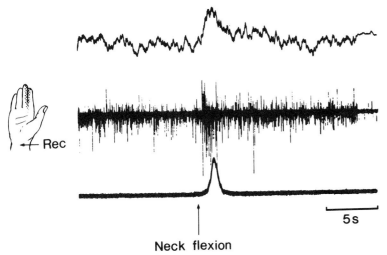

Figure 16–8. Recording from the right median nerve in a skin fascicle, with receptive field indicated. At the moment indicated by an arrow, the patient flexed her neck, which elicited Lhermitte's sign. The moment for the abnormal sensation was indicated by a grip force signal shown in the lower trace. Above is seen the multiunit burst in the neurogram and the integrated neurogram (time constant 0.5 second). (From Nordin M., Nyström B., Wallin U., et al. Ectopic sensory discharges and paresthesiae in patients with disorders of peripheral nerves, dorsal roots, and dorsal columns. *Pain* 20:231–245, 1984.)

5 s

Neck flexion

to assume from such correlations that certain functions are exclusively subserved in certain pathways. This is transparent from analysis of the reverse model: what are the remaining sensory functions if only one pathway remains intact? Almost complete cord transection sparing only one spinothalamic tract, in a human subject, resulted in remarkable preservation of several sensory modalities on both lower limbs: pain could be evoked by stimulation of both sides; light touch could be identified on both sides; passive joint movement could be detected on the ipsilateral side only; pinprick could be identified on the contralateral side only (Noordenbos and Wall, 1976). This key clinicopathologic correlation should lead to less rigidity in thinking about the sensory representations within ascending spinal pathways.

Positive Manifestations. Lhermitte's sign can be accepted as being due to ectopic mechanosensitive impulse generation from focally demyelinated spinal cord fibers (Nordin et al., 1984; Smith and McDonald, 1982) as illustrated in Figure 16–8. It is legitimate to regard ongoing paresthesias in spinal cord disease as reflecting ectopic *spontaneous* impulse generation, although this has not been confirmed. Further, the specific quality of these paresthesias does carry useful localizing value: tingling, pressure, or buzzing largely incriminating posterior columns and pain, warmth, cold, or itch incriminating spinothalamic tract origin (A. McArdle, 1967, personal communication). Paroxysmal positive sensory manifestations in patients with demyelinating disease probably belong in this context too (Matthews, 1975). Ongoing paresthesias or dysesthesias below the level of the lesion (central dysesthesia syndrome) may be prominent in patients with spinal cord injury. Quantitative sensory examination and neurophysiologic testing have revealed relative preservation of dorsal column functions with absence of spinothalamic system–mediated functions. Such afferent imbalance may be instrumental as a determinant of the abnormal sensory state, associated with cord or brain lesions (Berić et al., 1988; Leijon et al., 1989). On the other hand, in a patient with dysesthetic pain below the level of a

clinically *complete* traumatic spinal cord transection at C-5, abnormal single-unit activity was recorded in the somatosensory thalamus, suggesting spontaneous and evoked activity in thalamic neurons that have lost normal somatosensory input. Electrical stimulation of those regions of the thalamus can produce a sensation of pain (Lenz et al., 1988).

Chronic spontaneous pain after deafferentation deserves special comment. It is not at all uncommon in some lesions that affect primarily the peripheral nervous system but repercuss at the dorsal horn level. Chronic pain after spinal root avulsion is one example and postherpetic neuralgia probably another. The presumed mechanism is as follows: lesions of the primary sensory unit that sever its centrally directed axon (in dorsal root ganglia or dorsal roots), and thus anatomically deafferent second-order neurons, trigger plasticity changes in dorsal horn nociceptive neurons. These would be rendered either spontaneously active or responsive to subliminal fringe input otherwise suppressed under normal conditions. Neurophysiologic observations to support this view have been reported in animals (Lombard et al., 1979, 1981; Willis, 1990) and also in a paraplegic man (Loeser et al., 1968). Destructive microsurgery directed to the dorsal horn, the so-called dorsal root entry zone lesion, is reported to be encouragingly effective in these patients (Nashold and Ostdahl, 1979).

Axonal lesions of the peripheral branch of the primary sensory neuron have also been shown experimentally to upset the circuitry in dorsal horns and, in view of frequent failure of peripherally directed therapy against pain from nerve disease, it has been proposed that this situation also reflects secondary dorsal horn pathophysiology (Noordenbos and Wall, 1981). In the absence of anatomic injury to the primary sensory neuron, secondary central changes, in the form of altered activation pattern at cortical levels, have been demonstrated in arthritic rats with ongoing nociceptor input (Guilbaud et al., 1984), which is interesting in the context of chronic pain of nociceptive (rather than neuropathic) origin.

DISCRIMINATIVE SENSATION

Neurologists have traditionally obtained a measure of *tactile acuity* through the threshold for discrimination of two points in the skin. Microscopists and microneurographists have described a correspondence for such function in the varying concentrations of sensory end organs and receptive fields in different regions. Psychophysical experiments have emphasized that, over and above skin receptor density, the brain applies differential priorities, on a regional basis, for impulse detection and spatial or temporal discrimination. Together with the encoding variables at the periphery, these cortical decoding criteria obviously are crucial to determining tactile acuity (Ochoa and Torebjörk, 1983; Schady et al., 1983a,b).

Recognition of *texture* by active touch involves spatial displacements of skin relative to object, over time, and necessitates a dynamic and sensitive signaling system that can punctually register occurrence and recurrence of every physical encounter: it is probably exemplified by the RA and PC channels (see Table 16–1). On the other hand, recognition of *shape and consistency* has been thought to be resolved by the SA-I system from analysis of receptor characteristics coupled with the cognitive attributes of those channels (Darian-Smith and Oke, 1980; Ochoa and Torebjörk, 1983). Naturally, all these discriminative functions cooperate and are superimposed in everyday tactile discrimination tasks and may disintegrate with dysfunction at higher levels of the sensorium.

The pathophysiology of somatosensory cortex may be oversimplified as follows on the basis of its functional organization (Hyvärinen, 1982; Mountcastle, 1980; Werner and Whitsel, 1973) (see Chapters 49 and 50). The symptoms and signs of dysfunction, classically described by Critchley (1953), are listed in Table 16–2 in a tentative hierarchic order of dependence of the corresponding function on cortical inte-

Table 16–2. SEMIOLOGY OF PARIETAL CORTEX*

Inattention (extinction of simultaneous stimulus)

Asomatognosia (lack of recognition of internal and external space)

Astereognosia (inability to recognize palpated objects)
    Agraphesthesia
    Impaired two-point discrimination

Topagnosia (inability to localize)

Astathesthesia (inability to recognize limb position)
    Pseudoataxia

Akinesthesia (loss of directional sensitivity of skin and joints)

Loss of sense of movement

Hypoesthesia (increase of threshold or decrease of magnitude of sensation)

*Listed dysfunction appears contralaterally. Dominant hemisphere dysfunction (i.e., aphasia, tactile agnosia [bimanual astereognosis], and Gerstmann's syndrome) are not considered here in the context of somatic sensation.

gration (see also Chapters 51–56). Hypoesthesia may occur for any modality of superficial or deep mechanical or thermal somatosensation. Pain and vibration sense are affected least and only with more extensive lesions, conceivably because these modalities require relatively little spatial integration at the cortical level. Among functions of higher order, the mere sense of movement seems to be the least integration dependent because it is impaired late during disease. Directional kinesthesia is a more sensitive function, the basis of which has been demonstrated in the form of S-1 cortical units with specific unidirectional or multidirectional sensitivity (Gardner, 1984). The mechanism of astathesthesia is incompletely understood, as well as its relation to the phenomenon of pseudoataxia. The pathophysiology of topognosia probably involves defective capacity of demodulation or recomposition in the system of somatotopic cortical representation. Astereognosis is a more complex dysfunction, resulting from impaired resolution of macrogeometrics (size, shape), microgeometrics (roughness), other surface characteristics (thermal characteristics, friction), and the weight of objects (Johnson and Phillips, 1984; Roland, 1976). Inattention and asomatognosia apparently reflect disturbances of highly integrated parietal lobe functions (see also Chapters 54 and 56).

QUANTITATIVE SENSORY TESTS

For the purpose of documenting somatosensory status in a standardized and rigorous manner in patients, it is desirable to supplement the simple routine neurologic examination of sensation. Quantitative methods for examination of the somatosensory system introduce an element of precision to tests that are otherwise vague at both the stimulus level and the subjective sensory response level.

Precision is achieved at the response level through implementation of standard measurements of perception thresholds or of psychophysical suprathreshold magnitude estimation function. Precision at the level of stimulus can be achieved through equipment that delivers graded and measurable mechanical or thermal energies to sensory receptors. With the vibrameter, the thermal stimulator, and the algometer, the subjects essentially report on perception thresholds for various sensory modalities, rather than scaling subjective suprathreshold magnitude. These instruments enable refined noninvasive clinical tests to enrich the clinical sensory examination by introducing precision, particularly at the stimulus level.

It should be pointed out, however, that quantitative methods should be applied and interpreted on the basis of a thorough screening examination with conventional bedside tests for touch, discrimination (graphesthesia), pressure, pinprick, cold, and warmth. Isolated use of quantitative tests should be reserved for specific studies.

Vibrameter. Lindblom uses as stimulus a contin-

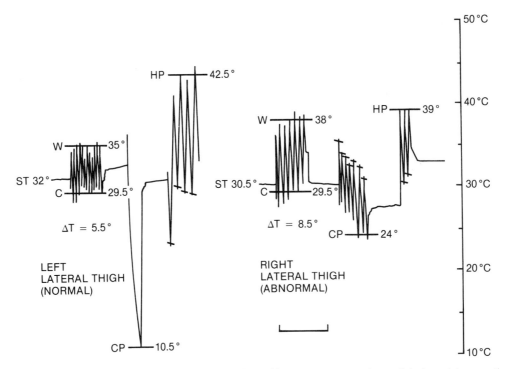

Figure 16–9. Records of cutaneous thermal sensitivity from a patient with a common type of neuralgia (meralgia paresthetica). The trace shows the interface temperature between the thermode and the skin during stimulation. The current, which drives the temperature from the resting skin temperature (ST) where there is no stimulus-evoked sensation, is switched by the patient several successive times, first at the perception for warmth (W) and cold (C). The ensuing peaks at W and C thus indicate the perception thresholds of warmth and cold, respectively. On the record from the control side *(left)*, these thresholds averaged about 35 and 29.5°C. The patient is then instructed to switch at the perception of pain on cold stimulation, and then for pain on warm stimulation. This gives estimates of the cold pain (CP) and heat pain (HP) thresholds. The right part of record, from center of painful skin, shows hypoesthesia for warmth (threshold at 38°C versus 35°C on the control side) and retained cold threshold. Suprathreshold cold stimulation quickly becomes painful, and the cold pain threshold leveled at 24°C (allodynia). Heat pain was signaled at a somewhat decreased temperature, 39°C versus 42.5°C on the control side (hyperalgesia). Time bar = 3 minutes; ΔT = threshold difference limen.

uous sinusoid vibration, the amplitude of which is monitored by means of a logarithmic potentiometer. The stimulus strength is given as the peak-to-peak displacement. This is recorded continuously and displayed digitally during the measurement. The procedure implies that the source of error that is caused by the variable tissue damping is controlled. The vibrator is hand-held and has an indicator of the pressure with which it is applied. The tremor of the examiner, as well as noise from other sources, can be avoided by filtering. Reference values for the vibration threshold, determined by the method of limits, are available for carpal, tibial, and tarsal stimulus sites (Goldberg and Lindblom, 1979).

The vibration threshold may be taken as a functional index of large-diameter afferent fibers. Compared with the conduction velocity, the vibration threshold is a more dynamic variable, enabling one to record transient phasic, as well as stationary, abnormalities of function. Either method can be more sensitive for the early diagnosis of nerve dysfunction. Vibrametry is used for assessment and follow-up of polyneuropathies and some mononeuropathies and spinal cord lesions (Lindblom and Tegnér, 1989). It can also be used in research projects in which vibratory sensitivity may be a relevant indicator (Lindblom and Meyerson, 1975).

Thermal Stimulator. The Marstock method, as recommended by Fruhstorfer et al. (1976), proves useful in that four measurements can quickly be estimated: the perception thresholds for warmth, cold, cold pain, and heat pain. In patients with peripheral nerve lesions, the shifts in warmth- or cold-specific thresholds indicate dysfunction of unmyelinated or small myelinated fibers, respectively (Hansson et al., 1991). The functions of these fiber populations are difficult to test with other methods. Furthermore, the Marstock method is useful to assess and analyze various types of disturbed thermosensation, which are common in both peripheral and central nervous system lesions, such as paradoxical cold or warm sensation. It is important to note that the method permits documentation of equivalents of positive sensory phenomena, such as thermal hyperalgesia and thermal allodynia (painful response to non-noxious temperatures), regardless of whether warm and cold thresholds are normal (Fig. 16–9). The combination of sensory loss (hypoesthesia) and exaggerated painful or dysesthetic sensations illustrated in Figure 16–9 is often seen in painful neuropathic lesions and is called *hyperpathia* (see Lindblom, 1985; Merskey, 1986).

Mechanical Pinch or Pressure Algometer. In addition to the information about thermal pain thresh-

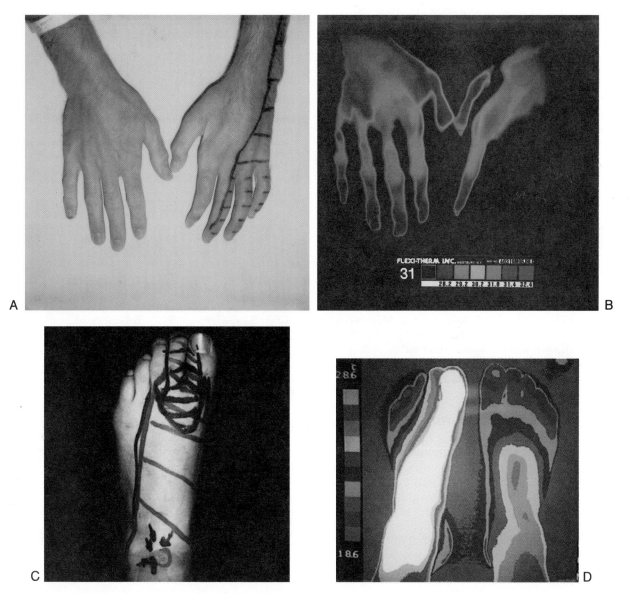

Figure 16–10. *(A* and *B)* Abnormal thermogram matching area of cutaneous sensory abnormality. In this case, the symptomatic patch of skin was hypoesthetic and relatively colder owing to *sympathetic denervation supersensitivity. (C* and *D)* After local anesthetic block of the left superficial and deep peroneal nerves at ankle level, striking warming developed in the anatomic skin nerve territories. The underlying paralytic vasodilatation caused by sympathetic efferent fiber block perfectly matched the area of cutaneous anesthesia *(hatched).*

olds that the thermal stimulator provides, information about mechanical pain threshold is useful. Estimates of mechanically evoked superficial or deep pain may be obtained using pinch pressure with a calibrated forceps or a blunt-ended pressure probe. Again, this allows documentation of not only hypoalgesia but also mechanical hyperphenomena (hyperalgesia and allodynia).

Thermography. As a complement to subjective changes in sensation volunteered by patients, useful visible documentation of matching abnormalities of skin temperature can be obtained via thermography (Color Fig. 16–10), which sensitively detects and precisely delineates deviations of skin temperature of neurogenic origin. Such abnormalities may reflect neurosecretory dysfunction, either altered sympathetic efferent function or antidromically determined release of neuropeptides from nociceptors. Four patterns can be recognized, two warm and two cold patterns, as follows (J. Ochoa, unpublished):

Paralytic vasodilatation caused by acute sympathetic vasoconstrictor deficit

Vasoconstriction from augmented somatosympathetic reflex activity

Vasogenic spasm after chronic vasoconstrictor denervation

Vasodilatation from antidromic nociceptor neurosecretion

Microneurography and Intraneural Microstimulation. Perhaps the most precise technique for dosage of afferent input is intraneural microstimulation (Torebjörk and Ochoa, 1980) combined with microneurography (see Vallbo et al., 1979). The combined approach allows the examiner to by-pass receptor adaptation, sensitization, and the various interactions arising from natural coactivation of receptors, while delivering any choice of patterned or monotonous impulse frequencies directly to the nerve fibers of identified kinds of afferent units. This method provides exquisite information about brain functions relating to decoding of sensory magnitude, quality, and localization of pure and specific sensory modalities. However, the method is invasive and time-consuming (Ochoa and Torebjörk, 1989; Torebjörk and Ochoa, 1990).

References

(Key references are designated with an asterisk.)

*Adrian E.D. The messages in sensory nerve fibres and their interpretation. *Proc. R. Soc.* B109:1–18, 1931.

Bender M.B., Stacy C., Cohen J. Agraphesthesia. *J. Neurol. Sci.* 53:531–555, 1982.

Berić A., Dimitrijević M.R., Lindblom U. Central dysesthesia syndrome in spinal cord injury patients. *Pain* 34:109–116, 1988.

Blumberg H., Jänig W. Neurophysiological analysis of efferent sympathetic and afferent fibers in skin nerves with experimentally produced neuromata. In Siegfried J., Zimmermann M., eds. *Phantom and Stump Pain*. Berlin, Springer-Verlag, pp. 15–31, 1981.

Borg K., Lindblom U. Increase of vibration threshold during wrist flexion in patients with carpal tunnel syndrome. *Pain* 26:211–219, 1986.

Buchthal F., Rosenfalck A. Sensory responses during recovery from local anaesthesia as related to sensory threshold. *Brain Res. (Special Issue)* 3:79–84, 1966.

Burgess P.R., Perl E.R. Cutaneous mechanoreceptors and nociceptors. In Iggo A., ed. *Handbook of Sensory Physiology*. Vol. 2. Berlin, Springer-Verlag, pp. 29–78, 1973.

Cline M., Ochoa J., Torebjörk H.-E. Chronic hyperalgesia and skin warming caused by sensitized C nociceptors. *Brain* 112:621–647, 1989.

Critchley M. *The Parietal Lobes*. London, Arnold, 1953.

Culp W., Ochoa J.L., Torebjörk H.E. Ectopic impulse generation in myelinated sensory nerve fibres in man. Phenomenology and attempts at biophysical interpretation. In Culp W., Ochoa J.L., eds. *Abnormal Nerves and Muscles as Impulse Generators*. New York, Oxford University Press, 1982.

Culp W.J., Ochoa J., Cline M., et al. Heat and mechanical hyperalgesia induced by capsaicin. Cross modality threshold modulation in human C nociceptors. *Brain* 112:1317–1331, 1989.

Darian-Smith T., Oke L. Peripheral neural representation of the spatial frequency of a grating moving at different velocities across the monkey's finger pad. *J. Physiol. (Lond.)* 309:117–133, 1980.

Desmedt J.E., ed. *Clinical Uses of Cerebral, Brainstem and Spinal Somatosensory Evoked Potentials. Progress in Clinical Neurophysiology*. Vol. 7. Basel, Karger, 1980.

Dyck P.J., Karnes J., O'Brien P.C., et al. Detection thresholds of cutaneous sensation in humans. In Dyck P.J., Thomas P.K., Lambert E.H., et al., eds. *Peripheral Neuropathy*. Vol.I. Philadelphia, Saunders, pp. 1103–1138, 1984.

Dykes R.W. Parallel processing of somatosensory information: a theory. *Brain Res. Rev.* 6:47–115, 1983.

Erlanger J., Gasser H.S. The compound nature of the action current of nerve as disclosed by the cathode ray oscilloscope. *Am.J. Physiol.* 70:624–666, 1924.

Erlanger J., Gasser H.S. The action potential in fibers of slow conduction in spinal roots and somatic nerves. *Am. J. Physiol.* 92:43–82, 1930.

Fechner G.T. *Elemente der Psychophysik*. Leipzig, 1860. Vol. 1 available in English translation as *Elements of Psychophysics*. New York, Rinehart and Winston, 1966.

*Fields H.L., Basbaum A.I. Anatomy and physiology of a descending pain control system. In Bonica J.J., Liebeskind J.C., Albe-Fessard D.G., eds. *Advances in Pain Research and Therapy*. New York, Raven Press, pp. 427–440, 1979.

Fruhstorfer H., Lindblom U. Sensibility abnormalities in neuralgic patients studied by thermal and tactile pulse stimulation. In von Euler C., Franzén O., Lindblom U., et al. *Somatosensory Mechanisms*. Wenner-Gren International Symposium Series. Vol. 41. London, Macmillan, pp. 353–361, 1984.

Fruhstorfer H., Lindblom U., Schmidt W.G. Method for quantitative estimation of thermal thresholds in patients. *J. Neurol. Neurosurg. Psychiatry* 39:1071–1075, 1976.

Gardner E.P. Cortical neuronal mechanisms underlying the perception of motion across the skin. In von Euler C., Franzén O., Lindblom U., et al., eds. *Somatosensory Mechanisms*. Wenner-Gren International Symposium Series. Vol. 41. London, Macmillan, pp. 93–112, 1984.

Gasser H.S. Conduction in nerves in relation to fiber types. *Proc. Assoc. Res. Nerv. Ment. Dis.* 15:35–59, 1934.

Gilliatt R.W. Sensory conduction studies in the early recognition of nerve disorders. *Muscle Nerve* 1:352, 1978.

Goldberg J.M., Lindblom U. Standardized method of determining vibratory perception thresholds for diagnosis and screening in neurological investigation. *J. Neurol. Neurosurg. Psychiatry* 42:793–803, 1979.

Guilbaud G. Peripheral and central electrophysiological mechanisms of joint and muscle pain. In Dubner R., Gebhart G.F., Bond M.R., eds. *Proceedings of the Vth World Congress on Pain*. Amsterdam, Elsevier, 201–215, 1988.

Guilbaud G., Lamour Y., Willer J.C. Organization of noxious and non-noxious inputs in SmI cortex: comparison in normal and in arthritic rats. In von Euler C., Franzén O., Lindblom U., et al., eds. *Somatosensory Mechanisms*. Wenner-Gren International Symposium Series. Vol. 41. London, Macmillan, pp. 81–92, 1984.

Halliday A.M. *Evoked Potentials in Clinical Testing. Clinical Neurology and Neurosurgery Monographs*. Vol. 3. Edinburgh, Churchill Livingstone, 1982.

Hansson P., Lindblom U., Lindström P. Graded assessment and classification of impaired temperature sensibility in patients with diabetic polyneuropathy. *J. Neurol. Neurosurg. Psychiatry* (in press).

*Holmes G. Sensation. In *Introduction to Clinical Neurology*. Edinburgh, E. and S. Livingstone, 1946.

Hyvärinen J. *The Parietal Cortex of Monkey and Man*. Berlin, Springer-Verlag, 1982.

*Iggo A., ed. *Handbook of Sensory Physiology*. Vol. II. *Somatosensory System*. Berlin, Springer-Verlag, 1973.

Johansson R., Vallbo A.B. Tactile sensibility in the human hand: relative and absolute densities of four types of mechanoreceptive units in glabrous skin. *J. Physiol. (Lond.)* 286:283–300, 1979.

Johnson K.O., Phillips J.R. Spatial and nonspatial neural mechanisms underlying tactile spatial discrimination. In von Euler C., Franzén O., Lindblom U., et al., eds. *Somatosensory Mechanisms*. Wenner-Gren International Symposium Series. Vol. 41. London, Macmillan, pp. 237–248, 1984.

Kaas J.H., Nelson R.J., Sur M., et al. Multiple representations of the body within the primary somatosensory cortex of primates. *Science* 204:521–523, 1979.

Knibestöl M., Vallbo A.B. Intensity of sensation related to activity of slowly adapting mechanoreceptive units in the human hand. *J. Physiol. (Lond.)* 300:251–267, 1980.

LaMotte R.H., Thalhammer J.G., Torebjörk H.E., Robinson C.J. Peripheral neural mechanisms of cutaneous hyperalgesia following mild injury by heat. *J. Neurosci.* 2:765–781, 1982.

Leijon G., Boivie J., Johansson I. Central post-stroke pain—neurological symptoms and pain characteristics. *Pain* 36:13–25, 1989.

Lenz F.A., Tasker R.R., Dostrovsky J.O., et al. Abnormal single-unit activity and responses to stimulation in the presumed ventrocaudal nucleus of patients with central pain. In Dubner R., Gebhart G.F., Bond M.R., eds. *Proceedings of the Vth World Congress on Pain*. Amsterdam, Elsevier, 157–164, 1988.

Levine J.D., Moskowitz M.A., Basbaum A.I. The contribution of neurogenic inflammation in experimental arthritis. *J. Immunol.* 135:843s–847s, 1985.

Lewis T., Pickering G.W., Rothschild P. Centripetal paralysis arising out of arrested blood flow to the limb, including notes on a form of tingling. *Heart* 16:1–32, 1931.

*Lindblom U. Assessment of abnormal evoked pain in neurological pain patients and its relation to spontaneous pain. A descriptive and conceptual model with some analytical results. In Fields H., Dubner R., Cervero F., eds. *Advances in Pain Research and Therapy*. Vol. 9. New York, Raven Press, pp. 409–423, 1985.

Lindblom U., Meyerson B.A. Influence on touch, vibration and cutaneous pain of dorsal column stimulation in man. *Pain* 1:257–270, 1975.

*Lindblom U., Tegnér R. Quantification of sensibility in mononeuropathy, polyneuropathy and central lesions. In Munsat T., ed. *Quantification of Neurological Deficit*. London, Butterworth, pp. 171–185, 1989.

Lindblom U., Verrillo R.T. Sensory functions in chronic neuralgia. *J. Neurol. Neurosurg. Psychiatry* 42:422–435, 1979.

Loesser J.D., Ward A.A., White L.E. Chronic deafferentation of human spinal cord neurons. *J. Neurosurg.* 29:48, 1968.

Loewenstein W.R. Mechano-electric transduction in the pacinian corpuscle. Initiation of sensory impulses in mechanoreceptors. In Loewenstein W.R., ed. *Handbook of Sensory Physiology*. Vol. 1. Principles of Receptor Physiology. Berlin, Springer-Verlag, pp. 269–290, 1971.

Lombard M.C., Nashold B.S. Jr., Pelissier T. Thalamic recordings in rats with hyperalgesia. In Bonica J.J., Liebeskind J.C., Albe-Fessard D.G., eds. *Advances in Pain Research and Therapy*. Vol. 3. New York, Raven Press, pp. 767–772, 1979.

Lombard M.C., Larabi Y., Albe-Fessard D. Electrophysiological study of cervical dorsal horn cells in partially deafferented rats. *Pain* 1(Suppl.):154, 1981.

Matthews W.B. Paroxysmal symptoms in multiple sclerosis. *J. Neurol. Neurosurg. Psychiatry* 38:617–623, 1975.

Merskey H. Pain terms. A current list with definitions and notes on usage. *Pain Suppl.* 3:215–221, 1986.

Moskowitz M.A., Henrickson B.M., Beyerl B.D. Trigeminovascular connections and mechanisms of vascular headache. In Vinken P.J., Bruyn G.W., Klawans H.L., eds. *Handbook of Clinical Neurology*. Vol. 48. Amsterdam, Elsevier, pp. 107–115, 1986.

Mountcastle V.B. Modality and topographic properties of single neurons of cat's somatic sensory cortex. *J. Neurophysiol.* 20:408–434, 1957.

Mountcastle V.B. The problem of sensing and the neural coding of sensory events. In Schmitt F.O., Quarton G., Melnechuk T., eds. *The Neurosciences: An Intensive Study Program*. New York, Rockefeller University Press, pp. 393–408, 1967.

*Mountcastle V.B. Neural mechanism in somesthesis. In Mountcastle V.B., ed. *Medical Physiology*. Vol. 1. 14th ed. St. Louis, Mosby, pp. 348–390, 1980.

Nashold B.S. Jr., Ostdahl R.H. Dorsal root entry zone lesions for pain relief. *J. Neurosurg.* 51:59–69, 1979.

Noordenbos W. *Pain*. Amsterdam, Elsevier, 1959.

Noordenbos W., Wall P.D. Diverse sensory functions with an almost totally divided spinal cord. A case of spinal cord transection with preservation of part of one anterolateral quadrant. *Pain* 2:185–195, 1976.

Noordenbos W., Wall P.D. Implications of the failure of nerve resection and graft to cure chronic pain produced by nerve lesions. *J. Neurol. Neurosurg. Psychiatry* 44:1068–1073, 1981.

Nordin M., Nyström B., Wallin V., et al. Ectopic sensory discharges and paresthesiae in patients with disorders of peripheral nerves, dorsal roots and dorsal columns. *Pain* 20:231–245, 1984.

Ochoa J. Pain in local nerve lesions. In Culp W.J., Ochoa J., eds. *Abnormal Nerves and Muscles as Impulse Generators*. New York, Oxford University Press, pp. 568–587, 1982.

Ochoa J. Peripheral unmyelinated units in man: structure, function, disorder, and role in sensation. In Kruger L., Liebeskind J.C., eds. *Advances in Pain Research and Therapy*. Vol. 6. New York, Raven Press, pp. 53–68, 1984.

Ochoa J., Mair W.G.P. The normal sural nerve in man. I. Ultrastructure and numbers of fibres and cells. *Acta Neuropathol.* 13:197–216, 1969.

Ochoa J., Noordenbos W. Pathology and disordered sensation in local nerve lesions: an attempt at correlation. In Bonica J.J., Liebeskind J.C., AlbeFessard D.G., eds. *Advances in Pain Research and Therapy*. Vol. 3. New York, Raven Press, pp. 67–90, 1979.

*Ochoa J., Torebjörk H.E. Paresthesiae from ectopic impulse generation in human sensory nerves. *Brain* 103:835–852, 1980.

*Ochoa J., Torebjörk H.E. Sensations evoked by intraneural microstimulation of single mechanoreceptor units innervating the human hand. *J. Physiol. (Lond.)* 342:633–654, 1983.

Ochoa J., Torebjörk E. Sensations evoked by intraneural microstimulation of identified C nociceptor fibres in human skin nerves. *J. Physiol. (Lond.)* 415:583–599, 1989.

Ochoa J., Torebjörk H.E., Culp W.J., et al. Abnormal spontaneous activity in single sensory nerve fibers in humans. *Muscle Nerve* 5:S74–S77, 1982.

Ochoa J., Torebjörk E., Culp W. Determinants of subjective attributes of normal cutaneous sensation and of paresthesiae from ectopic nerve impulse generation. In von Euler C., Franzén O., Lindblom U., et al., eds. *Somatosensory Mechanisms*. Wenner-Gren International Symposium Series. Vol. 41. London, Macmillan, pp. 379–387, 1984.

Ochoa J., Cline M., Dotson R., et al. Pain and paresthesias provoked mechanically in human cervical root entrapment (sign of Spurling). Single sensory unit antidromic recording of ectopic, bursting, propagated nerve impulse activity. In Pubols L.M., Sessle B.J., eds. *Effects of Injury on Trigeminal and Spinal Somatosensory Systems*. New York, Liss, pp. 389–397, 1987.

Rasminsky M. Ectopic generation of impulses and cross talk in spinal nerve roots of dystrophic mice. *Ann. Neurol.* 3:351–357, 1978.

Rasminsky M. Ephaptic transmission between single nerve fibres in the spinal nerve roots of dystrophic mice. *J. Physiol. (Lond.)* 305:151–169, 1980.

Roland P.E. Astereognosis. *Arch. Neurol.* 33:543–550, 1976.

Schady W., Torebjörk H.E., Ochoa J.L. Cerebral localization function from the input of single mechanoreceptive units in man. *Acta Physiol. Scand.* 119:277–285, 1983a.

Schady W., Torebjörk H.E., Ochoa J.L. Peripheral projections of nerve fibres in the human median nerve. *Brain Res.* 277:249–261, 1983b.

Seltzer Z., Devor M. Ephaptic transmission in chronically damaged peripheral nerves. *Neurology* 29:1061–1064, 1979.

Sinclair D.C. Cutaneous sensation and the doctrine of specific energy. *Brain* 78:584–614, 1955.

Sindou M., Quoex C., Baleydier C. Fiber organization at the posterior spinal cord-rootlet junction in man. *J. Comp. Neurol.* 153:15–26, 1974.

Smith K.J., McDonald W.I. Spontaneous and evoked electrical discharges from a central demyelinating lesion. *J. Neurol. Sci.* 55:39–47, 1982.

*Stevens S.S. On the psychophysical law. *Psychol. Rev.* 64:153–181, 1957.

Szolcsanyi J. A pharamacological approach to elucidation of the role of different nerve fibers and receptor endings in mediation of pain. *J. Physiol. (Paris)* 73:251–259, 1977.

Tegnér R., Borg J. The pathology of ligated nerves in relation to abnormal impulse generators. *Acta Physiol. Scand.* 133:589–590, 1988.

Torebjörk H.E., Hallin R.G. Perceptual changes accompanying controlled preferential blocking of A and C fibre responses in intact human skin nerves. *Exp. Brain Res.* 16:321–332, 1973.

Torebjörk H.E., Ochoa J. Specific sensations evoked by activity in single identified sensory units in man. *Acta Physiol. Scand.* 110:445–447, 1980.

Torebjörk H.E., Ochoa J.L. New method to identify nociceptor units innervating glabrous skin of the human hand. *Exp. Brain Res.* 81:509–514, 1990.

Torebjörk H.E., Ochoa J.L., McCann F.V. Paresthesiae: abnormal impulse generation in sensory nerve fibres in man. *Acta Physiol. Scand.* 105:518–520, 1979.

Towe A.L. Somatosensory cortex: descending influences on ascending systems. In Iggo A., ed. *Handbook of Sensory Physiology.* Vol. 2. *Somatosensory System.* Berlin, Springer-Verlag, pp. 701–718, 1973.

Tower S.S. Unit for sensory reception in cornea. *J. Neurophysiol.* 3:486–500, 1940.

Treede R.-D., Bromm B. Reliability and validity of ultra-late cerebral potentials in response to C-fibre activation in man. In Dubner R., Gebhart G.F., Bond M.R., eds. *Proceedings of the Vth World Congress on Pain.* Amsterdam, Elsevier, pp. 567–573, 1988.

Trevino D.L., Carstens E. Confirmation of the location of spinothalamic neurons in the cat and monkey by the retrograde transport of horseradish peroxidase. *Brain Res.* 98:177–182, 1975.

Vallbo A.B., Hagbarth K.E., Torebjörk H.E., et al. Somatosensory proprioceptive and sympathetic activity in human peripheral nerves. *Physiol. Rev.* 59:919–957, 1979.

*von Euler C., Franzén O., Lindblom U., et al., eds. *Somatosensory Mechanisms.* Wenner-Gren International Symposium Series. Vol. 41. London, Macmillan, 1984.

von Frey M. The distribution of afferent nerves in the skin. *J.A.M.A.* 47:645–648, 1906.

Wahrén L.K., Torebjörk E., Jørum E. Central suppression of cold-induced C fibre pain by myelinated fibre input. *Pain* 38:313–319, 1989.

Wall P.D., Gutnick M. Properties of afferent nerve impulses originating from a neuroma. *Nature* 248:740–743, 1974.

Weddell G. Somesthesis and the chemical senses. *Annu. Rev. Psychol.* 6:119–136, 1955.

Werner J., Whitsel L. Functional organization of the somatosensory cortex. In Iggo A., ed. *Handbook of Sensory Physiology.* Vol. 2. *Somatosensory System.* Berlin, Springer-Verlag, 1973.

Willis W.D. Jr. Electrophysiological evidence for a role of altered discharges of spinothalamic tract neurons in hyperalgesia. In Dimitrijević M.R., Wall P.D., Lindblom U., eds. *Recent Achievements in Restorative Neurology. 3. Altered Sensation and Pain.* Basel, Karger, 1990.

Yarnitsky D., Ochoa J.L. Release of cold-induced burning pain by block of cold-specific afferent input. *Brain* 113:893–902, 1990.

Zotterman Y. *Touch, Tickle and Pain. An Autobiography. Part Two.* Oxford, Pergamon Press, 1971.

Zotterman Y. Introduction. In Iggo A., ed. *Handbook of Sensory Physiology.* Vol. 2. *Somatosensory System.* Berlin, Springer-Verlag, 1973.

17

Pathophysiology of Neuronal and Axonal Degenerations

John W. Griffin
Paul N. Hoffman
Thomas O. Crawford

Slowly evolving degeneration of neurons underlies many of the heritable and sporadic disorders of the central nervous system, as well as most metabolic, heritable, and toxic neuropathies. In some disorders, such as Friedreich's ataxia and the axonal form of Charcot-Marie-Tooth disease, progressive *axonal* changes long precede perikaryal loss. In other disorders, including many cases of motor neuron disease, the clinical and pathologic features are dominated by subacutely evolving *perikaryal* degeneration, with the resulting loss of nerve fibers. This chapter reviews the pathophysiology of neuronal degenerations. It is useful to consider separately the major classes of axonal degeneration, including wallerian degeneration, abnormalities of caliber regulation, and distal axonal degeneration (dying-back) (Table 17–1). Primary involvement of the perikaryon is compared with the secondary changes that occur in response to axonal injury. Although these distinctions are conceptually helpful, the various classes of neuronal change are not mutually exclusive. The neuron is a single functional unit, and in many neuronal degenerations, elements of several of these changes can be found at various stages of the disease progression.

To introduce the topic of pathophysiology, the following discussion reviews the cellular organization of the perikaryon and the axon.

Perikaryal Organization

The neuron can properly be regarded as a highly differentiated secretory cell. Physicians are conditioned to think first of the relatively small amount of *external* secretion of neurotransmitters and modulators by neurons. In a few neurons, such as the neuroendocrine cells of the hypothalamus, external secretion represents a sizable metabolic commitment for the neuron. However, for most neurons, a process that might be termed *internal* secretion of proteins from the perikaryon into the axons and dendrites dwarfs the amount of external secretion in transmitter release. For example, the perikaryon of the large motor neuron probably secretes the equivalent of 25% of its volume into the axon daily, and a sizable volume must also enter the dendrites. These internally secreted proteins maintain and renew the cell processes.

Perikaryal structure reflects the synthetic requirements involved in maintenance of the cell processes (for review, see Price et al., 1984). Rather than metabolically inactive heterochromatin, dispersed euchromatin in which transcription occurs is the predominant form contained in the nucleus. The internal membrane system of the perikaryon is dominated by large blocks of granular endoplasmic reticulum. These blocks form the Nissl bodies, which are separated from each other by coiled channels composed mainly of cytoskeletal elements. The differences in staining between the Nissl bodies and the cytoskeletal channels produce the spotted or tigroid appearance with basophilic stains. The smooth membrane elements of the perikaryon and axon, synthesized in the granular endoplasmic reticulum, are processed through the Golgi apparatus where glycosylation occurs.

229

Table 17–1. CLASSIFICATION OF NEURONAL DEGENERATIONS

Class	Description	Examples	Pathophysiology
Axonal Degenerations			
Wallerian degeneration	Degeneration of distal stump of interrupted axons	Mechanical injury (transection or crush), vascular injury (tract degeneration after stroke)	Abrupt complete interruption of fast transport, degradation of axoplasm by calcium-activated proteases
Disorders of axonal caliber			
Axonal atrophy	Reduction in axonal caliber, loss of circularity and relatively thick myelin sheaths	Many chronic neuropathies (Charcot-Marie-Tooth disease, Friedreich's ataxia, uremia), stump of transected nerves, aging	*Reduction in amount* of neurofilament with transport or *maldistribution* of neurofilaments along the axon
Axonal swelling	Enlargment of the axon, with more nearly round fibers and relatively thin myelin sheaths	Neurofilamentous toxic neuropathies (2,5-hexanedione, carbon disulfide), amyotrophic lateral sclerosis, papilledema	Focal or multifocal accumulation of neurofilaments or other axonal organelles caused by impaired transport
Distal axonal degeneration	Wallerian-like loss of the distal regions of long fibers, with progression to involve more proximal regions	Most metabolic, toxic, and heritable neuropathies	Probably multiple mechanisms, including impairment in fast transport within the axon
Perikaryal Degenerations			
Primary			
Neuronal atrophy	Loss of perikaryal volume and subsequent death	Friedreich's ataxia and other heritable disorders	Unknown
Neurofibrillary	Accumulation of paired helical filaments and neurofilaments in the cell body (neurofibrillary tangles)	Alzheimer's disease, Pick's disease	Unknown
Secondary to axonal injury	Stereotyped morphologic and biochemical changes, including chromatolysis	Nerve injury; an element in the neuronal degeneration of spinal muscular atrophies and other degenerative disorders	Signal appears to be retrogradely transported

Axonal Organization

The cellular organization changes abruptly within the axon hillock. Three features distinguish the axon from the perikaryon. First, beyond the axon hillock, ribosomes and granular endoplasmic reticulum are absent. Instead, the internal membrane system of the axon is restricted to smooth membranes, including small vesicular structures and a racemose system of smooth membrane–bound cisternae and tubular structures. Second, several organelles contain different constituents or express different epitopes in the axon compared with the nerve cell body. For example, immunostaining has shown that the microtubule-associated protein MAP1 is abundant in the axon, whereas MAP2 predominates in the perikaryon and axon. Finally, compared with the coiled, complex cytoskeletal organization of the perikaryon, the axonal cytoskeleton is composed of highly organized parallel arrays of microtubules and neurofilaments, oriented in the long axis of the fiber (Fig. 17–1). The individual organelles are interconnected by numerous cross-linkers, or sidearms (Hirokawa, 1982). The only other organelles seen in normal axons include mitochondria and occasional prelysosomal profiles, including multivesicular bodies and dense bodies.

AXONAL TRANSPORT

Lacking ribosomes, the axon consequently lacks the capability for synthesis of proteins and other essential constituents. It instead utilizes continuous delivery of components synthesized within the perikaryon and delivered to it by specialized modes of intracellular motility, the axonal transport systems. Table 17–2 provides an overview of these transport systems.

The transport systems can be conveniently divided into two major classes. Slow transport carries cytoskeletal elements from the cell body down the axon at a rate ranging from 0.2 to 2 mm/day, varying with the species, the age of the animal, and the particular nerve (Hoffman et al., 1985; Lasek and Hoffman, 1976; Willard and Simon, 1981). There are no direct data for the rate of slow transport in humans, but in adult human nerve fibers, it is probable that the rate resembles that in other large mammals and approaches 1 mm/day. The major constituents of the slow phase of axonal transport are the cytoskeletal proteins of the axon. These proteins include tubulin, the protein subunit of microtubules, and the neurofilament proteins that form the neurofilament and contribute to its sidearms, or cross-linkers (Hirokawa,

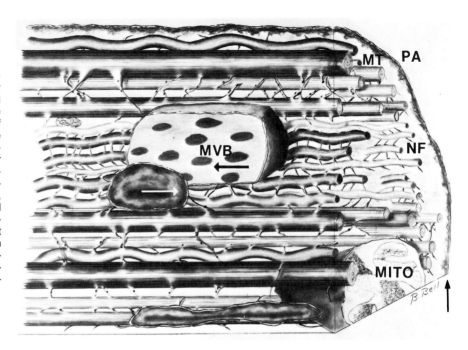

Figure 17–1. Schematic diagram of axoplasm. The axolemma is identified by the long arrows, and the periaxonal space, by PA. Note that most of the organelles in the axon are elements of the cytoskeleton. Microtubules (MT) are large and interconnected by long sidearms. Neurofilaments (NF) are smaller and less rigidly straight; they are interconnected by shorter, thicker cross-linkers. Note also the subaxolemmal fuzz, representing axonal spectrin (fodrin) and actin microfilaments. The vesicle identified by the white arrow is undergoing fast axonal transport and is interacting with microtubule sidearms. The adjacent multivesicular body (MVB) is undergoing retrograde transport. MITO = mitochondrion.

1982; Hoffman and Lasek, 1975; Willard and Simon, 1981). There is no direct evidence for retrograde transport of neurofilament proteins or tubulin in normal nerves, but in transected nerves with a retarded form of wallerian degeneration, neurofilaments accumulate in the most proximal segment of the distal stump (Glass and Griffin, 1991). This evidence suggests that cytoskeletal elements can undergo retrograde transport, at least in abnormal nerves.

In contrast, the fast transport system is clearly bidirectional, carrying membrane-bound vesicles both from the cell body down the axon (anterograde) and back toward the cell body (retrograde). The vesicles carried in an anterograde direction are predominantly 50–80 nm in diameter (Ellisman and

Table 17–2. AXONAL TRANSPORT SYSTEMS

Parameter	Fast Bidirectional		Intermediate (10–100 mm/day)	Slow	
	Anterograde (400 mm/day)	Retrograde (about 250 mm/day)		Component a (0.2–2 mm/day)	Component b (1–5 mm/day)
Constituents transported	50- to 80-nm vesicles with contents, including most transmission-related enzymes	Larger vesicles derived from endocytosis at nerve terminals	Mostly unknown; mitochondria	Cytoskeletal elements, including neurofilaments and tubulin	Glycolytic enzymes, actin
Mechanism of transport	Microtubule-based motility	Microtubule-based motility	Unknown	Unknown	Unknown
Distribution	Inserted into axolemma and synaptic terminal membrane	Returned to cell body	Unknown	Moves a continuous column of axoplasm	Uncertain
Means of turnover	Recycling and retrograde transport from terminal	Degradation in cell body	Unknown	Little breakdown en route; rapid proteolysis at nerve terminal	Unknown
Role	Renewal of synaptic terminal and axolemma; provision of large flux of membrane to allow for retrograde transport	Sampling of synaptic milieu	Unknown	Renewal of cytoskeleton; regulation of caliber	Provision of energy-related enzymes; rate limiting in regeneration

Lindsay, 1983), whereas those carried in a retrograde direction are larger and have features of prelysosomes (Tsukita and Ishikawa, 1980). These phases of transport should be regarded as part of a system of membrane recycling, occurring predominantly at the synaptic terminal. Fast transport renews axolemmal (Griffin et al., 1981; Tessler et al., 1980) and synaptic terminal membrane. Exocytosis, including transmitter release, is balanced by endocytosis. Some of the endocytotic vesicles, containing both endogenous neuronal smooth membrane and extracellular molecules taken up from the synaptic cleft, are transported back to the nerve cell body. Many of these retrogradely transported vesicles undergo degradation in the cell body, but some functionally important agents, such as nerve growth factor (NGF), are able to resist degradation and influence neuronal structure and biochemistry.

One axonal organelle, the neurofilament, requires special comment because of its importance in pathologic changes. The neurofilament is the neuronal form of a general class of 10-nm cytoskeletal intermediate filaments. In axons, neurofilaments are arranged in longitudinally oriented fascicles (Hirokawa, 1982). Each neurofilament is separated from its neighbor by about 45 nm and interconnected by innumerable sidearms, or cross-linkers. Each neurofilament is composed of three polypeptides, a 68-kd core; a 145-kd protein, which is wrapped in a helix around the core; and a 200-kd protein, which contributes to the cross-linkers (Lasek and Hoffman, 1976; Roots, 1983; Willard and Simon, 1981).

Mechanisms

The mechanisms of axonal transport are the subject of intensive research. In the case of slow transport, the mechanism remains uncertain. In addition, how much of the cytoskeleton is moving in an assembled form remains controversial. The structural hypothesis (Black and Lasek, 1980) held that the assembled cytoskeleton, including neurofilaments and microtubules, moved as a coherent structure. However, increasing evidence (Hirokawa et al., 1990; Hollenbeck, 1989, 1990; Nixon and Logvinenko, 1986; Watson et al., 1989) suggests that a large fraction of the assembled cytoskeleton may be stationary or moving slowly and that the stationary elements may be renewed by exchanges with the constituents of slow transport—either soluble subunits (particularly in the case of microtubules) or small bundles of neurofilaments.

In the case of the fast transport system, the underlying mechanisms are better delineated. Fast bidirectional transport is a microtubule-based system. This has been dramatically demonstrated by video microscopy of particle movement on single, isolated microtubules separated from extruded axoplasm (Schnapp et al., 1985; Vale et al., 1985). The force generation by microtubules requires ATP. Fast an-

terograde transport utilizes a specific protein, kinesin, that interacts with the microtubules to provide force and define the direction of movement. A different protein, brain dynein, is responsible for retrograde transport. Continued advances in the understanding of the mechanisms of transport are essential to further defining the pathophysiology of a variety of neuropathologic disorders.

Axonal Transport in Neuronal Disease

The axonal transport systems play at least three distinct roles in the pathophysiology of neuronal disease, as summarized in Table 17–3. First, the retrograde transport system may provide a route of entry for toxic and biologic agents—in effect, a "back door" to the central nervous system, which circumvents the blood-brain barrier. Many agents are known to bind to specific receptors in peripheral nerve terminals with high affinity, allowing their internalization. Such substances can be likened to saboteurs that outwit security systems by presenting acceptable identification to obtain access. For example, tetanus toxin, the neurotoxic protein produced in contaminated wounds by *Clostridium tetani*, binds to presynaptic motor nerve endings in neuromuscular junctions by interaction with its receptor, the ganglioside GD_{1b}. Such binding occurs both with locally produced toxin (Price et al., 1975; Schwab et al., 1979) and with hematogenously spread toxin (Price and Griffin, 1977), which reaches the synaptic cleft from the bloodstream. After internalization, the bound toxin is carried via retrograde transport at peak rates of about 250 mm/day to the nerve cell body. Although transport takes place in vesicles that form part of the neuronal lysosomal system, the toxin escapes degradation and passes trans-synaptically to the inhibitory presynaptic terminals that surround the neuronal perikaryon and proximal dendrites (Schwab et al., 1979). By preventing the release

Table 17–3. ROLES OF AXONAL TRANSPORT IN NEURONAL DISEASE

Role	Examples
Access to neuronal perikaryon via retrograde transport	Tetanus toxin; poliomyelitis and rabies viruses; doxorubicin (Adriamycin), ricin, and other agents of "suicide" transport
Delivery of axoplasm that is abnormal because of altered synthesis or gating in the perikaryon	Axonal atrophy and dying-back after axotomy; axonal degeneration after synthetic inhibition with doxorubicin
Abnormal delivery or removal of axoplasm because of primary changes in axonal transport	*Slow transport:* many disorders of axonal caliber; many types of neurofibrillary change *Fast transport:* many dying-back disorders

of inhibitory neurotransmitters from these sites, the toxin promotes unregulated firing of motor neurons and thereby produces the characteristic clinical manifestations of painful spasms of agonist and antagonist muscles. In fact, the early involvement of bulbar muscles (trismus, risus sardonicus) and axial muscles (opisthotonos) may reflect the short length of the relevant motor nerves, and hence the initial involvement of these neurons.

The second role of the transport systems in pathophysiology is as a passive carrier of abnormal or deficient axonal constituents, resulting from alterations in perikaryal synthesis or delivery to the axon. Examples of altered delivery (see Table 17–3) are discussed later.

Finally, it is likely that abnormalities of the transport systems themselves constitute the most common pathogenetically important role of the axonal transport systems in neuronal disorders. Within the past 10 years, a substantial literature has developed, as summarized in relation to specific pathologic changes later. By way of introduction, abnormalities of *slow* transport underlie or contribute to neurofilamentous changes and to several disorders of axonal caliber. In some models, the changes involve all of the constituents of slow transport; in others, the changes are confined to neurofilaments. In contrast, distal axonal degeneration is most closely associated with abnormalities in *fast* axonal transport within distal axons.

Any consideration of the pathophysiology of the axon requires recognition of the wide spectrum of axonal sizes, including calibers, lengths, and total volumes. Table 17–4 compares the length, caliber, and volume of the axons of representative small cortical interneurons and of large motor neurons in the sciatic nerve. The large motor axon is 10^4 greater than the interneuron in both axonal length and cross-sectional area; the axoplasmic volume is 10^8 greater. In addition, the relationship between perikaryal volume and axonal volume is strikingly different in the two neurons. In the interneuron, the axon has only 1% of the volume of the perikaryon, whereas in the motor neuron, the axonal volume exceeds the perikaryal volume by more than 1000-fold.

These different quantitative relationships are undoubtedly a factor in the different vulnerabilities of axons to disease processes. Axonal *length* is a key factor in vulnerability to the dying-back process of axons, whereas axonal *caliber* influences vulnerability in the neurofilamentous disorders and in axonal swelling and atrophy.

AXONAL DEGENERATION

Wallerian Degeneration

Wallerian degeneration is the prompt axonal breakdown that follows interruption of the axon. In the peripheral nervous system, wallerian degeneration normally follows a rapid time course. In humans, transection of a nerve results in electrical failure of the distal stump within 3–5 days. In most laboratory rodents, the distal stump fails within 6–20 hours and axoplasm is reduced to granular debris within 24–48 hours. The myelin sheath segments into ovoids of myelin that are gradually removed during the subsequent 2–3 weeks. In the central nervous system, the sequence is similar, although the timing is much slower. These basic cellular events were defined in the classic studies of Ramon y Cajal (1928). After the delineation of the axonal transport systems in the 1970s, wallerian degeneration came to be thought of as the simple consequence of interruption in continuous transport needed to maintain the axon. With the consequent breakdown of the axon, Schwann cells or glia were thought to dedifferentiate into phagocytes and remove myelin. In the past 5 years, wallerian degeneration has come to be appreciated as wonderfully rich and complex, with critical roles played by exogenous macrophages. Some classic morphologic studies (Ramon y Cajal, 1928) identified macrophages in degenerating nerves and central nervous system pathways, but the abundance and the early time of appearance were later revealed by immunocytochemical staining (Stoll et al., 1990). It is now clear that removal of myelin debris is profoundly retarded if macrophage recruitment and entry into nerve are prevented (Beuche and Friede, 1984, 1986; Lunn et al., 1989). As noted in Chapter 8, macrophage-derived factors are also required for initiation of a number of Schwann cell behaviors that characterize wallerian degeneration and subsequent axonal regeneration.

Distal Axonal Degeneration (Dying-Back)

The process of dying-back, as described by Cavanagh (1964), entails initial degeneration of the distal portions of the longest nerve fibers, with progression of the lesion to successively more proximal segments with time. In some models, caliber is a factor in vulnerability (Spencer and Schaumburg, 1976, 1977),

Table 17–4. AXONAL LENGTH, CALIBER, AND VOLUME COMPARISON

Cell Type	Perikaryal Diameter (μm)	Axonal Diameter (μm)	Axonal Length (μm)	Perikaryal Surface Area (μm²)	Axonal Surface Area (μm²)	Perikaryal Volume (μm²)	Axonal Volume (μm³)
Lumbar motor neuron	50	15	1.5×10^6	1.2×10^3	7×10^7	6.44×10^5	2.7×10^8
Interneuron	10	0.1	100	0.01	30	61	0.8

but dying-back is usually regarded as *length-dependent vulnerability*. Length-dependent vulnerability underlies the initial involvement of the feet and ankles and the loss of the ankle reflex in many axonal neuropathies. Schaumburg et al. (1974) demonstrated that the sequence of distal axonal degeneration often involves formation of foci of organelle accumulations within the distal axon, followed by wallerian-like degeneration distal to that site. The degenerative process thus proceeds in a stepwise fashion back toward the nerve cell body.

The pathophysiology of distal axonal degeneration is not fully understood in any condition. As with abnormalities in axonal caliber, potential deficits in maintenance of the distal axon could result from synthetic failure in the nerve cell body or from alterations in axonal transport. Early pathologic changes in the nerve cell body were noted in the experimental model of distal axonal degeneration produced by acrylamide exposure (Sterman, 1983), but specific perikaryal metabolic changes have not been convincingly demonstrated. In contrast, abnormalities of axonal transport have been found in acrylamide neuropathy and many other models. Both fast and slow axonal transport have been shown to be altered, but the most relevant changes probably are those of fast, ATP-dependent, microtubule-based transport. Several lines of evidence indicate that both anterograde and retrograde forms of fast axonal transport are disturbed in models of distal axonal degeneration, with more severe changes in the distal axon. In many models, the rate of fast axonal transport is maintained through much of the proximal region of the axon but is reduced within the distal axon (Jakobsen and Brimijoin, 1981; Sahenk and Mendell, 1981; Watson and Griffin, 1987). This reduction can be associated with multifocal accumulations of small particulate organelles, reflecting multifocal breakdown in organelle movement. The method by which fast transport is impaired undoubtedly varies in different disorders.

Disorders of Axonal Caliber

Alterations in axonal caliber, including axonal atrophy and axonal swelling, are probably the most common pathologic changes in neuronal disease. Axonal *atrophy* has been documented in a wide variety of peripheral nerve disorders, including both the axonal and demyelinating forms of Charcot-Marie-Tooth disease, uremic neuropathy, diabetic neuropathy, and a variety of toxic neuropathies (for review, see Dyck et al., 1984). In addition, atrophy appears to be a part of the aging process in both the peripheral and central nervous systems (Krinke et al., 1981). Focal or multifocal axonal *swellings* occur in amyotrophic lateral sclerosis (Carpenter, 1968; Delisle and Carpenter, 1984), in the neuritic plaques of Alzheimer's disease, and in certain heritable (Asbury et al., 1972) and toxic neuropathies, including

the glue-sniffing neuropathies (Korobkin et al., 1975; Spencer and Schaumburg, 1977). In many of these disorders, the axonal swellings are associated with distal axonal degeneration (dying-back), but changes in caliber may occur independently of axonal breakdown.

Changes in axonal caliber often reflect alterations in axonal neurofilament content. In normal axons, neurofilament content is closely correlated with axonal caliber, and the changes in disease can often be viewed as a failure of the normal mechanisms of neurofilament transport. In normal large axons, the cross-sectional axonal area is linearly related to neurofilament number (Hoffman et al., 1984); the only other organelle that occupies significant amounts of space is the microtubule (Hoffman et al., 1984). In small axons, microtubules are proportionately more numerous and thus play a role in determining axonal caliber, but in large fibers, neurofilaments outnumber microtubules by as much as 10- to 20-fold (Hoffman et al., 1984). It is now clear that spacing between neurofilaments is not fixed but can be altered in disease (Monteiro et al., 1990; Parhad et al., 1987). With these cautions in mind, a strong correlation remains between axonal caliber and neurofilament number.

Mechanisms

At least two mechanisms can produce altered neurofilament content in a given region of the axon: altered *amounts* of neurofilament undergoing transport and altered *kinetics* of neurofilament transport. The first mechanism entails *alteration in the quantity of neurofilaments delivered to the axon from the nerve cell body*, either by changes in neurofilament synthesis or by changes in gating into the axon. The best-studied mechanism of altering neurofilament delivery is by axotomy. In addition to structural changes in the neuronal perikaryon (described later), there is a decrease in the axonal caliber of the remaining proximal stump (Dyck et al., 1981; Hoffman et al., 1984) (Fig. 17–2). Throughout the evolution of this axonal atrophy, neurofilament density in the proximal stump remains normal. Hoffman et al. (1984) showed that, in transected rat sciatic nerves, the decrease in axonal caliber begins within 4 days after axotomy and is initially restricted to the most proximal region of the remaining proximal axonal stump. The atrophic segment subsequently spreads distally down the nerve at a rate of about 1.7 mm daily, closely corresponding to the rate of slow axonal transport in these animals (Fig. 17–3). This spatial and temporal sequence is of proximal-to-distal spread of axonal atrophy. This pattern correlates well with the observation that axotomy produces a prompt and selective reduction in the amount of neurofilament protein undergoing transport in the axon (Hoffman et al., 1985). Content of mRNA for the neurofilament proteins is markedly reduced (Hoffman et al., 1987), as is the relative labeling of newly synthesized neu-

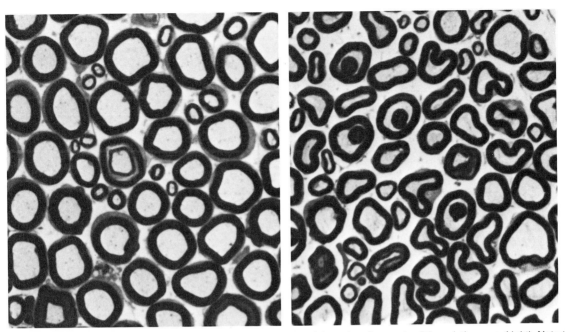

Figure 17–2. Comparison of the lumbar ventral roots in normal rats *(left)* and 2 weeks after crush of the sciatic nerve *(right)*. Note that after axotomy the axons undergo a reduction in caliber, reflecting a reduced amount of neurofilaments within slow transport. (From Hoffman P.N., Griffin J.W., Price D.L. Control of axonal caliber by neurofilament transport. Reproduced from the *Journal of Cell Biology*, 1984, vol. 99, pp. 705–714 by copyright permission of the Rockefeller University Press.)

rofilament proteins by radioactive amino acids. At the same time, mRNA content and the relative labeling of tubulin, actin, and a variety of other slow-component constituents are increased. Thus, the axonal atrophy after axotomy reflects a selective reduction in delivery to the axon of neurofilaments caused by a decrease in synthesis. Recovery of axonal caliber begins at times when functional reinnervation of muscle is occurring; if successful regeneration is blocked, caliber is not restored (Hoffman et al., 1984).

Studies using a variety of axonal neurotoxins have demonstrated that a similar type of axonal atrophy is a common and easily elicited change in peripheral nerve disease. For example, short-term administration of daily doses of acrylamide, an agent that induces distal axonal degeneration, produces proximal axonal atrophy (Gold et al., 1985). The means by which axonal disease results in altered perikaryal neurofilament synthesis is uncertain, but frank wallerian-like degeneration does not appear to be required.

The second mechanism of producing axonal atrophy is by inducing a *maldistribution of neurofilaments along the axon as a result of altered neurofilament transport*. The classic study of Weiss and Hiscoe (1948), the first direct demonstration of axonal transport, was based on mechanical obstruction of the proximal-to-distal movement of axoplasm. A gentle focal compression of nerve resulted in swelling of the axon proximal to the lesion and atrophy distally. Subsequent electron microscopic studies have shown that redundant neurofilaments accumulate proximal to the constriction, whereas the distal stump becomes relatively neurofilament poor, without changing neurofilament density (Friede, 1971). The precise dynam-

ics of this lesion remain incompletely understood: Baba et al. (1983) showed that vigorous nerve constrictions produce rapid atrophy all along the length of the distal stump. This pattern is difficult to explain solely by failure of renewal of axoplasm within the slow component and suggests that axoplasmic degradation is stimulated throughout the distal stump.

Distal axonal atrophy can also be produced by alterations in neurofilament transport. 3,3'-Iminodipropionitrile (IDPN) selectively impairs transport of the neurofilament proteins. Systemic intoxication (or administration) produces a paralysis of neurofilament migration all along large axons (Griffin et al., 1978, 1984). Neurofilament synthesis continues, so that newly synthesized neurofilaments are delivered to axons incapable of transporting them more distally. The result is a marked enlargement of the proximal axon, followed by gradual atrophy of the axon more distally, at least in part as a result of the failure to renew neurofilaments within the axoplasm (Clark et al., 1980). This combination of proximal axonal swelling and distal atrophy can be maintained for long periods by continuous administration of the toxin. However, when administration of the toxin is discontinued, the proximal swellings begin to migrate down the axon at rates up to 1 mm/day (Griffin et al., 1987) (Fig. 17–4). Susceptibility to these pathologic changes is a function of the (preintoxication) fiber caliber and thus of neurofilament content (Griffin et al., 1983c). Similar pathologic changes occur in some cases of motor neuron disease (Carpenter, 1968; Delisle and Carpenter, 1984) and in an animal model of motor neuron disease, hereditary canine spinal muscular atrophy. In this model, slow transport is retarded (Cork et al., 1982).

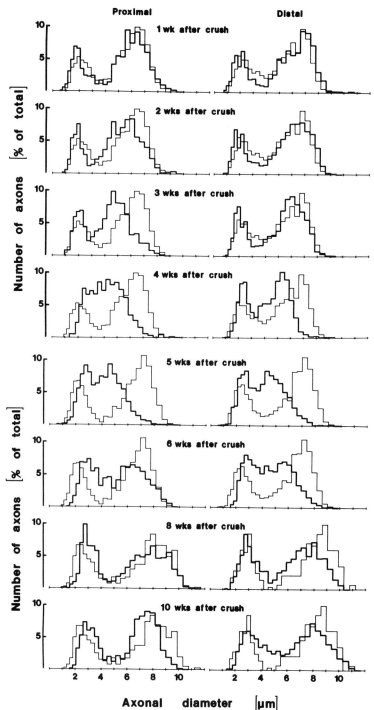

Figure 17–3. Spatial and temporal sequence of changes in the L-5 ventral roots of rats after sciatic nerve crush. The histograms of fiber diameters demonstrate the expected bimodal distributions; at each time after axotomy, the histograms on the left are from the proximal segment of the root, and those to the right, the distal. The thicker line represents histograms from the axotomized nerves, and the thinner line, from age-matched control animals. Note that atrophy begins first in the proximal segment, and appears later distally. Atrophy progresses centrifugally down these roots at a rate of 1.7 mm/day, reflecting the slow transport of axoplasm with reduced neurofilament content. The reduced neurofilament content is in turn due to reduced neurofilament synthesis in the perikaryon after axotomy. The return toward normal calibers, beginning at 6 weeks, is associated with reinnervation of the leg muscles. (From Hoffman P.N., Griffin J.W., Price D.L. Control of axonal caliber by neurofilament transport. Reproduced from the *Journal of Cell Biology*, 1984, vol. 99, pp. 705–714 by copyright permission of the Rockefeller University Press.)

A group of other chemical neurotoxins also produce neurofilamentous axonal swellings, but in general, these swellings begin in distal regions of the axon. Examples include 2,5-hexanedione (2,5-HD), the toxic metabolite involved in glue-sniffing neuropathy, and carbon disulfide intoxication. The effect of 2,5-HD intoxication is to speed the axonal transport of neurofilament proteins (Monaco et al., 1984); in this model, there is no change in synthesis of neurofilaments in the neuronal perikaryon (Watson et al., 1991). The distal accumulations of neurofilaments appear to reflect the accelerated transport down the axon. The biochemical mechanism by which IDPN and 2,5-HD alter neurofilament distribution is not known. Similar axonal pathologic change was found during slow wallerian degeneration in a heritable mouse model (J. Glass and J. W. Griffin, unpublished), suggesting that direct binding of the toxins to cytoskeletal elements need not be required. IDPN (Griffin et al., 1983a,c; Papasozomenos et al., 1982)

P   M   D

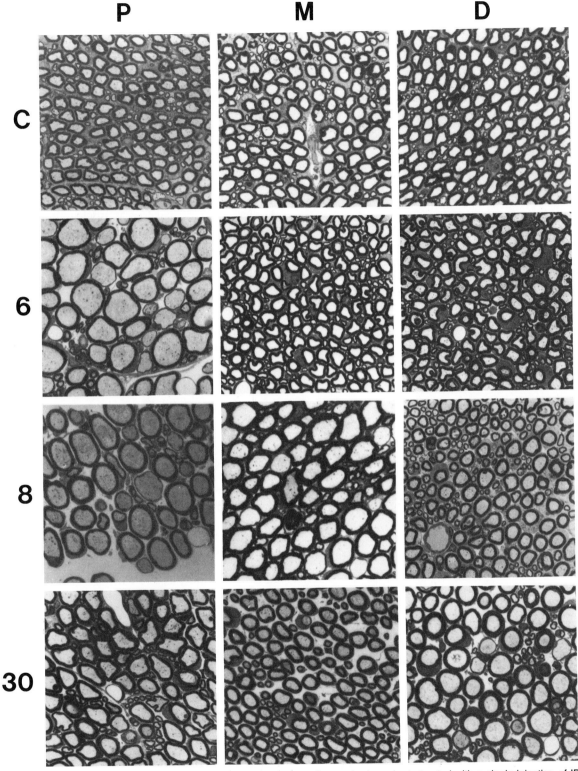

Figure 17–4. Light micrographs of cross-sections of the L-5 ventral root of normal rats and rats treated with a single injection of IDPN, an agent that selectively halts the normal slow transport of neurofilaments. For each root, the most proximal 3-mm segment (P) is to the left; the middle region (M) is in the center; and the distalmost segment (D) is to the right. C is a control animal; 6 = 6 days after IDPN administration; 8 = 8 days; 30 = 30 days. Note that, by 6 days, axonal swellings are present at the most proximal region of the ventral root in the IDPN-treated animals but are not in the middle or distal region. By 8 days, small swellings are beginning to appear at the middle region of the ventral root. By 30 days, swellings are most prominent in the distal region of the ventral root, and more proximal regions have undergone reduction in caliber. This sequence reflects the initial accumulation of neurofilaments in the most proximal portion of the ventral roots, owing to continued synthesis in the nerve cell body and delivery to axons whose neurofilament transport is blocked, followed by reversal of the block with time.

and 2,5-HD (Griffin et al., 1983b) have the ability to produce segregation of neurofilaments from microtubules within the axons; this may represent a structural basis for impaired neurofilament transport.

In summary, a variety of mechanisms, involving both altered neurofilament synthesis and altered neurofilament transport, can be invoked to explain alterations in axonal caliber. It is likely that the most common mechanism in human neurologic disease is the reduction of neurofilament synthesis leading to axonal atrophy. This hypothesis is consistent with the morphometric data in such diverse disorders as Charcot-Marie-Tooth disease type I, Friedreich's ataxia, and uremic neuropathy. In particular, in Charcot-Marie-Tooth disease, neurofilament density remains normal within the distal axons, but there is a marked reduction in neurofilament numbers (Nukada and Dyck, 1984). Because neurofilamentous axonal swellings are rarely seen in these disorders, it is likely that this reflects reduced neurofilament synthesis and delivery. This appears to be a part of generalized neuronal atrophy with reduction in perikaryal volume and distal axon degeneration. Because the relative vulnerability of axons to these processes depends on their original caliber (neurofilament content), it is appropriately termed *caliber-dependent vulnerability*.

Secondary Demyelination

Axonal caliber normally influences the amount of myelin formed in a given nerve fiber. Alterations in axonal caliber are eventually associated with demyelination. The seminal studies of Dyck and co-workers (1984) showed that, during sustained axonal atrophy, there is a sequence of loss of circularity of nerve fibers followed by paranodal demyelination and then segmental demyelination, with subsequent remyelination characterized by formation of multiple, shorter internodes. This sequence has been produced experimentally in the chronic axonal atrophy induced by permanent axotomy (Dyck et al., 1981), in atrophy distal to mechanical constriction of the nerve (Baba et al., 1983), and in the atrophic distal axon of IDPN-intoxicated animals. Morphometric data suggesting secondary demyelination have been found in Charcot-Marie-Tooth disease type I, uremic neuropathy, Friedreich's ataxia, and a variety of other disorders (Dyck et al., 1984). In some of these disorders, the repeated demyelination with onion bulb formation may come to dominate the pathologic changes. In the proximal regions of animals persistently exposed to IDPN, repeated demyelination and remyelination with formation of elaborate supernumerary Schwann cells (onion bulbs) have been demonstrated (Griffin and Price, 1981; Shimono et al., 1978). In such material, inspection of only one region at one point in time could produce the misleading impression of a primary demyelinating disorder.

PERIKARYAL DEGENERATIONS

Slowly evolving perikaryal degeneration and loss are the outstanding findings in a variety of neurodegenerative disorders; in none is the basis well understood. In most disorders, the perikaryon undergoes nonspecific changes. In some settings, such as Alzheimer's, Pick's, and Parkinson's diseases, the perikaryon undergoes cytoskeletal alterations, which are visible as a distinctive inclusion—neurofibrillary tangles in Alzheimer's disease, Pick bodies in Pick's disease, and Lewy bodies in Parkinson's disease.

The relationship of these alterations to the pathogenesis of neuronal loss is unclear in each case. In all these settings, an immunohistochemical finding is the staining of these inclusions with antibodies against ubiquitin (Leigh et al., 1989). In some cases (e.g., amyotrophic lateral sclerosis [Lowe et al., 1988]), immunohistochemical identification of ubiquitin provides an early marker of neuronal pathologic change. Ubiquitin is a low-molecular-weight protein that is implicated in the nonlysosomal breakdown of cellular proteins. Free exposure of a protein's NH_2 terminus, to which ubiquitin binds selectively, appears to commit the protein to degradation. Longer-lived proteins have the NH_2 terminus protected by $N\alpha$-acetylation or by tertiary folding of the end to the inside of a globular region (Hershko et al., 1984). That the distinctive perikaryal inclusions of the above and other diseases are labeled immunohistochemically with antibodies to ubiquitin suggests that these inclusions represent accumulation of cellular proteins that are resistant to proteolysis via the ubiquitin pathway.

One of the most important perikaryal reactions is accompanied by the histologic features of *chromatolysis*. This term has been applied to the changes seen in response to a wide variety of acute injuries but is best understood as the expression of the perikaryal response to axonal injury. In this setting, it may be more specifically termed the *axonal reaction* and may include all or any portion of the following morphologic features: perikaryal swelling and rounding; dispersion of granular endoplasmic reticulum (Nissl bodies) and formation of polyribosomes; displacement and deformation of the nucleus to a flattened position opposite the axon, with a concave face toward the inner aspect of the cell; and swelling or division of the nucleolus (Price and Porter, 1972). Associated with these perikaryal changes is a detachment of afferent synapses, proliferation of adjacent microglia, and swelling of neighboring astrocytes. There are physiologic changes in neuronal excitability. Among the numerous biochemical correlates of the axonal reaction are an increase in RNA synthesis. Specific mRNAs for tubulin, actin, and the growth-associated protein GAP-43 increase, whereas the synthesis and transport of neurofilament protein and transmission-related constituents, including transmitter-synthesizing enzymes, decrease.

Overall, the histologic changes of chromatolysis can be seen as a reordering of perikaryal synthetic priorities toward repair and regeneration. However, these morphologic features should not be considered synonymous with axonal repair. In some models, axonal regeneration can occur without histologic change in the perikarya. In other settings (e.g., in many central nervous system neurons and in motor neurons after ventral root evulsion), chromatolysis is marked and precedes neuronal degeneration. It is more accurate to consider chromatolysis the morphologic correlate of an injury response, during which axonal regeneration may be successful, unsuccessful, or aborted.

Attention has focused on the biologic features of normal neuronal death that appears to be invoked selectively during development. In early development, many regions have a surfeit of neurons in comparison with later times; the decrease in number is apparently well regulated and is normally confined to a brief duration. This natural cell death in the developing nervous system usually occurs just after axonal outgrowth to the target and thus provides a mechanism for the matching of target size with the innervating neuronal pool. It is generally thought that neurons may compete for some factor that is in limited supply within the target. This survival factor may be mediated either by physical contact with a restricted site on the target or by a diffusible substance.

The best-studied example of soluble trophic factor activity is the NGF dependency of certain neuronal populations. Cultured embryonic sympathetic neurons are dependent on low-concentration exposure to NGF for continued survival and growth. Removal of NGF from the media with anti-NGF antibodies leads to prompt neuronal degeneration. Interestingly, this degeneration can be prevented by inhibiting protein or RNA synthesis with specific inhibitors (Martin et al., 1988). This suggests that there is an endogenous "suicide" program within neurons that require active synthesis. Because NGF may be only one of many molecular trophic substances, the possibility exists that pathologic conditions characterized by selective neuronal degeneration may stem from abnormalities in specific trophic mechanisms.

References

Asbury A.K., Gale M.K., Cox S.C., et al. Giant axonal neuropathy: a unique case with segmental neurofilamentous masses. *Acta Neuropathol.* 20:237–247, 1972.

Baba M., Gilliatt R.W., Jacobs J.M. Recovery of distal changes after nerve constriction by a ligature. *J. Neurol. Sci.* 60:235–246, 1983.

Beuche W., Friede R.L. The role of non-resident cells in wallerian degeneration. *J. Neurocytol.* 13:767–796, 1984.

Beuche W., Friede R.L. Myelin phagocytosis in wallerian degeneration depends on silica-sensitive, bg/bg-negative and Fc-positive monocytes. *Brain Res.* 378:97–106, 1986.

Black M.M., Lasek R.J. Slow components of axonal transport: two cytoskeletal networks. *J. Cell Biol.* 86:616–623, 1980.

Carpenter S. Proximal axonal enlargement in motor neuron disease. *Neurology* 18:841–851, 1968.

Cavanagh J.B. The significance of the "dying back" process in human and experimental neurological diseases. *Int. Rev. Exp. Pathol.* 3:219–267, 1964.

Clark A.W., Griffin J.W., Price D.L. The axonal pathology in chronic IDPN intoxication. *J. Neuropathol. Exp. Neurol.* 39:42–55, 1980.

Cork L.C., Griffin J.W., Choy C., et al. Pathology of motor neurons in accelerated hereditary canine spinal muscular atrophy. *Lab. Invest.* 46:89–99, 1982.

Delisle M.B., Carpenter S. Neurofibrillary axonal swellings and amyotrophic lateral sclerosis. *J. Neurol. Sci.* 63:241–250, 1984.

Dyck P.J., Lais A.C., Karnes J.L., et al. Permanent axotomy, a model of axonal atrophy and secondary segmental demyelination and remyelination. *Ann. Neurol.* 6:575–583, 1981.

Dyck P.J., Nukada H., Lais A.C., et al. Permanent axotomy: a model of chronic neuronal and axonal atrophy, myelin remodeling and axonal degeneration. In Dyck P.J., Thomas P.K., Lambert E.H., et al., eds. *Peripheral Neuropathy.* 2nd ed. Philadelphia, Saunders, pp. 666–690, 1984.

Ellisman M.H., Lindsay J.D. The axoplasmic reticulum within myelinated axons is not transported rapidly. *J. Neurocytol.* 12:393–411, 1983.

Friede R.L. Changes in microtubules and neurofilaments in constricted, hypoplastic nerve fibers. *Acta Neuropathol.* 5(Suppl.):216–225, 1971.

Glass J., Griffin J.W. Neurofilament redistribution in transected nerves: evidence for bidirectional transport of neurofilaments. *J. Neurosci.* (in press).

Gold B.G., Griffin J.W., Price D.L. Slow axonal transport in acrylamide neuropathy: different abnormalities produced by single dose and continuous administration. *J. Neurosci.* 5:1755–1768, 1985.

Griffin J.W., Price D.L. Demyelination in experimental IDPN and hexacarbon neuropathies: evidence for an axonal influence. *Lab. Invest.* 45:130–141, 1981.

Griffin J.W., Hoffman P.N., Clark A.W., et al. Slow axonal transport of neurofilament proteins: impairment by β,β′-iminodipropionitrile administration. *Science* 202:633–635, 1978.

Griffin J.W., Price D.L., Drachman D.B., et al. Incorporation of axonally transported glycoproteins into axolemma during nerve regeneration. *J. Cell Biol.* 88:205–214, 1981.

Griffin J.W., Fahnestock K.E., Price D.L., et al. Cytoskeletal disorganization induced by local application of β,β′-iminodipropionitrile and 2,5-hexanedione. *Ann. Neurol.* 14:55–61, 1983a.

Griffin J.W., Fahnestock K.E., Price D.L., et al. Microtubule-neurofilament segregation produced by β,β′-iminodipropionitrile: evidence for association of fast axonal transport with microtubules. *J. Neurosci.* 3:557–566, 1983b.

Griffin J.W., Price D.L., Hoffman P.N. Neurotoxic probes of the axonal cytoskeleton. *Trends Neurosci.* 6:490–495, 1983c.

Griffin J.W., Anthony D.C., Fahnestock K.E., et al. 3,4-Dimethyl-2,5-hexanedione impairs the axonal transport of neurofilament proteins. *J. Neurosci.* 4:1516–1526, 1984.

Griffin J.W., Drucker N., Gold B.G., et al. Schwann cell proliferation and migration during paranodal demyelination. *J. Neurosci.* 7:682–699, 1987.

Hershko A., Heller H., Eytan E., et al. Role of the alpha-amino group of protein in ubiquitin-mediated protein breakdown. *Proc. Natl. Acad. Sci. U.S.A.* 81:7021–7025, 1984.

Hirokawa N. Cross-linker system between neurofilaments, microtubules, and membranous organelles in frog axons revealed by the quick-freeze, deep-etching method. *J. Cell Biol.* 94:129–142, 1982.

Hirokawa N., Sato-Yoshitake R., Yoshida T., et al. Brain dynein (MAP1C) localizes on both anterogradely and retrogradely transported membranous organelles in vivo. *J. Cell Biol.* 111:1027–1037, 1990.

Hoffman P.N., Lasek R.J. The slow component of axonal transport: identification of major structural polypeptides of the axon and their generality among mammalian neurons. *J. Cell Biol.* 66:351–366, 1975.

Hoffman P.N., Griffin J.W., Price D.L. Control of axonal caliber by neurofilament transport. *J. Cell Biol.* 99:705–714, 1984.

Hoffman P.N., Thompson G.W., Griffin J.W., et al. Changes in neurofilament transport coincide temporally with alterations in the caliber of axons in regenerating motor fibers. *J. Cell Biol.* 101:1332–1340, 1985.

Hoffman P.N., Cleveland D.W., Griffin J.W., et al. Neurofilament gene expression: a major determinant of axonal caliber. *Proc. Natl. Acad. Sci. U.S.A.* 84:3472–3476, 1987.

Hollenbeck P.J. The transport and assembly of the axonal cytoskeleton. *J. Cell Biol.* 108:223–227, 1989.

Hollenbeck P.J. Cytoskeleton on the move. *Nature* 343:408–409, 1990.

Jakobsen J., Brimijoin S. Axonal transport of enzymes and labeled proteins in experimental axonopathy induced by *p*-bromophenylacetylurea. *Brain Res.* 229:103–122, 1981.

Korobkin R., Asbury A.K., Sumner A.J., et al. Glue-sniffing neuropathy. *Arch. Neurol.* 32:158–162, 1975.

Krinke G., Suter J., Hess R. Radicular myelinopathy in aging rats. *Vet. Pathol.* 18:335–341, 1981.

Lasek R.J., Hoffman P.N. The neuronal cytoskeleton, axonal transport and axonal growth. In Goldman R., Pollard T., Rosenbaum J., eds. *Cell Motility*. Book C. *Microtubules and Related Proteins*. Cold Spring Harbor, NY, Cold Spring Harbor Laboratory, pp. 1021–1051, 1976.

Leigh P.N., Probst A., Dale G.E., et al. New aspects of the pathology of neurodegenerative disorders as revealed by ubiquitin antibodies. *Acta Neuropathol.* 79:61–72, 1989.

Lowe J., Lennox G., Jefferson D., et al. A filamentous inclusion body within anterior horn neurones in motor neurone disease defined by immunocytochemical localization of ubiquitin. *Neurosci. Lett.* 94:203–210, 1988.

Lunn E.R., Perry V.H., Brown M.C., et al. Absence of wallerian degeneration does not hinder regeneration in peripheral nerve. *Eur.J. Neurosci.* 1:27–33, 1989.

Martin D.P., Schmidt R.E., DiStefano P.S., et al. Inhibitors of protein synthesis and RNA synthesis prevent neuronal death caused by nerve growth factor deprivation. *J. Cell Biol.* 106:829–844, 1988.

Monaco S., Autilio-Gambetti L., Zabel D., et al. Giant axonal neuropathy: acceleration of neurofilament transport in optic axons. *Proc. Natl. Acad. Sci. U.S.A.* 82:920–924, 1984.

Monteiro M.J., Hoffman P.N., Gearhart J.D., et al. Expression of NF-1 in both neuronal and nonneuronal cells of transgenic mice: increased neurofilament density in axons without affecting caliber. *J. Cell Biol.* 111:1543–1557, 1990.

Nixon R.A., Logvinenko K.B. Multiple fates of newly synthesized neurofilament proteins: evidence for a stationary neurofilament network distributed nonuniformly along axons of retinal ganglion cell neurons. *J. Cell Biol.* 102:647–659, 1986.

Nukada H., Dyck P.J. Decreased axonal caliber and neurofilaments in hereditary motor and sensory neuropathy, type I. *Ann. Neurol.* 16:238–241, 1984.

Papasozomenos S.C., Yoon M., Crane R., et al. Redistribution of proteins of fast axonal transport following administration of β,β'-iminodipropionitrile: a quantitative autoradiography study. *J. Cell Biol.* 95:672–675, 1982.

Parhad I.M., Clark A.W., Griffin J.W. Effect of changes in neurofilament content on caliber of small axons: the IDPN model. *J. Neurosci.* 7:2256–2263, 1987.

Price D.L., Griffin J.W. Tetanus toxin: retrograde axonal transport of systemically administered toxin. *Neurosci. Lett.* 4:61–65, 1977.

Price D.L., Porter K.R. The response of ventral horn neurons to axonal transection. *J. Cell Biol.* 53:24–37, 1972.

Price D.L., Griffin J.W., Young A., et al. Tetanus toxin: direct evidence for retrograde intraaxonal transport. *Science* 188:945–947, 1975.

Price D.L., Griffin J.W., Hoffman P.N., et al. The response of motor neurons to injury and disease. In Dyck P.J., Thomas P.K., Lambert E.H., et al., eds. *Peripheral Neuropathy*. Vol. I. 2nd ed. Philadelphia, Saunders, pp. 732–759, 1984.

Ramon y Cajal S. *Degeneration and Regeneration of the Nervous System* (translated by R.M. May). London, Oxford University Press, 1928.

Roots B.I. Neurofilament accumulation induced in synapses by leupeptin. *Science* 221:971–972, 1983.

Sahenk Z., Mendell J.R. Acrylamide and 2,5-hexanedione neuropathies: abnormal bidirectional transport rate in distal axons. *Brain Res.* 219:397–405, 1981.

Schaumburg H.H., Wisniewski H.M., Spencer P.S. Ultrastructural studies of the dying-back process.I. Peripheral nerve terminal and axon degeneration in systemic acrylamide intoxication. *J. Neuropathol. Exp. Neurol.* 33:260–284, 1974.

Schnapp B.J., Vale R.D., Scheetz M.P., et al. Single microtubules from squid axoplasm support bidirectional movement of organelles. *Cell* 40:455–462, 1985.

Schwab M.E., Suda K., Thoenen H. Selective retrograde transynaptic transfer of a protein tetanus toxin subsequent to its retrograde axonal transport. *J. Cell Biol.* 82:798–810, 1979.

Shimono M., Imuzi K., Kuroiwa Y. 3,3'-Iminodipropionitrile induced centrifugal segmental demyelination and onion bulb formation. *J. Neuropathol. Exp. Neurol.* 37:375–386, 1978.

Spencer P.S., Schaumburg H.H. Central-peripheral distal axonopathy—the pathogenesis of dying-back polyneuropathies. In Zimmerman H., ed. *Progress in Neuropathology*. Vol.3. New York, Grune & Stratton, pp. 253–295, 1976.

Spencer P.S., Schaumburg H.H. Ultrastructural studies of the dying back process. III. The evolution of experimental peripheral giant axonal degeneration. *J. Neuropathol. Exp. Neurol.* 36:276–299, 1977.

Sterman A.B. Altered sensory ganglia in acrylamide neuropathy. Quantitative evidence of neuronal reorganization. *J. Neuropathol. Exp. Neurol.* 42:166–176, 1983.

Stoll G., Griffin J.W., Li C.Y., et al. Wallerian degeneration in the peripheral nervous system: participation of both Schwann cells and macrophages in myelin degradation. *J. Neurocytol.* 18:671–683, 1990.

Tessler A., Autilio-Gambetti A., Gambetti P. Axonal growth during regeneration: a quantitative autoradiographic study. *J. Cell Biol.* 87:197–203, 1980.

Tsukita S., Ishikawa H. The movement of membranous organelles in axons. Electron microscopic identification of anterogradely and retrogradely transported organelles. *J. Cell Biol.* 84:513–530, 1980.

Vale R.D., Schnapp B.J., Reese T.S., et al. Movement of organelles along filaments dissociated from the axoplasm of the giant squid axon. *Cell* 40:449–454, 1985.

Watson D.F., Griffin J.W. Vacor neuropathy: ultrastructural and axonal transport studies. *J. Neuropathol. Exp. Neurol.* 46:96–108, 1987.

Watson D.F., Hoffman P.N., Fittro K.P., et al. Neurofilament and tubulin transport slows along the course of mature motor axons. *Brain Res.* 477:225–232, 1989.

Watson D.F., Fittro K.P., Hoffman P.N., et al. Phosphorylation-related immunoreactivity and the rate of transport of neurofilaments in chronic 2,5-hexanedione intoxication. *Brain Res.* (in press).

Weiss P., Hiscoe H.B. Experiments on the mechanism of nerve growth. *J. Exp. Zool.* 107:315–395, 1948.

Willard M., Simon C. Antibody decoration of neurofilaments. *J. Cell Biol.* 89:198–205, 1981.

18

Pathophysiology of Nerve and Root Disorders

Gérard Said
P.K. Thomas

This chapter discusses the pathogenesis of the major symptoms and signs of diseases of the peripheral nervous system. The peripheral nervous system, defined anatomically by the presence of Schwann cells and the distinctive extracellular matrix that includes collagen, encompasses the spinal roots, the nerve trunks, the dorsal root and autonomic ganglia, and cranial nerves III through XII. Although the different pathologic processes that affect peripheral nerves may involve each of these major components of the peripheral nervous system to variable extents, the factors that determine the distribution of involvement in specific diseases are largely unknown.

The spinal roots, in particular, are predominantly involved in neuropathies such as the Guillain-Barré syndrome and some forms of experimental allergic neuritis. The reasons for the predilection of these neuropathies for the spinal roots are unknown but could be related to several anatomic features of the spinal roots: the relatively thin ensheathment of the roots by pia mater within the subarachnoid space, their sparse extracellular matrix, and their relatively less effective blood-nerve barrier.

Wallerian Degeneration

Any type of injury that causes axonal interruption leads to a sequence of changes in nerve fibers known as *wallerian degeneration*. The axonal segments distal to the site of axonal interruption survive for a few days and then disintegrate as they become deprived of the axonally transported components, essential for their structural maintenance and renewal, that are synthesized in the neuronal perikaryon. Axotomized Schwann cells in the nerve segment distal to the axonal transection manifest a transient phase of intense proliferation (for review, see Pleasure, 1989). Circulating macrophages enter the nerve segment distal to the trauma zone and assist resident Schwann cells in catabolizing myelin debris. Several weeks are required to remove all myelin debris from the distal segment. Fragmentation of the myelin sheath leads to formation of ovoids and balls of myelin within a few days after nerve transection and then of droplets of decreasing size. The size of myelin debris is useful in studies of nerve biopsy specimens to determine the age of the lesions, especially on isolated fiber preparations. Schwann cells in the distal nerve segment cease to assemble basal lamina and to express cell surface galactocerebroside. Schwann cell levels of mRNA for myelin proteins fall markedly, and the smaller amount of myelin P_0 protein that is synthesized distal to axonal transection is degraded rapidly in lysosomes. There is also an increase in expression of cell surface adhesion molecules and in the expression of nerve growth factor (NGF) receptors that are believed to display NGF in a manner optimal for support of regenerating axonal sprouts. Fibroblasts in the traumatized nerve segment and distal to it augment production of interstitial collagen, increasing the tensile strength of the damaged nerve and providing the collagenous framework required for axonal ensheathment by Schwann cells.

As regeneration proceeds, axonal growth cones penetrate the scar and extend into the tubular Schwann cell aggregates of the bands of Büngner. On reestablishment of contact with axonal sprouts, the Schwann cells that have proliferated after nerve transection assemble basal lamina, express surface galactocerebroside, and down-regulate NGF receptors and cell adhesion molecules. If the axon reaches a diameter sufficient to support myelination, usually greater than 1 μm, the Schwann cell is induced to synthesize myelin-associated glycoprotein and, later, myelin P_0 and myelin basic protein. In unmyelinated nerves, there is less proliferation of Schwann cells after axotomy than in myelinated fibers (Romine et al., 1976), suggesting that myelin debris may be the major trigger for Schwann cell mitosis. The degenerative changes that follow axonal interruption are usually succeeded by a sequence of reparative responses that, under ideal conditions, can lead to the restoration of peripheral nerve structure and function (Bray et al., 1981). Initially, several axonal branches grow from the proximal segment of the interrupted axons. One or more of these branches may succeed in growing along the bands of Schwann cells, as myelinated or unmyelinated, depending on axonal signals (Aguayo et al., 1976), and sustain their elongation toward their terminals. Recovery of nerve structure and function is usually most complete after crush injury in which the basal lamina sheaths of most fibers remains intact at the site of axonal interruption. In this situation, regenerating axons can be guided to their original targets. With lesions that transect nerve fibers and interrupt their basal laminae, functional recovery is often incomplete because of the mismatch between axons from the proximal stumps and the distal column of Schwann cells, even if the transected nerve stumps are closely apposed.

Regenerating axons can grow across gaps of several millimeters to reach the Schwann cells in the distal nerve stump. However, with gaps of longer distances or if the distal stump is removed, axonal growth becomes chaotic and neuromas result.

Axonopathy

Peripheral nervous system sensory and motor axons may exceed 1 m in length. Because peripheral nervous system axons lack ribosomes, the supply of essential structural proteins and enzymes to distal regions derived from the neuronal perikaryon must be transported through the axons for great distances. Neurons with long axons are particularly vulnerable to toxic or metabolic disturbances that compromise either perikaryal synthesis or transport of axonal proteins (Spencer et al., 1979). Such abnormalities result in degeneration starting at the most distal part of the axon and then progressing proximally. The term *dying-back* is often used to refer to such neuropathies. In humans, dying-back degeneration of fibers has been observed in diabetic neuropathy, in which it is often associated with axonal regeneration by distal sprouting (Said et al., 1983), and in Friedreich's ataxia (Said et al., 1986). In certain experimental toxic axonal neuropathies, such as those caused by hexacarbons, acrylamide, and carbon disulfide, accumulations of neurofilaments and other transported constituents of nerve at preterminal nodes of Ranvier are the earliest observable morphologic changes.

These changes are followed by wallerian-like degeneration of the distal part of the axon (Fig. 18–1). If the neuronal insult is temporary, the dying-back of distal axons can be followed by axonal regeneration with varying degrees of structural and functional repair. On the other hand, if the neuronal derangement is prolonged or severe, the degeneration may extend to the neuronal cell body with cell death. Patients recovering from central-peripheral distal ax-

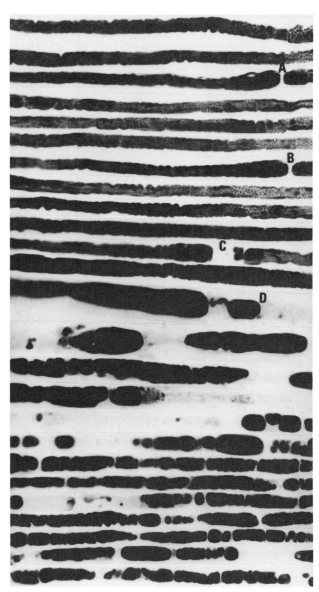

Figure 18–1. Consecutive segments of a nerve fiber isolated from the sciatic nerve of a rat intoxicated with acrylamide in drinking water for a month. The proximal end of the isolated segment is at the top left of the panel; the distal end, at the bottom right. The myelin sheath is stained black by postfixation with osmium tetroxide. A and B denote normal nodes of Ranvier. Node C is widened, and the fiber appears to be interrupted at D. Distal to D, the myelin sheath shows changes characteristic of wallerian degeneration, with ovoids and balls of degenerating myelin. Note the swelling of the fiber proximal to D caused by accumulation of neurofilaments. The incidence of such fibers is much higher in the distal sciatic nerves than proximally and increases with duration of the diet. Scale: 1 cm = 20 μm.

onopathies may be left with significant sensory and motor disturbances. Long axons are also more likely to sustain localized damage owing to trauma, ischemia, or other noxious influences. In amyloid neuropathy, for example, multifocal accumulations of amyloid in the endoneurium lead to distal degeneration of fibers (Said et al., 1984). The reason why unmyelinated and small myelinated fibers are predominantly affected in this condition is not known. In some axonal neuropathies, axonal atrophy and secondary segmental demyelination have been suggested (Dyck et al., 1984a,b). The observation that distal degeneration can also occur in central processes of neurons led Spencer and Schaumburg (1976, 1984) to introduce the term *central-peripheral distal axonopathy* to characterize more precisely many toxic axonal neuropathies (Schaumburg and Spencer, 1979).

In some experimental neuropathies, such as that caused by exposure to 3,3'-iminodipropionitrile (IDPN), such filamentous accumulations are found more proximally (Griffin and Price, 1980) and may be associated with distal axonal atrophy (Griffin et al., 1984). Axonal swelling is associated with segmental demyelination and Schwann cell proliferation, with onion bulb formations in spinal roots. There is no known example of such proximal axonopathy in humans. However, accumulation of neurofilaments occurs in the intraspinal segment of axons of motor neurons in amyotrophic lateral sclerosis.

Neuronal Degeneration

The primary destruction of nerve cell bodies can also lead to a loss of axons. In such neuronopathies, the pathologic changes resemble those of acute or chronic axonal degeneration.

Demyelination

The breakdown of myelin sheaths with relative preservation of axons (demyelination) was originally described by Gombault (1880) in experimental lead intoxication. Segmental demyelination, the pattern seen in individual myelinated fibers after the disintegration of the segment of myelin between two adjacent nodes of Ranvier, may begin in one of several ways. In the experimental demyelinating neuropathies caused by focal injection of diphtheria toxin (Allt and Cavanagh, 1969) or antiserum to galactocerebroside (Saida et al., 1979), myelin breakdown usually begins adjacent to the nodes of Ranvier or at the Schmidt-Lanterman incisures by destruction of layers of uncompacted myelin with extension to the remaining myelin sheath if there is a severe or prolonged insult to the Schwann cell. Intraneural injection of doxorubicin, an antineoplastic antibiotic that inhibits DNA-directed mRNA synthesis, induces degeneration of Schwann cells, resulting in a subacute, extremely severe demyelination. Focal

Schwann cell degeneration delays the remyelination that is not complete until at least 60–75 days postinjection (England et al., 1988). Electrophysiologic and morphologic studies showed that the incidence of fibers' undergoing axonal degeneration dramatically increased when high concentrations of doxorubicin were injected. In experimental demyelination induced by intraneural injection of demyelinating antisera (Saida et al., 1979), circulating macrophages are attracted to the site of injection within a few hours and removal of myelin debris is completed within a week after injection; the reason why removal of myelin debris is much more rapid in demyelination than in axonal degeneration is not clear. Remyelination occurs only after removal of myelin debris has been completed (Said et al., 1981a).

In the Guillain-Barré syndrome, which involves complex inflammatory-immune mechanisms (Hughes, 1990), and in experimental allergic neuritis (Lampert, 1969; Prineas, 1972), the initial myelin breakdown takes the form of invasion and phagocytosis of peripheral layers of myelin sheaths of normal appearance by macrophages, with subsequent removal of the whole damaged myelin sheath within a few days. In other instances, such as exposure to triethyltin (Graham et al., 1976), hexachlorophene (Towfighi et al., 1973), or tellurium, intramyelin edema with subsequent demyelination is observed (Fig. 18–2). Acute nerve compression also induces myelin abnormalities in the paranodal area (Ochoa et al., 1972).

Demyelination is also observed in the context of infectious diseases, including Chagas' disease, acquired immunodeficiency syndrome, cytomegalovirus neuropathy, tropical myeloneuropathy, Lyme disease–borreliosis, and the different forms of leprosy. In leprous neuropathies, demyelination may be related to degeneration of Schwann cells infected by *Mycobacterium leprae*, especially in the lepromatous form of the disease, or to release of products of activated macrophages in the endoneurium, especially in the tuberculoid form in which a delayed-type hypersensitivity reaction to *M. leprae* antigens occurs (reviewed in Said, 1990).

Demyelination in the peripheral nervous system was traditionally considered to imply a primary injury of the myelin-producing Schwann cells. It is now recognized that segmental demyelination can also be a response to axonal changes, in which the demyelination, which is termed secondary, is clustered in individual fibers. This phenomenon, which has been described in uremic neuropathy (Dyck et al., 1971), also occurs in Friedreich's ataxia (Dyck, 1984a; Said et al., 1986) and distal to chronic constriction (Baba et al., 1982). Conversely, axonal degeneration can accompany the demyelinating lesions of the Guillain-Barré syndrome (Asbury et al., 1969), experimental allergic neuritis (Madrid and Wisniewski, 1977), and the intraneural injection of demyelinating antisera (Said et al., 1981b). In such cases, the axonal lesions seem to be related to the

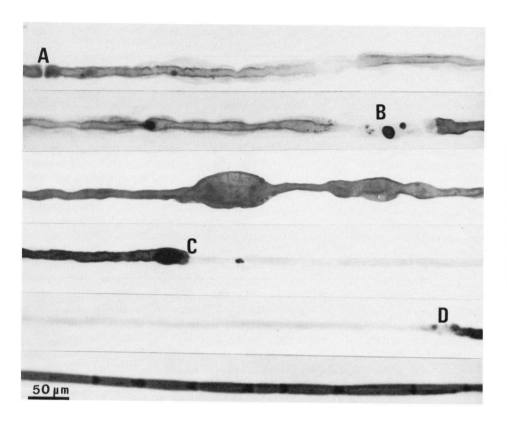

Figure 18–2. Segmental demyelination in tellurium-fed adult rats. Consecutive segments of a teased fiber from the sciatic nerve of a rat fed a diet containing 1.25% tellurium every day for 30 days. Intramyelinic edema is present between nodes B and C. The internode C-D is demyelinated. This is an example of demyelination caused by myelinopathy.

intensity of the inflammatory lesions rather than to the length of the demyelinated segments.

Re-ensheathment of the demyelinated segments usually follows peripheral nerve demyelination, both primary and secondary. After segmental demyelination, the internodal segments that were originally ensheathed by one Schwann cell are usually re-ensheathed by several Schwann cells, resulting in multiple, short internodes, as observed, for example, in the Guillain-Barré syndrome (Fig. 18–3). Within 10–14 days after acute demyelination, Schwann cells proliferate and approximately five times more Schwann cells are produced than are required to remyelinate the demyelinated area (Said et al., 1981a). Excessive Schwann cells that do not establish contact with an axon gradually disappear from the nerve, although with continued demyelination and remyelination, they accumulate around axons to produce a hypertrophic (onion bulb) neuropathy. Paranodal demyelination can be repaired by the insertion of a short intercalated segment of myelin formed by a single Schwann cell (Lubinska, 1958) or, if the myelin injury is slight, by extension from the original Schwann cell (Allt, 1969). The myelin sheaths of remyelinated segments are usually thinner, as well as shorter than normal (see Fig. 18–3).

SYMPTOMS OF NERVE AND ROOT DISORDERS

The major clinical manifestations of peripheral nerve and root disorders (for review, see Thomas,

1984) are motor weakness and incoordination; muscle atrophy; reflex attenuation or loss; sensory loss; disorders of sensation such as dysesthesias, paresthesias, and pain; and autonomic dysfunction. The nature and distribution of these clinical manifestations differ in the various nerve and root disorders and may provide some indication of the underlying cause.

Except for the most obvious extreme of total loss of motor and sensory function caused by axonal interruption or conduction block, the precise physiologic mechanisms giving rise to the symptoms of nerve and root disorders often remain a matter of speculation (see Chapter 3). Ectopic generation of nerve impulses undoubtedly has a role in production of some positive symptoms of peripheral nerve disease. Changes in secretion of neurotransmitters or putative trophic substances by injured nerve fibers may also be important, and increasing attention is being directed toward the possibility of changes in structure and function within the central nervous system in response to peripheral nerve injury.

Motor and Sensory Loss

Loss of muscle strength and sensation in peripheral nerve or spinal root disease can be caused by axonal interruption or degeneration or by conduction block in demyelinated fibers. However, the characteristic site of pathologic change is different in axonal and demyelinating neuropathies.

In axonal neuropathies, in which symptoms and

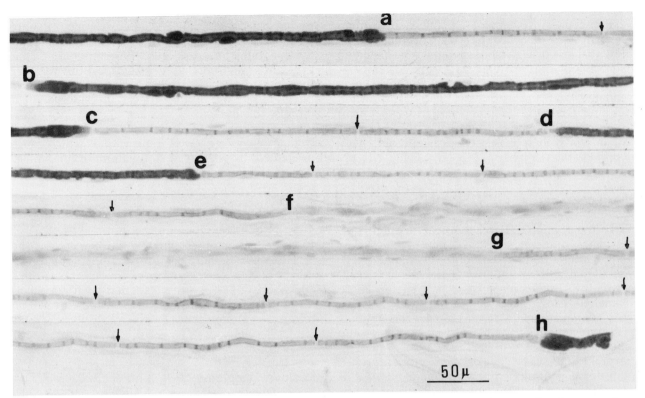

Figure 18–3. Demyelination and remyelination in the Guillain-Barré syndrome. Consecutive segments of a nerve fiber from a sural nerve biopsy from a patient with a demyelinative polyradiculoneuropathy of acute onset (Guillain-Barré syndrome). From top left to a, b-c, d-e, and distal to h, the original myelin sheath is still present. Segments a-b, c-d, e-f, and g-h are remyelinated. The newly formed nodes of Ranvier are shown by arrows. Note that the new internodes are much shorter than the original ones. The segment f-g is still demyelinated.

signs usually begin distally in the feet and then progress proximally, the clinical findings correlate well with both pathologic and physiologic findings in experimental neuropathies. In most experimental axonal neuropathies, the major pathologic alteration is found in the distal part of the peripheral nerves, affecting longer fibers before shorter fibers, and larger-diameter fibers before smaller-diameter fibers (Spencer and Schaumburg, 1976). Physiologic findings from animals with axonal neuropathies are consistent with this distal localization. For example, single-fiber studies in cats intoxicated with acrylamide have shown conduction failure near the terminals of both motor and sensory fibers with preserved normal conduction in the more proximal portion of these fibers (Sumner, 1980; Sumner and Asbury, 1975). The moderate decreases in conduction velocity sometimes found in compound action potential recordings from patients with axonal neuropathies are usually interpreted as reflecting preferential loss of large-diameter fibers rather than true slowing of conduction. However, the more marked reductions in conduction velocity observed in human hexacarbon neuropathies are attributed to the secondary demyelination associated with the axonal pathologic change (Korobkin et al., 1975).

In demyelinating neuropathies, motor and sensory loss may also be more severe distally than proximally, even though demyelinating lesions may affect both distal and proximal portions of peripheral nerves. If sites of demyelination are randomly distributed, longer fibers are more likely than shorter fibers to encompass a site of demyelination severe enough to cause conduction block and loss of effective conduction to and from the periphery.

The relationship of the decreased conduction velocity characteristic of demyelinated nerve to clinical manifestations of peripheral nerve disease is open to question. For example, patients who have completely recovered from acute demyelinating neuropathies can have persistently decreased nerve conduction velocities without any clinical deficit, except for absent ankle jerks. The argument that slowed conduction in demyelinated fibers is tolerated without clinical symptoms has been made more rigorously with respect to central nervous system demyelination (Rasminsky, 1973). Compensation for decreased peripheral conduction velocity, particularly in sensory systems, may demand some as yet unspecified adaptive responses of the central nervous system to temporally altered patterns of input.

Demyelinated fibers cannot transmit trains of impulses faithfully (McDonald and Sears, 1970; Rasminsky and Sears, 1972) at physiologic frequencies. This property may underlie abnormalities in sensory functions dependent on precise temporal coding of impulses and muscle fatigability found in some demyelinating neuropathies.

Predominant involvement of fibers of certain classes in some neuropathies may be reflected in preferential loss of sensations thought to be mediated by such fibers (e.g., early loss of pain and temperature sensation in amyloid neuropathy in which small myelinated and unmyelinated fibers are affected [Dyck and Lambert, 1969] and early loss of touch-pressure sensation and position sense in Friedreich's ataxia in which there is selective loss of large myelinated fibers [Dyck, 1984]).

Reflex Loss

Early loss of afferent nerve terminal function readily explains areflexia in axonal neuropathies. For example, after administration of the chemotherapeutic agent vincristine, the ankle jerks are lost early, whereas the H reflex response to only slightly more proximal electrical stimulation of the sciatic nerve is preserved (Guixheneuc et al., 1980). This implies initial involvement of the most distal portion of the Ia afferent fibers.

Several explanations have been advanced for reflex loss in demyelinating neuropathies. Gilliatt and Willison (1962) suggested that loss of reflexes in association with decreased conduction velocity may reflect temporal dispersion of afferent input to the spinal cord. If large-diameter fibers are preferentially affected, as occurs in neuropathies like that of Friedreich's ataxia, areflexia is probably due to loss of Ia afferent input; if small-diameter fibers are preferentially affected, as is known to occur with acute exposure to demyelinating antiserum to galactocerebroside (Lafontaine et al., 1982), areflexia could be due to loss of γ efferents. However, in neuropathies such as the Portuguese form of inherited amyloid neuropathy, in which unmyelinated and smaller-diameter myelinated fibers are preferentially affected (Dyck and Lambert, 1969), reflexes may be preserved until late in the course of the disease.

Muscle Atrophy

In patients with peripheral neuropathies, the presence or absence of muscle atrophy and electrical changes of denervation are usually used as criteria to distinguish between axonal and demyelinating neuropathies. Experimental denervation of muscle fibers leads to muscle atrophy and changes in the properties of the muscle fiber membrane such as partial loss of resting membrane potential, decreased sensitivity to the blocking action of tetrodotoxin on voltage-dependent sodium channels, development of extrajunctional acetylcholine receptors, and generation of spontaneous action potentials or fibrillations. There has been controversy concerning the mechanism of these changes. Several lines of experimental evidence (summarized by Purves and Lichtman, 1984) have been interpreted as indications that motor nerves have chemically mediated trophic influences on muscle fibers and that the effects of denervation are due to the interruption of these influences. However, there is also evidence to support the argument that loss of muscle activity itself is responsible for many if not all of the effects of denervation. If impulse conduction is blocked in the innervating nerve, normal muscle shows electrophysiologic changes characteristic of denervation, which can be prevented by electrical stimulation of the muscle (Lomo and Rosenthal, 1972).

Ataxia

Ataxia as a manifestation of peripheral nerve disease has traditionally been regarded as a manifestation of selective loss of proprioceptive input. Ropper and Shahani (1983) suggested that such ataxia, not invariably present in pure large-fiber neuropathies, may reflect an imbalance between loss of spindle and joint afferents.

Positive Symptoms of Peripheral Nerve Disease

The general classification of positive symptoms in neurologic disorders refers to symptoms reflecting an excess rather than a decrease of activity at some level of the nervous system. Before considering the clinical manifestations of positive symptoms in peripheral nerve disorders, some phenomenology of abnormal impulse generation in pathologic nerves is reviewed briefly.

In normal nerve fibers, impulses are ordinarily generated only at sensory nerve terminals or in cell bodies. In pathologic fibers, impulses may arise in the middle part of the axon and propagate toward both the central nervous system and the periphery (for reviews, see Rasminsky, 1983, 1984). Such ectopic impulses may arise spontaneously; may be associated with immediately antecedent, normally transmitted activity in the same fiber; or may be due to ephaptic interactions between adjacent fibers. Ectopic impulse generation has been demonstrated experimentally in the congenitally abnormally myelinated nerve fibers of dystrophic mouse spinal roots (Rasminsky, 1978) and in nerves demyelinated with lysolecithin (Calvin et al., 1982). However, this phenomenon is not an invariable consequence of demyelination, being little in evidence in nerve fibers demyelinated with diphtheria toxin (Bostock et al., 1983). Pathologic axons may be exquisitely mechanosensitive, generating ectopic impulses in response to mechanical stimuli that would be ineffective in normal fibers (Howe et al., 1977); and may fire repetitively at sites of pathologic change in response to single stimuli (Howe et al., 1976). Ephaptic transmission has been proved experimentally in dystrophic mouse spinal root axons (Huizar et al., 1975;

Rasminsky, 1980) and in experimental *Tullidora* neuropathy (Hernández-Cruz and Muñoz-Martínez, 1984). The mechanisms of ectopic impulse generation in pathologic nerve are unclear. Speculations center on changes both in ion channel distribution within pathologic axons and in extracellular potassium and calcium concentrations (Rasminsky, 1983).

A special case of ectopic impulse generation is that seen in experimental neuromas. Within a few days of acute injury to a peripheral nerve, sprouting neuroma fibers at the cut end become spontaneously active (Govrin-Lippmann and Devor, 1978; Wall and Gutnick 1974a,b). This spontaneous activity is largely confined to myelinated afferent units and has no fiber size predominance (Devor, 1983). At the peak of the activity, within the first 2 weeks after the acute injury, as many as 25% of the afferent fibers within a neuroma may be affected (Devor, 1983). Neuroma fibers are excited by mechanical stimulation (Wall and Gutnick, 1974a,b), pharmacologically by application of α-adrenergic agonists (Korenman and Devor, 1981), and by stimulation of sympathetic efferents (Devor and Jänig, 1981). Development of spontaneous excitability and adrenergic sensitivity can be depressed by application of the axoplasmic transport blockers colchicine or vinblastine to rat sciatic nerve proximal to the site of nerve injury (Devor and Govrin-Lippman, 1983). Devor (1983) speculated that the axon membrane in the sprouting fibers within neuromas differentiates to contain an excess of axoplasmically transported sodium and/or calcium channels and α-adrenergic receptors.

Wall and Devor (1983) showed that in normal rats there is a low level of ongoing spontaneous impulse activity arising from a small proportion (about 4–5%) of dorsal root ganglion cells of both myelinated and unmyelinated fibers. After nerve injury distal to the dorsal root ganglion, the proportion of dorsal root ganglion cells generating impulses in myelinated fibers is significantly increased (Burchiel, 1984; Wall and Devor, 1983). Injured fibers may thus have sites of ectopic impulse generation both in the vicinity of and remote from a nerve injury.

Some of the positive clinical phenomena affecting both motor and sensory function in peripheral nerve disorders may depend on the various manifestations of increased excitability of pathologic nerve fibers referred to earlier (see also Chapter 16).

Spontaneous Motor Unit Activity

Several clinical syndromes have been described in which continuous motor unit activity emanating from peripheral nerve is a prominent feature (reviewed in Auger et al., 1984; Rasminsky, 1984; Thomas, 1984). Accompanying manifestations include varying combinations of muscle stiffness weakness, atrophy, or hypertrophy; excessive sweating; dysphonia; and laryngeal spasm. The ectopic origin of the motor unit activity in peripheral nerve has been demonstrated by its elimination after administration of curare, by

its persistence during sleep and spinal anesthesia, and by the progressive reduction of activity with progressively more distal nerve blocks. In some cases, the ongoing motor unit activity is enhanced by voluntary muscle contraction, suggesting provocation of repetitive discharges by propagated action potentials ("neuromyotonia"). Axonal degeneration, demyelination, and normal nerve have been found in biopsy samples from individuals with variants of this syndrome. The excessive motor unit activity is often reduced or eliminated by treatment with anticonvulsant drugs such as diphenylhydantoin and carbamazepine.

Nielsen (1984) established that the motor discharges in hemifacial spasm are due to impulses arising in the facial nerve both spontaneously and by ephaptic excitation. Both the symptoms and the physiologic abnormality disappear after successful surgical decompression of the nerve, which is usually irritated by an ectatic blood vessel in the brain stem (Nielsen and Janetta, 1984). Other motor disorders that may also reflect ectopic impulse generation within peripheral nerve include spontaneous fasciculations, myokymia, muscle cramps, and tetany.

Positive and Distorted Sensory Symptoms

This rubric embraces a number of phenomena, such as paresthesia, dysesthesia, hyperesthesia, hyperalgesia, hyperpathia, and frank pain. The terminology is still confused. *Hyperesthesia* is an imprecise term that denotes an increased and unpleasant response to a non-noxious stimulus, such as touch; *dysesthesia* implies an abnormal sensory response, whether spontaneous or induced. The term *allodynia* has been advocated to denote a painful response to a stimulus that is normally nonpainful, and *hyperalgesia*, an increased response to a normally painful stimulus (Lindblom et al., 1986). Other researchers have used hyperalgesia more broadly to refer to a lowered threshold for pain stimulation and an increased magnitude of pain to suprathreshold stimuli (Cline et al., 1989). The latter phenomenon is observed in the syndrome of hyperpathia, in which the threshold for pain is increased but painful stimuli, especially if repetitive, are abnormally intense; the pain also spreads out from the site of stimulation.

Hyperalgesia from non-noxious stimuli can arise in myelinated fibers of large caliber, as it may be abolished by selectively blocking A fibers by pressure-ischemia (Campbell et al., 1988). Hyperalgesia can also arise from sensitized polymodal C fiber nociceptors. The application of capsaicin to skin reduces the temperature threshold for heat pain so that pain may occur spontaneously at normal skin temperatures. Both after capsaicin application and in some instances of nerve injury, the threshold for mechanically induced burning pain is temperature dependent (Cline et al., 1989; Culp et al., 1989). This has been referred to as cross-modality threshold modulation.

The advent of percutaneous microneurographic recording made it possible to correlate some subjective sensory phenomena with discharges recorded from single units or small groups of units in human peripheral nerves. Early studies using this technique showed that pain was associated with activation of small-diameter nociceptive afferents (Torebjörk and Hallin, 1974) and that postischemic paresthesias in normal individuals are associated with ectopic impulse generation in sensory myelinated fibers (Ochoa and Torebjörk, 1980). More recently, the technique was used to demonstrate a close correlation between ectopic discharges in various types of injured nerves and both painful and nonpainful paresthesias (Nordin et al., 1984; Nyström and Hagbarth, 1981; Ochoa et al., 1982). For example, the discharges recorded microneurographically from afferent peripheral nerve fibers during maneuvers that would compress a spinal root compromised by disc herniation resemble the discharges recorded from spinal root fibers in cats when pressure is applied to sites of chronic injury (Howe et al., 1977). Sensitized C fiber polymodal receptors were demonstrated by microneurography in acute experimental hyperalgesia in humans (Torebjörk et al., 1984).

Causalgia

Focal traumatic lesions to peripheral nerves are sometimes followed by the development of burning pain within the distribution of the injured nerve. This pain is characteristically associated with both hyperpathia and an increased threshold to light touch. Within the affected area, there may be poor localization, radiation, and summation of stimuli. The pain is characteristically exacerbated by emotional stress and other maneuvers associated with increased sympathetic outflow, such as urination or defecation.

There may be marked abnormalities of sympathetic tone in the affected part of the limb with tonic vasoconstriction or vasodilatation. The pain is frequently relieved by surgical or pharmacologic sympathetic block (Loh and Nathan, 1978). Classic hypotheses to explain causalgia invoked either involvement of sensory fibers traveling in sympathetic pathways or ephaptic cross-excitation between sympathetic outflow and nociceptive afferents, such cross-excitation occurring in neuromas (Seltzer and Devor, 1979). However, Devor (1983) suggested that much of the causalgia syndrome could be explained by the development of abnormal inward current conductances and ectopic α-adrenergic receptors in the region of nerve injury as described earlier. Catecholamines released from sympathetic efferents in the area of injury lead to abnormal afferent discharges that in turn are interpreted by the central nervous system as pain.

A distinction has been suggested (Asbury and Fields, 1984; Asbury and Gilliatt, 1984) between two types of neuropathic pain: (1) dysesthetic pain of classic causalgia, postherpetic neuralgia, and small-fiber neuropathies such as diabetes, in which pain is postulated to arise from stimulation of damaged or regenerating nociceptive fibers; and (2) nerve trunk pain associated with disorders such as spinal root compression and brachial neuritis in which pain is postulated to arise from stimulation of normal nociceptive endings of the nervi nervorum innervating inflamed or injured nerve trunks (Thomas, 1982).

Autonomic Dysfunction

Autonomic dysfunction is a feature of neuropathies in which small-diameter nerve fibers are affected. This can occur both in inherited disorders, such as the Riley-Day syndrome and familial amyloidosis in which there are profound decreases in the population of unmyelinated fibers, and in acquired neuropathies, such as those related to diabetes mellitus and primary amyloidosis. Autonomic hypofunction or hyperfunction can also occur in patients with the Guillain-Barré syndrome. The microneurographic demonstration that there are excessive bursts of sympathetic outflow in patients with Guillain-Barré syndrome with paroxysmal hypertension and tachycardia has been interpreted as evidence for lesions involving the afferent limb of the baroreflexes (Fagius and Wallin, 1983). Detailed discussion of the pathophysiology of autonomic dysfunction is found elsewhere in this volume (see Chapters 32, 33, and 39).

CENTRAL NERVOUS SYSTEM CHANGES

In conclusion, brief reference must be made to the accumulating evidence that peripheral nerve damage gives rise to changes in the central nervous system.

After axotomy, motor neurons undergo changes in membrane properties and alterations in synaptic input (Mendell, 1984). Persistence of such changes after regeneration of injured peripheral nerve could play a role in inhibiting full clinical recovery from motor deficits.

There are many sensory symptoms of peripheral nerve disorders that are not easily explained without postulating alterations in central processing of sensory input from the periphery. For example, phenomena such as poor localization of sensory stimuli, misperception of the nature of sensory stimuli, perception of innocuous stimuli as painful and persistent, and denervation pain do not readily lend themselves to explanation solely in terms of alterations in function in the periphery.

Several lines of evidence indicate that central processing of sensory input may be altered after peripheral nerve lesions (Nathan, 1983; Wall and Devor, 1982). Dramatic changes were observed in receptive fields of second- and higher-order sensory neurons in the spinal cord, the brain stem, the thalamus, and the somatosensory cortex after peripheral nerve injury (Devor and Wall, 1978, 1981a,b; Kass et al., 1983; McMahon and Wall, 1983). Changes also were observed in histochemical staining properties of primary afferent terminals within the spinal cord in animals subjected to peripheral nerve injury. After peripheral nerve section, there are changes in neuropeptides in the substantia gelatinosa: substance P (Barbut et al., 1981; Jessel et al., 1979) and somatostatin (McGregor et al., 1984) are depleted while vasoactive intestinal polypeptide is increased (McGregor et al., 1984). Although detailed elucidation of much of the pathophysiology of peripheral nerve injury or disease is still impossible, it is likely that changes in the central nervous system, such as those alluded to earlier, need to be invoked to provide a satisfactory explanation of many of the clinical symptoms.

References

(Key references are designated with an asterisk.)

Aguayo A.J., Epps J., Charron L., et al. Multipotentiality of Schwann cells in cross anastomosed and grafted myelinated and unmyelinated nerves. Quantitative microscopy and radioautography. *Brain Res.* 104:1–20, 1976.

Allt G. Repair of segmental demyelination in peripheral nerves: an electron microscope study. *Brain* 92:639–646, 1969.

Allt G., Cavanagh J.B. Ultrastructural changes in the region of the node of Ranvier in the rat caused by diphtheria toxin. *Brain* 92:459–468, 1969.

Asbury A.K., Arnason B.G., Adams R.D. The inflammatory lesion in idiopathic polyneuritis. Its role in pathogenesis. *Medicine (Baltimore)* 48:173–215, 1969.

Asbury A.K., Fields H.L. Pain due to peripheral nerve damage: an hypothesis. *Neurology (N.Y.)* 34:1587–1590, 1984.

Asbury A.K., Gilliatt R.W. The clinical approach to neuropathy. In Asbury A.K., Gilliatt R.W., eds. *Peripheral Nerve Disorders: A Practical Approach.* London, Butterworth, 1984.

*Asbury A.K., Johnson P.C. *Pathology of Peripheral Nerve.* Philadelphia, Saunders, 1978.

Auger R.G., Daube J.R., Gomez M.R., et al. Hereditary form of sustained muscle activity of peripheral nerve origin causing generalized myokymia and muscle stiffness. *Ann. Neurol.* 15:13–21, 1984.

Baba M., Fowler C.J., Jacobs J.M., et al. Changes in peripheral nerve fibres distal to a constriction. *J. Neurol. Sci.* 54:197–208, 1982.

Barbut D., Polak J.M., Wall P.D. Substance P in spinal cord dorsal horn decreases following peripheral nerve injury. *Brain Res.* 206:289–298, 1981.

Bostock H., Sears T.A., Sherratt R.M. The spatial distribution of excitability and membrane current in normal and demyelinated mammalian nerve fibres. *J. Physiol. (Lond.)* 341:41–58, 1983.

Bray G.M., Rasminsky M., Aguayo A.J. Interactions between axons and their sheath cells. *Annu. Rev. Neurosci.* 4:127–162, 1981.

Burchiel K.J. Effects of electrical and mechanical stimulation on two foci of spontaneous activity which develop in primary afferent neurons after peripheral axotomy. *Pain* 18:249–265, 1984.

Calvin W.H., Devor M., Howe J.F. Can neuralgias arise from minor demyelination? Spontaneous firing, mechanosensitivity, and after-discharge from conducting axons. *Exp. Neurol.* 75:755–763, 1982.

Campbell J.N., Raja S.N., Meyer R.A., et al. Myelinated afferents signal the hyperalgesia associated with nerve injury. *Pain* 32:89–94, 1988.

Cline M.A., Ochoa J., Torebjörk H.E. Chronic hyperalgesia and skin warming caused by sensitized C nociceptors. *Brain* 112:621–647, 1989.

Culp W.J., Ochoa J., Cline M., et al. Heat and mechanical hyperalgesia induced by capsaicin. Cross modality threshold modulation in human C nociceptors. *Brain* 112:1317–1332, 1989.

Devor M. Nerve pathophysiology and mechanisms of pain in causalgia. *J. Autonom. Nerv. Syst.* 7:371–384, 1983.

Devor M., Govrin-Lippmann R. Axoplasmic transport block reduces ectopic impulse generation in injured peripheral nerves. *Pain* 16:73–85, 1983.

Devor M., Jänig W. Activation of myelinated afferents ending in a neuroma by stimulation of the sympathetic supply in the rat. *Neurosci. Lett.* 24:43–47, 1981.

Devor M., Wall P.D. Reorganisation of spinal cord sensory map after peripheral nerve injury. *Nature* 275:75–76, 1978.

Devor M., Wall P.D. Plasticity in the spinal cord sensory map following peripheral nerve injury in rats. *J. Neurosci.* 1:679–684, 1981a.

Devor M., Wall P.D. The effect of peripheral nerve injury on receptive fields of cells in the cat spinal cord. *J. Comp. Neurol.* 199:277–291, 1981b.

Dyck P.J. Neuronal atrophy and degeneration predominantly affecting peripheral sensory and autonomic neurons. In Dyck P.J., Thomas P.K., Lambert E.H., et al., eds. *Peripheral Neuropathy.* 2nd ed. Philadelphia, Saunders, pp. 1557–1559, 1984.

Dyck P.J., Lambert E.H. Dissociated sensation in amyloidosis. *Arch. Neurol.* 20:480–507, 1969.

Dyck P.J., Johnson W.J., Lambert E.H., et al. Segmental demyelination secondary to axonal degeneration in uremic neuropathy. *Mayo Clin. Proc.* 46:400–431, 1971.

Dyck P.J., Nukada H., Lais A.C., et al. Permanent axotomy: a model of chronic neuronal degeneration preceded by axonal atrophy, myelin remodeling, and degeneration. In Dyck P.J., Thomas P.K., Lambert E.H., et al., eds. *Peripheral Neuropathy.* 2nd ed. Philadelphia, Saunders, pp. 666–690, 1984a.

*Dyck P.J., Thomas P.K., Lambert E.H., et al., eds. *Peripheral Neuropathy.* 2nd ed. Philadelphia, Saunders, 1984b.

England J.D., Rhee E.K., Said G., et al. Schwann cell degeneration induced by doxorubicin (Adriamycin). *Brain* 111:901–913, 1988.

Fagius J., Wallin B.G. Microneurographic evidence of excessive sympathetic outflow in the Guillain-Barré syndrome. *Brain* 106:589–600, 1983.

Gilliatt R.W., Willison R.G. Peripheral nerve conduction in diabetic neuropathy. *J. Neurol. Neurosurg. Psychiatry* 25:11–18, 1962.

Gombault A. Contribution à l'étude de la névrite parenchymateuse subaiguë et chronique. Névrite segmentaire périaxile. *Arch. Neurol.* 1:11–38, 177–190, 1880.

Govrin-Lippmann R., Devor M. Ongoing activity in severed nerves: source and variation with time. *Brain Res.* 159:406–410, 1978.

Graham D.I., DeJesus P.V., Pleasure D.E., et al. Triethyltin sulfate-induced neuropathy in rats. Electrophysiologic, morphologic and biochemical studies. *Arch. Neurol.* 33:40–48, 1976.

Griffin J.W., Price D.L. Proximal axonopathies induced by toxic chemicals. In Spencer P.S., Schaumburg H.H., eds. *Experimental and Clinical Neurotoxicology.* Baltimore, Williams & Wilkins, pp. 161–178, 1980.

Griffin J.W., Cork L.C., Hoffman P.N., et al. Experimental models of motor neuron degeneration. In Dyck P.J., Thomas P.K., Lambert E.H., et al., eds. *Peripheral Neuropathy.* 2nd ed. Philadelphia, Saunders, pp. 621–635, 1984.

Guiheneuc P., Ginet J., Groleau J.Y., et al. Early phase of vincristine neuropathy in man. *J. Neurol. Sci.* 45:355–366, 1980.

Hernández-Cruz A., Muñoz-Martinez E.J. Axon-to-axon transmission in *Tullidora* (buckthorn) neuropathy. *Exp. Neurol.* 84:533–548, 1984.

Howe J.F., Calvin W.H., Loeser J.D. Impulses reflected from dorsal root ganglia and from focal nerve injuries. *Brain Res.* 116:139–143, 1976.

Howe J.F., Loeser J.D., Calvin W.H. Mechanosensitivity of dorsal root ganglia and chronically injured axons: a physiological basis for the radicular pain of nerve root compression. *Pain* 3:25–41, 1977.

Hughes R.A.C. *The Guillain-Barré Syndrome.* Berlin, Springer-Verlag, 1990.

Huizar P., Kuno M., Miyata Y. Electrophysiological properties of spinal motoneurons of normal and dystrophic mice. *J. Physiol. (Lond.)* 248:231–246, 1975.

Jessel T., Tsunoo A., Kanazawa I., et al. Substance P: depletion in the dorsal horn of rat spinal cord after section of the peripheral processes of primary sensory neurons. *Brain Res.* 168:247–259, 1979.

Kaas J.H., Merzenich M.M., Killackey H.P. The reorganization of the somatosensory cortex following peripheral nerve damage in adult and developing mammals. *Annu. Rev. Neurosci.* 6:325–356, 1983.

Korenman E.M.D., Devor M. Ectopic adrenergic sensitivity in damaged peripheral nerve axons in the rat. *Exp. Neurol.* 72:63–81, 1981.

Korobkin R., Asbury A.K., Sumner A.J., et al. Glue-sniffing neuropathy. *Arch. Neurol.* 32:158–162, 1975.

Lafontaine S., Rasminsky M., Saida T., et al. Conduction block in rat myelinated fibres following acute exposure to anti-galacto-cerebroside serum. *J. Physiol. (Lond.)* 323:287–306, 1982.

Lampert P.W. Mechanism of demyelination in experimental allergic neuritis: electron microscopic studies. *Lab. Invest.* 20:127–138, 1969.

Lindblom U., Mersky H., Mumford J.M., et al. Pain terms: a current list with definitions and notes on usage. *Pain Suppl.* 3:S215–S221, 1986.

Loh L., Nathan P.W. Painful peripheral states and sympathetic blocks. *J. Neurol. Neurosurg. Psychiatry* 41:664–671, 1978.

Lomo T., Rosenthal J. Control of ACh sensitivity by muscle activity in the rat. *J. Physiol. (Lond.)* 221:493–513, 1972.

Lubinska L. "Intercalated" internodes in nerve fibres. *Nature* 181:957–958, 1958.

Madrid R.E., Wisniewski H.M. Axonal degeneration in demyelinating disorders. *J. Neurocytol.* 6:103–117, 1977.

McDonald W.I., Sears T.A. The effects of experimental demyelination on conduction in the central nervous system. *Brain* 93:583–598, 1970.

McGregor G.P., Gibson S.J., Sabate I.M., et al. Effect of peripheral nerve section and nerve crush on spinal cord neuropeptides in the rat: increased VIP and PHI in the dorsal horn. *Neuroscience* 13:207–216, 1984.

McMahon S.B., Wall P.D. Plasticity in the nucleus gracilis of the rat. *Exp. Neurol.* 80:195–207, 1983.

Mendell L.M. Modifiability of spinal synapses. *Physiol. Rev.* 64:260–324, 1984.

Nathan P.W. Pain and the sympathetic nervous system. *J. Autonom. Nerv. Sys.* 7:363–370, 1983.

Nielsen V.K. Pathophysiology of hemifacial spasm: I. Ephaptic transmission and ectopic excitation. *Neurology (N.Y.)* 34:418–426, 1984.

Nielsen V.K., Janetta P.J. Pathophysiology of hemifacial spasm: III. Effects of facial nerve decompression. *Neurology (N.Y.)* 34:891–897, 1984.

Nordin M., Nyström B., Wallin U., et al. Ectopic sensory discharges and paresthesiae in patients with disorders of peripheral nerves, dorsal roots and dorsal columns. *Pain* 20:231–245, 1984.

Nyström B., Hagbarth K.-E. Microelectrode recordings from transected nerves in amputees with phantom limb pain. *Neurosci. Lett.* 27:211–216, 1981.

Ochoa J., Torebjörk H.E. Paresthesiae from ectopic impulse generation in human sensory nerves. *Brain* 102:835–853, 1980.

Ochoa J., Fowler T.J., Gilliatt R.W. Anatomical changes in peripheral nerves compressed by a pneumatic tourniquet. *J. Anat.* 113:433–455, 1972.

Ochoa J., Torebjörk H.E., Culp W.J., et al. Abnormal spontaneous activity in single sensory nerve fibers in humans. *Muscle Nerve* 5:S74–S77, 1982.

Pleasure D. Biochemistry of neuropathy. In Siegel G.J., Agranoff B.W., Albers R.W., et al., eds. *Basic Neurochemistry: Molecular, Cellular, and Medical Aspects.* 4th ed. New York, Raven Press, pp. 685–696, 1989.

Prineas J.W. Acute idiopathic polyneuritis: an electron microscope study. *Lab. Invest.* 26:133–147, 1972.

Purves D., Lichtman J.W. *Principles of Neural Development.* Sunderland, MA, Sinauer Associates, 1984.

Rasminsky M. The effects of temperature on conduction in demyelinated single nerve fibers. *Arch. Neurol.* 28:287–292, 1973.

Rasminsky M. Ectopic generation of impulses and cross-talk in spinal nerve roots of "dystrophic" mice. *Ann. Neurol.* 3:351–357, 1978.

Rasminsky M. Ephaptic transmission between single nerve fibres in the spinal nerve roots of dystrophic mice. *J. Physiol. (Lond.)* 305:151–169, 1980.

Rasminsky M. Ectopic impulse generation in pathological nerve fibres. *Trends Neurosci.* 6:388–390, 1983.

Rasminsky M. Ectopic impulse generation in pathologic nerve fibers. In Dyck P.J., Thomas P.K., Lambert E.H., et al., eds. *Peripheral Neuropathy.* 2nd ed. Philadelphia, Saunders, pp. 911–918, 1984.

Rasminsky M., Sears T.A. Internodal conduction in undissected demyelinated nerve fibres. *J. Physiol. (Lond.)* 227:323–350, 1972.

Romine J.S., Bray G.M., Aguayo A.J. Schwann cell multiplication after crush injury of unmyelinated fibres. *Arch. Neurol.* 33:49–54, 1976.

Ropper A.H., Shahani B. Proposed mechanism of ataxia in Fisher's syndrome. *Arch. Neurol.* 40:537–538, 1983.

Said G. Studies on the mechanisms of nerve lesions in leprous neuropathies. In McKhann G., ed. *Childhood Neuropathy. New Issues in Neurosciences.* Vol.2. New York, Wiley, pp. 85–94, 1990.

Said G., Duckett S., Sauron B. Proliferation of Schwann cells in tellurium-induced demyelination in young rats. *Acta Neuropathol.* 53:173–179, 1981a.

Said G., Saida, K., Saida T., et al. Axonal lesions in acute experimental demyelination: a sequential teased nerve fiber study. *Neurology (N.Y.)* 31:413–421, 1981b.

Said G., Slama G., Selva J. Progressive centripetal degeneration of axons in small fiber diabetic polyneuropathy. *Brain* 106:791–807, 1983.

Said G., Ropert A., Faux N. Length-dependent degeneration of fibers in Portuguese amyloid polyneuropathy: a clinicopathological study. *Neurology (N.Y.)* 34:1025–1032, 1984.

Said G., Marion M.-H., Selva J., et al. Hypotrophic and dyingback nerve fibers in Friedreich's ataxia. *Neurology* 36:1292–1299, 1986.

Saida K., Saida T., Brown M.J., et al. In vivo demyelination induced by intraneural injection of anti-galactocerebroside serum: a morphologic study. *Am. J. Pathol.* 95:99–110, 1979.

Schaumburg H.H., Spencer P.S. Clinical and experimental studies of distal axonopathy—a frequent form of brain and nerve damage produced by environmental chemical hazards. *Ann. N. Y. Acad. Sci.* 329:14–29, 1979.

Seltzer Z., Devor M. Ephaptic transmission in chronically damaged peripheral nerves. *Neurology (Minneap.)* 29:1061–1064, 1979.

Spencer P.S., Schaumburg H.H. Central and peripheral distal axonopathy—the etiology of dying-back polyneuropathies. *Progr. Neuropath.* 3:253–295, 1976.

Spencer P.S., Schaumburg H.H. Experimental models of primary axonal disease induced by toxic chemicals. In Dyck P.J., Thomas P.K., Lambert E.H., et al., eds. *Peripheral Neuropathy.* 2nd ed. Philadelphia, Saunders, pp. 636–649, 1984.

Spencer P.S., Sabri M.I., Schaumburg H.H., et al. Does a defect in energy metabolism cause axonal degeneration in polyneuropathies? *Ann. Neurol.* 5:501–507, 1979.

Sumner A.J. Axonal polyneuropathies. In Sumner A.J., ed. *The Physiology of Peripheral Nerve Disease.* Philadelphia, Saunders, pp. 340–357, 1980.

Sumner A.J., Asbury A.K. Physiological studies of the dying-back phenomenon. I. Effects of acrylamide on muscle stretch afferents. *Brain* 98:91–100, 1975.

Thomas P.K. Pain in peripheral neuropathy: clinical and morphological aspects. In Culp W.J., Ochoa J., eds. *Abnormal Nerves and Muscles as Impulse Generators.* New York, Oxford University Press, 1982.

Thomas P.K. Symptomatology and differential diagnosis of peripheral neuropathy. Clinical features and differential diagnosis. In Dyck P.J., Thomas P.K., Lambert E.H., et al., eds. *Peripheral Neuropathy.* 2nd ed. Philadelphia, Saunders, pp. 1169–1190, 1984.

Torebjörk H.E., Hallin R.G. Identification of afferent C units in intact human skin nerves. *Brain Res.* 67:387–403, 1974.

Torebjörk H.E., LaMotte R.H., Robinson C.V. Peripheral neural correlates of magnitude of cutaneous pain and hyperalgesia. *J. Neurophysiol.* 51:325–339, 1984.

Towfighi J., Gonatas N.K., McCrea L. Hexachlorophene neuropathy in rats. *Lab. Invest.* 29:428–436, 1973.

Wall P.D., Devor M. Consequences of peripheral nerve damage in the spinal cord and in neighboring intact peripheral nerves. In Culp W.J., Ochoa J., eds. *Abnormal Nerves and Muscles as Impulse Generators.* New York, Oxford University Press, 1982.

Wall P.D., Devor M. Sensory afferent impulses originate from dorsal root ganglia as well as from the periphery in normal and nerve injured rats. *Pain* 17:321–339, 1983.

Wall P.D., Gutnick M. Ongoing activity in peripheral nerves. The physiology and pharmacology of impulses originating from a neuroma. *Exp. Neurol.* 45:580–593, 1974a.

Wall P.D., Gutnick M. Properties of afferent nerve impulses originating from a neuroma. *Exp. Neurol.* 45:580–593, 1974b.

19

Disorders of Peripheral Nerve

Arthur K. Asbury
Shawn J. Bird

The basic pathologic processes affecting peripheral nerve and root, the semiology of neuropathic disorders, and their current pathophysiologic explanations are fully described in Chapter 18. The first purpose of this chapter is to build on that base by providing an overview of the wide array of peripheral neuropathies that affect humans. Disorders of peripheral nerve exhibit such a bewildering and complex set of manifestations that it is difficult for the physician to know where to begin and how to proceed. Therefore, the second purpose is to develop a logical approach and assessment scheme (summarized in Figure 19–1) that guides the examiner to correct diagnostic and management decisions.

GENERAL DESCRIPTION OF NEUROPATHIC SYNDROMES

The prototypic picture of polyneuropathy occurs with acquired toxic or metabolic neuropathic states. The first noticeable symptoms tend to be sensory and consist of tingling, prickling, burning, or band-like dysesthesias in the balls of the feet, in the tips of the toes, or in a general distribution over the soles. Symmetry of symptoms and findings in a distal graded fashion is the rule, but occasionally dysesthesias appear in one foot a brief time before the other or may be more pronounced in one foot. Some care and judgment must be exercised to avoid confusion with mononeuropathy multiplex, in which sensory symptoms tend to appear in the distribution of individual digital nerves, either in the hand or the foot.

With worsening of polyneuropathy, weakness, pansensory deficit, and loss of tendon jerks spread centripetally and symmetrically and may eventually involve the torso and axial structures in addition to the limbs. Numbness and imbalance (negative symptoms) are the hallmarks of sensory loss but are often accompanied by positive symptoms, including pain. As a rule, pain in polyneuropathy is dysesthetic and is experienced distally, but there is frequently also a nerve trunk component, which is deep and aching in character and is experienced proximally (Asbury, 1990; Asbury and Fields, 1984).

When sensory disturbance ascends to midthigh in the legs and above the elbows in the arms, a tent-shaped area of hypoesthesia on the lower abdomen may often be demonstrated. This grows broader and the apex extends rostrally toward the sternum as the neuropathy worsens. This tent-shaped sensory disturbance on the anterior torso is a nerve length–dependent phenomenon in this situation, involving the segmental truncal nerves. It can be mistaken for a sensory deficit of spinal cord origin if care is not taken to check for a sensory level on the back and to outline carefully the area of deficit. Similarly, in the most extreme cases, hypoesthesia at the crown of the scalp may be present and can spread in radial directions to both the trigeminal and upper cervical distributions. This is also a nerve length–dependent phenomenon but is seen only in the most severe and advanced cases.

Variations on the overall pattern and sequence of progressive polyneuropathy are manifold. They include alterations in the rate of evolution of symptoms, the course, and the eventual degree of severity; the presence or absence of positive motor and sensory symptoms; the symmetry of features and their distribution in terms of proximal versus distal, arms versus legs, and motor versus sensory; the relative proportion of dysfunction attributable to large-fiber

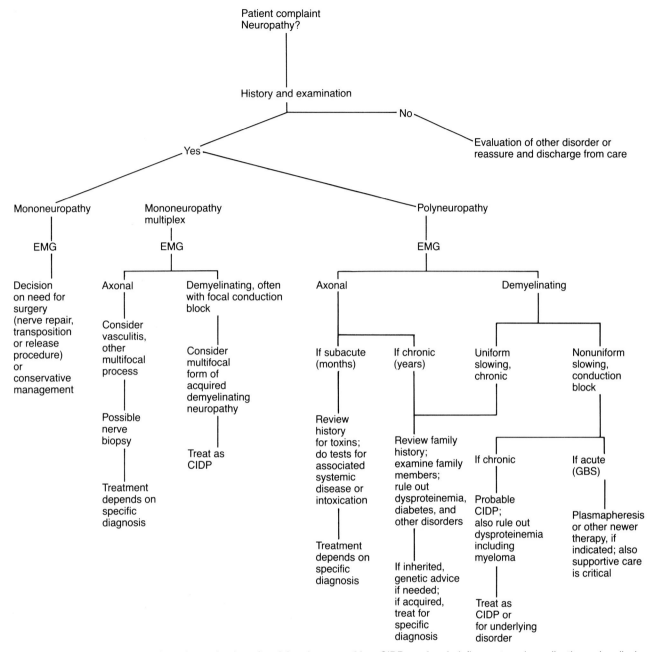

Figure 19–1. Flow chart approach to the evaluation of peripheral neuropathies. CIDP = chronic inflammatory demyelinating polyradiculo-neuropathy; EMG = electromyography; GBS = Guillain-Barré syndrome. (Data from Asbury A.K. New aspects of disease of the peripheral nervous system. In Isselbacher K.T., Adams R.D., eds. *Harrison's Principles of Internal Medicine.* Update 4. New York, McGraw-Hill, pp. 211–219, 1983.)

deficit and to small-fiber deficit; and the determination, mainly by electrodiagnostic examination, of axonal versus demyelinating processes.

ASSESSMENT AND DIAGNOSIS OF NEUROPATHY

Symptoms and Signs

Clues to diagnosis of peripheral neuropathies often lie in unnoted or readily forgotten events occurring weeks or months before the onset of symptoms. Inquiry should be made about recent viral illnesses; other systemic symptoms; institution of new medications; potentially toxic exposures to solvents, pesticides, or heavy metals; the occurrence of similar symptoms in family members or co-workers; habits concerning alcohol ingestion; and the presence of known underlying medical disorders. It is also useful to ask patients if they would otherwise feel well if free of their neuropathic symptoms to determine the presence or absence of underlying systemic illness.

It is important to learn how symptoms first appeared. Even with distal polyneuropathies, symptoms may appear in the sole of one foot a few days or a week before appearing in the other, but usually the patient describes a distal graded disturbance that moves evenly and symmetrically in centripetal fashion. Tingling dysesthesias appear in the fingertips only when similar symptoms have reached the level of the knees. It is most important to determine whether symptoms first appeared in the distribution of individual digital nerves involving only one-half of a digit at a time and then gradually spread to become coalescent. This pattern of onset raises strong suspicions of a multifocal process (mononeuropathy multiplex) such as might be encountered with a systemic vasculitis or cryoglobulinemia.

Evolution of neuropathy ranges from rapid worsening during the course of a few days to an indolent process extending many years. Polyneuropathies with a slowly progressive course lasting more than 5 years are most likely to be genetically determined, particularly if the major manifestations are distal atrophy and weakness with few or no positive sensory symptoms. Exceptions are diabetic polyneuropathy and paraproteinemic neuropathies, in which the progression may be insidious for 5–10 years and most of the manifestations are sensory. Axonal degenerations of toxic or metabolic origin tend to evolve during several weeks to a year or longer, and the rate of progression of demyelinating neuropathies is highly variable, ranging from a few days in Guillain-Barré syndrome (GBS) to many years in others.

If major fluctuations occur in the course of neuropathy, two possibilities are brought to mind: (1) relapsing forms of neuropathy and (2) repeated toxic exposures. Slow fluctuation in symptoms taking place for weeks or months (reflecting changes in the activity of neuropathy) should not be confused with daily variation or diurnal undulation of symptoms. The latter are common to all neuropathic disorders. An example is carpal tunnel syndrome, in which dysesthesias may be prominent at night but absent during the day.

In polyneuropathies, the findings can be expected to be symmetric on both sides of the body. If only one foot slaps when the patient walks, the process is not symmetric and the possibility of a multifocal process is raised. In addition, in acquired symmetric polyneuropathies, the muscles of extension and abduction tend to be weakened to a greater extent than the muscles of flexion and adduction. Hence, weakness in lower legs often affects the peroneal and anterior tibial muscles, with attendant footdrop, more than the gastrocnemius group or foot invertors. In most polyneuropathies, the legs are more severely affected than the arms, and the distal muscles more than the proximal ones. There are exceptions, as in lead neuropathy, in which manifestations of bilateral wristdrop may predominate, and occasionally in porphyric neuropathy, in which the arms may be more affected than the legs, and proximal muscles more than distal. Proximal patterns of sensory deficit may occur rarely, sparing distal extremities and involving

proximal limbs and torso, as in analphalipoproteinemic neuropathy and porphyric neuropathy.

Palpation of nerve trunk to detect enlargement is a frequently forgotten part of the neurologic examination. In mononeuropathies, the entire course of the nerve trunk in question should be explored manually for focal thickening, the presence of neurofibroma, point tenderness, Tinel's phenomenon (generation of a tingling sensation in the sensory territory of the nerve by tapping along the course of the nerve trunk), and elicitation of pain by putting the nerve trunk on stretch. In leprous neuritis, fusiform thickening of nerve trunks is frequent, and beading of nerve trunks may be encountered in amyloid polyneuropathy. Certain genetically determined neuropathies of the hypertrophic variety may be attended by uniform thickening of all nerve trunks, often to the caliber of a clothesline or larger.

Most neuropathies involve nerve fibers of all sizes, but on occasion, selective damage to large or to small fibers predominates. In a polyneuropathy affecting mainly small fibers, diminished pinprick and temperature sensation, often with burning painful dysesthesias, may predominate, along with autonomic dysfunction but with relative sparing of motor power, balance, and tendon jerks. Selected cases of amyloid and distal diabetic polyneuropathies fall into this category (M.J. Brown et al., 1976; Dyck and Lambert, 1969; Said et al., 1984). In contrast, large-fiber polyneuropathy is characterized by areflexia, imbalance, relatively minor cutaneous sensory deficit, and variable but often severe motor dysfunction.

Electrodiagnosis

The next step is electrodiagnostic examination. It is not generally possible to make the distinction between axonal and demyelinating disorders on clinical examination alone, and electrodiagnostic analysis is particularly useful. The distinction between primarily demyelinating neuropathy and one that is primarily axonal is crucial because of the differing approaches to diagnosis and management. If, in a particular instance of progressive polyneuropathy of subacute or chronic evolution, the electrodiagnostic findings are those of an axonopathy, a long list of metabolic states and exogenous toxins comes into consideration (Tables 19–1 and 19–2). If the course is protracted for several years, it raises the likelihood of the neuronal (axonal) form of peroneal muscular atrophy (hereditary motor-sensory neuropathy type II [HMSN-II], or Charcot-Marie-Tooth disease type II [CMT-II]); family members must be examined and additional attention given to the family history.

Alternatively, if the electrodiagnostic findings are more indicative of primary demyelination of nerve, the approach is entirely different. The possibilities then include acquired demyelinating neuropathy, thought to be immunologically mediated, and genetically determined neuropathies, some of which are

Table 19–1. POLYNEUROPATHY ASSOCIATED WITH SYSTEMIC DISEASES*

Systemic Disease	Occurrence	Axonal			Demyelinating			Sensory Versus Motor	Autonomic	Comment
		Ac	Sub	Chr	Ac	Sub	Chr			
Diabetes mellitus	C	−	±	+	−	±	+	S, SM, rarely M	± to +	Mixed axonal-demyelinating disease often seen; (see Table 19–4; also Dyck et al., 1987b)
Uremia	S'	±	+	+	−	−	−	SM	±	Controllable with proper dialysis; curable with successful renal transplant
Porphyria (three types)	R	+	±	−	−	−	−	M	± to +	May be proximal > distal and may have atypical proximal sensory deficits
Hypoglycemia	R	±	+	+	−	−	−	M	−	Usually with insulinoma; arms often > legs; ? anterior horn cells affected
Vitamin deficiency, excluding B$_{12}$	S'	−	+	+	−	−	−	SM	±	Involves at least thiamine, pyridoxine, folate, pantothenic acid; probably others
Vitamin B$_{12}$ deficiency	S'	−	±	+	−	−	−	S	−	Peripheral nerve involvement variable; often overshadowed by myelopathy
Chronic liver disease	S'	−	−	−	−	−	+	S or SM	−	Usually mild or subclinical
Primary biliary cirrhosis	R	−	±	+	−	−	−	S	−	Epineurial and subperineurial xanthomatous deposits
Primary systemic amyloidosis	R	−	±	+	−	−	−	SM	+	Also seen with amyloidosis associated with myeloma or macroglobulinemia (Kelly et al., 1979)
Hypothyroidism	R	−	−	−	−	±	+	S	−	May respond to thyroid replacement (Dyck and Lambert, 1970)
Chronic obstructive pulmonary disease	S'	−	±	+	−	−	−	S or SM	−	Often subclinical; may compound toxic neuropathy caused by almitrine
Acromegaly	R	−	−	+	−	−	−	S	−	Carpal tunnel syndrome also frequent (Low et al., 1974)
Malabsorption (sprue, celiac disease)	S'	−	±	+	−	−	−	S or SM	±	Basis for neuropathy unclear; deficiency suspected
Carcinoma (sensory)	R	−	+	+	−	−	−	Pure S	−	Carcinomatous sensory neuronopathy; due to gangliitic neuropathy; mostly breast carcinoma; paraneoplastic; relatively rare
Carcinoma (sensorimotor)	S'	−	+	+	−	−	−	SM	±	Sensorimotor axonal neuropathy; mostly with lung carcinoma; more common than pure sensory, but still infrequent
Carcinoma (late)	C	−	+	+	−	−	−	S > M	±	Mild, late axonal neuropathy, probably related to weight loss and wasting (Hawley et al., 1980)
Carcinoma (demyelinating)	S'	−	−	−	+	+	±	SM	−	Acute or relapsing demyelinating neuropathy sometimes seen with carcinoma
Lymphoma, including Hodgkin's	S'	−	+	+	+	+	±	See earlier	±	Same as carcinomatous types, although pure sensory type is even rarer
Polycythemia vera	R	−	±	+	−	−	−	S	−	Also many central nervous system manifestations; often shooting pains in limbs (Yiannikas et al., 1983)

Table continued on following page

marked by uniform and drastic slowing of nerve conduction velocities.

With these considerations in hand, one can construct a flow chart (see Fig. 19–1) that summarizes the clinical and electrodiagnostic approach to the evaluation and management of a neuropathic disorder. Using this scheme, the clinician determines for each patient the tempo, distribution, severity and functional impairment, and other features discussed earlier, making a clinical judgment as to whether the problem represents a mononeuropathy, mononeuropathy multiplex, or a polyneuropathy. Often, this

Table 19–1. POLYNEUROPATHY ASSOCIATED WITH SYSTEMIC DISEASES* *Continued*

Systemic Disease	Occurrence	Axonal			Demyelinating			Sensory Versus Motor	Autonomic	Comment
		Ac	Sub	Chr	Ac	Sub	Chr			
Multiple myeloma, lytic type	S'	−	±	+	−	−	−	S, M or SM	±	Symptomatic neuropathy uncommon, subclinical neuropathy frequent
Multiple myeloma,† osteosclerotic or solitary plasmacytoma	S'	−	−	±	−	±	+	SM		Although many show severe slowing of nerve conduction velocity, this may be secondary demyelination (Mendell et al., 1985; Ohi et al., 1985)
Benign monoclonal gammopathy	S'									
IgA		−	±	+	−	−	−	SM	−	IgM κ (or occasionally λ) may bind to
IgG		−	±	+	−	−	±	SM	−	myelin-associated glycoprotein or ?
IgM		−	−	−	−	±	+	SM	−	ganglioside
Macroglobulinemia	R	−	−	±	−	−	+	SM	−	Usually but not always axonal
Cryoglobulinemia	R	−	±	+	−	−	−	SM	−	May be mononeuropathy multiplex in presentation

*− = absent; ± = sometimes; + = usual; R = rare; S' = sometimes; C = common; S = sensory; M = motor; SM = sensorimotor; Ac = acute; Sub = subacute; Chr = chronic; Ig = immunoglobulin.
†Some cases associated with POEMS syndrome (see text; Nakanishi et al., 1984).

distinction is obvious. With the clinical and electrodiagnostic information in hand, the clinician can narrow the differential diagnostic possibilities and management options to only a few. The remainder of this chapter deals with the details of this general formulation.

Electrodiagnosis is a key part of the evaluation of any neuropathy (see Fig. 19–1). For example, it allows one to be certain about the presence or absence of sensory deficit when this is unclear from clinical examination alone. It provides information about the distribution of subclinical findings, thus sharpening the diagnostic focus. The general concerns, more fully discussed elsewhere (Asbury, 1980), that may be posed by the clinician to the electrodiagnostician, include the following:

1. The distinction between disorders primary to nerve or to muscle
2. The distinction between root involvement and more distal nerve trunk involvement
3. The distinction between generalized polyneuropathic processes and widespread multifocal nerve trunk involvement
4. The confirmation of a clinical impression that a particular neuropathic disorder is purely motor or purely sensory, which often suggests that the primary process is a neuronopathy
5. The distinction between upper and lower motor neuron weakness
6. The distinction, in a given generalized polyneuropathic process, between a primary demyelinating neuropathy and an axonal degeneration
7. The assessment, in both primary axonal and demyelinating neuropathies, of many factors bearing on the nature, activity, and likely prognosis of the neuropathy
8. The assessment, in mononeuropathies, of the site of the lesion and its major effect on nerve

fibers, especially the distinction between conduction block and wallerian degeneration
9. The characterization of disorders of the neuromuscular junction
10. The identification, often in muscle of normal bulk and strength, of chronic partial denervation, fasciculations, and myotonia
11. The analysis of cramp, and its distinction from physiologic contracture

Nerve Biopsy

A note should be added on the diagnostic utility of cutaneous nerve biopsy. There are relatively few indications for this invasive technique. The main one is in asymmetric and multifocal neuropathic disorders producing a clinical picture of mononeuropathy multiplex, the basis of which is still unclear after other laboratory investigations are complete. Diagnostic considerations include vasculitis, amyloidosis, leprosy, and occasionally sarcoidosis. Many authorities (Dyck and Arnason, 1984; McCombe et al., 1987) recommend cutaneous nerve biopsy as part of the diagnostic evaluation of suspected chronic inflammatory demyelinating polyradiculoneuropathy (CIDP). Additionally, nerve biopsy is helpful when one or more cutaneous nerves are palpably enlarged. Another clinical application is in establishing the diagnosis in some genetically determined pediatric disorders such as metachromatic leukodystrophy, Krabbe's disease, giant axonal neuropathy, and infantile neuroaxonal dystrophy. In all of these recessively inherited diseases, both the central nervous system and the peripheral nervous system are affected.

There is a tendency to carry out sural nerve biopsy in distal symmetric polyneuropathies of subacute or

Table 19–2. POLYNEUROPATHY ASSOCIATED WITH DRUGS OR ENVIRONMENTAL TOXINS*

	Axonal			Demyelinating			Sensory Versus Motor	Autonomic	CNS	Comment
	Ac	*Sub*	*Chr*	*Ac*	*Sub*	*Chr*				
Drug										
Almitrine (respiratory stimulant)	–	+	+	–	–	–	S > M	–	–	Used in chronic respiratory insufficiency
Amiodarone (antiarrhythmic)	–	–	+	–	–	+	SM	–	–	Dose-dependent neuropathy, reversible by decreasing dose; lysosomal dense body accumulation
Aurothioglucose (antirheumatic)	±	±	–	+	+	–	SM	–	–	Idiosyncratic reaction, ? immune mediated (Katrak et al., 1980)
Cisplatin (antineoplastic)	–	+	+	–	–	–	S	–	–	Severe sensory neuropathy, ? neuronopathy; also ototoxicity; dose related
Dapsone (dermatologic including leprosy)	–	±	+	–	–	–	M	–	–	Dose-related pure motor neuropathy
Dideoxycytidine; dideoxyinosine (antiviral)	–	+	+	–	–	–	S > M	–	–	Probable axonopathy; probably dose related; drugs used in trials for human immunodeficiency virus type 1 infection
Disulfiram (antialcohol)	±	+	+	–	–	–	SM	–	±	Usually occurs after months of treatment
Hydralazine (antihypertensive)	–	±	+	–	–	–	S > M	–	–	Pyridoxine antagonist; only rarely neurotoxic
Isoniazid (antituberculous)	–	±	+	–	–	–	SM	±	–	Pyridoxine antagonist; in slow acetylators
Metronidazole (antiprotozoal)	–	–	±	–	–	–	S	–	+	Dose-related central-peripheral distal axonopathy
Misonidazole (radiosensitizer)	–	±	+	–	–	–	S	–	+	Neurotoxicity is the limiting factor
Nitrofurantoin (urinary antiseptic)	–	±	+	–	–	–	SM	–	–	Generally total dose related; presence of renal failure may enhance toxicity
Perhexilene (antiarrhythmic)	–	–	±	–	–	+	SM	±	–	Dose-related neuropathy; lysosomal dense body accumulation
Phenytoin (anticonvulsant)	–	–	+	–	–	–	S > M	–	–	Large-fiber neuropathy, mild, after 20–30 y of phenytoin use
Suramin (antineoplastic)				+	+	–	SM	+	–	Rapidly evolving neuropathy mimicking GBS; conduction block prominent (La Rocca et al., 1990)
Taxol (antineoplastic)	+	+	–	–	±	–	S > M	–	–	Dose-related neuropathy; dysesthetic (Lipton et al., 1989)
Thalidomide (antileprous)	–	–	+	–	–	–	S > M	±	+	Red skin and brittle nails; also teratogenic; recovery from neuropathy poor
L-Tryptophan (health food additive)	–	+	+	–	–	–	SM	±	–	This or a congener is cause of eosinophilia-myalgia syndrome
Vincristine (antineoplastic)	–	+	+	–	–	–	S > M	–	–	Mild sensory neuropathy is nearly universal, hands > feet; motor signs should prompt cessation of treatment

Table continued on following page

Table 19–2. POLYNEUROPATHY ASSOCIATED WITH DRUGS OR ENVIRONMENTAL TOXINS* *Continued*

	Axonal			Demyelinating			Sensory Versus Motor	Autonomic	CNS	Comment
	Ac	Sub	Chr	Ac	Sub	Chr				
Toxin										
Acrylamide (flocculant, grouting agent)	−	±	+	−	−	−	S > M	±	+	Large-fiber neuropathy; sensory ataxia
Arsenic (herbicide, insecticide)	±	+	+	−	−	−	SM	±	±	Skin changes and Mee lines in nails; if acute intoxication, many systemic effects
Buckthorn (toxic berry)	−	−	−	+	+	−	SM	−	−	Only occurs where berries grow; may mimic GBS
Carbon disulfide (CS₂) (industrial)	−	−	+	−	−	+	SM	−	+	Neurofilamentous accumulation in axons; demyelinating features are secondary
γ-Diketone hexacarbons (solvents)	−	±	+	−	−	+	SM	±	+	Same features as CS₂; these solvents in restricted use
Dimethylamino-propionitrile (industrial)	−	−	+	−	−	−	S > M	+	−	Small-fiber neuropathy with prominent bladder symptoms and impotence in males
Diphtheria	−	−	−	+	+	−	SM	−	−	Clinically rare; can be confused with GBS
Inorganic lead	−	−	+	−	−	−	M > S	−	±	Selective motor neuropathy with prominent wristdrop
Organophosphates	−	±	+	−	−	−	SM	−	+	Brain and spinal cord are also affected, the latter irreversibly
Pryidoxine (vitamin)	−	±	+	−	−	−	S	−	−	Usually occurs with megadose intake; may occur with only 300 mg/d
Thallium (rat poison)	−	+	+	−	−	−	SM		+	Also alopecia, Mee lines in nails; ? selective damage to neural mitochondria

*− = absent; ± = sometimes; + = usual; S = sensory; M = motor; SM = sensorimotor; Ac = acute; Sub = subacute; Chr = chronic; CNS = central nervous system.

chronic evolution. This practice is discouraged, unless all other diagnostic measures have been exhausted and the condition continues to worsen. Nerve biopsy in polyneuropathies may also be useful as part of an approved research protocol when the biopsy provides crucial information not otherwise obtainable.

POLYNEUROPATHY

The classification of polyneuropathies has become increasingly complex as the capacity to discriminate new subgroups and identify new associations with toxins and systemic disorders is enhanced. Further, the grasp of the pathophysiologic basis for the clinical phenomena observed in neuropathy has increased rapidly (see Chapter 18). Despite descriptive advances and improved understanding of the mechanisms of phenomena, little progress has been made in illuminating the fundamental pathogenetic events in nervous tissue that eventuate in any of the poly-

neuropathies, either clinical or experimental. Some tentative speculations have been put forward to explain toxic and metabolic polyneuropathies (Ohi et al., 1985; see also Chapter 17), but future progress probably depends on gaining better knowledge of the normal metabolic economy of the lower motor and primary sensory neuron.

Detailed consideration of every polyneuropathy cannot be undertaken here, but it is useful to summarize the important features of each major grouping of polyneuropathies.

Acute Axonal Polyneuropathy

If one uses the term acute to mean evolution during days, acute polyneuropathies are relatively uncommon. Included are porphyric neuropathy and massive intoxications, often suicidal or homicidal in intent. For example, an individual receiving a large amount (100 mg) of arsenous oxide becomes violently ill in a few hours, with vomiting, diarrhea, and circulatory collapse. In 1–3 days, serious renal liver failure ensues, and between 14 and 21 days, polyneuropathy appears and evolves rapidly, often as the systemic disorder abates. Progression occurs for 2–3 weeks, but recovery takes place over months after a plateau period.

Subacute Axonal Polyneuropathy

Subacute, meaning to evolve in weeks, characterizes many instances of toxic and metabolic polyneuropathy, but perhaps even more of these are chronic (months) in evolution (see Tables 19–1 and 19–2 for possibilities). Management in almost all instances involves removing the offending agent or treating the associated systemic disorder.

Chronic Axonal Polyneuropathy

The category of chronic axonal polyneuropathy includes many more types of polyneuropathy, primarily because the term chronic subsumes neuropathies that have progressed for as short a period as 6 months to as long as 60 years. Diabetic polyneuropathy and the polyneuropathies associated with dysproteinemias are important examples, but both usually also demonstrate some features of demyelination. Inherited neuropathies are perhaps the most common disorders in this category. As a rough approximation, slow worsening for more than 5 years; absence of positive symptoms, mainly motor deficit; and absence of systemic disorder all favor a genetically determined neuropathy. Although these are mostly autosomal dominant in inheritance pattern (HMSN-II), X-linked varieties are known, including a form phenotypically resembling dominantly inherited HMSN and also adrenomyeloneuropathy. To complete the picture, an array of rare autosomal recessive neuropathies occurs in childhood (Table 19–3), including autosomal recessive forms of HMSN-I and -II.

Acute Demyelinating Polyneuropathy

For all practical purposes, acute demyelinating polyneuropathy is synonymous with GBS (see later). Other acute demyelinating polyneuropathies are rare and include buckthorn berry intoxication and diphtheritic polyneuritis (see Table 19–2). In addition, acute solvent inhalation neuropathy (huffer's neuropathy) may closely mimic GBS, as may suramin-induced polyneuropathy (La Rocca et al., 1990).

Subacute Demyelinating Polyneuropathy

Subacute demyelinating neuropathies are heterogeneous in origin, although all are acquired. Most common is a relapsing and remitting neuropathy, a form of CIDP, which has many clinical features in common with GBS but differs from GBS in tempo, course, and paucity of triggering events. Previously mentioned toxins (buckthorn berry, diphtheria toxin) may also induce a picture of widespread subacute demyelination of peripheral nerve (see Table 19–2).

Chronic Demyelinating Polyneuropathy

Although more common than the subacute neuropathies, chronic polyneuropathy with demyelinating features encompasses a wide diversity of disorders, the most common of which is CIDP (see later). Others that may have demyelinating features are hereditary neuropathies and acquired neuropathies associated with diabetes mellitus, dysproteinemias, other metabolic states, and some chronic intoxications. To complicate matters, many of these disorders present an electrodiagnostic picture of mixed axonal-demyelinating findings. Frequently, it is difficult, if not impossible, to determine which process, axonal degeneration or demyelination, is the primary event. Aspects of many of these neuropathies are alluded to in Tables 19–1 to 19–3 and in the following sections.

OTHER PATTERNS OF NEUROPATHY

Mononeuropathy

Mononeuropathies are characterized by focal involvement of a single nerve trunk and therefore imply a local causation. Direct trauma, compression, and entrapment are the usual causes. Compressive or entrapment neuropathies most commonly involve the median nerve in the carpal tunnel, the ulnar nerve at the ulnar groove or in the cubital tunnel, the radial nerve at the spiral groove, and the peroneal nerve at the fibular head. However, they may also occur at any site where a nerve is subjected to mechanical trauma. Diabetics may develop isolated nerve infarction. Less commonly, isolated nerve lesions may reflect sarcoidosis, single neurofibromas or schwannomas, or a rare embolic infarction.

In the absence of a history of trauma to the nerve trunk, factors favoring conservative management include sudden onset; no motor deficit; few or no sensory findings, even though pain and sensory symptoms might be present; and no evidence of substantial axonal degeneration by electrodiagnostic studies. Factors favoring surgical intervention include a chronic and progressive course, neurologic deficit on examination (particularly a motor deficit), and electrodiagnostic evidence that the lesion has produced a significant degree of wallerian degeneration. Excellent reviews of compression and entrapment neuropathies include those of W.F. Brown

Table 19–3. GENETICALLY DETERMINED NEUROPATHIES*

Genetic Disorder	Inheritance Pattern	Age at Onset	Basic Process	Other Features	Other Systems Involved	Metabolic Defect	Comment
Peroneal muscular atrophy type I (HMSN-I, CMT-I)	Dominant	Decades 1–3	Demyelination	Hypertrophic changes with onion bulb formation; marked decrease in NCV	Pes cavus, congenital hip problems	Unknown	Most families link to chromosome 17 (HMSN-Ia); some families link to Duffy locus on chromosome 1 (HMSN-Ib)
Peroneal muscular atrophy type II (HMSN-II; CMT-II)	Dominant	Decades 3–5	Axonal	Marked decrease in NAP; NCV slowly decreased	Fewer have pes cavus	Unknown	Same as HMSN-I
Hereditary amyloid neuropathies	Dominant	Decades 3–4	Axonal	Small-fiber involvement; endoneurial amyloid deposition	Some families— cornea; dysautonomia often prominent	Prealbumin is major protein of amyloid fibril	Many different point mutations now known
Hereditary sensory neuropathy type I	Dominant	Decades 1–3	Neuronopathy	DRG neurons selectively involved	Sensorineural deafness, some families	Unknown	Frequent distal mutilation hands and feet
Porphyric neuropathy	Dominant	Adult life	Axonal	Neuropathy part of attacks; may be recurrent	Widespread cellular abnormality	Enzyme defects in porphyrin pathway	Acute intermittent porphyria, variegate porphyria, and erythropoietic porphyria
Hereditary liability to pressure palsy	Dominant	Decades 2–3	? Demyelination	Tomaculous changes in myelin	—	Unknown	Ulnar, peroneal, and brachial plexus involvement particularly
Fabry's disease	X-linked	Young males	Neuronopathy	Sensory neuronopathy, small DRG neurons	Kidney, skin lung	Accumulation of ceramide trihexoside	Neuropathy painful; often die of renal failure
Peroneal muscular atrophy (CMT-X) (Phillips et al., 1985)	X-linked	Decades 1–3	Axonal or demyelination	Heterozygote females may have symptoms	—	Unknown	Localizes to long arm of X chromosome
Adrenomyelo-neuropathy	X-linked	Young males	? Axonal	Mild neuropathy, spastic paraparesis, baldness, hypogonadism	Adrenal cortex, cerebral white matter, spinal cord	Accumulation of very long chain fatty acids	Phenotypic variant of adrenoleukodystrophy
Hereditary sensory neuropathy type II	Recessive	Decades 1–3	Neuronopathy	DRG neurons selectively involved	—	Unknown	May be less severe than type I
Déjérine-Sottas neuropathy (HMSN-III)	Recessive	1st decade	Demyelination	Hypertrophic change with onion bulb formation	May be retarded	Unknown	Marked nerve trunk enlargement
Refsum's disease	Recessive	1st or 2nd decade	Demyelination	Hypertrophic change with onion bulb formation	Retinitis pigmentosa, ichthyosis, sensorineural deafness	Defect in α oxidation of β-methyl fatty acids	Low phytanate diet, plasmapheresis therapy
Ataxia-telangiectasia	Recessive	Decades 1 or 2	Axonal	Neuropathy moderate	Cell nuclear aneuploidy, skin and scleral telangiectasia, cerebellar atrophy, immunopathy	Basic defect unknown	High incidence of early neoplasia
Hereditary tyrosinemia	Recessive	1st decade	Axonal	Acute, severe neuropathy	Hepatic failure and renal disease	Defect of fumaryl-acetoacetate hydrolase	Attacks resemble crises of neuropathic porphyria (Mitchell et al., 1990)
Anaphalipo-proteinemia	Recessive	Decades 1 or 2	Axonal	Small sensory fibers; unusual sensory pattern	Tonsillar hypertrophy; possibly hepatosplenomegaly	Absent high-density lipoprotein	Severity and pattern of neuropathy variable
Abetalipo-proteinemia	Recessive	Decades 1 or 2	Neuronopathy	Large DRG neurons	Retinitis; acanthocytosis of red blood cells	Absence of all lipoprotein containing apoB	Proprioceptive disturbance marked, minimal small-fiber deficit
Giant axonal neuropathy	Recessive	1st decade	Axonal	Massive segmental accumulation of neurofilaments	Slowly progressive encephalopathy with Rosenthal fibers	Generalized disorder of 10-nm filaments	Intermediate filament masses in other cell types

Table 19–3. GENETICALLY DETERMINED NEUROPATHIES* *Continued*

Genetic Disorder	Inheritance Pattern	Age at Onset	Basic Process	Other Features	Other Systems Involved	Metabolic Defect	Comment
Metachromatic leukodystrophy	Recessive	1st decade	Demyelination	Schwannopathy with cerebroside accumulation	Cerebral white matter disease predominates	Defect of arylsulfatase A	Infantile, juvenile, and adult-onset forms
Globoid cell leukodystrophy	Recessive	1st decade	Demyelination	Schwannopathy with galactocerebroside accumulation	Cerebral white matter disease predominates	Defect of β-galactosidase	Characteristic clefts in Schwann cell cytoplasm by electron microscopy
Friedreich's ataxia	Recessive	1st decade	Axonal	Spinocerebellar and corticospinal tracts involved; also primary sensory neuron	Cardiomyopathy usual cause of death	Controversial	Ataxia both sensory and cerebellar

*NAP = nerve action potential; NCV = nerve conduction velocity; DRG = dorsal root ganglion; HMSN = hereditary motor-sensory neuropathy; CMT = Charcot-Marie-Tooth disease.

(1987), Dawson et al. (1990), Gilliatt and Harrison (1984), Stewart (1987), and Stewart and Aguayo (1984).

Mononeuropathy Multiplex

The term *mononeuropathy multiplex* means simultaneous or sequential involvement of individual noncontiguous nerve trunks, either partially or completely, evolving during days to years. Because the disease process underlying mononeuropathy multiplex involves peripheral nerves in a multifocal and random fashion, there is a tendency, as worsening occurs, for the neurologic deficit to become less patchy and multifocal and more confluent and symmetric. Some patients initially have a distal symmetric neuropathy (Kissel et al., 1985). Attention to the pattern of early symptoms is therefore important in making the judgment that a particular neuropathy is indeed a mononeuropathy multiplex.

After the diagnosis is established, the next question is whether the process is primarily axonal or primarily demyelinating. Our experience indicates that almost one-third of all adults with the clinical syndrome of mononeuropathy multiplex have clear-cut findings of a demyelinating disorder, usually with multiple foci of persistent conduction block by electrodiagnostic examination. More intensive study of this subgroup (Lewis et al., 1982) suggests that the multifocal demyelinating neuropathy represents part of the spectrum of CIDP. Management of this multifocal subgroup is the same as for CIDP (see later).

The remaining two-thirds of patients with mononeuropathy multiplex exhibit axonal involvement, heterogeneously distributed, by electrodiagnostic examination. Although ischemia is suspected as the basis for neuropathy in these patients, only about one-half can be shown to have a systemic vasculitis affecting the vasa nervorum. The cause of the others remains undetermined, even on follow-up, and the basis for mononeuropathy multiplex in these cases is uncertain.

In individuals for whom vasculitic change in the vasa nervorum can be demonstrated, any of a large number of underlying disorders may be responsible. The primary vasculitides of the polyarteritis nodosa group constitute the most frequent cause, followed closely by vasculitis occurring in the course of connective tissue disorders. In descending order of frequency, these disorders are rheumatoid arthritis, systemic lupus erythematosus, and mixed connective tissue disease. As many as one-third of patients with vasculitis on nerve biopsy have nonsystemic vasculitic neuropathy, in which the vasculitic process is limited to peripheral nerve (Dyck et al., 1987a). This disorder represents an organ-specific form of leukocytoclastic angiitis analogous to the benign cutaneous vasculitis limited to skin. No clinical or serologic evidence of systemic involvement can be demonstrated, the course is relatively benign compared with that of a systemic vasculitis, and aggressive immunosuppression is seldom required. Other rarer causes of mononeuropathy multiplex caused by nerve ischemia from occlusion of the vasa nervorum include mixed cryoglobulinemia, Sjögren's syndrome, Wegener's granulomatosis, progressive systemic sclerosis, Churg-Strauss allergic granulomatosis, and hypersensitivity angiitis. Management of the neuropathy in each instance is predicated on the appropriate treatment of the responsible disease.

Pure Motor Neuropathy

In an exclusively lower motor neuron syndrome, the diagnostic possibilities are few (Bird, 1990). These disorders may be in the form of motor neuropathies or neuronopathies, which are often clinically indistinguishable. The syndrome of multifocal motor neuropathy (MMN) with conduction block has been described (Parry and Clarke, 1988). Other forms of lower motor neuron disease without conduction block may be distinct from amyotrophic lateral sclerosis. There are also acquired lower motor neuron disorders resulting from various toxic or infectious agents, such as lead, dapsone, and poliovirus. Hereditary disorders include the hereditary motor neuropathies (spinal muscular atrophy), hexosaminidase A deficiency, and porphyric neuropathy.

In some neuropathic disorders, motor dysfunction is the predominant abnormality. These disorders include acute inflammatory demyelinating polyneuropathy (GBS), some forms of CIDP, HMSN, and diphtheritic neuropathy. However, sensory involvement is usually evident in these disorders on clinical or electrophysiologic examination. Disorders of presynaptic neuromuscular transmission, such as the Lambert-Eaton myasthenic syndrome, tick paralysis, and organophosphate intoxication, may be confused clinically with motor neuropathies but can be distinguished electrodiagnostically.

Patients with MMN with conduction block were previously likely to have been considered to have purely motor CIDP or lower motor neuron forms of amyotrophic lateral sclerosis. However, this syndrome may be distinguished from these and other disorders by distinctive clinical, electrophysiologic, and immunologic features. Clinically, MMN is characterized by asymmetric, distally predominant limb weakness with no bulbar, upper motor neuron, or sensory involvement. The electrophysiologic hallmark of this disorder is multifocal conduction block limited to motor nerves. Unlike the case with CIDP, cerebrospinal fluid protein is typically normal, and few patients with MMN appear to respond to corticosteroid therapy. In some patients, aggressive immunosuppression with cyclophosphamide may result in improvement. Although the syndrome is defined by clinical and electrophysiologic criteria, many of those with MMN may have high titers of antiganglioside antibodies, particularly anti-GM$_1$ antibodies (Pestronk et al., 1990). Some patients with a lower motor neuron syndrome without multifocal conduction block may also have elevated antiganglioside titers. It is unclear whether this latter group represents a number of heterogeneous disorders or if conduction block was present but not identified electrophysiologically. The relationship between motor neuron syndromes and antibodies to gangliosides is intriguing, but no causal role has been established. These antibodies may be pathogenic; alternatively, they may be markers of autoimmune reactivity in general and not directly involved in the pathogenesis. As a third possibility, they may represent a secondary consequence of the disease process. Although there appears to be an association between certain lower motor neuron syndromes and high titers of anti-GM$_1$ antibodies, the clinical significance of these antibodies, particularly in low titers, remains uncertain.

Pure Sensory Neuropathy and Neuronopathy

In many neuropathies, the manifestations are primarily sensory. The predominant fiber type involved (large or small diameter) may be helpful in identifying the underlying disorder. Selective damage to small sensory fibers, with diminished pain-temperature sensation and autonomic dysfunction, occurs with certain axonal neuropathies, most commonly in association with diabetes. Other possibilities include amyloid polyneuropathies, sensory perineuritis, neuropathy associated with hyperlipidemia or primary biliary cirrhosis, leprous neuritis, or acquired immunodeficiency syndrome (AIDS)–associated neuropathy. Neuropathy caused by ciguatera toxin (reef fish poisoning) and chronic metronidazole or misonidazole use may present in a similar fashion. There are relatively few causes of large-fiber sensory neuropathy that are manifested by proprioceptive loss with ataxia. These are primarily demyelinating polyneuropathies, such as the rare sensory variant of CIDP and certain dysproteinemic neuropathies (anti–myelin-associated glycoprotein [MAG] antibody associated). Most patients with this clinical picture have sensory neuronopathies in which the primary pathologic event is in the dorsal root ganglion or trigeminal cell bodies. However, the clinical picture may be indistinguishable from that in sensory neuropathies.

Sensory neuronopathies are usually distinct and recognizable. Clinically, they cause symmetric acral, body-wide sensory loss and areflexia in contradistinction to the length-dependent changes seen in most axonal neuropathies. Unlike the case with sensory axonal neuropathies, there is little likelihood of recovery. This is because of the irreplaceable loss of sensory cell bodies. The type of sensory disturbance also reflects the size of the sensory neurons involved and the rate of progression. When small fibers are prominently involved or the course is acute or subacute, positive symptoms (pain and dysesthesias) occur frequently. Loss of large sensory neurons results in sensory ataxia and proprioceptive loss, pseudoathetosis, and areflexia. In all of these disorders of sensory neurons, a motor component is absent clinically. Electrodiagnostic study demonstrates reduced or absent sensory nerve action potentials with normal motor conduction studies. A minor degree of chronic partial denervation may be seen as a subclinical feature but is not prominent.

The rate of progression varies greatly, from acute to chronic, and may be helpful in arriving at the appropriate diagnosis (Asbury and Brown, 1990). Acute sensory neuronopathies evolve dramatically over days, and some cases may be related to the use of semisynthetic penicillins (Sterman et al., 1980). In other instances, no apparent cause is found, or the case is related to a disorder that usually causes a subacute sensory neuronopathy. Subacute sensory neuronopathies are most commonly associated with malignancy and Sjögren's syndrome or are idiopathic. Paraneoplastic sensory neuronopathy occurs mainly with small cell lung carcinoma. A specific antibody (anti-Hu) that binds to a 35- to 40-kd protein present in the nuclei of most neurons (including those of the dorsal root ganglia), and also in small cell lung carcinoma, is present in high titers in patients with this form of paraneoplastic sensory neuronopathy (Dalmau et al., 1990). When present, this antibody is considered to be an excellent diagnostic marker and is likely involved in the pathogenesis of the disorder as well. Although neuropathy associated with Sjögren's syndrome is most commonly in the form of polyneuropathy, a small subgroup of patients have a subacute sensory neuronopathy that can mimic the paraneoplastic disorder (Griffin et al., 1990). In both the paraneoplastic form and that associated with primary Sjögren's syndrome, the onset of sensory neuronopathy typically precedes the manifestations or diagnosis of the associated disorders.

Certain neurotoxins affect primarily the sensory system and in high doses result in subacute neuronopathy. These include cisplatin, pyridoxine (vitamin B_6), and taxol. Chronic sensory neuronopathies, evolving for years, may be inherited (hereditary sensory neuropathies). A subgroup of patients exhibit progressive idiopathic disorders that may be chronic or subacute. Some of these are associated with circulating paraproteins, particularly those that bind to MAG.

Autonomic Neuropathies

Autonomic disturbances often accompany neuropathic processes involving small myelinated and unmyelinated fibers. Neuropathies that may result in clinically prominent or even predominant autonomic abnormalities include those with diabetes mellitus and primary amyloidosis, the GBS, and inherited disorders such as the Riley-Day syndrome and familial amyloidosis. Pandysautonomia may be seen idiopathically or as a paraneoplastic disorder (McLeod, 1990).

Sudomotor abnormalities result in anhidrosis, hyperhidrosis, or heat intolerance. Loss of autonomic innervation to other organ systems may lead to specific patterns of dysfunction, including orthostatic hypotension, urinary retention, urinary frequency and incontinence, sexual impotence, gastrointestinal motility disorders, and pupillary abnormalities. The function and dysfunction of these various systems are discussed fully in Chapters 32 through 36.

Plexopathy

Brachial plexus lesions, which are usually unilateral, are relatively common and are readily distinguishable clinically from upper limb mononeuropathies (Mumenthaler, 1984). The usual causes are direct trauma to the plexus, cervical rib or bands (Gilliatt, 1984), malignant infiltration or compression (Kori et al., 1981), brachial neuritis (neuralgic amyotrophy) (England and Sumner, 1987), and damage from therapeutic radiation. As an approximation, injury to the upper plexus, which arises from C5-7

roots, results from particular types of trauma (arm jerked downward), brachial neuritis, and radiation damage. Findings localizing to the lower plexus, which arises from C8–T1 roots, are likely to be due to malignant infiltration, other types of trauma (arm jerked upward), and cervical rib or bands. Lederman and Wilbourn (1984) pointed out that malignant involvement of the brachial plexus is more likely to occur with pain, Horner's syndrome, and a subacute course; whereas radiation damage to the brachial plexus is more likely to exhibit paresthesias without pain, an indolent progression, and more prominent electrodiagnostic findings.

SPECIAL CATEGORIES OF NEUROPATHY

Hereditary Neuropathies

The major characteristics of the highly variegated group of hereditary neuropathies are summarized in Table 19–3. Some generalizations can be made. With the exception of the porphyric neuropathies, hereditary neuropathies have insidious onset of neuropathic dysfunction and indolent progression during years or decades. Most of these diseases are quite rare, with the striking exception of the dominantly inherited peroneal muscular atrophies (HMSN-I and -II, or CMT-I and -II). In peroneal muscular atrophy, phenotypic expression is often variable, so that affected family members of a propositus may have no symptoms and minimal neurologic findings but (in HMSN-I) may still show severe reduction of nerve conduction velocity.

Molecular genetic linkage studies of large kinships with autosomal dominantly inherited polyneuropathy and slow nerve conduction (HMSN-I) indicated genetic heterogeneity (Chance et al., 1990; Defesche et al., 1990; Timmerman et al., 1990; Vance et al., 1989). In a few families, the disease locus is tightly linked to the Duffy blood group locus on chromosome 1 (HMSN-Ib), but in many more families, the neuropathy locus is linked to markers in the pericentromeric region of chromosome 17 (HMSN-Ia). Different disease loci may exist on chromosome 17 (Chance et al., 1990), and some families do not evidence linkage to markers on either chromosome 1 or 17. Cloning specific disease-related genes for HMSN-I may be accomplished soon.

Acquired Neuropathies

Diabetic Neuropathies

Classifications of the neuropathies of diabetes have been put forward (M.J. Brown and Asbury, 1984; Bruyn and Garland, 1970; Dyck et al., 1987b; Thomas and Eliasson, 1984). (For a thorough monograph devoted to diabetic neuropathy, see Dyck et al., 1987b.) The classification in Table 19–4 is a variation

Table 19–4. CLASSIFICATION OF DIABETIC
NEUROPATHIES

Symmetric
1. Distal primarily sensory polyneuropathy
   a. Mainly large fibers affected
   b. Mixed*
   c. Mainly small fibers affected*
2. Autonomic neuropathy
3. Chronically evolving proximal motor neuropathy*†

Asymmetric
1. Rapidly evolving proximal motor neuropathy*†
2. Cranial mononeuropathy†
3. Truncal neuropathy*†
4. Entrapment neuropathy in the limbs

*Often painful.
†Recovery, partial or complete, is likely.

of these schemes. All of these cases do not fit neatly into a single category and may have features of several. By far the most common neuropathy is the distal primarily sensory polyneuropathy. Its occurrence appears to be mainly a function of the duration of diabetes, and its progress is insidious, probably remaining subclinical for years.

Distal symmetric polyneuropathy in diabetes is difficult to manage. An occasional patient with previous poor glycemic control can exhibit marked improvement of sensory function and lessening of pain if the diabetes is closely regulated. Such cases are not common, but optimal glycemic control remains the mainstay of treatment. The role of aldose reductase inhibitors in preventing the complications of diabetes mellitus is still unsettled.

Pathogenesis of diabetic polyneuropathy is also a subject of controversy. Unspecified metabolic derangements were previously postulated, but both Dyck et al. (1986) and Johnson et al. (1986) put forward evidence that endoneurial vascular factors also were at play. Low and colleagues (1987) demonstrated nerve hypoxia in experimental settings; altered myoinositol metabolism in peripheral nerves of diabetics is thought to be important (Greene and Lattimer, 1987), and nonenzymatic glycosylation of endoneurial structures may also play a role (Brownlee et al., 1988). How and whether all of these factors converge to damage peripheral nerve insidiously in diabetes during a period of time remains uncertain. Ischemia of nerve has also been suggested as the basis for many of the focal and multifocal neuropathies that occur in diabetes mellitus. Fortunately, most affected patients recover in months to a year or two without specific intervention other than attention to glycemic control. The management of entrapment neuropathies in diabetic patients is the same as for patients without diabetes.

Neuropathies with Other Systemic Metabolic Disorders

Uremia. Uremic polyneuropathy is a subacute or chronic motor-sensory polyneuropathy that occurs in the setting of long-standing renal failure. It has been extensively and critically reviewed (Bolton and Young, 1990). The polyneuropathy can be stabilized or prevented by adequate dialysis, unless the neuropathy is already advanced. Successful renal transplantation usually reverses the neuropathy, often with complete recovery. Pathologically, the neuropathy is marked by axonal atrophy, secondary demyelination, and eventual axonal degeneration in a centripetal pattern. Although neither a specific neurotoxin nor other mechanism for the polyneuropathy has been identified, there is pathophysiologic evidence of axolemmal dysfunction (decreased resting membrane potential, sodium channel abnormality, and slowing impulse propagation) (Nielsen, 1974).

Hepatic Disorders. The most common neuropathy associated with hepatic disorders is a mild, usually asymptomatic demyelinating polyneuropathy that occurs in a majority of individuals with chronic hepatic failure of diverse causes. Usually, the systemic liver disorder is of much greater consequence than the mild, often subclinical neuropathy. In childhood cholestatic liver disease, a progressive and severe large-fiber sensory neuropathy with sensory ataxia may result from secondary vitamin deficiency. In addition, in acute or chronic viral hepatitis, GBS may occur intercurrently and is presumably triggered by the viral infection. Finally, in primary bilary cirrhosis, cutaneous sensory neuropathies, often painfully dysesthetic, are recognized.

Chronic Respiratory Insufficiency. Although a relatively inconsequential axonal polyneuropathy has been recognized in advanced chronic obstructive pulmonary disease, it was not considered of clinical importance until almitrine, a respiratory stimulant, was introduced into the management of hypoxemic pulmonary disease. It is now clear that almitrine frequently induces a toxic polyneuropathy, but it is not known whether the underlying polyneuropathy of chronic respiratory insufficiency is additive to the toxic effects.

Critical Illness Polyneuropathy. Bolton and colleagues have written extensively on the subacute axonal polyneuropathy that occurs in severely ill patients in intensive care units who have multiple organ failure, sepsis, hypoalbuminemia, peripheral edema, and often profound weakness and wasting (Zochodne et al., 1987). This polyneuropathy, which may be severe enough to require mechanical ventilation, affects almost half of critically ill patients who have sepsis persisting longer than 2 weeks.

Toxic and Nutritional Neuropathies

Many therapeutic agents, chemicals, and nutritional deficiencies can cause a distal symmetric polyneuropathy with a length-dependent loss of sensory, reflex, and motor functions (see Table 19–2). Alcoholic polyneuropathy results from long-standing abuse and is likely due to malnutrition and associated vitamin deficiencies, although a direct toxic effect may also play a role. Neuropathy caused by deficiencies of water-soluble vitamin (particularly thiamine, pyridoxine, folate, and pantothenic acid) is also seen occasionally in anorexic individuals or those with malabsorption. The myelopathy of vitamin B$_{12}$ deficiency usually clinically overshadows the variably present polyneuropathy. Deficiency of fat-soluble vitamin E, usually from malabsorption, results in sensory ataxia from large-fiber involvement.

The neuropathies that occur with the use of antineoplastic agents are dose dependent and, if severe, may limit treatment. Neuropathogenic agents include vincristine and vinblastine, cisplatin, and newer products such as suramin (LaRocca et al., 1990) and taxol (Lipton et al., 1989). Vincristine inhibits microtubule assembly in axons, whereas taxol, a plant alkaloid, promotes microtubule assembly. In tissue culture, this latter effect results in abnormal bundles of microtubules. Both mechanisms disrupt normal cell functions, including axoplasmic transport, and may produce neuropathy. A number of other drugs, heavy metals, and industrial toxins produce polyneuropathy (see Table 19–2). A sensorimotor neuropathy is commonly a prominent manifestation of the epidemic illness eosinophilia-myalgia syndrome. This disorder is characterized by myalgia, eosinophilia, and various systemic manifestations. Eosinophilia-myalgia syndrome has been convincingly associated with the consumption of L-tryptophan and may be the result of a contaminant in the manufactured product. Sural nerve biopsies have demonstrated axonal degeneration with perineurial, and occasionally endoneurial, fibrosis and perivascular cell infiltrates (Heiman-Patterson et al., 1990). The exact pathogenesis of the neuropathy is unknown. The subacute neuropathy may be severe and has resulted in respiratory failure and death. There is no known effective therapy.

Selective involvement of large sensory neurons (sensory neuronopathy) by neurotoxins is a less common pattern than is distal symmetric sensorimotor polyneuropathy. Cisplatin, pyridoxine, and taxol are important examples of agents that cause this presentation. Dose-response studies using pyridoxine (Xu et al., 1989) demonstrated that the same neurotoxin can cause a neuronopathy in large doses but an indolent distal sensory axonal neuropathy in smaller doses. Megadose pyridoxine given to rats resulted in a neuronopathy with necrosis of dorsal root ganglion cells and centrifugal axonal degeneration, whereas chronic low-dose administration produced a neuropathy with perikaryal and axonal atrophy. This model supports the concept that a sublethal sensory neuronal lesion underlies the pathogenesis of at least some types of toxic neuropathy.

Inflammatory Vascular Disorders

Inflammatory vascular disorders may cause an axonal sensorimotor polyneuropathy or mononeuropathy multiplex. This is seen most commonly with vasculitides, connective tissue diseases, and sarcoidosis. Although some patients may have systemic manifestations of the underlying disease, it is common for the neuropathy to be the presenting feature. Neuropathy may occur in up to half of those with a primary vasculitis, such as polyarteritis nodosa. Allergic granulomatous angiitis (Churg-Strauss) may be associated with eosinophilia and asthma; hypersensitivity angiitis frequently involves skin in addition to nerve. Granulomatous vasculitis of nerve, respiratory tract, and kidneys is characteristic of Wegener's granulomatosis. Other connective tissue disorders, such as rheumatoid arthritis and systemic lupus erythematosus, are frequently associated with necrotizing angiitis of nerve. Neuropathy is less often a feature of mixed connective tissue disease, scleroderma, and Sjögren's syndrome. Sjögren's syndrome may also be manifest as a sensory and autonomic neuropathy, as a sensory neuronopathy, or with cranial mononeuropathies (particularly trigeminal). Sarcoidosis may produce a granulomatous polyneuropathy or polyradiculopathy. As discussed earlier, isolated vasculitis of peripheral nerve (nonsystemic vasculitic neuropathy) is important to recognize because of its relatively benign prognosis. Quantitative immunohistochemical analyses of nerve biopsy specimens from patients with vasculitis suggested that the primary mechanism of injury is a direct T cell–mediated cytotoxic process (Kissel et al., 1989). No differences are seen between those with systemic vasculitides and those with isolated nerve vasculitis. The neuropathies associated with human immunodeficiency virus (HIV) infection are discussed in Chapter 98.

Dysproteinemic Neuropathies

An association between polyneuropathy and both myeloma and macroglobulinemia has been recognized for many years. Although multiple myeloma with either lytic or diffuse osteoporotic bone lesions is commonly encountered, it is associated with clinically overt polyneuropathy relatively infrequently (approximately 5% of cases). These neuropathies are sensorimotor, may be severe, and generally do not reverse with successful suppression of the myeloma. Electrodiagnostic and pathologic features are consistent with a process of axonal degeneration in most cases (see Table 19–1).

In contrast, myeloma with osteosclerotic features, although representing only 3% of all myelomas, is associated with a polyneuropathy in almost one-half of cases. It is characterized by single or multiple osteosclerotic lesions on radiographic skeletal survey. These neuropathies seem to be different from those linked to multiple myeloma (Ohi et al., 1985) in that they (1) often respond to radiation or removal of the primary lesion, (2) are demyelinating in character, (3) associate with different monoclonal proteins and light chains (almost all λ as opposed to mostly κ in multiple myeloma), and (4) frequently manifest other systemic findings. These include skin thickening, hyperpigmentation, hypertrichosis, organomegaly, endocrinopathy, anasarca, papilledema, and clubbing of fingers, the whole constellation being referred to as POEMS (polyneuropathy, organomegaly, endocrinopathy, M protein, and skin changes), polyneuropathy, endocrinopathy, paraproteinemia, or Crow-Fukase syndrome (Bardwick et al., 1980; Nakanishi et al., 1984). Diagnosis is confirmed by biopsy of the osteosclerotic lesion.

A monoclonal gammopathy of undetermined significance is found in up to 5–10% of patients with a polyneuropathy of unknown cause. This immunoglobulin M (IgM) serum spike, usually modest in size and with κ light chain, is associated with a demyelinating neuropathy, which often has a protracted course and indolent progression. In about one-quarter to one-half of cases, the monoclonal serum protein binds to normal human peripheral myelin, specifically to MAG (Latov et al., 1988). In other rare instances, the IgM protein binds to certain gangliosides or glycoproteins. The MAG-associated neuropathies are clinically and electrophysiologically homogeneous (Kelly, 1990; Kelly et al., 1988). This distinct syndrome is characterized by indolently progressive, predominantly large-fiber sensory abnormalities (loss of proprioception, ataxia, and areflexia) and to a lesser degree loss of pain and temperature modalities and weakness. Immunocytochemical studies show binding of IgM to nerve obtained from these patients at biopsy or autopsy, but in a pattern different from that seen after incubation of nerve with the IgM serum. Incubated nerves show uniform staining of the entire expanse of compact myelin sheath, but in vivo deposited IgM can be demonstrated to localize more selectively, probably at sites of myelin splitting (Mendell et al., 1985). The myelin-splitting phenomenon is only seen in MAG-associated neuropathies. Whether the IgM bound to nerve in vivo plays a role in damaging the nerve is still a vexing question, although plasmapheresis has been successful in treating some patients with MAG-associated neuropathy.

Neuropathy Caused by Infectious Agents

Leprosy is a common cause of neuropathy worldwide (Sabin and Swift, 1975). *Mycobacterium leprae* organisms readily invade Schwann cells in cutaneous nerve twigs, particularly those associated with unmyelinated nerve fibers. Two major forms of leprous neuritis are recognized, tuberculoid and lepromatous, which actually represent the extremes of a spectrum of disease, with dimorphous leprosy (patchy and multifocal involvement of skin and nerve) being intermediate. Tuberculoid (high-resistance) leprosy is restricted to a single patch of hypoesthetic or anesthetic skin in any location. The skin patch is frequently thickened, reddened, or hypopigmented. If a superficially placed nerve trunk,

typically a cutaneous nerve, courses just beneath the area of affected skin, it may be engulfed in the inflammatory reaction, resulting in an associated mononeuropathy. Such a nerve may be palpably enlarged and beaded. Lepromatous (low-resistance) leprosy is marked by immunologic tolerance and widespread skin thickening, cutaneous anesthesia, and anhidrosis, sparing only the warmest parts of the body, notably the axilla, the groin, and beneath the scalp hair. Motor signs (focal weakness and atrophy) result from damage to mixed nerves lying close to the skin, particularly median, ulnar, peroneal, and facial nerves. Management of leprous neuritis is complex, involving extensive patient education, protection of insensitive parts, and protracted, perhaps lifelong, therapy with dapsone and adjunctive drugs such as rifampin and clofazimine.

Peripheral nerve disease is a late manifestation of infection with the tick-borne spirochete *Borrelia burgdorferi* (Lyme disease) (Halperin et al., 1990). In addition to cranial neuropathy and polyradiculopathy, sensorimotor polyneuropathy is common in a large percentage of untreated patients. It is predominantly sensory and generally mild. The neuropathic abnormalities are reversible, clinically and electrophysiologically, with antibiotic therapy. It is rarely, if ever, associated with a demyelinating neuropathy.

Neuropathy is common with HIV infection and occurs in several forms, depending on the stage of the infection (Parry, 1989). GBS or CIDP may be the presenting feature of previously asymptomatic HIV infection. The clinical and electrophysiologic features are similar to those with GBS or CIDP without HIV seropositivity, but lymphocytic pleocytosis is often more prominent in the cerebrospinal fluid (Cornblath et al., 1987). These neuropathies are likely autoimmune because they are uncommon in AIDS patients who are severely immunocompromised and they respond to plasmapheresis or corticosteroids. Whether nerve infection by the virus plays a direct role or facilitates an immune response against myelin is unclear. Neuropathy in the form of CIDP or mononeuropathy multiplex may be seen in patients with the AIDS-related complex. In those patients with multifocal axonal degeneration, overt vasculitis has been occasionally reported. A distal symmetric sensory-predominant polyneuropathy is the most common neuropathic syndrome in persons with AIDS. The pathogenesis is suspected to be due to infection with HIV but this is not proved. Improvement with zidovudine has been reported. Polyradiculopathy, often as a cauda equina syndrome, is seen in those with AIDS and is most often due to cytomegalovirus infection. Ganciclovir, an acyclovir analogue, has been effective therapy in this latter disorder.

Herpes zoster is a sensory neuritis characterized by acute inflammation of one or more dorsal root ganglia and is caused by varicella-zoster virus infection. Lancinating pain and hyperalgesia in the skin of affected dermatomes occur for 3–4 days, followed by the appearance of herpetic eruption in the same distribution. Painful raised blisters on reddened bases characterize the eruption. If the inflammatory process spreads to involve adjacent motor roots of anterior horns of the cord, segmental motor weakness and wasting appear. Paralysis of the oculomotor nerves may occur in conjunction with ophthalmic division involvement of the trigeminal ganglion (ophthalmoplegic zoster). Facial paralysis may occur with involvement of the geniculate ganglion and herpetic eruption on the ipsilateral tympanic membrane or external canal (Ramsay Hunt syndrome). In a small proportion of cases, pain does not subside in a few weeks as expected but persists indefinitely as a dysesthetic, hyperpathic postherpetic neuralgia. This sequence is most common in herpes zoster ophthalmicus. Management includes the use of tricyclic antidepressants (amitriptyline) or of carbamazepine.

Guillain-Barré Syndrome

GBS is an acute, frequently severe and fulminant polyneuropathy (Arnason, 1984). It occurs at a rate of one case per million population per month, or approximately 3500 cases per year in North America. In more than two-thirds of cases, a viral infection, either clinically overt or evidenced by serum titer rise, precedes the onset of neuropathy by 1–3 weeks. Herpesvirus (cytomegalovirus, Epstein-Barr virus) infection accounts for a large proportion of virus-triggered cases. A surgical procedure precedes by 1–4 weeks another 5–10% of cases (Arnason and Asbury, 1968), and GBS appears to occur on a background of lymphoma, including Hodgkin's disease, and lupus erythematosus more frequently than is attributable to chance alone. Although the weight of evidence suggests that GBS is immune mediated (see McFarlin, 1990), the immunopathogenesis remains obscure. In 1976–1977, a flurry of some 500 cases followed the national swine influenza vaccination program in the United States, which exceeded by several-fold the baseline incidence expected in this period among the vaccinees. The epidemiologic features of this outbreak have been analyzed (Safranek et al., 1991).

The clinical features of GBS typically include areflexic motor paralysis with mild sensory disturbance coupled with acellular rise in total protein level in the cerebrospinal fluid by the end of the first week of symptoms. The diagnostic criteria (Asbury et al., 1978) promulgated for the purposes of field surveys are generally accepted. Most patients with GBS require hospitalization, and about one-third need ventilatory assistance at some point during the illness. Prognosis is good; approximately 85% of patients make complete or nearly complete recovery in time. The mortality rate is 3–4%.

The most important factors in determining prognosis of GBS are (1) the age of the patient, (2) the severity in terms of the necessity for respiratory assistance, (3) the severity of the electrodiagnostic findings when the patient is first seen, and (4) whether plasmapheresis is carried out (McKhann et al., 1988). Plasmapheresis, if done in the first 2–3 weeks of illness, shortens the time to regain the capacity to walk unassisted (Guillain-Barré Syndrome Study Group, 1985), may lessen the maximal deficit (French Cooperative Group in Plasma Exchange in Guillain-Barré Syndrome, 1987), and may also lessen the degree of residual dysfunction. Other therapeutic approaches under investigation include high-dose intravenous immunoglobulin (Kleyweg et al., 1988) and pulsed high-dose intravenous corticosteroids (Hughes et al., 1991, study in progress in London).

Chronic Inflammatory Demyelinating Polyradiculoneuropathy

CIDP, a relatively common neuropathy, has many features in common with GBS, such as widespread, often patchy, demyelination of sensory and motor nerves and roots; elevated cerebrospinal fluid protein levels; and a probable immunopathologic basis. Differences from GBS include slower evolution and time course, relative paucity of antecedent events, less inflammatory cell infiltrate in nerve tissue (Barohn et al., 1989), and lack of demyelinating activity in patient serum when tested in experimental systems. Two major subgroups can be recognized, a relapsing group with an average age of onset of 27 years and a progressive or monophasic group with mean age of onset of 51 years (McCombe et al., 1987).

Management of CIDP has been based on the use of corticosteroids, other more potent immunosuppressants (azathioprine, cyclophosphamide) in selected cases, and plasmapheresis. High-dose intravenous immunoglobulin has been beneficial in some cases (van Doorn et al., 1990).

Miscellany

Ischemia of nerve severe enough to produce clinical symptoms has as its basis widespread compromise of blood flow in the vasa nervorum. Typically, this is the result of small-vessel disease involving the vasa nervorum directly, as occurs with vasculitis, rather than large-vessel disease. Clinically, widespread vasa nervorum diseases produce mononeuropathy multiplex, which electrodiagnostically has the features of a patchy axonal process. Occasionally, occlusion of a proximal limb artery or shunting of flow results in an axonal neuropathy in all distal nerves of the limb. In the arms, this ischemic monomelic neuropathy is most often the result of arteriovenous shunt placement for hemodialysis.

Cold exerts deleterious effects on peripheral nerve directly, without an intermediate step of ischemia being necessary. Cold injury to nerve occurs after prolonged exposure, usually of limb or limbs, to moderately low temperatures, as with immersion of the feet in seawater; actual freezing of tissue is not required. Axonal degeneration of myelinated fibers is the pathologic expression of cold injury (Nukada et al., 1981; Peyronnard et al., 1977). Physiologic studies have suggested that the most pronounced changes may be localized to the distal portion of the nerve at the nerve fiber-receptor junction (Carter et al., 1988). Frequently, limbs affected by cold injury to nerve show sensory deficit and dysesthesias, cutaneous vasomotor instability, painfulness, and marked sensitivity to minimal cold exposure, which persists for many years (Suri et al., 1978). The pathophysiology of this phenomenon is uncertain.

Trophic changes accompanying severe neuropathy deserve mention. The array of observable changes in completely denervated muscle, bone, and skin, including hair and nails, is well known, if incompletely understood. It is unclear what portion of the changes are due purely to denervation versus those caused by disuse, immobility, lack of weight bearing, and particularly recurrent, unnoticed painless trauma. Considerable evidence favors the view that ulceration of skin, poor healing, tissue resorption, neurogenic arthropathy, and mutilation are the result of repeated heedless injury to insensitive parts. As such, this sequence of events is avoidable with proper care and monitoring (Brand and Ebner, 1969; Sabin and Swift, 1975).

References

(Key references are designated with an asterisk.)

Arnason B.G.W. Acute inflammatory demyelinating polyradiculoneuropathies. In Dyck P.J., Thomas P.K., Lambert E.H., et al., eds. *Peripheral Neuropathy.* 2nd ed. Philadelphia, Saunders, pp. 2050–2100, 1984.

Arnason B.G.W., Asbury A.K. Idiopathic polyneuritis after surgery. *Arch. Neurol.* 18:500–507, 1968.

Asbury A.K. The clinical view of neurosmuscular electrophysiology. In Sumner A.J., ed. *The Physiology of Peripheral Nerve Disease.* Philadelphia, Saunders, pp. 484–491, 1980.

Asbury A.K. New aspects of disease of the peripheral nervous system. In Isselbacher K.J., Adams R.D., eds. *Harrison's Principles of Internal Medicine.* Update 4. New York, McGraw-Hill, pp. 211–219, 1983.

Asbury A.K. Pain in generalized neuropathies. In Fields H.L., ed. *Pain Syndromes in Neurology.* London, Butterworth, pp. 131–142, 1990.

Asbury A.K., Brown M.J. Sensory neuronopathy and pure sensory neuropathy. *Curr. Opin. Neurol. Neurosurg.* 3:708–711, 1990.

Asbury A.K., Fields H.L. Pain due to peripheral nerve damage: an hypothesis. *Neurology* 34:1587–1590, 1984.

*Asbury A.K., Gilliatt R.W., eds. *Peripheral Nerve Disorders: A Practical Approach.* London, Butterworth, 1984.

Asbury A.K., Arnason B.G., Karp H.R., et al. Criteria for diagnosis of Guillain-Barré syndrome. *Ann. Neurol.* 3:565–567, 1978.

Bardwick P.A., Zvaifler M.H., Gill G.N., et al. Plasma cell neoplasia with polyneuropathy, organonegaly, endocrinopathy, M protein and skin changes: the POEMS syndrome. *Medicine* 59:311–322, 1980.

Barohn R.J., Kissel J.T., Warmolts J.R., et al. Chronic inflammatory demyelinating polyradiculoneuropathy: clinical characteristics, course, and recommendations for diagnostic criteria. *Arch. Neurol.* 46:878–884, 1989.

Bird S.J. Pure motor neuropathy. *Curr. Opin. Neurol. Neurosurg.* 3:704–707, 1990.

*Bolton C.F., Young G.B. *Neurological Complications of Renal Failure.* London, Butterworth, 1990.

Brand P.W., Ebner J.D. Pressure sensitive devices for denervated hands and feet. *J. Bone Joint Surg. [Am.]* 51:109–116, 1969.

Brown M.J., Asbury A.K. Diabetic neuropathy. *Ann. Neurol.* 15:2–12, 1984.

Brown M.J., Martin J.R., Asbury A.K. Painful diabetic neuropathy—a morphometric study. *Arch. Neurol.* 33:164–171, 1976.

Brown W.F. The place of electromyography in the analysis of traumatic peripheral nerve lesions. In Brown W.F., Bolton C.F., eds. *Clinical Electromyography.* Stoneham, Butterworth, pp. 159–175, 1987.

Brownlee M., Cerami A., Vlassara H. Advanced glycosylation end products in tissue and the biochemical basis of diabetic complications. *N. Engl. J. Med.* 318:1315–1321, 1988.

Bruyn G.W., Garland H. Neuropathies of endocrine origin. In Vinken P.J., Bruyn G.W., eds. *Handbook of Clinical Neurology.* Vol. 8. Amsterdam, North Holland, pp. 29–71, 1970.

Carter J.L., Shefner J.M., Krarup C. Cold-induced peripheral nerve damage: involvement of touch receptors of the foot. *Muscle Nerve* 11:1065–1069, 1988.

Chance P.F., Bird T.D., O'Connell P., et al. Genetic linkage and heterogeneity in type I Charcot-Marie-Tooth disease (hereditary motor and sensory neuropathy type I). *Am. J. Hum. Genet.* 47:915–925, 1990.

Cornblath D.R., McArthur J.C., Kennedy P.E., et al. Inflammatory demyelinating peripheral neuropathies associated with human T-cell lymphotrophic virus type III infection. *Ann. Neurol.* 21:32–40, 1987.

Dalmau J., Furneaux H.M., Gralla R.J., et al. Detection of the anti-Hu antibody in the serum of patients with small cell lung cancer: a quantitative Western blot analysis. *Ann. Neurol.* 27:544–552, 1990.

Dawson D.M., Hallett M., Millender L.H. *Entrapment Neuropathies.* 2nd ed. Boston, Little, Brown, pp. 1–484, 1990.

Defesche J.C., Hoogendijk J.E., de Visser M., et al. Genetic linkage of hereditary motor and sensory neuropathy type I (Charcot-Marie-Tooth disease) to markers of chromosomes 1 and 17. *Neurology* 40:1450–1453, 1990.

Dyck P.J., Arnason B.G.W. Chronic inflammatory demyelinating polyradiculoneuropathy. In Dyck P.J., Thomas P.K., Lambert E.H., et al., eds. *Peripheral Neuropathy.* 2nd ed. Philadelphia, Saunders, pp. 2101–2114, 1984.

Dyck P.J., Lambert E.H. Dissociated sensation in amyloidosis: compound action potential, quantitative histologic and teased-fiber, and electron microscopic studies of sural nerve biopsies. *Arch. Neurol.* 20:490–507, 1969.

Dyck P.J., Lambert E.H. Polyneuropathy associated with hypothyroidism. *J. Neuropathol. Exp. Neurol.* 29:631–658, 1970.

*Dyck P.J., Thomas P.K., Lambert E.H., et al., eds. *Peripheral Neuropathy.* 2nd ed. Philadelphia, Saunders, 1984.

Dyck P.J., Karnes J., O'Brien P.C., et al. The spatial distribution of fiber loss in diabetic polyneuropathy suggests ischemia. *Ann. Neurol.* 19:440–449, 1986.

Dyck P.J., Benstead T.J., Conn D.L., et al. Nonsystemic vasculitic neuropathy. *Brain* 110:843–853, 1987a.

Dyck P.J., Karnes J., O'Brien P.C. Diagnosis, staging, and classification of diabetic neuropathy and association with other complications. In Dyck P.J., Thomas P.K., Asbury A.K., et al., eds. *Diabetic Neuropathy.* Philadelphia, Saunders, pp. 36–44, 1987b.

England J.D., Sumner A.J. Neuralgic amyotrophy: an increasingly diverse entity. *Muscle Nerve* 10:60–68, 1987.

French Cooperative Group in Plasma Exchange in Guillain-Barré Syndrome. Efficiency of plasma exchange in Guillain-Barré syndrome: role of replacement fluids. *Ann. Neurol.* 22:753–761, 1987.

Gilliatt R.W. Thoracic outlet syndromes. In Dyck P.J., Thomas P.K., Lambert E.H., et al., eds. *Peripheral Neuropathy.* 2nd ed. Philadelphia, Saunders, pp. 1409–1424, 1984.

Gilliatt R.W., Harrison M.J.G. Nerve compression and entrapment. In Asbury A.K., Gilliatt R.W., eds. *Peripheral Nerve Disorders: A Practical Approach.* London, Butterworth, pp. 243–286, 1984.

Greene D.A., Lattimer S.A. Altered myo-inositol metabolism in diabetic nerve. In Dyck P.J., Thomas P.K., Asbury A.K., et al., eds. *Diabetic Neuropathy.* Philadelphia, Saunders, pp. 289–298, 1987.

Griffin J.W., Cornblath D.R., Alexander E., et al. Ataxic sensory neuropathy and dorsal root ganglionitis associated with Sjogren's syndrome. *Ann. Neurol.* 27:304–315, 1990.

Guillain-Barré Syndrome Study Group. Plasmapheresis and acute Guillain-Barré syndrome. *Neurology* 35:1096–1104, 1985.

Halperin J., Luft B.J., Volkman D.J., et al. Lyme neuroborreliosis: peripheral nervous system manifestations. *Brain* 113:1207–1221, 1990.

Hawley R.F., Cohen M.H., Saini N., et al. The carcinomatous neuromyopathy of oat-cell lung cancer. *Ann. Neurol.* 7:65–72, 1980.

Heiman-Patterson T.D., Bird S.J., Parry G.J., et al. Peripheral neuropathy associated with eosinophilia-myalgia syndrome. *Ann. Neurol.* 28:522–528, 1990.

Johnson P.C., Doll S.C., Cromey D.W. Pathogenesis of diabetic neuropathy. *Ann. Neurol.* 19:450, 1986.

Katrak S.M., Pollock M., O'Brien C.P., et al. Clinical and morphological features of gold neuropathy. *Brain* 103:671–687, 1980.

Kelly J.J. The electrodiagnostic findings in polyneuropathies associated with IgM monoclonal gammopathies. *Muscle Nerve* 13:1113–1117, 1990.

Kelly J.J., Kyle R.A., O'Brien P.C., et al. The natural history of peripheral neuropathy in primary systemic amyloidosis. *Ann. Neurol.* 6:1–7, 1979.

Kelly J.J., Adelman L.S., Barkman E., et al. Polyneuropathies associated with IgM monoclonal gammopathies. *Arch. Neurol.* 45:1355–1359, 1988.

Kissel J.T., Slivka A.P., Warmolts J.R., et al. The clinical spectrum of necrotizing angiopathy of the peripheral nervous system. *Ann. Neurol.* 18:251–257, 1985.

Kissel J.T., Reithman J.L., Omerza J., et al. Peripheral nerve vasculitis: immune characterization of vascular lesions. *Ann. Neurol.* 25:291–297, 1989.

Kleyweg R.P., van der Meché F.G.A., Meulstee J. Treatment of Guillain-Barré syndrome with high-dose gammaglobulin. *Neurology* 38:1639–1641, 1988.

Kori S.H., Foley K.M., Posner J.B. Brachial plexus lesions in patients with cancer: 100 cases. *Neurology* 31:45–50, 1981.

LaRocca R.V., Meer J., Gilliatt R.W., et al. Suramin-induced polyneuropathy. *Neurology* 40:954–960, 1990.

Latov N., Hays A.P., Sherman W.H. Peripheral neuropathy and anti-MAG antibodies. *Crit. Rev. Neurobiol.* 3:301–332, 1988.

*Layzer R.B. *Neuromuscular Manifestations of Systemic Disease.* Contemporary Neurology Series.* Vol. 25. Philadelphia, Davis, 1984.

Lederman R.J., Wilbourn A.J. Brachial plexopathy: recurrent cancer or radiation? *Neurology* 34:1331–1335, 1984.

Lewis R.A., Sumner A.J., Brown M.J., et al. Multifocal demyelinating neuropathy with persistent conduction block. *Neurology* 32:958–964, 1982.

Lipton R.B., Apfel S.C., Dutcher J.P., et al. Taxol produces a predominantly sensory neuropathy. *Neurology* 39:368–373, 1989.

Low P.A., McLeod J.G., Turtle J.R., et al. Peripheral neuropathy in acromegaly. *Brain* 97:139–147, 1974.

Low P.A., Tuck R.R., Takeuchi M. Nerve micro-environment in diabetic neuropathy. In Dyck P.J., Thomas P.K., Asbury A.K., et al., eds. *Diabetic Neuropathy.* Philadelphia, Saunders, pp. 266–278, 1987.

McCombe P.A., Pollard J.D., McLeod J.G. Chronic inflammatory demyelinating polyradiculoneuropathy: a clinical and electrophysiological study of 92 cases. *Brain* 110:1617–1630, 1987.

McFarlin D.E. Immunological parameters in Guillain-Barré syndrome. *Ann. Neurol.* 27(Suppl.):S25–S29, 1990.

McKhann G.M., Griffin J.W., Cornblath D.R., et al. Guillain-Barré Syndrome Study Group: plasmapheresis and the Guillain-Barré syndrome: analysis of prognostic factors and the effect of plasmapheresis. *Ann. Neurol.* 23:347–353, 1988.

McLeod J.G. Autonomic dysfunction in peripheral nerve disease. In Bannister R., ed. *Autonomic Failure.* London, Oxford University Press, pp. 607–623, 1990.

Mendell J.R., Sahenk Z., Whitaker J.N., et al. Polyneuropathy and IgM monoclonal gammopathy: studies on the pathogenetic role of anti–myelin-associated-glycoprotein antibody. *Ann. Neurol.* 17:243–254, 1985.

Mitchell G., Larochelle J., Lambert M., et al. Neurologic crises in hereditary tyrosinemia. *N. Engl. J. Med.* 322:432–437, 1990.

Mumenthaler M. Brachial plexus neuropathies. In Dyck P.J.,

Thomas P.K., Lambert E.H., et al., eds. *Peripheral Neuropathy.* 2nd ed. Philadelphia, Saunders, pp. 1383–1393, 1984.

Nakanishi T., Sobue I., Toyokura Y., et al. The Crow-Fukase syndrome: a study of 102 cases in Japan. *Neurology* 34:712–720, 1984.

Nielsen V.K. The peripheral nerve function in chronic renal failure: X. Decremental nerve conduction in uremia? *Acta Med. Scand.* 196:83, 1974.

Nukada H., Pollock M., Allpress S. Experimental cold injury to peripheral nerve. *Brain* 104:779–811, 1981.

Ohi T., Kyle R.A., Dyck P.J. Axonal attenuation and secondary segmental demyelination in myeloma neuropathies. *Ann. Neurol.* 17:255–261, 1985.

Parry G.J. Peripheral neuropathies associated with human immunodeficiency virus infection. *Ann. Neurol.* 23(Suppl.):S49–S53, 1988.

Parry G.J., Clark S. Multifocal acquired demyelinating neuropathy masquerading as motor neuron disease. *Muscle Nerve* 11:103–107, 1988.

Pestronk A., Chaudhry V., Feldman E.L., et al. Lower motor neuron syndromes defined by patterns of weakness, nerve conduction abnormalities, and high titers of antiglycolipid antibodies. *Ann. Neurol.* 27:316–326, 1990.

Peyronnard J.M., Pedneault M., Aguayo A.J. Neuropathies due to cold: quantitative studies of structural changes in human and animal nerves. *Excerpta Med. Int. Congr. Ser.* 434:308–329, 1977.

Phillips L.H., Kelly T.E., Schnatterly P., et al. Hereditary motor-sensory neuropathy (HMSN): possible X-linked dominant inheritance. *Neurology* 35:498–502, 1985.

Sabin T.D., Swift T.R. Leprosy. In Dyck P.J., Thomas P.K., Lambert E.H., eds. *Peripheral Neuropathy.* Philadelphia, Saunders, pp. 1166–1198, 1975.

Safranek T.J., Lawrence D.N., Kurland L.T., et al. Reassessment of the association between Guillain-Barré syndrome and receipt of swine influenza vaccine in 1976–1977: results of a two-state study. *Am. J. Epidemiol.* 133:1–12, 1991.

Said G., Ropert A., Faux N. Length-dependent degeneration of fibers in Portugese amyloid polyneuropathy. *Neurology* 34:1025–1032, 1984.

*Schaumburg H.H., Spencer P.S., Thomas P.K. *Disorders of Peripheral Nerves. Contemporary Neurology Series.* Vol. 24. Philadelphia, Davis, 1983.

*Spencer P.S., Schaumburg H.H., eds. *Experimental and Clinical Neurotoxicology.* Baltimore, Williams & Wilkins, 1980.

Sterman A.B., Schaumburg H.H., Asbury A.K. The acute sensory neuronopathy syndrome: a distinct clinical entity. *Ann. Neurol.* 7:354–358, 1980.

Stewart J.D. *Focal Peripheral Neuropathies.* New York, Elsevier, 1987.

Stewart J.D., Aguayo A.J. Compression and entrapment neuropathies. In Dyck P.J., Thomas P.K., Lambert E.H., et al., eds. *Peripheral Neuropathy.* 2nd ed. Philadelphia, Saunders, pp. 1435–1457, 1984.

Sumner A.J., ed. *The Physiology of Peripheral Nerve Disease.* Philadelphia, Saunders, 1980.

Suri M.L., Vijayan G.P., Puri H.C., et al. Neurological manifestations of frostbite. *Indian J. Med. Res.* 67:292–299, 1978.

Thomas P.K., Eliasson S.G. Diabetic neuropathy. In Dyck P.J., Thomas P.K., Lambert E.H., et al., eds. *Peripheral Neuropathy.* 2nd ed. Philadelphia, Saunders, pp. 1773–1810, 1984.

Timmerman V., Raeymaekers P., DeJonghe P., et al. Assignment of the Charcot-Marie-Tooth neuropathy type 1 (CMTa) gene to 17p11.2-p12. *Am. J. Hum. Genet.* 47:680–685, 1990.

Vance J.M., Nicholson G.A., Yamaoka L.H., et al. Linkage of Charcot-Marie-Tooth neuropathy type 1a to chromosome 17. *Exp. Neurol.* 104:186–189, 1989.

van Doorn P.A., Brand A., Strengers P.F.W., et al. High-dose intravenous immunoglobulin treatment in chronic inflammatory demyelinationg polyneuropathy: a double-blind, placebo-controlled, crossover study. *Neurology* 40:209–212, 1990.

Xu Y., Sladky J.T., Brown M.J. Dose-dependent expression of neuropathy after experimental pyridoxine intoxication. *Neurology* 39:1077–1083, 1989.

Zochodne D.W., Bolton C.F., Wells G.A., et al. Critical illness polyneuropathy. A complication of sepsis and multiple organ failure. *Brain* 110:819–941, 1987.

20

The Myotatic Unit and Its Disorders

David Burke
James W. Lance

The term *myotatic reflex* was coined by Liddell and Sherrington (1924) as an alternative for "reflexes produced by muscle stretch." Basically, similar reflex mechanisms are brought into play by various maneuvers, such as overt muscle stretching, halting a shortening contraction, electrically stimulating afferent fibers from muscle, stimulating muscle receptors by vibration, and in opposite sense, muscle unloading. As a general term, myotatic is preferable to proprioceptive, because in Sherrington's classification, proprioceptive reflexes included those of vestibular origin. The myotatic unit comprises those neural elements essential for the myotatic reflex—muscle receptors and their afferent fibers, spinal pathways, motor neurons, and muscle (Fig. 20–1). In this chapter, emphasis is placed on data that are relevant to or have been obtained from human subjects.

MUSCLE RECEPTORS AND THEIR INNERVATION

Skeletal muscle makes up the largest sensory organ in the body. Myotatic reflexes depend on the activity of mechanoreceptors, and of these, only the muscle spindle and the Golgi tendon are considered in detail. However, their afferent fibers constitute only about 20% of the 1500 afferents coming from the triceps surae muscles of the cat (Kniffki et al., 1981). Most of the remainder come from undifferentiated free nerve endings, responsive to nociceptive, thermal, or mechanical stimuli. There are also some that probably contribute to the cardiorespiratory responses to exercise. These afferents are small and slowly conducting, the majority being unmyelinated (called group IV muscle afferents), the rest being small myelinated fibers (mainly group III and some group II).

Natural movement is accompanied by active and passive changes in length of all muscles acting on the moving joint, by distortion of joint capsule, and by deformation of skin. The afferent activity generated by movement comes from all of these sources. The activity of receptors other than the muscle spindle and the Golgi tendon organ does not contribute directly to myotatic reflexes, but it can modulate transmission in myotatic reflex pathways and alter the excitability of α and γ motor neurons. In pathologic states, such as spasticity, a normally innocuous afferent volley from these receptors can produce reflex activity such as flexor spasms.

Muscle Spindle

Spindle counts vary for different muscles (for example, more than 1300 have been found in the

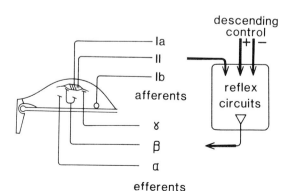

Figure 20–1. The components of the myotatic unit.

human quadriceps femoris [Voss, 1971]). The muscle spindle consists of 2–12 specialized muscle fibers enclosed in a connective tissue capsule, lying in parallel with the contractile fibers of the muscle (Fig. 20–1). The capsule makes the spindle fusiform (spindle shaped). The specialized muscle fibers inside the capsule are called *intrafusal* and generate negligible force when activated by their motor fibers, which are termed *fusimotor* (for terminology, see Table 20–1). In cats and humans, the intrafusal muscle fibers can be divided into three types (for reviews, see Banks et al., 1981; Boyd, 1980). On average, each spindle contains four fibers in which the nuclei form a chain along the middle portion of the muscle fiber (hence, nuclear chain fiber). There are two types of fiber in which the nuclei are grouped at the center of the fiber (nuclear bag fibers). The two types of bag fiber are called bag 1 and bag 2, and each spindle commonly has one of each.

There are two types of sensory receptor on the spindle. The primary ending consists of branches of a large myelinated afferent axon (group Ia afferent), forming spirals around the center of each intrafusal muscle fiber. The secondary endings are found on slightly more polar regions of, almost exclusively, the nuclear chain intrafusal fibers and are formed by the branches of 1–5 myelinated fibers of smaller diameter (group II afferents). The mechanical (viscoelastic) properties of the intrafusal muscle fibers determine the patterns of response of the afferent terminals lying on them (Boyd, 1980). The polar regions of the bag 1 fiber have high viscosity and, initially, resist stretch, which is therefore absorbed by the innervated central region. The resulting abrupt onset and gradual relaxation of the deformation imposed on the terminals of the primary ending pro-

duce a dynamic burst of impulses in the Ia afferent, superficially resembling a response to the velocity (and/or acceleration) of movement. The bag 2 fiber has more elastic tissue associated with it and responds to stretch more uniformly throughout its length, as do chain fibers. These intrafusal fibers give the primary and secondary endings a discharge proportional to the extent of stretch (Boyd, 1980; Matthews, 1972, 1981).

Each intrafusal muscle fiber receives a motor innervation, usually from more than one motor axon. Such polyneuronal innervation is peculiar to intrafusal muscle, occurring with contractile (extrafusal) muscle fibers only in the neonate or during early stages of reinnervation. In amphibia, muscle spindles receive their motor innervation from branches of the efferent axons directed to the contractile (extrafusal) muscle. These skeletofusimotor neurons have become known as β motor neurons. In mammals, a separate motor control for muscle spindles has developed, although 20–30% of spindles also receive some β innervation (Emonet-Dénand et al., 1980). Motor neurons that innervate only muscle spindles are of relatively small size, have slowly conducting efferent axons, and are known as γ motor neurons. Fusimotor neurons, whether γ (i.e., exclusively fusimotor) or β (i.e., skeletofusimotor), can be classified as dynamic or static by their effects on the response of the primary spindle ending to large-amplitude stretch (Matthews, 1972). The type of effect is determined by the intrafusal fiber innervated by the fusimotor axon—hence, bag 1, dynamic; bag 2 or chain, static (Boyd, 1980, 1981; Matthews, 1981). Any one fusimotor axon may supply several spindles but has the same effect (dynamic or static) on all of the spindles that it innervates, an effect mediated by producing a local stiffening of the intrafusal muscle fiber so that more of the stretch is transmitted to the regions innervated by the afferent terminals.

Primary and secondary endings are extremely sensitive to stretch of small amplitude, measured in tens or hundreds of micrometers. In this range, the responses to stretch are linear. The primary ending is more sensitive, but its dynamic response is qualitatively similar to that of the secondary ending (Matthews, 1972, 1981). Dynamic and static fusimotor neurons may *reduce* spindle sensitivity to stretch of low amplitude, extending the linear range into larger amplitudes (Hulliger et al., 1977; see also Matthews, 1981). Traditional views of fusimotor-spindle function in health and disease do not incorporate these properties and are therefore seriously flawed. Indeed, past emphasis on concepts derived from large-amplitude stretch may have directed attention away from what could be a major biologic role of the muscle spindle, namely, to produce reflex compensation not for externally applied changes in length of large amplitude but for small irregularities in the programing or performance of movement (Binder and Stuart, 1980).

It is worth noting that there are some anatomic differences between human and feline spindles, and

Table 20–1. SPINDLE TERMINOLOGY

Intrafusal Muscle Fibers		
Bag 1	1/spindle	Dynamic
Bag 2	1/spindle	Static
Chain	3–5/spindle	Static
Sensory Receptors		
Primary	On all fibers	Dynamic and static
Secondary	Chain fibers only	Static
Afferent Fibers		
Group Ia	From primary ending	Dynamic and static
Group II	From secondary endings	Static (Note: only with large-amplitude stretch)
Fusimotor Fibers		
γ	Intrafusal muscle only (bag 1, bag 2, and chain)	Dynamic or static
β	Intrafusal and extrafusal muscle (bag 1, long chain)	Dynamic or static
Adequate Stimuli		
Stretch	i.e., external change in length	
Fusimotor activity	i.e., internal change in length	

human group I afferents have much slower conduction velocities (D. Burke and Gandevia, 1990). In addition, there are marked differences in size and length of reflex pathways. The precise mode of operation of the fusimotor system must differ in cat and human subjects, even if the ultimate goal of the fusimotor-spindle mechanism is the same. Direct recordings have been made from spindle afferents in conscious human subjects to clarify a number of issues relevant to human disease (for reviews, see D. Burke, 1981; Vallbo et al., 1979). These recordings suggest the following:

1. Spindles in relaxed muscles, flexors or extensors, behave as if there is little background fusimotor drive.
2. Spindle endings are sensitive to tendon percussion, vibration, and other forms of stretch in the absence of fusimotor drive.
3. Fusimotor neurons innervating a muscle are activated when that muscle contracts voluntarily.
4. Fusimotor neurons innervating a nonactive muscle are not normally activated significantly when another muscle is contracted, such as when tendon jerks are reinforced in the Jendrassik maneuver.
5. The fusimotor system is not normally used to modify the strength of myotatic reflexes (for example, it is not responsible for the potentiation produced by the Jendrassik maneuver).

The γ motor neurons of the cat have been shown to receive extensive reflex inputs from peripheral afferents (although they lack a monosynaptic Ia pathway), indicating that fusimotor drive can be modulated by the sensory activity generated during movement (Taylor and Prochazka, 1981). The situation seems to be similar in human subjects: cutaneous mechanoreceptors can reflexly excite γ motor neurons through a spinal reflex pathway, which is subject to supraspinal control (Aniss et al., 1990). Loss of control of this reflex pathway could contribute to flexor spasms in the paraplegic and loss of manual dexterity in the hemiplegic.

Golgi Tendon Organ

Golgi tendon organs are almost as plentiful as muscle spindles. The tendon organ is an encapsulated receptor containing nerve endings in collagenous fascicles into which 5–15 muscle fibers insert (Barker, 1974). Contraction of these muscle fibers distorts the afferent endings, which are branches of a large, myelinated, rapidly conducting afferent fiber called the group Ib afferent. The 5–15 muscle fibers that insert into a tendon organ usually come from different motor units, without bias for any particular motor unit type (Proske, 1981; Reinking et al., 1975).

It is a fallacy that tendon organs are found mainly in tendons and are thus in series with the whole muscle. As represented diagrammatically in Figure 20–1, the majority line the aponeuroses of origin and

insertion, with less than 10% in the tendon proper (Barker, 1974; Proske, 1981). An individual tendon organ lies in series only with the 5–15 motor units that have a muscle fiber inserting into it, being in parallel with the remainder (Houk and Henneman, 1967; Houk et al., 1980). Tendon organs are exquisitely sensitive to the contraction of their in-series motor units, having a threshold for discharge of only a few milligrams (Houk and Henneman, 1967; Houk et al., 1980; Reinking et al., 1975). Therefore, some tendon organs are probably activated even in the weakest of contractions. Tendon organs are not part of an overload protection mechanism, which is mobilized when contraction force exceeds some safe level. Rather the total discharge from the tendon organs in a muscle grows with the strength of contraction. On the other hand, tendon organs are generally silent in relaxed muscle. They usually remain so during passive stretch, provided the muscle does not contract, because (1) they are not in the tendon in direct line with the increase in passive force and (2) the component of passive force transmitted to a tendon organ is not delivered to the nerve terminals as effectively as the active force generated by contraction of an inserting muscle fiber. The sole function of a tendon organ is to monitor muscle contraction: it is a misnomer to call it a stretch receptor. Together, the tendon organ and the muscle spindle are capable of providing the nervous system with all the information required to calibrate movement—length and force. As it happens, they can have opposite reflex effects on the motor neuron pool. However, they are not biologic opposites; their functional roles in the programing and reflex modulation of movement are complementary.

The issues discussed earlier are relevant to the *clasp-knife phenomenon*, an inhibitory response that was previously attributed to tendon organs. Tendon organs are undoubtedly mobilized as a reflex contraction increases in strength and certainly have an inhibitory effect on the motor neuron pool (provided that their reflex pathways within the spinal cord remain operative [see later]). However, tendon organs cannot produce a persisting, complete suppression of the reflex contraction, as occurs with the clasp-knife phenomenon in the quadriceps muscles of spastic patients (D. Burke and Lance, 1973). Other inhibitory inputs must be responsible, perhaps a number operating together, such as spindle group II afferents (Bessou et al., 1984; D. Burke and Lance, 1973), nonspindle group II and III muscle afferents (Iles et al., 1989; Rymer et al., 1979), and joint afferents (Baxendale and Ferrell, 1981). Indeed, in spinal animals such afferents share a common reflex pathway, inhibiting extensor motor neurons and facilitating flexor motor neurons, hence flexion reflex afferents (Eccles and Lundberg, 1959).

SPINAL REFLEX EFFECTS

Spinal reflexes represent only one function of the inputs from group Ia, spindle group II, and group Ib afferents. All of these afferents project to higher centers, including the cerebral cortex, where they may be used in long-loop reflexes and in the programming of movement (Desmedt, 1980). In addition, group Ia afferents contribute significantly to kinesthetic sensations such as joint position sense (Matthews, 1981; McCloskey, 1978). By and large, human joint afferents do not adequately encode joint movement (D. Burke et al., 1988), much as in the cat. However, when muscle spindles are prevented from playing any role in kinesthesia, receptors in the joint do contribute to the residual movement awareness (Ferrell et al., 1987).

Group Ia afferents from spindle primary endings have an overall excitatory effect on the motor neuron pool of the homonymous muscle and its synergists, and an inhibitory effect on the antagonist pool (Fig. 20–2). The excitatory effects are produced through a number of pathways: monosynaptic, oligosynaptic, and possibly polysynaptic (Schomburg and Behrends, 1978; Watt et al., 1976; see also Jankowska, 1979; Jankowska et al., 1981). The amount of monosynaptic excitation is related to motor neuron size, being greatest in low-threshold (slow, type S) motor neurons and weakest in high-threshold (fast fatigable, type FF) motor neurons (Fleshman et al., 1981). Each group Ia afferent has an excitatory monosynaptic connection with almost every motor neuron in the homonymous pool, the percentage of connectivity being highest (100%) with low-threshold (type S) motor neurons and lowest (87%) with high-threshold (type FF) motor neurons (Fleshman et al., 1981). As indicated in Table 20–2, the Ia monosynaptic input

Table 20–2. α MOTOR NEURON AND MOTOR UNIT PROPERTIES*

Parameter	Classification		
Motor Neuron Property			
Cell size	Small	Intermediate	Large
Recruitment threshold	Low	Intermediate	High
Ia monosynaptic input	Strongest	Intermediate	Weakest
Axonal conduction velocity	Slow	Fast	Fast
Motor Unit Physiology			
Type	S	FR	FF
Twitch contraction time	Slow	Fast	Fast
Twitch or tetanic force	Low	Intermediate/ high	High
Fatigability	Very low	Low	High
Muscle Fiber Histochemistry			
Type	I (SO)	IIA (FOG)	IIB (FG)
Myosin ATPase	Low	High	High
Glycolytic/ glycogenolytic	Low	High	High
Oxidative	High	Medium/high	Low

*Individual properties overlap between different types.

is therefore stronger for type S motor neurons (R. E. Burke, 1981), the corollary for humans being that the ankle jerk and H reflex appear more in soleus (predominantly type S) than in gastrocnemius (mixed). Human group Ia afferents also project to different motor neuron pools, across joints (Mao et al., 1984), and may produce oligosynaptic excitation in homonymous and synergistic motor neuron pools (Malmgren and Pierrot-Deseilligny, 1988a) in addition to the monosynaptic excitation. Cutaneous inputs affect transmission in the oligosynaptic pathway (Malmgren and Pierrot-Deseilligny, 1988b), and transmission is facilitated at the onset of a voluntary contraction (Baldissera and Pierrot-Deseilligny, 1989). An upper motor neuron lesion would impair this source of reflex feedback.

The reciprocal group Ia inhibition of antagonists involves a disynaptic pathway, the interneuron of which (the Ia inhibitory interneuron) acts as an integrating center, being activated by other primary afferents and by descending pathways (including the corticospinal tract) and inhibited by collaterals from homonymous Renshaw cells (Figs. 20–2 and 20–3). At the onset of a voluntary contraction and while it is increasing, the reciprocal inhibitory pathway from agonist to antagonist is opened and that from antagonist to agonist is closed (Crone et al., 1987). In upper motor neuron lesions, supraspinal facilitation of transmission in the inhibitory circuit may be lost, and accordingly, Ia disynaptic (reciprocal) inhibition from forearm extensors to forearm flexors is reduced in patients with hemiplegic spasticity but not those with flaccidity (Nakashima et al., 1989; see also

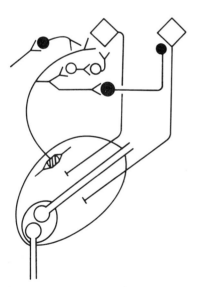

Figure 20–2. Group Ia reflex connections. The group Ia afferent makes monosynaptic and polysynaptic excitatory connections with homonymous motor neurons and a disynaptic inhibitory connection with the antagonistic motor neuron pool. The monosynaptic pathway can be inhibited presynaptically by an interneuron that depolarizes the afferent terminals. Open circles = excitatory interneurons; forked = excitatory (depolarizing) synapses; large filled circles = inhibitory interneurons; small filled circle = inhibitory (hyperpolarizing) synapse.

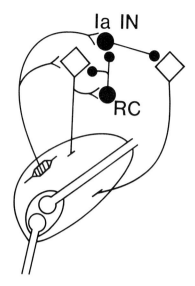

Figure 20–3. Renshaw cell (RC) actions. Renshaw cells are activated by recurrent collaterals of α motor neurons and inhibit the parent motor neuron pool. They also inhibit the Ia inhibitory interneurons (Ia IN) responsible for reciprocal inhibition of the antagonist pool. They therefore tend to curtail agonist contraction and disinhibit the antagonist, as would be required in a cyclic movement such as walking.

Yanagisawa et al., 1976, for studies on the hemiplegic leg). In spinal humans, reciprocal inhibition from soleus to tibialis anterior is enhanced (Ashby and Wiens, 1989), possibly contributing to difficulty in activating the flexors voluntarily. In writer's cramp and other dystonias, there is no defect in the Ia disynaptic inhibitory pathway (Nakashima et al., 1989).

The monosynaptic pathway can be modulated by a phenomenon known as *presynaptic inhibition*. In this situation, interneurons depolarize the terminals of the group Ia afferent fiber so that the partially depolarized afferent terminal releases less transmitter at its synapse on the motor neuron (see Fig. 20–2). The responsible interneurons are fed by a variety of peripheral inputs, including Ia afferent fibers from various related muscles—agonists, synergists, and particularly antagonists (Berardelli et al., 1987; Iles and Roberts, 1987). Normally, there appears to be a background level of presynaptic inhibition that can be turned up or down. For example, at the onset of a voluntary contraction, presynaptic inhibition of excitatory Ia pathways to the agonist is reduced (Hultborn et al., 1987). In human spinal shock, there is evidence of overactivity of presynaptic inhibitory mechanisms (Ashby et al., 1974). In established spasticity caused by cerebral or spinal lesions, comparable studies suggest that presynaptic inhibitory mechanisms are suppressed (Ashby et al., 1974, 1980; Delwaide, 1971; Iles and Roberts, 1986; Nakashima et al., 1989). Interestingly, a depression of presynaptic inhibition from forearm extensors to forearm flexors appears to occur in patients with writer's cramp and other dystonias, and this is the first

objective physiologic defect to be demonstrated in these disorders (Nakashima et al., 1989).

Group Ib afferent activity produces inhibition of homonymous and synergistic motor neuron pools through disynaptic and trisynaptic circuits in which the Ib volley excites interneurons that inhibit the motor neuron pool. The Ib inhibitory interneuron receives inputs from cutaneous afferent fibers (both inhibitory and excitatory [Bergego et al., 1981; Pierrot-Deseilligny et al., 1981]); and also excitatory collaterals from Ia afferents (Jankowska, 1979). Supraspinal control of this interneuron is affected through at least four descending pathways—corticospinal and rubrospinal, which excite the interneuron, so enhancing transmission in the Ib inhibitory pathway, and two systems that arise from the bulbar reticular formation and suppress transmission of group Ib inhibition by inhibiting the Ib inhibitory interneuron. In patients with spasticity, transmission in the Ib inhibitory interneuron is depressed (Delwaide and Oliver, 1988), further evidence that the Golgi tendon organ plays no role in the clasp-knife phenomenon (Burke and Lance, 1973; see earlier).

The reflex effects of group II afferents from secondary spindle endings have not been fully clarified, and adequate techniques have not been developed to study their effects in human subjects. Initially, they were thought to produce inhibition of extensor motor neurons and facilitation of flexor motor neurons, a flexion reflex pattern (Eccles and Lundberg, 1959; Laporte and Bessou, 1959). More recently, it has been suggested that they produce significant homonymous excitation, even in extensor motor neurons (Matthews, 1969, 1972, 1981). Spindle group II afferents do produce monosynaptic excitation of motor neurons, but this is less frequent and of lower amplitude than that produced by group Ia afferents and does not vary significantly with motor neuron size (Munson et al., 1982). All other group II reflex circuits contain a number of interneurons. It is quite probable that the same afferent could have opposing effects on the one motor neuron pool, dependent on which reflex circuit is chosen by supraspinal centers to be appropriate for a particular task (see Holmqvist and Lundberg, 1961).

Modulation of myotatic reflexes is possible on the output side of the reflex arc, through an inhibitory interneuron known as the Renshaw cell. This interneuron is activated by a branch of the motor axon and feeds back predominantly onto the active motor neuron pool and its synergists to produce recurrent inhibition (see Fig. 20–3). The Renshaw cell also suppresses activity in the Ia inhibitory interneuron directed to the antagonistic pool, so decreasing the reciprocal Ia inhibition from the active myotatic unit to its antagonist (see Fig. 20–3). The excitability of the Renshaw cell is subject to supraspinal control: for example, a voluntary contraction suppresses Renshaw cell activity to the active motor neuron pool and allows reciprocal Ia inhibition of the antagonist (Hultborn and Pierrot-Deseilligny, 1979). The latter helps prevent myotatic reflex activity in the antagonist as it is stretched in a voluntary movement. In spastic patients, the level of recurrent inhibition produced by Renshaw cells is normal or increased but the ability to modulate the inhibition is lost (Katz and Pierrot-Deseilligny, 1982). A defect in recurrent inhibition therefore cannot be responsible for the exaggerated tendon jerks and increased muscle tone of the spastic state, although it could contribute to a loss of motor control when the patient attempts to move.

α MOTOR NEURONS AND RECRUITMENT

Whether activated reflexly or voluntarily, slowly or rapidly, the α motor neurons of human subjects are recruited in a reproducible sequence (see Desmedt, 1981). Small motor neurons (type S, slow twitch, fatigue resistant) are recruited first, then the large—initially, type FR (fast twitch, fatigue resistant), and finally, type FF (fast twitch, fatigue sensitive). This orderly pattern of recruitment follows that predicted by Henneman's (1957, 1981) size principle. Subsequent experimenters have been able systematically to alter the normal pattern of recruitment using cutaneous stimuli (Garnett and Stephens, 1981), but their findings do not invalidate the basic principle of orderly recruitment or its clinical utility. Type S motor neurons innervate muscle fibers that stain poorly for myosin ATPase and are rich in oxidative enzymes but poor in glycolytic and glycogenolytic enzymes. At the other extreme, type FF units stain stongly for myosin ATPase and are poor in oxidative enzymes but have high levels of glycolytic and glycogenolytic enzymes. The muscle fiber's enzyme content determines contraction time (myosin ATPase), resistance to fatigue (oxidative enzymes), and ability to perform brief intense work in the absence of oxygen (glycolytic and glycogenolytic enzymes). These properties, summarized in Table 20–2, are homogeneous for all muscle fibers of a single motor unit and are imposed by the innervating motor neuron. Enzyme stains constitute an important component of the histologic assessment of muscle biopsy specimens.

The gradation of force depends on rate modulation of active motor units as well as motor unit recruitment and derecruitment (Buchthal and Schmalbruch, 1980; R.E. Burke, 1981). In slowly increasing or steady contractions, individual motor neurons are recruited when the contraction level reaches threshold for that unit. At its threshold, the discharge of a motor neuron is usually slow and irregular. With increasing contraction strength, the discharge rate becomes more regular and increases in frequency as more units are recruited. For low-threshold motor neurons, the discharge rate rarely exceeds 10 Hz. For higher-threshold motor neurons, the discharge rates may exceed 40 Hz in maximal efforts, but achievement of such rates necessitates reflex support from muscle spindles in the contracting muscle, driven by activation of the fusimotor system (Bongiovanni and

Hagbarth, 1990; Gandevia et al., 1990). If a normal subject makes a rapid phasic (ballistic) contraction, there is a near-synchronous activation of motor units of all sizes, with peak discharge rates transiently exceeding 100 Hz. Such rates cannot be sustained even with maximal efforts.

With fatigue, there is a slowing of contraction and relaxation times of muscle so that lower motor unit firing rates are required to produce a fused tetanic contraction providing maximal available power (Bigland-Ritchie and Woods, 1984). These changes in motor unit twitch properties are paralleled by a decline in motor neuron firing rates, such that the achievable rates are sufficient to produce maximal available power. The decline in firing rate is determined by feedback from muscle receptors (Gandevia et al., 1990) and is due to disfacilitation of the motor neuron pool (caused by declining excitatory feedback from spindle afferents [Bongiovanni and Hagbarth, 1990]) and active inhibition (caused by excitation of intramuscular chemoreceptors with small afferent fibers [Bigland-Ritchie et al., 1986]).

As a result of immobilization, with the development of spasticity or parkinsonian rigidity, and in paraplegia, there may be changes in the discharge patterns of volitionally activated motor units and changes in their contractile properties (Edström, 1970; Hopf et al., 1974; Mayer et al., 1984; Young and Mayer, 1982; for review, see Desmedt, 1981). Indeed, Dietz and Berger (1984) suggested that the changes in contractile properties lead to increased stiffness and so contribute to the increase in tone typical of spasticity. This view has been supported by direct measurements of stiffness and electromyographic (EMG) activity in hemiparetic patients, with more stiffness than expected for the amount of EMG activity (Lee et al., 1987).

CLINICALLY USEFUL MYOTATIC REFLEXES

The tendon jerk, the H reflex, and the tonic vibration reflex are clinically useful myotatic reflexes that can be elicited readily in humans. They are much more complex than analogous reflexes in the cat, and this has not received adequate recognition in the past. It is virtually impossible in humans to generate a muscle afferent volley that is not significantly dispersed by the time it enters the spinal cord. Human afferent pathways are long and the conduction velocity of group I afferents is relatively slow (cat: range, 72–120 m/second [cf. Matthews, 1972]; humans: maximal velocity, 60–70 m/second [cf. D. Burke et al., 1983]). The electrical stimulus used for the H reflex of soleus activates afferents synchronously at the popliteal fossa and produces an afferent volley that reaches the motor neuron pool approximately 15 ms later, but the slowest Ia afferents in that volley probably arrive 9–10 ms after the fastest. In addition, it is impossible in human subjects to deliver electrical (or mechanical) stimuli so that they activate selectively only a restricted population of group Ia afferent fibers (D. Burke et al., 1983).

Direct muscle stretch is not required to produce a tendon jerk. Percussion on a muscle tendon sets up a decaying vibration wave that propagates in all directions from the percussion site, being transmitted particularly effectively by bone to muscle and skin remote from the site of impact (D. Burke et al., 1983; Lance and de Gail, 1965). Primary spindle endings are sensitive to this low-amplitude vibratory stretch, discharging at high frequency (up to 200 Hz) even in relaxed subjects—in whom there is little background fusimotor activity (D. Burke, 1981; Vallbo et al., 1979). Spread of the percussion wave to spindle endings in remote muscles may produce tendon jerks in muscles not directly stretched, particularly if the patient is tense or spastic (Lance, 1965; Lance and de Gail, 1965). Such reflex irradiation is therefore due to failure to restrict the stimulus to receptors in the percussed muscle, and this readily accounts for other reflex signs, such as the inverted supinator jerk and Hoffman's sign. As noted earlier, spindle endings are exquisitely sensitive to low-amplitude disturbances. However, as also noted, the major effect of fusimotor activity is to decrease the sensitivity of spindle endings to disturbances of small amplitude. If there were background fusimotor activity, it is unlikely that the spindle response to percussion would be enhanced (Morgan et al., 1984). It is therefore difficult to attribute tendon jerk hyperreflexia in spastic patients to overactivity of fusimotor neurons, as was once thought to be the case (for example, Dietrichson, 1971; Jansen, 1962; Rushworth, 1960). There is convincing evidence of abnormalities in spinal reflex pathways in spastic patients, but there is no convincing evidence that a fusimotor disorder contributes to the abnormal myotatic reflexes (D. Burke, 1983).

Percussion is not a clean stimulus, and the nervous system is therefore subjected to a highly dispersed afferent volley containing activity from a variety of muscle and cutaneous mechanoreceptors from a variety of sources. The rise time of the percussion-induced increase in excitability in the soleus motor neuron pool of human subjects is approximately 10 ms, with motor neuron discharge occurring in the last half of the rising phase (D. Burke et al., 1984). Given the existence of oligosynaptic pathways to motor neurons from group Ia and other afferents, it is inconceivable that oligosynaptic pathways do not contribute to the human ankle jerk.

The H reflex is produced by stimulating afferents in the motor nerve electrically, the presumption being that a pure group Ia afferent volley is set up. By stimulating afferent axons, the electrical stimulus by-passes receptor mechanisms to produce a reflex that is believed by many to be otherwise identical with the tendon jerk. This belief is fallacious and has resulted in erroneous conclusions in the clinical literature (see D. Burke, 1983). The afferent volleys set up by electrical stimuli and by tendon percussion are

not similar (Table 20–3), and the spinal reflex circuits engaged by the volleys are probably not identical. As with the tendon jerk, the assumption that the H reflex is exclusively monosynaptic is probably invalid (D. Burke et al., 1984).

The H reflex can be recorded from soleus in all normal subjects, on stimulation of the tibial nerve in the popliteal fossa (Fig. 20–4a). It can also be recorded from quadriceps and from forearm muscles, particularly if reflex excitability is raised by performing the Jendrassik maneuver or a weak voluntary contraction of the test muscle. Comparable reflexes can be recorded from other muscles, such as the tibialis anterior and thenar muscles (Fig. 20–5), if the subject performs a steady voluntary contraction and an averager is used (D. Burke et al., 1989). In general, however, the greater the ease of its elicitation in muscles other than soleus (and quadriceps), the more likely is reflex excitability to be high—either physiologically (a tense subject) or pathologically (a spastic patient). The major clinical use of H reflex testing is in assessing the integrity of the entire reflex arc in patients with peripheral nerve or nerve root disorders. In spasticity, attempts to quantitate the enhanced amplitude of the H reflex (e.g., by using H/M ratios) have not proved sufficiently reproducible within a subject or discriminative between subjects to be useful diagnostically.

Application of a vibrator oscillating at approximately 100 Hz to a muscle belly (de Gail et al., 1966; Lance, 1965) or muscle tendon (Hagbarth and Ek-

Table 20–3. AFFERENT VOLLEYS FOR ANKLE JERK AND H REFLEX

Parameter	Ankle Jerk	Soleus H Reflex
Stimulus	Percussion on the Achilles tendon	Electrical in popliteal fossa
*Activated Afferents**		
Type	Ia > II > Ib Cutaneous	Ia = Ib > II Cutaneous
Source	Throughout limb, including antagonist	Triceps surae Long flexor muscles Sural nerve skin Intrinsic muscles of foot Skin of sole of foot
Impulses	Multiple per afferent (interval <5 ms)	One per afferent
Degree of Ia Dispersion		
At popliteal fossa	>10–20 ms	Nil
At spinal cord	Great	9–10 ms
Rising Phase of Excitability Induced in Motor Neuron Pool†	About 10 ms	<4–5 ms

*Data from Burke D., Gandevia S.C., McKeon B. The afferent volleys responsible for spinal proprioceptive reflexes in man. *J. Physiol. (Lond.)* 339:535–552, 1983.
†Data from Burke D., Gandevia S.C., McKeon B. Monosynaptic and oligosynaptic contributions to human ankle jerk and H reflex. *J. Neurophysiol.* 52:435–448, 1984.

Figure 20–4. *(a)* The H reflex of soleus. The traces illustrate EMG activity of soleus in response to electrical stimulation of the tibial nerve in the popliteal fossa, using progressively increasing stimulus levels. The early potential (labeled M) is the direct response to activation of motor fibers. It increases until all motor axons have been stimulated. The second potential at about 30 ms (labeled H) is the H reflex response produced by the electrically evoked afferent volley. Initially, as the stimulus level increases, the H reflex potential increases, reflecting the greater size of the afferent volley. However, stimulation of motor fibers produces an antidromic volley, and this prevents transmission of the orthodromically conducted H reflex volley in these fibers. Hence, as the M wave increases, there is occlusion of the H reflex volley. *(b)* The F wave of abductor pollicis brevis. Supramaximal stimulation of the median nerve at the wrist (top trace, low gain) ensures that any late EMG potential is not a reflex potential (see earlier). In the next nine traces, at high gain, the large-amplitude early

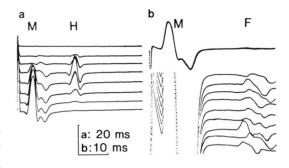

EMG potential is the supramaximal compound muscle action potential (M wave). The small late responses at about 30 ms (labeled F) are F waves. Note the variable shape and latency of successive F waves. Vertical calibration: 10 mV for *a* and top trace of *b*; 1 mV for the lower nine traces of *b*.

lund, 1965) produces a tonic reflex contraction of that muscle (the tonic vibration reflex), associated with inhibition of the antagonist (Fig. 20–6). In relaxed normal human subjects, the excitability of reflex pathways within the spinal cord is so low that only by vibration can a tonic myotatic reflex be produced. Even so, contraction strength normally increases slowly during a few seconds after its onset, and in some muscles spinal reflex circuits must be primed by a background voluntary contraction. Vibration is not a clean stimulus and cannot be applied such that

only primary spindle endings are activated. Nevertheless, it is possible to drive human primary spindle endings maximally by vibration, and the reflex changes so produced can probably be attributed to these receptors (D. Burke et al., 1976). In spastic patients, similar vibration evokes a reflex contraction that starts abruptly and rapidly achieves full development (D. Burke et al., 1972; Hagbarth and Eklund, 1968), as if reflex circuits within the spinal cord were fully active ab initio (Fig. 20–7). The tonic vibration reflex normally requires supraspinal potentiation of

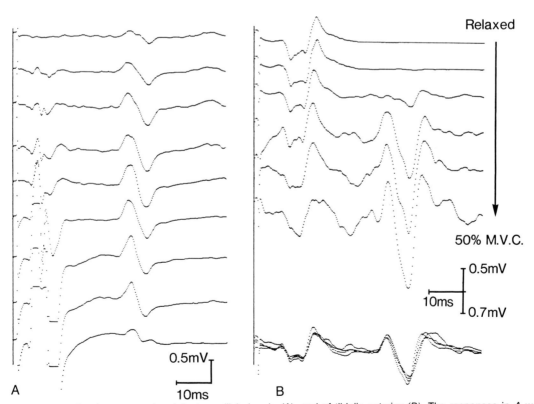

Figure 20–5. H reflexes of a thenar muscle, abductor pollicis brevis *(A)*, and of tibialis anterior *(B)*. The responses in *A* were recorded during a steady contraction in response to progressively increasing stimulus intensities delivered at 4 Hz. In *B*, a constant stimulus of 4 mA was delivered at 4 Hz during varying levels of background contraction, ranging from relaxed (upper trace) to 40–50% maximal voluntary power (sixth trace). The lowest traces contain four superimposed averages, recorded during a moderate background contraction. In *A* and *B*, each trace is the average of 128 responses. (From Burke D., Adams R.W., Skuse N.F. The effects of voluntary contraction on the H reflex of human limb muscles. *Brain* 112:417–433, 1989, by permission of Oxford University Press.)

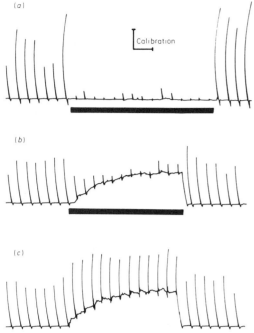

Figure 20–6. The reflex effects of muscle vibration in normal humans. *(a and b)* Vibration was applied to the belly of the quadriceps femoris muscle while the patellar tendon was percussed regularly every 5 seconds, producing knee jerks. In *b*, a tonic vibration reflex developed gradually; tendon jerks were suppressed. In *a*, the subject voluntarily controlled the tonic vibration reflex, but the tendon jerks were still suppressed. *(c)* The subject performed a slow voluntary contraction mimicking the time course of the reflex contraction in *b*. This did not suppress the tendon jerk. Calibrations: vertical, 0.4 kg for *a*, 0.6 kg for *b* and *c*; horizontal, 10 seconds. (From de Gail P., Lance J.W., Neilson P.D. Differential effects on tonic and phasic reflex mechanisms produced by vibration of muscles in man. *J. Neurol. Neurosurg. Psychiatry* 29:1–11, 1966.)

spinal circuits, mainly by vestibulospinal and reticulospinal pathways in the anterior quadrants of the spinal cord (Gillies et al., 1971). It cannot be elicited if spinal cord centers are isolated by spinal transection, except as a variable, often phasic response to vibration of large amplitude (Dimitrijević et al., 1977), in which case the reflex response may not be generated through myotatic reflex pathways.

In normal human subjects, vibration of muscle or tendon inhibits phasic myotatic reflexes such as the tendon jerk (see Fig. 20–6) and the H reflex (de Gail et al., 1966; Delwaide, 1971), a phenomenon that is multifactorial but includes presynaptic inhibition of the monosynaptic group Ia pathway (Ashby et al., 1980; Delwaide, 1971; Gillies et al., 1969). In patients with spasticity, no such inhibition can be demonstrated, the basic finding suggesting that presynaptic inhibitory mechanisms are suppressed in spasticity (Ashby et al., 1980; Delwaide, 1971; Iles and Roberts, 1986).

Normal subjects can voluntarily suppress the tonic vibration reflex with ease, by exerting a control over spinal reflex circuits. Spastic patients cannot (Hagbarth and Eklund, 1968). In patients suspected of having minimal motor disorders, such as spasticity,

dystonia, and choreoathetosis, the application of vibration can cause a deterioration in motor performance not seen in the normal subject. This can be demonstrated and recorded by asking the patient to draw a spiral (Archimedes' screw) with and without vibration.

THE F WAVE

The F wave is an artifact that never occurs in normal life. When stimulated electrically, a motor axon conducts an orthodromic discharge directly to the muscle (to produce the M wave) and an antidromic discharge back to the motor neuron's axon hillock (Fig. 20–8). Randomly, but on approximately 2–5% of occasions, the antidromically conducted impulse invades the cell's initial segment, discharges the motor neuron, and sets up an orthodromic impulse in the motor axon. This produces a late EMG potential in the relevant muscle at a latency dependent on conduction of an impulse centrally and then peripherally over the full length of the motor axon.

If a supramaximal stimulus is used, the antidromic volley in motor axons affects every motor axon, and this prevents any H reflex potentials from appearing in the EMG because the reflexly evoked orthodromic impulse in a motor axon collides with the antidromic impulse. Equally, however, the reflex discharge prevents the antidromic impulse from setting up an F wave, and consequently, F waves do not sample the lowest-threshold reflexly excitable motor neurons in muscles such as the soleus and thenar (D. Burke et al., 1989). For most muscles, supramaximal stimuli produce F waves in response to most stimuli, but the latency and shape of individual F wave EMG potentials vary because the discharge involves different motor neurons (see Fig. 20–4*b*).

The excitability of the motor neuron pool determines the ease of elicitation of F waves. Thus, if a subject is tense or performs a reinforcement maneuver (such as the Jendrassik maneuver) or suffers from spasticity, the prevalence of F waves is increased, and prolonged complex F waves, reflecting the discharge of multiple motor neurons, may occur. In patients with peripheral nerve abnormalities, the incidence of F waves tends to be low, and if there is significant chronic partial denervation, the duration of the F wave potentials may be increased, reflecting

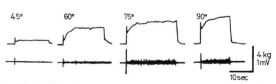

Figure 20–7. The tonic vibration reflex of the quadriceps femoris muscles of a spastic patient, recorded at different degrees of knee joint flexion. Upper trace: force. Lower trace: EMG. (From Burke D., Andrews C.J., Lance J.W. The tonic vibration reflex in spasticity, Parkinson's disease and normal man. *J. Neurol. Neurosurg. Psychiatry* 35:477–486, 1972.)

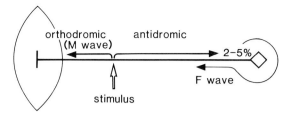

Figure 20–8. The mechanism of the F wave. Electrical stimulation of a motor axon produces an action potential that propagates orthodromically to the muscle (so producing a direct motor response, the M wave) and antidromically back to the motor neuron. On approximately 2–5% of occasions, the antidromic impulse invades the motor neuron cell body and sets up a discharge that propagates orthodromically back down the axon to the muscle, producing a late EMG potential, the F wave. Hence, the F wave latency plus the M wave latency equals twice the conduction time for the motor axon (neglecting the turn-around time at the motor neuron level).

the greater size of the intact motor units. In polyneuropathies and proximal lesions, such as the Guillain-Barré syndrome, latency measurements (correlated to or corrected for limb length or height) may reveal conduction slowing that cannot be detected in conventional motor conduction studies, performed on a restricted, purely distal segment of the nerve.

ABNORMALITIES OF THE MYOTATIC UNIT

Diminished Motor Neuron Activity

Withdrawal of Facilitation (Spinal Shock)

Spinal shock results from the sudden withdrawal of supraspinal facilitation of spinal circuits. In the acute phase of spinal shock in monkeys, the regional metabolic rate for glucose is diminished in the ventral gray matter caudal to the transection (Schwartzman et al., 1983), while metabolism in the cap of the dorsal horn is increased, probably because of the withdrawal of brain stem inhibition of flexor reflex pathways. Metabolism in layers VII and VIII, the site of inhibitory interneurons, remains unaltered.

In the cat, spinal shock is multifactorial and is associated with decreased excitability of interneurons, α motor neurons, and γ motor neurons (for reviews, see Barnes and Schadt, 1979; Mendell, 1984). It is sometimes said that the withdrawal of fusimotor activity is responsible for or contributes to spinal shock in humans. However, this is unlikely to be the major factor for the following reasons:

1. Cutaneous and autonomic reflex pathways may be as affected as the myotatic reflex.
2. Normal subjects who relax fully have no significant background fusimotor drive, even though their spindle endings are sufficiently sensitive that tendon percussion produces normal tendon jerks (D. Burke et al., 1981).
3. There is, as noted earlier, little evidence that the

fusimotor system operates as a gain-control mechanism for myotatic reflexes (see D. Burke, 1983).

Presumably the responsible mechanisms are multiple in humans, as in the cat; excessive presynaptic inhibition may be one factor (Ashby et al., 1974).

In some patients, the stage of spinal shock is quite brief, lasting only a few days, but in others, hyporeflexia persists long after the insult. The reasons for this are not known. Spinal lesions that develop slowly commonly by-pass the stage of spinal shock, gradually developing the hyperreflexia characteristic of spasticity. One month after spinal transection in the monkey, glucose metabolism in the ventral horns exceeds that found in controls (Schwartzman et al., 1983).

Loss of Reflex Activation

Any neuropathy affecting large sensory fibers abolishes tendon jerks by depriving motor neurons of group Ia afferent input. Tendon reflexes may be absent, even in the presence of a coexisting pyramidal lesion in conditions such as subacute combined degeneration and Friedreich's ataxia. Posterior root compression, for example, by extruded disc substance or tumor, impairs conduction in large-diameter fibers preferentially so that tendon reflexes may be lost before signs of small-fiber damage (loss of sensation to pinprick and temperature) become apparent. Compression of the spinal cord or intrinsic cord lesions interrupt the myotatic arc at the segmental level, thus abolishing tendon reflexes mediated by the appropriate segment.

Damage to the Motor Neuron

Acute anterior poliomyelitis is characterized by hypotonia and loss of tendon reflexes in the acute phase. In the chronic phase, reflexes remain impaired in proportion to loss of motor neurons and therefore to the degree of wasting and weakness in the affected segmental distribution. Patients who have recovered from poliomyelitis may experience progressive weakness in later life (Anderson et al., 1972; Mulder et al., 1972), probably owing to premature fall-out of previously "sick" motor neurons.

Spinal muscular atrophy assumes different forms at different ages. The congenital or infantile form (Werdnig-Hoffmann disease), one cause of the floppy infant syndrome, usually runs a progressive downhill course during the first year of life. Juvenile spinal atrophy (Kugelberg-Welander disease) is a heredofamilial cause of proximal muscular wasting, which runs a slowly progressive course from onset in childhood or adolescence to late middle age. By contrast, motor neuron disease is rarely encountered in adolescence and usually appears in late middle age, causing death in an average of 4 years from the onset of symptoms. It may affect first the cranial motor nuclei, with the exception of the ocular motor neurons (in progressive bulbar palsy) or spinal motor neurons (in progressive muscular atrophy), but signs of upper and lower motor neuron lesions are usually found together (in amyotrophic lateral sclerosis). Chronic spinal muscular atrophy may develop in later life, causing predominantly distal changes resembling the distribution in Charcot-Marie-Tooth disease.

Compression of ventral roots or of motor fibers in the cervical or lumbosacral plexuses causes segmental reflex changes, varying in intensity with the proportion of axons that fail to conduct the nerve impulse. Radiculopathies may be localized, as in brachial radiculopathy (neuralgic amyotrophy), or diffuse, as in Guillain-Barré disease. Motor polyneuropathies commonly cause distal wasting, weakness, and areflexia, which is more severe in the lower limbs.

Excessive Motor Neuron Activity

Withdrawal of Inhibition

Spasticity. Lesions of the upper motor neuron (the corticospinal tract and its accompanying corticoreticulospinal fibers) usually give rise to spasticity. Spasticity may be defined as "a motor disorder characterized by a velocity-dependent increase in tonic stretch reflexes (muscle tone) with exaggerated tendon jerks, resulting from hyperexcitability of the stretch reflex, as one component of the upper motor neuron syndrome" (Lance, 1980a). The other components are weakness, abnormal posture (as may occur in hemiplegic patients), and release of flexor reflexes, resulting in flexor spasms, the Babinski response, and the inhibition of the quadriceps stretch reflex responsible for the clasp-knife phenomenon (Lance, 1980b). The α motor neurons are hyperexcitable, and there are abnormalities in reflex transmission (see under Spinal Reflex Effects). On the other hand, there is no evidence that excessive fusimotor drive contributes to spasticity (for review, see D. Burke, 1983), although fusimotor dysfunction could contribute to lack of dexterity after upper motor neuron lesions caused by inability to activate fusimotor neurons voluntarily and/or inability to control reflex pathways operating on fusimotor neurons.

It is worth noting that muscle tone in spastic patients is dependent on both enhanced reflex activity and increased stiffness of spastic muscle (Dietz and Berger, 1984; Lee et al., 1987). Furthermore, studies of reflex activity in voluntarily contracting muscles have shown broadly similar stretch reflex dynamics in spastic and normal muscles, suggesting that the primary defect in spasticity is a lowered reflex threshold rather than abnormally increased velocity-dependent reflex responsiveness (Powers et al., 1989).

Spinal Rigidity. Destruction of inhibitory interneurons in the spinal gray matter may permit isolated motor neurons to become spontaneously active, a condition known as spinal rigidity, which has been reported in patients with spinal cord glioma (Rush-

worth et al., 1961) and spinal cord ischemia (Tarlov, 1967). The rigidity persists during rest and even during sleep.

Stiff-Man Syndrome. The term *stiff-man syndrome* was introduced by Moersch and Woltman (1956), who described 14 patients in whom progressive muscular rigidity, resembling chronic tetanus, began between the ages of 28 and 54 years. Stiffness appears particularly in the axial and lumbar girdle muscles and is aggravated by startle, which can induce painful spasms (Gordon et al., 1966). Congenital familial forms of stiff-man syndrome have been reported (Sander et al., 1980). The stiffness is abolished by sleep and by blockade of ventral roots (thus indicating a spinal origin), peripheral nerve, or neuromuscular junction. Meinck et al. (1984) reported that muscle spasms were evoked by various exteroceptive stimuli (acoustic, vestibular, and somatosensory). Myotatic reflexes were not enhanced and were suppressed normally by vibration of the Achilles tendon (unlike the situation in a patient reported by Isaacs, 1979). Because muscular rigidity was augmented by clomipramine (inhibiting neuronal uptake of serotonin and norepinephrine) and reduced by clonidine (inhibiting norepinephrine release by activating central α_2 adrenoceptors), Meinck et al. (1984) postulated that the condition was caused by the unbalanced action of medially descending noradrenergic brain stem pathways influencing the axial musculature. An autoimmune pathogenesis of this syndrome is suggested by the finding of autoantibodies to glutamic acid decarboxylase in a patient, who also had elevated levels of cerebrospinal fluid immunoglobulin in an oligoclonal pattern and type I diabetes (Solimena et al., 1988). This finding has been confirmed, but there are conflicting reports on the benefits of plasma exchange and immunosuppression (Harding et al., 1989; Vicari et al., 1989). The spasms of stiff-man syndrome respond to diazepam, baclofen, and sodium valproate (Spehlmann et al., 1981).

Tetanus. Tetanus toxin blocks postsynaptic inhibition of motor neurons and depresses long-latency reflexes, presumably by damage to interneurons, whereas short-latency excitatory reflexes are enhanced (Bratzlavsky and Vander Eecken, 1976). Reciprocal innervation is abolished so that antagonistic muscles contract together in producing muscular spasms. In addition to its central actions, which produce continuous motor neuron activity, tetanus toxin acts as a presynaptic blocking agent at the neuromuscular junction (Fernandez et al., 1983). In cephalic tetanus, a high local concentration of tetanus toxin can produce a lower motor neuron paralysis, whereas lesser concentrations in the brain stem cause muscular spasms in appropriate cranial muscles (Dastur et al., 1977). Chromatolysis of motor neurons can be demonstrated in dogs only when large doses of tetanus toxin are used (Tarlov et al., 1973).

Excessive Supraspinal Activation

In basal ganglia disorders such as Parkinson's disease and dystonia musculorum deformans, myotatic reflex pathways are essentially normal, although they are subjected to excessive supraspinal drive.

Excessive Spinal Activation

Segmental myoclonus, rhythmic or arrhythmic, can arise from various pathologic changes confined to the spinal cord (Marsden et al., 1981), resulting in involuntary repetitive contractions at approximately 1/second, usually of neighboring muscles, even antagonists, sharing common or adjacent segmental levels. The contractions may persist during sleep and may be unaffected by segmental reflex influences, although this is not so invariably.

Enhanced Motor Neuron Excitability

Fasciculation. *Fasciculation* is the name given to a spontaneous contraction of the muscle fibers composing a motor unit, which is visible as a muscle twitch through the skin. Muscle fasciculations may be seen and felt in otherwise normal people and are often remarkably persistent. They may be considered benign, unless they are accompanied by muscular wasting and weakness. Fasciculations are a prominent feature of motor neuron disease but can occur in almost any disorder of the lower motor neuron, particularly nerve root compression. In motor neuron disease, the ectopic neural discharge may arise at any point along a neuron from cell soma to nerve terminal (Roth, 1982; Wettstein, 1979), although workers differ in their estimates of the proportion originating proximally and distally.

Myokymia. Synchronous contraction of multiple motor units producing undulation of the muscle belly is known as *myokymia*. The condition is usually associated with disease of the lower motor neuron, is aggravated by voluntary muscle contraction, and may be associated with neuromyotonia.

Neuromyotonia. Delay in muscle relaxation after voluntary contraction originating from peripheral nerve rather than muscle is known as *pseudomyotonia* or *neuromyotonia* to distinguish it from myotonia caused by a disorder of the muscle membrane. Neuromyotonia has been reported in motor neuropathies, heredofamilial and sporadic, in association with fasciculation and myokymia (Lance et al., 1979). Other familial cases have been reported without peripheral neuropathy (Auger et al., 1984). The origin of the syndrome from peripheral nerve has been demonstrated by the persistence of muscle activity during general and spinal anesthesia, the graded diminution of spontaneous muscle activity with progressively more distal nerve blocks, and its abolition by curare (Wallis et al., 1970). As with fasciculation, ectopic neural discharges can be initiated throughout the length of the axon, down to and including its terminal arborization. Neuromyotonia responds well to treatment with carbamazepine or phenytoin.

Isaacs' Syndrome. Isaacs (1961) described two pa-

tients with progressive stiffness caused by continuous muscle fiber activity. The stiffness became more severe after voluntary muscle contraction and caused the patients to assume an abnormal posture. Muscular weakness, fasciculation, and areflexia suggest the presence of an underlying motor neuropathy, thus linking this condition with neuromyotonia. Like neuromyotonia, Isaacs' syndrome persists during general anesthesia, is abolished by neuromuscular blockade, and responds to phenytoin. The stiffness in Isaacs' syndrome persists despite peripheral nerve blockade and may be accentuated by pressure-ischemia produced by inflation of a sphygmomanometer, as in eliciting Trousseau's sign (Oda et al., 1989).

Continuous Motor Neuron Discharge of Proximal Origin. Seven members of a single family with constant muscle twitching and episodic stiffness were reported by Ashizawa et al. (1983). They differed from the patients described earlier in that continuous muscle activity disappeared during spinal anesthesia, indicating origin from the proximal part of the motor neuron.

References

(Key references are designated with an asterisk.)

Anderson A.D., Levine S.A., Gellert H. Loss of ambulatory ability in patients with old anterior poliomyelitis. *Lancet* 2:1061–1063, 1972.

Aniss A.M., Diener H.C., Hore J., et al. Reflex influences on muscle spindles in human pretibial muscles during standing. *J. Neurophysiol.* 64:671–679, 1990.

Ashby P., Wiens M. Reciprocal inhibition following lesions of the spinal cord in man. *J. Physiol. (Lond.)* 414:145–157, 1989.

Ashby P., Verrier M., Lightfoot E. Segmental reflex pathways in spinal shock and spinal spasticity in man. *J. Neurol. Neurosurg. Psychiatry* 37:1352–1360, 1974.

Ashby P., Verrier M., Carleton S. Vibratory inhibition of the monosynaptic reflex. In Desmedt J.E., ed. *Progress in Clinical Neurophysiology.* Vol. 8. *Spinal and Supraspinal Mechanisms of Voluntary Motor Control and Locomotion.* Basel, Karger, pp. 254–262, 1980.

Ashizawa T., Butler I.J., Harati Y., et al. A dominantly inherited syndrome with continuous motor neuron discharges. *Ann. Neurol.* 13:285–290, 1983.

Auger R.G., Daube J.R., Gomez M.R., et al. Hereditary form of sustained muscle activity of peripheral nerve origin causing generalized myokymia and muscle stiffness. *Ann. Neurol.* 15:13–21, 1984.

Baldissera F., Pierrot-Deseilligny E. Facilitation of transmission in the pathway of non-monosynaptic Ia excitation to wrist flexor motoneurones at the onset of voluntary movement in man. *Exp. Brain Res.* 74:437–439, 1989.

Banks R.W., Barker D., Stacey M.J. Structural aspects of fusimotor effects on spindle sensitivity. In Taylor A., Prochazka A., eds. *Muscle Receptors and Movement.* London, Macmillan, pp. 5–16, 1981.

Barker D. The morphology of muscle receptors. In Barker D., Hunt C.C., McIntyre A.K., eds. *Handbook of Sensory Physiology III. 2. Muscle Receptors.* New York, Springer-Verlag, pp. 1–190, 1974.

Barnes C.D., Schadt, J.C. Release of function in the spinal cord. *Prog. Neurobiol.* 12:1–13, 1979.

Baxendale R.H., Ferrell W.R. The effect of knee joint afferent discharge on transmission in flexion reflex pathways in decerebrate cats. *J. Physiol. (Lond.)* 315:231–242, 1981.

Berardelli A., Day B.L., Marsden C.D., et al. Evidence favouring presynaptic inhibition between antagonist muscle afferents in the human forearm. *J. Physiol. (Lond.)* 391:71–83, 1987.

Bergego C., Pierrot-Deseilligny E., Maziéres L. Facilitation of transmission in Ib pathways by cutaneous afferents from the contralateral foot sole in man. *Neurosci. Lett.* 27:297–301, 1981.

Bessou P., Joffroy M., Montoya R., et al. Effects of triceps stretch by ankle flexion on intact afferents and efferents of gastrocnemius in the decerebrate cat. *J. Physiol. (Lond.)* 346:73–91, 1984.

Bigland-Ritchie B.R., Woods J.J. Changes in muscle contractile properties and neural control during human muscular fatigue. *Muscle Nerve* 7:691–699, 1986.

Bigland-Ritchie B.R., Dawson N.J., Johansson R.S., et al. Reflex origin for the slowing of motoneurone firing rates in fatigue of human voluntary contractions. *J. Physiol. (Lond.)* 379:451–459, 1986.

Binder M.D., Stuart D.G. Motor unit–muscle receptor interactions: design features of the neuromuscular control system. In Desmedt J.E., ed. *Progress in Clinical Neurophysiology.* Vol. 8. *Spinal and Supraspinal Mechanisms of Voluntary Motor Control and Locomotion.* Basel, Karger, pp. 72–98, 1980.

Bongiovanni L.G., Hagbarth, K.-E. Tonic vibration reflexes elicited during fatigue from maximal voluntary contraction in man. *J. Physiol. (Lond.)* 423:1–14, 1990.

*Boyd I.A. The isolated mammalian muscle spindle. *Trends Neurosci.* 3:258–265, 1980.

Boyd I.A. The action of the three types of intrafusal fibre in isolated cat muscle spindles on the dynamic and length sensitivities of primary and secondary sensory endings. In Taylor A., Prochazka A., eds. *Muscle Receptors and Movement.* London, Macmillan, pp. 17–32, 1981.

Bratzlavsky M., Vander Eecken H. Medullary actions of tetanus toxin. *Arch. Neurol.* 33:783–785, 1976.

Buchthal F., Schmalbruch H. Motor unit of mammalian muscle. *Physiol. Rev.* 60:90–142, 1980.

Burke D. The activity of human muscle spindle endings in normal motor behavior. In Porter R., ed. *International Review of Physiology.* Vol. 25. *Neurophysiology IV.* Baltimore, University Park Press, pp. 91–126, 1981.

*Burke D. Critical examination of the case for or against fusimotor involvement in disorders of muscle tone. In Desmedt J.E., ed. *Motor Control Mechanisms in Health and Disease.* New York, Raven Press, pp. 133–150, 1983.

*Burke D., Gandevia S.C. The peripheral motor system. In Paxinos G., ed. *The Human Nervous System.* New York, Academic Press, pp. 125–145, 1990.

Burke D., Lance J.W. Studies of the reflex effects of primary and secondary spindle endings in spasticity. In Desmedt J.E., ed. *New Developments in Electromyography and Clinical Neurophysiology.* Vol.3. Basel, Karger, pp. 475–495, 1973.

Burke D., Andrews C.J., Lance J.W. The tonic vibration reflex in spasticity, Parkinson's disease and normal man. *J. Neurol. Neurosurg. Psychiatry* 35:477–486, 1972.

Burke D., Hagbarth K.-E., Löfstedt L., et al. The responses of human muscle spindle endings to vibration of non-contracting muscles. *J. Physiol. (Lond.)* 261:673–693, 1976.

Burke D., McKeon B., Skuse N.F. The irrelevance of fusimotor activity to the Achilles tendon jerk of relaxed humans. *Ann. Neurol.* 5:547–550, 1981.

Burke D., Gandevia S.C., McKeon B. The afferent volleys responsible for spinal proprioceptive reflexes in man. *J. Physiol. (Lond.)* 339:535–552, 1983.

Burke D., Gandevia S.C., McKeon B. Monosynaptic and oligosynaptic contributions to human ankle jerk and H reflex. *J. Neurophysiol.* 52:435–448, 1984.

Burke D., Gandevia S.C., Macefield G. Responses to passive movement of receptors in joint, skin and muscle of the human hand. *J. Physiol. (Lond.)* 402:347–361, 1988.

Burke D., Adams R.W., Skuse N.F. The effects of voluntary contraction on the H reflex of human limb muscles. *Brain* 112:417–433, 1989.

*Burke R.E. Motor units: anatomy, physiology and functional organization. In Brooks V.B., ed. *Handbook of Physiology.* Section 1. *The Nervous System.* Vol. II. *Motor Control.* Part 1. Bethesda, American Physiological Society, pp. 345–422, 1981.

Crone C., Hultborn H., Jespersen B., et al. Reciprocal Ia inhibition between ankle flexors and extensors in man. *J. Physiol. (Lond.)* 389:163–185, 1987.

Dastur F.D., Shahani M.T., Dastoor D.H., et al. Cephalic tetanus: demonstration of a dual lesion. *J. Neurol. Neurosurg. Psychiatry* 40:782–786, 1977.

de Gail P., Lance J.W., Neilson P.D. Differential effects on tonic and phasic reflex mechanisms produced by vibration of muscles in man. *J. Neurol. Neurosurg. Psychiatry* 29:1–11, 1966.

Delwaide P.J. *Étude Expérimentale de l'Hyperréflexie Tendineuse en Clinique Neurologique.* Brussels, Editions Arscia, 1971.

Delwaide P.J., Oliver E. Short-latency autogenic inhibition (IB inhibition) in human spasticity. *J. Neurol. Neurosurg. Psychiatry* 51:1546–1550, 1988.

*Desmedt J.E., ed. *Progress in Clinical Neurophysiology.* Vol. 8. *Spinal and Supraspinal Mechanisms of Voluntary Motor Control and Locomotion.* Basel, Karger, 1980.

*Desmedt J.E., ed. *Progress in Clinical Neurophysiology.* Vol. 9. *Motor Unit Types, Recruitment and Plasticity in Health and Disease.* Basel, Karger, 1981.

Dietrichson P. Phasic ankle jerk in spasticity and parkinsonian rigidity. *Acta Neurol. Scand.* 47:22–51, 1971.

Dietz V., Berger W. Interlimb coordination of posture in patients with spastic paresis. *Brain* 107:965–978, 1984.

Dimitrijević M.R., Spencer W.A., Trontelj J.V., et al. Reflex effects of vibration in patients with spinal cord lesions. *Neurology (Minneap.)* 27:1078–1086, 1977.

Eccles R.M., Lundberg A. Synaptic actions in motoneurones by afferents which may evoke the flexion reflex. *Arch. Ital. Biol.* 97:199–221, 1959.

Edström L. Selective changes in the sizes of red and white muscle fibers in upper motoneuron lesions and parkinsonism. *J. Neurol. Sci.* 11:537–550, 1970.

Emonet-Dénand F., Jami L., Laporte Y. Histophysiological observations on the skeleto-fusimotor innervation of mammalian spindles. In Desmedt J.E., ed. *Progress in Clinical Neurophysiology.* Vol. 8. *Spinal and Supraspinal Mechanisms of Voluntary Motor Control and Locomotion.* Basel, Karger, pp. 1–11, 1980.

Fernandez J.M., Ferrandiz M., Larrea L., et al. Cephalic tetanus studied with single fibre EMG. *J. Neurol. Neurosurg. Psychiatry* 46:862–866, 1983.

Ferrell W.R., Gandevia S.C., McCloskey D.I. The role of joint receptors in human kinaesthesia when intramuscular receptors cannot contribute. *J. Physiol. (Lond.)* 386:109–118, 1987.

Fleshman J.W., Munson J.B., Sypert G.W., et al. Rheobase, input resistance, and motor-unit type in medial gastrocnemius motoneurons in the cat. *J. Neurophysiol.* 46:1326–1338, 1981.

Gandevia S.C., Macefield G., Burke D., et al. Voluntary activation of human motor axons in the absence of muscle afferent feedback: the control of the deafferented hand. *Brain* 113:1563–1581, 1990.

Garnett R., Stephens J.A. Changes in recruitment threshold of motor units produced by cutaneous stimulation in man. *J. Physiol. (Lond.)* 311:463–473, 1981.

Gillies J.D., Lance J.W., Neilson P.D., et al. Presynaptic inhibition of the monosynaptic reflex by vibration. *J. Physiol. (Lond.)* 205:329–339, 1969.

Gillies J.D., Burke D.J., Lance J.W. Tonic vibration reflex in the cat. *J. Neurophysiol.* 34:252–262, 1971.

Gordon E.E., Januszko D.M., Kaufman L. A critical survey of stiff-man syndrome. *Am. J. Med.* 42:582–599, 1966.

Hagbarth K.-E., Eklund G. Motor effects of vibratory muscle stimuli in man. In Granit R., ed. *Muscular Afferents and Motor Control.* Stockholm, Almqvist and Wiksell, pp. 177–186, 1965.

Hagbarth K.-E., Eklund G. The effects of muscle vibration in spasticity, rigidity and cerebellar disorders. *J. Neurol. Neurosurg. Psychiatry* 31:207–213, 1968.

Harding A.E., Thompson P.D., Kocen R.S., et al. Plasma exchange and immunosuppression in the stiff man syndrome. *Lancet* 2:195, 1989.

Henneman E. Relation between size of neurons and their susceptibility to discharge. *Science* 126:1345–1346, 1957.

Henneman E. Recruitment of motoneurons: the size principle. In Desmedt J.E., ed. *Progress in Clinical Neurophysiology.* Vol. 9. *Motor Unit Types, Recruitment and Plasticity in Health and Disease.* Basel, Karger, pp. 26–60, 1981.

Holmqvist B., Lundberg A. Differential supraspinal control of synaptic actions evoked by volleys in the flexion reflex afferents in alpha motoneurones. *Acta Physiol. Scand.* 54(Suppl. 186):1–51, 1961.

Hopf H.C., Herbort R.L., Gnass M., et al. Fast and slow contraction times associated with fast and slow spike conduction of skeletal muscle fibres in normal subjects and in spastic hemiparesis. *Z. Neurol.* 206:193–202, 1974.

Houk J.C., Henneman E. Responses of Golgi tendon organs to active contractions of the soleus muscle of the cat. *J. Neurophysiol.* 30:466–481, 1967.

Houk J.C., Crago P.E., Rymer W.Z. Functional properties of Golgi tendon organs. In Desmedt J.E., ed. *Progress in Clinical Neurophysiology.* Vol. 8. *Spinal and Supraspinal Mechanisms of Voluntary Motor Control and Locomotion.* Basel, Karger, pp. 33–43, 1980.

Hulliger M., Matthews P.B.C., Noth J. Effects of static and of dynamic fusimotor stimulation on the response of Ia fibres to low frequency sinusoidal stretching covering a wide range of amplitudes. *J. Physiol. (Lond.)* 267:811–838, 1977.

Hultborn H., Pierrot-Deseilligny E. Changes in recurrent inhibition during voluntary soleus contractions in man studied by an H-reflex technique. *J. Physiol. (Lond.)* 297:229–251, 1979.

Hultborn H., Meunier S., Pierrot-Deseilligny E., et al. Changes in presynaptic inhibition of Ia fibres at the onset of voluntary contraction in man. *J. Physiol. (Lond.)* 389:757–772, 1987.

Iles J.F., Roberts R.C. Presynaptic inhibition of monosynaptic reflexes in the lower limbs of subjects with upper motoneuron disease. *J. Neurol. Neurosurg. Psychiatry* 49:937–944, 1986.

Iles J.F., Roberts R.C. Inhibition of monosynaptic reflexes in the human lower limb. *J. Physiol. (Lond.)* 385:69–87, 1987.

Iles J.F., Jack J.J.B., Kullmann D.M., et al. The effects of lesions on autogenetic inhibition in the decerebrate cat. *J. Physiol. (Lond.)* 419:611–625, 1989.

Isaacs H. A syndrome of continuous muscle-fibre activity. *J. Neurol. Neurosurg. Psychiatry* 24:319–325, 1961.

Isaacs H. Stiff man syndrome in a black girl. *J. Neurol. Neurosurg. Psychiatry* 42:988–994, 1979.

Jankowska E. New observations on neuronal organization of reflexes from tendon organ afferents and their relation to reflexes evoked from muscle spindle afferents. *Prog. Brain Res.* 50:21–36, 1979.

Jankowska E., McCrea D., Mackel R. Oligosynaptic excitation of motoneurones by impulses in group Ia muscle spindle afferents in the cat. *J. Physiol. (Lond.)* 316:411–425, 1981.

Jansen J.K.S. Spasticity—functional aspects. *Acta Neurol. Scand.* 38(Suppl. 3):41–51, 1962.

Katz R., Pierrot-Deseilligny E. Recurrent inhibition in patients with upper motoneurone lesions. *Brain* 105:103–124, 1982.

Kniffki K.-D., Mense S., Schmidt R.F. Muscle receptors with fine afferent fibers which may evoke circulatory reflexes. *Circ. Res.* 48(Suppl. 1):25–31, 1981.

Lance J.W. The mechanism of reflex irradiation. *Proc. Aust. Assoc. Neurol.* 3:77–80, 1965.

Lance J.W. Symposium synopsis. In Feldman R.G., Young R.R., Koella W.P., eds. *Spasticity: Disordered Motor Control.* Chicago, Year Book Medical Publishers, pp. 485–494, 1980a.

Lance J.W. The control of muscle tone, reflexes, and movement: Robert Wartenberg Lecture. *Neurology (N.Y.)* 30:1303–1313, 1980b.

Lance J.W., de Gail P. Spread of phasic muscle reflexes in normal and spastic subjects. *J. Neurol. Neurosurg. Psychiatry* 28:328–334, 1965.

Lance J.W., Burke D., Pollard J. Hyperexcitability of motor and sensory neurons in neuromyotonia. *Ann. Neurol.* 5:523–532, 1979.

Laporte Y., Bessou P. Modifications d'excitabilité de motoneurones homonymes provoquées par l'activation physiologique de fibres afférents d'origine musculaire du groupe II. *J. Physiol. (Paris)* 51:897–908, 1959.

Lee W.A., Boughton A., Rymer W.Z. Absence of stretch reflex gain enhancement in voluntarily activated spastic muscle. *Exp. Neurol.* 98:317–335, 1987.

Liddell E.G.T., Sherrington C.S. Reflexes in response to stretch (myotatic reflexes). *Proc.R. Soc. London Ser. B* 96:212–242, 1924.

Malmgren K., Pierrot-Deseilligny E. Evidence for non-monosynaptic Ia excitation of human wrist flexor motoneurones, possibly via propriospinal neurones. *J. Physiol. (Lond.)* 405:747–764, 1988a.

Malmgren K., Pierrot-Deseilligny E. Inhibition of neurones transmitting non-monosynaptic Ia excitation to human wrist flexor motoneurones. *J. Physiol. (Lond.)* 405:765–783, 1988b.

Mao C.C., Ashby P., Wang M., et al. Synaptic connections from large muscle afferents to the motoneurons of various leg muscles in man. *Exp. Brain Res.* 56:341–350, 1984.

Marsden C.D., Hallett M., Fahn S. The nosology and pathophysiology of myoclonus. In Marsden C.D., Fahn S., eds. *Movement Disorders. Neurology* 2. London, Butterworth, pp. 196–248, 1981.

Matthews P.B.C. Evidence that the secondary as well as the primary endings of the muscle spindles may be responsible for the tonic stretch reflex of the decerebrate cat. *J. Physiol. (Lond.)* 204:365–393, 1969.

*Matthews P.B.C. *Mammalian Muscle Receptors and Their Central Actions.* London, Arnold, 1972.

Matthews P.B.C. Evolving views on the internal operation and functional role of the muscle spindle. *J. Physiol. (Lond.)* 320:1–30, 1981.

Mayer R.F., Burke R.E., Toop J., et al. The effect of spinal cord transection on motor units in cat medial gastrocnemius muscles. *Muscle Nerve* 7:23–31, 1984.

*McCloskey D.I. Kinesthetic sensibility. *Physiol. Rev.* 58:763–820, 1978.

Meinck H.-M., Ricker K., Conrad B. The stiff-man syndrome: new pathophysiological aspects from abnormal exteroceptive reflexes and the response to clomipramine, clonidine and tizanidine. *J. Neurol. Neurosurg. Psychiatry* 47:280–287, 1984.

*Mendell L.M. Modifiability of spinal synapses. *Physiol. Rev.* 64:260–324, 1984.

Moersch F.P., Woltman H.W. Progressive fluctuating muscular rigidity and spasm ("stiff-man" syndrome): report of a case and some observations in 13 other cases. *Mayo Clin. Proc.* 31:421–427, 1956.

Morgan D.L., Prochazka A., Proske U. Can fusimotor activity potentiate the reponses of muscle spindles to a tendon tap? *Neurosci. Lett.* 50:209–215, 1984.

Mulder D.W., Rosenbaum R.A., Layton D.D. Late progression of poliomyelitis or forme fruste amyotrophic lateral sclerosis. *Mayo Clin. Proc.* 47:756–761, 1972.

Munson J.B., Sypert G.W., Zengel J.E., et al. Monosynaptic projections of individual spindle group II afferents to type identified medial gastrocnemius motoneurons in the cat. *J. Neurophysiol.* 48:1164–1174, 1982.

Nakashima K., Rothwell J.C., Day B.L., et al. Reciprocal inhibition between forearm muscles in patients with writer's cramp and other occupational cramps, symptomatic hemidystonia and hemiparesis due to stroke. *Brain* 112:681–697, 1989.

Oda K., Fukushima N., Shibasaki H., et al. Hypoxia-sensitive hyperexcitability of the intramuscular nerve axons in Isaacs' syndrome. *Ann. Neurol.* 25:140–145, 1989.

Pierrot-Deseilligny E., Bergego C., Katz R., et al. Cutaneous depression of Ib reflex pathways to motoneurones in man. *Exp. Brain Res.* 42:351–361, 1981.

Powers R.K., Campbell D.L., Rymer W.Z. Stretch reflex dynamics in spastic elbow flexor muscles. *Ann. Neurol.* 25:32–42, 1989.

Proske U. The Golgi tendon organ: properties of the receptor and reflex action of impulses arising from tendon organs. In Porter R., ed. *International Review of Physiology.* Vol. 25. *Neurophysiology IV.* Baltimore, University Park Press, pp. 127–171, 1981.

Reinking R.M., Stephens J.A., Stuart D.G. The tendon organs of cat medial gastrocnemius: significance of motor unit size and type for the activation of Ib afferents. *J. Physiol. (Lond.)* 250:491–512, 1975.

Roth G. The origin of fasciculations. *Ann. Neurol.* 12:542–547, 1982.

Rushworth G. Spasticity and rigidity: an experimental study and review. *J. Neurol. Neurosurg. Psychiatry* 23:99–117, 1960.

Rushworth G., Lishman W.A., Hughes J.T., et al. Intense rigidity of the arms due to isolation of motoneurones by a spinal tumour. *J. Neurol. Neurosurg. Psychiatry* 24:132–142, 1961.

Rymer W.Z., Houk J.C., Crago P.E. Mechanisms of the clasp-knife reflex studied in an animal model. *Exp. Brain Res.* 37:93–113, 1979.

Sander J.E., Layzer R.B., Goldsobel A.B. Congenital stiff-man syndrome. *Ann. Neurol.* 8:195–197, 1980.

Schomburg E.D., Behrends H.B. The possibility of phase dependent monosynaptic and polysynaptic Ia excitation to homonymous motoneurones during fictive locomotion. *Brain Res.* 143:533–537, 1978.

Schwartzman R.J., Eidelberg E., Alexander G.M., et al. Regional metabolic changes in the spinal cord related to spinal shock and later hyperreflexia in monkeys. *Ann. Neurol.* 14:33–37, 1983.

*Solimena M., Folli F., Denis-Donini S., et al. Autoantibodies to glutamic acid decarboxylase in a patient with stiff-man syndrome, epilepsy, and type I diabetes mellitus. *N. Engl. J. Med.* 318:1012–1020, 1988.

Spehlmann R., Norcross K., Rasmus S.C., et al. Improvement of stiff-man syndrome with sodium valproate. *Neurology (N.Y.)* 31:1162–1163, 1981.

Tarlov I.M. Rigidity in man due to spinal interneuron loss. *Arch. Neurol.* 16:536–543, 1967.

Tarlov I.M., Ling H., Yamada H. Neuronal pathology in experimental local tetanus. Clinical implications. *Neurology (Minneap.)* 23:580–591, 1973.

*Taylor A., Prochazka A., eds. *Muscle Receptors and Movement.* London, Macmillan, 1981.

*Vallbo Å.B., Hagbarth K.-E., Torebjörk H.E., et al. Somatosensory, proprioceptive, and sympathetic activity in human peripheral nerves. *Physiol. Rev.* 59:919–957, 1979.

Vicari A.M., Folli F., Pozza G., et al. Plasmapheresis in the treatment of stiff-man syndrome (letter). *N. Engl. J. Med.* 320:1499, 1989.

Voss V.H. Tabelle der absoluten und relativen Muskelspindelzahlen der menschlichen Skelettmuskulatur. *Anat. Anz.* 129:562–572, 1971.

Wallis W.E., Van Poznak A., Plum F. Generalized muscular stiffness, fasciculations and myokymia of peripheral nerve origin. *Arch. Neurol.* 22:430–439, 1970.

Watt D.G.D., Stauffer E.K., Taylor A., et al. Analysis of muscle receptor connections by spike triggered averaging: I. Spindle primary and tendon organ afferents. *J. Neurophysiol.* 39:1375–1392, 1976.

Wettstein A. The origin of fasciculations in motoneuron disease. *Ann. Neurol.* 5:295–300, 1979.

Yanagisawa N., Tanaka R., Ito Z. Reciprocal Ia inhibition in spastic hemiplegia of man. *Brain* 99:555–574, 1976.

Young J.L., Mayer R.F. Physiological alterations of motor units in hemiplegia. *J. Neurol. Sci.* 54:401–412, 1982.

The Brain and Motor Control

21

Central Mechanisms of Initiation and Control of Movement

Garrett E. Alexander
Mahlon R. DeLong

The ease with which humans and other primates are able to make coordinated musculoskeletal movements belies the complexity of the underlying computational problems. When analyzed mathematically, the process of translating the intended goal of a movement, such as reaching for an object in space, into an appropriate set of muscle activations requires a complex set of transformations, including sequential computations of (1) the trajectory of the hand in space; (2) the magnitudes and time courses of the trajectory-dictated joint displacements (inverse kinematics); (3) the magnitudes and time courses of the kinematics-dictated joint torques (inverse dynamics); (4) the muscle tensions necessary to achieve the required joint torques; and (5) the magnitude and timing of the neural inputs appropriate for achieving the required muscle tensions (Hildreth and Hollerbach, 1987; Saltzman, 1979). These computations must also take into account a number of complicating factors, including the reconciliation of multiple spatial frames of reference (i.e., retinocentric, head-centered, and body-centered coordinate systems for locating objects in external space and the separate,

multidimensional coordinate systems of joints and muscles), the dynamic interactions between articulated limb segments, and the highly nonlinear length-tension properties of muscle. The enormity of the problem is underscored by the rather limited success that engineers have had in developing robots that can interact successfully with a complex and changing environment. Measured against the relatively rigid, clumsy, and inefficient motor performance of even the most sophisticated of robots (Loeb, 1983), the highly adaptive motor capacities of humans and other primates are truly remarkable.

How, then, is motor control achieved in animals such as these? And how are their respective motor systems, with individual neurons operating at mere fractions of the speeds of conventional computers, able reliably, in fact vastly, to outperform computer-controlled robots on nearly any type of nonrepetitive task? Neither of these questions can be answered at present with any degree of certainty. It is important to be aware, however, that developments in neurobiology and related fields of research have begun to indicate that biologic solutions to the problem of motor control may differ in fundamental ways from the systematic, algorithmic solutions employed by roboticists and engineers. Thus, before the neurobiology of motor control is considered in any detail, it

Preparation of this review was made possible in part by grants from the National Institute of Neurological Disorders and Stroke (NS 17678, NS 15417, and NS 23160).

seems worthwhile to review some of the general characteristics that distinguish natural, brain-based motor systems from the computer-controlled systems used in robotics. Throughout this chapter, the focus, where possible, is on the motor systems of humans and other primates to maximize the potential relevance of these discussions to an understanding of various clinical disorders of motor control.

It has become commonplace to compare the operations of the brain and those of a digital computer and thus, for example, to speak of the motor system (or some of its parts) as being engaged in the storage and/or execution of various types of motor programs. Although appealing because of its apparent simplicity, this concept has not proved helpful in gaining insight into the mechanisms that underlie motor control. After all, programs require programmers, first to identify the appropriate algorithm (a fixed sequence of logical or mathematic operations) that is needed to solve a particular problem and then to implement that algorithm with a set of commands appropriate to the hardware on which the program is to be run. There are as yet no scientific theories of motor programming that explain how these theoretic programs might originate in the brain. This and other conceptual difficulties pose serious constraints on the heuristic value of the motor programming metaphor.

Another major difference between computer- and brain-based motor systems is in the latter's superior flexibility and adaptability in response to changing task demands. For example, one of the salient features of human motor behavior is the relative ease with which learned movements, even those with complicated trajectories such as drawing or writing, can be readily scaled in time and space, transferred between extremities, and adjusted for the use of hand-held tools, all with little or no practice. This uniquely biologic phenomenon of motor equivalence is well known, but its neural basis is poorly understood. Such a capacity for ready adaptability to changing task demands is, by comparison, virtually absent in conventional robots. One explanation for the ease with which subjects can modify previously learned movements is that motor control in humans and other primates may be organized primarily in terms of the spatial aspects of the task, rather than the kinematics or dynamics of the jointed limb (Bernstein, 1984; Hogan et al., 1987). In natural reaching to objects, the hand's trajectory tends to be straight and its velocity profile smooth and bell shaped, as would be expected if such movements were planned and controlled in terms of the coordinate system of external space (Abend et al., 1982; Morasso, 1981). Because of the complex relations between multijoint (wrist, elbow, shoulder) kinematics and hand trajectory, however, if spatially targeted movements were controlled primarily in terms of joint kinematics, even small degrees of incoordination among the joints involved could produce irregular and more curvilinear hand trajectories (Hogan et al., 1987). Observations such as these prompted several motor theorists to propose that goal-directed limb movements may

be organized primarily in terms of the target or goal of the movement, rather than the kinematic or dynamic features of the movement itself (Bernstein, 1984; Hollerbach, 1982). If so, one would expect to find neural representations within the motor system of some of the spatial aspects of learned motor tasks, and such representations have been demonstrated in several different motor areas in the monkey (Alexander and Crutcher, 1990b).

Another important difference between natural and artificial motor systems is the relative speed of their respective computing elements. Whereas modern computers can perform millions of sequential operations every second, neural systems are restricted to a few hundred at most (assuming combined synaptic and conduction delays of about 1–5 ms/step). Because the reaction times of primates, for example, are on the order of a quarter of a second, it has been estimated that less than a hundred sequential operations could be performed during a typical reaction time, if the brain were to operate like a conventional digital computer (J.A. Feldman and Ballard, 1982). This 100-step limit in biologic systems seems to preclude the solution of the earlier-outlined motor control problem by means of a conventional, serial algorithm. Arguments such as this have tended to reinforce the growing belief that biologic motor systems may solve the problem of motor control through mechanisms that differ radically from those employed in conventional robotics.

It is widely recognized that the functional architectures of brains in general, and of primate motor systems in particular, are highly parallel in nature. This sort of architecture may provide an important clue as to how such a complex problem as that of motor control can be solved in biologic systems so much more efficiently than is possible in most artificial systems that use a serial, algorithmic approach. However, it is just as important that biologic systems are self-organizing. That is, in biologic motor systems, performance tends to improve with practice, whereas such is not the case with artificial motor systems that are controlled by conventional computers. The neural basis of self-organization (or learning) in biologic motor systems is not known with certainty, but there is growing evidence concerning other parts of the nervous system that such effects may be based on activity-dependent modifications of synaptic strengths (Linsker, 1990). Models of neural networks with these properties are rapidly being developed and studied, and such connectionist or parallel distributed processing models of the motor system are perhaps the most plausible from the standpoint of what is already known about the anatomy and physiology of motor control. The essence of most connectionist models is that they are self-organizing, massively parallel networks in which learning is distributed throughout the system (being based on activity-dependent changes at each synapse). Information is thus stored not in discrete locations (e.g., as bytes of information) but rather in the overall pattern of variable-strength connections

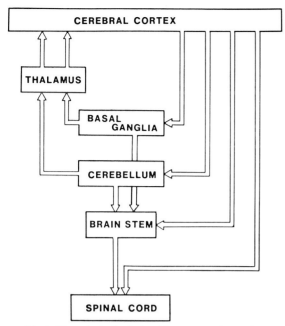

Figure 21–1. The principal relationships among the major components of the motor system. Note that the basal ganglia and the cerebellum may be viewed as key elements in two parallel, reentrant systems, which return their influences to the cortex through discrete and separate portions of the ventrolateral thalamus. This illustration also emphasizes the parallel projections of the cerebral cortex to multiple levels of the motor system.

OVERVIEW OF MOTOR SYSTEMS IN PRIMATES

Although the neuronal substrates of many reflexes and basic movement synergies are present at spinal levels, the supraspinal systems provide the complex modulatory control of segmental mechanisms necessary for adaptive and skilled motor acts. As indicated in Figure 21–1, the segmental motor apparatus within the spinal cord is influenced by two principal categories of descending pathways: those originating from the cerebral cortex and those arising from various brain stem nuclei, many of which are themselves recipients of descending cortical influences. The cortical motor fields (Fig. 21–2), whose descending projections modulate (both directly and indirectly) the output of the segmental motor apparatus, are influenced in turn by other cortical areas and by outputs from the cerebellum and the basal ganglia.

The basal ganglia and the cerebellum can each be viewed as parallel, *reentrant* networks that receive separate, but largely similar, inputs from various cortical areas (including motor, premotor, and somatosensory cortex) and return their own respective influences to specific, and largely separate, precentral motor areas via basal ganglia– and cerebellum-specific connections within the ventrolateral thalamus (see Fig. 21–1). This chapter examines, in sequence, the cortical areas involved in motor control; the corticospinal systems; the separate, reentrant motor pathways that pass respectively through the basal ganglia and the cerebellum; and the descending brain stem motor pathways. Before these suprasegmental systems are discussed, however, it is important to have a general understanding of the segmental motor apparatus and its intrinsic capabilities.

among neurons. The distributed representations inherent in such models are in keeping with the well-known fault tolerance in biologic motor systems (that is, the loss of one or a few neural elements involved in a particular motor pattern can be tolerated without significant loss of function) (Rumelhart et al., 1986). Moreover, models of this sort tend to mimic many of the characteristic features of human motor learning, such as the tendency to generalize or transfer skills across closely related motor patterns and to minimize conflicts between different motor patterns when they are learned together rather than in sequence (Grossberg and Kuperstein, 1989).

SEGMENTAL MOTOR APPARATUS

Among the basic motor patterns mediated by spinal mechanisms are phasic and tonic stretch re-

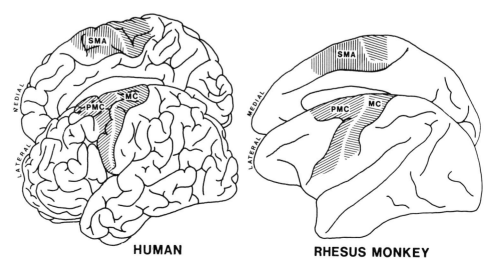

Figure 21–2. Locations of the motor and premotor fields in humans and rhesus monkey. In each case, the mesial aspect of the hemisphere has been projected as a mirror image. SMA = supplementary motor area; PMC = premotor cortex; MC = motor cortex.

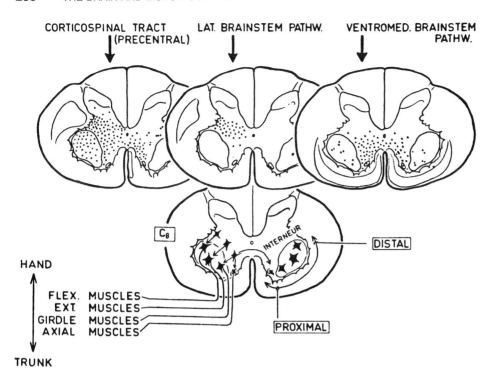

CORTICOSPINAL TRACT
(PRECENTRAL)

LAT. BRAINSTEM PATHW.

VENTROMED. BRAINSTEM
PATHW.

HAND

FLEX. MUSCLES
EXT. MUSCLES
GIRDLE MUSCLES
AXIAL MUSCLES

TRUNK

C_8 INTERNEUR DISTAL PROXIMAL

Figure 21–3. *(Upper)* The terminal distribution of the descending cortical and subcortical pathways in the lower cervical cord of the rhesus monkey. *(Lower)* A corresponding segment in the cat showing the organization of the projections from interneurons to motor neurons (the trajectories of the projections are not shown). (From Lawrence D.G., Kuypers H.G.J.M. The functional organization of the motor system in the monkey. II. The effects of lesions of the descending brain stem pathways. *Brain* 91:15–36, 1968, by permission of Oxford University Press.)

flexes, flexor withdrawal responses, crossed extensor reflexes, local supporting reactions, tonic neck and lumbar reflexes, and a number of more complex movement synergies, such as rhythmic stepping. It has been shown, for example, that the spinal cord isolated from descending influences is capable of supporting rhythmic stepping movements in cats suspended over a treadmill (for detailed review, see Forssberg, 1982). The isolated spinal locomotor generator produces appropriately timed stepping phases and phasically gates tactile reflex arcs to elicit differential effects of afferent input that are appropriate for each phase of the step cycle. Analysis of the ontogeny of bipedal locomotion in humans suggests that elements of the spinal locomotor generator may control the reflex stepping of neonates, with the supraspinal influences required for fully bipedal locomotion being gradually superimposed during the subsequent 2 years of development (Forssberg, 1985).

The segmental motor apparatus of the spinal cord consists of topographically organized pools of α and γ motor neurons, as well as local interneurons and intersegmental propriospinal neurons. Motor neurons are clustered within the ventral horn, in Rexed lamina IX, where they receive extensive monosynaptic and polysynaptic segmental inputs from muscles, joints, and skin. Although most supraspinal influences are mediated through spinal interneurons, spinal motor neurons in primates receive monosynaptic excitatory inputs from at least four descending systems, including the corticospinal, reticulospinal, rubrospinal, and vestibulospinal tracts. Monosynaptic inhibitory inputs to spinal motor neurons have been demonstrated from reticulospinal and medial vestibulospinal tracts. Interneurons and proprio-

spinal neurons are distributed throughout the intermediate zone, in laminae V–VII, and in a medial portion of the ventral horn, in lamina VIII. These groupings are illustrated in the lower portion of Figure 21–3.

Motor neurons that innervate the axial musculature are situated in an extreme ventromedial sector of lamina IX, whereas those that innervate the intrinsic extremity musculature are clustered within a dorsolateral sector. Motor neurons for the limb girdle musculature are located in an intermediate position. As shown in Figure 21–3, this ventromedial-dorsolateral gradient of proximal-distal representation is also maintained within the intermediate zone (laminae V–VIII) that contains the propriospinal neurons. Propriospinal neurons projecting to limb girdle and axial motor neurons tend to project for considerable distances above and below the segment of origin, thus influencing large groups of proximal muscles (Kuypers, 1981). By contrast, propriospinal neurons projecting to motor neurons that innervate the intrinsic muscles of the limb tend to project only short distances above and below the segment of origin, thereby influencing smaller, more restricted groups of distal muscles.

Propriospinal neurons are generally distinguished from other interneurons (such as Renshaw cells and Ia inhibitory interneurons) by their lack of intercalation into segmental reflex arcs and intrinsic feedback pathways. Studies with cats have shown that propriospinal neurons may receive direct projections from a variety of descending pathways (corticospinal, rubrospinal, tectospinal, and so on), as well as inputs from segmental afferent fibers (group Ia, Ib, II, and so on) (for extensive review, see Baldissera et al.,

1981). Anatomic studies with cats and monkeys revealed that propriospinal neurons give off intersegmental projections that run in the fasciculi proprii immediately surrounding the ventral horn (reviewed in Kuypers, 1981). These ascending and descending propriospinal projections appear to be topographically organized, terminating within restricted portions of the intermediate zone and the immediately adjacent ventral horn. Propriospinal neurons located in the dorsolateral portion of the intermediate zone project largely to dorsolateral portions of the ventral horn and the intermediate zone of other levels; correspondingly, the ventromedially placed propriospinal neurons eventually terminate in ventromedial portions of the ventral horn and the intermediate zone.

By virtue of their intersegmental connectivity and convergent inputs from supraspinal, intersegmental, and intrasegmental sources, propriospinal neurons seem well suited for their proposed roles in the relay of descending motor commands and the intersegmental coordination of complex movement synergies. Indeed, extensive studies of the C3-4 propriospinal system in cats (Lundberg, 1979) demonstrated that descending motor commands for rapid, synergic movements of the forelimb, such as those involved in reaching, are relayed through the propriospinal neurons of the upper cervical segments. On the other hand, descending commands controlling fine distal movements (e.g., the toe grasping required for food retrieval) appear to by-pass the propriospinal relays.

CORTICAL CONTROL OF MOVEMENT

In humans and other primates, motor control depends critically on the integrity of various motor fields within the cerebral cortex. Most are located within the frontal agranular cortex (i.e., those regions of cortex within the frontal lobe that lack a well-developed internal granular layer, or layer IV), but studies have shown that some of the cortical motor fields are actually located within bordering regions that traditionally had been considered part of the limbic system (Dum and Strick, 1991). The known motor fields encompass the primary motor cortex, which is coextensive with Brodmann area 4, and several premotor areas that lie either within area 6 (which extends across the medial and lateral surfaces of the hemisphere) or within adjoining cortex along the banks of the cingulate sulcus (including parts of areas 23 and 24) (Dum and Strick, 1991; Evarts, 1981; M. Wiesendanger, 1981). In humans, it is still customary to distinguish only two premotor areas: the premotor cortex, which lies on the lateral surface of the hemisphere immediately rostral to primary motor cortex, and the supplementary motor area (SMA), which also lies in front of the primary motor cortex but resides, for the most part, on the medial surface of the hemisphere (see Fig. 21–2). In monkeys, however, there is clear evidence of at least two premotor

areas located on the lateral convexity (the arcuate premotor and precentral motor areas) and at least three within the medial wall of the hemisphere (including the SMA within the medial frontal agranular cortex and two cingulate motor areas located within the cingulate sulcus). Each of these premotor fields is somatotopically organized, each projects directly to the primary motor cortex (establishing an anatomic basis for its designation as a premotor area), and all but one (the precentral motor area) have direct corticospinal projections that are comparable with those that arise from area 4 (Dum and Strick, 1991; Murray and Coulter, 1981). It seems reasonable to suspect that similar degrees of structural and functional differentiation must also exist within the premotor fields of humans, although there are obviously profound limitations on the precision with which such questions can be addressed directly in human subjects.

Functional analyses of the cortical motor fields in humans have been facilitated by imaging techniques that permit assessments of regional cerebral blood flow and regional oxidative metabolism and by electrical recordings of event-related cerebral potentials. During voluntary movements of a limb, focal increases in cerebral blood flow are seen within the contralateral primary motor cortex and within the SMA, usually on both sides (Fox et al., 1985; Roland, 1984; Roland et al., 1980). During the planning or preparation for a movement that is merely rehearsed but not executed, increases in blood flow are seen within the SMA and within the premotor cortex on the lateral surface of the hemisphere, but not within primary motor cortex (Roland et al., 1980).

Studies of event-related potentials in humans (Deecke et al., 1976; Neshige et al., 1988) suggest that early during the preparation for a voluntary movement (several hundred milliseconds before electromyographic [EMG] onset) both the SMA and primary motor cortex become active bilaterally, giving rise to the slow negative potential referred to as the readiness potential, or *Bereitschaftspotential*. In scalp recordings, the *Bereitschaftspotential* is centered on the vertex (Barrett et al., 1986; Deecke et al., 1976), but in subdural recordings, it has been shown to arise from discrete foci within the primary and supplementary motor areas (Neshige et al., 1988). After the *Bereitschaftspotential*, and approximately 250–400 ms before onset of EMG activity, a second potential can be discerned, the so-called negative slope. In scalp recordings, the negative slope is centered on the contralateral centroparietal region (Barrett et al., 1986), but in subdural recordings, it has been found to arise from separate foci within the supplementary motor and contralateral primary motor areas, with little or no involvement of the ipsilateral primary motor cortex (Neshige et al., 1988). After the negative slope is another, steeper, negative potential, the motor potential, which begins shortly (50–100 ms) before onset of EMG activity and continues (in the form of several subsets of potentials) throughout the movement. In both scalp and subdural recordings, the various components of the motor potential appear to arise exclusively from the contralateral primary motor and somatosensory cortices (Barrett et al., 1986; Deecke et al., 1976; Neshige et al., 1988).

Although the techniques available for functional studies in humans do not have the spatial or temporal resolution of the single-cell recording techniques that have been used to study motor physiology in behaving monkeys, the two approaches yielded results that are largely congruent. Thus, for example, during the preparation for movement, much higher proportions of neurons become active in the lateral premotor area and the SMAs than in the primary motor cortex, whereas the reverse is seen during movement execution (Alexander and Crutcher, 1990c; Tanji and Kurata, 1985; Wise, 1985).

Motor Cortex

Primary motor cortex is linked closely with the segmental motor apparatus via its direct corticospinal projections. It has been estimated that the motor cortex contributes approximately 40% of the corticospinal fibers that make up each human medullary pyramid. The motor cortex is influenced in turn by direct projections from the premotor areas and from somatosensory cortex and receives indirect subcortical input from the basal ganglia and the cerebellum. The motor cortex is thus often viewed as a summing point for influences conveyed from cortical and subcortical sensorimotor structures, as well as for those relayed from the periphery via the somatosensory cortex and parietal area 5. A major role of the motor cortex suggested by these and other considerations is to integrate a wide variety of cortical and subcortical inputs and, from this integrated information, to generate descending command signals that specify the distribution, timing, and magnitude of muscular activation.

Given the massive contribution of the motor cortex to the pyramidal tract, it is not surprising that the functions of this area are often viewed in terms of its pyramidal tract contribution, especially as reflected by the motor deficits that result from lesions of this pathway. A more direct and positive indication of the functions of the motor cortex has been obtained in studies of the activity of motor cortex pyramidal tract neurons (PTNs) in the behaving primate. These studies were pioneered by Evarts and colleagues (for detailed review, see Evarts, 1981). Motor cortex PTNs have been shown to discharge before the onset of muscular activity and to have properties similar in many respects to those of spinal α motor neurons, with patterns of discharge that are highly correlated with force and with the length and tension properties of muscles. The PTNs also exhibit rate modulation in relation to increasing force and are recruited in an orderly manner in relation to size. A direct action of PTNs on α motor neurons has been

demonstrated by spike-triggered averaging techniques (Cheney and Fetz, 1980).

Another function of the motor cortex appears to be the mediation of certain cutaneous and proprioceptive reflexes. In the monkey, input from deep and cutaneous receptors is directed to separate regions of the motor cortex (Strick and Preston, 1982). Sensory feedback to PTNs appears to operate in a manner similar to that found for α motor neurons, with the important added feature of modulation of the response in relation to the intention, or motor set, of the subject. Thus, unlike the case with the spinal stretch reflex arc, transmission through the transcortical reflex circuit depends on the subject's motor set. The motor cortex also appears to participate in input-output coupling of cutaneous reflexes. Transmission through this transcortical pathway appears to be modulated by input from the SMA. Studies with the monkey suggest that projections from the SMA to the motor cortex may have an inhibitory effect on motor cortex neuronal responses to spinal inputs (M. Wiesendanger, 1981). The release of this inhibitory control of motor cortex output in response to somatosensory input may explain why lesions of the SMA are frequently associated with involuntary grasping (so-called forced grasping) of objects that come in contact with the hand (Smith et al., 1981; M. Wiesendanger, 1981).

Although the functions of the motor cortex are partially reflected by the actions of its PTNs and the deficits resulting from lesions of the pyramidal tract, the role of the motor cortex in motor control is clearly not limited to its corticospinal output. The motor cortex also contributes substantial projections to the premotor cortex, the SMA, and the somatosensory cortex, as well as to the thalamus, the basal ganglia, and the cerebellum (via the pontine nuclei) (for reviews, see Carpenter, 1981; Humphrey, 1983). These additional outputs presumably serve to inform the target areas of the intended movement (corollary discharge) and to exert some influence on the outputs from these areas. Evidence in monkeys suggests that these non–pyramidal tract projections from the motor cortex are derived largely from separate populations of non-PTNs, rather than from PTN collaterals (Jones and Wise, 1977). Thus, the motor cortex appears to participate in the suprasegmental control of movement not only via the direct spinal projections of its PTNs but also through its numerous influences on other brain regions involved in motor control.

Premotor Cortex

Clinical and experimental studies with humans have suggested several roles for the premotor cortex of the lateral convexity (PMC). One role, which appears to be subserved particularly by its caudal part, is the control of proximal limb musculature and interlimb coordination (Freund, 1984; Freund and Hummelsheim, 1984; M. Wiesendanger, 1981). This is consistent with the anatomic evidence indicating heavy projections from this region to the medial pontomedullary reticular formation, whose spinal projections constitute the bulk of the ventromedial descending brain stem system (see under Brain Stem Descending Pathways). Studies with humans showed maximal increases in regional cerebral blood flow in PMC during voluntary movements that require sensory guidance (Roland et al., 1980). Other studies suggested that the more rostral portions of the PMC function as a higher motor association area. Lesions of this portion of the PMC may result in apraxia, perseveration, and disturbances in visuomotor tasks (M. Wiesendanger, 1981; Wise, 1985). Studies in the monkey showed that there are at least two anatomically distinct premotor areas on the lateral convexity and that both are somatotopically organized (Muakkassa and Strick, 1979). Studies of single-cell activity and of the behavioral effects of lesions provided evidence of involvement of the PMC in the preparation for specific movements (including the postural fixation required for limb movements), the modulation of transcortical reflexes, and the control of visually guided limb movements (M. Wiesendanger, 1981; Wise, 1985). It is noteworthy that the PMC appears to receive a major input from parietal area 7, which has been shown to participate in the control of visually guided arm movements in the mechanisms underlying directed attention (Lynch et al., 1977; Robinson et al., 1978).

Supplementary Motor Area

Penfield and Welch (1951) coined the term *supplementary motor area* for that portion of area 6, lying anterior to area 4 on the medial surface of the hemisphere, from which complex movements were evoked by electrical stimulation both in humans and in subhuman primates. Although earlier investigations focused largely on the role of the SMA in spasticity and the phenomenon of forced grasping, which often occurred after SMA lesions, renewed attention has been focused on the SMA because the aforementioned electrophysiologic and regional cerebral blood flow studies suggested a special role for this area in the planning of voluntary movements. A further perspective on the role of the SMA in high-level motor control was indicated by reports that SMA lesions in humans may lead to a severe poverty of movement (akinesia) and mutism (Damasio and VanHoesen, 1980; LaPlane et al., 1977; Masdeu et al., 1978).

It is noteworthy in this regard that a major output of the basal ganglia is directed (via the thalamus) to the SMA. It remains uncertain, however, whether the akinesia and mutism reported after lesions involving the SMA can be explained simply in terms of the loss of basal ganglia influences on the cerebral cortex. A role of the SMA in speech production, suggested by the reports of SMA lesions, is also supported by data from cerebral blood flow studies (Larsen et al., 1978) and from reports of vocalization and speech arrest induced by electrical stimulation of this region in humans (Penfield and Welch, 1951; Talairach and Bancaud, 1966).

Participation of the SMA in complex motor functions and the possible gating of the motor cortex is supported by single-cell recordings in the SMA of monkeys, which revealed changes in neuronal activity related not only to movement execution but also to the preparation for movement and motor set (see Tanji et al., 1980). Input to the SMA in the monkey comes from wide areas of the cortex, including prefrontal areas, motor cortex, PMC, somatosensory cortex, and parietal area 5, which is believed to be strongly involved in the tactile guidance of exploratory limb movements. These diverse inputs suggest that the SMA may act as a summing point for channeling a wide range of cortical influences into motor output. Some of these corticocortical connections may also play a role in the modulation of transcortical reflexes by the SMA (see earlier). It has been suggested that the SMA and the PMC, by virtue of their inputs from parietal and frontal association areas, may in some way mediate shifts in attention to various somatosensory stimuli.

Although considerable emphasis has been placed on influences from the SMA on the motor cortex, retrograde labeling studies indicate that the SMA also projects directly to the spinal cord (Biber et al., 1978; Murray and Coulter, 1981). Electrical stimulation of the SMA in conscious humans evoked simple as well as complex synergic movements that may be localized to head, arm, or leg (VanBuren and Fedio, 1976). Moreover, microstimulation and single-cell recording studies indicated that the SMA is somatotopically organized and that activation of the SMA may evoke discrete movements of the limbs (Alexander and Crutcher, 1990c; Macpherson et al., 1982). These findings suggest a role of this region in the control of distal as well as proximal portions of the limb (Macpherson et al., 1982) and a closer coupling between the SMA and the spinal motor mechanisms than was envisioned previously. Thus, it appears that the SMA may function not only to transmit motor commands to the motor cortex and to gate transcortical reflexes, but also as an output channel to influence directly the spinal cord and the brain stem in parallel with the motor cortex.

CORTICOSPINAL SYSTEMS

The corticospinal (or pyramidal) tract comprises direct projections to the spinal cord not only from multiple cortical motor areas (see earlier) but also from several somatosensory areas. The latter include primary somatosensory fields (areas 3, 1, and 2) and the somatosensory association area within adjacent area 5, as well as the supplementary sensory area (medial area 5) (Catsman-Berrevoets and Kuypers,

1976; Coulter and Jones, 1977; Coulter et al., 1979). In the human, approximately 1 million corticospinal fibers (compared with about 250,000 in the monkey) pass through each medullary pyramid, with 70–90% crossing in the motor decussation and continuing caudally as the *lateral* corticospinal tract and 10–30% remaining uncrossed and forming the *ventral* corticospinal tract (DeMyer, 1959). In higher primates, the corticospinal tract increases enormously in size, and the distribution of terminals within the spinal gray matter shifts ventrally to include the motor neuron pools, reflecting increased direct control of segmental output (Fig. 21–4). Comparative studies indicate that these pathways have emerged and been selectively strengthened in various species, especially primates, roughly in accordance with an increasing capacity for the execution of movements that are highly fractionated (that is, in which closely approximated structures, such as fingers, are moved in relative independence) (Kuypers, 1981). Selective lesions of the corticospinal pathway lead to the specific loss of ability to perform movements of this type. Contrary to what might have been expected, it seems that the capacity for making fractionated movements is not based on the corticospinal projections' being

organized in the same fashion as a telephone switchboard, with simple point-to-point mappings of cortical motor neurons onto spinal motor neurons. Instead, there appears to be an enormous amount of both convergence and divergence of connections between these two sets of neurons.

Thus, for example, injections of individual corticospinal axons with anatomic tracers showed that each axon can give rise to a surprisingly large number of terminal branches that diverge to innervate multiple separate spinal motor nuclei (Shinoda et al., 1981). Conversely, the ventral horn at a given level of the spinal cord may receive corticospinal inputs from several different cortical motor fields (Dum and Strick, 1991; Murray and Coulter, 1981). Studies using spike-triggered averaging (in which the action potentials of individual cortical motor neurons are correlated with rectified EMG activity recorded from a number of different muscles) showed that most corticospinal neurons appear to have direct, presumably monosynaptic connections with more than one muscle (Fetz and Cheney, 1980; Fetz et al., 1989). In most cases, the muscle field of a given cortical neuron is restricted to a relatively small number of functionally related muscles (generally two or three), and the amount of facilitation (or suppression) provided to each muscle is usually different (Lemon, 1988). In some cases, individual corticospinal neurons exerted reciprocal effects on muscles that are functional antagonists (e.g., flexors versus extensors of a finger) (Kasser and Cheney, 1985), and thus far there have been no reports of neurons that provide postspike facilitation to both agonists and antagonists of the same joint. The relative weakness of the postspike EMG facilitation that is associated with the activity of any single corticospinal neuron suggests that convergent input from many such cells is necessary for EMG activity to be initiated in a given motor unit (Fetz et al., 1989; Lemon, 1988). Corticospinal neurons that influence a particular muscle are often clustered together, but their individual motor fields may differ significantly from one another (i.e., although all of the cells within a cluster may influence a single muscle in common, they may each provide additional facilitation to different sets of functionally related muscles) (Lemon, 1988).

How, then, can the capacity for fractionated movements be explained in the face of the striking convergence and divergence of descending corticospinal projections from the various cortical motor fields? The answer is not yet known with any certainty, but one possibility is that the convergent corticospinal inputs to a given motor unit may be differentially strengthened (or weakened) by experience according to some type of hebbian synaptic learning rule (based on the temporal coincidence of presynaptic and postsynaptic activation) (Brown et al., 1990; Grossberg and Kuperstein, 1989; Rumelhart et al., 1986). This type of process could lead to the coordination of functionally related but spatially distributed corticospinal neurons, or clusters of such neurons, and thereby account for movement fractionation despite

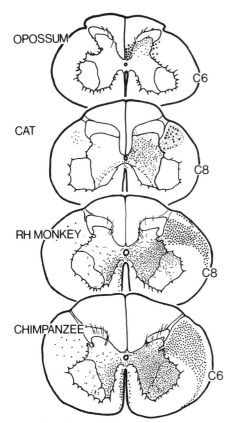

Figure 21–4. Distribution of corticospinal fibers from the left hemisphere to low cervical spinal gray matter in opossum, cat, rhesus monkey, and chimpanzee. (From Kuypers H.G.J.M. Anatomy of the descending pathways. In Brookhart J.M., Mountcastle V.B., Brooks V.B., eds. *Handbook of Physiology*. Section 1. *The Nervous System*. Vol. II. *Motor Control*. Part 1. Bethesda, American Physiological Society, pp. 597–666, 1981.)

the absence of one-to-one mapping between cortical and spinal motor neurons.

In many respects, the corticospinal projections originating in different cortical areas can be properly construed as constituting multiple parallel, but functionally differentiated, descending systems (for detailed review, see Humphrey, 1983). Corticospinal projections from cytoarchitectonically distinct cortical areas terminate in different portions of the spinal gray matter. In the monkey, for example, corticospinal fibers originating in areas 4 and 3a terminate within the intermediate zone and the motor nuclei of the ventral horn, whereas those from areas 2 and 5 terminate within different portions of the dorsal horn (Coulter and Jones, 1977; Kuypers and Brinkman, 1970). Thus, the anatomic organization of corticospinal projections from area 4 and adjoining area 3a is best suited for controlling motor output through direct connections with propriospinal neurons and motor neurons, whereas projections from parietal areas 2 and 5 to interneurons within the dorsal horn may allow for the modulation of ascending as well as intrasegmental transmission of somatosensory information.

The terminal fields of corticospinal fibers that project to interneurons and propriospinal neurons in the intermediate zone are topographically organized and overlap those of both the ventromedial and dorsolateral descending brain stem pathways (see later). In the monkey, for example, those parts of area 4 that represent the distal limb musculature project to the interneurons and short propriospinal neurons in the *dorsolateral* portions of the intermediate zone, whereas those that represent the proximal musculature project to the interneurons and long propriospinal neurons of the *ventromedial* portion of the spinal intermediate zone (Kuypers and Brinkman, 1970) (see Fig. 21-3).

Corticospinal fibers descending contralaterally in the lateral corticospinal tract terminate on interneurons of almost all categories, but especially on those related to motor neurons of distal muscles of the limb. In primates, the direct, monosynaptic corticospinal projections to motor neurons are likewise concentrated on the cells related to the distal extremity musculature. In addition, some corticospinal fibers descending ipsilaterally in the ventral corticospinal tract make connections on both sides of the cord with interneurons related to motor neurons of axial and girdle muscles.

Pyramidal Tract Syndrome

Although the combination of weakness, spasticity, and hyperreflexia (the upper motor neuron [UMN] syndrome—see later) that results from certain cortical and subcortical lesions in humans is sometimes referred to as the pyramidal tract syndrome, this use of the term is based on a common misconception of the effects of selective damage to the corticospinal (or pyramidal) tract. This view arose from clinical observations in patients with corticospinal lesions, in whom there is almost invariably associated damage to other descending systems. In fact, there has been only one anatomically verified case report of isolated destruction of the pyramidal tact in humans, and this patient did not develop spasticity (Bucy et al., 1964). Studies in monkeys repeatedly demonstrated that isolated pyramidal tract lesions are not accompanied by increased muscle tone or hyperreflexia (Bucy et al., 1966; Gilman and Marco, 1971).

In primates, the acute effects of disruption of the corticospinal system by pyramidotomy are profound but are followed by a remarkable degree of recovery (Gilman and Marco, 1971; Lawrence and Kuypers, 1968a; Tower, 1940). Immediately after selective destruction of both medullary pyramids, the limbs become hypotonic and severely weak, the arms more so than the legs. After several days, however, monkeys are able to stand unsupported, to walk, and to reach for food. By this time, movements of the trunk and the proximal portions of the limbs appear normal. Distal limb movements recover more slowly. Initially, the hand is held in an abnormal position and handling of objects is impaired. Eventually, there is a nearly full recovery of the use of limbs, including the hand, with the exception of a permanent loss of independent movements of the fingers. Similar results are associated with section of the corticospinal tracts at the level of the cerebral peduncle (Bucy et al., 1966). In humans, isolated damage to the corticospinal tract is associated with the appearance of the Babinski sign (Bucy et al., 1964).

Acute disruption of the primate corticospinal system is also associated with dramatic effects on muscle tone and deep tendon reflexes, both of which are reduced or absent in the contralateral extremities immediately after sectioning of the medullary pyramid (Gilman and Marco, 1971; Tower, 1940) or cerebral peduncle (Bucy et al., 1966) in monkeys. Within days to weeks after either procedure, however, muscle tone and reflexes show considerable recovery and usually return to normal. Spasticity is not seen after pure corticospinal tract lesions.

Upper Motor Neuron Syndrome

In contrast to the pyramidal tract syndrome, which is rarely encountered in humans, the UMN syndrome, characterized by weakness in association with spasticity and hyperreflexia, is a common clinical entity. After the immediate and transient period of hypotonia and depressed reflexes associated with acute UMN lesions, the deep tendon reflexes of the limbs gradually reappear and eventually become hyperactive, and increased tone develops (predominantly in the antigravity muscles) in response to stretch. The hypertonicity of spasticity is strongly velocity dependent.

The UMN syndrome is believed to result from

combined damage to the corticospinal and cortico-reticulospinal systems as a consequence of lesions that may involve cerebral cortex, internal capsule, brain stem, or spinal cord. Although it now seems clear that motor cortex lesions alone do not result in spasticity or hyperreflexia, it remains uncertain whether development of the UMN syndrome depends on additional damage to descending (cortico-reticulospinal) projections from PMC and/or from SMA. It was shown in monkeys (Gilman et al., 1974) that lesions confined to motor cortex did not result in spasticity but instead produced a pattern of weakness and hypotonia indistinguishable from that of the pyramidal tract syndrome, whereas lesions that included PMC as well as motor cortex resulted in a combination of weakness and spasticity that strongly resembled the human UMN syndrome. In this study, however, it was acknowledged that the PMC lesions undercut at least some of the fibers emanating from the SMA, leaving unresolved the relative contributions of PMC and SMA damage to the observed results.

Several reports (Coxe and Landau, 1965; Denny-Brown, 1966; Travis, 1955) indicated that selective SMA lesions in monkeys are followed by mild-to-moderate increases in muscle tone, particularly in flexors of the trunk and limbs, but the resulting hypertonia was noted by at least one investigator (Denny-Brown, 1966) to be of a plastic type that was quite distinct from that of spasticity. There have been indications that SMA lesions in humans are not associated with increased muscle tone (LaPlane et al., 1977; Penfield and Jasper, 1954), and it was reported that patients with lesions apparently restricted to PMC (from computed tomographic evidence) experienced selective proximal weakness in association with generalized spasticity (Freund and Hummelsheim, 1984).

Because of the inconsistencies among these various reports, it remains unresolved whether damage to descending projections from SMA and/or PMC regions is responsible for the development of spasticity in the UMN syndrome.

The increased deep tendon reflexes and velocity-dependent increases in muscle tone that are characteristic of spasticity are thought to represent enhancements of phasic and tonic stretch reflexes, respectively (Lance, 1980). Spasticity is believed to result primarily from direct increases in the excitability of α rather than γ motor neurons, because fusimotor drive has been shown not to exceed normal levels in spastic monkeys (Gilman et al., 1974) or humans (Hagbarth et al., 1973), and normal subjects whose muscle spindles are maximally activated by high-frequency muscle vibration do not have spasticity (Burke et al., 1976). In addition to velocity-dependent increases in muscle tone, spasticity is also associated with the so-called clasp-knife phenomenon, a length-dependent inhibition of extensor stretch reflexes (Lance, 1980). In the lower extremity, for example, increasing stretch of the quadriceps muscle is eventually followed by a sudden and persistent collapse

of resistance, with further stretch being unopposed. By contrast, in decerebrate rigidity, or in the rigidity associated with parkinsonism, there is continued, relatively uniform resistance to stretch throughout the entire joint excursion. It has been suggested (Burke et al., 1972) that the clasp-knife reaction results from damage to the dorsal reticulospinal tract, with consequent hyperreactivity of flexor reflex afferent arcs. If this explanation is correct, the occurrence of the clasp-knife phenomenon in spasticity of cortical or capsular origin might be attributable to the interruption of corticoreticular inputs to the dorsal reticulospinal system.

The UMN syndrome in humans is associated with reductions in the maximal force generated by individual motor units through voluntary effort (Tang and Rymer, 1981). This is reflected by alterations in force-EMG relationships and motor unit recruitment patterns. Thus, for the limb with UMN weakness, a larger than normal proportion of the motor neuron pool, including more high-threshold motor units, must be recruited to achieve a given level of force. This may account in part for the greater sense of effort and increased fatigability seen in patients with UMN weakness.

The motor performance deficits associated with the UMN syndrome appear to be attributable primarily to weakness and abnormalities in the recruitment of motor units rather than to interference from spasticity in the form of exaggerated stretch reflexes. EMG analyses have shown that impairments in rapid repetitive limb movements in patients with spasticity result from limited and prolonged recruitment of agonist motor units and not from the activation of antagonistic stretch reflexes (Sahrmann and Norton, 1977). Moreover, the elimination of spasticity by local fusimotor anesthesia has been shown not to resolve the motor performance deficits associated with UMN weakness (Landau et al., 1960). It should be emphasized in this regard that, in many patients, spasticity may be an asset, because it may provide an essential component for residual postural support. In fact, the treatment of spasticity (which is usually directed toward the relief of flexor spasms) may occasionally result in further motor impairment because of decreased postural support and increased fatigability.

REENTRANT CORTICAL-SUBCORTICAL CIRCUITS: CEREBELLUM AND BASAL GANGLIA

In parallel with the phylogenetic expansion of the neocortex and the emergence of the direct corticospinal systems, there has been increased development of two major reentrant systems centered on the *cerebellum* and the *basal ganglia*, both of which receive inputs from diverse cortical areas and convey their respective influences, in turn, to specific portions of the frontal cortex via discrete, nonoverlapping projections to the ventrolateral thalamus (see Fig. 21–1).

In relation to the million or so cortical PTNs that project directly to the human spinal cord, the cortical inputs to the cerebellum and the basal ganglia appear massive. It has been estimated, for example, that in humans there are approximately 16 million cortico-pontine axons from each hemisphere that converge on the nuclei of the basis pontis, whose projections are directed to the cortex and the deep nuclei of the cerebellum (Tomasch, 1969). The corticostriate projections appear to be even more substantial, as the human neostriatum has been estimated to contain approximately 110 million neurons per hemisphere (Schroder et al., 1975), compared with an estimated 12 million neurons receiving corticopontine projections in each half of the basis pontis (Tomasch, 1969).

Earlier concepts of the motor system were predicated on the belief that there was convergence of cerebellar and basal ganglia influences within the thalamus, with subsequent relay of these integrated influences to the motor cortex (Evarts and Thach, 1969; Kemp and Powell, 1971). There is considerable evidence, however, that the cerebellum and the basal ganglia send their respective outputs to separate thalamic regions, which in turn project to different frontal cortical fields (Asanuma et al., 1983; DeLong and Georgopoulos, 1981; Schell and Strick, 1984). In general, the cerebellum appears to play an important role in initiating movement and in specifying the patterns of muscular activation required for coordinated motor acts, whereas the basal ganglia appear to serve more of a role in specifying the direction of movements (regardless of muscle pattern) and in scaling the movement amplitude. For the purposes of this overview, some of the important similarities and differences between the basal ganglia and the cerebellum are outlined, in terms of their thalamocortical connections and their relationships with the segmental motor apparatus.

Anatomically, the cerebellum appears to be more directly related to spinal and brain stem areas concerned with movement than are the basal ganglia. For example, substantial input comes to the cerebellum directly from the spinal cord, whereas the basal ganglia receive sensory input only after processing by the sensorimotor cortex. Moreover, on the output side, the cerebellum sends heavy projections to brain stem nuclei that directly influence the segmental motor apparatus, and part of its projections to the thalamus are directed to a region (in the monkey, nucleus ventralis lateralis pars oralis) with direct connections to motor cortex.

Until recently, the basal ganglia were thought to exert little direct influence on brain stem nuclei with descending projections to the segmental motor apparatus, although the reciprocal connections between the basal ganglia output nuclei (globus pallidus pars interna [GPi] and substantia nigra pars reticulata [SNr]) and the brain stem tegmental pedunculopontine nuclei were well known (Edley and Graybiel, 1983). However, physiologic studies have begun to implicate the pediculopontine nucleus as a component of the mesencephalic locomotor region (see under Brain Stem Descending Pathways), which appears to exert important influences on the intrinsic locomotor pattern generators within the spinal cord (Garcia-Rill, 1986). There is also anatomic evidence in the rat indicating that a minority of pediculopontine nucleus neurons send direct projections to the cervical spinal cord (Spann and Grofova, 1989). The functional significance of these descending pathways is unclear, however, especially as they seem to be rather modest in comparison with the more robust projections along the reentrant basal ganglia–thalamocortical pathways.

In primates, the basal ganglia as a whole receive substantial topographic inputs from virtually the entire neocortex (Kunzle, 1975, 1977; Selemon and Goldman-Rakic, 1985; Yeterian and VanHoesen, 1978), whereas the cerebellum receives only sparse projections from cortical fields outside the premotor and sensorimotor areas (Dhanarajan et al., 1977; Humphrey et al., 1984; R. Wiesendanger et al., 1979). Although it was earlier suggested that the basal ganglia may play a major role in transmitting influences from cortical association areas to motor cortex, it now appears that influences from cortical association areas are routed through basal ganglia–thalamocortical circuits that are separate from and parallel to those carrying sensorimotor information and are returned to prefrontal rather than to motor or premotor areas (Alexander et al., 1986; DeLong and Georgopoulos, 1981).

The segregation of cerebellar and basal ganglia influences within the thalamus assumes considerable clinical importance in consideration of the rationale for stereotaxic approaches to the treatment of movement abnormalities such as tremor, rigidity, and dyskinesias. These neurosurgical procedures rest on the principle of interrupting transmission of abnormal activity originating from the basal ganglia, the cerebellum, and the thalamus to the precentral motor fields (for review, see DeLong and Georgopoulos, 1981). Although earlier surgical approaches were directed toward the interruption of basal ganglia output at the level of the globus pallidus or its efferent pathways, the most common target for such procedures presently is the ventrolateral thalamus, which receives both basal ganglia and cerebellar input. The most effective target site for the alleviation of tremor is generally believed to be the nucleus ventralis intermedius. The nucleus ventralis intermedius appears to be homologous to the monkey nucleus ventralis lateralis pars oralis and thus to be the recipient of cerebellar, but not basal ganglia, influences. By contrast, rigidity appears to respond more readily to lesions situated more rostrally in the thalamus in an area receiving basal ganglia output.

Basal Ganglia Motor Pathways

The reentrant motor pathways that pass through the basal ganglia constitute the basal ganglia–thalamocortical motor circuit (Fig. 21–5). In primates, the striatal portion of the motor circuit is largely coextensive with the putamen. This part of the striatum receives topographic projections from the primary motor cortex, the premotor cortex, and the SMA, as well as from the somatosensory cortex and area 5. These projections result in a somatotopic organization within the putamen that is preserved throughout

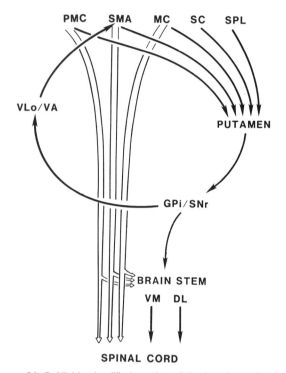

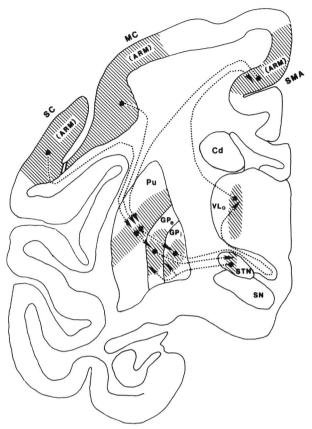

Figure 21–6. Somatotopic organization of the basal ganglia–thalamocortical motor circuit, showing the maintained somatotopy throughout the pathway. SMA = supplementary motor area; MC = primary motor cortex; SC = somatosensory cortex; VLo = thalamic nucleus ventralis lateralis pars oralis; GPe = globus pallidus pars externa; GPi = globus pallidus pars interna; SN = substantia nigra; STN = subthalamic nucleus; Cd = caudate nucleus; Pu = putamen.

Figure 21–5. Highly simplified version of the basal ganglia–thalamocortical motor circuit, illustrating the cortical reentrant properties, which are similar to those of the cerebellar circuits (see Fig. 21–8). The main route by which the basal ganglia are able to influence the segmental motor apparatus is via the cortical motor fields that receive thalamic input from the basal ganglia recipient zones (VLo and VA). There is increasing evidence that the basal ganglia also send descending projections to brain stem areas, which in turn project directly to the spinal cord, but these connections are of lesser magnitude and their functional significance is much less clear than that of the basal ganglia–thalamocortical circuitry. This figure should be compared with Figure 21–8, which depicts the cerebellar circuits. In each case, large areas of motor, premotor, and somatosensory cortex project to the respective basal ganglia or cerebellar input nuclei. The respective output nuclei of the basal ganglia and the cerebellum then project back to select target zones within the precentral motor areas. These projections are conveyed through separate subnuclei within the ventrolateral thalamus (VLo/VA for the basal ganglia, and area X and VPLo [not shown here; see Fig. 21–8] for the cerebellum). The outflow from the basal ganglia are centered predominantly on the supplementary motor area (SMA), but the basal ganglia also influence selected regions within the premotor cortex (PMC) and the motor cortex (MC). Conversely, the predominant output of the cerebellum is to portions of PMC and MC that are largely separate from those receiving basal ganglia influences. SC = somatosensory cortex; SPL = area 5 within the superior parietal lobule (somatosensory association cortex); VLo = thalamic nucleus ventralis lateralis pars oralis; VA = thalamic nucleus ventralis anterior; GPi = globus pallidus pars interna; SNr = substantia nigra pars reticulata; VM = ventromedial group of brain stem descending pathways; DL = dorsolateral brain stem descending pathways.

all subsequent stages of the motor circuit (Fig. 21–6). Thus, the putamen projects topographically to specific portions of both segments of the globus pallidus (globus pallidus pars externa [GPe] and GPi) as well as to the SNr. In turn, the respective motor portions of both GPi and SNr, which represent the basal ganglia output nuclei, send topographic projections to specific thalamic nuclei in the ventrolateral and the intralaminar thalamus. The motor circuit is closed by means of the thalamocortical projections from these thalamic regions to selected portions of the SMA, the premotor cortex, and the primary motor cortex.

Neurophysiologic studies have shown that individual neurons at all stages of the motor circuit are exquisitely tuned to different aspects of motor processing. Within each nuclear and cortical component of the circuit, some neurons code for the highest levels of motor processing, such as the coding of the intended limb movement in external spatial coordinates, whereas others code for much lower levels of motor processing, such as the precise pattern of required muscle activations. Some neurons within the motor circuit discharge exclusively during the preparation for movement, whereas other neurons discharge exclusively during movement execution. On average, neurons at cortical levels of the motor circuit tend to begin discharging somewhat earlier than those at subcortical levels, suggesting that activity within the motor circuit may be initiated within the precentral motor fields.

Organization of Basal Ganglia Circuitry

Like the other basal ganglia–thalamocortical circuits (Alexander et al., 1986), the motor circuit includes a *direct pathway* to the basal ganglia output nuclei that arise from inhibitory striatal (putaminal) efferents, which contain both γ-aminobutyric acid (GABA) and substance P. Activation of this pathway tends to disinhibit the thalamic stage of the circuit (Fig. 21–7). Each circuit also includes an *indirect pathway* that passes first to the GPe via striatal projection neurons that contain both GABA and enkephalin, then from GPe to the subthalamic nucleus (STN) via a purely GABAergic pathway, and finally

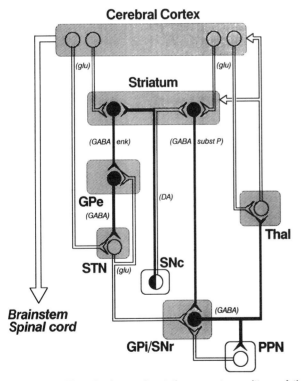

Figure 21–7. The circuitry and putative neurotransmitters of the basal ganglia–thalamocortical pathways, indicating the parallel direct and indirect pathways from the striatum to the basal ganglia output nuclei. The striatal component of the motor circuit is the putamen, and the thalamic component is the thalamic nuclei ventralis lateralis pars oralis and ventralis anterior pars parvocellularis. The cortical components are indicated in Figure 21–5. Inhibitory neurons are shown as filled circles, whereas excitatory neurons are unfilled. DA = dopamine; enk = enkephalin; GABA = γ-aminobutyric acid; glu = glutamate; PPN = pedunculopontine nucleus; SNc = substantia nigra pars compacta; Thal = thalamus. (From Alexander G.E., Crutcher M.D. Functional architecture of basal ganglia circuits: neural substrates of parallel processing. *Trends Neurosci.* 13:266–271, 1990.)

to the output nuclei via an excitatory, probably glutamatergic, projection from the STN. The high spontaneous discharge rate of most GPe neurons exerts a tonic inhibitory influence on the STN. Activation of the inhibitory GABA-enkephalin projection from the striatum tends to suppress the activity of GPe neurons and thereby to disinhibit the STN, thus increasing the excitatory drive on the output nuclei and increasing the inhibition of their efferent targets within the thalamus. The two striatal efferent systems thus appear to have opposing effects on the basal ganglia output nuclei and, accordingly, on the thalamic targets of basal ganglia outflow (Albin et al., 1989; Alexander and Crutcher, 1990a).

During the execution of specific motor acts, movement-related neurons within GPi and SNr may show either phasic increases or phasic decreases in their normally high rates of spontaneous discharge. Phasic *decreases* in GPi-SNr discharge may play a crucial role in motor control by disinhibiting the ventrolateral thalamus and thereby gating or facilitating cortically initiated movements (via excitatory thalamocortical connections), whereas phasic *increases* in GPi-SNr discharge may have the opposite effect.

The role of dopamine within the basal ganglia appears to be complex, and many issues remain unresolved. Dopaminergic inputs appear to have a net excitatory effect on striatal neurons that send GABA–substance P projections to the basal ganglia output nuclei (via the direct pathway) and a net inhibitory effect on those that send GABA-enkephalin projections to GPe (via the indirect pathway). Thus, in effect, the overall influence of dopamine within the striatum may be to reinforce any cortically initiated activation of a particular basal ganglia–thalamocortical circuit by both facilitating conduction through that circuit's direct pathway (which has a net excitatory effect on the thalamus) and suppressing conduction through the indirect pathway (which has a net inhibitory effect on the thalamus).

The role of acetylcholine in the striatum is not well understood. Clinically, dopamine and acetylcholine have antagonistic effects on many movement disorders, including Parkinson's disease. Acetylcholine appears to be the neurotransmitter for a class of large interneurons within the striatum. On the basis of the functional antagonism between acetylcholine and dopamine at the level of the striatum, it is speculated that these cholinergic neurons may have a selective excitatory influence on the GABA-enkephalin neurons of the indirect pathway.

Basal Ganglia Dysfunction: Hypokinetic and Hyperkinetic Disorders

Movement disorders associated with basal ganglia dysfunction constitute a spectrum of abnormalities that range from the *hypokinetic* disorders (of which Parkinson's disease is the best-known example) at one extreme to the *hyperkinetic* disorders (exemplified by Huntington's disease and hemiballismus) at the other (DeLong, 1990). Hypokinetic disorders are characterized by significant impairments in movement initiation (akinesia) and reductions in the amplitude and velocity of voluntary movements (bradykinesia). Hyperkinetic disorders, by contrast, are characterized by excessive motor activity in the form of involuntary movements (dyskinesias). The development of primate models of these disorders (induced by systemic or local administration of selective neurotoxins) has made it possible to clarify some of the pathophysiologic mechanisms underlying such diverse symptoms as the akinesia of parkinsonism and the involuntary movements of hemiballismus.

There is considerable evidence that shifts in the balance between activity in the direct and indirect pathways through the basal ganglia motor circuit may account for the hypokinetic and hyperkinetic features of basal ganglia disorders. Thus, in general, it appears that enhanced conduction through the indirect pathway leads to hypokinetic disorders (by increasing thalamic inhibition), whereas enhanced conduction through the direct pathway results in hyperkinetic disorders (by decreasing thalamic inhibition) (Albin et al., 1989; DeLong, 1990; see also Chapter 22).

There have been numerous approaches to the production of a suitable primate model of Parkinson's disease, but 1-methyl-4-phenyl-1,2,3,6-tetrahydropyridine (MPTP)–induced parkinsonism represents the first model with features that closely resemble the clinical, pathologic, and biochemical characteristics of the human disorder. Animals treated with MPTP exhibit signs virtually identical to those in humans with Parkinson's disease, including akinesia, bradykinesia, flexed posture, muscular rigidity, and postural tremor. MPTP-treated animals exhibit the pathologic hallmark of Parkinson's disease (i.e., loss of melanin-containing neurons of the pars compacta of the substantia nigra and resulting loss of dopamine in the striatum and the substantia nigra).

In monkeys with MPTP-induced parkinsonism, the neurons in both the subthalamic nucleus and the basal ganglia output nuclei (GPi and SNr) show increased rates of discharge. This is consistent with other evidence indicating that a loss of striatal dopamine should increase transmission through the indirect pathway and reduce transmission through the direct pathway. The overall effect of such imbalances is to increase the output from GPi-SNr, leading to excessive inhibition of thalamocortical neurons (DeLong, 1990).

Apart from parkinsonism, the basal ganglia disorder for which the neuropathologic substrate has seemed least in doubt is hemiballismus. In humans, vascular lesions restricted to the STN frequently result in involuntary, often violent movements of the contralateral limbs (termed *hemiballismus* because of the superficial resemblance of the movements to throwing motions). This disorder provides one of the clearest correlations in clinical neurology between localized pathologic change and movement abnormality. In addition to the proximal ballistic movements, these involuntary movements may take the form of more distal, irregular (choreiform), or more continuous writhing (athetoid) movements. Hemiballismus has been produced in monkeys by experimental lesions of the STN.

Until recently, this disorder was generally viewed as resulting from a release of GPi from an inhibitory control from the STN. However, there is evidence that the projections from STN to GPi are actually excitatory and probably glutamatergic. Neurophysiologic and metabolic imaging studies of experimental hemiballismus suggest that this condition results from a disinhibition of the ventrolateral thalamus related to reduced output from GPi associated with loss of excitatory STN-GPi projections.

There is evidence of a common mechanism underlying both the choreiform movements of Huntington's disease and the dyskinesias in hemiballismus. Early in the course of Huntington's disease, there is a selective loss of the striatal GABA-enkephalin neurons that give rise to the indirect pathway (Reiner et al., 1988). The consequent loss of inhibition of GPe neurons is expected to lead to excessive inhibition of STN neurons, and this functional inactivation of the STN could thus explain the choreiform motor disturbances in Huntington's disease that resemble those seen in hemiballismus (Albin et al., 1989; DeLong, 1990).

The phenomenon of levodopa (L-dopa)–induced dyskinesias (which occur during periods of dopamine excess associated with the pharmacologic treatment of Parkinson's disease) can be explained on a similar basis. That is, excessive dopaminergic inhibition of the striatal GABA-enkephalin neurons would lead to reduced excitatory input to GPi-SNr via the indirect pathway, and this effect would be compounded by excessive dopaminergic stimulation of the striatal GABA–substance P neurons that send inhibitory projections to GPi-SNr via the direct pathway.

Role of Basal Ganglia in Motor Control

Most theories of the role of the basal ganglia in normal motor control are based on the various deficits seen in Parkinson's disease. Thus, it has been variously suggested that the basal ganglia play a role in (1) movement initiation (because of the akinesia seen in Parkinson's disease); (2) the scaling of movement amplitude and/or velocity (because of the bradykinesia seen in Parkinson's disease); (3) the automatic execution of motor programs (because of the characteristic impairment of compound sequential or simultaneous movements in Parkinson's disease); or (4) corollary discharge involving comparison of efference copies of cortical motor commands with proprioceptive feedback from the movement itself (because of a characteristic tendency for subjects with Parkinson's disease to overestimate the magnitude of movements carried out in the absence of visual feedback). It is generally hazardous, however, to infer the normal function of a given brain structure from the deficits produced by lesions of that structure. At present, the role of the basal ganglia in normal motor control is uncertain, even though a great deal is known about the motor impairments that are associated with damage to these structures. It is clear, however, that the basal ganglia are positioned anatomically to influence nearly the entire frontal lobe and particularly the precentral motor areas. On the basis of current knowledge of the functional organization of the motor circuit, it seems plausible to suggest that the basal ganglia may play an important role in modulating motor patterns initiated at cortical levels by reinforcing currently selected patterns via the direct pathway and suppressing potentially conflicting patterns via the indirect pathway. Overall, this leads to a focusing of neural activity related to a cortically initiated movement in a fashion analogous to the inhibitory surround seen in various sensory systems.

Cerebellar Motor Pathways

Like the basal ganglia, the cerebellum influences various cortical motor areas via reentrant pathways that pass through the ventrolateral thalamus. The cerebellothalamocortical connections are indicated in Figure 21–8. The functional organization of the cerebellum and its role in normal and abnormal motor control are discussed in Chapter 23. The following is concerned primarily with the relationships between the cerebellum and other components of the motor system and not with more detailed aspects of its anatomy and physiology. The functional organization of the cerebellum corresponds largely to longitudinal divisions into the lateral, the intermediate, and the medial cerebellum. Each of the longitudinal subdivisions of the cerebellar cortex projects to separate components of the deep cerebellar nuclei. Thus, the Purkinje cells of the lateral cerebellum project to the dentate nucleus; those of the intermediate cerebellar cortex, to the interpositus nucleus; and those of the medial cerebellum, to the fastigial nucleus. Both the lateral and the intermediate cerebellum and their corresponding deep cerebellar nuclei have separate somatotopic representations. Both sets of structures are involved in the control of voluntary movements, but neurons within the dentate nucleus represent relatively high levels of motor processing (e.g., the abstract direction of movement independent of the specific patterns of muscle activations), whereas the neurons in the nucleus interpositus tend to represent lower processing levels (e.g., specifying the pattern and timing of muscle activations) (Brooks and Thach, 1981). Dentate neurons also tend to begin discharging somewhat earlier than their counterparts in the nucleus interpositus.

Unlike the case with basal ganglia, much of the cerebellum receives direct information from spinal levels and, in turn, sends projections directly to the spinal cord. The spinocerebellar projections, which

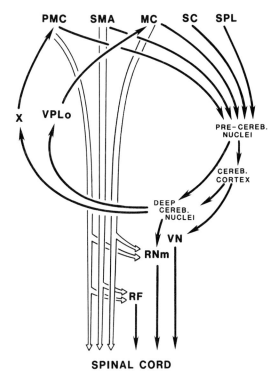

Figure 21–8. Principal relationships between key cerebellar structures and other components of the motor system. This illustration emphasizes the reentrant nature of the projections from the cerebellum to specific portions of the ventrolateral thalamus (area X and the oral portion of the ventral posterolateral nucleus [VPLo]), whose projections are returned to specific portions of the precentral cortex. In this highly schematic illustration, the precerebellar nuclei are intended to include the pontine nuclei as well as the parvocellular portions of the red nuclei and the inferior olivary nuclei. Note that the cerebellum exerts descending influences on the segmental motor apparatus of the spinal cord via projections to the magnocellular portion of the red nucleus (RNm) and the vestibular nuclei (VN). PMC = premotor cortex; SMA = supplementary motor area; MC = primary motor cortex; SC = somatosensory cortex; SPL = area 5 within the superior parietal lobule (somatosensory association cortex); RF = reticular formation.

are somatotopically organized, are directed primarily to the medial and the intermediate cerebellar cortex and deep nuclei, but some spinocerebellar projections are also conveyed to the medial portions of the lateral cerebellum. Likewise, the direct descending cerebellospinal projections arise primarily from the deep nuclei of the medial and the intermediate cerebellum (Ito, 1984).

The lateral cerebellum receives the bulk of its inputs from the pontine nuclei, which in turn receive massive projections from the cortical motor and premotor areas as well as from primary somatosensory cortex and the somatosensory association area (Dhanarajan et al., 1977). Unlike the striatal input nuclei of the basal ganglia, however, the pontine nuclei appear to receive relatively little input from other areas of cortex, such as the cortical association areas (R. Wiesendanger et al., 1979). The lateral cerebellum and, to some extent, the intermediate cerebellum are components in a cerebellothalamocortical circuit (see Fig. 21–8). Although the same cortical and sensory motor areas that project to the basal ganglia project also to the precerebellar nuclei (which include the pontine nuclei and the parvocellular red nucleus and inferior olivary nucleus), the thalamic nuclei that receive projections from the deep cerebellar nuclei project back to restricted target zones within the precentral motor areas. In general, these target zones within motor and premotor cortex are separate from those that receive basal ganglia projections (Schell and Strick, 1984), although there are some areas of overlap.

Dysfunction in Cerebellar Circuits: The Cerebellar Syndrome

Damage to the cerebellar cortex, the deep cerebellar nuclei, or the inferior olive tends to produce the same type of motor disturbances. The complete cerebellar syndrome consists of ataxia, dysmetria, and action tremor (Gilman et al., 1981). Complex movements tend to become decomposed into poorly coordinated submovements. The most striking effects of cerebellar lesions are a disruption of timing and a loss of accuracy. In simple movements, these deficits are correlated with delays in the onset of agonist EMG activity, and the duration of the agonist burst also tends to be prolonged. This leads to a characteristic overshooting of goal-directed movements. When this is coupled with the characteristic 3-Hz oscillations of goal-directed limb movements in cerebellar patients, the net effect is that of frank ataxia. Cerebellar patients also show characteristic reduction in muscle tone, associated with reductions in tonic stretch reflexes. These reductions in tonic stretch reflexes are thought to result from reduced excitatory drive to γ motor neurons, leading to reduced sensitivity of muscle spindles.

Role of Cerebellum in Motor Control

As for the basal ganglia, most theories of the role of the cerebellum in motor control are based on extrapolations from the motor effects of cerebellar lesions. Thus, the delay in movement initiation led some investigators to speculate that the cerebellum is involved in movement initiation, whereas other researchers argued that the timing deficits in cerebellar patients argue for a role of the cerebellum in controlling the sequencing of muscle activations required for smooth, coordinated movements (for discussion see Brooks and Thach, 1981). Other workers argued that the decomposition of complex movements into their constituent submovements argues for a role of the cerebellum in coordinating the disparate elements of a complex movement into a single, coordinated whole. Again, it is prudent to be circumspect about making functional attributions to a particular neural structure solely on the basis of the effects of lesions. After all, from that information alone one cannot be sure whether a behavioral impairment resulted from the loss of a function subserved by the damaged structure or from abnormal activity in the structures that remain.

Because of the highly ordered, almost geometric arrangements of cerebellar microarchitecture, many theorists have argued that the cerebellum functions like a neural computer. One of the more explicit formulations of this theory maintains that the primary role of the cerebellum is to effect the necessary coordinate transformations required for translating the goal of a movement in terms of the coordinates of external space into the multidimensional coordinates appropriate for controlling a multijointed limb (Pellionisz and Llinas, 1985). According to this view, the cerebellum is effectively hard-wired to carry out these transformations, much like a digital array processor.

Perhaps the most popular theory at present is that the primary role of the cerebellum is in motor learning. This is based on a variety of experimental evidence, including the loss of adaptation of the vestibulo-ocular reflex after lesions of the vestibulo-cerebellum. There are many versions of this theory, but one of the most prominent attempts to include a specific role of the climbing fibers in motor learning, arguing that the coincident occurrence of specific mossy fiber and climbing fiber input leads to semipermanent changes (i.e., learning) in the conductivity of mossy fiber–granule cell inputs to the Purkinje cells.

It must be emphasized, however, that much more is known about the nature of the motor disturbances associated with cerebellar lesions than about the normal role of the cerebellum in motor control. It seems reasonable, however, on the basis of reports about the results of lesions and neurophysiologic studies to infer that the cerebellum does play an important role in orchestrating the timing and sequencing of neuronal assemblies required for coordinated movement. That the cerebellum has a role in motor learning would also appear likely from a variety of evidence, but whether that role is unique to the cerebellum seems more doubtful. Evidence continues to accumulate that the motor system in particular, and the brain in general, is organized as a massively parallel, self-organizing system in which learning, at the synaptic level, is distributed throughout the system.

BRAIN STEM DESCENDING PATHWAYS

Information concerning the anatomic organization of the brain stem descending systems greatly exceeds the understanding of the functions of these systems. This is a clear reversal of the situation that existed 2–3 decades ago, when there was limited appreciation of the anatomic substrates of the dramatic effects on muscle tone and spinal reflexes elicited by lesions and electrical stimulation of various brain stem regions. As attention was directed to the functional properties of anatomically defined descending pathways, it became increasingly apparent that descending brain stem influences were characterized by far more specificity and a far greater complexity of organization than was previously suspected (for review, see Peterson, 1984). Moreover, there is substantial evidence that the descending brain stem systems participate not only in the modulation of segmental reflex pathways and the regulation of muscle tone, but also in the control of voluntary movements.

Although the corticospinal tracts in primates are often viewed as the primary pathways mediating voluntary control of movements, studies with the monkey after interruption of these pathways revealed a marked residual capacity for voluntary movement, which must be due to the activity of the remaining brain stem descending systems. Indeed, it appears that certain brain stem descending pathways, some of which are under cortical influence, may constitute the basic suprasegmental control systems on which the corticospinal systems are superimposed.

Brain Stem Influences on Muscle Tone and Posture

The mammalian central nervous system contains the neural substrates for a variety of righting and static postural reflexes that provide for specific, involuntary adjustments of the head and body in response to certain environmental and proprioceptive stimuli. In general, the righting reflexes consist of phasic motor responses that serve to return the organism to a normal starting position after its postural orientation has been disturbed either by external forces or by its own volitional movements (Magnus, 1926b). The static reflexes (which include tonic neck, lumbar, and labyrinthine reflexes; the crossed extensor reflex; and local supporting reactions) are characterized by fixed postural attitudes that are maintained for the duration of the inciting tactile, proprioceptive, or labyrinthine stimulus (Magnus, 1926a). With the exception of the optic righting reflex, which depends on inputs from visual cortex, and certain intrasegmental and intersegmental static reflexes that are organized at spinal levels, the righting and static postural reflexes are mediated principally by descending pathways that originate in the brain stem. In the conscious adult animal, and particularly in primates, these reflexes are suppressed or modulated by descending cortical and subcortical influences. In spite of this, however, each of the righting reflexes can be demonstrated in the intact monkey (Magnus, 1926b), and the static postural reflexes (tonic neck, lumbar, and labyrinthine) have even been demonstrated in normal adult humans, in whom they are largely subliminal but nevertheless detectable by careful EMG analyses (Tokizane et al., 1951).

Lesions of the brain stem may result in the release of static postural reflexes from cortical and subcortical control, leading to exaggerated changes in tone and posture in response to minimal environmental stimuli. Such effects were first described in detail by Sherrington (1898, 1909), who reported that transections of the midbrain at the intercollicular level, in primates and other mammals, resulted in a state he termed "decerebrate rigidity." Such decerebrate preparations were characterized by a strong extensor bias that affected the neck as well as the extremities, so that the head and limbs were thrust backward and held extended against gravity when the trunk was suspended in the prone position. Eventually it was determined that the decerebrate state could be produced by brain stem transections located at any level below the red nuclei but above the vestibular complex (Magnus, 1926a). With unilateral brain stem transections, the resulting extensor bias was restricted to the *ipsilateral* musculature. It was also found that decerebrate posturing was abolished on the same side below unilateral lesions of the vestibular nuclei (Magnus, 1926a). Even in his earliest reports, Sherrington emphasized that decerebrate rigidity was actually a reflex phenomenon, for he noted that sectioning the dorsal roots that supplied a particular limb abolished the rigidity in that limb, thus demonstrating that "the production and maintenance of decerebrate rigidity" depended on "centripetal impulses from peripheral sense organs of the limb" (Sherrington, 1898).

In humans, as in the monkey, although there may be varying degrees of associated spasticity and hyperreflexia, the decerebrate state per se is seldom characterized by fixed extensor posturing (M.H. Feldman, 1971; M.H. Feldman and Sahrmann, 1971); rather, the upper limbs often assume a slightly flexed position in the absence of external stimulation. Both upper and lower extremities tend to remain in any position to which they are moved by the examiner, a feature attributed to the combined release of lengthening and shortening reactions to muscle stretch (Sherrington, 1909). Transient decerebrate *extensor posturing*, with hyperextension of the head and neck, extension with adduction and internal rotation of the arms, and to a lesser extent, extension of the legs, is elicited most readily by nociceptive stimulation of the head or trunk. When applied to distal portions of the extremities, such stimuli tend to evoke *flexor withdrawal* of the stimulated limb, which may be accompanied by a *crossed extensor* reflex in the opposite extremity. In addition, local *supporting reactions* comparable with the reflex standing of the decerebrate monkey (Denny-Brown, 1966) may be elicited from the lower extremities of decerebrate humans (M.H. Feldman and Sahrmann, 1971). Asymmetric and symmetric *tonic neck reflexes* and *tonic labyrinthine reflexes* may also be evoked in exaggerated form in the decerebrate human or monkey (M.H. Feldman, 1971; M.H. Feldman and Sahrmann, 1971). For example, passive hyperextension of the neck in a supine, decerebrate patient increases the extensor drive to all four extremities through the additive effects of the symmetric tonic neck and tonic labyrinthine reflexes (Tokizane et al., 1951).

In sum, the decerebrate state associated with rostral brain stem dysfunction is characterized by lowered thresholds and increased response amplitudes for a variety of tonic postural reflexes. These limited residual capacities to respond to environmental stimuli are mediated in part by complex facilitory and inhibitory influences descending to spinal levels from pontomedullary structures released from more rostral inputs. The discussion that follows considers current concepts of the functional organization of some of these descending pontomedullary pathways.

Pontomedullary Projections to Spinal Cord

The *lateral vestibulospinal* tract originates mainly from the lateral vestibular nucleus of Deiter and descends ipsilaterally over the full extent of the cord (for detailed reviews, see Pompeiano, 1972; Wilson and Peterson, 1981). This pathway contributes to the mediation of both righting and tonic postural labyrinthine reflexes. Somatotopically organized projections from the lateral vestibular nucleus terminate mainly on the interneurons and propriospinal neurons in laminae VII and VIII, although physiologic evidence indicates that at least some of these fibers make monosynaptic contact with spinal motor neurons. The predominant effects of activation of the lateral vestibulospinal tract, at least in the cat, are monosynaptic and polysynaptic excitation of extensor motor neurons, and disynaptic and polysynaptic inhibition of flexor motor neurons. These influences are exerted on static γ motor neurons as well as α motor neurons. As noted earlier, vestibulospinal influences play an important role in the mediation of decerebrate rigidity, which is abolished in the ipsilateral limbs by lesions of the lateral vestibular nucleus or by interruption of the lateral vestibulospinal tract. The relative extensor hypertonus observed in decerebrate rigidity appears to result principally from release of the direct excitatory influences of vestibulospinal neurons on γ motor neurons that supply the static spindles of extensor muscles of the neck, trunk, and limbs (Pompeiano, 1972).

The *medial vestibulospinal* tract, which has both ipsilateral and contralateral components, originates from portions of the medial, lateral, and descending vestibular nuclei and descends only to midthoracic regions, distributing terminals to medial parts of laminae VII and VIII (Pompeiano, 1972; Wilson and Peterson, 1981). This pathway, like the lateral vestibulospinal tract, plays an important role in the mediation of labyrinthine righting and tonic postural reflexes. The medial vestibulospinal tract has been shown in the cat to contain both excitatory and inhibitory fibers that make monosynaptic contacts with motor neurons in the upper cervical segments (above the limb segments).

Stimulation of various parts of the pontomedullary reticular formation augments or suppresses segmental reflexes differentially through descending *reticulospinal pathways*. Early experiments (Magoun and Rhines, 1946; Rhines and Magoun, 1946) gave rise to the view that the pontomedullary reticulospinal system was organized in terms of a medially situated *inhibitory* system and a laterally adjacent *facilitory* system, defined according to the contrasting effects on motor activity that resulted from rather coarse electrical stimulation of the two regions. A short time later, however, evidence was presented (Gernandt and Thulin, 1955; Sprague and Chambers, 1954) that low-intensity stimulation of the pontomedullary reticular formation evoked more complex, usually reciprocal, movements of the extremities, rather than the pure suppression or facilitation of motor activity that had been reported with higher currents. The complex nature of reticulospinal influences on spinal motor mechanisms was further underscored by the demonstration in freely moving cats that microstimulation of a given locus within the medial medullary reticular formation results in the activation of either flexor or extensor muscles of a given limb, depending on the phase of the step cycle at which the stimulus is delivered (Drew and Rossignol, 1984).

Although the concept that the reticulospinal system is organized in terms of separate inhibitory and facilitory systems appears to be oversimplified (based as it is on results obtained in anesthetized or decerebrate animals that are incapable of demonstrating the functional complexities reported with less-compromised preparations), most of the studies of reticulospinal influences on tone and posture have been carried out from this perspective. Accordingly, the following account considers the reticulospinal pathways in terms of the provisional framework of inhibitory and facilitory systems, notwithstanding the aforementioned limitations of this approach. Currently, the single inhibitory reticulospinal system of Magoun and Rhines (1946) is thought to comprise at least four separate descending inhibitory systems, including the dorsal and ventral reticulospinal tracts, each derived from the medial pontomedullary reticular formation, and two monoaminergic inhibitory pathways derived from the noradrenergic locus ceruleus (and nucleus subceruleus) and the serotoninergic nuclei of the dorsal raphe (Lundberg, 1982).

The *dorsal reticulospinal* tract originates within the medial portion of the pontomedullary reticular formation, which corresponds roughly to the nucleus reticularis gigantocellularis of the medulla and the caudal portion of the nucleus reticularis pontis caudalis, and descends to spinal levels within the dorsolateral funiculus (Engberg et al., 1968). Tonic activity within the dorsal reticulospinal tract appears to contribute to decerebrate rigidity (in concert with the descending excitatory influences of the vestibulospinal system on extensor muscles) by suppressing flexor reflex afferent transmission through inhibition of segmental interneurons in the flexor reflex afferent arc (Lundberg, 1982). This effectively results in the activation of limb extensors and the inhibition of limb flexors. The release of flexor reflexes (manifested in its most extreme form by flexor spasms) that accompanies traumatic or functional transection of the spinal cord is thought to result from interruption of the dorsal reticulospinal pathway (Burke et al., 1972). Despite the foregoing evidence implicating the dorsal reticulospinal pathway in inhibitory mechanisms, it should be noted that stimulation of the medial pontomedullary reticular formation has also been shown to produce monosynaptic excitation of trunk and limb motor neurons (Peterson, 1979).

The *ventral reticulospinal* tract originates from roughly the same medial pontomedullary region as the dorsal reticulospinal tract but descends instead in the ventral funiculus (Lundberg, 1982; Magoun and Rhines, 1946). Activation of this pathway has been shown to abolish decerebrate rigidity, inhibit the tonic vibratory reflex, and suppress phasic stretch reflexes (deep tendon reflexes) in both flexors and extensors (Andrews et al., 1973a; Gilles et al., 1971; Magoun and Rhines, 1946). These effects appear to be mediated through a combination of postsynaptic inhibition of internuncial cells, presynaptic inhibition of Ia and Ib spinal afferent fibers via primary afferent depolarization, and the generation of monosynaptic, inhibitory postsynaptic potentials in spinal motor neurons (Lundberg, 1982). There is anatomic and physiologic evidence that this pathway is under cortical control and may provide the substrate for coordinated suppression of stretch reflexes that would otherwise interfere with smooth and rapid execution of volitional movements (Andrews et al., 1973b). The characterization of this pathway initially gave rise to the concept of the *corticoreticulospinal* system. In the monkey, the premotor cortex and the SMA constitute the principal sources of direct cortical input to the medial medullary reticular formation (Catsman-Berrevoets and Kuypers, 1976). It has been proposed that the increased tone and hyperreflexia that characterize spasticity may result from damage (at any level) to this system (Andrews et al., 1973b; Ashby et al., 1972; Gilman and Marco, 1971).

The other proposed inhibitory reticulospinal systems are two monoaminergic descending brain stem pathways that provide direct innervation to motor neuron pools at all levels of the cord (for detailed review, see Lundberg, 1982). *Noradrenergic* fibers arise from the locus ceruleus and the nucleus subceruleus and descend in the ventrolateral funiculus. *Serotoninergic* fibers arise from components of the pontomedullary raphe nuclei and descend in several pathways located within the lateral funiculus. Both the noradrenergic and the serotoninergic descending fibers appear to suppress flexor reflex afferent transmission. Activation of raphe-spinal fibers is also believed to result in excitation of spinal motor neurons. It has been proposed that the tonic inhibition of flexor reflex afferent transmission that accompanies decerebrate rigidity is mediated through the combined activity of the descending serotoninergic

system and the dorsal reticulospinal system (Lundberg, 1982).

The *facilitory reticulospinal* system is thought to arise from the pontomedullary reticular formation immediately adjacent to the cells of origin of the dorsal and ventral reticulospinal tracts. The pontine contribution to the facilitory system appears to include the nucleus reticularis pontis oralis and the rostral portion of the nucleus reticularis pontis caudalis, and the medullary contribution includes the laterally situated nucleus reticularis parvocellularis. Activation of this pathway at the level of the brain stem augments the tonic vibratory reflex both in flexors and in extensors (Andrews et al., 1973a) and leads to monosynaptic excitation of motor neurons innervating limb as well as axial muscles (Peterson, 1979).

Midbrain Projections to Spinal Cord

Several midbrain regions send direct projections to the segmental motor apparatus of the spinal cord. Perhaps the most thoroughly studied of the descending midbrain pathways is the *rubrospinal* tract, which arises from the magnocellular portion of the red nucleus. In the monkey, rubrospinal neurons receive direct *corticorubral* inputs from rostral parts of the leg and the arm representations of primary motor cortex, as well as from adjoining parts of premotor cortex. This and other evidence suggests that the corticorubrospinal system may participate in the control of voluntary movements of the hand and the foot, particularly those requiring simultaneous, synergistic actions of the digits, as in gripping and grip-releasing movements (Humphrey et al., 1984). The rubrospinal tract and the magnocellular portion of the red nucleus decline in size and importance in higher primates. In humans, there are only about 200 magnocellular neurons in the red nucleus (compared with approximately 1000 in the monkey), and the human rubrospinal tract does not appear to descend beyond the upper cervical segments (Nathan and Smith, 1982). Thus, the functional significance of this pathway in humans may be limited.

The *tectospinal* tract is largely crossed and descends only as far as the lower cervical segments. This pathway originates from portions of deep and intermediate layers of the superior colliculus that receive *corticotectal* projections from somatosensory cortex (Jones and Wise, 1977). Neurons in the deep layers of this part of the superior colliculus in cats respond to contralateral tactile stimulation of the head, neck, and upper extremity (Stein et al., 1976). The functional organization of the tectospinal pathway, with its topographically ordered visual, auditory, and somatosensory inputs, suggests that it may play an important role in facilitating visually guided head movements and in orienting the head and upper body (including the upper limb) toward relevant external stimuli (for review, see Coulter et al., 1979).

In the monkey, the *nucleus cuneiformis* and adjacent

midbrain tegmentum project directly to the spinal cord (Castiglioni et al., 1978). In cats, this region has been implicated in the supraspinal control of patterned locomotion. Low-intensity electrical stimulation of the mesencephalic locomotor region, which includes portions of the nucleus cuneiformis, gives rise to graded rhythmic treadmill walking in cats with precollicular postmamillary transections of the brain stem (Garcia-Rill et al., 1983; Orlovsky and Shik, 1976). Whether the direct spinal projections from nucleus cuneiformis play a role in the control of locomotion in primates is uncertain. If so, these might provide more discrete and direct mesencephalic influence on spinal locomotor mechanisms than exist in the cat, because the feline nucleus cuneiformis does not appear to project beyond the pontomedullary reticular formation (Garcia-Rill et al., 1983).

The *interstitiospinal* tract arises from the ipsilateral interstitial nucleus of Cajal and provides extensive projections to all levels of the cord (for review, see Castiglioni et al., 1978). The precise function of this pathway is not known, but it has been suggested that, because of its relationships with the medial longitudinal fasciculus and the oculomotor complex, the interstitiospinal tract may participate in the control of movements that involve rotation of the body around the longitudinal axis. It has been proposed that dysfunction of the interstitial nucleus may play a role in the genesis of spasmodic torticollis, but as yet there has been no neuropathologic confirmation of this suggestion (see Tarlov, 1970). It is noteworthy, however, that in the monkey, lesions of the ventromedial tegmentum that involve the interstitial nucleus may result in a disorder closely resembling spasmodic torticollis (Battista et al., 1976).

There is evidence in the monkey of additional direct spinal projections from several related midbrain nuclei, including the nucleus of Darkschevich, the oculomotor and supratrochlear nuclei, the Edinger-Westphal nuclei, and adjacent portions of the dorsomedial and ventromedial midbrain tegmentum (Castiglioni et al., 1978). The functional significance of these pathways, like that of the more familiar interstitiospinal tract, has yet to be determined.

Brain Stem Pathways in Voluntary Movements

In addition to their influences on posture, muscle tone, and segmental reflexes, the descending brain stem systems have a significant role in the control of voluntary movement. Indeed, it has been shown that the descending brain stem systems are capable of mediating a wide range of movements, even after removal of all direct corticospinal influences by bilateral pyramidotomy (Lawrence and Kuypers, 1968a,b; Tower, 1940). On the basis of their terminal distributions within the spinal gray matter, the pathways that originate in the brain stem and descend to

influence the spinal segmental motor apparatus have been grouped into *ventromedial* and *dorsolateral bulbospinal* systems (Kuypers and Lawrence, 1967; Lawrence and Kuypers, 1968a,b) (see Fig. 21–3). The functional significance of these groupings has been demonstrated by studies of the differential effects of lesions of each system on motor performance in primates.

The ventromedial system consists of descending fibers derived from the medial pontine and medullary reticular formation, certain vestibular nuclei (most importantly, the lateral vestibular nucleus), the superior colliculus, and the interstitial nucleus of Cajal. The ventromedial system terminates largely in the ventral and medial parts of the internuncial zone, which contains propriospinal neurons with long and intermediate-length axons that project to motor neurons innervating the limb girdle and axial musculature. This system thus seems well suited anatomically for synergic activation of relatively large numbers of proximal limb and trunk muscles, but lacking in the capacity for control of independent movements of the limb. It has been proposed (Lawrence and Kuypers, 1968b) that the ventromedial system may provide the basic substrate for movement and posture, on which those systems controlling distal, fractionated movements are superimposed.

The dorsolateral system consists of rubrospinal fibers derived principally from the magnocellular portion of the red nucleus, with additional descending contributions from the ventrolateral pontine tegmentum and the raphe nuclei of the lower brain stem. The dorsolateral system terminates in the dorsal and lateral parts of the spinal internuncial zone. This system appears anatomically to provide for a greater degree of control of the distal musculature than does the ventromedial system.

The suggestion that the ventromedial and dorsolateral brain stem descending systems may serve complementary roles in the control of voluntary movements is supported by studies in monkeys of the effects of lesions of the two systems (after recovery from bilateral pyramidotomies to eliminate direct corticospinal influences) (Lawrence and Kuypers, 1968a,b). Thus, lesions that interrupt the ventromedial pathways result in severe impairment of axial and proximal extremity movements and whole-body (limb-trunk) synergies, such as those used in righting, locomotion, and climbing, but leave distal extremity movements relatively unaffected. On the other hand, lesions that involve the dorsolateral pathways lead to impairment of fractionated distal extremity movements, such as those involved in grasping and manipulating small objects, with relative sparing of proximal limb movements and combined movements of body and limbs, such as are required for locomotion.

CONCLUDING REMARKS

The various cortical and subcortical systems concerned with motor control exhibit both hierarchic and parallel features. At the lowest level, the spinal cord is capable of coordinating a number of reflex activities and basic movement synergies. The segmental motor apparatus is influenced by a variety of pathways descending from brain stem and cortical regions that regulate transmission through spinal reflex arcs, modulate spinal mechanisms subserving basic movement synergies, and provide the substrates for voluntary control of discrete movements of individual body parts. The descending brain stem systems provide substantial control of muscle tone, posture, and movement, while being subject, in turn, to various controlling influences projected from cerebellum, basal ganglia, and cortex.

The degree of cortical control of motor functions increases markedly in higher primates. Primary motor cortex is closely related to the segmental motor apparatus by virtue of its direct projections to spinal motor neurons and interneurons and appears to play a major role in the execution of movement. The direct corticospinal systems appear essential for the execution of independent skilled movements of individual body parts, particularly of the distal extremities. The motor cortex appears to play a major role in motor control by (1) specifying the appropriate muscle synergies for a particular act, (2) determining the proper sequencing and timing of muscle activations, and (3) informing other components of the motor system of the intended output (by means of an efference copy or corollary discharge). The motor cortex also appears to mediate certain cutaneous and proprioceptive transcortical reflexes.

The premotor areas, including the SMA and the premotor cortex, are thought to play somewhat different roles. The SMA appears to be significant in the control of complex motor synergies and to modulate input-output coupling in the motor cortex. The SMA may also modulate spinal mechanisms directly via direct projections to the spinal cord. The premotor cortex appears not only to play a relatively specialized role in the control of proximal musculature but also to participate rather selectively in the control of movements that are triggered or guided by visual stimuli. Parietal areas 5 and 7 also participate in the control of movements. Area 5 appears to be preferentially involved in movements that are guided by tactile stimuli, whereas area 7 has been shown to play a role in selective attention and in the control of visually guided movements directed into extrapersonal space.

The large reentrant subcortical pathways involving the basal ganglia and the cerebellum provide input to the precentral motor fields by means of segregated pathways directed to specific cortical target zones. The two systems appear to operate largely in parallel, although each has been implicated in somewhat different aspects of motor control. In both cases, considerably more is known about the specific motor disturbances that are associated with selective damage to either system than about their respective contributions to motor control under normal conditions.

The distributed components of the motor system normally function in concert, and to a large extent in parallel, to generate coordinated movements. Damage to different regions may result in highly characteristic abnormalities of movement and posture. The manifestations of damage to the descending brain stem systems and corticospinal pathways and the precentral motor fields have been the focus of this overview. Chapters 22–26 explore in greater detail the functional organization of the cerebellum, the basal ganglia, and the cerebral cortex and the clinical expressions of pathologic changes within these structures.

Acknowledgment

In preparing the manuscript, we received valuable assistance from Barbara Zuckerman.

References

(Key references are designated with an asterisk.)

Abend W., Bizzi E., Morasso P. Human arm trajectory formation. *Brain* 105:331–348, 1982.

*Albin R.L., Young A.B., Penney J.B. The functional anatomy of basal ganglia disorders. *Trends Neurosci.* 12:366–375, 1989.

*Alexander G.E., Crutcher M.D. Functional architecture of basal ganglia circuits: neural substrates of parallel processing. *Trends Neurosci.* 13:266–271, 1990a.

Alexander G.E., Crutcher M.D. Neural representations of the target (goal) of visually guided arm movements in three motor areas of the monkey. *J. Neurophysiol.* 64:164–178, 1990b.

Alexander G.E., Crutcher M.D. Preparation for movement: neural representations of intended direction in three motor areas of the monkey. *J. Neurophysiol.* 64:133–150, 1990c.

*Alexander G.E., DeLong M.R., Strick P.L. Parallel organization of functionally segregated circuits linking basal ganglia and cortex. *Annu. Rev. Neurosci.* 9:357–381, 1986.

Andrews C., Knowles L., Hancock J. Control of the tonic vibration reflex by the brain stem reticular formation in the cat. *J. Neurol. Sci.* 18:217–226, 1973a.

Andrews C., Knowles L., Lance J.W. Corticoreticulospinal control of the tonic vibration reflex in the cat. *J. Neurol. Sci.* 18:207–216, 1973b.

Asanuma C., Thach T., Jones E.G. Distribution of cerebellar terminations in the ventral lateral thalamic region of the monkey. *Brain Res. Rev.* 5:237–265, 1983.

Ashby P., Andrews C., Knowles L., et al. Pyramidal and extrapyramidal control of tonic mechanisms in the cat. *Brain* 95:21–30, 1972.

Baldissera F., Hultborn H., Illert M. Integration in spinal neuronal systems. In Brookhart J.M., Mountcastle V.B., Brooks V.B., eds. *Handbook of Physiology.* Section 1. *The Nervous System.* Vol. II. *Motor Control.* Part 1. Bethesda, American Physiological Society, pp. 509–595, 1981.

Barrett G., Shibasaki H., Neshige R. Cortical potentials preceding voluntary movement: evidence for three periods of preparation in man. *Electroencephalogr. Clin. Neurophysiol.* 63:327–339, 1986.

Battista A.F., Goldstein M., Miyamoto T., et al. Effect of centrally acting drugs on experimental torticollis in monkeys. *Adv. Neurol.* 14:329–337, 1976.

Bernstein N. The problem of the interrelation of co-ordination and localization (originally published in *Arch. Biol. Sci.,* 38, 1935). In Whiting H.T.A., ed. *Human Motor Actions: Bernstein Reassessed.* Amsterdam, North Holland, pp. 77–119, 1984.

Biber M.P., Kneisley L.W., Lavail J.H. Cortical neurons projecting to the cervical and lumbar enlargements of the spinal cord in young and adult rhesus monkeys. *Exp. Neurol.* 59:492–508, 1978.

*Brooks V.B., Thach W.T. Cerebellar control of posture and movement. In Brookhart J.M., Mountcastle V.B., Brooks V.B., eds. *Handbook of Physiology*. Section 1. *The Nervous System*. Vol. II. *Motor Control*. Part 2. Bethesda, American Physiological Society, pp. 877–946, 1981.

Brown T.H., Kairiss E.W., Keenan C.L. Hebbian synapses: biophysical mechanisms and algorithms. *Annu. Rev. Neurosci.* 13:475–511, 1990.

Bucy P.C., Keplinger J.E., Siqueira E.B. Destruction of the "pyramidal tract" in man. *J. Neurosurg.* 21:285–298, 1964.

Bucy P.C., Ladpi R., Ehrlich A. Destruction of the pyramidal tract in the monkey. *J. Neurosurg.* 25:1–23, 1966.

Burke D., Knowles L., Andrews C., et al. Spasticity, decerebrate rigidity and the clasp-knife phenomenon: an experimental study in the cat. *Brain* 95:31–48, 1972.

Burke D., Hagbarth K.E., Lofstedt L., et al. The responses of human muscle spindle endings to vibration during muscle contraction. *J. Physiol. (Lond.)* 261:695, 1976.

Carpenter M.B. Anatomy of the corpus striatum and brain stem integrating systems. In Brookhart J.M., Mountcastle V.B., Brooks V.B., eds. *Handbook of Physiology*. Section 1: *The Nervous System*. Vol. II. *Motor Control*. Part 2. Bethesda, American Physiological Society, pp. 947–996, 1981.

Castiglioni A.J., Gallaway M.C., Coulter J.D. Spinal projections from the midbrain in monkey. *J. Comp. Neurol.* 178:329–346, 1978.

Catsman-Berrevoets C.E., Kuypers H.G.J.M. Cells of origin of cortical projections to dorsal column nuclei, spinal cord and bulbar medial reticular formation in the rhesus monkey. *Neurosci. Lett.* 3:245–252, 1976.

Cheney P.D., Fetz E.E. Functional classes of primate corticomotoneuronal cells and their relation to active force. *J. Neurophysiol.* 44:773–791, 1980.

Coulter J.D., Jones E.G. Differential distribution of corticospinal projections from individual cytoarchitectonic fields in the monkey. *Brain Res.* 129:335–340, 1977.

Coulter J.D., Bowker R.M., Wise S.P., et al. Cortical, tectal and medullary descending pathways to the cervical spinal cord. *Prog. Brain Res.* 50:263–274, 1979.

Coxe W.S., Landau W.M. Observations upon the effect of supplementary motor cortex ablation in the monkey. *Brain* 88:763–773, 1965.

Damasio A.R., VanHoesen G.W. Structure and function of the supplementary motor area. *Neurology (N. Y.)* 30:359, 1980.

Deecke L., Grozinger B., Kornhuber H.H. Voluntary finger movement in man: cerebral potentials and theory. *Biol. Cybern.* 23:99–119, 1976.

*DeLong M.R. Primate models of movement disorders of basal ganglia origin. *Trends Neurosci.* 13:281–285, 1990.

*DeLong M.R., Georgopoulos A.P. Motor functions of the basal ganglia. In Brookhart J.M., Mountcastle V.B., Brooks V.B., et al. eds. *Handbook of Physiology*. Section 1. *The Nervous System*. Vol. II. *Motor Control*. Part 2. Bethesda, American Physiological Society, pp. 1017–1061, 1981.

DeMyer W. Number of axons and myelin sheaths in adult human medullary pyramids. *Neurology (Minneap.)* 9:42–47, 1959.

Denny-Brown D. *The Cerebral Control of Movement*. Springfield, IL, Thomas, 1966.

Dhanarajan P., Ruegg D.G., Wiesendanger M. An anatomical investigation of the corticopontine projection in the primate (*Saimiri sciureus*): the projection from motor and somatosensory areas. *Neuroscience* 2:913–922, 1977.

Drew T., Rossignol S. Phase-dependent responses evoked in limb muscles by stimulation of medullary reticular formation during locomotion in thalamic cats. *J. Neurophysiol.* 52:653–675, 1984.

*Dum R.P., Strick P.L. Premotor areas: nodal points for parallel efferent systems involved in the central control of movement. In Humphrey D.R., Freund H.J., eds. *Motor Control: Concepts and Issues. Dahlem Konferenzen*. Chichester, Wiley, pp. 383–411, 1991.

Edley S.M., Graybiel A.M. The afferent and efferent connections of the feline nucleus tegmenti pedunculopontinus, pars compacta. *J. Comp. Neurol.* 217:187–215, 1983.

Engberg I., Lundberg A., Ryall R.W. Reticulospinal inhibition of transmission in reflex pathways. *J. Physiol. (Lond.)* 194:201–223, 1968.

Evarts E.V. Role of motor cortex in voluntary movements in primates. In Brookhart J.M., Mountcastle V.B., Brooks V.B., et al., eds. *Handbook of Physiology*. Section 1. *The Nervous System*. Vol. II. *Motor Control*. Part 2. Bethesda, American Physiological Society, pp. 1083–1120, 1981.

Evarts E.V., Thach W.T. Motor mechanism of the CNS: cerebrocerebellar interrelations. *Annu. Rev. Physiol.* 31:451–498, 1969.

Feldman J.A., Ballard D.H. Connectionist models and their properties. *Cognitive Sci.* 6:205–254, 1982.

Feldman M.H. The decerebrate state in the primate. I. Studies in monkeys. *Arch. Neurol.* 25:501–516, 1971.

Feldman M.H., Sahrmann S. The decerebrate state in the primate. II. Studies in man. *Arch. Neurol.* 25:517–525, 1971.

Fetz E.E., Cheney P.D. Postspike facilitation of forelimb muscle activity by primate corticomotoneuronal cells. *J. Neurophysiol.* 44:751–772, 1980.

Fetz E.E., Cheney P.D., Mewes K., et al. Control of forelimb muscle activity by populations of corticomotoneuronal and rubromotoneuronal cells. *Prog. Brain Res.* 80:437–449, 1989.

Forssberg H. Spinal locomotor functions and descending control. In Sjolund B.H., ed. *Brain Stem Control of Spinal Mechanisms*. New York, Elsevier, pp. 253–271, 1982.

Forssberg H. Ontogeny of human locomotor control. I. Infant stepping, supported locomotion and transition to independent locomotion. *Exp. Brain Res.* 57:480–493, 1985.

Fox P.T., Fox J.M., Raichle M.E., et al. The role of cerebral cortex in the generation of voluntary saccades: a positron emission tomographic study. *J. Neurophysiol.* 54:348–369, 1985.

Freund H.J. Premotor areas in men. *Trends Neurosci.* 7:481–483, 1984.

Freund H.J., Hummelsheim H. Premotor cortex in man: evidence for innervation of proximal limb muscles. *Exp. Brain Res.* 53:479–482, 1984.

Garcia-Rill E. The basal ganglia and the locomotor regions. *Brain Res. Rev.* 11:47–63, 1986.

Garcia-Rill E., Skinner R.D., Gilmore S.A., et al. Connections of the mesencephalic locomotor region (MLR). II. Afferents and efferents. *Brain Res. Bull.* 10:63–71, 1983.

Gernandt B.E., Thulin C.A. Reciprocal effects upon spinal motoneurons from stimulation of bulbar reticular formation. *J. Neurophysiol.* 18:113–129, 1955.

Gilles J.D., Burke D.J., Lance J.W. Supraspinal control of tonic vibration reflex. *J. Neurophysiol.* 34:302–309, 1971.

Gilman S., Marco L.A. Effects of medullary pyramidotomy in the monkey. I. Clinical and electromyographic abnormalities. *Brain* 94:495–514, 1971.

Gilman S., Lieberman J.S., Marco L.A. Spinal mechanisms underlying the effects of unilateral ablation of areas 4 and 6 in monkeys. *Brain* 97:49–64, 1974.

Gilman S., Bloedel J.R., Lechtenberg R. *Disorders of the Cerebellum*. Philadelphia, Davis, 1981.

Grossberg S., Kuperstein M. *Neural Dynamics of Adaptive Sensory-Motor Control*. New York, Pergamon Press, 1989.

Hagbarth K.E., Wallin B.G., Lofstedt L. Muscle spindle responses to stretch in normal and spastic subjects. *Scand. J. Rehab. Med.* 5:156–159, 1973.

Hildreth E.C., Hollerbach J.M. Artificial intelligence: computational approach to vision and motor control. In Mountcastle V.B., Plum F., Geiger S.R., eds. *Handbook of Physiology*. Section 1. *The Nervous System*. Vol. V. *High Functions of the Brain*. Part 2. Bethesda, American Physiological Society, pp. 605–642, 1987.

Hogan N., Bizzi E., Mussa-Ivaldi F.A., et al. Controlling multijoint motor behavior. *Exerc. Sport Sci. Rev.* 15:153–190, 1987.

Hollerbach J.M. Computers, brains and the control of movement. *Trends Neurosci.* 5:189–192, 1982.

Humphrey D.R. Corticospinal systems and their control by premotor cortex, basal ganglia, and cerebellum. In Rosenberg R.N., Willis W.D., eds. *The Clinical Neurosciences: Neurobiology*. New York, Churchill Livingstone, pp. 547–587, 1983.

Humphrey D.R., Gold R., Reed D.J. Sizes, laminar and topographic origins of cortical projections to the major divisions of the red nucleus in the monkey. *J. Comp. Neurol.* 225:75–94, 1984.

Ito M. *The Cerebellum and Neural Control*. New York, Raven Press, 1984.

Jones E.G., Wise S.P. Size, laminar and columnar distribution of efferent cells in the sensory-motor cortex of monkeys. *J. Comp. Neurol.* 175:391–437, 1977.

Kasser R.J., Cheney P.D. Characteristics of corticomotoneuronal postspike facilitation and reciprocal suppression of EMG activity in the monkey. *J. Neurophysiol.* 4:959–978, 1985.

Kemp J.M., Powell T.P.S. The connexions of the striatum and globus pallidus: synthesis and speculation. *Philos. Trans. R. Soc. Lond. [Biol.]* 262:441–457, 1971.

Kunzle H. Bilateral projections from precentral motor cortex to the putamen and other parts of the basal ganglia. An autoradiographic study in *Macaca fascicularis*. *Brain Res.* 88:195–209, 1975.

Kunzle H. Projections from the primary somatosensory cortex to basal ganglia and thalamus in the monkey. *Exp. Brain Res.* 30:481–492, 1977.

*Kuypers H.G.J.M. Anatomy of the descending pathways. In Brookhart J.M., Mountcastle V.B., Brooks V.B., et al., eds. *Handbook of Physiology*. Section 1. *The Nervous System*. Vol. II. *Motor Control*. Part 1. Bethesda, American Physiological Society, pp. 597–666, 1981.

Kuypers H.G.J.M., Brinkman J. Precentral projections to different parts of the spinal intermediate zone in the rhesus monkey. *Brain Res.* 24:29–48, 1970.

Kuypers H.G.J.M., Lawrence D.G. Cortical projections to the red nucleus and the brain stem in the rhesus monkey. *Brain Res.* 4:151–188, 1967.

Lance J.W. The control of muscle tone, reflexes, and movement: Robert Wartenberg lecture. *Neurology (N. Y.)* 30:1303–1313, 1980.

Landau W.M., Weaver R.A., Hornbein T.F. Fusimotor nerve function in man: differential nerve block studies in normal subjects and in spasticity and rigidity. *Arch. Neurol.* 3:10–23, 1960.

LaPlane D., Talairach J., Meininger V., et al. Clinical consequences of corticectomies involving the supplementary motor area in man. *J. Neurol. Sci.* 34:301–314, 1977.

Larsen B., Skinhoj E., Lassen N.A. Regional cortical blood flow variations in the right and left hemisphere during automatic speech. *Brain* 101:193–209, 1978.

Lawrence D.G., Kuypers H.G. The functional organization of the motor system in the monkey. I. The effects of bilateral pyramidal lesions. *Brain* 91:1–14, 1968a.

Lawrence D.G., Kuypers H.G. The functional organization of the motor system in the monkey. II. The effects of lesions of the descending brain stem pathways. *Brain* 91:15–26, 1968b.

*Lemon R. The output map of the primate motor cortex. *Trends Neurosci.* 11:501–506, 1988.

Linsker R. Perceptual neural organization: some approaches based on network models and information theory. *Annu. Rev. Neurosci.* 13:257–281, 1990.

Loeb G.E. Finding common ground between robotics and physiology (letter). *Trends Neurosci.* 6:203–204, 1983.

Lundberg A. Integration in a propriospinal motor centre controlling the forelimb in the cat. In Asanuma H., Wilson V.J., eds. *Integration in the Nervous System*. Tokyo, Igaku Shoin, pp. 47–64, 1979.

Lundberg A. Inhibitory control from the brain stem of transmission from primary afferents to motoneurons, primary afferent terminals and ascending pathways. In Sjolund B.H., ed. *Brain Stem Control of Spinal Mechanisms*. New York, Elsevier, pp. 179–224, 1982.

Lynch J.C., Mountcastle V.B., Talbot W.H., et al. Parietal lobe mechanisms for directed visual attention. *J. Neurophysiol.* 40:362–389, 1977.

Macpherson J.M., Marangoz C., Miles T.S., et al. Microstimulation of the supplementary motor area (SMA) in the awake monkey. *Exp. Brain Res.* 45:410–416, 1982.

Magnus R. Physiology of posture. Part I. *Lancet* 2:531–536, 1926a.

Magnus R. Physiology of posture. Part IIB. General static reactions of the mid-brain animal. *Lancet* 2:585–588, 1926b.

Magoun H.W., Rhines R. An inhibitory mechanism in the bulbar reticular formation. *J. Neurophysiol.* 9:165–171, 1946.

Masdeu J.C., Schoene W.C., Funkenstein H. Aphasia following infarction of the left supplementary motor area. *Neurology (Minneap.)* 28:1220–1223, 1978.

Morasso P. Spatial control of arm movements. *Exp. Brain Res.* 42:223–227, 1981.

Muakkassa K.F., Strick P.L. Frontal lobe inputs to primate motor cortex: evidence for four somatotopically organized "premotor" areas. *Brain Res.* 177:176–182, 1979.

Murray E.A., Coulter J.D. Organization of corticospinal neurons in the monkey. *J. Comp. Neurol.* 195:339–365, 1981.

Nathan P.W., Smith M.C. The rubrospinal and central tegmental tracts in man. *Brain* 105:223–269, 1982.

Neshige R., Luders H., Shibasaki H. Recording of movement-related potentials from scalp and cortex in man. *Brain* 111:719–736, 1988.

Orlovsky G.M., Shik M.L. Control of locomotion: a neurophysiological analysis of the cat locomotor system. *Int. Rev. Physiol.* 10:281–317, 1976.

Pellionisz A., Llinas R. Tensor network theory of the metaorganization of functional geometries in the central nervous system. *Neuroscience* 16:245–273, 1985.

Penfield W., Jasper H. *Epilepsy and the Functional Anatomy of the Human Brain*. Boston, Little, Brown, 1954.

Penfield W., Welch K. The supplementary motor area of the cerebral cortex. *Arch. Neurol. Psychiatry* 66:289–317, 1951.

Peterson B.W. Reticulo-motor pathways: their connections and possible roles in motor behavior. In Asanuma H., Wilson V.J., eds. *Integration in the Nervous System*. Tokyo, Igaku Shoin, pp. 185–200, 1979.

Peterson B.W. The reticulospinal system and its role in the control of movement. In Barnes C.D., ed. *Brainstem Control of Spinal Cord Function*. Orlando, FL, Academic Press, pp. 27–86, 1984.

Pompeiano O. Vestibulospinal relations: vestibular influences on gamma motoneurons and primary afferents. *Prog. Brain Res.* 37:197–232, 1972.

Reiner A., Albin R.L., Anderson K.D., et al. Differential loss of striatal projection neurons in Huntington disease. *Proc. Natl. Acad. Sci. U.S.A.* 85:5733–5737, 1988.

Rhines R., Magoun H.W. Brain stem facilitation of cortical motor response. *J. Neurophysiol.* 9:219–229, 1946.

Robinson D.L., Goldberg M.E., Stanton G.B. Parietal association cortex in the primate: sensory mechanisms and behavioral modulations. *J. Neurophysiol.* 41:910–932, 1978.

Roland P.E. Organization of motor control by the normal human brain. *Hum. Neurobiol.* 2:205–216, 1984.

Roland P.E., Larsen B., Lassen N.A., et al. Supplementary motor area and other cortical areas in organization of voluntary movements in man. *J. Neurophysiol.* 43:118–136, 1980.

Rumelhart D.E., McClelland J.L., PDP Research Group. *Parallel Distributed Processing: Explorations in the Microstructure of Cognition*. Cambridge, MA, M.I.T. Press, 1986.

Sahrmann S.A., Norton B.J. The relationship of voluntary movement to spasticity in the upper motor neuron syndrome. *Ann. Neurol.* 2:460–465, 1977.

Saltzman E. Levels of sensorimotor representation. *J. Math. Psych.* 20:91–163, 1979.

Schell G.R., Strick P.L. The origin of thalamic inputs to the arcuate premotor and supplementary motor areas. *J. Neurosci.* 4:539–560, 1984.

Schroder K.E., Hopf A., Lange H., et al. Morphemetrisch-statistische Strukturanalysen des Striatum, Pallidum und Nucleus subthalamicus beim Menschen. I. Striatum. *J. Hirnforsch.* 16:333–350, 1975.

Selemon L.D., Goldman-Rakic P.S. Longitudinal topography and interdigitation of cortico-striatal projections in the rhesus monkey. *J. Neurosci.* 5:776–794, 1985.

Sherrington C.S. Decerebrate rigidity, and reflex coordination of movements. *J. Physiol. (Lond.)* 22:319–322, 1898.

Sherrington C.S. On plastic tonus and proprioceptive reflexes. *Q. J. Exp. Physiol.* 2:109–156, 1909.

Shinoda Y., Yokota J., Futami T. Divergent projection of individual corticospinal axons to motorneurons of multiple muscles in the monkey. *Neurosci. Lett.* 23:7–12, 1981.

Smith A.M., Bourbonnais D., Blanchette G. Interactions between forced grasping and a learned precision grip after ablation of the supplementary motor area. *Brain Res.* 222:395–400, 1981.

Spann B.M., Grofova I. Origin of ascending and spinal pathways from the nucleus tegmenti pedunculopontinus in the rat. *J. Comp. Neurol.* 283:13–27, 1989.

Sprague J.M., Chambers W.W. Control of posture by reticular

formation and cerebellum in the intact, anesthetized and unanesthetized, and in the decerebrated cat. *Am. J. Physiol.* 176:52–64, 1954.

Stein B.E., Magalhães-Castro B., Kruger L. Relationship between visual and tactile representations in cat superior colliculus. *J. Neurophysiol.* 39:401–419, 1976.

Strick P.L., Preston J.B. Two representations of the hand in area 4 of a primate. II. Somatosensory input organization. *J. Neurophysiol.* 48:150–159, 1982.

Talairach J., Bancaud J. The supplementary motor area in man. *Int. J. Neurol.* 5:330–347, 1966.

Tang A., Rymer W.Z. Abnormal force-EMG relations in paretic limbs of hemiparetic human subjects. *J. Neurol. Neurosurg. Psychiatry* 44:690–698, 1981.

Tanji J., Kurata K. Contrasting neuronal activity in supplementary and precentral motor cortex of monkeys. I. Responses to instructions determining motor responses to forthcoming modalities. *J. Neurophysiol.* 53:129–141, 1985.

Tanji J., Taniguchi K., Saga T. Supplementary motor area: neuronal response to motor instructions. *J. Neurophysiol.* 43:60–68, 1980.

Tarlov E. On the problem of the pathology of spasmodic torticollis in man. *J. Neurol. Neurosurg. Psychiatry* 33:457–463, 1970.

Tokizane T., Murao M., Ogata T., et al. Electromygraphic studies on tonic neck, lumbar and labyrinthine reflexes in normal persons. *Jpn. J. Physiol.* 2:130–146, 1951.

Tomasch J. The numerical capacity of the human corticopontocerebellar system. *Brain Res.* 13:476–484, 1969.

Tower S.S. Pyramidal lesion in the monkey. *Brain* 63:39–90, 1940.

Travis A.M. Neurological deficiencies following supplementary motor area lesions in *Macaca mulatta. Brain* 78:155–174, 1955.

VanBuren J.M., Fedio P. Functional representation on the medial aspect of the frontal lobes in man. *J. Neurosurg.* 44:275–289, 1976.

*Wiesendanger M. Organization of secondary motor area of cerebral cortex. In Brookhart J.M., Mountcastle V.B., Brooks V.B., eds. *Handbook of Physiology.* Section 1. *The Nervous System.* Vol. II. *Motor Control.* Part 2. Bethesda, American Physiological Society, pp. 1121–1147, 1981.

Wiesendanger R., Wiesendanger M., Ruegg D.G. An anatomical investigation of the corticopontine projection in the primate (*Macaca fascicularis* and *Saimiri sciureus*). II. The projection from frontal and parietal association areas. *Neuroscience* 4:747–765, 1979.

Wilson V.J., Peterson B.W. Vestibulospinal and reticulospinal system. In Brookhart J.M., Mountcastle V.B., Brooks V.B., eds. *Handbook of Physiology.* Section 1. *The Nervous System.* Vol. II. *Motor Control.* Part 1. Bethesda, American Physiological Society, pp. 667–702, 1981.

Wise S.P. The primate premotor cortex: past, present, and preparatory. *Annu. Rev. Neurosci.* 8:1–19, 1985.

Yeterian E.H., VanHoesen G.W. Cortico-striate projections in the rhesus monkey: the organization of certain cortico-caudate connections. *Brain Res.* 139:43–63, 1978.

22

Motor Dysfunction and Movement Disorders

C. David Marsden

The field of movement disorders encompasses the conditions characterized by insufficient movement (Parkinson's disease and its variants) and excessive movement (the dyskinesias of tremor, chorea, myoclonus, tics, and dystonias). Many, but not all, are due to abnormal function of the basal ganglia. The role of the basal ganglia in normal motor control is discussed in Chapter 21, disorders of movement caused by cerebellar disease are reviewed in Chapter 23, and spasticity is addressed in Chapters 20 and 21. This chapter concentrates on the pathophysiology and clinical features of the other major classes of movement disorders.

Common focal brain diseases, such as stroke or tumor, rarely respect the anatomic boundaries of the basal ganglia. Usually, they infringe on adjacent structures, making it difficult to draw firm clinicopathologic conclusions. Focal lesions restricted to the basal ganglia are rare.

Degenerations of the brain affecting the basal ganglia also usually affect other structures. The most common, Parkinson's disease, undoubtedly causes severe disruption of basal ganglia function attributable to devastation of the zona compacta of the substantia nigra and of the adjacent ventral tegmental area. Loss of pigmented neurons in these regions leads to profound destruction of the dopamine pathways to the striatum. That from zona compacta to putamen is affected more than those to the caudate and to the ventral striatum. However, in Parkinson's disease, there also is loss of dopamine projections to selected areas of the cerebral cortex and perhaps to the spinal cord and of noradrenergic projections from the locus ceruleus to the cerebral cortex and elsewhere. In addition, in the later stages of the illness, a proportion of patients begin to exhibit signs of dementia, which now is thought to be a consequence, at least in part, of pathologic change of the substantia

innominata causing loss of cerebral cortical acetylcholine projections, as well as pathologic changes of cortical neurons themselves. Parkinson's disease, therefore, spreads beyond the confines of the basal ganglia.

Another well-known basal ganglia degeneration is Huntington's disease. Although the pathologic characteristic of this illness is gross atrophy of the caudate nucleus (more than the putamen and even more than the nucleus accumbens), there also is conspicuous cerebral cortical atrophy along with degeneration in the thalamus and the hypothalamus.

Human pathologic findings thus do not provide many examples of pure basal ganglia disease. Nevertheless, it is possible to distinguish two major motor consequences of basal ganglia damage (Marsden, 1984a):

1. The akinetic-rigid parkinsonian syndrome
2. Abnormal involuntary movements, or dyskinesias

THE AKINETIC-RIGID SYNDROME

Inability to move (akinesia), poverty of movement (hypokinesia), and slowness of movement (bradykinesia), associated with muscular rigidity, are common consequences of basal ganglia disease. These abnormalities of movement can be subsumed under akinesia. Akinesia, rest tremor, and rigidity are the hallmarks of Parkinson's disease. An akinetic-rigid syndrome also is seen in many other pathologic entities affecting the basal ganglia bilaterally (Table 22–1).

The akinetic-rigid syndrome occurs with lesions causing the following:

Abnormal dopaminergic input to the striatum, as

Table 22–1. CAUSES OF THE AKINETIC-RIGID
SYNDROME

Adults	Juveniles
Pure Parkinsonism	*Pure Parkinsonism*
Parkinson's disease	Wilson's disease
Postencephalitic parkinsonism	Hallervorden-Spatz disease
Drug-induced parkinsonism	Pallidal degenerations
	Juvenile Huntington's disease
Parkinsonism-Plus	Dopa-responsive dystonia-
Progressive supranuclear palsy	parkinsonism
Multiple system atrophy	
Olivopontocerebellar	
degeneration	
Striatonigral degeneration	
Shy-Drager syndrome	
Corticobasal degeneration	
Basal ganglia calcification	
Parkinsonism in Dementia	
Alzheimer's disease	
Pick's disease	
Creutzfeld-Jakob disease	
Cerebrovascular disease	
Multi-infarct	
Bingswanger's disease	
Head injury	
Anoxia	
Hydrocephalus	

in Parkinson's disease itself (or in drug-induced parkinsonism produced by dopamine receptor blockade by neuroleptic antipsychotic drugs)

Extensive damage to the striatum, as in the Westphal variant of Huntington's disease, Wilson's disease, or striatonigral degeneration

Damage to the output zones of the basal ganglia (i.e., the medial globus pallidus and the substantia nigra pars reticulata), as in progressive supranuclear palsy, the progressive pallidal degenerations, and Hallervorden-Spatz disease

Diffuse cerebral conditions, as Pick's disease, corticobasal degeneration, hydrocephalus, and cerebrovascular disease (attributable either to multiple cerebral infarcts or to subcortical vascular encephalopathy of Binswanger)

The general conclusion is that any pathologic change (or drug) that causes extensive bilateral disruption of the striatopallidal complex or its outputs can cause an akinetic-rigid syndrome.

Unilateral lesions can cause akinesia and rigidity of the contralateral body, as in the hemiparkinsonism seen in the early stages of Parkinson's disease and the rare symptomatic parkinsonism caused by cerebral tumor. However, bilateral damage causes more severe akinesia and rigidity, particularly of axial structures, and also produces another common feature of this syndrome, postural instability and locomotor difficulty.

Thus, the akinetic-rigid syndrome characteristic of many basal ganglia diseases includes a variety of motor disorders. Some of these may represent positive symptoms caused by release of abnormal activity in distant brain regions. By analogy, spasticity is a positive phenomenon attributable to release of spinal motor mechanisms from corticospinal and bulbospinal control. Rigidity (and rest tremor) probably falls into this category. Positive symptoms do not provide good evidence of the normal functions of the part of the brain that is damaged. Negative symptoms, by which is meant functions that are lost, on the other hand, do give some clues as to function. Loss of the ability to initiate and execute movement, loss of postural stability, and locomotor difficulty are the key negative symptoms of basal ganglia disease causing the akinetic-rigid syndrome.

The pathophysiology of these cardinal features of basal ganglia disease—akinesia, rigidity, postural change, and locomotor difficulty—is discussed separately. (Tremor is reviewed in Chapter 25.)

Characteristic Features

Akinesia

Most of the detailed studies of akinesia have been undertaken with patients with Parkinson's disease (Table 22–2).

Delay in initiation of movement is variable. The akinetic patient takes longer than normal to respond to external stimuli. For example, reaction times to visual stimuli are prolonged and more variable than normal (Evarts et al., 1981). However, on occasion, such patients can respond briskly (paradoxical kinesia). Delayed reactions are not thought to be the result of failure to perceive the stimulus, and patients with Parkinson's disease generally can improve reaction time if given a warning clue (Heilman et al., 1976), and they can correct their mistakes (Angel et al., 1970). Preparation for movement appears intact, for choice reaction times are not prolonged disproportionate to the delay in a simple reaction time. In addition, patients with Parkinson's disease can learn a new motor task, formulate an internal plan of that task, and move in anticipation of a known signal (Bloxham et al., 1984; Day et al., 1984). Thus, they

Table 22–2. DISORDERS OF MOVEMENT IN
PARKINSON'S DISEASE

Simple Movements
Delay in initiation
Slowness in execution
Inadequate initial agonist activity
Slowness in executing corrective action

Complex Movements
Slowness and fatigue of repetitive action
Inability to execute concurrent action
Inability to execute sequential action
Dependence on visual feedback
Freezing in course of action

Postural Movements
Loss of postural fixation
Loss of anticipatory postural flexes
Loss of righting reactions
Loss of protective reactions

can take predictive action, which means that they possess the capacity to select a sequence of motor programs in preparation to move. However, their performance is poor, and they are more dependent on visual feedback than are normal subjects (Cooke et al., 1978). Delayed motor reactions to predictable external stimuli, which is typical of Parkinson's disease, could be due to failure to prepare a movement known to be required in advance, a failure to hold that movement in store, or a failure to deliver the prepared stored motor program. There is some suggestion that preparation for movement may be impaired, for the early phase of the electroencephalographic *Bereitschaftspotential* preceding self-paced voluntary movement is abnormal in Parkinson's disease (Dick et al., 1989).

Slowness in execution of movement is attributed to an inability to deliver the correct initial motor command to the agonist muscle (Flowers, 1976; Hallett and Khoshbin, 1980). The correct muscle is chosen (i.e., the movement starts in the right direction), and the usual reciprocal relation between agonist and antagonist generally is preserved. However, the size of the initial electromyographic burst in the agonist, which starts the movement and gives its initial velocity, is too small. As a result, the patient moves to the point of aim slowly and usually undershoots (hypometria). The final position often is achieved by a repetitive series of small agonist bursts causing a sequence of incremental steps. The more difficult the task, the worse the performance is (Sanes, 1985). Why patients choose the wrong size of agonist burst to produce the required size and velocity of movement is uncertain. They know what is required and can deliver bigger agonist bursts in different circumstances, but there is a breakdown between perception of what is needed and the necessary motor output.

Difficulty with complex movements is typical of patients with Parkinson's disease who have particular problems in executing repetitive, concurrent, or sequential actions. Repetitive movements are undertaken increasingly slowly, and the amplitude of the action gets progressively smaller, as for example in micrographia (Margolin and Wing, 1983). Patients with Parkinson's disease have particular difficulty in executing two simultaneous motor acts or in switching from one motor act to another (Schwab et al., 1954). They commonly freeze in the middle of a motor sequence. Such problems with complex motor actions have been explored experimentally. Benecke et al. (1986, 1987) showed that patients with Parkinson's disease have added difficulty (expressed as extra slowness) when they try to execute two motor programs simultaneously with the same arm. In addition, they have added difficulty when attempting to execute two motor programs sequentially with the same or opposite arms. They perform the individual movements in sequence more slowly than when each is carried out alone, and the interval between the two movements is prolonged. The extra slowness in executing such a complex motor sequence is more closely related to the degree of clinical bradykinesia than to the slowness of single movements.

It is difficult to put all of these manifestations of akinesia into a single, simple framework, and there has been considerable speculation as to the pathophysiology of this symptom of basal ganglia disease (Brooks, 1975; Denny-Brown, 1962, 1968; Denny-Brown and Yanagasawa, 1976; Hassler, 1978; Marsden, 1982; Martin, 1967). Some investigators suggest that akinesia is due to a failure to focus attention on a particular motor pattern; others propose that it represents an inability to switch in a particular motor pattern or to switch from one motor pattern to another; still other researchers attribute all of these difficulties to an inability to activate the agonist muscle correctly. At present, no single explanation fully satisfies, and of course, there may be more than one pathophysiologic abnormality at work to cause the many manifestations of akinesia.

Another way of looking at the problem is to divide motor action into a series of events and to examine how akinesia affects each of these various phases of movement (Marsden, 1984b). Initially, there must be a perceptual process to decide how to act. There is no good evidence that this is an error in Parkinson's disease. Preparation for action then must be undertaken. This requires selection and sequencing of the motor programs necessary to execute the overall motor plan. Present evidence, such as it is, suggests that patients with Parkinson's disease can prepare for action in this way, although such preparation may be inaccurate. Finally, the motor plan must be executed. Here, patients with parkinsonism make mistakes. Although their basic motor programs are correct in general form, they are inaccurate in exact specification and initiation of agonist activity. They also have further difficulties in running a smooth sequence of motor programs. Complex actions requiring automatic execution of a motor plan, encompassing a number of sequential motor programs, may break down (Marsden, 1982).

In the end analysis, these problems of akinesia must result from abnormality of the message delivered from the basal ganglia to the premotor cortex and thence to the motor cortex. Until the nature of this message is known, the basis of akinesia is likely to remain uncertain.

Rigidity

The second major feature of the akinetic-rigid syndrome is muscle stiffness, appreciated by the examiner as a resistance to passive movement both in agonist and in antagonist and throughout the range of movement. Rigidity is most evident in flexor muscles of the neck, trunk, and limbs, thereby contributing to the characteristic flexed posture in Parkinson's disease. If tremor is superimposed, the rigidity may be broken up into "cogwheel" resistance. Rigidity contributes to, but is not the only explanation of, akinesia. This is all too evident after stereotaxic surgery for Parkinson's disease. A successful operation, placing a lesion in the ventrolateral nucleus of the thalamus, abolishes rigidity, but akinesia can persist and progress.

The pathophysiology of rigidity is uncertain. Initial explanations based on the suggestion that muscle spindles were overactive owing to excessive γ motor neuron drive have not been supported by direct recording from human muscle spindle afferents (Burke et al., 1977). However, most of such recordings have been from primary spindle afferents. Although tendon jerks (phasic stretch reflexes) are normal in Parkinson's disease, tonic stretch reflexes are increased (Andrews et al., 1972), and the behavior of secondary spindle afferents has not been established.

Another abnormality of stretch reflex function has been identified in Parkinson's disease. More than a decade ago, it was discovered that passive stretch of human and other primate muscles evokes not only the classic monosynaptic spinal stretch reflex but also later long-latency stretch reflexes. The latter may employ transcerebral, perhaps transcortical, stretch reflex pathways. Long-latency stretch reflexes are enhanced in patients with Parkinson's disease, particularly at low velocities of stretch (Rothwell et al., 1983b; Tatton and Lee, 1975). Long-latency stretch reflex pathways do not traverse the basal ganglia, so their exaggeration in Parkinson's disease probably represents a positive or release phenomenon. However, increased long-latency stretch reflexes cannot account for parkinsonian rigidity. They are evoked by fast stretch, whereas rigidity is best appreciated by slow muscle stretching. Enhanced long-latency stretch reflexes are characteristic of some types of myoclonus, where rigidity is not evident.

The explanation of rigidity must lie in the spinal response to slow or tonic muscle stretch. Most reflexes considered to be of spinal origin appear normal in Parkinson's disease. For instance, the tendon jerks, H reflex, and tonic vibration reflex are not altered; the excitability of anterior horn cells is not greatly increased; and presynaptic inhibition of spindle input as well as Renshaw cell–mediated recurrent inhibition appear intact (Delwaide, 1985). It seems most likely that the sensitivity of the complex spinal interneuronal machinery that controls anterior horn cell activity is altered in Parkinson's disease owing to defective supraspinal control. The basal ganglia modulate the activity of the spinal premotor machinery, both via control of cerebral premotor and motor systems and their descending corticospinal pathways, and via projections of basal ganglia directly to brain stem motor centers and bulbospinal systems. The successful relief of rigidity by stereotaxic lesions in the thalamic nuclei receiving pallidal input, which project to premotor areas, suggests that corticospinal projections are critical.

In summary, rigidity appears to be a consequence of overactive tonic stretch reflex mechanisms in the spinal cord, released from control by basal ganglia damage.

Postural Abnormalities

Patients with an akinetic-rigid syndrome exhibit two abnormalities of posture:

1. Postural deformity refers to the alterations of the position of limbs, neck, and trunk. The classic flexed posture of Parkinson's disease must represent the consequence of excessive activity in limb and trunk flexor muscles, compared with that in antagonist extensors. Such postural deformity therefore may be the result of the distribution of rigidity.
2. Loss of postural stability is another characteristic feature of many akinetic-rigid syndromes. It occurs after some years in Parkinson's disease but may be a presenting symptom of other illnesses, such as progressive supranuclear palsy and multiple system atrophy.

The position of the body in space, its posture, ultimately depends on the relative activity of muscles working against the forces of gravity. Changes in the balance of forces in agonists and antagonists alter posture, as is evident in the characteristic positions of the limbs in patients with spasticity or rigidity.

The maintenance of equilibrium, or postural stability, is another problem. A major human motor feat is to keep the center of gravity stable over the narrow base provided by the feet, in the face of external disturbances or shifts of position produced by voluntary movement (Martin, 1967). Some assistance is provided by the mechanical stiffness of the ankle joints, but a sequence of nervous reflexes also is required to prevent falling. Anticipatory postural reflexes occur even before the center of gravity shifts (Traub et al., 1980). When instability does occur, a collection of righting reflexes, some of peripheral origin such as the spinal stretch reflex, others generated centrally, come into play to protect balance (Nashner, 1966). If they fail, protective reactions are activated to reduce the consequences of a fall (Martin, 1967). All these mechanisms must be integrated with those of locomotion to allow normal safe gait.

Postural instability includes a number of phenomena. Patients with Parkinson's disease fall over (their immediate righting reactions are abnormal), and when they do, they fail to extend their arms to protect themselves (their later protective reactions are deficient) (Martin, 1967). Righting reactions themselves are complex. Anticipatory postural reflexes, which take place before the center of gravity shifts, are abnormal in Parkinson's disease (Dick et al., 1986; Traub et al., 1980). Subsequent compensatory righting reflexes also are inadequate.

It is uncertain whether all these abnormalities of postural stability are due to basal ganglia damage alone or to more widespread pathologic alteration. The difficulty is that they tend to appear relatively late in the course of Parkinson's disease, when many parts of the brain are likely to be affected. In other diseases with widespread pathologic change, postural instability is an early feature. Another observation is that postural instability is not improved by stereotactic thalamic lesions that relieve rigidity and tremor. However, some authors have attributed control of postural reaction specifically to the basal ganglia (Martin, 1967).

In summary, postural deformity and postural instability are characteristic of the akinetic-rigid syndrome. Postural instability results from loss of anticipatory postural reflexes, of compensatory righting reflexes, and of protective reactions.

Locomotor Difficulty

Walking or running necessitates (1) the execution of relatively stereotyped alternating limb movements, (2) adaptation of this locomotor pattern to expected and unexpected external conditions using afferent information, and (3) maintenance of equilibrium by stabilization of the center of gravity by postural adjustment. These three facets of walking must be integrated to produce balanced locomotion.

Early debates about the neural control of locomotion centered on whether it was produced by central pattern generators or by peripheral feedback, whereby activity in one group of muscles stimulates receptors that in turn activate the next group, and so on as a reflex chain (Brown, 1914).

Experimental work, particularly in the cat, has established the existence of locomotor generators. The deafferented, decerebrate cat can be made to walk on a treadmill. Even the spinal cat can walk. Thus the cat's spinal cord and brain stem must contain central pattern generators capable of producing locomotion (Grillner, 1975, 1981; Grillner and Zangger, 1975; Shik and Orlovsky, 1976). These lower locomotor centers are less powerful in primates, especially in humans.

Central locomotor generators obviously are under the control of peripheral afferents and descending motor commands in the intact animal (Grillner, 1975). Thus, decerebrate cats can change walking speed if that of the treadmill is altered. Descending influences include those from cerebral cortex and basal ganglia. The decerebrate cat does not initiate walking spontaneously. If the transection is made higher, above the subthalamus, however, spontaneous walking does occur, and electrical stimulation of the subthalamus can initiate locomotion. In the classic intercollicular decerebrate preparation, locomotion can be initiated by stimulation of a region of the midbrain and the lateral region of the pons. Thus, various crucial areas (the subthalamic locomotor region and the pontine locomotor region) appear necessary to initiate walking. Presumably they do so by issuing instructions to the spinal locomotor generators, which are under local reflex control (Pierrot-Deseilligny et al., 1983). Again, how far these observations apply to humans is uncertain. Such locomotor regions themselves must be under control from the cerebral cortex, via corticobulbar pathways, to allow

conscious control of walking. Finally, the cerebellum provides analysis of incoming peripheral afferent signals and controls brain stem locomotor centers.

From this brief background on the complexity of the neural organization of walking, it is obvious that gait can be compromised by damage to virtually any part of the neuraxis. The walk of a patient with parkinsonism is diagnostic (Knutsson, 1972). The flexed bowed individual has difficulty in starting. The feet may not move at all or may mark time without forward movement. Eventually, the patient may get going with a rush of little steps, only to be halted frozen to the spot, particularly when attempting to turn or pass through a doorway. While the patient with parkinsonism is walking, the arms do not swing, the body remains flexed, and there is a tendency to fall (Nutt et al., 1983). Sometimes, the pace uncontrollably speeds up, and the patient cannot stop until she or he meets a firm object.

Such a gait is not, however, specific for Parkinson's disease (defined pathologically by Lewy body degeneration of specific brain stem nuclei, in particular the substantia nigra). A parkinsonian gait is evident in many other conditions (e.g., progressive supranuclear palsy, multiple system atrophy, and drug-induced parkinsonism) known to affect the basal ganglia to cause an akinetic-rigid syndrome. A more or less identical gait can be seen in patients with cerebrovascular disease; some have multiple small infarcts in many cerebral regions, including the basal ganglia; others may have the characteristic periventricular white matter change of Binswanger's encephalopathy on computed tomography or magnetic resonance imaging. A similar gait disturbance also may be seen in long-standing hydrocephalus, in which ventricular enlargement may cause damage to the periventricular white matter.

Pathophysiology

Experimental studies in subhuman primates on the anatomic and functional organization of the basal ganglia have given fresh insight into the pathophysiology of the akinetic-rigid syndrome. In particular, it is possible to produce a remarkable replica of Parkinson's disease in a variety of primate species by administration of the neurotoxin 1-methyl-4-phenyl-1,2,3,6-tetrahydropyridine (MPTP). MPTP (or rather the toxic metabolite 1-methyl-4-phenylpyridinium ion [MPP$^+$]) selectively destroys the dopaminergic neurons of the substantia nigra. The way in which MPTP produces such nigrostriatal degeneration has been studied extensively. On entry into the brain, it is metabolized by monoamine oxidase B via MPDP to MPP$^+$ in glia. MPP$^+$ is concentrated and retained in dopaminergic neurons via active uptake and binding to neuromelanin. MPP$^+$ finally kills nigral neurons by inhibition of mitochondrial energy metabolism.

In the monkey rendered parkinsonian by MPTP

treatment, basal ganglia neuronal activity has been studied using the 2-deoxyglucose method, which identifies presynaptic nerve terminal activity. The changes observed in MPTP-treated primates are as follows (M.A. Mitchell et al., 1989).

There is increased activity of γ-aminobutyric acid (GABA)–ergic (colocalized with enkephalin) projections from the striatum (especially the putamen) to the lateral pallidal segment. Consequently, there is inhibition of GABAergic neurons projecting from the lateral pallidum to the subthalamus. As a result, there is increased activity of excitatory glutamatergic subthalamic projections to the medial pallidal segment. The medial pallidal neurons therefore are driven by excessive subthalamic input; they also receive a direct GABAergic inhibitory input from the striatum (colocalized with substance P), whose activity appears to be decreased. As a consequence of both inputs, medial pallidal GABAergic neuronal activity is increased, inhibiting its thalamic targets. Finally, there is presumed to be reduced excitatory thalamic drive to premotor cortical regions. These changes may be the cause of the poverty of movement and, perhaps, rigidity of Parkinson's disease.

In parallel to these changes in striatopallidal modulation of premotor cortical motor function, there are changes in descending striatopallidal control of brain stem motor centers that project to the spinal cord. It must be recalled that the substantia nigra pars reticulata is homologous to the medial pallidal segment. Nigra reticulata has major projections to the superior colliculus concerned with the control of certain classes of eye movement and to other brain stem centers (for example, the pedunculopontine nucleus) concerned with the control of posture and locomotion. In the parkinsonian MPTP-treated primate, activity in basal ganglia outputs to the pedunculopontine nucleus is greatly increased. Alterations in these brain stem influences from the basal ganglia may be responsible for eye movement defects, postural instability, and locomotor difficulty of Parkinson's disease.

DYSKINESIAS

Basal ganglia diseases also cause a variety of abnormal involuntary movements. Dyskinesias can be divided into five general categories for clinical purposes: (1) tremors, (2) chorea and ballismus, (3) myoclonus, (4) tics, and (5) dystonias.

Of pathologic tremors (see Chapter 25), only parkinsonian rest tremor can be attributed with confidence to basal ganglia abnormality. Myoclonus is not a conspicuous feature of basal ganglia disease but usually arises as a result of cerebral cortical, cerebellar, brain stem, or spinal cord disorders. Tics may be due to abnormal function of the basal ganglia, but there is no sound pathologic evidence of this assumption, which is based mainly on pharmacologic grounds. Accordingly, further discussion is focused

on parkinsonian rest tremor, chorea, hemiballismus, and dystonia.

Parkinsonian Rest Tremor

As with rigidity, rest tremor appears to be a positive release phenomenon attributable to abnormal function of the thalamus. Many observers have recorded thalamic neuronal activity at the time of stereotaxic surgery for Parkinson's disease. Bursts of activity can be detected in phase with tremor beats in an area of the ventrolateral thalamus corresponding to nucleus ventralis intermedius. Such thalamic tremor bursts also are seen in the absence of visible tremor, suggesting that they are the cause rather than the consequence of the tremor.

Typical rest tremor can be produced experimentally in the monkey by causing lesions in midbrain ventromedial tegmental area (Poirier et al., 1975). To be effective, such lesions must damage several structures, including the ventral component of the superior cerebellar peduncle, the descending rubral systems, and the substantia nigra and its efferents. Lesions confined to the superior cerebellar peduncle and red nucleus cause ataxia without tremor, but if such animals are given dopamine antagonist drugs, rest tremor appears. Lesions confined to the substantia nigra cause neither ataxia nor tremor. The effective lesion presumably causes deafferentation of the thalamus, from which tremor bursts again can be recorded in the experimental animal. Similar bursts of discharge, related to tremor activity, can be recorded in the motor cortex, and the tremor itself is abolished by lesions of the cortical motor neuron pathway (but not by lesions confined to the pyramidal pathway or by peripheral deafferentation) (Lamarre and Joffroy, 1979).

These data suggest that rest tremor is due to unrestrained thalamic activity driving motor cortex and cortical motor neuron pathways to generate rhythmic spinal motor neuron discharge at about 5 Hz. Peripheral influences appear to play only a small part in rest tremor. Deafferentation of a limb does not reliably abolish rest tremor, and it is difficult to reset such tremor by a peripheral disturbance (Lee and Stein, 1981).

Chorea

Chorea is distinguished from other dyskinesias by the continuous flow of abnormal movements, which are random in timing and distribution (Marsden et al., 1983). Each choreic movement consists of brief fragments of muscle contraction. If chorea affects distal limb muscles, the amplitude of each movement is relatively small; if proximal muscles are affected, the movements are large and wild, or ballistic. Hemiballismus refers to hemichorea affecting proximal limb muscles (see later). The patient with chorea often walks in characteristic fashion. The gait is unsteady, with unexpected lurches, swaying, and halts, producing a superficial impression of ataxia. Sudden unexpected movements of the trunk and arms often require the patient to walk on a wide base to prevent falling, and turning is difficult. The length of step is irregular, for the leg may suddenly swing too far or in the wrong direction. The derivation of chorea from the Latin *choreus* alludes to the dancing gait of such patients.

Chorea in Huntington's disease is attributed to severe damage to the striatum. There is profound loss of GABAergic striatopallidal projection neurons. Those projecting to the lateral pallidal segment are more severely affected initially (Reiner et al., 1988). Occasionally, focal striatal lesions, such as stroke or tumor, cause contralateral chorea. However, in many illnesses producing symptomatic chorea, for example, Sydenham's disease, thyrotoxicosis, polycythemia rubra vera, and the various forms of cerebral arteritis, it is impossible to identify focal pathologic change as the cause of this dyskinesia. It may be that specific hormonal or immunologic effects on the striatum are responsible for chorea in these conditions, but this is speculation. What is known, however, is that dopamine agonist drugs can provoke chorea when administered to patients with Parkinson's disease and that dopamine antagonist drugs can reduce chorea. Chorea thus appears to be the opposite of the akinetic-rigid syndrome. The latter is confidently attributed to striatal dopamine deficiency, whereas the former appears to be due to overactivity of striatal dopaminergic mechanisms.

Chorea and the akinetic-rigid syndrome also have opposite effects on muscle tone. Whereas in the latter there is rigidity with exaggerated long-latency stretch reflexes, in chorea there is hypotonia with reduced long-latency stretch reflexes (Noth et al., 1983).

Why damage in the striatum, be it structural or pharmacologic, should cause chorea is not clear. Choreic movements often appear to be fragments of normal movement, appearing in inappropriate circumstances and lacking any purpose. There is a hint that they may be determined by peripheral stimuli, which in ordinary circumstances would be ignored. One hypothesis of basal ganglia function is that these structures normally filter the mass of cortical input they receive to select movement appropriate to the circumstances. Striatal damage might prevent normal suppression of unwanted motor responses to external stimuli, resulting in chorea.

Newer insights into the pathophysiology of chorea have derived from analysis of experimental hemichorea or hemiballismus and levodopa dyskinesias (see later). These studies have reinforced the view that chorea and ballismus are similar in origin.

Hemiballismus

Hemiballismus is unusual among basal ganglia movement disorders in that it can be attributed to a focal lesion of the subthalamic nucleus or its connections (Martin, 1967). A focal vascular lesion, or rarely a tumor, in this region causes the characteristic sudden and unpredictable, wild swinging movements of the contralateral shoulder and hip, associated with less dramatic distal chorea. A similar disorder can be produced in monkeys by lesions in the same site or by injection of GABA antagonist into the subthalamic nucleus (Crossman et al., 1984, 1988). At first sight, the latter effect appears contradictory. Antagonism of the inhibitory pathway from the lateral pallidal segment to the subthalamus should produce subthalamic overactivity. However, injection of GABA antagonists into the subthalamus produces contralateral hemiballismus after a delay. Initially, there is indeed increased activity of subthalamic neurons; however, this is followed by depolarization blockade and hemiballismus appears during this latter period.

The subthalamic nucleus is related reciprocally to the lateral segment of the globus pallidus and projects to both the medial segment of the globus pallidus and the pars reticulata of substantia nigra. Thus, it is in a position to gate the major outputs of the striatopallidal complex. Chorea and hemiballismus of the contralateral limbs can also be provoked by infusion of GABA antagonists into the lateral pallidal segment. This is interpreted as being due to inhibition of the GABAergic striopallidal pathway, causing increased activity in the GABAergic pathway from lateral pallidum to the subthalamus, with consequent inhibition of the subthalamus. Similar contralateral chorea or hemiballismus also can be produced by infusion of the glutamate antagonist kynurenic acid into the medial pallidum, presumably owing to blockade of subthalamopallidal excitatory drive.

Hemiballismus produced experimentally in the monkey by a lesion in the subthalamic nucleus can be reduced or abolished by lesions in medial globus pallidus, the ventrolateral nucleus of the thalamus, or the motor cortex (Carpenter et al., 1950). Hemiballismus thus is seen as the result of loss of subthalamic control of pallidal output to motor cortex via ventrolateral thalamus.

The alterations in neuronal activity in the basal ganglia in experimental hemichorea or hemiballismus induced by infusion of GABA antagonists into the lateral pallidum or subthalamus have been investigated using the 2-deoxyglucose method (I.J. Mitchell et al., 1985a,b). GABA antagonist injections into the lateral pallidum abolish the actions of the inhibitory pathway from the striatum to the lateral pallidum and cause increased activity in the inhibitory GABAergic pathway from the lateral pallidum to the subthalamus. Resulting inhibition of subthalamic excitation of the medial pallidum reduces activity of pallidothalamic pathways that normally suppress ventrolateral thalamic neurons. The overall result is increase of thalamic drive to premotor cortical areas, which is presumed to result in contralateral chorea and hemiballismus mediated by corticospinal and corticobulbar systems.

The clinical difference between chorea and ballismus is best explained by their different pathologic features. Acute destruction of the subthalamus produces the most massive disruption of the subthalamopallidal system, resulting in gross contralateral dyskinesias affecting both proximal and distal muscles. Chorea in Huntington's disease is due to gradual multifocal destruction of the striatum, causing restricted and regionally localized loss of striatopallidal pathways; as a consequence, there is a topographically restricted increase in some pallidosubthalamic pathways. The result is more focal and localized chorea. In both chorea and ballismus, however, the fundamental abnormality is underactivity of subthalamic drive to the medial pallidum and of pallidothalamic systems. These changes are the opposite of those seen in experimental Parkinson's disease.

An interesting confirmation of this general scheme comes from the study of levodopa-induced dyskinesias in parkinsonian MPTP-treated primates (Crossman, 1990). As in human Parkinson's disease, levodopa not only restores mobility but also induces a range of dyskinesias in MPTP-treated animals, in particular chorea, dystonias, and stereotypies. Levodopa-induced chorea is characterized by a partial reversal of the metabolic changes evident in 2-deoxyglucose studies in parkinsonian MPTP-treated animals. Activity in pathways from the striatum to the lateral pallidum is decreased, presumably owing to increased dopaminergic inhibition of this striatopallidal GABAergic (and enkephalinergic) system. Consequently, there is increased inhibitory activity in the GABAergic pathway from lateral pallidum to subthalamus. Again, the findings in animals exhibiting levodopa-induced chorea are the converse of those seen in the parkinsonian state. One surprising result, however, is that there is a considerable increase in 2-deoxyglucose activity in the medial pallidum in animals with levodopa-induced chorea. This cannot be due to subthalamopallidal activity, for this activity is reduced. Rather, it must reflect increased activity in direct striatal projections to the medial pallidum, stimulated by dopamine derived from levodopa. The end product of these changes is reduced activity of medial pallidal neurons projecting to thalamus (and pedunculopontine nucleus). Consequently, there is increased thalamocortical action. In confirmation of these concepts, stereotaxic thalamotomy has been found to reduce or abolish levodopa-induced chorea in MPTP-treated primates.

Dystonia

The characteristic feature of dystonia is the presence of prolonged muscle spasms that distort the limbs and axial structures into typical dystonic postures. If such spasms are repetitive, dystonic movements occur; if they are sustained, dystonic postures are maintained. There is disagreement over the relation of dystonia to athetosis. Athetosis originally was used to describe distal limb movements and postures, whereas torsion dystonia referred to proximal limb and axial movements and postures. The difficulty is illustrated by those researchers who claim that athetosis is no more than distal dystonia, whereas other investigators believe that torsion dystonia is proximal and axial athetosis. For purposes of this chapter, dystonia describes both types of abnormal movements and postures.

The syndrome of torsion dystonia can affect most muscles of the body (although those controlling eye movement and the sphincters are spared). Spasms can affect the orbicularis oculi muscle (blepharospasm), the jaw and mouth (oromandibular dystonia), the neck (spasmodic torticollis), the larynx (spasmodic dysphonia), the trunk (axial dystonia), and the arms (dystonic writer's cramp). The legs commonly are affected in children to produce any type of gait disturbance, some of which may be so bizarre that they defy description and often arouse the suspicion of hysteria. The most typical is the tendency for the foot to plantar flex and invert, and for the great toe to extend, as it approaches the floor. Other variants include flexion of the whole leg as it is advanced, contortions of the hips and trunk, and hopping or even crawling activities, all in the absence of other signs that might explain such difficulties.

The dystonias comprise a number of primary often familial conditions and many symptomatic or secondary types attributable to known diseases. Among the primary dystonias, those commencing in childhood and adolescence often become generalized (affecting the whole body) or segmental (affecting major adjacent body parts). Primary dystonias with onset in adult life usually remain focal (e.g., blepharospasm, oromandibular dystonia, spasmodic torticollis, axial dystonia, and writer's cramp). Most cases of familial dystonia commence in early life and are inherited as autosomal dominant traits with reduced penetrance. Most cases of primary adult-onset focal dystonia are sporadic.

The characteristic features of dystonia are (1) excessive cocontraction of antagonist muscles during voluntary movement, (2) overflow of contraction to remote muscles not normally employed in voluntary movement, and (3) spontaneous spasms of cocontraction. All contribute to the typical picture of dystonic movements and postures (Rothwell et al., 1983a; Yanagisawa and Goto, 1971).

The abnormal cocontraction of agonist and antagonist muscles in dystonia and the overflow to distant muscles suggest some breakdown in the normal mechanisms of reciprocal inhibition, but why this occurs is not known. It has been shown that the classic disynaptic 1a reciprocal inhibitory pathway is intact in those with arm dystonia, but the later phase of reciprocal inhibition attributed to presynaptic inhibition is defective (Nakashima et al., 1989a). Presumably, this is due to defective supraspinal control of these spinal mechanisms. Similar defective inhibition in interneuronal pathways has been shown for the R2 component of the blink reflex in blepharospasm (Berardelli et al., 1985) and for exteroceptive neck muscle reflexes in torticollis (Nakashima et al., 1989b). It appears that the interneuronal inhibitory networks in brain stem and spinal cord are underfunctioning to cause the spontaneous and action-induced muscle spasms and overflow characteristic of dystonia. This appears to be the consequence of defective descending control from the brain. For reasons discussed later, the critical abnormality is believed to be an abnormality of basal ganglia control of brain stem motor centers that project to these bulbar and spinal interneuronal motor mechanisms.

In many patients with dystonia, particularly those in whom the illness is inherited, no histologic pathologic abnormality has been documented in the brain. Such patients are believed to have abnormal basal ganglia function, perhaps biochemical in origin, because the dysfunctions are identical with those in diseases known to cause basal ganglia damage. Dystonia is seen in patients with, for example, Wilson's disease, Hallervorden-Spatz disease, a variety of metabolic disorders, and mitochondrial encephalomyopathies. In all these conditions, there is overt basal ganglia damage.

Occasionally, focal unilateral lesions, usually vascular or tumor, may cause contralateral dystonia (Marsden et al., 1985; Narbonna et al., 1984). Such lesions may be in the striatum (particularly putamen), the globus pallidus, or the thalamus. These lesions appear to distort the motor output from basal ganglia to motor cortex. Yet other individuals with similarly placed lesions may not exhibit dystonia.

It has proved difficult to provoke dystonia in experimental primates either by localized lesions in the basal ganglia or by injection of drugs into the striatopallidal complex. As a result, there are fewer clues to the pathophysiology of dystonia compared with what is known about chorea or hemiballismus and parkinsonism. Present theories concentrate on differential effects on the direct striatomedial pallidal GABAergic (substance P) pathway and the indirect striatolateral pallidal GABAergic (enkephalinergic)–subthalamomedial pallidal system. In levodopa-induced dystonia in MPTP-treated parkinsonian monkeys, there is thought to be not only reduced subthalamomedial pallidal excitation (the substrate of chorea) but also marked direct striatomedial pallidal inhibition. However, this is but a crude hypothesis and much more research is required to unravel the mysteries of the pathophysiology of dystonia.

MAJOR DILEMMAS

The student of the basal ganglia evidently is faced with much that is inexplicable. A few paradoxes can be highlighted.

1. Why do different pathologic lesions in similar zones of the basal ganglia produce such diverse effects? For example, abnormal function of the striatum can cause an akinetic-rigid syndrome (dopamine deficiency in Parkinson's disease), chorea (striatal degeneration in Huntington's disease), or dystonia (striatal lesions caused by stroke or tumor). Perhaps this difficulty will be resolved by clearer understanding of the microcircuitry of the basal ganglia.

2. Why do similar pathologic lesions in different zones produce the same movement disorder? For example, dystonia may be produced by a vascular lesion in the striatum, the globus pallidus, or the thalamus. Again, greater understanding of the internal organization of the basal ganglia may explain this problem.

3. Why do similar pathologic lesions in the same part of the basal ganglia sometimes cause a movement disorder but in other patients have no such effect? For example, a vascular lesion in the region of the globus pallidus may or may not produce contralateral dystonia. This may be because the exact anatomic extent of the lesion differs in the two cases. Another possible explanation is that attempts at regeneration cause reorganization of basal ganglia function. The concept is given some credence by the frequent delay in appearance of movement disorders after basal ganglia insults. Such delayed onset is seen, for example, in the akinetic-rigid syndrome that follows carbon monoxide poisoning and the dystonia that occurs after perinatal brain injury.

4. Why does one disease affecting the basal ganglia cause such a variety of movement disorders? For example, Wilson's disease may produce tremor (of various types), an akinetic-rigid syndrome, dystonia, or a mixture of these problems. Indeed, it is characteristic of many different diseases affecting the basal ganglia that they may cause a variety of clinical pictures.

Answers to these and other similar questions must await further understanding of the basal ganglia.

References

Andrews C.J., Burke D., Lance J.W. The response to muscle stretch and shortening in parkinsonian rigidity. *Brain* 95:795–812, 1972.

Angel R.W., Alston W., Higgins J.R. Control of movement in Parkinson's disease. *Brain* 93:1–14, 1970.

Benecke R., Rothwell J.C., Dick J.P.R., et al. Performance of simultaneous movements in patients with Parkinson's disease. *Brain* 109:739–757, 1986.

Benecke R., Rothwell J.C., Dick J.P.R., et al. Disturbances of sequential movements in patients with Parkinson's disease. *Brain* 110:361–379, 1987.

Berardelli A., Rothwell J.C., Day B.L., et al. Pathophysiology of blepharospasm and oromandibular dystonia. *Brain* 108:593–608, 1985.

Bernstein N. *The Coordination and Regulation of Movements.* Oxford, Pergamon Press, 1967.

Bloxham C.A., Mindel T.A., Frith C.D. Initiation and execution of predictable and unpredictable movements in Parkinson's disease. *Brain* 107:371–384, 1984.

Brooks V.B. Roles of cerebellum and basal ganglia in initiation and control of movements. *Can. J. Neurol. Sci.* 2:265–277, 1975.

Brown T.G. The intrinsic factors in the act of progression in the mammal. *Proc. R. Soc. Lond. [Biol]* 84:308–319, 1914.

Burke D., Hagbarth K-E., Wallin B.G. Reflex mechanisms in parkinsonian rigidity. *Scand. J. Rehab. Med.* 9:15–23, 1977.

Carpenter M.B., Whittier J.R., Mettler F.A. Analysis of choreoid hyperkinesia in the rhesus monkey. Surgical and pharmacological analysis of hyperkinesia resulting from lesions in the subthalamic nucleus of Luys. *J. Comp. Neurol.* 92:293–332, 1950.

Cooke J.D., Brown J.D., Brooks V.B. Increased dependence on visual information for movement control in patients with Parkinson's disease. *Can. J. Neurol. Sci.* 5:413–415, 1978.

Crossman A.R. A hypothesis on the pathophysiological mechanisms that underlie levodopa- or dopamine agonist–induced dyskinesia in Parkinson's disease: implications for future strategies in treatment. *Mov. Disord.* 5:100–108, 1990.

Crossman A.R., Sambrook M.A., Jackson A. Experimental hemichorea/hemiballismus in the monkey. Studies on the intracerebral site of action in a drug-induced dyskinesia. *Brain* 107:579–596, 1984.

Crossman A.R., Mitchell I.J., Sambrook M.A., et al. Chorea and myoclonus in the monkey induced by GABA-antagonism in the lentiform complex: the site of drug action and a hypothesis of the neural mechanisms of chorea. *Brain* 111:1211–1233, 1988.

Day B.L., Dick J.P.R., Marsden C.D. Patients with Parkinson's disease can employ a predictive motor strategy. *J. Neurol. Neurosurg. Psychiatry* 47:1299–1306, 1984.

Delwaide P.J. Are there modifications in spinal cord functions of parkinsonian patients? In Delwaide P.J., Agnoli A., eds. *Clinical Neurophysiology in Parkinsonism.* Amsterdam, Elsevier, pp. 19–32, 1985.

Denny-Brown D. *The Basal Ganglia and Their Relation to Disorders of Movement.* London, Oxford University Press, 1962.

Denny-Brown D. Clinical symptomatology of diseases of the basal ganglia. In Vinken P.J., Bruyn G.W., eds. *Handbook of Clinical Neurology.* Vol. 6. *Diseases of the Basal Ganglia.* Amsterdam, North Holland, pp. 133–211, 1968.

Denny-Brown D., Yanagasawa N. The role of the basal ganglia in the initiation of movement. *Res. Publ. Assoc. Res. Nerv. Ment. Dis.* 55:115–149, 1976.

Dick J.P.R., Rothwell J.C., Berardelli A., et al. Associated postural adjustments in Parkinson's disease. *J. Neurol. Neurosurg. Psychiatry* 49:1378–1385, 1986.

Dick J.P.R., Rothwell J.C., Day B.L., et al. *Bereitschaftspotential* is abnormal in Parkinson's disease. *Brain* 112:233–244, 1989.

Evarts E.V., Teravainen H., Calne D.B. Reaction time in Parkinson's disease. *Brain* 104:167–186, 1981.

Flowers K.A. Visual "closed loop" and "open loop" characteristics of voluntary movement in patients with parkinsonism and intention tremor. *Brain* 99:269–310, 1976.

Grillner S. Locomotion in vertebrates: central mechanisms and reflex interaction. *Physiol. Rev.* 55:247–304, 1975.

Grillner S. Control of locomotion in bipeds, tetrapods and fish. In Brooks V.B., ed. *Handbook of Physiology.* Section 1. *The Nervous System.* Vol. II. *Motor Control.* Part 2. Bethesda, American Physiological Society, pp. 1179–1236, 1981.

Grillner S., Zangger P. How detailed is the central pattern generation for locomotion? *Brain Res.* 88:367–371, 1975.

Hallet M., Khoshbin S. A physiological mechanism of bradykinesia. *Brain* 103:301–304, 1980.

Hassler R. Striatal control of locomotion, intentional actions and of integrating and perceptive activity. *J. Neurol. Sci.* 36:187–224, 1978.

Heilman K.M., Bowers D., Watson R.T., et al. Reaction times in Parkinson's disease. *Arch. Neurol.* 33:139–140, 1976.

Innman V.T. Human locomotion. *Can. Med. Assoc. J.* 94:1047–1054, 1966.

Knutsson E. An analysis of parkinsonian gait. *Brain* 95:475–486, 1972.

Lamarre Y., Joffroy A.J. Experimental tremor in monkey: activity of thalamic and precentral cortical neurons in the absence of feedback. *Adv. Neurol.* 24:109–122, 1979.

Lee R.G., Stein R.B. Resetting of tremor by mechanical perturbations. A comparison of essential tremor and parkinsonian tremor. *Ann. Neurol.* 10:523–531, 1981.

Margolin D.I., Wing A.M. Agraphia and micrographia: clinical manifestations of motor programming and performance disorders. *Acta Psychol.* 54:263–283, 1983.

Marsden C.D. The mysterious motor functions of the basal ganglia. *Neurology (N.Y.)* 32:514–539, 1982.

Marsden C.D. Motor disorders in basal ganglia disease. *Hum. Neurobiol.* 2:245–250, 1984a.

Marsden C.D. Which motor disorder in Parkinson's disease indicates the true motor function of the basal ganglia? *Ciba Found. Symp.* 107:225–237, 1984b.

Marsden C.D., Obeso J.A., Rothwell J.C. Clinical neurophysiology of muscle jerks: myoclonus, chorea and tics. In Desmedt J.E., ed. *Motor Control Mechanisms in Health and Disease.* New York, Raven Press, pp. 865–881, 1983.

Marsden C.D., Obeso J.A., Zarranz J.J., et al. The anatomical basis of symptomatic dystonia. *Brain* 108:463–483, 1985.

Martin J.P. *The Basal Ganglia and Posture.* London, Pitman Medical, 1967.

Mitchell I.J., Jackson A., Sambrook M.A., et al. Common neural mechanisms in experimental chorea and hemiballismus in the monkey. Evidence from 2-deoxyglucose autoradiography. *Brain Res.* 339:346–350, 1985a.

Mitchell I.J., Sambrook M.A., Crossman A.R. Subcortical changes in the regional uptake of ^{3}H-2-deoxyglucose in the brain of the monkey during experimental choreiform dyskinesia elicited by injection of a gamma-aminobutyric acid antagonist into the subthalamic nucleus. *Brain* 108:421–438, 1985b.

Mitchell M.A., Clarke C.E., Boyce S., et al. Neural mechanisms underlying parkinsonian symptoms based upon regional uptake of 2-deoxyglucose in monkeys exposed to 1-methyl-4-phenyl-1,2,3,6-tetrahydropyridine. *Neuroscience* 32:213–226, 1989.

Nakashima K., Rothwell J.C., Dy B.L., et al. Reciprocal inhibition between forearm muscles in patients with writer's cramp and other occupational cramps, symptomatic hemidystonia and hemiparesis due to stroke. *Brain* 112:681–697, 1989a.

Nakashima K., Thompson P.D., Rothwell J.C., et al. An exteroceptive reflex in the sternocleidomastoid muscle produced by electrical stimulation of the supraorbital nerve in normal subjects and patients with spasmodic torticollis. *Neurology* 39:1354–1358, 1989b.

Narbonna J., Obeso J.A., Tunon T., et al. Hemidystonia secondary to localised basal ganglia tumour. *J. Neurol. Neurosurg. Psychiatry* 47:704–709, 1984.

Nashner L.M. Adapting reflexes controlling the human posture. *Exp. Brain Res.* 26:59–72, 1966.

Noth J., Friedman H.H., Podoll K. Absence of long-latency reflexes to imposed finger displacements in patients with Huntington's disease. *Neurosci. Lett.* 35:97–100, 1983.

Nutt J.G., Nashner L.M., Horack F.B. Why do Parkinson patients fall? *Ann. Neurol.* 14:136, 1983.

Pierrot-Deseilligny E., Bergego C., Mazieres L. Reflex control of bipedal gait in man. In Desmedt J.E., ed. *Motor Control Mechanisms in Health and Disease.* New York, Raven Press, pp. 699–716, 1983.

Poirier L.J., Pechadre J.C., Larochelle L., et al. Stereotaxic lesions and movement disorders in monkeys. *Adv. Neurol.* 10:5–22, 1975.

Reiner A., Albin R.L., Anderson K.D., et al. Differential loss of striatal projection neurons in Huntington's disease. *Proc. Natl. Acad. Sci. U.S.A.* 85:5733–5737, 1988.

Rothwell J.C., Obeso J.A., Day B.L., et al. Pathophysiology of dystonias. In Desmedt J.E., ed. *Motor Control Mechanisms in Health and Disease.* New York, Raven Press, pp. 851–863, 1983a.

Rothwell J.C., Obeso J.A., Traub M.M., et al. The behaviour of the long-latency reflex in patients with Parkinson's disease. *J. Neurol. Neurosurg. Psychiatry* 46:35–44, 1983b.

Sanes J.N. Information processing deficits in Parkinson's disease during movement. *Neuropsychologia* 23:381–392, 1985.

Schwab R.S., Chaftez M.E., Walker S. Control of two simultaneous voluntary motor acts in normals and parkinsonism. *Arch. Neurol.* 72:591–598, 1954.

Shik M.L., Orlovsky G.N. Neurophysiology of locomotor automatism. *Physiol. Rev.* 56:465–501, 1976.

Tatton W.G., Lee R.G. Evidence for abnormal long-loop reflexes in rigid parkinsonian patients. *Brain Res.* 100:671–676, 1975.

Traub M.M., Rothwell J.C., Marsden C.D. Anticipatory postural reflexes in Parkinson's disease and other akinetic rigid syndromes and in cerebellar ataxia. *Brain* 103:393–412, 1980.

Yanagisawa N., Goto A. Dystonia musculorum deformans. Analysis with electromyography. *J. Neurol. Sci.* 13:39–65, 1971.

23

Cerebellum and Motor Dysfunction

Sid Gilman

The cerebellum is responsible for the maintenance of posture and for the smoothly integrated coordination of movements, both simple and complex. It is needed for movements requiring an accurate estimate of the goal in time and space toward which a movement is executed. The cerebellum functions together with the cerebral cortex in the control of movement, and, together with other parts of the nervous system, it is involved in the adjustment of muscle responses to stretch. The cerebellum is needed for the development and performance of motor skills.

Lesions of the cerebellum delay the initiation of movement and lead to clumsiness of movement but do not prevent the execution of movement. With cerebellar injury, muscles that normally act together lose their capacity to do so. Movements then deteriorate into incomplete or inaccurate forms, producing errors of force, velocity, and timing. Muscle strength may be diminished somewhat but is not lost. Cerebellar lesions alone do not disrupt sensation in the body or cognitive abilities.

The nature of cerebellar deficits can be understood best from the perspective of the normal anatomic, physiologic, and pharmacologic organization of the cerebellum. Accordingly, in this chapter the structure and function of the cerebellum are discussed before the disorders of cerebellar function resulting from disease are described. A number of excellent reviews and monographs on the cerebellum have been published (Bloedel and Courville, 1981; Bloedel et al., 1984; Brooks and Thach, 1981; Gilman et al., 1981; Ito, 1984, 1989; King, 1988; Palay and Chan-Palay, 1982).

CEREBELLAR ANATOMY

Lobar and Lobular Divisions

The cerebellum consists of a central longitudinal structure, the vermis, and two hemispheres (Fig. 23–

1). The intermediate zone between the vermis and the lateral part of the hemisphere on each side is called the paravermis. The cerebellar cortex is divided by fissures into three major lobes, the anterior, the posterior, and the flocculonodular. The primary fissure separates the anterior and posterior lobes, and the postnodular fissure divides the posterior and flocculonodular lobes. Additional shallow fissures subdivide the anterior and posterior lobes into a series of transverse lobules. The lobules have been given proper names and also identified with a numbering system (Gilman et al., 1981) (see Fig. 23–1).

From comparative anatomic studies, the cerebellum has been subdivided into three component parts, the archicerebellum, the paleocerebellum, and the neocerebellum (Brodal, 1981). The archicerebellum consists of the flocculonodular lobe; the paleocerebellum comprises the vermis of the anterior lobe plus the pyramis, uvula, and paraflocculus; and the neocerebellum involves the lateral parts of the cerebellum, including most of the hemispheres and the middle portion of the vermis (see Fig. 23–1). The divisions of the cerebellum from comparative anatomic studies correspond reasonably well to the sites of termination of the afferents projecting to the cerebellum (Brodal, 1981) (Fig. 23–2). Vestibular afferents project heavily into the flocculonodular lobe (the archicerebellum), so the term *vestibulocerebellum* has been applied to this lobe. The major afferent projections from the spinal cord (Kitamura and Yamada, 1989) terminate in the vermis (the paleocerebellum), leading to the term *spinocerebellum* for this region. The projections from the pons terminate in the cerebellar hemispheres, and the term *pontocerebellum* is used for the hemispheres. This system of nomenclature has been useful, but it is somewhat misleading because the anatomic locations of the termination sites do not describe completely the sites

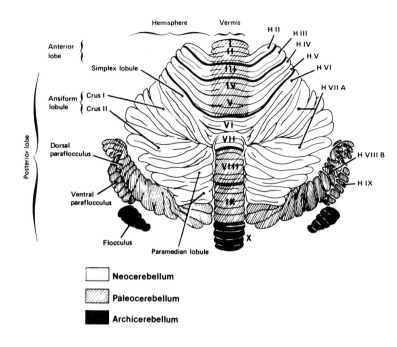

Figure 23–1. Diagram of the cerebellar cortex of the monkey shown "unfolded" to project the cerebellar cortex onto a single plane. The three components of the cerebellum based on phylogenetic considerations are shown with shading. The names of the lobules are given at the left and Larsell's numerical nomenclature is superimposed on vermal structures and listed at the right. Note that part of the vermis (lobules VI and VII) is actually a component of the neocerebellum. (From Gilman S., Bloedel J.R., Lechtenberg R. *Disorders of the Cerebellum.* Philadelphia, Davis, 1981.)

activated physiologically (Brodal and Brodal, 1985; Gilman et al., 1981; Suzuki and Keller, 1988a,b).

From the clinical perspective, the most useful conception of the overall organization of the cerebellum came from the notion that the cerebellum consists functionally of a series of sagittal zones (Gilman et al., 1981). Three zones were identified initially: a vermal zone containing cerebellar cortical efferent neurons projecting to the fastigial nucleus; a paravermal zone with neurons projecting to the interposed nuclei; and a lateral zone including the most lateral region of the anterior lobe and the lateral portion of the hemispheres, which contain cortical

neurons projecting to the lateral (dentate) nucleus (Fig. 23–3*A*). Many subsequent studies have confirmed this idea, and the number of identifiable zones has been expanded substantially (Voogd, 1969, 1982) (Fig. 23–3*B*).

Microscopic Anatomy

A strikingly uniform structure throughout, the cerebellar cortex consists of an outer molecular layer, a Purkinje cell layer, and an inner granular layer (Fig. 23–4). The molecular layer contains two types

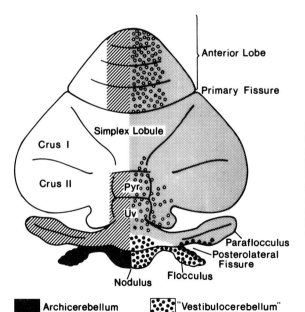

Figure 23–2. Diagram of the mammalian cerebellum. *(Left)* Components of the cerebellum based on phylogenetic considerations. *(Right)* Components of the cerebellum based on the sites of termination of major afferent systems for the spinal cord (spinocerebellum), vestibular system (vestibulocerebellum), and cerebral cortex via the pontine nuclei (pontocerebellum). The components of the cerebellum based on these considerations do not show complete congruence. In addition, the physiologic effects of activating afferent sources project far beyond the anatomic boundaries indicated in this diagram. (Modified from Brodal A. *Neurological Anatomy in Relation to Clinical Medicine.* 3rd ed. New York, Oxford University Press, 1981.)

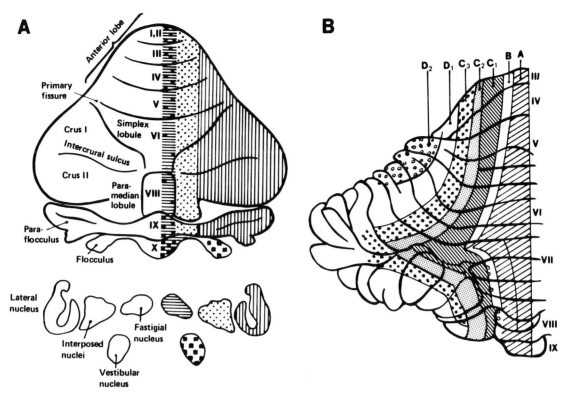

Figure 23–3. Diagrams of the zonal organization of the cerebellum. In the upper part of *A*, the cerebellum is divided into three sagittal zones, each of which connects with the deep cerebellar or vestibular nucleus shown in the lower part of *A*. This pattern of organization was obtained from studies of the projections of Purkinje cells onto the cerebellar nuclei in cats. *(B)* Results of studies of the zonal organization of the cerebellum in ferrets. Comparable but not identical zones have been shown in anatomic studies of the corticonuclear projections in cats. (*A* adapted from Jansen J., Brodal A. Experimental studies on the intrinsic fibers of the cerebellum. II. The cortico-nuclear projections. *J. Comp. Neurol.* 73:267–321, 1940. *B* adapted from Voogd J. The importance of fibre connections in the comparative anatomy of the mammalian cerebellum. In Llinás, R., ed. *Neurobiology of Cerebellar Evolution and Development*. Chicago, American Medical Association, pp. 493–514, 1969. Copyright 1969, American Medical Association.)

of interneurons (basket cells and stellate cells), the dendrites of Purkinje cells and Golgi cells, parallel fibers, and several types of collateral fibers. The Purkinje cell layer contains the Purkinje cell bodies. The granular layer consists of granule cells, Golgi cells, and numerous fibers.

Mossy Fibers

The inputs to the cerebellum are mediated over three distinctive types of fibers: mossy, climbing, and monoaminergic (Gilman et al., 1981). These fibers give collateral projections to the deep cerebellar nuclei before terminating within the cerebellar cortex (Gerrits and Voogd, 1987; Van der Want et al., 1987). The mossy fiber afferents originate in a large number of regions outside the cerebellum, including the spinocerebellar tracts of the spinal cord (Gerrits et al., 1985) and the pontine (Gerrits and Voogd, 1986), vestibular (Carleton and Carpenter, 1983), and reticular (Gerrits and Voogd, 1987) nuclei. Mossy fiber afferents enter the cerebellum through all three cerebellar peduncles and project to the granular layer. Mossy fibers make synaptic contact with granule cells and terminate in either simple or complex formations termed *mossy fiber rosettes*. These rosettes make syn-

aptic contact with the dendrites of granule cells and Golgi cells. In the rosettes, mossy fibers also make synaptic connection with other elements forming cerebellar glomeruli, which consist of mossy fiber rosettes, the dendrites of granule cells, and Golgi cell axons and dendrites. Granule cell axons ascend to the molecular layer, where they bifurcate and form parallel fibers, which run longitudinally along each folium. Each parallel fiber makes synaptic contact with as many as 500 Purkinje cells, and each Purkinje cell receives the convergent projections of more than 200,000 parallel fibers. Parallel fibers also make synaptic connection with the interneurons of the cerebellar cortex, stellate cells, basket cells, and Golgi cells.

Climbing Fibers

These fibers originate in the inferior olivary nucleus, cross the midline, and ascend through the cerebellar white matter to the molecular layer, where they form multiple synaptic contacts with the dendritic trees of Purkinje cells. These fibers give collateral projections to the deep cerebellar nuclei before terminating within the cerebellar cortex (Buisseret-Delmas, 1988a,b; Van der Want and Voogd, 1987;

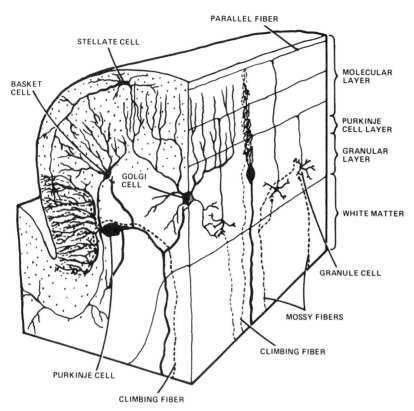

Figure 23–4. Diagram in perspective of the principal elements of the cerebellar cortex. Incoming mossy fibers make synaptic connections with granule cells, which give rise to parallel fibers. Climbing fibers ascend directly to connect with the dendrites of Purkinje cells. Stellate cells make contact with the dendrites of Purkinje cells, and basket cells connect with the somas of Purkinje cells. Parallel fibers connect with all three types of interneurons: stellate, basket, and Golgi cells. Golgi cell axons make synaptic connections with mossy fiber rosettes and granule cell dendrites. Golgi cell dendrites make contact with mossy fibers, parallel fibers, and recurrent collaterals of Purkinje cells. (Modified from Eccles J.C., Ito M., Szentágothai J. *The Cerebellum as a Neuronal Machine*. New York, Springer-Verlag, 1967.)

Van der Want et al., 1989). Each Purkinje cell receives synaptic input from only one climbing fiber, but a single climbing fiber can bifurcate within a folium and project to more than one Purkinje cell. Climbing fiber collaterals make contact with Purkinje cell dendrites and other cerebellar cortical neurons, including stellate cells, basket cells, and Golgi cells.

Aminergic Afferent Projections

Neuronal aminergic afferents constitute an input system to the cerebellum separate from mossy fibers and climbing fibers and include noradrenergic, dopaminergic, and serotoninergic afferents. The locus ceruleus contains noradrenergic neurons with axons projecting into the cerebellum through the superior cerebellar peduncle (Pickel et al., 1974) and terminating in all parts of the cerebellar cortex (Hökfelt and Fuxe, 1969). These fibers make synaptic contact with Purkinje cell dendrites in the molecular layer (Bloom et al., 1971) and with granule cell dendrites in the superficial part of the granular layer (Kimoto et al., 1981). Dopaminergic fibers arising in the ventral mesencephalic tegmentum project to the interposed and lateral cerebellar nuclei and to the Purkinje cell and granule cell layers of the cerebellar cortex (Simon et al., 1979).

Serotoninergic afferents arising in the raphe nuclei of the brain stem project to all lobules of the cerebellum except possibly lobule IV. These fibers terminate in both the molecular and granular layers

(Takeuchi et al., 1982), forming (1) terminals within the granular layer appearing similar to those of mossy fibers, (2) extensive branches through the molecular layer similar to parallel fiber branches, and (3) terminals distributed diffusely through the molecular and granular layers.

Purkinje Cells and Interneurons of the Cerebellar Cortex

Purkinje cells constitute the sole output projection neurons for the cerebellar cortex. These cells are aligned in a single layer in the cerebellar cortex and have a unique pattern of dendritic arborization. This arborization contains primary, secondary, and tertiary branches forming a flat plate oriented perpendicular to the long axis of the folium. Purkinje cells receive synaptic contacts from parallel fibers, climbing fibers, stellate cells, and basket cells. Purkinje cell axons project to the vestibular and deep cerebellar nuclei and to other elements in the cerebellar cortex (Umetani et al., 1986). In coursing through the granular layer or immediately after entering white matter, Purkinje cell axons give rise to one or more recurrent collaterals (Bishop, 1988). These ascend to the Purkinje cell layer and form supra- and infraganglionic plexuses above and below the Purkinje cell layer, respectively. Collaterals of Purkinje cell axons form synapses with basket and Golgi cells (Bishop and O'Donoghue, 1986; O'Donoghue et al., 1989).

Superficial stellate cells are located in the outer two-thirds of the molecular layer of the cerebellar cortex. These interneurons receive input from parallel fibers and make synaptic connections on the basilar dendrites and, in some instances, the somas of Purkinje cells. Basket cells, or deep stellate cells, are located in the molecular layer just superficial to the Purkinje cell layer. Basket cell dendrites receive connections from parallel fibers and axon collaterals of Purkinje cells. Basket cells form a dense plexus of axons in the shape of a basket around the body and axon hillock of Purkinje cells. Golgi cells contain two dendritic ramifications, one in the granular layer, the other in the molecular layer. Golgi cell dendrites make contact with mossy fibers in the granular layer and with parallel fibers and recurrent collaterals of Purkinje cells in the molecular layer. Golgi cell axons project to the cerebellar glomerulus, where they make contact with mossy fiber rosettes and granule cell dendrites.

Projections of the Deep Cerebellar Nuclei

Axons emerging from the deep cerebellar nuclei project through the superior and inferior cerebellar peduncles (Fig. 23–5). Fibers in the superior cerebellar peduncle originate in all cerebellar nuclei, including the fastigial. These form an ascending pathway terminating in the upper brain stem and a descending pathway projecting to the medulla (Chan-Palay, 1977). Axons in the inferior cerebellar peduncle project from the fastigial nucleus to the vestibular nuclei and the pontomedullary reticular formation. Some neurons in the fastigial and interpositus nuclei project directly to the spinal cord (Asanuma et al., 1980, 1983). In addition to projections outside the cerebellum, all the cerebellar nuclei send axon collaterals into the cerebellar cortex (Dietrichs, 1983).

All cerebellar nuclei send axons to the inferior olivary nucleus (Ikeda et al., 1989; Legendre and Courville, 1987). The nucleo-olivary fibers are collaterals of nucleofugal axons ascending into the upper

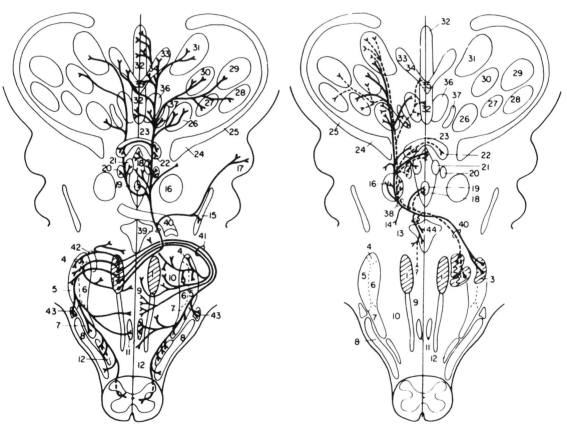

Figure 23–5. Diagram of the efferent connections of the cerebellar nuclei. *(Left)* Fastigial nucleus. *(Right)* Interpositus and lateral (dentate) nuclei. Numbers are identified as follows: 1 indicates the fastigial nucleus; 2, nucleus interpositus anterior; 2', nucleus interpositus posterior; 3, lateral (dentate) nucleus; 4, superior vestibular nucleus; 5, lateral vestibular nucleus; 6, medial vestibular nucleus; 7, inferior (descending) vestibular nucleus; 8, lateral reticular nucleus; 9, medial bulbar reticular formation; 10, lateral bulbar reticular formation; 11, perihypoglossal nuclei; 12, nucleus parasolitarius; 13, descending limb of the brachium conjunctivum; 14, pontine reticular formation; 15, lateral lemniscal nucleus; 16, red nucleus; 17, superior colliculus; 18, periaqueductal gray; 19, Edinger-Westphal nucleus; 20, interstitial nucleus; 21, nucleus of Darkshevich; 22, posterior commissure nucleus; 23, posterior commissure; 24, field of Forel; 25, reticular nucleus; 26, center median nucleus; 27, ventral posteromedial nucleus; 28, ventral posterolateral nucleus; 29, lateral posterior nucleus; 30, ventral lateral nucleus; 31, ventral anterior nucleus; 32, midline nuclei; 33, central lateral nucleus; 34, paracentral nucleus; 35, central medial nucleus; 36, ventromedial nucleus; 37, parafascicular nucleus; 38, crossed ascending limb of branchium conjunctivum; 39, accessory brachium conjunctivum; 40, brachium conjunctivum; 41, hook bundle; 42, direct fastigiobulbar tract; 43, group x of Brodal and Pompeiano; 44, tegmental reticular nucleus. (From Ito M. *The Cerebellum and Neural Control.* New York, Raven Press, p. 143, 1984.)

brain stem (Dietrichs and Walberg, 1985, 1986; Dietrichs et al., 1985). The cerebellar nuclei also project into the pontine gray, nucleus reticularis tegmenti pontis, lateral reticular nucleus, and other reticular nuclei, all of which are sources of mossy fiber afferents to the cerebellar nuclei and cortex (Ito, 1984).

The Fastigial Nucleus

This nucleus sends efferent fibers through three major pathways: (1) the hook bundle, (2) direct fastigiobulbar fibers, and (3) the accessory brachium conjunctivum (Carpenter and Batton, 1982). The hook bundle contains fibers from the caudal portion of the fastigial nucleus that cross the midline, loop around the brachium conjunctivum, and, by way of the inferior cerebellar peduncle, reach the medulla oblongata. In the cat and rat, these fibers terminate in the four major vestibular nuclei (Carleton and Carpenter, 1983), cell groups f and x, and nucleus parasolitarius (Ross et al., 1981). In the cat, neurons distributed throughout the fastigial nucleus project through the hook bundle to the pontomedullary reticular formation (Ito, 1984). Neurons in the rostral part of the fastigial nucleus project through the hook bundle to the lateral reticular nucleus (Ito, 1984). In the monkey, fastigioreticular fibers originate in the rostral regions of the fastigial nucleus, cross in the hook bundle and project to the nucleus reticularis gigantocellularis, dorsal paramedian reticular nucleus, magnocellular part of the lateral reticular nucleus (Batton et al., 1977), nucleus reticularis tegmenti pontis, and raphe nuclei (Asanuma et al., 1983). Long fastigiospinal fibers project through the hook bundle to the contralateral side of the spinal cord (Fukushima et al., 1977).

The direct fastigiobulbar projection arises in the rostral part of the fastigial nucleus and terminates in the ipsilateral four vestibular nuclei and the reticular formation (Ito, 1984).

The accessory brachium conjunctivum contains projections originating in the caudal half of the fastigial nucleus that cross within the cerebellum and emerge through the contralateral superior cerebellar peduncle (Batton et al., 1977). These axons terminate within the superior colliculus bilaterally, the nucleus of the posterior commissure, the nucleus of Darkshevich, and the interstitial nucleus of Cajal (Sugimoto et al., 1982). Projections from the fastigial nucleus also terminate bilaterally in the thalamic nucleus ventralis lateralis (Asanuma et al., 1983) and in the septum, hippocampus, amygdala (Heath, 1973), locus ceruleus, and substantia nigra (Snider et al., 1976).

The Interpositus Nucleus

The projections of this nucleus are divided into anterior and posterior components based on their site of origin in the nucleus. The anterior interpositus nucleus projects through the superior cerebellar pe-

duncle to the red nucleus (Angaut et al., 1986), thalamus, nucleus reticularis tegmenti pontis, pontine nuclei (McCrea et al., 1978), superior colliculus (Uchida et al., 1983), anterior and posterior pretectal nuclei (Sugimoto et al., 1982), and oculomotor nucleus (Gacek, 1977). The posterior interpositus nucleus projects through the dorsal portion of the superior cerebellar peduncle and across the midline to the medial border of the red nucleus, and to the superior colliculus, zona inserta, lateral part of the nucleus ventralis lateralis, medial region of the nucleus ventralis posterior lateralis, and lateral part of the nucleus ventralis anterior (Sugimoto et al., 1982; Uchida et al., 1983).

The Lateral (Dentate) Nucleus

The lateral cerebellar nucleus projects through the brachium conjunctivum to the red nucleus and terminates in the rostral (parvocellular) third of the nucleus. The terminal fields of the lateral nuclear projection in the red nucleus are at least partially separate from those of the interpositus projection, which are found in the magnocellular part of the red nucleus (Asanuma et al., 1983). The lateral cerebellar nucleus projects to the medullary reticular formation through the descending limb of the superior cerebellar peduncle, terminating on reticulospinal neurons. Other projections of the ascending fibers of the lateral nucleus reach the superior colliculus, pretectum (Sugimoto et al., 1982), and thalamic nuclei ventralis posterior lateralis and ventralis lateralis (Thach and Jones, 1979).

CEREBELLAR FUNCTION

The Synaptic Actions of Cerebellar Neurons

The synaptic effects of the various cellular elements of the cerebellum are now understood in considerable detail, and the relationships are simple (Eccles et al., 1967). Mossy fiber and climbing fiber afferents to the cerebellum are excitatory, but monoaminergic afferents are inhibitory (Figs. 23–6 and 23–7). The axons of granule cells (parallel fibers) are excitatory (see Fig. 23–6). The interneurons within the cerebellum, basket cells, stellate cells, and Golgi cells, are inhibitory (Figs. 23–6 and 23–8). The output neurons of the cerebellar cortex, Purkinje cells, are inhibitory or disfacilitatory (see Fig. 23–7). Nuclear neurons are probably excitatory (see Fig. 23–7).

The output neurons of the cerebellar cortex, Purkinje cells, can be excited by both climbing fiber and mossy fiber inputs. Climbing fibers form excitatory synapses directly with the dendritic trees of Purkinje cells (see Fig. 23–7). Collaterals of climbing fibers also excite the deep cerebellar nuclei and the interneurons of the cerebellar cortex. The excitatory mossy fiber input is mediated after a synaptic connection

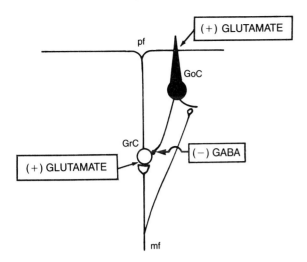

Figure 23–6. Diagram of the neuronal connections between mossy fibers, granule cells, parallel fibers, and Golgi cells. Inhibitory neurons are shown in black and inhibitory synaptic connections are indicated with a (−). Excitatory neurons are shown unshaded and excitatory synaptic connections are indicated with a (+). The most likely candidates for neurotransmitter substances at each synaptic connection are indicated. mf = mossy fiber; pf = parallel fiber; GrC = granule cell; GoC = Golgi cell; GABA = γ-aminobutyric acid.

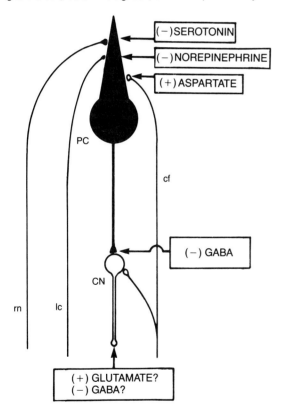

Figure 23–7. Diagram of the neuronal connections between Purkinje cells and deep cerebellar nuclear cells, climbing fibers, and aminergic afferent projections. Inhibitory neurons are shown in black and inhibitory synaptic connections are indicated with a (−). Excitatory neurons are shown unshaded and excitatory synaptic connections are indicated with a (+). Candidates for neurotransmitter substances at each synaptic connection are indicated. The ? indicates that evidence concerning the neurotransmitters is preliminary. PC = Purkinje cell; rn = raphe nucleus projection; lc = locus ceruleus projection; CN = cerebellar (or vestibular) nucleus cell; cf = climbing fiber; GABA = γ-aminobutyric acid.

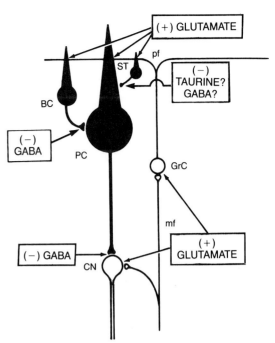

Figure 23–8. Diagram of the neuronal connections between mossy fibers, granule cells, cerebellar nuclear cells, parallel fibers, Purkinje cells, stellate cells, and basket cells. Inhibitory neurons are shown in black and inhibitory synaptic connections are indicated with a (−). Excitatory neurons are shown unshaded and excitatory synaptic connections are indicated with a (+). Candidates for neurotransmitter substances at each synaptic connection are indicated. The ? indicates that evidence concerning the neurotransmitters is preliminary. mf = mossy fiber; CN = cerebellar (or vestibular) nucleus cell; GrC = granule cell; pf = parallel fiber; ST = stellate cell; BC = basket cell; PC = Purkinje cell; GABA = γ-aminobutyric acid.

by granule cells (see Fig. 23–8). Parallel fibers, formed from the bifurcated axons of granule cells, provide an excitatory input to the dendritic spines of Purkinje cells. Parallel fibers also excite the three types of interneurons: stellate cells, basket cells, and Golgi cells (see Figs. 23–6 and 23–8). Stellate cells and basket cells inhibit the dendrites and somas of Purkinje cells, respectively (see Fig. 23–8). Both parallel fibers and mossy fibers activate Golgi cells, and these in turn inhibit granule cells (see Fig. 23–6). Purkinje cells have inhibitory or disfacilitatory effects on neurons in the deep nuclei of the cerebellum and the vestibular nuclei (see Fig. 23–7). Collaterals of Purkinje cells inhibit the interneurons of other Purkinje cells.

Activation of Purkinje cells over the mossy fiber–granule cell–parallel fiber route causes Purkinje cell firing with spikes of simple configuration (Eccles et al., 1967). Stimulation of Purkinje cells by climbing fiber input results in a powerful excitation of Purkinje cells that is termed the *climbing fiber response.* This response consists of an initial spike followed by a long-lasting depolarization, with two to six superimposed wavelets termed *complex spikes* (Fig. 23–9).

Projections from the locus ceruleus have inhibitory synaptic effects on Purkinje cells (Moises and Wood-

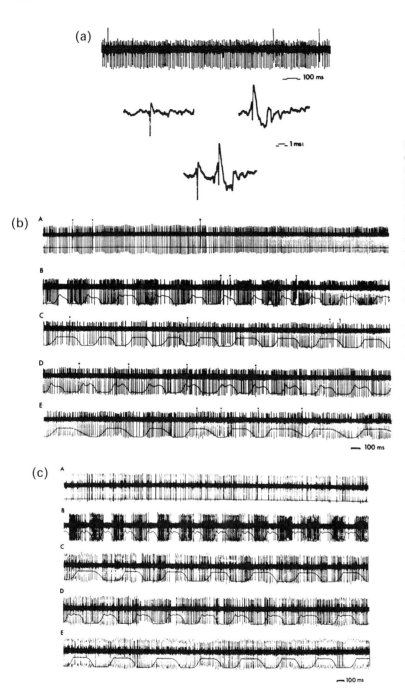

Figure 23–9. *(a)* Maintained discharge of a Purkinje cell recorded extracellularly in the awake monkey showing a simple *(left)* and complex *(right)* spike potential. The slow trace at the top shows the different patterns of discharge of the simple and complex spikes and the fast traces on the bottom show their different shapes. *(b)* Discharge of a Purkinje cell with a monkey immobile *(A)* and during movement of the ipsilateral wrist *(B)*, the ipsilateral shoulder *(C)*, the contralateral wrist *(D)*, and the contralateral shoulder *(E)*. The line below the unit discharge represents movements of the manipulandum lever. For wrist movements, up indicates flexion and down indicates extension. For shoulder movements, up indicates a pushing movement and down a pulling movement. The simple spike shows changes in discharge frequency in a consistent relationship to movements of the ipsilateral wrist but not to other movements. The complex spike, indicated with dots, shows no obvious relation to the movement. *(c)* Discharge of a dentate nucleus neuron with the monkey still *(A)* and during movement at the ipsilateral wrist *(B)*, the ipsilateral shoulder *(C)*, the contralateral wrist *(D)*, and the contralateral shoulder *(E)*. The line below the unit discharge represents movement of the manipulandum lever. For wrist movements, up indicates flexion and down indicates extension. For shoulder movements, up indicates a pushing movement and down indicates a pulling movement. Neuronal discharge is related to movement of the ipsilateral wrist, less so to movement of the ipsilateral shoulder, and not at all consistently to movement of the contralateral arm. (From Thach W.T. Discharge of Purkinje and cerebellar nuclear neurons during rapidly alternating arm movement in the monkey. *J. Neurophysiol.* 31:785–797, 1968.)

ward, 1980), and the effects are duplicated by application of norepinephrine (Freedman and Hoffer, 1975). Projections from the raphe nuclei form a dense network in the granular layer but may make contact with Purkinje cell dendrites. Electrical stimulation of the raphe nuclei decreases Purkinje cell discharge, and iontophoretic application of serotonin, which is thought to be the mediator of neurons projecting from the raphe nucleus, decreases the spontaneous discharge of Purkinje cells (Bloom et al., 1972).

The Neurotransmitters of the Cerebellum

Mossy Fibers

Only a few of the neurotransmitters of the cerebellum have been identified. The neurotransmitters of the mossy fibers are unknown, but a number of candidates have been identified. Acetylcholine was thought to be one of them, but more recent studies make this unlikely (Neustadt et al., 1988). Acetylcholine may provide innervation of cerebellar capillaries and microvessels (Estrada et al., 1983). Glutamate is probably a neurotransmitter of the mossy fiber–granule cell synapse as well as the mossy fiber collaterals to the deep cerebellar nuclei (Fagg and Foster, 1983; Fonnum, 1984; Greenamyre et al., 1984; Monaghan et al., 1986). Glutamate receptors have been found on granule cells (Garthwaite and Brodbelt, 1989; Greenamyre et al., 1984), and glutamate-like immunoreactivity has been demonstrated in mossy fibers (Clements et al., 1987). The mossy fiber synaptic connection acts on both *N*-methyl-D-aspartate

(NMDA) and non-NMDA receptors on granule cells (Garthwaite and Brodbelt, 1989). Moreover, levels of glutamate-binding sites are reduced in animals (McBride and Ghetti, 1988) and humans (Albin and Gilman, 1990; Tsiotos et al., 1989) with depletion of the granule cell layer. Other candidate neurotransmitters for the synaptic connections of the mossy fibers are γ-aminobutyric acid (GABA), substance P (Inagaki et al., 1982; Korte et al., 1980), somatostatin (Inagaki et al., 1982), enkephalin, cholecystokinin, and secretogranin.

Granule Cells

Considerable evidence indicates that glutamate is a neurotransmitter released from the axon terminals of granule cells (i.e., parallel fibers) (Fagg and Foster, 1983; Fonnum, 1984; Greenamyre et al., 1984) (see Fig. 23–6). Glutamate released from parallel fibers probably acts only at non-NMDA receptors at synapses with Purkinje cells but at both NMDA and non-NMDA receptors at synapses with inhibitory interneurons (Garthwaite and Beaumont, 1989). The conclusion that glutamate is a neurotransmitter of the parallel fibers is based on the observations that (1) glutamate levels are markedly reduced in animals (McBride and Ghetti, 1988) and humans (Albin and Gilman, 1990; Tsiotos et al., 1989) with reduced numbers of granule cells, (2) glutamate-like immunoreactivity is seen in parallel fibers (Clements et al., 1987), (3) glutamate is released from synaptosomal preparations of rat cerebellum (Levi and Gallo, 1986), and (4) iontophoretic application of glutamate reproduces the parallel fiber–induced excitation of Purkinje cells (Ito, 1984). Some parallel fibers may utilize neurotransmitters other than glutamate because not all granule cells or parallel fibers show glutamate-like immunoreactivity (Clements et al., 1987).

Climbing Fibers

Asparate is thought to be an important neurotransmitter of the climbing fibers (Matute et al., 1987; Wenthold et al., 1986) (see Fig. 23–7). Injury to climbing fibers by intoxication with 3-acetylpyridine reduces substantially the aspartate content of rat cerebellum (Rea et al., 1980). In addition, D-[³H]aspartate is transported retrograde along climbing fibers from the cerebellum to the inferior olive (Matute et al., 1987; Wiklund et al., 1984) and potassium-induced, calcium-dependent release of D-[³H]aspartate is reduced after destruction of climbing fibers (Wiklund et al., 1982, 1984). Moreover, aspartate is released from climbing fibers in cerebellar slices (Toggenburger et al., 1983). Finally, aspartate is reduced in the cerebellar cortex of patients with olivary degeneration associated with the dominant form of inherited olivopontocerebellar atrophy (Perry et al., 1977). Other candidate neurotransmitters of the climbing fibers are homocysteic acid, adenosine,

somatostatin, enkephalin, cholecystokinin, and secretogranin.

Cerebellar Cortical Interneurons

Substantial evidence indicates that Golgi cells utilize GABA as an inhibitory neurotransmitter (Mugnaini and Oertel, 1985) (see Fig. 23–6). [³H]GABA is taken up by Golgi cells (Hökfelt and Ljungdahl, 1975). Presynaptic Golgi axon terminals are rich in glutamate decarboxylase, the key enzyme in formation of GABA (McLaughlin et al., 1974), and show high-affinity uptake of GABA (Wilkin et al., 1974). In addition, the localization of GABA-like immunoreactivity in Golgi cell terminals (Ottersen et al., 1988) and the localization of GABA receptor–like immunoreactivity (Meinecke et al., 1989; Somogyi et al., 1989) are compatible with the idea that Golgi cells utilize GABA as a transmitter.

There is strong evidence that basket cells use GABA as an inhibitory neurotransmitter (Mugnaini and Oertel, 1985) (see Fig. 23–8). [³H]GABA is taken up by basket cells (Hökfelt and Ljungdahl, 1975), and iontophoretic application of GABA inhibits the discharge of Purkinje cells (Okamoto and Sakai, 1981). The GABA antagonists bicuculline and picrotoxin block the basket cell inhibition of Purkinje cells (Dupont et al., 1979). Glutamate decarboxylase occurs in basket cell endings around Purkinje cells (Oertel et al., 1981), and the localization of GABA receptor–like immunoreactivity (Meinecke et al., 1989; Somogyi et al., 1989) provides supportive evidence.

There is evidence that GABA mediates stellate cell inhibition of Purkinje cells (Mugnaini and Oertel, 1985), but there is also evidence that taurine may mediate stellate cell inhibition (see Fig. 23–8). Taurine exerts potent inhibitory effects on Purkinje cells, and taurine sensitivity is higher in the dendrites (where stellate cells make contact) than in the somas of Purkinje cells (Fredrickson et al., 1978). Administration of TAG, an agent that blocks the actions of taurine but not those of GABA, interferes with the stimulus-induced actions of stellate cells on Purkinje cells (Okamoto et al., 1983). Reduced taurine content is associated with agenesis of stellate cells after x-irradiation (Nadi et al., 1977). There is also evidence that taurine may not be a major neurotransmitter of the stellate cells; most studies of taurine histochemistry show weak or no staining of stellate cells (Madsen et al., 1985; Magnusson et al., 1988).

Purkinje Cells

Strong evidence implicates GABA as an inhibitory neurotransmitter of Purkinje cells (Ito, 1984; Mugnaini and Oertel, 1985) (see Fig. 23–7). Iontophoretic application of GABA mimics the action of Purkinje cells by inducing membrane hyperpolarization in Deiters neurons. The GABA inhibitors picrotoxin and bicuculline block Purkinje cell inhibitory actions. Deiters nucleus has a high GABA content, particularly in the dorsal region, which receives Purkinje cell inhibition, and the GABA content is decreased in the dorsal part of Deiters nucleus after chronic ablation of the cerebellar cortex. Electrical stimulation of the cerebellar cortex releases GABA into the fourth ventricle, presumably by liberating it at Purkinje cell axon terminals. Levels of glutamate decarboxylase activity are closely associated with the density of Purkinje cell axon terminals in the cerebellum and vestibular nuclei (Chan-Palay et al., 1979). In mice with degeneration of Purkinje cells, the GABA content of the cerebellar nuclei falls by 50% (Roffler-Tarlov et al., 1979). The localization of GABA-containing terminals (Mugnaini and Oertel, 1985) and GABA receptors (Wamsley and Palacios, 1984) provides supportive evidence.

Motilin, a polypeptide found in the gastrointestinal tract of various species (Yanaihara et al., 1980), has also been found in Purkinje cells (Nilaver et al., 1982). The possibility that it serves as a neurotransmitter has not yet been explored. Inositol 1,4,5-triphosphate, which mediates the effects of several neurotransmitters, has been found to act in Purkinje cells at the site of the endoplasmic reticulum (Ross et al., 1989).

Nuclear Cells

The neurotransmitters of the nuclear cells have not been determined with certainty. There is substantial evidence that GABA is a neurotransmitter released by nuclear cells projecting back to the cerebellar cortex (Batini et al., 1989) and nuclear cells connecting with the inferior olivary nuclei (Angaut and Sotelo, 1987, 1989; de Zeeuw et al., 1989). There is less compelling evidence for other transmitters of the deep cerebellar nuclei. Acetylcholine may be a neurotransmitter of the cerebellothalamic and cerebellorubral pathways (Nieoullon and Dusticier, 1981); however, iontophoretic application of acetylcholine has little effect on the excitability of neurons in the red nucleus (Ito, 1984). Other studies suggest that glutamate may be a neurotransmitter of cerebellothalamic and cerebellorubral pathways and that acetylcholine may function in the presynaptic control of glutamatergic nerve endings (Nieoullon et al., 1984) (see Fig. 23–7).

Cerebellar Neuronal Activity During Motor Tasks

The Functions of Nuclear and Purkinje Cells

Our understanding of cerebellar function has been greatly enhanced by microelectrode studies of neural unit activity in animals trained to perform motor tasks involving movements at a single joint (Bava et al., 1983; Chapman et al, 1986; Schieber and Thach, 1985a,b). In the awake monkey sitting quietly, neu-

rons of the dentate and interposed nuclei discharge steadily at high rates, with nuclear cells discharging at about half the rate of Purkinje cells (Thach, 1970a,b, 1978) (see Fig. 23–9). As the monkey performs conditioned movements of the arms, the discharge frequencies of both nuclear cells and Purkinje cells alternate between values higher and lower than the resting frequencies. The discharge patterns are time locked to the patterns of movement (Thach, 1970a,b). Nuclear cells and Purkinje cells of the same (intermediate) sagittal cerebellar zone show similar times of change in frequency in relation to the movement, and the initial change in frequency is an increase for both types of neurons (Thach, 1970a,b). These findings suggest that mossy fiber inputs stimulate the discharge of both nuclear cells and Purkinje cells (Brooks and Thach, 1981). This conclusion is supported by studies of neural unit activity in monkeys during startle movements provoked by loud sounds and bright lights (Mortimer, 1975). In this situation, on the average, dentate and interposed nuclear cells change discharge frequency before changes in Purkinje cell activity, suggesting that the Purkinje cell inhibits the output of the nuclear cell and that mossy fiber inputs activate both.

Several studies of single-unit activity in the cerebellar nuclei during whole-arm reaching movements revealed a less direct relationship between the details of muscle movement and unit activity than did the studies of single-joint movement (Grimm and Rushmer, 1974; MacKay, 1988a,b; Robertson and Grimm, 1975). In these studies, most nuclear neurons discharged in the same pattern and at about the same rate for all movement trajectories (MacKay, 1988a). Moreover, cerebellar nuclear activities during certain movements were similar although the movements were performed in opposite directions (MacKay, 1988a,b; Schieber and Thach, 1985a,b). In contrast, a study utilizing vectorial representations of the relation of unit activity to movement direction demonstrated that many Purkinje, interpositus, and dentate neurons discharge in relation to the direction of whole-arm reaching movements (Fortier et al., 1989; see also Frysinger et al., 1984, and Wetts et al., 1985). Additional investigations are needed to clarify the discrepancies in these studies.

The overall conclusion of studies of unit activity in awake animals is that mossy fiber inputs furnish excitatory drive for nuclear cells in relation to motor tasks (Brooks and Thach, 1981). The mossy fiber input to the cerebellar cortex constitutes a side loop consisting of a mossy fiber–granule cell–parallel fiber Purkinje cell circuit with related inhibitory interneurons (Ito, 1984). The inhibitory cerebellar cortical side loop appears to function in the inhibitory feed-forward control of nuclear cell discharge, intended in some way to modulate the excitation that mossy fiber inputs provide to nuclear cells.

Initiation of Movement

In monkeys flexing and extending a wrist in response to a light signal, the onsets of changes in discharge of dentate and interpositus neurons overlap considerably, but dentate neurons generally change much earlier than interpositus neurons and the peak alteration in dentate neuronal discharge occurs long before electromyographic activity appears (Thach, 1970b). The peak change of activity in interpositus neurons occurs with the onset of electromyographic activity. Thus, the dentate nucleus is involved earlier than the interpositus nucleus in this particular task, in tasks involving the elbow (Chapman et al., 1986; MacKay, 1988b), and in whole-arm movements (MacKay 1988a). In similar studies, neuronal activity was recorded in the dentate nucleus and motor cortex in monkeys alternately flexing and extending a wrist (Thach, 1975). The times of change in frequency of dentate and motor cortical neurons and of electromyographic activity form large overlapping distributions, but significant timing differences do occur. The median change in dentate nucleus activity occurs before the median change in motor cortex activity, and alterations in motor cortex neuronal discharge develop before electromyographic activity. This finding, along with the results of related studies (Beaubaton and Trouche, 1982; Spidalieri et al., 1983), supports the general idea that dentate neuronal activity excites activity in the motor cortex. The "motor set," that is, the preparation for a motor act, has a strong influence on the responsiveness of dentate neurons (Strick, 1983), and these neurons are strongly coupled to visuomotor behavior (Stein, 1986).

Interpositus nucleus neurons show a median change in activity at about the time that flexion-extension movements about the wrist begin (Schieber and Thach, 1985a,b; Thach, 1970a, 1978), and interpositus neurons change in discharge frequency after an alteration in frequency of motor cortex neurons in a visual reaction time task (Thach, 1978). Interpositus neurons respond quickly to limb perturbation of the monkey holding a static position (Thach, 1978). Interpositus neurons discharge in direct relationship to specific features of limb muscle activity during ambulation movements (Schwartz et al., 1987). The interpositus nucleus also appears to be involved in controlling the arrest of movement (Otero, 1976). These observations suggest that the interpositus nucleus may be involved in ongoing movement and that this involvement is independent of the initiation of movement.

Duration of Movement

The discharge of cerebellar neurons correlates with the duration of movement for a variety of tasks, including locomotion (Armstrong and Edgley, 1984a,b; Schwartz et al., 1987), limb movements (Fortier et al., 1989; MacKay, 1988a,b), and rhythmic movements of limb and body (Arshavsky et al., 1983, 1984). Cerebellar neurons, particularly those in lobules VI and VII of the posterior vermis, discharge in relationship to eye movements, head movements,

and retinal image velocity signals (Suzuki and Keller, 1988a,b). For limb movements, the dentate nucleus and the related portions of the cerebellar hemisphere appear to be concerned with the early stages of movement, including formulation and initiation (Schwartz et al., 1987; Thach, 1978). In contrast, the interposed nuclei and the associated portions of intermediate cerebellar cortex are involved in the electromyographic activity and possibly the kinematics of limb movement (MacKay, 1988a,b; Schwartz et al., 1987). During locomotion, dentate nuclear discharge is not closely coupled with stepping movements, but it is responsive to perturbations involving arrest and resumption of locomotion (Schwartz et al., 1987). In contrast, the discharge of interposed neurons is tightly coupled to the muscle activity patterns in locomotion, including coupling of unit discharge to a specific phase of the step cycle (Schwartz et al., 1987). In contrast, the discharge of interposed neurons is tightly coupled to the muscle activity patterns in locomotion, including coupling of unit discharge to a specific phase of the step cycle (Schwartz et al., 1987). Perturbations of the step cycle do not alter these phase relationships.

The studies just described are compatible with the idea that dentate neurons initiate activity in the motor cortex (Thach, 1978). Interpositus neurons discharge later in the course of movement; their activity appears to be strongly dependent on signals initiated in the limbs and transmitted over spinocerebellar pathways; and their activity may help to stop movement. Both the dentate and interpositus nuclei appear to be involved in posture control, but the tonic discharge of the interpositus nucleus appears more clearly related to the force of muscular contraction than that of the dentate nucleus (Brooks and Thach, 1981).

Type of Movement

A number of investigations have been concerned with the types of movement that the cerebellum controls. The accumulated evidence indicates that the cerebellum is involved in movement initiation and termination and in the control of slow simple, rapid simple (ballistic), self-terminated simple, slow ramp, and compound movements and in maintained postures (holds) and compound postural adjustments (Brooks and Thach, 1981).

Movement Force, Velocity, Position, and Direction

Many investigators have attempted to determine the degree to which the cerebellum controls individual aspects of movement such as force, velocity, position, and direction. During wrist flexion and extension, many Purkinje, interpositus, and dentate neurons discharge in relation to wrist movements and to the posture of the wrist at the end of the movements (Thach, 1970a,b, 1978). The discharge is correlated with the direction of movement (Fortier et al., 1989; Frysinger et al., 1984; Wetts et al., 1985) and with the pattern of muscle activity during prehension as well as wrist flexion and extension (Frysinger et al., 1984; Wetts et al., 1985). The activity of Purkinje, interpositus, and dentate neurons is correlated with the velocity of movement (Frysinger et al., 1984; Mano and Yamamoto, 1980; Wetts et al., 1985). A tentative interpretation of these studies is that dentate neurons behave as though they were signaling for movement to occur without regard to the individual characteristics of movement; the interpositus nucleus appears to be involved in the control of movement velocity; and the fastigial nucleus evidently monitors movement as it occurs.

Other studies support these interpretations. In monkeys trained to move a limb in a certain direction when signaled to do so by a perturbation of the limb, interpositus discharge correlates with limb perturbation, whereas dentate discharge correlates with the intended movement of the limb (Strick, 1978). In monkeys trained to move a handle from one of three positions to another, a load was placed alternately against flexion and extension of the wrist and the handle was perturbed during the holds by briefly doubling the load (Thach, 1978). In this paradigm, neurons in the interpositus nucleus appear to discharge in relation to the pattern of muscle activity, force, and velocity. Neurons in the dentate nucleus and lateral cerebellum are activated in correlation with joint position and the direction of the intended movement regardless of which muscles hold the joint or direct the movement (Brooks and Thach, 1981). Some neurons in the dentate nucleus may discharge in anticipation of the direction of the movement without any contraction of the muscles involved. These neurons appear to be involved in the planning of movements in connection with neurons in the precentral region of the cerebral cortex.

Representation of Body Parts in the Cerebellum

Several studies in awake animals have been concerned with the representation of body parts within the cerebellum (Brooks and Thach, 1981; Fortier et al., 1989; MacKay, 1988a,b; Suzuki and Keller, 1988a,b). These studies have shown that Purkinje cells and the nuclear cells to which they project are activated with movement at one or several joints and are arranged in a topographic pattern that shows some tendency toward a somatotopic distribution. These findings are generally compatible with the results of studies in anesthetized animals showing that body parts are represented in the cerebellum as a "fractured mosaic" (Ito, 1984; Logan and Robertson, 1986; Robertson, 1985; Robertson and Elias, 1988).

Control of α and γ Motor Neurons

Many investigations have supported the possibility that the cerebellum controls separately the activity of

α and γ motor neurons (Mano and Yamamoto, 1980; Schieber and Thach, 1985a,b). The advantage of this capability is that it makes it possible to "set" the muscle spindle apparatus for the correct amount of feedback during muscular actions requiring highly skilled motions.

MOTOR LEARNING AND THE FUNCTION OF THE CLIMBING FIBER

As mentioned earlier, Purkinje cells generate two types of spikes, simple and complex. Simple spikes are generated mainly by input from granule cells and complex spikes mainly by input from climbing fibers (see Fig. 23–9). Thus, complex spike activity is an index of climbing fiber discharge. Studies attempting to correlate climbing fiber discharge with motor activity have not revealed any simple relationships (Brooks and Thach, 1981). Moreover, the discharge frequency of complex spikes has not been clearly associated with limb movement in one direction as opposed to another. Complex spikes may occur repeatedly toward the end of some movements of long duration; however, they discharge with a low frequency compared with simple spikes and are not apparently influenced by the subsequent occurrence of simple spike activity. Purkinje cell output modulation appears to be mainly under the control of mossy fiber input to the cerebellar cortex. Despite the lack of correlation between complex spike activity and motor activity, climbing fiber input to the cerebellum seems critical for cerebellar function. Destroying the inferior olive or its climbing fibers results in motor deficits qualitatively similar to those caused by removing the entire cerebellum (Murphy and O'Leary, 1971).

Currently, the most attractive idea about climbing fiber function is that it has a conditioning effect on Purkinje cells that is essential for normal cerebellar function (Albus, 1971; Ito, 1984; Marr, 1969). Moreover, climbing fiber function is central to a hypothesis concerning motor learning (Ito, 1984, 1989). According to this hypothesis, the cerebellum consists of an excitatory main line pathway through the deep cerebellar and vestibular nuclei, along with an inhibitory cerebellar cortical side path that influences the nuclei. The flow of information through the main line can be adjusted by adding more or less inhibition to the nuclei from the cortical Purkinje cells. The discharge of climbing fibers makes the adjustment, strengthening or weakening the influence of various synapses in the cerebellar cortical pathways converging on the Purkinje cell. A plastic change in synaptic activity is thought to result from this. Several studies have provided support for this idea:

1. Recording simple and complex spike activity in awake monkeys performing a familiar task interrupted by a novel task (Gilbert and Thach, 1977) (Fig. 23–10)

2. Training animals behaviorally to change the gain of the vestibulo-ocular reflex (Lisberger, 1984), with reversal of the change after cerebellar ablation (Ito, 1984)
3. Altering the synaptic effect of parallel fiber activation through electrical pairing of mossy fiber input with climbing fiber input (Ito, 1984)
4. Demonstrating that inferior olive lesions induce long-lasting functional modification of Purkinje cells (Benedetti et al., 1984)
5. Developing long-term depression by simultaneous stimulation of climbing fibers and parallel fibers but not by stimulation of either climbing fibers or parallel fibers alone (Ito, 1989)

The idea that the cerebellum functions as a learning network capable of plastic changes was proposed by Marr (1969) and later amended by Albus (1971) and Fujita (1982). Marr proposed that a parallel fiber–Purkinje cell synapse increases its transmission efficacy to a maximal amount if the parallel fiber is active at about the same time as the climbing fiber input to the Purkinje cell. Albus proposed that the parallel fiber–Purkinje cell synapse would be depressed during conjunctive climbing fiber stimulation. He emphasized the divergence of mossy fibers onto numerous granule cells and considered the cerebellum to be similar to a simple perceptron, that is, a pattern recognizer with learning capability. Fujita modified the Marr and Albus models to incorporate an adaptive filter model dealing with the temporal pattern of impulse trains. The Fujita model assumes that the mossy fiber–granule cell relay acts as a phase converter in association with the Golgi cell, which functions as a leaky integrator. Gilbert (1975) suggested that climbing fiber action is responsible for the formation of short-term memory, which is converted to long-term memory by noradrenergic input from the locus ceruleus to the Purkinje cell. Transient functional plasticity may be turned into a permanent memory through a long-term change in synaptic morphology.

Ito (1989) developed the thesis that long-term depression, a form of synaptic plasticity, is an important memory element for cerebellar motor learning. Repetitive stimulation of parallel fibers along with climbing fibers leads to a long-lasting depression of transmission from parallel fibers to the Purkinje cell. Long-term depression includes an early phase of about 10 minutes followed by a later phase. Ito suggests that long-term depression may participate in adaptive control of the vestibulo-ocular reflex (Ito, 1982; Nagao, 1988), the optokinetic eye movement response (Nagao, 1988), classical conditioning of the eye blink reflex (Thompson, 1986), responses to perturbation of locomotion (Matsukawa and Udo, 1985), postural compensation (Amat, 1983), and certain forms of voluntary movement (Eckmiller, 1987; Stone and Lisberger, 1986). Motor learning has been found to be deficient in patients with chronic cerebellar disease (Sanes et al., 1990).

DISORDERS OF CEREBELLAR FUNCTION

Localization of Disease Processes in the Cerebellum

Although the anatomy of the cerebellar cortex appears to be uniform throughout its structure, regional specificity results from the input-output relations of the various parts of the cerebellum (Dichgans and Diener, 1986; Gilman et al., 1981). For the clinician wishing to understand the localization of cerebellar function, the cerebellum should be viewed as a sagittally oriented structure containing three zones on each side: midline, intermediate, and lateral (Gilman et al., 1981). The midline zone consists of the anterior and posterior parts of vermal cortex, the fastigial nucleus, and the associated input and output projections. The discharge of neural units in the midline zone appears to reflect the force and velocity of movements as they occur. Although the connections of the midline zone are complex, the major afferents originate in the spinal cord and in the brain stem reticular and vestibular nuclei and the major efferents project to vestibulospinal and reticulospinal neurons. Many of these afferent and efferent projections are concerned with posture, locomotion, the position of the head in relation to the trunk, and the control of extraocular movements (Gilman et al., 1981). Correspondingly, the clinical signs resulting from midline cerebellar disease consist of disordered stance and gait (Maurice-Williams, 1975), truncal titubation (Gilman et al., 1981), rotated postures of

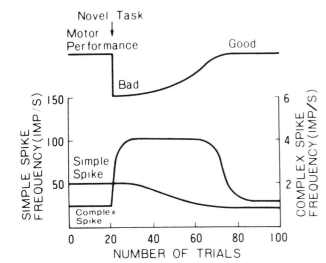

Figure 23–10. Purkinje cell responses to introduction of a novel task. A monkey was trained to move a handle in a horizontal arc by flexing or extending the wrist to a central position and attempting to hold it there despite flexor and extensor loads applied to the handle. With known loads, motor performance and discharge frequencies of simple spikes and complex spikes were steady. When the extensor load was increased from a known level of 300 g to a novel load of 450 g (arrow), motor performance deteriorated and then, over the next 40–60 trials, improved substantially. Simple spike activity decreased but complex spike activity increased markedly. (From Gilbert P.F.C., Thach W.T. Purkinje cell activity during motor learning. *Brain Res.* 128:309–328, 1977.)

the head (Amici et al., 1976), and disturbances of extraocular movements (Leigh and Zee, 1983). Some authors consider the flocculus, nodulus, and uvula as a separate group, the vestibulocerebellum (Dichgans, 1984; Dichgans and Diener, 1984, 1986). In the past, dysarthria has been considered a sign of midline cerebellar disease, but this disorder may be linked to lesions of the cerebellar hemispheres, particularly the left (Lechtenberg and Gilman, 1978).

The intermediate zone of the cerebellum consists of the paravermal region of the cerebellar cortex and the interposed nuclei on each side. Major afferents to this zone arise in many structures, including the spinal cord, brain stem, and cerebral cortex. Similarly, efferent projections reach both rostral and caudal regions of the nervous system. Neuronal activity in this region appears to be involved in the control of movement velocity, force, and the pattern of muscle activity. Thus far, patients with disease strictly limited to the intermediate zone have not been reported. Accordingly, the clinical disorders related to disease of this zone have been linked with those related to disease of the lateral zone.

The lateral zone of the cerebellum consists of the cerebellar hemisphere and the dentate nucleus of each side. This zone receives input from a number of sources, particularly the cerebral cortex via relay nuclei in the pons and the brain stem reticular nuclei. The lateral zone sends projections to the brain stem and thalamic structures that engage both forebrain and spinal levels of the central nervous system. Neural units in this zone of the cerebellum are involved in the planning of movements in connection with neurons in the precentral region of the cerebral cortex. The abnormalities resulting from lesions of the lateral zone are related chiefly to voluntary movements and consist of hypotonia, dysarthria, dysmetria, dysdiadochokinesia, excessive rebound, impaired check, kinetic and static tremors, decomposition of movements, past-pointing, and eye movement disorders (Gilman et al., 1981).

The Significance of Certain Neurologic Symptoms

Ito (1984) presented evidence that three major principles govern the characteristics of cerebellar control mechanisms: open-loop, multivariable, and adaptive learning. An open-loop control system as applied to the nervous system is a reflex arc lacking feedback. A multivariable control system is one that sets relationships for multiple inputs and outputs. Adaptive learning control systems are those that adjust their responses to maintain optimal performance under changing circumstances. Ito viewed the symptoms of cerebellar lesions as resulting from impaired function of the open-loop and multivariable controls associated with loss of adaptive learning capability for acquiring or restoring motor skills. He attributed dysmetria and delayed movement initia-

tion to failure of open-loop motor control. Dysmetria represents inaccuracy of a goal-directed movement that is normally performed in a predictive manner without feedback correction. Delayed movement initiation indicates the disordered function of an open-loop control mechanism for which there is no time for feedback correction. Ito viewed incoordination as a disturbance in multivariable control, which is needed to integrate the component parts of compound movements.

Studies of Cerebellar Function with Positron Emission Tomography

Positron emission tomography has made it possible to study cerebellar function in both normal control subjects and patients with cerebellar disease (Gilman et al., 1988). Local cerebral metabolic rate has been studied with positron emission tomography and fluorodeoxyglucose in patients with an adult-onset cerebellar disease, olivopontocerebellar atrophy (Gilman et al., 1988). The results demonstrated a marked decrease of metabolic rate in the cerebellum and brain stem of the patients in comparison with age- and sex-matched normal control subjects. The degree of hypometabolism was related to the severity of the speech disorder (Kluin et al., 1988) and the clinical neurologic impairment (Rosenthal et al., 1988). Studies of patients with alcoholic cerebellar degeneration revealed hypometabolism in the anterior superior aspects of the cerebellar vermis and in the medial rostral aspects of the frontal lobe (Gilman et al., 1990a). Studies of patients with Friedreich's ataxia demonstrated cerebral glucose hypermetabolism early in the course of the disease, with a return toward normal levels later (Gilman et al., 1990b).

The Clinical Signs of Cerebellar Disease

Abnormalities of Stance and Gait

The most common clinical signs of cerebellar disease are abnormalities of standing and walking (Amici et al., 1976). With disease of the midline zone of the cerebellum, these abnormalities usually appear without corresponding disturbances in the coordinated movements of the other limbs when tested separately. With disease of the lateral zone, difficulty in standing and walking occurs along with disorders of movement of the other limbs. The stance is usually on a broad base, and there may be a severe truncal tremor that can evolve into titubation. Postural abnormalities may occur, especially if the cerebellar disorder is long in duration. These abnormalities consist of scoliosis, elevation or depression of a shoulder, and a pelvic tilt. Postural abnormalities of marked degree generally occur more frequently with disease of the lateral than with disease of the midline zone of the cerebellum. Unequal degrees of hypotonia affecting the truncal musculature probably account for this. During walking, truncal instability may be manifested by falls to the right, left, forward, or backward in individual patients (Holmes, 1922). Walking consists of a series of steps irregularly placed, some too far forward, some not sufficiently far forward, and some too far to the left or right. The legs are often lifted too high during ambulation. Gait deficits can be enhanced by various maneuvers, including walking in tandem or walking on the heels, the toes, or backward. The side toward which a patient falls, swerves, drifts, or leans does not indicate with certainty the side of a cerebellar lesion. Ataxia of gait with unimpaired limb coordination otherwise occurs with injury to the anterior superior portion of the cerebellar vermis and is the hallmark of the cerebellar disturbance resulting from nutritional and alcoholic damage to the nervous system (Victor et al., 1989). Lesions of the flocculonodular lobe also are associated with disorders of stance and gait, often in association with multidirectional nystagmus and head rotation (Gilman et al., 1981).

Titubation

This consists of a rhythmic tremor of the body or head, appearing as a rocking motion forward and backward, from side to side, or in a rotatory movement and usually occurring several times per second. The tremor of the head usually is associated with a distal static tremor of the fingers and wrist.

Rotated or Tilted Postures of the Head

These postures can result from cerebellar disease and are associated with disease of the vermis or the flocculonodular lobule. The direction of a head tilt, that is, the side to which the occiput points, does not have localizing significance with respect to the side of the cerebellar pathologic change (Gilman et al., 1981).

Disturbances of Extraocular Movements

Cerebellar disease involving the midline zone results in numerous and varied abnormalities of oculomotor function, including saccadic dysmetria, impaired smooth pursuit, gaze-evoked nystagmus, rebound nystagmus, downbeat nystagmus, postsaccadic drift, vestibulo-ocular reflex cancellation, inappropriate vestibulo-ocular reflex, and fixation suppression of caloric nystagmus (Leigh and Zee, 1983). Disease of the lateral zones of the cerebellum can result in a wide variety of oculomotor abnormalities, including dysmetric saccades, impaired smooth pursuit, fixation abnormalities, postsaccadic drift, gaze-evoked nystagmus, rebound nystagmus, downbeat nystagmus, and positional nystagmus (Leigh and Zee, 1983).

Decomposition of Movement

Disease in the lateral zone of the cerebellum results in abnormalities of both simple and compound movements (Flament and Hore, 1986; Gilman et al., 1981; Hallett et al., 1975). Simple movements consist of changes of posture or movements restricted to one joint or plane and may be slow or rapid. The slowest simple movements, consisting of changes of posture about one joint and lasting 1 second and longer, are produced by agonist muscle contraction alone, without participation by antagonist muscles. The fastest (ballistic) simple movements also result from agonist muscle contraction alone. Other simple movements result from a triphasic pattern consisting of two agonist bursts separated by an antagonist burst (Brooks and Thach, 1981). Slow self-terminated simple movements are frequently studied in monkeys. These movements rely on external visual or auditory cues for feedback guidance to reach their end points, but with practice these movements are made faster and become independent of external cues. Compound movements involve a change of posture at two or more joints. The lateral zone of the cerebellum participates in many aspects of the control of both simple and compound movements, including movement initiation (Brooks and Thach, 1981), current control of ongoing movement (Marsden et al., 1977), and termination (braking) of movement (Vilis and Hore, 1980).

Cerebellar lesions impair the control of simple movements, both slow (Beppu et al., 1984) and rapid (Flament and Hore, 1986; Holmes, 1922). Muscular contractions under both isotonic and isometric conditions are affected (Flament and Hore, 1988; Mai et al., 1988, 1989) (Fig. 23–11), and the execution of serial movements is impaired (Inhoff et al., 1989). Self-terminated simple movements are abnormal after cerebellar lesions in that movement initiation is delayed (Hallett et al., 1975) and braking is abnormal (Vilis and Hore, 1980). Ballistic movements are carried out abnormally after cerebellar lesions (Spidalieri et al., 1983). Injury to the cerebellar hemispheres results in deterioration of compound arm movements with decomposition into their constituent parts. This leads to errors of direction, delay in the initiation of one portion of the compound movement, and an excessive trajectory with movement (Brooks and Thach, 1981; Miall et al., 1987). Lateral cerebellar dysfunction also influences long-latency stretch reflexes (Diener and Dichgans, 1986; Diener et al., 1984; Marsden et al., 1978). The disorders of movement with cerebellar disease result from a variety of abnormalities, including disturbances in the central commands that initiate movements and in the regulation of proprioceptive feedback (Hore and Flament, 1988) (Fig. 23–12).

Dysmetria

Dysmetria is a disturbance of the trajectory or placement of a body part during active movements.

Figure 23–11. Effects of inactivation by cooling of cerebellar dentate and interposed nuclei on tracking task performance with extension movements at the elbow under isotonic and isometric conditions for three monkeys (MI, PA, and DU). Fifteen superimposed position (two left columns) and torque (two right columns) records are shown under control conditions and during cooling. Note the tremulous movements induced by cooling under both isotonic and isometric conditions. A torque of 0.026 N m opposed the isotonic movements in MI and PA and a torque of 0.056 N m was provided in DU. Calibrations: position, 15°; torque (targets), 0.027 N m in monkey MI, 0.033 N m in PA, 0.061 N m in DU. (From Flament D., Hore J. Comparison of cerebellar intention tremor under isotonic and isometric conditions. *Brain Res.* 439:179–186, 1988.)

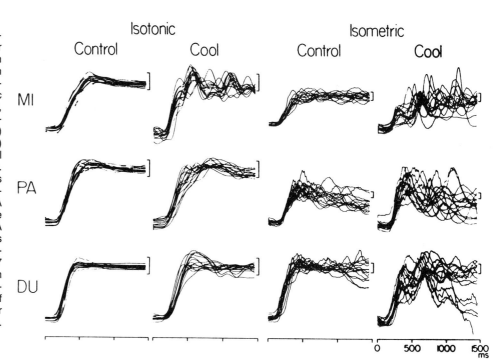

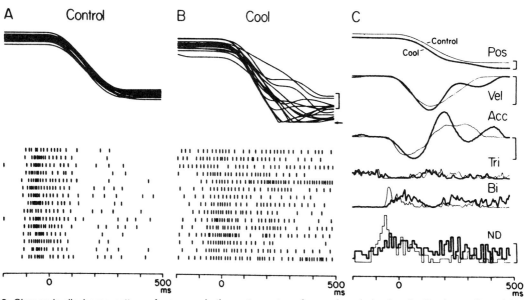

Figure 23–12. Change in discharge pattern of a neuron in the motor cortex of a monkey during inactivation by cooling of the contralateral dentate and interpositus nuclei. *(A)* Records of 15 trials of a flexion movement at the elbow with the limb position shown in the upper trace and the associated neural discharge records in the raster display. *(B)* Records of 15 trials of a flexion movement at the elbow during cerebellar nuclear cooling. Note the disturbances of position control and the changes in pattern of the discharge of the motor cortex neuron. The arrow indicates a mechanical stop limiting manipulandum excursion. *(C)* Averages of eight control movements (thin line) and eight movements during cooling (thick line), showing position (Pos), velocity (Vel), acceleration (Acc), triceps (Tri), and biceps (Bi) electromyograms and histograms of the neuronal discharge (ND) of the motor cortex neuron. All records are synchronized to movement onset at time 0 ms. Calibrations: position, 12°; velocity, 200°/second; acceleration, 2000°/second; neural discharge, five spikes. All records are for the same animal and the same motor cortex neuron. (From Hore J., Flament D. Changes in motor cortex neural discharge associated with the development of cerebellar limb ataxia. *J. Neurophysiol.* 60:1285–1302, 1988.)

Hypometria refers to a trajectory in which the body part falls short of its goal, and hypermetria indicates a trajectory in which the body part extends beyond its goal.

Dysdiadochokinesia and Dysrhythmokinesia

Dysdiachokinesia is a manifestation of the decomposition of movement occurring in cerebellar disease appearing with alternating or fine repetitive movements. To test for dysdiadochokinesia the patient taps one hand with the other, rapidly placing the palmar and dorsal surfaces alternately upward. When this is performed quickly, deficits appear in the rate of alternation and in the completeness of the sequence. The patient cannot produce regularly syncopated movements, and the hand may be supinated or pronated incompletely. Opposing each finger in rapid succession against the thumb of the same hand will demonstrate finer deficits in coordination. Alternate tapping of the heel and toe on the floor also will reveal deficits in movements of the feet. Dysrhythmokinesia is a disorder of the rhythm of rapidly alternating movements. This can be evoked by asking the patient to tap out a rhythm such as three rapid beats followed by one delayed beat. The rhythm is distorted with cerebellar lesions.

Ataxia

Ataxia is a term used to describe various problems with movement that result chiefly from the combined effects of dysmetria and decomposition of movement. With decomposition of movement, errors occur in the sequence and speed of the component parts of a movement. The result is lack of speed and skill in acts requiring the smoothly coordinated activity of several muscles. Movements previously fluid and accurate become halting and imprecise. Other terms used for the abnormalities of movement observed with cerebellar disease are asynergia and dyssynergia. These terms indicate that the patient is unable to perform the various components of a movement at the right time in the appropriate space.

Check and Rebound

Impaired check and excessive rebound are related signs of cerebellar injury. To examine for abnormal check, the examiner asks the patient to maintain the arms extended forward in space while the examiner taps the wrists strongly enough to displace the arms. The patient keeps the eyes shut and the hands pronated. A small displacement should result in a rapid, accurate return to the original position in a normal subject. With injury to the cerebellum, a light tap to the wrist results in a large displacement of the affected arm followed by an overshoot beyond the original position. Return to the original position is achieved by oscillation of the arm around its initial position. Wide excursion of the affected arm results from impaired check. Excessive rebound results in overshoot beyond the original position. Impaired check can also be assessed by forcefully pulling on the patient's forearm while the patient flexes the elbow. On releasing the forearm abruptly, the examiner will evoke an unchecked contraction of the arm and the patient will strike his or her chest with the hand or wrist. The basic phenomenon underlying impaired check is the inability to stop abruptly an ongoing movement.

Tremor

Cerebellar dysfunction results in static and kinetic tremors (Cole et al., 1988; Flament and Hore, 1988; Gilman et al., 1981; Hore and Flament, 1986). The term *intention tremor* is widely used but is ambiguous, usually referring to the tremor that occurs with limb movement. The term *kinetic tremor* is preferable. Static tremor can be demonstrated by observing a patient with the arms extended parallel to the floor with the hands open. Often this position can be sustained steadily for several seconds, but then a rhythmic oscillation occurs, generated at the shoulder. Studies suggest that static tremor is driven by stretch-evoked peripheral feedback to the cerebral cortex (Flament et al., 1984; Hore and Flament, 1986). A kinetic tremor, usually affecting the proximal musculature exclusively in cerebellar disease, can be brought out by having the patient perform the finger-to-nose and heel-to-shin tests.

Dysarthria

Patients with disease restricted to the cerebellum develop an ataxia of speech characterized by imprecise consonants, excessive and equalized stress patterns, irregular articulatory breakdowns, distorted vowels, prolonged phonemes, prolonged intervals, and slowness of rate, as well as excessive loudness variations, pitch breaks, and voice tremor (Kluin et al., 1988). Cerebellar disease alone does not lead to strained, strangled speech, which appears to result from corticobulbar disease (Gilman and Kluin, 1984).

Abnormalities of Muscle Tone

Hypotonia (decreased resistance to passive muscular extension) can result from lateral cerebellar lesions, usually acutely after cerebellar injury, with decreased abnormality over time (Holmes, 1922). Associated pendular deep tendon reflexes may be seen. Tonic stretch reflexes induced by muscle vibration (Lance et al., 1966) are abnormal in patients with cerebellar disorder and appear to be related to clinical hypotonia. Hypotonia has been found in monkeys after complete cerebellectomy (Gilman, 1969), in the ipsilateral limbs after unilateral cerebellar ablation (Gilman, 1969), and after lesions of the cerebellar

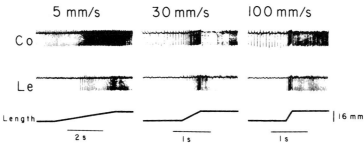

Figure 23–13. Effects of 16 mm of extension of the gastrocnemius muscle at three velocities on the discharge of a gastrocnemius muscle spindle primary afferent before (Co) and immediately after a cryogenic lesion (Le) of the ipsilateral fastigial nucleus. Trace of ramp displacement of muscle is below unit activity. Note that the spindle primary afferent is firing without applied extension of the muscle. The muscle afferent discharge frequency increases rapidly with extension of the muscle and, at maintained full extension, falls abruptly to a rate dependent on the new muscle length. With cooling of the ipsilateral fastigial nucleus, a decrease of the static components of the response occurs, but the discharge at peak frequency is not affected. (From Kornhauser D., Bromberg M.B., Gilman S. Effects of lesions of fastigial nucleus on static and dynamic responses of muscle spindle primary afferents in the cat. *J. Neurophysiol.* 47:977–986, 1982.)

nuclei (Growdon et al., 1967). Hypotonia is most marked in the extensor muscles of monkeys with cerebellar lesions, but it decreases with time and is replaced by tonic flexion of the affected limbs (Gilman et al., 1981). Hypotonia does not appear in cats and dogs after cerebellar ablation; these animals develop marked extensor rigidity with opisthotonos. The extensor rigidity of dogs and cats with cerebellar ablation is termed α *rigidity* because it persists after section of the dorsal roots, which abolishes decerebrate γ rigidity (Gilman et al., 1981).

The cerebellum manipulates the linkage of α and γ motor neurons in the performance of movements. Inactivation of the cerebellar cortex in the cat by cooling results in a decrease of muscle spindle afferent excitability (Gilman et al., 1981). In the decerebellate monkey, muscle spindle primary afferents are defective in function, showing raised thresholds and depressed static and dynamic sensitivities (Gilman, 1969). Muscle spindle secondary afferents, however, show essentially normal responses. Hypotonia appears to be related to the muscle spindle abnormalities. Cerebellectomy in the cat reduces muscle spindle sensitivity to static extension and a variety of natural external inputs (Gilman and McDonald, 1967a), with greater abnormalities affecting afferents with high conduction velocity than with low conduction velocity (Gilman and McDonald, 1967b) and with low baseline rates of γ motor neuron firing (Gilman and Ebel, 1970). The reason is that cerebellar lesions result in defective γ motor neuron regulation of muscle spindle output (Gilman et al., 1981). Thus, γ motor neurons having synaptic connection with spindle receptors innervated by afferent fibers of high conduction velocity receive a falsely low indication of static muscle length. The decrease of fusimotor activity leading to abnormalities in muscle spindle function is an important factor in the pathogenesis of cerebellar hypotonia. Although the decrease of fusimotor activity after cerebellar lesions results from abnormal function of a long reflex loop through the precentral cortex (Gilman et al., 1971, 1974), vestibulospinal and reticulospinal pathways also appear to be involved because lesions of the fastigial nucleus

markedly decrease muscle spindle activity (Kornhauser et al., 1982) (Fig. 23–13).

Other Disturbances Related to Cerebellar Function

Although cerebellar disease is not thought to affect cognitive function, there is some evidence that the cerebellum may be involved in the pathogenesis of a severe cognitive disorder. Hypoplasia of neocerebellar vermal lobules VI and VII has been found in magnetic resonance scans of patients with autism, a developmental disorder that results in severe deficits of language, social, and cognitive function (Courchesne et al., 1988). Some additional evidence suggests that the cerebellum may be involved in higher cerebral cortical functions (Botez et al., 1989; Bracke-Tolkmitt et al., 1989; Leiner et al., 1986).

References

(Key references are designated with an asterisk.)

Albin R.L., Gilman S. Autoradiographic localization of inhibitory and excitatory amino acid neurotransmitter receptors in human normal and olivopontocerebellar atrophy cerebellar cortex. *Brain Res.* 552:37–45, 1990.

Albus J.S. A theory of cerebellar function. *Math. Biosci.* 10:25–61, 1971.

Amat J. Interaction between signals from vestibular and forelimb receptors in Purkinje cells of the frog vestibulocerebellum. *Brain Res.* 278:287–290, 1983.

Amici R., Avanzini G., Pacini L. Cerebellar tumors. *Monogr. Neural. Sci.* 4:1–112, 1976.

Angaut P., Sotelo C. The dentato-olivary projection in the rat as a presumptive GABAergic link in the olivo-cerebello-olivary loop. An ultrastructural study. *Neurosci. Lett.* 83:227–231, 1987.

Angaut P., Sotelo C. Synaptology of the cerebello-olivary pathway. Double labelling with anterograde axonal tracing and GABA immunocytochemistry in the rat. *Brain Res.* 479:361–365, 1989.

Angaut P., Batini C., Billard J.M., et al. The cerebellorubral projection in the rat: retrograde anatomical study. *Neurosci. Lett.* 68:63–68, 1986.

Armstrong D.M., Edgley S.A. Discharges of Purkinje cells in the paravermal part of the cerebellar anterior lobe during locomotion in the cat. *J. Physiol. (Lond.)* 352:403–424, 1984a.

Armstrong D.M., Edgley S.A. Discharges of nucleus interpositus neurones during locomotion in the cat. *J. Physiol. (Lond.)* 351:411–432, 1984b.

Arshavsky Y.I., Gelfand I.M., Orlovsky G.N. The cerebellum and control of rhythmical movements. *Trends Neurosci.* 6:417–422, 1983.

Arshavsky Y.I., Orlovsky G.N., Popova L.B. Activity of cerebellar Purkinje cells during fictitious scratch reflex in the cat. *Brain Res.* 290:33–41, 1984.

Asanuma C., Thach W.T., Jones E.G. Nucleus interpositus projection to spinal interneurons in monkeys. *Brain Res.* 191:245–248, 1980.

Asanuma C., Thach W.T., Jones E.G. Brainstem and spinal projections of the deep cerebellar nuclei in the monkey, with observations on the brainstem projections of the dorsal column nuclei. *Brain Res. Rev.* 5:299–322, 1983.

Batini C., Biusseret-Delmas C., Compoint C., et al. The GABAergic neurones of the cerebellar nuclei in the rat: projections to the cerebellar cortex. *Neurosci. Lett.* 99:251–256, 1989.

Batton R.R., Jayaraman A., Ruggiero D., et al. Fastigial efferent projections in the monkey: an autoradiographic study. *J. Comp. Neurol.* 174:281–306, 1977.

Bava A., Grimm R.J., Rushmer D.S. Fastigial unit activity during voluntary movement in primates. *Brain Res.* 288:371–374, 1983.

Beaubaton D., Trouche E. Participation of the cerebellar dentate nucleus in the control of a goal-directed movement in monkeys. *Exp. Brain Res.* 46:127–138, 1982.

Benedetti P., Montarolo P.G., Rabacchi S. Inferior olive lesion induces long-lasting functional modification in the Purkinje cells. *Exp. Brain Res.* 55:368–371, 1984.

Beppu H., Suda M., Tanaka R. Analysis of cerebellar motor disorders by visually guided elbow tracking movements. *Brain* 107:787–809, 1984.

Bishop G.A. A quantitative analysis of the recurrent collaterals derived from Purkinje cells in zone x of the cat's vermis. *J. Comp. Neurol.* 247:17–31, 1988.

Bishop G.A., O'Donoghue D.L. Heterogeneity in the pattern of distribution of the axonal collaterals of Purkinje cells in zone b of the cat's vermis: an intracellular HRP study. *J. Comp. Neurol.* 253:483–499, 1986.

*Bloedel J.R., Courville J. Cerebellar afferent systems. In Brooks V.B., ed. *Handbook of Physiology.* Section 1. *The Nervous System.* Vol. II. *Motor Control.* Part 2. Bethesda, American Physiological Society, pp. 735–829, 1981.

*Bloedel J.R., Dichgans J., Precht W., eds. *Cerebellar Functions.* Berlin, Springer-Verlag, 1984.

Bloom F.E., Hoffer B.J., Siggins G.R. Studies on norepinephrine-containing afferents to Purkinje cells of rat cerebellum. I. Localization of the fibers and their synapses. *Brain Res.* 25:501–521, 1971.

Bloom F.E., Hoffer B.J., Siggins G.R., et al. Effects of serotonin on central neurons: microiontophoretic administration. *Fed. Proc.* 31:97–106, 1972.

Botez M.I., Botez T., Elie R., et al. Role of the cerebellum in complex human behavior. *Ital. J. Neurol. Sci.* 10:291–300, 1989.

Bracke-Tolkmitt R., Linden A., Canavan A.G.M., et al. The cerebellum contributes to mental skills. *Behav. Neurosci.* 103:442–446, 1989.

*Brodal A. *Neurological Anatomy in Relation to Clinical Medicine.* 3rd ed. New York, Oxford University Press, 1981.

Brodal A., Brodal P. Observations on the secondary vestibulocerebellar projections in the macaque monkey. *Exp. Brain Res.* 58:62–74, 1985.

*Brooks V.B., Thach W.T. Cerebellar control of posture and movement. In Brooks V.B., ed. *Handbook of Physiology.* Section 1. *The Nervous System.* Vol. II. *Motor Control.* Part 2. Bethesda, American Physiological Society, pp. 877–946, 1981.

Buisseret-Delmas C. Sagittal organization of the olivocerebello-nuclear pathway in the rat. I. Connections with the nucleus fastigii and the nucleus vestibularis lateralis. *Neurosci. Res.* 5:475–493, 1988a.

Buisseret-Delmas C. Sagittal organization of the olivocerebello-nuclear pathway in the rat. II. Connections with the nucleus interpositus. *Neurosci. Res.* 5:494–512, 1988b.

Carleton S.C., Carpenter M.B. Afferent and efferent connections of the medial, inferior and lateral vestibular nuclei in the cat and monkey. *Brain Res.* 278:29–51, 1983.

Carpenter M.B., Batton R.R. Jr. Connections of the fastigial nucleus in the cat and monkey. *Exp. Brain Res.* 6(Suppl.):250–291, 1982.

*Chan-Palay V. *Cerebellar Dentate Nucleus: Organization, Cytology and Transmitters.* New York, Springer-Verlag, 1977.

Chan-Palay V., Palay S.L., Wu J.-Y. Gamma-aminobutyric acid pathways in the cerebellum studied by retrograde and anterograde transport of glutamic acid decarboxylase antibody after in vivo injections. *Anat. Embryol.* 157:1–14, 1979.

Chapman C.E., Spidalieri G., Lamarre Y. Activity of dentate neurons during arm movements triggered by visual, auditory and somesthetic stimuli in the monkey. *J. Neurophysiol.* 55:203–226, 1986.

Clements J.R., Monaghan P.L., Beitz A.J. An ultrastructural description of glutamate-like immunoreactivity in the rat cerebellar cortex. *Brain Res.* 421:343–348, 1987.

Cole J.D., Philip H.I., Sedgwick E.M. Stability and tremor in the fingers associated with cerebellar hemisphere and cerebellar tract lesions in man. *J. Neurol. Neurosurg. Psychiatry* 51:1558–1568, 1988.

Courchesne E., Yeung-Courchesne R., Press G.A., et al. Hypoplasia of cerebellar vermal lobules VI and VII in autism. *N. Engl. J. Med.* 318:1349–1354, 1988.

de Zeeuw C.I., Holstege J.C., Ruigrok T.J.H., et al. Ultrastructural study of the GABAergic, cerebellar, and mesodiencephalic innervation of the cat medial accessory olive: anterograde tracing combined with immunocytochemistry. *J. Comp. Neurol.* 284:12–35, 1989.

Dichgans J. Clinical symptoms of cerebellar dysfunction and their topodiagnostical significance. *Hum. Neurobiol.* 2:269–279, 1984.

Dichgans J., Diener H.-C. Clinical evidence for functional compartmentalization of the cerebellum. In Bloedel J.R., Dichgans J., Precht W., eds. *Cerebellar Functions.* Berlin, Springer-Verlag, 1984.

Dichgans J., Diener H.-C. Different forms of postural ataxia in patients with cerebellar diseases. In Bles W., Brandt T., eds. *Disorders of Posture and Gait.* Amsterdam, Elsevier, 1986.

Diener H.-C., Dichgans J. Long loop reflexes and posture. In Bles W., Brandt T., eds. *Disorders of Posture and Gait.* Amsterdam, Elsevier, 1986.

Diener H.-C., Dichgans J., Bacher M., et al. Characteristic alterations of long-loop "reflexes" in patients with Friedreich's disease and late atrophy of the cerebellar anterior lobe. *J. Neurol. Neurosurg. Psychiatry* 47:679–685, 1984.

Dietrichs E. The cerebellar corticonuclear and nucleocortical projections in the cat as studied with anterograde and retrograde transport of horseradish peroxidase. V. The posterior lobe vermis and the flocculonodular lobe. *Anat. Embryol. (Berl.)* 167:449–462, 1983.

Dietrichs E., Walberg F. The cerebellar nucleo-olivary and olivo-cerebellar projections in the cat as studied with anterograde and retrograde transport in the same animal after implantation of crystalline WGA/HRP. II. The fastigial nucleus. *Anat. Embryol. (Berl.)* 173:253–261, 1985.

Dietrichs E., Walberg F. The cerebellar nucleo-olivary and olivo-cerebellar projections in the cat as studied with anterograde and retrograde transport in the same animal after implantation of crystalline WGA/HRP. III. The interposed nuclei. *Brain Res.* 373:373–383, 1985.

Dietrichs E., Walberg F., Nordby T. The cerebellar nucleo-olivary and olivo-cerebellar projections in the cat as studied with anterograde and retrograde transport in the same animal after implantation of crystalline WGA/HRP. I. The dentate nucleus. *Neurosci. Res.* 3:52–70, 1985.

Dupont J.L., Crepel F., Delhaye-Bouchaud N. Influence of bicuculline and picrotoxin on reversal properties of excitatory synaptic potentials in cerebellar Purkinje cells of the rat. *Brain Res.* 173:577–580, 1979.

Eccles J.C., Ito M., Szentágothai J. *The Cerebellum as a Neuronal Machine.* New York, Springer-Verlag, 1967.

Eckmiller R. Neural control of pursuit eye movements. *Physiol. Rev.* 67:797–857, 1987.

Estrada C., Hamel E., Krause D.N. Biochemical evidence for cholinergic innervation of intracerebral blood vessels. *Brain Res.* 266:261–270, 1983.

Fagg G.E., Foster A.C. Amino acid neurotransmitters and their pathways in the mammalian central nervous system. *Neuroscience* 9:701–719, 1983.

Flament D., Hore J. Movement and electromyographic disorders associated with cerebellar dysmetria. *J. Neurophysiol.* 55:1221–1233, 1986.

Flament D., Hore J. Comparison of cerebellar intention tremor under isotonic and isometric conditions. *Brain Res.* 439:179–186, 1988.

Flament D., Vilis T., Hore J. Dependence of cerebellar tremor on proprioceptive but not visual feedback. *Exp. Neurol.* 84:314–325, 1984.

Fonnum F. Glutamate: a neurotransmitter in mammalian brain. *J. Neurochem.* 42:1–11, 1984.

Fortier P.A., Kalaska J.F., Smith A.M. Cerebellar neuronal activity related to whole-arm reaching movements in the monkey. *J. Neurophysiol.* 62:198–211, 1989.

Fredrickson R.C.A., Neuss M., Morzorati S.L., et al. A comparison of the inhibitory effects of taurine and GABA on identified Purkinje cells and other neurons in the cerebellar cortex of the rat. *Brain Res.* 145:117–126, 1978.

Freedman R., Hoffer B.J. Phenothiazine antagonism of the noradrenergic inhibition of cerebellar Purkinje neurons. *J. Neurobiol.* 6:277–288, 1975.

Frysinger R.C., Bourbonnaes D., Kalaska J.F., et al. Cerebellar cortical activity during antagonist cocontraction and reciprocal inhibition of forearm muscles. *J. Neurophysiol.* 51:32–49, 1984.

Fujita M. Adaptive filter model of the cerebellum. *Biol. Cybern.* 45:195–206, 1982.

Fukushima K., Peterson B.W., Uchino Y.U., et al. Direct fastigiospinal fibers in the cat. *Brain Res.* 126:538–542, 1977.

Gacek R.R. Location of the brainstem neurons projecting to the oculomotor nucleus in the cat. *Exp. Neurol.* 57:725–749, 1977.

Garthwaite J., Beaumont P.S. Excitatory amino acid receptors in the parallel fibre pathway in rat cerebellar slices. *Neurosci. Lett.* 107:151–156, 1989.

Garthwaite J., Brodbelt A.R. Synaptic activation of N-methyl-D-aspartate and non–N-methyl-D-aspartate receptors in the mossy fibre pathway in adult and immature rat cerebellar slices. *Neuroscience* 29:401–412, 1989.

Gerrits N.M., Voogd J. The nucleus reticularis tegmenti pontis and the adjacent rostral paramedian reticular formation: differential projections to the cerebellum and the caudal brain stem. *Exp. Brain Res.* 62:29–45, 1986.

Gerrits N.M., Voogd J. The projection of the nucleus reticularis tegmenti pontis and adjacent regions of the pontine nuclei to the central cerebellar nuclei in the cat. *J. Comp. Neurol.* 258:52–69, 1987.

Gerrits N.M., Voogd J., Nas W.S.C. Cerebellar and olivary projections of the external and rostral internal cuneate nuclei in the cat. *Exp. Brain Res.* 57:239–255, 1985.

Gilbert P.F.C. How the cerebellum could memorise movements. *Nature* 254:688–689, 1975.

Gilbert P.F.C., Thach W.T. Purkinje cell activity during motor learning. *Brain Res.* 128:309–328, 1977.

Gilman S. The mechanism of cerebellar hypotonia. An experimental study in the monkey. *Brain* 92:621–638, 1969.

Gilman S., Ebel H.C. Fusimotor neuron responses to natural stimuli as a function of prestimulus fusimotor activity in decerebellate cats. *Brain Res.* 21:367–384, 1970.

Gilman S., Kluin K. Perceptual analysis of speech disorders in Friedreich disease and olivopontocerebellar atrophy. In Bloedel J.R., Dichgans J., Precht W., eds. *Cerebellar Functions.* Berlin, Springer-Verlag, pp. 148–163, 1984.

Gilman S., McDonald W.I. Cerebellar facilitation of muscle spindle activity. *J. Neurophysiol.* 30:1495–1512, 1967a.

Gilman S., McDonald W.I. Relation of afferent fiber conduction velocity to reactivity of muscle spindle receptors after cerebellectomy. *J. Neurophysiol.* 30:1513–1522, 1967b.

Gilman S., Marco L.A., Ebel H.C. Effects of medullary pyramidotomy in the monkey. II. Abnormalities of muscle spindle afferent responses. *Brain* 94:515–530, 1971.

Gilman S., Lieberman J.S., Marco L.A. Spinal mechanism underlying the effects of unilateral ablation of areas 4 and 6 in monkeys. *Brain* 97:49–64, 1974.

*Gilman S., Bloedel J.R., Lechtenberg R. *Disorders of the Cerebellum.* Philadelphia, Davis, 1981.

Gilman S., Markel D.S., Koeppe R.A., et al. Cerebellar and brainstem hypometabolism in olivopontocerebellar atrophy detected with positron emission tomography. *Ann. Neurol.* 23:223–230, 1988.

Gilman S., Adams K., Koeppe R.A., et al. Cerebellar and frontal hypometabolism in alcoholic cerebellar degeneration studied with positron emission tomography. *Ann. Neurol.* 28:775–785, 1990a.

Gilman S., Junck L., Markel D.S., et al. Cerebral glucose hypermetabolism in Friedreich's ataxia detected with positron emission tomography. *Ann. Neurol.* 28:750–757, 1990b.

Greenamyre J.T., Young A.B., Penney J.B. Jr. Quantitative autoradiographic distribution of L-[³H]glutamate binding sites in the rat central nervous system. *J. Neurosci.* 4:2133–2144, 1984.

Grimm R.J., Rushmer D.S. The activity of dentate neurons during an arm movement sequence. *Brain Res.* 71:309–326, 1974.

Growdon J.H., Chambers W.W., Liu C.N. An experimental study of cerebellar dyskinesia in the rhesus monkey. *Brain* 90:603–632, 1967.

Hallett M., Shahani B.T., Young R.R. EMG analysis of patients with cerebellar deficits. *J. Neurol. Neurosurg. Psychiatry* 38:1163–1169, 1975.

Heath R.G. Fastigial nucleus connections to the septal region in monkey and cat: a demonstration with evoked potentials of a bilateral pathway. *Biol. Psychiatry* 6:193–196, 1973.

Hökfelt T., Fuxe K. Cerebellar monoamine nerve terminals, a new type of afferent fiber to the cortex cerebelli. *Exp. Brain Res.* 9:63–72, 1969.

Hökfelt T., Ljungdahl Å. Uptake mechanisms as a basis of the histochemical identification and tracing of transmitter-specific neuron populations. In Cowan W.M., Cuneod M., eds. *The Use of Axonal Transport for Studies of Neuronal Connectivity.* Amsterdam, Elsevier, pp. 249–305, 1975.

Holmes G. The Croonian lectures on the clinical symptoms of cerebellar disease and their interpretation. *Lancet* 1:1177–1182, 1231–1237; 2:59–65, 111–115, 1922.

Hore J., Flament D. Evidence that a disordered servo-like mechanism contributes to tremor in movements during cerebellar dysfunction. *J. Neurophysiol.* 56:123–136, 1986.

Hore J., Flament D. Changes in motor cortex neural discharge associated with the development of cerebellar limb ataxia. *J. Neurophysiol.* 60:1285–1302, 1988.

Ikeda Y., Noda H., Sugita S. Olivocerebellar and cerebelloolivary connections of the oculomotor region of the fastigial nucleus in the macaque monkey. *J. Comp. Neurol.* 284:463–488, 1989.

Inagaki S., Shiosaka S., Takatsuki K., et al. Ontogeny of somatostatin-containing neuron system of the rat cerebellum including its fiber connections: an experimental and immunohistochemical analysis. *Dev. Brain Res.* 3:509–527, 1982.

Inhoff A.W., Diener H.-C., Rafal R.D., et al. The role of cerebellar structures in the execution of serial movements. *Brain* 112:565–581, 1989.

Ito M. Cerebellar control of the vestibulo-ocular reflex—around the flocculus hypothesis. *Annu. Rev. Neurosci.* 5:275–296, 1982.

*Ito M. *The Cerebellum and Neural Control.* New York, Raven Press, 1984.

Ito M. Long-term depression. *Annu. Rev. Neurosci.* 12:85–102, 1989.

Kimoto Y., Tohyama M., Satoh K., et al. Fine structure of rat cerebellar noradrenaline terminals as visualized by potassium permanganate "in situ perfusion" fixation method. *Neuroscience* 6:47–58, 1981.

*King J.S., ed. *New Concepts in Cerebellar Neurobiology.* New York, Liss, 1988.

Kitamura T., Yamada J. Spinocerebellar tract neurons with axons passing through the inferior or superior cerebellar peduncles. *Brain Behav. Evol.* 34:133–142, 1989.

Kluin K.J., Gilman S., Markel D.S., et al. Speech disorders in olivopontocerebellar atrophy correlate with positron emission tomography findings. *Ann. Neurol.* 23:547–554, 1988.

Kornhauser D., Bromberg M.B., Gilman S. Effects of lesions of fastigial nucleus on static and dynamic responses of muscle spindle primary afferents in the cat. *J. Neurophysiol.* 47:977–986, 1982.

Korte G.E., Reiner A., Karten H.J. Substance P–like immunoreactivity in cerebellar mossy fibers and terminals in the red-eared turtle, *Chrysemys scripta elegans. Neuroscience* 5:903–914, 1980.

Lance J.W., Degail P., Nielson P.D. Tonic and phasic spinal cord mechanisms in man. *J. Neurol. Neurosurg. Psychiatry* 29:535–544, 1966.

Lechtenberg R., Gilman S. Speech disorders in cerebellar disease. *Ann. Neurol.* 3:285–290, 1978.

Legendre A., Courville J. Origin and trajectory of the cerebello-olivary projection: an experimental study with radioactive and fluorescent tracers in the cat. *Neuroscience* 21:877–891, 1987.

Leigh R.J., Zee D.S. *The Neurology of Eye Movements.* Philadelphia, Davis, 1983.

Leiner H.C., Leiner A.L., Dow R.S. Does the cerebellum contribute to mental skills? *Behav. Neurosci.* 100:443–454, 1986.

Levi G., Gallo V. Release studies related to the neurotransmitter role of glutamate in the cerebellum: an overview. *Neurochem. Res.* 11:1627–1642, 1986.

Lisberger S.G. The latency of pathways containing the site of motor learning in the monkey vestibulo-ocular reflex. *Science* 225:74–76, 1984.

Logan K., Robertson L.T. Somatosensory representation of the climbing fiber system in the rat. *Brain Res.* 372:290–300, 1986.

MacKay W.A. Unit activity in the cerebellar nuclei related to arm reaching movements. *Brain Res.* 442:240–254, 1988a.

MacKay W.A. Cerebellar nuclear activity in relation to simple movements. *Exp. Brain Res.* 71:47–58, 1988b.

Madsen S., Ottersen O.P., Storm-Mathisen J. Immunocytochemical visualization of taurine: neuronal localization in the rat cerebellum. *Neurosci. Lett.* 60:255–260, 1985.

Magnusson K.R., Madl J.E., Clements J.R., et al. Colocalization of taurine- and cysteine sulfinic acid decarboxylase–like immunoreactivity in the cerebellum of the rat with monoclonal antibodies against taurine. *J. Neurosci.* 8:4551–4564, 1988.

Mai N., Bolsinger P., Avarello M., et al. Control of isometric finger force in patients with cerebellar disease. *Brain* 111:973–998, 1988.

Mai N., Diener H.-C., Dichgans J. On the role of feedback in maintaining constant grip force in patients with cerebellar disease. *Neurosci. Lett.* 99:340–344, 1989.

Mano N., Yamamoto K. Simple-spike activity of cerebellar Purkinje cells related to visually guided wrist tracking movement in the monkey. *J. Neurophysiol.* 43:713–728, 1980.

Marr D. A theory of cerebellar cortex. *J. Physiol. (Lond.)* 202:437–470, 1969.

Marsden C.D., Merton P.A., Morton H.B., et al. Disorders of movement in cerebellar disease in man. In Rose F., ed. *The Physiological Aspects of Clinical Neurology.* Oxford, Blackwell Scientific Publications, pp. 179–199, 1977.

Marsden C.D., Merton P.A., Morton H.B., et al. The effect of lesions of the central nervous system on long-latency stretch reflexes in the human thumb. *Prog. Clin. Neurophysiol.* 4:334–341, 1978.

Matsukawa T., Udo M. Responses of cerebellar Purkinje cells to mechanical perturbations during locomotion of decerebrate cats. *Neurosci. Res.* 2:393–398, 1985.

Matute C., Wiklund L., Streit P., et al. Selective retrograde labeling with D-[³H]-aspartate in the monkey olivocerebellar projection. *Exp. Brain Res.* 66:445–447, 1987.

Maurice-Williams R.S. Mechanisms of production of gait unsteadiness by tumors of the posterior fossa. *J. Neurol. Neurosurg. Psychiatry* 38:143–148, 1975.

McBride W.J., Ghetti B. Changes in the content of glutamate and GABA in the cerebellar vermis and hemispheres of the Purkinje cell degeneration (pcd) mutant. *Neurochem. Res.* 13:121–125, 1988.

McCrea R.A., Bishop G.A., Kitai S.T. Morphological and electrophysiological characteristics of projection neurons in the nucleus interpositus of the cat cerebellum. *J. Comp. Neurol.* 181:397–420, 1978.

McLaughlin B.J., Wood J.G., Saito K., et al. The fine structural localization of glutamate decarboxylase in synaptic terminals of rodent cerebellum. *Brain Res.* 76:377–391, 1974.

Meinecke D.L., Tallman J., Rakic P. GABA_A/benzodiazepine receptor–like immunoreactivity in rat and monkey cerebellum. *Brain Res.* 493:303–319, 1989.

Miall R.C., Weir D.J., Stein J.F. Visuo-motor tracking during reversible inactivation of the cerebellum. *Exp. Brain Res.* 65:455–464, 1987.

Moises H.C., Woodward D.J. Potentiation of GABA inhibitory action in cerebellum by locus coeruleus stimulation. *Brain Res.* 182:327–344, 1980.

Monaghan P.L., Beitz A.J., Larson A.A., et al. Immunocytochemical localization of glutamate-, glutaminase- and aspartate aminotransferase–like immunoreactivity in the rat deep cerebellar nuclei. *Brain Res.* 363:364–370, 1986.

Mortimer J.A. Cerebellar responses to teleceptive stimuli in alert monkeys. *Brain Res.* 83:369–390, 1975.

Mugnaini E., Oertel W.H. An atlas of the distribution of GABAergic neurons and terminals in the rat CNS as revealed by GAD immunohistochemistry. In Bjorklund A., Hökfelt T., eds. *Handbook of Chemical Neuroanatomy.* Vol. 4. *GABA and Neuropeptides in the CNS.* Amsterdam, Elsevier, pp. 436–608, 1985.

Murphy M.G., O'Leary J.L. Neurological deficit in cats with lesions of the olivocerebellar system. *Arch. Neurol.* 24:145–157, 1971.

Nadi N.S., McBride W.J., Aprison M.H. Distribution of several amino acids in regions of the cerebellum of the rat. *J. Neurochem.* 28:453–455, 1977.

Nagao S. Behavior of floccular Purkinje cells correlated with adaptation of horizontal optokinetic eye movement response in pigmented rabbits. *Exp. Brain Res.* 73:489–497, 1988.

Neustadt A., Frostholm A., Rotter A. On the cellular localization of cerebellar muscarinic receptors: an autoradiographic analysis of weaver, reeler, Purkinje cell degeneration and staggerer mice. *Brain Res. Bull.* 20:163–172, 1988.

Nieoullon A., Dusticier N. Decrease in choline acetyltransferase activity in the red nucleus of the cat after cerebellar lesion. *Neuroscience* 6:1633–1641, 1981.

Nieoullon A., Kerkerian L., Dusticier N. High affinity glutamate uptake in the red nucleus and ventrolateral thalamus after lesion of the cerebellum in the adult cat: biochemical evidence for functional changes in the deafferented structures. *Exp. Brain Res.* 55:409–419, 1984.

Nilaver G., Defendini R., Zimmerman E.A., et al. Motilin in the Purkinje cell of the cerebellum. *Nature* 295:597–598, 1982.

O'Donoghue D.L., King J.S., Bishop G.A. Physiological and anatomical studies of the interactions between Purkinje cells and basket cells in the cat's cerebellar cortex: evidence for a unitary relationship. *J. Neurosci.* 9:2141–2150, 1989.

Oertel W.H., Schmechel D.E., Mugnaini E., et al. Immunocytochemical localization of glutamate decarboxylase in rat cerebellum with a new antiserum. *Neuroscience* 6:2715–2735, 1981.

Okamoto K., Sakai Y. Inhibitory actions of taurocyamine, hypotaurine, homotaurine, taurine and GABA on spike discharges of Purkinje cells, and localization of sensitive site, in guinea pig cerebellar slices. *Brain Res.* 206:371–386, 1981.

Okamoto K., Kimura H., Sakai Y. Evidence for taurine as an inhibitory neurotransmitter in cerebellar stellate interneurons: selective antagonism by TAG (6-aminomethyl 3-methyl-4H,1,2,4-benzothiadiazine-1,1-dioxide). *Brain Res.* 265:163–168, 1983.

Otero J.B. Comparison between red nucleus and precentral neurons during learned movement in the monkey. *Brain Res.* 101:37–46, 1976.

Ottersen O.P., Storm-Mathisen J., Somogyi P. Colocalization of glycine-like and GABA-like immunoreactivities in Golgi cell terminals in the rat cerebellum: a postembedding light and electron microscopic study. *Brain Res.* 450:342–353, 1988.

*Palay S.L., Chan-Palay V., eds. The cerebellum. New vistas. *Exp. Brain. Res.* 6(Suppl.):1–637, 1982.

Perry T.L., Currier R.D., Hansen S., et al. Aspartate-taurine imbalance in dominantly inherited olivopontocerebellar atrophy. *Neurology (Minneap.)* 27:257–261, 1977.

Pickel V.M., Segal M., Bloom F.E. A radioautographic study of the efferent pathways of the nucleus locus coeruleus. *J. Comp. Neurol.* 155:15–42, 1974.

Rea M.A., McBride W.J., Rohde R.H. Regional and synaptosomal levels of amino acid neurotransmitters in the 3-acetylpyridine deafferented rat cerebellum. *J. Neurochem.* 34:1106–1108, 1980.

Robertson L.T. Somatosensory representation of the climbing fiber system in the rostral intermediate cerebellum. *Exp. Brain Res.* 61:73–86, 1985.

Robertson L.T., Elias S.A. Representations of the body surface by climbing fiber responses in the dorsal paraflocculus of the cat. *Brain Res.* 452:97–104, 1988.

Robertson L.T., Grimm R.J. Responses of primate dentate neurons to different trajectories of the limb. *Exp. Brain Res.* 23:447–462, 1975.

Roffler-Tarlov S., Beart P.M., O'Gorman S., et al. Neurochemical and morphological consequences of axon terminal degeneration in cerebellar deep nuclei of mice with inherited Purkinje cell degeneration. *Brain Res.* 168:75–95, 1979.

Rosenthal G., Gilman S., Koeppe R.A., et al. Motor dysfunction in olivopontocerebellar atrophy is related to cerebral metabolic rate studied with positron emission tomography. *Ann. Neurol.* 24:414–419, 1988.

Ross C.A., Ruggiero D.A., Reis D.J. Afferent projections to cardiovascular portions of the nucleus of the tractus solitarius in the rat. *Brain Res.* 223:402–408, 1981.

Ross C.A., Meldolesi J., Milner, T.A., et al. Inositol 1,4,5-triphosphate receptor localized to endoplasmic reticulum in cerebellar Purkinje neurons. *Nature* 339:468–470, 1989.

Sanes J.N., Dimitrov B., Hallett M. Motor learning in patients with cerebellar dysfunction. *Brain* 113:103–120, 1990.

Schieber M.H., Thach W.T. Trained slow tracking. I. Muscular production of wrist movement. *J. Neurophysiol.* 54:1213–1227, 1985a.

Schieber M.H., Thach W.T. Trained slow tracking. II. Bidirectional discharge patterns of cerebellar nuclear, motor cortex, and spindle afferent neurons. *J. Neurophysiol.* 54:1228–1270, 1985b.

Schwartz A.B., Ebner T.J., Bloedel J.R. Responses of interposed and dentate neurons to perturbations of the locomotor cycle. *Exp. Brain Res.* 67:323–338, 1987.

Simon H., Le Moal M.L., Calas A. Efferents and afferents of the ventral tegmental-A10 region studied after local injection of [³H]leucine and horseradish peroxidase. *Brain Res.* 178:17–40, 1979.

Snider R.S., Maiti A., Snider S.R. Cerebellar pathways to ventral midbrain and nigra. *Exp. Neurol.* 53:714–728, 1976.

Somogyi P., Takagi H., Richards J.G., et al. Subcellular localization of benzodiazepine/GABA$_A$ receptors in the cerebellum of rat, cat, and monkey using monoclonal antibodies. *J. Neurosci.* 9:2197–2209, 1989.

Spidalieri G., Busby L., Lamarre Y. Fast ballistic arm movements triggered by visual, auditory, and somesthetic stimuli in the monkey. II. Effects of unilateral dentate lesion on discharge of precentral cortical neurons and reaction time. *J. Neurophysiol.* 50:1359–1379, 1983.

Stein J.F. Role of the cerebellum in the visual guidance of movement. *Nature* 323:217–221, 1986.

Stone L.S., Lisberger S.G. Detection of tracking errors by visual climbing fiber inputs to monkey cerebellar flocculus during pursuit eye movements. *Neurosci. Lett.* 72:163–168, 1986.

Strick P.L. Cerebellar involvement in "volitional" muscle reponses to load changes. *Prog. Clin. Neurophysiol.* 4:85–93, 1978.

Strick P.L. The influence of motor preparation on the response of cerebellar neurons to limb displacements. *J. Neurosci.* 3:2007–2020, 1983.

Sugimoto T., Mizuno N., Uchida K. Distribution of cerebellar fiber terminals in the midbrain visuomotor areas: an autoradiographic study in the cat. *Brain Res.* 238:353–370, 1982.

Suzuki D.A., Keller E.L. The role of the posterior vermis of monkey cerebellum in smooth-pursuit eye movement control. I. Eye and head movement–related activity. *J. Neurophysiol.* 59:1–18, 1988a.

Suzuki D.A., Keller E.L. The role of the posterior vermis of monkey cerebellum in smooth-pursuit eye movement control. II. Target velocity–related Purkinje cell activity. *J. Neurophysiol.* 59:19–40, 1988b.

Takeuchi Y., Kimura H., Sano Y. Immunohistochemical demonstration of serotonin-containing nerve fibers in the cerebellum. *Cell Tissue Res.* 226:1–12, 1982.

Thach W.T. Discharge of cerebellar neurons related to two maintained postures and two prompt movements. I. Nuclear cell output. *J. Neurophysiol.* 33:527–536, 1970a.

Thach W.T. Discharge of cerebellar neurons related to two maintained postures and two prompt movements. II. Purkinje cell output and input. *J. Neurophysiol.* 33:537–547, 1970b.

Thach W.T. Timing of activity in cerebellar dentate nucleus and cerebral motor cortex during prompt volitional movement. *Brain Res.* 88:233–241, 1975.

Thach W.T. Correlation of neural discharge with pattern and force of muscular activity, joint position, and direction of the intended movement in motor cortex and cerebellum. *J. Neurophysiol.* 41:654–676, 1978.

Thach W.T., Jones E.G. The cerebellar dentatothalamic connection: terminal field, lamellae, rods and somatotopy. *Brain Res.* 169:168–172, 1979.

Thompson R.F. The neurobiology of learning and memory. *Science* 233:941–947, 1986.

Toggenburger G., Wiklund L., Henke H., et al. Release of endogenous and accumulated exogenous amino acids from slices of normal and climbing fibre–deprived rat cerebellar slices. *J. Neurochem.* 41:1606–1613, 1983.

Tsiotos P., Plaitakis A., Mitsacos A., et al. L-Glutamate binding sites of normal and atrophic human cerebellum. *Brain Res.* 481:87–96, 1989.

Uchida K., Mizuno N., Sugimoto T., et al. Direct projections from the cerebellar nuclei to the superior colliculus in the rabbit: an HRP study. *J. Comp. Neurol.* 216:319–326, 1983.

Umetani T., Tabuchi T., Ichimura R. Cerebellar corticonuclear and corticovestibular fibers from the posterior lobe of the albino rat, with comments on zones. *Brain Behav. Evol.* 29:54–67, 1986.

Van der Want J.J.L., Voogd J. Ultrastructural identification and localization of climbing fiber terminals in the fastigial nucleus of the cat. *J. Comp. Neurol.* 258:81–90, 1987.

Van der Want J.J.L., Gerrits N.M., Voogd J. Autoradiography of mossy fiber terminals in the fastigial nucleus of the cat. *J. Comp. Neurol.* 258:70–80, 1987.

Van der Want J.J.L., Wiklund L., Guegan M., et al. Anterograde tracing of the rat olivocerebellar system with *Phaseolus vulgaris* leucoagglutinin (PHA-L). Demonstration of climbing fiber collateral innervation of the cerebellar nuclei. *J. Comp. Neurol.* 288:1–18, 1989.

Victor M., Adams R.D., Collins G.C. *The Wernicke-Korsakoff Syndrome and Related Neurologic Disorders Due to Alcoholism and Malnutrition.* 2nd ed. Philadelphia, Davis, 1989.

Vilis T., Hore J. Central neural mechanisms contributing to cerebellar tremor produced by limb perturbations. *J. Neurophysiol.* 43:279–291, 1980.

Voogd J. The importance of fibre connections in the comparative anatomy of the mammalian cerebellum. In Llinás R., ed. *Neurobiology of Cerebellar Evolution and Development.* Chicago, American Medical Association, pp. 493–514, 1969.

Voogd J. The olivocerebellar projection in the cat. *Exp. Brain Res.* 6(Suppl.):134–161, 1982.

Wamsley J.K., Palacios J.M. Amino acid and benzodiazepine receptors. In Bjorklund A., Hökfelt T., Kuhar M.J., eds. *Handbook of Chemical Neuroanatomy*. Vol. 3. *Classical Transmitters and Transmitter Receptors in the CNS*. Amsterdam, Elsevier, pp. 352–385, 1984.

Wenthold R.J., Skaggs K.K., Altschuler R.A. Immunocytochemical localization of aspartate aminotransferase and glutaminase immunoreactivities in the cerebellum. *Brain Res.* 363:371–375, 1986.

Wetts R., Kalaska J.F., Smith A.M. Cerebellar nuclear cell activity during antagonist cocontraction and reciprocal inhibition of forearm muscles. *J. Neurophysiol.* 54:231–244, 1985.

Wiklund L., Toggenburger G., Cuénod M. Aspartate: possible neurotransmitter in cerebellar climbing fibers. *Science* 216:78–79, 1982.

Wiklund L., Toggenburger G., Cuénod M. Selective retrograde labelling of the rat olivocerebellar climbing fiber system with D-[^{3}H]aspartate. *Neuroscience* 13:441–468, 1984.

Wilkin G., Wilson J.E., Balázs R., et al. How selective is high affinity uptake of GABA into inhibitory nerve terminals? *Nature* 252:397–399, 1974.

Yanaihara N., Yanaihara C., Nagai K., et al. Motilin-like immunoreactivity in porcine, canine, human and rat tissues. *Biomed. Res.* 1:76–83, 1980.

24

Pharmacologic Aspects of Motor Dysfunction

Anne B. Young
John B. Penney, Jr.

A great deal of progress has been made over the past several decades in our understanding of the anatomy, physiology, and pharmacology of the motor system. The chemical neurotransmitters of many of the pathways known to be involved in motor function have been identified, and drugs are available that can either promote or suppress the function of these neurotransmitter substances. In this chapter the neurochemical anatomy and neuropharmacology of these pathways are reviewed. In addition, the chemical pathology of certain common motor disorders is discussed.

NEUROCHEMISTRY OF MOTOR PATHWAYS

Cerebral Cortex and Corticofugal Pathways

The importance of the cerebral cortex in motor control increases as one ascends the phylogenetic scale. Lesions of the cerebral cortex or of its output fibers affect the function of lower motor neurons in the spinal cord and lead to spasticity and impairment of fine motor control in humans (Kuypers, 1981). Cortical fiber projections have been mapped in detail, and cortical influences on motor neurons involve two nearly parallel fiber systems. The lateral corticospinal (or pyramidal) tract is a direct pathway to the spinal cord and thence to motor neurons, whereas the corticobulbar tract is the first part of an indirect and more integrative corticospinal pathway involving brain stem relay neurons, which in turn project to the spinal cord as subcortical descending tracts. These descending brain stem motor pathways in-clude the reticulospinal, vestibulospinal, rubrospinal, and descending, noradrenergic, dopaminergic, and serotoninergic pathways (Kuypers, 1981).

Electrophysiologic and anatomic studies of both carnivores and primates show that pyramidal tract fibers give rise to branches ending in thalamus, striatum, brain stem, and spinal cord that have excitatory synaptic actions (Kuypers, 1981). Fibers of cortical origin that do not travel in the pyramidal tract also make excitatory connections in the brain stem (Lawrence and Kuypers, 1968). In the primate, most pyramidal tract fibers arise from precentral Brodmann areas 4 and 6. Most of the remaining pyramidal tract fibers rise from parietal cortex. The origin of nonpyramidal corticobulbar fibers is similar (Kuypers, 1981).

Various possible neurotransmitters have been screened for their ability to mimic the normal synaptic excitatory responses evoked by cortical and pyramidal stimulation. L-Glutamate was found to be a potent excitatory agent when applied iontophoretically to the neurons in cerebral cortex, caudate nucleus, and red nucleus that are normally excited by cortical or pyramidal tract stimulation (Altman et al., 1976; Stone, 1988). L-Aspartic acid and DL-homocysteic acid also are effective excitatory agents at some of these sites. Excitatory amino acid antagonists such as glutamate diethyl ester and 2-amino-7-phosphonoheptanoic acid block some components of the excitation produced by either cortical stimulation or iontophoretic application of some amino acids (Altman et al., 1976; Herrling, 1985; Stone, 1988). In the cat, the corticocaudate excitation appears to be mediated by a quisqualate or kainate subtype of excitatory amino acid receptor and not the N-methyl-D-aspartate (NMDA) subtype (Herrling, 1985). Acetylcholine is excitatory at some sites but not at sites in the red nucleus; furthermore, there are low levels of acetylcholine and its associated synthetic enzyme, choline acetyltransferase, at sites where iontophoretically applied acetylcholine is ineffective (McLennan, 1969). Thus acetylcholine is an unlikely candidate for neurotransmitter of corticofugal neurons. The other major excitatory transmitter in the nervous system, substance P, is unlikely to be the neurotransmitter of corticofugal fibers because it is not found in cell bodies in layer V of cerebral cortex and has no known projections paralleling the pyramidal tract (Ljungdahl et al., 1978).

In addition to electrophysiologic studies, biochemical studies have established a strong correlation between markers for L-glutamate and the corticofugal fiber system. The primary biochemical markers for putative glutamatergic fibers are glutamate levels, high-affinity glutamate uptake into synaptosomes (isolated presynaptic terminals), calcium-dependent glutamate release from tissues, and retrograde transport of tritiated D-aspartate in selective pathways (Fonnum, 1984; McGeer and McGeer, 1989). These techniques have been applied to studies of various corticofugal pathways. Results of these studies are summarized in Table 24–1. Corticofugal fibers to ventrolateral thalamus, striatum, red nucleus, pons, and spinal cord have all been associated with glutamate or a glutamate-like substance (Fagg and Foster, 1983; Fonnum, 1984; Young et al., 1981, 1983).

Basal Ganglia

Striatum

The basal ganglia are important for the control of movement. Disorders of movement such as chorea, parkinsonism, athetosis, dystonia, and hemiballismus are thought to be caused by diseases of the basal ganglia.

The basal ganglia (the caudate nucleus, putamen, nucleus accumbens, pallidum, subthalamic nucleus, and substantia nigra) are deep nuclei that have a large number of interconnections and also a number of important afferent and efferent connections. One of the major afferent pathways is from the cerebral cortex and is thought to be glutamatergic (Fig. 24–1) (Fonnum, 1984; Graybiel and Ragsdale, 1983). Each area of cerebral cortex, from the most primitive olfactory structure to the most highly organized association cortex, has projections to the putamen, the caudate nucleus, the nucleus accumbens, or the outer layers of olfactory tubercle (anterior perforated substance) (Parent, 1986). These nuclei (the striatum) all have similar histochemical appearances and neurochemical properties (Graybiel and Ragsdale, 1983). Each region of striatum recieves somatotopically organized input from the cerebral cortex and sends somatotopically organized output to the medial globus pallidus, substantia nigra pars reticulata, and ventral pallidum (Switzer et al., 1982).

The more dorsal parts of the striatum (caudate nucleus and putamen) play an important role in the modulation of motor behavior (Albin et al., 1989; DeLong and Georgopoulos, 1981; Penney and Young, 1983). This behavior is mediated via input from motor, sensory, and association cortex. Caudate and putamen differ in function largely because the

Table 24–1. PUTATIVE EXCITATORY AMINO ACID PATHWAYS INVOLVED IN MAMMALIAN MOTOR FUNCTION

Pathway	Methods Used to Provide Evidence
Cerebral cortex to	
Thalamus	Uptake, electrophysiology
Striatum	Uptake, release, levels, electrophysiology
Substantia nigra	Uptake
Red nucleus	Uptake
Pontine nuclei	Uptake, release
Spinal cord	Uptake
Cerebellar	
Parallel fibers	Uptake, levels, release, electrophysiology
Climbing fibers	Uptake, levels, release

Data from reviews by Fagg and Foster (1983), Fonnum (1984), and McGeer and McGeer (1989).

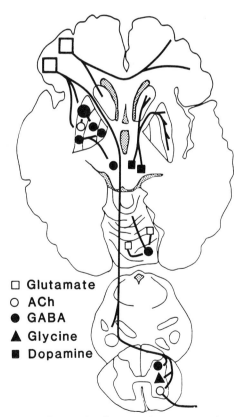

□ Glutamate
○ ACh
● GABA
▲ Glycine
■ Dopamine

Figure 24–1. Schematic diagram of neurotransmitter pathways involved in motor function in human brain. Filled symbols denote putative inhibitory pathways and open symbols denote putative excitatory pathways. Sections represent horizontal slices through human brain at the level of the caudate, putamen, external and internal globus pallidus, substantia nigra, and cerebellum; the level of the pons; and the level of the spinal cord.

projections they receive come from different areas of cortex. The caudate and putamen in turn project to the lateral segment of the globus pallidus, medial globus pallidus, and substantia nigra pars reticulata (Carpenter, 1981). The lateral global pallidus projects to the subthalamic nucleus, which in turn projects back to medial global pallidus and substantia nigra pars reticulata (Carpenter, 1981). Medial global pallidus and substantia nigra pars reticulata have major projections to the ventral lateral pars oralis and ventral medial nuclei of the thalamus (Carpenter, 1981; DeLong and Georgopoulos, 1981). These thalamic nuclei then project to premotor and supplementary motor cortex (Schell and Strick, 1984). This corticostriatopallidothalamocortical pathway is important in the selection and execution of complex motor behaviors. Disruption of the pathway causes abnormalities in the sequencing and smooth execution of various motor programs (Albin et al., 1989; Penney and Young, 1983).

A second major input to the striatum comes from dopaminergic cells of the ventral midbrain (Gerfen et al., 1987; Graybiel, 1989; Ungerstedt, 1971). Dopamine influences the corticostriatocortical feedback circuit by modulating the activity and processing of basal ganglia.

Further afferent pathways to the striatum come from the intralaminar nuclei of the thalamus, the raphe nucleus, and the locus ceruleus. The intralaminar nuclei have excitatory connections with striatal neurons, but the transmitter of this pathway is unknown. The neurotransmitter of the raphe nucleus is serotonin and that of the locus ceruleus is norepinephrine. Both serotonin and norepinephrine are involved in motor function but to a much lesser extent than dopamine.

There is a complex internal organization of the striatum. Many neurotransmitters are found in high concentration in the caudate and putamen, including acetylcholine, γ-aminobutyric acid (GABA), substance P, enkephalin, dynorphin, somatostatin, dopamine, serotonin, norepinephrine, and glutamate (Graybiel and Ragsdale, 1983). Anatomic evidence points to subcompartmentation of the striatum into clusters, patches, or "islands" of high neuronal density and a less dense surrounding "matrix." Histochemical studies in carnivores and primates have shown that the cell patches are associated with regions of light staining for acetylcholinesterase that have been termed *striosomes*. Developmentally, all the cells in the patches have the same birth date. Early in development, the patches appear as dark regions of acetylcholinesterase staining on a light background and are associated with bundles of dopamine fibers, terminals, and high levels of opiate receptor binding. Later, the surrounding areas develop dense staining, leading to the final pattern of a cholinesterase dark matrix with superimposed lighter-staining patches. As this adult pattern appears, dopamine inputs to the remaining areas of striatum develop (Graybiel and Ragsdale, 1983).

The patch and matrix differ in their connections as well. Studies with rodents indicate that patches receive input from deep layers of cortex, particularly prefrontal, and matrix receives input from more superficial layers of cortex, particularly in motor-sensory areas (Gerfen, 1989). In rodents and primates, the dopaminergic input to patch comes from the densocellular zone of the substantia nigra, whereas dopaminergic inputs to matrix come from more diffuse parts of pars compacta, the retrorubral area and the ventral tegmental area (Gerfen et al., 1987; Graybiel, 1989). Patch efferents go back to the densocellular zone of substantia nigra pars compacta, whereas matrix efferents go to both zones of globus pallidus and the substantia nigra pars reticulata (Albin et al., 1989; Gerfen, 1984; Parent, 1986).

The most numerous cell type in the striatum is the so-called medium spiny neuron as defined in Golgi studies. This neuronal type contains high concentrations of glutamic acid decarboxylase, the enzyme that is rate limiting in the synthesis of the inhibitory neurotransmitter GABA. Medium spiny neurons have also been associated with enkephalin-like, dynorphin-like, and substance P–like immunoreactivity. Indeed, these transmitter substances have been colocalized with glutamic acid decarboxylase in many caudate neurons (Oertel et al., 1983; Penny et al., 1986). A smaller number of large aspiny neurons have also been found in Golgi preparations of striatum. These neurons contain choline acetyltransferase–like immunoreactivity and are thought to use acetylcholine as their transmitter (Phelps et al., 1985). A population of small aspiny neurons is also present that contain somatostatin (DiFiglia and Aronin, 1982).

The output from the caudate and putamen comes from the medium-sized spiny neurons. Most of these striatal output cells send their axons to the lateral globus pallidus, the medial globus pallidus, or the substantia nigra pars reticulata but not to all three areas (see Fig. 24–1) (Gimenez-Amaya and Graybiel, 1990; Parent, 1986). GABA, however, is used as a neurotransmitter of fibers to all three projection areas. Substance P and dynorphin cells project predominantly to the medial globus pallidus and the substantia nigra pars reticulata, with only very minor projections to lateral globus pallidus. Enkephalin output is predominantly to the lateral globus pallidus and the ventral pallidum with minor projections to the substantia nigra pars reticulata and the medial globus pallidus. Somatostatin and acetylcholine cells are thought to be interneurons within the striatum (Albin et al., 1989).

Lateral Globus Pallidus and Subthalamic Nucleus

The cells of the lateral globus pallidus are large, polymorphic neurons. The vast majority appear to be projection neurons. The cells contain glutamic acid decarboxylase–like immunoreactivity and use GABA as a neurotransmitter (Young and Penney, 1984). They project to the subthalamic nucleus and the substantia nigra. Their primary inputs come from the striatum and the subthalamic nucleus (Carpenter, 1981).

The projections of the lateral globus pallidus to the subthalamic nucleus are somatotopically arranged, and the lateral globus pallidus in turn receives somatotopically arranged projections from the subthalamic nucleus and striatum (Parent, 1986). The subthalamic nucleus is situated ventral to the lateral portion of thalamus and dorsal to the substantia nigra (Carpenter, 1981). It receives input from the cerebral cortex and from the lateral globus pallidus. The input from cerebral cortex is excitatory and probably glutamatergic. The GABAergic input from the lateral globus pallidus is inhibitory (Young and Penney, 1984). The rostral, lateral, and ventral portions of the subthalamic nucleus project to the lateral globus pallidus. The medial, caudal, and dorsal portions of the nucleus project to the medial globus pallidus and the substantia nigra pars reticulata. The cells of the subthalamic nucleus are probably excitatory and glutamatergic (Nakanishi et al., 1987; Smith and Parent 1988). The subthalamic nucleus seems to be the source of excitatory drive to the globus pallidus and the substantia nigra pars reticulata. Lesions of the subthalamic nucleus result in hemiballismus or chorea. The enkephalin-GABA striatopallidal efferents probably serve to disinhibit the subthalamic nucleus, and when the enkephalin-GABA cells are not functional, the subthalamic nucleus is excessively inhibited by the lateral pallidum. Damage to the striatal enkephalin cells may be the cause of the chorea seen in Huntington's disease (HD) (Albin et al., 1989).

Medial Globus Pallidus

The known afferents to the medial globus pallidus come from the caudate and putamen as well as from the subthalamic nucleus. The cells of the medial globus pallidus are GABAergic and inhibitory (Penney and Young, 1983). They project to the magnocellular portion of the ventral lateral nucleus (pars oralis) of the thalamus. The latter area of thalamus does not receive major inputs from other subcortical structures and it, in turn, projects to supplementary motor cortex (Schell and Strick, 1984).

Substantia Nigra

Pars Reticulata

The substantia nigra pars reticulata and the medial globus pallidus, which are separated developmentally by the internal capsule, are thought to be similar structures (DeLong and Georgopoulos, 1981). Cells in the substantia nigra pars reticulata are GABAergic. They receive input from the striatum and the subthalamic nucleus. These neurons have extensive dendritic fields that interact with the dendritic fields of the substantia nigra pars compacta neurons. Substantia nigra pars reticulata neurons have extensive axon collaterals that feed back onto other reticulata neurons as well as onto pars compacta neurons (Young and Penney, 1984). Pars reticulata neurons project either to ventromedial thalamus or to the superior colliculus and the brain stem reticular formation (Beckstead and Frankfurter, 1982). It is thought that the projection to superior colliculus is an important pathway in the eye movement disorders seen in basal ganglia disease (Albin et al., 1989). Ventromedial thalamic neurons project diffusely to layer I of frontal cortex (Herkenham, 1979).

Pars Compacta

The neurons of the pars compacta have been studied extensively. These are pigmented cells in the rostral midbrain that contain dopamine and melanin. They have extensive dendritic trees that extend into the pars reticulata. Their projections have been described. There are also dopaminergic projections to the nucleus accumbens, but those projections come primarily from the dopamine neurons in the adjacent ventral tegmental area (Graybiel, 1989). The cells of the compacta receive glycinergic input, presumably from interneurons, and GABAergic input from axon collaterals of the pars reticulata neurons. The dopamine cells also receive noradrenergic and serotoninergic input from the raphe nucleus and the locus ceruleus.

Cerebellum

The cerebellum is a highly structured area of the nervous system overlying the brain stem. The neuroanatomy and neurophysiology of the cerebellum are well known and are reviewed in Chapter 23. There are five neuronal types within the cerebellar cortex, and four of these are inhibitory. The inhibitory cells include the well-known Purkinje cell, the stellate and basket cells of the molecular layer, and the Golgi cell, which is contained primarily in the granule cell layer. The sole excitatory neuron in the cerebellum is the granule cell.

Input to the cerebellar cortex comes from mossy fibers and from climbing fibers. The transmitter of the mossy fibers is unknown; that of the climbing fibers is thought to be aspartate (Fagg and Foster, 1983) except for the portion of fibers that are noradrenergic and come from the locus ceruleus. The mossy fibers synapse on granule cells and Golgi cells in the granule cell layer. The climbing fibers synapse directly on Purkinje cells. The granule cells project to the molecular layer and branch to form the parallel fibers with synapses on the dendritic spines of multiple Purkinje cells. The neurotransmitter of the granule cells is thought to be glutamate (Young et al., 1974); all the other cerebellar cortical cells appear to use GABA (Schulman, 1983). The basket and stellate cells are influenced by both granule cell and climbing fiber input and modify the behavior of the Purkinje cells. The Purkinje cells are the sole output cells of the cerebellar cortex and are GABAergic and inhibitory on the deep nuclei of cerebellum. Peptide neuromodulators are also contained in cerebellar neurons. Motilin-like immunoreactivity is located in some Purkinje cells, and enkephalin is located in some Golgi cells and mossy fibers (Schulman, 1983).

The deep nuclei (dentate, emboliform, globos, and fastigial nuclei) have some direct projections to the spinal cord but primarily project to neurons in the reticular formation, vestibular nuclei, red nucleus, and thalamus. The neurotransmitter of the deep cerebellar nuclei is unknown but is excitatory and, possibly, glutamate.

Spinal Cord

The anatomy of the spinal cord is complex and will not be reviewed in detail here. Only the aspects pertinent to motor pharmacology will be touched on. The large motor neurons of the ventral horn contain high concentrations of choline acetyltransferase and use acetylcholine as a neurotransmitter (Houser et al., 1983). They are influenced directly and indirectly by numerous descending pathways and by various afferent systems. Multiple inhibitory and excitatory interneuronal systems in the spinal cord have been studied as well (Baldissera et al., 1981; Grillner and Dubuc, 1988).

The amino acid glycine is thought to be the neurotransmitter of the so-called Ia inhibitory interneurons, which receive input from both descending pathways and peripheral Ia afferents (Fig. 24–2). These interneurons mediate reciprocal inhibition during reflex action and coordinated motor activity. Glycine is also thought to be the neurotransmitter of the Renshaw cells, which mediate recurrent inhibition in the ventral horn. Two infamous toxins act by blocking the actions of glycine and causing marked hyperreflexia at all levels of the nervous system. Tetanus toxin, a product of *Clostridium tetani*, prevents the release of glycine from presynaptic terminals. Strychnine is a potent alkaloid that antagonizes the action of glycine at its receptor (Young and Macdonald, 1983).

In the spinal cord, GABA is also an important inhibitory neurotransmitter. GABA interneurons in the dorsal horn of the spinal cord receive excitatory input from primary afferents at one level and then synapse directly on the axon terminals of primary afferents from an adjacent level (Hunt, 1983). At these axoaxonic synapses, GABA depolarizes the axon terminals and inhibits release from the primary afferent. GABA can thus modulate the activity of sensory input. This process is called *presynaptic inhibition*.

Excitatory glutamatergic and aspartatergic neurons are also thought to exist in spinal cord (Davidoff et al., 1967), but their connections are less well known (Davidoff, 1985). Descending glutamate inputs have

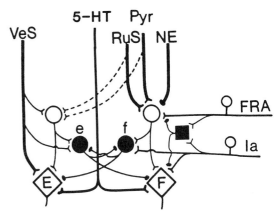

Figure 24–2. Supraspinal and afferent inputs to GABAergic interneurons and reciprocal Ia interneurons of the lumbar spinal cord. Open circles denote excitatory interneurons; filled circles, glycinergic inhibitory interneurons; filled square, a GABAergic inhibitory interneuron. The descending vestibulospinal (VeS), rubrospinal (RuS), pyramidal tract (Pyr), and descending serotonin (5-HT) pathways are excitatory, and the descending norepinephrine pathway (NE) is inhibitory. A primary muscle spindle afferent (Ia) is shown projecting to a GABAergic interneuron, a flexor motor neuron (F), and a flexor-coupled Ia interneuron (f). Similar projections exist to the extensor motor neurons (E) and extensor-coupled interneurons (e) but are not shown here. The flexor reflex afferents (FRA) project indirectly to ipsilateral flexor motor neurons and flexor-coupled Ia interneurons. (Modified from Young A.B., Macdonald R.L. Glycine as a spinal cord neurotransmitter. In Davidoff R.A., ed. *Handbook of the Spinal Cord*. New York, Marcel Dekker, pp. 1–43, 1983 by courtesy of Marcel Dekker Inc.)

not been defined in terms of their specific cellular connections. However, it is thought that corticofugal (glutamatergic) fibers synapse directly on motor neurons as well as on GABA, glycine, and other interneurons (Baldissera et al., 1981).

Descending catecholamine and serotonin pathways also play a role in the control of spinal reflex mechanisms (Anderson, 1983; Marshall, 1983). Noradrenergic input to spinal cord interneurons is important in the control of flexor reflex afferent input (see Fig. 24–2) as well as in controlling tonic and phasic γ motor neurons (Anderson, 1983; Grillner and Dubuc, 1988). Descending serotonin pathways affect motor neuron activity and increase motor reflexes in flexor and extensor muscles (Grillner and Dubuc, 1988; Marshall, 1983).

Neuropeptides are found in high concentrations in the spinal cord. Immunoreactivity for many peptides is found in the small-diameter unmyelinated primary afferent fibers and in the substantia gelatinosa of the spinal cord (Hunt, 1983). The role of these neuropeptides in motor function is unknown. Further study of the role of peptides in spinal cord is warranted.

NEUROPHARMACOLOGY OF MOTOR DISORDERS

Spasticity

Spasticity is an abnormality of tone characterized by increased resistance to passive manipulation of a joint. In particular, it is a velocity-dependent increase in tone that is followed by a relaxation phase. It is thus characterized by the so-called clasp-knife phenomenon. Spasticity arises from interruption of the corticospinal tract at any level between the cerebral cortex and the spinal cord. The increased tone seen in spasticity caused by damage above the cervical spinal cord is characterized by increased flexor tone in the upper extremities with flexion at the elbow and at the wrist and increased extensor tone in the lower extremity with increased extension at the knee and ankle. Concomitant with the tone changes are a number of other symptoms and signs. Deep tendon reflexes become hyperactive, and clonus can often be elicited at the affected joints. In patients with spinal cord or brain stem lesions, abnormal flexor or extensor spasms can be elicited by cutaneous stimulation. These spasms cause painful contraction of the muscles in the affected limb (see also Chapters 20 and 21).

The neurochemistry of spasticity has been studied only to a limited extent. There is evidence that glutamate is a neurotransmitter of the corticospinal tract (Fonnum, 1984; Young et al., 1983). There have, however, been no studies of calcium-dependent glutamate release, high-affinity glutamate uptake, or glutamate receptors in cases of spasticity. The pharmacology of glutamatergic systems is limited. Many glutamate agonist drugs are neurotoxins and convulsants. Thus, therapies directed toward glutamate replacement have not received much attention. Glycine has been found to enhance activity at the NMDA subtype of excitatory amino acid receptor, and blockers of NMDA receptors or the glycine modulatory site may be useful muscle relaxants (Turski et al., 1987). Drugs that block the function of glutamate at its receptors have been synthesized and are being evaluated for their potential as anticonvulsant and muscle relaxant medications. Few of these substances have been looked at in models of spasticity.

The drug baclofen, which interacts with a specific subtype of GABA receptor, the $GABA_B$ receptor (Bowery et al., 1984), is an inhibitor of glutamate release (Potashner, 1978). Baclofen is beneficial in the treatment of spasticity (Davidoff, 1985). There may be supersensitive glutamate receptors on motor neurons in spasticity to account for the drug's effectiveness. Glutamate supersensitivity would result in increased responsiveness to the glutamate pathways that are still intact, such as primary afferents and local interneuron circuits. Thus, baclofen may act by reducing glutamate release at the spinal cord level and suppressing segmental reflexes (Davidoff, 1985). Alternatively, baclofen may alter the release of other neurotransmitters from other descending or afferent pathways such as the descending noradrenergic or serotonin ones (Bowery et al., 1984).

The GABA interneurons in dorsal and intermediate gray of spinal cord that mediate the presynaptic inhibition of primary afferent input are underactive in spasticity (Delwaide, 1973). Many of the current therapies for spasticity have been directed at increasing GABAergic function in the nervous system (Davidoff, 1985). Benzodiazepines have also been used because benzodiazepine receptors have been closely linked to GABA receptors at all levels of the nervous system. However, GABAergic agonists and benzodiazepines tend to be nondiscriminatory in their effect on spasticity. Dosages that reduce tone in the spastic limbs also cause sedation and ataxia and provide only minimal relief from flexor spasms and clonus (Landau, 1974). Although the spinal cord GABA interneurons appear to be physiologically underactive in spasticity, no one has found increased GABA or benzodiazepine receptors in spinal cords of spastic animals or humans.

The other major inhibitory interneuron in spinal cord, the glycine interneuron, mediates postsynaptic inhibition and reciprocal Ia inhibition. Animal studies indicate that glycine levels, uptake, and turnover are decreased in the spinal cord in spasticity (Hall et al., 1979). In spastic humans, physiologic studies suggest that the glycine interneurons are underactive (Delwaide, 1973). Furthermore, although glycine crosses the blood-brain barrier poorly, systemic administration of glycine to spastic patients and animals has proved beneficial (Davidoff, 1985). Unfortunately, no potent glycine agonists have been produced that can cross the blood-brain barrier and be used in the treatment of spasticity.

An important but often underemphasized part of spasticity is the role of descending catecholamine (Marshall, 1983) and serotonin (Anderson, 1983) pathways in the regulation of reflex activity and tone. Animal studies indicate that catecholamines are important in regulating flexor reflex afferent pathways and overall reflex mechanisms at the spinal cord level (Grillner and Dubuc, 1988). Lesions of the corticospinal tract above the brain stem, which spare the brain stem serotonin and catecholamine nuclei (raphe nuclei, locus ceruleus, and substantia nigra), result frequently in increased tone of the clasp-knife variety and clonus but rarely in flexor or extensor spasms. In these patients, the descending catecholamine and serotonin pathways may be relatively overactive. One therapeutic approach has been to antagonize noradrenergic responses in such cases using α-adrenergic antagonists (Davidoff, 1985; Mai, 1978). $α_2$-Adrenergic agonists have also been found effective in the treatment of spasticity (Hutchinson, 1989).

In patients with primary brain stem or spinal cord lesions, the descending catecholamine pathways are often interrupted. In these patients, descending adrenergic input is presumably deficient, particularly because animal studies suggest that catecholamine, dopamine, and serotonin receptor levels are increased in spinal cord below the level of a cord lesion (Anderson, 1983; Marshall, 1983). Thus adrenergic and dopaminergic agonists may be effective for relief of such symptoms as flexor and extensor spasms. These drugs could be used in combination with drugs that have overall effects on tone, such as baclofen or the benzodiazepines, to ameliorate the symptoms of spasticity.

In summary, much work needs to be done to understand the underlying neurochemistry of spasticity. However, each symptom of spasticity may have a unique pathophysiology that must be treated selectively. Thus, symptoms such as increased tone and clonus may be alleviated most effectively by drugs that block glutamate and noradrenergic function or augment GABA and glycine function. Patients with prominent flexor or extensor spasms may best be treated with drugs that augment noradrenergic function.

The Choreas

Huntington's Disease

HD is a dominantly inherited disorder characterized by progressive intellectual dysfunction and abnormal involuntary movements (see Chapter 87). The neuropathology of HD is characterized by severe neuronal loss and gliosis in the caudate and putamen (de la Monte et al., 1988; Roos, 1986; Vonsattel et al., 1985). There is also some cell loss in globus pallidus, substantia nigra pars reticulata, thalamus, and cortex. The observed neurotransmitter abnormalities in Huntington's disease are what one would expect with profound loss of nerve cells in the caudate and putamen (Perry et al., 1973; Young and Penney, 1984). There are decreases in GABA, glutamic acid decarboxylase, substance P, angiotensin-converting enzyme, and enkephalin levels locally in the caudate and putamen and in their projection areas, globus pallidus and substantia nigra pars reticulata. Because the inputs to caudate and putamen from the locus ceruleus, dorsal raphe nucleus, and substantia nigra pars compacta are relatively spared in HD, the striatal concentrations of norepinephrine, serotonin, and dopamine on a per gram basis are increased.

Concentrations of three peptides, somatostatin, neurotensin, and thyrotropin-releasing hormone, appear to be increased in the striatum of HD patients (Martin, 1984; Nemeroff et al., 1983). The role of these peptides in striatal function is unknown. The increase in observed somatostatin levels appears to reflect in part sparing of a class of striatal neurons in the disease process (Ferrante et al., 1985). The findings may have important implications for the pathophysiology of this disorder.

The receptor changes seen in brains in HD are again consistent with loss of nerve cell bodies in the caudate and putamen (Young and Penney, 1984). In the caudate and putamen, there are large decreases in glutamate, muscarinic cholinergic, GABA, benzodiazepine, opiate, and dopamine receptor levels. In the immediate striatal projection areas GABA receptor levels are increased in the globus pallidus and the pars reticulata, consistent with the development of denervation supersensitivity. The number of ben-

zodiazepine-binding sites also changes in parallel with the GABA receptor alterations. New evidence suggests that the earliest lesions in HD are loss of glutamate receptors and striatopallidal enkephalin neurons (Albin et al., 1990).

Although the neurochemistry of HD has been well defined, the treatment of this disorder has been much less rewarding than the treatment of Parkinson's disease. Currently the most commonly used agents are the neuroleptic agents that block dopamine receptors (Shoulson, 1984). This treatment is most effective early in the disease, when dopamine receptor levels are presumably not significantly reduced. The use of GABAergic agents has not led to any substantial improvement in symptoms in HD despite the profound loss of GABA in HD (Shoulson, 1984). The fact that the GABA output cells to the pallidum and the substantia nigra pars reticulata make synapses on other GABA cells that project from the globus pallidus and pars reticulata to the thalamus may in part explain the lack of utility of these agents. With two sequential GABA neurons, restoration of GABAergic function in the striatopallidal system may be counterbalanced by simultaneous augmentation of pallidothalamic GABA pathways. Alternatively, replacement of GABA may not be sufficient to restore the complex pattern of activity in interconnections and projections required for normal movement.

Hemiballismus

Hemiballismus is a unilateral movement disorder characterized by high-amplitude, proximal arrhythmic jerks of the affected arm and/or leg. It is accompanied by distal smaller-amplitude choreic movements. Hemiballismus is caused by lesions in the subthalamic nucleus (Carpenter, 1981). This disorder can arise from inflammatory lesions, stroke, or tumor involvement in the nucleus. Because the neurotransmitter of the subthalamic nucleus is probably glutamatergic, no specific therapies are available for hemiballismus. Neuroleptic agents are commonly used with variable success. Alternatively, high doses of benzodiazepines have been given to suppress the movements. Often drugs are ineffective, and patients have died from exhaustion with the disorder. If patients survive, the amplitude and the frequency of the movements tend to decrease, and the patient may be left with only mild or moderate choreiform movements (see also Chapter 22).

Tardive Dyskinesia

Tardive dyskinesia is a drug-induced movement disorder that occurs in patients being treated with agents that block dopamine receptors, such as the phenothiazines, butyrophenones, and thioxanthenes (Tarsy and Baldessarini, 1984). The elderly and those given prolonged high-dose treatment are the most susceptible. The primary etiology of this disorder is unknown, although changes in the dopamine receptor and in striatal GABAergic systems have been suggested (Fibiger and Lloyd, 1984; Tarsy and Baldessarini, 1984). Postmortem studies of patients who died with tardive dyskinesia have suggested equivocal changes in dopamine receptors. Dopamine receptor blockade in animals results in increased cholinergic and GABAergic turnover in striatum, but markers of GABAergic function may be decreased in tardive dyskinesia. Current therapies are directed primarily at decreasing dopamine synthesis, storage, and release with drugs such as reserpine, tetrabenazine, low-dose ergot alkaloids, or clonidine (Goetz and Klawans, 1984). Lecithin and certain GABAergic agents have also been used in attempts to augment both cholinergic and GABAergic function (Tarsy and Baldessarini, 1984; Thaker et al., 1990).

Other Choreas

Sydenham's chorea (one of the primary manifestations of rheumatic fever) and chorea gravidarum are seen rarely now. Sydenham's chorea is typically seen weeks to months after the other symptoms of rheumatic fever. Virtually nothing is known about the neurochemistry of either condition. Neuroleptics have been used for treatment.

Parkinsonism

Drug-Induced Parkinsonism

The classic triad of parkinsonian symptoms are bradykinesia, rigidity, and tremor. Neuroleptic agents (such as the phenothiazines and butyrophenones) and other dopamine-blocking drugs such as metoclopramide (Reglan) (Indo and Ando, 1982) have been found to produce parkinsonian symptoms. Drug-induced parkinsonism is common because of the wide use of neuroleptic agents in the treatment of mental illness. The propensity for a neuroleptic agent to produce parkinsonism is related to the potency of the drug in blocking dopamine receptors and inversely to the potency of the drug in blocking muscarinic cholinergic receptors (Snyder et al., 1974). Certain classes of neuroleptics (the atypical neuroleptics) produce few parkinsonian side effects. In general, these atypical agents have been found to affect mesolimbic dopamine pathways from the ventral tegmental area with few effects on the substantia nigra pars compacta neurons (Chiodo and Bunney, 1983; White and Wang, 1983). The neurochemical and receptor changes underlying these differential effects on pars compacta versus ventral tegmental neurons are under investigation. In the future, drugs may be produced that have effects primarily on the mesolimbic dopamine system with few or no effects on the nigrostriatal system.

Idiopathic Parkinsonism

Parkinson's disease is characterized by a loss of dopamine neurons in the substantia nigra pars com-

pacta (see also Chapters 22 and 86). Loss of these neurons can be caused by viruses, atherosclerotic disease, manganese intoxication, N-methyl-4-phenyl-1,2,3,6-tetrahydropyridine (MPTP) ingestion (David et al., 1979; Langston et al., 1983), and unknown (idiopathic) factors. The disease is characterized by large decreases in striatal concentrations of dopamine, homovanillic acid (the major metabolite of dopamine), and tyrosine hydroxylase (the rate-limiting enzyme in dopamine synthesis). There are also changes in dopamine receptors in Parkinson's disease (Rinne, 1982; Young and Penney, 1984). Two types of dopamine receptors have been defined: D_1 and D_2 (Creese et al., 1983; Seeman, 1983). Both types have a state with relatively low affinity for agonists and one with high affinity for agonists. The D_1 receptor is linked to and stimulates the enzyme adenylate cyclase in the striatum. The D_2 receptor inhibits this enzyme. The D_2 receptor has high affinity for the various neuroleptic drugs, such as the phenothiazines, butyrophenones, and thioxanthenes. D_2 receptors are thought to mediate the antipsychotic and extrapyramidal motor effects of these drugs. There is evidence that D_1 receptor activation is necessary for normal D_2 receptor activation (Walters et al., 1987). There are also dopamine D_2 autoreceptors that control the release of dopamine from dopamine terminals. Agonists at the autoreceptor decrease dopamine release; antagonists promote release. Dopamine itself, several of the ergot alkaloids (apomorphine, bromocriptine, pergolide, and lisuride), and the neuroleptics interact potently with these autoreceptors. Thus, at extremely low doses, dopamine agonists may make parkinsonian symptoms worse.

In the brains of patients with Parkinson's disease, the D_1 receptor levels are reduced to 20–30% of those seen in normal caudate nucleus and putamen (Rinne, 1982). The functional significance of this change is unknown. The D_2 receptor levels, on the other hand, are significantly increased in brains of untreated patients who die of Parkinson's disease (Lee et al., 1978; Rinne, 1982). This change is thought to be due to an attempt by the brain to compensate for the major dopamine deficit in this disease.

Dopamine affects striatal GABA and cholinergic function (Albin et al., 1989). Therefore, other treatment strategies in Parkinson's disease have been to block cholinergic function with anticholinergic agents and to modify GABAergic function. Although anticholinergic agents are useful, to date no GABAergic drugs have been found effective. Various other receptors and neurotransmitter substances are altered in Parkinson's disease, but currently no other specific drug therapies have been found useful in treating the disease. In fact, the most potent antiparkinsonian drug is levodopa in combination with a peripherally acting dopa decarboxylase inhibitor such as carbidopa or benserazide (the combinations are Sinemet or Madopar, respectively).

Until recently, all treatment for Parkinson's disease has been symptomatic. Preliminary evidence now suggests that selegiline (deprenyl, Eldepryl), a selective inhibitor of monoamine oxidase type B, may slow down the deterioration of dopamine neurons (Parkinson Study Group, 1989; Tetrud and Langston, 1989). By inhibiting monoamine oxidase type B, the drug may protect against protoxins activated by the enzyme or against the hydroxyl radicals produced by the enzyme reactions.

Cerebellar Degenerations

Little is known about the neurochemistry of the cerebellar degenerations, although some measurements have been made in patients post mortem. There appear to be abnormalities in glutamate and aspartate levels in the spinal cord of patients who die with Friedreich's ataxia (Butterworth and Giguere, 1982; Huxtable et al., 1979). Abnormalities in other amino acid levels have also been seen, but the relevance of these changes to the pathophysiology of the spinocerebellar degenerations is unknown. Likewise, the neurochemistry of most of the olivopontocerebellar atrophies is unknown. However, abnormalities of glutamate dehydrogenase levels have been observed in fibroblasts and lymphocytes from patients with the recessive type IV olivopontocerebellar atrophy (Duvoisin et al., 1983; Plaitakis et al., 1982). Plasma levels of glutamate and aspartate were increased after a glutamate load in these cases. It has been suggested that these increased glutamate levels may be neurotoxic to neurons, resulting in accelerated neuronal cell death in the areas of brain with high concentrations of glutamate receptors. Neurochemical studies of the brains of patients who die with olivopontocerebellar atrophy have shown prominent receptor changes (Albin and Gilman, 1990; Kish et al., 1989; Makowiec et al., 1990).

Treatment of cerebellar ataxia with pharmacologic agents has been disappointing. Numerous trials with β-adrenergic blockers, GABAergic agonists, and other drugs have not resulted in substantial relief of cerebellar symptoms. The cholinergic agonist physostigmine may offer some relief (Kark et al., 1981). Isoniazid has been reported to be effective in selected cases of ataxia (Sabra et al., 1982), but the effects are not dramatic. The rationale for using isoniazid is that it inhibits the synthesis of GABA as well as its degradation by interfering with the vitamin B_6 cofactors necessary for the activity of glutamate decarboxylase and GABA transaminase. In animals, low doses of isoniazid raise GABA levels and high doses lower them (see also Chapter 23).

CONCLUSION

Much is known about the neurochemistry of the motor system but much also remains to be learned before ideal therapies for motor disorders are available. There has been accelerated acquisition of information concerning the synaptic circuitry, neurochemistry, and neuropharmacology of pathways involved in motor function. Further breakthroughs and innovation in the pharmacotherapy of movement disorders can be expected. Additional investigations of postmortem tissues and more sophisticated studies of the functional anatomy of transmitter-specific pathways in living humans with techniques such as positron emission tomography will further enhance our knowledge.

References

(Key references are designated with an asterisk.)

Albin R.L., Gilman S. Autoradiographic localization of inhibitory and excitatory amino acid neurotransmitter receptors in human normal and olivopontocerebellar atrophy cerebellar cortex. *Brain Res.* 522:37–45, 1990.

*Albin R.L., Young A.B., Penney J.B. The functional anatomy of basal ganglia disorders. *Trends Neurosci.* 12:366–375, 1989.

Albin R.L., Young A.B., Penney J.B., et al. Abnormalities of striatal projection neurons and N-methyl-D-aspartate receptors in presymptomatic Huntington's disease. *N. Engl. J. Med.* 322:1293–1298, 1990.

Altman H., ten Bruggeneate G., Picklemann P., et al. Effects of glutamate, aspartate and two presumed antagonists on feline rubrospinal neurons. *Pflugers Arch.* 364:249–255, 1976.

Anderson E.G. The serotonin system in the spinal cord. In Davidoff R.A., ed. *Handbook of the Spinal Cord.* Vol. I. *Pharmacology.* New York, Marcel Dekker, pp. 241–328, 1983.

Baldissera F., Hultborn, H., Illert M. Integration in spinal neuronal systems. In Brooks V.B., ed. *Handbook of Physiology.* Section 1. *The Nervous System.* Vol. II. *Motor Control.* Bethesda, American Physiological Society, pp. 509–595, 1981.

Beckstead R.M., Frankfurter A. The distribution and some morphological features of substantia nigra neurons that project to the thalamus, superior colliculus and pedunculopontine nucleus in the monkey. *Neuroscience* 7:2377–2388, 1982.

Bowery N.G., Price G.W., Hudson A.L., et al. GABA receptor multiplicity. *Neuropharmacology* 23:219–231, 1984.

Butterworth R., Giguere J.-F. Selective spinal cord amino acid abnormalities in Friedreich's ataxia. *Soc. Neurosci. Abstr.* 8:152, 1982.

*Carpenter M.B. Anatomy of the corpus striatum and brainstem integrating systems. In Brooks V.B., ed. *Handbook of Physiology.* Section 1. *The Nervous System.* Vol. II. *Motor Control.* Bethesda, American Physiological Society, pp. 947–995, 1981.

Chiodo L.A., Bunney B.S. Typical and atypical neuroleptics: differential effects of chronic administration on the activity of A9 and A10 midbrain dopaminergic neurons. *J. Neurosci.* 3:1607–1619, 1983.

Creese I., Sibley D.R., Hamblin M.W., et al. The classification of dopamine receptors: relationship to radioligand binding. *Annu. Rev. Neurosci.* 6:43–71, 1983.

David G.C., Williams A.C., Markey S.P., et al. Chronic parkinsonism secondary to intravenous injection of meperidine analogues. *Psychiatry Res.* 1:249–254, 1979.

Davidoff R.A. Antispasticity drugs: mechanisms of action. *Ann. Neurol.* 17:107–116, 1985.

Davidoff R.A., Graham L.T. Jr., Shank R.P., et al. Changes in amino acid concentrations associated with loss of spinal interneurons. *J. Neurochem.* 14:1025–1031, 1967.

de la Monte S.M., Vonsattal J.-P., Richardson E.P. Morphometric demonstration of atrophic changes in the cerebral cortex, white matter, and neostriatum in Huntington's disease. *J. Neuropathol. Exp. Neurol.* 47:516–525, 1988.

*DeLong M.R. Georgopoulos A.P. Motor functions of the basal ganglia. In Brooks V.B., ed. *Handbook of Physiology.* Section 1. *The Nervous System.* Vol. II. *Motor Control.* Bethesda, American Physiological Society, pp. 1017–1061, 1981.

Delwaide P.J. Human monosynaptic reflexes and presynaptic inhibition. In Desmedt J.E., ed. *New Developments in Electromyography and Clinical Neurophysiology.* Vol. 3. Basel, Karger, pp. 508–522, 1973.

DiFiglia M., Aronin N. Ultrastructural features of immunoreactive somatostatin neurons in the rat caudate nucleus. *J. Neurosci.* 2:1267–1274, 1982.

Duvoisin R.C., Chokroverty S., Lepore F., et al. Glutamate dehydrogenase deficiency in patients with olivopontocerebellar atrophy. *Neurology (N.Y.)* 33:1322–1326, 1983.

Fagg G.E., Foster A.C. Amino acid neurotransmitters and their pathways in the mammalian central nervous system. *Neuroscience* 9:701–719, 1983.

Ferrante R.J., Kowall N.W., Beal M.F., et al. Selective sparing of a class of striatal neurons in Huntington's disease. *Science* 230:561–563, 1985.

Fibiger H.C., Lloyd K.G. Neurobiological substrates of tardive dyskinesia: the GABA hypothesis. *Trends Neurosci.* 7:462–464, 1984.

Fonnum F. Glutamate: a neurotransmitter in mammalian brain. *J. Neurochem.* 42:1–11, 1984.

Gerfen C.R. The neostriatal mosaic: compartmentalization of corticostriatal input and striatonigral output. *Nature* 311:461–464, 1984.

Gerfen C.R. The neostriatal mosaic: striatal patch-matrix organizations related to cortical lamination. *Science* 246:385–388, 1989.

Gerfen C.R., Herkenham M., Thibault J. The neostriatal mosaic. II. Patch- and matrix-directed mesostriatal dopaminergic and non-dopaminergic systems. *J. Neurosci.* 7:3935–3944, 1987.

Gimenez-Amaya J.M., Graybiel A.M. Compartmental origins of the striatopallidal projection in the primate. *Neuroscience* 34:111–126, 1990.

Goetz C.G., Klawans H.L. Tardive dyskinesia. *Neurol. Clin.* 2:605–614, 1984.

*Graybiel A.M. Dopaminergic and cholinergic systems in the striatum. In Crossman A.R., Sambrook M.A., eds. *Neural Mechanisms in Disorders of Movement,* London, Libbey, pp. 3–16, 1989.

*Graybiel A.M., Ragsdale C.W. Jr. Biochemical anatomy of the striatum. In Emson P.C., ed. *Chemical Neuroanatomy.* New York, Raven Press, pp. 427–504, 1983.

Grillner S., Dubuc R. Control of locomotion in vertebrates: spinal and supraspinal mechanisms. *Adv. Neurol.* 47:425–453, 1988.

Hall P.V., Smith J.E., Lane J., et al. Glycine and experimental spinal spasticity. *Neurology (Minneap.)* 29:262–267, 1979.

Herkenham M. The afferent and efferent connections of the ventromedial thalamic nucleus in the rat. *J. Comp. Neurol.* 153:487–518, 1979.

Herrling P.L. Pharmacology of the corticocaudate excitatory postsynaptic potential in the cat: evidence for its mediation by quisqualate or kainate receptors. *Neuroscience* 14:417–426, 1985.

Houser C.R., Crawford G.D., Barber R.P., et al. Organization and morphological characteristics of cholinergic neurons: an immunocytochemical study with a monoclonal antibody to choline acetyltransferase. *Brain Res.* 266:97–119, 1983.

Hunt S.P. Cytochemistry of the spinal cord. In Emson P.C., ed. *Chemical Neuroanatomy.* New York, Raven Press, pp. 53–81, 1983.

Hutchinson D.R. Modified release tizanidine: a review. *J. Int. Med. Res.* 17:565–573, 1989.

Huxtable R., Azari J., Reisine T., et al. Regional distribution of amino acids in Friedreich's ataxia brains. *Can. J. Neurol. Sci.* 6:255–258, 1979.

Indo T., Ando K. Metoclopramide-induced parkinsonism—clinical characteristics of 10 cases. *Arch. Neurol.* 39:494–496, 1982.

Kark R.Z., Pieter B., Maria M.R., et al. Double-blind, triple-crossover trial of low doses of oral physostigmine in inherited ataxias. *Neurology* 31:288–292, 1981.

Kish S.J., Li P.P., Robaitaille Y., et al. Cerebellar [³H]inositol-1,4,5-triphosphate binding is markedly decreased in human olivopontocerebellar atrophy. *Brain Res.* 489:473–376, 1989.

*Kuypers H.G.J.M. Anatomy of the descending pathways. In Brooks V.B., ed. *Handbook of Physiology.* Section 1. *The Nervous System.* Vol. II. *Motor Control.* Bethesda, American Physiological Society, pp. 597–665, 1981.

Landau W.M. Spasticity: the fable of a neurological demon and the emperor's new therapy. *Arch. Neurol.* 31:217–219, 1974.

Langston J.W., Ballard P., Tetrud J.W., et al. Chronic parkinsonism in humans due to a product of meperidine-analog synthesis. *Science* 219:979–980, 1983.

Lawrence D.G., Kuypers H.G.J.M. The functional organization of the motor system in the monkey. II. The effects of lesions of the descending brain-stem pathways. *Brain* 91:15–36, 1968.

Lee T., Seeman P., Rajput A., et al. Receptor basis for dopaminergic supersensitivity in Parkinson's disease. *Nature* 273:59–61, 1978.

Ljungdahl A., Hökfelt T., Nilsson G. Distribution of substance P–like immunoreactivity in the central nervous system of the rat. I. Cell bodies and nerve terminals. *Neuroscience* 3:861–943, 1978.

Mai J. Depression of spasticity of alpha-adrenergic blockade. *Acta Neurol. Scand.* 57:65–76, 1978.

Makowiec R.L., Albin R.L., Cha J.J., et al. Two types of quisqualate receptors are decreased in human olivopontocerebellar atrophy cerebellar cortex. *Brain Res.* 523:309–312, 1990.

Marshall K.C. Catecholamines and their actions in the spinal cord. In Davidoff R.A., ed. *Handbook of the Spinal Cord.* Vol. I. *Pharmacology.* New York, Marcel Dekker, pp. 275–328, 1983.

Martin J.B. Huntington's disease: new approaches to an old problem. The Robert Wartenberg lecture. *Neurology (N.Y.)* 34:1059–1072, 1984.

McGeer P.L., McGeer E.G. Amino acid neurotransmitters. In Siegel G.J., Albers R.W., Agranoff B.W., et al., eds. *Basic Neurochemistry.* 4th ed. Boston, Little Brown, pp. 311–332, 1989.

McLennan H. Cholinesterase in the feline red nucleus. *Int. J. Neuropharmacol.* 8:489–490, 1969.

Nakanishi H., Kita H., Kitai S.T. Intracellular study of rat substantia nigra pars reticulata neurons in an in vitro slice preparation: electrical membrane properties and response characteristics to subthalamic stimulation. *Brain Res.* 437:45–55, 1987.

Nemeroff C.B., Youngblood W.W., Mamberg P.J., et al. Regional brain concentrations of neuropeptides in Huntington's chorea and schizophrenia. *Science* 221:972–975, 1983.

Oertel W.H., Riethmuler G., Mugnaini E., et al. Opioid peptide–like immunoreactivity localized in GABAergic neurons of rat neostriatum and central amygdaloid nucleus. *Life Sci.* 33(Suppl.):73–76, 1983.

Parent A. *Comparative Neurobiology of the Basal Ganglia.* New York, Wiley, 1986.

Parkinson Study Group. Effect of deprenyl on the progression of disability in early Parkinson's disease. *N. Engl. J. Med.* 321:1364–1371, 1989.

*Penney J.B., Young A.B. Speculations on the functional anatomy of basal ganglia disorders. *Annu. Rev. Neurosci.* 6:73–94, 1983.

Penny G.R., Afsharpour S., Kitai S.T. The glutamate decarboxylase–, leucine enkephalin–, methionine enkephalin–, and substance P–immunoreactive neurons in the neostriatum of the rat and cat: evidence for partial population overlap. *Neuroscience* 17:1011–1045, 1986.

Perry T.L., Hansen S., Kloster M. Huntington's chorea: deficiency of gamma-aminobutyric acid in brain. *N. Engl. J. Med.* 288:337–342, 1973.

Phelps P.E., Houser C.R., Vaughn J.E. Immunocytochemical localization of choline acetyltransferase within the rat neostriatum: a correlated light and electron microscopic study of cholinergic neurons and synapses. *J. Comp. Neurol.* 238:286–307, 1985.

Plaitakis A., Berl S., Yahr M.D. Abnormal glutamate metabolism in an adult-onset degenerative neurological disorder. *Science* 216:193–196, 1982.

Potashner S.J. Baclofen: effects on amino acid release. *Can. J. Physiol. Pharmacol.* 56:150–154, 1978.

Rinne U.K. Brain neurotransmitter receptors in Parkinson's disease. In Marsden C.D., Fahn S., eds. *Movement Disorders.* London, Butterworth, pp. 59–74, 1982.

Roos R.A.C. Neuropathology of Huntington's chorea. In Vinken P.I., Bruyn G.W., Klawans H.L., eds. *Handbook of Clinical Neurology.* Vol. 49. Amsterdam, Elsevier, pp. 315–326, 1986.

Sabra A.F., Hallet M., Sudarsky L., et al. Treatment of action tremor in multiple sclerosis with isoniazid. *Neurology (N.Y.)* 32:912–914, 1982.

Schell G.R., Strick P.L. The origin of thalamic inputs to the arcuate premotor and supplementary motor areas. *J. Neurosci.* 4:539–560, 1984.

Schulman J.A. Chemical neuroanatomy of the cerebellar cortex. In Emson P.C., ed. *Chemical Neuroanatomy.* New York, Raven Press, pp. 209–228, 1983.

Seeman P. Nomenclature of central and peripheral dopaminergic sites and receptors. *Biochem. Pharmacol.* 31:2563–2568, 1983.

Shoulson I. Huntington's disease: a decade of progress. *Neurol. Clin.* 2:515–526, 1984.

Smith Y., Parent A. Neurons of the subthalamic nucleus in primates display glutamate but not GABA immunoreactivity. *Brain Res.* 453:353–356, 1988.

Snyder S.H., Greenberg D., Yamamura H.I. Antischizophrenic drugs and brain cholinergic receptors: affinity for muscarinic sites predicts extrapyramidal effects. *Arch. Gen. Psychiatry* 31:58–61, 1974.

Stone T.W. NMDA receptors and ligands in the vertebrate CNS. *Prog. Neurobiol.* 30:333–368, 1988.

Switzer R.C., Hill J., Heimer L. The globus pallidus and its rostroventral extension into the olfactory tubercle of the rat: a cyto and chemoarchitectural study. *Neuroscience* 7:1891–1904, 1982.

Tarsy D., Baldessarini R.J. Tardive dyskinesia. *Annu. Rev. Med.* 35:605–623, 1984.

Tetrud J.W., Langston J.W. The effect of deprenyl (selegiline) on the natural history of Parkinson's disease. *Science* 245:519–522, 1989.

Thaker G.K., Nguyen J.A., Strauss M.E., et al. Clonazepam treatment of tardive dyskinesia: a practical GABA mimetic strategy. *Am. J. Psychiatry* 147:445–451, 1990.

Turski L., Klockgether T., Sontag K.-H., et al. Muscle relaxant and anticonvulsant activity of 3-(($\pm$)-2-carboxypiperazin-4-yl)propyl-1-phosphonic acid, a novel N-methyl-D-aspartate antagonist, in rodents. *Neurosci. Lett.* 73:143–148, 1987.

Ungerstedt U. Stereotaxic mapping of the monamine pathways in the rat brain. *Acta Physiol. Scand. Suppl.* 367:1–48, 1971.

Vonsattel J.-P., Myers R.H., Stevens T.J., et al. Neuropathological classification of Huntington's disease. *J. Neuropathol. Exp. Neurol.* 44:559–577, 1985.

Walters J.R., Bergstrom D.A., Carlson J.H., et al. D1 dopamine receptor activation required for postsynaptic expression of D2 agonist effects. *Science* 236:719–722, 1987.

White F.J., Wang R.T. Differential effects of classical and atypical antipsychotic drugs on A9 and A10 dopamine neurons. *Science* 221:1054–1056, 1983.

Young A.B., Macdonald R.L. Glycine as a spinal cord neurotransmitter. In Davidoff R.A., ed. *Handbook of the Spinal Cord.* New York, Marcel Dekker, pp. 1–43, 1983.

Young A.B., Penney J.B. Neurochemical anatomy of movement disorders. *Neurol. Clin.* 2:417–433, 1984.

Young A.B., Oster-Granite M.L., Herndon R.M., et al. Glutamic acid: selective depletion by viral-induced granule cell loss in hamster cerebellum. *Brain Res.* 73:1–13, 1974.

Young A.B., Penney J.B., Bromberg M.B. Decreased glutamate uptake in subcortical areas deafferented by sensorimotor cortical ablation in the cat. *J. Neurosci.* 1:241–249, 1981.

Young A.B., Penney J.B., Dauth G.W., et al. Glutamate or aspartate as a possible neurotransmitter of cerebral corticofugal fibers in the monkey. *Neurology (N.Y.)* 33:1513–1516, 1983.

25

Tremor

Robert R. Young

Tremor, the simplest and most common movement disorder, is not one entity; it is simply a neurologic symptom or sign that was originally defined clinically by inspection of the patient. In his essay "The shaking palsy," Sir James Parkinson (1817) said: "Tremor can indeed only be considered as a symptom, although species of it must be admitted." In the second century AD, Galen divided tremors into two species: that occurring at rest and that seen during movement. Since then, many more complicated classifications of tremor have been promulgated. A contemporary classification will be presented later, but for interesting historical reviews of earlier categorizations, see Brumlik and Yap (1970) and Hubble et al. (1989). For the present discussion, tremor is defined as a more or less rhythmic movement disorder, the mechanical oscillation having a relatively constant period in any one clinical setting. Electromyographic (EMG) activity in clinically significant tremors is typically grouped into bursts that are also rhythmic. Tremors often arise because of abnormal behavior of distal limb musculature and, at any one joint, movement tends to be in only one plane.

Various tremors began to be categorized and defined objectively about 100 years ago when movement transducers were first used to record them. Whether tremor occurred at rest or during action had always been obvious clinically, but neurologists could then subdivide tremor on the basis of frequency. Although tremors can clinically be termed coarse and slow or fine and fast, it is not possible to be accurate about tremor frequency without the use of some recording device. Perhaps for historical reasons, an overemphasis on a tremor's frequency as its sole or major diagnostic criterion has persisted. A tremor's frequency is not a particularly reliable clue to its type; the frequencies have too much overlap and variability (Elble, 1986).

With the development of clinical EMG and related physiologic techniques during the past 45 years, more precise categorization of tremors has been pos-

sible. Several illustrative examples of these advances will be mentioned now and explained later. In patients with Parkinson's disease, bursts of EMG activity responsible for tremor at rest alternate between flexor and extensor muscles in the forearm, whereas bursts of EMG activity responsible for essential-familial or enhanced physiologic tremors in the same patients with Parkinson's disease tend to occur synchronously in antagonist muscle groups (Shahani and Young, 1976). Although clinically significant tremors are accompanied by clear bursts of EMG activity, the smallest-amplitude subclinical tremors are not; physiologic tremor can thus be differentiated from enhanced physiologic tremor (definitions to follow). Within the last 20 years, semimicroelectrode recordings have been made from human muscle spindle primary afferents (microneurography) (Vallbo et al., 1979). These recordings have shown that enhanced physiologic tremor is not accompanied by α-γ coactivation (Hagbarth and Young, 1979; Young and Hagbarth, 1980), whereas tremor at rest (Hagbarth et al., 1975a,b) and essential-familial tremor are.

More recent computer manipulations of mechanical and EMG data provide ready quantification of tremor amplitude and frequency and their fluctuations with time. Freund's computer assessment of changes in muscle force output frequencies with the passage of time, fatigue, and so forth (Freund et al., 1984) are called muscle activity spectra, and he suggested that they may permit one to monitor activity within a motor neuron pool without recording EMG. Further examples of the utility of such techniques for tremor analysis will be given during the discussions of pathophysiology.

The use of clinical neurophysiologic methods of tremor analysis inevitably led to conflict between newer categorizations of tremor and those drawn from earlier clinical observations. On the one hand, tremor can be recorded in situations in which it is not visible clinically (physiologic tremor, ballistocardiac tremor, or subclinical tremor in certain patients with Parkinson's disease). On the other hand, clinical phenomena that had been called tremor (for example, the flapping tremor of asterixis or cerebellar intention tremor) can now be seen as quite distinct and different from the usual sorts of tremor. The latter observations suggest that such disorders should be categorized independently and not included among tremors. Modern reclassifications of tremor are not just academic exercises; they are essential because, as with other common neurologic symptoms, tremors can be discussed and treated rationally only after they have been subdivided into functionally and therapeutically coherent groups.

These functional categories, which had typically been defined clinically, are now being further subdivided and/or amalgamated, sometimes more on physiologic than on clinical grounds. For example, at least four separate types of tremor can be seen in patients with Parkinson's disease (Young, 1985), and there are two separate EMG types of essential-familial tremor. In contrast, a single tremor type can now be recognized in different clinical settings, whereas previously it would have been considered a different type of tremor in each setting. Essential-familial tremor may appear in patients with Parkinson's disease or in those with Charcot-Marie-Tooth familial neuropathy, and there is no need to have a separate category (i.e., Roussy-Lévy tremor; Yudell et al., 1965) for essential-familial tremor seen in the latter situation, for example. Essential-familial tremor should be treated as such wherever it is found (Young, 1982).

Finally, many tremors with different names, such as nervous tremor, adrenergic tremor, or withdrawal tremor, can usefully be grouped together as enhanced physiologic tremors (Young, 1984a). Examples are given in the following text.

The advent of tremor-specific therapies (Hubble et al., 1989; Young and Shahani, 1979a) has assisted in the categorization of tremors and has reinforced the utility and even the apparent reality of the present categories. Some therapies, such as thalamotomy and propranolol, are less specific; others, such as levodopa and primidone, are more specific. That is, the former are effective against several types of tremor, whereas the latter are each useful only in the treatment of one type. If we had more unequivocal understanding of neuropharmacology, therapeutic efficacy, particularly with specific treatments, should afford considerable insight into tremor pathophysiology.

As knowledge of tremors has deepened, areas of scientific endeavor previously untapped by neurologists have become important for explication of the various pathophysiologies of tremors. Such areas include β-adrenergic receptor function, robotics, muscle and limb mechanics or kinetics, and statistical analysis of motor unit discharge patterns, particularly synchronization of discharge, as stochastic point processes. Areas needing more fundamental work have also been identified, such as autonomic inner-

vation of skeletal muscle fibers and spinal mechanisms that normally function to desynchronize discharges in a motor neuron pool. Discussions to follow should exemplify the possibility that detailed analyses of tremor will lead to new and unexpected insights into fundamental aspects of the motor system.

NONTREMORS

In addition to movement disorders such as tardive dyskinesia and choreoathetosis, which are rarely confused with tremor, there are situations in which tremor is suspected but in which, on more careful evaluation, something else proves to be the trouble. One of these is a nervous patient who feels "trembly" internally, nothing being visible or recordable. Another, sensory ataxia, caused by lesions affecting peripheral nerves or central structures such as dorsal columns, ventrobasal thalamus, or parietal cortex, is a nonrhythmic, proximal greater than distal disorder of movement. Its awkward irregularity is not particularly tremulous; in fact, the involuntary slow movements or instabilities of posture are more apt to be confused with the slow, primarily proximal oscillations in multiple planes more appropriately termed cerebellar ataxia or dysmetria than intention tremor. In addition to oscillatory ataxias, lesions of the cerebellar system (spinocerebellar or other inputs, the cerebellum itself, or its outflow pathways) are sometimes associated with a rhythmic titubation of head and trunk. This may be considered a true cerebellar tremor but usually is not difficult to recognize and categorize as titubation. However, when titubation is present in complex settings, such as with severe multiple sclerosis or cerebral palsy or after a bad head injury, it can be difficult to differentiate from other tremors of head, neck, and shoulder girdle.

Nontremors also include myoclonus of different types, but most frequently negative myoclonus or asterixis is confused with tremor (Young and Shahani, 1986) (see also Chapters 22 and 109). The brief irregular jerky movements of asterixis are due to brief involuntary pauses in background EMG activity, and even when frequent, they are not truly rhythmic. Most patients in a general hospital who, at first glance, are thought to be tremulous will, on more thorough study, not be found to have a tremor at all; EMG studies will document the presence of asterixis. Their asterixis, if bilateral as it usually is, will be due to one of many metabolic encephalopathies. Unilateral asterixis, on the other hand, is a sign of a structural central nervous system (CNS) lesion that may otherwise be inconspicuous. The most discrete lesion that produces unilateral asterixis is a ventrolateral thalamotomy (Young et al., 1976). Any anticonvulsant in excessive amounts will produce bilateral asterixis, whereas normal therapeutic levels of an anticonvulsant can, in the presence of an appropriately localized albeit asymptomatic cerebral lesion, produce unilateral asterixis on the side opposite to the brain lesion.

Muscular weakness, whether of peripheral or central origin, may be associated with involuntary irregularities of contraction that are rarely confused with tremor. These abnormal movements may be of several types:

1. Action fasciculations, as when only a few giant motor units remain functional in a muscle after polio or with motor system disease
2. Pauses in contraction that are longer than those seen with asterixis (sometimes caused by lapses in concentration)
3. Other nontremulous irregularities of tonic motor neuron discharge

Clonus (Desmedt, 1978) and shivering are two phenomena that meet the criteria for tremor but, because of the peculiar and obvious clinical context of each, should be considered independently.

Patterns of EMG activity in all these nontremors are irregular and much more chaotic than in the tremors to be discussed.

NORMAL TREMORS

Normal tremors are present in all human beings but do not produce symptoms. Such tremors were not recognized before the advent of mechanical recordings and, because they are not associated with synchronization or grouping of motor unit discharges, cannot be recognized on EMG recordings either. Early investigators were surprised to find that even in the absence of clinical tremor, their mechanical recordings did not consist of a flat line (Brumlik and Yap, 1970). Even when muscles are truly at rest without any EMG activity, they and the limbs are continuously being oscillated, albeit with excursions of extremely low amplitude, by vibrations transmitted from the large vessels in the chest and abdomen consequent upon periodic ejection of blood from the heart. At one time, these vibrations were recorded and used diagnostically by cardiologists as the ballistocardiogram. This *ballistocardiac effect* produces larger-amplitude limb tremors when cardiac output is increased but, because of their extremely low amplitude even then, has no known neurologic significance. Although it is obviously a tremor at rest, ballistocardiac tremor has nothing to do with Parkinson's disease; the tremor at rest seen in the latter condition does not correspond to a larger version of the former.

Whenever muscles are activated by recruitment of their motor neurons, larger-amplitude, somewhat irregular oscillations of that limb can be recorded. Although these movements are an order of magnitude larger than the ballistocardiac tremor, they are still too small to be visible clinically. This *physiologic tremor* is not due to synchronization, grouping, or other abnormalities of motor unit discharges; the

EMG consists of a normal interference pattern without bursts of activity. The tremor is a passive mechanical movement in which the limb tends to vibrate like any second-order system at its natural frequency determined by its mass and the spring-like stiffness of its muscles and tendons (Freund and Dietz, 1978; Rack, 1978; Stiles, 1976; Young and Wiegner, 1985). It vibrates because it is being "forced" by only partially fused twitches of motor units that are contracting at a rate less than that required to produce a fused tetanus. Physiologic tremor is irregular in both amplitude and frequency (Fig. 25–1A and B). Different body parts tremble at different frequencies depending on their mass; for example, physiologic tremor at the wrist, in any one person, has a broad-frequency spectrum between 8 and 12 Hz, whereas in the fingers its frequency range is two or three times higher. From moment to moment, both the amplitude and frequency of physiologic tremor vary even at any one joint in one person. Some mechanical amplification technique is needed to make this normal tremor visible because its amplitude is usually considerably less than 0.1° at wrist or finger, for example (Hagbarth and Young, 1979).

ENHANCED PHYSIOLOGIC TREMORS

Although physiologic tremor is not visible clinically and therefore produces no symptoms, all normal subjects and all patients (except those with a peripheral neuropathy sufficient to abolish stretch reflexes; see later) do have tremors from time to time that are visible and clinically significant. These tremors have a number of causes (Table 25–1) and can usefully be categorized according to the cause—for example, stage fright, nervous tremor, and terbutaline tremor. On the other hand, they all represent an enhancement of the underlying physiologic tremor via operation of the spinal stretch reflex arc (see Lippold, 1970). That is, under a variety of circumstances, the amplitude of physiologic tremor increases and its frequency becomes much more monorhythmic (see Fig. 25–1F). The prototype *enhanced physiologic tremor* is that produced by β-adrenergic agents, particularly $β_2$ agonists such as are used in the therapy of asthma. Similar is the tremor produced by increases in circulating levels of endogenous epinephrine associated with anxiety, stage fright, or preparation for athletic or other combat. Other hyperadrenergic states are also associated with typical enhanced physiologic tremor—for example, thyrotoxicosis; withdrawal from alcohol, opiates, or sedatives; increased blood levels of nicotine (Shiffman et al., 1983), which releases catecholamines from the adrenal medulla; ingestion of levodopa, which is metabolized to catecholamines peripherally; ingestion of amphetamines; use of methylxanthines in coffee, tea, or colas (Dobmeyer et al., 1983; Robertson et al., 1978); fatigue and even nonfatiguing use of muscles; and hunger or hypoglycemia, which produces increased epi-

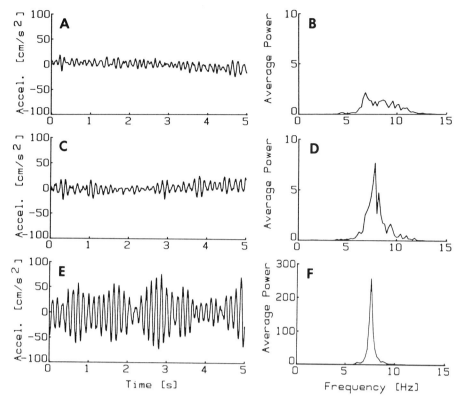

Figure 25–1. Physiologic and enhanced physiologic tremor. *(A, C,* and *E)* Wrist tremor in a normal subject is measured with an accelerometer 16 cm distal to the wrist with the subject seated comfortably, the arm supported, and the lightly splinted hand held horizontal against gravity. *(B, D,* and *F)* Spectral analysis plots (power-frequency histograms) of ten 5-s epochs of acceleration data, one epoch of which is shown to the left of each plot. The baseline tremor in an otherwise relaxed subject *(C, D)* is enhanced 90 min after ingestion of 5 mg terbutaline *(E, F)* and is reduced below baseline values 90 min after ingestion of 40 mg propranolol *(A, B).* Power is in arbitrary units; note the change of scale in *F,* where the power spectrum is also narrowed. Root mean square displacements of 10 successive epochs were *A,* 29 μm; *B,* 36 μm; and *C,* 150 μm. Of particular interest is the enhancement of physiologic tremor *(C* and *D* compared with *A* and *B)* in a subject who was under no stress and did not feel anxious. (Courtesy of Allen W. Wiegner, M.D., West Roxbury Veterans Administration Hospital, Boston.)

nephrine levels. Agents that produce similar tremors but with mechanisms less clear include lithium (Gaby et al., 1983), corticosteroids, and tricyclic antidepressants.

The precise mechanisms involved in production of enhanced physiologic tremors remain to be fully disclosed, but the following observations have been made. Human muscle spindle primary afferent (Ia) endings are sufficiently sensitive, particularly in contracting muscles with α-γ coactivation, to respond to each tiny stretch of the muscle produced by physiologic tremor. These tremor-induced bursts of Ia activity have been recorded microneurographically (Fig. 25–2*A*), but their entry into the spinal cord does not appear to affect discharge properties of the active

motor neurons in patients with simple physiologic tremor (Hagbarth and Young, 1979). On the other hand, hyperadrenergic states, fatigue, and so on (see Table 25–1) produce increased synchronization of discharge of independent motor neurons (Fig. 25–2*B*). This tendency to grouping of motor unit discharges is related, as both cause and effect, to increasingly prominent bursts of Ia activity in the afferent arc of the segmental stretch reflex (Young and Hagbarth, 1980). There appears to be a continuum between pure physiologic tremor at the one extreme in which the stretch reflex arc is not involved, at least on the efferent side, and full-blown, large-amplitude, enhanced physiologic tremors at the other extreme in which the stretch reflex arc is very much involved (Fig. 25–2*C*) (Young, 1984a).

Spindle primary endings are activated by the recurrent and cyclic stretches of muscle. As enhanced physiologic tremor develops, these Ia bursts produce reflex discharges from the motor neuron pool or, more precisely, alter the time of discharge of cells in the voluntarily active motor neuron pool so that EMG discharges occur in bursts with monosynaptic latency after each little stretch of the muscle. Each EMG burst produces contraction of muscle and is timed to do so at exactly the instant when the muscle is already being shortened by the next cycle of tremor. The muscle therefore shortens a little more than it would have without the EMG-induced contraction. To state it another way, these properly timed force pulses produce increased excursions at the joint involved with tremor in a manner similar to what happens with appropriately timed small force pulses

Table 25–1. CAUSES OF ENHANCED PHYSIOLOGIC TREMOR

β₂-Adrenergic agonists	Anxiety
Epinephrine	Excitement
Isoproterenol	Exercise
Metaproterenol	Fatigue
Terbutaline	Hypoglycemia
Amphetamines	Jendrassik's maneuvers
Levodopa	Muscle contraction
Lithium	Muscle vibration
Nicotine	Pheochromocytoma
Prednisone	Stress
Thyroid hormones	Thyrotoxicosis
Xanthines in	Withdrawal from
Coffee	Alcohol
Colas	Opiates
Tea	Sedatives

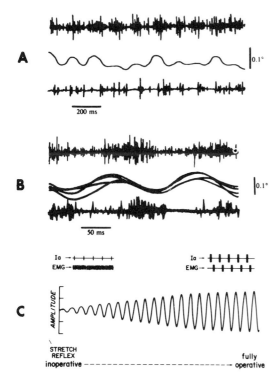

Figure 25–2. Muscle spindle and EMG correlates of physiologic and enhanced physiologic tremor. The upper traces in *A* and *B* are microneurographic recordings of afferent responses from muscle spindle primary (Ia) endings in a wrist flexor muscle of a normal subject at the beginning *(A)* and after 15 minutes *(B)* of holding the hand outstretched, palm up, against gravity. The middle trace of each is from a goniometer that records movement at the wrist, and the lower traces are EMG recordings from the same wrist flexor muscle. Calibrations for tremor amplitude are 0.1°. Time calibrations are 200 ms *(A)* and 50 ms *(B)*. *(A)* Single recording; *(B)* four superimposed sweeps. Note the extreme nonlinear sensitivity of Ia endings to the irregular, tiny muscle stretches produced by physiologic tremor in *A* and to the larger, more regular movements seen with enhanced physiologic tremor in *B*. Only in *B* ("fatigue tremor") are bursts of EMG activity synchronized to the tremor movements; the EMG potentials occur approximately 20 ms later than the Ia discharges. (*A* and *B* from Hagbarth K.-E., Young R.R. Participation of the stretch reflex in human physiological tremor. *Brain* 102:509–526, 1979, by permission of Oxford University Press.)

applied to the back of a child who is sitting on a playground swing. The timing of each force pulse is crucial. If the timing is appropriate, even small but rhythmically repeated force pulses can produce a large-amplitude excursion. Patients without operation of the segmental stretch reflex arc do not demonstrate enhanced physiologic tremors even under appropriate circumstances of adrenergic stimulation (Shahani, 1984). Peripheral β₂-adrenergic blockade also tends to reduce the amplitude of all of these enhanced physiologic tremors.

Marsden et al. (1967) first demonstrated the presence of tremorogenic β-adrenergic receptors in the human forearm. Sufficiently concentrated solutions of β agonists such as isoproterenol given intravenously produce a generalized enhanced physiologic tremor, but when dilute solutions of these agents are infused into a brachial artery, a typical enhanced

physiologic tremor appears only in that forearm in normal subjects or in patients with essential-familial tremor (Fig. 25–3) (Young et al., 1975). These β receptors, which appear to be β₂ in type, are within muscle but may also be on other structures in the forearm. β-Adrenergic stimulation of skeletal muscle produces effects on the contractile apparatus that vary, in part at least, with the histochemical or metabolic type of muscle fiber that is being studied (Bowman, 1980; Bowman and Nott, 1971). In human muscles, which are composed of mixtures of fiber types, adrenergic stimulation usually shortens the half-relaxation time and sometimes shortens the contraction time of a twitch (Marsden and Meadows, 1970; Young and Hagbarth, 1980). Because of the extreme nonlinear sensitivity of spindle Ia endings (see Hagbarth and Young, 1979; Matthews, 1977), they behave like accelerometers (Wiegner and Young, 1984) and tend to discharge sooner on the falling phase of a twitch or tremor cycle when it relaxes more quickly. This alters the timing of Ia input to spinal motor neurons.

In the same context, it is interesting to note that during muscle contraction as phosphocreatine stores are exhausted, lactic acid concentrations increase and half-relaxation time increases (McMahon, 1984). Adrenergic stimulation would tend to counteract the latter increase. In any case, changes in muscle mechanics in hyperadrenergic situations produce a more unfused contraction that would thus become more tremulous or twitch-like, whereas previously it had been more fused and tetanic. In addition, however, EMG activity in the adrenergically bathed muscles becomes grouped into bursts so that some afferent input from the limb must also have altered the discharge time of spinal motor neurons. Our hypothesis is that muscle spindle afferent discharge is altered by adrenergically induced changes in mechanical properties of the muscle (for a more detailed analysis, see Young and Wiegner, 1985). The altered timing with which these Ia afferent bursts reach the active motor neuron pool produces increased synchronization of discharge and, as outlined earlier, increased tremor.

In most if not all of the hyperadrenergic states mentioned earlier, systemically increased circulating levels of norepinephrine presumably affect all skeletal muscle fibers. Effects on extrafusal fibers have been well demonstrated but effects on intrafusal muscle fibers remain to be clarified (Young and Hagbarth, 1980). There may also be conditions with increased numbers of and/or sensitivity of intramuscular adrenergic receptors. Furthermore, catecholamines released locally in muscle may play a role in development of tremor. Catecholaminergic unmyelinated nerve fibers have been shown to end on skeletal muscle fibers in certain species and even to be present inside muscle spindles (Barker and Saito, 1981). These fibers are distinct from those that end on intramuscular blood vessels. The functional significance of the former fibers remains to be demonstrated, but they may play a role in the production

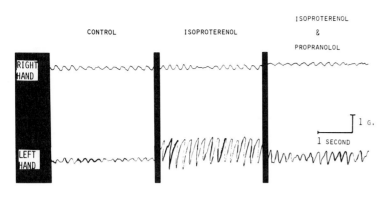

Figure 25–3. Tremors are additive. These accelerometer recordings are from the outstretched left and right hands of a patient with essential-familial tremor. Infusion of a dilute solution of a β_2 agonist (isoproterenol) into the left brachial artery (see Young et al., 1975) produces an unusually large-amplitude action tremor in the left forearm. This combination of pre-existing tremor and enhanced physiologic tremor is altered toward the control level by simultaneous intra-arterial infusion of propranolol. Calibrations are 1 second and 1 *g* acceleration. (From Young R.R. Tremor in relation to certain other movement disorders. In Findley L.J., Capildeo R., eds. *Movement Disorders: Tremors.* New York, Oxford University Press, pp. 463–472, 1984, by permission of Oxford University Press.)

of enhanced physiologic tremor. Not only after a muscle has become fatigued but also early during a sustained contraction, appropriately localized release of monoamines may be useful. As part of the flight-or-fight reaction, increased adrenergic stimulation of skeletal muscle apparently has survival value for the organism and species; during such stimulation, contractile strength is increased, endurance prolonged, and contractions made speedier. These improvements in muscle performance are, however, accompanied by a greatly increased metabolic rate, so in the interests of conservation of energy, adrenergic stimulation of muscle should be as restricted as possible, both in time and in terms of which muscles are involved. In addition to this adrenergically induced reduction in metabolic efficiency, enhanced physiologic tremors are another unavoidable side effect of such otherwise useful alterations in muscle activity.

ESSENTIAL-FAMILIAL TREMOR

Normal subjects, when they develop an action tremor of the outstretched hands consequent on increased adrenergic activity in skeletal muscle, temporarily look very much like patients with *essential-familial tremor*. However, the latter is a slowly progressive, idiopathic, permanent disorder, whereas with enhanced physiologic tremor the etiology is often clear and the tremor usually short lived. It is usually not misdiagnosed as essential-familial tremor. Nevertheless, the diagnostic situation unfortunately *is* complicated by the fact that patients with essential-familial tremor (or one of the parkinsonian tremors) temporarily develop a much larger tremor during hyperadrenergic situations such as those listed in Table 25–1. *Tremors are additive* (see Fig. 25–3), and the larger than usual tremor experienced by a patient with Parkinson's disease or essential-familial tremor when that patient is in a laboratory (see Fig. 25–1C), on stage, or otherwise frightened should be considered a combination of pre-existing tremor and enhanced physiologic tremor (Young 1982, 1983, 1984b). One may also refer to these temporarily larger

tremors as enhanced essential-familial tremor or enhanced parkinsonism tremor at rest.

Essential-familial tremor is an action tremor, the opposite of a tremor at rest; it occurs solely during activity of the limbs or body part in question. As opposed to the situation in Parkinson's disease, for example, no tremor occurs in the arms when a patient with essential-familial tremor is walking. However, orthostatic truncal tremor may be a subvariant of essential-familial tremor. The latter tremor may also involve speech, neck, face, or chin. Tremor may be apparent only with the limb in certain positions (e.g., hand supine or elbows flexed and abducted) or during certain complex activities such as shaving. Essential-familial tremor of the neck may sometimes be mistaken for torticollis, and it has been suggested that essential-familial tremor, rather than being a monosymptomatic condition as is generally believed, may actually be part of a more widespread CNS degenerative disorder that has a continuum of motor abnormalities ranging from torticollis at one extreme to essential-familial tremor at the other (Critchley, 1972). Although this is an interesting hypothesis, there are no statistical or other data to support it.

In a population survey of a rural county in Mississippi, Haerer et al. (1982) found an overall prevalence ratio for essential-familial tremor of 414.6 per 100,000 inhabitants. In Scandinavia, the prevalence ratio is 10–15 times larger (Larson and Sjögren, 1960; Rautakorpi et al., 1982), whereas in the Parsi community of India, it is five times larger (Bharucha et al., 1988). Epidemiologic studies of essential-familial tremor are difficult because it is often misdiagnosed or overlooked. Rautakorpi et al. (1982) found that only about 10% of such subjects had sought treatment for the tremor. Also, the tremor may not become symptomatic before late middle life. Essential-familial tremor is not uncommon; it may be the most frequent movement disorder (Hubble et al., 1989). It affects approximately 5 million people in North America and will by chance occur in patients with other illnesses.

Essential-familial tremor is best considered a monosymptomatic condition (is it an illness?), but it can certainly occur in patients with other neurologic illnesses such as Parkinson's disease and Charcot-

Marie-Tooth familial polyneuropathy (Hubble et al., 1989; Martinelli et al., 1987). There is no evidence that the occurrence of two of these disorders in the same patient is anything other than coincidental. For example, the progressive neuropathy with sensory ataxia described by Roussy and Lévy (1926) was *not* associated with tremor. The coexistence of familial tremor and Charcot-Marie-Tooth familial neuropathy in the same patient is simply an example of the unfortunate inheritance of two unrelated conditions and is not Roussy-Lévy syndrome as suggested earlier (Yudell et al., 1965). This coexistence does, however, emphasize the fact that essential-familial tremor is centrally driven and not dependent on the stretch reflex arc. Even in patients with severe neuropathies and no functional stretch reflex, essential-familial tremor has the same clinical appearance, neurophysiologic hallmarks, and therapeutic response to propranolol or alcohol as it does when it appears in isolation. It must be emphasized, therefore, that in contradistinction to enhanced physiologic tremor, essential-familial tremor is centrally driven and not mediated via the stretch reflex. Propranolol's beneficial effect in these patients with tremor and neuropathy must also be centrally mediated. There is no evidence for earlier assumptions that essential-familial is simply abnormally prominent physiologic tremor (Marshall, 1962) and that propranolol is effective in the former patients by means of peripheral actions (Marsden, 1984).

When essential-familial tremor affects distal upper extremities, as it usually does, its amplitude increases toward the end of projected movements in which the patient attempts to make an increasingly accurate arrival at the target. The percentage increase is less marked, however, than is the case with cerebellar ataxia, in which the terminal oscillation is so prominent. The latter movements are primarily proximal; no ataxia or dysmetria is seen with essential-familial tremor. Nevertheless, because of a superficial similarity between the two conditions, neurologists in the past sometimes referred to essential-familial tremor as a minor cerebellar tremor. It was earlier called Minor's tremor after a Russian neurologist who described it. No neuropathologic lesion in cerebellum or elsewhere has been recognized in rare postmortem examinations of patients with essential-familial tremor (Herskovits and Blackwood, 1969), and its neurochemistry is unknown. Its pathophysiology is also a mystery except for a few details noted in the preceding paragraph. No good animal models have been described (see reviews by Lamarre, 1975, 1984), but Brooks and Thach (1981) reported that lesions in the interpositus nucleus of the cerebellum in monkeys produce an action tremor with certain similarities to essential-familial tremor. However, unilateral cerebellar infarction was reported to be associated with disappearance of essential-familial tremor from the same side of the patient's body (Dupuis et al., 1989).

When there is a positive family history of this tremor, which is the case for roughly 50% of patients,

it is called familial; in the absence of such a family history, it is called essential. It appears to be an autosomal dominant trait (Herskovits et al., 1988). Although it can arise at any age, essential-familial tremor most commonly develops or becomes symptomatic in middle life and worsens with age. It may become prominent only when a patient is 60 or 70 years old and, in the latter circumstance, was formerly called senile tremor, but there seems no particular reason to use what has become a pejorative term. There is no clinical, electrodiagnostic, or pharmacologic difference among essential, familial, and senile tremors. To distinguish it from Parkinson's disease, it was formerly called benign essential tremor, but that is often not the case; it can produce considerable disability. When essential-familial tremor is prominent in childhood, diagnosis may be difficult because patients appear more restless or choreoathetotic than simply tremulous. They may even have shuddering attacks (Vanesse et al., 1976). Children with this disorder find, for example, that it is difficult to hold their heads still in the barber chair. By their middle to late teens, the restlessness will become clearly tremulous. Regardless of the age of patients with essential-familial tremor, one hears them complain that the harder they try to hold still or minimize the tremor, the worse it gets. This observation obviously provides an important clue to the pathophysiology of essential-familial tremor, but its significance in neurophysiologic terms is still unclear. It may simply be that with increased effort and concentration, generalized muscular tension and anxiety levels rise, both of which produce enhanced physiologic tremor, which then is added to the underlying essential-familial tremor. However, there is probably more to it than that.

In addition to brief increases in amplitude of essential-familial tremor with efforts to make a precise movement, tremor amplitude is also increased by any of the factors in Table 25–1 (except perhaps caffeine; see Koller et al., 1987) that produce enhanced physiologic tremor. The latter phenomenon (enhanced essential-familial tremor, or the fact that tremors are additive) (see Fig. 25–3) has led to widespread confusion in the literature between the two types of tremor. As illustrated in Figure 25–1, low-level enhanced physiologic tremor is often present in subjects being studied in tremor laboratories. Propranolol or other β blockers acutely diminish this component of tremor in normal subjects and in those with essential-familial or parkinsonian tremors. In many published studies, this reduction in enhanced physiologic tremor was mistaken for an effect directly on the underlying pathologic tremor.

Because the two types of tremor appear similar clinically and because he found their frequencies to decline with age, Marshall (1961, 1962) suggested that essential-familial tremor was simply a more prominent and persistent form of what he called physiologic tremor. By the latter he meant what is now called enhanced physiologic tremor, which he thought was due to failure of damping of oscillations within a movement servomechanism. As outlined earlier, a sort of oscillation involving the stretch reflex arc underlies enhanced physiologic tremor, but essential-familial tremor persists in patients with severe neuropathies and no demonstrable function of the stretch reflex. These two tremors are thus different and not merely two different amplitude ranges of the same tremor. Furthermore, when one separates out the patients with enhanced physiologic tremor, neither we nor Marsden et al. (1969) have been able to demonstrate a particularly linear relationship between frequency of essential-familial tremor and patients' ages. This separation of one action tremor from the other has also permitted a more rational therapy (see later).

Another difference between these two action tremors is that subjects in whom enhanced physiologic tremor is the only symptomatic disability can perform various functions without tremor in the absence of anxiety-provoking circumstances, asthma medications, and so on. Conversely, patients with essential-familial tremor find the tremor worse in public, but even in private with no particular anxiety the tremor continues to trouble them. Anxiolytic agents, tranquilizers, and sedatives have no particular effect on essential-familial tremor but may help reduce the enhancement of it by anxiety or stage fright. Although they alleviate anxiety, tranquilizers and alcohol also result in significant decrement in the ability of performing artists to function at a high level (Brantigan et al., 1979). Modest amounts of ethyl alcohol (a small glass of sherry, for example) usually produce a prompt and marked alleviation of essential-familial tremor (Growdon et al., 1975). Alcohol does so by actions on the central rather than peripheral nervous system; when concentrations of ethanol similar to those produced by drinking it are infused into the brachial artery, tremor in that limb is not reduced (Growdon et al., 1975). The amounts of oral ethanol required are not of a magnitude associated with even mild inebriation, and after several hours, when the serum level of alcohol falls, there is often a rebound increase in tremor amplitude. A significant number of chronic alcoholics, as many as 50% in some series (Lefebvre-D'Amour et al., 1978; Schroeder and Nasrallah, 1982), suffer from essential-familial tremor. This has led to the suggestion, by the lay public, that alcoholism produces tremor, a hypothesis that has never been proved. It seems likely that some of these alcoholics became addicted to that substance as a result of the fact that it ameliorates their tremor temporarily. The "morning after," when serum alcohol levels are low, is associated with considerable rebound increase in tremor amplitude, perhaps in part because of the hyperadrenergic withdrawal effects known to produce enhanced physiologic tremor. The tremor of delerium tremens is an extreme example of this. Nevertheless, alcohol in small amounts remains a useful symptomatic therapy in many patients (permitting them to eat out occasionally in a restaurant, for example) and should not be categorically proscribed. The risk of alcoholism in patients with essential-familial tremor appears to be acceptably low (Koller, 1983).

Centrally active β-adrenergic blocking agents such as propranolol, when taken several times a day on a continuous basis, are effective in reducing tremor amplitude in 75–80% of patients with essential-familial tremor (Winkler and Young, 1971, 1974). Treatment once a day with sustained-release propranolol may be even more effective (Cleeves and Findley, 1988). Such reductions are much more useful clinically in patients in whom the tremor produces its disability by interfering with the use of one or both upper extremities. In other patients, in whom tremor primarily affects the head and neck so that it produces a cosmetic rather than functional disability, propranolol therapy seems to be less effective. A single dose of propranolol (40 or 80 mg) taken about an hour before either a normal subject or a patient with essential-familial tremor gets up to speak in public, goes on stage, appears in front of a television camera, or the like markedly ameliorates the tremor associated with stage fright or performance anxiety.

Propranolol and other peripherally acting β-adrenergic antagonists are effective in this regard by virtue of their interference with the mechanisms described earlier that produce enhanced physiologic tremor (see Fig. 25–3). In patients with essential-familial tremor propranolol taken chronically therefore has two independent modes of action. It operates in the long run within the CNS on as yet poorly defined mechanisms to reduce the amplitude of essential-familial tremor, and it acts much more rapidly at intramuscular β receptors to reduce enhanced physiologic tremor associated with stress or anxiety. Propranolol and other β antagonists that pass the blood-brain barrier have central and peripheral actions, but many of the newer β blockers, the hydrophilic ones, tend not to enter the CNS. They are less useful than propranolol as an antitremor agent because they affect only peripheral β responses and even then, in the case of more cardioselective $β_1$ blockers such as atenolol or metoprolol, tend not to be as effective in blocking $β_2$ receptors in muscle. For a review, see Marsden (1984). Unfortunately, from an academic viewpoint, none of the available β-adrenergic blocking agents is completely selective. If such an agent were available, it could be used to define more accurately the tremorogenic receptors.

None of the β blockers can be used indiscriminately in patients with congestive heart failure, heart block, severe asthma, or, perhaps, insulin-dependent diabetes mellitus. In addition to side effects produced by interference with various β-adrenergic activities, β blockers, particularly centrally active ones, may produce fatigue, insomnia, depression, and a feeling of lassitude. Although they interfere with the fight-or-flight response, it has not been possible to demonstrate any deterioration in motor performance caused by agents such as propranolol during such demanding activities as are required by the public performance of a concert musician (Brantigan et al., 1979, 1982). Propranolol taken just before a performance improves it by reducing the physical manifestations of stage fright without reducing finesse or other skills needed to play well. On the other hand, propranolol and other β antagonist therapies do interfere with performance in sports, such as long-distance running, that require endurance rather than, or in addition to, particular muscular finesse and fine movements (Fellenius, 1983).

Different insights into the pathophysiology of essential-familial tremor are presumably provided by the observation that primidone is often effective in its therapy (Findley et al., 1985; Koller and Royse, 1986; O'Brien et al., 1981), whereas phenobarbital (one of primidone's major metabolites) (Sarso et al., 1988) and phenylethylmalonic acid (its other main metabolite) (Calzetti et al., 1981) are not effective in this respect. Primidone is often effective in remarkably small doses, such as 50 mg three times a day; rarely do patients require the usual adult antiepileptic dose of 250 mg three or four times a day. Many tremor patients are also remarkably sensitive to the sedative side effects of primidone or have an unusually severe adverse reaction to the first dose, with nausea, vomiting, ataxia, and giddiness. Primidone should therefore be started in extremely low doses (25 mg) at bedtime and increased gradually. There is as yet no understanding of the CNS pharmacologic mechanisms whereby ethanol, primidone, or propranolol relieves essential-familial tremor. For a discussion of other drugs that have not proved to be effective in treating essential-familial tremor, including calcium channel blockers and drugs involved in serotonin or γ-aminobutyric acid (GABA) metabolism, see Hubble et al. (1989).

Stereotaxic ventrolateral thalamotomy completely and permanently eliminates essential-familial tremor from the contralateral side of the body (for a review see Andrew, 1984) but does not affect enhanced physiologic tremor. How neurosurgical interruption of circuits mediating input to the motor system from both basal ganglia and cerebellum can produce relief of essential-familial tremor, parkinsonian tremor at rest, and rigidity without producing some profound deficit of motor performance is completely unknown. It has not yet been possible to demonstrate negative symptoms resulting from stereotaxic disruption of the circuits involved in the production of tremor; one has no idea what they do under normal circumstances. Presumably, certain central mechanisms responsible for these tremors share the same circuits, but that is not to say that essential-familial tremor is a forme fruste of Parkinson's disease (Barbeau and Pourcher, 1982; Critchley, 1949).

TREMORS WITH PARKINSON'S DISEASE

Patients with Parkinson's disease can have at least four different types of tremor (Delwaide and Gonce, 1988; Young, 1985). Like everyone else, they all have enhanced physiologic tremor when in stressful situations or exposed to other hyperadrenergic states. Some also have typical essential-familial tremor, which may be more prevalent in patients with Parkinson's disease than in the general population (Barbeau and Pourcher, 1982; Geraghty et al., 1985; Schwab and Young, 1971). On the other hand, Cleeves et al. (1988) found no clear link between essential-familial tremor and Parkinson's disease. It should be noted that about 10% of patients initially thought to have Parkinson's disease prove to have only essential-familial tremor, the former diagnosis being incorrect. Patients with Parkinson's disease may also have a tremor that is present only during writing and at no other time; nothing is known of its pathophysiology. Most commonly, however, they have a typical, almost pathognomonic tremor at rest. This term is somewhat of a misnomer because when patients are lying comfortably with their axial and proximal limb girdle muscles entirely relaxed, there is no tremor. On the other hand, when they are sitting at rest or even lying in an attitude of repose with postural contractions in axial and proximal muscles, an involuntary pill-rolling tremor of the hands and sometimes a similar tremor of the face, jaw, neck, and legs appears even though the patient thought those body parts were at rest. When the patient voluntarily uses the limb or changes its position, the tremor either disappears or is markedly reduced in amplitude. After a variable period, sometimes only a few seconds, tremor returns when the limb is held in a new position.

Tremor at rest is primarily an embarrassment rather than a handicap because it tends to disappear when the limb is used; however, in some patients it does produce functional disability. It may recur after a cup has been held near the mouth for a few seconds or when the patient is holding a newspaper. Most patients with Parkinson's disease either have a clinically obvious tremor at rest or a subclinical tremor that can be recorded electromyographically. Rare patients with Parkinson's disease, particularly early in the course of the illness, have no tremor at rest demonstrable by any clinical or laboratory technique.

The parkinsonian tremor at rest has a rather typical movement pattern when recorded with an accelerometer on the hand. Rather than having the clean sinusoidal quality seen in patients with essential-familial tremor, tremor at rest in a patient with Parkinson's disease has a more complex waveform that suggests that components of the tremor produced by different muscles in one upper extremity are slightly out of phase with one another (Fig. 25–4D). The EMG activity underlying this tremor is also quite typical even when one uses surface EMG recordings (Young, 1985; Young and Shahani, 1979a,b). Bursts of EMG activity occur at 4 or 5 Hz in flexors and extensors of the wrist, for example, but the activity in these antagonistic muscle groups is almost exactly 180° out of phase (see Fig. 25–4D). In fact, it has the same appearance as in normal subjects who

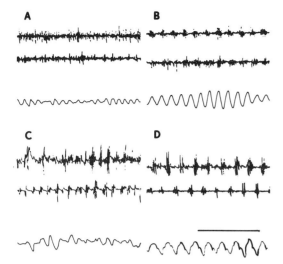

Figure 25–4. Different types of tremor. In each, the lower trace is an accelerometric recording from the outstretched hand, and the upper two traces are surface EMG recordings from wrist extensor (upper) and flexor (middle) muscle groups. *(A)* Physiologic tremor; there is no evidence of synchronization of EMG activity. *(B)* Essential-familial tremor; the movements are regular and EMG bursts occur simultaneously in antagonistic muscle groups. *(C)* Neuropathic tremor (Adams et al., 1972); movements are quite irregular and EMG bursts vary in timing between the two groups. *(D)* Parkinsonian tremor at rest; the movements are not smooth and EMG bursts alternate between antagonistic muscle groups. Calibration is 1 second.

alternately contract flexors and extensors to mimic a tremor at rest. In contrast, in most patients with essential-familial tremor, bursts of EMG activity occur more or less synchronously in antagonistic muscle groups (see Fig. 25–4B).

When one uses intramuscular electrodes to study the behavior of single motor units in patients with tremor at rest of Parkinson's disease, two rather specific abnormalities are seen (Fig. 25–5A). Any single motor unit, as it is recruited, rather than firing irregularly at frequencies between 4–5 and 8–10 Hz, suddenly begins to fire regularly at approximately 4 or 5 Hz, the tremor frequency. In addition, it may discharge as a doublet. That is, the same motor unit may fire twice within 20 or 30 ms and then not again for another one-fourth or one-fifth of a second. These high-frequency double discharges can be seen normally in association with phasic EMG activity (Logigian et al., 1988) or during a tonic contraction when tension is quickly increased. Doublets never occur normally four or five times a second. In addition to these abnormalities of single motor neuron discharge, when one studies the behavior of two independent motor units, striking synchronization is seen; the second motor unit to be recruited, usually the larger of the two, tends to fire in a time-locked fashion slightly after the first rather than independently of it as normally takes place. What one sees in the EMG bursts of patients with tremor at rest (see Fig. 25–5A) is therefore the following: single units firing once or as doublets at the tremor frequency and independent motor units being synchro-

nized to fire at almost the same instant during each burst. In patients with essential-familial tremor, single motor units also sometimes fire in the form of doublets. Synchronization of independent motor units is also present. However, the larger second motor unit to be recruited may fire either before or after the first one in any given burst, and the time between discharges of the two is much more variable from burst to burst than is the case with tremor at rest. To understand the pathophysiology of any of these abnormalities, much more research is needed

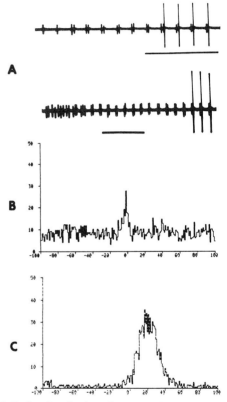

Figure 25–5. Synchronization of motor unit activity in tremor. *(A)* Needle EMG recordings from wrist extensor muscles of patients with Parkinson's disease. In each, force increases slowly from left to right. Note the normal discharge pattern of a single motor unit at the bottom left. Later, it and the single unit in the upper trace begin to discharge in an abnormally slow rhythmic fashion at the tremor frequency; each also frequently discharges doubly with an instantaneous firing frequency of about 50 Hz. Then as the next larger unit is recruited *(right)*, its discharge is synchronized with and follows that of the unit recruited earlier. Calibration is 1 second. *(B and C)* Cross-correlation histograms of the firing times of two single motor units in a normal subject before *(B)* and after *(C)* the development of enhanced physiologic tremor caused by fatigue. Abscissas are in milliseconds between discharges of the two units, and ordinates represent the number of discharges at each interval divided by the duration of the recording (units = Hz). Note in *B* that, apart from a relatively weak short-term synchronization of the two units about 0, they discharge independently of one another. In *C*, the unit discharges become strongly synchronized, with one tending to occur about 20 ms after the other. *(A from Young R.R. Tremor in relation to certain other movement disorders. In Findley L.J., Capildeo R., eds. *Movement Disorders: Tremors*. New York, Oxford University Press, pp. 463–472, 1984, by permission of Oxford University Press. *B* and *C* courtesy of M. Margaret Wierzbicka, M.D., West Roxbury Veterans Administration Hospital, Boston.)

into mechanisms controlling discharge of spinal motor neurons. Synchronization of discharges of independent motor neurons ordinarily does not take place (see Fig. 25–5B) despite the presence of various physiologic factors that would tend to promote it. CNS mechanisms are obviously normally active to prevent synchronization that appears under abnormal circumstances (Logigian et al., 1988). As seen in Figure 25–5C, synchronization can be quantified (Wiegner and Wierzbicka, 1987) and is not an all-or-nothing phenomenon as might be inferred from Figure 25–5A.

Stereotaxic ventrolateral thalamotomy effects a permanent cure of tremor at rest and rigidity in contralateral limbs of patients with Parkinson's disease (Andrew, 1984; Kelly et al., 1987). Medications that minimize enhanced physiologic tremor (peripheral β-adrenergic blocking agents, for example) reduce the enhancement of tremor amplitude found in patients with Parkinson's disease who become nervous or anxious (Koller and Herbster, 1987). Even patients sitting quietly during tremor recordings who do not feel particularly nervous have a little enhanced physiologic tremor that is quickly suppressed by propranolol or other β blockers (compare Fig. 25–1A and C). Because tremors are additive, propranolol therefore *does* reduce tremor in patients with Parkinson's disease but, despite contradictory reports in the literature because of confusion about which tremor was being treated, β blockers do not affect the amplitude of the underlying tremor at rest. To do that, one of the specific anti-Parkinson medications must be used. Older anticholinergic agents reduce the amplitude of tremor at rest but are only moderately effective in that regard. Now that CNS muscarinic acetylcholine receptor subtypes have been identified (Caulfield and Straughan, 1983), better therapeutic agents may become available. Levodopa also often reduces the amplitude of tremor at rest but is usually less effective in treating that symptom than in relieving akinesia. Bromocriptine is only slightly more effective as a therapy for tremor at rest than levodopa.

In summary, a really effective medical therapy for tremor at rest has not been discovered. Neither has the specific histopathologic or neurochemical abnormality responsible for tremor in Parkinson's disease as distinct from akinesia and rigidity been discovered. Nigral degeneration with striatal dopamine deficiency is probably related to tremor at rest, but correlations of the degree of these abnormalities with severity of tremor are less good than with akinesia or rigidity. Furthermore, tremor severity in a population of patients with Parkinson's disease seems to vary independently of the other symptoms. Finally, of eight patients with MPTP-induced parkinsonism, only four had mild tremor at rest and a proximal postural tremor was more prominent than the resting tremor (Burns et al., 1985). In these patients only nigrostriatal dopamine neurons are destroyed, whereas in naturally occurring Parkinson's disease, cell loss is also present in other CNS regions such as dorsal motor vagal nucleus, raphe nuclei, and even

the spinal cord. Perhaps lesions in these extranigral areas determine the extent and severity of tremor at rest. For further discussion see Jenner and Marsden (1988).

Neither essential-familial tremor nor parkinsonian tremor at rest is driven around the peripheral stretch reflex arc, as is the case with enhanced physiologic tremor. Patients with severe neuropathies or the occasional patients with dorsal rhizotomies continue to have the first two tremors but do not develop enhanced physiologic tremor. Neither of the former two tremors depends, therefore, on the stretch reflex arc for its maintenance. That is not to deny, however, that input from the limb influences these tremors. Perturbations such as stretch of muscle can reset the timing of each of these tremors and can also alter their amplitude (Lee and Stein, 1981). Inputs from peripheral sensory receptors interact with central tremor mechanisms but the latter are the prime movers.

Microneurographic recordings from human muscle spindle primary (Ia) fibers have demonstrated α-γ coactivation during tremor at rest (Hagbarth et al., 1975a,b) but not during enhanced physiologic tremor (Hagbarth and Young, 1979; Young and Hagbarth, 1980) (Fig. 25–6). In spinal reflexes such as tendon jerks, clonus, tonic stretch reflexes, tonic vibratory reflexes, and enhanced physiologic tremor, segmental afferent input from muscle spindles activates α but not γ motor neurons (so-called α-γ dissociation or pure α drive). On the other hand, with voluntary contractions of muscle and in tremor at rest, α and γ motor neurons are activated simultaneously, presumably to prevent muscle spindle insensitivity as extrafusal fibers contract (Vallbo, 1973; Vallbo et al., 1979). The α-γ coactivation is another example in which the outcome of normal voluntary descending cerebrospinal motor activity is similar to tremor at rest—microneurographic and EMG recordings from normal subjects imitating a tremor at rest are identical with those from patients with Parkinson's disease (Hagbarth et al., 1975a,b). One reasonable hypothesis is that tremor at rest is due to faulty operation (i.e., *release*) of cerebral motor centers, the output of which travels down to spinal motor neuron pools through normal pathways. Because both essential-familial and parkinsonian tremor at rest are alleviated by the same stereotactic thalamic lesion, one assumes there must be some overlap in the central mechanisms responsible for their production. This suggestion is also supported by the fact that patients with long-standing, mild, essential-familial tremor characteristically report an increase in that tremor as the first symptom of what turns out a year or so later to be the development of Parkinson's disease (Schwab and Young, 1971). Despite such hints, the pathophysiology of these tremors that arise within the CNS is virtually unknown. For an interesting explication of the following hypothesis, see the paper by Buzsaki et al. (1990). They suggested that parkinsonian tremor is due to network oscillations of thalamocortical cells because the striatal dopamine level is

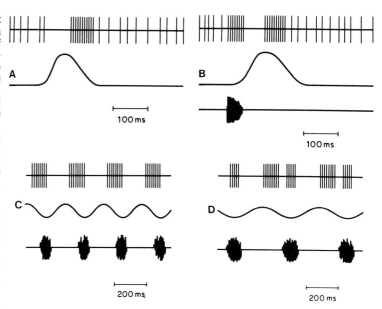

Figure 25–6. α-γ coactivation. The upper trace in each set of three drawings is meant to represent impulses in Ia fibers. The middle trace represents the change in length of the muscle containing those spindles (shortening is upward). The lower trace is EMG activity from the same muscle. (A) Electrically induced twitch of the extrafusal fibers; Ia endings, which fall silent as the muscle shortens, discharge in a burst as the muscle is passively stretched during the relaxation phase of the twitch. Calibration is 100 ms. In B there has been a voluntary twitch of the muscle. The EMG discharge producing that twitch is accompanied by a burst of Ia activity that reflects intrafusal contraction resulting from α-γ coactivation. Passive stretch produces a second burst of Ia activity during the relaxation phase of the twitch. Calibration is 100 ms. (C) Repetitive activity around the stretch reflex arc (clonus or enhanced physiologic tremor) in which each stretch of the muscle produces a burst of Ia activity followed shortly by an EMG burst. Note that there is only one burst of spindle activity per movement cycle; each burst has an origin similar to that in A. There is no evidence of intrafusal, α-γ–mediated contraction; this represents α-γ dissociation without γ activity. Calibration is 200 ms. (D) Either a voluntary tremor or the tremor at rest of Parkinson's disease. Each movement cycle is accompanied by two bursts of spindle discharges in B. One reflects α-γ coactivation and the other passive discharge during the relaxation phase. Calibration is 200 ms. (From Young R.R. Tremor in Parkinson's disease. In Delwaide P.J., Agnoli A., eds. *Clinical Neurophysiology in Parkinsonism*. Amsterdam, Elsevier, pp. 139–162, 1985.)

decreased, thereby enhancing the efficacy of GABAergic thalamopetal burst-promoting systems. They assumed that subcortical aminergic inputs to the thalamus act normally as antiburst or antioscillation mechanisms.

Paré et al. (1990) suggested that rhythmic low-threshold calcium spikes underlie tremor-related discharge of thalamic (VLa) neurons that receive inhibitory inputs from globus pallidus interna. Rhythmic output via VLa axons to premotor cortex and thence to motor cortex may activate motor programs ordinarily used to produce rapid alternating movements. In the same vein, Bergman et al. (1990) injected ibotenic acid into the subthalamic nucleus of monkeys with MPTP-induced parkinsonism. Lesions produced thereby in subthalamic nucleus "almost completely abolished" tremor in these monkeys. DeLong had demonstrated earlier that activity of subthalamic nucleus neurons was increased in such parkinsonian monkeys. The theory is that loss of striatal dopamine in Parkinson's disease produces excessive inhibitory activity from striatal neurons to globus pallidus externa. Increased inhibition there allows increased subthalamic nucleus activity, which then produces increased excitation of globus pallidus interna. As noted, this would increase inhibition of thalamus and thalamocortical neurons. This reduction in cortical activity could produce tremor as well as akinesia. Because the latter was also alleviated by lesions of subthalamic nucleus in the monkeys, akinesia may, after all, be a positive sign of motor dysfunction (and thereby amenable to ablation therapies) rather than a negative sign as has always been assumed.

NONPARKINSONIAN TREMORS AT REST

An occasional elderly patient has a tremor at rest of the face, jaw, and sometimes the hands. Although it looks exactly like that seen with Parkinson's disease, this tremor is unaccompanied by other symptoms of that illness and does not respond at all to levodopa or other antiparkinsonian therapy. The exact nature of this tremor at rest of the elderly is unknown. Is it caused by the same lesion that produces the identical-appearing tremor in Parkinson's disease, a lesion different from the nigral lesion?

Tremor at rest can also be seen with various cerebellar system lesions that produce titubation, as described earlier. Patients with the extrapyramidal lesions of Wilson's disease may also have a tremor at rest in the legs with a severe, proximal action tremor of the arms. Pathophysiologies of movement disorders in that condition are much more complex than the underlying biochemical cause and are not understood.

MISCELLANEOUS

Adams et al. (1972) first described a disabling action tremor in six patients with a relapsing, remitting, steroid-sensitive, demyelinating polyneuropathy. When the neuropathy improved, so did the tremor, and both worsened together when steroid administration was tapered. The tremor appeared to be particularly prominent when it was no longer possible, because of neuropathic deafferentation, to produce proprioceptive silent periods in ongoing muscle activity by electrical stimulation of the mixed muscle nerve. The EMG patterns underlying this neuropathic tremor (see Fig. 25–4C) are more irregular than those seen with essential-familial or parkinsonian tremor at rest and are neither consistently alternating nor synchronous in type. When complete deafferentation produces sensory ataxia but not a tremor, how does a neuropathy produce this tremor? One hypothesis is that neuropathic tremor is due to a peculiarly selective deafferentation in which muscle afferent input is deficient but joint position and other inputs remain functional. Smith et al. (1984) and Dalakas et al. (1984) have reported several similar patients.

Many older categorizations of tremor, for example, those using such classic clinical groupings as "toxic" (see Brumlik and Yap, 1970, pp. 8–9), are no longer useful. In that particular instance, too many separate types of tremor with completely different etiologies and fundamental mechanisms were grouped together—for example, alcoholic tremor, coffee-induced tremor, and the tremors produced by carbon monoxide, copper, manganese, or mercury poisoning. One expects and hopes our present categorizations will also be refined as fundamental pathophysiologic knowledge develops. Insight into the pathophysiology of various tremors obviously awaits progress in neurobiology of normal motor control. Perhaps our limited understanding of some of these tremors will provide clues or stimuli important to the progress of neurobiology in general.

Factitious or psychogenic tremors are sometimes the most difficult to recognize and treat. Recordings of tremor movements or acceleration may be useful in that situation. If the patient is distracted during measurements of tremor, frequency or amplitude or both may change in ways different from what one sees with pathologic tremors. Also, the patient can be asked to tap the nontremulous hand at frequencies other than that in the symptomatic hand. Often the movements in the latter then alter frequency to match the former.

CONCLUDING REMARKS

Each of the various tremor types is, as a first approximation, entirely different from all others and each must be considered separately. Knowledge of mechanisms responsible for production of enhanced physiologic tremors and for their pharmacotherapy is greater than for the tremor at rest of Parkinson's disease. The latter may have less to do with depopulation of substantia nigra pars compacta and striatal dopamine deficiency than was originally thought. The former is produced by β_2-adrenergic activation of muscle. Whereas knowledge of the pathophysiology of even these two tremors is sketchy, it is virtually nil for other tremors. In a review of the manifestations and management of these tremors, the best one can do is to describe their phenomenology as precisely as possible. Further clinical neurophysiologic research is under way into peripheral aspects such as muscle mechanics, limb kinetics, spindle primary afferent behavior, and mechanisms for synchronizing motor neuron discharge. However, it will probably not be possible to understand how centrally driven tremors arise until we understand a great deal more about the normal motor system in general and about muscle mechanics and single motor neuron discharge properties in particular.

Meanwhile, we do have sufficient knowledge to separate enhanced physiologic tremor from subclinical physiologic tremor and from essential-familial tremor. Although earlier authorities preferred to consider the latter tremor as simply a larger than normal physiologic tremor, that is now an untenable hypothesis. Enhanced physiologic tremors are driven around the stretch reflex arc; disappear in the presence of a severe neuropathy; do not show α-γ coactivation; are not affected by thalamotomy, primidone, and alcohol; and are immediately reduced in amplitude by selective peripheral-acting β_2-adrenergic antagonists. Essential-familial tremor does not depend on the stretch reflex arc for its appearance, continues unabated despite deafferentation, is cured by thalamotomy, is immediately alleviated by ethanol acting centrally, and is eventually reduced in amplitude by oral primidone, propranolol, or other centrally active β blockers. Physiologic tremor differs from enhanced physiologic tremor, which also differs from essential-familial tremor.

Finally, *tremors are additive*, so that enhanced physiologic tremor is often engrafted on a pre-existing essential-familial or parkinsonian tremor. To reduce confusion in the literature, for example, about what happens when a tremulous patient with Parkinson's disease takes propranolol (Koller and Herbster, 1987), and to ensure optimally effective therapies, each tremor must be considered in isolation.

Acknowledgments

Drs. Allen W. Wiegner and M. Margaret Wierzbicka have contributed substantially both to our understanding of tremor mechanisms and to our ability to quantify the mechanical and electromyographic correlates of tremor.

References

(Key references are designated with an asterisk.)

Adams R.D., Shahani B.T., Young R.R. Tremor in association with polyneuropathy. *Trans. Am. Neurol. Assoc.* 34:44–48, 1972.

Andrew J. Surgical treatment of tremor. In Findley L.J., Capildeo R., eds. *Movement Disorders: Tremor.* New York, Oxford University Press, pp. 339–351, 1984.

Barbeau A., Pourcher E. New data on the genetics of Parkinson's disease. *Can. J. Neurol. Sci.* 9:53–60, 1982.

Barker D., Saito M. Autonomic innervation of receptors and muscle fibres in cat skeletal muscle. *Proc. R. Soc. Lond. [Biol.]* 212:317–332, 1981.

Bergman H., Wichmann T., DeLong M.R. Reversal of experimental parkinsonism by lesions of the subthalamic nucleus. *Science* 249:1436–1438, 1990.

Bharucha N.E., Bharucha E.P., Bharucha A.E., et al. Prevalence of essential tremor in the Parsi community of Bombay, India. *Arch. Neurol.* 45:907–908, 1988.

Bowman W.C. Effects of adrenergic activators and inhibitors on skeletal muscles. *Handb. Exp. Pharm.* 54:47–128, 1980.

Bowman W.C., Nott N.W. Muscle tremor produced by sympathomimetic bronchodilators. *J. Pharm. Pharmacol.* 23(Suppl.):225, 1971.

Brantigan C.O., Brantigan T.A., Joseph N. The effect of beta blockade on stage fright: a controlled study. *Rocky Mt. Med. J.* 72:227–232, 1979.

Brantigan C.O., Brantigan T.A., Joseph N. Effect of beta blockade and beta stimulation on stage fright. *Am. J. Med.* 72:88–94, 1982.

Brooks V.B., Thach W.T. Cerebellar control of posture and movement. In Brooks V.B. ed. *Handbook of Physiology*. Section 1. *The Nervous System*. Vol. II. *Motor Control*. Part 2. Bethesda, American Physiological Society, pp. 877–946, 1981.

Brumlik J., Yap C.-B. *Normal Tremor*. Springfield, IL, Thomas, 1970.

Burns R.S., LeWitt P.A., Ebert M.H., et al. The classical syndrome of striatal dopamine deficiency—parkinsonism induced by 1-methyl-4-phenyl-1,2,3,6-tetrahydropyridine (MPTP). *N. Engl. J. Med.* 312:1418–1421, 1985.

Buzsaki G., Smith A., Berger S., et al. Petit mal epilepsy and parkinsonian tremor: hypothesis of a common pacemaker. *Neuroscience* 36:1–14, 1990.

Calzetti S., Findley L., Risani F., et al. Phenylethylmalonamide in essential tremor. *J. Neurol. Neurosurg. Psychiatry* 44:932–934, 1981.

Caulfield M., Straughan D. Muscarinic receptors revisited. *Trends Neurosci.* 6:73–75, 1983.

Cleeves L., Findley L. Propranolol and propranolol-LA in essential tremor: a double-blind comparative study. *J. Neurol. Neurosurg. Psychiatry* 51:379–381, 1988.

Cleeves L., Findley L., Koller W. Lack of association between essential tremor and Parkinson's disease. *Ann. Neurol.* 24:23–26, 1988.

Critchley E. Clinical manifestations of essential tremor. *J. Neurol. Neurosurg. Psychiatry* 35:365–372, 1972.

Critchley M. Observations on essential (heredofamilial) tremor. *Brain* 72:113–139, 1949.

Dalakas M.C., Teravainen H., Engel W.K. Tremor as a feature of chronic relapsing and dysgammaglobulinemic polyneuropathies. Incidence and management. *Arch. Neurol.* 41:711–714, 1984.

Delwaide P.J., Gonce M. Pathophysiology of Parkinson's signs. In Jankovic J., Tolosa E., eds. *Parkinson's Disease and Movement Disorders*. Baltimore, Urban & Schwarzenberg, pp. 59–73, 1988.

*Desmedt J.E. ed. *Physiological Tremor, Pathological Tremor and Clonus. Progress in Clinical Neurophysiology*. Vol. 5. Basel, Karger, 1978.

Dobmeyer D.J., Stine R.A., Leier C.V., et al. The arrhythmogenic effects of caffeine in human beings. *N. Engl. J. Med.* 308:814–816, 1983.

Dupuis M.J.M., Delwaide P.J., Boucqucy D., et al. Homolateral disappearance of essential tremor after cerebellar stroke. *Mov. Disord.* 4:180–187, 1989.

Elble R.J. Physiologic and essential tremor. *Neurology* 36:225–231, 1986.

Fellenius E. Muscle fatigue and beta-blockers—a review. *Int. J. Sports Med.* 4:1–8, 1983.

*Findley L.J., Capildeo R., eds. *Movement Disorders: Tremor*. New York, Oxford University Press, 1984.

Findley L.J., Cleeves L., Calzetti S. Primidone in essential tremor of the hands and head: a double blind controlled clinical study. *J. Neurol. Neurosurg. Psychiatry* 48:911–915, 1985.

Freund H.-J., Dietz V. The relationship between physiological and pathological tremor. In Desmedt J.E., ed. *Physiological Tremor, Pathological Tremor and Clonus. Progress in Clinical Neurophysiology*. Vol. 5. Basel, Karger, pp. 66–89, 1978.

Freund H.-J., Hefter H., Hoemberg V., et al. Differential diagnosis of motor disorders by tremor analysis. In Findley L.J., Capildeo R., eds. *Movement Disorders: Tremor*. New York, Oxford University Press, pp. 27–35, 1984.

Gaby N.S., Lefkowitz D.S., Israel J.R. Treatment of lithium tremor with metoprolol. *Am. J. Psychiatry* 140:593–595, 1983.

Geraghty J.J., Jankovic J., Zetusky W.J. Association between essential tremor and Parkinson's disease. *Ann. Neurol.* 17:329–333, 1985.

Growdon J.H., Shahani B.T., Young R.R. The effect of alcohol on essential tremor. *Neurology (Minneap.)* 25:259–262, 1975.

Haerer A.F., Anderson D.W., Schoenberg B.S. Prevalence of essential tremor. *Arch. Neurol.* 39:750–751, 1982.

Hagbarth K.-E., Young R.R. Participation of the stretch reflex in human physiological tremor. *Brain* 102:509–526, 1979.

Hagbarth K.-E., Wallin G., Löfstedt L. Muscle spindle activity in man during voluntary fast alternating movements. *J. Neurol. Neurosurg. Psychiatry* 38:625–635, 1975a.

Hagbarth K.-E., Wallin G., Löfstedt L., et al. Muscle spindle activity in alternating tremor of parkinsonism and in clonus. *J. Neurol. Neurosurg. Psychiatry* 38:636–641, 1975b.

Herskovits E., Blackwood W. Essential (familial, hereditary) tremor. A case report. *J. Neurol. Neurosurg. Psychiatry* 32:509–511, 1969.

Herskovits E., Figueroa E., Mangone C. Hereditary essential tremor in Buenos Aires (Argentina). *Arq. Neuro-Psiquiatr.* 46:238–247, 1988.

*Hubble J.P., Busenbark K.L., Koller W.C. Essential tremor. *Clin. Neuropharmacol.* 12:453–482, 1989.

Jenner P., Marsden C.D. MPTP-induced parkinsonism as an experimental model of Parkinson's disease. In Jankovic J., Tolosa E., eds. *Parkinson's Disease and Movement Disorders*. Baltimore, Urban & Schwarzenberg, pp. 37–48, 1988.

Kelly P.J., Ahlekog J.E., Goeres S.J., et al. Computer-assisted stereotactic ventralis lateralis thalamotomy with microelectrode recording in patients with Parkinson's disease. *Mayo Clin. Proc.* 62:655–664, 1987.

Koller W.C. Alcoholism in essential tremor. *Neurology (N.Y.)* 33:1074–1076, 1983.

Koller W.C., Herbster G. Adjuvant therapy of parkinsonian tremor. *Arch. Neurol.* 44:921–923, 1987.

Koller W.C., Royse V. Efficacy of primidone in essential tremor. *Neurology* 36:121–124, 1986.

Koller W.C., Cone S., Herbster G. Caffeine and tremor. *Neurology* 37:169–172, 1987.

Lamarre Y. Tremorgenic mechanism in primates. In Meldrum B.S., Marsden C.D., eds. *Primate Models of Neurological Disorders*. New York, Raven Press, pp. 23–34, 1975.

Lamarre Y. Animal models of physiological, essential and parkinsonian-like tremors. In Findley L.J., Capildeo R., eds. *Movement Disorders: Tremor*. New York, Oxford University Press, pp. 183–194, 1984.

Larsson T., Sjögren T. Essential tremor—a clinical and genetic population study. *Acta Psychiatr. Neurol. Scand.* 36(Suppl. 144):1–176, 1960.

Lee R.G., Stein R.B. Resetting tremor by mechanical perturbations: a comparison of essential tremor and parkinsonian tremor. *Ann. Neurol.* 10:523–531, 1981.

Lefebvre-D'Amour M., Shahani B.T., Young R.R. Tremor in alcoholic patients. In Desmedt J.E., ed. *Physiological Tremor, Pathological Tremor and Clonus. Progress in Clinical Neurophysiology*. Vol. 5. Basel, Karger, pp. 160–164, 1978.

Lippold O.C.J. Oscillation in the stretch reflex arc and the origin of the rhythmical 8–12 c/s component of physiological tremor. *J. Physiol. (Lond.)* 206:359–382, 1970.

*Logigian E.L., Wierzbicka M.M., Bruyninckx F., et al. Motor unit synchronization in physiologic, enhanced physiologic, and voluntary tremor in man. *Ann. Neurol.* 23:242–250, 1988.

*Marsden C.D. Origins of normal and pathological tremor. In Findley L.J., Capildeo R., eds. *Movement Disorders: Tremor*. New York, Oxford University Press, pp. 37–84, 1984.

Marsden C.D., Meadows J.C. The effect of adrenaline on the contraction of human muscle. *J. Physiol. (Lond.)* 207:429–448, 1970.

Marsden C.D., Foley T.H., Owen D.A.L., et al. Peripheral beta-adrenergic receptors concerned with tremor. *Clin. Sci.* 33:53–65, 1967.

Marsden C.D., Meadows J.C., Lange G.W., et al. Variation in human physiological finger tremor with particular reference to changes with age. *Electroencephalogr. Clin. Neurophysiol.* 27:169–178, 1969.

Marshall J. The effect of aging upon physiological tremor. *J. Neurol. Neurosurg. Psychiatry* 24:14–17, 1961.

Marshall J. Observations on essential tremor. *J. Neurol. Neurosurg. Psychiatry* 25:122–125, 1962.

Martinelli P., Gabellini A.S., Gulli M.R., et al. Different clinical features of essential tremor: a 200 patient study. *Acta Neurol. Scand.* 75:106–111, 1987.

Matthews P.B.C. *Mammalian Muscle Receptors and Their Central Actions*. Baltimore, Williams & Wilkins, 1977.

McMahon T.A. *Muscles, Reflexes and Locomotion*. Princeton, Princeton University Press, pp. 44–45, 1984.

O'Brien M.D., Upton A.R., Toseland P.A. Benign familial tremor treated with primidone. *Br. Med. J.* 282:178–180, 1981.

Paré D., Curro'Dossi R., Steriade M. Neuronal basis of the parkinsonian resting tremor: a hypothesis and its implications for treatment. *Neuroscience* 35:217–226, 1990.

Parkinson J. An Essay on the Shaking Palsy (1817). *Med. Classics* 2:964–997, 1937.

Rack P.M.H. Mechanical and reflex factors in human tremor. In Desmedt J.F., ed. *Physiological Tremor, Pathological Tremor and Clonus. Progress in Clinical Neurophysiology*. Vol. 5. Basel, Karger, pp. 17–27, 1978.

Rautakorpi I., Takala J., Marttila R.J., et al. Essential tremor in a Finnish population. *Acta Neurol. Scand.* 66:58–67, 1982.

Robertson D., Froelich J.C., Carr R.K. Effects of caffeine on plasma activity, catecholamines and blood pressure. *N. Engl. J. Med.* 298:181–186, 1978.

Roussy G., Lévy G. Sept cas d'une maladie familiale particulière. *Rev. Neurol. (Paris)* 2:427–450, 1926.

Sasso E., Perucca E., Calzetti S. Double-blind comparison of primidone and phenobarbital in essential tremor. *Neurology* 38:808–810, 1988.

Schroeder D., Nasrallah H.A. High alcoholism rate in patients with essential tremor. *Am. J. Psychiatry* 139:1471–1473, 1982.

Schwab R.S., Young R.R. Non-resting tremor in Parkinson's disease. *Trans. Am. Neurol. Assoc.* 96:305–307, 1971.

Shahani B.T. Tremor associated with peripheral neuropathy. In Findley L.J., Capildeo R., eds. *Movement Disorders: Tremor*. New York, Oxford University Press, pp. 389–398, 1984.

Shahani B.T., Young R.R. Physiological and pharmacological aids in the different diagnosis of tremor. *J. Neurol. Neurosurg. Psychiatry* 39:772–783, 1976.

Shiffman S.M., Gritz E.R., Maltese J., et al. Effects of cigarette smoking and oral nicotine on hand tremor. *Clin. Pharmacol. Ther.* 33:800–805, 1983.

Smith I.S., Furness P., Thomas P.K. Tremor in peripheral neuropathy. In Findley L.J., Capildeo R., eds. *Movement Disorders: Tremor*. New York, Oxford University Press, pp. 399–406, 1984.

Stiles R.N. Frequency and displacement amplitude relations for normal hand tremor. *J. Appl. Physiol.* 40:44–54, 1976.

Vallbo A.B. Muscle spindle afferent discharge from resting and contracting muscles in normal human subjects. In Desmedt J.E., ed. *New Developments in Electromyography and Clinical Neurophysiology*. Basel, Karger, pp. 251–262, 1973.

Vallbo A.B., Hagbarth K.-E., Törebjork H.E., et al. Somatosensory, proprioceptive, and sympathetic activity in human peripheral nerves. *Physiol. Rev.* 59:919–957, 1979.

Vanesse M., Bedard P., Andermann F. Shuddering attacks in children: an early clinical manifestation of essential tremor. *Neurology* 26:1027–1030, 1976.

Wiegner A.W., Wierzbicka M.M. A method for assessing significance of peaks in cross-correlation histograms. *J. Neurosci. Methods* 22:125–131, 1987.

Wiegner A.W., Young R.R. EMG, Ia and stretch reflex activity during damped hand oscillations in man. *Soc. Neurosci. Abstr.* 10:637, 1984.

Winkler G.F., Young R.R. The control of essential tremor by propranolol. *Trans. Am. Neurol. Assoc.* 96:66–68, 1971.

Winkler G.F., Young R.R. Efficacy of chronic propranolol therapy in action tremors of the familial, senile or essential varieties. *N. Engl. J. Med.* 290:984–988, 1974.

Young R.R. Essential-familial and other action tremors. *Semin. Neurol.* 2:386–391, 1982.

Young R.R. Enhanced physiological tremor in Parkinson's disease. In Yahr M.D., ed. *Current Concepts of Parkinson's Disease and Related Disorders*. Princeton, Excerpta Medica, pp. 56–72, 1983.

Young R.R. Physiological and enhanced physiological tremor. In Findley L.J., Capildeo R., eds. *Movement Disorders: Tremor*. New York, Oxford University Press, pp. 127–134, 1984a.

Young R.R. Tremor in relation to certain other movement disorders. In Findley L.J., Capildeo R., eds. *Movement Disorders: Tremor*. New York, Oxford University Press, pp. 463–472, 1984b.

*Young R.R. Tremor in Parkinson's disease. In Delwaide P.J., Agnoli A., eds. *Clinical Neurophysiology in Parkinsonism*. Amsterdam, Elsevier, pp. 139–162, 1985.

Young R.R., Hagbarth K.-E. Physiological tremor enhanced by manoeuvres affecting the segmental stretch reflex. *J. Neurol. Neurosurg. Psychiatry* 43:248–256, 1980.

Young R.R., Shahani B.T. Pharmacology of tremor. *Clin. Neuropharmacol.* 4:139–156, 1979a.

Young R.R., Shahani B.T. Single unit behavior in human muscle afferent and efferent systems. In Poirier L.J., Sourkes T.L., Bedard P.J., eds. *The Extrapyramidal System and Its Disorders*. New York, Raven Press, pp. 178–183, 1979b.

Young R.R., Shahani B.T. Asterixis—one type of negative myoclonus. In Fahn S., Marsden C.D., Van Woert M., eds. *Myoclonus*. New York, Raven Press, pp. 137–156, 1986.

*Young R.R., Wiegner A.W. Tremor. In Swash M., Kennard C., eds. *Scientific Basis of Clinical Neurology*. Edinburgh, Churchill Livingstone, pp. 116–132, 1985.

Young R.R., Growdon J.H., Shahani B.T. Beta-adrenergic mechanisms in action tremor. *N. Engl. J. Med.* 298:950–953, 1975.

Young R.R., Shahani B.T., Kjellberg R.N. Unilateral asterixis produced by a discrete CNS lesion. *Trans. Am. Neurol. Assoc.* 101:306–307, 1976.

Yudell R., Dyck P.J., Lambert E.H. A kinship with the Roussy-Lévy syndrome. *Arch. Neurol.* 13:432–440, 1965.

26

Oculomotor Control: Normal and Abnormal

R. John Leigh
David S. Zee

An approach to understanding eye movements best begins by examining the ways in which they serve vision (Leigh and Zee, 1991). Conjugate eye movements may be classified according to their function (Table 26–1). All eye movements serve the needs of vision and are aimed at ensuring optimal visual acuity. A prerequisite of clear vision is that images of objects be held relatively steady on the retina. Vestibular and optokinetic eye movements work together to keep the image of the world stationary on the retina during head rotation; pursuit eye movements also contribute. By producing compensatory slow phases in the orbit that are equal and opposite to head movements, these reflexes ensure that gaze (eye position in space) can be held constant during head rotation and clear vision can be preserved. Saccadic, pursuit, and vergence eye movements change gaze so that images of objects of interest are brought to or kept on the fovea, where visual resolution is highest. Saccades rapidly bring onto the fovea the image of an object detected in the periphery; pursuit movements keep on the fovea the image of an object that is already moving. Vergence movements rotate the eyes in opposite directions so that the images of a single object are simultaneously placed on the foveas. For single, binocular vision, the images of an object must stimulate corresponding retinal elements, and alignment of the visual axes must be correct to within a few minutes of arc.

In this chapter, we first discuss the normal and abnormal control of conjugate eye movements and then turn to mechanisms of ocular alignment and disorders causing diplopia.

OCULOMOTOR CONTROL SIGNALS

To interpret abnormal ocular motility it is helpful to understand the way the central nervous system normally controls eye movements (Leigh and Zee, 1991; D.A. Robinson, 1981). To do this one must know the normal patterns of innervation for moving the eyes to change gaze accurately and for holding the eyes steady to maintain gaze on a stationary object of interest (Henn et al., 1982a,b; Hepp et al., 1989; D.A. Robinson, 1978; Van Gisbergen and Van Opstal, 1989). The major hindrance to rotation of the globe is orbital viscosity because the moment of inertia of the globe is relatively small. For rapid eye movements (saccades and quick phases of nystagmus), a powerful contraction of the extraocular muscles is necessary to overcome viscous drag. This is accomplished by a phasic increase in the frequency of neural discharge that is called the pulse of innervation. Once the eyes are brought to their new position they must be held there against the elastic restoring forces of the orbital tissues, which tend to return the globe to the primary position. Preventing this centripetal drift requires a steady contraction of the extraocular muscles. This is produced by a constant, tonic level of neural activity called the step of innervation. The oculomotor control signal for saccadic eye movements is this pulse-step of innervation (Fig. 26–1). This pattern of activity is reflected in the characteristics of the discharge of both ocular motor neurons and the eye muscles themselves.

The immediate premotor command for the saccadic

Supported by National Institutes of Health grant EY06717, the Department of Veterans Affairs, and the Evenor Armington Fund (to Dr. Leigh) and by National Institutes of Health grant EY01849 (to Dr. Zee). We are grateful to Ms. Holly A. Stevens for editorial assistance.

Table 26–1. A FUNCTIONAL CLASSIFICATION OF HUMAN EYE MOVEMENTS

Class of Eye Movement	Main Function
Visual fixation	To hold the image of a stationary object on the fovea when the head is stationary
Vestibular	To hold images of the seen world steady on the retina during brief head rotations
Optokinetic	To hold images of the seen world steady on the retina during sustained head rotation
Smooth pursuit	To hold the image of a moving target on the fovea
Nystagmus quick phases	To reset the eyes during prolonged rotation and direct gaze toward the oncoming visual scene
Saccade	To bring images of objects of interest onto the fovea
Vergence	To move the eyes in opposite directions so that images of a single object are placed simultaneously on both foveas

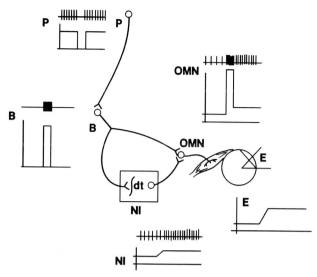

Figure 26–2. Relationship between pause cells (P) and burst cells (B) during saccades. Pause cells cease discharging just before each saccade, allowing the burst cells to generate the pulse. The pulse is integrated by the neural integrator (NI) to produce the step. The pulse and step combine to produce the innervational change on the ocular motor neurons (OMN) that produces the saccadic eye movement (E). Vertical lines represent individual discharges of neurons. Underneath the schematized neural (spike) discharge is a plot of discharge rate versus time. (From Leigh R.J., Zee D.S. *The Neurology of Eye Movements*. 2nd ed. *Contemporary Neurology Series*. Philadelphia, Davis, 1991.)

pulse is generated by burst neurons, which for horizontal saccades lie within the pontine paramedian reticular formation and for vertical saccades lie within a structure of the mesencephalon called the rostral interstitial nucleus of the medial longitudinal fasciculus (riMLF). Burst neurons discharge at high frequencies beginning just before and time locked to the saccade itself. Otherwise they are silent because of inhibitory inputs from pause neurons, which are located between the rootlets of the abducens nerve in nucleus raphe interpositus (Büttner-Ennever and Büttner, 1988; Büttner-Ennever et al., 1988). Pause neurons discharge tonically except during saccades, when they pause and allow burst neurons to generate a saccade.

The step of innervation is thought to be created by a neural gaze-holding network or neural integrator that integrates, in the mathematical sense, the saccadic eye velocity command to produce the appropriate position-coded information for the oculomotor

neurons. The medial vestibular nucleus and the adjacent nucleus prepositus hypoglossi are critically important for the neural integration of horizontal oculomotor signals (Cannon and Robinson, 1987). The flocculus of the cerebellum also contributes (Zee et al., 1981). For integration of vertical oculomotor signals, the interstitial nucleus of Cajal probably supplements the medial vestibular and prepositus nuclei (Fukushima et al., 1990). All types of versional eye movements require a step component of innervation to hold gaze at the end of a movement. Experimental evidence suggests that one integrator is shared by the versional eye movement systems (Cannon and Robinson, 1987). Figure 26–2 shows schematically the relationship between burst neurons, pause neurons, and the neural integrator for the generation of saccadic commands.

CONTROL OF HORIZONTAL CONJUGATE GAZE

The abducens nucleus itself is the site of assembly of the premotor commands for horizontal conjugate eye movements (Büttner-Ennever and Büttner, 1988; Henn et al., 1982a). The nucleus contains two types of neurons: abducens motor neurons, with axons that innervate the lateral rectus muscle, and abducens internuclear neurons, with axons that project, via the contralateral medial longitudinal fasciculus (MLF), to the medial rectus subdivision of the con-

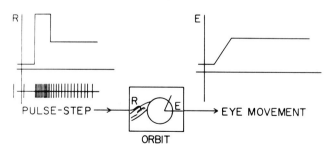

Figure 26–1. Neural signal for a saccade. *(Right)* Eye movement; E is eye position in the orbit, and the abscissa scale represents time. *(Left)* Neural signal sent to the extraocular muscles to produce the saccade. The vertical lines indicate the occurrence of action potentials of an ocular motor neuron. The graph above is a plot of the neuron's discharge rate (R) against time. It shows the neurally encoded pulse (velocity command) and step (position command). (From Leigh R.J., Zee D.S. *The Neurology of Eye Movements*. 2nd ed. *Contemporary Neurology Series*. Philadelphia, Davis, 1991.)

tralateral oculomotor nucleus (Fig. 26–3). Lesions of the abducens nucleus, therefore, cause a conjugate gaze palsy, an inability to move the eyes beyond the midline with any type of ipsilaterally directed versional eye movement (saccadic, pursuit, optokinetic, or vestibular). Lesions of the MLF, on the other hand, deprive the ipsilateral medial rectus of its innervation during versional eye movements. This leads to paresis of adduction during conjugate gaze but with intact adduction during convergence—internuclear ophthalmoplegia (INO) (Gamlin et al., 1989). If a "conjugate" gaze palsy is not perfectly conjugate, a coexisting abducens nerve lesion (abduction affected more than adduction) is suggested. A brain stem lesion affecting one abducens nucleus and the adjacent MLF causes paralysis of both ipsi-

lateral conjugate gaze and adduction of the ipsilateral eye. The only remaining movement during attempted conjugate gaze is abduction of the contralateral eye. This is the "one-and-a-half" syndrome (Pierrot-Deseilligny et al., 1981; Wall and Wray, 1983). A unilateral abducens nerve palsy combined with a bilateral INO also causes a one-and-a-half syndrome.

How do saccadic, pursuit, and vestibular commands reach the abducens nucleus? The velocity commands for horizontal saccades come from burst cells located in the pontine paramedian reticular formation adjacent to the abducens nucleus. Lesions here impair ipsilateral saccades, but vestibular slow phases and smooth pursuit may be spared (Hanson et al., 1986; Henn et al., 1984; Johnston and Sharpe, 1989; Kommerell et al., 1987; Pierrot-Deseilligny et al., 1984). This is because vestibular inputs and pursuit commands reach the abducens nucleus by direct projections from the vestibular nuclei; only if these pathways are involved, in addition to the lesion, will vestibular or pursuit movements also be affected. The output of the neural integrator (the step [tonic] component for versional eye movements) appears to reach the abducens nucleus via projections from the nucleus prepositus hypoglossi and the medial vestibular nucleus (see Fig. 26–3). Mesencephalic lesions, too, may affect horizontal eye movements, presumably by interrupting descending pathways carrying higher-level commands. A deficit in contralateral saccades and ipsilateral pursuit is the usual finding (Zackon and Sharpe, 1984).

The excitatory command for the horizontal vestibulo-ocular reflex comes from the contralateral vestibular nuclear complex. When the head is still, neurons in the right and left vestibular nuclei discharge tonically at the same rate. During horizontal head rotation the lateral semicircular canal in one labyrinth is stimulated and the lateral canal in the other is inhibited. This creates an imbalance between the discharge rates of the right and left vestibular nuclei; activity increases on one side and decreases on the other. The difference encodes head velocity and provides the command that generates the slow phase of vestibular nystagmus.

During sustained, constant-velocity head rotations, peripheral vestibular signals no longer encode head velocity accurately, as the cupula of the semicircular canal slowly returns to its initial position. Visual (optokinetic) inputs, however, also reach the vestibular nuclei, and by supplanting the fading labyrinthine signal they help sustain nystagmus. This tight relationship between optokinetic and vestibular eye movements is reflected in the finding of abnormalities of optokinetic responses after peripheral or central vestibular lesions. Because smooth pursuit tracking movements also contribute to the generation of slow phases during optokinetic stimulation, the optokinetic response is best judged by measuring optokinetic afternystagmus, a prolonged, slowly decaying nystagmus that occurs after the lights are turned off following full-field optokinetic stimulation. Op-

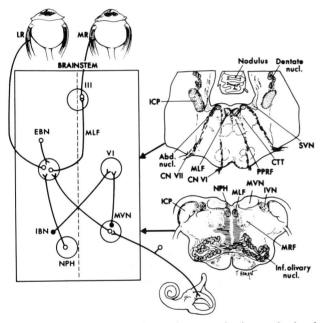

Figure 26–3. Anatomic pathways important in the synthesis of horizontal versional eye movements. The abducens nucleus (VI) contains abducens motor neurons that innervate the ipsilateral lateral rectus muscle (LR) and abducens internuclear neurons with axons that ascend in the contralateral medial longitudinal fasciculus (MLF) to make contact with medial rectus (MR) motor neurons in the contralateral third nerve nucleus (III). From the horizontal semicircular canal, primary vestibular afferents project mainly to the medial vestibular nucleus (MVN), where they synapse and then send an excitatory connection to the contralateral abducens nucleus and an inhibitory projection to the ipsilateral abducens nucleus. (An ipsilateral projection, via the ascending tract of Deiters, is not shown.) Saccadic inputs reach the abducens nucleus from ipsilateral excitatory burst neurons (EBN) and contralateral inhibitory burst neurons (IBN). Eye position information (the output of the neural integrator) reaches the abducens nucleus from neurons within the nucleus prepositus hypoglossi (NPH) and adjacent MVN. The anatomic sections at the right correspond to the level of the arrowheads on the schematic at the left. Abd. nucl. = abducens nucleus; CN VI = abducens nerve; CN VII = facial nerve; CTT = central tegmental tract; ICP = inferior cerebellar peduncle; IVN = inferior vestibular nucleus; Inf. olivary nucl. = inferior olivary nucleus; PPRF = pontine paramedian reticular formation; MRF = medullary reticular formation; SVN = superior vestibular nucleus. (From Leigh R.J., Zee D.S. *The Neurology of Eye Movements*. 2nd ed. *Contemporary Neurology Series*. Philadelphia, Davis, 1991.)

tokinetic afternystagmus is the best measure of the action of the portion of the optokinetic response generated via the vestibular nuclei.

CONTROL OF VERTICAL CONJUGATE GAZE

Mesencephalic structures are important for vertical eye movements (Fig. 26–4) (Büttner-Ennever and Büttner, 1988; Büttner-Ennever et al., 1982; Pierrot-

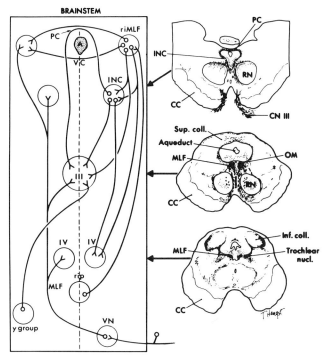

Figure 26–4. Anatomic pathways important in the synthesis of vertical and torsional, versional eye movements. Vestibular inputs from the vertical semicircular canals synapse in the vestibular nucleus (VN) and ascend in the medial longitudinal fasciculus (MLF) and brachium conjunctivum (not shown) to make contact with neurons in the trochlear nucleus (IV), oculomotor nucleus (III), interstitial nucleus of Cajal (INC), and rostral interstitial nucleus of the medial longitudinal fasciculus (riMLF). The riMLF, which lies in the prerubral fields, also receives an input from omnipause neurons of the nucleus raphe interpositus (rip), which lies in the pons. The riMLF contains saccadic burst cells that project ipsilaterally to the motor neurons of III and IV and send an axon collateral to INC. Connections between the right and left riMLF may pass in or near the posterior commissure (PC) and ventral commissure (VC). Cells in INC that may encode vertical eye position (contributing to the neural integrator) also project to III and IV: projections to the elevator subnuclei (innervating the superior rectus and inferior oblique muscles) pass above the aqueduct of Sylvius (A) in the posterior commissure; projections to the depressor subnuclei (innervating the inferior rectus and superior oblique) pass ventrally. Signals contributing to vertical smooth pursuit and eye-head tracking reach III from the y group via the brachium conjunctivum and a crossing ventral tegmental tract. The anatomic sections at the right correspond to the level of the arrowheads of the schematic at the left. CC = crus cerebri; CN III = oculomotor nerve; RN = red nucleus; Sup. coll. = superior colliculus; Inf. coll. = inferior colliculus; OM = oculomotor nucleus. (From Leigh R.J., Zee D.S. *The Neurology of Eye Movements.* 2nd ed. *Contemporary Neurology Series.* Philadelphia, Davis, 1991.)

Deseilligny et al., 1982). The vertical premotor saccadic command arises in burst cells located in the riMLF. This structure is ventral to the sylvian aqueduct in the prerubral fields at the junction of the midbrain and thalamus. The normal function of the vertical burst cells in the riMLF probably depends on ascending inputs from the pontine paramedian reticular formation because bilateral caudal pontine lesions cause abnormalities of vertical saccades (Hanson et al., 1986; Henn et al., 1984). The riMLF projects predominantly ipsilaterally to the nuclei of cranial nerves III and IV (Büttner-Ennever and Büttner, 1988). Each riMLF is connected to its counterpart, probably by the posterior and ventral commissures. Bilateral lesions of the riMLF in monkeys and in humans produce a predominant deficit of downward saccades or paralyze all vertical saccades. More dorsal lesions, in the posterior commissure, produce specific deficits in upward gaze: Parinaud's syndrome (Keane, 1990).

The velocity commands for vertical vestibular and pursuit commands and the vertical eye position command, in part, ascend to the midbrain in the MLF and brachium conjunctivum. Thus, bilateral INO causes not only bilateral paresis of adduction but also abnormalities of the vertical vestibulo-ocular reflex, vertical smooth pursuit, and vertical gaze holding (Evinger et al., 1977; Ranalli and Sharpe, 1988).

HIGHER-LEVEL CONTROL OF SACCADES

In the monkey, several cortical areas in parietal and frontal cortex have been shown to contribute to the control of saccadic eye movements (Tusa et al., 1986). In parietal area 7a (part of the inferior parietal lobule), neurons that respond to visual stimuli are also influenced by the direction of gaze (i.e., eye position in the orbit). These neurons may contribute to a transformation of retinal inputs to signals encoding the position of a target with respect to the head (Andersen et al., 1989). In the adjacent cortex of the lateral intraparietal sulcus are neurons that show presaccadic activity and encode the "motor error" command necessary for programming a saccade. The lateral intraparietal sulcus projects to both the frontal eye fields and the superior colliculus.

The frontal lobes contain three areas that contribute to the control of saccadic eye movements: frontal eye fields (FEFs), supplementary eye fields, and dorsolateral prefrontal cortex. The FEFs (part of area 8) contain a subpopulation of neurons that discharge before voluntary saccades to seen or remembered visual targets (Bruce and Goldberg, 1985). Microstimulation of this area elicits contralateral saccades. The supplementary eye fields, which lie in the dorsomedial frontal lobes, contribute to programming of saccades as part of complex or learned behaviors (Mann et al., 1988; Schlag and Schlag-Rey, 1987). The dorsolateral prefrontal cortex seems important for programming saccades to remembered target locations (Boch and Goldberg, 1989; Funahashi et al., 1989).

Lesions of these frontal lobe regions produce subtle behavioral deficits. Monkeys with a chronic FEF lesion show a specific defect in the ability to generate saccades to remembered targets (Deng et al., 1986). Patients who have undergone excision of portions of the frontal lobes, as treatment for epilepsy, are unable to suppress unwanted saccades to a novel stimulus presented in the contralateral visual field (Guitton et al., 1985). In addition, such patients show prolonged latency of saccades made to predictable target jumps (Sharpe, 1986).

All three frontal areas project to brain stem structures important in saccadic programming via parallel descending pathways (Leichnetz, 1981; Stanton et al., 1988a,b). Although direct projections from frontal cortex to the pontine reticular formation do exist, at least in the monkey, indirect projections via the superior colliculus seem more important. Subcortical frontal lesions produce increased latency of contralateral saccades, independent of any visual field defect (Pierrot-Deseilligny et al., 1987).

The superior colliculus has superficial, intermediate, and deep layers (D.L. Robinson and McClurkin, 1989; Sparks and Hartwich-Young, 1989). The superficial layers receive inputs from the optic tract and visual cortex. The intermediate and deep layers of the superior colliculus contain neurons that, when electrically stimulated, produce saccadic eye movements; they receive inputs from the lateral intraparietal sulcus and the FEFs. The FEFs send a direct projection to the superior colliculus but also an indirect projection via the caudate nucleus and the pars reticulata of the substantia nigra. The latter, indirect pathway is composed of two serial inhibitory links: a phasically active caudate-nigral inhibition and a tonically active nigrocollicular inhibition (Hikosaka and Wurtz, 1989; Hikosaka et al., 1989). If the FEFs cause caudate neurons to discharge, the nigrocollicular inhibition is removed and the superior colliculus is able to activate a saccade (see later). Thus, disease affecting the caudate could impair the ability to make saccades in complex tasks. Conversely, disease affecting the pars reticulata of the substantia nigra might disinhibit the superior colliculus and so cause excessive, inappropriate saccades. Such a combination of deficits is encountered in patients with disease of the basal ganglia, such as Huntington's disease (Lasker et al., 1987). In addition to these descending pathways, the eye fields of the frontal lobes have reciprocal connections with the intralaminar thalamic nuclei (Schlag-Rey and Schlag, 1984); the role of the latter in the control of saccadic eye movements has yet to be clearly defined. Lesions of the posterior thalamus that presumably involve frontotectal pathways, combined with collicular lesions, cause a hypometria of saccades to contralateral targets (Albano and Wurtz, 1982). Combined lesions of the FEFs and superior colliculus produce a profound, enduring deficit in ocular motility (Schiller et al., 1980). Such deficits are probably due to loss of both

of the major descending pathways that trigger saccades: the pathways that mediate saccades to novel visual stimuli and the pathways that are involved in programming of internally generated voluntary saccades.

CONTROL OF SMOOTH PURSUIT

In monkeys, a subdivision of the visual system is concerned with the perception of motion. It starts with retinal ganglion cells that project to the magnocellular layers of the lateral geniculate nucleus (Livingstone and Hubel, 1988). Some striate cortex neurons respond to moving visual stimuli, but they have small visual fields and are unable to encode motion of complex visual stimuli such as might occur in natural surroundings. Further information processing occurs in the middle temporal visual area, to which striate cortex projects. Neurons in this area respond to the speed and direction of target motions in three dimensions (Komatsu and Wurtz, 1988). Discrete lesions of the middle temporal area in monkeys produce a scotoma for motion in the affected visual field (Dürsteler and Wurtz, 1988). The consequences are that saccades can still be made accurately to stationary targets in the affected visual field, but moving stimuli cannot be tracked accurately by saccades or smooth pursuit (Dürsteler and Wurtz, 1988).

The middle temporal visual area projects to the adjacent medial superior temporal visual area; neurons here not only encode moving visual stimuli but also carry an eye movement signal (Newsome et al., 1988). Lesions of the medial superior temporal area cause a deficit of horizontal smooth pursuit for targets moving toward the side of the lesion. In addition, a retinotopic deficit for motion detection, similar to that with middle temporal visual area lesions, is present for targets in the contralateral visual hemifield (Dürsteler and Wurtz, 1988).

Human homologues of the middle temporal and medial superior temporal visual areas have been suggested (Leigh, 1989). In addition, a descending pathway for smooth pursuit has been postulated (Pierrot-Deseilligny et al., 1989). This pathway runs ipsilaterally through the retrolenticular portion of the internal capsule and posterior portion of the cerebral peduncle to reach the dorsolateral pontine nuclei (Suzuki et al., 1990). The latter nuclei also receive inputs from a portion of the FEFs that is probably concerned with smooth pursuit (Leichnetz, 1989). The dorsolateral pontine nuclei project to the flocculus, uvula, and dorsal vermis of the cerebellum, which in turn project to the oculomotor nuclei via the vestibular nuclei (Fig. 26–5). Lesions at various sites along this descending pursuit pathway produce predominant deficits of ipsilateral, horizontal smooth pursuit (Pierrot-Deseilligny et al., 1989).

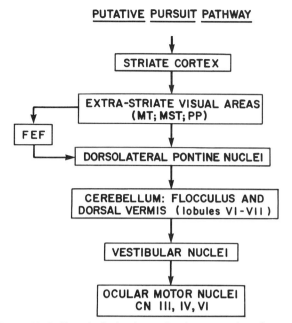

PUTATIVE PURSUIT PATHWAY

STRIATE CORTEX

EXTRA-STRIATE VISUAL AREAS
(MT; MST; PP)

FEF

DORSOLATERAL PONTINE NUCLEI

CEREBELLUM: FLOCCULUS AND
DORSAL VERMIS (lobules VI-VII)

VESTIBULAR NUCLEI

OCULAR MOTOR NUCLEI
CN III, IV, VI

Figure 26–5. Hypothetical scheme for the generation of smooth pursuit eye movements. The pathway starts with striate cortex, which received inputs from the lateral geniculate nuclei (indicated by topmost arrow). MT = middle temporal visual area; MST = medial superior temporal visual area; PP = posterior parietal cortex; FEF = frontal eye fields. (From Leigh R.J., Zee D.S. *The Neurology of Eye Movements*. 2nd ed. *Contemporary Neurology Series*. Philadelphia, Davis, 1991.)

CEREBELLAR INFLUENCES ON EYE MOVEMENTS

The cerebellum plays an important role in both immediate on-line and long-term adaptive oculomotor control (Berthoz and Melvill Jones, 1985; Leigh and Zee, 1991). The latter refers to the mechanisms that ensure that eye movements remain appropriate to their stimulus in normal development and aging as well as disease. The vestibulocerebellum, especially the flocculus, contains a group of Purkinje cells that discharge in relation to the velocity of the eyes moving in space (gaze velocity) during smooth pursuit tracking, with the head either still or moving. Other cells discharge in relation to saccades or to the position of the eyes in the orbit. Three distinct cerebellar syndromes have been identified as the result of studies of discrete lesions.

Lesions of the flocculus impair smooth visual tracking—both smooth pursuit with the head still and steady fixation of a target rotating with the head (Zee et al., 1981). The latter, called cancellation of the vestibulo-ocular reflex, is comparable to fixation suppression of caloric nystagmus. Floccular lesions also cause horizontal gaze–evoked nystagmus, which implicates the vestibulocerebellum in the normal function of the neural integrator. Other signs of flocculectomy are downbeat nystagmus, rebound nystagmus, and postsaccadic drift or glissades (see under Disorders of Saccadic Eye Movements).

Lesions of the nodulus and adjacent uvula cause a prolongation of the vestibular response. If monkeys with such lesions are placed in darkness, periodic alternating nystagmus may develop (Waespe et al., 1985).

Lesions of the dorsal vermis (lobules IV–VII) and the underlying fastigial nuclei cause saccadic dysmetria, especially hypermetria of centripetal (centering) saccades (Optican and Robinson, 1980; Selhorst et al., 1976).

The cerebellum—especially the flocculus—also plays an important role in mediating the adaptive capabilities of the oculomotor system (Berthoz and Melvill Jones, 1985). Floccular lesions interfere with the adaptive capability of maintaining the accuracy of vestibular eye movements as well as preventing postsaccadic drift (Lisberger et al., 1984; Optican et al., 1986). For example, when normal subjects wear reversing prisms (so that the seen world moves in the same direction as head rotation), they undergo an adaptive reprogramming of their vestibulo-ocular reflex. They learn to generate slow phases in the same direction as head rotation even when rotated in complete darkness. Patients with cerebellar disorders show deficits in this adaptive capability (Yagi et al., 1981).

DISORDERS OF SACCADIC EYE MOVEMENTS

Abnormalities of saccades can be divided into disorders of accuracy, velocity, latency, and stability. Furthermore, they can be analyzed as disorders of the saccadic innervational commands—the pulse, the step, and the match between the pulse and the step (Fig. 26–6). For optimal performance the saccadic pulse must be of the appropriate amplitude (approximately height × width) to ensure that the saccade is accurate, and of the appropriate height to ensure that the saccade is of high velocity. The saccadic pulse and step must be perfectly matched to prevent drift of the eyes after the saccade. A change in amplitude of the pulse creates saccadic overshoot or undershoot—saccadic dysmetria. This sign is characteristic of disorders of the dorsal vermis or the fastigial nuclei of the cerebellum, although it appears with lesions in other parts of the nervous system. In Wallenberg's syndrome, for example, a specific pattern of saccadic dysmetria occurs. Saccades overshoot to the side of the lesion and undershoot away from the side of the lesion, and with attempted purely vertical saccades there is an inappropriate horizontal component toward the side of the lesion. With lesions of the superior cerebellar peduncle, the opposite pattern occurs: saccades overshoot opposite to the side of the lesion (Ranalli and Sharpe, 1986).

A decrease in the height of the saccadic pulse causes slow saccades. Normally, saccades follow a relatively invariant relationship between peak velocity and amplitude. Slow horizontal saccades usually imply disease affecting the horizontal burst cells in

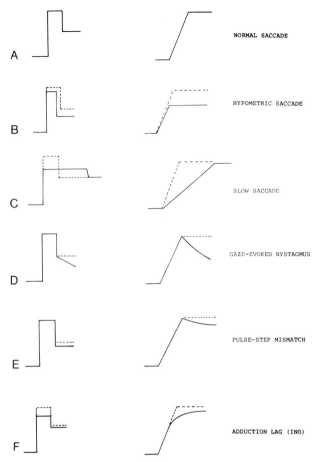

Figure 26–6. Disorders of the saccadic pulse and step. Innervation patterns are shown on the left, eye movements on the right. Dashed lines indicate the normal response. *(A)* Normal saccade. *(B)* Hypometric saccade: pulse amplitude (width × height) is too small but pulse and step are matched appropriately. *(C)* Slow saccade: decreased pulse height with normal pulse amplitude and normal pulse-step match. *(D)* Gaze-evoked nystagmus: normal pulse, poorly sustained step. *(E)* Pulse-step mismatch (glissade): step is relatively smaller than pulse. *(F)* Adduction lag: pulse amplitude is reduced, and step also is too small. (From Leigh R.J., Zee D.S. *The Neurology of Eye Movements.* 2nd ed. *Contemporary Neurology Series.* Philadelphia, Davis, 1991.)

the pons, such as olivopontocerebellar atrophy. Slow vertical saccades usually imply disease affecting the vertical burst cells of the midbrain, such as progressive supranuclear palsy. A mismatch in size between the pulse and the step produces brief (several hundred millisecond) postsaccadic drift or glissades. Postsaccadic drift occurs with disease of the vestibulocerebellum. The combination of slow, hypometric saccades and postsaccadic drift also occurs with INO, ocular motor nerve palsies, myasthenia gravis, and ocular myopathies.

Disorders of saccadic initiation lead to an increase in saccadic latency (the normal saccadic latency is about 200 ms). Often an associated head movement or a blink is needed to help initiate the saccade. Impaired saccadic initiation has been reported in patients with a variety of conditions including frontal

or parietal lobe lesions, congenital or acquired oculomotor apraxia, Huntington's disease, progressive supranuclear palsy, and Alzheimer's disease (for a review see Leigh and Zee, 1991).

Inappropriate saccades disrupt steady fixation (Abel et al., 1984) (Fig. 26–7). They include square wave jerks, small-amplitude (up to 5°) saccades that take the eyes off target and are followed within 200 ms by a corrective saccade. Square wave jerks may occur in normal, elderly subjects or in patients with cerebral hemisphere lesions, but they are especially prominent in progressive supranuclear palsy and in cerebellar disease (Sharpe et al., 1982). Square wave jerks may be an exaggeration of the microsaccades that occur in normal individuals during fixation and can be most easily detected by ophthalmoscopy when the patient is instructed to fixate a target seen with the other eye. Macro–square wave jerks (10–40° in amplitude) have been observed in multiple sclerosis and olivopontocerebellar atrophy. Macrosaccadic oscillations consist of sequences of markedly hypermetric saccades, separated by a normal intersaccadic interval (several hundred milliseconds), that continually overshoot the target. This causes a prominent

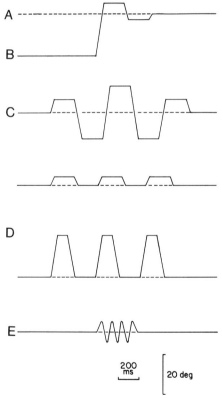

200 ms | 20 deg

Figure 26–7. Saccadic oscillations. *(A)* Dysmetria: inaccurate saccades. *(B)* Macrosaccadic oscillations: hypermetric saccades about the position of the target. *(C)* Square wave jerks: small, uncalled-for saccades away from and back to the position of the target. *(D)* Macro–square wave jerks: large, uncalled-for saccades away from and back to the position of the target. *(E)* Ocular flutter: to-and-fro, back-to-back saccades without an intersaccadic interval. (From Leigh R.J., Zee D.S. *The Neurology of Eye Movements.* 2nd ed. *Contemporary Neurology Series.* Philadelphia, Davis, 1991.)

back-and-forth oscillation about the point of fixation. Macrosaccadic oscillations reflect an increase in saccadic system gain (the saccade amplitude–target displacement relationship). They are typically found in patients with lesions in the midline deep cerebellar nucleus (Selhorst et al., 1976).

Saccadic oscillations without an intersaccadic interval (back-to-back, to-and-fro saccades) are called ocular flutter when they are limited to the horizontal plane and opsoclonus when they are multidirectional (horizontal, vertical, and torsional). Either type of oscillation may occur in patients with various types of encephalitis, as a remote effect of neuroblastoma or other tumors, and in association with toxins. Such oscillations are typically brought out by a change in gaze, eye closure, or an associated blink. Flutter and opsoclonus may reflect a disorder of saccadic pause neurons (Zee and Robinson, 1979), although other explanations are possible (Leigh and Zee, 1991; Ridley et al., 1987). Voluntary nystagmus is another example of saccadic oscillations without an intersaccadic interval.

DISORDERS OF SMOOTH PURSUIT

Low-velocity, inadequate pursuit is a common oculomotor finding. It is often a side effect of medications such as sedatives and anticonvulsants. It also occurs with disease of the cerebellum or of the brain stem in, for example, progressive supranuclear palsy. Smooth pursuit capability also decreases with age.

An imbalance of pursuit "tone" has been hypothesized as the cause of the nystagmus that occurs with cerebral hemispheral lesions. There is a slow constant drift of the eyes toward the side of the intact hemisphere, and pursuit of targets moving toward the side of the lesion is impaired. Disturbances of smooth pursuit caused by hemispheric lesions were described earlier.

"Reversal" of smooth pursuit may be seen in some patients with congenital nystagmus: the smooth eye movements are directed opposite to the motion of the target (Halmagyi et al., 1980a). A similar reversal occurs with optokinetic stimulation of the posterior retina of the albino rabbit, an animal with anomalies of the visual pathways. It has been speculated that the reversed pursuit in patients with congenital nystagmus may also be due to aberrant visual-oculomotor connections.

Abnormalities of smooth pursuit are usually accompanied by commensurate disturbance of tracking of smoothly moving targets with combined movements of eye and head. This is tested by asking the patient to fixate a target rotating with the head. If cancellation (fixation suppression) of the vestibulo-ocular reflex is intact, no nystagmus is seen and the eyes remain stationary in orbit. When pursuit is defective, cancellation is also impaired and nystagmus appears.

MECHANISMS OF NYSTAGMUS

Nystagmus is a repetitive, to-and-fro movement of the eyes. When pathologic, it reflects abnormalities in the mechanisms that hold images steady on the retina: the vestibular, optokinetic, and pursuit systems and the neural integrator. A disturbance of any of these mechanisms may cause drifts of the eyes—the slow phases of nystagmus—during attempted steady fixation. Corrective quick phases of saccades then reset the eyes.

Constant-velocity drifts of the eyes (Fig. 26–8A) with corrective quick phases produce jerk nystagmus, which is usually caused by an imbalance of vestibular or possibly optokinetic or pursuit drives. Lesions of the peripheral vestibular apparatus (laby-

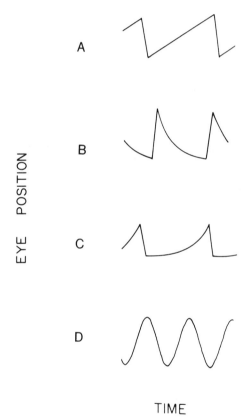

Figure 26–8. Four common slow-phase waveforms of nystagmus. *(A)* Constant-velocity drift of the eyes. This occurs in nystagmus caused by peripheral or central vestibular disease and also with lesions of the cerebral hemisphere. The added quick phases give a sawtooth appearance. *(B)* Drift of the eyes back from an eccentric orbital position toward the midline (gaze-evoked nystagmus). The drift has a negative exponential time course, with decreasing velocity. This waveform reflects an unsustained eye position signal caused by an impaired neural integrator. *(C)* Drift of the eyes away from the primary position with a positive exponential time course (increasing velocity). This waveform suggests an unstable neural integrator and is encountered in congenital nystagmus and in cerebellar disease. *(D)* Pendular nystagmus. Quick phases may be superimposed on this sinusoidal oscillation. Pendular nystagmus is encountered as a type of congenital nystagmus and with acquired disease. (From Leigh R.J., Zee D.S. *The Neurology of Eye Movements.* 2nd ed. *Contemporary Neurology Series.* Philadelphia, Davis, 1991.)

rinth or nerve VIII) usually cause a mixed horizontal-torsional nystagmus with slow phases directed toward the side of the lesion. Because smooth pursuit is preserved, peripheral vestibular nystagmus is suppressed during fixation. This may be evaluated at the bedside by using the ophthalmoscope; when the fixating eye is transiently covered, drifts of the optic disc and retinal vessels may appear or increase in velocity if there is an underlying vestibular imbalance. Frenzel goggles can also be used to remove fixation and bring out nystagmus. Nystagmus induced by a change in head position is frequently due to degenerative changes in labyrinth—benign positional vertigo—but may also be due to central disease (see Chapter 31). In particular, purely vertical positional nystagmus is suggestive of a posterior fossa lesion.

Nystagmus caused by disease of central vestibular connections may be purely torsional, purely vertical (downbeat or upbeat), or purely horizontal, or it may have a pattern that mimics that of peripheral vestibular lesions (Baloh and Yee, 1989). Smooth pursuit is usually also affected, so the velocity of slow-phase drift of central vestibular nystagmus does not diminish with fixation. Downbeat nystagmus in primary position usually reflects disease at the craniocervical junction, such as the Arnold-Chiari malformation or degenerative lesions of the cerebellum. Upbeat nystagmus in primary position occurs with lesions at the pontomedullary or pontomesencephalic junction or in the fourth ventricle (A. Fisher et al., 1983). Downbeat nystagmus is usually increased by convergence or lateral gaze. Purely torsional nystagmus usually reflects intrinsic brain stem involvement in the vestibular nuclei (Noseworthy et al., 1988) or lesions in the vestibulocerebellum. Periodic alternating nystagmus (horizontal jerk nystagmus that changes direction every 2 minutes) is a form of central vestibular nystagmus (Leigh et al., 1981) and can be created experimentally by removing the cerebellar nodulus (Waespe et al., 1985). It can be successfully treated with baclofen (Halmagyi et al., 1980b).

Nystagmus on attempted eccentric gaze and with slow phases that show a declining exponential time course (see Fig. 26–8B) is due to an unsustained eye position command. This is gaze-evoked nystagmus, and it commonly occurs as a side effect of certain medications, especially anticonvulsants, hypnotics, and tranquilizers; with disease of the cerebellar flocculus; or, in the brain stem, with lesions in the nucleus prepositus hypoglossi and medial vestibular nuclei. The latter structures are frequently involved in Wernicke's encephalopathy and account for the gaze-evoked nystagmus and vestibular paresis. With prolonged eccentric gaze, gaze-evoked nystagmus may damp and actually change direction. This is centripetal nystagmus (Leech et al., 1977). It is often followed by rebound nystagmus when the eyes return to the primary position; slow phases are directed toward the prior position of eccentric gaze. Rebound nystagmus usually coexists with other cerebellar eye signs (Bondar et al., 1984; Hood, 1981).

Latent nystagmus also has slow phases with exponentially decreasing velocity (Dell'Osso et al., 1979). Latent nystagmus appears when one eye is occluded; then both eyes drift conjugately so that the slow phases of the viewing eye are directed toward the nose. Latent nystagmus is commonly associated with strabismus and is acquired early in life but does not imply any underlying neurologic disease.

Nystagmus with slow phases that show an increasing exponential time course (see Fig. 26–8C) are typical of congenital nystagmus and may be due to instability of smooth pursuit or gaze-holding mechanisms (Optican and Zee, 1984). Congenital nystagmus is usually horizontal, accentuated by attempted fixation, diminished by convergence or active eyelid closure, associated with a head turn, and sometimes accompanied by reversed smooth pursuit. Occasionally, acquired lesions of the cerebellum produce nystagmus with slow phases that have increasing exponential waveforms.

Pendular nystagmus consists of a slow phase that is a sinusoidal oscillation (see Fig. 26–8D) rather than a unidirectional drift. Quick phases may be superimposed. Congenital nystagmus often appears pendular, although the slow-phase waveform of the nystagmus is usually not a true sinusoid and the nystagmus becomes a jerk at extremes of horizontal gaze. Acquired pendular nystagmus may be a manifestation of multiple sclerosis or a sequel to brain stem infarction with inferior olivary hypertrophy (the syndrome of palatomyoclonus) (Gresty et al., 1982; Nakada and Kwee, 1986). Acquired pendular nystagmus may have both horizontal and vertical components, and the amplitude and phase relationships of the two sine waves determine the trajectory taken by the eyes. For example, the trajectory is oblique if the sine waves are in phase and, more commonly, elliptical (or circular) if they are 90° out of phase. Acquired pendular nystagmus is frequently disconjugate and may even be horizontal in one eye and vertical in the other.

So-called convergence-retraction nystagmus, which occurs with midbrain lesions and usually coexists with upgaze paralysis (Parinaud's syndrome), actually consists of asynchronous adducting saccades (Keane, 1990; Ochs et al., 1979). Cocontraction may also occur, causing the eyes to retract into the orbit. See-saw nystagmus (one eye goes up, the other down) occurs with midbrain lesions and may be related to an imbalance in activity in structures that receive projections from the labyrinthine otolith organs (Kanter et al., 1987). Skew deviation and the ocular tilt reaction (one half cycle of see-saw nystagmus) may also be manifestations of otolith and especially utricular imbalance (Hedges and Hoyt, 1982). Skew deviation occurs with lesions in the medulla and the pons as well as the midbrain and may be part of an ocular tilt reaction (Brandt and Dieterich, 1987).

Dissociated nystagmus, which is greatest or present only in the abducting eye, commonly occurs in INO. The mechanism of abducting nystagmus in

Table 26–2. PULLING ACTIONS OF THE EXTRAOCULAR MUSCLES WITH THE EYE IN PRIMARY POSITION

Muscle	Primary Action	Secondary Action	Tertiary Action
Lateral rectus	Abduction	—	—
Medial rectus	Adduction	—	—
Superior rectus	Elevation	Intorsion	Adduction
Inferior rectus	Depression	Extorsion	Adduction
Superior oblique	Intorsion	Depression	Abduction
Inferior oblique	Extorsion	Elevation	Abduction

INO is unknown, and a number of hypotheses have been proposed (Leigh and Zee, 1991). In some patients this nystagmus is due to an adaptive increase in innervation to the medial rectus motor neurons of the paretic eye (Zee et al., 1987). Although an adaptive increase in saccadic innervation might help adduct the weak eye, because of Hering's law of equal innervation, it would also lead to abduction overshoot and nystagmus in the other eye. Alternatively, abducting nystagmus may occur because the MLF lesion interrupts a descending pathway to contralateral abducens motor neurons. Finally, dissociated nystagmus in INO may reflect asymmetric gaze-evoked nystagmus resulting from involvement of structures outside but adjacent to the MLF. It is possible that in a patient with INO, one or more of these mechanisms are responsible for the dissociated nystagmus.

OCULAR ALIGNMENT: ANATOMIC AND PHYSIOLOGIC PRINCIPLES

Cranial nerves III, IV, and VI supply the extraocular muscles, lid, and pupils. (Disorders of the pupils are considered in Chapter 34.) The 12 muscles that move the eyes carry out a precisely coordinated act, and it is not surprising that diplopia is a relatively common neurologic symptom. To identify which muscle weakness is causing diplopia, the neurologist must understand the relevant physiologic principles. To localize the lesion causing the muscle weakness, the anatomy of the courses of cranial nerves III, IV, and VI must be known.

The Extraocular Muscles

The primary pulling directions of the six extraocular muscles, when the eye is in primary position, are summarized in Table 26–2. The lateral rectus always abducts and the medial rectus always adducts the eye, but the actions of the vertical muscles depend on the starting position of the eye. The vertical recti and the oblique muscles pull the globe in both vertical and cyclotorsional directions. Because cyclotorsional movements of the eye are harder to interpret and compare at the bedside than are vertical movements, it is important to test the vertical recti and oblique muscles with the eye in a position that will cause the

muscle in question to have primarily a vertical action. Thus, to test the vertical recti, bring the eye first into the abducted position; to test the oblique muscle, bring the eye first into the adducted position.

The fibers of the extraocular muscles have certain histologic and histochemical differences from those of limb muscles (Spencer and Porter, 1988). As each muscle is traced anteriorly, two parallel layers are formed. The more peripheral or "orbital" layer of extraocular muscle is composed predominantly of singly innervated "coarse" fibers that have a rich microvasculature and are well suited to the sustained contractions necessary for steady fixation. The more central or "global" portion of extraocular muscle is composed of "granular" fibers that are relatively poor in oxidative enzymes and mitochondria, coarse fibers (similar to those of the orbital layers), and "fine" fibers that may be of the nontwitch type. Both orbital and global layers may contain multi-innervated fibers. Lennerstrand (1975) showed that multi-innervated fibers in the cat can develop a fused contraction at firing rates one-quarter of those necessary to produce maximal force. All muscle fibers contract for all functional types of eye movement (D.A. Robinson, 1978). However, the more fatigue-resistant fibers are well suited for holding steady fixation, and the global, fast-twitch fibers are more effective for moving the eye rapidly to a new orbital position (Scott and Collins, 1973). These differences become important, for example, when attempting to interpret the abnormal eye movements of myasthenia gravis.

The Courses of the Oculomotor Nerves

The anatomy of the oculomotor, trochlear, and abducens nerves is summarized in Figures 26–3, 26–4, 26–9, and 26–10 and is reviewed in more detail by Leigh and Zee (1991). The abducens nucleus lies in the floor of the fourth ventricle, where it is capped by the genu of the facial nerve. Because the abducens nucleus contains both motor neurons destined for the sixth nerve and internuclear neurons destined for the MLF, a lesion of the abducens nucleus causes an ipsilateral total gaze palsy. The abducens motor neurons leave the medial aspect of the nucleus and descend through the pontine tegmentum, passing through the medial lemniscus and lateral to the cortical spinal tract to emerge at the caudal border of the pons. Here the sixth nerve lies close to the

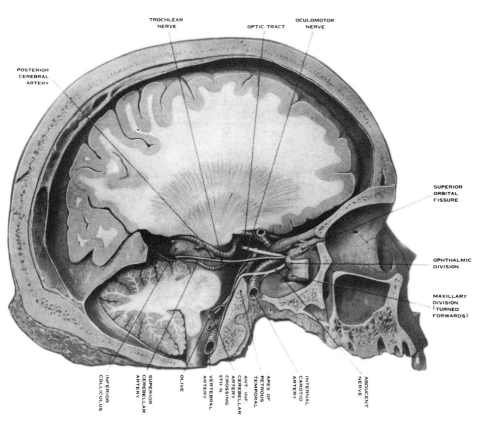

Figure 26–9. Parasagittal view of the intracranial courses of the third, fourth, and sixth cranial nerves. (From Warwick R. *Wolff's Anatomy of the Eye and Orbit.* 7th ed. Philadelphia, Saunders, 1976.)

anterior inferior cerebellar artery. The nerve then passes nearly vertically, running along the clivus through the prepontine cistern, where it is close to the inferior petrosal sinus. It then penetrates the dura medial to the trigeminal nerve and passes under the petroclinoid ligament. The abducens nerve then courses forward in the body of the cavernous sinus, lying lateral to the internal carotid artery and medial to the ophthalmic division of the trigeminal nerve. For a short part of its course, the abducens nerve carries pupillosympathetic fibers (Parkinson et al., 1978). It then enters the orbit through the superior orbital fissure to innervate the lateral rectus muscle.

The trochlear nucleus lies at the level of the inferior colliculus in the midbrain. Its fibers pass dorsally around the central gray and decussate completely in the anterior medullary velum to emerge from the dorsal aspect of the brain stem. The fourth nerve then passes laterally around the upper pons lying between the superior cerebellar and posterior cerebral arteries. It then runs forward on the free edge of the tentorium for 1–2 cm and penetrates the dura of the tentorium to enter the cavernous sinus. Here it initially lies laterally and below the third nerve. It enters the orbit through the superior orbital fissure, where it lies above the levator palpebrae superioris and passes to the medial aspect of the orbit to supply the superior oblique muscle.

The oculomotor nucleus sends fibers to extraocular muscles, to the levator palpebrae superioris, pupillary constrictor, and ciliary body. The oculomotor nucleus is a paired structure; its anatomy is sum-

marized in Figure 26–10. The classic scheme of Warwick (1953), shown in Figure 26–10*A*, has been modified by Büttner-Ennever and Akert (1981) on the basis of studies with tracer techniques. The latter authors demonstrated that the medial rectus neurons (see Fig. 26–10*B*, top) are distributed in three areas, A, B, and C. Neurons in all three locations receive inputs from the internuclear neurons of the contralateral abducens nucleus via the MLF (see Fig. 26–10*B*, bottom). Projections from the oculomotor nucleus are ipsilateral except those to the superior rectus, which are totally crossed, and those to the levator palpebrae superioris, which are both crossed and uncrossed.

From the nucleus, fascicles of the oculomotor nucleus pass ventrally through the MLF, red nucleus, substantia nigra, and medial part of the cerebral peduncle to emerge as rootlets in the interpeduncular fossa. At this point the oculomotor nerve runs forward between the posterior cerebral artery and the superior cerebellar artery. It passes through the basal cistern close to the temporal lobe uncus and over the petroclinoid ligament to gain the lateral wall of the cavernous sinus. Here, parasympathetic pupillary fibers lie peripherally in the dorsomedial part of the nerve as it passes forward and divides into superior and inferior rami. These both pass through the superior orbital fissure, the superior ramus supplying the superior rectus and levator palpebrae muscles and the inferior ramus supplying the medial rectus, inferior rectus, and inferior oblique muscles and the ciliary ganglion.

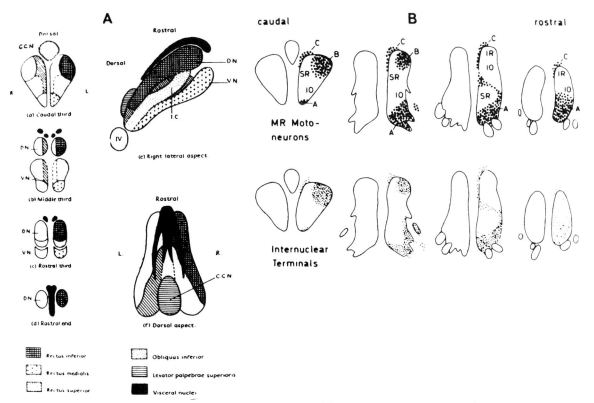

Figure 26–10. Anatomy of the oculomotor complex. *(A)* Warwick's scheme based on retrograde degeneration studies. CCN = caudal central nucleus; DN = dorsal nucleus; IC = intermediate nucleus; IV = trochlear nucleus; VN = ventral nucleus; R = right; L = left. *(B)* Scheme of Büttner-Ennever and Akert, based on radioactive tracer techniques. *(Top)* The medial rectus (MR) motor neurons, identified by injecting isotope into medial rectus muscle, lie in three groups, A, B, and C. IO = inferior oblique; IR = inferior rectus; SR = superior rectus. *(Bottom)* The same three areas also receive inputs from abducens internuclear neurons as demonstrated by injecting isotope into the contralateral sixth nerve nucleus. (*A* from Warwick R. Representation of the extra-ocular muscles in the oculomotor nuclei of the monkey. *J. Comp. Neurol.* 98:449–503, 1953. *B* from Büttner-Ennever J.A., Akert K. Medial rectus subgroups of the oculomotor nucleus and their abducens internuclear input in the monkey. *J. Comp. Neurol.* 197:17–27, 1981.)

CLINICAL TESTING OF DIPLOPIA: PHYSIOLOGIC PRINCIPLES

The range of movement of each eye can be tested independently with the other eye covered (ductions), and thus the direction of any limitation of movement can be correlated with the pulling action of a muscle (see Table 26–2). There are, however, many advantages to comparing the movements of the two eyes with both of them viewing (versions) as the subject is asked to fixate a target in the various positions of gaze. The nine cardinal positions of gaze include primary position, secondary positions (adduction, abduction, elevation, depression), and tertiary positions (combined horizontal and vertical movements from primary positions). In interpreting such testing, it is important to bear in mind several physiologic principals. First, Sherrington (1894) proposed that whenever an agonist muscle (e.g., the lateral rectus) contracts, the antagonist muscle (e.g., the medial rectus) commensurately relaxes. In other words, the agonist and antagonist do not cocontract; this is called the law of reciprocal innervation. Second, the extraocular muscles are arranged in yoke pairs (e.g., the right lateral rectus and the left medial rectus),

and the members of a yoke pair must receive equal innervation so that the eyes move together. This is Hering's law of motor correspondence. Although the way in which the extraocular muscles interact is quite complicated (for example, even during a simple horizontal movement, all the extraocular muscles contribute [Boeder, 1961]), these two principles can be effectively applied to testing for extraocular muscle paresis. Third, as noted at the outset, each retinal element localizes the visual stimulus that falls on it in a specific visual direction. If images from a single object fall on disparate or noncorresponding retinal elements of each eye, that object will be localized in two different directions. Fourth, the image of an object of interest is preferentially brought to the fovea, where it can be seen best, by a saccadic eye movement. Fifth, many normal subjects may develop a deviation of the visual axes when sensory fusional mechanisms (vergence) are temporarily interrupted by covering one eye; this is a phoria or latent deviation of the visual axis. Because the eyes still obey Hering's law and move together, the deviation is constant in all directions of gaze and is called concomitant (or comitant). If the amount of deviation between the visual axes changes with the direction of gaze, the deviation is called nonconcomitant and usually points to weakness of an extraocular muscle or mechanical hindrance in the orbit.

A clinical system for diplopia testing is summarized in Table 26–3 and is discussed in more detail by Leigh and Zee (1991). After looking for head tilts or turns, visual acuity, visual fields, pupils, and eyelids should be checked as preliminaries to testing ocular motility. Establishing the range of movement of each eye while the other is covered (ductions) and with both eyes viewing (versions) may reveal limitation of movement caused by extraocular muscle palsy. It is often useful to ask the patient to follow a penlight and to note the relative positions of the two corneal reflections with the eyes in each field of gaze. Further testing is, however, often required to elucidate the deficit. Such methods include subjective tests and cover tests.

Subjective tests depend on the patient's report of the subjective visual direction of images from one test object for each eye. If both images lie on corresponding retinal elements—for example, both foveas—the object will be reported to lie in the same visual direction. If the two images lie on noncorresponding retinal elements (Fig. 26–11), the object may appear to lie in two visual directions and the patient will report diplopia. Two further principles are important in this type of testing: (1) the images are maximally separated when the patient looks into the direction of action of the paretic muscle and (2) the target seen by the paretic eye is projected more peripherally (see Fig. 26–11). The red glass and the Maddox rod help the patient identify which image corresponds to the paretic eye. The Lancaster red-green test (Lancaster, 1939; Zee et al., 1984) enables the direction of the principal visual axis (line connecting the fovea with the fixation point) to be determined for each eye in each field of gaze. The patient wears a pair of goggles, conventionally with

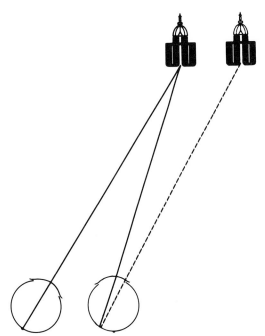

Figure 26–11. Disparate retinal images. The image of a distant object lies on the fovea of the left eye but, because of an esotropia (e.g., as in right lateral rectus palsy) the image in the right eye lies medial to the right fovea. Each retinal element corresponds to a specific subjective visual direction. Consequently, the subject localizes the same object in two different directions and experiences diplopia. The broken line indicates the perceived direction of the false image. (From Leigh R.J., Zee D.S. *The Neurology of Eye Movements*. 2nd ed. *Contemporary Neurology Series*. Philadelphia, Davis, 1991.)

a red filter in front of the right eye and a green filter in front of the left eye. Thus, the patient can see the image of a red light with the right eye and the image of a green light with the left eye. This test prevents fusional vergence. Red and green images are projected onto a screen in front of the patient from two flashlights, one emitting a red light and the other a green light. The examiner holds one flashlight and the patient holds the other. The separation of the red and green images on the screen in each of the nine cardinal positions of gaze is measured and represents the deviation of the visual axes.

Cover tests demand less cooperation by the patient than does the red glass or the Maddox rod. Cover tests depend on the principle that when one eye is required to fix on an object, it preferentially does so with the fovea. (Certain exceptions to this rule, caused by anomalous retinal correspondence, occur in congenital strabismus.) If the principal visual axis is not directed toward the object, an eye movement (saccade) will be necessary to move the image of the object, toward the fovea. The detection and estimated size of this corrective saccade ("movement of redress") provide an indication of misalignment of the visual axes.

The cover test (Fig. 26–12) reveals a tropia, a misalignment of the visual axes when both eyes are viewing. The patient is instructed to fix on a target

Table 26–3. A SUMMARY SCHEME FOR DIPLOPIA TESTING

Preliminary examinations
    Look for head tilts and turns
    Check visual acuity and visual fields
    Examine pupils and eyelids

Determine range of movement
    First, with one eye viewing (ductions)
    Second, with both eyes viewing (versions)

Use subjective tests to estimate amount of diplopia in the nine cardinal positions of gaze
    Red glass test
    Maddox rod
    Lancaster red-green test

Use the cover test to examine the tropia in the nine cardinal positions of gaze (prisms can be used to measure the deviation; see Von Noorden, 1990)

For vertical deviations, use the Bielschowsky head-tilting test

Systematically examine dynamic characteristics of the different functional classes of eye movement (Leigh and Zee, 1991)

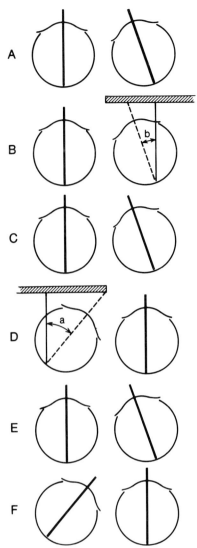

Figure 26–12. The cover test. *(A)* Initially, with both eyes viewing, there is an esotropia (right eye turned in). *(B)* When the cover is placed before the nonfixating right eye, no movement occurs, nor does it occur when *(C)* the cover is removed. *(D)* When the left eye is covered, the right eye must fixate the target and a movement of redress occurs. Note that the deviation of the sound eye, under cover (the secondary deviation, *a*) is greater than that of the primary deviation under cover (primary deviation, *b*). When the cover is removed, either *(E)* the left eye again takes up fixation or *(F)* the paretic eye continues to fixate if the patient is an "alternate fixator." (From Leigh R.J., Zee D.S. *The Neurology of Eye Movements.* 2nd ed. *Contemporary Neurology Series.* Philadelphia, Davis, 1991.)

that requires a visual discrimination (e.g., an *E*) and ensures a fixed accommodative state. The fixation target should be at distance, but testing with a near target is sometimes also necessary. First, with the eyes in primary position, cover the right eye and look for a movement of the uncovered left eye (movement of redress). If no movement of the left eye is seen when the right eye is covered, remove the cover and then cover the left eye, looking for a movement of redress of the right eye. For horizontal deviations, exotropia points to medial rectus weakness and esotropia to lateral rectus weakness. Repeat

this test with the eyes brought into the nine cardinal positions of gaze by rotating the head while the eyes fixate on the same target. In this way, the field of gaze in which the deviation is maximal can be determined.

Testing for Vertical Strabismus with the Bielschowsky Head-Tilting Test

After a paralytic strabismus has been present for some months, changes in the innervation and mechanical properties of the muscles occur so that the deviation no longer increases when the eyes look into the direction of action of the paretic muscle. This so-called spread of comitance can be particularly troublesome in the diagnosis of vertical muscle palsies. In this situation, noting any change of a vertical deviation as the patient tilts the head (ear to shoulder) to the right or to the left can often be helpful (Bielschowsky, 1940). Classically, with a superior oblique palsy, the deviation is increased when the patient's head is tilted to the side of the palsy and reduced with a head tilt to the opposite side (Fig. 26–13).

TOPOLOGIC DIAGNOSIS OF OCULOMOTOR NERVE PALSIES

Whereas knowledge of physiologic principles is essential in deducing which extraocular muscles are weak and thus which nerves are involved, anatomic knowledge allows the clinician to determine the site of the responsible lesion. Specifically, determination of involvement of other cranial nerves or of descending pathways is essential for proper localization. Causes of palsies of cranial nerves VI, IV, and III are summarized in Tables 26–4, 26–5, and 26–7, respectively.

Etiology of Abducens Nerve Palsy

Disease affecting the abducens nucleus causes an ipsilateral conjugate gaze palsy (Bennett and Savill, 1889; Meinberg et al., 1981; Pierrot-Deseilligny and Goasquen, 1984). This is because the abducens nucleus contains not only abducens motor neurons (bound for the sixth nerve) but also abducens internuclear neurons that pass into the contralateral MLF and so reach the contralateral medial rectus subnucleus (Büttner-Ennever and Akert, 1981; Maciewicz and Spencer, 1977) (see Fig. 26–3). Hereditary gaze palsies and Möbius' syndrome (horizontal gaze palsy, facial diplegia, and associated developmental anomalies) are probably due to failure of development of the abducens nucleus (Mellinger and Gomez, 1977). Duane's retraction syndrome is more common. This condition is characterized by narrowing of the palpebral fissure on adduction (retraction) and (1)

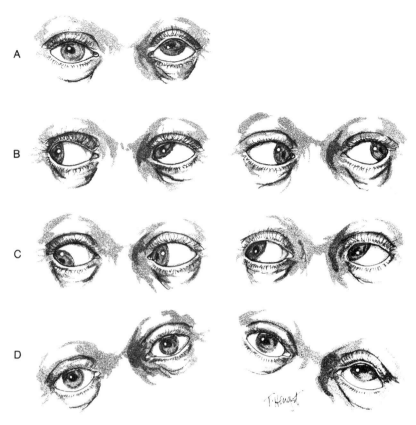

A

B

C

D

Figure 26–13. Diagnosis of vertical ocular deviation. The steps in diagnosis of a left superior oblique palsy are shown. *(A)* In primary position there is a left hypertropia. *(B)* This deviation becomes worse in right gaze, implying weakness of the right superior rectus or left superior oblique. *(C)* With the eyes in right gaze, the deviation is worse on looking down, implying weakness of the left superior oblique muscle. *(D)* The Bielschowsky head-tilting test. When the head is tilted to the left, there is exaggeration of the left hypertropia. (From Leigh R.J., Zee D.S. *The Neurology of Eye Movements*. 2nd ed. *Contemporary Neurology Series*. Philadelphia, Davis, 1991.)

limitation of abduction but full adduction (type I), (2) limitation of adduction but full abduction (type II), or (3) limitation of both abduction and adduction (type III). Some cases of Duane's syndrome are acquired, for example, through orbital injury, but in most patients the syndrome is due to abnormal development of the abducens nucleus. Thus, at autopsy, one patient who had a unilateral, left, type I Duane's syndrome had no left sixth nerve and the lateral rectus muscle was innervated by branches of the oculomotor nerve (Miller et al., 1982). The brain stem of this patient showed a normal right abducens nucleus but the left abducens nucleus contained less than half as many neurons as the right; these remaining cells were thought to be internuclear neurons. Duane's syndrome should be differentiated from other causes of sixth nerve palsy that require investigation. Patients with Duane's syndrome seldom complain of diplopia. The syndrome occurs more frequently in females and affects the left eye more than the right.

Lesions of the fascicles of the abducens nerve usually also involve structures through which the nerve passes. For example, sixth nerve palsy may be accompanied by ipsilateral facial weakness and contralateral hemiplegia (Millard-Gubler syndrome). Common pathologies at this site are infarction, demyelination, and tumor (Keane, 1976). Within its subarachnoid course, the sixth nerve may be involved along with other cranial nerves by infective or neoplastic meningitis, chordoma, or enlarged ectatic basilar aneurysm (Table 26–4).

Table 26–4. CAUSES OF ABDUCENS NERVE PALSY*

Nucleus
    Congenital gaze palsy and Möbius' syndrome
    Duane's syndrome (some cases)
    Infarction
    Tumor
    Wernicke's encephalopathy

Fascicular
    Infarction
    Demyelination
    Tumor

Subarachnoid
    Meningitis (infective and neoplastic)
    Trauma
    Subarachnoid hemorrhage
    Cerebellopontine angle and clivus tumor
    Aneurysm—ectatic basilar artery or berry aneurysm

Petrous
    Infection of petrous tip or mastoid
    Trauma
    Expanding supratentorial lesion
    After lumbar puncture

Cavernous sinus and superior orbital fissure
    Tumor (nasopharyngeal carcinoma, pituitary
      adenoma, meningioma)
    Aneurysm
    Cavernous sinus thrombosis
    Carotid—cavernous sinus thrombosis
    Dural arteriovenous malformation
    Infectious, including herpes zoster

Localization uncertain
    Infarction (often in association with diabetes or
      hypertension)

*See the following references: Galetta and Smith, 1989; Keane, 1976; Rush and Younge, 1981.

Table 26–5. CAUSES OF TROCHLEAR NERVE PALSY*

Nuclear and fascicular
  Trauma
  Hemorrhage or infection
  Demyelination

Subarachnoid
  Trauma
  Tumor
  Neurosurgical complication
  Meningitis

Cavernous sinus and superior orbital fissure
  Tumor
  Aneurysm
  Herpes zoster
  Tolosa-Hunt syndrome

Localization uncertain
  Infarction (often in association with diabetes or
    hypertension)

*See the following references: Mansour and Reinecke, 1986; Younge and Sutula, 1977.

As the abducens nerve rises and passes over the petrous bone, it lies close to the fifth nerve. These adjacent nerves may be involved by infection of the petrous bone causing diplopia and facial pain—Gradenigo's syndrome (Symonds, 1944); deafness commonly coexists.

Within the cavernous sinus the sixth nerve may be involved with carotid aneurysm, carotid-cavernous fistula, dural arteriovenous shunts (Leonard et al., 1984), or tumors. Abducens palsy here may be accompanied by Horner's syndrome (caused by involvement of adjacent oculosympathetic fibers) or involvement of other cranial nerves in the cavernous sinus.

Abducens nerve palsy should always be differentiated from myasthenia gravis, convergence spasm (spasm of the near triad [Griffin et al., 1976]), and diseases of the orbit (see Table 26–9).

Etiology of Trochlear Nerve Palsy

Involvement of the trochlear nucleus is rare, and the most common site of involvement is the subarachnoid course of the nerve. Here the fourth nerves emerge together from the anterior medullary velum. Thus, bilateral fourth nerve palsy after blunt head trauma is most likely due to contrecoup forces transmitted to the emerging nerves by the free edge of the tentorium. The nerves may also be involved in their subarachnoid course by tumor or as a consequence of neurosurgical procedure (Table 26–5).

Within the cavernous sinus, involvement of the trochlear nerve by tumor or aneurysm is usually accompanied by involvement of adjacent cranial nerves. Herpes zoster ophthalmicus may involve any oculomotor nerve (Archambault et al., 1988), but involvement of the trochlear nerve may reflect the common connective sheath that it shares with the first division of the trigeminal nerve (Lavin et al.,

1984). In many cases of trochlear nerve palsy, no cause can be found (Younge and Sutula, 1977), although sometimes diabetes or hypertension is associated.

Superior oblique palsy should be differentiated from involvement of other vertical extraocular muscles, skew deviation, or restrictive disease of the orbit. The Bielschowsky head-tilting test and forced duction tests help in making the diagnosis.

Etiology of Oculomotor Nerve Palsy

Lesions of the nucleus of the third nerve are rare and, when they occur, are often associated with involvement of structures important for vertical conjugate gaze (Bogousslavsky and Regli, 1983). Based on the anatomic scheme of Warwick (see Fig. 26–10A), Daroff (1970) suggested certain clinical criteria for diagnosis of nuclear third nerve palsy. Büttner-Ennever and Akert (1981) have demonstrated more than one location for medial rectus neurons (Fig. 26–10B), and it seems unlikely that medial rectus paralysis (unilateral or bilateral) is the sole manifestation of a nuclear third nerve palsy. With this modification, Daroff's criteria are summarized in Table 26–6. Confirmation of this scheme depends on clinicopathologic correlation. Zackon and Sharpe (1984) reported binocular paralysis of elevation with a unilateral oculomotor nucleus lesion. This supports the experimental evidence that crossing axons from one superior rectus subnucleus pass through the fellow subnucleus of the other side (Bienfang, 1975). Whether unilateral paralysis of depression in association with midbrain signs represents an isolated

Table 26–6. DIAGNOSIS OF NUCLEAR OCULOMOTOR NERVE PALSY*

Obligatory nuclear lesions
  Unilateral third nerve palsy with contralateral superior rectus
    paresis and bilateral partial ptosis
  Bilateral third nerve palsy associated with spared levator
    function (internal ophthalmoplegia may be present or
    absent)

Possible nuclear lesions
  Bilateral total third nerve palsy
  Bilateral ptosis
  An isolated weakness of any single muscle *except* the levator
    and medial rectus muscles

Conditions that cannot be due to nuclear lesions
  Unilateral third nerve palsy, with or without internal
    involvement, associated with normal contralateral superior
    rectus function
  Unilateral internal ophthalmoplegia
  Unilateral ptosis
  Isolated unilateral or bilateral medial rectus weakness

*In the absence of pupillary involvement, ocular myasthenia must always be ruled out.

Modified from Daroff R.B. Ocular manifestations of brainstem and cerebellar dysfunction. In Smith J.L., ed. *Neuro-ophthalmology*. Vol. 5. Symposium of the University of Miami and Bascom Palmer Eye Institute. Hallandale, FL, Huffman, pp. 104–118, 1970.

lesion of one inferior rectus subnucleus (Warren et al., 1982) remains controversial (Smith, 1982).

Fascicular third nerve lesions usually also involve adjacent structures. Claude's syndrome consists of third nerve palsy, contralateral cerebellar ataxia, and tremor; it is due to involvement of the red nucleus and its cerebellar connections. Weber's syndrome consists of third nerve palsy and contralateral hemiplegia, the latter caused by involvement of one cerebral peduncle. Benedikt's syndrome combines third nerve palsy, contralateral ataxia, and contralateral hemiplegia; if vertical gaze impairment is also present, it is referred to as Nothnagel's syndrome. Fascicular lesions may lead to a pattern of weakness that mimics effects of more distal lesions (Ksiazek et al., 1989).

In its subarachnoid course, the third nerve may be compressed by aneurysm, usually from the posterior communicating artery and sometimes from the basilar artery (Trobe et al., 1978) (Table 26–7). In such cases only rarely is the pupil affected alone; ptosis and external ophthalmoplegia usually coexist. With posterior communicating aneurysms, third nerve palsy may occur in the setting of subarachnoid hemorrhage, but another presentation is of acute diplopia with facial or orbital pain but without evidence of subarachnoid hemorrhage. The latter cases must be differentiated from third nerve palsy resulting from diabetes or hypertension, in which cerebral arteriography is not indicated. In the past, pupil involvement was used to identify patients who harbor an aneurysm, but more recent evidence has shown that this sign is fallible, particularly at the time of the patient's presentation (Kissel et al., 1983). Pupil-sparing third nerve palsies require careful observation for a week before a decision can be made concerning arteriography. After that time, third nerve palsy with complete pupillary sparing is only rarely due to aneurysm (Keane, 1983). Partial pupillary involvement may be grounds for an arteriogram (Klingele et al., 1983). In the future, magnetic resonance arteriography (Ross et al., 1989) may become the method of choice for identifying such aneurysms.

At least some cases of third nerve infarction, usually in association with diabetes, hypertension, or collagen-vascular disease, involve the subarachnoid portion of the nerve. Another site is within the cavernous sinus. Such "medical third nerve palsies" usually are acute in onset, are preceded by facial or orbital pain, and are characterized by total or relative sparing of the pupil (for a review see Nadeau and Trobe, 1983).

At the tentorial edge the third nerve may be compressed by the uncus of the temporal lobe during cerebral herniation. Pupillary dilatation may be the first warning of such herniation (Plum and Posner, 1980).

Within the cavernous sinus the oculomotor nerve may be compressed by aneurysm or tumor. With carotid aneurysm, about half of all patients suffer pain in the face; abducens and trochlear palsies may coexist. Sparing of the pupil is more common with cavernous sinus than with posterior communicating aneurysms. This difference may be due to less frequent involvement of the inferior division of the oculomotor nerve, which carries the pupillomotor fibers (Nadeau and Trobe, 1983). An alternative explanation is that there is a coexistent sympathetic and parasympathetic paresis (Meadows, 1959). Tumors in the region of the cavernous sinus often grow slowly and pain is not a usual feature (Trobe et al., 1978). Often multiple cranial nerves are involved. A relatively common finding with such slowly progressive processes is aberrant regeneration of the oculomotor nerve (Boghen et al., 1979). This is characterized by anomalous synkinetic movements; most commonly the lid elevates during adduction or depression of the eye (Hepler and Cantu, 1967). Aberrant regeneration of the third nerve also occurs after trauma, aneurysm (Cox et al., 1979), and congenital third nerve palsy (Miller, 1977).

As the oculomotor nerve passes through the superior orbital fissure it divides into superior and inferior branches; isolated involvement of either ramus has been reported (Derakhshan, 1978; Susac and Hoyt, 1977).

Table 26–7. CAUSES OF OCULOMOTOR NERVE PALSY*

Nuclear
    Congenital hypoplasia
    Infarction
    Tumor

Fascicular
    Infarction
    Tumor

Subarachnoid
    Aneurysm of posterior communicating or basilar arteries
    Meningitis—infectious or neoplastic
    Nerve infarction (often in association with diabetes or hypertension)
    Tumor

At the tentorial edge
    Uncal herniation
    Trauma

Cavernous sinus and superior orbital fissure
    Aneurysm
    Tumor (pituitary adenoma, meningioma, nasopharyngeal carcinoma)
    Nerve infarction (often in association with diabetes or hypertension)
    Pituitary infarction
    Cavernous sinus thrombosis
    Carotid cavernous fistula
    Infections, including herpes zoster
    Tolosa-Hunt syndrome

Orbit
    Trauma
    Tumor

Localization uncertain
    Migraine

*See the following references: Green et al., 1964; Nadeau and Trobe, 1983; Rush and Younge, 1981.

Etiology of Multiple Oculomotor Nerve Palsies

The main causes of multiple oculomotor nerve palsies are trauma, basal arachnoiditis and tumor infiltrations, lesions within the cavernous sinus (where the three nerves are adjacent), and generalized neuropathies (Table 26–8).

The clinical characteristics of aneurysm and tumors of the cavernous sinus region were discussed earlier. Spread of nasopharyngeal carcinoma to this region may cause painful ophthalmoplegia, the most commonly affected oculomotor nerve being the abducens (Rosenbaum and Seaman, 1955). One other condition that is localized in this area is a low-grade inflammatory disorder of the cavernous sinus called Tolosa-Hunt syndrome (Campbell and Okazaki, 1987; Hunt et al., 1961; Tolosa, 1954). It is a disease of middle or later life, and the presenting complaints are retro-orbital pain and diplopia. The third or sixth nerve or combinations of oculomotor nerves may be involved. Sensation over the first two divisions of the trigeminal nerve may be impaired. Slight proptosis and impairment of visual acuity may occur. Carotid arteriography may show narrowing of the intracavernous portion of the artery and is required to exclude aneurysm or tumor. Corticosteroid medications usually produce a prompt improvement.

The third, fourth, and sixth cranial nerves may be involved as part of a generalized neuropathy associated with toxins or the Guillain-Barré syndrome. The Miller Fisher variant of the latter condition consists

Table 26–8. CAUSES OF MULTIPLE OCULOMOTOR NERVE PALSIES*

Brain stem
  Tumor
  Infarction

Subarachnoid
  Meningitis (infective and neoplastic)
  Trauma
  Clivus tumor
  Aneurysm—ectatic basilar artery
  Sarcoidosis

Cavernous sinus and superior orbital fissure
  Aneurysm
  Tumor (pituitary adenoma, meningioma, nasopharyngeal
    carcinoma)
  Cavernous sinus thrombosis
  Pituitary infarction
  Carotid-cavernous fistula
  Sphenoid sinus mucocele
  Infections (herpes zoster)
  Tolosa-Hunt syndrome

Orbital
  Trauma
  Tumor
  Mucormycosis

Localization uncertain
  Post-inflammatory neuropathy (Guillain-Barré and
    Miller Fisher syndromes)

*See the following references: Rucker, 1966; Rush and Younge, 1981.

Table 26–9. DIFFERENTIAL DIAGNOSIS OF OCULAR MOTOR NERVE PALSIES

Concomitant strabismus

Disorders of vergence, especially spasm of the near triad

Brain stem disorders causing abnormal prenuclear inputs
  (e.g., skew deviation)

Myasthenia gravis

Restrictive ophthalmopathy (e.g., Brown's superior oblique
  tendon sheath syndrome)

Trauma (e.g., blow-out fracture of the orbit)

Ophthalmic Graves' disease

Orbital metastases

Orbital pseudotumor

Orbital infections (e.g., trichinosis)

Disease affecting extraocular muscle*
  Oculopharyngeal dystrophy
  Myotubular myopathy
  Myotonic dystrophy

Kearns-Sayre syndrome*

*For reviews of these conditions see Berenberg et al., 1977; Drachman, 1975; and Petty et al., 1986.

of ophthalmoplegia, areflexia, and ataxia (M. Fisher, 1956). The pattern of ophthalmoparesis may sometimes suggest central involvement, mimicking gaze palsies or internuclear ophthalmoplegia. Whether the central nervous system is involved in Fisher's syndrome is a matter of controversy (Meienberg and Ryffel, 1983). However, at least some of the disorders of ocular motility reported in Fisher's syndrome can be ascribed to central adaptive responses to a peripheral palsy (Zee and Yee, 1977).

Disorders of Ocular Alignment Not Related to Disease of the Oculomotor Nerves

Table 26–9 summarizes the various central and peripheral disorders that may mimic oculomotor palsies. Concomitant strabismus, in which the deviation is constant for all fields of gaze, is most commonly encountered in children but may occasionally present in adulthood—for example, after one eye has been patched for ophthalmic reasons. Spasm of the near triad (convergence spasm) occurs in hysterical patients and can usually be detected by careful observation of the pupils and by demonstration of a full range of eye movements with one eye viewing or in response to rapid, passive head turns (Griffin et al., 1976). Certain brain stem disorders may cause ocular misalignment because of a disturbance of prenuclear inputs. Examples are certain cases of internuclear ophthalmoplegia and vertical skew deviation. Diagnosis in such cases depends on documentation of accompanying oculomotor and other brain stem signs (see Leigh and Zee, 1991, for a review). When diplopia is due to myasthenia gravis, characteristic findings are fatigue brought on by sustained upward or lateral gaze and involvement of extraocular muscles supplied by more than one nerve. Ptosis is common. Quantitative studies of saccadic metrics before and after injection of edrophonium (Schmidt et al., 1980; Yee et al., 1976) are more reliable and sensitive in diagnosing myasthenia than are the cover tests or the Lancaster red-green test. Restrictive ophthalmopathy includes congenital conditions such as Brown's syndrome, in which the adducted eye cannot be elevated (Wilson et al., 1989), sequelae of orbital trauma, and inflammatory conditions. Forced duction testing will help determine that strabismus is due to mechanical hindrance rather than muscle weakness (Von Noorden, 1990). Thyroid ophthalmopathy characteristically causes impaired elevation and extortion of the eye on abduction (Dresner and Kennerdell, 1985). Thyroid function tests may be abnormal and computed tomography of the orbit may demonstrate enlarged extraocular muscles (Hallin and Feldon, 1988). Progressive limitation of ocular motility, accompanied by ptosis, is a feature of a number of dystrophic processes (see Table 26–9). Diplopia is not a common complaint in these conditions.

References

(Key references are designated with an asterisk.)

Abel L.A., Traccis, S., Dell'Osso L.F., et al. Square wave oscillation. The relationship of saccadic intrusions and oscillations. *Neuro-ophthalmology* 4:21–25, 1984.

Albano J.E., Wurtz R.H. Deficits in eye position following ablation of monkey superior colliculus, pretectum, and posterior-medial thalamus. *J. Neurophysiol.* 43:318–337, 1982.

Andersen R.A. Visual and eye movement functions of the posterior parietal cortex. *Annu. Rev. Neurosci.* 12:377–403, 1989.

Archambault P., Wise J.S., Rosen J., et al. Herpes zoster ophthalmoplegia. Report of six cases. *Neuro-ophthalmology* 8:185–191, 1988.

Baloh R.W., Yee R.D. Spontaneous vertical nystagmus. *Rev. Neurol. (Paris)* 145:527–532, 1989.

Bennett A.H., Savill T. A case of permanent conjugate deviation of the eyes and head, the result of a lesion limited to the sixth nucleus; with remarks on associated lateral movements of the eyeballs, and rotation of the head and neck. *Brain* 12:102–116, 1889.

Berenberg R.A., Pellock J.M., DiMauro S., et al. Lumping or splitting? Ophthalmoplegia-plus or Kearns-Sayre syndrome? *Ann. Neurol.* 1:37–54, 1977.

*Berthoz A., Melvill Jones G., eds. *Reviews of Oculomotor Research.* Vol. 1. *Adaptive Mechanisms in Visual-Vestibular Interactions.* Amsterdam, Elsevier, 1985.

Bielschowsky A. *Lectures on Motor Anomalies.* Hanover, NH, Dartmouth College Publications, 1940.

Bienfang D.C. Crossing axons in the third nerve nucleus. *Invest. Ophthalmol.* 14:927–930, 1975.

Boch R.A., Goldberg M.E. Participation of prefrontal neurons in the preparation of visually guided eye movements in the rhesus monkey. *J. Neurophysiol.* 61:1064–1084, 1989.

Boeder P. The cooperation of extraocular muscles. *Am. J. Ophthalmol.* 51:469–481, 1961.

Boghen D., Chartrand J.P., LaFlamme J.P., et al. Primary aberrant third nerve regeneration. *Ann. Neurol.* 6:415–418, 1979.

Bogousslavsky J., Regli F. Nuclear and prenuclear syndromes of the oculomotor nerve. *Neuro-ophthalmology* 3:211–216, 1983.

Bondar R.L., Sharpe J.A., Lewis A.J. Rebound nystagmus in olivocerebellar atrophy: a clinicopathological correlation. *Ann. Neurol.* 15:474–477, 1984.

Brandt T., Dieterich M. Pathological eye-head coordination in roll: tonic ocular tilt reaction in mesencephalic and medullary lesions. *Brain* 110:644–666, 1987.

Bruce C.J., Goldberg M.E. Primate frontal eye fields: single neurons discharging before saccades. *J. Neurophysiol.* 53:603–635, 1985.

Büttner-Ennever J.A., Akert K. Medial rectus subgroups of the oculomotor nucleus and their abducens internuclear input in the monkey. *J. Comp. Neurol.* 197:17–27, 1981.

Büttner-Ennever J.A., Büttner U. The reticular formation. In Büttner-Ennever J.A., ed. *Reviews of Oculomotor Research.* Vol. 2. *Neuroanatomy of the Oculomotor System.* Amsterdam, Elsevier, pp. 119–176, 1988.

Büttner-Ennever J.A., Büttner U., Cohen B., et al. Vertical gaze paralysis and the rostral interstitial nucleus of the medial longitudinal fasciculus. *Brain* 105:125–149, 1982.

Büttner-Ennever J.A., Cohen B., Pause M., et al. Raphe nucleus of the pons containing omnipause neurons of the oculomotor system in the monkey, and its homologue in man. *J. Comp. Neurol.* 267:307–321, 1988.

Campbell R.J., Okazaki H. Painful ophthalmoplegia (Tolosa-Hunt variant): autopsy findings in a patient with necrotizing intracavernous carotid vasculitis and inflammatory disease of the orbit. *Mayo Clin. Proc.* 62:520–526, 1987.

Cannon S.C., Robinson D.A. Loss of the neural integrator of the oculomotor system from brain stem lesions in monkey. *J. Neurophysiol.* 57:1383–1409, 1987.

Cox T.A., Wurster J.B., Godfrey W.A. Primary aberrant oculomotor regeneration due to intracranial aneurysm. *Arch. Neurol.* 36:570–571, 1979.

Daroff R.B. Ocular manifestations of brainstem and cerebellar dysfunction. In Smith J.L., ed. *Neuro-ophthalmology.* Vol. 5. Symposium of the University of Miami and Bascom Palmer Eye Institute. Hallandale, FL, Huffman, pp. 104–118, 1970.

Dell'Osso L.F., Schmidt D., Daroff R.B. Latent, manifest latent, and congenital nystagmus. *Arch. Ophthalmol.* 97:1877–1885, 1979.

Deng S.Y., Goldberg M.E., Segraves M.A., et al. The effect of unilateral ablation of the frontal eye fields on saccadic performance in the monkey. In Keller E.L., Zee D.S., eds. *Adaptive Processes in Visual and Oculomotor Systems.* Oxford, Pergamon Press, pp. 208–210, 1986.

Derakhshan I. Superior branch palsy of the oculomotor nerve with spontaneous recovery. *Ann. Neurol.* 4:478–479, 1978.

Drachman D.A. Ophthalmoplegia plus: a classification of the disorders associated with progressive external ophthalmoplegia. In Vinken P.J., Bruyn G.W., eds. *Handbook of Clinical Neurology.* Vol. 22. *System Disorders and Atrophies.* Part II. New York, American Elsevier, pp. 203–216, 1975.

Dresner S.C., Kennerdell J.S. Dysthyroid orbitopathy. *Neurology* 35:1628–1634, 1985.

Dürsteler M.R., Wurtz R.H. Pursuit and optokinetic deficits following chemical lesions of cortical areas MT and MST. *J. Neurophysiol.* 60:940–965, 1988.

Evinger L.C., Fuchs A.F., Baker R. Bilateral lesions of the medial longitudinal fasciculus in monkeys: effects on the horizontal and vertical components of voluntary and vestibular induced eye movements. *Exp. Brain Res.* 28:1–20, 1977.

Fisher A., Gresty M., Chamers B., et al. Primary position upbeating nystagmus. A variety of central positional nystagmus. *Brain* 106:949–964, 1983.

Fisher M. An unusual variant of acute idiopathic polyneuritis (syndrome of ophthalmoplegia, ataxia and areflexia). *N. Engl. J. Med.* 255:57–65, 1956.

Fukushima K., Fukushima J., Harada C., et al. Neuronal activity related to vertical eye movement in the region of the interstitial nucleus of Cajal in alert cats. *Exp. Brain Res.* 79:43–64, 1990.

Funahashi S., Bruce C.J., Goldman-Rakic P.S. Mnemonic coding of visual space in the monkey's dorsolateral prefrontal cortex. *J. Neurophysiol.* 61:331–349, 1989.

Galetta S.L., Smith J.L. Chronic isolated sixth nerve palsies. *Arch. Neurol.* 46:79–82, 1989.

Gamlin P.D.R., Gnadt J.W., Mays L.E. Lidocaine-induced unilateral internuclear ophthalmoplegia: effects on convergence and conjugate eye movements. *J. Neurophysiol.* 62:82–95, 1989.

Green W.R., Hackett E.R., Schlezinger N.S. Neuroophthalmologic evaluation of oculomotor nerve paralysis. *Arch. Ophthalmol.* 72:154–167, 1964.

Gresty M.A., Ell J.J., Findley L.J. Acquired pendular nystagmus: its characteristics, localizing value and pathophysiology. *J. Neurol. Neurosurg. Psychiatry* 45:431–439, 1982.

Griffin J.F., Wray S.H., Anderson D.P. Misdiagnosis of spasm of the near reflex. *Neurology* 26:1018–1020, 1976.

Guitton D., Buchtel H.A., Douglas R.M. Frontal lobe lesions in man cause difficulties in suppressing reflexive glances and in generating goal-directed saccades. *Exp. Brain Res.* 58:455–472, 1985.

Hallin E.S., Feldon S.E. Graves' ophthalmopathy: I. Simple CT estimates of extraocular muscle volume. *Br. J. Ophthalmol.* 72:674–677, 1988.

Halmagyi G.M., Gresty M.A., Leech J. Reversed optokinetic nystagmus (OKN): mechanism and clinical significance. *Ann. Neurol.* 7:429–435, 1980a.

Halmagyi G.M., Rudge P., Gresty M.A., et al. Treatment of periodic alternating nystagmus. *Ann. Neurol.* 8:609–611, 1980b.

Hanson M.R., Hamid M.A., Tomsak R.L., et al. Selective saccadic palsy caused by pontine lesions: clinical, physiological, and pathological correlations. *Ann. Neurol.* 20:209–217, 1986.

Hedges T.R., Hoyt W.F. Ocular tilt reaction due to an upper brainstem lesion: paroxysmal skew deviation, torsion, and oscillation of the eyes with head tilt. *Ann. Neurol.* 11:537–540, 1982.

*Henn V., Büttner-Ennever J.A., Hepp K. The primate oculomotor system. I. Motoneurons. *Hum. Neurobiol.* 1:77–85, 1982a.

*Henn V., Hepp K., Büttner-Ennever J.A. The primate oculomotor system. II. Premotor system. *Hum. Neurobiol.* 1:87–95, 1982b.

Henn V., Land W., Hepp K., et al. Experimental gaze palsies in monkeys and their relation to human pathology. *Brain* 107:619–636, 1984.

Hepler R.J., Cantu R.C. Aneurysms and third nerve palsies: ocular status of survivors. *Arch. Ophthalmol.* 77:604–608, 1967.

Hepp K., Henn V., Vilis T., et al. Brainstem regions related to saccade generation. In Wurtz R.H., Goldberg M.E., eds. *Reviews of Oculomotor Research.* Vol. 3. *The Neurobiology of Saccadic Eye Movements.* Amsterdam, Elsevier, pp. 105–212, 1989.

Hikosaka O., Wurtz R.H. The basal ganglia. In Wurtz R.E., Goldberg M.E., eds. *Reviews of Oculomotor Research.* Vol. 3. *The Neurobiology of Saccadic Eye Movements.* Amsterdam, Elsevier, pp. 257–281, 1989.

Hikosaka O., Sakamoto M., Usi S. Functional properties of monkey caudate neurons. I. Activities related to saccadic eye movements. *J. Neurophysiol.* 61:780–798, 1989.

Hood J.D. Further observations on the phenomenon of rebound nystagmus. *Ann. N. Y. Acad. Sci.* 374:532–539, 1981.

Hunt W.E., Meagher J.N., LeFever H.E., et al. Painful ophthalmoplegia. *Neurology (Minneap.)* 11:56–62, 1961.

Johnston J.L., Sharpe J.A. Sparing of the vestibulo-ocular reflex with lesions of the paramedian pontine recticular formation. *Neurology* 39:876, 1989.

Kanter D.S., Ruff R.L., Leigh R.J., et al. See-saw nystagmus and brainstem infarction. MRI findings. *Neuro-ophthalmology* 7:279–283, 1987.

Keane J. Bilateral sixth nerve palsy. Analysis of 125 cases. *Arch. Neurol.* 33:681–683, 1976.

Keane J.R. Aneurysms and third nerve palsies. *Ann. Neurol.* 14:696–697, 1983.

Keane J.R. The pretectal syndrome: 206 patients. *Neurology* 40:684–690, 1990.

Kissel J.T., Burde R.M., Klingele T.G., et al. Pupil-sparing oculo-

motor palsies with internal carotid–posterior communicating artery aneurysms. *Ann. Neurol.* 13:149–154, 1983.

Klingele T.G., Burde R.J., Kissel J.T., et al. Pupil-sparing oculomotor palsy. *Ann. Neurol.* 14:698, 1983.

Komatsu H., Wurtz R.H. Relation of cortical areas MT and MST to pursuit eye movements. I. Localization and visual properties of neurons. *J. Neurophysiol.* 60:580–603, 1988.

Kommerell G., Henn V., Bach M., et al. Unilateral lesion of the paramedian pontine reticular formation. Loss of rapid eye movements with preservation of vestibulo-ocular reflex and pursuit. *Neuro-ophthalmology* 7:93–98, 1987.

Ksiazek S.M., Repka M.Z., Maguire A., et al. Divisional oculomotor nerve paresis caused by intrinsic brainstem disease. *Ann. Neurol.* 26:714–718, 1989.

Lancaster W.B. Detecting, measuring, plotting and interpreting ocular deviations. *Arch. Ophthalmol.* 22:867–880, 1939.

Lasker A.G., Zee D.S., Hain T.C., et al. Saccades in Huntington's disease: initiation defects and distractability. *Neurology* 37:364–370, 1987.

Lavin P.J.M., Younkin S.G., Kori S.H. The pathology of ophthalmoplegia in herpes zoster ophthalmicus. *Neuro-ophthalmology* 4:75–80, 1984.

Leech J., Gresty M.A., Hess K., et al. Gaze failure, drifting eye movements, and centripetal nystagmus in cerebellar diseases. *Br. J. Ophthalmol.* 61:774–781, 1977.

Leichnetz G.R. The prefrontal cortico-oculomotor trajectories in monkey: a possible explanation for the effects of stimulation lesion experiments on eye movements. *J. Neurol. Sci.* 49:387–396, 1981.

Leichnetz G.R. Inferior frontal eye field projections to the pursuit-related dorsolateral pontine nucleus, and middle temporal areas (MT) in the monkey. *Visual Neurosci.* 3:171–180, 1989.

Leigh R.J. The cortical control of ocular pursuit movements. *Rev. Neurol. (Paris)* 145:605–612, 1989.

*Leigh R.J., Zee D.S. *The Neurology of Eye Movements.* 2nd ed. Philadelphia, Davis, 1991.

Leigh R.J., Robinson D.A., Zee D.S. A hypothetical explanation for periodic alternating nystagmus: instability in the optokinetic-vestibular system. *Ann. N. Y. Acad. Sci.* 374:619–635, 1981.

Lennerstrand G. Motor units in eye muscles. In Lennerstrand G., Bach-y-Rita P., eds. *Basic Mechanisms of Ocular Motility and Their Clinical Implications.* New York, Pergamon Press, pp. 119–143, 1975.

Leonard T.J.K., Moseley I.F., Sanders M.D. Ophthalmoplegia in carotid cavernous sinus fistula. *Br. J. Ophthalmol.* 68:128–134, 1984.

Lisberger S.G., Miles F.A., Zee D.S. Signals used to compute errors in the monkey vestibulo-ocular reflex: possible role of the flocculus. *J. Neurophysiol.* 52:1140–1153, 1984.

Livingstone M., Hubel D. Segregation of form, color, movement, and depth: anatomy, physiology, and perception. *Science* 240:740–749, 1988.

Maciewicz R.J., Spencer R.F. Oculomotor and abducens internuclear pathways in the cat. In Baker R., Berthoz A., eds. *Control of Gaze by Brain Stem Neurons.* New York, Elsevier, pp. 99–108, 1977.

Mann S.E., Thau R., Schiller P.H. Conditional task-related responses in monkey dorsomedial frontal cortex. *Exp. Brain Res.* 69:460–468, 1988.

Mansour A.M., Reinecke R.D. Central trochlear palsy. *Surv. Ophthalmol.* 30:279–297, 1986.

Meadows S.P. Intracavernous aneurysms of the internal carotid artery. *Arch. Ophthalmol.* 65:566–574, 1959.

Meienberg O., Ryffel E. Supranuclear eye movement disorder in Fisher's syndrome of ophthalmoplegia, ataxia and areflexia. *Ann. Neurol.* 40:402–405, 1983.

Meienberg O., Büttner-Ennever J.A., Kraus-Ruppert R. Unilateral paralysis of conjugate gaze due to a lesion of the abducens nucleus. *Neuro-ophthalmology* 2:47–51, 1981.

Mellinger J.F., Gomez M.R. Agenesis of the cranial nerves. In Vinken P.J., Bruyn G.W., eds. *Handbook of Clinical Neurology.* Vol. 30. *Congenital Malformations of the Brain and Skull.* Part I. New York, Elsevier, pp. 395–414, 1977.

Miller N.R. Solitary oculomotor nerve palsy in childhood. *Am. J. Ophthalmol.* 83:106–111, 1977.

Miller N.R., Kiel S.A., Green W.R., et al. Unilateral Duane's retraction syndrome (type I): a clinical pathological case report. *Arch. Ophthalmol.* 100:1468–1472, 1982.

Nadeau S.E., Trobe J.D. Pupil sparing in oculomotor palsy: a brief review. *Ann. Neurol.* 13:143–148, 1983.

Nakada T., Kwee I.L. Oculopalatal myoclonus. *Brain* 109:431–441, 1986.

Newsome W.T., Wurtz R.H., Komatsu H. Relation of cortical areas MT and MST to pursuit eye movements. II. Differentiation of retinal from extraretinal inputs. *J. Neurophysiol.* 60:604–620, 1988.

Noseworthy J.H., Ebers G.C., Leigh R.J., et al. Torsional nystagmus: quantitative features and possible pathogenesis. *Neurology* 38:992–994, 1988.

Ochs A., Stark L., Hoyt W.F., et al. Opposed adducting saccades in convergence-retraction nystagmus. A patient with sylvian aqueduct syndrome. *Brain* 102:497–508, 1979.

Optican L.M., Robinson D.A. Cerebellar-dependent adaptive control of the primate saccadic system. *J. Neurophysiol.* 44:1058–1076, 1980.

Optican L.M., Zee D.S. A hypothetical explanation of congenital nystagmus. *Biol. Cybern.* 50:119–134, 1984.

Optican L.M., Zee D.S., Miles F.A. Floccular lesions abolish adaptive control of post-saccadic ocular drift in primates. *Exp. Brain Res.* 64:596–598, 1986.

Parkinson D., Johnston J., Chaudhuri A. Sympathetic connections to the fifth and sixth cranial nerves. *Anat. Rec.* 191:221–226, 1978.

Petty R.K.H., Harding A.E., Morgan-Hughes J.A. The clinical features of mitochondrial myopathy. *Brain* 109:915–938, 1986.

Pierrot-Deseilligny C., Goasguen J. Isolated abducens nucleus damage due to histiocytosis X. *Brain* 107:1019–1032, 1984.

Pierrot-Deseilligny C., Chain F., Serdaru M., et al. The "one-and-one-half" syndrome. Electro-oculographic analyses of five cases with deductions about the physiological mechanisms of lateral gaze. *Brain* 104:665–669, 1981.

Pierrot-Deseilligny C., Chain F., Gray F., et al. Parinaud's syndrome. Electro-oculographic and anatomical analyses of six vascular cases with deductions about vertical gaze organization in the premotor structures. *Brain* 105:667–696, 1982.

Pierrot-Deseilligny C., Goasguen J., Chain F., et al. Pontine metastasis with dissociated bilateral horizontal gaze paralysis. *J. Neurol. Neurosurg. Psychiatry* 47:159–164, 1984.

Pierrot-Deseilligny C., Rivaud S., Penet C., et al. Latencies of visually guided saccades in unilateral hemispheric cerebral lesions. *Ann. Neurol.* 21:138–148, 1987.

Pierrot-Deseilligny C., Rivaud S., Samson Y., et al. Some instructive cases concerning the circuitry of ocular smooth pursuit in the brainstem. *Neuro-ophthalmology* 9:31–42, 1989.

Plum F., Posner J.B. *The Diagnosis of Stupor and Coma.* 3rd ed. Philadelphia, Davis, 1980.

Ranalli P.J., Sharpe J.A. Contrapulsion of saccades and ipsilateral ataxia: a unilateral disorder of the rostral cerebellum. *Ann. Neurol.* 20:311–316, 1986.

Ranalli P.J., Sharpe J.A. Vertical vestibulo-ocular reflex, smooth pursuit and eye-head tracking dysfunction in internuclear ophthalmoplegia. *Brain* 111:1299–1317, 1988.

Ridley A., Kennard C., Schlotz C.L., et al. Omnipause neurons in two cases of opsoclonus associated with oat cell carcinoma of the lung. *Brain* 110:1699–1709, 1987.

Robinson D.A. The functional behavior of the peripheral oculomotor apparatus: a review. In Kommerell G., ed. *Disorders of Ocular Motility. Neurophysiological and Clinical Aspects.* Munich, Bergmann, pp. 43–61, 1978.

*Robinson D.A. Control of eye movements. In Brooks V.B., ed. *Handbook of Physiology.* Bethesda, American Physiological Society, 1981.

Robinson D.L., McClurkin J.W. The visual superior colliculus and pulvinar. In Wurtz R.H., Goldberg M. E., eds. *The Neurobiology of Saccadic Eye Movements.* Amsterdam, Elsevier, pp. 337–360, 1989.

Rosenbaum H.E., Seaman W.B. Neurologic manifestations of nasopharyngeal tumors. *Neurology* 5:868–874, 1955.

Ross J.S., Masaryk T.J., Modic M.T., et al. Magnetic resonance angiography of the extracranial carotid arteries and intracranial vessels: a review. *Neurology* 39:1369–1376, 1989.

Rucker C.W. The causes of paralysis of the third, fourth and sixth cranial nerves. *Am. J. Ophthalmol.* 61:1293–1298, 1966.

Rush J.A., Younge B.R. Paralysis of cranial nerves III, IV, and VI. Cause and prognosis in 1,000 cases. *Arch. Ophthalmol.* 99:76–79, 1981.

Schiller P.H., True S.D., Conway J.L. Deficits in eye movements following frontal eye-field and superior colliculus ablations. *J. Neurophysiol.* 44:1175–1189, 1980.

Schlag J., Schlag-Rey M. Evidence for a supplementary eye field. *J. Neurophysiol.* 57:179–200, 1987.

Schlag-Rey M., Schlag J. Visuomotor functions of central thalamus in monkey. I. Unit activity related to spontaneous eye movements. *J. Neurophysiol.* 51:1149–1174, 1984.

Schmidt D., Dell'Osso L.F., Abel L.A., et al. Myasthenia gravis: dynamic changes in saccadic waveform, gain and velocity. *Exp. Neurol.* 68:365–377, 1980.

Scott A.B., Collins C.C. Division of labor in human extraocular muscle. *Arch. Ophthalmol.* 90:319–322, 1973.

Selhorst J.B., Stark L., Ochs A.L., et al. Disorders in cerebellar ocular motor control. II. Macrosaccadic oscillations: an oculographic, control system, and clinico-anatomical analysis. *Brain* 99:509–522, 1976.

Sharpe J.A. Adaptation to frontal lobe lesions. In Keller E.L., Zee D.S., eds. *Adaptive Processes in Visual and Oculomotor Systems.* Oxford, Pergamon Press, pp. 239–246, 1986.

Sharpe, J.A., Herishanu Y.O., White O.B. Cerebral square wave jerks. *Neurology (N.Y.)* 32:57–62, 1982.

Sherrington C.S. Experimental note on two movements of the eyes. *J. Physiol. (Lond.)* 17:27–28, 1894.

Smith J. L. The "nuclear third" question. *Neuro-ophthalmology* 2:61–63, 1982.

*Sparks D.L., Hartwich-Young R. The deep layers of the superior colliculus. In Wurtz R.H., Goldberg M.E., eds. *Reviews of Oculomotor Research.* Vol. 3. *The Neurobiology of Saccadic Eye Movements.* Amsterdam, Elsevier, pp. 213–255, 1989.

Spencer R.F., Porter J.D. Structural organization of the extraocular muscles. In Büttner-Ennever J.A., ed. *Reviews of Oculomotor Research.* Vol. 2. *Neuroanatomy of the Oculomotor System.* Amsterdam, Elsevier, pp. 33–79, 1988.

Stanton G.B., Goldberg M.E., Bruce C.J. Frontal eye field efferents in the macaque monkey. I. Subcortical pathways and topography of striatal and thalamic terminal fields. *J. Comp. Neurol.* 271:473–492, 1988a.

Stanton G.B., Goldberg M.E., Bruce C.J. Frontal eye field efferents in the macaque monkey. II. Topography of terminal fields in midbrain and pons. *J. Comp. Neurol.* 271:493–506, 1988b.

Susac J.O., Hoyt W.F. Inferior branch palsy of the oculomotor nerve. *Ann. Neurol.* 2:335–339, 1977.

Suzuki D.A., May J.G., Keller E.L., et al. Visual motion response properties of neurons in dorsolateral pontine nucleus of alert monkey. *J. Neurophysiol.* 63:37–59, 1990.

Symonds C.P. A discussion of cranial nerve palsies associated with otitis. *Proc. R. Soc. Med.* 37:386, 1944.

Tolosa E. Periarteritic lesions of the carotid siphon with the clinical features of carotid infraclinoid aneurysm. *J. Neurol. Neurosurg. Psychiatry* 17:300–302, 1954.

Trobe J.D., Glaser J.S., Quencer R.C. Isolated oculomotor paralysis. The product of saccular and fusiform aneurysms of the basilar artery. *Arch. Ophthalmol.* 96:1236–1240, 1978.

Tusa R.J., Zee D.S., Herdman S.J. Effects of unilateral cerebral cortical lesions on ocular motor behavior in monkeys: saccades and quick phases. *J. Neurophysiol.* 56:1590–1625, 1986.

Van Gisbergen J.A.M., Van Opstal A.J. Models. In Wurtz R.H., Goldberg M.E., eds. *Reviews of Oculomotor Research.* Vol. 3. *The Neurobiology of Saccadic Eye Movements.* Amsterdam, Elsevier, pp. 69–101, 1989.

Von Noorden G.K. *Burian–Von Noorden's Binocular Vision and Ocular Motility.* 4th ed. St. Louis, Mosby, 1990.

Waespe W., Cohen B., Raphan T. Dynamic modification of the vestibulo-ocular reflex by nodulus and uvula. *Science* 228:199–202, 1985.

Wall M., Wray S.H. The one-and-a-half syndrome: a study of 20 cases and review of the literature. *Neurology* 33:971–980, 1983.

Warren W., Burde R.M., Klingele T.G., et al. Atypical oculomotor paresis. *Neuro-ophthalmology* 2:13–18, 1982.

Warwick R. Representation of the extra-ocular muscles in the oculomotor nuclei of the monkey. *J. Comp. Neurol.* 98:449–503, 1953.

Wilson M.E., Eustis H.S. Jr., Parks M.M. Brown's syndrome. *Surv. Ophthalmol.* 34:153–172, 1989.

Yagi T., Shimizu M., Sekine S., et al. New neurotological test for detecting cerebellar dysfunction. Vestibulo-ocular reflex changes with horizontal vision-reversal prisms. *Ann. Otol. Rhinol. Laryngol.* 90:276–280, 1981.

Yee R.D., Cogan D.G., Zee D.S., et al. Rapid eye movements in myasthenia gravis. II. Electro-oculographic analysis. *Arch. Ophthalmol.* 94:1465–1472, 1976.

Younge B.R., Sutula F. Analysis of trochlear nerve palsies. Diagnosis, etiology and treatment. *Mayo Clin. Proc.* 52:11–18, 1977.

Zackon D.H., Sharpe J.A. Midbrain paresis of horizontal gaze. *Ann. Neurol.* 16:495–504, 1984.

Zee D.S., Robinson D.A. A hypothetical explanation of saccadic oscillations. *Ann. Neurol.* 5:405–414, 1979.

Zee D.S., Yee R.D. Abnormal saccades in paralytic strabismus. *Am. J. Ophthalmol.* 83:112–114, 1977.

Zee D.S., Yamazaki A., Butler P.H., et al. Effects of the ablation of flocculus and paraflocculus on eye movement in primate. *J. Neurophysiol.* 46:878–899, 1981.

Zee D.S., Chu F.C., Optican L.M., et al. Graphic analysis of paralytic strabismus with the Lancaster red-green test. *Am. J. Ophthalmol.* 97:587–592, 1984.

Zee D.S., Hain T.C., Carl J.R. Abduction nystagmus in internuclear ophthalmoplegia. *Ann. Neurol.* 21:383–388, 1987.

Cranial Nerves and Their Disorders

27

Smell and Taste and Their Disorders

Richard L. Doty
Charles P. Kimmelman
Ronald P. Lesser

All environmental nutrients and airborne chemicals required for life enter the human body by means of the nose and the mouth. Olfaction and taste monitor the intake of such materials and determine the flavor and palatability of foods and beverages. In addition, these primary senses warn of toxins, such as spoiled food, leaking natural gas, polluted air, and smoke, and serve as diagnostic indicators for a number of serious diseases, including Alzheimer's disease and some forms of parkinsonism. Despite such important functions, however, the chemical senses have been generally disregarded from a medical perspective and are often not tested. Such neglect does not stem from a want of patients experiencing chemosensory problems; for example, data from the National Ambulatory Medical Care Survey suggest that, for 1975 and 1976 combined, 435,000 visits to physicians' offices occurred in which a major presenting complaint was chemosensory in nature (Report of the Panel on Communicative Disorders to the National Advisory Neurological and Communicative Disorders and Stroke Council, 1979).

This chapter summarizes key aspects of the anatomy and physiology of the olfactory and gustatory systems and presents techniques for their clinical

Supported by grant RO1 AG 08148 from the National Institute on Aging and grant PO1 00161 from the National Institute on Deafness and Other Communication Disorders.

assessment. Emphasis is placed on the sensory evaluation of olfactory function and on the pathophysiology of this system, because olfactory disorders are much more common than gustatory ones, and most complaints of taste dysfunction are in fact due to olfactory anomalies.

OLFACTION

Anatomy and Physiology of Olfaction

Odorants are detected intranasally by specialized receptor cells in the olfactory epithelium and, in some cases, by free nerve endings from the ophthalmic and maxillary divisions of the trigeminal nerve within the nasal epithelium. In addition, some inhaled chemicals are detected by nerve endings within the pharynx and the oral cavity, such as those associated with the glossopharyngeal and vagal nerves. Qualitative odor sensations are mediated by the cranial nerve I receptors; the sensations mediated by the other nerves are primarily those of the common chemical sense, such as warmth/coolness, sharpness, and irritation (Doty et al., 1978; Silver and Moulton, 1982).

The human olfactory neuroepithelium is located in the superior nasal cavity and encompasses a portion of the superior turbinate, the superior nasal septum, and the region of the cribriform plate. Contrary to textbook descriptions, this 2- to 5-cm² region is rarely visually distinct from the surrounding respiratory epithelium. At least four main cell types are found in this region: bipolar olfactory receptor cells, microvillar cells, sustentacular or supporting cells, and basal cells (Moran et al., 1982b) (Fig. 27–1).

The first of these cell types—the primary olfactory receptor cell—numbers approximately 6 million in humans. Each of these bipolar flask-shaped neurons bears a slender rod, which enlarges at the surface of the epithelium into the olfactory knob or vesicle, from which 10–30 cilia project (Fig. 27–2). Odorant receptor sites are found on these hair-like processes. The cilia often have the standard 9 + 2 arrangement of microtubules in their basal segments, although variations occur (e.g., 9 + 3 and 9 + 4). Because they generally lack dynein arms, active motility is believed to be absent (Moran et al., 1982b).

The second of these cell types—the microvillar cell—contains microvilli that project into the mucus.

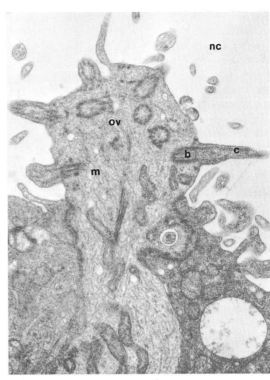

Figure 27–2. Longitudinal section through an olfactory vesicle (ov). b = basal body; c = olfactory cilium; m = microtubules; nc = nasal cavity. (× 22,110.) (From Moran D.T., Rowley J.C., Jafek B.W., et al. The fine structure of the olfactory mucosa in man. *J. Neurocytol.* 11:721–746, 1982. Published by Chapman & Hall.)

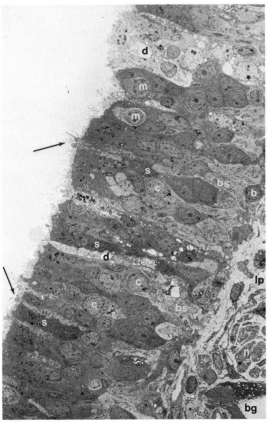

Figure 27–1. Low-power electron micrograph (× 670) of a longitudinal section through a biopsy specimen of human olfactory mucosa taken from the nasal septum. Four cell types are indicated: ciliated olfactory receptors (c), microvillar cells (m), supporting cells (s), and basal cells (b). The arrows point to ciliated olfactory knobs of the bipolar receptor cells. d = degenerating cells; bs = base of the supporting cells; lp = lamina propria; n = nerve bundle, bg = Bowman gland. (From Moran D.T., Rowley J.C., Jafek B.W., et al. The fine structure of the olfactory mucosa in man. *J. Neurocytol.* 11:721–746, 1982. Published by Chapman & Hall.)

These rotund cells are located adjacent to the primary bipolar cells in a 1:10 ratio and bear no cilia (Moran et al., 1982a) (see Fig. 27–1). The function of these cells is unknown, although a study using horseradish peroxidase tracer indicates that they send axons into the olfactory bulb, suggesting a sensory function (Rowley et al., 1989).

The third of these cell types—the sustentacular cell—is distributed throughout the olfactory region in contact with the other cell types and with one another, forming the matrix of the epithelium. These cells contribute to the production of mucus and may serve pinocytotic uptake and enzymatic degradation functions. In addition, they probably insulate the primary olfactory receptor cells from one another and may regulate the potassium concentration in the extracellular space near the receptor cells (Walz and Hertz, 1983).

The last of these four cell types—the basal cell—serves as the stem cell for the other cells in the olfactory epithelium, including the bipolar receptor cells. These cells are located near the lamina propria during their resting stage (see Fig. 27–1) and undergo major morphologic and functional changes during differentiation. The capacity of the bipolar receptor cell neuron to regenerate continuously from the basal cells or from cells in a compartment immediately above them (e.g., see Yamagishi et al., 1989) is a unique property of the olfactory neuroepithelium

(Graziadei, 1973). This property may explain the phenomenon of the delayed return of olfactory function in some persons after viral insult to the olfactory neuroepithelium. However, some fully differentiated olfactory receptor cells can be quite long lived, and, under nonpathologic conditions the receptor cell turnover may largely represent newly formed cells that fail to establish synapses within the olfactory bulb (Hinds et al., 1984).

The unmyelinated axons of the primary receptor cells traverse the lamina propria, form fine bundles sheathed by Schwann cells (which course through the cribriform plate), and enter the olfactory bulb, synapsing in spheric masses of neuropile termed *glomeruli* (Fig. 27–3). These complex structures consist of interwoven processes of the receptor cell axons with mitral, tufted, and periglomerular cell dendrites or processes. Because many more neurons enter glomeruli than leave them, they are a focus of a high degree of convergence of information (A.C. Allison and Warwick, 1949). These spheric structures are a key component of all olfactory systems, being present even in insects (MacLeod, 1971; Shepherd, 1972).

As can be seen in Figure 27–3, the mitral and tufted cells are large second-order neurons with primary dendrites entering the glomeruli and with secondary dendrites terminating in various regions of the bulb. These cells give off collaterals along their centrally directed course that interact with granule

cells and cells within the periglomerular and external plexiform layer regions. The mitral and tufted cell axons form the lateral olfactory tract, which projects to more central brain regions, including the anterior olfactory nucleus, the prepiriform cortex, the periamygdaloid cortex, the olfactory tubercle, the nucleus of the lateral olfactory tract, and the corticomedial nucleus of the amygdala (for details on central projections, see Brodal, 1981; Haberly and Price, 1977; Kretteck and Price, 1977a,b, 1978; MacLeod, 1971; Powell et al., 1965).

The mitral and tufted cells are involved in complex reverberating circuits in which negative feedback and positive feedback occur. For example, mitral cells can modulate their own output via the stimulation of granule cells (which are inhibitory to them) or via stimulation of excitatory inputs within the external plexiform layer. Reciprocal inhibition between neighboring mitral or tufted cells presumably results in sharpening the contrast between adjacent channels, similar to that seen in visual and tactile pathways (MacLeod, 1971).

Although the manner in which specific olfactory information is conveyed via the first-order neurons is not well understood, the initial component of the olfactory code is mediated by a large ensemble of sensory cells, each of which conveys a fraction of the information that signifies the nature of the odorant (Lancet, 1986). Odorants absorb into the mucus covering the olfactory epithelium and diffuse (alone or in conjunction with carrier proteins) to the cilia and terminal processes of olfactory receptor cells, where they bind to proteinaceous receptor sites located on one or both of these structures (Rhein and Cagan, 1981). This process leads, at least for some odorants, to the activation of a membrane-bound G protein, which in turn induces an adenylate cyclase–mediated increase in intracellular cyclic AMP (cAMP) (Jones and Reed, 1989; Menevse et al., 1977; Pace et al., 1985). As in other senses, intensity is coded, in part, by the relative frequency of firing in the afferent neurons (cf. Drake et al., 1969; Osterhammel et al., 1969). Interestingly, and as would be expected from the aforementioned observations, the perceived intensity of some odors to humans is correlated with the degree to which they induce adenylate cyclase activity in ciliary preparations (Doty et al., 1990). Odor quality is presumably coded via some type of a cross-fiber pattern, because individual olfactory receptor cells respond to a wide range of odorants, have response spectra that do not completely overlap, exhibit different types of responses to applied stimulants (e.g., although most receptor cells evidence excitatory responses, some evidence inhibitory responses, and others, on-off responses), and have highly overlapping response spectra (Mair and Gesteland, 1980; Sicard and Holley, 1984).

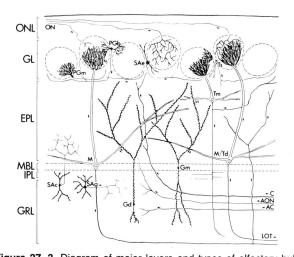

Figure 27–3. Diagram of major layers and types of olfactory bulb neurons in the mammalian olfactory bulb, as based on stained Golgi's material. Main layers are indicated on left as follows: ONL = olfactory nerve layer; GL = glomerular layer; EPL = external plexiform layer; MBL = mitral body layer; IPL = internal plexiform layer; GRL = granule cell layer. ON = olfactory nerves; PGb = periglomerular cells with biglomerular dendrites; PGm = periglomerular cell with monoglomerular dendrites; SAe = short-axon cell with extraglomerular dendrites; M = mitral cell; M/Td = displaced mitral or deep tufted cell; Tm = middle tufted cell; Ts = superficial tufted cell; Gm = granule cell with cell body in mitral body layer; Gd = granule cell with cell body in deep layers; SAc = short-axon cell of Cajal; SAg = short-axon cell of Golgi; C = centrifugal fibers; AON = fibers from anterior olfactory nucleus; AC = fibers from anterior commissure; LOT = lateral olfactory tract. (From Shepherd G.M. Synaptic organization of the mammalian olfactory bulb. *Physiol. Rev.* 52:864–917, 1972.)

Clinical Evaluation of Olfactory Function

Olfactory distortion or loss arises from a number of causes, including intranasal pathologic conditions (e.g., sinusitis, rhinitis), mechanical obstruction of the nasal airways, environmental or industrial pollutants, aging, and various medical and psychologic conditions (e.g., Alzheimer's disease, Parkinson's disease, Korsakoff's psychosis, and cystic fibrosis) (Amoore, 1986; 1988a,b; 1989b; Doty, 1979; Doty and Frye, 1989; Doty et al., 1984b; Schiffman, 1983; Schwartz et al., 1989) (Table 27–1). Overall incidence of smell loss after head injuries is approximately 7%, although this figure is much higher in cases of severe injury (ranging from 30 to 80% [cf. Sumner, 1976]). In the past, olfactory disorders were rarely examined quantitatively, largely because of the lack of standardized assessment procedures. Fortunately, significant progress has been made in the area of clinical measurement of olfactory function, permitting more detailed clinical discription of olfactory disturbances.

Classification of Olfactory Disorders

Both the patient's complaint and the objective sensory diagnosis can be adequately classified within the following schema:

Table 27–1. EXAMPLES OF DISORDERS REPORTED TO BE ASSOCIATED WITH OLFACTORY DYSFUNCTION

Endocrine	**Nutritional**
Adrenocortical insufficiency	Chronic renal failure
Cushing's syndrome	Cyanocobalamin (vitamin B_{12})
Diabetes mellitus	deficiency
Hypothyroidism	Korsakoff's psychosis
Kallmann's syndrome	
Primary amenorrhea	**Psychiatric**
Pseudohypoparathyroidism	Depression
Turner's syndrome	Olfactory reference syndrome
	Schizophrenia
Local Diseases and Mechanical	
Obstruction of Airways	**Tumors**
Adenoid hypertrophy	Intracranial
Allergic rhinitis	Aneurysms of the anterior
Atrophic rhinitis (ozena)	communicating bifurcation
Bronchial asthma	Frontal lobe glioma
Deformity caused by trauma	Hydrocephalus
Exposure to toxic chemicals	Internal carotid aneurysms
Leprosy	extending over the
Malignant disease of paranasal	pituitary fossa
sinuses with extension into	Neuroblastoma
nasal cavities	Suprasellar meningioma
Nasal polyposis	Sphenoid ridge meningioma
Sinusitis	Other meningiomas
Sjögren's syndrome	Intranasal
Tumors of nasopharynx with	Adenocarcinoma
extension into nasal cavities	Inverted papilloma
Vasomotor rhinitis	Melanoma
	Squamous cell carcinoma
Neurologic	
Alzheimer's disease	**Viral and infectious**
Epilepsy	Acute viral hepatitis
Head trauma	Herpes simplex
Huntington's chorea	Influenza-like infections
Intracranial surgery	
Korsakoff's psychosis	
Multiple sclerosis	
Parkinson's disease	

Data from Doty R.L. A review of olfactory dysfunctions in man. *Am. J. Otolaryngol.* 1:57–79, 1979; and Schiffman S.S. Taste and smell in disease. *N. Engl. J. Med.* 308:1275–1279, 1337–1343, 1983.

General (or total) anosmia—inability to detect any qualitative olfactory sensations

Partial anosmia—ability to detect some, but not all, qualitative olfactory sensations

General (or total) hyposmia—decreased sensitivity to all odorants

Partial hyposmia—decreased sensitivity to some, but not all, odorants

Dysosmia—either a distortion in the perception of an odor (e.g., the presence of an unpleasant odor when a normally pleasant odor is being smelled) or the presence of an odor that occurs in the absence of active smelling or sniffing behavior (sometimes termed an olfactory hallucination)

General (or total) hyperosmia—increased sensitivity to all odors

Partial hyperosmia—increased sensitivity to only some odors

Agnosia—inability to recognize an odor sensation, even though olfactory sensory processing, language, and general intellectual functions are sufficiently intact so that the recognition failure is not due to deficits in one or more of these functions

Separate determination of the patient's complaint and the objectively determined sensory disorder is important, because the two do not always coincide. Although other classification schemes are utilized in the literature (e.g., dysosmia is sometimes used as a generic term under which the other classes fall), the terminology just given suffices to categorize the vast majority of olfactory complaints and dysfunctions.

Sensory Assessment of Olfactory Function

Quantitative assessment of olfactory function is essential for a number of reasons: first, to establish the validity of the patient's complaint; second, to characterize the exact nature of the problem (which is critical for establishing a diagnosis); and third, to monitor objectively the efficacy of any interventions or treatments. In addition, some tests of smell function provide means for detecting malingering (cf. Doty, 1989; Doty et al., 1984a,b). Such detection is particularly important in litigation cases, as a number of courts have awarded sizable sums of money for loss of olfactory function.

Psychophysical procedures remain the primary means by which olfactory function is assessed in the clinic, even though certain electrophysiologic techniques offer the theoretic advantage of not being dependent on a patient's verbal response (e.g., averaged evoked potentials) (for review, see Doty, 1991). Controversy surrounds the validity of olfactory evoked potentials and other odorant-induced changes in electrophysiologic measures (e.g., heart rate changes), as they are highly variable and their neural origin is difficult to determine (cf. T. Allison and Goff, 1967; Lorig, 1989; Plattig and Kobal, 1979;

D.B. Smith et al., 1971). Although psychophysical responses can be obtained from subjects injected intravenously with an odorant (a potentially useful means of assessing the presence of intact cranial nerve I function in persons with nasal diseases that prevent testing with airborne odorants), the physiologic basis of this phenomenon is controversial (Maruniak et al., 1983), and sound normative data are not available for the interpretation of such tests.

The first step in assessing olfactory function is to determine the degree to which qualitative olfactory sensations are present. For this assessment, we routinely use a 40-item microencapsulated ("scratch 'n sniff") smell test (termed the University of Pennsylvania Smell Identification Test; commercially available from Sensonics, Inc., Haddonfield, NJ). This test is highly reliable (test-retest reliability is .95 [cf. Doty et al., 1984a, 1989b]), allows the classification of patients into discrete categories of dysfunction, provides a percentile score of a patient's performance relative to age- and sex-matched controls, and has procedures for detecting malingering. Scores on this test reflect both gross and subtle olfactory problems associated with current and previous smoking behavior (Frye et al., 1990) and numerous neurologic diseases (e.g., Alzheimer's disease, Korsakoff's psychosis, and Parkinson's disease [Fig. 27–4]) and correlate highly with the levels of certain catecholamine metabolites in the cerebrospinal fluid of some patient groups (e.g., $r \approx .90$ with the lumbar levels of 3-methoxy-4-hydroxyphenylglycol in patients with Korsakoff's psychosis [cf. Mair et al., 1983]). The relationship between age and the scores on this standardized test is presented in Figure 27–5, which shows the pattern of smell loss in the elderly (Doty et al., 1984b). It is also apparent from this illustration that, on the average, women score higher on this test than men.

A second step in assessing smell function is to determine the absolute level of an odorant that the patient can detect. Although air-dilution olfactometry is the method of choice in presenting stimuli for such an assessment, it is not practical in the typical clinical setting. An alternative approach is to present odorants diluted in a liquid diluent (e.g., odorless mineral oil) via small vessels held over the nose (i.e., "sniff bottles"). We most commonly use the rose-like odorant phenyl ethyl alcohol for such a test, because it is pleasant smelling at higher concentrations, elicits relatively little trigeminal activity, and is easily dissolved in most diluents (Doty et al., 1978; 1984a). Although several psychophysical procedures can be used to establish a threshold estimate, a modified ascending single staircase procedure is preferable, because higher concentrations are initially avoided (minimizing adaptation effects) and a stable measure can be established with a minimal number of trials (see Cornsweet, 1962; Doty et al., 1984a; Ghorbanian et al., 1983).

Although detection threshold values typically agree with results obtained from smell identification tests, in some instances patients who fail identification tests perform normally on detection tests. However, the reverse rarely occurs. Because some patients can use subtle non–cranial nerve I cues to obtain low detection thresholds, the results of the identification test are weighted more heavily in ascertaining a sensory diagnosis than are those from the threshold test. Care must be taken in making this judgment, however, because an odor identification test can be sensitive to distortions of smell function that are unaccompanied by changes in the detection threshold, including some forms of agnosia. Even though such conditions are rare compared with uncomplicated smell losses caused by viruses and nasal obstruction, they must be kept in mind in cases in which central nervous system damage is known or suspected.

On rare occasion, it is useful to evaluate unilateral olfactory function by occluding each nostril. However, the patency of the nasal airways cyclically fluctuates in most persons (the so-called nasal cycle) and the majority of olfactory disorders occur bilaterally, including the dysfunction associated with Parkinson's disease (Doty et al., 1991c).

Although a number of other procedures are avail-

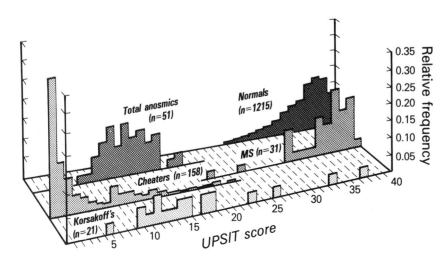

Figure 27–4. Frequency distribution of scores on the University of Pennsylvania Smell Identification Test (UPSIT) for five groups of subjects. MS = multiple sclerosis. (Reprinted with permission from *Physiol. Behav. [Monograph]*, vol. 32, Doty R.L., Shaman P., Dann M., Development of the University of Pennsylvania Smell Identification Test: a standardized microencapsulated test of olfactory function, Copyright 1984, Pergamon Press.)

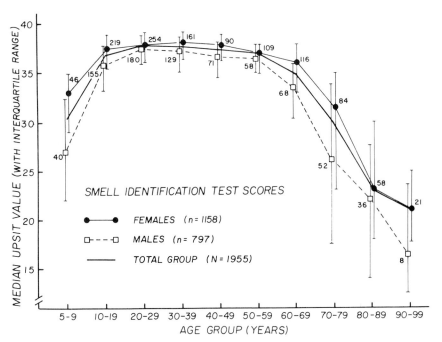

Figure 27-5. Scores on the University of Pennsylvania Smell Identification Test as a function of age in a large heterogeneous group of subjects. Numbers by data points indicate sample sizes. (From Doty, R.L., Shaman P., Applebaum S.L., et al. Smell identification ability: changes with age. *Science* 226:1441–1443, 1984. Copyright 1984 by the AAAS.)

able for assessing olfactory function, such as magnitude estimation and multidimensional scaling, more research is needed to determine whether they contribute substantially to the clinical information obtained by the aforementioned tests. Procedures such as magnitude estimation, although quite economical of time, share with thresholds the problem of marked between-subject variability, and—depending on the odorant used—may not be as sensitive to a number of subject-related variables as detection threshold measures (cf. Berglund et al., 1971; R.L. Doty, unpublished observations).

Medical Examination and Treatment of Patients with Olfactory Disorders

The aim of the medical evaluation is to identify the cause of the olfactory dysfunction and to correct the problem, if possible. The patient's history is extremely important in arriving at a diagnosis. The physician needs to assess the pattern of loss (sudden onset, gradual), its duration (days, months, years), preceding events (e.g., head trauma, viral infection), and any accompanying medical disorders (e.g., nutritional defect, neurologic conditions [e.g., parkinsonism]). Specific nasal symptoms, especially epistaxis, nasal pain, rhinorrhea, and obstruction, should be elicited; these may direct attention to an inflammatory or neoplastic disorder. A history of allergy or nasal polyps is important, because these disorders can lead to olfactory dysfunction. A family history of other chemosensory or neurologic diseases should be sought; environmental exposure to irritants and chemicals should be reviewed with the patient.

During the physical examination, the physician should pay special attention to the nose and the upper respiratory tract. This necessitates endoscopic examination of the nasal cavity, the meati, the septum, and the sinus ostia. Small polyps may be found, which otherwise would have gone undetected. A nasopharyngeal neoplasm or its metastasis to the neck may be discovered. Neurologic examination of the orbital contents and the cranial nerves may direct attention to a lesion of the skull base. Although a severely deviated nasal septum may play a role in olfactory dysfunction (Leopold, 1988), most septal deviations are unrelated to the ability to smell.

The following laboratory studies are recommended when clinically indicated: complete blood count with white blood cell differential count, serum levels of calcium and angiotensin-converting enzyme (may be elevated in sarcoidosis), erythrocyte sedimentation rate (may be elevated in inflammatory disorders, such as Wegener's granulomatosis), serologic tests for syphilis, and serum levels of glucose and creatinine. Imaging studies of the nose, paranasal sinuses, and cranial contents are critical to the evaluation. This is best done with computed tomography or magnetic resonance imaging in the axial, coronal and/or sagittal planes. Biopsy of the olfactory neuroepithelium has been performed in the research setting but is not done routinely in the clinic (Lovell et al., 1982).

After all information is gathered, a diagnosis is reached. Usually, the cause of the olfactory dysfunction is (1) obstruction of odorant access to the neuroepithelium by inflammation or, rarely, neoplasm; (2) damage to the olfactory neuroepithelium; or (3) damage to the central olfactory pathways. Obstructive problems can result from allergic rhinitis, nasal polyps, chronic rhinosinusitis, and benign or malignant nasal neoplasms. Overuse and abuse of topical nasal sprays (as in rhinitis medicamentosa) is also seen. Direct injury to the neuroepithelium can be caused by nasal or skull base surgery, external trauma, topical or systemic effects of drugs (cocaine, aminoglycoside antibiotics), and most commonly, viruses, such as herpes simplex and influenza.

Trauma, although capable of shearing the fine nerve filaments of cranial nerve I from the olfactory bulb at the cribriform plate, can also have central causes (Sumner, 1976), and animal research has revealed that intracranial hemorrhage can lead to degeneration of the olfactory epithelium without transection of the olfactory nerve (Nakashima et al., 1984b). It is generally believed that long-standing cases of anosmia not caused by intranasal disease or blockage are likely permanent and untreatable with current therapies.

Of considerable significance to the neurologist are the findings that Alzheimer's disease, Korsakoff's psychosis, Huntington's chorea, idiopathic Parkinson's disease, and the parkinsonism-dementia complex of Guam are accompanied by clear-cut alterations in smell function (Doty et al., 1987, 1988b, 1989a, 1991a,b,c; Mair et al., 1983; Moberg et al., 1987; Peabody and Tinklenberg, 1985; Ward et al., 1983). Such alterations are consistent, in several of these conditions, with known biochemical and morphologic anomalies in brain regions associated with olfaction, including the primary and secondary olfactory pathways (Esiri and Wilcock, 1984; Reyes et al., 1986). Indeed, lesions within the olfactory system appear to be among the first pathologic changes to occur in Alzheimer's disease (Hyman et al., 1984), and punctate lesions in monoamine-rich regions of the brain stem and diencephalon of patients with Korsakoff's psychosis likely relate to the previously noted correlation between their smell identification test scores and lumbar cerebrospinal fluid levels of 3-methoxy-4-hydroxyphenylglycol (Mair et al., 1983). Interestingly, MPTP-induced parkinsonism is unaccompanied by major olfactory dysfunction (Doty et al., 1991b).

It is also significant that a variety of intracranial tumors can influence smell function (for review see Doty, 1979). For example, it has been estimated that 20% of the tumors of the temporal lobe or lesions of the uncinate convolution produce olfactory disturbances, usually in the form of unpleasant smell hallucinations (e.g., Furstenberg et al., 1943).

Most authors believe that olfactory auras occur in association with temporal lobe seizures (Daly, 1958b; Holmes, 1927; Jackson, 1869, 1880; Penfield and Kristiansen, 1951; Weiser et al., 1985). Gloor et al. (1982), elaborating on this, suggested that the mesiotemporal limbic structures, but not the temporal neocortex, were essential for such symptoms. Auras have been variously described and include smells resembling burning oil (Penfield and Kristiansen, 1951), peaches, lemons (Daly, 1975), blood (Daly, 1958a), and "something to do with animals" (Gloor et al., 1982).

Howe and Gibson (1982) reviewed 273 patients with complex partial seizures. Only 22 had olfactory and 9 had gustatory hallucinations with their seizures. Six had both. Three of these were proved to have gliomas, and one, an arteriovenous malformation. These authors pointed out that, overall, the frequency of tumors in this group was not higher than would be expected in patients with temporal lobe epilepsy.

Studies of patients undergoing surgical treatment of intractable psychomotor seizures suggested that the amygdala is an essential element for the elaboration of olfactory auras and that amygdalotomy can eliminate such hallucinatory phenomena (Andy et al., 1975). For example, Chitanondh (1966) reported successful treatment of seven patients with seizure disorders, olfactory hallucinations, and psychiatric problems by stereotaxically placed amygdalotomies and that "stereotaxic amygdalotomy has a dramatic effect upon olfactory seizures, auras and hallucinations. It is a safe surgical procedure and can be done without neurological deficit."

Although few detailed psychophysical studies of olfactory function have been performed in patients receiving amygdalotomies, there is some indication that bilateral amygdaloid lesions have at least some adverse effect on odor differentiation and identification (Andy et al., 1975). Clearly, unilateral excision of 5–7 cm of the anterior temporal lobe for intractable epilepsy has detrimental effects on odor quality discrimination, immediate and delayed recognition memory, ability to match an odor to its visually or haptically presented source, and the verbal identification of odors (Eskenazi et al., 1983). However, odor detection ability per se appears to be unimpaired, and the benefits derived from the elimination of olfactory hallucinations and seizure activity by such procedures appear considerable.

It is possible to characterize routinely most olfactory problems quantitatively and to use this information, along with that obtained from the history and the physical examination, to determine the cause of the dysfunction. Unfortunately, with the exception of odorant access problems within the nose and those rare cases in which dysosmia is associated with clear-cut seizure disorders, meaningful treatments are not available for most olfactory problems. Although zinc and vitamin therapies have been suggested in the literature, there is no compelling evidence that these therapies are effective, except in cases in which frank zinc or vitamin deficiences exist. Even though some dysosmias are reportedly cured by periodic anesthetization of the olfactory receptor region, most dysosmias remit spontaneously, and such treatment often provides only temporary relief. Extremely debilitating, long-standing, severe dysosmia may be amenable to treatment either by resection of one or both olfactory bulbs (Kaufman et al., 1988) or by operative destruction of segments of the olfactory neuroepithelium (Leopold et al., 1990).

GUSTATION

Patients commonly fail to distinguish between flavor and taste and often report loss of taste sensation in the presence of normal sweet, sour, bitter, and salty responsiveness. Although true loss of gustatory function exists, it is rare, as taste responsiveness is mediated bilaterally by four nerves within the oral cavity, as indicated in the next section. Thus, a number of studies report that less than 1% of head injury patients exhibit true taste loss, as compared with more than 7% overall for loss of olfactory function (Sumner, 1976). In our experience, strange taste sensations (i.e., dysgeusias) are much more common than taste losses or decrements per se.

Anatomy and Physiology of Taste

The peripheral receptors for taste—the taste buds—are round epithelial structures consisting of slender cells arranged like the segments of a grapefruit (Fig. 27–6C). The long axis of the taste bud is perpendicular to the surface of the epithelium. The superficial portion of the bud is marked by an excavation, the taste pit, into which the microvilli of the sensory cells project. Several cell types are discernible within the taste bud. Thus, histologic studies reveal light and dark cells that bear microvilli that project into the taste pit. There is also a light cell with a club-like ending, as well as basal cells (Murray, 1973). These different cell types are presumed to represent different stages of generation and degeneration of the sensory taste cells. Cell turnover is thought to occur during a 10-day interval, at least in the rat (Beidler and Smallman, 1965).

As in the olfactory system, somatosensory sensations (e.g., stinging, burning, cooling, and sharpness) can be induced by some oral stimulants via trigeminal afferents located on the tongue and throughout the oral cavity. Although, in a strict

sense, one cannot view this type of stimulation as being taste, such stimulation is critical in determining the overall gestalt of flavor, such as that experienced when eating spicy foods like chili.

Taste buds are located in the oral cavity on the soft palate and tongue, the pharynx, the larynx, and the esophagus. The largest number are on the surface of the tongue, being associated with visible protuberances termed *papillae*. Of the four types of papillae—fungiform, foliate, circumvallate, and filiform—only the first three harbor taste buds. The location of these types of papillae varies, with the circumvallate papillae being arranged in an inverted V at the border between the anterior two-thirds and the posterior one-third of the tongue. The club-like fungiform papillae are scattered on the anterior two-thirds of the tongue, and the foliate papillae are located on the lateral border of the posterior middle third of the tongue (Fig. 27–6A).

Up to 200 taste buds are present in each circumvallate papilla, whereas far fewer buds are present in each of the other types. The pores of the circumvallate taste buds open into a furrow or moat, separating each papilla from the surrounding tissue. Secretions from the glands of von Ebner enter this moat, which acts as a container for the taste solutions. Taste buds associated with the foliate papillae are similarly positioned within the walls of furrows, unlike the taste buds in the fungiform papillae, which are positioned within a small opening at their top (Fig. 27–6B).

The innervation of the taste buds is complex. The afferent fibers from the buds within the fungiform papillae and from trigeminal nerve endings enter the lingual nerve. The taste fibers subsequently join the chorda tympani nerve, which merges with the facial nerve in the temporal bone. These fibers enter the brain stem with the nervus intermedius. The taste buds of the circumvallate and foliate papillae are subserved by fibers traveling directly to the brain stem with the glossopharyngeal nerve, although the anterior folds of the foliate papillae may be inner-

Figure 27–6. (*A* and *B*) Distribution of taste buds on the human tongue. Taste buds of the fungiform and foliate papillae are innervated by cranial nerve VII. Those of the circumvallate papillae are innervated by cranial nerve IX. Cranial nerve V carries nontaste somatosensory sensations. See text for details. (*C*) Fine structure of taste bud. 1 and 2 = presumably supporting cells that secrete materials into the lumen of the bud; 3 = sensory receptor cell; 4 = basal cell from which the other cell types arise. (Modified from Shepherd G.M. *Neurobiology.* New York, Oxford University Press, 1983.)

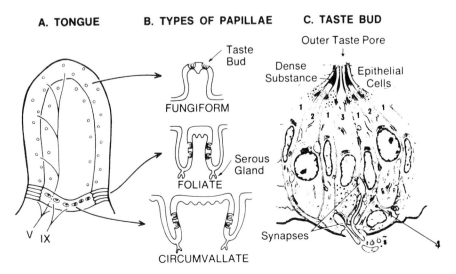

A. TONGUE

B. TYPES OF PAPILLAE

C. TASTE BUD

Taste Bud

FUNGIFORM

Serous Gland

FOLIATE

CIRCUMVALLATE

V IX

Outer Taste Pore

Dense Substance

Epithelial Cells

Synapses

vated by the chorda tympani nerve in some species. The afferents from taste buds on the palate travel with the greater superficial petrosal nerve, which joins the facial nerve at the geniculate ganglion. Taste buds of the larynx and the esophagus are subserved primarily by vagal afferents.

The peripheral gustatory nerve fibers enter the brain stem and project to the nucleus of the tractus solitarius, which begins in the rosterolateral medulla and extends caudally along the ventral border of the vestibular nuclei. Chorda tympani fibers synapse rostral to the glossopharyngeal fibers. The central relays for the receptors on the palate probably project to the region innervated by the chorda tympani, and those for the receptors subserved by the vagus, to a region caudal to the projection of the glossopharyngeal.

The taste fibers subsequently project from the nucleus of the tractus solitarius to the pontine parabrachial nuclei (at least in the rat). From there, two divergent pathways arise. One synapses in the thalamus and continues to the cortical gustatory area. There may also be direct connections that by-pass the thalamus. The second pathway from the parabrachial nuclei distributes broadly to the ventral forebrain. Although little is known about these pathways in the human, there is physiologic evidence that the primary cortical area for taste in other primates is located deep in the parietal operculum and adjacent parainsular cortex (see Norgren, 1984).

Hausser-Hauw and Bancaud (1987) provided clinical evidence that supports this conclusion in a group of 30 patients who manifested gustatory hallucinations during epileptic seizures. Such symptoms could have resulted from seizures of parietal or temporal origin or occur after electrical stimulation of the hippocampus, the amygdala, the rolandic or parietal operculum, or the first or second temporal convolutions. However, whereas they were intermixed with other symptoms in the case of temporal lobe seizures, they occurred as isolated or prominent symptoms in the case of parietal seizures or parietal or rolandic stimulation. One of their patients and one described by Penfield and Faulck (1955) reported resolution of gustatory symptoms after resections of the parietal operculum. However, Hausser-Hauw and Bancaud (1987) noted that 4% of 305 patients with temporal lobe seizures, but only 2% of 309 patients with suprasylvian seizures and 3% of 102 patients with suprasylvian and infrasylvian seizures, reported gustatory symptoms; they suggested that reorganization of cortical pathways in patients with temporal lobe epilepsy accounted for the discrepancy. An alternative possibility, suggested by Gloor et al. (1982), is that activation of mesiotemporal structures is necessary before symptoms such as taste achieve experiential immediacy. Hausser-Hauw and Bancaud (1987) reviewed the physiologic and anatomic evidence, which supports the presence of taste pathway projections to the amygdala, particularly its central nucleus. Such a pathway might provide an additional explanation for the observations of Gloor et al. (1982).

As in the case of olfaction, taste intensity in humans has been shown to correlate with the magnitude of the neural response (as measured electrophysiologically from the chorda tympani nerve bundle as it crosses the tympanic membrane) (Diamant et al., 1965). The nature of quality coding is more complex, and there are proponents of both labeled line and cross-fiber patterning theories. Other investigators believe that this distinction is artificial and subsume labeled line theory within a cross-fiber patterning theory. Regardless of such theoretic distinctions, there is evidence at the level of the first-order neuron for reasonably discrete classes of neurons (within a broadly tuned population of cells) that can be identified as responding best to specific tastants. For example, there are sweet-sensitive fibers in the hamster chorda tympani nerve that increase their firing rates more vigorously to sucrose than to other tastants (Frank, 1973). Analogous cell types are seen for stimulants representing nonsweet taste categories. However, recordings in taste-related neurons in the brain stem suggest that the central fibers are much more broadly tuned than are the first-order neurons (D.V. Smith et al., 1983). It is noteworthy that substances have been discovered that selectively alter taste perceptions. For example, miraculin, a glycoprotein from the berry of the African shrub *Syncepalum dilcificum*, produces an alteration of all sour tastes to a sucrose-like sweetness. Gymnemic acid, an extract from the leaves of the Indian plant *Gymnema sylvestre,* can block the perception of sweet sensation (and the corresponding electrophysiologic activity) without significantly altering the perception of the other taste qualities (for review of taste modifiers, see Kurihara, 1971).

Clinical Evaluation of Taste Function

Numerous factors influence normal gustatory function. It should be re-emphasized, however, that most patients with the complaint of loss of taste evidence, on psychophysical examination, normal taste function and abnormal smell function. For this reason, it is useful to use the term *flavor* in describing the complex synthesis of gustatory, olfactory, and somatosensory sensations. Whole-mouth taste deficits are uncommon.

Many of the same conditions that are associated with olfactory disturbances are also reported to influence taste function. For example, taste disorders have been reported after head trauma, zinc deficiency, adrenocortical insufficiency, and viral infections (Table 27–2). In addition, however, taste disturbances appear to be present much more frequently than olfactory ones as a result of the use of pharmacologic agents, such as antirheumatic drugs, antiproliferative drugs, and substances bearing a sulfhydryl group (e.g., penicillamine and captopril). Although the mechanisms responsible for such phenomena are poorly understood, a number of taste stimuli can elicit taste perceptions when injected into the bloodstream, analogous to the intravascular olfaction phenomenon discussed earlier (Bradley, 1973).

Deficiency (as in Sjögren's syndrome) or hyperviscosity of saliva leads, in time, to lessened taste acuity, presumably as the result of accompanying decreases in the number of papillae and taste buds and possible functional alteration in the remaining taste buds (Brightman, 1977). Whether such morphologic alterations in humans are due to the elimination of lubricating or trophic activity from the saliva is not known. In our experience, neither artificial saliva nor water mouthwashes have proved successful in restoring normal taste function in patients with xerostomia. However, systematic research is needed to ascertain whether such materials can improve taste function in certain types of xerostomia.

Post-traumatic ageusia is much less common than post-traumatic anosmia. Ageusia to one or more of the primary taste modalities is believed to occur in less than 1% of persons with major head injury (Sumner, 1976). Although the literature is scant, the prognosis for post-traumatic ageusia is far better than for post-traumatic anosmia. Considerable controversy exists regarding the underlying cause of most head trauma–related cases of ageusia, because general ageusia should theoretically be nearly impossible to induce. Unfortunately, many of the reports of ageusia in the literature are based on the patient's report rather than on the results of sound psychophysical testing, so they may not reflect the true incidence of this problem and, in some instances, may actually be mislabeled cases of anosmia (Deems et al., 1991).

Complaints of taste loss or distortion are commonly reported in various carcinomas. For example, squamous cell carcinoma of the mucous membranes of the upper aerodigestive tract can interfere with taste by direct destruction of receptors and neural pathways. Malnutrition associated with these tumors can also lead to ageusia. Significant increases in recognition thresholds for bitter in patients with metastatic carcinomas and decreases in such thresholds for sour in breast cancer patients were reported (Settle et al., 1979). Radiation therapy alters taste bud cell turnover and can affect taste function, although return after radiation treatment has been observed (Conger, 1973).

Gustatory symptoms have been reported in association with epileptic seizures for more than a century (Daly, 1958a; Gowers, 1909; Holmes, 1927; Jackson, 1990; Wieser et al., 1985). Daly (1975) suggested that such sensations reflect those basic to taste (sweet, acid, bitter, and salty), although sweet tastes seem to occur less frequently. Tastes have been described as peculiar, rotten (Penfield and Kristiansen 1951), sweet—along with a pungent odor (Daly, 1958b), or like a cigarette, rotten apples, or vomitus (Hausser-Hauw and Bancaud, 1987). However, as noted earlier, many of the latter tastes likely represent smell sensations that are miscategorized as tastes by both the patients and their physicians.

Although taste acuity declines with age, the perceptual decrease is not as marked as that seen for olfaction (Cowart, 1981; Weiffenbach, 1984; Weiffenbach et al., 1982). Nonetheless, in conjunction with the loss seen in the sense of smell, such decrements may lead to anorexia, weight loss, and malnutrition in some of the elderly.

Classification of Taste Disorders

As for olfactory disorders, we classify the patient's complaint and the results of sensory tests separately. The terms we use for such classification are as follows:

Total ageusia—lack of taste sensation to all tastants
Partial ageusia—lack of taste sensation to some tastants

Table 27–2. EXAMPLES OF DISORDERS REPORTED TO BE ASSOCIATED WITH GUSTATORY DYSFUNCTION

Endocrine	**Autoimmune**	**Nutritional**
Adrenocortical insufficiency	Pemphigus	Cachexia
Congenital adrenal hyperplasia	Sjögren's syndrome	Chronic renal failure
Panhypopituitarism		Cirrhosis of the liver
Cushing's syndrome	**Local Alterations of Taste Buds or Papillae**	Niacin (vitamin B$_3$) deficiency
Cretinism	Chemicals, drugs	Zinc deficiency
Hypothyroidism	Xerostomia	
Diabetes mellitus		**Psychiatric**
Turner's syndrome	**Neurologic**	Depression
Pseudohypoparathyroidism	Bell's palsy	Schizophrenia
	Epilepsy	
Inflammatory	Familial dysautonomia	**Tumors**
Infections	Head trauma	Oral cavity cancer
Candidiasis	Middle ear operations with manipulation or	Base of skull neoplasia
Gingivitis	damage to chorda tympani	
Herpes simplex	Multiple sclerosis	
Periodontitis	Raeder's paratrigeminal syndrome	
Sialadenitis		

Data from Doty R.L. A review of olfactory dysfunctions in man. *Am. J. Otolaryngol.* 1:57–79, 1979; and Schiffman S.S. Taste and smell in disease. *N. Engl. J. Med.* 308:1275–1279, 1337–1343, 1983.

Total hypogeusia—lessened sensation to all tastants

Partial hypogeusia—lessened sensation to tastants representing one to three of the four major taste qualities

Hypergeusia—heightened smell ability

Dysgeusia—the presence of a strange or distorted taste sensation

Sensory Assessment of Taste Function

Numerous procedures have been developed for evaluating gustatory function, although few data are available concerning their reliability or validity. We find that taste tests in which drops of stimulus are applied to the tongue are less than satisfactory in some instances, because the area stimulated is difficult to control and often the stimulus volume is not large enough to induce a reliable response. Although electrogustometric procedures can be of use in establishing gross neural deficit, they have limited use in the clinic, as the results obtained are dependent on the electrodes selected (electrical taste may be an iontophoretic phenomenon) and not all taste qualities can be reliably elicited. Furthermore, subtle alterations in taste function cannot be measured by these techniques. In general, when direct current is used, a sour taste is evoked if the anode is applied to the tongue. Current reversal brings about a less distinct response described variously as soap-like, metallic, or bitter. Sweet sensations are rarely, if ever, elicited using an electrical stimulus.

The initial test we use for assessing gustatory function incorporates a concentration series of suprathreshold tastants representing sweet, sour, bitter, and salty tastes. In this whole-mouth sip-and-spit test developed by R. Gregg Settle, the patient

1. Swishes 10 ml of solution in his or her mouth
2. Indicates the taste quality of each stimulus
3. Scales the perceived intensity of each stimulus using a fully anchored nine-point category scale (1 = no taste; 9 = extremely strong taste)
4. Rates the perceived pleasantness of each stimulant on a similar nine-point scale (1 = dislike extremely; 9 = like extremely)

Five concentrations of sucrose, citric acid, sodium chloride, and caffeine are presented in counterbalanced order twice during the test, and deionized water rinsings are interspersed between stimulus presentations. This test reveals gross abnormalities of taste function, is easy for the patient to perform, and is reasonably economical of time, in that all four taste qualities can be evaluated in half the time required to obtain a single taste threshold. The hedonic rating serves both as a measure of perceptual affect (the chemical senses seem particularly focused on affect) and as a means of assessing gustatory function in a rare class of patients who deny perceiving taste intensity, yet evidence the ability to taste via correct quality of classification of stimuli and normal pleasantness functions.

If a taste problem is suspected on the basis of suprathreshold taste testing, patient report, or apparent etiology, we additionally determine single staircase gustatory detection thresholds analogous to those performed in olfaction. For these tests, the aforementioned four tastants are used, and abnormality is assumed when a patient's threshold value falls beyond two standard deviations from that of a healthy control group.

Regional (quadrant) taste testing is indicated when damage to one or more of the individual nerves innervating the taste buds is suspected. Although such tests are easy to perform on the front of the tongue, it is sometimes difficult to deposit a taste stimulus accurately on the back of the tongue, given its depth within the oral cavity and the stimulation of the gag reflex. In most cases, tastants can be micropipetted into the region, although stimulus spread can be a problem. Although it is possible to confine the stimulus spread by using small pieces of filter paper soaked in the taste solution, stimulus contact is not always adequate and difficulties are encountered in retrieving the small pieces of filter paper. For such regional testing, it is useful to employ an automated micropipette to present suprathreshold concentrations of the four target tastants in a forced-choice paradigm with deionized water rinsing between trials.

Medical Examination and Treatment of Patients with Gustatory Disorders

Dysfunction of the taste system can be due to one or more causes, including the following:

1. Oral medical problems that release bad-tasting materials (e.g., gingivitis and sialadenitis)
2. The use of different types of metals in fillings and dental appliances, which results in intraoral current gradients sensed by the taste system
3. Transport problems of tastants to the taste buds (e.g., caused by dryness of the oral cavity and by damage of the taste pores or the papillae)
4. Destruction or loss of the taste buds themselves
5. Damage to one or more of the neural pathways innervating the taste buds
6. Central neural factors

In addition to performing the standard history and physical examination mentioned under Medical Examination and Treatment of Patients with Olfactory Disorders, we palpate and examine the tongue carefully to detect signs of scaring, inflammation, atrophy of papillae, or neoplasm. Although not done routinely, biopsy of circumvallate or fungiform papillae for detailed microscopic examination has proved useful in determining whether pathologic changes are present in taste bud tissue. In cases of suspected salivary gland disease, we obtain a biopsy specimen of minor salivary gland tissue in the lower lip to determine the presence of lymphoepithelial lesion (indicative of Sjögren's syndrome). In cases in which the basis of the dysfunction cannot be ascribed to peripheral factors, we obtain appropriate radiographs to rule out central nervous system tumors or lesions.

Treatment is straightforward in cases in which decreased salivation or local oral pathologic alteration caused by dental factors is the basis of a dysgeusia or hypogeusia. Saliva can be supplemented by various salivary substitutes. Nutritional deficiencies can be corrected. Radiation-induced xerostomia may improve with time. In some cases, flavor enhancers can be of at least some benefit.

CONCLUDING REMARKS

The chemical senses of taste and smell determine, in large part, the flavor of foods and beverages and warn of fire, dangerous fumes, leaking gas, spoiled foods, and polluted environments. Disorders of these senses often result from accidents, disease states, medical interventions, aging, and exposure to a number of environmental pollutants and can serve as important indicators of a number of diseases. This chapter briefly reviewed the anatomy and physiology of these senses, some etiologic factors responsible for their dysfunction, and information regarding their evaluation and management. It was specifically noted that most patients with complaints of taste loss have, in fact, olfactory dysfunction and that true taste loss is relatively rare.

References

(Key references are designated with an asterisk.)

Allison A.C., Warwick R.T.T. Quantitative observations on the olfactory system of the rabbit. *Brain* 72:186–197, 1949.

Allison T., Goff W.R. Human cerebral evoked responses to odorous stimuli. *Electroencephalogr. Clin. Neurophysiol.* 22:558–560, 1967.

*Amoore J.E. Effects of chemical exposure on olfaction in humans. In Barrow C.S., ed. *Toxicology of the Nasal Passages.* Washington, DC, Hemisphere Publishing, pp. 155–190, 1986.

Andy O.J., Jurko M.F., Hughes J.R. The amygdala in relation to olfaction. *Confin. Neurol.* 37:215–222, 1975.

Beidler L.M., Smallman R.L. Renewal of cells within taste buds. *J. Cell Biol.* 27:263–272, 1965.

Berglund B., Berglund U., Ekman G., et al. Individual psychophysical functions for 28 odorants. *Percept. Psychophys.* 9:379–384, 1971.

Bradley R.M. Electrophysiological investigations of intravascular taste using perfused rat tongue. *Am. J. Physiol.* 224:300–304, 1973.

Brightman V.J. Disordered oral sensation and appetite. In Kare M.R., Maller O., eds. *The Chemical Senses and Nutrition.* New York, Academic Press, pp. 363–380, 1977.

Brodal A. *Neurological Anatomy in Relation to Clinical Medicine.* New York, Oxford University Press, 1981.

Chitanondh H. Stereotaxic amygdalotomy in the treatment of olfactory seizures and psychiatric disorders with olfactory hallucination. *Confin. Neurol.* 27:181–196, 1966.

Conger A.D. Loss and recovery of taste acuity in patients irradiated to the oral cavity. *Radiat. Res.* 53:338–347, 1973.

Cornsweet T.N. The staircase method in psychophysics. *Am. J. Psychol.* 75:485–491, 1962.

Cowart B.J. Development of taste perception in humans: sensitiv-

ity and preference throughout the life span. *Psychol. Bull.* 90:43–71, 1981.

Daly D. Ictal affect. *Am. J. Psychiatry* 115:97–108, 1958a.

Daly D. Uncinate fits. *Neurology* 8:250–260, 1958b.

Daly D.D. Ictal clinical manifestations of complex partial seizures. *Adv. Neurol.* 2:57–83, 1975.

Deems D.A., Doty R.L., Settle R.G., et al. Smell and taste disorders: a study of 750 patients from the University of Pennsylvania Smell and Taste Center. *Arch. Otolaryngol. Head Neck Surg.* 117:519–528, 1991.

Diamant H., Oakley B., Strom L., et al. A comparison of neural and psychophysical responses to taste stimuli in man. *Acta Physiol. Scand.* 64:67–74, 1965.

*Doty R.L. A review of olfactory dysfunctions in man. *Am. J. Otolaryngol.* 1:57–79, 1979.

Doty R.L. *The Smell Identification Test Administration Manual.* 2nd ed. Haddonfield, NJ, Sensonics, 1989.

Doty R.L. Olfactory psychophysics. In Laing D.G., Doty R.L., Breipol W., eds. *The Human Sense of Smell.* New York, Springer-Verlag, in press.

Doty R.L., Frye R. Influence of nasal obstruction on smell function. *Otolaryngol. Clin. North Am.* 22:398–411, 1989.

Doty R.L., Brugger W.E., Jurs P.C., et al. Intranasal trigeminal stimulation from odorous volatiles: psychometric responses from anosmic and normal humans. *Physiol. Behav.* 23:373–380, 1978.

Doty R.L., Shaman P., Applebaum S.L., et al. Smell identification ability: changes with age. *Science* 226:1441–1443, 1984a.

Doty R.L., Shaman P., Dann M. Development of the University of Pennsylvania Smell Identification Test: a standardized microencapsulated test of olfactory function. *Physiol. Behav. (Monograph)* 32:489–502, 1984b.

Doty R.L., Reyes P., Gregor T. Presence of both odor identification and detection deficits in Alzheimer's disease. *Brain Res. Bull.* 18:597–600, 1987.

Doty R.L., Deems D.A., Frye R., et al. Olfactory sensitivity, nasal resistance, and autonomic function in the multiple chemical sensitivities (MCS) syndrome. *Arch. Otolaryngol. Head Neck Surg.* 114:1422–1427, 1988a.

Doty R.L., Deems D., Stellar S. Olfactory dysfunction in Parkinson's disease: a general deficit unrelated to neurologic signs, disease stage, or disease duration. *Neurology* 38:1237–1244, 1988b.

Doty R.L., Riklan M., Deems D.A., et al. The olfactory and cognitive deficits of Parkinson's disease: evidence for independence. *Ann. Neurol.* 25:166–171, 1989a.

Doty R.L., Ugrawal U., Frye R.E. Evaluation of the internal consistency reliability of the fractionated and whole University of Pennsylvania Smell Identification Test (UPSIT). *Percept. Psychophys.* 45:381–384, 1989b.

Doty R.L., Kreiss D., Frye R.E. Odor intensity: correlation with odorant-sensitive adenylate cyclase activity in cilia from frog olfactory receptor cells. *Brain Res.* 527:130–134, 1990.

Doty R.L., Perl D.P., Steele J., et al. Odor identification deficit of the parkinsonism-dementia complex of Guam: equivalence to that of Alzheimer's and idiopathic Parkinson's disease. *Neurology* 41(Suppl. 2):77–80, 1991a.

Doty R.L., Singh A., Tetrude J., et al. Lack of olfactory dysfunction in MPTP-induced parkinsonism. (submitted b).

Doty R.L., Stern M.B., Pfeiffer C., et al. Bilateral olfactory dysfunction in early stage medicated and unmedicated idiopathic Parkinson's disease. *J. Neurol. Neurosurg. Psychiatry* (in press c).

Drake B., Johansson, B., von Sydow E., et al. Quantitative psychophysical and electrophysiological data on some odorous compounds. *Scand. J. Psychol.* 10:89–96, 1969.

Esiri M.M., Wilcock P.K. The olfactory bulbs in Alzheimer's disease. *J. Neurol. Neurosurg. Psychiatry* 47:56–60, 1984.

Eskenazi B., Cain W.S., Novelly R.A., et al. Olfactory functioning in temporal lobectomy patients. *Neuropsychologia* 21:365–374, 1983.

Frank M. An analysis of hamster afferent taste nerve response functions. *J. Gen. Physiol.* 61:588–618, 1973.

Frye R.E., Schwartz B., Doty R.L. Dose-related effects of cigarette smoking on olfactory function. *J.A.M.A.* 263:1233–1236, 1990.

Furstenberg A.C., Crosby E., Farrior B. Neurologic lesions which influence the sense of smell. *Arch. Otol.* 48:529–530, 1943.

Ghorbanian S.N., Paradise J.L., Doty R.L. Odor perception in children in relation to nasal obstruction. *Pediatrics* 72:510–516, 1983.

Gloor P., Olivier A., Quesney L.F., et al. The role of the limbic system in experiential phenomena of temporal lobe epilepsy. *Ann. Neurol.* 12:129–144, 1982.

Gowers W.R. The Hughlings-Jackson lecture on special sense discharges from organic disease. *Brain* 32:303–326, 1909.

Graziadei P.P.C. The ultrastructure of vertebrate olfactory mucosa. In Friedmann I., ed. *The Ultrastructure of Sensory Organs.* Oxford, Elsevier, pp. 267–305, 1973.

Haberly L.B., Price J.L. The axonal projection patterns of the mitral and tufted cells of the olfactory bulb in the rat. *Brain Res.* 129:152–157, 1977.

Hausser-Hauw C., Bancaud J. Gustatory hallucinations in epileptic seizures. Electrophysiological, clinical and anatomical correlates. *Brain* 110:339–359, 1987.

*Hinds J.W., Hinds P.L., McNelly N.A. An autoradiographic study of the mouse olfactory epithelium: evidence for long-lived receptors. *Anat. Rec.* 210:375–383, 1984.

Holmes G. Local epilepsy. *Lancet* 1:957–962, 1927.

Howe J.C., Gibson J.D. Uncinate seizures and tumors, a myth reexamined. *Ann. Neurol.* 12:227, 1982.

Hyman B.T., Van Hoesen G.W., Damasio A.R., et al. Alzheimer's disease: cell-specific pathology isolates the hippocampal formation. *Science* 225:1168–1170, 1984.

Jackson J.H. (1869) A study of convulsions. In Taylor J., ed. *Selected Writings of John Hughlings Jackson.* London, Hodder and Stoughton, pp. 8–36, 1931.

Jackson J.H. (1880) On right or left-sides spasm at the onset of epileptic paroxysms, and on crude sensation warnings, and elaborate mental states. In Taylor J., ed. *Selected Writings of John Hughlings Jackson.* London, Hodder and Stoughton, pp. 308–317, 1936.

Jones D.T., Reed R.R. G$_{OLF}$: an olfactory neuron specific–G protein involved in odorant signal transduction. *Science* 244:790–795, 1989.

Kaufman M.D., Lassiter R.R.L., Shenoy B.V. Paroxysmal unilateral dysosmia: a cured patient. *Ann. Neurol.* 24:450–451, 1988.

Krettek J.E., Price J.L. Projections from the amygdaloid complex and adjacent olfactory structures to the entorhinal cortex and to the subiculum in the rat and cat. *J. Comp. Neurol.* 172:723–752, 1977a.

Krettek J.E., Price J.L. The cortical projections of the mediodorsal nucleus and adjacent thalamic nuclei in the rat. *J. Comp. Neurol.* 171:157–191, 1977b.

Krettek J.E., Price J.L. Amygdaloid projections to subcortical structures within the basal forebrain and brainstem in the rat and cat. *J. Comp. Neurol.* 178:225–254, 1978.

Kurihara K. Taste modifiers. In Beidler L.M., ed. *Handbook of Sensory Physiology.* Vol. IV. *Chemical Senses.* Part 2. *Taste.* New York, Springer-Verlag, pp. 362–378, 1971.

*Lancet D. Vertebrate olfactory reception. *Annu. Rev. Neurosci.* 9:329–355, 1986.

Leopold D.A. The relationship between nasal anatomy and human olfaction. *Laryngoscope* 98:1232–1238, 1988.

Leopold D.A., Youngentaub S.L., Schwob J.E., et al. Successful treatment of phantosmia with preservation of olfaction (abstract 185). Twelfth Annual Meeting of the Association for Chemoreception Sciences, Sarasota, FL, April 18–22, 1990.

Lorig T.S. Human EEG and odor response. *Prog. Neurobiol.* 33:387–398, 1989.

Lovell M.A., Jafek B.W., Moran D.T., et al. Biopsy of human olfactory mucosa: an instrument and a technique. *Arch. Otolaryngol.* 108:247–249, 1982.

*MacLeod P. Structure and function of higher olfactory centers. In Beidler L., ed. *Handbook of Sensory Physiology.* Vol. IV. *Olfaction.* New York, Springer-Verlag, pp. 182–204, 1971.

*Mair R.B., Gesteland R.C. Process in olfactory reception. In Breuer M.M., ed. *Cosmetic Science.* New York, Academic Press, pp. 83–123, 1980.

Mair R.B., McEntee W.J., Doty R.L. Olfactory perception in Korsakoff's psychosis: correlation with brain noradrenergic activity. *Neurology* 33(Suppl. 2):64–65, 1983.

Maruniak J.A., Silver W.L. Moulton D.G. Olfactory receptors respond to bloodborne odorants. *Brain Res.* 265:312–316, 1983.

Menevse A., Dodd G., Poydner T.M. Evidence for the specific involvement of cyclic AMP in the olfactory transduction mechanism. *Biochem. Biophys. Res. Commun.* 77:671–677, 1977.

Moberg P.J., Pearlson G.D., Speedie L.J., et al. Olfactory recognition: differential impairments in early and late Huntington's and Alzheimer's disease. *J. Clin. Exp. Neuropsychol.* 9:650–664, 1987.

Moran D.T., Rowley J.C., Jafek, B.W. Electron microscopy of human olfactory epithelium reveals a new cell type: the microvillar cell. *Brain Res.* 253:39–46, 1982a.

*Moran D.T., Rowley J.C., Jafek B.W., et al. The fine structure of the olfactory mucosa in man. *J. Neurocytol.* 11:721–746, 1982b.

Murray R.G. The ultrastructure of taste buds. In Friedman I., ed. *The Ultrastructure of Sensory Organs.* New York, Elsevier North Holland Biomedical Press, pp. 1–81, 1973.

Nakashima T., Kimmelman C.P., Snow J.B. Jr. Effect of olfactory nerve section and hemorrhage on the olfactory neuroepithelium. *Surg. Form* 35:562–564, 1984a.

Nakashima T., Kimmelman C.P., Snow J.B. Jr. Structure of human fetal and adult olfactory neuroepithelium. *Arch. Otolaryngol.* 110:641–646, 1984b.

*Norgren R. Central neural mechanisms of taste. In Darien-Smith I., ed. *Handbook of Physiology.* Secion 1. *The Nervous System.* Vol. 3. *Sensory Processes.* Bethesda, American Physiological Society, 1984.

Osterhammel P., Terkildsen K., Zilstorff K. Electro-olfactograms in man. *J. Laryngol. Otol.* 83:731–733, 1969.

Pace U., Hanski E., Salmon Y. et al. Odorant-sensitive adenylate cyclase may mediate olfactory reception. *Nature* 316:255–258, 1985.

Peabody C.A., Tinklenberg J.R., Olfactory deficits and primary degenerative dementia. *Am. J. Psychiatry* 142:524–525, 1985.

Penfield W.G., Kristiansen K. Epileptic seizure patterns. Springfield, IL, Thomas, 1951.

Penfield W., Faulk M.E. The insula: further observations on its function. *Brain* 78:445–470, 1955.

Plattig K.-H., Kobal G. Spatial and temporal distribution of olfactory evoked potentials and techniques involved in their measurement. In Lehmann D., Callaway E., eds. *Human Evoked Potentials.* New York, Plenum Publishing, 1979.

Powell T.P.S., Cowan W.M., Raisman G. The central olfactory connexions. *J. Anat.* 99:791–813, 1965.

Report of the Panel on Communicative Disorders to the National Advisory Neurological and Communicative Disorders and Stroke Council. June 1, 1979. Washington, DC, U.S. Public Health Service, NIH Publication No. 81–1914, 1979.

Reyes P.F., Golden G.T., Fagel P.L., et al. The prepiriform cortex in dementia of the Alzheimer type. *Arch. Neurol.* 44:644–645, 1987.

Rhein L.D., Cagan R.H. Role of cilia in olfactory recognition. In Cagan R.H., Kare M.R., eds. *Biochemistry of Taste and Olfaction.* New York, Academic Press, pp. 47–68, 1981.

Rowley J.C. III, Moran D.T., Jafek B.W. Peroxidase backfills suggest the mammalian epithelium contains a second morphologically distinct class of bipolar sensory neuron: the microvillar cell. *Brain Res.* 502:387–400, 1989.

*Schiffman S.S. Taste and smell in disease. *N. Engl. J. Med.* 308:1275–1279, 1337–1343, 1983.

*Schwartz B., Doty R.L., Frye R.E., et al. Olfactory function in chemical workers exposed to acrylate and methacrylate vapors. *Am. J. Public Health* 79:613–618, 1989.

Settle R.G., Quinn M.R., Brand J.G., et al. Gustatory evaluation of cancer patients: preliminary results. In van Eys J., Nichols B.L., Seeling M.S., eds. *Nutrition and Cancer.* New York, Spectrum Publications, 1979.

*Shepherd G.M. Synaptic organization of the mammalian olfactory bulb. *Physiol. Rev.* 52:864–917, 1972.

Shepherd G.M. *Neurobiology.* New York, Oxford University Press, 1983.

Sicard G., Holley A. Receptor cell responses to odorants: similarity and differences among odorants. *Brain Res.* 292:283–296, 1984.

Silver W.L., Moulton D.G. Chemosensitivity of rat nasal trigeminal receptors. *Physiol. Behav.* 28:927–931, 1982.

Smith D.B., Allison T., Goff W.R., et al. Human odorant evoked responses: effect of trigeminal or olfactory deficit. *Electroencephalogr. Clin. Neurophysiol.* 30:313–317, 1971.

Smith D.V., van Buskirk R.L., Travers J.B., et al. Coding of taste stimuli by hamster brain stem neurons. *J. Neurophysiol.* 50:541–558, 1983.

*Sumner D. Disturbance of the senses of smell and taste after head injuries. In Vinken P.J., Bruyn G.W., eds. *Handbook of Clinical Neurology. Injuries of the Brain and Skull.* Part II. New York, American Elsevier, pp. 1–25, 1976.

Walz W., Hertz L. Functional interactions between neurons and astrocytes. II. Potassium homeostasis at the cellular level. *Prog. Neurobiol.* 20:133–183, 1983.

Ward C.D., Hess W.A., Calne D.B. Olfactory impairment in Parkinson's disease. *Neurology (N.Y.)* 33:943–946, 1983.

Weiffenbach J.M. Taste and smell perception in aging. *Gerontology* 3:137–146, 1984.

Weiffenbach J.M., Baum B.J., Burghauser R. Taste thresholds: quality specific variations with human aging. *J. Gerontol.* 32:372–377, 1982.

Weiser H.G., Hailemariam S., Regard M., et al. Unilateral limbic epileptic status activity: stereo EEG, behavioral and cognitive data. *Epilepsia* 26:19–29, 1985.

Yamagishi M., Nakamura H., Takahashi S., et al. Olfactory receptor cells: immunocytochemistry for nervous system–specific proteins and re-evaluation of their precursor cells. *Arch. Histol. Cytol.* 52(Suppl.):375–381, 1989.

28

Pathophysiology of Vision

Christopher Kennard
K.H. Ruddock

Human visual function can be investigated non-invasively by psychophysical methods, which require observer participation, and by objective methods, which usually involve the recording of electrical potentials with surface electrodes. This chapter reviews briefly the structural and functional organization of the mammalian visual system and describes psychophysical and objective techniques applicable to the examination of abnormal human vision. Finally, the pathophysiology of a number of different classes of abnormal vision is discussed.

THE PRIMATE VISUAL PATHWAYS: GROSS OVERALL STRUCTURE

The eye forms an optical image of the visual field on the retina, which projects topographically to the lateral geniculate nucleus (LGN) and thence to the striate cortex (Brodmann area 17; visual area V1) in the occipital lobe, and also to the superficial layers of the superior colliculus (Fig. 28–1). The striate cortex projects in turn to multiple areas in the pre-striate cortex (Brodmann areas 18 and 19), each carrying a map of the visual field, and the superior colliculus projects to the cortex via the pulvinar. The collicular and striate projections converge onto the inferior parietal lobe (Brodmann area 7). Noteworthy features of retinal projections to the brain are

1. The separate projections of the two visual half-fields, on each side of the vertical meridian, to the contralateral hemisphere
2. Fibers from the two eyes that do not converge until after the first synapse in the striate cortex
3. The large magnification of the cortical representation of the macular visual area relative to the periphery
4. The central area in which the fields of view of the two eyes overlap, thereby providing stereoscopic function

The two hemispheric projections are connected by fibers that course via the corpus callosum and synapse at the boundary region (the representation of the field around the vertical meridian) between the various field maps. Severance of the callosal fibers causes degeneration at the boundaries between the different visual areas, designated V1 to V6 (Zeki, 1970, 1978). Other retinal projections include those to the pretectal region and the accessory optic tract (Pasik and Pasik, 1971).

Ablation studies suggest that the retinal projection to the striate cortex mediates fine discrimination of stimulus variables such as spatial form (i.e., defining what is seen), whereas the projection to the colliculus controls eye movements made in response to light stimulation (i.e., defining where it is located). Damage to the striate cortex in humans usually results in permanent blindness for stimuli presented in corresponding field areas, but recovery of visual function after ablation of the striate cortex occurs in nonhuman primates that receive postoperative training (Cowey, 1967; Pasik and Pasik, 1971; Weiskrantz, 1972). Ablation of localized regions in either the superior colliculus or the striate cortex of the macaque causes temporary disturbances of function consistent with malfunction in "where" and "what" channels, respectively, but subsequent recovery occurs. Ablation of corresponding regions of both projection areas, however, leads to permanent blindness for light stimuli located within the corresponding visual field area (Mohler and Wurtz, 1977).

FUNCTIONAL ORGANIZATION OF MAMMALIAN VISION

Retinal Processing

Early stages of visual processing, including phototransduction, have been studied mainly in lower vertebrates, and such studies provide important ev-

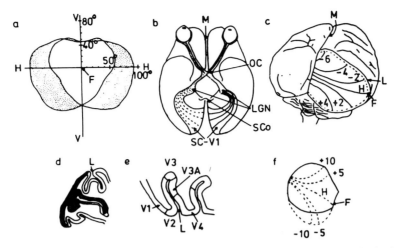

Figure 28–1. *(a)* The visual fields for the two eyes, plotted relative to the fixation point F. H denotes the horizontal meridian, and V, the vertical meridian. The clear area denotes the region of binocular overlap of the two visual fields. *(b)* The primate visual pathways from below. OC = optic chiasma; LGN = lateral geniculate nucleus; SC-V1 = striate visual cortex, or visual area V1; SCo = superior colliculus; M = midline. *(c)* View of the macaque brain from the rear lower right, showing the mapping onto the cortex of the visual field. The line H denotes the mapping of the horizontal meridian with the fovea mapped at F. Other lines denote the mapping of lines drawn in the left half-field, parallel to and at angles (e.g., 2°) above (+) or below (−) the horizontal meridian. L = lunate sulcus; M = midline. *(d)* Cross-section cut parallel to the midline through the macaque striate cortex showing the lunate sulcus (L) and visual area V1 *(shaded)*. Note the inner region of V1, which corresponds to the mapping of the peripheral field onto the calcarine fissure. *(e)* Cross-section cut perpendicularly to the midline through area V1, showing also the prestriate areas (e.g., V2). L = lunate sulcus. *(f)* Mapping of the visual field onto the surface of the superior colliculus. H denotes the locus of the horizontal meridian, and other loci are the mappings of lines drawn parallel to, but (e.g., 5°) above (+) and below (−) the horizontal meridian. (*c* modified from LeVay S., Hubel D.H., Wiesel T.N. The pattern of ocular dominance columns in macaque visual cortex revealed by a reduced silver stain. *J. Comp. Neurol.* 159:559–576, 1975. *e* modified from Zeki S. Interhemispheric connections of pre-striate cortex of monkey. *Brain Res.* 19:63–75, 1970. *f* modified from Cynader M., Berman M. Receptive field organisation of monkey superior colliculus. *J. Neurophysiol.* 35:187–201, 1972.)

idence regarding the origin of the electroretinogram (e.g., Rodieck, 1973). The receptive field of a visual neuron is defined as the retinal area within which presentation of a light stimulus changes the electrophysiologic activity of the cell, and neurons at different levels of the visual pathways exhibit central and surrounding regions that generate mutually antagonistic responses. Consequently, these neurons re-

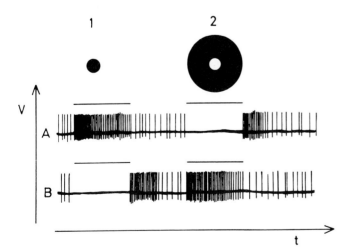

Figure 28–2. Schematic response patterns for retinal ganglion cells, with voltage (V) displayed against time (t). (A) On-center ganglion cell, showing responses to (1) a spot of light centered on the recording electrode and (2) a surround annulus. (B) Off-center ganglion cell, again showing responses to (1) a central spot and (2) surround annulus.

spond strongly to local changes in stimulus contrast, but weakly to change in overall illumination, as is illustrated for retinal ganglion cells (Fig. 28–2).

Rod photoreceptors mediate scotopic responses under low ambient lighting, whereas at higher (photopic) illuminations, cone photoreceptors provide high spatial resolution and color vision. There is considerable species variation in the relative numbers of rods and cones, and this is reflected in the electrophysiologic responses recorded from retinal neurons. Ganglion cell responses in cat and monkey are classified into three principal classes, X, Y, and W, corresponding to the β, α, and γ plus δ morphologic groups, respectively (Stone, 1983).

X and Y ganglion cells have circularly symmetric, antagonistic receptive fields (consisting of center and surround), and a light spot presented at the receptive field center elicits a response at *stimulus on* in about half the cells and at *stimulus off* in the remainder (see Fig. 28–2). These two groups therefore respond to light spots of opposite contrast polarity. *X-type cell* responses are characterized as follows:

1. Receptive field centers are small (i.e., they have a high-frequency spatial response).
2. Responses tend to be sustained during light stimulation (i.e., they have low-pass temporal frequency response).
3. Responses are frequently wavelength selective.
4. There is linear interaction between signals arising

in the center and the surrounding region of the receptive field.

5. They have a slow conduction velocity along fine fibers.

In contrast, for *Y-type cells*

1. Receptive field centers are large, giving low-frequency spatial responses.
2. Responses tend to exhibit strong transients at stimulus on or stimulus off (i.e., they have band-pass temporal frequency response).
3. They respond equally to all stimulus wavelengths (luminance response).
4. They exhibit nonlinear interaction between the receptive field center and surrounding area.
5. They have a fast conduction velocity along thicker fibers.

In the macaque, the group of ganglion cells identified anatomically as Pβ, which yields X-type responses, projects to the parvocellular (numbered III–VI) layers of the LGN, whereas a second group, Pα, with Y-type responses, projects to the magnocellular (numbered I and II) layers of the LGN (Perry et al., 1984). A heterogeneous group of cells, designated Pγ and Pε, corresponding to the W-type response group, projects to the superior colliculus, which also receives input from Y-type Pα ganglion cells (Marrocco, 1978; Perry and Cowey, 1984). Separate projection streams from parvocellular and magnocellular layers of the LGN can be traced through the striate and prestriate cortical areas (Zeki and Shipp, 1988). There is also evidence of a sparse direct projection from the LGN to the prestriate cortical areas (Benevento and Yoshida, 1981; Fries, 1981).

Cortical Processing

In cortical area V1, many neurons are binocularly driven and possess elongated receptive fields, responding to bar- or edge-shaped stimuli oriented within some 20° of a preferred direction. There are two principal functional classes of *orientation-selective neuron,* called simple and complex (Hubel and Wiesel, 1962, 1968), and their responses are illustrated in Figure 28–3. In addition, there are specialized regions of the striate cortex that possess monocularly driven neurons with nonoriented receptive fields, the responses of which are frequently wavelength selective (Gouras, 1974; Livingstone and Hubel, 1984).

Area V1 is organized into columns of cells with the same eye dominance and independently into columns showing sequential changes in orientation selectivity. Neurons in each of the visual areas V1 to V6 tend to be selectively responsive to a particular stimulus variable. Many neurons in V1 respond specifically to spatial pattern, whereas 60% in V2 are sensitive to retinal disparity of images in the two eyes, as required for stereoscopic depth discrimination (Hubel and Wiesel, 1970). Some 90% of neurons

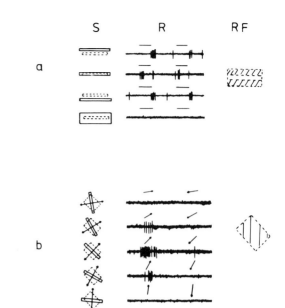

Figure 28–3. Responses of striate cortical neurons. The left column (S) denotes the stimulus *(solid lines)* marked in relation to the receptive field *(dashed lines)*; the middle column (R) denotes the response trace plotted as voltage against time, with arrows above the trace denoting direction of movement; and the right column (RF) denotes the (enlarged) receptive field of the cell, with hatched areas corresponding to areas antagonistic to the clear areas. *(a)* Simple cell; note that responses are selective for the width of the stimulus bar. The stationary stimulus is presented during the time interval indicated by the horizontal bars in R. *(b)* Complex cell; note that responses are selective for the orientation and direction of movement of the stimulus bar. (Modified from Hubel D.H., Wiesel T.N. Receptive fields and functional architecture of monkey striate cortex. *J. Physiol. [Lond.]* 195:215–243, 1968.)

in area V3 are sensitive to stimulus orientation, whereas about 60% of those in V4 are sensitive to stimuli of a given color appearance as opposed to spectral composition, and their large receptive fields, combined with the complex retinotopic mapping of V4, may mediate constant color appearance under changes in illumination (Zeki, 1980). In areas V5 and V6, neurons are predominantly sensitive to movement in a specific direction (Zeki, 1978). Neurons in the superficial layers of the *superior colliculus* are selectively sensitive to flashed or moving light stimuli, have large receptive fields with no orientation selectivity, and receive both rod- and cone-mediated inputs (Goldberg and Wurtz, 1972; Marrocco and Li, 1977).

Light-sensitive neurons of the *posterior parietal cortex* fire in response to visually evoked saccades, and their firing is facilitated by attentive fixation. They respond to fast-moving targets and have large receptive fields, sometimes extending into the contralateral half-field (Mountcastle, 1981). Neurons that respond to highly specific visual stimuli such as faces have been observed in the superior temporal sulcus of the macaque (Perrett et al., 1982). The organization of the multiple interconnections between the different visual cortical areas was reviewed by Zeki and Shipp (1988).

The separate retinal projection to V1 and to the superior colliculus, the subdivision of these projections into parallel channels (e.g., the X, Y, and W optic nerve fibers), and the multiple cortical field maps, each responding selectively to a given stimulus variable, are all significant for the interpretation of abnormal visual function (see under Objective Methods of Studying Human Vision).

PSYCHOPHYSICAL METHODS FOR THE EXAMINATION OF HUMAN VISUAL FUNCTION

Threshold illumination (I_t) for detection of a target (e.g., a circular spot of light as used in plotting visual fields) provides the simplest measure of visual function. I_t depends on many factors, including target size and duration, retinal adaptation, the background field illumination, and stimulus wavelength (Fig. 28–4). *Spectral sensitivities* recorded at the fovea and in the extrafoveal dark-adapted retina reveal photopic, V_λ (cone-mediated) and scotopic, V'_λ (rod-mediated) functions, respectively, corresponding to the retinal distributions of the two photoreceptor classes. Pre-

retinal light losses increase with observer age (Ruddock, 1972), and the ages of defective and control groups should be carefully matched. Color vision is mediated by three classes of cone, with peak absorptions at 420, 535, and 565 nm, and can be investigated by color-matching and by two-color increment threshold methods (Stiles, 1978; Wright, 1946). These methods yield responses closely related to the cone absorption spectra, and special methods are required for the investigation of postreceptor chromatic mechanisms.

Spatial and temporal responses are frequently represented by sensitivity functions for threshold detection of periodic stimuli (Fig. 28–5). These response functions depend on the mean retinal illumination, extending to high frequencies as average illumination increases. The temporal modulation response curves (see Fig. 28–5*b*) change from low pass to band pass as retinal illumination increases, and the overall shape of these functions is markedly dependent on the configuration of the visual field used in their measurement (Kelly, 1972). *The spatial contrast sensitivity* function comprises two components, the low-pass response of the ocular media, and a band-pass response arising in the neural channels, and the latter is modified by disorders of the neural path-

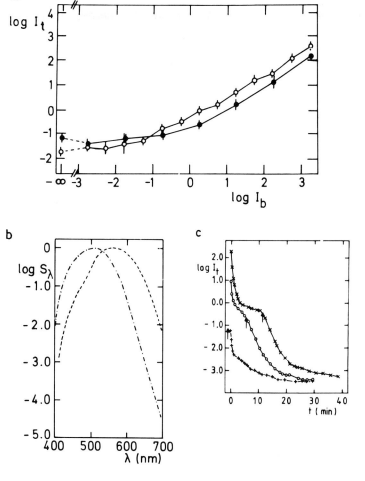

Figure 28–4. Illumination level (I_t) for detection of a test flash, illustrating the effects of changing a number of different variables. *(a)* I_t plotted against background illumination (I_b) (both expressed in log trolands). The circular target (diameter 1°) was superimposed centrally on the circular background field (diameter 7°) and flashed for 0.5 second every second. Data for two subjects. *(b)* Relative spectral sensitivity (S_λ) defined as E_λ^{-1}, where E_λ is the energy flux required for detection of a monochromatic test flash, plotted against the test wavelength (λ). V_λ (– – –) is the standard photopic (cone) response, and V'_λ (–·–·–), the standard scotopic (rod) response function. *(c)* I_t (log trolands) plotted against time (t) after 2-min adaptation to light illumination: 5.25 log trolands (×), 4.15 log trolands (o), and 2.17 log trolands (+). The violet test flash appeared colorless at times longer than those marked by the arrow on each plot and were then detected by rod vision.

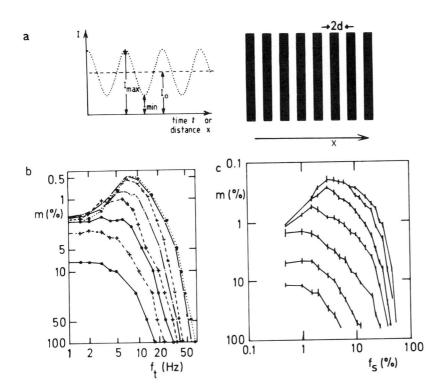

Figure 28–5. Temporal and spatial modulation sensitivity functions for the normal human eye. *(a)* Definition of modulation (m) equal to $(I_{max} - I_{min})/2I_o$ for a sinusoid stimulus of average illumination I_o; illumination (I) is plotted against time (t) or distance (x). The spatial frequency (f_s) of a sinusoidal grating (drawn schematically as a square wave grating) is defined as $(2d)^{-1}$. *(b)* Temporal response functions, with percentage of modulation for detection of a sinusoidally flickering target plotted against the flicker frequency (f_t). Each curve refers to a different mean illumination level, the values being, in order of increasing cut-off frequency at m = 100%, 0.375, 1, 3.75, 10, 37.5, 100, 1000, and 10,000 trolands. *(c)* Spatial response functions, with percentage of modulation (or contrast) for threshold detection of a one-dimensional grating plotted against the grating spatial frequency (f_s). Each curve refers to a different mean illumination level, increasing in steps of × 10 from 0.0009 to 900 trolands as the cut-off frequency increases. (*b* modified from de Lange, H. Research into the dynamic nature of the human fovea cortex systems. *J. Opt. Soc. Am.* 48:777–789, 1958. *c* modified from van Nes, F.L., Bouman M.A. Spatial modulation function in the human eye. *J. Opt. Soc. Am.* 57:401–406, 1967.)

ways. These transfer functions represent threshold response characteristics for the whole visual system. The speed of transmission of signals along the visual pathways increases as the illumination level rises, which corresponds to the increase in temporal frequency response (see earlier). This provides an explanation for the Pulfrich (1922) phenomenon, which occurs when a neutral density filter is placed over one eye. In this case, a pendulum swinging in a plane perpendicular to the line of sight appears to move in an elliptic path toward and away from the observer; placing the filter over the left eye gives clockwise rotation, and over the right eye, anticlockwise rotation. The effect occurs because the difference between transmission times of signals from the two eyes is equivalent to a disparity in the retinal locations on the two retinas, and this is interpreted as a change in stereoscopic depth. Under voluntary fixation, the eyes are subject to small, rapid involuntary eye movements, and if these are compensated artificially (visual stabilization), visual sensations fade rapidly, within a few seconds (Ditchburn, 1973).

Psychophysical methods have been developed for measurement of responses arising in *single response channels*. I_t for detection of a circular target moving across a modulated background field is dependent on the modulation frequency, and measurements with a variety of background configurations reveal response functions describing two visual channels. Each is characterized by a spatial and temporal response function and both spatial responses are circularly symmetric (Fig. 28–6).

Of these two spatiotemporal (ST) channels, that designated ST1 has smaller spatial dimensions and low-pass (i.e., sustained) temporal response, whereas

that designated ST2 has a larger receptive field and band-pass (i.e., transient) temporal response. The ST1 and ST2 channels correspond to X and Y electrophysiologic mechanisms, respectively (Ruddock, 1983). An analysis of spatial contrast sensitivity functions, recorded with both steady and flickering lights, led Wilson and Bergen (1979) to postulate the existence of four response channels, two sustained and two transient, with the two former corresponding closely in spatial properties to the ST1 channel. A second method relies on selective adaptation induced by spatially periodic patterns (gratings), which raises threshold for detection of a target with spatial characteristics similar to those of the adaptation pattern (Fig. 28–6b and c). Threshold increases significantly only when the adaptation and target gratings are oriented within 20° of each other, and when their spatial frequencies differ by a factor of less than 2 (Blakemore and Campbell, 1969). The tuning curve always peaks at the test grating frequency; thus, there are multiple channels tuned to different spatial frequencies or bar widths. Adaptation effects occur when the gratings are presented to different eyes, indicating that they arise in binocularly controlled mechanisms. The dark and light bars of the target can be adapted independently, which implies separate processing of positive and negative contrast. The properties of these orientation-selective channels correlate closely with those of orientation-sensitive electrophysiologic units in area V1.

Stereoscopic vision requires fusion of disparate images on the two retinas. Fine stereoscopic depth discrimination is measured with pairs of vertically oriented bars, and global fusion of stereoscopic images is examined with random dot stereograms (Ju-

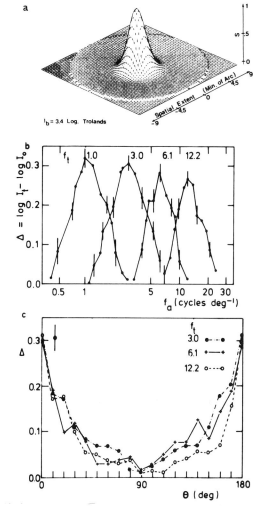

tors, processing is said to be serial (Fig. 28–7b and c). Considerable attention has been paid to the detection of different stimulus features, such as orientation and color, when they are presented in conjunction (Treisman, 1988) and to the parametric limits at which parallel processing is no longer possible (Alkhateeb et al., 1990; Javadnia and Ruddock, 1988). The method has been applied in the examination of visual dysfunctions involving higher visual centers, such as visual agnosia and developmental dyslexia.

OBJECTIVE METHODS OF STUDYING HUMAN VISION

Three measurements involving surface electrodes have proved of value. The *electro-oculogram*, measured by placing an electrode on either side of the eye, determines dipole potential changes that occur as a consequence of voluntary eye movements. The *electroretinogram*, which is recorded between a corneal electrode and a reference electrode placed on the forehead, has been valuable in the detection of retinal diseases (Ikeda, 1982). *Visual evoked potentials* are measured between a recording electrode placed near the inion and a reference electrode placed on the forehead. They are of particular value in determining delays in signal transmission to the occipital lobe and in establishing cortical responses to pattern stimuli (Regan, 1985). They have also been used to demonstrate that the abnormal pattern of decussation that occurs in optic nerve fibers of nonhuman albinos is present in human albinos (Apkarian et al., 1983; Creel et al., 1974). Measurement of the pupillary reflex to light has also provided important information about the effects of central lesions on activity in the visual pathways (Alexandridis, 1985). (See Chapter 123.)

Figure 28–6. *(a)* Spatial distribution of sensitivity (S) for the spatiotemporal channel 1 response mechanism, which is circularly symmetric. *(b)* The difference (Δ) between log threshold illumination (log I_o) for detection of a test grating after 2-min adaptation to a uniform field and that (log I_t) after 2-min adaptation to a grating of spatial frequency (f_s) plotted against f_s. Values are given for four test gratings, the spatial frequencies of which are given with the data (e.g., 6.1 cycles/degree). *(c)* Δ (as defined in b) plotted against the relative orientation angle (θ) between the test and adaptation gratings. The test and adaptation gratings were matched in spatial frequency, and data are given for three frequencies. (Modified with permission from *Vision Res.*, vol. 13, Maudarbocus A.Y., Ruddock K.H., Non-linearity of visual signals in relation to shape-sensitive adaptation responses, Copyright 1973, Pergamon Press.)

ACQUIRED AND CONGENITAL DISTURBANCES OF THE VISUAL PATHWAYS

The neurologic causes of visual disturbance produce their effects through damage to nerve fibers or neurons, which may be diffuse (as in certain genetically determined disorders such as Friedreich's ataxia) or focal (as in tumors). Damage to the visual pathways results in a variety of structural and functional abnormalities of nerve fibers, the particular combination found being determined by the nature of the disease process.

Degeneration (resulting from ganglion cell loss or interruption of axons by severe compression, trauma, or infarction), of course, abolishes transmission. The resulting visual loss is persistent, although it can to

lesz, 1971), the fusion of which produces a separation in depth of pattern and background from the unstructured images presented to each eye.

Visual search involves the ability to detect visually a target element embedded in a number of identical distractor elements, from which it is distinguished by a parametric difference such as relative orientation (Fig. 28–7a), which can be measured in terms of the response time for target detection. Two response modes are usually distinguished. Parallel processing is said to occur when the response time is independent of the number of distractors, whereas when response time increases with the number of distrac-

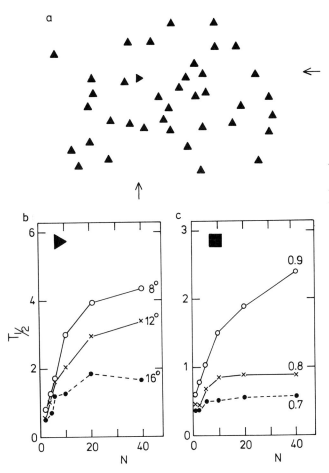

Figure 28–7. *(a)* A typical field used for visual search measurements. The target, indicated by the arrows, is distinguished from the 40 identical distractor elements by its relative orientation. *(b)* The time taken for 50% probability of detecting a target ($T_{1/2}$) is plotted against the number of distractor elements (N). A distractor element is illustrated at the top left of each plot, and the target was rotated, relative to the distractors, through the angle denoted to the left of each data set. Note that the $T_{1/2}$ values depend strongly on the orientation of the distractors. *(c)* As *b*, but the target is changed in magnification relative to the distractor elements. The side length of the target, expressed relative to the distractor value of 1.0, is given with each set of data. Note that for larger parametric differences between the target and the distractors, $T_{1/2}$ is independent of N (parallel processing), whereas for smaller differences, $T_{1/2}$ is proportional to N (serial processing).

some extent be compensated when the fiber loss is incomplete (McDonald, 1982). *Demyelination* (which occurs focally in multiple sclerosis or at the site of compression by tumor [Clifford-Jones et al., 1985]) is associated with a variety of morphologic abnormalities ranging from partial- or full-thickness demyelination confined to the paranodal region of individual internodes to full-thickness loss over many consecutive internodes. In keeping with this range of morphologic abnormalities, there are, as in the peripheral nervous system (see Chapter 18), a variety of abnormalities of conduction, including complete block, partial block with slowed conduction and impairment of the ability to transmit trains of impulses at physiologic frequencies, thermolability of conduction, spontaneous activity, and enhanced mechanosensitivity (McDonald and Sears, 1970; Smith and McDonald, 1980).

The symptoms of lesions of the visual pathways depend ultimately on the conduction defects. Although some symptoms, such as the color distortions of optic neuritis, cannot yet be accounted for with certainty by the known pathophysiology of central axons, others can. For example, the thermolability of conduction in partially demyelinated fibers provides a sufficient explanation for exercise-induced deterio-

ration of vision in multiple sclerosis (*Uhthoff's phenomenon*): increases of temperature of as little as 0.5°C in the physiologic range may convert partial to complete conduction block in experimentally demyelinated peripheral nerve fibers, and a reversible decline in amplitude of the visual evoked potential has been demonstrated during exercise in patients experiencing Uhthoff's phenomenon (Persson and Sachs, 1981). The Pulfrich effect is seen in optic neuritis (Rushton, 1975) and may account for the difficulty that some patients experience in negotiating traffic because of their inability to judge the changing position of moving vehicles.

Phosphenes (i.e., spots or flashes of light perceived in the absence of luminous stimuli) can originate in many different sites along the visual pathways and can be accounted for by abnormal discharges. They can also be produced by electrical stimulation of the striate and prestriate cortical areas (Brindley and Lewin, 1968; Foerster, 1929). At the retinal level, mechanical pressure on the eye can produce phosphenes sufficiently intense to be seen in a brightly lit room, and in the elderly, they may occur during eye movements, particularly in myopes. They occur in optic neuritis, especially during eye movement (Davis et al., 1976), probably on the basis of the hyperexcitability of demyelinated nerve fibers; the same properties can account for the phosphenes experienced with tumors involving the visual pathways (McDonald, 1982). Ischemia of nerve cells and fibers results in spontaneous discharge, which can account for the phosphenes seen with ischemia of the occipital cortex in migraine, embolism, and infarction.

When conduction is blocked by demyelination or abolished by degeneration in bundles of nerve fibers, characteristic defects in the *visual fields* are produced, the form of which depends on the localization of the causative lesion in the visual pathways (Fig. 28–8). Interesting phenomena may occur in patients with such field defects; for example, subjects with bitemporal hemianopia as a consequence of pituitary adenomas report overlapping or separation of the surviving nasal half-fields, an effect referred to as the hemifield slide phenomenon (Kirkham, 1972).

Lesions in the occipital lobe result in the development of a homonymous hemianopia, which is rapid when it is due to infarction but slow when due to tumors. During such slow development, the field defect spreads inward from the periphery and color is affected before disturbances either for form or for black-and-white objects. The homonymous hemianopia or quadrantanopia so resulting may or may not spare the macula field (central 2–3°). This sparing, found usually in posterior cerebral artery occlusion, is due to two factors. First, the occipital pole containing the macular field representation has a rich anastomotic network between terminal branches of the middle cerebral artery and the posterior cerebral artery, resulting in sparing of a portion of the blood supply. Second, it has been shown experimentally (Bunt and Minckler, 1977; Stone et al., 1973) that there is a vertically oriented median strip centered on the fovea in which retinal ganglion cells project either ipsilaterally or contralaterally. It has been shown that ipsilaterally projecting cells in and around

the fovea can generate 2–3° of bilateral representation in the geniculocortical pathways, because they are intermingled with contralaterally projecting cells on the nasal side of the foveal pit (Fukuda et al., 1989; Leventhal et al., 1988). Bilateral occipital lobe anoxia or infarction results in cortical blindness, which may be accompanied by the patient's emphatic denial of blindness in the face of gross evidence to the contrary (Anton's syndrome). Recovery of function may occur to a variable extent. Usually, light discrimination returns first, then spatial perception, and finally color perception, although selective recovery of any of these functions can occur (Warrington, 1984).

The critical site of the visual disturbance has not been identified in congenital disorders such as amblyopia and albinism. *Amblyopia* is characterized by loss of spatial resolution not associated with any lesion of the visual pathways, which cannot be rectified by refractive correction. Abnormal vision during childhood that affects one eye, attributable either to squint (strabismus) or to a large refractive error in one eye (anisometropia), causes amblyopia in that eye. Stimulus deprivation of one eye during early development in cat or monkey leads to reduced innervation of area V1 by fibers projecting from the deprived eye, and consequently, fewer neurons in area V1 are driven by that eye (Wiesel, 1982). Human amblyopes tend to suppress the inappropriate images arising in their defective eye, which leads to effects similar to those observed in visually deprived animals. Precortical effects are also observed in cats with surgically induced strabismus. Thus, the receptive fields of X-type ganglion cells and LGN neurons are coarser in the strabismic than in the normal projection pathway, apparently because the normal refinement of these fields that occurs during development is arrested at the time of surgery (Ikeda, 1980). In contrast, Y-type cells in the strabismic pathway have essentially normal receptive fields.

Albinism, the failure to manufacture melanin be-

Figure 28–8. Patterns of visual field loss (indicated in black on right diagrams) resulting from lesions in visual pathways at sites labeled A to G. The A indicates optic nerve lesions result in a central scotoma *(left)* or arcuate defects *(right)*; B, optic nerve lesions just before the chiasm produce junctional scotoma owing to ipsilateral optic nerve involvement with the inferior contralateral crossing fibers *(dashed line)*; C, chiasm lesions produce a bitemporal hemianopia; D, optic tract lesions result in incongruous hemianopic defects; E and F, lesions of the optic radiation result in either homonymous quadrantinopia or hemianopia, depending on the extent and location of the lesion (upper quadrant, temporal lobe; lower quadrant, parietal lobe); G, lesions of the striate cortex produce a homonymous hemianopia, sometimes with macular sparing, particularly in the case of vascular disturbances.

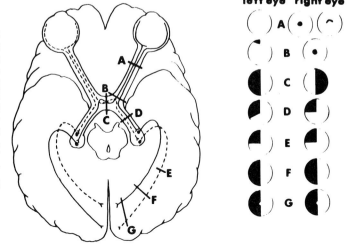

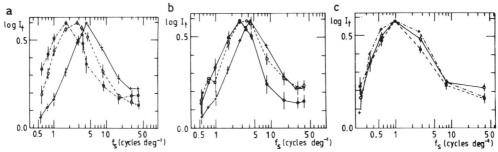

Figure 28–9. *(a)* Normalized spatial frequency response curves for the spatiotemporal channel 1 mechanism, measured for 6 normal subjects *(crosses)* and for the normal eyes *(open circles)* and defective eyes *(closed circles)* of 12 strabismic amblyopes. The shift to low spatial frequency of the amblyopic data denotes an increase in spatial size. Both the normal and defective eyes are affected, the latter more significantly. *(b)* As *a*, but for six normal subjects *(crosses)* and six refractive amblyopes (normal eyes, *open circles*; defective eyes, *closed circles*). *(c)* Normalized spatial frequency responses of the spatiotemporal channel 2 mechanism. Mean data for six normal subjects *(crosses)* and for the normal *(full circles)* and defective eyes *(open circles)* of nine amblyopes (seven strabismic and two refractive). Note that all three sets of data are similar.

cause of an inherited deficiency of tyrosinase, is associated with abnormal optic nerve projections, owing to an abnormally high proportion of fibers crossing at the chiasma (Guillery and Kaas, 1971). Consequently, albinos should experience diplopia, which they appear to overcome by a tendency to suppress the neural responses arising in one eye; thus, a situation equivalent to that of monocular deprivation pertains.

FUNCTIONAL ABNORMALITIES ASSOCIATED WITH NEUROLOGIC DISORDERS OF THE VISUAL PATHWAYS

Related groups of abnormal responses are discussed together, and their occurrence and expression among the different classes of visual disorder are described.

Incremental Threshold Illumination for Detection of a Light Flash

I_t is raised in retinal disorders such as retinitis pigmentosa, diabetic retinopathy, and senile macular degeneration (Greenstein et al., 1983). The increases for foveal detection are similar in each of these disorders, and the implied loss of light sensitivity is postreceptoral in origin. I_t is raised in the affected eyes of subjects with previous retrobulbar neuritis (Burde and Gallin, 1975) and is also subject to abnormally large scatter (Harms, 1976), which in subjects with multiple sclerosis is more pronounced at high overall illumination (Patterson et al., 1980). Threshold variability may explain the flickering on and off experienced by some patients with multiple sclerosis when targets are located in certain areas of the visual field (Ellenberger and Ziegler, 1980; Frisén and Hoyt, 1974). Patients with optic neuritis also exhibit fatigue effects during prolonged visual testing (Sunga and Enoch, 1970).

Recovery of Dark Adaptation After Bleaching

This may be prolonged by diseases affecting the photoreceptors, pigment epithelium, or adjacent choroid in subjects who manifest no significant loss of visual activity. Prolongation is caused by delayed regeneration of the photopigment and occurs in diseases such as senile macular degeneration, pigment epithelial detachment, central serous retinopathy, and diabetic retinopathy (Chilaris, 1962; Haegerstrom-Portnoy et al., 1983; Severin et al., 1967).

Spatial Vision

Amblyopes have reduction in both conventional and Vernier acuity measured with gratings (Freeman et al., 1972; Levi and Klein, 1982) and exhibit losses in contrast threshold sensitivity, which for some strabismic amblyopes occur at all spatial frequencies and for others are restricted to low frequencies (Hess and Howell, 1977). The ST1 spatial responses of amblyopic eyes are shifted to low frequencies relative to the normal response, whereas the ST2 responses are normal (Fig. 28–9). This correlates with the electrophysiologic evidence that in kittens X-type ganglion cells have enlarged receptive field centers after surgically induced strabismus, whereas Y-type ganglion cells are unaffected (Ikeda, 1980). The ST1 responses of normal eyes in amblyopes subject to extensive patching treatment are also displaced to low spatial frequencies. Both ST1 and ST2 spatial responses in an albino subject were displaced to low frequencies, but detection of beats between high-frequency gratings established that his low visual acuity arose postreceptorally (Barbur et al., 1980a). Abnormal spatial functions have also been reported by Wilson et al. (1988). Vernier acuity in the normal eye of subjects who had monocular deprivation in childhood sometimes exceeds that of normal vision, apparently because a greater cortical area can be innervated by the spared eye (Freeman and Bradley, 1980).

Changes in contrast threshold sensitivity functions are observed in many neurologic disorders (Arden, 1978) and may occur in the absence of acuity loss. In subjects with multiple sclerosis, contrast sensitivity losses occur for different ranges of spatial frequency in different subjects, sometimes without corresponding reduction in visual acuity, and may be indicative of selective impairment of specific spatial channels (Regan et al., 1977) (Fig. 28–10). Loss of contrast sensitivity in patients with multiple sclerosis is frequently restricted to specific grating orientation (Regan et al., 1980) and such effects appear to reflect changes in orientation-specific cortical mechanisms. High-frequency contrast sensitivity losses are found in diabetic retinopathy (Arundale, 1978; Sjöstrand and Frisén, 1977) and modified contrast thresholds were reported for subjects with blurred vision as a result of occipital and right parietal lesions (Bodis-Wollner and Diamond, 1976). Effects for the latter group, like those for patients with multiple sclerosis, occur at different spatial frequencies in different subjects and are not always accompanied by reduction in Snellen acuity.

Central lesions can give rise to a number of disturbances of visual function, which involve higher levels of pattern recognition. *Visual agnosia* is defined as the inability to recognize visually objects or their photographic representations, even though visual resolution is normal and other sensory discriminations are fully retained. In accordance with Lissauer's (1890) original description, two general categories of visual agnosia are usually distinguished, namely apperceptive and associative, which are differentiated by the inability in the former to copy objects or drawings. The condition is rare, with only 4 cases found in 415 patients with posterior cortical lesions (Hecaen and Angelergues, 1962) and 1 partial case in 114 patients with unilateral brain damage (De

Renzi et al., 1968). Although reservations have been expressed regarding the existence of visual agnosia, a number of well-documented cases have been described in the last 20 years or so. Apperceptive agnosia usually involves diffuse bilateral cortical damage, frequently resulting from inhalation of toxic fumes, whereas patients with associative agnosia display a variety of lesions. The condition can occur in combination with other visual disturbances, including those discussed here, and is sometimes associated with an inability to integrate local features, themselves recognized correctly, into a percept of an entire scene. The response characteristics of some 40 published cases have been summarized by Ruddock (1991), and the theoretic issues raised by the condition have been discussed by Hecaen and Albert (1978), Bauer and Rubens (1985), and Warrington (1984) (see also Chapter 54).

More specific disturbances of pattern recognition have also been identified. Bodamer (1947) introduced the term *prosopagnosia* to describe the inability to recognize faces or their representations. Although prosopagnosia can occur in isolation, it is also observed in conjunction with other functional deficits, such as achromotopsia and visual agnosia. An inability to distinguish between objects belonging to other object categories, such as buildings, animals, and vehicles, is often demonstrated by persons with prosopagnosia. It is suggested that prosopagnosia involves a disturbance of the ability to recognize the historical context of a given object, whereas the capacity to recognize the generic class of an object is preserved (Damasio et al., 1982). In visual agnosia, the latter is also lost. A detailed account of prosopagnosia is given in Chapter 54.

Inability to read when other visual functions are preserved is called *acquired dyslexia*, or *alexia*, and in its pure form, it does not involve inability to write. The underlying cause was first identified by Dejerine (1892) as a lesion of the dominant (left) hemisphere

Figure 28–10. Percentage contrast (C) required for threshold detection of grating, plotted against the spatial frequency (f_s) of the grating. Data show responses for the two eyes of strabismic subjects *(upper curves)*. The lower curves show the ratios (R) of the sensitivities for the two eyes, plotted against f_s, and the bar symbols on the abscissa show the standard deviations of the differences. *(a)* Data for a subject showing sensitivity with losses extending to low spatial frequencies. *(b)* Data for a subject with sensitivity losses for intermediate spatial frequencies. (Modified from Regan D., Silver R., Murray T.H. Visual acuity and contrast sensitivity in multiple sclerosis: hidden visual loss. *Brain* 100:563–579, 1977, by permission of Oxford University Press.)

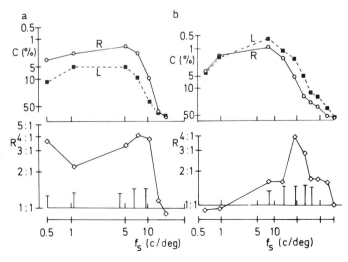

combined with damage to the splenium of the corpus callosum, which disrupts the pathways connecting the intact right visual cortex to the left angular gyrus. Consequently, there is no input to the speech center in the dominant hemisphere, and the hemispheric lesion usually gives rise to hemianopia of the contralateral half-field. In developmental dyslexia, difficulties in reading occur that are less severe than those observed in alexia but that also appear to involve abnormalities of the dominant hemisphere (Galaburda et al., 1985). Although a number of visual functional abnormalities have been described in association with developmental dyslexia, there is considerable dispute about their contribution to the reading difficulties.

There are a variety of abnormalities in the perception of position and orientation within the visual environment associated with central lesions. Such errors of visuospatial function can affect the visual localization of objects, the judgment about their relative size and distance from the patient, and the ability to touch objects (Holmes, 1918b); and they can be restricted to a single hemisphere, thereby demonstrating topographic mapping of the functions (Cole et al., 1962; Riddoch, 1935). The critical lesions for this defect occur in the region of the occipitoparietal parietal boundary (Holmes and Horrax, 1919; Ross Russell and Bharucha, 1978). Disruption of stereoscopic vision may also occur, in addition to these other abnormalities (Holmes and Horrax, 1919; Riddoch, 1917).

Some patients with central lesions exhibit loss of topographic functions, such as finding their way around a familiar environment, learning new routes, and identifying place locations on a map. Such disorders frequently occur in combination with other disorders, such as visual agnosia and prosopagnosia, and they have been identified as class-specific agnosias, akin to prosopagnosia (Landis et al., 1986).

Stereoscopic visual function is sensitive to imbalance in responses of the two eyes during development; thus both amblyopes and albinos experience loss of both fine stereoscopic depth discrimination and global stereoscopy. There is also reduction in interocular transfer of various visual adaptation effects, which are normally so transferred in normal vision, and the degree of binocular transfer is related to the stereoacuity (Mitchell and Ware, 1974).

Subjects with a split optic chiasm have bitemporal hemianopias (see Fig. 28–8) and are blind to stimuli located beyond the fixation point, which are imaged onto the nasal retina. Nonetheless, such subjects possess normal stereoscopic depth discrimination for objects located in front of the fixation point (Blakemore, 1970). Split brain subjects, with the callosal fibers severed, have no stereoscopic depth discrimination along the visual axis, and thus callosal fibers appear to contribute to stereoscopic function and presumably mediate that function in cases of split chiasm (Mitchell and Blakemore, 1970). Loss of stereoscopic function, particularly of global stereoscopy, is one of the most frequently observed visual defects

and can be restricted to targets located behind the fixation point or to those located in front of it (Jones, 1977; Richards, 1970).

Temporal Responses

Responses of amblyopic subjects to flicker and target movement are normal (Grounds et al., 1983; Hess et al., 1978; Miles, 1949; but see Wood and Kulikowski, 1978). In contrast, subjects with multiple sclerosis exhibit reduced critical flicker fusion (Titcome and Willison, 1961), reduced resolution between double flashes (Galvin et al., 1976), and increased latency in the affected eye, as established psychophysically (Heron et al., 1974), by evoked potentials (Halliday et al., 1972), and by the resulting Pulfrich effect (Rushton, 1975). Temporal modulation functions measured for subjects with retrobulbar neuritis, retinopathy, or cranial trauma were depressed to an extent that depended on stimulus conditions and on the development of the condition (Meyer et al., 1983) (Fig. 28–11).

Grossly disturbed detection of target movement was discovered in a subject with bilateral damage involving the lateral temporal occipital cortex (Zihl et

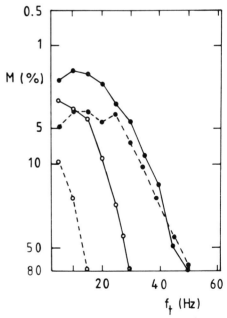

Figure 28–11. de Lange temporal response functions (see Fig. 28–8) for subjects with visual defects, with percentage modulation (M) for threshold detection of a flickering target plotted against the flicker frequency (f_t). The target was circular, of diameter 1° and mean luminance 200 candelas/m². Data for the right eye *(open circles, solid line)* and left eye *(open circles, dashed line)* of a subject with retrobulbar neuritis and for a subject with retinal toxicity from ethambutol, before toxicity *(filled circles, solid line)* and in the third month *(filled circles, dashed line)* at a level of 15 mg/kg. (Modified from Meyer J.J., Reyu P., Bousquet A., et al. An automatic intermittent light stimulator to record flicker perceptive thresholds in patients with retinal disease. In Breinin G.M., Siegel I.M., eds. *Advances in Diagnostic Visual Optics.* Berlin, Springer-Verlag, pp. 173–179, 1983.)

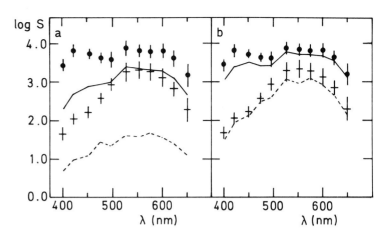

Figure 28–12. Spectral sensitivity (S), defined as in Figure 28–4*b*, for detection of a monochromatic test plotted against the flash wavelength. The circular test flash (diameter, 1°) was presented on a white background (1000 trolands; color temperature, 3200 K). The test was presented either as a 0.5-second flash or as a 25-Hz flickering target. Solid lines mean data for 0.5-second flash for 30 eyes affected by retrobulbar neuritis *(a)*, and for 26 eyes contralateral to the affected eyes *(b)*. Dashed lines mean data for 25-Hz flashing target for 30 eyes affected by retrobulbar neuritis *(a)*, and for 26 eyes contralateral to the affected eyes *(b)*. The error bars refer to 30 normal eyes recorded for 0.5-Hz flashes *(open circles)* and 25-Hz flicker *(crosses)*. (Modified from Alvarez S.L., King-Smith P.E. Dichotomy of psychophysical responses in retrobulbar neuritis. *Ophthalmic Physiol. Opt.* 4:101–105, 1984.)

al., 1983). This selective loss of function involved failure to perceive (1) movement in depth, (2) target movement at velocities above 10°, (3) the movement after effect, and (4) φ motion, although movement of acoustic and tactile stimuli was detected normally. Lesions of the parieto-occipital boundary region cause neglect of sensory stimuli located contralaterally to the lesion (Bender, 1946) and in extreme cases, visual stimuli fade completely within 1 second under voluntary fixation. In one subject, targets moving at more than 8°/second were detected normally, whereas detection of slower-moving targets was impaired (Holliday et al., 1985).

Acquired Color Vision Defects

These differ from congenital defects in the high incidence of discrimination losses involving blue and blue-green stimuli, in the unstable nature of the defects, and in the fact that they are restricted to one eye, although rare unilateral congenital defects occur (B.G. Bender et al., 1972; Judd, 1948). Acquired defects are usually classified, according to performance on screening tests designed for the detection of congenital defects, as yellow-blue or red-green according to the color confusions experienced. Kollner (1912) attributed blue-yellow defects to diseases of the ocular media and retina and red-green defects to diseases of the optic nerve, but there are many exceptions to this rule. Francois and Verriest (1968) tabulated results for 1179 eyes, involving 92 separate diseases. They identified four classes of color vision deficiency:

1. General loss of hue discrimination
2. Type I red-green deficiency, in which the photopic V_λ function deviates toward the scotopic V'_λ function
3. Type II red-green deficiency, in which the photopic V_λ function is normal
4. Blue-yellow deficiency

Class 2 defects predominate in macular dystrophy; class 3, in retrobulbar neuritis; and class 4, in glau-

coma and diabetic retinopathy. Methods have been developed for the study of postreceptoral mechanisms involved in acquired color vision deficiencies. For example, King-Smith and Carden (1976) determined spectral sensitivity functions for targets flashed at 1 and 25 Hz, the former testing X-type chromatic channels and the latter Y-type flicker-sensitive channels. Such measurements demonstrate that, for some subjects with retrobulbar neuritis, impaired responses are restricted to the chromatic mechanisms, whereas for others, there are additional losses affecting the flicker-sensitive mechanisms (Alvarez and King-Smith, 1984) (Fig. 28–12).

Achromatopsia

Achromatopsia, the complete absence of hue discrimination, occurs in subjects with lesions of the occipitotemporal and/or lingual gyrus (Meadows, 1974b). Positron emission tomographic studies have confirmed that the lingual and/or fusiform gyrus is the homologue of the macaque V4 (Lueck et al., 1989). Achromatopsia is restricted to the contralateral hemifield in unilateral lesions (Albert et al., 1975; M.B. Bender and Kanzer, 1939). Color discrimination losses in subjects recovering from cortical blindness occur independently of losses in spatial acuity, shape discrimination, and spatial localization (Warrington, 1984). Abnormal visual function in colored, particularly red, lights has been described for a subject who has normal vision for black-and-white stimuli (Hendricks et al., 1981). Threshold sensitivity, visual acuity, and critical flicker fusion are dramatically reduced in red light and visual responses are suppressed for up to 12° away from a red target (Fig. 28–13). This subject can identify stereoimages in two-color random dot stereograms (Julesz, 1971), even though the red component pattern is completely unresolved, thus establishing dissociation of color vision and stereoscopy. No structural correlate of this defect has been found.

Residual Visual Function

Localized damage to the human striate cortex causes a permanent scotoma in the corresponding

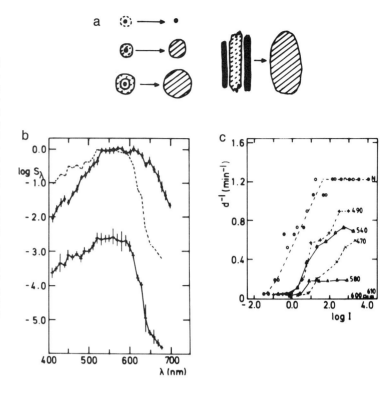

Figure 28–13. Data for subject M.W. with abnormal inhibitory responses to colored stimuli. *(a)* Targets consisting of black and red areas, the latter denoted by the regions covered by broken lines *(left)* and their appearance as drawn by M.W. *(right)*. In his drawings, the hatched areas appeared steely gray and the black areas appeared as drawn. Note the spread of the steely-gray area beyond the area of the red stimulus, and the associated suppression of the black areas. *(b)* Relative spectral sensitivity (S_λ) for detection of a monochromatic circular target (diameter, 1°) presented for 0.5 second every 1 second, plotted against target wavelength. Crosses: data for M.W. ($\pm$ 1 SE); circles: data for a normal subject. The dashed curved line represents M.W.'s data displaced upward for comparison. *(c)* Resolution at the threshold for detection of a grating expressed as d^{-1}, where d is the width in minutes of the grating bars, plotted against the average illumination of the grating (100% modulated). N = data for normal subject, recorded for wavelengths 610 nm *(filled circles)* and 540 nm *(open circles)*. Other data for subject M.W., recorded for different wavelengths as denoted, in nanometers. Note M.W.'s low resolution for gratings of wavelengths 610 and 600 nm.

visual field area (Holmes, 1918a; Teuber et al., 1960), and complete blindness in two subjects with extensive cortical damage was described by Brindley et al. (1969). Riddoch (1917), however, reported that some subjects detect flashed or moving targets located within scotomata associated with cortical damage. Pöppel et al. (1973) and Perenin and Jeannerod (1978) found that hemianopic subjects can locate, by either eye movements or hand pointing, targets presented within the blind hemifield, and Weiskrantz et al. (1974) showed that, in forced choice experiments, a hemianope discriminated orientation and spatial structure of patterns presented to his blind hemifield. As the light stimuli elicited no conscious sensations, these responses were termed *blindsight* (Weiskrantz, 1980). A capacity for color discrimination has also been observed in some patients (Stoerig, 1987).

Blindsight, or residual vision, frequently involves the detection and localization of transient (flashed or moving) lights presented to the blind hemifield, without discrimination of stimulus variables such as size, shape, and color (Barbur et al., 1980b; Blythe et al., 1987) (Fig. 28–14). Cooperative interactions between normal and blind regions of the visual field have been demonstrated in a number of responses, including φ motion (Blythe et al., 1986) and reaction times in the detection of a light flash (Marzi et al., 1984), and in the tilt of the perceived vertical meridian after adaptation to a rotating pattern (Pizzamiglio et al., 1984). The incidence of residual visual capacities in patients with lesions has been variously estimated as 20% (Blythe et al., 1987) to 100% (Pizzamiglio et al., 1984). The pupillary reflex can be recorded for light stimulation of the blind hemifield and under

certain conditions is similar to the normal response (Barbur and Forsyth, 1986).

Residual vision that occurs within areas of the visual field classified as blind by normal parametric methods is usually attributed to activity in the retinocollicular projection pathway. The feature of such visual function common to all patients, namely, the capacity to detect and locate transient stimuli, is consistent with activity in a "where" rather than "what" projection pathway. It has been argued that such residual vision is caused by light scattered into the normal hemifield (Campion et al., 1983), but many response features, including cooperative interactions between normal and blind regions of the visual field, are inconsistent with this explanation. Zihl and von Cramon (1985) found that training improved blindsight performance and increased the blindfield area within which blindsight can be achieved.

Other Disturbances of Visual Perception

Polyopia, the perception of multiple images, is associated with mainly right-sided occipital lesions and can be experienced with either eye. The relationship between the secondary image and the true image may be either constant or changing, and the multiple images may or may not overlap. M.B. Bender (1945) described four cases and attributed the phenomenon to impaired fixation, but Meadows (1973) showed that shifts in fixation were inadequate to describe the effect. The false image or images usually occur in visual field regions where perceived image brightness is raised and, in some cases, may

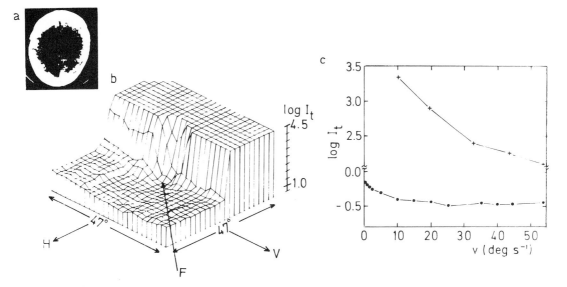

Figure 28–14. Data for a hemianope with traumatic damage to the left hemisphere. *(a)* Computed tomographic scan, showing that the left striate cortex is damaged. *(b)* Threshold illumination (I_t) recorded over the central 47° square of the retina, for the detection of a circular target (1.2° diameter) presented statically to the subject. H and V denote the vertical and horizontal meridians, respectively, and F, the fovea. Note the sudden increase in I_t to the right of the vertical meridian, with sparing around the fovea; the plateau to the right denotes the maximal light level available at which the target was still undetected. *(c)* I_t for detection of a circular target (diameter, 5.7°) located 30° off axis, plotted against target velocity (v), which was directed along the horizontal meridian. + = data for hemianope's blind hemifield; · = data for a normal subject.

be related to epileptic activity (M.B. Bender and Sobin, 1963). Polyopia is observed rarely during electrical stimulation of the visual cortex (Brindley and Lewin, 1968). An even rarer phenomenon is that of episodic *inverted vision*, usually associated with lesions in the parieto-occipital region, vestibulocerebellar system, or frontal lobes (Solms et al., 1988).

The term *palinopsia* is applied both to the abnormal prolongation of visual images after offset of a light stimulus and to the paroxysmal or episodic reappearance of images in the absence of immediate and appropriate light stimuli. The two types of palinopsia have different characteristics, the former occurring systematically, with the duration of the afterimage increasing with increase in the illumination level or duration of the stimulus (Kinsbourne and Warrington, 1963) (Fig. 28–15), whereas the latter is unpredictable in occurrence and independent of the brightness of the original stimulus (M.B. Bender, 1963; M.B. Bender et al., 1968; Critchley, 1951). Episodic palinopsia is usually observed during the evolution or resolution of a homonymous field defect, predominantly arising from lesions in the right posterior cerebral hemisphere. These images appear not to be associated with sensory seizures or psychogenic elaboration and are probably a type of release hallucination (M.B. Bender et al., 1968; Cummings et al., 1982). The possibility of drug-induced palinopsis was reported in relation to *trazodone* (Hughes and Lessell, 1990).

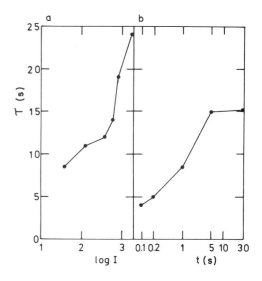

Figure 28–15. The time (τ) for which the afterimage of a white light stimulus raises threshold for detection of a white light test flash in a subject with palinopsia. For subjects with normal vision, detection of the target recovers within 0.1 second of the offset of the stimulus. Thresholds are plotted in *a* as a function of the illumination level of the eliciting stimulus (in log trolands), the stimulus being viewed for 5 seconds, and *b* as a function of the duration of the eliciting stimulus, which was of illumination 2.8 log trolands. The stimulus that elicited the afterimage was circular, of diameter 30°, and the target was also circular, of diameter 3.8°. (Modified from Blythe I.M., Bromley J.M., Ruddock K.H., et al. A study of systematic visual perseveration involving central mechanisms. *Brain* 109:661–675, 1986, by permission of Oxford University Press.)

In *visual illusory spread*, there is visual perseveration in the spatial domain. There is an extension of the visual perception over an area greater than that excited by the object presented to the observer (Critchley, 1951).

Visual hallucinations occur under many circumstances such as drug withdrawal, anoxia, and schizophrenia, in addition to those related to focal neurologic disease. Lesions in the occipital or temporal lobes may give rise to simple (e.g., light glares and lines [Lance, 1976]) or complex (Kolmel, 1985) hallucinations. Although occasionally such hallucinations may be due to epileptic discharges (Penfield and Perot, 1963), another mechanism may be a release phenomenon in which visual cortical areas are deprived of normal visual impulses, resulting in release of cortical activity that normal visual inputs keep suppressed (Cogan, 1973; Lepore, 1990).

References

(Key references are designated with an asterisk.)

Albert M.L., Reches A., Silverberg R. Hemianopic colour blindness. *J. Neurol. Neurosurg. Psychiatry* 38:546–549, 1975.

Alexandridis E. *The Pupil*. Berlin, Springer-Verlag, 1985.

Alkhateeb W.F., Morris R.J., Ruddock K.H. Effect of stimulus complexity on simple spatial discriminations. *Spatial Vis.* 5:129–141, 1990.

Alvarez S.L., King-Smith P.E. Dichotomy of psychophysical responses in retrobulbar neuritis. *Ophthalmic Physiol. Opt.* 4:101–105, 1984.

Apkarian P., Reits D., Spekreijse H., et al. A decisive electrophysiological test for human albinism. *Electroencephalogr. Clin. Neurophysiol.* 55:513–531, 1983.

Arden G.B. The importance of measuring contrast sensitivity in cases of visual disturbance. *Br. J. Ophthalmol.* 62:198–209, 1978.

Arundale K. Investigation into the variation of human contrast sensitivity with age and ocular pathology. *Br. J. Ophthalmol.* 68:213–215, 1978.

Barbur J.L., Forsyth P.M. Can the pupil be used as a measure of the visual input associated with the geniculo-striate pathway? *Clin. Vision Sci.* 1:107–111, 1986.

Barbur J.L., Holliday I.E., Ruddock K.H., et al. Spatial characteristics of movement detection mechanisms in human vision. III. Subjects with abnormal visual pathways. *Biol. Cybernet.* 37:99–105, 1980a.

Barbur J.L., Ruddock K.H., Waterfield V.A. Human visual responses in the absence of the geniculo-calcarine projection. *Brain* 103:905–928, 1980b.

Barbur J.L., Forsyth P.M., Findlay J.M. Human saccadic eye movements in the absence of geniculocalcarine projection. *Brain* 111:63–82, 1988.

Bauer R.M., Rubens A.B. Agnosia. In Heilman K.M., Valenstein, E., eds. *Clinical Neuropsychology*. Oxford, Oxford University Press, pp. 187–241, 1985.

Bender B.G., Ruddock K.H., de Vries de Mol E.C., et al. The colour vision characteristics of an observer with unilateral defective colour vision: results and analysis. *Vision Res.* 12:2036–2057, 1972.

Bender M.B. Polyopia and monocular diplopia of cerebral origin. *Arch. Neurol. Psychiatry* 54:323–338, 1945.

*Bender M.B. Changes in sensory adaptation time and after sensation with lesions of parietal lobe. *Arch. Neurol. Psychiatry* 55:299–319, 1946.

Bender M.B. Disorders in visual perception. In Halpern L., ed. *Problems of Dynamics in Neurobiology*. Jerusalem, Port Press, pp. 319–375, 1963.

Bender M.B., Kanzer M. Dynamics of homonymous hemianopias and preservation of central vision. *Brain* 62:404–421, 1939.

Bender M.B., Sobin A.J. Polyopia and palinopsia in homonymous half-fields of vision. *Trans. Am. Neurol. Assoc.* 88:56–62, 1963.

Bender M.B., Feldman M., Sobin A.J. Palinopsia. *Brain* 91:321–338, 1968.

Benevento L.A., Yoshida K. The afferent and efferent organization of the lateral geniculo-prestriate pathways in macaque monkey. *J. Comp. Neurol.* 203:455–474, 1981.

Blakemore C.B. Binocular depth perception and the optic chiasm. *Vision Res.* 10:43–47, 1970.

Blakemore C., Campbell F.W. On the existence of neurons in the human visual system sensitive to the orientation and size of retinal images. *J. Physiol. (Lond.)* 203:237–260, 1969.

Blythe I.M., Bromley J.M., Kennard C., et al. Visual discrimination of target displacement remains after damage to the striate cortex in humans. *Nature* 320:619–621, 1986.

Blythe I.M., Kennard C., Ruddock K.H. Residual vision in patients with retrogeniculate lesions of the visual pathways. *Brain* 11:887–905, 1987.

Bodamer J. Die Prosop-Agnosie. *Arch. Psychiatr. Nervenkr.* 179:6–54, 1947.

Bodis-Wollner I., Diamond S.P. The measurement of spatial contrast sensitivity in cases of blurred vision associated with cerebral lesions. *Brain* 99:693–710, 1976.

Brindley G.S., Lewin W.S. The sensations produced by electrical stimulation of the visual cortex. *J. Physiol. (Lond.)* 196:479–493, 1968.

Brindley G.S., Gautier-Smith P.C., Lewin W. Cortical blindness and the functions of the non-geniculate fibres of the optic tracts. *J. Neurol. Neurosurg. Psychiatry* 32:259–264, 1969.

Bunt A.H., Minckler D.S. Foveal sparing. *Arch. Ophthalmol.* 95:1445–1447, 1977.

Burde R.M., Gallin P.F. Visual parameters associated with recovered retrobulbar optic neuritis. *Am. J. Ophthalmol.* 79:1034–1037, 1975.

Campion J., Latto R., Smith Y.M. Is blindsight an effect of scattered light, spared cortex and near-threshold vision? *Behav. Brain Sci.* 6:423–486, 1983.

Chilaris G.A. Recovery time after macular illumination as a diagnostic and prognostic test. *Am. J. Ophthalmol.* 53:311–314, 1962.

Cleland P.G., Saunders M., Rosser R. An unusual case of visual perseveration. *J. Neurol. Neurosurg. Psychiatry* 44:262–263, 1981.

Clifford-Jones R.E., MacDonald W.E., Landon D.N. Chronic optic nerve compression: an experimental study. *Brain* 108:241–262, 1985.

Cogan D.G. Visual hallucinations as release phenomena. *Albrecht von Graefes Arch. Klin. Exp. Ophthalmol.* 188:139–150, 1973.

Cole M., Schutta H.S., Warrington E.K. Visual disorientation in homonymous half-fields. *Neurology (Minneap.)* 12:257–263, 1962.

Cowey A. Perimetric study of field defects in monkeys after cortical and retinal ablation. *Q. J. Exp. Psychol.* 19:232–235, 1967.

Creel D., Witkop C.J. Jr., King R.A. Asymmetric visually evoked potentials in human albinos: evidence for visual system anomalies. *Invest. Ophthalmol.* 13:430–440, 1974.

Critchley M. Types of visual perseveration. Palinopsia and illusory visual spread. *Brain* 74:267–299, 1951.

Cummings M.D., Syndulko K., Goldberg Z., et al. Palinopsia reconsidered. *Neurology (N.Y.)* 32:444–447, 1982.

Cynader M., Berman M. Receptive field organisation of monkey superior colliculus. *J. Neurophysiol.* 35:187–201, 1972.

Damasio A.R., Damasio H., van Hoesen G.W. Prosopagnosia: anatomic basis and behavioral mechanisms. *Neurology (N.Y.)* 32:331–341, 1982.

Davis F.A., Bergen D., Schauf C. Movement phosphenes in optic neuritis: a new clinical sign. *Neurology (Minneap.)* 26:1100–1104, 1976.

Dejerine J. Contribution à l'étude anatomopathologique et clinique des différentes variétés de cécité verbale. *Mem. Soc. Biol.* 4:61–90, 1892.

de Lange H. Research into the dynamic nature of the human fovea cortex systems. *J. Opt. Soc. Am.* 48:777–789, 1958.

De Renzi E., Faglioni P., Spinnler H. The performance of patients with unilateral brain damage on face recognition tasks. *Cortex* 4:17–34, 1968.

Ditchburn R.W. *Eye Movement and Visual Perception*. Oxford, Clarendon Press, 1973.

Ellenberger C., Ziegler T. The Swiss cheese visual field of time varying abnormalities of vision after "recovery" from optic neuritis. In Smith J.L., ed. *Neuro-ophthalmology Focus 1980.* New York, Masson, pp. 175–179, 1980.

*Foerster O. Beiträge zur Pathophysiologie der Sehbahn und der Sehsphäre *J. Psychol. Neurol. Lpz.* 39:463–485, 1929.

François J., Verriest G. Nouvelles observations de déficiences acquises de la discrimination chromatique. *Ann. Oculist.* 201:1097–1114, 1968.

Freeman R.D., Bradley A. Monocularly deprived humans: non deprived eye has super normal Vernier acuity. *J. Neurophysiol.* 43:1645–1653, 1980.

Freeman R.D., Mitchell D.E., Millodot M. A neural effect of partial deprivation in humans. *Science* 175:1384–1386, 1972.

Fries W. The projection from the lateral geniculate nucleus to the prestriate cortex of the macaque monkey. *Proc. R. Soc. Lond. [Biol.]* 213:73–80, 1981.

Frisén L., Hoyt W.F. Insidious atrophy of retinal nerve fibres in multiple sclerosis. *Arch. Ophthalmol.* 70:403–422, 1974.

Fukuda Y., Sawai H., Watanabe M., et al. Nasotemporal overlap of crossed and uncrossed retinal ganglion cell projections in the Japanese monkey (*Macaca fuscata*). *J. Neurosci.* 9:2352–2373, 1989.

Galaburda A.M., Sherman G.F., Rosen G.D., et al. Developmental dyslexia: four consecutive patients with cortical anomalies. *Ann. Neurol.* 18:222–223, 1985.

Galvin R.J., Regan D., Heron J.R. Impaired temporal resolution of vision after acute retrobulbar neuritis. *Brain* 99:255–268, 1976.

Goldberg M.E., Wurtz R. Activity of the superior colliculus in behaving monkeys. 1. Visual receptive fields of single neurons. *J. Neurophysiol.* 35:542–559, 1972.

Gouras P. Opponent-colour cells in different layers of foveal striate cortex. *J. Physiol. (Lond.)* 238:583–602, 1974.

Greenstein V.C., Hood D.C., Siegel I.M., et al. A psychophysical technique for testing explanations of sensitivity loss due to retinal disease. In Breinin G.M., Siegel I.M., eds. *Advances in Diagnostic Visual Optics.* Berlin, Springer-Verlag, pp. 218–224, 1983.

Grounds A.R., Holliday I.E., Ruddock K.H. Two spatiotemporal filters in human vision. 2. Selective modification in amblyopia, albinism and hemianopia. *Biol. Cybern.* 47:191–201, 1983.

Guillery R.W., Kaas J.H. A study of normal and congenitally abnormal retino-geniculate projections in cat. *J. Comp. Neurol.* 143:73–79, 1971.

Haegerstrom-Portnoy G., Adams A.J., Brown B., et al. Dynamics of visual adaptation are altered in vascular disease. In Breinin G.M., Siegel I.M., eds. *Advances in Diagnostic Visual Optics.* Berlin, Springer-Verlag, pp. 225–231, 1983.

Halliday A.M., McDonald W.I., Mushin J. Delayed visual evoked response in optic neuritis. *Lancet* 1:982–985, 1972.

Harms H. Role of perimetry in assessment of optic nerve dysfunction. *Trans. Ophthalmol. Soc. U. K.* 96:363–367, 1976.

Hecaen H., Albert M.L. Disorders of visual perception. In Hecaen H., Albert M.L., eds. *Human Neuropsychology.* New York, Wiley, pp. 176–247, 1978.

Hecaen H., Angelergues R. Agnosia for faces (prosopagnosia). *Arch. Neurol. Psychiatry* 7:92–100, 1962.

Hendricks I.M., Holliday I.E., Ruddock K.H. A new class of visual defect, spreading inhibition elicited by chromatic light stimuli. *Brain* 104:813–840, 1981.

Heron J.R., Regan D., Milner B.A. Delay in visual perception in unilateral optic atrophy after retrobulbar neuritis. *Brain* 97:69–78, 1974.

Hess R.F., Howell E.R. The threshold contrast sensitivity function in strabismic amblyopia: evidence for a two type classification. *Vision Res.* 17:1049–1055, 1977.

Hess R.F., Howell E.R., Kitchin J.E. On the relationship between pattern and movement perception in strabismic amblyopia. *Vision Res.* 18:375–377, 1978.

Holliday I.E., Kennard C., Ruddock K.H. Rapid fading of visual sensations in a subject with a parietal-occipital tumour. *Ophthalmic Physiol. Opt.* 5:149–156, 1985.

Holmes G. Disturbances of vision by cerebral lesions. *Br. J. Ophthalmol.* 2:353–384, 1918a.

Holmes G. Disturbances of visual orientation. *Br. J. Ophthalmol.* 2:449–468, 1918b.

Holmes G., Horrax G. Disturbances of spatial orientation and visual attention with loss of stereoscopic vision. *Arch. Neurol. Psychiatry* 1:385–407, 1919.

Hubel D.H., Wiesel T.N. Receptive fields, binocular interaction and functional architecture in the cat's visual cortex. *J. Physiol. (Lond.)* 160:106–154, 1962.

*Hubel D.H., Wiesel T.N. Receptive fields and functional architecture of monkey striate cortex. *J. Physiol. (Lond.)* 195:215–243, 1968.

Hubel D.H., Wiesel T.N. Cells sensitive to binocular depth in area 18 of the macaque monkey cortex. *Nature* 225:41–43, 1970.

Hughes M.S., Lessell S. Trazodone-induced palinopsia. *Arch. Ophthalmol.* 108:398–400, 1990.

Ikeda H. Visual acuity—its development and amblyopia. *J. R. Soc. Med.* 73:546–555, 1980.

Ikeda H. Clinical electroretinography. In Halliday M., ed. *Evoked Potentials in Clinical Testing.* London, Churchill Livingstone, pp. 569–594, 1982.

Javadnia A., Ruddock K.H. The limits of parallel processing in the visual discrimination of orientation and magnification. *Spatial Vis.* 3:97–114, 1988.

Jones R. Defects of stereo vision. *J. Physiol. (Lond.)* 264:621–640, 1977.

Judd D.B. Colour perceptions of deuterenopic and protanopic observers. *J. Res. Natl. Bur. Stand.* 41:247–271, 1948.

Julesz B. *Foundations of Cyclopean Perception.* Chicago, University of Chicago Press, 1971.

Kelly D.H. Flicker. In Jameson D., Hurvich L.M., eds. *Handbook of Sensory Physiology.* Vol. II/4. *Visual Psychophysics.* Berlin, Springer-Verlag, pp. 273–302, 1972.

King-Smith P.E., Carden D. Luminance and opponent colour contributions to visual detection and adaptation and to temporal and spatial integration. *J. Opt. Soc. Am.* 66:709–717, 1976.

Kinsbourne M., Warrington E.K. A study of visual perseveration. *J. Neurol. Neurosurg. Psychiatry* 26:468–475, 1963.

Kirkham T.H. The ocular symptomology of pituitary tumours. *Proc. R. Soc. Med.* 65:517–518, 1972.

Kollner H. *Die Störungen des Farbensinnes, ihre klinische Bedeutung und ihre Diagnose.* Berlin, Karger, 1912.

Kolmel H.W. Complex visual hallucinations in the hemianopic field. *J. Neurol. Neurosurg. Psychiatry* 48:29–38, 1985.

Lance J.W. Simple formed hallucinations confined to an area of a specific visual field. *Brain* 99:719–734, 1976.

Landis T., Cummings J.R., Benson D.F., et al. Loss of topographic familiarity in environmental agnosia. *Arch. Neurol.* 43:132–136, 1986.

Lepore F.E. Spontaneous visual phenomena with visual loss. *Neurology* 40:444–447, 1990.

LeVay S., Hubel D.H., Wiesel T.N. The pattern of ocular dominance columns in macaque visual cortex revealed by a reduced silver stain. *J. Comp. Neurol.* 159:559–576, 1975.

Leventhal A.G., Ault S.J., Vitek D.J. The nasotemporal division in private retina: the neural bases of macular sparing and splitting. *Science* 240:66–67, 1988.

Levi D.M., Klein S. Hyperacuity and amblyopia. *Nature* 298:268–270, 1982.

Lissauer H. Ein Fall von Seelenblindheit nebst einen Beitrag zur Theorie derselben. *Arch. J. Psychiatry* 21:222–270, 1890.

Livingstone M.S., Hubel D.H. Anatomy and physiology of a colour system in the primate visual cortex. *J. Neurosci.* 4:309–356, 1984.

Lueck C.J., Zeki S., Friston K.J., et al. The colour centre in man. *Nature* 349:386–389, 1989.

Marrocco R.T. Conduction velocities of afferent input to superior colliculus in normal and decorticate monkey. *Brain Res.* 140:155–158, 1978.

Marrocco R.T., Li R.H. Monkey superior colliculus: properties of single cells and their afferent inputs. *J. Neurophysiol.* 40:844–860, 1977.

Marzi C.A., Tassinari G., Aglioti S., et al. Spatial summation across the vertical meridian in hemianopics: a test of blind sight. *Neuropsychologia* 24:749–758, 1984.

Maudarbocus A.Y., Ruddock K.H. Non-linearity of visual signals in relation to shape-sensitive adaptation responses. *Vision Res.* 13:1713–1737, 1973.

McDonald W.I. The symptomatology of tumours of the anterior visual pathways. *J. Can. Neurol. Sci.* 1:381–390, 1982.

McDonald W.I., Sears T.A. The effects of experimental demyelination on conduction in the central nervous system. *Brain* 93:583–598, 1970.

Meadows J.C. A case of monocular polyopia. *J. Neurol. Sci.* 18:249–253, 1973.

Meadows J.C. The anatomical basis of prosopagnosia. *J. Neurol. Neurosurg. Psychiatry* 37:489–501, 1974a.

Meadows J.C. Disturbed perception of colours associated with localised cerebral lesions. *Brain* 97:615–632, 1974b.

Meyer J.J., Reyu P., Bousquet A., et al. An automatic intermittent light stimulator to record flicker perceptive thresholds in patients with retinal disease. In Breinin G.M., Siegel I.M., eds. *Advances in Diagnostic Visual Optics.* Berlin, Springer-Verlag, pp. 173–179, 1983.

Miles P.W. Flicker fusion frequency in amblyopia ex anopsia. *Am. J. Ophthalmol.* 32:225–231, 1949.

Mitchell D.E., Blakemore C. Binocular depth perception and the corpus callosum. *Vision Res.* 10:49–54, 1970.

Mitchell D.E., Ware C. Interocular transfer of a visual after effect in normal and stereoblind humans. *J. Physiol. (Lond.)* 236:707–721, 1974.

Mohler C.W., Wurtz R.H. Role of striate cortex and superior colliculus in visual guidance of saccadic eye-movements in monkeys. *J. Neurophysiol.* 40:74–94, 1977.

Mountcastle V.B. Functional properties of the light sensitive neurons of the posterior parietal cortex and their regulation by state controls: influence on excitability of interested fixation and angle of gaze. In Pompeiano O., Ajmore Marsam C., eds. *Brain Mechanisms and Perceptual Awareness.* New York, Raven Press, 1981.

Pasik T., Pasik P. The visual world of monkeys deprived of striate cortex: effective stimulus parameters and the importance of the accessory optic system. *Vision Res.* 3(Suppl.):419–435, 1971.

Patterson V.H., Foster D.H., Heron J.R. Variability of visual threshold in multiple sclerosis. Effect of background luminance on frequency of seeing. *Brain* 103:139–147, 1980.

Penfield W., Perot P. The brain's record of auditory and visual experience. *Brain* 86:595–696, 1963.

Perenin M.T., Jeannerod J.M. Visual function within the hemianopic field following early cerebral hemidecortication in man 1. Spatial localisation. *Neuropsychologia* 16:1–13, 1978.

Perrett D.I., Rolls E.T., Caan W. Visual neurones responsive to faces in the monkey temporal cortex. *Exp. Brain Res.* 47:329–342, 1982.

Perry V.H., Cowey A. Retinal ganglion cells that project to the superior colliculus and pretectum in the macaque monkey. *Neuroscience* 12:1125–1137, 1984.

Perry V.H., Oehler R., Cowey A. Retinal ganglion cells that project to the dorsal lateral geniculate nucleus of the macaque monkey. *Neuroscience* 12:1101–1123, 1984.

Persson H.E., Sachs V. Visual evoked potentials elicited by pattern reversal during provoked visual impairment in multiple sclerosis. *Brain* 104:369–382, 1981.

Pizzamiglio L., Antonucci G., Francia A. Response of the cortically blind hemifields to a moving visual scene. *Cortex* 20:89–99, 1984.

Pöppel E., Held R., Frost D. Residual visual function after brain wounds involving the central visual pathways in man. *Nature* 243:295–296, 1973.

Pulfrich C. von. Die Stereoskopie im Dienste der isochromen und heterochromen Photometrie. *Naturwissenschaften* 10:553–564, 569–574, 695–601, 714–722, 735–743, 751–761, 1922.

*Regan D. Evoked potentials in diagnosis. In Swash M., Kennard C., eds. *Scientific Basis of Clinical Neurology.* Edinburgh, Churchill Livingstone, pp. 358–370, 1985.

Regan D., Silver R., Murray T.H. Visual acuity and contrast sensitivity in multiple sclerosis: hidden visual loss. *Brain* 100:563–579, 1977.

Regan D., Whitlock J.A., Murray T.J., et al. Orientation—specific losses of contrast sensitivity in multiple sclerosis. *Invest. Ophthalmol. Vis. Sci.* 19:324–328, 1980.

Richards W. Stereopsis and stereo blindness. *Exp. Brain Res.* 10:380–388, 1970.

Riddoch G. Dissociation of visual perceptions due to occipital injuries with especial reference to appreciation of movement. *Brain* 40:15–57, 1917.

Riddoch G. Visual disorientation in homonymous half-fields. *Brain* 58:376–382, 1935.

Rodieck R.W. *The Vertebrate Retina.* San Francisco, Freeman, 1973.

Ross Russell R.W., Bharucha F. The recognition and prevention of border zone cerebral ischaemia during cardiac surgery. *Q. J. Med.* 47:303–323, 1978.

Ruddock K.H. Light transmission through the ocular media and macular pigment and its significance for psychophysical investigation. In Jameson D., Hurvich L.M., eds. *Handbook of Sensory Physiology.* Vol. II/4. *Visual Psychophysics.* Berlin, Springer-Verlag, pp. 455–469, 1972.

*Ruddock K.H. Visual mechanisms for the analysis of spatial pattern. *Ophthalmic Physiol. Opt.* 3:93–119, 1983.

Ruddock K.H. Spatial vision after cortical lesions. In Regan D.M., ed. *Vision and Visual Dysfunction.* Vol. 10. *Spatial Vision.* London, Macmillan, pp. 261–289, 1991.

Rushton D. Use of the Pulfrich pendulum for detecting abnormal delay in the visual pathway in multiple sclerosis. *Brain* 98:283–296, 1975.

Severin S.L., Tour R.L., Kershaw R.H. Macular function of the photostress test. *Arch. Ophthal. (Chicago)* 77:163–167, 1967.

Sjöstrand J., Frisén L. Contrast sensitivity in macular disease: a preliminary report. *Acta Ophthalmol. (Kbh.)* 55:507–514, 1977.

Smith K.J., McDonald W.I. Spontaneous and mechanically evoked activity due to a central demyelinating lesion. *Nature* 286:154–155, 1980.

Solms M., Kaplan-Solms K., Saling M., et al. Inverted vision after frontal lobe disease. *Cortex* 24:499–509, 1988.

Stiles W.S. *Mechanisms of Colour Vision.* London, Academic Press, 1978.

Stoerig P. Chromacity and achromacity: evidence for a functional differentiation in visual field defects. *Brain* 110:869–886, 1987.

*Stone J. *Parallel Processing in the Visual System.* New York, Plenum Publishing, 1983.

Stone J., Leicester J., Sherman S.M. The naso-temporal division of the monkey's retina. *J. Comp. Neurol.* 150:333–348, 1973.

Sunga R.N., Enoch J.M. Further perimetric analysis of patients with lesions of the visual pathways. *Am. J. Ophthalmol.* 70:402–422, 1970.

Teuber H.L., Battersby W.S., Bender M.B. *Visual Field Defects After Penetrating Missile Wounds of the Brain.* Cambridge, MA, Harvard University Press, 1960.

Titcombe A.F., Willison R.G. Flicker fusion in multiple sclerosis. *J. Neurol. Neurosurg. Psychiatry* 24:260–265, 1961.

Treisman A. Features and objects. The fourteenth Bartlett memorial lecture. *Q. J. Exp. Psychol.* 40A:201–237, 1988.

van Nes F.L., Bouman M.A. Spatial modulation function in the human eye. *J. Opt. Soc. Am.* 57:401–406, 1967.

Warrington E.K. Visual deficits associated with occipital lobe lesions in man. In *Scripta Varia.* 54. Vatican City, Pontificia Academy of Sciences, 1984.

Weiskrantz L. Behavioural analysis of the monkey's visual nervous system. *Proc. R. Soc. Lond. [Biol.]* 182:427–455, 1972.

Weiskrantz L. Varieties of residual visual experience. *J. Exp. Psychol.* 32:365–386, 1980.

Weiskrantz L., Warrington E.K., Sanders M.D., et al. Visual capacity in the hemianopic field following a restricted occipital ablation. *Brain* 97:709–718, 1974.

Wiesel T.N. Post-natal development of the visual cortex and the influence of the environment. *Nature* 299:583–591, 1982.

Wilson H.R., Bergen J.R. A four mechanism model for threshold spatial vision. *Vision Res.* 19:19–32, 1979.

Wilson H.R., Mets M.B., Nagy S.E., et al. Spatial frequency and orientation tuning of visual mechanisms in the human albino. *Vision Res.* 28:991–999, 1988.

Wood I.C.J., Kulikowski J.J. Pattern and movement detection in patients with reduced visual acuity. *Vision Res.* 18:331–334, 1978.

Wright W.D. *Researches on Normal and Defective Colour Vision.* London, Kimpton, 1946.

Zeki S. Interhemispheric connections of pre-striate cortex of monkey. *Brain Res.* 19:63–75, 1970.

*Zeki S. Uniformity and diversity of structure and function in rhesus monkey prestriate visual cortex. *J. Physiol. (Lond.)* 277:273–290, 1978.

Zeki S.M. Representation of colours in the cerebral cortex. *Nature* 284:412–418, 1980.

Zeki S., Shipp S. The functional logic of cortical connections. *Nature* 335:311–317, 1988.

Zihl J. "Blindsight": improvement of visually guided eye movements by systematic practice in patients with cerebral blindness. *Neuropsychologia* 18:71–77, 1980.

Zihl J., von Cramon D. Visual field recovery from scotoma in patients with post-geniculate damage: a review of 55 cases. *Brain* 108:335–365, 1985.

Zihl J., von Cramon D., Mai N. Selective disturbance of movement vision after bilateral brain damage. *Brain* 106:313–340, 1983.

29

Diseases of the Optic Nerve

W. Ian McDonald
David Barnes

The fibers constituting the optic nerve originate in the retina and terminate in the lateral geniculate nucleus and the superior colliculus. They may be involved by disease in any part of their course, resulting in a variety of symptoms, of which the most common is visual loss (Table 29–1). Precise early diagnosis is crucial because a number of conditions that are potentially curable can cause blindness if treatment is delayed. The key to successful management is a systematic approach to the problem.

APPROACH TO THE PATIENT

Two questions need to be answered: *where* is the lesion causing visual impairment, and *what* is its pathologic nature? A few points are worthy of special comment.

Clinical Assessment

A scrupulously detailed account of the onset and progression of visual symptoms is essential, because it provides clues to the localization and the extent of the lesion and to its pathologic nature. There are four main patterns of visual impairment.

1. *Transient*, which is usually associated with a vascular mechanism
2. *Abrupt and persistent*, which is also usually due to a vascular cause
3. *Acute or subacute and spontaneously reversible*, which usually reflects a demyelinating process
4. *Chronic and progressive*, which is usually due to compression

It is, however, important to emphasize that there are exceptions to these generalizations, which is impor-

tant in planning investigation. The history must also include inquiry into the presence of symptoms attributable to concomitant involvement of the structures in the neighborhood of the optic nerve and chiasm, which provide useful evidence of localization. In particular, inquiry should be made about nasal sinus disease and pituitary and hypothalamic dysfunction.

The clinical examination is directed toward documenting the severity of the visual loss and the localization and extent of the lesion causing it (Table 29–2). The visual acuity, corrected either with a pinhole or by refraction, provides an essential baseline. The visual fields provide the most important single piece of localizing information (see Chapter 28). Both white and colored objects should be used because, for reasons that are not altogether clear, defects caused by damage to optic nerve fibers are often more readily detected with red than with white objects: relative luminance alone does not appear to account for the phenomenon (Mullen and Plant, 1986). Although this observation remains valid for the clinical assessment of color vision in diseases of the optic nerve, research suggests that, for compressive lesions at least, the blue-yellow axis of color perception is affected earlier than is the red-green axis (M. Potts, unpublished observations). Color vision should be tested with each eye separately because the earliest clinical evidence of damage to the optic nerve is often a change in color perception. Unilateral impairment with relatively preserved visual acuity (better than 6/24 [20/80]) is good evidence of optic nerve as opposed to retinal damage and, if congenital color blindness can be excluded as a result of previous examination, bilateral impairment indicates bilateral disease. The observations that may be helpful in detecting subclinical involvement of the optic nerve are as follows:

Disc swelling
Disc pallor

Table 29–1. SYMPTOMS OF OPTIC NERVE DISEASE

Attributable to Optic Nerve Fiber Damage
Visual loss
    Transient
    Abrupt and persistent
    Acute or subacute and permanent
    Acute or subacute and spontaneously reversible
    Progressive
Phosphenes

Neighborhood Symptoms
Pain
Sensory disturbance in the face
Diplopia
Endocrine symptoms

Slits in the retinal fiber layer
Relative afferent pupillary defect
Impairment of color vision
Abnormal visual evoked potentials (VEPs)
A lesion on magnetic resonance imaging (MRI)
    scan

The position of the eye in the orbit should be recorded accurately because the existence and direction of proptosis provides useful localizing information about tumors. Examination of the upper six cranial nerves may provide clues to localization: unilateral anosmia may accompany a subfrontal meningioma and involvement of the oculomotor and fifth nerves is common in lesions involving the orbital fissure and cavernous sinus.

The second stage in the assessment of patients with visual failure involves the performance of routine investigations, which should be carried out in all cases, and the selection of special procedures, which may provide definitive evidence of localization and clues to the pathologic nature of the lesion.

Although the systematic application of these principles leads to a specific diagnosis in a majority of cases, an appreciable number of patients remain undiagnosed at presentation. All such patients must be followed regularly until the cause of the visual loss is established. Failure to abide by this rule may lead to unnecessary loss of sight.

ISCHEMIC OPTIC NEUROPATHY

Acute anterior ischemic optic neuropathy is relatively common. Its pathologic basis is infarction of the optic nerve head. In most cases a specific cause

Table 29–2. CLINICAL ASSESSMENT OF
VISUAL IMPAIRMENT

History and family history
Corrected visual acuity
Visual fields and color vision
Examination of eye, orbit, pupils, and fundus
Examination of cranial nerves I–VIII
Examination of postnasal space and ears
General medical examination

is not found. Hypertension and evidence of arteriosclerosis elsewhere are frequent, and diabetes is occasionally present. Acute ischemic optic neuropathy may occur with polycythemia or migraine and may follow massive gastrointestinal hemorrhage. The most important condition (because of the therapeutic implications) with which it occurs is giant cell arteritis (see Chapter 80). In the latter, ischemic optic neuropathy may occur in isolation or in combination with central retinal artery occlusion.

The condition usually occurs after the fifth decade. The onset is abrupt and usually painless, and the visual loss commonly reaches its peak immediately. The visual acuity is variably and not necessarily severely affected, depending on the distribution of the infarction and the corresponding field loss, which is often sectorial with an arcuate component, reflecting the anterior location of the lesion. Inferior nasal defects are most common, but central scotomata are not infrequent (Boghen and Glaser, 1975). Fundal examination reveals a swollen optic disc with peripapillary linear (nerve fiber layer) hemorrhages. In the uncomplicated form of ischemic optic neuropathy, the retinal arterioles appear normal, an important distinction from central retinal artery occlusion. Within a few days, the disc, while still swollen, starts to become pale. Fluorescein angiography shows marked leakage at the disc, usually with evidence of underperfusion of parts of it. The VEP is reduced in amplitude and may be delayed (Halliday and McDonald, 1981; Hennerici et al., 1977). Limited recovery is possible, but the greater part of the field loss usually persists. Treatment is that of the underlying illness; no specific therapy is beneficial. If giant cell arteritis is suspected, prompt treatment with steroids is essential (see Chapter 80).

In the chronic progressive form of ischemic optic neuropathy, visual deterioration may continue for a month or more (Borchert and Lessell, 1988; Drance, 1976). This disorder may respond to optic nerve decompression (Sergott et al., 1989). Occasionally, ischemic optic neuropathy affects the posterior portion of the optic nerve, which is relatively resistant to ischemia. In most of these patients, however, an obvious cause exists, such as a shower of emboli or systemic hypotension (Rizzo and Lessell, 1987; Weinstein et al., 1989).

Simultaneous bilateral anterior ischemic optic neuropathy is extremely uncommon, although patients with a previous attack in one eye may notice symptoms in both eyes together when the second eye later becomes affected. Beri et al. (1987) did not find a single definite case of simultaneous bilateral involvement in a large study of both arteritic and nonarteritic anterior ischemic optic neuropathy. However, we have seen a few patients in whom the changes of acute ischemic optic neuropathy were present in both eyes. Thus, although it is rare, either simultaneous or closely sequential bilateral involvement of the eyes does occur.

OPTIC NEURITIS

The term *optic* or *retrobulbar neuritis* is used to refer to a syndrome characterized clinically by subacute visual loss associated with a central scotoma. Vision recovers spontaneously over a matter of weeks. The term may be used in connection with specific diseases (e.g., syphilis or herpes zoster), but when used without qualification, the cause is usually unknown and, if the patient recovers, it is assumed that the underlying pathologic process was that of demyelination. In childhood, bilateral optic neuritis is sometimes preceded by an infection such as measles, chickenpox, mumps, and infectious mononucleosis, and the presence in some cases of other fleeting neurologic abnormalities suggests that the visual symptoms may be the most obvious manifestation of a more widespread encephalomyelitis (Parkin et al., 1984). A similar picture is seen rarely in adults. Optic neuropathy may be associated with sinusitis, and prompt treatment of the sinus disease can lead to recovery of visual function (Awerbuch et al., 1989). The association with infected mucocele of the sphenoid sinus is discussed later.

Little information is available about the pathologic features of optic neuritis, except when it occurs in multiple sclerosis. Under these circumstances, the predominant pathologic change is demyelination with relative preservation of the axons; some axons are, however, always lost and this is reflected in the ophthalmologically visible slit-like defects in the nerve fiber layer of the retina (Frisén and Hoyt, 1974). There is a marked astrocytic gliosis. Remyelination is scanty at postmortem examination in multiple sclerosis (Prineas and Connell, 1979). The completeness of clinical and electrophysiologic recovery after optic neuritis in childhood raises the possibility, however, that remyelination may be more extensive in younger patients (Kriss et al., 1988). Similar pathologic changes probably occur in other forms of optic neuritis that have clinical and evoked potential features similar to those in multiple sclerosis.

Optic neuritis commonly occurs in young adults, but can occur in early childhood and rarely even in the eighth decade. Women are more commonly affected than men. The onset is usually with blurring and/or dimness of vision often preceded or accompanied by discomfort in the affected eye, particularly on eye movement. The visual loss usually increases during days or a week or two and persists for several weeks. Visual impairment is often more marked in bright surroundings. Phosphenes, often precipitated by eye movement or occasionally by a sudden noise (Page et al., 1982), may be experienced by up to one-third of patients (see Chapter 28).

On examination, the visual acuity is variably impaired; it may fall to no perception of light without necessarily implying a poor visual prognosis. The characteristic field defect is a central scotoma, but it is important to realize that other defects may be found early and late in the course: a sector defect at the onset may evolve into a typical central scotoma, and fine arcuate scotomata are a common residual defect (Frisén and Hoyt, 1974). The optic disc is swollen in rather less than 50% of patients with disease in the acute stage, presumably depending on the propinquity of the lesion to the nerve head. Hemorrhages are exceptional and never profuse. Sheathing of the peripheral retinal venules and/or focal leakage of fluorescein occurs in about one-quarter of patients (Lightman et al., 1987). Cells can be detected in the media with the slit lamp in about 10% of cases, but frank uveitis is rare.

The characteristic abnormality in the pattern VEP in optic neuritis is a substantial delay in the P100 with a well-preserved waveform (Halliday et al., 1972). Other abnormalities can occur and overall 90% of patients have abnormal VEPs (Halliday and McDonald, 1981). In 90% of these, the abnormality is persistent. The cerebrospinal fluid is often normal, but in about 25% of patients, oligoclonal bands are present (Nikoskelainen et al., 1980). Fluorescein angiography shows modest leakage from the disc.

MRI of the optic nerves in acute optic neuritis has provided important insights into the relationship between the visual disturbance and the lesion responsible, which can be visualized in more than 80% of cases (D.H. Miller et al., 1988a; Youl et al., 1991). Enhancement of the lesion with the contrast agent gadolinium–diethylenetriamine pentaacetic acid indicates the presence of blood-nerve barrier damage and inflammation (Fig. 29–1). Optic disc swelling is particularly associated with anterior lesions on MRI, although mild swelling may sometimes occur with lesions as far back as the optic canal. Poor visual outcome (worse than 6/12 [20/40]) is associated with more extensive lesions and with those situated in the optic canal. These findings have obvious implications for rationalizing the use of steroids in optic neuritis.

Recovery usually takes place during weeks, and the visual acuity returns to 6/12 (20/40) or better in 90% of patients; the mechanisms involved have been discussed in detail elsewhere (McDonald, 1983). They probably include dispersal of edema from regions of relative restriction of the optic nerve, such as in the scleral and optic canals; restoration of conduction by remyelination; development of conduction in persistently demyelinated fibers; and adaptive synaptic changes compensating for nerve fiber degeneration. The relative importance of each of these mechanisms in different patients and at different ages is unknown.

In a few patients, a sense of disequilibrium attributable to the Pulfrich effect (see Chapter 28) may be troublesome. Return or worsening of symptoms with exercise or a hot bath may occur, particularly in those patients who later develop multiple sclerosis. The pathophysiologic mechanisms underlying these phenomena are discussed in Chapter 28.

An important aspect of prognosis is the risk of multiple sclerosis. This risk was found to be about 75% 15 years after isolated attacks of optic neuritis in the United Kingdom (Francis et al., 1987). The

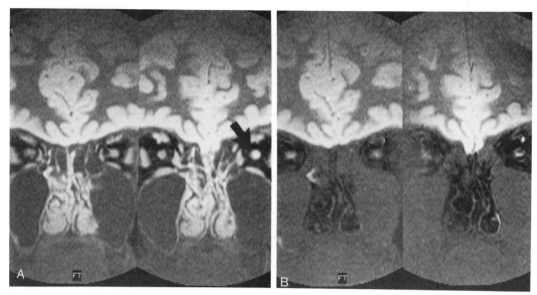

Figure 29–1. Coronal T1-weighted MRI scan of the optic nerves in acute left-sided optic neuritis. *(A)* Unenhanced image showing abnormally high signal in the affected nerve *(arrow)*. *(B)* After injection of gadolinium–diethylenetriamine pentaacetic acid, the signal from the affected, but not the unaffected, optic nerve is markedly diminished because of enhancement after leakage of the dye through the abnormal blood-nerve barrier.

reported figures, however, vary widely. For example, the risk was 8% in Japan (Isayama et al., 1982), 45% in Denmark (Sandberg-Wollheim et al., 1990), and 58% in Massachusetts (Rizzo and Lessell, 1988). A number of factors, including patient selection, the racial origin and geographic location of the patients, and the length of follow-up, probably contribute to these variations. The influence of latitude remains unclear, but high frequencies of progression to multiple sclerosis are not seen in lower latitudes. The risk appears to be significantly higher for women than for men (Rizzo and Lessell, 1988), for those with age at onset between 21 and 40 years (Hely et al., 1986), and for patients with cerebrospinal fluid oligoclonal bands at presentation (Moulin et al., 1983; Sandberg-Wollheim et al., 1990).

There is conflicting evidence concerning the importance of various human leukocyte antigen (HLA) phenotypes: Hely et al. (1986) observed that the risk was increased in DR2- and B7-positive patients. Although Francis et al. (1987) did not confirm this observation, DR3 did confer increased risk, especially in combination with DR2. The overall influence of recurrence of optic neuritis on the progression to multiple sclerosis remains unclear, but Sandberg-Wollheim et al. (1990) found that, if the time between episodes is taken into account, there is a significantly increased risk in patients with an early (median interval, 7.5 months) recurrence.

The MRI findings in the brain are also prognostic: D.H. Miller et al. (1988b) found that, in patients with clinically isolated optic neuritis, associated brain lesions were associated with a relative risk of 6.8 of multiple sclerosis occurring within a year.

The diagnosis of optic neuritis is not usually difficult. Ischemic optic neuropathy may be a problem in older patients; fluorescein angiography is, however, often helpful when the patient is seen in the acute stages. Central serous retinopathy may cause confusion when the optic disc is normal. However, there is often an associated visual distortion and macular edema may be visible ophthalmoscopically. Fluorescein angiography usually confirms the diagnosis by showing single-point leakage into the subretinal space.

Uniocular visual disturbances indistinguishable from optic neuritis are occasionally an early feature of the vasculitides, including Behçet's disease, sicca syndrome, and systemic lupus erythematosus. The optic nerves may be involved in human immunodeficiency virus–positive individuals (Winyard et al., 1989). The correct diagnosis is important, as many causes, such as syphilitic perineuritis and cryptococcosis, are treatable.

Because tumors can rarely cause a syndrome resembling optic neuritis (McDonald, 1982), it is important that all patients should have computed tomography (CT) or MRI when there are any atypical clinical or investigative features. Errors in diagnosis can be minimized if the physician is alert to discrepancies in the clinical picture, such as failure to remit, unusual features in the onset or course, onset after 50 years of age, and the presence of neurologic abnormalities in the upper cranial nerves not attributable to multiple sclerosis. High-resolution CT or MRI should be performed whenever there is doubt about the diagnosis.

There is no convincing evidence that therapy influences the visual outcome of optic neuritis, although treatment with steroids or adrenocorticotrophin probably shortens the duration of visual loss (Gould et al., 1977) and is therefore indicated in bilateral optic neuritis and in unilateral optic neuritis when there is poor vision in the unaffected eye. The association of poor visual outcome with more extensive lesions and with those in the optic canal raises the question of whether this subgroup should always be treated with steroids. A trial is indicated.

Bilateral Optic Neuritis

Simultaneous involvement of both eyes is uncommon in adults. Multiple sclerosis may follow, although some patients may show no signs of dissemination of lesions even after more than 30 years (Parkin et al., 1984). Whether some of these cases are sporadic examples of Leber's hereditary optic neuropathy (LHON) awaits clarification using mitochondrial DNA (mtDNA) analysis (see later). The prognosis for vision appears to be poor in late-onset bilateral cases.

Chronic Optic Neuritis

Slowly progressive optic neuritis is on rare occasions the presenting feature of multiple sclerosis (Ormerod and McDonald, 1984), which may declare itself only years later. It cannot be emphasized too strongly that most cases of progressive visual loss attributable to optic neuropathy are due to potentially curable tumors and that the diagnosis of chronic optic neuritis must be made only after careful exclusion of other conditions.

Optic Neuritis in Childhood

Simultaneously bilateral optic neuritis in childhood carries a good visual prognosis. Kriss et al. (1988) found the risk of multiple sclerosis to be approximately 15% after 9 years, and their findings did not support the suggestion that the risk is higher in unilateral cases.

HEREDITARY OPTIC NEUROPATHIES

Leber's Hereditary Optic Neuropathy

The best known (but not most common) form of hereditary optic neuropathy is that associated with the name of Leber. The observation that LHON is maternally transmitted led to the suggestion that it may be due to a defect of mtDNA, which is inherited exclusively from the mother. Wallace et al. (1988) supported this hypothesis by demonstrating a point mutation at position 11778, a highly conserved site of mtDNA, in 9 of 11 pedigrees with LHON. This mutation in a gene for one subunit of NADH:coenzyme Q reductase (a complex of the respiratory chain) causes the loss of a restriction site for the endonuclease *Sfa*NI. A subsequent study of British pedigrees with LHON found the same point mutation in 50% of patients (Holt et al., 1989), although a different abnormality of mtDNA could not be excluded in the remainder. The mechanisms by which respiratory chain abnormalities might cause the clinical manifestations of LHON are unknown. Environmental factors such as cigarette smoking may be important, although MRI shows abnormal optic nerve signal in LHON but not in tobacco-alcohol amblyopia, suggesting that they are different pathologic processes (Kermode et al., 1989).

Patients with typical LHON usually present in the third and fourth decades. Of white patients with LHON, 80% are male, and of Japanese patients, 60% are male. The first symptom is usually blurring of vision, commonly bilaterally. If one eye is affected first, the second is usually involved within a month, although intervals of more than 1 year have been recorded (Carroll and Mastaglia, 1979). The acuity usually falls to 6/60 (20/200) or less during 2–3 weeks; complete blindness is rare. Field defects are at first centrocecal, but rapidly expand to become large bilateral central scotomata. The fundi show a characteristic appearance in the first week or two: the discs are abnormally pink and markedly swollen; the adjacent retinal nerve fibers are also swollen, probably as a result of stasis of axoplasmic flow at the nerve head. At this stage, there is a marked increase in the number of small vessels, producing a vasculitic appearance (Fig. 29–2); hemorrhages are, however, trivial or absent (Nikoskelainen et al., 1983; Smith et al., 1973). The vascular changes have been observed in individuals at risk for up to 3 years before the development of visual symptoms (Nikoskelainen et al., 1982); they disappear, however, after the onset of visual loss and the disc becomes pale. LHON rarely presents with insidious visual failure.

The demonstration of the mutation of mtDNA discussed earlier may prove to have important implications for the management and prognosis of patients with LHON. Although severe visual loss is usually permanent, up to 25% of patients show useful recovery to 6/12 (20/40) or better, and these individuals appear not to have the mutation. Furthermore, the proportion of mtDNA that is abnormal in any individual may correlate with the severity of disease and the risk of transmission by carrier females. Follow-up studies of affected and carrier individuals should clarify these issues and provide a basis for accurate genetic counseling.

The presence of abnormal mtDNA in the brain may explain the cerebral abnormalities that are occasionally associated with LHON (Wallace, 1970) and that may resemble mitochondrial encephalopathy. Parker et al. (1989) reported abnormal NADH:coenzyme Q reductase activity in several members of the same family, some of whom had clinically typical LHON, and others, mitochondrial encephalopathy (although they did not have the 11778 mutation).

Hitherto, LHON could only be diagnosed with

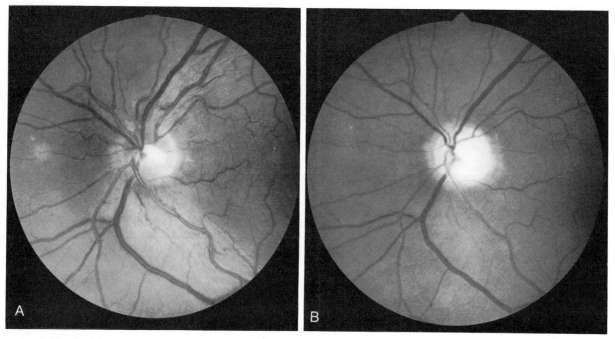

Figure 29–2. The fundal appearances in LHON. *(A)* Acutely, the disc is markedly swollen and is surrounded by abnormal telangiectatic vessels. *(B)* The same eye, 18 months later, shows optic atrophy and persistence of telangiectatic vessels.

certainty in the presence of a characteristic family history. The diagnosis can now be made in isolated cases if the 11778 mtDNA mutation is present, although absence of the mutation does not exclude it. The vasculitic fundal appearances were at first thought to be specific, but have since been described in cone dystrophy in which, however, visual loss develops insidiously. Retinal vascular disease is common in retinal receptor dystrophies generally and may give rise to retinal edema and optic nerve swelling (A.C. Bird, unpublished observations). The disorder most likely to be confused with LHON is acute bilateral optic neuritis, in which fluorescein angiography reveals leakage at the disc, whereas in Leber's disease, despite gross disc swelling, the permeability to fluorescein is normal.

No treatment has proved effective so far. It has sometimes been argued that steroids should be used in the acute stage to minimize optic nerve fiber damage, but there is no convincing evidence that they do so. If they are used, the course should be of limited duration. Hydroxocobalamin and L-cystine have both been advocated, but we have not seen benefit from either. Surgical decompression of the optic nerve has been advocated in Japan (Imachi, 1969), but the procedure is not without risk and has not come into general use.

Dominantly Inherited Optic Atrophy

Dominantly inherited optic atrophy is probably the most common form of inherited optic atrophy seen in the United Kingdom and the United States. The visual impairment is often first noticed at school age

or may be discovered accidentally, for example, when an affected individual fails a vision test for a driving license. Only exceptionally are the acuities less than 6/36 (20/120). The discs are pale and may show a rather characteristic pie-shaped excavation temporally. Field defects are often hard to demonstrate but when present are centrocecal or sometimes apparently bitemporal in form, the latter leading to confusion with chiasmal compression. The blue field may be smaller than the red, which is opposite to the normal state of affairs, reflecting the blue-yellow dyschromatopia (Smith, 1972). Dominantly inherited optic atrophy may rarely be associated with deafness (Kollarits et al., 1979).

There is usually little change in the visual impairment over the years, but because acuities on average tend to be lower in older patients, it has been suggested that exceptionally there may be some deterioration. No specific treatment is available. As in all patients with visual impairment, every effort should be made to achieve the best possible vision by correcting refractive errors and making use of appropriate low vision aids.

Other Inherited Optic Atrophies

Isolated recessive optic atrophy has been described but is rare. Another rarity is optic atrophy in association with diabetes insipidus, diabetes mellitus, deafness, and renal abnormalities (the Wolfram syndrome [Cremers et al., 1977]). Because several components of the syndrome are treatable, its recognition is more important than its rarity might suggest. Optic atrophy may be found in association with both dominantly and recessively inherited neurodegenerative disorders (see Chapter 88).

TOXIC, NUTRITIONAL, AND METABOLIC AMBLYOPIA

A large number of toxic substances can produce visual loss. The clinical syndromes range from acute and permanent blindness (as in methyl alcohol intoxication) to chronic and insidious, although potentially reversible, visual impairment (as in intoxication with ethambutol). The topic was excellently reviewed by N.R. Miller (1982).

Subacute visual loss with central or centrocecal scotomata can occur with chronic ethanol ingestion and smoking. The clinical features of this syndrome were well reviewed by Krumsiek et al. (1985). In the United Kingdom, the use of certain dark pipe tobaccos is particularly associated with amblyopia. The fundus is usually normal at presentation; there is marked impairment of color vision and there are afferent pupillary defects. The pattern VEP is reduced in amplitude, and the flash-evoked electroretinogram is subnormal (Ikeda et al., 1978).

The mechanism of the visual loss is not fully understood. There is some evidence for a defect in cyanide metabolism, but the issue is unresolved (Foulds and Pettigrew, 1977; Potts, 1973). Whatever the pathogenesis, clinical and electrophysiologic recovery usually follows treatment with large doses of hydroxocobalamin (Foulds and Pettigrew, 1977; Ikeda et al., 1978). It is often difficult for the patient to stop smoking, and in such cases, a monthly maintenance dose (hydroxocobalamin, 1 mg) is often prescribed.

A syndrome of subacute bilateral visual loss is well recognized in young black persons. It was originally recognized in Jamaica, but a similar syndrome occurs in young Bahamans, Cubans, Puerto Ricans, and Jamaicans who have lived in the United States for years before the onset of visual disturbance (Glaser, 1990). We have seen it in fit, educated native black Africans in whom there was no evidence of nutritional deficiency and ingestion of toxic substances was denied. The clinical picture is indistinguishable from that occasionally seen in white patients, some of whom later have multiple sclerosis, but a majority do not, even after lengthy follow-up (Parkin et al., 1984). The nosological status of these syndromes remains uncertain.

The optic nerves may be involved in other metabolic disorders, including vitamin B_{12} deficiency, diabetes, and uremia. Although clinical diabetic optic neuropathy is rare, a subclinical increase in the VEP latency (often with reduced amplitude) is found in most patients, compromising the usefulness of this test in diabetics suspected of having multiple sclerosis (Puvanendran et al., 1983). The incidence of anterior ischemic optic neuropathy is increased in diabetics, and young diabetic men in particular are prone to a recurrence in the fellow eye (Beri et al., 1987).

Uremic patients are susceptible to a variety of insults to the optic nerves, including toxic (e.g., deferoxamine), ischemic, and infectious (Hamed et al., 1989) optic neuropathies. More specifically, the term *uremic optic neuropathy* refers to the bilateral visual loss with swelling of the optic nerve heads that occasionally develops in severely uremic individuals. Knox et al. (1988) recommended treatment with dialysis and steroids, after which useful vision is restored in many patients. Investigations are usually unhelpful, but the possibility of cryptococcal meningitis must be borne in mind in immunocompromised individuals. A lumbar puncture should therefore be performed after CT in appropriate cases.

INFILTRATIONS OF THE OPTIC NERVE

The optic disc swelling of papilledema is associated with obstruction to axoplasmic flow (Tso and Hayreh, 1977a,b). Swelling, usually associated with visual loss, can also result from infiltration of the disc by abnormal tissue in glioma and in systemic disorders such as leukemia, lymphoma, sarcoidosis, and metastatic carcinoma. Infiltration of the optic discs is often unilateral. Such swelling must be distinguished from that produced by drusen—which often appear as small, rounded, glinting masses which autofluoresce on or at the edge of the disc—and from elevated discs with abnormally branched and tortuous vessels; it has been suggested that the swelling under these circumstances is due to the presence of buried drusen. Visual loss in association with drusen is exceptional, but does occur (Sanders et al., 1971). The differential diagnosis of unilateral swelling of the optic disc is discussed by Glaser (1990) and Sanders and Sennhenn (1980).

DIFFUSE ORBITAL DISEASE

The optic nerve may be involved in disease processes primarily affecting other tissues in the orbit, including muscle and connective tissue.

Orbital cellulitis is rare but is usually curable if treatment is prompt and vigorous. The onset is acute, with severe pain, proptosis, erythema of the lids, and limitation of eye movement. The patient is obviously ill. There is often clinical or radiologic (especially CT) evidence of sinusitis. The CT scan may reveal swelling of the muscles. Posterior spread of infection may lead to meningitis and septic *cavernous sinus thrombosis*. This grave complication is often heralded by stupor progressing to coma. Hemiparesis caused by infarction and subdural empyema may occur. Optic disc swelling is not prominent but the retinal veins are often distended, and the CT scan may show irregular masses produced by distention of the superior ophthalmic vein (Clifford-Jones et al.,

1982). Although orbital cellulitis can undoubtedly occur without sinus thrombosis, the reverse probably does not apply. The distinction is of little practical importance because both conditions require prompt and intensive antibiotic therapy. The possible benefits of anticoagulants are probably outweighed by the risk of hemorrhage, and their use is best avoided.

Subacute orbital cellulitis is produced occasionally by mucormycosis in debilitated patients with diabetes. A striking clinical sign is gangrene of the hard palate, which arises from occlusion of the vessels supplying the mucosa and the bone by fungal elements. The condition has a poor prognosis, but occasionally can be treated effectively by amphotericin B with or without surgery (Lehrer et al., 1980).

In addition to these specific forms of organismal orbital inflammation, unilateral or bilateral proptosis and ophthalmoplegia with varying amounts of pain can occur with vasculitis (including polyarteritis and Wegener's granulomatosis), sarcoidosis, and a group of inflammatory disorders within which several clinical syndromes are recognized. Transitional cases occur, however. This confusing topic has been excellently reviewed by Jakobiec and Jones (1979).

The *Tolosa*, or *Tolosa-Hunt*, *syndrome*, in which the optic nerve may be affected, producing severe visual loss, resembles orbital cellulitis in presenting acutely with severe periocular pain and ophthalmoplegia, often (though not invariably) accompanied by proptosis, conjunctival edema, and involvement of cranial nerve V. Constitutional disturbance may be marked but the sensorium is clear. A raised white blood cell count and erythrocyte sedimentation rate, although they occur, are exceptional and other evidence of infection is absent. A CT scan often reveals thickening of one or more of the external ocular muscles (Fig. 29–3), which has led to the use of the term *orbital myositis*. MRI may show abnormal soft tissue in the cavernous sinus (Goto et al., 1990). These imaging appearances correspond to the pathologic finding of nonspecific inflammatory tissue in the orbit and the cavernous sinus. The condition may remit spontaneously after a few weeks, and it is not uncommon to obtain a past history of one or more similar self-limited episodes. If there is no evidence of infection, it is appropriate to treat the patient with high doses of steroids. The pain is often relieved within hours. If it is not, the diagnosis should be reviewed and the possibility of other causes, such as intracranial aneurysm should be considered.

Orbital pseudotumor is a chronic nonspecific inflammatory syndrome. It is often painful, sometimes severely so. Pathologically, there may be marked lymphocytic infiltration; this can lead to confusion with lymphoma, which occasionally causes isolated proptosis (Fowler et al., 1975). CT often reveals marked enlargement of the extraocular muscles and occasionally shows abnormal tissue extending intracranially, making differentiation from lymphoma still more difficult. Visual loss occurs, although infrequently, probably as a result of compression of the optic nerves by the enlarged muscles. A similar

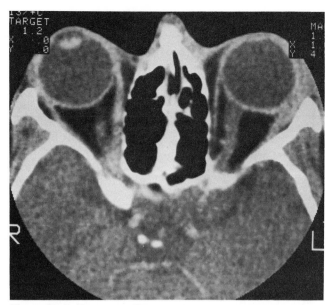

Figure 29–3. Transverse CT scan of the orbits in the Tolosa-Hunt syndrome. There is bilateral proptosis with thickening of particularly the right medial and left lateral rectus muscles. There is also abnormal tissue at the right orbital apex.

picture may be seen in *dysthyroid eye disease*, in which, however, pain is exceptional and other evidence of present or past Graves' disease is usually present. In both conditions, the enlargement of the external ocular muscles may be extreme, leading to compression of the optic nerve at the orbital apex. The visual impairment may be reversed with steroids, but it is often difficult to wean the patient from them. Radiotherapy may be helpful in intractable cases of orbital pseudotumor. Surgical decompression is preferable in dysthyroid eye disease when sight is threatened.

COMPRESSION OF THE ANTERIOR VISUAL PATHWAYS

Tumors are of course the most common cause of compression of the optic nerve, the incidence of different types varying in different parts of its course. The absolute frequency of the various tumors is difficult to determine because of variations in the source and mode of referral of patients to different centers.

The pathologic characteristics of tumors encountered in the orbit were dealt with excellently by Henderson (1973), and of intracranial tumors by Russell and Rubinstein (1989). In contrast to the extensive literature on the histopathologic features of the neoplasms themselves, that on the morphologic changes induced in the nerve fibers on which the symptoms depend is small. It is clear that severe chronic compression results in degeneration. It is equally clear from the reversibility of symptoms in many patients that other processes must be involved. The topic was reviewed by Clifford-Jones et al. (1985) in the light of an experimental study of the morphologic consequences of optic nerve compression. In essence, they found that a degree of compression that produces partial impairment of optic nerve function is characterized by a focal, predominantly demyelinating lesion with preservation of continuity of a majority of the axons. Remyelination occurs and can commence while the nerve is still compressed; some of the new myelin segments, still subject to pressure, show evidence of secondary breakdown. The relationship between these morphologic changes, disordered conduction, and the symptoms of compression of the anterior visual pathways was reviewed by McDonald (1982) and Clifford-Jones et al. (1985) and is summarized in Chapter 28.

Orbital Tumors

In adult life, extrinsic tumors are much more common than intrinsic tumors involving the orbital portion of the optic nerve. Among the former, the commonest, excluding metastases, are cavernous hemangioma, meningioma, and neurofibroma. In all three, the usual history is of slowly progressive visual failure. Quite severe visual loss may first be discovered accidentally when the good eye is closed while rubbing it to remove a foreign body. A dull ache may be present, but pain is not usually prominent, except with malignant tumors. Examination provides good evidence for the site of the tumor. An arcuate component to a scotoma and retinal folds visible ophthalmoscopically suggest an anterior location. Pure central scotomata not breaking out of the periphery are uncommon but do occur. Tumors enlarging within the muscle cone produce an axial proptosis, as may an intracranial sphenoid wing meningioma. It is important to appreciate, however, that small tumors situated at the orbital apex may produce severe visual loss before proptosis develops. The optic disc may be swollen or atrophic.

A striking form of transient visual loss is sometimes seen with orbital tumor (Bradbury et al., 1987). The patient may complain of temporary loss of sight at one or other extreme of gaze. Under such circumstances, the affected pupil dilates and becomes fixed to direct and consensual stimulation by light. Vision and the pupillary reflexes return when the eyes are recentered. Fluorescein angiography in the deviated position shows that the retinal blood flow is arrested. The absence of the consensual reflex indicates that the ciliary body is also ischemic. The retinal circulation returns with centering of the globe to reveal the characteristic changes of the chronically swollen optic disc. Although usually encountered with optic nerve sheath meningioma, we have seen this phenomenon with optic nerve glioma and extrinsic tumors. Presumably, in each case the ophthalmic artery is temporarily occluded because of relative restriction of its movement in relation to the more rigid tumor.

High-resolution CT and MRI are both useful investigations for suspected orbital tumor. The multiplanar capability and superior ability to resolve the site and extent of orbital lesions of MRI make it the modality of choice when available (Eidelberg et al., 1988), although CT may be required to detect calcification or bony changes. The pattern VEP is often reduced in amplitude, and the waveform is distorted; marked delay is unusual but does occur (McDonald, 1982). Half-field stimulation may be helpful in the early detection of chiasmal involvement causing damage to nerve fibers from the other eye.

Optic Nerve Glioma

Orbital optic nerve glioma is uncommon in adult life but does occur (Wulc et al., 1989). In contrast to the case with chiasmal glioma (Hoyt et al., 1973), this tumor is usually slow growing, and operative intervention can be delayed until useful vision is lost or posterior extension of the tumor threatens to make removal technically problematic.

Optic nerve glioma in childhood presents special problems. Pathologically the tumors are of low grade, most being pilocytic astrocytomas (Russell and Rubinstein, 1989). The rate of growth of the tumors varies widely, and they are known occasionally to regress spontaneously (Borit and Richardson, 1982). Patients usually have proptosis and the consequences of visual loss, including squint (Wright et al., 1989a). The optic disc may be pale or swollen, sometimes with tumor extending forward into the vitreous. Optociliary shunt vessels may be seen, as with long-standing meningiomas. Neurofibromatosis is present in about half the patients. The tumors are often also present intracranially at the time of presentation, although whether they extend actively from the orbit to involve the intracranial structures or whether they are of multicentric origin is not established. Precocious puberty and other endocrine disturbances may result from hypothalamic involvement. A curious form of eye movement disorder, see-saw nystagmus, is sometimes seen. Unfortunately, the extent of the tumors cannot be predicted reliably from clinical and investigative evidence. Microscopic evidence of tumor at the peripheral cut end of the optic nerve resected at its junction with the chiasm may be found even when visual fields, pattern VEPs with half-field stimulation, CT scans, and inspection at operation have given no indication of chiasmal involvement. MRI may prove to be more useful: we have seen abnormal signal in involved optic nerves even before swelling had begun to develop. The management of these tumors is discussed later.

Optic Nerve Sheath Meningioma

Optic nerve sheath meningioma is most commonly found in middle life but may occur at any age. Interestingly, the overall female preponderance of optic nerve sheath meningioma is reversed in patients younger than 30 years (Wright et al., 1989b). Visual loss and modest proptosis are the most common initial symptoms, and pain is unusual. The disc is either atrophic or swollen, and about 25% of patients have optociliary shunt vessels. The diagnosis, which is based on the clinical and radiologic findings, is usually straightforward. CT shows thickening, often irregular, of the optic nerve, sometimes with "tramline" calcification. In about 20% of patients, however, the distinction between an extrinsic and an intrinsic tumor cannot be made by CT, but the use of MRI reduces this proportion to less than 10%. Many optic nerve sheath meningiomas occurring in middle life and later never require treatment.

Hitherto, if follow-up suggested the need for intervention, surgery was undertaken, even though useful vision could rarely be preserved: radiotherapy was thought to be ineffective in these tumors. Kennerdall et al. (1988) reported their experience of 39 optic nerve sheath meningiomas. Six were confined to the orbit and showed an excellent response to radiotherapy alone, with preservation of vision. They concluded that radiotherapy slows tumor growth and is preferable to surgery in patients with declining vision or a constricting field. Surgical intervention is required only for cosmetic reasons or if the lesion is heading intracranially, in which case radiotherapy may be a useful adjunct. The findings of Kennerdall et al. (1988) are supported by our own limited experience.

Wright et al. (1989a,b) highlighted the difficult problems associated with the management of orbital optic nerve tumors in patients younger than 40 years. These problems arise because it is now apparent that in younger patients, particularly men under 30 years, optic nerve sheath meningiomas are more aggressive and invasive than those occurring in later life: in patients between 30 and 40 years, they behave in an intermediately aggressive fashion. Differentiation from the more benign gliomas is obviously of great importance and is possible in most patients, particularly when MRI is available. Wright et al. (1989a) recommended that all suspected optic nerve sheath meningiomas in patients younger than 30 years should be explored as soon as possible via a transfrontal cranio-orbitotomy because of the risk of incurable intracranial extension. If frozen section examination confirms the diagnosis, the lesion and the entire optic nerve should be removed. When vision is poor, excision of the tumor is indicated, regardless of investigational findings because it might be a meningioma and the operation has a low morbidity. When useful vision remains, conservative management is appropriate if imaging suggests a glioma or if the nature of the tumor is unknown. Such patients should be observed carefully at 3- to 6-month intervals, depending on progress, and surgery should be undertaken if the behavior or imaging characteristics of the lesion suggest either active glioma or meningioma. The role of radiotherapy in glioma is uncertain, and we restrict its use to patients with severe bilateral progressive visual loss.

Compression in the Optic Canal

The optic nerve nearly fills the bony canal and is therefore particularly vulnerable in this part of its course. Meningiomas may enter it from either the intracranial or the orbital ends. Nasopharyngeal carcinoma often concomitantly involves cranial nerves III, IV, V, and VI. In some individuals, there are bony defects in the lateral wall of the canal (Young, 1924); the optic nerve is then vulnerable to compression from mucocele (McDonald, 1982). The soft tissue component of tumors within the canal is often invisible on CT scans, its presence being indicated only by widening of the canal. This sign is often missed unless special care is taken to use bone windows. MRI is probably more sensitive for detecting and delineating tumors extending into the canal (Eidelberg et al. 1988). Rarely, the optic nerve is chronically compressed by abnormal bone in Paget's disease and fibrous dysplasia, and acutely compressed by hematoma after frontal trauma, for which steroids or early surgical decompression may be beneficial (Guy et al., 1989), although permanent visual impairment is likely.

Compression of the Intracranial Optic Nerve and Chiasm

The common causes of compression in this region are pituitary tumor, craniopharyngioma, meningioma, and aneurysm of the terminal carotid and anterior communicating arteries. Less common are chordoma and, in childhood, dysgerminoma. The symptoms are influenced by both the pathologic nature of the tumor and its location. Most patients usually have progressive visual loss, especially from the temporal side when the central part of the chiasm is involved. It is important from the point of view of management to appreciate that there may be accelerated deterioration during a week or two in patients with craniopharyngiomas, sphenoid mucoceles, and pituitary tumors. Occasionally, the latter cause an abrupt onset of visual loss accompanied by severe headache when infarction occurs; the cerebrospinal fluid may then be bloodstained. Spontaneously remitting visual loss indistinguishable from that caused by acute optic neuritis can occur with meningioma involving the intracranial optic nerve (McDonald, 1982). The mechanism is uncertain but may be related to the occurrence of infarction of part of the tumor with attendant reversible swelling. Aneurysm is not infrequently associated with spontaneous fluctuations in visual acuity and in form and extent of field loss for days or even minutes; such rapid events presumably have a vascular basis (McDonald, 1982). Phosphenes may occur but are of little or no localizing value (Weinberger and Grant, 1940).

Chiasmal compression is associated with certain characteristic visual disturbances (Kirkham, 1972; Nachtigäller and Hoyt, 1970; see Chapter 28). Some are due to a failure to maintain a stable relationship between the surviving nasal fields: vertical slip (hemifield slide) leads to a tendency in reading for the patient to drop prematurely to a lower line. With horizontal slip, words or letters run into each other or conversely letters are omitted or duplicated within a word (e.g., "door" may become "dor" or "dooor"). Patients with bitemporal field loss may find difficulty threading a needle or cutting fingernails even when the visual acuity is well preserved; objects behind the point of fixation fall into the blind temporal fields and become invisible—postfixational blindness. Testing for this phenomenon can be useful in detecting a small bitemporal scotomatous defect.

Headache, often referred to the vertex, is common in patients with pituitary tumors but is not usually severe. Aneurysm may be accompanied by severe pain with vascular characteristics and may be temporarily relieved by carotid compression.

Clinical evidence of the localization and extent of masses in this region is provided by the visual field defects and involvement of neighboring structures. The variety and significance of the field defects are described in Chapter 28. Here it should be noted in addition that partial superior bitemporal quadrantic defects may be found in association with congenital tilting of the optic discs. Such defects have no pathologic significance. Pituitary tumors often produce endocrine symptoms (see Chapter 40), although the latter can arise from secondary involvement of the pituitary or the hypothalamus by other tumors. Subfrontal meningioma may betray its presence by unilateral anosmia. Aneurysm or tumor involving the cavernous sinus often affects cranial nerve V, producing impairment of the corneal reflex or sensory loss in the face. There may be an oculomotor palsy, sometimes with evidence of aberrant reinnervation.

Investigation

Plain radiographs may still be a useful part of the preliminary assessment, although CT and MRI are the investigations of choice. If the pituitary fossa is normal, a chiasmal syndrome is unlikely to be due to a tumor of the gland. Craniopharyngiomas show calcification on CT scan in 70–93% of children and 30–67% of adults (Sorva et al., 1987). Although MRI cannot demonstrate calcification directly, it is better for determining tumor extent and detecting multiloculation that, when seen, is diagnostically useful. A minority of craniopharyngiomas arise from within the pituitary fossa. Curvilinear calcification may be seen in large aneurysms, which may erode the fossa from the side, mimicking primary intrasellar lesions. Meningiomas in this region often produce an increase in bone density, which is particularly helpful in diagnosing meningiomas en plaque, which may have little or no visible soft tissue component. Meningiomas can often be differentiated from pituitary lesions

by their tendency to creep over the edge of the fossa and produce underlying hyperostosis. It is therefore important to request CT bone windows if some of these lesions are not to be missed. Destruction of the clivus suggests a chordoma.

Although high-resolution CT readily detects tumors in this region, MRI offers several advantages. First, the extent of the tumor is usually better appreciated. Second, the chiasm is usually well seen, and the degree of compression can be assessed. Third, in our experience, MRI has replaced the need for preoperative angiography in most patients with pituitary tumor, as the major vessels are well shown, although angiography is occasionally performed if there is doubt after MRI. Fourth, enhancement with gadolinium may show extension of tumor not visible by other means. CT is superior to MRI for detecting bony changes and demonstrating the anatomy of the relevant sinuses before operation. The two imaging modalities therefore remain complementary in the assessment of these patients. VEP examination with half-field stimulation is often helpful in defining the localization and extent of the tumor, especially in the early stages (Halliday and McDonald, 1981).

Treatment

The approach to the treatment of a tumor of the pituitary gland that compresses the anterior visual pathways depends on whether or not it is a prolactinoma. If it is, the initial treatment is with bromocriptine, but the patients must be followed for the duration of this treatment with visual field examination and determination of prolactin levels: a small proportion of patients with prolactinomas treated in this way are cured. Even if surgery is indicated for a large prolactinoma, some surgeons advise a short preoperative course of bromocriptine. Women receiving this drug should be followed particularly carefully during pregnancy because of the risk of sudden tumor enlargement. Although some physicians have advised the use of bromocriptine in other types of pituitary tumor, we have seen a number of patients with progressive visual deterioration after initial modest improvement. Surgery, usually with postoperative radiotherapy, is the recommended treatment for nonprolactinomas causing chiasmal compression. The transsphenoidal approach is preferred, unless the direction of tumor extension out of the fossa precludes removal by this route. Even then, some surgeons debulk large tumors transsphenoidally before going on to a transfrontal resection.

Radical surgery for craniopharyngiomas should be performed if possible, followed by radiotherapy if removal is incomplete. Most meningiomas should be removed as soon as possible, the exceptions being en plaque lesions without an appreciable space-occupying component, and cavernous sinus meningiomas, which are not usually resectable but which fortunately tend to progress rather slowly. The role of radiotherapy in these, and in incompletely removed lesions, remains to be established. Aneurysms should be dealt with on their merits: large lesions tend to contain much clot and rupture only infrequently.

One of the remarkable features of the surgical treatment of tumors of the anterior visual pathways is the speed with which initial improvement may occur, and the completeness of recovery in some cases, even when nerve fiber loss and optic atrophy are appreciable (Kayan and Earl, 1975). The mechanisms were reviewed by Clifford-Jones et al. (1985). Although the management of some of the more important lesions that may compress the anterior visual pathways is described earlier, a full account is beyond the scope of this chapter. Certain principles should, however, be emphasized. The first is that, despite the fluctuations already mentioned, the course is generally downhill. Second, the longer a tumor compresses the visual pathways, the more limited is recovery. Third, there is the question of the fitness of the patient to withstand one or another form of intracranial surgery. Finally, as illustrated by the management of young-onset orbital optic nerve sheath meningioma, there are special considerations in relation to the compressing mass—its pathologic nature, its natural history, and its location. The decision by the physician as to whether to treat and what form of treatment to recommend must take all these factors, together with the preferences and particular skills of his or her neurosurgical colleagues, into account.

References

(Key references are designated with an asterisk.)

Awerbuch G., Labadie E.L., Van Dalen J.T. Reversible optic neuritis secondary to paranasal sinusitis. *Eur. Neurol.* 29:189–193, 1989.

Beri M., Klugman M.R., Kohler J.A., et al. Anterior ischemic optic neuropathy. VII. Incidence of bilaterality and various influencing factors. *Ophthalmology* 94:1020–1028, 1987.

*Boghen D.R., Glaser J.S. Ischaemic optic neuropathy. The clinical profile and natural history. *Brain* 98:689–708, 1975.

Borchert M., Lessell S. Progressive and recurrent nonarteritic anterior ischemic optic neuropathy. *Am. J. Ophthalmol.* 106:443–449, 1988.

Borit A., Richardson E.P. Jr. The biological and clinical behaviour of pilocytic astrocytomas of the optic pathways. *Brain* 105:161–187, 1982.

Bradbury P.G., Levy I.S., McDonald W.I. Transient uniocular visual loss on deviation of the eye in association with intraorbital tumours. *J. Neurol. Neurosurg. Psychiatry* 50:615–619, 1987.

Carroll W.M., Mastaglia F.L. Leber's optic neuropathy. A clinical and visual evoked potential study of affected and asymptomatic members of a six generation family. *Brain* 102:559–580, 1979.

Clifford-Jones R.E., Ellis C.J.K., Stephens J.M., et al. Cavernous sinus thrombosis. *J. Neurol. Neurosurg. Psychiatry* 45:1092–1097, 1982.

Clifford-Jones R.E., McDonald W.I., Landon D.N. Chronic optic nerve compression. An experimental study. *Brain* 108:241–262, 1985.

Cremers C.W.J.R., Wijdeveld P.G.A.B., Pinckers A.J.L.G. Juvenile diabetes mellitus, optic atrophy, hearing loss, diabetes insipidus, atonia of the urinary tract and bladder, and other abnormalities (Wolfram syndrome). *Acta Neurol. Scand. Suppl.* 264:3–16, 1977.

Drance S.M. Ischaemic optic neuropathy. *Trans. Ophthalmol. Soc.* 96:415–417, 1976.

Eidelberg D., Newton M.R., Johnson G., et al. Chronic unilateral optic neuropathy: a magnetic resonance study. *Ann. Neurol.* 24:3–11, 1988.

Foulds W.S., Pettigrew A.R. Tobacco alcohol amblyopia. In Brockhurst R.J., Boruchoff S.A., Hutchinson B.T., et al., eds. *Controversy in Ophthalmology*. Philadelphia, Saunders, pp. 851–865, 1977.

Fowler T.J., Earl C.J., McAllister V.L., et al. Tolosa-Hunt syndrome. The dangers of an eponym. *Br. J. Ophthalmol.* 59:149–154, 1975.

Francis D.A., Compston D.A.S., Batchelor J.R., et al. A reassessment of the risk of multiple sclerosis developing in patients with optic neuritis after extended follow-up. *J. Neurol. Neurosurg. Psychiatry* 50:758–765, 1987.

Frisén L., Hoyt W.F. Insidious atrophy of retinal nerve fibres in multiple sclerosis. *Arch Ophthalmol.* 92:91–97, 1974.

Glaser J.S. *Neuroophthalmology*. 2nd ed. Philadelphia, Lippincott, p. 118, 1990.

Goto Y., Hosokawa S., Goto I., et al. Abnormality in the cavernous sinus in three patients with Tolosa-Hunt syndrome: MRI and CT findings. *J. Neurol. Neurosurg. Psychiatry* 53:231–234, 1990.

Gould E.S., Bird A.C., Leaver P.K., et al. Treatment of optic neuritis by retrobulbar injection of triamcinolone. *Br. Med. J.* 1:1495–1497, 1977.

Guy J., Sherwood M., Day A.L. Surgical treatment of progressive visual loss in traumatic optic neuropathy. *J. Neurosurg.* 70:799–801, 1989.

Halliday A.M., McDonald W.I. Visual evoked potentials. In Stalberg E., Young R.R., eds. *Neurology. Clinical Neurophysiology*. Vol. 1. London, Butterworth, pp. 228–258, 1981.

Halliday A.M., McDonald W.I., Mushin J. Delayed visual evoked response in optic neuritis. *Lancet* 1:982–985, 1972.

Hamed L.M., Winyard K.E., Glaser J.S., et al. Optic neuropathy in uraemia. *Am. J. Ophthalmol.* 108:30–35, 1989.

Hely M.A., McManis P.G., Doran T.J., et al. Acute optic neuritis: a prospective study of risk factors for multiple sclerosis. *J. Neurol. Neurosurg. Psychiatry* 49:1125–1130, 1986.

*Henderson J.W. *Orbital Tumors*. Philadelphia, Saunders, p. 705, 1973.

Hennerici M., Wenzel D., Freund H-J. The comparison of small-size rectangle and checkerboard stimulation for the evaluation of delayed visual evoked responses in patients suspected of multiple sclerosis. *Brain* 100:119–136, 1977.

Holt I.J., Miller D.H., Harding A.E. Genetic heterogeneity and mitochondrial DNA heteroplasmy in Leber's hereditary optic neuropathy. *J. Med. Genet.* 26:739–743, 1989.

Hoyt W.F., Meshel L.G., Lessell S., et al. Malignant optic glioma of adulthood. *Brain* 96:121–132, 1973.

Ikeda H., Tremain K.E., Sanders M.D. Neurophysiological investigation in optic nerve disease: combined assessment of the visual evoked response and electroretinogram. *Br. J. Ophthalmol.* 62:227–239, 1978.

Imachi J. Neurosurgical treatment of Leber's optic atrophy and its pathogenetic relationship to arachnoiditis. In Brunette J., Barbeau A., eds. *Progress in Neuroophthalmology*. Amsterdam, Excerpta Medica, pp. 121–127, 1969.

Isayama Y., Takahashi T., Shimoyoma T., et al. Acute optic neuritis and multiple sclerosis. *Neurology (N.Y.)* 32:73–76, 1982.

Jakobiec F.A., Jones I.S. Orbital inflammations. In Jones I.S., Jakobiec F.A., eds. *Diseases of the Orbit*. New York, Harper & Row, pp. 187–267, 1979.

*Kayan A., Earl C.J. Compressive lesions of the optic nerves and chiasm. Pattern of recovery of vision following surgical treatment. *Brain* 98:13–28, 1975.

Kennerdall J.S., Maroon J.C., Malton M., et al. The management of optic nerve sheath meningiomas. *Am. J. Ophthalmol.* 106:450–457, 1988.

Kermode A.G., Plant G.T., Miller D.H., et al. Tobacco-alcohol amblyopia and Leber's optic neuropathy: magnetic resonance imaging findings. *J. Neurol. Neurosurg. Psychiatry* 52:147, 1989.

Kirkham T.H. The ocular symptomatology of pituitary tumours. *Proc. R. Soc. Med.* 65:517–518, 1972.

Knox D.L., Hanneken A.M., Hollows F.C., et al. Uraemic optic neuropathy. *Arch. Ophthalmol.* 106:50–54, 1988.

Kollarits C.R., Pinheiro M.L., Swann E.R., et al. The autosomal dominant syndrome of progressive optic atrophy and congenital deafness. *Am. J. Ophthalmol.* 87:789–792, 1979.

Kriss A., Francis D.A., Cuendet F., et al. Recovery after optic neuritis in childhood. *J. Neurol. Neurosurg. Psychiatry* 51:1253–1258, 1988.

Krumsiek J., Kruger C., Patzold U. Tobacco-alcohol amblyopia neuro-ophthalmological findings and clinical course. *Acta Neurol. Scand.* 72:180–187, 1985.

Lehrer R.I., Howard D.H., Sypherd P.S., et al. Mucormycosis. *Ann. Intern. Med.* 93:93–108, 1980.

Lightman S., McDonald W.I., Bird A.C., et al. Retinal venous sheathing in optic neuritis. *Brain* 110:405–414, 1987.

*McDonald W.I. The symptomatology of tumours of the anterior visual pathways. The 1981 Silversides Lecture. *Can. J. Neurol. Sci.* 9:381–390, 1982.

*McDonald W.I. Doyne Lecture. The significance of optic neuritis. *Trans. Ophthalmol. Soc. U. K.* 103:230–246, 1983.

Miller D.H., Newton M.R., van der Poel J.C., et al. Magnetic resonance imaging of the optic nerve in optic neuritis. *Neurology* 38:175–179, 1988a.

Miller D.H., Ormerod I.E.C., McDonald W.I., et al. The early risk of multiple sclerosis after optic neuritis. *J. Neurol. Neurosurg. Psychiatry* 51:1569–1571, 1988b.

*Miller N.R. *Walsh and Hoyt's Clinical Neuroophthalmology.* Vol. 1. 4th ed. Baltimore, Williams & Wilkins, 1982.

Moulin D., Paty D.W., Ebers G.C. The predictive value of cerebrospinal fluid electrophoresis in "possible" multiple sclerosis. *Brain* 106:809–816, 1983.

Mullen K.T., Plant G.T. Colour and luminance vision in optic neuritis. *Brain* 109:1–14, 1986.

Nachtigäller H., Hoyt W.F. Störungen des Seheindruckes bei bitemporaler Hemianopsie und Verschiebung der Sehachsen. *Klin. Monatsbl. Augenheilk.* 156:821–836, 1970.

Nikoskelainen E., Frey H., Salmi A. Prognosis of optic neuritis and measles virus antibodies. *Ann. Neurol.* 9:545–550, 1980.

*Nikoskelainen E., Hoyt W.F., Nummelin K. Ophthalmoscopic findings in Leber's hereditary optic neuropathy. I. The fundus findings in asymptomatic family members. *Arch. Ophthalmol.* 100:1597–1602, 1982.

Nikoskelainen E., Hoyt W.F., Nummelin K. Ophthalmoscopic findings in Leber's hereditary optic neuropathy. II. The fundus findings in affected family members. *Arch. Ophthalmol.* 101:1059–1068, 1983.

Ormerod I.E.C., McDonald W.I. Multiple sclerosis presenting with progressive visual failure. *J. Neurol. Neurosurg. Psychiatry* 47:943–946, 1984.

Page N.G.R., Bolger J.P., Sanders M.D. Auditory evoked phosphenes in optic nerve disease. *J. Neurol. Neurosurg. Psychiatry* 45:7–12, 1982.

Parker W.D., Oley C.A., Parks J.K. A defect in mitochondrial electron-transport activity (NADH-coenzyme Q oxidoreductase) in Leber's hereditary optic neuropathy. *N. Engl. J. Med.* 320:1331–1333, 1989.

Parkin P.J., Heirons R., McDonald W.I. Bilateral optic neuritis. A long-term follow up. *Brain* 107:951–964, 1984.

Potts A.M. Tobacco amblyopia. *Surv. Ophthalmol.* 17:313–331, 1973.

Prineas J., Connell F. Remyelination in multiple sclerosis. *Ann. Neurol.* 5:22–31, 1979.

Puvanendran K., Devathasan G., Wong P.K. Visual evoked responses in diabetes. *J. Neurol. Neurosurg. Psychiatry* 46:643–647, 1983.

Rizzo J.F., Lessell S. Posterior ischaemic optic neuropathy during general surgery. *Am. J. Ophthalmol.* 103:808–811, 1987.

Rizzo J.F., Lessell S. Risk of developing multiple sclerosis after uncomplicated optic neuritis: a long-term prospective study. *Neurology* 38:185–190, 1988.

Russell D.S., Rubinstein L.J. *Pathology of Tumours of the Nervous System.* 5th ed. London, Arnold, 1989.

Sandberg-Wollheim M., Bynke H., Cronqvist S., et al. A long-term prospective study of optic neuritis: evaluation of risk factors. *Ann. Neurol.* 27:386–393, 1990.

Sanders M.D., Gay A.J., Newman M. Haemorrhagic complications of drusen of the optic disc. *Am. J. Ophthalmol.* 71:204–217, 1971.

Sanders M.D., Sennhenn R.H. Differential diagnosis of unilateral optic disc oedema. *Trans. Ophthalmol. Soc. U.K.* 100:123–131, 1980.

Sergott R.C., Cohen M.S., Bosley T.M., et al. Optic nerve decompression may improve the progressive form of nonarteritic ischaemic optic neuropathy. *Arch. Ophthalmol.* 107:1743–1754, 1989.

Smith D.P. Diagnostic criteria in dominantly inherited juvenile optic atrophy: a report of three new families. *Am. J. Optom.* 49:183–200, 1972.

Smith J.L., Hoyt W.F., Susac J.O. Ocular fundus in acute Leber's optic atrophy. *Arch. Ophthalmol.* 90:349–354, 1973.

Sorva R., Jaaskinen J., Heiskanen O. Craniopharyngioma in children and adults. Correlations between radiological and clinical manifestations. *Acta Neurochir.* 89:3–9, 1987.

Tso M.O.M., Hayreh S.S. Optic disc edema in raised intracranial pressure: III. A pathologic study of experimental papilledema. *Arch. Ophthalmol.* 95:1448–1457, 1977a.

Tso M.O.M., Hayreh S.S. Optic disc edema in raised intracranial pressure: IV. Axoplasmic transport in experimental papilledema. *Arch. Ophthalmol.* 95:1458–1462, 1977b.

Wallace D.C. A new manifestation of Leber's disease and a new explanation for the agency responsible for its unusual pattern of inheritance. *Brain* 93:121–132, 1970.

Wallace D.C., Singh G., Lott M.T., et al. Mitochondrial DNA mutation associated with Leber's hereditary optic neuropathy. *Science* 242:1427–1430, 1988.

Weinberger I.M., Grant F.C. Visual hallucinations and their neuro-optical correlates. *Arch. Ophthalmol.* 32:166–199, 1940.

Weinstein J.M., Morris G.L., ZuRhein G.M., et al. Posterior ischaemic optic neuropathy due to *Aspergillus fumigatus*. *J. Clin. Neuro. Ophthalmol.* 9:7–13, 1989.

Winyard K.E., Hamed L.M., Glaser J.S. The spectrum of optic nerve disease in human immunodeficiency virus infection. *Am. J. Ophthalmol.* 107:373–380, 1989.

Wright J.E., McNab A.A., McDonald W.I. Optic nerve glioma and the management of optic nerve tumours in the young. *Br. J. Ophthalmol.* 73:967–974, 1989a.

Wright J.E., McNab A.A., McDonald W.I. Primary optic nerve sheath meningioma. *Br. J. Ophthalmol.* 73:960–966, 1989b.

Wulc A.E., Bergin D.J., Barnes D., et al. Orbital optic nerve glioma in adult life. *Arch. Ophthalmol.* 107:1013–1016, 1989.

Youl B.D., Miller D.H., MacManus D.G., et al. Optic nerves show gadolinium enhancement in early optic neuritis. *Neuroradiology* 33(Suppl.):129–130, 1991.

Young G. Retrobulbar neuritis of sphenoidal sinus origin. *J. Laryngol. Otol.* 39:381–383, 1924.

30

Disorders of Hearing

Linda M. Luxon

The eighth cranial nerve lies in the internal auditory meatus of the petrous portion of the temporal bone and is unique in subserving two sensory functions: hearing and balance. This chapter is concerned with auditory function; vestibular disorders are fully covered in Chapter 31.

ANATOMY AND PHYSIOLOGY

Sound is transduced by the hair cells of the organ of Corti into neural activity, which is transmitted along the cochlear division of the eighth cranial nerve. This nerve consists of fibers from three types of neurons (Fig. 30–1) (Spoendlin, 1984): (1) afferent neurons, which lie in the spiral ganglion and connect the cochlea to the brain stem; (2) efferent olivococh-

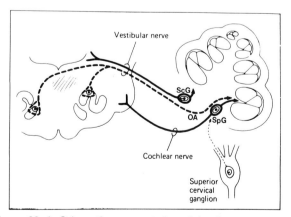

Figure 30–1. Schematic representation of the three components innervating the cochlea. Heavy line, afferent neuron; heavy interrupted line, efferent olivocochlear neuron; fine interrupted line, autonomic adrenergic neuron. ScG = Scarpa ganglion; OA = Oort anastomosis; SpG = spiral ganglion. (From Spoendlin H. Primary neurons and synapses. In Friedmann I., Ballantyne J., eds. *Ultrastructural Atlas of the Inner Ear*. London, Butterworth, pp. 133–164, 1984.)

lear neurons, which originate in the superior olivary complex; and (3) autonomic adrenergic neurons, which originate in the cervical sympathetic trunk and innervate the cochlea.

In the human, there are approximately 30,000 afferent cochlear neurons, with myelinated axons each consisting of about 50 lamellae, and 4–6 μm in diameter. This histologic structure forms the basis of a uniform conduction velocity, which is an important functional feature. Throughout the length of the auditory nerve, there is a tonotopic arrangement of afferent fibers, with "basal" fibers wrapped over the centrally placed "apical" fibers in a twisted rope-like fashion.

Spoendlin (1978) identified two types of afferent neurons in the spiral ganglion on the basis of morphologic differences:

Type I cells (95%) are bipolar and have myelinated cell bodies and axons that project to the inner hair cells.
Type II cells (5%) are monopolar with unmyelinated axons and project to the outer hair cells of the organ of Corti.

Each inner hair cell is innervated by about 20 fibers, each of which synapses on only one cell. In contrast, each outer hair cell is innervated by approximately six fibers, and each fiber branches to supply approximately 10 cells (Fig. 30–2).

The efferent cochlear supply originates as a group of approximately 500 fibers, which emerge from the brain stem in the vestibular nerve and cross over to the auditory nerve via the Oort bundle. Approximately 80% of the efferent fibers originate in the contralateral superior olivary complex, whereas the remainder arise ipsilaterally (Rasmussen, 1942). Within the cochlea, the fibers divide into (1) an inner spiral group, which arises primarily ipsilaterally and synapses with the afferent neurons to the inner hair cells, and (2) a more numerous outer radial group,

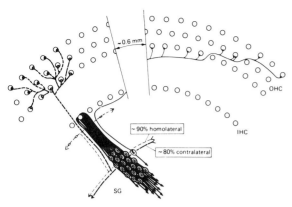

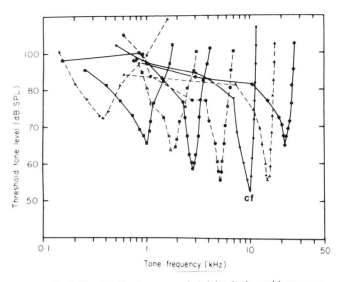

Figure 30–2. Horizontal innervation scheme of the organ of Corti of the cat. OHC = outer hair cell; IHC = inner hair cell; SG = spiral ganglion; solid lines = afferent nerve fibers; thick interrupted lines = efferent nerve fibers to outer hair cells; thin interrupted lines = efferent nerve fibers to inner hair cells; 0.6 mm = average length of the basal spiral course of the outer spiral fibers. (From Spoendlin H. Primary neurons and synapses. In Friedmann I., Ballantyne J., eds. *Ultrastructural Atlas of the Inner Ear*. London, Butterworth, pp. 133–164, 1984.)

Figure 30–4. Family of tuning curves for eight single cochlear nerve fibers of the guinea pig. CF = characteristic frequency. (From Evans E.F. Pathophysiology of hearing. In Lutman M.E., Haggard M.P., eds. *Hearing Science and Hearing Disorders*. London, Academic Press, pp. 61–80, 1983.)

which arises mainly contralaterally and synapses directly with the outer hair cells (Fig. 30–3).

On entering the brain stem, the auditory nerve bifurcates to send a branch to each of the dorsal and ventral divisions of the cochlear nuclei. The tonotopic arrangement of fibers, which was identified in the auditory nerve, is preserved, with basal fibers projecting dorsally and apical fibers projecting ventrally.

By inserting fine microelectrodes into single cochlear nerve fibers of anesthetized animals, the pattern of response of individual fibers to different audio frequencies and intensities has been identified and plotted as a tuning curve (Fig. 30–4). There is a minimal threshold at one frequency, the characteristic or best frequency, but the threshold rises sharply for frequencies above and below this level (Pickles, 1982). Single auditory nerve fibers therefore appear to behave as band-pass filters. The basilar membrane vibrates preferentially to different frequencies, at different distances along its length, and the fre-

quency selectivity of each cochlear nerve fiber is similar to that of the inner hair cell to which the fiber is connected. Thus, each cochlear nerve fiber exhibits a tuning curve covering a different range of frequencies from its neighboring fiber (Evans, 1979). By this mechanism, complex sounds are broken down into component frequencies (frequency resolution) by the filters of the inner ear. Kemp (1978) showed that the ear not only receives sounds but also generates auditory activity, and it has been postulated that this activity may in some way provide positive feedback and enhance the sensitivity and sharpness of tuning of the auditory filters.

PATHOPHYSIOLOGY

Sensory degeneration and neural degeneration do not occur independently (Johnsson, 1974), and there is a good correlation between the extent and severity of hair cell loss and nerve degeneration in the osseous spiral lamina. Complete degeneration of the end organ is associated with severe loss of afferent neurons, but the cochlear efferent fibers remain intact. If the supporting elements of the organ of Corti survive, cochlear neural degeneration is delayed despite severe hair cell loss (Hinojosa and Lindsay, 1980).

Experimentally, many noxious stimuli (e.g., ischemia, hypoxia, mechanical trauma, surgical interference, noise trauma, and drugs) have been shown to produce outer hair cell damage before inner hair cell damage, and single auditory fiber studies have indicated that auditory sensitivity is lost and frequency resolution decreased by such noxious agents (Pickles, 1982). Other studies have documented a reduction in the spontaneous activity of the auditory nerve

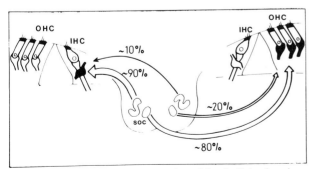

Figure 30–3. Schematic representation of the ipsilateral and contralateral efferent nerve supply from the superior olivary complex. OHC = outer hair cell; IHC = inner hair cell; SOC = superior olivary complex. (From Spoendlin H. Primary neurons and synapses. In Friedmann I., Ballantyne J. eds. *Ultrastructural Atlas of the Inner Ear*. London, Butterworth, pp. 133–164, 1984.)

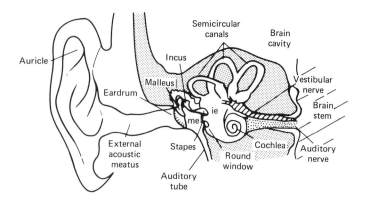

Figure 30–5. Diagram of external ear, middle ear (me), inner ear (ie), and eighth cranial nerve (Adapted from Moore B.C.J. *Introduction to the Psychology of Hearing.* London, Macmillan, p. 14, 1977.)

after hair cell damage (Liberman and Kiang, 1978). These pathophysiologic changes have been demonstrated to be associated with the loss of frequency resolution and reduced threshold sensitivity, which are characteristic of sensorineural hearing loss. Sensitivity may be improved with amplification, but frequency resolution cannot—hence the complaint of the patient: "Please do not shout; I can hear you. Speak clearly."

Primary neuronal degeneration as a cause of sensorineural hearing loss has been considered rare, but Suga and Lindsay (1976) found this to be the most prominent histopathologic change in the temporal bones of 17 aged patients. It would therefore appear that purely neural hearing loss may occur, but more often, clinically pathologic changes of the cochlea result in changes in both the sensory and the neural elements, which makes a clinical distinction between end-organ and/or eighth cranial nerve damage extremely difficult. Clinically, pathologic alteration of the cochlear nerve may be associated with hearing loss or tinnitus or both.

Hearing loss may be divided into two types: conductive and sensorineural. Conductive hearing loss is secondary to pathologic changes of the middle ear (Fig. 30–5), whereas sensorineural hearing loss results most commonly from cochlea, less commonly from auditory nerve, and rarely from central auditory dysfunction.

For the clinician attempting to differentiate sensorineural loss of cochlear origin from that of neural origin, two pathophysiologic phenomena are important: loudness recruitment and abnormal auditory adaptation. In 1948, Dix et al. reported that *loudness recruitment* (an abnormally rapid increase in loudness, with an increase in the intensity of the stimulus) is consistently associated with disorders affecting the hair cells of the organ of Corti, whereas it is characteristically absent in deafness related to structural damage of the cochlear nerve fibers. Loudness of the stimulus depends on the total activity within the auditory nerves. As the stimulus intensity rises, the number of fibers activated is initially small while only the frequency-specific segments of the tuning curves are activated, but the number increases abruptly when the tails of the tuning curves are encountered

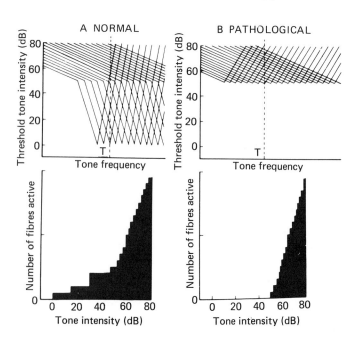

Figure 30–6. A neural explanation of loudness recruitment. Loudness in the abnormal ear grows with intensity after the threshold is reached, because the tips of the tuning curves are missing. (From Evans E.F. The sharpening of cochlea frequency selectivity in the normal and abnormal cochlea. *Audiology* 14:419–442, 1979.)

(Fig. 30–6A). In the pathologic ear (Fig. 30–6B), the tuning curves of the cochlear nerve fibers are less sharp than normal, and there is therefore greater overlap of effective frequency ranges. Thus, when the fibers are stimulated by a frequency above the elevated threshold, the increase in the number of fibers activated for a given increase in stimulus level is greater than normal. The perceived loudness of the sound therefore grows more steeply with intensity than normal. In addition, pathologic nerve fibers exhibit a greater than normal increase of activity with intensity after the threshold has been reached. The relative importance of these two mechanisms in the phenomenon of loudness recruitment is not known.

Abnormal auditory adaptation was first documented by Gradenigo in 1893, who reported that patients with acoustic tumors could hear a maximally vibrating tuning fork for only a few seconds. Classically, patients with an eighth cranial nerve disorder exhibit marked auditory adaptation, in contrast to patients with cochlear hearing loss, who do not show this derangement. Adaptation refers to the slow decrease in discharge frequency with time, which is observed after an initial burst of neural activity in response to an adequate stimulus applied to the end organ. In the presence of neural dysfunction, although the initial response may be normal or near-normal, the response to a continuous stimulus cannot be maintained at the normal level. Clinically, if a continuous tone is presented to either ear, the patient perceives that the tone fades during a given period, and there is said to be abnormal auditory adaptation or *tone decay* (see later).

Tinnitus may be defined as the perception of sound that originates from within the head rather than from the external world. The conditions with which tinnitus is associated and the proposed mechanisms by which tinnitus originates are legion, but in most instances the pathophysiology of the symptom remains obscure. Tinnitus is frequently but not always associated with hearing impairment, and the proposed pathophysiologic mechanisms include decoupling in the stereocilia of the hair cells; misinterpretation of auditory neural activity by higher auditory centers; and self-sustaining oscillation of the basilar membrane, consequent on the evoked cochlear mechanical response (McFadden, 1982). The mechanisms implicating the cochlear nerve are briefly reviewed here.

One popular theory is that of an abnormality of spontaneous resting activity of primary auditory nerve fibers, either as a result of hypo- or hyperexcitability of damaged hair cells or as a direct consequence of some derangement of the primary neurons themselves. Single-fiber studies with animals that have been subjected to ototoxic stimuli (noise, drugs, or mechanical trauma) that are known to produce tinnitus in humans have revealed conflicting results. Liberman and Kiang (1978) showed reduced spontaneous rates in cats after intense noise exposure, whereas Schmiedt and co-workers (1980) showed increased spontaneous discharge rates of primary auditory fibers in gerbils after noise exposure. This difference may merely reflect species variation in the lesions produced by noise and emphasizes the need for an acceptable animal model of tinnitus.

Møller (1984) expounded the theory that tinnitus, in some instances, may be the result of derangement of the temporal pattern of auditory nerve discharges. He proposed that damage to the myelin sheath between auditory nerve fibers may allow ephaptic transmission (cross-talk) between adjacent nerve fibers, as previously proposed in cases of hemifacial spasm and trigeminal neuralgia (Jannetta, 1977; Kumagami, 1974) (see Chapter 3). Møller noted that the root entry zone of cranial nerves is particularly sensitive to mechanical pressure and emphasized that the auditory nerve is covered by central myelin for 15–20 mm (Bridger and Farkashidy, 1980), compared with only a few millimeters for the fifth and seventh cranial nerves. He concluded that the eighth cranial nerve is particularly vulnerable to damage to the myelin sheath.

Another less well documented mechanism for the development of tinnitus is a derangement of the efferent fibers of the eighth cranial nerve that produces aberrant auditory behavior (McFadden, 1982).

Unilateral tinnitus is a frequent early symptom of a tumor affecting the eighth cranial nerve (Brackmann, 1981), which is commonly associated with unilateral hearing loss. It is assumed that these cochlear symptoms are due to compression of the auditory nerve as the tumor on the vestibular division of the eighth cranial nerve grows in size. Little is known of tinnitus in other eighth cranial nerve disorders, although Jannetta (1975, 1980) reported relief of tinnitus after decompression of blood vessels pressing on the eighth cranial nerve.

Investigation

Investigation of the auditory system to identify eighth cranial nerve lesions should be accompanied by appropriate assessment of the vestibular system, because anatomically the two systems are intimately related from the peripheral labyrinth to the brain stem (see Fig. 30–5). Standard vestibular investigation allows differentiation of peripheral labyrinthine and eighth cranial nerve lesions from more central vestibular lesions; Pfaltz (1969) has emphasized the diagnostic importance of galvanic stimulation of the vestibular system. On the basis of his work in Menier's disease, he maintained that "the galvanic test is the only diagnostic procedure allowing differentiation of an end-organ lesion from a lesion of the peripheral neuron."

In attempting to identify a sensorineural hearing loss of auditory nerve origin, it is necessary to exclude cochlear and central auditory pathologic changes (Berlin, 1976). For the common clinical task of differentiating primary cochlear from eighth cranial nerve dysfunction, it is generally accepted that an auditory test battery is required (Grant, 1981), including threshold assessment, a test of abnormal auditory adaptation, a test of recruitment (most commonly by means of acoustic reflex measurements), speech audiometry, and electrophysiologic assessment.

Audiometry

Pure-Tone Audiometry. In this most widely available quantitative test of hearing threshold, electrically generated pure tones are delivered by an earphone or bone conductor, and the minimal intensity audible to a patient is recorded at frequencies between 125 and 8000 Hz. Thresholds in patients with cochlear nerve dysfunction may range from normal in the early stages to total hearing loss in the later stages. A unilateral, or asymmetric (between the two ears), sensorineural hearing loss requires careful investigation to exclude a vestibular schwannoma.

Békésy's Audiometry. In this self-recording form of audiometry (Békésy, 1947), the patient adjusts the intensity of a continuous or a pulsed tone to a level that is just audible as it sweeps across the test range of frequencies. The results provide information on auditory threshold, recruitment, and abnormal auditory adaptation. Jerger (1960) classified four diagnostic categories (Fig. 30–7). In eighth cranial nerve dysfunction, the diagnostic sensitivity may be increased by conducting the tests at a comfortable level of loudness rather than at the threshold level. In

addition, further diagnostic information may be obtained by comparing a forward sweep of the test frequencies with a backward sweep, and the following criteria are considered to provide good evidence of an eighth cranial nerve lesion, particularly at 500 and 1000 Hz (Jerger et al., 1972):

1. 10-dB separation across at least two octaves
2. 30-dB separation across at least one octave
3. 50-dB separation across at least one-half of an octave

Tests of Abnormal Auditory Adaptation

Tests of abnormal auditory adaptation are of particular value in identification of eighth cranial nerve lesions (Morales-Garcia and Hood, 1972). At threshold levels, the tone decay test may fail to identify eighth cranial nerve lesions, and certain workers therefore favor the suprathreshold adaptation test (Jerger and Jerger, 1975). A pure tone of 100 dB is presented to the test ear for 60 seconds and the patient is asked to signal as long as the test tone is heard. If on two occasions the tone decays, the test is repeated with a pulsed tone. If the pulsed tone is heard but the continuous tone decays, the test result is considered to be positive for a neural lesion.

Abnormal auditory adaptation may also be measured by using Békésy's audiometry (see Fig. 30–7) and by measuring acoustic reflex decay (see later).

Tests of Loudness Recruitment

Equal Loudness Balance Test. In unilateral hearing loss, the equal loudness balance test of Fowler (1936) is the most simple test for recruitment. Pure tones of the same frequency but different intensities are delivered alternately to the left and right ears until the patient signals that the tones appear to be of equal loudness in each ear. The intensity levels of tones giving a sensation of equal loudness are plotted right ear against left ear (Fig. 30–8). The presence or absence of recruitment may then be judged.

Loudness Discomfort Levels. In bilateral hearing impairment, determination of loudness discomfort levels provides a valuable means of assessing recruitment (Hood and Poole, 1966). The tests are carried out by using a standard audiometer at the time of the threshold assessment. Short tones of increasing intensity at each frequency are presented until the sound becomes uncomfortably loud. In the normal subject, this level is about 100 dB. In cochlear disease, loudness discomfort levels are often normal, and with increasing degrees of deafness, the threshold curve and the loudness discomfort level approach each other. In nerve fiber lesions, loudness recruitment is absent and loudness discomfort levels are markedly elevated (Fig. 30–9).

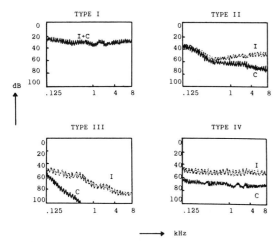

Figure 30–7. Diagram illustrating Jerger's classification of Békésy's tracings. Type I: the continuous (C) and pulsed (I, for interrupted pulse) tracings overlap throughout the recording—characteristic of normal ears and conduction disorders. Type II: pulsed and continuous tracings overlap at low frequencies, but at about 1.5 kHz they separate by 5–20 dB for the remainder of the test frequency range—characteristic of cochlear dysfunction. Type III: the continuous tracing drops away abruptly from the pulsed tracing almost as soon as the test begins—characteristic of severe abnormal auditory adaptation and almost pathognomonic of a retrocochlear lesion. Type IV: the continuous tracing runs below the pulsed tracing throughout the recording, showing some abnormal auditory adaptation even at low frequencies—most commonly seen in retrocochlear lesions.

Acoustic Reflex Measurements

The stapedius muscles contract bilaterally in response to a loud sound directed to either ear (Fig.

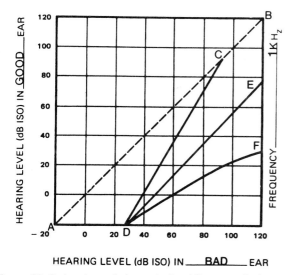

Figure 30–8. Loudness balance tests. AB = results in normal subject; DC = incomplete recruitment of cochlear origin. DE = in the absence of recruitment with a cochlear pathology; DF = in the presence of loudness reversal in the case of an acoustic neuroma. (From Luxon L.M. Diseases of the eighth cranial nerve. In Dyck P.J., Thomas P.K., Lambert E.H., et al. eds. *Peripheral Neuropathy.* 2nd ed. Philadelphia, Saunders, pp. 1300–1336, 1984.)

30–10). This contraction alters the acoustic impedance (i.e., the resistance to the passage of sound) of the middle ear, which may be measured by using an impedance bridge (Fig. 30–11). The minimal intensity of sound at a given frequency that produces contraction of the stapedius muscle is known as the *acoustic reflex threshold*. In eighth cranial nerve lesions, this reflex threshold is commonly elevated or absent (Fig. 30–12), but caution must be exercised in interpreting the results, because abnormalities of reflex thresholds may be found in disorders of the middle ear, seventh and eighth cranial nerves, cochlea, and brain stem (Wiley and Block, 1984). Characteristic patterns of ipsilateral and contralateral reflexes are, however, observed for different pathologic sites (Fig. 30–13). Decay of the stapedial reflex, which is a measure of abnormal auditory adaptation, is another feature observed in patients with eighth cranial nerve lesions. If a pure tone is presented continuously for 15 seconds, the reflex amplitude rapidly falls (Anderson et al., 1970), particularly at 500 and 1000 Hz.

Speech Audiometry

Classically, poor speech discrimination is reported in eighth cranial nerve disorders, but this result is by no means invariable (Dix, 1974). Many methods of determining the threshold of speech reception have been recorded. In 1971, Jerger and Jerger described a speech discrimination test using monosyllabic word lists, which would appear to differentiate between cochlear and eighth cranial nerve lesions by means of a "roll-over" ratio (Fig. 30–14). By this means, cochlear losses with maximal roll-over ratios of 0.40 were clearly separated from eighth cranial nerve lesions, in which the lowest ratio was 0.45. Jerger and Hayes (1977) reported another speech test in which a comparison of the results of phonemically balanced speech material and synthetic sentence material enabled identification of eighth cranial nerve disorders.

Electrophysiologic Tests

Electrophysiologic tests have provided a major advance in the last 2 decades in the identification and location of pathologic change in the auditory system.

Evoked Otoacoustic Emissions. Evoked otoacoustic emissions are low-level acoustic signals of cochlear origin, which can be recorded within the external auditory meatus in response to stimulation of the cochlea by clicks or short tone bursts. They are thought to reflect biomechanical activity within the outer hair cells of the organ of Corti and may lead to an objective means of differentiating cochlear from retrocochlear hearing loss (Kemp et al., 1990).

Brain Stem Auditory Evoked Responses. These evoked responses are obtained by averaging a series of potentials that are thought to be generated from the major processing centers of the auditory system in response to a repetitive sound stimulus (see Chapter 123). Although there is no uniform agreement as to the exact site of origin of each wave observed, the most generally accepted anatomic correlates are illustrated in Figure 30–15. However, Møller and coworkers (1988) suggested that both wave I and wave II reflect auditory nerve activity and that wave III is the earliest potential generated in the brain stem. They proposed that wave II reflects activity within

Figure 30–9. Loudness discomfort levels (L). *(A)* In a normal subject. *(B)* In a patient with a cochlear lesion. *(C)* In a patient with a neural lesion.

A

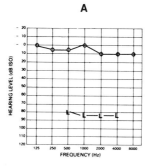

B

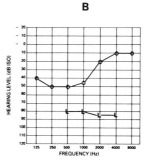

C

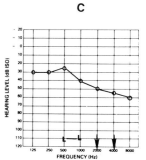

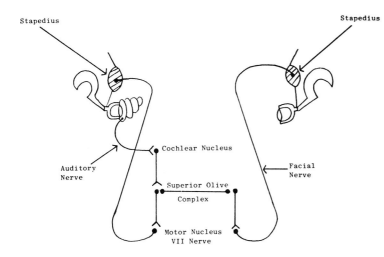

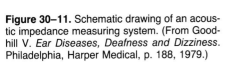

Figure 30–10. Diagram of the anatomic pathways of the stapedial reflex. (From Luxon L.M. Diseases of the eighth cranial nerve. In Dyck P.J., Thomas P.K., Lambert E.H., et al., eds. *Peripheral Neuropathy*. 2nd ed. Philadelphia, Saunders, pp. 1300–1336, 1984.)

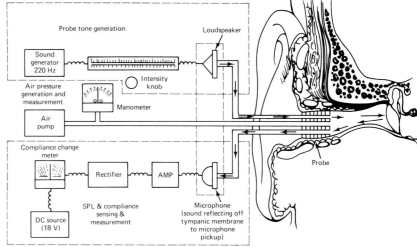

Figure 30–11. Schematic drawing of an acoustic impedance measuring system. (From Goodhill V. *Ear Diseases, Deafness and Dizziness*. Philadelphia, Harper Medical, p. 188, 1979.)

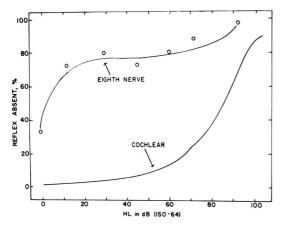

Figure 30–12. Diagram to illustrate stapedial reflex results in eighth cranial nerve and cochlear pathology. HL = hearing level. (From Jeger J., Hayes D. Clinical use of acoustic impedance testing in audiologic diagnosis. In Beagley H.A., ed. *Audiology and Audiological Medicine*. Vol. 2. New York, Oxford University Press, p. 718, 1981.)

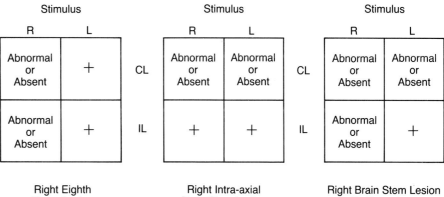

Figure 30–13. Patterns of stapedial reflex responses in eighth cranial nerve and brain stem lesions. CL = contralateral reflex; IL = ipsilateral reflex.

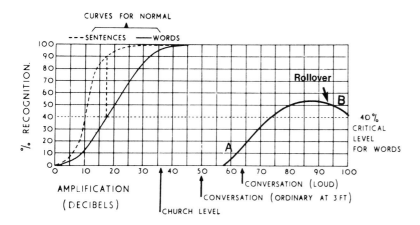

Figure 30–14. Speech discrimination curve for a normal subject and a patient with acoustic neuroma (AB) demonstrating a roll-over phenomenon. Roll-over ratio = (maximal score − minimal score)/maximal score, up to 110 dB. SPL = sound pressure level above roll-over point.

Figure 30–15. Diagram illustrating the anatomic correlates of the waves observed in the brain stem electrical response. (From Duane D.D. A neurological perspective of central auditory dysfunction. In Keith R.W., ed. *Central Auditory Dysfunction*. Orlando, FL, Grune & Stratton, p. 11, 1977. With permission of Psychological Corporation.)

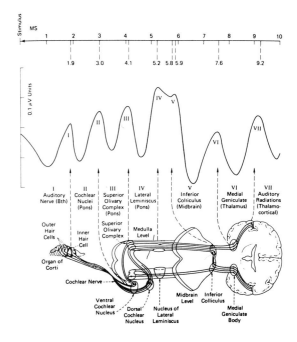

the intracranial portion of the auditory nerve, which thus explains the prolonged latency between peaks I and II in patients with surgically confirmed vascular compression of the eighth cranial nerve (Møller et al., 1986) and in patients with hereditary motor-sensory neuropathy type I (Charcot-Marie-Tooth disease) (Garg et al., 1982).

The brain stem auditory evoked response is highly reproducible in a given subject and shows little variation among normal subjects. Various parameters of this response may be studied to identify dysfunction, but in practice, latency abnormalities, particularly of wave V, appear to be the most consistent parameter (Clemis and Mitchell, 1977; Selters and Brackmann, 1977). In patients with retrocochlear hearing loss, there is a consistent interaural difference in the latency of wave V (Fig. 30–16), whereas in patients with cochlear lesions and loudness recruitment, there is a progressive disappearance, at high intensity of stimulation, of the interaural difference in the latency of wave V, which is observed at low intensities of stimulation. A further common finding in eighth cranial nerve disorders is the presence of wave I in the absence of wave V (Starr and Hamilton, 1976). In evaluating these disorders, Prasher (1982) demonstrated the value of interwave latency measurements, particularly the wave I–V interval. To identify wave I, a technique of combining brain stem responses with electrocochleography was used (Fig. 30–17). Prasher's initial study suggests

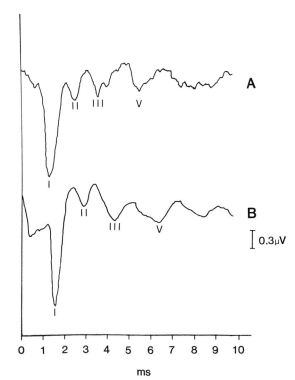

Figure 30–17. Combined electrocochleography and brain stem evoked response illustrating the prolonged wave I–V interval in a patient with a left acoustic neurinoma (A is the tracing for the normal right ear and B is the tracing for the abnormal left ear).

that this combined approach greatly improves the detection rate of eighth cranial nerve lesions.

Electrocochleography is the measurement of the electrical output of the cochlea and eighth cranial nerve in response to an auditory stimulus. Although a widened action potential (Eggermont and Odenthal, 1977) and preservation of the cochlear microphonic potential (Gibson and Beagley, 1976) have been reported in patients with schwannomas, these findings are not diagnostic. However, a unique electrocochleographic finding in 30% of patients with schwannomas is the presence of an action potential complex in the absence of subjective hearing (Morrison et al., 1976).

DISORDERS OF THE EIGHTH CRANIAL NERVE

Congenital and Hereditary Lesions

Congenital and hereditary sensorineural hearing loss is a common entity and occurs as a solitary finding or as part of a syndrome. Histopathologic studies are rare, but the following account outlines what is known of eighth cranial nerve pathologic changes in this group of disorders.

Congenital and hereditary hearing loss may be divided broadly into (1) failure of normal development of the auditory system secondary to aplasia or

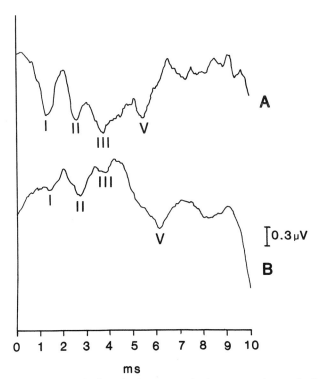

Figure 30–16. Auditory brain stem evoked responses in a patient with a left acoustic neurinoma, with A the tracing for the normal right ear and B the tracing for the abnormal left ear. An interaural difference in the latency of wave V is seen.

chromosomal aberrations, and (2) degeneration after development, either an isolated auditory defect or in association with other abnormalities.

Four main types of inner ear aplasia have been described, three of which are associated with eighth cranial nerve abnormalities:

1. *Michel's defect*—complete absence of the otic capsule and eighth cranial nerve
2. *Mondini's defect*—incomplete development of the bony and membranous labyrinths, with dysgenesis of the spiral ganglion
3. *Scheibe's defect*—membranous cochleosaccular dysplasia, with atrophy of both divisions of the eighth cranial nerve

The rare trisomies of group D and E chromosomes are chromosomal aberrations that affect the auditory labyrinth, and absence of the spiral ganglion has been documented.

After development, isolated inner ear dysfunction is usually consequent on degeneration of the stria vascularis and/or cochlear end organ (Gacek, 1971; Lindsay, 1973), but an associated secondary phenomenon is a reduction of nerve fibers in the modiolus.

Secondary degeneration of the auditory nerve has been reported in association with other defects in many syndromes (Table 30–1). The Arnold-Chiari malformation is a congenital deformity in which the brain stem and the cerebellum are elongated downward into the cervical canal. In a large series of cases (Rydell and Pulec, 1971), 20% of patients were found to suffer auditory and/or vestibular symptoms. The authors postulated stretching of the lower cranial nerves, including the eighth cranial nerve, as relative changes in the brain stem position occur with age, or alternatively, with pressure on the eighth cranial nerve as it is bent over the edge of the porus acusticus.

Clinically and pathologically, there is considerable overlap of the various syndromes of inherited spinal degeneration, ataxias, and neuropathies, and the association of hearing loss and vestibular abnormalities with these disorders is well recognized. A number of degenerative neurologic disorders, under the new system of nomenclature, would fall within the category of *multisystem atrophy*, a term that encom-

Table 30–1. CONGENITAL OR INHERITED SYNDROMES ASSOCIATED WITH DOCUMENTED AUDITORY NERVE ABNORMALITIES

Anencephaly (Lindsay, 1973)
Treacher Collins syndrome (Lindsay, 1973)
Preauricular pit–cervical fistula–hearing loss syndrome (Fitch et al., 1976)
Wildervanck's syndrome (Wildervanck, 1963)
Usher's syndrome (F.R. Nager, 1927)
Kearns-Sayre syndrome (Lindsay and Hinojosa, 1976)
Waardenburg's syndrome (Fisch, 1959)
Pendred's syndrome (Hvidberg-Hansen and Jorgensen, 1968)
Alport's syndrome (Johnsson and Arenburg, 1981)
Spinocerebellar degeneration and ataxias (see text)

passes degenerative disorders including progressive autonomic failure, atypical parkinsonism, and cerebellar ataxia in association with a multiplicity of other features including optic nerve atrophy, peripheral neuropathy, dementia, epilepsy, myoclonus, hearing loss, and vestibular dysfunction (Duvoisin, 1987; Harding, 1981).

In 1974, Spoendlin reported his classic study of the temporal bones of two sisters with Friedreich's ataxia and concluded that "the most striking features are selective and extensive damage to the neurons of the eighth nerve, whereas the peripheral receptor organs, such as the organ of Corti and the vestibular sensory epithelia, remain unaffected." Igarashi and co-workers (1982) confirmed these observations. A clinical study of four patients with Friedreich's ataxia (Satya-Murti et al., 1980) also found evidence of primary eighth cranial nerve damage on the basis of audiometric and brain stem evoked potential studies. Subsequent brain stem evoked potential studies in Friedreich's ataxia revealed inconsistent results (Ell et al., 1984; Shanon et al., 1981), which probably reflects variable involvement of the eighth cranial nerve and the brain stem in this disease.

Hearing loss in association with dominantly inherited late-onset cerebellar ataxia has been reported but is rare (Harding, 1982), whereas 14% of patients with idiopathic late-onset cerebellar ataxia had a hearing loss (Harding, 1981). The site of the auditory lesion could not be identified because no audiometric data were available.

As early as 1951, Denny-Brown reported a case of hereditary sensory neuropathy with deafness, which at postmortem examination revealed "thin auditory nerves." Subsequently, a histopathologic study of a patient with Roussy-Lévy syndrome with hearing loss (Sylvester, 1972) identified degeneration of spiral ganglion cells as the cause of the hearing loss. Hallpike et al. (1980) reported a case of afferent neuropathy associated with deafness, in which temporal bone studies revealed severe degeneration of the cochlear fibers and cells of the spiral ganglion. In this latter case the etiology was uncertain, but a hereditary neuropathy was considered to be the most likely diagnosis.

Hearing loss has been reported in the hereditary motor and sensory neuropathies, but more recent work suggests that it is more common than was previously appreciated (Perez et al., 1988; Raglan et al., 1987). Audiologic evaluation, including electrophysiologic assessment, has indicated eighth cranial nerve dysfunction in these disorders (Satya-Murti et al., 1979). Abnormal auditory brain stem evoked responses were identified in patients with normal hearing (Perez et al., 1988; Raglan et al., 1987), which supports eighth cranial nerve involvement, and Perez and co-workers drew attention to the particularly prolonged interval between wave I and wave II, which Garg and co-workers (1982) had earlier suggested was compatible with dysfunction of this nerve.

Hearing loss has also been reported with a number

of inherited muscle disorders, including facioscapulohumeral muscular dystrophy (Brouwer et al., 1990), spinal muscular atrophy (Boltshauser et al., 1989), and myotonic dystrophy (Wright et al., 1988), but audiometric investigations suggest that the hearing loss is of cochlear origin. Moreover, in mitochondrial cytopathy, hearing loss has been documented in 25% of a group of 66 patients (Morgan-Hughes et al., 1982). However, in a case report the hearing loss has been associated with loudness recruitment and normal brain stem evoked responses, which suggests a cochlear lesion (Petty et al., 1986), although in the Kearns-Sayre syndrome, which is a variant of mitochondrial cytopathy, Lindsay and Hinojosa (1976) documented advanced secondary cochlear nerve degeneration.

From these clinical and histopathologic studies, it would seem likely that a proportion of the inherited neurologic degenerative disorders are associated with hearing loss related to cochlear nerve involvement.

Trauma

The eighth cranial nerve may be damaged by mechanical trauma, barotrauma, or surgical intervention. Severe head injury may result in temporal bone fracture. In longitudinal fractures the eighth cranial nerve is not usually affected, but in transverse fractures the vestibule of the inner ear and the roof of the internal auditory meatus are frequently affected, which produces total auditory and vestibular failure as a result of hemorrhage, tearing, and/or stretching of the nerve fibers. In 40–50% of this latter group, the facial nerve is also affected. The prognosis of hearing loss depends on the extent of damage to the eighth cranial nerve, and improvement generally occurs within the first 3–4 weeks, although there are reports of improvement up to 6 months later.

Less severe injuries may result in concussion of the inner ear with concomitant secondary neural degeneration (Schuknecht, 1974). The prognosis in this situation is uncertain; some reports note marked improvement, whereas others describe progressive deterioration (Lindsay and Zajtchuk, 1970). Penetrating wounds to the skull, such as gunshot wounds, may affect the eighth cranial nerve in the internal auditory meatus. Barotrauma producing decompression sickness is an increasingly common problem in divers and may affect the eighth cranial nerve.

Infection

Bacterial, viral, and mycotic infections may damage the eighth cranial nerve by direct invasion of the organism along nerves and vessels of the internal auditory meatus, secondary to meningoencephalitis. Labyrinthine damage may also occur as a result of blood-borne infection.

Bacterial Infection

Bacterial meningitis, producing profound hearing loss, is most commonly seen in neonates and young children (Lindsay, 1973). *Streptococcus pneumoniae, Neisseria meningitidis,* and *Haemophilus influenzae* commonly produce complete sensory and/or neural destruction, which may be impossible to differentiate except histopathologically. The long-term prognosis of meningitic hearing loss is poor, but if sufficient auditory nerve function remains, the cochlear implant provides a new and effective form of management.

Although *tuberculous meningitis* is now rare in Western societies, it should be considered in the immigrant, the debilitated (e.g., alcoholics), and the immunosuppressed populations. Morrison (1975) reported two young adults with hearing loss caused by multiple arachnoid adhesions affecting the eighth cranial nerve, secondary to tuberculous meningitis. The common complicating ototoxic effect of antituberculous medication had been excluded in these two cases.

The need for vigilance in the diagnosis of syphilis has also been emphasized. Although labyrinthine involvement is common in syphilis, eighth cranial nerve dysfunction, usually as a result of *syphilitic meningitis*, is rare. Morrison (1975) reported three patients with acute syphilitic meningitis and hearing loss attributable to eighth cranial nerve involvement. The diagnosis may be confirmed by elevated protein levels and cell counts as well as by positive serologic tests of the cerebrospinal fluid. These findings are in contrast to the situation in the more common entity of syphilitic labyrinthitis, in which relatively normal cerebrospinal fluid findings are the rule. Adequate antisyphilitic therapy is mandatory, and at least one additional lumbar puncture is necessary to assess the efficacy of therapy. Despite adequate treatment, the prognosis for recovery from syphilitic eighth cranial nerve dysfunction must be guarded.

Tick-borne infections caused by *Borrelia burgdorferi,* or the European *Borrelia* spirochete, have been identified as giving rise to central nervous system disease including meningoencephalitis and cranial neuritis. Rosenhall and co-workers (1988) studied 73 patients with a primary complaint of vertigo and identified serologic evidence of *Borrelia* infection in 10, 4 of whom had an associated sensorineural hearing loss. The authors concluded that eighth cranial nerve damage as a result of this infection was possible.

Two aggressive bacterial conditions affecting the eighth cranial nerve deserve mention. *Petrositis* results from chronic labyrinthine infection that extends into the apical portion of the petrous temporal bone, affecting the abducent nerve and trigeminal ganglion and giving rise to a Gradenigo syndrome, with otitis media, paralysis of the ipsilateral lateral rectus muscle, and pain behind the ipsilateral eye. Involvement of the eighth cranial nerve may also produce vertigo and hearing loss. *Malignant otitis externa* usually results from an infection with *Pseudomonas aeruginosa* in a debilitated patient. The junction of the cartilaginous and osseous portions of the external auditory canal is invaded, and infection spreads through the adjacent structures. Eighth cranial nerve involvement has been reported (Dinapoli and Thomas, 1971). Prolonged treatment with carbenicillin or gentamicin has improved the prognosis for this condition.

Viral Infection

Viral infection may also affect the inner ear by direct invasion along the nerves and vessels of the internal auditory meatus. Lindsay (1973) demonstrated marked infiltration by lymphocytes and histiocytes of the eighth cranial nerve, the neural remnants in the modiolus of the cochlea, and branches of the vestibular nerve. Schuknecht and Kitamura (1981), in a case of recurrent vestibular symptoms, demonstrated histopathologic changes in the eighth cranial nerve similar to those of a reported case of herpes zoster oticus (Zajtchuk et al., 1972) and therefore postulated a viral effect on the vestibular division of the eighth cranial nerve. Extrapolation of this theory suggests that viral infection may be responsible in certain cases of sensorineural hearing loss, as a result of involvement of the auditory division of the eighth cranial nerve (Sando et al., 1977).

The Ramsay Hunt syndrome, or *herpes zoster oticus,* would appear to be a clear-cut example of a mononeuritis of the eighth cranial nerve. A deep burning pain in the ear is followed within a few days by a vesicular eruption in the external auditory canal and on the concha. Subsequently, hearing loss and vertigo develop, with or without seventh cranial nerve involvement. Blackley and co-workers (1967) documented marked perivascular, perineural, and intraneural round cell infiltration in the seventh and eighth cranial nerves in this condition. It is of interest that careful assessment of auditory and vestibular function in patients with *Bell's palsy* frequently reveals objective evidence of eighth cranial nerve dysfunction (Rauchbach and Stroud, 1975), and as serologic evidence of viral infection is frequently found in Bell's palsy, it has been postulated that the primary pathology is a viral mononeuritis multiplex (Sandstedt et al., 1981).

In the last decade, acquired immunodeficiency syndrome has emerged as a major transmissible disorder with protean manifestations. A patient with this disorder in whom unilateral sudden sensorineural hearing loss was a prominent symptom was reported (Real et al., 1987). The pathophysiology of the hearing loss was not clarified, but the authors hypothesized that the human T cell lymphotrophic virus type III may directly involve the spiral ganglion or acoustic division of the eighth cranial nerve or that an opportunistic pathogen, such as herpes zoster varicellosus, may invade the neural components in an immunosuppressed patient and cause temporary or permanent neuropathy. An alternative explanation is that the hearing loss is related to an opportunistic meningitis, for example, cryptococcal meningitis.

Mycotic Disease

Cryptococcosis and coccidioidomycosis may produce basilar meningitis, with involvement of the cranial nerves including the eighth (Maslan et al., 1985). Confirmation of the diagnosis depends on identification of the fungal antigen in the cerebrospinal fluid and use of complement fixation, latex agglutination, or immunofluorescence techniques.

Rickettsial Infection

Dolan and co-workers (1986) reported hearing loss in association with Rocky Mountain spotted fever and postulated that the lesion may be a vasculitis involving the auditory nerve.

Vascular Disease

The vertebrobasilar circulation supplies the peripheral labyrinth, eighth cranial nerve, and brain stem. Ischemia may therefore produce an auditory deficit as a result of dysfunction at more than one level in the auditory system. The majority of reports of hearing loss of vascular origin tend to implicate primary cochlear damage with secondary neural hearing loss (Belal, 1980; Gussen, 1976; Kimura and Perlman, 1958). Morrison (1975) quoted a case of sudden unilateral loss of eighth cranial nerve function in a patient with heart block who had experienced two previous cerebrovascular episodes. This diagnosis should be considered in patients with a clear history of ischemic cardiovascular disease, hypertension, or vertebrobasilar ischemia. Indeed, one study (Susmano and Rosenbush, 1988) suggests that unexplained hearing loss may be an early marker of vascular disease. Other less common causes of arterial occlusion that may affect the eighth cranial nerve include the subclavian steal syndrome, polycythemia, emboli, arteritis, the hypercoagulation syndrome, and cardiopulmonary by-pass surgery.

Aneurysms and vascular loops of the anterior inferior cerebellar artery may compress the eighth cranial nerve and give rise to vestibular and auditory symptoms. The clinical picture is indistinguishable from that related to any other cerebellopontine angle lesion, and the correct diagnosis is made by use of angiography or magnetic resonance imaging (Moseley, 1988; Phelps and Lloyd, 1982). Other intracranial aneurysms, such as posterior communicating artery aneurysm, may also produce sudden sensorineural hearing loss (Colclasure, 1981).

Neoplasia

Vestibular schwannomas, which are more commonly but incorrectly known as acoustic neurinomas, account for 10% of intracranial tumors and more than 75% of cerebellopontine angle lesions (Gonzalez-Revilla, 1948). Although most of the tumors arise from the superior division of the vestibular nerve, deafness and tinnitus are the most frequent presenting symptoms (Pulec et al., 1971). Reviewing 200 patients with such tumors, Johnson (1968) reported that only 42% showed a classic retrocochlear hearing loss (see earlier), whereas abnormal brain stem evoked responses occurred in approximately 95% of surgically proven cases (Josey et al., 1980). All patients with unilateral sensorineural deafness, bilateral asymmetric sensorineural deafness, or unexplained unilateral tinnitus must be investigated to exclude a small vestibular schwannoma. Vestibular investigation frequently reveals an ipsilateral canal paresis on caloric testing (Dix, 1974), with or without a directional preponderance, depending on the degree of brain stem or cerebellar involvement. Conventional radiography may reveal funneling of the internal auditory meatus in cases of vestibular schwannoma, but normal radiologic results do not exclude pathologic changes. The definitive procedure for the identification of small tumors is magnetic resonance imaging (Moseley, 1988).

Bilateral tumors may occur with both forms of autosomal dominant neurofibromatosis: peripheral neurofibromatosis, or von Recklinghausen's disease, and central neurofibromatosis. The second condition is much rarer (Kanter et al., 1980). It most commonly occurs in a young adult with bilateral hearing loss, but unlike the case with unilateral tumors, tinnitus is less common. In unilateral cases, the tumor tends to displace the facial and cochlear nerves anteriorly so that they lie as a flattened ribbon-like structure across the tumor. In bilateral disease, the tumor is usually a lobulated mass through which the cochlear and facial nerves pass. Thus, not surprisingly, although reports of hearing preservation after excision of unilateral tumors continue to increase, little success has been reported for bilateral cases because of invasion of the cochlear nerve by the tumor.

The 8th cranial nerve may also be compressed, rarely, by schwannomas on the 5th, 7th, 9th, or 11th cranial nerves, but after vestibular schwannomas, meningiomas and epidermoid cysts of the cerebellopontine angle are the most common tumors at this site.

The internal auditory meatus is a frequent site of metastatic tumor within the temporal bone; secondary deposits, particularly from breast, kidneys, lung, stomach, larynx, prostate, and thyroid gland, may affect the eighth cranial nerve by compression (Schuknecht et al., 1968). Paparella and co-workers (1973) reported that 11 of 25 patients with various forms of leukemia showed infiltration of the eighth cranial nerve on temporal bone examination. Deafness caused by involvement of this nerve in carcinomatous and lymphomatous meningitis is common (Beal, 1990). Deafness has been reported rarely in association with carcinomatous neuropathy (Denny-Brown, 1948; Henson et al., 1954) and carcinomatous sub-

acute cerebellar degeneration (Brain and Wilkinson, 1965). McGill (1976) described a case of oat cell carcinoma of the lung with carcinomatous encephalomyelitis and severe unilateral deafness and vertigo secondary to atrophy of the cochlear nerve, ganglion cells, and ipsilateral cochlear nuclei of the brain stem.

Metabolic Disease

Diabetes Mellitus. Certain abnormalities affecting the eighth cranial nerve have been documented: Jorgensen (1964) and Kovar (1973) reported thickening of the walls of the vasa nervorum; Makishima and Tanaka (1971) reported atrophy of the spiral ganglion; and Kovar (1973) noted demyelination and axonal beading of the eighth cranial nerve. Despite these observations, Colletti and co-workers (1985) established cochlear involvement in 87% of 120 diabetics by using Békésy's audiometry and stapedial reflex measurements. Abnormalities of stapedial reflex parameters such as latency and rise time indicated additional eighth cranial nerve and brain stem abnormalities in 34% of their patients. These workers suggested that the diverse results previously reported in the literature are best explained on the basis of differences in the sensitivity and the interpretation of the various audiologic tests used.

Uremia. Bergstrom and co-workers (1973) linked the hearing loss in renal disease with uremic polyneuropathy, despite the fact that this neuropathy rarely affected the cranial nerves. In a case report, Lucien and Jacob (1987) documented a bilateral sensorineural hearing loss with stapedial reflex threshold decay and abnormal brain stem evoked responses indicating eighth cranial nerve dysfunction in a patient with uremia. Seven weeks after dialysis, the hearing loss had improved and the nerve abnormalities had returned to normal. Despite this evidence, other temporal bone studies in renal disease have identified cochlear abnormalities (Oda, 1974), and it must be presumed that auditory symptoms in acquired renal disease have a multifactorial etiology.

Temporal Bone Disorders

Otosclerosis. Otosclerosis is a disorder of the bony labyrinth that usually manifests itself by immobilization of the stapes and produces a conductive hearing loss. However, Sando et al. (1974), on the basis of temporal bone studies, postulated that otosclerotic foci may compress neural elements within the bony labyrinth to produce the sensorineural component of the hearing loss that may be observed in some cases of otosclerosis.

Paget's Disease. Auditory and vestibular symptoms are well recognized in this condition. A bilateral sensorineural hearing loss is generally observed, but a conductive component may be present. On the basis of histopathologic studies, Lindsay and Suga

(1976) demonstrated severe degeneration of the auditory nerve. Subsequently, Applebaum and Clemis (1977) demonstrated encroachment of the internal auditory meatus by Paget-type bone, with compression of the cochlear division of the eighth cranial nerve. No other cochlear abnormality was observed. It would therefore seem that, although the pathogenesis of audiovestibular symptoms may be multifactorial in Paget's disease (including fracture of the labyrinthine capsule, vascular disturbances, and degeneration of the sensory elements), neural degeneration is probably the primary mechanism.

Fibrous Dysplasia. In fibrous dysplasia, skeletal aberrations are associated with endocrinopathy and abnormal pigmentation of the skin and mucous membranes. It is rarely associated with hearing loss of eighth cranial nerve origin (G.T. Nager et al., 1982).

Osteopetrosis. This group of uncommon genetic disorders is characterized by increased skeletal density and abnormalities of bone modeling. Encroachment on the cochlear nerve may produce sensorineural hearing loss, and work by Miyamoto et al. (1980) suggested that symptoms of seventh and eighth cranial nerve damage may be the first indication of such disease.

Toxic Disorders

Drugs. Many drugs are known to produce cochlear damage, but thalidomide has been demonstrated to produce aplasia of the eighth cranial nerve in association with a Michel aplasia of the inner ear (Jorgensen et al, 1964). Vincristine sulfate has been demonstrated to produce bilateral cochlear nerve damage (Mahajan et al., 1981). Silverstein et al. (1967) have postulated that salicylates, which are highly concentrated in the perilymph, may interfere with the enzymatic activity of the hair cells or the cochlear neurons, or both.

Alcohol. Ylikoski et al. (1981) identified extensive degeneration of both myelinated and unmyelinated nerve fibers in the cochlear and vestibular divisions of the eighth cranial nerve in a chronic alcoholic patient with a marked peripheral neuropathy. In general, however, cranial nerve involvement in chronic alcoholic neuropathy is rare, and it has been suggested that the neuropathy is perhaps more related to accompanying malnutrition rather than to the direct toxic effect of alcohol.

Chemicals. Poisoning with both lead and mercury produces auditory and vestibular symptoms, although the underlying pathophysiologic mechanism is unclear. Experiments (Gozdzik-Zolnierkiewicz and Moszynski, 1969) demonstrated segmental demyelination and axonal degeneration of the eighth cranial nerve in 75% of animals receiving intraperitoneal injections of 1% lead acetate solution. No abnormalities were observed in the end organs or ganglion cells. However, this finding cannot be extrapolated to humans, and no other temporal bone studies are available.

Autoimmune Disorders

A number of reports in the literature document the occurrence of sudden retrocochlear loss in immune disorders. Morrison (1975) reported a 2-year-old boy who became acutely ill after a measles vaccination and on recovery was subtotally deaf in the right ear. He also reported a 17-year-old girl who developed a retrocochlear hearing loss with vestibular symptoms after a hypersensitivity reaction to ampicillin. A good recovery was made with large doses of corticosteroids. Wendt and Burks (1981) reported a 28-year-old woman who developed encephalomyeloradiculoneuropathy after a minor influenza-like illness that was associated with central nervous system abnormalities, including a profound bilateral hearing loss, which was attributed to eighth cranial nerve involvement. In another 28-year-old woman, a bilateral hearing loss associated with diffuse neurologic impairment was observed after infection with *Mycoplasma pneumoniae* (Rothstein and Kenny, 1979). Encephaloradiculoneuropathy may be the result of an abnormal immune response to a preceding infection, vaccination, or insect sting. Such a mechanism may explain reports of sudden deafness after antitetanus serum and tetanus toxoid vaccinations.

In many autoimmune disorders, including Hashimoto's disease, polyarteritis nodosa, Wegener's granulomatosis, rheumatoid arthritis, and Cogan's syndrome, lesions of the cochlear nerve have been postulated (Stephens et al., 1982), but there are few temporal bone studies to support this hypothesis. In Cogan's syndrome, the most consistent histopathologic finding is diffuse degeneration of all neural elements of the inner ear (Smith, 1970; Wolff et al., 1965), and in a case of severe polyarteritis, McNeil et al. (1952) also demonstrated bilateral vestibular and cochlear nerve lesions with degenerative changes, loss of myelin, and fragmentation of axons. However, a subsequent temporal bone report (Gussen, 1977) identified primary cochlear abnormalities in polyarteritis.

Neurologic manifestations of sarcoidosis occur in only 5% of patients with this disorder. A granulomatous meningitis directly infiltrates the cranial nerves, and the eighth nerve is the fourth most commonly affected (Jahrsdoerfer et al., 1981). The hearing loss may be fluctuating and may be the initial manifestation of neurologic sarcoidosis.

Demyelination

Vestibular dysfunction is well recognized in multiple sclerosis, but auditory symptoms are less clearly defined. Clinically, the hearing loss is frequently unilateral, and, given the complexity and crossings of the auditory nerve fibers within the central nervous system, the lesion is most probably in the intramedullary auditory nerve or cochlear nucleus (Barratt et al., 1988). Support for this view is provided by Miller et al. (1988), who showed enhanced magnetic resonance imaging lesions at both root entry zones in a patient with multiple sclerosis who had acute deafness. The proximal part of the eighth cranial nerve is supported by glial tissue, and it has also been postulated that plaques of demyelination may affect this region. This hypothesis has been supported by early pathologic studies (Brock and Gagel, 1933) and by some clinical studies (Citron et al., 1963; Hennenbert, 1966; Rose and Daly, 1964). However, on the basis of a single temporal bone study, Ward et al. (1965) were unable to identify any eighth cranial nerve lesion in a patient with multiple sclerosis, and in a large study of 61 patients with multiple sclerosis, Noffsinger and associates (1972) were unable to correlate vestibular and auditory abnormalities, making an eighth cranial nerve lesion unlikely.

Eighth cranial nerve demyelination has not been well documented in the Guillain-Barré syndrome, although a report of two patients, one of whom had a hearing loss, identified bilaterally prolonged wave I latencies in auditory evoked potentials that improved on clinical recovery. These findings suggest that acoustic nerve conduction abnormalities from demyelination may occur in the Guillain-Barré syndrome (Nelson et al., 1988).

References

(Key references are designated with an asterisk.)

Anderson H., Barr B., Wedenberg E. The early detection of acoustic tumours by the stapedial reflex test. In Wolstenholm G.L.W., Knight J., eds. *Sensorineural Hearing Loss*. London, Churchill Livingstone, pp. 275–294, 1970.

Appelbaum E., Clemis J. Temporal bone histology of Paget's disease with sensorineural hearing loss and narrowing of the internal auditory canal. *Laryngoscope* 87:1753–1759, 1977.

Barratt H.J., Miller D., Rudge P. The site of the lesion causing deafness in multiple sclerosis. *Scand. Audiol.* 17:67–71, 1988.

Beal M.F. Multiple cranial nerve palsy—a diagnostic challenge. *N. Eng. J. Med.* 322:461–463, 1990.

Békésy G.V. A new audiometer. *Acta Otolaryngol.* 35:411–422, 1947.

Belal A. Pathology of vascular sensorineural hearing impairment. *Laryngoscope* 90:1831–1839, 1980.

Bergstom L., Jenkins P., Sando I., et al. Hearing loss in renal disease: clinical and pathological studies. *Ann. Otol. Rhinol. Laryngol.* 82:555–576, 1973.

Berlin C. New developments in evaluating central auditory mechanism. *Ann. Otol. Rhinol. Laryngol.* 85:833–841, 1976.

Blackley B., Friedmann I., Wright L. Herpes zoster auris with facial nerve palsy and auditory nerve symptoms. A case report with histological findings. *Acta Otolaryngol. (Stockh.)* 63:533–550, 1967.

Boltshauser E., Lang W., Spillmann T., et al. Hereditary distal muscular atrophy with vocal cord paralysis and sensorineural hearing loss: a dominant form of spinal muscular atrophy? *J. Med. Genet.* 26:105–108, 1989.

Brackmann D.E. Panel discussion. *J. Laryngol. Otol. Suppl.* 4:143–144, 1981.

Brain L., Wilkinson M. Subacute cerebellar degeneration associated with neoplasms. *Brain* 88:465–478, 1965.

Bridger M.W.M., Farkashidy J. The distribution of neuro-glia and Schwann cells in the 8th nerve of man. *J. Laryngol. Otol.* 94:1353–1362, 1980.

Brock W., Gagel O. Rechtsoeitiger kleinhimbrucjenwinkel Tumour. Multiple Sklerose. Ein falsche Diagnose. *Arch. Ohren. Nasen. Kehlkopfheilkd.* 143:227–229, 1933.

Brouwer O.F., Ruys C.J.M., Brand R., et al. Hearing loss in facioscapulohumeral muscular dystrophy. *J. Neurol.* 237:1:S56, 1990.

Citron L., Dix M.R., Hallpike C.S., et al. A recent clinico-pathological study of cochlear nerve degeneration resulting from tumour pressure and disseminated sclerosis with particular reference to the finding of normal threshold sensitivity for pure tone. *Acta Otolaryngol. (Stockh.)* 56:330–337, 1963.

Clemis J.D., Mitchell C. Electrocochleography and brainstem responses used in the diagnosis of acoustic tumours. *J. Otolaryngol.* 6:447–459, 1977.

Colclasure J.B., Graham S.S. Intracranial aneurysm occurring as sensori-neural hearing loss. *Otolaryngol. Head Neck Surg.* 89:283–287, 1981.

Colletti V., Fiorino F.G., Sittoni V., et al. Auditory evaluation in diabetes mellitus. *Adv. Audiol.* 3:121–132, 1985.

Denny-Brown D. Primary sensory neuropathy with muscular changes associated with carcinoma. *J. Neurol. Neurosurg. Psychiatry* 11:73–87, 1948.

Denny-Brown D. Hereditary, sensory radiculoneuropathy. *J. Neurol. Neurosurg. Psychiatry* 14:237–252, 1951.

Dinapoli R.P., Thomas J.E. Neurologic aspects of malignant otitis externa: report of three cases. *Mayo Clin. Proc.* 46:339–344, 1971.

Dix M.R. The vestibular acoustic system. In Vinken P.J., Bruyn B.W., eds. *Handbook of Clinical Neurology*. Vol. 16. New York, American Elsevier, p. 301, 1974.

*Dix M.R., Hallpike C.S., Hood J.D. Observations upon the loudness recruitment phenomenon, with special reference to the differential diagnosis of disorders of the internal ear and 8th nerve. *Proc. R. Soc. Med.* 41:516–526, 1948.

Dolan S., Everett E.D., Renner L. Hearing loss in Rocky Mountain spotted fever (letter). *Ann. Intern. Med.* 104:285, 1986.

Duvoisin R.C. The olivopontocerebellar atrophies. In Marsden C.D., Fahn S., eds. *Movement Disorders II*. London, Butterworth, pp. 249–271, 1987.

Eggermont J.J., Odenthal D. Potentialities of clinical electrocochleography. *Clin. Otolaryngol.* 2:275–286, 1977.

Ell J., Prasher D., Rudge P. Neuro-otological abnormalities in Freidreich's ataxia. *J. Neurol. Neurosurg. Psychiatry* 47:26–32, 1984.

*Evans E.F. Single unit studies of the mammalian auditory nerve. In Beagley H.A., ed. *Auditory Investigation: The Scientific and Technological Basis*. New York, Oxford University Press, 1979.

Fisch L. Deafness as part of an hereditary deafness syndrome. *J. Laryngol.* 73:355–382, 1959.

Fitch M., Lindsay J.R., Srolovitz H. Temporal bone in the preauricular pit–cervical fistula–hearing loss syndrome. *Ann. Otol. Rhinol. Laryngol.* 85:268–375, 1976.

Fowler E.P. A method for the early detection of otosclerosis: a study of sounds well above threshold. *Arch. Otolaryngol.* 24:731–741, 1936.

Gacek R.R. The pathology of hereditary sensorineural hearing loss. *Ann. Otol. Rhinol. Laryngol.* 80:289–298, 1971.

Garg P., Markand O.M., Bustion P.S. Brainstem auditory evoked response in hereditary motor-sensory neuropathy: site of origin of wave II. *Neurology (N.Y.)* 32:1017–1019, 1982.

Gibson W.P.R., Beagley H. Electrocochleography in the diagnosis of acoustic neuroma. *J. Laryngol. Otol.* 90:127–139, 1976.

Gonzalez-Revilla A. Differential diagnosis of tumors at the cerebello-pontine recess. *Bull. Johns Hopkins Hosp.* 83:187–212, 1948.

Gozdzik-Zolnierkiewicz T., Moszynski B. VIIIth nerve in experimental lead poisoning. *Acta Otolaryngol. (Stockh.)* 68:85–89, 1969.

Gradenigo G. Clinical signs of affectations of the auditory nerve. *Arch. Otolaryngol.* 22:213–215, 1893.

Grant J.M. Audiological diagnosis of cochlear versus 8th nerve site of lesion. *J. Otolaryngol. Soc. Aust.* 5:86–88, 1981.

Gussen R. Sudden deafness of vascular origin: a human temporal bone study. *Ann. Otol. Rhinol. Laryngol.* 85:94–100, 1976.

Gussen R. Polyarteritis nodosa and deafness: a human temporal bone study. *Arch. Otorhinolaryngol.* 217:263–271, 1977.

Hallpike C.S., Harriman D.G.F., Wells C.E.C. A case of afferent neuropathy and deafness. *J. Laryngol. Otol.* 94:945–964, 1980.

Harding A.E. "Idiopathic" late onset cerebellar ataxia: a clinical and genetic study of 36 cases. *J. Neurol. Sci.* 51:259–271, 1981.

Harding A.E. The clinical features and classification of the late onset autosomal dominant cerebellar ataxias. A study of the 11 families, including descendants of "the Drew family of Walworth." *Brain* 105:1–28, 1982.

Hennebert D. Auditory adaptation in multiple sclerosis. The clinical value of the threshold tone decay test. *Acta Neurol. Belg.* 66:263–266, 1966.

Henson R., Russell, D.S., Wilkinson M. Carcinomatous neuropathy and myopathy: a clinical and pathological study. *Brain* 77:82–121, 1954.

Hinojosa R., Lindsay J.R. Profound deafness, associated sensory and neural degeneration. *Arch. Otolaryngol.* 106:193–209, 1980.

Hood J.D., Poole J.P. The tolerable limit of loudness: its clinical and physiological significance. *J. Acoust. Soc. Am.* 40:47–53, 1966.

Hvidberg-Hansen J., Jorgensen M.B. The inner ear in Pendred's syndrome. *Acta Otolaryngol. (Stockh.)* 66:129–135, 1968.

Igarashi M., Miller R.H., O-Uchi T., et al. Temporal bone findings in Friedreich's ataxia. *ORL J. Otorhinolaryngol. Relat. Spec.* 44:146–155, 1982.

Jahrsdoerfer R.A., Thompson E.G., Johns M.M.E., et al. Sarcoidosis and fluctuating loss. *Ann. Otol. Rhinol. Laryngol.* 90:161–163, 1981.

Jannetta P.J. Neurovascular cross-compression in patients with hyperactive dysfunction symptoms of the 8th cranial nerve. *Surg. Forum* 26:467–469, 1975.

Jannetta P.J. Observation on the aetiology of trigeminal neuralgia, hemifacial spasm, acoustic nerve dysfunction and glossopharyngeal neuralgia. Definite microsurgical treatment and results in 117 patients. *Neurochirurgia (Stuttg.)* 20:145–154, 1977.

Jannetta P.J. Neurovascular decompression in cranial nerve and systemic disease. *Am. J. Surg.* 192:518–524, 1980.

Jerger J. Békésy audiometry in analysis of auditory disorders. *J. Speech Hear. Res.* 3:275–287, 1960.

Jerger J., Hayes D. Diagnostic speech audiometry. *Arch. Otolaryngol.* 103:216–222, 1977.

Jerger J., Jerger S. Diagnostic significance of PB word functions. *Arch. Otolaryngol.* 93:573–580, 1971.

Jerger J., Jerger S. A simplified tone decay test. *Arch. Otolaryngol.* 101:403–407, 1975.

Jerger J., Jerger S., Maudlin L. The forward-backward discrepancy in Békésy audiometry. *Arch. Otolaryngol.* 96:400–406, 1972.

Johnson E.W. Auditory findings in 200 cases of acoustic neuromas. *Arch. Otolaryngol.* 88:598–603, 1968.

Johnsson L.J. Sequence of degeneration of Corti's organ and its first order neurons. *Ann. Otol. Rhinol. Laryngol.* 83:294–303, 1974.

Johnsson L.J., Arenburg I.K. Cochlear abnormalities in Alport's syndrome. *Arch. Otolaryngol.* 107:340–349, 1981.

Jorgensen M.B. Changes of ageing in the inner ear and in the inner ear of diabetes mellitus—histological studies. *Acta Otolaryngol. (Stockh.) Suppl.* 188:125–128, 1964.

Jorgensen M.B., Kristensen H.K., Buch N.H. Thalidomide induced aplasia of the inner ear. *J. Laryngol.* 78:1095–1101, 1964.

Josey A.F., Jackson G.G., Glasscock M.E. Brainstem evoked response audiometry in confirmed eighth nerve tumors. *Am. J. Otrolaryngol.* 1:285–290, 1980.

Kanter W.R., Eldridge R., Fabricant R., et al. Central neurofibromatosis with bilateral acoustic neuroma: genetic, clinical and biochemical distinctions from peripheral neurofibromatosis. *Neurology (N.Y.)* 30:851–859, 1980.

Kemp D.T. Stimulated acoustic emissions from within the human auditory system. *J. Acoust. Soc. Am.* 64:1386–1391, 1978.

Kemp D.T., Ryan S., Bray B. A guide to the effective use of otoacoustic emissions. *Ear Hear.* 11:93–105, 1990.

Kimura R., Perlman H.B. Arterial obstruction of the labyrinth; 1) cochlear changes. *Ann. Otol. Rhinol. Laryngol.* 67:5–40, 1958.

Kovar M. The inner ear in diabetes mellitus. *Otorhinolaryngology* 35:42–57, 1973.

Kumagami H. Neuropathological findings of hemifacial spasm and trigeminal neuralgia. *Arch. Otolaryngol.* 99:60–64, 1974.

Liberman N.C., Kiang N.Y. Acoustic trauma in cats. *Acta Otolaryngol. Suppl.* 358:1–63, 1978.

Lindsay J.R. Profound childhood deafness. Inner ear pathology. *Ann. Otol. Rhinol. Laryngol.* 82:(Suppl. 5):1–121, 1973.

Lindsay J.R., Hinojosa R. Histopathologic features of the inner ear associated with Kearns-Sayre syndrome. *Arch. Otolaryngol.* 102:747–752, 1976.

Lindsay J.R., Suga R. Paget's disease and sensorineural deafness. Temporal bone histology of Paget's disease. *Laryngoscope* 86:1029–1042, 1976.

Lindsay J.R., Zajtchuk J. Concussion of the inner ear. *Ann. Otol. Rhinol. Laryngol.* 79:699–709, 1970.

Lucien J.C.A., Jacob M.M. Hearing loss in a uraemic patient, indications of involvement of the VIII nerve. *J. Laryngol. Otol.* 101:492–496, 1987.

Mahajan S.L., Ideda Y., Myers T., et al. Acute acoustic nerve palsy associated with vincristine therapy. *Cancer* 47:2404–2406, 1981.

Makishima K., Tanaka K. Pathological changes of the inner ear and central auditory pathways in diabetes. *Ann. Otol. Rhinol. Laryngol.* 80:218–228, 1971.

Maslan M.J., Graham M.D., Flood L.M. Cryptococcal meningitis: presentation as sudden deafness. *Am. J. Otol.* 6:435–437, 1985.

McFadden D. *Tinnitus: Fact, Theory and Treatment.* Washington, National Academy Press, 1982.

McGill P. Carcinomatous encephalomyelitis with auditory and vestibular manifestations. *Ann. Otol. Rhinol. Laryngol.* 85:120–126, 1976.

McNeil N.F., Berke M., Reingold I.M. Polyarteritis nodosa causing deafness in an adult. *Ann. Intern. Med.* 37:1253–1267, 1952.

Miller D.H., Rudge P., Johnson G., et al. Serial gadolinium enhanced magnetic resonance imaging in multiple sclerosis. *Brain* 111:927–939, 1988.

Miyamoto R.T., House W.F., Brackmann D.E. Neuro-otological manifestations of the osteopetroses. *Arch. Otolaryngol.* 106:210–214, 1980.

Møller A.R. Pathophysiology of tinnitus. *Ann. Otol. Rhinol. Laryngol.* 93:39–44, 1984.

Møller A.R., Jannetta A.P.J., Sekhar L.N. Diagnosis and surgical treatment of disabling positional vertigo. *J. Neurosurg.* 64:21–28, 1986.

Møller A.R., Jannetta A.P.J., Sekhar L.N. Contributions from the auditory nerve to the brain-stem auditory evoked potentials (BAEPs): results of intracranial recording in man. *Electroencephalogr. Clin. Neurophysiol.* 71:198–211, 1988.

Morales-Garcia C., Hood J.D. Tone decay test in neuro-otological diagnosis. *Arch. Otolaryngol.* 96:231–247, 1972.

Morgan-Hughes J.A., Hayes D.J., Clark J.B., et al. Mitochondrial encephalomyopathies: biochemical studies in two cases revealing defects in the respiratory chain. *Brain* 105:553–582, 1982.

*Morrison A.W. *Management of Sensorineural Deafness.* London, Butterworth, 1975.

Morrison A.W., Gibson W.P.R., Beagley H. Transtympanic electrocochleography in the diagnosis of retrocochlear tumours. *Clin. Otolaryngol.* 1:153–167, 1976.

Moseley I. *Magnetic Resonance Imaging in Disorders of Nervous System.* Oxford, Blackwell, 1988.

Nager F.R. Zur Histologie der Taubstummheit bei Retinitis pigmentosa. *Beitr. Pathol. Anat. Allg. Pathol.* 77:288–303, 1927.

Nager G.T., Kennedy G.W., Kopstein E. Fibrous dysplasia: a review of the disease and its manifestation in the temporal bone. *Ann. Otol. Rhinol. Laryngol. Suppl.* 92:1–52, 1982.

Nelson K.R., Gilmore R.L., Massey A. Acoustic nerve conduction abnormalities in Guillain-Barré syndrome. *Neurology* 38:1263–1266, 1988.

*Noffsinger D., Olsen W.O., Carhart R., et al. Auditory and vestibular aberrations in multiple sclerosis. *Acta Otolaryngol. Suppl. (Stockh.)* 303:1–63, 1972.

Oda M. Labyrinthine pathology of chronic renal failure patients treated with haemodialysis and kidney transplantation. *Laryngoscope* 83:1489–1506, 1974.

Paparella M.M., Berlinger N.T., Oda M., et al. Otological manifestations of leukemia. *Laryngoscope* 83:1510–1526, 1973.

Perez H., Vílchez J., Sevilla T., et al. Audiologic evaluation in Charcot-Marie-Tooth disease. *Scand. Audiol. Suppl.* 30:211–213, 1988.

Petty R.K.H., Harding A.E., Morgan-Hughes J.A. The clinical features of mitochondrial myopathy. *Brain* 109:915–938, 1986.

Pfaltz C.R. The diagnostic importance of the galvanic test in otoneurology *Pract. Oto-Rhino-Laryngol.* 31:193–203, 1969.

*Phelps P.D., Lloyd G.A.S. High resolution air, CT meatography: the demonstration of normal and abnormal structures in the cerebellopontine system and internal auditory meatus. *Br. J. Radiol.* 55:19–22, 1982.

*Pickles J.O. The auditory nerve. In *Introduction to the Physiology of Hearing.* London, Academic Press, pp. 71–106, 1982.

Prasher D. *Studies of Early Auditory Evoked Potentials and Their Clinical Applications.* Ph.D. thesis, University of London, 1982.

Pulec J.L., House W.F., Britton B.H., et al. A system of management of acoustic neuroma based on 364 cases. *Trans. Am. Acad. Ophthalmol. Otolaryngol.* 75:48–55, 1971.

Raglan E., Prasher D.K., Trinder E., et al. Auditory function in hereditary motor and sensory neuropathy (Charcot-Marie-Tooth disease). *Acta Otolaryngol. (Stockh.)* 103:50–55, 1987.

Rasmussen G.L. An efferent cochlear bundle (abstract). *Anat. Rec.* 82:441, 1942.

Rauchbach E., Stroud M.H. Vestibular involvement in Bell's palsy. *Laryngoscope* 85:1396–1398, 1975.

Real R., Thomas M., Gerwin J.M. Sudden hearing loss and acquired immunodeficiency syndrome. *Otolaryngol. Head Neck Surg.* 97:409–412, 1987.

Rose R.M., Daly J.F. Reversible temporary threshold shift in multiple sclerosis. *Laryngoscope* 75:424–428, 1964.

Rosenhall U., Hanner P., Kaijser B. Borrelia infection and vertigo. *Acta Otolaryngol. (Stockh.)* 106:111–116, 1988.

Rothstein T.L., Kenny G.E. Cranial neuropathy, myeloradiculopathy and myositis complications of *Mycoplasma pneumoniae* infection. *Arch. Neurol.* 36:476–477, 1979.

Rydell R.E., Pulec J.L. Arnold-Chiari malformation. *Arch. Otolaryngol.* 94:8–12, 1971.

Sando I., Hemenway W.G., Miller D.R. Vestibular pathology in otosclerosis: temporal bone histopathological report. *Laryngoscope* 84:593–605, 1974.

Sando I., Harada. T., Loehr A., et al. Sudden deafness. Histopathologic correlation in temporal bone. *Ann. Otol. Rhinol. Laryngol.* 86:269–279, 1977.

Sandstedt P., Hyden B., Odkvist L. Bell's palsy—part of a polyneuropathy? *Acta Neurol. Scand.* 64:66–73, 1981.

Satya-Murti S., Cacace A., Hanson P.A. Abnormal auditory evoked potentials in hereditary motor-sensory neuropathy. *Ann. Neurol.* 5:445–448, 1979.

Satya-Murti S., Cacace A., Hanson P.A. Auditory dysfunction in Friedreich's ataxia. Result of spiral degeneration. *Neurology (N.Y.)* 30:1047–1053, 1980.

Schmiedt R., Zwislocki J.J., Hammernik R.P. Effects of hair cell lesions on responses of cochlear nerve fibres, (1) lesions, tuning curves, two-tone inhibition and responses to trapezoidal wave patterns. *J. Neurophysiol.* 43:16–30, 1980.

Schuknecht H.F. *Pathology of the Ear.* Cambridge, MA, Harvard University Press, 1974.

Schuknecht H.F., Kitamura K. Vestibular neuritis. *Ann. Otol. Rhinol. Laryngol. Suppl.* 90:1–19, 1981.

Schuknecht H.F., Allam A.F., Murakami Y. Pathology of secondary malignant tumors of the temporal bone. *Ann. Otol. Rhinol. Laryngol.* 77:5–22, 1968.

*Selters W.A., Brackmann D.E. Acoustic tumour detection with brainstem evoked electric response audiometry. *Arch. Otolaryngol.* 103:181–187, 1977.

Shanon E., Mordechai Z., Himelfarb, M.D., et al. Auditory function in Friedreich's ataxia: electrophysiological study of a family. *Arch. Otolaryngol.* 197:254–256, 1981.

Silverstein H., Bernstein J., Davies D. Salicylate ototoxicity: a biochemical and electrophysiological study. *Ann. Otol. Rhinol. Laryngol.* 76:118–128, 1967.

Smith J.L. Cogan's syndrome. *Laryngoscope* 80:121–132, 1970.

*Spoendlin H.H. Optic and cochleo-vestibular degenerations in hereditary ataxias. Temporal bone pathology in two cases of Freidreich's ataxia with vestibulo-cochlear disorders. *Brain* 97:41–48, 1974.

Spoendlin H.H. The afferent innervation of the cochlea. In Naunton R.F., Fernandex C., eds. *Evoked Electrical Activity in the Auditory Nervous System.* London, Academic Press, pp. 21–39, 1978.

*Spoendlin H.H. Primary neurons and synapses. In Friedmann I., Ballantyne J., eds. *Ultrastructural Atlas of the Inner Ear.* London, Butterworth, pp. 133–164, 1984.

Starr A., Hamilton A.E. Correlation between confirmed site of neurological lesions and abnormalities of far field auditory brainstem responses. *Electroencephalogr. Clin. Neurophysiol.* 41:595–608, 1976.

Stephens S.D.G., Luxon L.M., Hinchcliffe R. Immunological disorders and auditory lesions. *Audiology* 21:128–148, 1982.

Suga S., Lindsay J.R. Histopathological observations of presbycusis. *Ann. Otol. Rhinol. Laryngol.* 85:169–184, 1976.

Susmano A., Rosenbush S.W. Hearing loss and ischemic heart disease. *Am. J. Otol.* 9:403–408, 1988.

Sylvester P.E. Spinocerebellar degeneration, hormonal disorder, hypogonadism and mental deficiency. *J. Ment. Defic. Res.* 16:203–214, 1972.

Ward P.H., Cannon D., Lindsay J.R. The vestibular system in multiple sclerosis. *Laryngoscope* 75:1031–1047, 1965.

Wendt J.S., Burks J.S. An unusual case of encephalomyeloradiculoneuropathy in a young woman. *Arch. Neurol.* 38:726–727, 1981.

Wildervanck L.G. Perceptive deafness associated with split hand and foot syndrome: a new syndrome? *Acta Genet. (Basel)* 13:161–169, 1964.

Wiley P.L., Block M.G. Acoustic and non-acoustic reflex patterns in audiological diagnosis. In Sholmo Silman S., ed. *The Acoustic Reflex, Basic Principles and Clinical Application.* Orlando, FL, Academic Press, pp. 388–411, 1984.

Wolff D., Bernard W.G., Tsutsumi S., et al. The pathology of Cogan's syndrome causing profound deafness. *Ann. Otol. Rhinol. Laryngol.* 74:507–520, 1965.

Wright R.B., Glantz R.H., Butcher J. Hearing loss in myotonic dystrophy. *Ann. Neurol.* 23:202–203, 1988.

Ylikoski J.S., House J.W., Hernandez I. Eighth nerve alcoholic neuropathy. A case report with light and electron microscopic findings. *J. Laryngol. Otol.* 95:631–642, 1981.

Zajtchuk J.P., Matz G.J., Lindsay J.R. Temporal bone pathology in herpes oticus. *Ann. Otol. Rhinol. Laryngol.* 81:331–338, 1972.

31

Vertigo and Dizziness

Thomas Brandt

Vertigo, the displeasing distortion of static gravitational orientation or the erroneous perception of self-motion or object motion, is not a clinical entity but a multisensory syndrome, which is induced by either physiologic (motion) stimulation or pathologic dysfunction. Management includes pharmacologic and physical therapy as well as surgery and psychotherapy. Influenced by the pharmaceutic industry, physicians tend to overestimate the benefit of antivertiginous drugs. These have only three clear indications for symptomatic relief of nausea and vertigo: in acute peripheral vestibulopathy, in acute brain stem or archicerebellar lesions near the vestibular nuclei, and for prevention of motion sickness.

Vertigo usually implies a mismatch among inputs from the sensory systems subserving static and dynamic spatial orientation as well as posture: vestibular, visual, and somatosensory. These systems are mutually interactive and redundant in that orientation, posture, and locomotion are guided by simultaneous reafferent cues. The functional ranges of the individual systems overlap, enabling them to compensate partially for each other's deficiencies. The intensity of the vertigo is a function of the mismatch and is increased if the intact sensory systems are eliminated, such as with eye closure during pathologic vestibular vertigo (Fig. 31–1).

Vertigo may thus be induced by physiologic stimulation (height vertigo, motion sickness) or pathologic dysfunction of any of the stabilizing sensory systems. The symptoms of vertigo include sensory qualities identified as vestibular, visual, and somatosensory. As distinct from one's perception of self-motion during natural locomotion, the vertigo experience is linked to impaired perception of a stationary environment; this perception is mediated by central nervous system processes known as space constancy mechanisms. Loss of the outside stationary reference system required for orientation and postural regulation contributes to the distressing admixture of both self-motion and surround motion. Four typical forms

of vertigo symptoms serve as a guide for differential diagnosis (Fig. 31–2):

1. Attacks of rotational vertigo
2. Sustained rotational vertigo
3. Positional vertigo
4. Dizziness with postural imbalance

Physiologic and clinical vertigo syndromes are commonly characterized by a combination of phenomena involving perceptual, oculomotor, postural, and vegetative manifestations: vertigo, nystagmus, ataxia, and nausea (Brandt and Daroff, 1980a; Honrubia and Brazier, 1982) (Fig. 31–3). These four manifestations correlate with different aspects of vestibular function and emanate from different sites within the central nervous system. The vertigo itself results from a disturbance of corticospatial orientation. Nystagmus is produced by a direction-specific imbalance in the vestibulo-ocular reflex (VOR), which activates brain stem neuronal circuitry. Vestibular ataxia (or postural imbalance) is caused by inappropriate or abnormal activation of monosynaptic and polysynaptic vestibulospinal pathways. Finally, the unpleasant vegetative effects of nausea and vomiting relate to chemical activation of the medullary vomiting center. Under certain conditions, these distressing symptoms may be preceded by a pleasurable vegetative sensation, presumably mediated through the limbic system, accounting for the popularity of carnival rides and the like.

PERIPHERAL VESTIBULAR NERVE AND LABYRINTHINE VERTIGO SYNDROMES

The three most common peripheral vestibular vertigo syndromes, in order of frequency, are benign paroxysmal positioning vertigo, vestibular neuritis, and Meniere's disease. A distinction should be made between positional and positioning vertigo. Benign

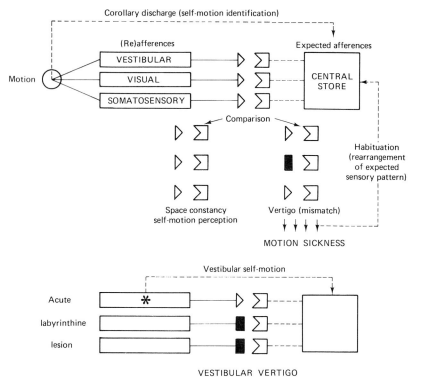

Figure 31–1. Diagram of the sensory conflict or the neural mismatch concept of motion sickness *(top)* and vertigo caused by unilateral vestibulopathy *(bottom)*. An active movement leads to stimulation of the sensory organs, whose messages are compared with a multisensory pattern of expectation calibrated by earlier experience of motions (central store). The pattern of expectation is prepared either by the efference copy signal, which is emitted parallel to and simultaneously with the motion impulse, or by vestibular excitation during passive transportation in vehicles. If sensory stimulation acting at the time and the pattern of expectation are in agreement, self-motion is perceived, while space constancy is maintained. If, for example, there is no adequate visual report of motion, because the field of view is filled with stationary environmental contrasts (e.g., reading in car), a sensory mismatch occurs. With repeated stimulation, motion sickness is induced through summation; the repeated stimulation leads to a rearrangement of the stored pattern of expectation, however, so that a habituation to the initially challenging stimulation is attained within days. An acute unilateral labyrinthine dysfunction causes vertigo because the self-motion sensation induced by the vestibular tone imbalance is contradicted by vision and the somatosensors.

paroxysmal positioning vertigo is caused by cupulo-lithiasis onto the cupula of the posterior canal. It is precipitated by rapid head tilt, which evokes an enhanced postrotatory *positioning* response, rather than a *positional* response. Two other disorders may be frequent but are less easy to diagnose: perilymph fistulas, which necessitate tympanoscopy to demonstrate perilymph leakage, and neurovascular compression syndromes (vestibular paroxysmia), for which there is no pathognomonic test. Positional vertigo has been described as a consequence of vestibular nerve compression by intracranial blood vessels (Jannetta et al., 1984). It may manifest with classic symptoms of Meniere's disease (Møller, 1988). Hesitation is highly justifiable (Brandt, 1991), because retromastoid craniectomy for microvascular decompression is the recommended management. The remainder of the peripheral vestibular syndromes are comparatively less frequent but arise from a more varied assortment of causes and pathologic changes (Table 31–1).

Acute Unilateral Peripheral Vestibulopathy (Vestibular Neuritis)

The chief symptom of the common unilateral labyrinthine lesion (also known as vestibular neuritis) is the acute onset of prolonged severe rotational vertigo associated with spontaneous nystagmus, postural imbalance, and nausea without concomitant auditory dysfunction. Caloric testing invariably shows ipsilateral hyporesponsiveness (horizontal semicircular ca-

nal paresis). Epidemic occurrence and a few autopsy studies that exhibited cell degeneration of one or more vestibular nerve trunks (Schuknecht and Kitamura, 1981) support viral vestibular nerve site origin, similar to that of Bell's palsy or sudden unilateral hearing loss. The condition mainly affects the age group of 30–60 years without preference for sex (Dix and Hallpike, 1952) with a natural history of gradual recovery within 1–6 weeks.

Normal vestibular end organs generate a tonic resting firing frequency equal from the two sides that is transmitted to the vestibular nuclei via vestibular nerves. Pathologic processes involving an end organ alter its firing frequency, thereby creating a tone imbalance. The imbalance causes most of the manifestations of the vertigo syndrome. The symptoms abate when the tone is re-equalized by either peripheral restitution (70–80% of the patients) or central compensation. The possibility that the three semicircular canals and the otoliths (utricle and saccule) may be separately involved in partial labyrinthine lesions is suggested by the occasional observation of an acute unilateral vestibulopathy (horizontal canal paresis) and a benign paroxysmal positioning vertigo (functional cupulolithiasis of the posterior canal) simultaneously in the same ear of a patient (Büchele and Brandt, 1988).

In vestibular neuritis, the fast phase of the rotational spontaneous nystagmus as well as the initial perception of apparent body motion is directed away from the side where the lesion is, and the postural reactions initiated by vestibulospinal reflexes are usually opposite to the direction of vertigo; these result

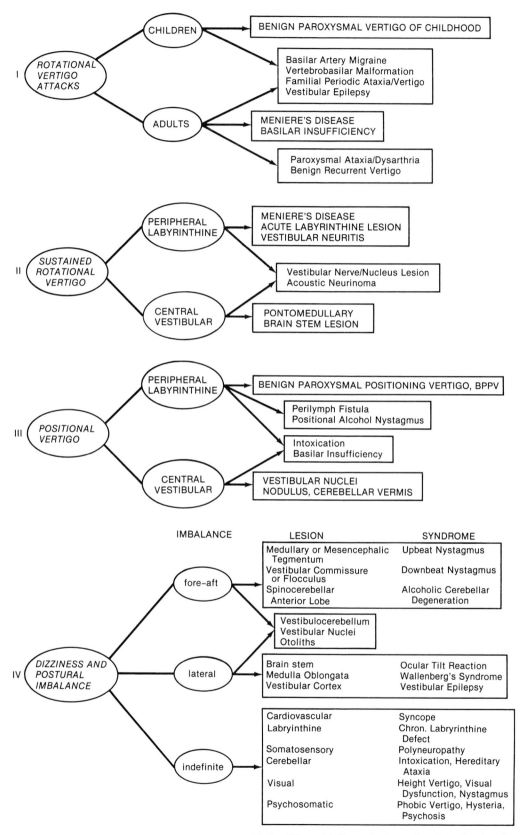

Figure 31–2. Four typical forms of vertigo symptoms serve as a guide for differential diagnosis: I, attacks of rotational vertigo; II, sustained rotational vertigo; III, positional vertigo; IV, dizziness with postural imbalance.

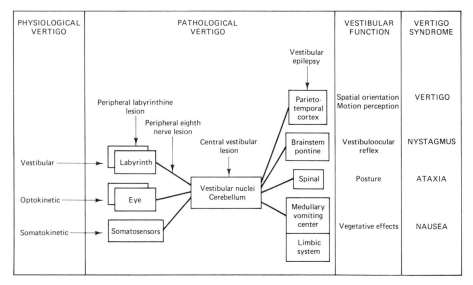

Figure 31–3. Classification and origin of different types of physiologic and pathologic vertigo commonly characterized by a combination of phenomena involving perceptual, oculomotor, postural, and vegetative manifestations. (From Brandt T., Daroff R. B. The multisensory physiological and pathological vertigo syndromes. Reprinted with permission from *Annals of Neurology*, 7:195–203, 1980.)

in both the Romberg fall and past-pointing toward the side with the lesion (Table 31–2). The nystagmus is typically reduced in amplitude by fixation and enhanced by eye closure or Frenzel's (high plus) lenses. Gaze nystagmus in the direction of spontaneous nystagmus as well as a significant directional preponderance of optokinetic nystagmus may be another consequence of the peripheral lesion and not due to involvement of the brain stem or cerebellum.

Management

During the first 1–3 days when nausea is prominent, vestibular sedatives such as the antihistamine dimenhydrinate (Dramamine), 50–100 mg every 6 hours, or the anticholinergic scopolamine (Transderm-Scop), 0.6 mg, can be administered parenterally for symptomatic relief, with the major side effect being general sedation.

The capacity to antagonize acetylcholine by competitive inhibition is the only known similarity among the drugs to counter labyrinthine vertigo and motion sickness. The most probable sites of primary action are the synapses of vestibular nuclei that exhibit a reduced discharge and diminished neuronal action to body rotation. These drugs should not be given longer than nausea lasts because they prolong the time necessary to achieve central compensation. A further mode of treatment is physical therapy with the Cawthorne-Cooksey (Cawthorne, 1944) exercises modified according to the knowledge of vestibular physiology (Table 31–3). Vestibular exercises consist mainly of eye, head, and body movements designed to provoke a sensory mismatch; they enhance compensation by facilitating central recalibration, although the symptoms initially are uncomfortable.

Animal experiments have shown that exercises promote central compensation of spontaneous nystagmus and postural imbalance. Compensation requires profound reorganization of commissural brain stem connections between the vestibular nuclei; the spinocerebellar posterior vermis probably has a more direct functional linkage to the vestibulospinal system, whereas archicerebellar flocculus, uvula, and nodulus are connected more directly to the vestibulo-oculomotor system (Igarashi, 1984). Pharmacologic and metabolic studies suggest that the state of central compensation for a peripheral vestibular lesion is both dynamic and fragile (Zee, 1985): alcohol, phenobarbital, chlorpromazine, diazepam, and adrenocorticotropin antagonists retard compensation; caffeine, amphetamines, and adrenocorticotropin accelerate compensation; cholinomimetics, cholinesterase inhibitors, adrenergic agents, γ-aminobutyric acid agonists, and alcohol may (re)produce decompensation.

Benign Paroxysmal Positioning Vertigo

In benign paroxysmal positioning vertigo, initially described by Bárány in 1921, attacks of rotational vertigo and concomitant positioning nystagmus are precipitated by head extension as well as by lateral head tilt toward the affected ear. It is the most common cause of vertigo in the elderly and is due to cupulolithiasis of the posterior semicircular canal. There is frequently a natural history of spontaneous recovery and the possibility of a most effective mechanical therapy by positioning maneuvers on a serial basis.

Schuknecht (1969) proposed that degenerated material from the utricular macula gravitates and becomes attached to the cupula of the posterior canal, which is situated directly inferior to the utricle when the head is upright. The posterior semicircular canal thus serves as a receptacle for the detached sediment. The cupula, normally of equal specific gravity with the endolymph and a transducer of only angular accelerations, then theoretically should become sen-

Table 31–1. VERTIGO IN VESTIBULAR NERVE AND LABYRINTHINE DISORDERS

Site	Syndrome	Mechanism
Labyrinth	Frequent (unilateral or bilateral)	
	Benign paroxysmal positioning vertigo	Cupulolithiasis
	Meniere's disease	Endolymphatic hydrops
	Perilymph fistula	Pathologic elasticity of bony labyrinth
	Less frequent (unilateral or bilateral)	
	Ototoxic drugs	Hair cell and peripheral neuron damage
	Labyrinthitis	Viral or bacterial
	Delayed endolymphatic hydrops	Impaired endolymph resorption after labyrinthitis or trauma
	Otosclerosis	Damage to sensory cells
	Vestibular atelectasis	Collapse of ampullae and utricle walls
	Vascular	Ischemia of superior part of vestibular labyrinth
	Hyperviscosity syndrome	Venous obstruction
	Autoimmune inner ear disease	Vasculitis and inflammation
	Congenital (genetic or intrauterine factors)	Aplasia, malformation
Vestibular nerve	Frequent	
	Vestibular neuritis	Viral vestibular nerve inflammation
	Acoustic neurinoma (and other cerebellopontine angle tumors)	Compression of the nerve (and of central vestibular structures)
	Disabling positional vertigo (vestibular paroxysmia)	Neurovascular compression
	Less frequent	
	Herpes zoster oticus	Vestibular nerve inflammation
	Polyneuropathy	Vascular, toxic, or inflammatory
	Vascular (e.g., diabetes mellitus)	Vestibular nerve ischemia
	Meningeosis carcinomatosa	Tumor infiltration
	Paget's disease	Compression of the vestibular nerve

sitive to changes in head position relative to the gravitational vector. Because the symptoms of benign paroxysmal positioning vertigo are compatible with the cupulogram of an ampullofugal stimulation of the posterior canal of the undermost ear (Schmidt, 1985), it is more likely that the heavy cupula creates an overexcitability of the posterior canal to angular accelerations in the specific plane. Thus, benign paroxysmal positioning vertigo constitutes a post-rotatory positioning rather than a positional vertigo syndrome (Brandt, 1990). The hypothesis of cupulolithiasis, which was proved histologically, may also explain the fatigability of the manifestations. The detached particles might be dispersed from the cupula into the endolymphatic space.

Rotational vertigo and nystagmus begin after a latency of seconds after head tilt toward the affected ear and subside after 10–60 seconds and ultimately abate, even with maintenance of the precipitating position. The nystagmus, best seen with Frenzel's glasses to avoid fixation suppression, is horizontal rotary, with the fast phase beating toward the undermost ear; the nystagmus beats upward (toward the forehead) when gaze is directed toward the uppermost ear (Fig. 31–4). When the patient returns to the seated position, the vertigo and nystagmus may recur in the opposite direction. Constant repetition of this maneuver results in ever-lessening symptoms. Head extension at upright stance causes a vestibulospinal ataxia, with the direction of fall toward the affected ear and forward. In the initial course of the disease, patients may also have other

Table 31–2. FUNCTIONAL CLASSIFICATION OF LABYRINTHINE LESIONS

Semicircular Canal Type	Otolith Type
Spontaneous rotational vertigo (self-motion and/or surround motion toward fast phase of nystagmus)	Sensation of tilt or levitation; to-and-fro or linear vertigo (mostly dependent on head position or acceleration)
Postural imbalance, laterotorsion, tendency to fall and past-pointing in direction opposite to vertigo	Postural imbalance with ipsiversive deviation of the postural vertical and subjective visual vertical (opposite in direction to vertigo), ataxic gait
Spontaneous nystagmus, primarily contraversive and horizontal rotary	Diminished ocular counter-rolling on head tilt, spontaneous cyclorotation of the eyes and skew deviation
Visual slip of environment after rapid head movements caused by impaired VOR	Vibration oscillopsia (reduced visual acuity during walking); somatosensory sensation of walking on pillows
Homolateral horizontal canal paresis with canal irrigation; normal responses with vertical canal dysfunction	Equal caloric responses
Severe nausea	Moderate nausea

Table 31–3. PHYSICAL THERAPY FOR ACUTE, UNILATERAL LABYRINTHINE LESIONS

Clinical Stage	Physical Exercise	Strategy
I. **Approximately days 1–3** Nausea Spontaneous nystagmus with fixation	No exercise: bed rest Head immobilization Eyes closed	Prevent falls Avoid active head accelerations leading to cross-coupled effects Avoid visual-vestibular mismatch
II. **Approximately days 2–5** No spontaneous nausea Incomplete suppression of spontaneous nystagmus by fixation straight ahead	Exercise in bed supine and sitting 1. Fixation straight ahead; voluntary saccades and eccentric gaze-holding (10, 20, and 40° horizontal/vertical); reading exercise Smooth pursuit (finger movements or pendulum ± 20–40°, 20–60°/s) Active head oscillations with fixation of a stationary target at 1-m distance (0.5–2 Hz; ± 20–30°; yaw—pitch—roll) 2. First balance exercise—free sit and stance and guided gait (eyes open/eyes closed)	Visual control of stabilization of gaze in space by suppressing spontaneous nystagmus through voluntary fixation impulse (retinal slip) Visually guided control of target fixation Provoke vestibular stimuli for recalibration of VOR under visual control of retinal slip of viewed target Circulatory training, prophylaxis of thrombosis
III. **Approximately days 4–7** Suppression of spontaneous nystagmus with fixation straight ahead, but continued gaze nystagmus in the direction of fast phase, and spontaneous nystagmus with Frenzel's glasses	1. Static stabilization: four-point stance; stance on one knee and one foot; upright stance (eyes open/eyes closed; head upright/head extension) 2. Dynamic stabilization: Smooth pursuit and head oscillation exercises at free stance as described above Exercises with rope, ball, and club under fixation (eye and head) of the instrument (sitting/standing/walking)	Recalibrate visuovestibulospinal reflexes for postural control and eye-hand coordination at free body movements
IV. **Approximately weeks 2–3** No spontaneous vertigo Weak spontaneous nystagmus with Frenzel's glasses	Complex balance exercise; successive increase in difficulty above the demands for postural control under daily life conditions	Expose the subjectively recovered patient increasingly to unstable body positions to facilitate rearrangement and recruitment of control capacities

From Brandt T. Episodic vertigo. In Rakel R. E., ed. *Conn's Current Therapy*. Philadelphia, Saunders, pp. 841–847, 1991.

symptoms of otolithic vertigo with normal head upright position, and especially of the somatosensory sensation of walking on pillows (see Table 31–2). The latter is probably due to the actual unequal heavy loads of the two utricular otoliths and is compensated centrally within 1–3 weeks.

Etiologic conditions associated with benign paroxysmal positioning vertigo are head (labyrinthine) trauma, infections, stapedectomy, and most often, aging. The initial occurrence is usually experienced on awakening in the morning rather than on first lying down.

Management

The mechanism of cupulolithiasis led us to contrive a mechanical therapy by challenging these patients with precipitating head positions on a repeated and serial basis (see Fig. 31–4) to promote the loosening and ultimate dispersion of the degenerated otolithic material from the cupula (Brandt and Daroff, 1980b). Certainly such a regimen should be undertaken for 2–4 weeks in all patients with unremitting benign paroxysmal positioning vertigo in whom a surgical procedure is contemplated. In the rare patients refractive to prolonged physical therapy, surgical tran-section of the posterior ampullary nerve via a middle ear approach can be considered (Gacek, 1978). This operation provides relief of vertigo; it is, however, not easy to locate the particular semicircular canal nerve surgically, and sensorineural hearing loss is a possible complication. Drug therapy with anti–motion sickness medications has not proved particularly efficacious.

Meniere's Disease

The syndrome first described by Meniere in 1861 is characterized by fluctuating hearing loss, tinnitus, and prolonged decrescendo nystagmus-vertigo attacks for hours caused by endolymphatic hydrops and periodical ruptures in the membranes separating endolymph from perilymph, which subsequently cause intermediate potassium palsy of vestibular nerve fibers (Dohlmann, 1976). The condition chiefly affects the 30- to 50-year-old age group. There is irregular frequency of attacks and a tendency to bilateral involvement but spontaneous amelioration after years or decades.

The hydrops may result from either insufficient fluid resorption in the endolymphatic sac or acquired

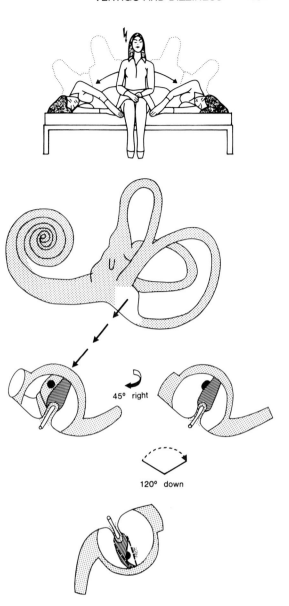

Figure 31–4. Mechanism of cupulolithiasis, the most probable cause of benign paroxysmal positioning vertigo. Inorganic heavy particles detached from the otoconial layer (by degeneration or head trauma) gravitate to and become settled on the cupula of the posterior semicircular canal. The heavy material causes a specific gravity differential between the cupula and the endolymph with postrotatory overexcitability. After rapid head tilt toward the affected ear or after head extension, when the posterior semicircular canal is moved in the specific plane of stimulation, an ampullofugal deflection of the cupula occurs with a rotational vertigo and concomitant nystagmus. The therapeutic protocol is as follows: the patients are seated with their eyes closed and are tilted laterally with the lateral aspect of their occiputs resting on the bed to ensure proper plane-specific stimulation of the posterior semicircular canal. They remain in their position until the evoked vertigo subsides or for at least 30 seconds and then sit up for another 30 seconds before assuming the opposite head-down position for another 30 seconds. This sequence of positional changes is repeated about five times on a serial basis several times daily. (From Brandt T. Episodic Vertigo. In Rakel R. E., ed. *Conn's Current Therapy*. Philadelphia, Saunders, pp. 841–847, 1991.)

blocking within the endolymphatic duct. The cause is still unknown, although scarring labyrinthitis can lead to endolymphatic hydrops. Because the disease progresses from the pars inferior (cochlear duct) to the pars superior (semicircular canals, utricle) of the labyrinth, auditory dysfunction is more likely to precede vestibular symptoms. Audiometry is helpful in diagnosis, particularly when reversibility of hearing deficits becomes apparent with administration of dehydrating agents such as oral glycerol. The typical attack is experienced as an initial sensation of fullness of the ear, a hearing decrement, and tinnitus before rotational vertigo; postural imbalance, nystagmus, and nausea follow within minutes. Because no pathognomonic test is available, diagnosis may remain uncertain in the early stage of the disease, particularly in the case of monosymptomatic and episodic dysfunction. Rarely, *vestibular drop attacks* (indistinguishable from basilar drop attacks) may occur, when

sudden changes in fluid pressure cause inadequate otolith–end-organ stimulation with a reflex-like vestibulospinal loss of postural tone (Black et al., 1982).

Management

Antivertiginous drugs (see under Acute Unilateral Peripheral Vestibulopathy [Vestibular Neuritis]) counteract vertigo and nausea in an acute attack. Fewer than 5% of patients ultimately require surgical treatment, because the success of regular endolymphatic sac shunt operations was shown to be a placebo effect (Thomson et al., 1981). The histamine derivative betahistine hydrochloride (Vasomotal, Aequamen), 8 mg three times daily, has been advocated as the drug of first choice. Intratympanic treatment with ototoxic antibiotics such as gentamicin sulfate (Refobacin), 8–24 mg instilled daily via a plastic tube inserted behind the annulus via the transmeatal approach, is obviously able to damage selectively the secretory epithelium (and thereby to improve endolymphatic hydrops) before significantly affecting vestibular and cochlear function. Instillations (up to 10 days), therefore, should be stopped when daily audiograms or a check of spontaneous nystagmus by use of Frenzel's glasses indicates end-organ dysfunction.

For patients in whom more conservative procedures have failed, selective destructive surgical techniques have been proposed, such as middle fossa vestibular nerve section as well as ultrasonic or cryosurgical vestibular destruction, to preserve serviceable hearing function. Because this surgical approach does not affect the pathologic hydrops mechanism and therefore does not prevent ongoing fluctuating hearing loss, there is an obvious tendency for it to be less often considered. Indication for surgical damage becomes even more doubtful if one takes into account the relatively benign natural history of the disease, with a spontaneous remission rate of about 80% within 5 years. The ideal but rare patient for whom to contemplate surgical labyrinthectomy has unilateral Meniere's disease with frequent vertigo or drop attacks but without functional hearing remaining on the affected side. Particularly in elderly patients, ablative surgical procedures may cause long-lasting postural imbalance, owing to the reduced capability of central compensation of the postoperative vestibular tone imbalance.

Perilymph Fistula

Perilymph fistulas may lead to episodic vertigo and sensorineural hearing loss owing to a pathologic elasticity of the bony labyrinth, usually at the round or oval window. A history of trauma (or physical exertion), with subsequent vertigo and hearing loss, and a positional nystagmus of short latency but long duration, which is not as violent as in benign paroxysmal positioning vertigo, should lead the physician to suspect a fistula. Some fistulas appear as a solely otolithic vertigo with periodic head motion intolerance, gait ataxia, and distressing tilt sensations on head tilt. Even though some typical clinical vascular and pressure fistula tests are useful, a definite diagnosis can be made only by exploratory tympanotomy, which sometimes demonstrates pumping of the stapes when the patient performs the Valsalva maneuver.

The combination of vertigo, eye movements, and postural instability (either semicircular canal or otolith type) induced by high-intensity auditory stimulation in congenitally deaf patients and those with labyrinthine fistulas (e.g., luxated stapes footplate) is known as the *Tullio phenomenon*.

Management

In the acute case, medical treatment is universally recommended because most often these fistulas heal spontaneously and the results of surgical interventions are not encouraging (Singleton et al., 1978). Medical care consists of absolute bed rest with head elevation for 5–10 days; avoidance of straining, sneezing, or coughing; and use of stool softeners. If symptoms persist for 3–4 weeks, exploratory tympanotomy is indicated under local anesthesia, with the Valsalva maneuver or gentle palpation of the footplate to make the leak apparent. For patching the fistula, perichondrial graft from the tragus is superior to fat.

Acoustic Neurinomas

Acoustic neurinomas (schwannomas), which mostly arise from the vestibular part of cranial nerve VIII in the internal auditory canal, initially present with unilateral hearing loss (see Chapter 30). In later stages, they cause vertigo, nystagmus, and postural imbalance because, as the acoustic neurinomas increase in size, the brain stem structures that subserve central compensation of the progressive peripheral nerve damage are compressed.

Positional and Positioning Vertigo and Nystagmus

Positional and positioning vertigo and nystagmus syndromes can be attributed to either peripheral or central vestibular dysfunction (Table 31–4). The most common form is benign paroxysmal positioning vertigo. Positional vertigo is a characteristic symptom in perilymph fistulas, Meniere's disease, and vestibular atelectasis. Other labyrinthine manifestations, such as positional alcohol nystagmus (Fig. 31–5), positional nystagmus with macroglobulinemia, and nystagmus caused by heavy water or glycerol ingestion, occur because of a specific gravity differential be-

Table 31–4. POSITIONAL AND POSITIONING VERTIGO AND NYSTAGMUS

Central vestibular (pontomedullary brain stem or vestibulocerebellum)
  Positional downbeat nystagmus
  Central positional nystagmus without major vertigo
  Central positional vertigo with nystagmus
  Basilar insufficiency

Vestibular nerve
  Neurovascular compression (disabling positional vertigo)

Peripheral labyrinth
  Benign paroxysmal positioning vertigo
  Cupula-endolymph gravity differential (buoyancy mechanism)
    Positional alcohol vertigo and nystagmus
    Positional heavy water nystagmus
    Positional glycerol nystagmus
    Positional nystagmus with macroglobulinemia
  Perilymph fistula
  Meniere's disease
  Vestibular atelectasis
  (Physiologic head extension vertigo or bending-over vertigo)

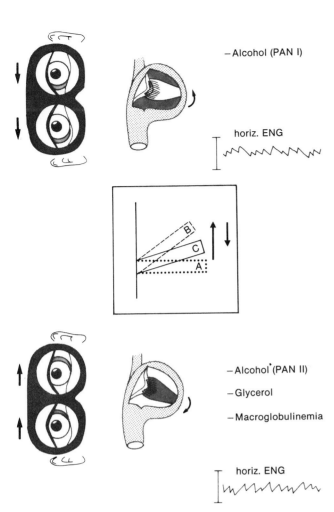

Figure 31–5. Positional alcohol nystagmus. Ingestion of water-soluble molecules with different specific weights, such as alcohol, heavy water, or glycerol, causes a specific gravity differential between the cupula and the endolymph (buoyancy mechanism), with positional nystagmus and vertigo. During the resorption phase of alcohol, nystagmus beats toward the undermost ear (PAN I, with the cupula relatively lighter than the endolymph). Positional nystagmus beats toward the uppermost ear during alcohol-reduction phase (PAN II), as well as in glycerol-, heavy water–, and macroglobulinemia-induced positional nystagmus (with the cupula relatively heavier than the endolymph). The gravity-dependent deflection force on the cupula (*inset*, B) must be greater than the physiologic restoring force (*inset*, C) for the positional nystagmus to last as long as the precipitating head position is maintained. horiz. ENG = horizontal electronystagmogram.

extension. Experimental extirpation of the nodulus in the cat causes postural downbeat nystagmus (Fernandez et al., 1960), which has been confirmed by clinical experience (Kattah et al., 1984). Physiologically, the nodulus may have an inhibitory influence on the gain of the vertical otolith-ocular reflex, and lesional postural downbeat nystagmus is abolished by additional bilateral labyrinthectomy.

Positional Alcohol Nystagmus and Vertigo

A major reason why the semicircular canals selectively transduce angular acceleration and not gravitational position is that the cupula (housed in the ampulla of the canals, and in which the hair cells are embedded) has the same specific gravity as endolymph. Alcohol is lighter than endolymph, and when blood levels approach 40 mg/100 ml, alcohol diffuses into the cupula, rendering it lighter than endolymph and thereby transforming the semicircular canals into gravity-sensitive receptors (Money et al., 1974). Nystagmus and vertigo then occur when the subject lies down. In phase I of positional alcohol nystagmus, the nystagmus beats toward the undermost ear. With time, blood alcohol diffuses into endolymph, restoring its specific gravity to that of the cupula. There is then a silent period, beginning between 3½ and 5 hours after cessation of alcohol ingestion, when positional vertigo is absent. Alcohol selectively diffuses out of the cupula before it leaves the endolymph. This causes the cupula to be transiently denser than the endolymph, thus initiating phase II, which begins between 5 and 10 hours after cessation of drinking, when the blood level drops to about 20 mg/100 ml. In positional alcohol nystagmus phase II, nystagmus beats to the uppermost ear. Positional vertigo may persist until all the alcohol eventually leaves the endolymph, but this may not transpire until many hours after the blood alcohol level has reached zero. Phase II is usually associated with motion sickness and is a major concomitant of the hangover. The morning-after drink of alcohol may indeed re-equalize the specific gravities and lessen, albeit transiently, the untoward symptoms. A similar mechanism may enable macroglobulinemia to alter specific gravity of the cupula and create positional nystagmus (Keim and Sachs, 1975).

Traumatic Vertigo

Traumatic vertigo is among the most frequent sequelae associated with head and neck injuries and barotrauma (Table 31–5). Central vestibular vertigo syndromes caused by brain stem dysfunction (concussion, hemorrhage) and classic paroxysmal positioning vertigo are well recognized. The peripheral end organs and vestibular nerves may also be affected by temporal bone fractures or hemorrhages into the endolymphatic and perilymphatic space (e.g., perilymph fistulas). Patients often describe

tween the cupula and the endolymph (buoyancy mechanism). Central positional vertigo has at least three forms: positional downbeat nystagmus (caused by nodulus), positional nystagmus without concurrent vertigo, and positional vertigo with nystagmus. They always indicate dysfunction (disinhibition) of the infratentorial connections between vestibular nuclei and vestibulocerebellar structures (Brandt, 1990). The finding of positional downbeat nystagmus with only slight vertigo with the patient in the head-hanging position indicates a vestibulocerebellar nodulus lesion and may be related to downbeat nystagmus syndrome, which also shows activation on head

Table 31–5. VERTIGO AFTER HEAD AND/OR NECK INJURY

Site	Syndrome	Mechanism
Labyrinth	Otolithic vertigo	Loosening of otoconia
	Benign paroxysmal positioning vertigo	Cupulolithiasis
	Loss of labyrinthine function	Temporal bone fractures, concussion, or hemorrhage
	Perilymph fistula	Round or oval window rupture, temporal bone fracture or hemorrhage
Vestibular nerve	Loss of vestibular function	Concussion or hemorrhage
Brain stem or vestibulocerebellum	All central vestibular vertigo syndromes (downbeat or upbeat nystagmus, ocular tilt reaction, central positional nystagmus and vertigo, and others)	Concussion or hemorrhage
Cervical	Whiplash vertigo (not a clear entity)	Not known (vascular compression ? neuromuscular ? neurovascular ?)
	Cervical vertigo ?	
Psychogenic	Phobic postural vertigo	Anxious introspection causes dissociation between efference and efference copy
	Secondary gain factors	

their post-traumatic vertigo as a head motion intolerance and unsteadiness in gait similar to walking on pillows. Because these symptoms resemble those of otolith dysfunction, one might speculate that this vulnerable accelerometer is affected by trauma (Brandt and Daroff, 1980a). Otoconia is easily dislodged by linear accelerations, resulting in unequal loads on the macula beds and a tonus imbalance between the two otoliths (Brandt, 1991). Vertigo resulting from barotrauma is mostly of peripheral labyrinthine origin (alternobaric vertigo, round or oval window fistulas) or part of the decompression sickness.

CENTRAL VESTIBULAR VERTIGO

Central vestibular vertigo syndromes are caused, in the majority of cases, by dysfunction induced by a lesion, but a small proportion result from pathologic excitation of various structures, ranging from the vestibular nuclei to the vestibular cortex (vestibular epilepsy, paroxysmal dysarthria and ataxia in multiple sclerosis) (Table 31–6). Most of the patients have an intra-axial, paramedian infratentorial lesion, especially of the pontomedullary tegmentum, involving vestibular nuclei connections to vestibulocerebellar structures. A preliminary classification of vestibular

Table 31–6. CENTRAL VESTIBULAR VERTIGO SYNDROMES

Site	Syndrome	Mechanism
Vestibular cortex	Vestibular epilepsy	Simple partial seizures
Thalamus	Ocular tilt reaction	Paramedian thalamic infarction, hemorrhage
	Thalamic astasia	Posterolateral thalamic lesions
Vestibulocerebellum		
Flocculus	Downbeat nystagmus vertigo	Disinhibition of vertical VOR in pitch
Nodulus	Positional downbeat nystagmus	Inappropriate otolith-canal interaction ?
Vestibular nuclei	Central positional vertigo and/or nystagmus	Inappropriate otolith-canal interaction ?
Vestibulocerebellar loop ?		
Mesodiencephalic brain stem	Ocular tilt reaction	Tone imbalance of VOR in roll
	Upbeat nystagmus vertigo	Tone imbalance of vertical VOR in pitch
Pontomedullary brain stem	Paroxysmal dysarthria/ataxia in multiple sclerosis	Transversally spreading ephaptic axonal activation
	Pseudo–vestibular neuritis	Vestibular nerve root plaque in multiple sclerosis, lacunar infarction
	Ocular tilt reaction	Graviceptive pathway lesion with tone imbalance of VOR in roll
	Downbeat nystagmus vertigo	Tone imbalance of VOR in pitch
Medullary	Upbeat nystagmus vertigo	Tone imbalance of VOR in pitch
	Paroxysmal vertigo evoked by lateral gaze or head position	Vestibular nuclei lesion ?
Brain stem and cerebellum	Pseudo–vestibular neuritis	Ischemia of superior labyrinth, vestibular nerve, vestibular nuclei (AICA or PICA infarction)
	Lateropulsion in Wallenberg's syndrome	Ischemic lesion–induced deviation of subjective vertical
	Familial periodic vertigo	Hereditary, metabolic ?
	Encephalitis with predominant vertigo	Viral infection
	Epidemic vertigo	Viral infection

brain stem syndromes may be attempted (Brandt, 1991), according to the three major functional planes of the VOR:

Disorders of VOR in horizontal (yaw) plane	Pseudo–vestibular neuritis (partial AICA or PICA infarction; multiple sclerosis plaques)
Disorders of VOR in sagittal (pitch) plane	Downbeat nystagmus and vertigo Upbeat nystagmus and vertigo
Disorders of VOR in frontal (roll) plane	Ocular tilt reaction (lateropulsion?)

In this context, disorders of the VOR are not limited to those affecting eye movements but include those affecting the vestibulospinal reflexes and perception, because the VOR, perception, and control of posture are intimately and inextricably connected. Central vestibular syndromes are the cause of the vertigo in up to 25% of patients whose main complaint is vertigo. The proportion is greater if one includes all the cerebellar and brain stem disorders in which vertigo is a secondary symptom.

Vestibular Epilepsy

Vestibular seizures (vertiginous epilepsy) are caused by focal discharges from either the temporal lobe or the parietal association cortex (Schneider et al., 1968), which receives bilateral vestibular projections from the ipsilateral thalamus. The patient experiences a sudden rotational or linear vertigo accompanied by contraversive body or head and eye rotation. The symptom lasts only several seconds and may be associated with mild nausea but rarely with vomiting. Tinnitus, often unilateral, and contralateral paresthesias may precede or accompany the vertigo. Contraversive epileptic nystagmus may occur. An aura, temporal lobe seizures, or absences may also be experienced as episodic vertigo by the patient (for treatment, see Chapter 72). Vertiginous epilepsy should be distinguished from vestibulogenic epilepsy (Barac, 1968). This is a variety of sensory-evoked epilepsy, either partial complex or grand mal, induced by peripheral labyrinthine stimulation (caloric irrigation or spinning).

The combination of nonepileptic paroxysmal dysarthria, vertigo, and ataxia is a well-known manifestation of multiple sclerosis. The suggested mechanism of the attacks is a transversally spreading ephaptic activation of adjacent axons within a partially demyelinated lesion in fiber tracts of the pontine tegmentum involving the brachium conjunctivum (Osterman and Westerberg, 1975). Carbamazepine is the most effective treatment and results in complete disappearance of the attacks in most cases. Paroxysms of vertigo and ataxia have also been described as familial periodic ataxia with autosomal dominant inheritance. Acetazolamide (Diamox), a potent drug for prevention of periodic paralysis, is also effective in preventing periodic ataxia and vertigo (Zasorin et al., 1983).

Basilar Insufficiency

Nystagmus, vertigo, and postural imbalance induced when the head is maximally rotated and/or extended while standing and terminated abruptly by returning the head to a neutral upright position are frequently reported experiences. Clinicians usually attribute these symptoms to intermittent basilar insufficiency caused by a functional compression of the vertebral artery, particularly in elderly patients with atheroma or with cervical spondylosis and osteophytes narrowing the transverse foramina.

Transient attacks of vertigo of central origin are the most common early symptom of basilar insufficiency because of the steep pressure gradient from the aorta to the terminal pontine arteries, which are long, tenuous, circumferential arteries and therefore provide a most vulnerable blood supply for the vestibular nuclei (Williams and Wilson, 1962). The possibility cannot be excluded that transient ischemia of the labyrinths may also contribute, because blood supply originates from the same source. Experimental studies on blood flow in cadavers reveal that extreme head positions may reduce flow through one or another of the vertebral or carotid vessels (Toole and Tucker, 1960).

Thus, vestibular vertigo and ataxia and drop attacks can undoubtedly be precipitated by extreme extension or rotation of the neck, at least when a partial obstruction of the arteries combines with a sudden fall of systemic blood pressure (e.g., in a patient rising from a chair and looking up). An association of dysfunctions that convinces the clinician of the diagnosis is that of vertigo with visual illusions, field defects, diplopia, drop attacks (see also under Meniere's Disease) or motor symptoms.

Apart from basilar insufficiency, however, symptoms of to-and-fro vertigo and postural imbalance occur frequently in healthy people (e.g., elicited by overhead work while standing on an unstable wobbling ladder or in situations in which visual cues conflict with proprioceptive input [looking up at moving clouds]). Such *physiologic head extension vertigo* with measurably increased postural sway must be related to a functional deficiency of the otoliths, which are beyond their optimal functional range in the offending head-extended or bending-over position (Brandt and Daroff, 1980a). The physiologic instability related to this head position can be determined by attempting to balance on one foot with one's eyes closed and head extended as compared with the neutral head position. Simple training of postural balance improves body sway activity and therefore postural stability within days by 30–50%

owing to multimodal sensorimotor rearrangement (Brandt et al., 1981).

Basilar Artery Migraine

Whereas basilar insufficiency is a disease of the elderly, sudden attacks of basilar artery migraine occur predominantly in adolescent girls (Bickerstaff, 1961). Vertigo, nystagmus, and ataxia are key symptoms of the aura lasting from minutes to 1 hour and are frequently combined with other signs of dysfunction within the basilar and posterior cerebral artery territory: dysarthria, perioral and distal limb paresthesias, drop attacks, and scotomata or visual hallucinations as well as loss of consciousness or global amnesia. The accompanying but usually subsequent headache is predominantly occipital.

Typically, there is a family history of migraine; attacks exhibit an obvious relation to the menstrual cycle; additional classic migraine attacks may occur in the same patient, and with increasing age, basilar artery migraine tends to become a rare event.

The simple vascular hypothesis that aura dysfunctions are due to vasoconstriction and transient ischemia, whereas headache is caused by excessive dilatation of dural and extracranial vessels, is not generally accepted and may be further substantiated by results of biochemical investigations on platelet function, prostaglandins, the serotininergic raphe system, and opioid receptors. Benign paroxysmal vertigo of childhood, paroxysmal torticollis in infancy, and benign recurrent vertigo in adults are also regarded as typical manifestations of migraine, even without the apparently obligatory headache.

Downbeat Nystagmus Vertigo

The combination of postural instability, oscillopsia, and downbeat nystagmus in the primary or lateral position of gaze is a well-defined clinical sign, almost specific for a structural lesion of the paramedian craniocervical junction (Cogan, 1968; see Chapter 26).

The suggested and appealing mechanism of a downward pursuit defect (Zee et al., 1974) cannot explain ataxia. It was questioned by Baloh and Spooner (1981) who assumed "that downbeat nystagmus is a type of central vestibular nystagmus resulting from an imbalance in the central vertical vestibulo-ocular pathways, due either to a lesion in the floor of the 4th ventricle between the vestibular nuclei (which interrupts the tonic excitatory activity to the inferior recti), or to a bilateral lesion of the flocculus (which leads to an increase in tonic excitatory activity to the superior recti due to a disinhibition)." Both lesions have been demonstrated to cause downbeat nystagmus in animals. Because static head tilt, however, mainly modulates the intensity of the nystagmus, otolith function is probably involved rather than there being a solely semicircular canal–related cause.

About 30% of the cases are due to Arnold-Chiari malformation and basilar invagination. Other etiologic conditions associated with downbeat nystagmus are drug intoxication, multiple sclerosis, vascular disease, alcoholic cerebellar degeneration, brain stem tumors, hematomas, encephalitis, magnesium depletion, and communicating hydrocephalus.

The clinical oculomotor abnormalities are the following: downbeat nystagmus is present in darkness, as well as with fixation; amplitude and slow-phase velocity increase on lateral gaze or with head extension; and downward pursuit is saccadic. The retinal slip in downbeat nystagmus is misinterpreted as motion of the visual scene (distressing oscillopsia) because the involuntary ocular movements that override fixation are not associated with an appropriate efference copy signal. Oscillopsia is a permanent symptom, but the amplitude of the illusory motion is smaller than the net retinal slip caused by the nystagmus. Postural imbalance is particularly apparent for the fore-aft body sway with a tendency to fall backward (compensation of the lesional forward vertigo, which corresponds to downbeat nystagmus). The patients' pathologic postural sway, with eyes open, is dependent on the direction of gaze; it increases with increasing nystagmus amplitudes and is pathophysiologically caused by a combination of both a direction-specific vestibulocerebellar ataxia and a reduced visual stabilization owing to the nystagmus (Büchele et al., 1983).

Management

Physical balance training improves postural instability significantly. A surgical suboccipital decompression in Arnold-Chiari malformation because of the compression of the herniating cerebellum against the caudal brain stem may gradually improve some of the distressing symptoms. It is our recent experience that baclofen may effectively suppress downbeat as well as upbeat nystagmus.

Upbeat Nystagmus Vertigo

The combination of postural instability, oscillopsia, upbeat nystagmus in the primary position of gaze, and saccadic upward pursuit analogous to downbeat nystagmus most probably is a defect of the vertical VOR, caused by the same etiologic conditions. Because the manifestations are typically modulated by otolithic input caused by static head tilt, upbeat nystagmus is also a kind of positional nystagmus in a broader sense. Two separate intra-axial brain stem lesions, in the tegmentum of the pontomesencephalic and the pontomedullary junction near the perihypoglossal nuclei (Fig. 31–6), are implicated in the provocation of this syndrome (Fisher et al., 1983), whereas there is not sufficient evidence that the

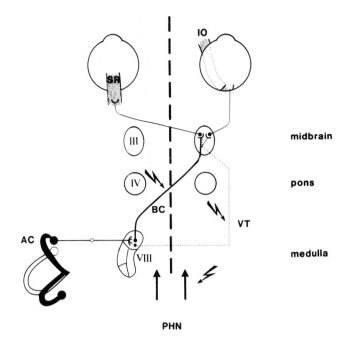

Figure 31-6. Upbeat nystagmus. Schematic representation of the three-neuron excitatory reflex arc from the anterior semicircular canal (AC), the superior vestibular nucleus (VIII), and the brachium conjunctivum (BC) to the contralateral oculomotor nucleus (III), the superior rectus muscle (SR), and the inferior oblique muscle (IO). Furthermore, the excitatory ventral tegmental pathway (VT) is depicted, which connects the superior vestibular nucleus with the contralateral oculomotor nucleus. An ascending pathway from the perihypoglossal nuclei (PHN) in the medulla possibly modulates the tone of vertical VOR. The *zigzag arrows* indicate the lesions of the brachium conjunctivum, the ventral tegmental pathway, and the perihypoglossal connection, which may produce upbeat nystagmus.

anterior cerebellar vermis is involved. A ventral tegmental pathway may also be of functional significance (Ranalli and Sharpe, 1988).

Upbeat nystagmus may be associated with severe vertigo-ataxia and nausea, particularly initially; depending on the cause, the natural history frequently shows a gradual improvement or disappearance, as opposed to the situation with downbeat nystagmus, which is usually a permanent sign.

Ocular Tilt Reaction

The ocular tilt reaction is an oculocephalic synkinesis with the triad of ipsilateral head tilt, ocular torsion, and skew deviation, experimentally elicited by Westheimer and Blair (1975) by electrical stimulation of the rostral midbrain tegmentum in the region of the interstitial nucleus of Cajal. Single cases have been reported with ocular tilt reaction as a transient phenomenon after inadvertent labyrinth destruction during stapedectomy and paroxysmal events in multiple sclerosis or brain stem abscess.

Administering carbamazepine or baclofen may possibly have therapeutic benefit (Hedges and Hoyt, 1982).

Head tilt, ocular torsion, and skew deviation must be attributed to a fundamental pattern of active roll motion based on graviceptive innervation. The contraversive head and eye tilt with utricular nerve stimulation is probably compensatory, as is the ipsilateral tilt with a lesion of the otolith (Fig. 31–7). Pathologic ocular tilt reaction involves a deviation of the internal representation of the gravitational vector and subjective vertical. A similar mechanism causes ocular tilt reaction and lateropulsion with body deviation and fall toward the side with the lesion in Wallenberg's syndrome (Brandt and Dieterich, 1987), whereas unilateral mesodiencephalic lesions (paramedian thalamic infarctions) cause contraversive ocular tilt reaction (Halmagyi et al., 1990). This points to the existence of a crossed graviceptive pathway between the vestibular nuclei and the contralateral interstitial nucleus of Cajal.

NONVESTIBULAR VERTIGO SYNDROMES

Nonvestibular (sensory) vertigo syndrome refers to visual and somatosensory vertigo. In a strict sense,

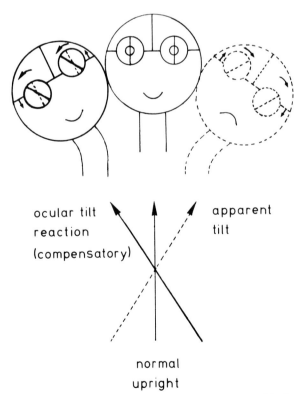

Figure 31-7. The ocular tilt reaction is a synkinesis of ipsilateral head tilt, ocular torsion, and skew deviation caused by processes of the rostral midbrain tegmentum or dorsolateral medulla. It involves a deviation of the internal representation of gravitational vector (subjective vertical) and probably reflects compensation with respect to perceived orientation.

such a distinction is not correct because convergence of multisensory inputs at various levels of the central vestibular system sometimes makes it impossible for neurons as well as for conscious perception to differentiate clearly among vestibular, somatosensory, and visual stimulation (Dichgans and Brandt, 1978).

VISUAL VERTIGO

Viewing a moving large visual display characteristically induces within seconds an apparent body motion opposite in direction to pattern motion and a visuospinal postural destabilization in an objectively stationary subject. Tilting the head during an optokinetically induced sense of self-rotation (circularvection) elicits optokinetic Coriolis' effects indistinguishable from the well-known true vestibular cross-coupled effects.

Slight visual vertigo and measurable postural instability occur with gradual changes of visual acuity (whether spectacles are used or not) or in anisometropia or unilateral aphakia when spectacle magnification causes an insurmountable problem for perception (Paulus et al., 1984).

The sudden onset of an extraocular muscle paresis induces ocular vertigo with perceptual illusions and oscillopsia during voluntary eye and head movements and also affects locomotion and balance, which gradually improve with training. The impairment of motor control can be attributed to an acute sensory deficiency of visual localization of objects in egocentric coordinates, which is usually calculated from both the position of the target on the retina and the awareness of eye position in the head. Paretic deviation of normal eye position caused by the lack of the afferent extraretinal information results in a dissociation of the subjective visual and somatosensory straight-ahead orientation, producing a mismatch that is responsible for the direction-specific distortion of locomotion (Brandt, 1984) (Fig. 31–8).

CERVICAL VERTIGO

Cervical vertigo is unlike other vertigo syndromes and has been controversial. Neck afference not only assists the coordination of eye, head, and body but also affects spatial orientation and control of posture. This implies that stimulation of or lesions in these structures could produce cervical vertigo. In fact, unilateral local anesthesia of the upper dorsal cervical roots induces ataxia and nystagmus in animals and ataxia without nystagmus in humans (DeJong and Bles, 1986). Cervical vertigo, if it exists outside these experimental conditions, is obviously characterized by ataxia and unsteadiness of gait rather than by a clear rotational or linear vertigo.

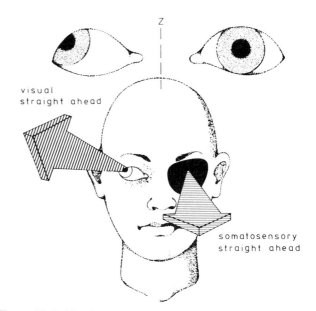

Figure 31–8. Visual vertigo with sudden onset of an extraocular muscle paresis. Paretic deviation of normal eye position caused by the lack of afferent extraretinal information results in a dissociation of the subjective visual and somatosensory straight-ahead orientation. A mismatch occurs that is responsible for the direction-specific distortion of locomotion and reaching movements.

VERTIGO IN CHILDREN

In the pediatric and adolescent age group, vertigo is less common than in adults, but because of the variety of presentations and underlying causes, it is a diagnostic challenge (Balkany and Finkel, 1986; Britton and Block, 1988). The most important episodic vertigo syndromes in childhood and adolescence are benign paroxysmal vertigo of childhood, basilar artery migraine, perilymph fistulas, secondary Meniere's disease, and the rare familial periodic vertigo. Sustained severe rotational vertigo caused by an acute unilateral vestibular loss occurs with labyrinthitis, with vestibular neuritis, or after head trauma. In the latter, postconcussion otolithic vertigo and typical benign paroxysmal positioning vertigo may also occur. Various rare genetic and embryopathic labyrinth malformations cause unilateral or bilateral loss of auditory and/or vestibular function (Baloh and Honrubia, 1990).

Benign paroxysmal vertigo in childhood was first described by Basser (1964). It is characterized by attacks of sudden rotational vertigo lasting seconds to minutes associated with nystagmus and postural imbalance. Age at onset is within the first 4 years of life; attacks disappear spontaneously between the ages of 5 and 8 years. This condition and also benign paroxysmal torticollis of infancy are regarded as migraine equivalents because a significant proportion of these children experience common migraine in later life or have a positive family history.

Differential diagnosis includes vestibular epilepsy, posterior fossa tumor, psychogenic dizziness, and familial periodic vertigo with onset in early childhood (White, 1969).

PSYCHOGENIC VERTIGO

Vertigo is a subjective complaint in schizophrenia, depressive illness, hysteria, and anxiety neurosis (Table 31–7). The use of Frenzel's lenses helps to establish the psychogenic cause if rotational vertigo occurs without concomitant nystagmus and if the eyes converge while the patient describes the sensation of vertigo.

Phobic Vertigo. With its characteristic panic attacks, phobic vertigo is one of the most frequent vertigo syndromes and tends to incapacitate the patient in his or her occupational and social activities. Neurotic acrophobia results when physiologic height vertigo induces a conditioned phobic reaction, which is characterized by a dissociation between the objective and the subjective risk of falling. Although this dissociation is typically experienced by the acrophobic (fearful of heights) patient, he or she cannot resist the impulse to shun heights. Agoraphobia (fear of wide open spaces) may also be initiated by the physiologic impairment of visual control of body sway consequent on the increasing distance to stationary objects in the visual environment as long as it mainly involves subjective postural imbalance in wide open spaces. Panic attacks and phobic vertigo syndromes encompass a neurotic compulsive structure of personality with an attitude of anxious expectation as well as the stimulus situation, which provokes the attacks and is often uncomfortable even for healthy subjects.

Psychotherapy is directed toward in vivo desensitization procedures such as successive approximation to the feared situation or flooding without a graduated approach.

Phobic Postural Vertigo. A syndrome of phobic postural vertigo attacks that is distinguishable from agoraphobia and acrophobia has been described. Among my patients, it was the third most common cause of vertigo. It is characterized by the combination of initial vertigo with subjective postural and gait instability and the fear of impending death (Brandt, 1990). Patients complain of vertigo rather than anxiety and feel physically ill. The illusory perception (vertigo) can be explained by the hypothesis that an impairment of the space constancy mechanism in these patients leads to partial uncoupling of the efference copy for active head movements. Vertigo and postural instability, according to the patients' reports, can also occur without anxiety. Experience so far seems to indicate that the initial results of psychotherapy are favorable.

PHYSIOLOGIC STIMULATION VERTIGO

Physiologic stimulation vertigo is defined as vertigo induced by external stimulation of the normal vestibular, visual, or somatosensory system (Brandt and Daroff, 1980a).

Motion Sickness

Motion sickness is induced during passive locomotion in vehicles and is generated either by unfamiliar body acceleration, to which the person has therefore not adapted, or by an intersensory mismatch involving conflicting vestibular and visual stimuli. For simple body oscillations, the incidence of motion sickness decreases as the frequency of oscillation increases. Infants are highly resistant to motion sickness, but thereafter, up to about 12 years of age, children are more susceptible than adults. Dynamic spatial orientation of infants is not affected by visual-vestibular mismatches (Brandt, 1984).

Physical prevention of motion sickness involves vestibular training to promote central habituation (see Fig. 31–1), as well as head fixation and head position during stimulation to avoid cross-coupling effects (Table 31–8). Motion sickness is significantly reduced when ample peripheral vision of the stationary surroundings is provided during vehicle acceleration. Conversely, the symptoms are heightened in closed ship cabins or while reading and, to a lesser extent, while simply sitting in the back seat of a moving vehicle. This creates a visual-vestibular conflict, in which the vestibular signals of acceleration are contradicted by visual information of a seemingly stationary environment. Anti–motion sickness drugs such as scopolamine and dimenhydrinate are effective in preventing both vestibular and optokinetic motion sickness. In cases of exceptionally severe motion sickness, combinations of either D-amphetamine sulfate and L-scopolamine hydrobromide or promethazine and D-amphetamine provide far better protection than any single drug.

Physiologic Height Vertigo

Height vertigo, a visually induced syndrome that is commonly experienced on the top of high struc-

Table 31–7. FORMS OF PSYCHOGENIC VERTIGO

Vertigo as a symptom in
  Anxiety neurosis
  Depression
  Hysteria
  Psychosis
  Post-traumatic syndrome
  Deliberate simulation
Vertigo as a defined syndrome in
  Phobic postural vertigo
  Agoraphobia
  Acrophobia
Psychogenic overlay of organic vertigo syndromes in
  Predisposed personalities
  Manifest psychiatric disorders
  Deliberate aggravation of symptoms (inflation)

Table 31–8. PHYSICAL PREVENTION OF MOTION SICKNESS

Strategy	Mechanisms
Chronic	
Vestibular training: repetitive exposure to stimuli during active head movements	Acceleration-specific central habituation
Simulator training	Using the benefit of positive visual-vestibular habituation transfer
Acute	
Head fixation	Avoidance of additional acceleration and cross-coupling, e.g., Coriolis' effects
Head position (relative to gravity vector):	Using the benefit of the natural habituation for head–Z axis accelerations
Ship: supine	
Car: supine, head in driving direction	
Helicopter: sitting	
Counterbalance of vehicle-induced body motions	
Visual control of vehicle motion. If not possible: eyes closed	Avoidance of visual-vestibular mismatch

tures, is manifested by a subjective instability of posture and locomotion, coupled with a fear of falling and vegetative symptoms, which spontaneously remit after termination of the inducing stimulus. Physiologic postural instability accompanying height vertigo conditions is caused by a geometrically explainable (Fig. 31–9) visually induced postural im-

balance, when the distance between the observer and the nearest stationary object contrasts in the environment exceeds a critical limit (Bles et al., 1980; Brandt et al., 1980).

Susceptible subjects should avoid the free upright stance in critical situations at high altitudes. This is done intuitively by grasping for stationary framework

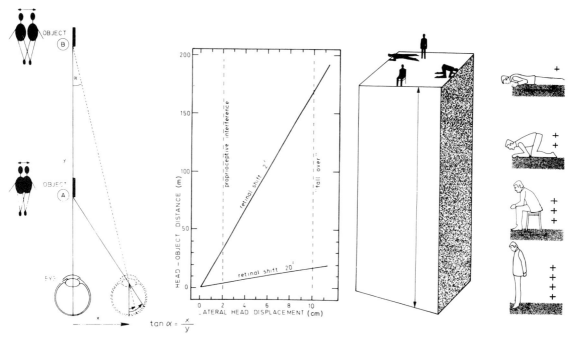

Figure 31–9. Mechanism of physiologic height vertigo, being a distance vertigo caused by visual destabilization of postural balance when the distance between the observer's eye and the nearest visible stationary contrasts becomes critically large (Brandt et al., 1980). Geometric analysis *(left)* indicates that, to be visually detected, body sway must increase with increasing distance between the eyes and the nearest stationary contrast. Angular displacements α on the retina, caused by a lateral head displacement, are smaller the greater is the distance y to the object. Diagram shows relationship between head-object distances (y) and lateral head displacement (x) for a given retinal displacement threshold of either 2 or 20 minutes of arc. However, because postural regulation involves the multiloop control, additional proprioceptive cues may alter sway amplitudes as well. Thus, a visually induced (measurable) postural imbalance causes physiologic vertigo and introduces a real danger of falling from a high position. This mechanism is affected by additional cognitive and psychologic factors mainly responsible for height anxiety. The magnitude of subjective height vertigo is related to body position and is at its maximum when the person is in upright stance where it is comparatively difficult to maintain postural balance *(right)*.

or leaning against a wall for support. When looking down, one should obtain stationary cues from nearby contrasts in the peripheral visual field. Staring at moving objects such as clouds increases the danger of falling because additional postural destabilization through linear vection may be induced. One should avoid long exposure times, because height vertigo usually takes several seconds to develop. Looking through binoculars is dangerous because it restricts the visual field and introduces the unusual magnification factor to which the observer has not yet become adjusted. Body and head position should be adjusted to the gravitational vector because vision receives a relatively greater sensorial weight (which is undesirable) if the otoliths are displaced beyond their optimal working range by extreme head tilt. It may also be true on the basis of other observations that the feet should be firmly planted on an "earth horizontal" surface.

References

(Key references are designated with an asterisk.)

Balkany T.J., Finkel R.S. The dizzy child. *Ear Hear.* 7:138–142, 1986.

*Baloh R.W., Honrubia V. *Clinical Neurophysiology of the Vestibular System.* Philadelphia, Davis, 1990.

Baloh R.W., Spooner J.W. Downbeat nystagmus: a type of central vestibular nystagmus. *Neurology (N.Y.)* 31:304–310, 1981.

Barac B. Vertiginous epileptic attacks and so-called "vestibulogenic seizures." *Epilepsia* 9:137–144, 1968.

Bárány R. Diagnose von Krankheitserscheinungen im Bereiche des Otolithenapparates. *Acta Otolaryngol.* 2:434–437, 1921.

Basser L.S. Benign paroxysmal vertigo of childhood. *Brain* 87:141–152, 1964.

Bickerstaff E.R. Basilar artery migraine. *Lancet* 1:15–18, 1961.

Black F.O., Effron M.Z., Burns D.S. Diagnosis and management of drop attacks of vestibular origin: Tumarkin's otolithic crisis. *Otolaryngol. Head Neck Surg.* 90:256–262, 1982.

Bles W., Kapteyn T.S., Brandt T., et al. The mechanism of physiological height vertigo: II. Posturography. *Acta Otolaryngol.* 89:534–540, 1980.

Brandt T. Visual vertigo and acrophobia. In Dix M.R., Hood J.D., eds. *Vertigo.* New York, Wiley, pp. 439–466, 1984.

Brandt T. Positional and positioning vertigo and nystagmus. *J. Neurol. Sci.* 95:3–28, 1990.

*Brandt T. *Vertigo, Its Multisensory Syndromes.* London, Springer-Verlag, 1991.

Brandt T., Daroff R.B. The multisensory physiological and pathological vertigo syndromes. *Ann. Neurol.* 7:195–203, 1980a.

Brandt T., Daroff R.B. Physical therapy for benign paroxysmal positional vertigo. *Arch. Otolaryngol.* 106:484–485, 1980b.

Brandt T., Dieterich M. Pathological eye-head coordination in roll: tonic ocular tilt reaction in mesencephalic and medullary lesions. *Brain* 110:649–666, 1987.

Brandt T., Arnold F., Bles W., et al. The mechanism of physiological height vertigo: I. Theoretical approach and psychophysics. *Acta Otolaryngol.* 89:513–523, 1980.

Brandt T., Krafczyk S., Malsbenden I. Postural imbalance with head extension: improvement by training as a model for ataxia therapy. *Ann. N. Y. Acad. Sci.* 374:636–649, 1981.

Britton B.H., Block L.D. Vertigo in the pediatric and adolescent age group. *Laryngoscope* 96:139–146, 1988.

Büchele W., Brandt T. Vestibular neuritis, a horizontal semicircular canal paresis? *Adv. Otorhinolaryngol.* 42:157–161, 1988.

Büchele W., Brandt T., Degner D. Ataxia and oscillopsia in downbeat-nystagmus vertigo syndrome. *Adv. Otorhinolaryngol.* 30:291–297, 1983.

Cawthorne T. The physiologic basis for head exercises. *J. Chart. Soc. Physiother.* 106–107, 1944.

Cogan D.G. Down-beat nystagmus. *Arch. Ophthalmol.* 80:757–768, 1968.

DeJong J.M.B.V., Bles W. Cervical dizziness and ataxia. In Bles W., Brandt T., eds. *Disorders of Posture and Gait.* Amsterdam, Elsevier, pp. 185–206, 1986.

Dix M.R., Hallpike C.S. The pathology, symptomatology and diagnosis of certain common disorders of the vestibular system. *Proc. R. Soc. Med.* 45:341–354, 1952.

*Dix M.R., Hood J.D., eds. *Vertigo.* New York, Wiley, 1984.

Dichgans J., Brandt T. Visual-vestibular interaction: effects on self-motion perception and postural control. In Held R., Leibowitz H.W., Teuber H.-L., eds. *Handbook of Sensory Physiology.* Vol. VIII. *Perception.* Berlin, Springer-Verlag, pp. 755–804, 1978.

Dohlmann G.F. On the mechanism of the Meniere attack. *Arch. Otorhinolaryngol. (N.Y.)* 212:301–307, 1976.

Fernandez C., Alzate R., Lindsay J.R. Experimental observations on postural nystagmus. II. Lesions of the nodulus. *Ann. Otol.* 69:94–114, 1960.

Fisher A., Gresty M., Chambers B., et al. Primary position up-beating nystagmus: a variety of central positional nystagmus. *Brain* 106:949–964, 1983.

Gacek R.R. Further observations on posterior ampullary nerve transection for positional vertigo. *Ann. Otol. Rhinol. Laryngol.* 87:300–306, 1978.

Halmagyi G.M., Brandt, T., Dietrich M, et al. Tonic contraversive ocular tilt reaction due to unilateral mesodiencephalic lesion. *Neurology* 40:1503–1509, 1990.

Hedges T.R. III, Hoyt W.F. Ocular tilt reaction due to an upper brainstem lesion: paroxysmal skew deviation, torsion and oscillation of the eyes with head tilt. *Ann. Neurol.* 11:537–540, 1982.

*Honrubia V., Brazier M.A.B., eds. *Nystagmus and Vertigo.* London, Academic Press, 1982.

Igarashi M. Vestibular compensation. *Acta Otolaryngol. (Stockh.)* 406:78–82, 1984.

Jannetta P.J., Møller M.B., Møller A.R. Disabling positional vertigo. *N. Engl. J. Med.* 310:1700–1705, 1984.

Kattah J.C., Kolsky M.P., Luessenhop A.J. Positional vertigo and the cerebellar vermis. *Neurology* 34:527–529, 1984.

Keim R.J., Sachs G.B. Positional nystagmus in association with macroglobulinemia. *Ann. Otol. Rhinol. Laryngol.* 84:223–227, 1975.

Meniere P. Nouveaux documents relatifs aux lésions de l'oreille interne caractérisés par des symptômes de congestion cérébrale apoplectiforme. *Gazette Médicale (Paris)* 16:239–240, 1861.

Møller M.D. Controversy in Meniere's disease: results of micro-vascular decompression of the eighth nerve. *Ann. J. Otol.* 9:60–63, 1988.

Money K.E., Myles W.S., Hoffert D.M. The mechanism of positional alcohol nystagmus. *Can. J. Otolaryngol.* 3:302–313, 1974.

Osterman P.O., Westerberg C.-E. Paroxysmal attacks in multiple sclerosis. *Brain* 98:189–202, 1975.

Paulus W.M., Straube A., Brandt T. Visual stabilization of posture: physiologial stimulus characteristics and clinical aspects. *Brain* 107:1143–1163, 1984.

Ranalli P.J., Sharpe J.A. Upbeat nystagmus and the ventral tegmental pathway of the upward vestibulo-ocular reflex. *Neurology* 38:1329–1330, 1988.

Schmidt C.L. Zur Pathophysiologie des peripheren, paroxysmalen benignen Lagerungsschwindels (BPPV). *Laryngol. Rhinol. Otol. (Stuttg.).* 64:146–155, 1985.

Schneider R.C., Calhoun H.D., Crosby E.C. Vertigo and rotational movement in cortical and subcortical lesions. *J. Neurol. Sci.* 6:493–516, 1968.

Schuknecht H.F. Cupulolithiasis. *Arch. Otolaryngol.* 90:765–778, 1969.

Schuknecht H.F., Kitamura K. Vestibular neuritis. *Ann. Otol. Rhinol. Laryngol.* 90(Suppl. 78):1–19, 1981.

Singleton G.T., Post K.N., Karlan M.S., et al. Perilymph fistulas: diagnostic criteria and therapy. *Ann. Otol. Rhinol. Laryngol.* 87:797–803, 1978.

Thomson J., Bretlau P., Tos M., et al. Placebo effect in surgery for Meniere's disease. *Arch. Otolaryngol.* 107:271–277, 1981.

Toole J.F., Tucker H. Influence of head position upon cerebral circulation. *Arch. Neurol.* 2:616–623, 1960.

Westheimer G., Blair S.M. The ocular tilt reaction—a brain-stem oculomotor routine. *Invest. Ophthalmol.* 14:833–839, 1975.

White J.C. Familial periodic nystagmus, vertigo and ataxia. *Arch. Neurol.* 20:276–280, 1969.

Williams D., Wilson T.G. The diagnosis of the major and minor syndromes of basilar insufficiency. *Brain* 85:741–774, 1962.

Zasorin N.L., Baloh R.W., Myers L.B. Acetazolamide-responsive episodic ataxia syndrome. *Neurology (N.Y.)* 33:1212–1214, 1983.

Zee D.S. The management of patients with vestibular disorders. In Barber H.O., Sharpe J.A., eds. *Vestibular Disorders.* Chicago, Year Book Medical Publishers, pp. 254–277, 1988.

Zee D.S., Friendlich A.R., Robinson D.A. The mechanism of downbeat nystagmus. *Arch. Neurol.* 30:227–237, 1974.

Bodily Functions

32

Vasomotor Function and Dysfunction

Roger R. Tuck
James G. McLeod

Concentric smooth muscle is present in the walls of all blood vessels except capillaries. Changes in the tone of vascular smooth muscle can alter arterial blood pressure, venous blood pressure, and regional blood flow by affecting the caliber and distensibility of the vessels. Vasomotor tone is controlled mainly by neural reflexes, although it is also influenced by local metabolic conditions (e.g., acidosis), locally released substances (e.g., substance P), or circulating vasoactive substances (e.g., angiotensin). This chapter is primarily concerned with reflex control of vasomotor tone.

INNERVATION OF BLOOD VESSELS

Noradrenergic Vasomotor Nerves

Vascular smooth muscle is innervated by postganglionic, noradrenergic sympathetic nerve fibers that form a dense plexus of fine terminals of diameter about 0.5 μm in the adventitial layer of the vessel wall. Very few sympathetic nerve terminals penetrate the smooth muscle layer of the media. At intervals, the nerve terminals form varicosities of diameter 1–2 μm that contain numerous synaptic vesicles and mitochondria. The surface of the varicosities that face the smooth muscle cells is not covered by Schwann cell membrane and is separated from the smooth muscle cells by a gap of about 100 nm for arterioles and small arteries, and 1000–2000 nm for large arteries (Burnstock, 1975). In general, the density of sympathetic nerve terminals is high in precapillary sphincters, arterioles, and small arteries and is relatively low in large arteries and veins. The muscular veins of the portal-mesenteric system have a relatively dense sympathetic nerve supply (Burnstock, 1975).

Vascular smooth muscle cells respond to circulating catecholamines as well as to norepinephrine released by the sympathetic nerve terminals. Arterioles and small arteries with a relatively dense sympathetic innervation are less influenced by circulating catecholamines than are large arteries and veins (Burnstock, 1975).

The relative importance of circulating catecholamines in the control of vasomotor tone is not well understood. It may be of little significance except in such stressful situations as those induced by heavy exercise, fear, or hypotension.

Stimulation of the sympathetic nerve supply to blood vessels releases norepinephrine from the nerve terminals, usually causing contraction of the smooth muscle in the vessel walls by activating adrenoreceptors on their surface (Bevan et al., 1980) (Table 32–1). The receptors on most arteries and arterioles are selectively activated by phenylephrine and blocked by prazosin; these are designated α_1 adrenoreceptors. There is experimental evidence that smooth muscle of resistance vessels and veins also possesses adrenoreceptors of another subtype, resembling prejunctional α_2 receptors that are activated by clonidine and blocked by yohimbine, although their functional significance is uncertain (Hoffman and Lefkowitz, 1980; Vanhoutte and Shepherd, 1984).

Most vascular smooth muscle cells also possess a group of adrenoreceptors that, when activated, cause

Table 32–1. ADRENERGIC RECEPTORS FOUND ON VASCULAR SMOOTH MUSCLE

Classification	Selective Agonist	Selective Antagonist	Distribution	Effect of Activation on Vascular Smooth Muscle	Functional Significance
α_1	Phenylephrine	Prazosin	Most vascular smooth muscle	Contraction	Control of regional blood flow and vascular resistance; reflex control of arterial blood pressure
α_2	Clonidine	Yohimbine	Human digital arteries; possibly mainly in small resistance vessels	Contraction	Unknown
β_1	None	Atenolol	Renal and coronary arteries	Relaxation	Unknown
β_2	Salbutamol	Butoxamine	Most vascular smooth muscle	Relaxation	Maintenance of nutritional blood flow to certain tissues during α-adrenergic vasoconstriction

smooth muscle relaxation and vasodilatation. These receptors are classified as β_2 and are activated selectively by β-adrenergic agents, such as isoprenaline. The relatively weak β-adrenergic effect of norepinephrine on vascular smooth muscle is normally masked by its potent α-adrenergic properties but can be demonstrated during sympathetic nerve stimulation when α receptors are blocked pharmacologically. The blood vessels of certain regions of the face in some animals respond to sympathetic stimulation by dilating, presumably because of the relatively large proportion of β receptors on these vessels (Vanhoutte and Shepherd, 1984).

Vasodilatation may occur in some tissues, such as skeletal muscle, during sympathoadrenal stimulation because of the effect of circulating epinephrine on vascular smooth muscle β_2 receptors. This effect may be important in the maintenance of regional nutritional blood flow to certain organs in times of increased sympathetic activity (Vanhoutte and Shepherd, 1984).

Non-Noradrenergic Vasomotor Nerves

Acetylcholine, purines, polypeptides, and amines (other than norepinephrine) have been identified in nerves that supply vascular smooth muscle (Burnstock and Griffith, 1988) (Table 32–2). Many of these substances satisfy most or all of the criteria for a neurotransmitter. It is likely that most, if not all, vascular nerve terminals contain and release two or more neurotransmitters, a phenomenon known as *cotransmission.*

Acetylcholine

Release of acetylcholine by vasomotor nerve fibers causes smooth muscle relaxation and vasodilatation. The distribution of cholinergic vasomotor fibers and their functional significance in humans is unclear, but they may play a significant role in the control of

blood flow in skeletal muscle, erectile tissue, uterus, hair, tongue, skin, and salivary glands (Burnstock, 1980). Acetylcholine may cause relaxation of vascular smooth muscle by prejunctional inhibition of norepinephrine release from sympathetic fibers or by releasing endothelium-derived releasing factor, a potent smooth muscle relaxant.

Purines

ATP exists in some perivascular nerve terminals and acts as a neurotransmitter by way of two classes of purinoreceptors (Burnstock, 1980); it causes vasodilatation of some blood vessels and constriction of others. In the latter, ATP and norepinephrine may be released as cotransmitters from the same nerve terminals. The role of purinergic nerves has not been clarified in humans.

Peptides

Several peptides are found in vasomotor nerve fibers and are believed to affect vasomotor tone. Substance P, calcitonin gene–related peptide, and vasoactive intestinal polypeptide cause vasodilatation, whereas neuropeptide Y is a potent vasocon-

Table 32–2. PROBABLE NONADRENERGIC VASOACTIVE NEUROTRANSMITTERS

Neurotransmitter	Major Effect on Vascular Smooth Muscle	
	Contraction	*Relaxation*
Acetylcholine		+
ATP	+	+
Substance P		+
Calcitonin gene–related peptide		+
Vasoactive intestinal polypeptide		+
Neuropeptide Y	+	
Dopamine		+
Serotonin	+	

strictor. Like ATP, the role of vasoactive peptidergic neurotransmitters is unclear. Increased vasomotor sensitivity to calcitonin gene–related peptide has been found in the hands of patients with Raynaud's phenomenon, thus raising the possibility that disordered peptidergic vasomotor nerves may cause disease (Shawket et al., 1989).

Amines

The vascular smooth muscle of digital skin and the kidneys contains dopaminergic nerve fibers that cause vasodilatation when stimulated. Dopaminergic renal nerves have complex effects on renal tubular function and the release of angiotensin and aldosterone, as well as renal blood flow. Dopamine-mediated vasodilatation of the digital skin possibly protects against cold injury.

Serotonin has been found in vascular nerves in a number of tissues, including the cerebral arteries. Release of serotonin by these fibers is thought to cause vasoconstriction, which may be important in the pathogenesis of migraine and cerebral vasospasm and may play a role in the regulation of cerebral blood flow.

REFLEX CONTROL OF VASOMOTOR TONE

Resistance and Capacitance Vessels

Arterial blood pressure is directly proportional to both peripheral vascular resistance and cardiac output and is maintained within a narrow range by reflex control of these two variables. Peripheral resistance depends on the tone of smooth muscle in the small arteries, arterioles, and precapillary sphincters, which are collectively known as *resistance vessels*. Cardiac output is a function of heart rate and stroke volume. The latter is regulated by the venous return to the heart, which in turn is influenced by the tone of the smooth muscle of the venous system, particularly the veins of the abdominal viscera. These vessels are known as the *capacitance vessels* (Folkow and Neil, 1971).

Baroreflexes

Changes in arterial blood pressure are detected by specialized receptors (baroreceptors) located primarily in the carotid sinuses and in the aortic arch. The arterial baroreceptors are of two types: type 1 receptors consist of a few relatively thin myelinated fibers that run together for some distance before forming a diffuse arborization in a large loose plexus; type 2 receptors consist of a single thick myelinated fiber that arborizes, the fine end branches terminating in neurofibrillar end plates (Kirchheim, 1976). Impulses generated by the baroreceptors are conveyed to the nucleus of the tractus solitarius by afferent fibers in the glossopharyngeal (carotid sinus branch) and vagus nerves (Fig. 32–1) and are integrated in the brain stem with signals from the hypothalamus, cerebral hemispheres, and elsewhere (Kirchheim, 1976; Korner, 1980).

The baroreflexes provide a negative feedback control mechanism that maintains systemic blood pressure at a relatively constant level. When systemic blood pressure rises, an increase in the frequency of impulses from the baroreceptors results in increased efferent vagal activity and a fall in the heart rate, and a decrease in activity in the efferent sympathetic

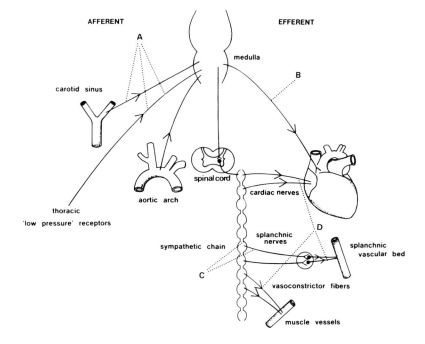

Figure 32–1. Diagrammatic representation of the baroreflex pathways controlling vasomotor tone and heart rate. (Modified from Lance J.W., McLeod J.G. *A Physiological Approach*. I. *Clinical Neurology*. 3rd ed. London, Butterworth, 1981.)

preganglionic and postganglionic vasomotor nerve fibers, which causes a reduction in vasomotor tone. Therefore both peripheral vascular resistance and the cardiac stroke volume diminish, causing a reflex fall in arterial blood pressure. When systemic pressure falls, the reflex decrease in efferent vagal activity produces an increase in heart rate. Increased sympathetic activity causes vasoconstriction and an increase in peripheral vascular resistance, which tend to reverse the fall in blood pressure. It has been demonstrated in humans by direct recording that muscle sympathetic nerve fiber activity increases in response to (1) a fall in blood pressure (Delius et al., 1972a); (2) changes in posture from lying to sitting and standing (Burke et al., 1977); (Fig. 32–2) and (3) the application of lower-body negative pressure, which is thought to unload intrathoracic low-pressure volume receptors (Sundlof and Wallin, 1978).

The splanchnic vascular bed plays an important part in human blood pressure regulation (Low et al., 1975; McLeod, 1980). There is a decrease in hepatic blood flow upon assuming the upright posture that is abolished by splanchnicectomy (Wilkins et al., 1951). Other studies, in which lower-body negative pressure has been applied to normal subjects, have confirmed the importance of the splanchnic vascular bed in human blood pressure control and have indicated that decreased splanchnic conductance accounts for approximately one-third of the reduction in total vascular conductance that occurs during the procedure (Rowell et al., 1972). Low-pressure baroreceptors in the cardiopulmonary region may be responsible for initiating splanchnic and forearm vasoconstriction (Johnson et al., 1974). Further evidence of the importance of the mesenteric vascular bed is that sympathectomy has little influence on blood pressure control unless the splanchnic nerves are sectioned (Wilkins et al., 1951); also, patients with spinal cord lesions do not develop significant postural hypotension unless the lesion is above the level of the splanchnic out-flow at T-6 (Guttmann and Whitteridge, 1947). Constriction of venous capacitance beds may cause a redistribution of blood

during postural changes, but it does not appear to be an essential part of the compensatory vascular response for maintenance of systemic arterial blood pressure in the upright position (Samueloff et al., 1966).

Venoarteriolar Reflex

There is evidence that in humans and other animals subcutaneous and muscle blood flow is partly controlled by local sympathetic reflexes (Henriksen, 1977). An increase in transmural venous pressure results in a reduction in subcutaneous and muscle blood flow. During head-up tilting, this response is not affected by spinal epidural anesthesia, which blocks baroreflex-mediated efferent sympathetic outflow, but is abolished by local infiltration with lidocaine or phentolamine and by applying external pressure to the limb, which reduces transmural pressure (Henriksen, 1977; Skagen et al., 1982). This vasoconstrictor response to increased vascular transmural pressure is probably mediated by stretch receptors in the walls of veins that, when stimulated, activate a local sympathetic nerve reflex causing constriction of regional arterioles. The venoarteriolar reflex may contribute to as much as 45% of the increased vascular resistance that occurs on assuming the upright posture (Henriksen, 1977).

TESTS OF VASOMOTOR FUNCTION
(Tables 32–3 and 32–4)

Effect of Change of Posture on Arterial Blood Pressure

In normal individuals, systolic blood pressure may rise or fall in response to standing or tilting. Diastolic pressure usually rises by a few millimeters of mercury. A fall of greater than 15 mm Hg in the systolic blood pressure and 5 mm Hg in the diastolic blood pressure on standing or tilting is probably abnormal

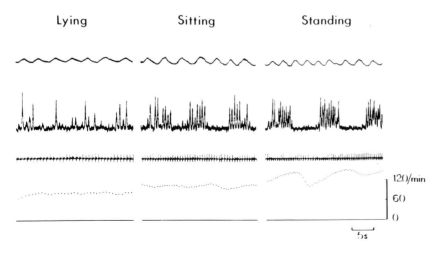

Lying   Sitting   Standing

Figure 32–2. Muscle sympathetic nerve activity obtained by intraneural recording. Sympathetic nerve activity is greatest in the standing position and least in the supine position. Traces from above are respiratory movement (inspiration upward), mean voltage muscle sympathetic nerve activity, electrocardiogram, and heart rate. (From Burke D., Sundlof G., Wallin B.G. Postural effects on muscle nerve sympathetic activity in man. *J. Physiol. [Lond.]* 272:399–414, 1977. With permission.)

Table 32–3. CLINICAL TESTS OF VASOMOTOR CONTROL

Test	Normal Response	Part of Reflex Arc Tested
Change of posture—tilt from horizontal to vertical posture	Fall in BP* ≤15/5 mm Hg Reduction in blood flow in cutaneous, muscular, and splanchnic beds	Afferent and efferent limbs
Lower-body negative pressure	As above	As above
Valsalva's maneuver	Phase I: rise in BP Phase II: gradual reduction of BP to plateau, tachycardia Phase III: fall in BP Overshoot of BP, bradycardia	Afferent and efferent limbs
Inspiratory gasp	Peripheral vasoconstriction in skin vessels	Afferent and efferent limbs
Isometric exercise	Increase in BP, diastolic ≥15 mm Hg (male), ≥8 mm Hg (female) Increase in heart rate Increased blood flow through exercising muscles Increased venomotor tone	Sympathetic efferent pathways
Cold pressor test	Increase in BP Increase in heart rate Reduction in cutaneous blood flow	Sympathetic efferent pathways
Emotional stress	Increase in BP Increase in heart rate Reduction in cutaneous blood flow	Sympathetic eferent pathways
Axon reflex	Increased cutaneous blood flow (flare response)	Cutaneous afferent fibers
Infusion of pressor drugs	Rise in blood pressure Slowing of heart rate	Adrenergic receptors Afferent and efferent limbs

*BP = arterial blood pressure.

(Johnson and Spalding, 1974). Postural hypotension can be detected by measuring the arterial blood pressure with a cuff when the subject is in the supine position and for several minutes after the subject assumes an upright posture, but it is recorded more reliably with an arterial cannula and pressure transducer (Fig. 32–3). Noninvasive methods of continuous blood pressure recording are now available.

Lower-Body Negative Pressure

The effect of gravity on the circulation that follows assumption of an upright position can be simulated by the application of lower-body negative pressure with the subject in the supine position (Bannister et al., 1967). In normal subjects, up to 40 mm Hg of lower-body negative pressure causes a fall in systolic pressure of less than 10 mm Hg (Bennett et al., 1980) and a decrease in forearm and splanchnic blood flow, which are due to increased vascular resistance in the forearm and splanchnic circulation (Johnson et al., 1974; Rowell et al., 1972). Muscle sympathetic nerve activity is increased during lower-body negative pressure (Sundlof and Wallin, 1978). These changes are believed to be due to the unloading of low-pressure intrathoracic baroreceptors, which results in increased efferent sympathetic vasomotor activity. In patients with idiopathic orthostatic hypotension and in some patients with diabetes mellitus (with or without postural hypotension), there is a marked fall in systolic blood pressure and little or no increase in

Table 32–4. NONINVASIVE BEDSIDE TESTS OF CARDIOVASCULAR REFLEXES

Test	Normal Responses	Part of Reflex Arc Tested
Change in posture (vertical tilt)	Fall in BP* ≤15/5 mm Hg	Afferent and efferent limbs
Isometric exercise (sustained hand grip)	Increased diastolic BP ≥15 mm Hg (male), ≥8 mm Hg (female)	Sympathetic efferent pathways
Valsalva's ratio (ratio of longest to shortest heart period during Valsalva's maneuver)	≥1.4†	Afferent and efferent limbs
Heart rate response to standing (30:15 ratio)	≥1.04†	Afferent and parasympathetic efferent limbs
Heart rate variation with respiration (sinus arrhythmia)	Maximum exceeds minimal heart rate ≥15† beats/minute	Vagal afferent and efferent limbs

*BP = arterial blood pressure.
†These control values vary with the age of the subject.

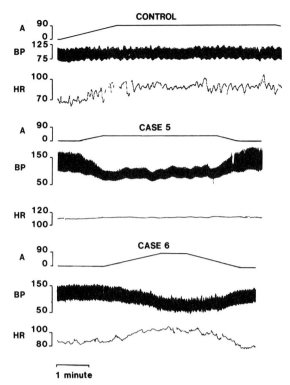

Figure 32–3. Arterial blood pressure and heart rate recorded from a healthy subject and from two patients with Guillain-Barré syndrome during tilting. Both patients had orthostatic hypotension and one (case 5) had a fixed heart rate. A = angle of tilt; BP = arterial blood pressure, mm Hg; HR = heart rate, beats per minute. (From Tuck R.R., McLeod J.G. Autonomic dysfunction in Guillain-Barré syndrome. *J. Neurol. Neurosurg. Psychiatry* 44:983–990, 1981.)

forearm vascular resistance during lower-body negative pressure because of impaired afferent vagal and efferent sympathetic activity (Bannister et al., 1967; Bennett et al., 1980).

Effect of a Test Meal on Blood Pressure

In normal subjects, ingestion of a test meal results in a fall in total peripheral resistance and forearm blood flow, an increase in cardiac output, and no change in arterial blood pressure. In patients with chronic autonomic failure, there is a rapid and prolonged fall in blood pressure after a test meal, with no change in forearm or skin blood flow (Mathias et al., 1989).

Valsalva's Maneuver

The changes in heart rate and arterial blood pressure in response to attempted forced expiration against a closed glottis or mouthpiece provide a useful screening test for abnormalities of control of vasomotor tone (Sharpey-Schafer, 1956). The transient changes of arterial blood pressure that accompany Valsalva's maneuver can be detected only if blood pressure is recorded from an arterial cannula or from a digital artery using a servo-plethysmomanometer, a noninvasive device that faithfully records transmural arterial pressure changes (Molhoek et al., 1984). However, useful clinical information about the state of reflex cardiovascular control can also be obtained from a record of changes in heart rate alone (Levin, 1966).

The test should be standardized. A widely used protocol involves having the subject breathe forcefully into a mouthpiece, which is connected to a mercury manometer, and maintaining an expiratory pressure of 40 mm Hg for 10 seconds (Bannister et al., 1977). The increased intrathoracic pressure is transmitted to the arterial system where a brief elevation of blood pressure is observed (phase I) (Fig. 32–4). The reduction in venous return to the heart reduces both cardiac output and mean arterial blood pressure (phase II), which are associated with a tachycardia related to increased cardiac sympathetic activity. When the maneuver is stopped, the reduced intrathoracic pressure is recorded as a stepped fall in the arterial blood pressure (phase III). The increased cardiac output that accompanies the rise in venous return to the heart, plus the increased peripheral vascular resistance that is due to increased vasomotor sympathetic activity, causes a marked rise in arterial blood pressure (phase IV), which is accompanied by a reflex vagally induced bradycardia.

In normal subjects, the ratio of the longest RR interval occurring after the maneuver to the shortest

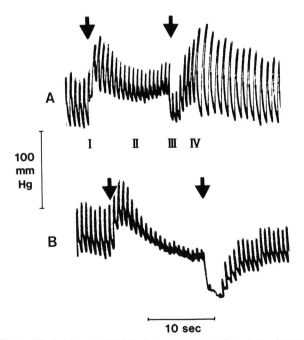

Figure 32–4. Intra-arterial blood pressure recording during Valsalva's maneuver from a healthy subject (A) and from a patient with amyloid neuropathy (B). The four phases of the blood pressure response are indicated by Roman numerals. In the patient, there is no overshoot of blood during phase IV of the maneuver. (From McLeod J.G. Autonomic nervous system. In Sumner A.J., ed. *The Physiology of Peripheral Nerve Disease.* Philadelphia, Saunders, pp. 432–483, 1980.)

interval during the maneuver is known as the Valsalva ratio (Levin, 1966). It usually exceeds 1.4, but the control value decreases with age. A lower ratio is usually indicative of impaired autonomic nervous control of the heart and blood vessels, although low values may be recorded in patients with congenital or acquired cardiopulmonary disease.

When efferent sympathetic vasoconstrictor activity is impaired, there is no overshoot of blood pressure in phase IV and consequently no bradycardia even if the baroreceptors, their afferent nerve supply, the vasomotor center, and the vagus nerves to the heart are all intact. Unless blood pressure is recorded continuously during Valsalva's maneuver, it is impossible to decide whether absence of the reflex bradycardia in phase IV is due to impaired efferent sympathetic vasomotor activity or to abnormal vagal function (see Fig. 32–4).

Emotional Stress

Emotional stress in the form of mental arithmetic results in an increase in heart rate of about 20% and mean arterial pressure of 15% (Ludbrook et al., 1975) and in an increase in cutaneous sympathetic nerve activity (Delius et al., 1972b). An unexpected loud noise or painful stimulus has similar effects on arterial blood pressure and pulse because of increased sympathetic vasomotor nerve activity. These tests are used to evaluate the sympathetic efferent pathway, because they do not involve activation of the afferent limb of the reflex arc. However, some normal individuals may have no response to these stimuli (Johnson and Spalding, 1974).

Inspiratory Gasp

A sudden inspiratory gasp causes peripheral vasoconstriction that is impaired or absent in patients with peripheral neuropathy resulting from amyloidosis or diabetes mellitus (Low et al., 1983). Because it is present in patients with cervical cord lesions above the sympathetic outflow to the hand, the reflex pathway passes mainly through the spinal cord (Gilliatt et al., 1948).

Isometric Exercise

An increase in heart rate, arterial blood pressure, and cardiac output occurs during sustained isometric contraction of a group of muscles (Lind et al., 1964). In healthy subjects, administration of phentolamine (an α-adrenergic antagonist) blocks the pressor response, thus indicating that there is an increase in vasomotor tone during isometric exercise (Freyschuss, 1970). The cardiovascular response to isometric exercise is mediated partly by a reflex, the afferent limb of which consists of small-diameter fibers that are activated by metabolic or mechanical changes in contracting muscles, and partly by a central command (Ewing, 1983; Freyschuss, 1970; Goodwin et al., 1971). An increase in diastolic pressure of at least 15 mm Hg in males and 8 mm Hg in females occurs after 5 minutes of sustained hand grip at 30% of the maximal voluntary effort (Ewing et al., 1974). In patients with diabetic and other autonomic neuropathies, the pressor response may be reduced or absent (Ewing, 1983; Ewing et al., 1974).

Cold Pressor Test

The application of a cold stimulus to the neck or hand elicits a rapid reduction in forearm and skin blood flow and an increase in arterial blood pressure in the majority of normal subjects. The response is believed to be reflex—the afferent side of which consists of pain and temperature fibers in the skin, and the efferent side of the sympathetic vasoconstrictor fibers (Jamieson et al., 1971).

Axon Reflex

A painful thermal, electrical, or mechanical stimulus, or the intradermal injection of histamine results in local redness at the site of injury or injection that is due to vasodilatation. This is followed 15–30 seconds later by further vasodilatation in the skin up to a radius of 15 mm around the site of injury (flare response). The latter effect is due to stimulation of collateral branches of afferent pain fibers that causes vasodilatation possibly by releasing ATP or substance P (Burnstock, 1977, 1980). The axon reflex can be assessed objectively by iontophoresing acetylcholine into the skin and measuring the accompanying change in skin blood flow with a laser Doppler flowmeter (Parkhouse and Le Quesne, 1988). The flare response is abolished by lesions of sensory nerves to the area of skin being tested and in disorders affecting sensory pain fibers, even though autonomic fibers may be intact (Johnson and Spalding, 1964).

Cutaneous and Muscle Blood Flow

Although changes in skin temperature have been used to assess variation in cutaneous blood flow in response to various stimuli, they may be misleading. Reflex changes in skin blood flow in response to such stimuli as local cooling or heating or a deep inspiration can be assessed more reliably with heat flow discs (Johnson, 1965) or with laser Doppler velocimetry (Low et al., 1983). Skin blood flow in the hand and forearm can be measured quantitatively by using venous occlusion plethysmography and strain-gauge plethysmography (Clarke et al., 1958) or by measuring the clearance rate of radioactive isotopes from the skin (Harris et al., 1952; Neilsen, 1972).

Cutaneous venomotor tone can be measured by occluding the arterial supply to a limb and inserting a needle that is connected to a pressure transducer into a superficial vein (Delius and Kellerova, 1971). Such maneuvers as a sudden deep inspiration or mental stress that result in increased arteriolar tone have a similar but longer lasting effect on venomotor tone.

Muscle blood flow can be measured by using venous occlusion or strain-gauge plethysmography in the forearm. However, this method gives only approximate results because skin and nerve blood flow both contribute to the total forearm blood flow. Other methods for measuring skeletal muscle blood flow include isotope clearance techniques (Harris et al., 1952), measurement of changes in muscle temperature (Blair et al., 1959), and measurement of the degree of oxygen desaturation of blood in the deep veins that drain forearm muscles (Roddie et al., 1957). Such invasive techniques are of value in physiologic studies but have limited application in the routine assessment of patients with disorders of vasomotor tone control.

Infusion of Pressor Drugs

Infusion of known amounts of norepinephrine induces a pressor response that is greater in patients with orthostatic hypotension secondary to neurologic disease than in normal subjects. This phenomenon occurs in patients with lesions of central autonomic pathways and both preganglionic and postganglionic sympathetic vasomotor nerves (Low et al., 1975; Mathias et al., 1976; Polinsky et al., 1981). The slope of the response curves relating blood pressure to plasma norepinephrine (or norepinephrine dose) is increased in such patients. A shift to the left of the curve suggests that denervation hypersensitivity is present as a result of a postganglionic lesion (Polinsky et al., 1981).

Heart Rate

Measurement of variations in heart rate in response to stimuli that influence baroreceptor activity may provide useful additional information about autonomic vasomotor control (Ewing, 1983) (see Table 32–4). The Valsalva ratio, described earlier in this section, is one such measurement. Another is the 30:15 ratio, which is the ratio of the 30th RR interval recorded after the patient stands from the supine position to the 15th interval. This ratio is age dependent, but it usually exceeds 1.04. Like the Valsalva ratio, the 30:15 ratio is reduced when abnormalities of the baroreflex arc are present. Lesions of the baroreceptor afferents, sympathetic efferents, and vagus nerves affect both ratios. In patients with isolated vagus nerve lesions, reflex control of vasomotor tone may be normal.

Measurement of changes in the RR interval during quiet or deep breathing is a useful index of cardiac vagal parasympathetic function. Although this measurement does not provide direct information about reflex vasomotor control, an abnormal result raises the possibility of a widespread disorder of the autonomic nervous system. Several methods of quantitating the variation in RR interval with respiration have been devised. The heart rate variation in normal subjects taking deep breaths at the rate of six per minute is at least 15 beats per minute (Ewing, 1983).

Baroreceptor function can be assessed quantitatively by studying the relationship between the RR interval (heart period) and arterial blood pressure. Pharmacologic agents, such as glyceryl trinitrate and phenylephrine, which do not directly affect heart rate, are given intravenously to lower or raise blood pressure that is measured by direct intra-arterial recording. After injection of the drug, each successive RR interval can be plotted against the systolic pressure of the preceding pulse during a change in blood pressure (Smyth et al., 1969). Alternatively, the RR interval can be measured when the blood pressure has reached a steady state (Korner et al., 1974). Both methods give a measure of baroreflex sensitivity that is reduced in patients with disorders of reflex cardiovascular control, such as diabetes mellitus and Guillain-Barré syndrome (Low et al., 1975; Tuck and McLeod, 1981) (Fig. 32–5).

NEUROLOGIC DISORDERS AFFECTING VASOMOTOR CONTROL

Neurologic diseases affecting vasomotor control are legion (Appenzeller, 1982; Bannister, 1988), and

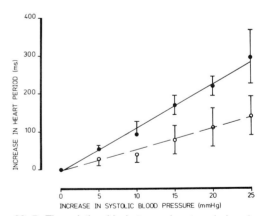

Figure 32–5. The relationship between heart period and systolic blood pressure after intravenous injections of phenylephrine. The closed circles represent the means of the pooled data from five healthy subjects and the open circles the means of the pooled data from seven patients with Guillain-Barré syndrome. Vertical bars represent ± 1 SEM. The slopes of the regression lines are 12 ms/mm Hg for the healthy subjects and 5.7 ms/mm Hg for the patients, which is significantly less than the control mean ($P < .01$). The result demonstrates reduced sensitivity of the blood pressure–heart rate component of the baroreflex in patients with Guillain-Barré syndrome. (From Tuck R.R., McLeod J.G. Autonomic dysfunction in Guillain-Barré syndrome. *J. Neurol. Neurosurg. Psychiatry* 44:983–990, 1981.)

Table 32–5. NEUROLOGIC DISEASES THAT CAUSE HYPERTENSION OR POSTURAL HYPOTENSION AS A RESULT OF IMPAIRMENT OF VASOMOTOR CONTROL

Disease	Manifestation of Impaired Vasomotor Control		Presumed Site of Lesion Causing Impairment of Vasomotor Control				
					Efferent Sympathetic Fibers		Baro-receptor Afferents
	Hyper-tension	Orthostatic Hypotension	Vasomotor Center	Spinal Cord	Preganglionic	Postganglionic	
A. Central nervous system							
Progressive autonomic failure (including Shy-Drager syndrome; idiopathic orthostatic hypotension)	–	+	–	+	+	+	+
Spinal cord lesion	+	+	–	+	–	–	–
Wernicke's encephalopathy	–	+	–	+	+	+	–
Holmes-Adie syndrome	–	+	–	–	+	+	+
Tabes dorsalis	–	+	–	–	–	–	+
B. Peripheral nervous system							
Diabetes	–	+	–	–	+	+	+
Guillain-Barré syndrome	+	+	–	–	+	–	+
Acute autonomic neuropathy	–	+	–	–	+	+	+
Amyloidosis	–	+	–	–	+	+	+
Porphyria	+	+	–	–	+	+	+
Uremia	–	+	–	–	+	+	+
Hereditary sensory and autonomic neuropathy type III*	–	+	–	–	+	+	–
Hereditary sensory and autonomic neuropathy type V*	–	+	–	–	+	–	–
Paraneoplastic carcinomatous neuropathy	–	+	–	–	+	+	–
Vincristine neuropathy	–	+	–	–	–	+	–
Perhexiline neuropathy			Unknown	Unknown			
Thallium toxicity	+	–	–	–	–	–	+
C. Other							
Dopamine β-hydroxylase deficiency	–	+	–	–	–	+	–
Tetanus	+	–	?+	?+	–	–	–
Poliomyelitis	+	+	+	–	–	–	–

*From Dyck P.J. Neuronal atrophy and degeneration predominantly affecting peripheral sensory and autonomic nerves. In Dyck P.J., Thomas P.K., Lambert E.H., et al., eds. *Peripheral Neuropathy.* 2nd ed. Philadelphia, Saunders, pp. 1557–1599, 1984.

the most important of these are summarized in Table 32–5. Johnson and Lambie deal with autonomic disorders, including those with vasomotor dysfunction, in Chapter 39. Gilliatt and Roberts consider disordered vasomotor control in syncopal states in Chapter 73.

References

(Key references are designated with an asterisk.)

*Appenzeller O. *The Autonomic Nervous System: An Introduction to Basic and Clinical Concepts.* 3rd ed. Amsterdam, Elsevier North Holland Biomedical Press, 1982.

*Bannister R. *Autonomic Failure. A Textbook of Clinical Disorders of the Autonomic Nervous System.* 2nd ed. New York, Oxford University Press, 1988.

Bannister R., Ardill L., Fentem P. Defective autonomic control of blood vessels in idiopathic orthostatic hypotension. *Brain* 90:725–746, 1967.

Bannister R., Sever P., Gross M. Cardiovascular reflexes and biochemical responses in progressive autonomic failure. *Brain* 100:327–344, 1977.

Bennett T., Hosking D.J., Hampton J.R. Cardiovascular responses to graded reductions of central blood volume in normal subjects and in patients with diabetes mellitus. *Clin. Sci.* 58:193–200, 1980.

*Bevan J.A., Bevan R.D., Duckles S.P. Adrenergic regulation of

vascular smooth muscles. In Bohr D.F., Somlyo A.P., Sparks H.V., eds. *Handbook of Physiology.* Section 2. *The Cardiovascular System.* Vol. II. Bethesda, American Physiological Society, pp. 515–566, 1980.

Blair D.A., Golenhofen K., Seidel W. Muscle blood flow during emotional stress. *J. Physiol. (Lond.)* 149:61P–62P, 1959.

Burke D., Sundlof G., Wallin B.G. Postural effects on muscle nerve sympathetic activity in man. *J. Physiol. (Lond.)* 272:399–414, 1977.

Burnstock G. Innervation of vascular smooth muscle: Histochemistry and electron microscopy. *Clin. Exp. Pharmacol. Physiol. Suppl* 2:7–20, 1975.

Burnstock G. Autonomic neuro-effector junctions-reflex vasodilatation of the skin. *J. Invest. Dermatol.* 69:47–57, 1977.

Burnstock G. Cholinergic and purinergic regulation of blood vessels. In Bohr D.F., Somlyo A.P., Sparks H.V., eds. *Handbook of Physiology.* Section 2. *The Cardiovascular System.* Vol. II. Bethesda, American Physiological Society, pp. 567–612, 1980.

*Burnstock G., Griffith S.G. *Noradrenergic Innervation of Blood Vessels.* Vol. 1. *Putative Neurotransmitters.* Boca Raton, FL, CRC Press, 1988.

Clarke, R.S.S., Ginsburg J., Hellon R.F. Use of the strain gauge plethysmograph in assessing the effect of certain drugs on the blood flow through the skin and muscle of the human forearm. *J. Physiol. (Lond.)* 140:318–326, 1958.

Delius W., Kellerova E. Reaction of arterial and venous vessels in the human forearm and hand to deep breath or mental strain. *Clin. Sci.* 40:271–282, 1971.

Delius W., Hagbarth K.-E., Hongell A. et al. Manoeuvres affecting sympathetic outflow in human muscle nerves. *Acta Physiol. Scand.* 84:172–186, 1972a.

Delius W., Hagbarth K.-E., Hongell A., et al. Manoeuvres affecting sympathetic outflow in human skin nerves. *Acta Physiol. Scand.* 84:172–186, 1972b.

Ewing D.J. Practical bedside investigation of diabetic autonomic failure. In Bannister R., ed. *Autonomic Failure.* New York, Oxford University Press, pp. 370–405, 1983.

Ewing D.J., Irving J.B., Kerr F., et al. Clarke B.F. Cardiovascular responses to sustained handgrip in normal subjects and in patients with diabetes mellitus: a test of autonomic function. *Clin. Sci.* 46:295–306, 1974.

Folkow B., Neil E. *Circulation.* New York, Oxford University Press, 1971.

Freyschuss U. Cardiovascular adjustment to somatomotor innervation. *Acta Physiol. Scand. Suppl.* 342, 1970.

Gilliatt R.W., Guttmann L., Whitteridge D. Inspiratory vasoconstriction in patients after spinal injuries. *J. Physiol. (Lond.)* 107:67–75, 1948.

Goodwin G.M., McCloskey D.I., Mitchell J.H. Cardiovascular and respiratory responses to changes in central command during isometric exercise at constant muscle tension. *J. Physiol. (Lond.)* 219:40–41P, 1971.

Guttmann L., Whitteridge D. Effects of bladder distension on autonomic mechanisms after spinal cord injuries. *Brain* 70:361–404, 1947.

Harris R., Martin A.J., Williams H.S. Correlation of skin temperature and circulatory changes in muscle and subcutaneous tissue of the hand during trunk heating. *Clin. Sci.* 11:429–440, 1952.

Henriksen O. Local sympathetic reflex mechanisms in regulation of blood flow in human subcutaneous tissue. *Acta Physiol. Scand. Suppl.* 450:7–48, 1977.

Hoffman B.B., Lefkowitz R.J. Alpha-adrenergic receptor subtypes *N. Engl. J. Med.* 302:1390–1396, 1980.

Jamieson G.G., Ludbrook J., Wilson A. Cold hypersensitivity in Raynaud's phenomenon. *Circulation* 44:254–264, 1971.

Johnson J.M., Rowell L.B., Niederberger M., et al. Human splanchnic and forearm vasoconstrictor responses to reduction in right atrial and aortic pressures. *Circ. Res.* 34:515–524, 1974.

Johnson R.H. Some vasomotor changes in temperature regulation in man. *Bibl. Anat.* 7:288–293, 1965.

Johnson R.H., Spalding J.M.K. Progressive sensory neuropathy in children. *J. Neurol. Neurosurg. Psychiatry* 27:125–130, 1964.

*Johnson R.H., Spalding J.M.K. *Disorders of the Autonomic Nervous System.* Oxford, Blackwell Scientific Publications, 1974.

Kirchheim H.R. Systemic arterial baroreceptor reflexes. *Physiol. Rev.* 56:100–176, 1976.

Korner P.I. Central nervous system control of autonomic cardiovascular function. In Bohr D.F., Somlyo A.P., Sparks H.V., eds. *Handbook of Physiology.* Section 2. *The Cardiovascular System.* Vol. I. Bethesda, American Physiological Society, pp. 691–739, 1980.

Korner P.I., West M.J., Shaw J.B., et al. "Steady-state" properties of the baroreceptor-heart rate reflex in essential hypertension in man. *Clin. Exp. Pharmacol. Physiol.* 1:65–76, 1974.

Levin A.B. A simple test of cardiac function based upon the heart rate changes induced by the Valsalva maneuver. *Am. J. Cardiol.* 18:90–99, 1966.

Lind A.R., Taylor S.H., Humphreys P.W., et al. The circulatory effects of sustained voluntary muscle contraction. *Clin. Sci.* 27:229–244, 1964.

Low P.A., Neumann C., Dyck P.J., et al. Evaluation of skin vasomotor reflexes using laser Doppler velocimetry. *Mayo Clin. Proc.* 58:583–592, 1983.

Low P.A., Walsh J.C., Huang C.-Y., et al. The sympathetic nervous system in diabetic neuropathy. *Brain* 98:341–356, 1975.

Ludbrook J., Vincent A., Walsh J.A. Effects of mental arithmetic on arterial pressure and hand blood flow. *Clin. Exp. Pharmacol. Physiol. Suppl.* 2:67–70, 1975.

Mathias C.J., Frankel H.L., Christensen N.J., et al. Enhanced pressor response to noradrenaline in patients with cervical spinal cord transection. *Brain* 99:757–770, 1976.

McLeod J.G. Autonomic nervous system. In Sumner A.J., ed. *The Physiology of Peripheral Nerve Disease.* Philadelphia, Saunders, pp. 432–483, 1980.

Mathias C.J., da Costa D.F., Fosbraey P., et al. Cardiovascular, biochemical and hormonal changes during food-induced hypotension in chronic autonomic failure. *J. Neurol. Sci.* 94:255–269, 1989.

Molhoek G.P., Wesseling K.H., Settels J.J., et al. Evaluation of the Penà servo-plethysmo-manometer for the continuous, noninvasive measurement of finger blood pressure. *Basic Res. Cardiol.* 79:598–609, 1984.

Neilsen S.L. Measurement of blood flow in adipose tissue from the washout of xenon-133 after atraumatic labelling. *Acta Physiol. Scand.* 84:187–196, 1972.

Parkhouse N., Le Quesne P.M. Quantitative objective assessment of peripheral nociceptive C fibre function. *J. Neurol. Neurosurg. Psychiatry,* 51:28–34, 1988.

Polinsky R.J., Kopin I.J., Ebert M.H., et al. Pharmacologic distinction of different orthostatic hypotension syndromes. *Neurology (N.Y.)* 31:1–7, 1981.

Roddie K., Shepherd J.T., Whelan R.F. The vasomotor nerve supply to the skin and muscle of the human forearm. *Clin. Sci.* 16:67–74, 1957.

Rowell L.B., Detry J.M., Blackman J.R., et al. Importance of the splanchnic vascular bed in human blood pressure regulation. *J. Appl. Physiol.* 32:213–220, 1972.

Samueloff S.L., Browse N.L., Shepherd J.G. Response of capacity vessels in human limbs to head up tilt and suction on lower body. *J. Appl. Physiol.* 21:47–61, 1966.

Sharpey-Schafer E.P. Circulatory reflexes in chronic disease of the afferent nervous system. *J. Physiol. (Lond.)* 134:1–10, 1956.

Shawket S., Dickerson C., Hazleman B., et al. Selective suprasensitivity to calcitonin–gene-related polypeptide in the hands in Raynaud's phenomenon. *Lancet* 2:1354–1356, 1989.

Skagen K., Haxholdt O., Henriksen O., et al. Effect of spinal sympathetic blockade upon postural changes of blood flow in human peripheral tissues. *Acta Physiol. Scand.* 114:165–170, 1982.

Smyth M.S., Sleight P., Pickering G.W. Reflex regulation of arterial blood pressure during sleep in man. A quantitative method of assessing baroreflex sensitivity. *Circ. Res.* 24:109–121, 1969.

Sundlof G., Wallin B.G. Effect of lower body negative pressure on muscle sympathetic nerve activity. *J. Physiol. (Lond.)* 287:525–532, 1978.

Tuck R.R., McLeod J.G. Autonomic dysfunction in Guillain-Barré syndrome. *J. Neurol. Neurosurg. Psychiatry* 44:983–990, 1981.

Vanhoutte P.M., Shepherd J.T. Autonomic nerves to the systemic blood vessels. In Dyck P.J., Thomas P.K., Lambert E.H., et al., eds. *Peripheral Neuropathy.* 2nd ed. Philadelphia, Saunders, pp. 300–326, 1984.

Wilkins R.W., Culbertson J.W., Inglefinger F.J. The effect of splanchnic sympathectomy in hypertensive patients upon estimated hepatic blood flow in the upright as contrasted with the horizontal posture. *J. Clin. Invest.* 30:312–317, 1951.

33

Sudomotor Function and Dysfunction

Phillip A. Low

Advances have been made in three areas of sudomotor physiology. First, noninvasive tests of sudomotor function have been developed and applied to the evaluation of autonomic neuropathies. Second, the function of sudomotor receptors is being elucidated. The third area is the interest being shown in dynamic aspects of sudomotor function.

This chapter focuses first on normal sudomotor function. This discussion is followed by a description of certain noninvasive tests of sudomotor function and their applications and a section devoted to sudomotor dysfunction.

THE HUMAN SWEAT GLAND

There are two types of sweat glands, eccrine and apocrine. The apocrine sweat gland is of no importance neurologically and is not considered further in this chapter. The eccrine sweat glands are simple tubular glands that extend down from the epidermis to the lower dermis. The lower portion is a tightly coiled secretory apparatus consisting of two types of cells. One is a dark basophilic cell that secretes mucous material and the other a light acidophilic cell that is responsible for the passage of water and electrolytes. Surrounding the secretory cells are myoepithelial cells; contraction of the latter is thought to aid the expulsion of sweat. The eccrine secretion is a clear, watery fluid containing about 0.5% solids, mainly sodium chloride (normal values average 17 mEq/L). These glands receive a rich supply of blood vessels and sympathetic nerve fibers but are unusual in that sympathetic innervation is cholinergic. The full complement of eccrine glands develops in the embryonic state, and no new glands develop after birth. The distribution of eccrine glands shows re-gional differences (Table 33–1), with the greatest density in the palms and soles. Density varies from 400/cm² on the palm to about 80/cm² on the thighs and upper arm. The total numbers are approximately 2 to 5 million.

The sweat gland's major function is thermoregulatory. It does not perform any significant excretory function, although some electrolytes, urea, and a few other substances may be eliminated by the gland in the process of secretion of water for cooling.

SUDOMOTOR NEUROANATOMY

Thermoreceptors are present in the preoptic-anterior hypothalamus area, skin, viscera, and spinal cord. In addition to the spinothalamic tract, afferent pathways ascend as multisynaptic fibers in lateral spinal cord to the reticular formation of the brain stem and finally to the hypothalamus and thalamus. These signals are integrated in the posterior hypothalamus where a set point is established.

Efferent pathways are shown in Figure 33–1. Crossed and uncrossed fibers from the hypothalamus travel via the tegmentum of the pons and the lateral reticular substance of the medulla to the intermediolateral column. The major efferent pathways in humans to the spinal cord are thought to be the reticulospinal tracts.

The intermediolateral column neurons are cholinergic and synapse with the postganglionic sympathetic neurons at the paravertebral sympathetic ganglia. The latter supply the eccrine sweat glands (Fig. 33–2). There are about 5000 preganglionic neurons per segment of thoracic cord in humans, with an attrition rate of 5–7% per decade (Low and Dyck, 1977, 1978; Low et al., 1977).

479

Table 33–1. REGIONAL DISTRIBUTION AND OUTPUT OF SWEAT GLANDS IN MALES IN RESPONSE TO GENERALIZED HEATING

Area	Sweat Gland Density (Number/cm^2)	Sweat output (μl/cm^2/min)	Sweat Output/Gland (μl/gland/min)
Forehead	237	1.17	0.005
Chest	84	1.36	0.016
Abdomen	99	0.86	0.009
Scapula	91	0.76	0.008
Lumbar region	88	0.61	0.007
Anterior deltoid	115	0.40	0.003
Forearm (lateral)	111	0.61	0.006
Hand (dorsum)	240	0.30	0.001
Thigh (lateral)	85	0.71	0.008
Leg (posterior)	82	0.64	0.008
Foot (dorsum)	183	0.34	0.002
Mean	129	0.71	0.007

Adapted from Thomson M.L. A comparison between the number and distribution of functioning eccrine sweat glands in Europeans and Africans. *J. Physiol. (Lond.)* 123:225–233, 1954; and Weiner J.S. The regional distribution of sweating. *J.Physiol. (Lond.)* 104:32–40, 1945.

Sudomotor dermatomes are less precise than sensory dermatomes, because a single ganglion receives fibers from five or six preganglionic levels and skin is multi-innervated. Approximate sudomotor dermatomes are T1-2, ipsilateral face; T2-6, upper limb; T5-12, trunk; T10–L3, lower limb. As a rule, concordance of sudomotor dermatomes is good where postganglionic fibers enter the nerve trunk but poor proximal to that.

THERMOREGULATION

It has become well established that the afferent inputs include not only the hypothalamic temperature sensor but important extrahypothalamic sensors as well (Cabanac, 1975). The best-recognized extrahypothalamic temperature sensor is the spinal cord, but abdominal viscera and skin also contain effective temperature sensors. When core temperature is clamped near the sweating threshold (for instance, by placing heat exchangers into chronically implanted arteriovenous shunts in primates), skin heating alone evokes a sweat response. In warm human subjects whose core temperature is held constant, skin heating evokes a reflex sweat response (Wyss et al., 1974). Different skin areas vary in their thermosensitivities and make different contributions to the mean skin temperature. For instance, the scrotum of the goat, ram, and pig and the nose of the rabbit are exceptionally sensitive. In humans, the face accounts for 21% of input to the mean skin temperature; chest and back, 21%; abdomen, 17%; thighs 15%; upper arms, 12%; lower legs, 8%; and forearm, 6%. There is also a phasic response to heating that disappears in seconds and is followed by a more protracted and important sudomotor response.

Single-unit recordings have yielded evidence of summation, inhibition, and facilitation of afferent inputs. The integration of these inputs provides a set or reference point and the development of efferent outputs (Hardy, 1980).

In cats and dogs, all evidence points to the absolute requirement for diencephalic structures for effective defense against body cooling and heating. All parts of the forebrain, except the hypothalamus and the medial thalamus, may be removed without seriously compromising thermoregulation. These findings almost certainly apply to humans as well. In the spinal human, slight thermal sweating may occur as a spinal reflex, which is of little value in thermoregulation.

The effector side of thermoregulation comprises sweating, shivering, and vasomotor changes. These mechanisms are responsible for (1) evaporative heat loss, (2) direct heat exchange by radiation and convection between the skin and the environment, and (3) variations in skin blood flow. The mechanisms are modified by behavioral changes regulating mainly activity and clothing. Much research has been conducted on nonshivering thermogenesis and diet-induced thermogenesis (Hales, 1984), but their roles in adult human subjects remain to be established.

DERMATOMAL RECRUITMENT OF SWEATING

The supine human subject responds to a rise in ambient temperature with a dermatomal recruitment of sweating (Table 33–2). The palm, sole, and axilla sweat at room temperature. Sweating in other skin areas is progressively recruited in the following order: dorsum of foot, calf, thigh, trunk, upper extremity, and finally the face; however, significant individual variations occur. There is also no parallel between onset of sweating and a sense of warmth. The sense of warmth appears successively on the forehead, chest, arm, forearm, hand, abdomen, thigh, leg, and foot when the room is heated.

SWEATING REFLEXES

Axon Reflex

The administration of acetylcholine to subcutaneous tissue by intradermal injection or iontopho-

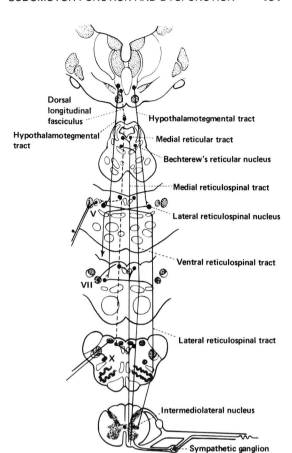

Figure 33–1. The probable efferent pathways of thermoregulatory sweating in humans. (From List C.F., Peet M.M. Sweat secretion in man. V. Disturbances of sweat secretion with lesions of the pons, medulla and cervical portion of cord. *Arch. Neurol. Psychiatry* 42:1098–1127, 1939.)

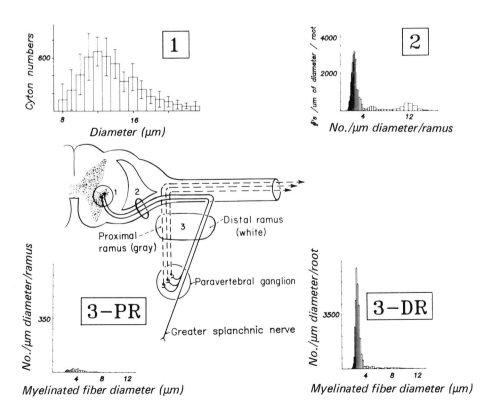

Figure 33–2. Diameter histogram of T-7 intermediolateral column cell bodies (1), ventral root myelinated fibers (2), gray ramus (3-PR), and white ramus (3-DR) of normal human subjects. (Adapted from Low P.A. Quantitation of autonomic responses. In Dyck P.J., Thomas P.K., Lambert, E.H., et al., eds. *Peripheral Neuropathy*. Vol. I. 2nd ed. Philadelphia, Saunders, pp. 1139–1165, 1984.)

Table 33–2. INSENSIBLE SWEATING AND DERMATOMAL RECRUITMENT OF THERMOREGULATORY SWEATING

| Area | Sensory Dermatome | Insensible Sweating (μl/cm^2/min) | Sweating Threshold (°C) | | Usual Order of Recruitment |
			Air Temperature	Skin Temperature	
Foot (dorsum)	L-5, S-1	0.02	26–27	32–33	1
Lateral calf	L-5	0.02	27	33.1	2
Medial calf	L-4				3
Lateral thigh	L-2	0.03	28		4
Medial thigh	L2-3		28		5
Abdomen	T-10	0.02	29	34.3	6
Dorsum hand	C6-8	—	30	—	7 or 8
Chest	T-5	0.01	30	34.7	7 or 8
Ulnar forearm	T-1	0.02	32	35.2	11
Radial forearm	C-6		33		12
Medial arm	T-2	0.01	33	35.5	11
Lateral arm	C-5, C-6		33		12
Forehead	V-1	0.05	33	34.8	9
Cheek	V-2	0.05	34	35.1	10
Palm	C6–T1	0.11	<room temperature		
Sole	S-1	0.09	<room temperature		

Adapted from Hertzman A.B., Randall W.C., Peiss C.N., et al. Regional rates of evaporation from the skin at various environmental temperatures. *J. Appl. Physiol.* 5:153–161, 1952; and Burch G.E., Sodeman W.A. Regional relationships of rate of water loss in normal adults in subtropical climate. *Am. J. Physiol.* 138:603–609, 1943.

resis results in two responses. Acetylcholine binds to the M$_3$ receptor (equivalent to M$_{2B}$ [ileal]) on the eccrine sweat gland to evoke the sweat response. This muscarinic response is evoked by acetylcholine and pilocarpine and is only slightly inhibited by the nicotinic antagonist hexamethonium. The second response is the axon reflex. Acetylcholine binds to the nicotinic receptor on the postganglionic sympathetic terminal to activate the axon. The impulse travels retrogradely to a branch point, then orthogradely. At the neuroglandular junction, acetycholine is released and binds to the M$_3$ receptor on a second population of sweat glands. The axon reflex is blocked by hexamethonium and is not evoked by the muscarinic agonist pilocarpine. When the axon reflex and the muscarinic responses are simultaneously recorded after subcutaneous acetylcholine administration, there is a latency difference of approximately 3 seconds that reflects the axonal conduction time and the delay at the neuroglandular junction.

The axon reflex appears to be mediated entirely by sympathetic postganglionic fibers and is lost days to weeks after postganglionic sympathectomy. The somatic sensory neuron does not appear to participate in the reflex, because electrical stimulation of the dorsal root in the cat does not activate this reflex. In contrast, stimulation of ventral spinal root, which contains the sympathetic postganglionic outflow, causes sweating in its area of supply.

Somatosympathetic Reflexes

Somatosympathetic reflexes have been well studied in experimental animals, especially the cat (Sato and Schmidt, 1973), and have spinal, medullary, and supramedullary components. The reflex is elicited by stimulation of myelinated low-threshold cutaneous afferents (group II and, to a lesser degree, group III) or of high-threshold muscle afferents (group III and, to a lesser extent, group II). Unmyelinated afferents (group IV) from both skin and muscle nerves also evoke sympathetic reflex discharges (C reflex). There is a period of postexcitatory depression. The spinal component is restricted to segments near the afferent input, in contrast to the diffuse outflow of supraspinal reflexes. The skin potential component of these somatosympathetic reflexes (thought to derive in large part from sweat gland epithelium) has been studied in experimental animals and in humans. Although all three components appear to contribute to the response, the most important reflex pathway appears to be supramedullary. Powerful modulating influences are exerted by the spinal cord, brain, and afferent input. The efferent pathway courses from the posterior hypothalamus to the spinal cord via the ventrolateral portions of the brain stem.

After peripheral nerve section, skin potentials are no longer obtainable in the affected dermatome on direct or reflex stimulation. After sympathectomy, skin potentials are also lost, but only temporarily, and return in 4–6 months.

STIMULUS OF SWEATING

Eccrine sweating is normally evoked by thermal, emotional, and gustatory stimuli. The major sensor of thermoregulatory sweating in humans is probably in the preoptic-anterior hypothalamic area, although spinal cord, skin, and visceral sensors also contribute. These sensors respond to warming.

Emotional sweating is induced by anxiety, fear, embarrassment, excitement, and mental stress. Sweating evoked by these stimuli is more prominent in the palms of the hands, the soles of the feet, the axilla, and the forehead at room temperature. When dynamic recordings of the sweat response to raising the ambient temperature and to mental arithmetic are recorded at multiple skin areas (including the axilla, the palm, and the chest) simultaneously, it appears that differences between emotional sweating and thermoregulatory sweating are quantitative rather than qualitative (Sugenoya et al., 1982). A sweat response to mental arithmetic is present in all skin areas after the thermal threshold is reached. Because the threshold is lower in areas of emotional sweating, a sweat response to both heating and such stimuli as mental arithmetic is obtained at room temperature. As ambient temperature is raised, thermoregulatory sweating *and* emotional sweating are present in other skin areas, and the responses in all areas tend to occur synchronously. The Δ sweat response/Δ temperature is lower in the areas of emotional sweating, so that the thermoregulatory sweat response progressively lags behind other skin areas with continued heat. These two observations of (1) reduced threshold and (2) reduced Δ sweat response/Δ temperature explain the clinical differences in emotional sweating.

Gustatory sweating is defined as sweating that is accompanied by flushing in the head and face in response to food, especially spicy or acidic food. This form of sweating may occur in normal persons, but it is not usually obvious. By contrast, prominent gustatory sweating is seen after nerve injury.

Excercise is a powerful stimulus to the sweat response. One mechanism of its action is elevation of the core temperature. However, other mechanisms are highly likely, as indicated by the following observations (Robinson, 1980):

1. Sweating begins within 5 minutes of exercise before core or skin temperature rises.
2. Cessation of sweating after exercise occurs before rectal temperature begins to fall.
3. In human subjects who are warm and sweating, the rate of sweating increases within 1–2 seconds after commencement of vigorous work.
4. This sweating begins to decrease within 1–2 seconds after cessation of the work.

The nature of the additional mechanisms is uncertain. An interplay of a rise in core temperature and exercise may sensitize the hypothalamus to deep cutaneous sensors in venous plexuses draining working muscles. The abrupt sweat gland responses, however, precede temperature changes in working muscle and may be due to proprioceptive reflexes or, possibly, irradiation of impulses from the motor tracts in the brain stem that act reflexly through the thermoregulatory center (Robinson, 1980).

FACTORS THAT AFFECT THE SWEAT RESPONSES

Apart from the effective stimuli of sweating described earlier, a number of factors modulate the sweat response. These factors are noted in Table 33–3.

TESTS OF SUDOMOTOR FUNCTION

Numerous tests of sudomotor function have been devised. They differ in the nature of the stimulus and the methods used to monitor the sweat response (Low, 1984). A summary of tests of sudomotor function, along with references to studies that detail methodology, is shown in Table 33–4. Four tests—thermoregulatory sweat test (TST), quantitative sudomotor axon reflex test (QSART), Silastic skin imprint method, and skin potential recordings (peripheral autonomic skin potential)—are described here in some detail (see Fig. 33–3).

Thermoregulatory Sweat Test

The TST is a sensitive qualitative test of sudomotor function that requires little sophisticated equipment and provides important information on the pattern and degree of sweat loss. The original method by Guttmann involved the application of quinizarin indicator onto dry skin. The presence of sweating causes a change in the indicator from brown to violet. Quinizarin is not readily available and is allergenic. Alizarin red S may be substituted for quinizarin (Low et al., 1975); skin reactions are rare. Thermal stimulation using heat cradles or sweat cabinets can be used. The latter is more efficient, because heat is applied to the head as well. When heat is not applied to the head, the latency to thermoregulatory sweating is delayed. Fealey et al. (1989) suggested that the commonly used end point of a rise in oral tempera-

Table 33–3. FACTORS THAT AFFECT THE SWEAT RESPONSE

Parameter	Comments
Factors that increase the sweat response	
Male sex	Increased volume per unit sweat gland
Race (black > white)	Difference quite mild
Acclimatization	Increased gain (sweating/temperature); reduced sweat sodium content
Circadian rhythm	Higher in PM
Seasonal variation	Greater response in winter
Alcohol and drugs	Cutaneous vasodilation; reduced hypothalamic set point
Factors that reduce the sweat response	
Skin pressure	Mechanoreceptor stimulation–> inhibition of local sympathetic efferents
Hydromeiosis	Water on skin surface that reduces sweating rate
Dehydration	Reduced skin blood flow
Hyperosmolarity	Reduced skin blood flow
Cold stimulus	Reflex inhibition of sudomotor activity

Table 33–4. METHODS TO MEASURE SWEAT OUTPUT IN HUMAN SUBJECTS

Test	Principle	Reference
Minor's method	Iodine–alcohol–castor oil application; sweat droplets turn violet-black.	List and Peet (1938)
Sweat imprint method	Soft impression mold shows sweat imprint.	Kennedy et al. (1984)
Guttmann's method	Indicator powder; sweat turns powder purple.	Guttman (1947), Low et al. (1975)
Tannic acid method	Sweat droplet is seen as a brown dot.	Silverman and Powell (1945)
Starch paper–iodine paint	Hard copy of number 1.	Randall (1946)
Starch-iodine paper	Same as number 5 but no need to paint with iodine.	MacMillan and Spalding (1969)
Skin resistance recording	Sweating causes reduction in skin resistance.	Richter (1946)
Prism method	Sweat droplets are seen through prism.	Netsky (1948)
Conductivity change	Humidity increase changes conductivity of silk fiber coated with a salt.	Darrow (1927)
Sudorometer	Humidity change is detected.	Low et al. (1983)
Skin potential recording	Somatosympathetic activity evokes skin potential.	Shahani et al. (1984)

ture of 1°C is satisfactory, provided that (1) the resting core temperature is above 36.5°C and (2) the subject is not dehydrated. It is essential that the subject has not taken anticholinergic agents, including antihistamine, antidepressant, and some antiparkinsonian drugs for 48 hours before the test.

There are several distinctive abnormal sweat patterns (Tables 33–5 and 33–6). It is also necessary to recognize the normal range of sweat patterns. Anhidrosis or hypohidrosis is common in pressure points, scars, and areas subject to stretch or friction, and distal anhidrosis may occur infrequently in the female. The disadvantages of the test are its inability to distinguish among postganglionic, preganglionic, and central lesions; its discomfort; the qualitative nature of the information obtained; and the staining of clothing.

A semiquantitative approach to TST has been developed (Fealey et al., 1989). The percentage of total-body surface involved is determined by charting the areas of sweating followed by planimetric determination of the body surface affected. The study is done with the aid of the Dubois formula. The percentage of anhidrosis can then be estimated to mon-itor the course of a peripheral or central autonomic sudomotor dysfunction.

Quantitative Sudomotor Axon Reflex Test

The structure underlying QSART is the postganglionic sympathetic sudomotor axon. The involved physiologic mechanism is a local axon reflex (Figs. 33–3 and 33–4); the setup to measure QSART is shown in Figure 33–4. A key component of QSART is the multicompartmental sweat cell (see Fig. 33–4). During iontophoresis of acetylcholine, the nerve terminals in compartment C are stimulated. Impulses pass antidromically along the sympathetic C fiber to a branch point (see Fig. 33–1), then orthodromically to evoke a sweat response with a latency of 1–2 minutes. The axon reflex–mediated sweating occupies an area 3–5 cm in diameter. A stream of nitrogen gas of low constant humidity and controlled flow rate evaporates sweat droplets from compartment A. This stream of altered humidity and thermal mass is sensed, and data are reduced by a sudorometer and a computer console with A to D converter and

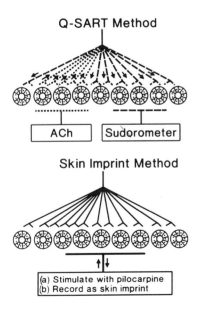

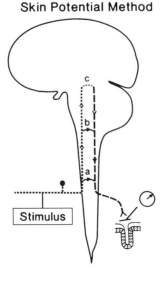

Figure 33–3. Diagram of neural pathways for the QSART, the skin imprint (Silastic) method, and skin potential recordings (a, b, and c refer to the spinal, bulbar, and suprabulbar components of somatosympathetic reflexes, respectively). ACh = acetylcholine.

Table 33–5. HYPERHIDROSIS

Pattern	Examples	Site*	Mechanisms
Distal	Thallium, arsenic neuropathy	P	Damaged spontaneously active postganglionic sweat fibers
Perilesional	Nerve irritation cord lesion	Postg. C	As above
Gustatory	Diabetic neuropathy	Postg.	Denervation with aberrant regeneration
	Seventh cranial nerve lesion	Postg.	
Causalgia	Partial sciatic nerve lesion	Postg.	Damaged spontaneously active postganglionic sweat fibers
Reflex sympathetic dystrophy	After minor injury	Postg. ? C	Sympathetic hyperactivity and other mechanisms
Compensatory	Postsympathectomy	Postg.	Reduced number of innervated sweat glands
	Central lesions	C	
Episodic generalized	Idiopathic	? C	Unknown mechanism
	Associated with agenesis of corpus callosum and hypothermia	C	Uncertain; ? episodic hypothalamic discharge
Palmar hyperhidrosis		C	Unknown
Hemihyperhidrosis	Poststroke	C	? irritation of sympathetic pathways
	Idiopathic	C	Exaggerated response to psychic stimulation

*P = peripheral; Postg. = postganglionic; C = central.

software to generate a sweat response that is read as output in microliters per square centimeter.

Standard recording sites are the proximal foot, the proximal leg (lateral aspect, 5 cm distal to the fibular head), the distal leg (medial aspect, 5 cm proximal to the medial malleolus), and the medial forearm (75% of the distance from the ulnar epicondyle to the pisiform bone).

There are now several recognized abnormal QSART patterns (see Fig. 33–3). The response may be (1) normal, (2) reduced, (3) absent, (4) excessive, or (5) persistent. Short latencies are common with patterns 4 and 5. Pattern 5, consisting of persistent sweat response when the stimulus ceases, is often seen in painful diabetic and other neuropathies, in

mild neuropathies, and in florid reflex sympathetic dystrophy.

QSART recordings have been done in many neuropathies, including diabetic neuropathy, multiple system atrophy, progressive autonomic failure, Sjögren's syndrome, Lambert-Eaton myasthenic syndrome, atopic dermatitis, aging, and distal small-fiber neuropathy.

The directly stimulated sweat response is thought to be muscarinic, and the axon reflex response, nicotinic. It is possible to record both the muscarinic and nicotinic responses. The axon reflex response is recorded as just noted. At the end of 10 minutes of recording, the capsule is removed, the skin is dried, and a dry capsule with compartment C (direct com-

Table 33–6. ANHIDROSIS AND HYPOHIDROSIS*

Pattern	Examples	Site	Mechanisms
Distal	Neuropathies (most)	Postg.	Postganglionic sympathetic failure
Global with acral sparing	IOH	C (mainly)	Preganglionic sympathetic failure
	Shy-Drager syndrome		
Global or segmental without acral sparing	Panautonomic neuropathy	Postg.	Postganglionic sympathetic failure
	Tangier's disease	Postg.	Postganglionic sympathetic failure
	CIA	Postg.	Postganglionic sympathetic failure
	Amyloid neuropathy	Preg. and postg.	Combined preganglionic and postganglionic failure
	IOH: Shy-Drager syndrome	Preg. and Postg.	
	CIA	Preg.	Preganglionic sympathetic failure
	Absence of sweat gland	Sweat gland	Preganglionic sympathetic failure Congenital absence
Dermatomal	Diabetic radiculopathy	Radicular	Postganglionic sympathetic failure
	Ulnar neuropathy	Nerve	Postganglionic sympathetic failure
	Leprotic neuropathy	Nerve	Postganglionic sympathetic failure
	Leprotic neuropathy	Nerve twig	Postganglionic sympathetic failure
	Sympathectomy	Rami; ganglia	Preganglionic or postganglionic lesion
Hemianhidrosis	Cerebral infarction	C	Interruption of central sympathetic outflow
	Spinal cord tumor		
Skin disease associated	Dermatophytosis	Sweat gland	Plugging of sweat duct

*Postg. = postganglionic; C = central; CIA = chronic idiopathic anhidrosis; Preg. = preganglionic; IOH = idiopathic orthostatic hypotension.

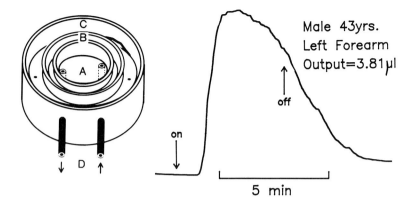

Male 43yrs.
Left Forearm
Output=3.81μl

Figure 33–4. QSART sweat cell *(left)* and QSART response *(right)*. The sweat response in compartment A is evoked in response to acetylcholine iontophoresis in compartment C. Compartment B is an air gap. Sweating causes a change in humidity of the nitrogen stream (D), which is sensed and plotted *(right)*.

5 min

partment) connected to sudorometer C is attached. The response is from directly stimulated sweat glands. The axon reflex response can be evoked by acetylcholine and nicotine but not by pilocarpine (a muscarinic agonist); it can be blocked by hexamethonium. Interestingly, pilocarpine or pirenzepine (an M_1 antagonist) inhibits the acetylcholine-evoked axon reflex response. Because pilocarpine is also an M_1 antagonist, it is likely that axon reflex response inhibition is due to M_1 antagonism, thus suggesting that muscarinic receptors modulate the nicotinic response.

Skin Silastic Imprint Method

Kennedy and colleagues (1984) published a detailed quantitative study in which they measured the number and size of sweat droplets by an imprint method. They stimulated sweating by iontophoresis of pilocarpine and recorded from the same population of sweat glands (see Fig. 33–1). The number and diameter distribution of sweat droplets can be quantitated from the sweat imprint. Sweat histogram abnormalities correlate well with impairment to pinprick perception (Kennedy et al., 1984). The method appears to detect reliably sweat gland failure in diabetic neuropathy. Results from the Kennedy study agree well with the QSART (Low et al., 1983); the sweat gland does not obey Cannon's law of denervation (i.e., the denervated end organ is supersensitive to its physiologic neurotransmitter). In preliminary work, the author has found that the diameter distribution of sweat droplets may be shifted in the direction of large-diameter droplets in chronic mild to moderate denervation.

Skin Potential Recordings

Recordings of skin resistance (galvanic skin response) and potential have been in continuous use since the end of the 19th century. Neural pathways for the reflex are described previously in the section on sweating reflexes and Figure 33–3. However, skin potential recordings to detect sympathetic sudomotor

deficit in the peripheral neuropathies and central autonomic deficits have been popularized more recently (Shahani et al., 1984). The recording electrodes are commonly electrode pairs (1 cm in diameter) applied to the dorsal and ventral surfaces of the foot, hand, or thighs. The stimulus might be an inspiratory gasp, a cough, a loud noise, an electric shock, or a stroke of the skin. Indeed, any form of somatic stimulation or psychic stress may evoke a response. The sources of the skin potential are the sweat gland and the epidermis.

The major advantage of the method is its simplicity; it can be used in any electromyography laboratory. The disadvantages are its variability and the tendency of the responses to habituate. The responses vary with the recording system, composition of the electrolyte paste, stimulus frequency, age of the patient, temperature, stress, status of central structures, and effects of hormones and drugs (Low, 1984). Skin potential abnormalities have been found in some patients with diabetic neuropathy. Skin potential recording correlates with QSART but can be considerably less sensitive than QSART. This test is unlikely to be objective enough to serve as a useful quantitative tool in clinical trials.

Comparison of Methods to Measure Sudomotor Activity (Table 33–7)

These tests provide different information and may be complementary. The sweat imprint method is a good and reliable quantitative test of sweat gland density and droplet diameter distribution of the directly stimulated sweat gland. QSART, in contrast, provides a dynamic quantitation of sweat output; it appears to detect sudomotor failure with greater sensitivity than the sweat imprint method. QSART fails when there is a lesion of the nicotinic receptor, the axon, or the sweat gland. The sweat imprint abnormality occurs only when the sweat gland fails secondary to denervation. Dynamic sudorometry is also capable of determining persistent sweat activity and studying somatosympathetic reflexes.

The TST is a straightforward, simple test that provides important information on the distribution

Table 33–7. COMPARISON OF FOUR METHODS TO MEASURE SUDOMOTOR ACTIVITY

Parameter	QSART	Silastic Imprint	PASP*
Principle	Axon reflex	Sweat gland M_3 Receptor activation	Somatosympathetic Pathway
Stimulus	Acetylcholine	Pilocarpine	Various
Receptor	Nicotinic	Muscarinic	Sensory
Pathway			
Afferent	Sympathetic C	Nil	Groups II and III
Efferent	Sympathetic C	Nil	Sympathetic B and C
Effector	Sweat gland	Sweat gland and epithelium	Sweat gland secretion
Response			
Latency	Long (1–2 min)	<QSART	Brief (seconds)
Turn on	Rapid	Rapid	Rapid
Turn off	Relatively fast	Extremely slow	Fast
(1–2 min)	(>2 h)	(Seconds)	
Neuropathy detection	Very sensitive	Sensitive	Sensitive
Advantages	Sensitive	Sensitive	Standard EMG equipment
	Reproducible	Reproducible	Variable (habituation)
	Accurate	Accurate	Less accurate
	Quantitative	Quantitative	Qualitative
Disadvantages	Time-consuming	Time-consuming	Habituation of response
	Special equipment	Special equipment	
	Rare problem with thick skin	Rare problem with thick skin	Many factors may affect response
Dynamic recording	Yes	No	Yes
Sweat histogram	No	Yes	No

*PASP = peripheral autonomic surface potential; EMG = electromyography.

of sweat activity. Because of the sampling problems inherent in quantitative tests, such as the Silastic and QSART recordings (which record from minute areas of skin), the TST provides important complementary information. Diabetic neuropathy appears to be characterized by multifocal nerve involvement; for instance, the patient with diabetic thoracic radiculopathy may have a diagnostic TST pattern but lack distal anhidrosis and have a normal Silastic or QSART recording. TST and QSART in combination can be used to define the site of the lesion causing anhidrosis (preganglionic versus postganglionic).

The skin potential recordings are dynamic, but the test is subject to great variability because it readily habituates and is a function of many factors. It has an evolving role in the electromyography laboratory but is unsuitable for clinical trials.

Postganglionic sympathetic efferents in awake human subjects may be recorded from skin by using microneurographic techniques. Skin sympathetic activity is quite different from muscle sympathetic activity in that it is not baroreflex sensitive. Instead, it is markedly sensitive to emotional stimuli and to temperature changes (Bini et al., 1980).

SUDOMOTOR DISORDERS

Hyperhidrosis

Hyperhidrosis (see Table 33–5) may result (1) from excessive activity of abnormal sudomotor nerve fibers, (2) from compensatory hyperactivity of a normally innervated but reduced population of eccrine sweat glands, (3) perhaps from muscarinic receptor

hypersensitivity, and (4) from altered central regulation. Damaged peripheral nerve, especially small-diameter fibers, are prone to fire spontaneously. Factors enhancing spontaneous activity include increased sympathetic drive, α-adrenergic activation, mechanostimulation, and nerve microenvironmental perturbations, such as hyperkalemia. The peripheral neuropathies, especially the toxic and certain metabolic ones (e.g., thallium, arsenic, or acrylamide poisoning and painful diabetic neuropathy), may have a phase of distal hyperhidrosis, coldness, and pain. Nerve root or plexus irritation may result in a phase of hyperhidrosis followed by an anhidrotic lesion with surrounding hyperhidrosis. A less pronounced perilesional hyperhidrosis may occur with a spinal cord lesion at the edge of the sensory loss, thus suggesting that central mechanisms may also be involved.

Gustatory sweating follows a partial nerve lesion and may occur in diabetic neuropathy. The sweating is thought to result from fiber damage with aberrant regeneration so that a taste stimulus, which would normally not induce sweating, results in excessive sweating.

A cardinal feature of reflex sympathetic dystrophy is an increased sympathetic effect with hyperhidrosis. The mechanisms of sympathetic hyperactivity are uncertain. Suggested mechanisms are (1) ephaptic transmission between sensory and sympathetic efferents, (2) spontaneous activity of damaged sudomotor fibers, (3) altered nerve microenvironment, and (4) hyperactivity of the spinal internuncial pool. In causalgia, nerve damage and spontaneous activity are present. The roles of these other mechanisms are less clear.

When a large portion of eccrine sweat glands is

denervated peripherally or centrally, the remaining glands undergo increased sweat secretion and compensatory hyperhidrosis results. This phenomenon may occur with central structural lesions as in cerebral infarction or brain tumors or after head trauma. Peripheral denervation after extensive sympathectomy may result in compensatory hyperhidrosis. Extensive sweat gland disease may also impose an increased secretory burden on remaining sweat glands.

Hypohidrosis and Anhidrosis

Distal anhidrosis (see Table 33–6) is commonly seen in the peripheral neuropathies and is almost invariably due to postganglionic denervation. When more widespread anhidrosis occurs (e.g., in some cases of amyloid, diabetic, and inflammatory neuropathy), the sweat loss is often asymmetric and there may be a significant component of preganglionic anhidrosis.

Global anhidrosis (see Table 33–6) may be preganglionic (as in multiple system atrophy) or peripheral (as in acute panautonomic neuropathy, progressive autonomic failure, and Tangier's disease). Global anhidrosis with sparing of hands and feet is usually central and may frequently occur in progressive autonomic failure and multiple system atrophy.

Lesions of peripheral nerve (root, plexus, trunk, or twigs) usually result in sweat impairment of dermatomal distribution. The anhidrosis resulting from sympathectomy has been well described. A complete interruption of sympathetic efferent pathways from the hypothalamus to the intermediolateral column of the spinal cord results in hemianhidrosis. Most lesions of the brain stem or the spinal cord, such as syringomyelia or neoplasms, however, result in incomplete hemianhidrosis because sympathetic efferent bundles are not well compacted.

Skin lesions of various types may damage sweat glands or plug sweat ducts with resulting anhidrosis; sometimes this is associated with compensatory hyperhidrosis of the remaining sweat glands.

THE FUTURE

Three areas of development hold particular promise. The first is the application of quantitative sudorometry in monitoring one aspect of peripheral nerve function, the postganglionic sympathetic neuron. The use of multiple recording sites makes it possible to define the severity and distribution of sympathetic failure in the neuropathies. This can result in a determination of the natural history of neuropathic disorders and their responses to therapy. A second area of development relates to an improved definition of sudomotor receptor function through the use of

autoradiography of sweat glands and in vivo receptor pharmacology in human subjects. The third area is the exploitation of dynamic sudorometry to study somatosympathetic reflexes. There is sympathetic activation by somatic stimuli. Sympathetic traffic may modulate cutaneous pain thresholds by operating through both rapidly and slowly acting mechanisms. In humans, sympathetic activity may exacerbate the pain of reflex sympathetic dystrophy and sympathetic block may alleviate the pain and hyperalgesia. The dynamic interactions await further study.

References

(Key references are designated with an asterisk.)

Bini G., Hagbarth K.E., Hynninen P., et al. Thermoregulatory and rhythm-generating mechanisms governing the sudomotor and vasoconstrictor outflow in human cutaneous nerves. *J. Physiol. (Lond.)* 306:537–552, 1980.

*Cabanac M. Temperature regulation. *Annu. Rev. Physiol.* 37:415–439, 1975.

Darrow C.W. Sensory, secretory and electrical changes in the skin following body excitation. *J. Exp. Psychol.* 10:197–226, 1927.

Fealey R.D., Lagerlund T.D., Low P.A. Thermoregulatory sweating abnormalities in diabetes mellitus. *Mayo Clin. Proc.* 64:617–628, 1989.

Guttmann L. The management of the quinizarin sweat test (QST). *Postgrad. Med. J.* 23:353–366, 1947.

Hales J.R.S., ed. *Thermal Physiology.* New York, Raven Press, 1984.

*Hardy J.D. Body temperature regulation. In Mountcastle V.B., ed. *Medical Physiology.* 14th ed. St. Louis, Mosby, pp. 1417–1445, 1980.

*Kennedy W.R., Sakuta M., Sutherland D., et al. Quantitation of sweating deficiency in diabetes mellitus. *Ann. Neurol.* 15:482–488, 1984.

List C.F., Peet M.M. Sweat secretion in man. I. Sweating responses in normal persons. *Arch. Neurol. Psychiatry* 39:1228–1237, 1938.

*Low P.A. Quantitation of autonomic responses. In Dyck P.J., Thomas P.K., Lambert E.H., et al., eds. *Peripheral Neuropathy.* Vol. I. 2nd ed. Philadelphia, Saunders, pp. 1139–1165, 1984.

Low P.A., Dyck P.J. Splanchnic preganglionic neurons in man. II. Morphometry of myelinated fibers of T7 ventral spinal root. *Acta Neuropathol.* 40:219–225, 1977.

Low P.A., Dyck P.J. Splanchnic preganglionic neurons in man. III. Morphometry of myelinated fibers of rami communicantes. *J. Neuropathol. Exp. Neurol.* 37:734–740, 1978.

*Low P.A., Walsh J.C., Huang C.Y., et al. The sympathetic nervous system in diabetic neuropathy: a clinical and pathological study. *Brain* 98:341–356, 1975.

Low P.A., Okazaki H., Dyck P.J. Splanchnic preganglionic neurons in man. I. Morphometry of preganglionic cytons. *Acta Neuropathol.* 40:55–61, 1977.

*Low P.A., Caskey P.E., Tuck R.R., et al. Quantitative sudomotor axon reflex test in normal and neuropathic subjects. *Ann. Neurol.* 14:573–580, 1983.

MacMillan A.L., Spalding J.M.K. Human sweating response to electrophoresed acetylcholine: a test of postganglionic sympathetic function. *J. Neurol. Neurosurg. Psychiatry* 32:155–160, 1969.

Netsky M.G. Studies on sweat secretion in man. I. Innervation of the sweat glands of the upper extremity; newer methods of studying sweating. *Arch. Neurol. Psychiatry* 60:279–287, 1948.

Randall W.C. Sweat gland activity and changing patterns of sweat secretion on the skin surface. *Am. J. Physiol.* 147:391–398, 1946.

Richter C.P. Instructions for using the cutaneous resistance recorder, or "dermometer," on peripheral nerve injuries, sympathectomies, and paravertebral blocks. *J. Neurosurg.* 3:181–191, 1946.

Robinson S. Physiology of muscular exercise. In Mountcastle V.B., ed. *Medical Physiology.* 14th ed. St. Louis, Mosby, pp. 1387–1416, 1980.

*Sato A., Schmidt R.F. Somatosympathetic reflexes: Afferent fibers, central pathways, discharge characteristics. *Physiol. Rev.* 53:916–947, 1973.

Shahani, B.T., Halperin J.J., Boulu P., et al. Sympathetic skin response—a method of assessing unmyelinated axon dysfunction in peripheral neuropathies. *J. Neurol. Neurosurg. Psychiatry* 47:536–542, 1984.

Silverman J.J., Powell V.E. A simple technic for outlining the sweat patterns. *War Med.* 7:178–180, 1945.

Sugenoya J., Ogawa T., Asayama M., et al. Occurrence of mental and thermal sweating on the human axilla. *Jpn. J. Physiol.* 32:717–726, 1982.

Wyss C.R., Brengelmann G.L., Johnson J.M., et al. Control of skin blood flow, sweating and heart rate: role of skin versus core temperature. *J. Appl. Physiol.* 36:726–733, 1974.

34

Pupillary Function and Dysfunction

James J. Corbett
H. Stanley Thompson

The iris is a fenestrated, muscular diaphragm that regulates the amount of light entering the eye. This diminutive autonomic muscle system works, with the ciliary muscle, to bring objects into sharp focus on the retina. The iris sphincter muscles are innervated by cholinergic fibers, and the radial dilator muscle fibers are supplied by adrenergic nerves. Not only does the pupil move in response to light and to near stimuli, but its size is influenced by the state of wakefulness, emotional tone, pain, and medications.

Pupils tend to be large in the young and become smaller with age. When one pupil is bigger than the other, but the responses of both to light, dark, and near stimuli are normal, the pupillary inequality is known as *simple anisocoria* (Loewenfeld, 1977). Simple anisocoria is often misinterpreted as an abnormality. In a normal population, 20% showed a simple anisocoria of at least 0.4 mm in dim light (Lam et al., 1987).

ANATOMY OF THE PUPILLARY PATHWAYS

Parasympathetic System

The pupil sphincter consists of about 50 motor units, segmentally innervated by postganglionic cholinergic fibers that originate in the ciliary ganglion. This ganglion is well named because most of its neurons send fibers to the ciliary muscle to change the shape of the lens, and only about 3% go to the iris sphincter. Preganglionic cholinergic fibers originate in the Edinger-Westphal nucleus. Segmental distortions of the pupil described in midbrain lesions imply that sectors of the iris sphincter muscle are represented topographically in the midbrain (Selhorst and Hoyt, 1976). The preganglionic fibers travel on the periphery of the oculomotor nerve, first dorsally, then mesially, and finally inferiorly as they enter the cavernous sinus and then pass through the superior orbital fissure with the inferior branch of the oculomotor nerve. These fibers synapse in the ciliary ganglion, which lies about 1 cm behind the globe between the lateral rectus muscle and the optic nerve. From the ganglion the short ciliary nerves pierce the sclera and run in the suprachoroidal space to innervate the ciliary muscle and iris sphincter.

Sympathetic System

Sympathetic fibers innervate the pupillary dilator muscle and Müller muscle in the upper and lower lid. The postganglionic fibers originate in the superior cervical ganglion. The central (first-order) and preganglionic (second-order) fibers traverse a long path beginning in the posterolateral hypothalamus. The axons travel through the periaqueductal gray, pons, and posterolateral medulla and then descend to the upper thoracic–lower cervical spinal cord, where they synapse in the intermediolateral cell column with the preganglionic fibers. These "second-order neurons" traverse the apex of the lung and, after dipping down in the ansa subclavia, ascend along the common carotid to the superior cervical ganglion. Ganglionic synapses are cholinergic. Fibers from the superior cervical ganglion follow the external carotid to innervate the sweat glands and the vasoconstrictor muscles of the arterioles of the face or ascend on the internal carotid to the cavernous sinus, where they condense, briefly travel on the abducens nerve, and then transfer to the ophthalmic division of the trigeminal and enter the orbit.

The Light Reflex

The light reflex is initiated in photoreceptor cells of the retina and traverses two intraretinal synapses to the retinal ganglion cell layer. The fibers of the retinal ganglion cells travel in the optic nerve, chiasm, and tract, where they separate, with some fibers going to the lateral geniculate to subserve vision and some, carrying pupilloconstrictor impulses, entering the dorsolateral aspect of the mesencephalon via the brachium of the superior colliculus. These mesencephalic fibers synapse in the pretectal nuclei, hemidecussate, and pass around the periaqueductal gray to the Edinger-Westphal nucleus. This completes the afferent limb of the reflex arc.

A light shining on either retina causes both pupils to constrict, producing both a direct and a consensual response (Fig. 34–1). This is the result of the double hemidecussation of the pupillomotor fibers: they cross at the chiasm and again at the pretectum. When one eye is tested at a time, and especially when the nasal retina is stimulated, a tiny, clinically insignificant anisocoria is produced. Occasionally, a slightly larger, clinically detectable asymmetry of pupil size is seen on illumination of one eye. This asymmetry is called a *consensual deficit*; this visible contraction anisocoria occurs in only a small percentage of the population and seldom causes clinical confusion.

BEDSIDE CLINICAL EXAMINATION OF THE PUPIL

It is useful for the examiner to divide the pupillary examination into two parts: the efferent and the afferent systems. Efferent defects produce anisocoria; afferent defects do not.

Detecting Efferent Defects

Parasympathetic Defects. In a darkened room, ask the patient to look in the distance, and shine the hand light from below onto both eyes at once. Note any pupillary inequality. Bring the light closer to the patient's face and closer to the patient's line of sight but keep both eyes illuminated or, alternatively, turn the room lights on. If this produces (or increases) an anisocoria, then suspect the larger pupil of having a weak iris sphincter and consider third nerve palsy, traumatic iridoplegia, anticholinergic medication, Adie's syndrome, or other parasympathetic lesions.

Sympathetic Defects. Start in the same way as just described with a hand light in a darkened room. If both pupils constrict and the inequality decreases slightly as the light is made brighter, then suspect the smaller pupil of having a weak dilator muscle. Look for the signs of Horner's syndrome. The pupillary asymmetry might also be a simple anisocoria. It is characteristic of Horner's syndrome that when the lights are turned out the affected pupil dilates much more slowly than the normal pupil. This is called *dilation lag* of the smaller pupil.

Detecting Afferent Defects

With a bright hand light in a darkened room, start in the same way as for efferent defects (see earlier). If the pupils are approximately equal in size and are both reactive to light, proceed with the alternating light test (Levatin's swinging flashlight test, 1959). The patient is seated comfortably in a dimly lit or darkened room (the darkness increases the amplitude of the pupillary response to light). The patient is asked to look into the distance and to keep both eyes wide open. The examiner should be comfortable and should be able to see the pupils clearly. It is easier to make decisions about pupil reactions when the irises are a light color and the pupils are large. Older patients with small pupils are more difficult to assess because of the small amplitude of the iris movements.

Using a bright hand light with an even beam, for example, a Welch-Allyn Halogen 3.5 V Finhoff transilluminator with a fresh bulb, proceed as follows:

1. *Check for an impaired light reaction.* If either pupil reacts poorly to light (an output defect), all obser-

Figure 34–1. The normal latency between illumination of the pupil and constriction is 250 ms. The amplitude of constriction is a function of the number of working ganglion cells or axons. Notice that both pupils are the same size and that the hippus is synchronous in the two eyes, suggesting it is of central origin.

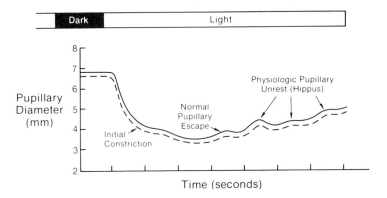

vations should be made in the eye with the better light reaction.

2. *Check for an anisocoria.* Small pupils let in less light and large pupils let in more. If neither pupil is smaller than 3 mm in light, then any anisocoria of less than 1.0 mm (in light) can be disregarded, at least with respect to an afferent defect induced by the pupillary inequality.

3. *Start alternating the light* from one eye to the other at a steady rate. Keep the light just below the visual axis and at a constant distance from each eye; illuminate each eye for about one full second and then switch the light quickly to the other eye.

4. *Observe the illuminated eye.* If reaction of the pupils is relatively weak when one eye is stimulated and better when the other is stimulated, there is an afferent defect relative to the good eye, or a *relative afferent pupillary defect* (RAPD). This pupillomotor input asymmetry can be measured by reducing the stimulus intensity to the better eye until both eyes have matched light reactions.

Even when light and accommodation are steady, the normal pupil fluctuates in size. This restlessness of the pupil is called *hippus* and is most evident in young people in moderate light. During the 19th century, hippus was regarded as a clonus of the pupil and its clinical associations were dutifully noted, but it is now generally acknowledged to be nothing more than physiologic pupillary unrest (H.S. Thompson et al., 1971a).

Relative Afferent Pupillary Defect

Galen clearly understood 1800 years ago that the pupils did not behave normally when one eye was blind. He found this to be a clinically useful observation. The normal eye has a brisk pupillary response to light, whereas the eye with optic nerve or retinal damage has a slower, less complete reaction to the same intensity of light; the worse the visual loss, the worse the pupil's reaction (Fig. 34–2). This asymmetry of light response is an RAPD, also known as a Marcus Gunn pupil, and is sometimes called a positive swinging flashlight test (Levatin, 1959). This sign ranks with optic atrophy as an important objective clinical sign of damage to the optic nerve. If both eyes are equally damaged, an asymmetry of pupillary input is not seen. Bilateral damage to the anterior visual system is usually asymmetric and produces an RAPD in the eye with the greater visual loss. The magnitude of the RAPD is proportional to the visual field defect.

The RAPD becomes a so-called amaurotic pupil when no amount of light shining in the affected eye causes the pupil to constrict. Much has been written about amaurotic pupils' being larger than their normal mates, but this may be due to the presence of a simple anisocoria. A larger pupil in an amaurotic eye may also be due to ischemic or traumatic iris damage related to whatever caused the amaurosis, such as more general ocular ischemia, acute glaucoma, or trauma. In short, an afferent pupillary defect does not by itself produce anisocoria; therefore, an amau-

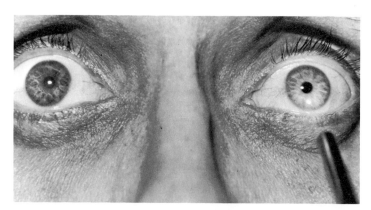

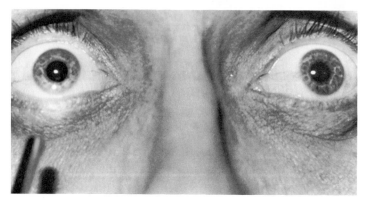

Figure 34–2. The relative afferent pupillary defect (RAPD) is found in diseases of the retina and optic nerve and in asymmetric chiasmal and optic tract damage. It does not occur in corneal, lenticular, or vitreous disease or in functional visual loss (hysteria). A small RAPD is seen in about 60% of persons with suppression amblyopia but is not related to the severity of visual deficit (Portnoy et al., 1983). The upper photograph shows the normal reaction of both pupils when the left is illuminated, and the lower photograph shows the RAPD when the right eye is illuminated.

rotic pupil should not be larger than its mate. If it is, there is usually some plausible explanation (H.S. Thompson, 1966).

Measurement of the Relative Afferent Pupillary Defect

The ability to measure an RAPD attaches added value to the sign. It can then be followed in successive examinations. Neutral density filters of 0.3, 0.6, 0.9, or 1.2 log units or a combination of these can be placed over the normal eye to induce an afferent defect that will balance the defect found in the affected eye (H.S. Thompson et al., 1981). Interobserver variability is low, and reproducibility is high (H.S. Thompson and Corbett, 1989).

An RAPD of 0.3–0.6 log units of neutral density filter is seen with some regularity in optic tract lesions (Bell and Thompson, 1978). The RAPD is always seen in the eye with the greater visual field loss. In a complete homonymous hemianopia, this is the eye with the temporal field loss (i.e., contralateral to the tract lesion).

The Dark Response

When the lights are turned off the pupils rapidly dilate by a combination of sphincter inhibition and contraction of the radial pupillary dilating muscles. Paradoxical contraction of the pupil sphincter in response to darkness is seen in some patients with congenital achromatopsia and in some with congenital stationary night blindness. The cause of this reaction is unclear, but in a child with nystagmus and poor vision such a pupillary finding is compelling evidence for a congenital abnormality of the retina as the explanation for visual loss (Barricks et al., 1977).

Reaction of the Pupil to Near Stimuli

The pupils react to a near target by becoming smaller. At the same time, the eyes converge and accommodation occurs; the lens become thicker as the ciliary muscle constricts. This coordinated response of the lens, pupil, and ocular motility to a near stimulus is organized in the mesencephalon. The amplitude of pupil constriction to near stimuli is essentially the same as that to light. The anatomic substrate of the near response is less well delineated, but the pathway is generally assumed to enter the Edinger-Westphal nucleus from the ventral side, whereas the light response fibers approach the nucleus from its dorsal side.

Damage to the retina, optic nerve, chiasm, optic tract, or dorsal midbrain results in a defect in one or both light reactions but leaves the near reaction intact. This accounts for one form of so-called light-near dissociation, in which the pupils react better to near than to light (H.S. Thompson, 1984) (see the later section on midbrain disorders of pupil function).

LOCALIZATION OF PARASYMPATHETIC PUPILLARY DEFECTS

Lesions in the brain stem can damage the third nerve nucleus directly or its axonal projections passing through the red nucleus to condense in the interpeduncular fossa. Damage to the mesencephalon rarely affects the pupil without also affecting ocular motility. Compression damage to the periaqueductal gray substance results in the sylvian aqueduct syndrome. Here, the pupils are mid-dilated, are frequently unequal in size, and react poorly to light but respond well to near stimuli, because the afferent light fibers are damaged but the fibers mediating the near response are spared.

Within the subarachnoid space, the third nerve is susceptible to compression by aneurysm, tumor, or uncal herniation. The pupillary fibers, peripherally located in the third nerve, are said to be particularly susceptible to compression. The rule of thumb that separates compression of the third nerve from other oculomotor palsies according to whether the pupil is dilated or not has been challenged (Kissel et al., 1983; Nadeau and Trobe, 1983), but it is still a valuable clinical rule.

In the cavernous sinus, the parasympathetic fibers to the sphincter and the sympathetic fibers to the dilators may be affected together, resulting in a mid-fixed pupil. This combination is decidedly uncommon and its existence difficult to prove. Compression or invasion of the third nerve by lesions of the most anterior cavernous sinus may spare the pupil because, at that point, the pupil fibers are already at the lowest part of the inferior branch of the oculomotor nerve.

The pupillary fibers in the orbit travel with the nerve to the inferior oblique and can be damaged in their preganglionic, ganglionic (ciliary ganglion), or postganglionic segments as a result of trauma (e.g., blow-out fractures, surgery), infection (e.g., herpes zoster ophthalmicus), tumor, or ischemia (e.g., diabetic partial third nerve palsy).

Pupillary Changes with Aberrant Regeneration of the Oculomotor Nerve

A fixed, dilated pupil in complete third nerve palsy that is due to trauma, aneurysm, or compression may eventually become a pupil that does not react to light but may constrict when the eye moves, especially up and in (Ohno and Mukuno, 1973). This is caused by aberrant regeneration of nerve fibers. Fibers that had previously innervated extraocular muscles now innervate the pupil sphincter. This produces one form of light-near dissociation.

Adie's Tonic Pupil

The tonic pupil is a special case of intraorbital parasympathetic ganglionic or postganglionic damage. At first, the light response is impaired, the pupil is enlarged, and accommodation is paralyzed. Although some strength often returns to the accommodation mechanism, the light reaction of the pupil does not recover and the near response is often tonic and exaggerated. Adie's tonic pupil is usually unilateral, but with the passage of time the other eye is frequently affected. Adie's tonic pupil is seen almost three times more often in women than in men and is most frequent in the 20- to 40-year-old group; mean age at onset is 32 years. In addition to the pupillary abnormalities, muscle stretch reflexes are frequently lost (H.S. Thompson, 1979). Involvement of the other pupil occurs at a rate of about 4% per year (H.S. Thompson, 1977).

Because the sphincter undergoes parasympathetic postganglionic denervation in Adie's syndrome, the pupil becomes sensitive to weak solutions of cholinergic drugs (e.g., 0.1% pilocarpine or 2.5% methacholine) (Bourgon et al., 1978; H.S. Thompson, 1972). Segments of the iris sphincter show no light reaction (Fig. 34–3). Aberrantly innervated segments receiving their supply from nerves previously destined for the ciliary muscle respond to near efforts with a slow, strong tonic contraction. Acutely, the Adie's pupil is larger than normal in light. The anisocoria is harder to appreciate in the dark. After some months or years, the pupil gradually shrinks in diameter until it actually can be the smaller of the two pupils and the anisocoria may not be appreciated in light.

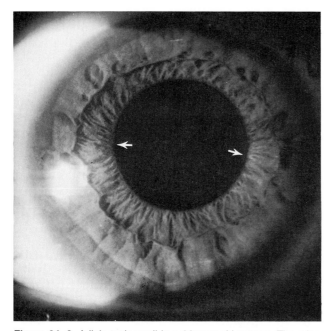

Figure 34–3. Adie's tonic pupil in a 36-year-old woman. The edge of the iris puckers at the 9 o'clock and the 3 o'clock positions in reaction to light. The edge of the iris is otherwise devoid of contraction.

Many patients with long-standing Adie's syndrome are affected bilaterally, with pupils that react poorly to light but well to near stimuli. These pupils may be mistaken for Argyll Robertson pupils but they react tonically to the near effort, whereas Argyll Robertson pupils constrict and redilate briskly to near stimuli.

Diagnosis of Adie's pupil is established by the following findings: (1) a pupil, usually enlarged, reacting poorly or not at all to light, the remaining light reaction being segmental; (2) weak and often slow changes of focusing in the affected eye; (3) supersensitivity to weak cholinergic drugs; (4) a better near response than light reaction, often slow and tonic; (5) depressed or absent muscle stretch reflexes in one or more limbs.

Adie's syndrome is easily the most common cause of a unilateral weak pupillary light reaction in ambulatory patients. Every neurologist should be able to recognize it.

Any unexplained, patchy loss of muscle stretch reflexes warrants a second, closer look at the pupils. An ophthalmoscope or otoscope may provide the magnification needed to see segmental light reactions of the iris sphincter.

Pathology of Adie's Pupil

Postmortem studies of four patients with Adie's syndrome revealed neuron loss in the ciliary ganglion and nodules of Nageotte. Some dorsal root ganglia showed similar changes. There were fewer fibers in the afferent limb of the spinal roots and paucity of short ciliary nerves, thus corroborating the neuronal loss (Harriman, 1970; Selhorst et al., 1984). These findings are consistent with a degenerative, rather than an inflammatory-infectious, cause.

The generic form of tonic pupil can be produced in humans by any damage to the ciliary ganglion or to postganglionic fibers. Ischemic injury (e.g., diabetes and ischemic orbitopathy) and trauma (surgical or orbital injury) regularly produce examples of tonic pupils, but patients with these injuries have none of the other progressive systemic features of Adie's syndrome. Bilateral tonic pupils have been reported with generalized forms of dysautonomia, such as acute autonomic neuropathy or idiopathic orthostatic hypotension.

The clinical usefulness of postganglionic denervation supersensitivity testing has been challenged by Jacobson (1990) and Ponsford et al. (1982); cholinergic supersensitivity in preganglionic lesions was found in both of these studies.

Pharmacologic Blockade: Medication-Induced Mydriasis

The unilaterally fixed dilated pupil may signal serious neurologic problems, such as early herniation of the temporal lobe. The ominous portent of this sign has not been lost on the misguided medical attention-seeker. Intentional instillation of mydriatics produces the appearance of mydriasis as a result of early compression of the third nerve. Separating these patients from those with compressive lesions requires only the administration of two drops of 1% pilocarpine in both eyes (H.S. Thompson et al., 1971b); 1% pilocarpine produces prompt and marked miosis in the normal pupil and in the denervated pupil but will not appreciably move a pupil dilated with an anticholinergic drug. The most common cause of this clinical dilemma today is the use of retroauricular scopalamine-containing patches to treat dizziness. These patches frequently itch or locally irritate the skin. Picking at the patch by the wearer contaminates the fingers with the belladonna alkaloids, and rubbing the eye then causes pupil dilation. Some antiperspirants apparently contain the anticholinergic drug propantheline bromide (Pro-Banthine). In farming country, unilateral or bilateral dilation may occur when there is accidental ocular contamination with jimsonweed, which contains stramonium. Bilateral fixed pupils are a regular occurrence when atropine is used parenterally during surgery or cardiac resuscitation.

Whether accidental or deliberate, the appearance of a widely dilated pupil, fixed to light and near stimuli and accompanied by no other signs of oculomotor nerve palsy, should strongly suggest medication-induced mydriasis.

HORNER'S SYNDROME

The effects of sympathetic denervation were experimentally described by Pourfour du Petit in 1761 and again by Claude Bernard in the 1850s, as well as by others. S. Weir Mitchell, who had studied with Bernard, described the typical clinical picture of sympathetic denervation in a wounded Civil War soldier (Mitchell et al., 1864). Nonetheless, it remained a relatively unrecognized clinical condition until Horner's clinical report of 1869.

Unilateral damage to the sympathetic nervous system at the central, preganglionic, or postganglionic level produces (1) narrowing of the lid fissure that is caused by relaxation of the retracting (Müller) muscles in both upper and lower lids; (2) miosis that results from loss of the dilator innervation and muscle tone; (3) anhidrosis of varying distribution, depending on the level of the lesion; (4) transient conjunctival injection that is caused by loss of conjunctival vasoconstrictor tone; and (5) transient ocular hypotension that is due to loss of adrenergic stimulation of the ciliary body.

The cardinal features of Horner's syndrome, miosis and ptosis, clinically outweigh all other features (Fig. 34–4). The ptosis is never profound enough to occlude the visual axis, and the miosis is never pinpoint; anisocoria may actually be quite minimal when the patient is examined in room light. The miosis is

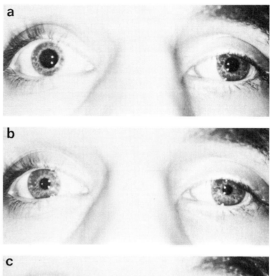

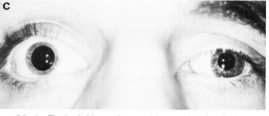

Figure 34–4. Typical Horner's syndrome. *(a)* In darkness, the anisocoria is most prominent; the ptosis, although more marked than usual, does not occlude the visual axis. *(b)* In light, anisocoria is all but gone. This emphasizes the need to examine pupils in reduced illumination. *(c)* At 45 minutes after instillation of two drops of 10% cocaine in both eyes. The right, unaffected, pupil is widely dilated. Although the left pupil is wider, it is less dilated than the right. This confirms the diagnosis of Horner's syndrome.

not intense because the pupil is small owing to failure of pupil dilators; there is no sphincter spasm. Sweating deficits can be evaluated with quinazarine, starch-iodine, or thermographic testing (see Chapter 33). It is rarely necessary to resort to these tests, because the combination of the patient's history, associated neurologic or physical signs and symptoms, and pharmacologic examination of the pupil should establish the location of the lesion with reasonable certainty. In occasional cases, the tests may be helpful (Morris et al., 1984).

Cocaine drops establish the diagnosis of Horner's syndrome (Table 34–1). A lesion at any site in the sympathetic pathway decreases the tonic output of norepinephrine into the neuroeffector junction. Cocaine acts by blocking the reuptake of norepinephrine, with consequent flooding of the synaptic cleft. This causes the dilator muscle to contract and the pupil to dilate. If norepinephrine is not being liberated into the cleft, as occurs with Horner's syndrome, the pupil does not dilate. Hydroxyamphetamine, by discharging norepinephrine from the nerve terminal, establishes whether the final neuron in the arc is affected. If it is damaged, the pupil will not dilate (H.S. Thompson, 1972). If, on the other hand, the first or second neuron is damaged, the third neuron still produces norepinephrine, which can be dis-

Table 34–1. PHARMACOLOGIC TESTING IN HORNER'S SYNDROME*

	Effect of Drug		
Drug	*Central Lesion*	*Preganglionic Lesion*	*Postganglionic Lesion*
Cocaine 4–10% (blocks reuptake of norepinephrine)	Affected pupil fails to dilate	Affected pupil fails to dilate	Affected pupil fails to dilate
Hydroxyamphetamine 1% (promotes release of norepinephrine from terminal axon, if present)	Dilates both pupils	Dilates both pupils	Affected pupil fails to dilate
Phenylephrine 1%	Dilates both pupils equally	Dilates both pupils	Affected pupil dilates more widely than normal pupil

*Two drops of the drug are instilled into each eye. After 45 minutes the reaction is observed. The cocaine test establishes the diagnosis of Horner's syndrome. Use of hydroxyamphetamine establishes that the lesion is postganglionic. The response to phenylephrine is based on the fact that a postganglionic lesion has denervation supersensitivity. This drug is used to show that the dilator muscle and its receptors are not damaged and that there is no mechanical impediment to pupil dilation, thus confirming the postganglionic denervation as the cause of the failure to dilate to cocaine and hydroxyamphetamine. Again, there is probably modest supersensitivity in preganglionic lesions, but postganglionic lesion denervation shows more.

charged by hydroxyamphetamine (H.S. Thompson and Mensher, 1971). It is not possible to distinguish, by drop testing, between lesions of the first and second neurons.

An earlier test for denervation sensitivity was a weak solution of epinephrine (1:1000). The concentrations were so weak that the results were often inconclusive. For this reason, the authors use 1% phenylephrine. It dilates the normal pupil a little, but the pupil with postganglionic denervation is clearly larger.

Another test that may be helpful in establishing the diagnosis of Horner's syndrome is dilation lag (Pilley and Thompson, 1975). When the pupillodilator muscle is not working properly, the pupil dilates only as a result of sphincter inhibition, whereas the normal pupil is also actively pulled open by the tone in the dilator muscle. As a result, the speed of dilation differs between the two sides; the Horner's pupil lags behind the normal pupil as they dilate in the dark. In a young patient with a light-colored iris, this dilation lag can be appreciated clinically (Fig. 34–5). If this observation is unequivocal, the diagnosis of Horner's syndrome stands on firmer ground.

Nonetheless, the standard test used to establish the presence or absence of Horner's syndrome is cocaine eye drops.

Pseudo–Horner's Syndrome: An Example of Simple Anisocoria

Unless it is already certain that the patient has acquired ptosis and miosis because of sympathetic denervation, the cocaine test should be used. It may save time, money, and embarrassment by preventing a needless search for serious disease in a patient with pseudo–Horner's syndrome (B.M. Thompson et al., 1982). Because about 20% of the population has anisocoria (Loewenfeld, 1977; this is only a brief introduction to the pupil and a description of simple anisocoria) and about 15% of the population has measurable asymmetry between the two palpebral fissures, the combination of miosis and ptosis on the same side occurs in about 3–4% of the population (Meyer, 1947). The causes of miosis and ptosis are found in Table 34–2. An "apparent" Horner's syndrome (pseudo–Horner's syndrome) in the context

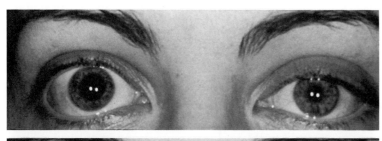
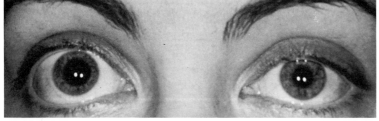

Figure 34–5. Dilation lag in Horner's syndrome. The upper photograph, taken at 5 seconds, shows the normal right pupil almost maximally dilated (compare the upper and lower photographs), whereas the Horner pupil dilates slowly. The lower photograph is taken at 15 seconds. The Horner pupil is smaller at 5 seconds than at 15 seconds because the dilator muscles are not actively dilating the pupil.

Table 34–2. CAUSES OF PTOSIS AND MIOSIS

Ptosis	Miosis

Myogenic
    Chronic progressive external ophthalmoplegia
    Myasthenia gravis
    Topical steroid eye drops
	Adie's pupil (old)
	    Light-near dissociation
	    Segmental iris sphincter palsy
	    Tonic near response
	    Cholinergic supersensitivity

Neurogenic
    Horner's syndrome
    Oculomotor nerve palsy
	Argyll Robertson pupil
	    Light-near dissociation
	    Serologic findings of syphilis

Mechanical
    Inflammatory (edema, allergy, chalazion,
        hordeolum, blepharitis, conjunctivitis)
    Cicatricial
    Tumor (lid, orbit)
    Blepharochalasis
	Sympathetic denervation
	    Dilation lag
	    Failure to dilate with cocaine

Levator dehiscence-disinsertion syndrome
    Aging
    Inflammation (ocular, lids, orbit)
    Surgery (ocular, orbital)
    Trauma
	Simple anisocoria
	    No dilation lag
	    Normal dilation with cocaine

	Iridocyclitis
	    Cells and flare in anterior chamber
	    Keratic precipitates
	    Posterior synechiae
	    "Stiffness" of iris

Pseudoptosis
    Dermatochalasis
    Duane's retraction syndrome
    Microphthalmosphthisis bulbi
    Enophthalmos
    Pathologic lid retraction of the opposite eye
    Chronic (old) Bell's palsy
    Voluntary blepharospasm
    Hypotropia
	Drug-induced iris sphincter spasm
	    History of exposure to miotic drops

of other neurologic symptoms may falsely suggest more extensive disease or prompt unwarranted diagnostic conclusions.

LESIONS IN THE SYMPATHETIC PATHWAY

Central Neuron

Central Horner's syndrome almost always occurs as part of a more extensive neurologic syndrome. Most commonly seen in Wallenberg's lateral medullary syndrome or with bilateral "pontine" miosis as a feature of pontine infarct or hemorrhage, central Horner's syndrome may also be seen with thalamic lesions (Carmel, 1968). Pontine miosis is probably a combination of bilateral loss of sympathetic tone and spastic miosis resulting from the loss of inhibition of the Edinger-Westphal nucleus. Sympathetic lesions alone never produce pinpoint pupils.

Preganglionic Sympathetic Lesions

Damage to the preganglionic fibers may occur as a result of thoracic surgical trauma, encroachment by pulmonary sulcus tumors (Pancoast's syndrome), trauma to the brachial plexus or carotid sheath, or aneurysms of the aorta or the subclavian artery as may occur with thoracic injuries (Grimson and

Thompson, 1979; Keane 1979). Cocaine testing establishes the presence of Horner's syndrome, and pupillary dilation after use of hydroxyamphetamine drops indicates that the lesion is not in the postganglionic neuron.

Postganglionic Horner's Syndrome

The most common form of Horner's syndrome seen in the outpatient department is an isolated third neuron sympathetic defect (Grimson and Thompson, 1979). First and second neuron Horner's syndrome, because of associated conditions, is more commonly encountered in the inpatient service. Postganglionic Horner's syndrome may occur with cluster headache; permanent oculosympathetic paralysis is seen in 10–25% of these patients. Transient, recurrent episodes of ptosis and miosis occur even more commonly in patients with cluster headache. Carotid artery dissection produces a characteristic constellation of continuous neck, jaw, tooth, ear, and tongue pain; ageusia; face or head pain; and ipsilateral postganglionic Horner's syndrome (Fisher, 1982). An isolated postganglionic Horner's syndrome is often benign and may be due to nothing more than ischemia or compression of the paracarotid sympathetic pathway as a result, perhaps, of vasospasm. The investigation of an "isolated" Horner's syndrome largely depends on where the lesion is placed and requires the use of associated clinical and radiologic findings and the results of pharmacologic testing.

Congenital Horner's Syndrome

Classically associated with Dejerine-Klumpke paralysis that is due to brachial plexus stretch, congenital Horner's syndrome is actually a rarity in this setting. More than one-half of children with congenital Horner's syndrome have no history of birth trauma, or the trauma is perinatal and surgical. Neuroblastoma in the mediastinum or primary in the cervical sympathetics is an occasional cause. The neurologic examination is almost always normal. Characteristics of congenital Horner's syndrome include hypochromia of the affected iris and postganglionic localization with hydroxyamphetamine testing, in addition to all of the classic features of sympathetic denervation. Less commonly, there is ipsilateral facial anhidrosis and impaired facial vasodilation (Fig. 34–6). Pharmacologic testing with hydroxyamphetamine in these patients produces no pupil dilation, which reflects transsynaptic dysgenesis of the postganglionic neurons in those patients whose lesions are clearly preganglionic (Weinstein et al., 1980).

EPISODIC AND UNEXPLAINED FORMS OF ANISOCORIA

The *tadpole pupil* is a brief segmental pupillary distortion lasting 1–5 minutes that is probably due to segmental spasm of the dilator muscle. Patients frequently experience minor local discomfort during episodes. Of 26 patients with tadpole pupil, concurrent Horner's syndrome was found in 11 patients and Adie's tonic pupil in 4. These episodic distortions were not accompanied by any serious neurologic problems, but migraine was a definite feature in 11 patients (H.S. Thompson et al., 1983).

Cyclic oculomotor spasms occur on the background of oculomotor paresis. They are thought to be the result of central and peripheral rearrangements following postnatal or congenital third nerve palsies. An intermittent miosis occurs when the lid is open and mydriasis when the lid is dropped. The diagnosis of this uncommon condition depends on careful examination and should be considered in a patient with a history of intermittent ptosis (Loewenfeld and Thompson, 1975).

Periodic miosis and *mydriasis* may be seen rarely in patients with cervical or spinal cord lesions in whom sympathetic inhibition (Horner's syndrome) may alternate for brief periods with sympathetic overactivity consisting of mydriasis, a wider palpebral fissure, and hyperhidrosis on the side of the lesion (Kline et al., 1984). Episodes of mydriasis may occasionally be a feature of migraine, or they may be unexplained. Whether the larger or the smaller pupil is abnormal, the patient requires careful examination in both bright and dim illumination (Woods et al., 1984) so that simple anisocoria can be ruled out.

Rarely, patients may experience unilateral episodes of pupillary sphincter irritability of one eye that results in recurrent dimming of vision. The cause is not known (H.S. Thompson and Corbett, 1980). *Sphincter spasm* is occasionally a clinical problem for the neurologist when a patient has iridocyclitis or is taking pilocarpine for glaucoma.

Convergence spasm is commonly seen in tense and suggestible patients. Visual blurring or diplopia is accompanied by constriction of both pupils and obvious estotropia. This may be mistaken for an acquired bilateral lateral rectus paresis, myasthenia gravis, or an unusual oculomotor synkinesis. Intermittent bilateral miosis, particularly in dim illumination, immediately alerts the examiner that the patient is voluntarily converging, and this accounts for the esotropia, miosis, and blurred vision.

Behr was sufficiently vague about his observations (on what has been called *Behr's pupil*) that it is hard to say in retrospect just what he meant. For many years, it was assumed that he had described a large contraction anisocoria of the contralateral pupil that occurred in patients with clean damage to the optic tract. Modern observation has failed to confirm this. Now it appears that he was probably saying that there was an afferent defect in the eye contralateral to a tract lesion, in which case he may turn out to have been correct. *Tournay's phenomenon*, dilation of the pupil of the abducted eye on extreme lateral gaze, is of no diagnostic use (Sharpe and Glaser, 1974).

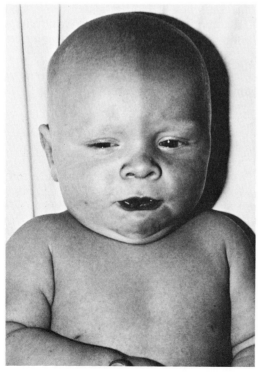

Figure 34–6. Characteristic failure of vasodilation on the side of a patient with congenital Horner's syndrome. The right side of the face is pallid, whereas the left side and the rest of the body are vasodilated and hyperemic. This reaction occurred after anticholinergic eye drops were administered but was also seen when the infant was fed via a bottle.

Pupillary Abnormalities in Seizures

Bilateral mydriasis in children having petit mal seizures is well recognized (Jammes, 1980). Dilation of the pupil of one eye contralateral to the hemisphere of focal cortical seizure activity has also been described (Zee et al., 1974). These pupils react poorly to light. Rarely, intermittent Horner's syndrome has been associated with psychomotor seizures (Afifi et al., 1990).

MIDBRAIN DISORDERS OF PUPILLARY FUNCTION

The dorsal mesencephalic location of the incoming light fibers and the ventral location of fibers that carry the near response provide anatomic separation of these two functions. Lesions to the afferent limb with no damage to the near reaction result in dissociation of the pupil reaction to light and near stimuli, which in light should be equal (H.S. Thompson, 1984).

Argyll Robertson Pupils

First described in 1869 by Douglas Argyll Robertson, these small pupils react poorly to light but react briskly to near stimuli. They are the hallmark of damage in the pretecto-oculomotor tract and central nervous system syphilis (Loewenfeld, 1970). Since the original description of Argyll Robertson pupils, a similar light-near dissociation has been described in association with other disorders, many of which have peripheral neuropathy as a feature. Damage to postganglionic fibers can produce tonic pupils that tend to become small as years pass. Distinguishing between bilateral old Adie's pupils and Argyll Robertson pupils may be difficult. Pupils that are small and react better to near stimuli than to light should be considered a sign of syphilis until fluorescent treponemal antibody absorption test proves otherwise. Any bilateral impairment of the light reaction warrants serologic studies.

Another midbrain lesion causing light-near dissociation is compression of the dorsal midbrain, such as by pinealoma, aneurysms of the vein of Galen, or dilated third ventricle (H.S. Thompson, 1984). The pupils are mid-dilated and may be slightly unequal, and the light reflex is depressed but the near response remains unaffected. This loss of light reflex with mid-dilated pupils may be the earliest sign of dorsal mesencephalic compression (Seybold et al., 1971). Midbrain corectopia, yet another central pupil defect, first described in 1906 by Kinnier Wilson, may be a feature of mesencephalic lesions that disrupt central cholinergic cells or fibers but leave others intact (Selhorst and Hoyt, 1976).

References

(Key references are designated with an asterisk.)

Afifi A.K., Corbett J.J., Thompson H.S., et al. Seizure-induced miosis and ptosis: association with temporal lobe magnetic resonance imaging abnormalities. *J. Child Neurol.* 5:142–146, 1990.

Barricks M.E., Flynn J.T., Kushner B.J. Paradoxical pupillary responses in congenital stationary night blindness. *Arch. Ophthalmol.* 95:1800–1804, 1977.

Bell R.A., Thompson H.S. Relative afferent pupillary defect in optic tract hemianopias. *Am. J. Ophthalmol.* 85:538–540, 1978.

Bourgon P., Pilley S.F.J., Thompson H.S. Cholinergic supersensitivity of the iris sphincter in Adie's tonic pupil. *Am. J. Ophthalmol.* 85:373–377, 1978.

Carmel P.W. Sympathetic defects following thalamotomy. *Arch. Neurol.* 18:378–387, 1968.

Fisher C.M. The headache and pain of spontaneous carotid dissection. *Headache* 23:60–65, 1982.

*Grimson B., Thompson H.S. Horner's syndrome: overall view of 120 cases. In Thompson H.S., ed. *Topics in Neuro-Ophthalmology.* Baltimore, Williams & Wilkins, pp. 151–156, 1979.

Harriman D.G.F. Pathological aspects of Adie's syndrome. *Adv. Ophthalmol.* 23:55–73, 1970.

Jacobson D.M. Pupillary responses to dilute pilocarpine in preganglionic 3rd nerve disorders. *Neurology* 40:804–808, 1990.

Jammes J.L. Fixed dilated pupils in petit mal attacks. *Neuro-Ophthalmology* 1:155–159, 1980.

*Keane J.R. Oculosympathetic paresis. Analysis of 100 hospitalized patients. *Arch. Neurol.* 36:13–15, 1979.

Kissel J.T., Burde R.M., Klingele T.G., et al. Pupil-sparing oculomotor palsies with internal carotid-posterior communicating artery aneurysms. *Ann. Neurol.* 13:149–154, 1983.

Kline L.B., McCluer S.M., Bonikowski F.P. Oculosympathetic spasm with cervical spinal cord injury. *Arch. Neurol.* 41:61–64, 1984.

*Lam B.L., Thompson H.S., Corbett J.J. The prevalence of simple anisocoria. *Am. J. Ophthalmol.* 104:69–73, 1987.

Levatin P.A. Pupillary escape in disease of the retina or optic nerve. *Arch. Ophthalmol.* 62:768–779, 1959.

Loewenfeld I.E. The Argyll Robertson Pupil, 1869–1969. A critical survey of the literature. In Schwartz B., ed. *Syphilis and the Eye.* Baltimore, Williams & Wilkins, 1970.

*Loewenfeld I.E. "Simple, central" anisocoria: a common condition seldom recognized. *Trans. Am. Acad. Ophthalmol. Otolaryngol.* 83:832–834, 1977.

*Loewenfeld I.E., Thompson H.S. Oculomotor paresis with cyclic spasms. A critical review of the literature and a new case. *Surv. Ophthalmol.* 20:81–124, 1975.

Meyer B.C. Incidence of anisocoria and difference in size of palpebral fissures in five hundred normal subjects. *Arch. Neurol. Psychiatry* 57:464–469, 1947.

*Miller N.R. *Walsh and Hoyt's Clinical Neuro-Ophthalmology.* Vol. 2. 4th ed. Baltimore, Williams & Wilkins, 1985.

Mitchell S.W., Morehouse G.R., Keen W.W. Jr. *Gunshot Wounds and Other Injuries to Nerves.* Philadelphia, Lippincott, 1864.

Morris J.G.L., Lee J., Lim C.L. Facial sweating in Horner's syndrome. *Brain* 107:751–758, 1984.

*Nadeau S.E., Trobe J.D. Pupil sparing in oculomotor palsy: a brief review. *Ann. Neurol.* 13:143–148, 1983.

Ohno S., Mukuno K. Studies on synkinetic pupillary phenomena resulting from aberrant regeneration of the third nerve. *Jpn. J. Clin. Ophthalmol.* 27:229–239, 1973.

*Pilley S.J.F., Thompson H.S. Pupillary dilatation lag in Horner's syndrome. *Br. J. Ophthalmol.* 59:731–735, 1975.

Ponsford J.R., Bannister R., Paul E.A. Methacholine responses in third nerve palsy and Adie's syndrome. *Brain* 105:583–597, 1982.

Portnoy J.Z., Thompson H.S., Lennarson L., et al. Pupillary defects in amblyopia. *Am. J. Ophthalmol.* 96:609–614, 1983.

Selhorst J.B., Hoyt W.F. Midbrain corectopia. *Arch. Neurol.* 33:193–195, 1976.

Selhorst J.B., Madge G., Ghatak N.R. The neuropathology of Holmes-Adie syndrome (abstract). *Ann. Neurol.* 16:138, 1984.

Seybold M.E., Yoss R.E., Hollenhorst R.W., et al. Pupillary

abnormalities associated with tumors of the pineal gland. *Neurology (Minneap.)* 21:232–237, 1971.

Sharpe J.A., GLaser J.S. Tournay's phenomenon, a reappraisal of anisocoria in lateral gaze. *Am. J. Ophthalmol.* 77:250–255, 1974.

*Thompson B.M., Corbett J.J., Kline L.B., et al. Pseudo-Horner's syndrome. *Arch. Neurol.* 39:108–111, 1982.

*Thompson H.S. Afferent pupillary defects: Pupillary findings associated with defects of the afferent arm of the pupillary light reflex arc. *Am. J. Ophthalmol.* 62:620–650, 1966.

Thompson H.S. Diagnostic pupillary drug tests. In Blodi F.D., ed. *Current Concepts in Ophthalmology.* Vol. 3. St. Louis, Mosby, pp. 76–90, 1972.

Thompson H.S. Adie's syndrome: some new observations. *Trans. Am. Ophthalmol. Soc.* 75:587–626, 1977.

Thompson H.S., ed. *Topics in Neuro-Ophthalmology.* Baltimore, Williams & Wilkins, pp. 93–123, 1979.

Thompson H.S. The pupil. In Moses R., ed. *Adler's Physiology of the Eye.* St. Louis, Mosby, 1980.

Thompson H.S. Light-near dissociation of the pupil. *Ophthalmologica* 189:21–23, 1984.

Thompson H.S., Corbett J.J. Spasms of the iris sphincter. *Ann. Neurol.* 8:547–549, 1980.

*Thompson H.S., Corbett J.J. Swinging flashlight test (letter). *Neurology* 38:154–156, 1989.

Thompson H.S., Mensher J.H. Adrenergic mydriasis in Horner's syndrome: the hydroxyamphetamine test for diagnosis of postganglionic defects. *Am. J. Ophthalmol.* 72:472–480, 1971.

Thompson H.S., Francheschetti A.T., Thompson P.M. Hippus. A history of the word. *Am. J. Ophthalmol.* 71:1116–1120, 1971a.

*Thompson H.S., Newsome D.A., Loewenfeld I.E. The fixed dilated pupil. *Arch. Ophthalmol.* 86:21–27, 1971b.

*Thompson H.S., Corbett J.J., Cox T.A. How to measure the relative afferent pupillary defect. *Surv. Ophthalmol.* 26:39–42, 1981.

Thompson H.S., Zackon D.H., Czarnecki J.S.C. Tadpole-shaped pupils caused by segmental spasm of the iris dilator muscle. *Am. J. Ophthalmol.* 96:467–477, 1983.

*Weinstein J.M., Zweifel T.J., Thompson H.S. Congenital Horner's syndrome. *Arch. Ophthalmol.* 98:1074–1078, 1980.

Wilson S.A.K. Ectopia pupillae in certain mesencephalic lesions. *Brain* 29:524–536, 1906.

Woods D., O'Connor P.S., Fleming R. Episodic unilateral mydriasis and migraine. *Am. J. Ophthalmol.* 98:229–234, 1984.

Zee D.S., Griffin J., Price D.L. Unilateral pupillary dilatation during adversive seizures. *Arch. Neurol.* 30:403–405, 1974.

35

Sexual Dysfunction in Neurologic Disease

Christopher D. Betts
Christopher G. Fowler
Clare J. Fowler

Sexual disability is a common feature of nervous system disease but one often ignored by neurologists. In part, this is due to mutual reticence and a commendable respect for the patient's privacy—there are still many occasions when there should be no intrusion into this delicate area. In addition, sexual problems tend to be neglected because they are overshadowed by other handicaps that attract higher clinical priorities.

Sexual failure, most commonly failure of penile erection in men, may profoundly damage self-esteem and is a potential source of marital disharmony. Even against a background of more obviously crippling disability, impotence can cause severe distress. The recent introduction of intracorporeal vasoactive drugs for treatment of erectile failure has proved highly successful in neurologic patients. Even when this and other physical treatments are inappropriate, almost all patients can benefit from explanation and counseling.

PHYSIOLOGY OF ERECTION

The genital organs, in common with the lower urinary tract, are innervated by three sets of peripheral nerves: (1) sacral parasympathetic (pelvic nerve), (2) thoracolumbar sympathetic (hypogastric and lumbar sympathetic chain), and (3) somatic (pudendal nerves). The peripheral innervation of the genitalia is complex; an excellent detailed review is given by de Groat (1988). In 1863, Eckhard discovered that stimulation of the pelvic nerves in dogs resulted in erection, and the nerves stimulated, assumed to be parasympathetic, became generally known as nervi erigentes. It is now known that the pelvic nerves may contain sympathetic as well as parasympathetic fibers; the parasympathetic fibers are still considered to be the main effectors of penile erection, but there is also evidence for a sympathetic erectile pathway via the hypogastric nerves (Bors and Comarr, 1960).

Parasympathetic Innervation

The parasympathetic efferent fibers to the penis arise from the S2-4 spinal cord segments, and the preganglionic fibers pass via the pelvic nerves to the pelvic plexus. The nerve branches of the pelvic plexus that innervate the corpora cavernosa have been named the *cavernous nerves*; their precise location in humans was described by Lepor et al. (1985). These nerves are small and difficult to identify at operation, and they are vulnerable during pelvic surgery or in traumatic disruption of the membranous urethra (Morehouse et al., 1972).

Sympathetic Innervation

Penile preganglionic sympathetic fibers arise from neurons in the gray matter from the T11–L2 spinal cord segments. The sympathetic nerves reach the genitalia by three pathways: the hypogastric nerves, the pelvic nerves, and the pudendal nerves. Some of the sympathetic fibers synapse in the paravertebral chain ganglia, whereas others synapse in the pelvic plexus.

501

Pelvic Plexus

This plexus is a confluence of nervous tissue that lies in the fascia on either side of the rectum and lower urinary tract. It is an important site for the integration and relay of autonomic pathways to the genitalia, bladder, and rectum. Entering the plexus are preganglionic fibers (sympathetic and parasympathetic) and sympathetic postganglionic fibers. The small cavernous nerves, passing from the plexus to innervate the corpora cavernosum and the spongiosum, take a course close to the prostate gland and the membranous urethra. Operative techniques to avoid these nerves during pelvic surgery have been described, and the risk of iatrogenic impotence may be reduced (Walsh and Donker, 1982).

Somatic Innervation

The pudendal nerve arises from the S2-4 segments of the spinal cord. Motor branches to the bulbospongiosus and ischiocavernosus muscles are important in sexual function. The dorsal nerve of the penis, a terminal branch of the pudendal nerve, is the sensory nerve of the glans and penile skin. Most of the sensory nerves to the glans have free endings, and sensation is thought to be conducted by small A δ or C fibers (Halata and Munger, 1986). Studies of paraplegic patients after spinal cord injuries have shown that bilateral sectioning of the pudendal nerves eliminates the reflex erections that occur in response to tactile stimulation (Bors and Comarr, 1960).

Neural Control of Erection

Formerly, the parasympathetic and sympathetic fibers to the corpora cavernosa were assumed to have antagonistic actions, with parasympathetic activity producing tumescence and sympathetic activity producing detumescence. This scheme retains some validity, although it is now recognized to be an oversimplification. Studies with paraplegic patients have demonstrated the importance of sympathetic fibers within the hypogastric nerves for mediation of erection. Lower motor neuron lesions affecting the sacral spinal cord abolish reflex erections to penile stimulation, but psychogenic erections are preserved. Cord lesions above T-11 generally abolish pyschogenic erections, but reflex erections remain. In normal circumstances, it is likely that both parasympathetic and sympathetic pathways act synergistically in the mediation of erection.

The presence of cholinergic nerves in the penis has been clearly demonstrated by histochemical techniques, but acetylcholine is unlikely to be the only transmitter involved in erection. Certainly, there is evidence that neuropeptide cotransmitters act with acetylcholine, but the importance of these substances is uncertain (Burnstock, 1986).

Mechanism of Erection

The exact mechanism of erection remains incompletely understood. Present evidence suggests that both an increase in arterial blood flow and an increase in venous resistance are important in producing and sustaining tumescence. On the basis of measurements of arterial blood flow and intracavernous pressure, five phases of penile erection are now recognized (Lue and Tanagho, 1988): initial filling, tumescence, full erection, rigid erection, and detumescence.

During the initial filling phase, arterial dilatation increases the blood inflow rate with peak velocities on the order of 30 cm/second. The intracavernous pressure begins to increase only during the second phase of erection (tumescence). As the pressure rises, the flow rate decreases; when the intracavernous pressure exceeds the diastolic pressure, inflow occurs only during systole. The penis rapidly expands during this phase of tumescence, which merges into the full erection phase when intracavernous pressure may approach 80% of the systolic blood pressure. The arterial flow is less than during the tumescence phase but still greater than that in the flaccid state.

In the rigid erection phase, contraction of the ischiocavernous muscle is thought to further increase venous resistance, which results in a rise in the intracavernous pressure above systolic blood pressure. During this rigid erection phase, the flow of blood in and out of the corpora virtually ceases. Fatigue of the ischiocavernous muscle limits the duration of this erectile phase to only a few minutes. Although contraction of the ischiocavernous muscle may account for increased venous resistance in this later stage of erection, the mechanism for increased resistance in the early phases of tumescence is not known. In some impotent patients with erectile failure, abnormal venous drainage can be demonstrated by using contrast medium (cavernography) during papaverine-induced erection. Controversy exists over the significance of these "venous leaks."

Detumescence is thought to be mediated by sympathetic adrenergic nerves. The initial process may involve expulsion of blood from the cavernosal spaces by contraction of cavernosal smooth muscle. During detumescence, the arterial flow returns to the flaccid state level.

Reflex and Pyschogenic Erections

Erection during sexual activity is primarily an involuntary reflex response to psychogenic and tactile genital stimulation. Supraspinal and spinal pathways are involved in the mediation of psychogenic erections; spinal pathways alone can mediate tactile reflex erections. As described earlier, sympathetic erectile pathways via the hypogastric nerves may preserve psychogenic erections in patients with lesions of the roots or sacral cord segments who have lost the ability to achieve reflex erections.

Higher Control of Penile Erection

Psychogenic erections are induced by memory or visual, auditory, olfactory, and imaginative stimuli with erotic content. Many of the data concerning the cerebral representation of penile erection come from work carried out on monkeys. These studies demonstrate the importance of limbic and hypothalamic pathways, particularly the medial preoptic anterior hypothalamic area (Dua and MacLean, 1964). In humans, Meyers (1962) reported two cases in which bilateral sectioning of the ansa lenticularis to relieve myoclonus resulted in postoperative impotence and loss of libido in the patients. These iatrogenic lesions involved areas analogous to regions in the monkey brain in which electrical stimulation may produce erections. Temporal lobe lesions and epilepsy have been associated with loss of erectile ability.

There is evidence from the work of MacLean and his colleagues (1963) and from more recent immunocytochemical studies that the important descending pathways concerned with erection pass through the medial forebrain bundle to the midbrain tegmental region and then via the ventrolateral pons and lateral funiculus of the cord to the lumbosacral centers associated with erectile function.

Information regarding the spinal pathways concerned with sexual function has resulted mainly from the study of patients with cord lesions after anterolateral cordotomy for pain relief (Hyndman and Wolkin, 1943). Although most such patients lose primarily erection and ejaculation, some may lose only orgasmic sensation while erection and ejaculation are preserved. The afferent tracts, described by Brindley (1985) as conducting "erotically coloured genital sensation," probably travel adjacent to the spinothalamic tracts.

Ejaculation

Normal antegrade ejaculation first requires the emission of semen and secretions from the vasa deferentia and seminal vesicles into the posterior urethra. Ejaculation involves closure of the bladder neck, relaxation of the external sphincter, and contraction of the bulbocavernous and ischiocavernous muscles in rhythmic propulsive waves. Emission and bladder neck closure are under sympathetic control, whereas the somatic, perineal branch of the pudendal nerve produces contraction of these muscles and ejaculation. The sympathetic fibers concerned with emission are thought to pass by way of the hypogastric nerves. Brindley (1986) has reported the use of a hypogastric nerve stimulator as a means of achieving seminal emission in paraplegic patients. These stim-

ulators may also cause erections, thus providing further evidence for a sympathetic erectile pathway.

NEUROPHYSIOLOGY OF FEMALE SEXUAL FUNCTION

Little is known about the neurophysiology of the female sexual response beyond what may be deduced from the innervation of the genitalia. As in the male, the somatic nerve supply to the female perineum is via the pudendal nerve and its perineal branch that supplies sensory fibers to the vulva and motor fibers to the superficial perineal muscles. The other terminal branch, the dorsal nerve of the clitoris, is purely sensory and innervates the cavernous tissue of the clitoris.

The vaginal secretion and swelling of the clitoris that occur in the arousal phase are under parasympathetic control. Orgasm is associated with contraction of circumvaginal muscles (Graber and Kline-Graber, 1979), but the neurophysiology of this is essentially unknown. The smooth muscle of the fallopian tubes and uterus are innervated by sympathetic fibers, but the part, if any, that this plays in the overall female sexual response remains a mystery.

NEUROLOGIC DISEASES THAT CAUSE SEXUAL DYSFUNCTION

Small-Fiber Peripheral Neuropathy and Autonomic Neuropathy

The peripheral nerve fibers that mediate control of sexual function are part of the autonomic nervous system and are composed of either unmyelinated or small myelinated nerve fibers. A generalized peripheral neuropathy involving small fibers, therefore, results in damage to the peripheral autonomic nervous system. Much less commonly, a subacute or acute-onset neuropathy may be confined to the peripheral autonomic nervous system (Brown and Asbury, 1984). Failure of penile erection is an early and almost inevitable feature of both types of neuropathy, although ejaculation is often remarkably preserved. Little or nothing is known of the effect of small-fiber neuropathy on female sexual function.

Small-fiber neuropathy occurs most commonly in diabetes, but it may also be a feature of alcoholic or uremic neuropathy. Rare causes of autonomic impairment that are due to small-fiber neuropathy include amyloidosis, Fabry's disease, and some of the hereditary sensory autonomic neuropathies (McLeod, 1988). Many patients with hereditary sensory autonomic neuropathy do not reach adult life; if they do, they may be too incapacitated to complain of erectile failure, but this is not inevitably the case.

Impotence and Diabetes

Estimates of the prevalence of erectile failure in diabetics vary considerably, but it is generally agreed that the incidence is significantly increased. Rubin and Babbott (1958) reported a 25% incidence in diabetics between 30 and 34 years old; the incidence rose to more than 50% in those over the age of 50 years. Another study found that 40% of insulin-dependent diabetics between the ages of 18 and 50 years may be so affected (Faerman et al., 1974).

Diabetic autonomic neuropathy often accompanies the generalized distal sensorimotor neuropathy of diabetes. Less commonly, it can occur in a relatively pure form in younger patients with juvenile-onset diabetes (Brown and Asbury, 1984). In general, the neuropathy of diabetes is length dependent, and the defect is maximal in the longest fibers.

Impotence is now thought to be the earliest clinical manifestation of autonomic neuropathy. According to the length principle, the autonomic fibers to the feet are most likely to be affected first, but the resulting deficit is initially asymptomatic. Defects of cardiac innervation and control of blood pressure occur relatively late, which may explain the fact that tests of autonomic function that were based on cardiovascular reflex responses failed to reveal an abnormality in diabetic men with impotence as an isolated symptom (Ewing et al., 1973).

The confusion about the extent of the neurogenic component in the pathogenesis of impotence in diabetics has arisen from ill-advised attempts to use neurophysiologic measurements of the bulbocavernous reflex to detect neuropathy. This reflex is the contraction of the bulbocavernous muscle that occurs in response to squeezing the glans penis. The latency of the response can be measured by using a needle electrode to record an electromyogram (EMG) from the bulbocavernous or urethral sphincter muscle in response to electrical stimulation of the dorsal nerve of the penis. The reflex is mediated by afferent and efferent fibers in the pudendal nerve that pass through an oligosynaptic reflex arc at S2-4 spinal segment levels (Vodusek and Janko, 1990). The reflex is mediated by the largest-diameter myelinated fibers in the pudendal nerve, and the minimal latency of the response is recorded. Herein lies the fallacy of using this measurement to assess small-fiber neuropathy. Although the mechanism of erectile failure in small-fiber neuropathy is uncertain, it seems likely that loss of parasympathetic innervation of the corpora cavernosa is important; therefore, measurement of minimal latency of a reflex arc subserved by heavily myelinated fibers has little relevance to the underlying problem. Indeed, several series have confirmed that abnormalities of the bulbocavernous reflex are not universally present in impotent diabetics who, on clinical grounds, are thought to have neurogenic erectile failure (Desai et al., 1988; Ertekin and Reel, 1976; Fowler et al., 1988a).

Unfortunately, a neurophysiologic test of the innervation of the penis does not yet exist, and neurophysiologic testing in the investigation of small-nerve fiber disease in generalized neuropathy is limited. Currently, the best estimate of the integrity of small myelinated and unmyelinated afferent fibers can be obtained by measuring the sensory thresholds for warming and cooling; warming is conveyed by unmyelinated fibers and cooling by small myelinated fibers (Fowler et al., 1988b). Small-fiber neuropathy can be detected by using a device that quantitates these sensations. From this, it can be concluded that if impotence occurs in a patient suspected of having small-fiber neuropathy, more relevant information can be obtained by testing perception of warming and cooling on the soles of the feet than by measuring the latency of the bulbocavernous reflex (Table 35-1) (Fowler et al., 1988a).

Small-fiber neuropathy may, however, be only part of the explanation for the high incidence of impotence in diabetes. An association between retinopathy and erectile failure in diabetics has been observed (McCulloch et al., 1984), and the observation that higher doses of intracorporeal papaverine are required in diabetics than in patients with impotence from central nervous system disease supports the view that erectile failure may be due in some part to coexistent small-vessel pathology. In other patients, occlusive large-vessel disease may also impair penile blood flow.

Impotence in Chronic Renal Failure

Impotence is common in patients with chronic renal failure, particularly those who are maintained on dialysis, in whom an incidence of greater than 30% has been reported (Sherman, 1975). Early involvement of small, unmyelinated fibers has been shown in uremic neuropathy (Lindblom and Tegner, 1985), and defective autonomic function has been demonstrated in patients undergoing long-term di-

Table 35-1. BULBOCAVERNOUS REFLEX LATENCY IN DIABETIC MEN WITH IMPOTENCE

Age (y)	Bulbocavernous Reflex Latency (ms)	Thermal Thresholds (°C)	
		Cooling	Warming
29	46*	3.6*	>6.0*
46	35.6	4.0*	>6.0*
65	46*	0.8	>6.0*
54	Absent*	1.1	>6.0*
48	Absent*	0.5	>6.0*
50	32	1.0	>6.0*
40	33	4.0*	>6.0*
65	34.5	1.3*	>6.0*
54	39.6	2.3*	>6.0*
38	38.4	1.1	>6.0*

*Indicates an abnormal result in testing bulbocavernous reflex latency and sensory threshold for warming and cooling of the feet in 10 diabetic patients, with clinical histories suggesting organic erectile failure, who responded well to intracorporeal papaverine (see Fowler et al., 1988a).

alysis (Ewing and Winney, 1975). Neuroendocrine, chemical, and psychologic factors, however, are also important. Renal failure is associated with a low serum testosterone level, high luteinizing hormone and follicle-stimulating hormone levels, and a poor response of serum testosterone to exogenous gonadotropins. This pattern of hormonal abnormality suggests a primary problem of testicular function.

After transplantation, testosterone levels rise, and patients may report an improvement in libido and erectile function (Baumgarten et al., 1977). However, in some patients impotence develops again after transplantation. This presumably results from alterations in penile blood flow as a consequence of the graft's taking its blood supply from the iliac vessels or, alternatively, to drug therapy after surgery.

Impotence and Alcoholism

Impotence in alcoholics is probably due to a combination of autonomic neuropathy and central hormonal and psychogenic factors. Studies of autonomic nervous system function in alcoholics have shown that peripheral sympathetic vasomotor control is relatively well preserved until peripheral neuropathy reaches an advanced state, although there may be an early involvement of postganglionic sympathetic fibers (Low et al., 1975). Duncan et al. (1980) showed vagal neuropathy in chronic alcoholics that results in abnormalities of cardiovascular reflexes.

Endocrine dysfunction occurs in chronic alcoholism with hypogonadism and gynecomastia, but testosterone levels are usually normal (Johnson, 1988). Recording nocturnal penile tumescence demonstrated normal erections in 50% of a small group of impotent alcoholics, and it was concluded that psychogenic factors were common in this disorder (Tan et al., 1984).

Multiple System Atrophy

Impotence is an early symptom of Shy-Drager syndrome and was described as a feature of the original cases by Shy and Drager (1960). Bannister and Oppenheimer (1972) reported its onset to predate that of other symptoms by up to 4 years. The observation has been corroborated in many other reports of case histories of this disorder (Quinn, 1989). Less is known about the prevalence of impotence when multiple system atrophy is manifested as a disorder with less pronounced symptoms of autonomic failure. However, the introduction of sphincter EMG to recognize anterior horn cell loss affecting the Onuf nucleus (see Chapter 36) in patients with parkinsonism (Eardley et al., 1989) has demonstrated a close correlation between abnormal sphincter EMG findings and a history of impotence. Indeed, a history of preserved potency should perhaps cast some doubt over a diagnosis of multiple system atrophy. The

effect of this disorder on female sexual activity is unknown.

Erectile failure in multiple system atrophy is complete, and all erections cease over a period of some months. This happens to men in their early 40s or 50s who are otherwise well, and the impotence is commonly ascribed to "early aging," stress, or depression. The correct organic diagnosis, even if given only retrospectively, often comes as a relief to a patient and his partner.

Response to intracorporeal injections of papaverine are good unless postural hypotension is extreme. In this case, it is recommended that the patient lie down for the injection to restore blood pressure.

Multiple Sclerosis

Sexual Dysfunction in Men

In their survey of a population in Newcastle with multiple sclerosis (MS), Miller et al. (1965) found a disturbance of erection in 60% of the men. A study from the Mayo Clinic reported an incidence of sexual dysfunction of 26% in men with MS who also had urinary symptoms (Ivers and Goldstein, 1963). Impotence is rarely an isolated presenting symptom of MS (P.C. Gautier-Smith, personal communication) but is frequently part of a complex of symptoms, particularly if these reflect an underlying cord lesion. Despite the high incidence of impotence in MS, there have been few studies of the problem.

In 1969, Vas studied a group of 37 men with MS, 17 of whom had impotence. All were still able to walk without the aid of a cane and were evaluated by the Kurtzke MS Disability Scale as grade 5 or less. The impotent patients were segregated into those with total or partial impotence. Total impotence was associated with a longer history of demyelinating disease, a higher overall Kurtzke disability score, and greater disability of bowel and bladder function than in patients with partial impotence or those still potent. Sudomotor function was examined by using quinizarin powder sprayed on the whole body, front and then back. Those totally impotent did not sweat below the waist, whereas those partially impotent perspired normally on the face, upper limbs, trunk, groin, and perineum but not on the lower limbs. The lack of a dermatomal pattern for anhidrosis was attributed to the lesions being in the central nervous system, possibly within the lateral horns of the dorsolumbar cord. A point of particular interest from this study was the observed variation in sexual potency that occurred in four patients: sexual function in two men improved and in two others deteriorated during the 2-year period of study.

More recently, Kirkeby et al. (1988) studied a group of impotent men with MS who had responded to an advertisement in a Danish MS newsletter. In all 29 men, penile arterial inflow and venous outflow study results were normal. In 26, the pudendal-evoked potential was found to be abnormal, and the bulbocavernous reflex was also abnormal in 8 of the men. The former finding is consistent with demyelination affecting ascending pathways within the cord, whereas the abnormal bulbocavernous reflex indicates an additional conus lesion. Nocturnal penile tumescence and rigidity were also studied in these patients, and one-third of the patients were found to have at least one erection in the course of two nights. It was concluded from this study that vasomotor control is probably unaffected in such patients but that cerebral modulation of erections is defective. The response to low dosages of intracorporeal papaverine was good in the majority of these patients.

Sexual Dysfunction in Women

The incidence of sexual problems in female patients with MS has been reported at 39% (Lilius et al., 1976), 52% (Lundberg, 1978), 56% (Valleroy and Kraft, 1984), and 73.9% (Minderhoud et al., 1984). Despite the evidence for sexual dysfunction in female patients, there has been remarkably little research on this aspect of MS. In comparison with male sexual problems, which are now more openly recognized in routine clinical practice, female sexual problems are infrequently discussed.

Lilius et al. (1976) sent a questionnaire to 302 patients with MS; responses indicated that the main female sexual problems encountered were loss of libido (27%) and loss of orgasm (33%). Valleroy and Kraft (1984) also examined sexual problems in 217 men and women with MS by means of a questionnaire. More than one-half of their patients were ambulatory without aids and 75% did not use a wheelchair. Sexual problems were reported by 56% of the women, and the most commonly occurring complaints were decreased sensation, decreased libido, decreased frequency or loss of orgasm, and difficulty with arousal. The study also showed that loss of mobility was not significantly associated with sexual dysfunction, but bladder dysfunction and spasticity seemed to be associated. Valleroy and Kraft concluded that sexual problems would be expected in at least 50% of female patients regardless of the degree of mobility.

The study by Minderhoud et al. (1984) was restricted to partially ambulant patients who were compared with an age-matched control group. In patients younger than 50 years of age, disturbances of sexual function were found in 73.9% of females compared with 71.4% of male patients and 18.7% of the control group. The problems were described as serious in 19.6% of patients. The symptoms reported were dyspareunia (8%) and disturbances of lubrication and orgasm (21 and 48%, respectively). Only a few female patients (3%) thought that the importance of sexual activity had decreased since the onset of the disease. In this study, there was no relationship between the incidence of sexual dysfunction and the degree of motor disturbance, age, or duration of the illness, but bladder dysfunction was again associated with disturbances of sexual function.

There have been few reports regarding the specific management of female sexual problems in MS. Management should include counseling not only for sexual difficulties but also for problems related to pregnancy, childbirth, and family upbringing. This topic is beyond the scope of this chapter, but there does appear to be a need for trained personnel to provide marital, sexual, and family counseling for female patients with MS.

Cortical Causes of Sexual Dysfunction

Cerebral lesions may affect sexual behavior and result in either habitual or paroxysmal changes, the latter occurring as focal epileptic phenomena. The exact site of lesions that produce such effects has been less clearly defined than the loci that control bladder function, probably because sexual behavior reflects more diffuse interactions between cortical and subcortical areas. Frontal lesions may diminish inhibition and thus result in inappropriate sexual behavior, but temporal lesions are associated most clearly with alterations in sexual activity.

Temporal Lobe Epilepsy, Hyposexuality, and Impotence

Early animal experiments showing that bitemporal lobectomy could result in profound changes in sexual behavior were exemplified by the Klüver and Bucy study of monkeys. These rhesus monkeys had both temporal lobes, as well as the uncus and hippocampus, removed. The monkeys exhibited "psychic blindness," a tendency to examine everything by oral contact, a tendency to react to all visual stimuli, a change in emotional behavior, and a gross increase in sexual activity (Klüver and Bucy, 1939). A somewhat unconvincing case of this syndrome in humans was reported in a man who underwent bilateral temporal lobectomy and then showed a tendency to have increased erections and to masturbate (Terzian and Dalle Ore, 1955).

Gastaut and Collomb (1954) noted a striking hyposexuality in several hundred patients with psychomotor seizures; in a systematic study of 36 patients, they confirmed the observation. These authors emphasized the global hyposexuality observed in the patients. In addition to a lack of desire for intercourse, these patients displayed a complete loss of sexual interest and curiosity. Patients with other types of epilepsy did not show these phenomena. Similarly, Saunders and Rawson (1970), in a study of 100 male epileptics living at home, found disturbances of sexual behavior confined to those with temporal lobe epilepsy.

Blumer and Walker (1967) looked at the effect of temporal lobe epilepsy on sexual behavior and the effect of lobectomy. They studied 26 patients with unilateral temporal lobe abnormalities who had undergone lobectomy. Eleven of the patients were hyposexual, and two of these patients (adult males) had become completely impotent within a year of the onset of seizures. These patients were concerned about their asexual attitudes, in contrast to the patients whose epilepsy had commenced when they were prepubescent; the latter patients had long-standing hyposexuality and were "satisfied with their sexual quiescence and erotically apathetic way of life." After surgery, changes in sexuality showed some correlation with improvement in seizure control. Four patients continued to have seizures and remained hyposexual, four had lessening of seizure frequency and a variable degree of awakening of sexuality, and three had a period of hypersexuality after operation and then returned to their former apathy when seizures recurred.

Hierons and Saunders (1966) reported 15 patients with impotence, all of whom had evidence of damage to the temporal lobes. Twelve patients had temporal lobe epilepsy at some time while they were impotent; three men were impotent for a period of 6–9 months preceding the development of epilepsy, and during this period no drugs were taken. In four patients, an increase in the dose of drugs brought the epilepsy under control, and impotence improved at the same time. These authors stated that in these patients "libido was probably normal," and the difficulty was a failure to obtain or maintain an erection. The series of Saunders and Rawson (1970) included seven similar patients.

The proposed mechanism of this effect is that discharges in the anterior temporal lobes put the limbic system into a state of excitation, which results in suppression of sexual function. The laterality is not important.

Alternatively, hyposexuality of some men with temporal lobe epilepsy may reflect a neuroendocrine deficiency. A study by Spark et al. (1984) showed that 11 of 16 hyposexual men had previously unrecognized temporal lobe epilepsy. These men presented because of diminished libido and impotence of secondary onset that had persisted for 2–10 years. In 11 patients, a diagnosis of temporal lobe epilepsy was established on the basis of electroencephalogram findings, although D.F. Scott and Prior (1984) questioned the electroencephalogram changes described in the report. In 4 of these 11 men, serum testosterone levels were persistently low, whereas 2 others had hyperprolactinemia. The remaining five patients with temporal lobe epilepsy had normal sex hormone levels. The most effective treatment for these men was to treat the epilepsy with anticonvulsant medication.

The role of anticonvulsants in causing impotence has been questioned. Of 12 patients with temporal lobe epilepsy and abnormal sexual behavior, in only 1 patient was reduced libido thought to be due to anticonvulsant medication. The remaining 67 patients with nontemporal forms of epilepsy but taking similar doses of anticonvulsants showed no evidence of disturbed sexual behavior (Saunders and Rawson, 1970).

More recently, the question of interaction between anticonvulsant medication and sex hormones in institutionalized patients with chronic epilepsy was studied, and a clear relationship between low sexual drive and decreased testosterone was demonstrated (Toone et al., 1983). However, this study was not able to establish a clear relationship between plasma levels of individual anticonvulsants and either hormonal or behavioral changes, and no attempt was made to divide the patients according to type of epilepsy.

Despite what appears in the literature to be a quite convincing association between temporal lobe epilepsy and primary hyposexuality or secondary impotence, those closely involved in the day-to-day management of patients with temporal lobe epilepsy remain doubtful that the relationship is causal, and the effect of anticonvulsant therapy on sexual drive and behavior remains difficult to elucidate (Toone, 1986).

Hypersexuality

Studies of series of patients with temporal lobe epilepsy have shown that interictal heterosexual hypersexuality is rare (Gastaut and Collomb, 1954). Taylor (1969) likewise reported hypersexuality in only 1 of 100 patients with temporal lobe epilepsy he studied, although 3 other patients in his series, 2 of whom were institutionalized, masturbated in public.

Sexual Seizures

The relationship between seizures and sexual experiences is complicated. There have been several reports of seizures brought on by intercourse (Gautier-Smith, 1980; Taylor 1969).

Saunders and Rawson (1970) found a single patient (among 100 male epileptics) who exposed himself and was arrested, but they were unconvinced of a relationship between this event and the patient's epilepsy. Currier et al. (1971) reported three patients and reviewed others in the literature in whom sexual behavior was considered to be due to "lack of inhibition related to postictal confusional period of temporal lobe seizures, possibly occurring as a response to activation of temporal lobe sexual connections with the limbic system and hypothalamus during the seizure."

Deviation

Bizarre sexual behavior has been reported in association with temporal lobe epilepsy. Most remarkable is the frequently cited case of a man with temporal lobe epilepsy who had a sexual fetish associated with shining safety pins and was cured by a temporal lobectomy (Mitchell et al., 1954).

THE MANAGEMENT OF ERECTILE DYSFUNCTION

Until recently, the investigation of erectile dysfunction was dominated by the need to identify patients in whom there was a purely psychologic cause. These patients could then be steered away from the drastic surgical treatment reserved for those in whom an organic pathology was firmly established. The advent of intracorporeal injection therapy changed this approach by offering an alternative means of both testing and treating impotence.

Psychologic Factors

Psychogenic impotence has been treated within a variety of psychosexual therapeutic models. Unfortunately, such therapy is extremely time-consuming, expensive, and not infrequently unsuccessful. This high rate of failure is partly due, no doubt, to the complexity of the psychodynamics involved, but it has also become increasingly clear that a mixed etiology, with both psychologic and organic components, is much more common in erectile failure than was formerly thought. The availability of a ready means of inducing erections has led to a more pragmatic approach to management with a willingness to use drug treatment even when a psychologic dimension to the problem is recognized (Brindley and Gingell, 1988). The emphasis, therefore, has moved away from costly and often unsatisfactory investigations, such as nocturnal penile tumescence studies, that were used to confirm the profound and absolute impotence of organic disease.

It is certainly true that psychogenic impotence may occur within the context of organic disease, and this is particularly so in neurologic disease. Physical disability, urinary and fecal incontinence, and mental changes may play a part, but the distortion of marital and family life caused by the illness is also of great importance. The hallmark of organic impotence is often considered to be a global lack of erections in any circumstances, including during masturbation, fantasy, and intercourse, and on waking. However, this may not apply in nervous system disease, such as MS, in which the ability to have an erection may wax and wane with the disease, and erections, although present, may be partial and insufficient for intercourse (Vas, 1969). Furthermore, in patients with spinal cord lesions that prevent psychogenic erections, the occurrence of reflex erections may complicate the picture. It can therefore be difficult to distinguish these apparent variabilities of erectile performance from the intermittency of psychogenic impotence; because erections can be induced pharmacologically in both psychogenic and neurogenic impotence, a successful response to intracorporeal injection does not distinguish between the two.

Patients who report the occurrence of good erections in some situations but not in others should ideally receive psychosexual assessment and therapy. In practice, because facilities for this treatment are inadequate, many patients in whom a psychologic cause is suspected must be content with general advice from their physicians or information and help from patient support groups, such as Sexual Problems of the Disabled (SPOD), which is active in the United Kingdom. When this is not enough, it may be reasonable to consider a physical means to improve sexual function.

Intracorporeal Injection Therapy

The production of penile erection by intracorporeal injection of papaverine was reported by Virag (1982), and the effectiveness of other vasoactive agents was demonstrated by Brindley (1983). These drugs produce erection in normal men and those with psychogenic and neurogenic impotence, but they are relatively ineffective in patients whose impotence is due to arterial or venous disease. Failure to respond can therefore be used to identify the latter group, who require vascular investigations and possibly surgical treatment. The successful induction of erection in an impotent patient raises the possibility of using intracorporeal injections for treatment (Brindley, 1986; Virag et al., 1984; Zorgniotti and Lefleur, 1985).

Diagnostic intracorporeal injections are usually given after evaluation of the patient in a urologic clinic. It is customary to start with a small dose of papaverine (15 mg in our clinic) injected deep into the dorsolateral aspect of one corpus cavernosum close to the base of the penis. The site is massaged to disperse the drug and pressure applied to avoid local bruising. A small starting dose is particularly important in neurologic disease in which an exaggerated and prolonged response is occasionally seen. If this fails to produce an erection, the patient should return for larger doses of papaverine (up to a maximum of 80 mg/2 ml). Alternatively, phentolamine (0.5–1 mg) may be added to potentiate the effect of papaverine.

The response in neurologic patients is often good. Of 30 patients with MS and impotence treated in our clinic, 15 patients (50%) responded to an injection of 20 mg of papaverine, 14 responded to a larger dose, and only 1 was unable to obtain an erection considered adequate for intercourse.

Those who get a successful erection in the clinic may be taught to administer the injection themselves. Alternatively, if the patient is too disabled to do this himself, a partner may be taught the technique. The effectiveness of intracorporeal papaverine seems to be augmented by sexual stimulation, and a lesser dose of the drug may be sufficient when the circumstances are suitably erotic. If there is a prominent psychologic element to the problem, the confidence engendered by a successful drug-induced erection may effect a prolonged cure and make further injections unnecessary. The short-term results of autoinjection or injection by the partner seem to be good. Twenty-seven of our patients with MS who had successful erections on test injection have been willing to learn the technique. Whether they will continue in the long term remains to be seen.

Unfortunately, this treatment has side effects. Prolonged erections, amounting to priapism, can occur, but they seem to be infrequent if care is taken to minimize the dose given. In our series, prolonged erections were more common in wheelchair-bound patients. The explanation for this is obscure.

All patients who are getting intracorporeal injections must be given instructions so that they can receive prompt treatment, usually by sugical aspiration or an antidote, such as metaraminol, if needed. Pain at the injection site, bruising, bleeding, and paresthesia have been described but are usually minor. A greater worry is the development of fibrous plaques within the penis. Anecdotal reports of the occurrence of extensive fibrosis of the erectile tissue that resembles severe Peyronie's disease in these patients are a cause for some alarm. A patient who is to undertake self-injection must be asked to sign a consent form, and possible side effects, complications, and treatment alternatives must be fully discussed before this form is signed. The patient should also be advised to limit the frequency of injection, and a limit of twice-weekly usage seems reasonable. It also makes sense for the treatment to be under control of a urologist, who can treat acute complications if they arise.

Penile Prostheses

When intracorporeal injection therapy is contraindicated or fails, the use of a surgically implanted prosthesis can be considered. There are two main types: the malleable (Small, 1978) and the much more life-like, but more complex, inflatable devices (F.B. Scott et al., 1979).

A penile prosthesis is implanted within the corpora cavernosa in a procedure that irrevocably destroys the erectile tissue. Failure of the prosthesis thus removes the possibility of other forms of treatment. Such failure may be due to sepsis, extrusion of the implant, or, in the case of an inflatable prosthesis, a mechanical disaster in the prosthesis itself (Pryor, 1988). Furthermore, the implant may become an embarrassment to those men whose disease advances until their general disability precludes sexual activity. In short, great care is needed before offering a penile prosthesis to a patient with progressive neurologic disease.

An alternative to both injection therapy and implant surgery is the use of ingenious external devices.

The Correctaid is a semirigid Silastic condom that acts as an external splint. The Erecaid induces tumescence by means of a vacuum and sustains it by a ring tourniquet at the penile base. These and other similar devices appear to help many users and their partners to attain sexual satisfaction (Wiles, 1988). They have the significant advantage of being free from serious adverse effects. However, they are expensive and are currently sold directly to the public by the manufacturers.

Failure of Orgasm and Ejaculation

Primary anorgasmia is uncommon in men (Brindley, 1985). Although it is occasionally seen in patients with other diseases that affect the central nervous system, secondary failure of orgasm is a particular problem of the young spinal cord–injured male. Depending on the level and completeness of injury, up to three-fourths of these men retain the capacity for uncontrolled reflex erection that, in 25% of the patients, is sufficient for penetration. Failure of ejaculation, on the other hand, is found in up to 70% of those with varying degrees of spinal cord injury and is virtually universal when transection is complete. In addition, these patients may undergo urologic surgery to the bladder neck that secondarily impairs their ability to ejaculate.

Vibrator-induced ejaculation can be used to obtain semen for artificial insemination. It is ineffective in patients with lesions between L-2 and S-1, as is the ejaculation induced by intrathecal anticholinesterase. Electroejaculatory techniques, used for years in animal husbandry, have also been applied to men. The largest series is described by Brindley (1981), who was able to obtain semen in either an antegrade or a retrograde fashion in up to 70% of patients studied. A major advantage of the technique is that, unlike vibratory and chemically induced emissions, electroejaculation can be obtained during the 6 months after injury, or during the period of spinal shock. At this time, the quality of the semen is better because the testicular changes characteristic of chronic spinal cord injury have yet to occur. The technique is painful, however, and a general anesthetic is needed unless the patient has no pain sensation below L-1.

Failure of seminal emission with a normal sensation of ejaculation is usually due to retrograde ejaculation that can be confirmed by microscopy of a postejaculation urine sample. It can be caused by any disease or drug that interferes with the competence of the bladder neck or the integrity of its sympathetic inflow. It most commonly results from destruction of the bladder neck in prostatic surgery or from section of the sympathetic nerves during retroperitoneal operations; it is rarely a symptom of primary neurologic disease. The results of drug treatment of retrograde ejaculation are extremely variable, but treatment with imipramine (25 mg three times a day) may be worthwhile.

References

(Key references are designated with an asterisk.)

Bannister R., Oppenheimer D.R. Degenerative diseases of the nervous system associated with autonomic failure. *Brain* 95:457–474, 1972.

Baumgarten, S.R., Lindsay G.K., Wise G.J. Fertility problems in renal transplant patients. *J. Urol.* 118:991–993, 1977.

Blumer D., Walker A.E. Sexual behaviour in temporal lobe epilepsy. *Arch. Neurol.* 16:7–43, 1967.

*Bors E., Comarr A.E. Neurological disturbances in sexual function with special reference to 529 patients with spinal cord injury. *Urol. Surg.* 10:191–222, 1960.

Brindley G.S. Electroejaculation: its technique, neurological implication and uses. *J. Neurol. Neurosurg. Psychiatry* 44:9–18, 1981.

Brindley G.S. Cavernosal alpha-blockade: a new technique for investigating and treating erectile impotence. *Br. J. Psychiatry* 143:332–337, 1983.

*Brindley G.S. Pathophysiology of erection and ejaculation. In Whitfield H.N., Hendry W.F., eds. *Textbook of Genitourinary Surgery.* Edinburgh, Churchill Livingstone, pp. 1083–1093, 1985.

Brindley G.S. Maintenance treatment of erectile impotence by cavernosal unstriated muscle relaxant injection. *Br. J. Psychiatry* 149:210–215, 1986.

Brindley G.S., Gingell J.C. Treatment of erectile impotence by intracavernosal injection of drugs that relax smooth muscle. In Gingell C., Abrams P., eds. *Controversies and Innovations in Urological Surgery.* London, Springer-Verlag, pp. 409–414, 1988.

Brown M.J., Asbury A.K. Diabetic neuropathy. *Ann. Neurol.* 15:2–12, 1984.

Burnstock G. The changing face of autonomic neurotransmission. *Acta Physiol. Scand.* 126:67–91, 1986.

Currier R.D., Little S.C., Sness J.F. Sexual seizures. *Arch. Neurol.* 25:260–266, 1971.

*de Groat W.C., Steers W.D. Neuroanatomy and neurophysiology of penile erection. In Tanagho E.A., Lue T.F., McClure R.D., eds. *Contemporary Management of Impotence and Infertility.* Baltimore, Williams & Wilkins, pp. 3–27, 1988.

Desai K.M., Dembny K., Morgan H., et al. Neurophysiological investigation of diabetic impotence. Are sacral response studies of value? *Br. J. Urol.* 61:68–73, 1988.

Dua S., MacLean P.D. Localization of penile erection in medial frontal lobe. *Am. J. Physiol.* 207:1425–1434, 1964.

Duncan G., Johnson R.H., Lambie D.G., et al. Evidence of vagal neuropathy in chronic alcoholics. *Lancet* 2:1053–1056, 1980.

Eardley I., Quinn N.P., Fowler C.J., et al. The value of urethral sphincter electromyography in the differential diagnosis of parkinsonism. *Br. J. Urol.* 64:360–362, 1989.

Ertekin C., Reel F. Bulbocavernosus reflex in normal men and patients with neurogenic bladder and/or impotence. *Br. J. Urol.* 28:1–15, 1976.

Ewing D.J., Winney R. Autonomic function in patients with chronic renal failure on intermittent haemodialysis. *Nephron* 15:424–429, 1975.

Ewing D.J., Campbell I.W., Burt A.A., et al. Vascular reflexes in diabetic autonomic neuropathy. *Lancet* 2:1354–1356, 1973.

Faerman I., Glocer I., Fox D., et al. Impotence and diabetes. Histological studies of the autonomic nervous fibers of the corpora cavernosa in impotent diabetic males. *Diabetes* 23:971–976, 1974.

Fowler C.J., Ali Z., Kirby R.S., et al. The value of testing for unmyelinated fibre, sensory neuropathy in diabetic impotence. *Br. J. Urol.* 61:63–67, 1988a.

Fowler C.J., Sitzoglou K., Ali Z., et al. The conduction velocities of peripheral nerve fibres conveying sensations of warming and cooling. *J. Neurol. Neurosurg. Psychiatry* 51:1164–1170, 1988b.

Gastaut H., Collomb H. Étude du comportement sexuel chez les épileptiques psychomoteurs. *Ann. Med. Psychol. (Paris)* 12:657–696, 1954.

Gautier-Smith P.C. Atteinte des fonctions cérébrales et troubles du comportement sexuel. *Rev. Neurol. (Paris)* 136:311–319, 1980.

Graber B., Kline-Graber G. Female orgasm: role of pubococcygeus muscle. *J. Clin. Psychiatry* 40:348–351, 1979.

Halata Z., Munger B. The neuroanatomical basis for the proto-pathic sensibility of the human penis. *Brain Res.* 371:205–230, 1986.

Hierons R., Saunders M. Impotence in patients with temporal lobe lesions. *Lancet* 2:761–764, 1966.

Hyndman O.R., Wolkin J. Anterior cordotomy. Further observations on the physiological results and the optimum manner of performance. *Arch. Neurol. Psychiatry* 50:129–148, 1943.

Ivers R.R., Goldstein N.P. Multiple sclerosis: a current appraisal of symptoms and signs. *Mayo Clin. Proc.* 38:457–466, 1963.

Johnson R.J. Autonomic failure in alcoholics. In Bannister R., ed. *Autonomic Failure.* Oxford, Oxford University Press, pp. 690–714, 1984.

Kirkeby H.J., Poulsen E.U., Petersen T., et al. Erectile dysfunction in multiple sclerosis. *Neurology* 38:1366–1371, 1988.

Klüver H., Bucy P.C. Preliminary analysis of the functions of the temporal lobes in monkeys. *Arch. Neurol. Psychiatry* 42:979–1000, 1939.

Lepor H., Gregerman M., Crosby R., et al. Precise localization of the autonomic nerves from the pelvic plexus to the corpora cavernosa: a detailed anatomical study of the adult male pelvis. *J. Urol.* 133:207–212, 1985.

Lilius H.G., Valtonen E.J., Wikstrom J. Sexual problems in patients suffering from multiple sclerosis. *Scand. J. Soc. Med.* 4:41–44, 1976.

Lindblom U., Tegner R. Thermal sensitivity in uremic neuropathy. *Acta Neurol. Scand.* 71:290–294, 1985.

Low P.A., Walsh J.C., Huang C.Y., et al. The sympathetic nervous system in alcoholic neuropathy. A clinical and pathological study. *Brain* 98:357–364, 1975.

*Lue T.F., Tanagho E.A. Hemodynamics of erection. In Tanagho E.A., Lue T.F., McClure R.D., eds. *Contemporary Management of Impotence and Infertility.* Baltimore, Williams & Wilkins, pp. 28–38, 1988.

Lundberg P.O. Sexual dysfunction in patients with multiple sclerosis. *Sex. Disability* 1:218–222, 1978.

MacLean P.D., Denniston R.H., Dua S. Further studies on cerebral representation of penile erection: caudal thalamus, midbrain and pons. *J. Neurophysiol.* 26:273–293, 1963.

McCulloch D.K., Young R.J., Prescott R.J., et al. The natural history of impotence in diabetic men. *Diabetologia* 26:437–440, 1984.

McLeod J.G. Autonomic dysfunction in peripheral nerve disease. In Bannister R., ed. *Autonomic Failure.* Oxford, Oxford University Press, pp. 607–623, 1988.

Meyers R. Three cases of myoclonus alleviated by ansotomy, with a note on post operative alibido and impotence. *J. Neurosurg.* 19:71–81, 1962.

Miller H., Simpson C.A., Yeates W.F. Bladder dysfunction in multiple sclerosis. *Br. Med. J.* 1:1265–1269, 1965.

Minderhoud J.M., Leehuis J.G., Kremer J., et al. Sexual disturbances arising from multiple sclerosis. *Acta Neurol. Scand.* 70:299–306, 1984.

Mitchell W., Falconer M.A., Hill D. Epilepsy with fetishism relieved by temporal lobectomy. *Lancet* 2:626–630, 1954.

Morehouse D.D., Belitsky P., MacKinnon K. Rupture of the posterior urethra. *J. Urol.* 107:255–258, 1972.

Pryor J.P. Penile prostheses. In Gingell C., Abrams P., eds. *Controversies and Innovations in Urological Surgery.* London, Springer-Verlag, 1988.

Quinn N. Multiple system atrophy—the nature of the beast. *J. Neurol. Neurosurg. Psychiatry* (Special Suppl.):78–89, 1989.

Rubin A., Babbott D. Impotence and diabetes mellitus. *J.A.M.A.* 168:498–500, 1958.

Saunders M., Rawson M. Sexuality in male epileptics. *J. Neurol. Sci.* 10:577–583, 1970.

Scott D.F., Prior F.P. Temporal lobe epilepsy and hyposexuality (letter). *Lancet* 1:743, 1984.

Scott F.B., Byrd G.J., Karacan I., et al. Erectile impotence treated with an inflatable implantable prosthesis; five years of clinical experience. *J.A.M.A.* 241:2609–2612, 1979.

Sherman F.P. Impotence in patients with chronic renal failure on dialysis: its frequency and etiology. *Fertil. Steril.* 26:221–223, 1975.

Shy G., Drager G. A neurological syndrome associated with orthostatic hypotension. *Arch. Neurol.* 2:511–527, 1960.

Small M.P. The Small-Carrion penile prosthesis. *Urol. Clin. North Am.* 5:549–561, 1978.

Spark R.F., Wills C.A., Royal H. Hypogonadism, hyperprolactinaemia, and temporal lobe epilepsy in hyposexual men. *Lancet* 1:413–417, 1984.

Tan E.T.H., Johnson R.H., Lambie D.G., et al. Erectile impotence in chronic alcoholics. *Alcoholism* 8:297–301, 1984.

Taylor D.C. Sexual behaviour and temporal lobe epilepsy. *Arch. Neurol.* 21:510–516, 1969.

Terzian H., Dalle Ore G. Syndrome of Klüver-Bucy reproduced in man by bilateral removal of the frontal lobes. *Neurology* 5:373–380, 1955.

*Toone B.K. Sexual disorders in epilepsy. In Pedley T.A., Meldrum B.S., eds. *Recent Advances in Epilepsy*. Edinburgh, Churchill Livingstone, pp. 233–259, 1986.

Toone B.K., Wheeler M., Nanjee M., et al. Sex hormones, sexual activity and plasma anticonvulsant levels in male epileptics. *J. Neurol. Neurosurg. Psychiatry* 46:824–826, 1983.

Valleroy M.L., Kraft G.K. Sexual dysfunction in multiple sclerosis. *Arch. Phys. Med. Rehabil.* 65:125–128, 1984.

*Vas C.J., Sexual impotence and some autonomic disturbances in men with multiple sclerosis. *Acta Neurol. Scand.* 45:166–184, 1969.

Virag R. Intracavernous injection of papaverine for erectile failure (letter). *Lancet* 2:938, 1982.

Virag R., Frydman D., Legman M., et al. Intracavernous injection of papaverine as a diagnostic and therapeutic method in erectile failure. *Angiology* 35:79–87, 1984.

Vodusek D.B., Janko M. The bulbocavernosus reflex. *Brain* 113:813–820, 1990.

Walsh P.C., Donker P.D. Impotence following radical prostatectomy: insight into etiology and prevention. *J. Urol.* 128:492–497, 1982.

Wiles P.G. Successful non-invasive management of erectile impotence in diabetic men. *Br. Med. J.* 296:161–162, 1988.

Zorgniotti A.W., Lefleur R.S. Auto-injection of the corpus cavernosum with a vasoactive drug combination for vasculogenic impotence. *J. Urol.* 133:39–41, 1985.

36

Bladder Dysfunction in Neurologic Disease

Clare J. Fowler
Christopher D. Betts
Christopher G. Fowler

Neurogenic bladder dysfunction has attracted less attention from neurologists than its problems merit, for both practical and intellectual reasons. On the one hand, there are few physical signs to be elicited and the relevant clinical investigations have been in the hands of the urologist. On the other hand, there is almost complete failure of attempts to interpret the few symptoms in terms of the complex underlying pathophysiology.

Normal bladder function requires the integrated activity of the autonomic and somatic nervous systems. Because the neural pathways that subserve the many reflexes of detrusor and sphincter function extend from the frontal lobes to the sacral spinal cord (Fig. 36–1), neurogenic causes of bladder disorders result from lesions at many levels of the neuraxis. However, little is known about the central neural connections of the lower urinary tract and, consequently, descriptions of bladder neurophysiology usually cover its peripheral innervation in much greater detail. In neurologic clinics, patients with central nervous system disorders more commonly present with troublesome bladder symptoms, and an understanding of the central neural control is therefore of greater clinical relevance.

NEURAL CONTROL OF BLADDER FUNCTION

Structure of the Detrusor and Sphincter Muscles

The main bulk of the bladder smooth muscle is arranged so that when it contracts the bladder emp-

ties. The arrangement of the detrusor fibers in the region of the bladder neck differs between the sexes; males have a circular distribution and the fibers form an effective bladder neck sphincter, whereas in females the fibers are arranged longitudinally or obliquely and there is no equivalent internal sphincter (Gosling et al., 1987).

The urethral sphincter, the rhabdosphincter, is composed of circularly oriented, predominantly type 1 (slow-twitch), striated muscle fibers (Gosling et al., 1981). In men, the rhabdosphincter is just distal to the prostate; in women, it surrounds most of the much shorter urethra. The rhabdosphincter is anatomically distinct from the sheet of muscles that form the pelvic floor.

Innervation of the Bladder and Sphincter

Parasympathetic Innervation (Pelvic Nerves)

The principal motor supply of the detrusor comes from parasympathetic preganglionic neurons, with cell bodies in the intermediolateral columns of the cord between S-2 and S-4. The preganglionic neurons emerge from the cord with the anterior spinal roots and send axons via the pelvic nerves to the pelvic parasympathetic plexus. This is a fine network in the adventitia that covers the bladder and rectum. Short postganglionic fibers travel from the plexus to innervate pelvic organs.

There is no postjunctional specialization between the postganglionic fibers and the smooth muscle of the detrusor. Instead, the postganglionic fibers have

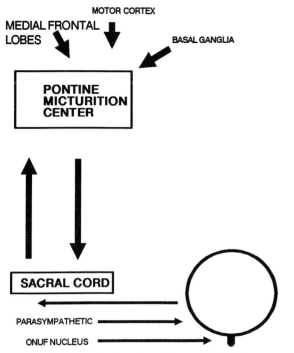

Figure 36–1. Diagram showing the major neurologic influences on control of bladder function.

diffuse varicosities along their lengths that contain vesicles from which acetylcholine is released (Burnstock, 1986). Although in some species noncholinergic-nonadrenergic transmitters are also present, their existence in humans is doubtful.

Sympathetic Innervation (Hypogastric Nerves and Sacral Sympathetic Chain)

The role of the sympathetic nervous system in human micturition remains unclear. Certainly, lumbar sympathectomy alone does not interfere with continence or voiding, although it commonly leads to retrograde ejaculation. The mammalian bladder receives sympathetic innervation from the thoracolumbar sympathetic chain via the hypogastric nerves. The bladder neck in males has a rich noradrenergic innervation, and sympathetic activity during ejaculation causes closure of the bladder neck to prevent retrograde ejaculation.

Somatic Innervation (Pudendal Nerves)

The striated muscle of the urethral sphincter is the only part of the urinary tract to receive a somatic innervation. Onufrowicz (1899) described a nucleus in the ventral horn of the spinal cord at S-2, S-3, and S-4. This nucleus, commonly known as the Onuf nucleus, contains the cell bodies of the motor neurons that innervate both the anal and the urethral sphincters. They are of smaller diameter than other anterior horn cells, but a study of the synaptology of these motor neurons in the cat has shown them to

be skeletomotor rather than part of the preganglionic parasympathetic perineal innervation (Pullen, 1988).

Motor fibers from these cells pass from the roots of S-2, S-3, and S-4 into the pudendal nerves, which during their course through the pelvis give off branches to the anal sphincter and the perineal branch to the striated urethral sphincter. Electromyographically, motor units from the striated sphincter are similar to those from skeletal muscle but of slightly lower amplitude (Chantraine, 1966; Fowler et al., 1984).

Sensory Innervation of the Lower Urinary Tract

The majority of afferent nerves are unmyelinated and end in the suburothelial plexus, where there are no specialized sensory endings (Gosling et al., 1987; Morrison, 1987). Because many of these fibers contain substance P, ATP, or calcitonin gene–related peptide and their release may alter muscle excitability, these plexus fibers may be regarded as sensory-motor nerves rather than purely sensory (Burnstock, 1990). There is evidence for the presence of capsaicin-sensitive nerves in the human bladder (Maggi et al., 1989).

The three sets of peripheral nerves (thoracolumbar sympathetic, sacral parasympathetic, and pudendal) all contain afferent nerve fibers. The afferent fibers that pass in the pelvic nerve and carry the sensation of bladder distention seem to be the most important to normal bladder function (George and Dixon, 1986). The afferent axons are of two types: unmyelinated C fibers and small myelinated A δ fibers.

The role of the hypogastric afferents is uncertain, but they may transmit some sensation of bladder distention and pain. The pudendal somatic afferents transmit sensations of flow of urine, pain, and temperature from the urethra and project to similar areas in the sacral spinal cord as bladder afferents. This overlap suggests the possibility of important areas in the sacral cord for viscerosomatic integration.

Nathan and Smith (1951), in a study of patients who had undergone anterolateral cordotomy, concluded that the ascending pathways from the bladder and urethra travel in the spinothalamic tracts. Spinobulbar fibers in the dorsal columns may also be important for the transmission of afferent information.

Central Neural Connections

Pontine Micturition Center

The importance of the pons for the control of micturition was first recognized by Barrington (1925). A nucleus in the dorsal tegmentum has been identified as a coordinating center, and de Groat (1990) suggested that it operates as a switching point acting on a spinobulbar or long-loop reflex (Figs. 36–2 and

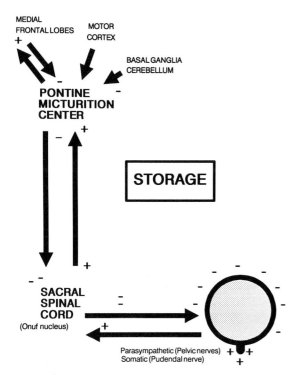

Figure 36–2. Diagram (as in Fig. 36–1) showing neural pathways that are active in bladder storage.

36–3). This switch is controlled by cerebral input and toggles between the bladder's reservoir and voiding states (de Groat, 1990). During the filling phase, pelvic nerve efferent activity is inhibited. When the bladder is appropriately full and micturition is con-

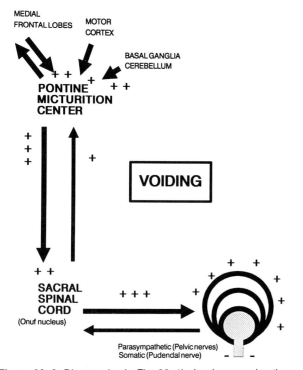

Figure 36–3. Diagram (as in Fig. 36–1) showing neural pathways that are active in voiding.

venient, higher centers exert an excitatory influence on the pontine micturition center, the long-loop reflex is facilitated, and pelvic nerve activity increases to produce detrusor contraction.

Suprapontine Influences on the Pontine Micturition Center

Higher centers, in particular the medial frontal lobes and basal ganglia, appear to act on the pontine micturition center, mostly in an inhibitory manner (see Fig. 36–2). Thus, lesions in these areas or in their connections with the pontine micturition center result in a reduced inhibition and hyperreflexia of the detrusor. When voiding occurs, it is properly coordinated with sphincter relaxation preceding detrusor contraction.

PHYSIOLOGY OF THE NORMAL BLADDER

Storage of Urine

As the normal bladder fills, contraction of the detrusor muscle is inhibited. In addition, there is an active process of compliance whereby fibers increase in length without a proportional increase in force. As a result, the rise in intravesical pressure during bladder filling does not exceed 10 cm H_2O and the detrusor is said to be stable (International Continence Society, 1981).

Detrusor inhibition requires intact pathways between the sacral cord and the pontine micturition center (see Fig. 36–2). Facilitation of activity in the striated urethral sphincter also occurs during filling. Thus, while intravesical pressure is low and urethral closure pressure high, the bladder is continent. A more marked increase in the activity of the rhabdosphincter occurs when intravesical pressure rises with abdominal straining.

Voiding

Voiding is normally a voluntary act resulting in the coordinated relaxation of the urethral sphincter and contraction of the detrusor. The stimulus to void comes from bladder distention, signaled by stretch-sensitive afferents (see Fig. 36–3). At the initiation of micturition, there is a prevoiding drop of urethral pressure that occurs 5–15 seconds before detrusor contraction (Tanagho and Miller, 1970): if combined sphincter electromyographic (EMG) and urodynamic studies are performed, the first observable change is silence on the EMG channel. Although the initiation of voiding is a voluntary act, complete bladder emptying depends on suppression of sphincter activity throughout the period of detrusor contraction until the bladder is completely empty. It has been proposed that this reflex is triggered by flow of urine in the proximal urethra.

BLADDER DYSFUNCTION IN NEUROLOGIC DISEASE

Suprapontine Causes of Disordered Bladder Function

Frontal Lobe Lesions

Andrew and Nathan (1964) identified areas of the medial frontal lobes that are important in the control of micturition and, to a lesser extent, defecation (Fig. 36–4). Of 10 patients with frontal tumors, 8 patients had precipitate micturition with or without warning and 7 of these were unable to stop micturition once it had started. Cystometry showed a rise in intravesical pressure on filling that would now be called hyperreflexia. Two patients were in urinary retention, presumably because of a failure of voluntary initiation of the voiding reflex.

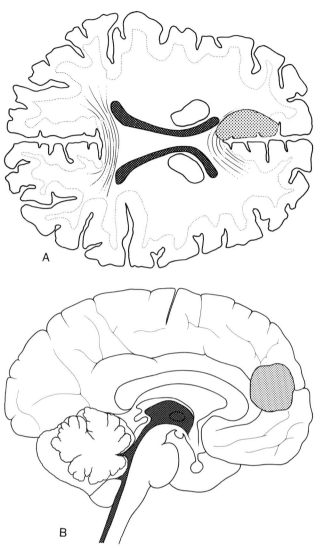

Figure 36–5. The site of lesions in medial frontal lobes that can result in disturbance of bladder function.

After studying these patients and others with non-neoplastic frontal lesions, the authors deduced that the cortical loci controlling micturition are in the superomedial part of the frontal lobes in the region of the anterior cingulate gyrus and the adjacent part of the superior frontal gyrus (see Fig. 36–4). Also important are white matter tracts that run to and from the genu of the corpus callosum. A lesion involving the anterior part of the genu, by disrupting connections between the medial parts of the frontal lobes, may thus effectively cause a bilateral deficit (Fig. 36–5). Because the bladder disorder can be improved by excision of the causative lesion and also because of the area of the brain involved, the disorder may be the result of a positive phenomenon, as suggested by Maurice-Williams (1974).

A study by Ueki (1960) of patients with brain tumors reported a higher incidence of disturbance of micturition with frontally located tumors than with tumors in other parts of the cerebral hemispheres.

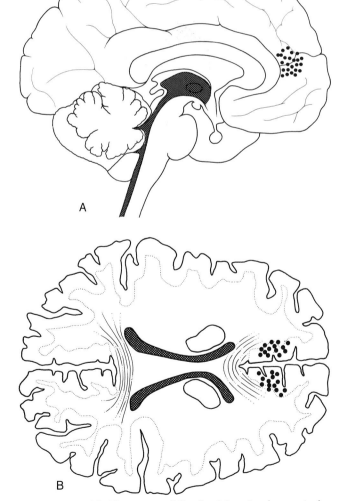

Figure 36–4. *(A)* The areas of the frontal cortex known to be important in the control of micturition. *B* was drawn on a horizontal section from the figures in Andrew and Nathan (1964), with kind advice from Dr. Peter Nathan.

Similar findings were reported by Maurice-Williams (1974); 14% of patients with frontal tumors had urinary frequency, urgency, and incontinence. In 100 consecutive patients with intracranial tumors, no instances of this syndrome were found with non-frontal tumors.

Hydrocephalus

Dilatation of the frontal horns and subependymal edema in active hydrocephalus involve the same areas of the frontal lobes that were identified by Andrew and Nathan as important in bladder control (see Figs. 36–4 and 36–6). Urinary incontinence is one of the triad of symptoms that characterizes normal-pressure hydrocephalus (Hakim and Adams, 1965). Although it has been said that urinary incontinence is the last of the three symptoms to appear, Fisher (1982) claimed that each symptom can appear independently of the others and that it is possible to have incontinence of urine and feces in the absence of gait and mental changes. The underlying bladder pathophysiology has been demonstrated to be detrusor hyperreflexia (Ahlberg et al., 1988), resulting in urgency and frequency about which the patient is appropriately concerned, provided there is not also marked intellectual deterioration.

Successful shunting that ameliorates the other symptoms of this disorder also improves incontinence. Cystometry carried out before and after a 50-ml cerebrospinal fluid tap showed a reduction of bladder hyperreflexia within 2–3 hours (Ahlberg et al., 1988). This remarkably rapid change in bladder behavior, as ventricular dilatation is reduced, indicates that the hyperreflexia must be due to conduction block in important neural pathways stretched by expanded frontal horns.

Pontine Lesions

The exact pontine location of the nuclei that constitute the micturition center is uncertain in humans. In animals, precise areas within the pons have been located. In rats, the important area seems to be the lateral dorsal tegmental nucleus; in cats the important site is in the region of the locus ceruleus (de Groat, 1975; Satoh et al., 1978). Despite the now considerable electrophysiologic, pharmacologic, and neuroanatomic evidence in animals relating to the presence of a pontine micturition center, there are few clinical reports of humans with urinary dysfunction resulting from pontine lesions. This may be due to the often life-threatening nature of pontine lesions in humans.

In 1901, Czyhlarz and Marburg reported two cases of pontine pathology associated with urinary retention. Holman (1926) reported eight patients with tumors closely related to the pons that were associated with either difficult micturition or complete urinary retention. At that time, despite Barrington's (1925) work, the importance of the pons in the control of micturition was not appreciated, and Holman proposed that lesions within the region of the pons may interrupt pathways from a higher micturition center.

A study by Ueki (1960) of the site of brain tumors causing disturbance of micturition showed that 77% of pontine lesions in the study resulted in such disturbance. The bladder dysfunction was called dysuria, by which the author meant "retardation and retardation with protraction" of micturition; this might now be called hesitancy and retention. It appears that whereas frontal tumors cause incontinence, pontine lesions are more likely to cause symptoms of hesitancy and retention. Renier and Gabreels (1980) reported that 12 of 17 children with pontine

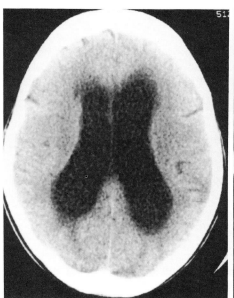
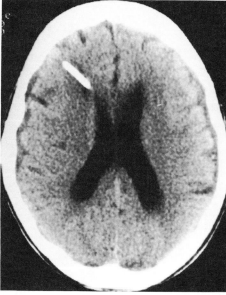

Figure 36–6. Computed tomographic scans of a patient with hydrocephalus before *(left)* and after *(right)* shunting. The patient was incontinent before the shunt.

gliomas had difficult and delayed micturition with episodes of complete retention.

de Groat (1990) showed that γ-aminobutyric acid, enkephalins, acetylcholine, and dopamine act as neurotransmitters in the pontine micturition center and that pharmacologic manipulation of these transmitters can alter bladder capacity in animals. This raises the possibility that alterations in levels of neurotransmitters may be important in degenerative neurologic diseases.

Spinal Cord Lesions

Lesions between the pontine center and the sacral cord interrupt pathways that are inhibitory to the detrusor (see Fig. 36–2), as well as those that coordinate normal sphincter-detrusor action (see Fig. 36–3). Several pathophysiologic effects are possible. These disorders may occur alone or in combination, as shown in Table 36–1.

Hyperreflexic Bladder. The definition of detrusor hyperreflexia, according to the International Continence Society (1981), is an overactivity resulting from disturbance of the neural control mechanisms. Loss of the normal inhibition from higher centers results in detrusor contractions during bladder filling. The contractions may occur spontaneously, or they may be provoked by some action, such as coughing; suprapubic tapping; or changing position from lying to standing. Typical symptoms include urgency of micturition and urge incontinence.

Detrusor-Sphincter Dyssynergia. A simultaneous contraction of sphincter and detrusor during the voiding phase is known as detrusor-sphincter dyssynergia. The failure of the sphincter to relax correctly results in obstructed voiding, an interrupted urinary stream, incomplete emptying, and high intravesical pressures. These abnormalities may lead to upper tract dilatation and renal damage.

Poorly Sustained Detrusor Contraction. Abnormal hyperreflexic contractions may be poorly sustained and, in combination with a degree of dyssynergia, result in incomplete emptying.

Increased Postmicturition Residual Volume. A high postmicturition residual volume in a hyperreflexic bladder means that little additional filling is required to provoke a detrusor contraction. The patient complains of frequently passing small volumes of urine. Poor bladder emptying is the disorder of bladder function most amenable to treatment if the patient or caregiver can perform intermittent catheterization, and the major effort in management should be directed to recognition of this disorder.

Spinal Cord Injury

A variable period of "spinal shock" follows acute spinal injury; during this period, the bladder is acontractile. Commonly, reflex activity of the detrusor returns within days or weeks and some degree of bladder function appears that may show a combination of disordered activities (see Table 36–1). The persistence of a hypocontractile or acontractile bladder in a minority of such patients remains a mystery. Poor bladder emptying after spinal injury may be due to detrusor-sphincter dyssynergia or poorly sustained detrusor contraction. Even when dyssynergia is suspected, attempts to improve bladder emptying by sphincterotomy may not always be successful. This failure has led to the suggestion that additional "occult" lesions at the sacral level may cause poor detrusor contractility (Light et al., 1987). However, Lucas and Thomas (1989) failed to find any correlation between the return of somatic conus reflexes (anal and bulbocavernous reflexes) and patterns of bladder function in the acute phase of spinal injury. Although Beric et al. (1987) demonstrated abnormal lumbosacral-evoked responses recorded over T-12, L-3, and S-1 in patients with acontractile bladders, Lucas and Thomas (1990) were unable to reproduce this finding.

Subsacral Lesions

Damage to the lowest part of the spinal cord, the conus and the cauda equina, has an unpredictable effect on bladder function because of the mixture of upper and lower motor neuron defects that may ensue.

Tethered Cord

Although a tethered cord usually produces symptoms in the growing child, the onset of bladder problems may be delayed into adult life and present considerable diagnostic difficulties at that time.

Pang and Wilberger (1982) reported on the clinical and radiologic features of a series of 23 adult patients with tethered cord. The mean age at onset was 33 years, and the most common complaint was pain felt bilaterally either in the lower back or perineal region. Sensorimotor defects in the legs were not always present, and over one-half of the patients had bladder symptoms. Urodynamic studies showed a small hyperreflexic bladder slightly more often than a large-capacity, hypocontractile one. All patients had radiologic evidence of lumbosacral spina bifida on plain x-ray films, but a myelogram or computed tomographic myelography was required to demonstrate the details of the underlying conus anomaly. Surgical intervention abolished pain in the majority of pa-

Table 36–1. PATHOPHYSIOLOGIC CONSEQUENCES OF A SPINAL LESION BETWEEN THE PONTINE MICTURITION CENTER AND THE SACRAL CORD

Hyperreflexic bladder
Detrusor-sphincter dyssynergia
Poorly sustained contractions
Abnormally high postmicturition residual volume

tients, but there was little improvement in bladder function.

Urologists see many patients in whom a diagnosis of idiopathic detrusor instability is made in the absence of any overt neurologic defects. The question as to what extent these patients should be further investigated to exclude a tethered cord remains a vexing one (Galloway and Tainsh, 1985).

Cauda Equina Lesions

Damage to the sacral roots S2-4, either within the spinal canal or extradurally, results in a lower motor neuron disorder of bladder function. Voluntary initiation of micturition is lost because the neural mechanisms for driving detrusor contraction are absent. The bladder becomes atonic, or hypotonic if the denervating injury is partial (Pavlakis et al., 1983a). Bladder compliance may also be impaired because it is an active process that requires intact neural pathways.

Although normal sensation of bladder stretch is lost, some awareness of pain may still be present as a result of afferent pathways in the sympathetic fibers conveyed by the hypogastric nerves. The striated urethral sphincter may be denervated (Fowler et al., 1984; Pavlakis et al., 1983a), and urethral closure will then be impaired. Continence may be preserved by the elastic tissues of the bladder neck as long as the intravesical pressures remain low, but stress incontinence is likely when the intravesical pressure rises.

Cauda equina lesions may result from trauma, metastases to the lumbar spine, or intradural tumors. Central protrusion of lumbar discs (L2-3, L3-4) is a common cause of damage to the cauda equina (Jennett, 1956). However, Lafuente et al. (1985) have drawn attention to the phenomenon of sacral sparing that can occur with cauda equina compression from a central disc prolapse. An unusual and poorly understood cauda equina syndrome can also occur in long-standing ankylosing spondylitis (Bartleson et al., 1983).

Perineal Nerve Injury and Stress Incontinence

Stress incontinence is the leakage of urine into the urethra that occurs during coughing, straining, laughing, and exercise, when a rise of intra-abdominal pressure is transmitted to the bladder contents. It is usually prevented by phasic recruitment of motor units in the striated urethral sphincter in response to sudden rises in intra-abdominal pressure. Stress incontinence occurs if there is a denervating lesion of the pelvic floor or sphincter, such as that resulting from injury of the perineal branch of the pudendal nerve (Swash et al., 1985). The increased incidence of stress incontinence in parous women has been shown by Swash and colleagues to be caused by a stretch injury of the peripheral pudendal nerve during childbirth (Snooks et al., 1984); an increase in fiber density in pubococcygeus muscle (Smith et al., 1989) can be demonstrated by single-fiber electromyography. The neurologic deficit that causes stress incontinence affects only the innervation of the sphincter and pelvic floor but leaves the innervation of the detrusor intact.

Stress incontinence in a man is a significant neurologic complaint that indicates a lower motor neuron lesion of S2-4.

NEUROLOGIC DISEASES THAT AFFECT BLADDER FUNCTION

Multiple Sclerosis

More than one-half of patients with multiple sclerosis have a persistent problem with bladder control (Miller et al., 1965; Van Poppel et al., 1983). Because neuroregulation of vesicosphincteric function requires intact function of long tracts of the neuraxis, it is not surprising that disruption of important physiologic pathways for bladder control result from the diffuse central nervous system lesions of this disease. However, demyelination affecting the spinal cord is probably the major determinant of impaired bladder control.

The most common symptoms are frequency and urgency of micturition, although in milder cases frequency alone may occur. Urgency presumably reflects hyperreflexic detrusor contractions. Urge incontinence occurs if the hyperreflexic contractions are extremely strong, if the pelvic floor has been denervated by nerve stretch injury in childbirth, or if the patient has poor mobility and is unable to reach a toilet in time. Not infrequently, patients with pronounced pyramidal disability describe urgency of micturition precipitated by rising from a sitting position.

Despite unwanted urgency and frequency, patients may also experience difficulty in initiating voluntary micturition, thus indicating interruption of bulbospinal pathways. Hesitancy of micturition is not uncommon, but frank retention is unusual. Patients frequently describe a poor urine stream that may be interrupted (Fig. 36–7) or may stop prematurely so that they get up from the toilet only to find that they need to go again within a few minutes. This probably reflects the detrusor-sphincter dyssynergia that accompanies spinal cord disease (see Table 36–1). Some patients are conscious of incomplete bladder emptying, although others who have this problem to the same degree remain unaware of it. Because an increased postmicturition residual can be managed by clean intermittent self-catheterization, this is a particularly important finding (see the later section on treatment).

Table 36–2 summarizes several urodynamic studies of the bladder disorder in multiple sclerosis. A hy-

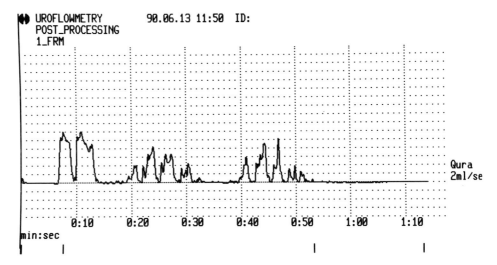

Figure 36–7. Urine flow rate of a patient with multiple sclerosis.

perreflexic detrusor is the most common finding, although most studies also report a variable incidence of hyporeflexic or areflexic bladders. Interruption of pathways between the pontine micturition center and the sacral cord would be expected to produce hyperreflexia. Hyporeflexia or areflexia is unexplained and will probably remain so until better ways of testing the neural pathways to the detrusor muscle itself are available.

In Table 36–2, the estimated incidence of detrusor-sphincter dyssynergia is quite variable; this may reflect the technical difficulty of demonstrating the disorder. To obtain EMG recordings from the urethral sphincter during urodynamic voiding studies, the patient should ideally have bladder and rectal catheters for pressure measurements, as well as a needle electrode in the urethral sphincter while attempting to void. The obvious difficulties this procedure imposes on the patient have led to recordings being made from alternative sites, such as the anal sphincter or the pelvic floor. It may still prove difficult to obtain an adequate EMG signal without electrical interference from other equipment, particularly if the study is being performed with x-ray screening. Detrusor-sphincter dyssynergia is a feature of subpontine spinal damage and, theoretically, would be expected to be present in all patients with neurologic deficits in the lower limbs.

Several studies have shown that it is not possible to predict the urodynamic findings in individual patients from their symptoms (Blaivas et al., 1979; Goldstein et al., 1982; Gonor et al., 1985; Petersen and Pedersen, 1984), and it has been taught that urodynamic assessment of these patients is essential in planning correct management. This is a counsel of perfection. In practice, treatment options are usually limited to treatment of hyperreflexia by drugs and improvement of bladder emptying by catheterization. The appropriateness of these measures is usually apparent from less rigorous investigations (see the later section on treatment).

There is some debate as to the risk of upper tract damage in patients with multiple sclerosis. Blaivas and Barnalias (1984) have identified those most at

Table 36–2. SUMMARY OF URODYNAMIC FINDINGS IN PATIENTS WITH MULTIPLE SCLEROSIS

		% Patients with		
Reference	Number of Patients	*Hyperreflexia*	*Hyporeflexia*	*Detrusor-Sphincter Dyssynergia*
Andersen and Bradley (1976a)	52	63	33	30
Ketelaer et al. (1977)	100	49		86
Bradley (1978)	302	62	34	72
Schoenberg et al. (1979)	39	74		50
Blaivas et al. (1979)	41	56	40	27
Piazza and Diokono (1979)	27	85	13	50
Beck et al. (1981)	46	87		
Philp et al. (1981)	52	99	0	88
Goldstein et al. (1982)	84	76		50
Van Poppel et al. (1983)	160	66	24	33
Awad et al. (1984)	39	67		51
Petersen and Pedersen (1984)	88	82	16	41
Hassouna et al. (1984)	70	70	18	75
Gonor et al. (1985)	64	78	20	12

risk as being young men with severe detrusor-sphincter dyssynergia. However, upper tract damage leading to renal impairment seems to be less common in multiple sclerosis than in spinal cord trauma. The explanation for this is uncertain, but it may be that poor bladder compliance is unusual in multiple sclerosis. In men, it is probably advisable to perform a renal ultrasound scan to look for dilatation every 3–4 years, but this is unnecessary in women.

Tropical Spastic Paraplegia

Tropical spastic paraplegia occurs in people from the West Indies. It is now known to result from meningoencephalitis after infection by a retrovirus, human T cell lymphotrophic virus type I. As might be expected in a spinal cord disorder, urinary symptoms are a common feature; in one series, they were estimated to be present in 88% of patients (Shibasaki et al., 1988). Patients have frequency, urgency, and urge incontinence, and urodynamic investigations show a combination of disorders (see Table 36–1).

Parkinson's Disease

The neurodegenerative processes of Parkinson's disease involve the neural mechanisms that control bladder function, and frequency and urgency are common (Murnaghan, 1961). Most urodynamic studies have shown a high incidence of detrusor hyperreflexia (Andersen and Bradley, 1976b; Pavlakis et al., 1983b; Porter and Bors, 1971). This may result from loss of the physiologic inhibition exerted by the basal ganglia on the pontine micturition center (Lewin et al., 1967) or from changes in neurotransmitters within the pontine micturition center itself (de Groat, 1990). However, clinical studies have shown no consistent change in detrusor hyperreflexia with a therapeutic response to either levodopa (Fitzmaurice et al., 1985) or apomorphine (Christmas et al., 1988); the hyperreflexia can be either reduced or exaggerated when the patient is "on."

There also appears to be an abnormality of sphincter function in Parkinson's disease. Galloway (1983) and Pavlakis and associates (1983b) have suggested that this is a bradykinesia of sphincter relaxation. The finding by Christmas et al. (1988) of a significant increase in urinary flow rates in the same patient before and after an injection of apomorphine (in combination with domperidone) supports this hypothesis (Fig. 36–8).

Bladder symptoms in patients with Parkinson's disease present considerable difficulties in management. Flow rates measured before and after apomorphine provide a method that can be used in elderly males with Parkinson's disease to distinguish patients with neurologically impaired voiding from those with benign prostatic hypertrophy causing obstructed voiding. It is well recognized that these

patients do badly after surgery (Staskin et al., 1988). Treatment by reducing hyperreflexia with drugs and by alleviating incomplete bladder emptying by intermittent catheterization (see the later section on treatment) is probably the best option.

Multiple System Atrophy

The term *multiple system atrophy* (MSA) is applied to a number of disease entities that have a common pathologic expression of neuronal atrophy in a variety of overlapping combinations (see Chapter 35). Originally thought to be an uncommon condition, in which the patient presents predominately with orthostatic hypotension and autonomic failure, the disorder is now recognized as having protean manifestations (Bannister, 1988). It can occur with features of Shy-Drager syndrome, cerebellar ataxia, or atypical parkinsonism. Disturbances of continence and micturition invariably accompany the other neurologic changes in Shy-Drager syndrome and may constitute the presenting symptom. The incidence of incontinence in other forms of MSA such as olivopontocerebellar atrophy or atypical parkinsonism, is not known, but when disturbances of bladder function develop they may occur later than in the Shy-Drager presentation.

Urodynamic investigations of patients with Shy-Drager syndrome have demonstrated detrusor hyperreflexia, loss of the micturition reflex, and large residual urine volumes but no evidence of detrusor-sphincter dyssynergia (Kirby et al., 1986; Lockhart et al., 1981). A decrease in bladder compliance may be marked in advanced cases. Denervation of the sphincters can be demonstrated electromyographically; it is due to cell loss in the Onuf nucleus, which is a particular feature of this disease (Kirby et al., 1986; Sakuta et al., 1978).

MSA affects sites that are involved in the neural control of micturition at several levels. The resultant picture of bladder dysfunction observed in a patient at any one time reflects a balance produced by various deficits, and this explains why the bladder dysfunction may alter considerably with progression of the disease.

Kirby et al. (1986) pointed out that the cell loss that had been observed to affect pontine and dorsal vagal nuclei occurred in areas precisely equivalent to the detrusor motor nuclei in experimental animals. This correlates well with the observation that many of these patients are unable to initiate voluntary micturition. Loss of cells in the sacral intermediolateral column is also a pathologic feature of MSA, and these cells are thought to be the preganglionic parasympathetic neurons that innervate the detrusor muscle. Thus, poor detrusor contraction with large residual volumes is a feature of the bladder disorder in this disease.

Selective cell loss of the anterior horn cells in the Onuf nucleus characterizes the condition and results

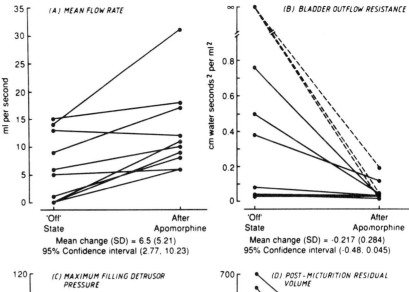

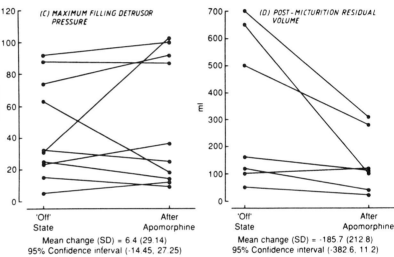

Figure 36–8. Measurements of flow rates before and after apomorphine therapy in patients with Parkinson's disease. (From Christmas T.J., Kempster P.A., Chapple C.R., et al. Role of subcutaneous apomorphine in parkinsonian voiding dysfunction. *Lancet* 2:1451–1453, 1988.)

in denervation of the striated muscle of the sphincters. This has become the basis of a neurophysiologic test to recognize MSA. Sakuta et al. (1978) demonstrated EMG changes of the anal sphincter in patients with MSA and compared these with the findings in patients with motor neuron disease. Kirby et al. (1986) examined motor units in the urethral sphincter and demonstrated marked prolongation and increased polyphasia of potentials that indicated recent reinnervation. Systematic analysis of sphincter EMG is now used to differentiate patients with MSA who present with atypical parkinsonism from those with idiopathic Parkinson's disease (Eardley et al., 1989) (Fig. 36–9).

Correct management of bladder dysfunction in patients with MSA can provide significant improvement in symptoms. A mistaken diagnosis of bladder outflow obstruction resulting from prostatic enlargement often leads to prostatectomy early in the course of the disease and leaves many of these men incontinent. Prostatectomy destroys the bladder neck, and the denervation that occurs in MSA means that continence can no longer be maintained by the rhab-

dosphincter. Because patients may have several years of active life before becoming disabled by progress of the disease, it is clearly important to recognize the disease and avoid surgery. Postmicturition residual volumes in these patients may be between 200 and 400 ml; bladder function can be greatly improved if the patients learn to perform intermittent self-catheterization (see the later section on treatment). Unstable contractions may also be a feature, particularly in the early stages of the disease, and timely treatment with either oxybutynin or terodiline can have a beneficial effect.

Neurologic Causes of Urinary Retention

Disease of the S2-4 roots can damage the motor and sensory pathways that innervate the detrusor, pelvic floor, and sphincters. The clinical picture is a combination of urinary retention and stress incontinence with altered sensation over the saddle area.

Transient urinary retention has been described in patients thought to have had a viral sacral myelora-

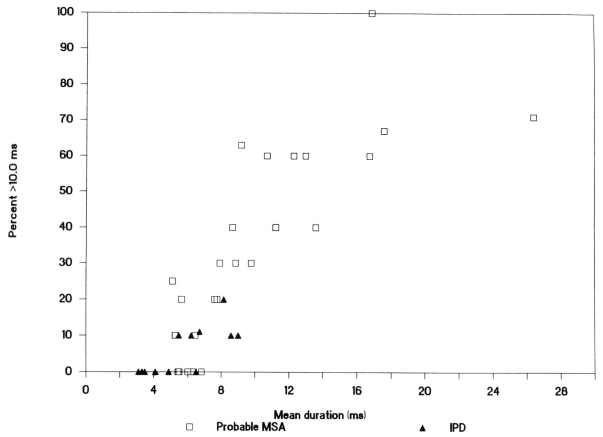

Figure 36–9. Motor unit analysis in MSA and idiopathic Parkinson's disease (IPD). (From Eardley I., Quinn N.P., Fowler C.J., et al. The value of urethral sphincter electromyography in the differential diagnosis of parkinsonism. *Br. J. Urol.* 64:360–362, 1989.)

diculitis. Herbaut et al. (1987) described three patients with this condition in whom urinary retention lasted for 7–15 days and did not recur. The authors stressed the importance of recognizing the minor concomitant neurologic abnormalities that reflect sacral root damage; all three of their patients had raised protein and lymphocytosis in the cerebrospinal fluid. Herpes simplex sacral radiculopathy with urinary retention is well recognized with herpetic vesicles on the perineum (Oates and Greenhouse, 1978) and is seen on the bladder wall at cystoscopy.

Urinary Retention in Women

A study of the patients with acute urinary retention admitted over a 9-month period to six Copenhagen hospitals found a ratio of men to women of 13:1 (Klarskov et al., 1987). The incidence of retention in women in this study was estimated as 7 per 100,000.

The anatomy of the female outflow tract is such that some women are able to void simply by relaxation of the sphincter and pelvic floor, without generating any significant rise in detrusor pressure. Difficult or obstructed voiding is highly abnormal, and four possible mechanisms should be considered:

1. Urethral strictures in women are rare, but they may be a late result of trauma during parturition or be associated with vulval atrophy in the elderly.

2. Detrusor-sphincter dyssynergia may cause urinary retention; however, because this disorder is likely to result from an interruption of neural pathways between the pontine micturition center and the sacral cord, clinical signs and symptoms of spinal cord disease are present and the accompanying bladder hyperreflexia is likely to produce urgency and frequency in addition to retentive symptoms. (A diagnosis of multiple sclerosis is often considered in young women with urinary retention, even if it is an isolated complaint, but in one author's experience [C.J. Fowler] this has never proved to be the case.)

3. Loss of contractility of the detrusor muscle may be due to injury of the S3-4 roots, which can result in bladder denervation, an atonic bladder, and urinary retention. Some accompanying sacral sensory loss may be expected, and EMG of either sphincter shows the changes of denervation and reinnervation (Fowler and Kirby, 1986).

4. The most common cause of urinary retention in young women is a condition, until recently thought to be psychogenic, in which retention occurs without any accompanying neurologic abnormalities. Urethral sphincter EMG reveals abnormal myotonic-like activity (so-called complex

repetitive discharges and decelerating bursts) that seems to impair sphincter relaxation.

Abnormal Electromyographic Activity of the Urethral Sphincter, Voiding Dysfunction, and Polycystic Ovaries

Abnormal sphincter EMG activity was first proposed as the cause of urinary retention in five women by Fowler and Kirby in 1985. These women had no symptoms of sacral root lesion or autonomic disturbance: anal sphincter control was normal, and they had no disturbance of perineal sensation. Each patient had undergone extensive neurologic investigation without any abnormality being found. Urethral sphincter EMG recorded with a fine concentric needle electrode revealed spontaneous activity, at that time erroneously called pseudomyotonia.

Further detailed examination of this EMG activity showed it to consist of activity that had been recognized by Dyro et al. (1983) as complex repetitive discharges and other, remarkable activity that had a pronounced decelerating component to it and was therefore called *decelerating bursts*. The sound produced by decelerating bursts is highly reminiscent of myotonic discharges and had led to its misnaming as pseudomyotonia (Butler, 1979). Butler aptly pointed out the similarity between the sound of this activity and underwater recordings of schools of whales calling to each other across the ocean.

With the use of a single-fiber EMG needle, analysis of jitter of the complexes showed it to be so low as to indicate that the complexes were the result of ephaptic transmission between muscle fibers (Fowler et al., 1985). This type of activity can be recorded from the urethral sphincter in disturbed bladder function other than urinary retention (Butler, 1979; Dyro et al., 1983; Fowler et al., 1988), but, conversely, it is the most common EMG finding in young women with isolated urinary retention (Fig. 36–10). The activity is confined to the urethral sphincter; skeletal muscle and anal sphincter EMG activity is normal.

The observation that patients with retention and abnormal EMG activity sometimes had the appearances typical of Stein-Leventhal syndrome led to a study to examine the incidence of polycystic ovaries in these patients. Ultrasonography of 22 women with voiding difficulties and abnormal sphincter EMG activity showed that 14 (64%) had polycystic ovaries; of the remaining 8 women, 4 had histories of significant ovarian pathology (Fowler et al., 1988).

The current speculative hypothesis of these associated findings is that the relative progesterone deficiency that occurs in polycystic ovaries reduces membrane stability in the striated muscle of the urethral sphincter. Pelvic floor muscles are known to show sexual differentiation (Beersiek et al., 1979), and immunohistochemical studies of the striated muscle of the urethral sphincter have shown it to be surrounded by a ring of material that is positive for vasoactive intestinal polypeptide (Crowe et al., 1985).

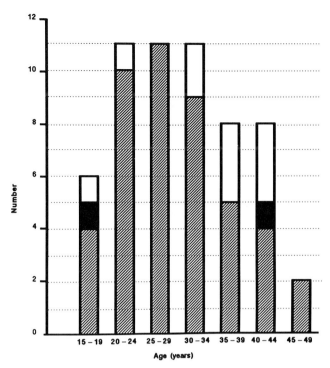

Figure 36–10. Urethral sphincter EMG findings in 57 women with urinary retention. The hatched rectangles indicate the number of women in whom profuse, abnormal spontaneous EMG activity was recorded (i.e., complex repetitive and decelerating burst discharges). The black rectangles represent those in whom changes of denervation and reinnervation were found, and the open rectangles indicate women with retention in whom sphincter EMG was normal.

The possibilities exist that some hormonally peculiar feature of this muscle renders it alone susceptible to development of the abnormal EMG activity that reflects ephaptic transmission between muscle fibers and that the presence of multiple complex repetitive discharge generators in the muscle impairs its normal relaxation.

INVESTIGATION OF BLADDER DYSFUNCTION IN NEUROLOGIC DISEASE

The basic aims of management of the neurogenic bladder are to minimize the risk to renal function that results from a failure of bladder emptying and to improve symptoms that arise from detrusor hyperreflexia. Elaborate investigations are not usually helpful in deploying the limited range of treatment options available. In practice, investigation can be confined to simple tests that help to establish failure of bladder emptying and its consequences and those that demonstrate the presence of bladder instability. Urologic conditions, such as benign prostatic hypertrophy and urolithiasis, affect patients with neurologic disease at least as frequently as those without neurologic disorders, and it may be necessary to exclude these conditions, especially in elderly patients. Investigation of hematuria, persistent urinary infection, or pyuria is best undertaken by a urologist.

A midstream specimen of urine for culture, a plain abdominal x-ray film to detect renal tract calcification, and routine biochemical assays as a guide to renal function are indicated initially in most patients.

Assessment of the Upper Urinary Tract

Intravenous urography provides an anatomic assessment of the kidneys and ureters, as well as giving limited information about renal function. If there is upper tract dilatation, a Tc 99m diethylenetriamine-pentaacetic acid renogram confirms the presence of obstruction. In neurologic patients, obstruction is usually at the level of the external urethral sphincter and results from detrusor-sphincter dyssynergia. Isotope renography also gives valuable information about differential renal function. Ultrasound examination of the urinary tract avoids exposure to ionizing radiation and provides anatomic information about the upper urinary tract similar to that provided by intravenous urography.

Detection of Detrusor Hyperreflexia

Simple filling cystometry is usually sufficient to detect detrusor hyperreflexia. The intravesical pressure is measured by means of a pressure transducer connected to a small-caliber urethral catheter while a second catheter is used to fill the bladder with fluid. The normal bladder can accommodate even the unphysiologically high rates of filling used in most urodynamic laboratories (60 ml/minute or more) without a rise in pressure until bladder capacity is almost reached. When there is detrusor hyperreflexia, the unstable smooth muscle contracts spontaneously during filling with a sharp rise in intravesical pressure. These contractions are not voluntarily suppressible, although the patient may be able to avoid incontinence by voluntarily contracting the external urethral sphincter. The contractions are usually associated with a feeling of urgency of micturition, and incontinence may occur.

A more ominous urodynamic finding is of a sustained and progressive rise in intravesical pressure during filling. This lack of bladder compliance is characteristic of spinal cord lesions and results in a persistently high intravesical pressure that endangers renal function.

If radiopaque fluid is used during the filling cystometrogram (videocystometry), the changing morphology of the bladder can be monitored by fluoroscopy and correlated with intravesical pressure changes.

Assessment of Bladder Emptying

Measurement of the urine flow rate during voiding is noninvasive and is easy with modern flowmeters.

The pattern of flow, the voided volumes, and the maximal and average urine flow rates provide useful information about the patient's detrusor function. A sharply interrupted stream in a patient with spinal cord disease is likely to be caused by detrusor sphincter dyssynergia and may be associated with a significant residual urine volume (see Fig. 36–7).

The most accurate measure of residual urine volume is obtained by passing a catheter into the bladder after voiding and measuring the amount of urine drained. This can often be done during cystometry. An alternative method is to compute the bladder volume after voiding from an ultrasound scan. This has the advantage of being noninvasive and allows repeated measurements to be made.

Neurophysiologic Investigations

Neurophysiologic techniques applied to the sphincters and pelvic floor provide a means of assessing the innervation of these structures that are otherwise somewhat inaccessible to examination. Although many neurourologic studies have employed neurophysiologic investigations as research tools, the role of such tests in clinical investigations to determine management is now well established.

It has been argued that urethral sphincter EMG is mandatory in the investigation of women with urinary retention (Fowler and Kirby, 1986). Demonstration of denervation and reinnervation of the sphincters in patients with prominent urinary symptoms and extrapyramidal disorders is an important finding that favors diagnosis of MSA (Eardley et al., 1989). The limitations of the bulbocavernous reflex in the investigation of impotence that is suspected to be a result of small-fiber neuropathy is discussed in Chapter 35, but measurement of the response can assist in diagnosing suspected sacral root lesions. A cortically recorded response to stimulation of the pudendal nerve is as easily obtained as a response to stimulation of a tibial nerve, but its value over the latter to demonstrate spinal cord disease that causes bladder symptoms remains to be demonstrated. A combination of these tests can be used to investigate patients suspected of having neurogenic bladder disorders, but limitations of the tests in terms of assessing detrusor innervation must be kept in mind.

TREATMENT OF URINARY SYMPTOMS IN NEUROLOGIC DISEASE

Renal failure is an important cause of morbidity and mortality in patients with spinal injuries and congenital cord lesions but is uncommon in progressive neurologic disease. In patients with mild urinary symptoms and no evidence of upper urinary tract complications, the inconvenience and possible side effects of treatment must be weighed against the likely benefits.

Medical Treatment of Impaired Bladder Emptying

When urologic causes for impaired bladder emptying have been excluded, the cause of significant residual urine in patients with neurologic diseases is usually either deficient detrusor contraction or detrusor sphincter dyssynergia. Both factors may operate in patients with spinal cord disease. Attempts to stimulate detrusor contraction or sphincter relaxation by drugs are largely futile, and most patients need some mechanical form of bladder drainage.

Intermittent Catheterization

Intermittent catheterization was first proposed as an alternative to a long-term indwelling catheter in patients who had spinal injuries (Guttmann and Frankel, 1966), and this technique has transformed the management of neurogenic bladder disorders. The method was originally described as an aseptic procedure performed by medical staff but was shown by Lapides et al. (1974) to be equally safe when using a clean but nonsterile technique. Clean intermittent self-catheterization has become a widely established technique practiced by patients as a means of improving bladder emptying, and it is equally applicable to children and the elderly (Webb et al., 1990).

Intermittent catheterization is performed by the patient or caregiver four or five times during a 24-hour period. The frequency of catheterization is often best determined by the patient, but the volume drained on each occasion generally should be less than 500 ml. A nurse specialist or continence adviser is normally responsible for providing information and teaching the technique. It is more difficult for females to learn to do this initially, and a mirror is useful at first. Although many patients first react with revulsion when this form of treatment is proposed, the majority master the method with adequate advice and training.

It has been the authors' experience that patients with residual volumes consistently more than 100 ml are most likely to benefit from clean intermittent self-catheterization. The degree of benefit depends on the volume of urine that can be held within the bladder before incontinence occurs. A weak urethral sphincter or severe detrusor hyperreflexia reduces the functional capacity of the bladder and compromises the symptomatic benefit to be gained from the technique. However, anticholinergic drugs to diminish detrusor hyperreflexia and increase capacity are often used in combination with intermittent self-catheterization.

Urinary infection is a surprisingly infrequent complication of this procedure. By draining the residual urine from the bladder, the incidence of symptomatic urinary infection may actually be reduced, although asymptomatic bacteriuria may be a more frequent finding. Manual dexterity is an important factor and can determine a patient's ability to carry out clean intermittent self-catheterization, but good eyesight does not seem to be an essential requirement. Many patients find it useful to talk to another patient who has already mastered the technique.

Medical Treatment of Detrusor Hyperreflexia

The inability of the bladder to hold normal volumes of urine in patients with neurologic diseases is usually the result of uninhibited detrusor contractions (detrusor hyperreflexia). The severity of symptoms is quite variable among patients and usually reflects differences in the amount of urine the bladder can hold before hyperreflexic contractions occur.

Many patients benefit from an explanation of their symptoms in relation to the neurologic problem. The completion of frequency-volume charts that record the number of incontinent episodes helps to assess the magnitude of the problem. The charts are also useful in evaluating the response to treatment and enable the patient to become aware of factors that influence the urinary symptoms.

Drug treatment is the most usual means of managing detrusor hyperreflexia. Of the many pharmacologic agents that have been used to reduce bladder hyperreflexia, the most effective have been those with predominantly anticholinergic properties. Propantheline is the most well-established anticholinergic in clinical use and has been shown in clinical trials to be effective in reducing hyperreflexia (Blaivas et al., 1980). However, side effects, including dry mouth, impaired accommodation, and constipation, often limit its clinical use. Imipramine, one of the tricyclic antidepressants, has a marked anticholinergic action that is sometimes useful in the treatment of detrusor hyperreflexia.

Propantheline and imipramine have largely been overtaken by agents aimed specifically at altering bladder function. Oxybutynin chloride, more widely used in the United States, is both a potent anticholinergic with a high affinity for muscarinic receptors in bladder tissue and a smooth muscle relaxant (Gajewski and Awad, 1986). Terodiline has been shown to have both anticholinergic and calcium antagonistic action on detrusor muscle (Andersson et al., 1984). Both drugs are moderately effective in reducing hyperreflexic contractions, but the dosage is limited by anticholinergic side effects. Dry mouth and constipation are the most frequent side effects, but impairment of accommodation can occur and must not be mistaken for deteriorating optic nerve function in multiple sclerosis.

Both oxybutynin and terodiline may potentiate a tendency to incomplete bladder emptying and urinary retention; when detrusor-sphincter dyssynergia is suspected, the residual urine volume should be measured before commencing either drug. If the residual volume is more than 100 ml, the patient should probably be taught clean intermittent self-catheterization before the anticholinergic is commenced. If the residual volume is in the range of 50–100 ml, the patient should be prepared for the possibility of needing clean intermittent self-catheterization, depending on the effects of the anticholinergic on bladder emptying.

Chronic Indwelling Catheter

Because of poor hand function and lack of a suitable caregiver, clean intermittent catheterization may be impossible for some patients. It may also be unsuitable for patients whose dominant bladder dysfunction is hyperreflexia. Under these circumstances and despite the disadvantages, an indwelling catheter may be the only means of ensuring adequate urinary drainage and personal hygiene.

The main complications of long-term catheterization are leakage alongside the catheter, intermittent blockage of the catheter, and chronic urinary infection. Stone formation may occur in association with the presence of the catheter and infection. Treatment of infection with antibiotics and antiseptic washouts is unlikely to be complete and may lead to colonization of the urinary tract with resistant organisms. Bypassing around the catheter is a common problem, usually as a result of uninhibited detrusor contractions, and is logically first managed with anticholinergic medication. The use of increasingly larger catheters with bigger balloons is best avoided. The larger balloons are likely to worsen the degree of detrusor instability, and large catheters can result eventually in a grossly patulous urethra.

Surgical Treatment of Urinary Dysfunction in Neurologic Disease

Surgery has little part to play in the management of most patients with bladder dysfunction in neuro-

Table 36–3. SURGERY FOR UROLOGIC DISORDERS

Operations to Improve Bladder Emptying
By improved drainage
External sphincterotomy or stenting of sphincter
Suprapubic catheterization
Urinary conduit diversion
Continent diversion
By stimulating detrusor contraction
Brindly anterior sacral root stimulator implant
Operations to Improve Bladder Storage
By reducing intravesical pressure
Cystodistention
Bladder transection
Phenol injection
Posterior sacral root section
Augmentation and substitution cystoplasty
By controlling bladder outlet
Bladder neck suspension
Artificial sphincter

logic disease. This is especially true of those suffering from progressive conditions, unless such a condition is compounded by a correctable urologic problem. Surgery is generally reserved for those patients in whom medical management fails to stop deterioration in renal function or for those with particularly disabling symptoms that cannot be controlled by medical means. Surgery may also be indicated for patients with intractable incontinence resulting from sphincter weakness. Various surgical procedures with different aims have been devised (Table 36–3).

References

Ahlberg J., Norlen L., Blomstrand C., et al. Outcome of shunt operation on urinary incontinence in normal pressure hydrocephalus predicted by lumbar puncture. *J. Neurol. Neurosurg. Psychiatry* 51:105–108, 1988.

Andersen J.T., Bradley W.E. Bladder and urethral innervation in multiple sclerosis. *Br. J. Urol.* 48:193–198, 1976a.

Andersen J.T., Bradley W.E. Cystometric, sphincter and electromyelographic abnormalities in Parkinson's disease. *J. Urol.* 116:75–78, 1976b.

Andersson K.-E., Sundwall A., Ulmsten V., eds. Terodoline in the treatment of urinary frequency and motor urge incontinence. *Scand. J. Urol. Nephrol. Suppl.* 87:13, 1984.

Andrew J., Nathan P.W. Lesions of the anterior frontal lobes and disturbances of micturition and defaecation. *Brain* 87:233–262, 1964.

Awad S.A., Gajewski J.B., Sogbein S.K., et al. Relationship between neurological and urological status in patients with multiple sclerosis. *J. Urol.* 132:499–502, 1984.

Bannister R., ed. *Autonomic Failure: A Textbook of Clinical Disorders of the Autonomic Nervous System.* Oxford, Oxford University Press, 1988.

Barrington F.J.F. The effect of lesions of the hind and midbrain on micturition in the cat. *Q. J. Physiol.* 15:82–102, 1925.

Bartleson J.D., Cohen M.D., Harrington T.M., et al. Cauda equina syndrome secondary to long-standing ankylosing spondylitis. *Ann. Neurol.* 14:662–668, 1983.

Beck R.P., Warren K.G., Whitman P. Urodynamic studies in female patients with multiple sclerosis. *Am. J. Obstet. Gynecol.* 139:273–276, 1981.

Beersiek F., Parks A.G., Swash M. Pathogenesis of anorectal incontinence: a histometric study of the anal musculature. *J. Neurol. Sci.* 42:111–127, 1979.

Beric A., Dimitrijevic M.R., Light J.K. A clinical syndrome of rostral and caudal spinal injury: neurological, neurophysiological and urodynamic evidence for occult sacral lesion. *J. Neurol. Neurosurg. Psychiatry* 50:600–606, 1987.

Blaivas J.G., Barnalias G.A. Detrusor-external sphincter dyssynergia in men with multiple sclerosis: an ominous urologic condition. *J. Urol.* 131:91–94, 1984.

Blaivas J.G., Bhimani G., Labib K.B. Vesicourethral dysfunction in multiple sclerosis. *J. Urol.* 122:342–347, 1979.

Blaivas J.G., Labib K.B., Michalik S.J., et al. Cystometric response to propantheline in detrusor hyperreflexia: therapeutic implications. *J. Urol.* 124:259–262, 1980.

Bradley, W.E. Urinary bladder dysfunction in multiple sclerosis. *Neurology (Minneap.)* 28:9(Part 2):52–58, 1978.

Burnstock G. The changing face of autonomic neurotransmission. *Acta Physiol. Scand.* 126:67–91, 1986.

Burnstock G. Innervation of bladder and bowel. In Bock G., Whelan J., eds. *Neurobiology of Incontinence.* Chichester, Wiley, pp. 2–14, 1990.

Butler W.J. Pseudomyotonia of the periurethral sphincter in women with urinary incontinence. *J. Urol.* 122:838–840, 1979.

Chantraine A. Electromyographie des sphincters striés urétal et anal humains. Etude descriptive et analytique. *Rev. Neurol. (Paris)* 115:396–403, 1966.

Christmas T.J., Kempster P.A., Chapple C.R., et al. Role of subcutaneous apomorphine in parkinsonian voiding dysfunction. *Lancet* 2:1451–1453, 1988.

Crowe R., Light J.K., Chilton C.P., et al. Vasoactive intestinal polypeptide (VIP)—immunoreactive nerve fibres associated with the striated muscle of the human external urethral sphincter. *Lancet* 1:47–48, 1985.

Czyhlarz E.V., Marburg O. Ueber cerebrale Blasenstörungen. *Jahrb. Pyschiatr. Neurol.* 20:134–174, 1901.

de Groat W.C. Nervous control of the urinary bladder of the cat. *Brain Res.* 87:201–211, 1975.

de Groat W.C. Central neural control of the lower urinary tract. In Bock G., Whelan J., eds. *Neurobiology of Incontinence.* Chichester, Wiley, pp. 27–42, 1990.

Dyro F.M., Bauer S.B., Hallett M., et al. Complex repetitive discharges in the external urethral sphincter in a pediatric population. *Neurourol. Urodynam.* 2:39–44, 1983.

Eardley I., Quinn N.P., Fowler C.J., et al. The value of urethral sphincter electromyography in the differential diagnosis of parkinsonism. *Br. J. Urol.* 64:360–362, 1989.

Fisher C.M. Hydrocephalus as a cause of disturbances of gait in the elderly. *Neurology (N.Y.)* 32:1358–1363, 1982.

Fitzmaurice H., Fowler C.J., Rickards D., et al. Micturition disturbance in Parkinson's disease. *Br. J. Urol.* 57:652–656, 1985.

Fowler C.J., Kirby R.S. Abnormal electromyographic activity (decelerating burst and complex repetitive discharges) in the striated muscle of the urethral sphincter in women in retention. *Br. J. Urol.* 57:67–70, 1985.

Fowler C.J., Kirby R.S. Electromyography of the urethral sphincter in women with urinary retention. *Lancet* 1:1455–1456, 1986.

Fowler C.J., Kirby R.S., Harrison M.J.G., et al. Individual motor unit analysis in the diagnosis of disorders of urethral sphincter innervation. *J. Neurol. Neurosurg. Psychiatry* 47:637–641, 1984.

Fowler C.J., Kirby R.S., Harrison M.J.G. Decelerating burst and complex repetitive discharges in the striated muscle of the urethral sphincter associated with urinary retention in women. *J. Neurol. Neurosurg. Psychiatry* 48:1004–1009, 1985.

Fowler C.J., Christmas T.J., Chapple C.R., et al. Abnormal electromyographic activity of the urethral sphincter, voiding dysfunction, and polycystic ovaries: a new syndrome? *Br. Med. J.* 297:1436–1438, 1988.

Gajewski J.B., Awad S.A. Oxybutinin versus probantheline in patients with multiple sclerosis and detrusor hyperreflexia. *J. Urol.* 135:966–968, 1986.

Galloway N.T.M. Urethral sphincter abnormalities in parkinsonism. *Br. J. Urol.* 55:691–693, 1983.

Galloway N.T.M., Tainsh J. Minor defects of the sacrum and neurogenic bladder dysfunction. *Br. J. Urol.* 57:154–155, 1985.

George N.J.R., Dixon J.S. Normal sensation of the lower urinary tract. In George N.J.R., Gosling J.A., eds. *Sensory Disorders of the Bladder and Urethra.* London, Springer-Verlag, pp. 7–17, 1986.

Goldstein I., Siroky M.B., Sax D.S., et al. Neurourologic abnormalities in multiple sclerosis. *J. Urol.* 128:541–545, 1982.

Gonor S.E., Carroll D.J., Metcalfe J.B. Vesical dysfunction in multiple sclerosis. *Urology* 25:429–431, 1985.

Gosling J.A., Dixon J.S., Critchley H.O.D., et al. A comparative study of the human external sphincter and periurethral levator ani muscles. *Br. J. Urol.* 53:35–41, 1981.

Gosling J.A., Dixon J.S., Humpherson J.A., eds. *Functional Anatomy of the Urinary Tract: An Integrated Text and Colour Atlas.* Edinburgh, Churchill Livingstone, 1987.

Guttmann L., Frankel H. The value of intermittent catheterisation in the early management of traumatic paraplegia and tetraplegia. *Paraplegia* 4:63–84, 1966.

Hakim S., Adams R.D. The special clinical problem of symptomatic hydrocephalus with normal cerebrospinal fluid pressure. *J. Neurol. Sci.* 2:307–327, 1965.

Hassouna M., Lebel M., Elhilali M. Neurologic correlation in multiple sclerosis. *Neurourol. Urodynam.* 3:73–77, 1984.

Herbaut A.G., Voordecker P., Monseu G., et al. Benign transient urinary retention. *J. Neurol. Neurosurg. Psychiatry* 50:354–355, 1987.

Holman E. Difficult urination associated with intracranial tumours of the posterior fossa. A physiologic and clinical study. *Arch. Neurol. Psychiatry* 15:371–380, 1926.

International Continence Society. Fourth report on the standardisation of terminology of lower urinary tract. *Br. J. Urol.* 53:333–335, 1981.

Jennett P. A study of 25 cases of compression of the cauda equina by prolapsed intervertebral discs. *J. Neurol. Neurosurg.* 19:109–116, 1956.

Ketelaer P., Leruitte A., Vereecken R.L. Striated urethral and anal sphincter electromyography during cystometry in multiple sclerosis. *Electromyogr. Clin. Neurophysiol.* 17:427–434, 1977.

Kirby R., Fowler C.J., Gosling J., et al. Urethro-vesical dysfunction in progressive autonomic failure with multiple system atrophy. *J. Neurol. Neurosurg. Psychiatry* 49:554–562, 1986.

Klarskov P., Andersen J.T., Asmussen C.F., et al. Acute urinary retention in women: a prospective study of 18 consecutive cases. *Scand. J. Urol. Nephrol.* 21:29–31, 1987.

Lafuente D.J., Andrew J., Joy A. Sacral sparing with cauda equina compression from central lumbar intervertebral disc prolapse. *J. Neurol. Neurosurg. Psychiatry* 48:579–581, 1985.

Lapides J., Diokno A.C., Lowe B.S., et al. Follow up on unsterile, intermittent self-cathertization. *J. Urol.* 111:184–187, 1974.

Lewin R.J., Dillard G.V., Porter R.W. Extrapyramidal inhibition of the urinary bladder. *Brain Res.* 4:301–307, 1967.

Light J.K., Beric A., Wise P.G. Predictive criteria for failed sphincterotomy in spinal cord injury. *J. Urol.* 138:1201–1204, 1987.

Lockhart J.L., Webster G.D., Sheremata W., et al. Neurogenic bladder dysfunction in the Shy-Drager syndrome. *J. Urol.* 126:119–121, 1981.

Lucas M.G., Thomas D.G. Lack of relationship of conus reflexes to bladder function after spinal cord injury. *Br. J. Urol.* 63:24–27, 1989.

Lucas M.G., Thomas D.G. Lumbosacral evoked potentials and vesicourethral function with chronic suprasacral spinal cord injury. *J. Neurol. Neurosurg. Psychiatry* 53:982–986, 1990.

Maggi C.A., Barbanti G., Santicciolo P., et al. Cystometric evidence that capsaicin-sensitive nerves modulate the afferent branch of micturition reflex in humans. *J. Urol.* 142:150–154, 1989.

Maurice-Williams R.S. Micturition symptoms in frontal tumours. *J. Neurol. Neurosurg. Psychiatry* 37:431–436, 1974.

Miller H., Simpson C.A., Yeates W.K. Bladder dysfunction in multiple sclerosis. *Br. Med. J.* 1:1265–1269, 1965.

Morrison J.F.B. Sensations arising from the lower urinary tract. In Torrens M., Morrison J.F.B., eds. *The Physiology of the Lower Urinary Tract.* London, Springer-Verlag, pp. 89–132, 1987.

Murnaghan G.F. Neurogenic disorders of the bladder in parkinsonism. *Br. J. Urol.* 33:403–409, 1961.

Nathan P.W., Smith M.C. The centripetal pathway from the bladder and urethra within the spinal cord. *J. Neurol. Neurosurg. Psychiatry* 14:262–280, 1951.

Oates J.K., Greenhouse P.R.D.H. Retention of urine in anogenital herpetic infection. *Lancet* 1:691–692, 1978.

Onufrowicz B. Notes on the arrangement and function of the cell groups in the sacral region of the spinal cord. *J. Nerv. Ment. Dis.* 26:498–504, 1899.

Pang D., Wilberger J.E. Tethered cord syndrome in adults. *J. Neurosurg.* 57:32–47, 1982.

Pavlakis A.J., Siroky M.B., Goldstein I. Neurourologic findings in conus medullaris and cauda equina injury. *Arch. Neurol.* 40:570–573, 1983a.

Pavlakis A.J., Siroky M.B., Goldstein I., et al. Neurourologic findings in Parkinson's disease. *J. Urol.* 129:80–83, 1983b.

Petersen T., Pedersen E. Neurourodynamic evaluation of voiding dysfunction in multiple sclerosis. *Acta Neurol. Scand.* 69:402–411, 1984.

Philp T., Read D.J., Higson R.H. The urodynamic characteristics of multiple sclerosis. *Br. J. Urol.* 53:672–675, 1981.

Piazza D.H., Diokono A.C. Review of neurogenic bladder in multiple sclerosis. *Urology* 14:33–35, 1979.

Porter R.W., Bors E. Neurogenic bladder in parkinsonism, effect of thalamotomy. *J. Neurosurg.* 34:27–32, 1971.

Pullen A.H. Quantitative synaptology of feline motorneurones to external anal sphincter muscle. *J. Comp. Neurol.* 269:414–424, 1988.

Renier W.O., Gabreels F.J.M. Evaluation of diagnosis and non-surgical therapy in 24 children with a pontine tumour. *Neuropaediatrie* 11:262–273, 1980.

Sakuta M., Nakanishi T., Toyokura Y. Anal muscle electromyograms differ in amyotrophic lateral sclerosis and Shy-Drager syndrome. *Neurology (Minneap.)* 28:1289–1293, 1978.

Satoh K., Shimizu N., Tohyama M., et al. Localization of the micturition reflex center at dorsolateral pontine tegmentum of the rat. *Neurosci. Lett.* 8:27–33, 1978.

Schoenberg H.W., Gutrich J., Banno J. Urodynamic patterns in multiple sclerosis. *J. Urol.* 122:648–650, 1979.

Shibasaki H., Endo C., Kuroda Y., et al. Clinical picture of HTLV-I associated myelopathy. *J. Neurol. Sci.* 87:15–24, 1988.

Smith A.R.B., Hosker G.L., Warrell D.W. The role of partial denervation of the pelvic floor in aetiology of genitourinary prolapse and stress incontinence of urine. A neurophysiological study. *Br. J. Obstet Gynaecol.* 96:24–28, 1989.

Snooks S.J., Setchell M., Swash M., et al. Injury to innervation of pelvic floor sphincter musculature in childbirth. *Lancet* 2:546–550, 1984.

Staskin D.S., Vardi Y., Siroky M.A. Post-prostatectomy incontinence in the parkinsonian patient: the significance of poor voluntary sphincter control. *J. Urol.* 140:117–118, 1988.

Swash M., Snooks S.J., Henry M. Unifying concept of pelvic floor disorders and incontinence. *J. R. Soc. Med.* 78:906–911, 1985.

Tanagho E.A., Miller E.R. Initiation of voiding. *Br. J. Urol.* 42:175–183, 1970.

Ueki K. Disturbances of micturition observed in some patients with brain tumour. *Neurol. Med. Chir.* 2:25–33, 1960.

Van Poppel H., Vereecken R.L., Leruitte A. Neuro-muscular dysfunction of the lower urinary tract in multiple sclerosis. *Paraplegia* 21:374–379, 1983.

Webb R.J., Lawson A.L., Neal D.E. Clean intermittent self-catheterisation in 172 adults. *Br. J. Urol.* 65:20–23, 1990.

37

Food Intake and Its Disorders

Paul R. McHugh

Only occasional examples of obesity fall to neurologists to manage and to study. Most obese patients are construed by clinicians as having a behavioral disruption with a complex psychologic cause involving personal and biologic issues that are difficult to unravel. Such patients are referred to internists or psychiatrists. A classification that distinguishes among the obese and some appreciation of physiologic controls on feeding now offer the possibility that more definite neural mechanisms and sites of pathology may bring more of these conditions into the ambit of neurology. At the moment, such basic information is only emerging, but it encourages a brief section in this text.

CLINICAL CONDITIONS

Three varieties of human obesity can be distinguished by aspects of the manifestations and causes: (1) lifelong "essential" obesity, (2) adult-onset obesity, and (3) syndromic obesity. The last variety has traditionally been the focus of neurologic interest. Intriguingly, it now provides opportunities for a consideration of brain mechanisms in the etiology of all these disorders.

Lifelong Essential Obesity

These patients report that their overweight status appeared when they were children. It increased along with their growth spurt at puberty and, in women, may also have increased with each preg-

Supported by National Institutes of Health grant 2-RO1 AM 19302.

nancy. These individuals eventually attain massive obesity with body weights of 150–250% or more above the ideal. All efforts at weight reduction prove ultimately futile. They lose weight with dieting and focused attention on food consumption, only to have massive obesity return gradually after they leave such a program. A sense that their body weight is "set" higher than in others derives from this experience of regular recovery of their obesity when vigilance is relaxed and the natural sequence of hunger and satiety are permitted free rein (Krotkiewski et al., 1977).

The fat distribution in these individuals is over the entire body; thus, even their forearms share in the obesity. These individuals constitute a minority of people who are overweight, but they represent a large number among those troubled by secondary clinical problems, such as diabetes mellitus, osteoarthritis, hypoventilation, and the pickwickian syndrome.

The most fruitful hypothesis of the underlying mechanism is that of Hirsch and Knittle (1970). These investigators demonstrated that in lifelong obesity, the patient has an increase in the number of fat cells in the body (hyperplasia), as well as an increase in the fat content of each cell (hypertrophy). The increase in the number of cells occurs early in life. In experimental animals at least, such hyperplasia can be provoked by overfeeding early in life. In humans, overfeeding in infancy may be one mechanism, but genetic factors are more likely to be crucial (Garn and Clark, 1976). Genetic strains of obese mice have been discovered (Ingalls et al., 1950) and may represent the best models for studying the fundamental disorder. Stunkard has provided the best evidence for genetics in human obesity in two separate studies (Stunkard et al., 1986a,b).

People with lifelong obesity usually seek medical

care either after discerning the refractory nature of their obesity or because of secondary symptoms that interfere with their general health. Success in treatment with dietary management has been poor. Quite clearly, they are burdened for life with the tendency to regain weight after a program of treatment related simply to dietary control. It is the appreciation of the deterministic aspect of this problem that has led physicians to attempt quite heroic measures to relieve the craving for food.

Such measures have included intestinal bypass procedures and the operative shrinkage of gastric capacity. Although there are no figures on any reduced morbidity or mortality among the operated obese, these procedures do produce loss of approximately 50% of the excess weight.

It has become clear that complicated and biologically based issues are critical components of this condition. Hedonism and gluttony do not explain this disorder. These people are victims of an increased intensity in the natural drive for food that is expressed even when bodily stores are full. They display this excessive motivation throughout their lives.

Adult-Onset Obesity

This condition is much more common than lifelong obesity. It appears in individuals who are of average weight until middle life (age 25–40) and then begin to gain weight. This form of obesity seems to be most related to dietary habits, particularly a high caloric intake, combined with a progressively more sedentary life. Animal experiments mimicking this obesity study the so-called snack food diets in rats. Rats gain weight rapidly on a variety of tasty high-fat foods, such as candy, cookies, and sweetened milk. They gain 2.5 times as much as controls, particularly if they have no access to activity wheels. The effectiveness of the diet is greater in older animals (Sclafani and Springer, 1976).

This form of weight gain in adult humans is common, particularly in affluent societies. Perhaps its most intriguing feature is its responsiveness to social attitudes. Excess weight has been acceptable in certain historical periods, but at other times it has been considered to be repulsive, at least by the upper social strata, and thus has diminished in occurrence (Goldblatt et al., 1965; Silverstone, 1968).

Although the weight gain in such people can be quite massive, the accumulation of fat seems to have a predilection for the trunk and proximal portions of the extremities. A central "middle-aged spread" is most typical, and little fat accumulates on the forearms or ankles. This distribution also matches Hirsch's observation that adult-onset obesity is produced by fat cell hypertrophy rather than by an increase in the number of fat cells throughout the body (Hirsch and Knittle, 1970).

Like essential obesity, this obesity produces risks to health and increases the risk for such conditions as diabetes mellitus, cardiac disorders, and orthopedic problems related to weight bearing. These secondary disturbances relate in large part to metabolic consequences of obesity that do not differ among the various obesity conditions, particularly the resistance to insulin or glucose utilization both in fat and in muscle cells. Insulin resistance relates directly to fat cell size and is inducible with weight gain and reversible with weight reduction.

Reduction in body weight is desirable in these people, as well as in the lifelong obese, and may be slightly easier for them to achieve. A program with sensible dietary management, education about nutrition and exercise, behavioral therapy, and group support as provided by assemblages of like-minded individuals, such as Weight Watchers and TOPS (Take Off Pounds Sensibly), seems to have some success in this group (Stunkard and Brownell, 1979; Stunkard and Penick, 1979). Adult-onset obesity may reflect a failure to reduce caloric intake along with the natural sedentariness of aging, rather than an excessive hunger drive, but we are still far from finding mechanisms that would define the pathologic problem.

Syndromic Obesity (Table 37–1)

The recognition by neurologists that obesity can be a symptom of disease, and particularly of disease in the nervous system, emerged at the turn of the century with the publication of two classic clinical cases, one by Babinski in 1900, the other by Fröhlich in 1901. These examples were noted to occur with pathologic lesions in the region of the pituitary and hypothalamus. It was the achievement of Erdheim (1906) to demonstrate with particular cases that an obesity syndrome with weight gains up to and

Table 37–1. OBESITY SYNDROMES

Hypothalamic Disorders
Tumors
    Craniopharyngioma
    Other intrinsic hypothalamic tumors
Hypothalamic inflammation
    Sarcoidosis
    Intrinsic hypothalamic abscess
Hydrocephalus
Traumatic injury to the hypothalamus

Identifiable Genetic Syndromes
Prader-Willi syndrome
Laurence-Moon-Biedl syndrome
Fröhlich's syndrome (adiposogenital syndrome)

Endocrine Disorders
Hypothyroidism
Cushing's disease (hyperadrenocorticism)
Stein-Leventhal syndrome
Pseudohypoparathyroidism

Medication-Induced Obesity
Phenothiazines
Tricyclic antidepressants

greater than 50 kg could occur in individuals who develop lesions restricted to the region of the hypothalamus, but sparing the pituitary.

As with all localized neurologic syndromes, the particular nature of the pathologic lesion can be anything that is capable of distorting and destroying hypothalamic tissue. Neoplasms (e.g., craniopharyngiomas, hamartomas, local gliomas); inflammatory processes, such as sarcoidosis, tuberculosis, arachnoiditis, and traumatic injuries; leukemic infiltrations; and aneurysms of the internal carotid artery have all been noted. Overeating and obesity constitute the regular symptoms, and other neurologic, behavioral, and endocrine changes can accompany them. The patients may be demented, apathetic, or sleepy, depending on the invasion of neighboring regions of the brain. They may show hypopituitarism and diabetes insipidus if the pituitary or its links to the hypothalamus are disrupted. They almost always have hyperinsulinemia, and, like some animals with lesions in similar regions, they may become aggressive and threatening. Reeves and Plum (1969) reported a patient with a hypothalamic neoplasm whose massive overeating and increasing obesity were accompanied by rage tendencies so severe that she could scarcely be approached by doctors or nurses if she was not eating or food was not being brought to her. Bray and Gallagher (1975) provided a superb and thorough review of the literature on this human disorder.

The hypothalamic pathologies usually appear after childhood, but a few genetic and chromosomal disorders (e.g., Laurence-Moon-Biedl syndrome and Prader-Willi syndrome) produce obesity along with a number of other neurologic abnormalities, including mental retardation. The obesity appears in early childhood, even in infancy, in association with overeating.

In all of these conditions, it is apparent that the obesity is a result of disruption of the customary regulation of feeding behavior by a neurologic process. The driven character of food intake and its frequent relationship to advancing cerebral pathology identify these individuals as subjects for investigation of the neural mechanisms of food regulation. They also exemplify the reason for assuming a nonjudgmental view of anomalies of food motivation and its control in the other obesity states.

The syndromic obesity, however, can be massive in degree, and the food intake of these patients may be close to continuous. Constant supervision and locking of food closets and refrigerators may be required to restrain them. As the obesity and bodily weight increase, all the secondary metabolic and structural problems emerge as with the other obesity conditions. The social and interpersonal problems in syndromic obesity can be worse than in the other conditions because of the intensity and persistence of the overeating. The obesity often becomes so great as to hamper movement and, along with the other often crippling neurologic symptoms, renders these patients totally disabled.

Treatment and prognosis depend on the accessibility of the underlying pathology to therapeutic control. Healing of inflammation or infection and removal of neoplasms, when possible, can lead to recovery. The mechanisms disrupting behavior in the genetic and chromosomal syndromes remain unknown. Treatment for these syndromes and the incurable hypothalamic syndromes is purely symptomatic and includes efforts to reduce access to calories and the use of surgical procedures, including vagotomy (Kral, 1983).

Cancer Anorexia

Although this chapter focuses on the issues of overeating, a section briefly dealing with a disorder of underfeeding is appropriate. It illustrates the same problems of our basic ignorance of mechanisms in the face of dramatic and even life-threatening changes in behavior.

Most examples of undereating are symptomatic of some major bodily illness, such as cancer, liver disease, infectious disorders, or metabolic disease, and the term *cancer anorexia* is commonly used. The behavior is appropriately entitled anorexia by the subjective feelings of lack of appetite and even revulsion for food that trouble the patients. The discernment, during the last decade, of a circulating factor tied to these disorders has greatly enhanced our appreciation of them (Cerami et al., 1985). This factor is called *cachectin* and is identical with tumor necrosis factor (Beutler et al., 1985); it acts presumptively on the area postrema to produce anorexia (Oliff, 1988). It is clear now that this anorexic state is associated with specific bodily metabolic changes that are quite distinct from starvation (Fong et al., 1989). The overriding question—now a major focus of research—is how to address the fitness of this combination of features (metabolic changes and reduction in food intake) to a bodily response to cancer and other debilitating conditions (McHugh et al., 1989).

Anorexia Nervosa

Anorexia nervosa is a disorder that affects young women primarily, usually beginning between the ages of 14 and 17 but occasionally found earlier in life or even up to age 40 or 50. No postmenopausal examples of true anorexia nervosa have been identified. The patient's symptoms begin with a loss of weight that is usually first noticed by the parents, who, on inquiring, are told by the patient that the weight loss is a result of dieting to improve appearance. Menstruation is soon interrupted; in fact, cessation of menses may be the first symptom of the illness. The patient often practices physical exercise to speed up the loss of weight. This weight loss can be extremely rapid, with the patient losing up to 25% of body weight within 2 or 3 months. Occasionally, the patient uses other methods, such as vomiting and laxatives, to increase weight loss.

Along with a preoccupation with body weight, the patient may change in personality. She becomes depressed, impatient, and irritable. Relations with her family become awkward and strained, with the parents uncertain as to whether to confront her behavior or to avoid a conflict and let "nature take its course." Eventually, however, with malnutrition appearing and the patient becoming weak and obviously emaciated, the parents usually take charge and bring the patient to a physician.

When first seen, usually by an internist, the patient is an obviously thin person, who most often discounts her behavior by pointing out that she is just following the lead of contemporary women in being concerned about her weight and appearance. The patient's face is gaunt, and her arms and legs seem bony and extremely thin. Her hands and feet are cold and blue, blood pressure is low, and the heart rate has slowed to 50 or 60 beats/minute. There often is an excessive growth of downy hair over the back, cheeks, forearms, and legs (lanugo hair).

Although the patient may admit that she is worried about her body weight and that she fears fatness and fears losing control over her eating, it becomes progressively more apparent that her picture of herself is distorted. She views herself fatter (or at least less thin) than she actually is.

We are still uncertain of the etiology of this condition. The term anorexia nervosa implies that the individual has little appetite; actually, her appetite can be intense, and she may be preoccupied with resisting and overcoming the urge to eat. Occasionally, the urge becomes so great that the patient succumbs to a binge of eating, after which she may induce vomiting to rid herself of the ingested calories. Only when the starvation is advanced does the patient begin to notice that she has little or no appetite.

Evidence that there is some particular functional disorder of the hypothalamus or other parts of the nervous system related to feeding behavior is only indirect, but it derives from the great excess of females with this disorder; its appearance at puberty; its regular association with menstrual abnormalities, sometimes preceding the loss of weight; and its persistence even to death in some patients.

However, it is far from proved that this is a neurologic disorder and not a psychogenic disorder, there being almost as much suggestive evidence that psychogenic features are important, including the increase in the incidence of anorexia nervosa in societies in which thinness is valued. The appearance of anorexia nervosa more commonly among ballet dancers and models who work to reduce their body weight and the frequent association of anorexia nervosa with distressed and disturbed family relationships also suggest a psychogenic contribution to etiology (Garner and Garfinkel, 1980).

The possibility that anorexia nervosa represents an aspect of affective disorder has also been suggested

(Cantwell et al., 1977). Affective disorder is frequent among family members of these patients, and certainly depression and depressive-like personalities may accompany the illness. A publication by Garfinkel and Garner (1987) gives clear directions about the utility of antidepressant treatments in some of these patients, and a multicenter double-blind study (Halmi et al., 1986) confirmed some efficacy for antidepressants.

Anorexia nervosa, however, remains something of an etiologic mystery. It may be that there is a heterogeneous combination of psychogenic and central nervous system factors in the developing woman—a combination of events that is hard to unravel to discern what is necessary and sufficient from patient to patient (Garfinkel et al., 1980). The neurologist's major problem with anorexia nervosa, however, is to understand the motivated behavior of feeding that is so deranged in these patients.

Because the mechanism of this condition is not understood, the treatment is purely symptomatic, and Andersen's book (1985) can be recommended. First, the problem is to win the patient's cooperation. Usually, the patient needs to be admitted to the hospital where restoration of body weight to normal by refeeding can be carried out in a supportive environment. Much of the refeeding of the patient is accomplished by nurses who win the patient's trust and gradually persuade the patient to take food and to see the issue as an illness that is dominating them.

Recovery of weight is accomplished by giving the patient 1500 calories (6.3 MJ) daily and within a few days persuading her to take full meals with supplements to reach an intake between 3500 and 4000 calories (14.6 and 16.7 MJ) daily.

After recovery of weight, the treatment of the patient has to be individualized. Psychologic and supportive treatments are directed to any emotional problems that may have been found, either in the patient or in the family. Long-term support is usually required to sustain the body weight. Like all symptomatic treatments, however, the long-term prognosis is more problematic than the short-term prognosis. In the short term, it is usually possible to get the patient to regain normal weight, and certainly death from malnutrition that formerly occurred, before vigorous refeeding was employed, is no longer part of the prognosis.

However, relapses requiring readmission to the hospital occur in almost 50% of patients, particularly those who have been severely malnourished. With persistence in the treatment and the readmission of patients to the hospital, many of them do recover completely after a course of illness that may run 3–4 years (Andersen et al., 1983).

CONSIDERATION OF FEEDING DISORDERS AS PROBLEMS IN MOTIVATION

Neural controls on feeding may be approached in a fashion similar to that used in motor and sensory studies. Such an approach may seek neural mechanisms tied to metabolic events. But this approach, essentially a search for a fundamental lesion in the integrative pathways of the body, has power only when there is a reasonably clear understanding of how elements of brain and body are tied together for a purpose.

The availability of such a basic paradigm is the reason why the neurology of motor-sensory function so outstrips the neurology of motivation. Thus, the conceptual neurologic approach that defines the anatomic localization of a pathologic lesion along a pathway from sensory affector to motor effector has focused and permitted the accumulation of information, and it is now the standard knowledge of clinical neurologists in explaining signs, symptoms, and courses of motor and sensory disorders. Neurologists lack any such fundamental organizing principles tying structure to function in the motivation of food intake (or any other motivated behavior, for that matter). Even though there is a locus in the hypothalamus where lesions disrupt aspects of this behavior, there is a minimum of information about the neural connections that are disrupted by lesions at this site or even what aspect of behavior is fundamental to the syndromes (is it too much hunger to too little satiety?). The laboratory work now proceeding is an attempt to develop some basic information from these neurologic beginnings that may (but certainly not yet) elucidate the nature of the feeding disturbance with hypothalamic disease. This work, of course, offers hope of illuminating the obesities that occur without coarse brain pathology—lifelong obesity, adult-onset obesity, and the peculiar states of food refusal associated with cancer and anorexia nervosa.

PHYSIOLOGIC PSYCHOLOGY OF FOOD INTAKE

Productive work has been carried out in the laboratory during the last several decades, and it does emerge from the clinical information. The first and most dramatic demonstration followed directly from the classic neurologic reports of an obesity syndrome with hypothalamic lesions. This clinical observation prompted first Hetherington and Ranson (1940) and then Tepperman et al. (1943) to produce lesions in the hypothalamus of the rat with the stereotactic instrument. With lesions restricted to the ventromedial hypothalamus in rats (and many other species), there is the prompt appearance of overeating and massive weight gain: hypothalamic hyperphagia.

This replication of the clinical syndrome in the laboratory made it accessible to analysis and encouraged further study. Here was an approach to the neural control of motivated drive that could be manipulated and by means of which mechanisms could be experimentally investigated.

There is great increase in food intake after ventro-medial hypothalamic lesions. This extra food is the major cause of body weight gain. Some, but not all, of the increased food intake is provoked by increased insulin secretion with lesions in this region. The weight gain in animals is not perpetual. Rather, there is an increase for several weeks (dynamic phase) and then a stabilizing of body weight (static phase), during which the food intake is reduced (Tepperman et al., 1943). If by dietary restraint the body weight sustained in the static phase is reduced, then the dynamic phase will reappear and the animal will overeat again to regain the high stable level if it is given free access to food.

It is not clear that humans with hypothalamic lesions have similar dynamic and static phases relating body weight and food intake. But the resemblance of this description to that seen in the lifelong obese and the syndromic obesities is obvious, suggesting that in them, the linkages between body stores and hypothalamic mechanisms are such as to "set" the weight higher than normal.

In fact, the concept of just what is deranged with hypothalamic lesions has changed over time with ongoing research. The original opinion (Hetherington and Ranson, 1940) was that metabolic alterations provoked the obesity. Tepperman et al. (1943) demonstrated overeating to be the prime cause for obesity, and Stellar (1954) proposed that the ventromedial hypothalamus might constitute a "satiety" center. The overeating would then be the result of a disruption in satiety—the natural inhibition on food intake produced by food itself. This conception seemed to be supported by Anand and Brobeck's observation in 1951 that lesions more lateral in the hypothalamus cause rats to stop eating and lose weight. The lateral hypothalamus, it was thought, might contain a "feeding" center reciprocating in its control over the motivation to eat with the ventromedial satiety center in response to food need and replenishment.

Such conceptualizations, in part encouraged by the wish for an overarching vision of the brain mechanisms in motivation, reached too far and may have brought out an explanatory concept prematurely. If one is strict about the term satiety, it means the inhibition on food intake produced by food itself. The overeating in the dynamic phase of weight gain after ventromedial hypothalamic lesions, however, is not explained by any deficit in response to food intake. Nutrients infused into overeating animals reduce their food intake as much as and no less than do such infusions in intact animals (McHugh et al., 1975).

Eventual weight stabilization suggests that the overeating seems to be provoked by a drive tied to body weight and perhaps to stores of body fat. The ventromedial hypothalamic lesion provokes a longer-term disruption of control of nutrition than is implied by the concept of a satiety deficit.

A similar implication can be derived from the results found in animals with lateral hypothalamic lesions. They appear to drop their body weight by avoiding food but eat again when a lower body weight is reached. Although the relationships between the hypothalamus and the body are still under investigation, the opinion that centers for satiety and feeding control have been discovered in the brain has been replaced by the appreciation that the hypothalamic regions function to influence body weight by stimulating or inhibiting food intake, rather than controlling the daily sequences of feeding activity as implied by such terms as a satiety center. The temptation to leap for simplifications of this problem is great. Mechanisms and their relationships remain elusive.

This laboratory work on the hypothalamus, however, did confirm that some human obesity syndromes derive from neural lesions in a similar site. It also established conclusively that the pituitary gland is not the site of the disruption provoking this behavior and that advancing the knowledge of the hypothalamus, its anatomy, and its linkages is needed for a better understanding of nutrition and body weight. However, much of the current physiologic psychology has turned to seek inputs to the brain and hypothalamus that might provide the information on which the brain acts for purposes of motivational and nutritional control.

The body weight status is a relatively stable feature in humans and in animals. There are bufferings of metabolism and activity that, in part, sustain this stability, but the energy intake and output tend to settle in adulthood, as well. The Framingham Epidemiological Study (Gordon and Kannel, 1973) showed that the majority of people display weight swings of 5–10 kg during 18 years of follow-up. This was a greater swing than other investigators had expected, but given the huge amounts of food ingested and the relative slowness of the alterations, any imbalance in energy consumed amounts to but 2% of that ingested (James, 1976).

There must be quite remarkable physiologic control on both intake and expenditure of energy, and as Garrow (1978) stated, "Hypothalamic reflexes are buried under layers of conditioning, cognitive and social factors." Nonetheless, pathology in the hypothalamus can provoke an increase in food consumption and a new body weight far in excess of the stable baseline.

Physiologic psychology has more recently been redirected toward the body in seeking "peripheral" controls on the "central" mechanisms. This was a return to themes that had been active in feeding studies before the hypothalamic discoveries. Walter Cannon (Cannon and Washburn, 1912), in particular, had focused his attention on the stomach and how its state of repletion might influence hunger and satiety.

Much of the focus of work has been on what inhibits food intake in ways distinct from making an animal sick. Perhaps the most thoroughly developed are studies of the contribution of the first portions of the gastrointestinal tract to satiety. Here anatomic structures, hormones, and food ingestion are seen to relate, and there is an emerging sense of their role in nutritional control.

Energy ingestion, regardless of body weight, is itself quite regulated. A dilution of the food energy leads to an increase in the volume of food consumed (Fomon et al., 1969), and an increase in energy expenditure leads to a compensatory increase in food consumed (Mayer et al., 1954). This responsiveness of daily food intake to the character of the nutrients and the energy needs must depend on a number of bodily systems, some, yet to be discerned, in the brain and others in the periphery that are tied to stomach, intestine, liver, and metabolism.

A variety of experimental designs have emerged to illuminate one or a set of such functions. For example, in monkeys, it is possible to show an inhibition on food intake that is precise when a preload of nutrients is infused into the stomach (McHugh and Moran, 1978). Eating is reduced by the amount of energy supplied in the preload. This occurs equally well for a preload delivered just before the animal's mealtime, when the satiating effect of the preload must depend, in part, on its effects on the stomach, as for a preload delivered 20 hours before mealtime, when effect cannot depend on the stomach directly because the preload will have passed through in the 20 hours. This influence of preloads on behavior is equally effective in obese and in normal animals and can even be demonstrated in animals that are gaining weight because of hypothalamic lesions. The mechanisms for these phenomena of feeding control remain obscure.

Finally, the ingestion of calories is accomplished in meals and the capacity of the organism to take a meal is primarily limited by the stomach. There is evidence that the stomach empties its contents in a calorically regulated fashion such that within certain limits, regardless of the character of the contents, they are delivered at a calorie-constant rate (Brener et al., 1983; Hunt and Stubbs, 1975; McHugh and Moran, 1979). The distention of the stomach could influence the size of a meal, and the rate of emptying of the nutrients into the intestine could influence the duration of the intermeal interval and thus the frequency of meals.

Body weight, daily caloric intake, and meal patterns are the controllable and related variables in the search for a set of mechanisms that could be the site of pathology and illuminate the behavior of food intake in normal and obese people.

Perhaps the most intriguing observation of the past decade was the demonstration that the hormone cholecystokinin (CCK) inhibits food intake when given to rats (Gibbs et al., 1973), monkeys (Gibbs et al., 1976), and humans (Kissileff et al., 1981). Interest in this observation derived from two aspects. First, CCK is an intestinal hormone released from the small intestine when food enters. That such a hormone might act to inhibit the intake of food itself had the attraction of being a plausible biologic feedback system. Second, CCK and receptors for CCK are plentiful in the central nervous system and in the hypothalamus. Here might be a circulating messenger from the periphery to the brain for controlling the feeding drive.

Much work has been accomplished during the two decades since the satiety function of CCK was discerned. In particular, it seems clear that much of the behavioral effect is satiety and not sickness or sedation, although it is likely that sickness can be provoked with high doses of exogenous CCK. The best evidence for this opinion has derived from the availability of CCK antagonists that can provoke increased food consumption, presumably from interference with endogenous CCK.

Issues for investigation, however, derived from efforts to determine the mechanism for CCK action. The initial thought was that the central nervous system receptors constitute the site of action of CCK released from the intestine. This idea, however, faced the problem that circulating CCK probably does not cross the blood-brain barrier at such sites as the hypothalamus. More likely, brain-derived CCK and circulating intestine-derived CCK may have different, even unrelated, functions. In fact, two quite distinct receptor systems for CCK have been discerned and distinguished by their specificity and location (Moran et al., 1986).

A second problem for conceptualizing the mechanism of CCK and satiety derives from the natural sequences of food intake. Food in humans and other nonruminants is taken in meals during which the behavior of feeding is sustained until, with a variable but usually considerable intake, satiety intervenes and food intake ceases. It is difficult to visualize how an intestinal hormone that is released promptly on the entrance of food into the gastrointestinal tract could act in such a pattern.

A proposed hypothesis was derived from the fact that one of CCK's physiologic functions is to inhibit gastric emptying. Therefore, some aspect of the hormone's satiety action might be indirect and derive from the effect of gastric inhibition on the state of the stomach during food intake. When a fasted animal eats, some food passes promptly into the intestine, provoking the secretory release of CCK. The hormone inhibits gastric emptying and thus facilitates distention of the stomach that occurs with continuing feeding. Feeding will stop when the stomach is distended and visceral afferent impulses are registered in the central nervous system (McHugh, 1979).

Some confirmation of this hypothesis has emerged. First, doses of CCK that are subthreshold for feeding inhibition in fasted animals act to inhibit feeding if the same doses are combined with a water load in the stomach that is retained by the inhibitory influence of CCK on gastric emptying (Moran and McHugh, 1982). Second, if the branches of the vagus nerve that carry afferent fibers from the stomach are cut, then CCK is much less effective as a satiety agent (G.P. Smith et al., 1981). Third, specific CCK receptors are found on the circular muscle of the pylorus and nowhere else in the gastrointestinal

tract, thus providing a location for CCK's inhibition on gastric emptying that promotes gastric distention during feeding (G.T. Smith et al., 1984). It now seems clear that CCK must be appreciated as a hormone that fits into meal taking. By inhibiting gastric emptying, CCK seems to be a hormone that helps to define and delimit meals. It is not a factor crucial to long-term nutritional control, as in body weight control or caloric regulation, but rather is a mealtime link in a chain of gastrointestinal events that coordinates feeding behavior with the filling and emptying of the stomach.

That circulating CCK may have effects on feeding other than an indirect action via its influence on gastric emptying is suggested by the presence of receptors at central nervous system sites where the blood-brain barrier is "permeable"—the area postrema (Moran et al., 1986). The CCK receptors here are different from other brain receptors in being quite specific for CCK itself. This is an identical specificity to the receptors on the pylorus. CCK at the area postrema and neighboring nucleus tractus solitarius may amplify visceral sensory input from the stomach and intestine through the vagus nerve, because it is the central entry site of vagal afferents. The area postrema may also be a site for sedation and for sickness that may be prompted by large amounts of circulating CCK produced by excess of food in the intestine.

It is uncertain how this or any other peripheral controls on the brain will explain human feeding disorders. We cannot show any of the power of clinical explanation from these studies as that revealed with hypothalamic experiments. Yet, there is emerging a conception of structures and functions, on which not only suggestions for pathology may rest but also a clear understanding of the interrelationships of behavior and the body in health and normal functioning. This is a new frontier in neurology and with its exploration will come a clearer understanding of some of the most obvious aspects of human brain function, motivated drives, to the service of which much motor sensory activity is directed.

References

(Key references are designated with an asterisk.)

*Anand B.K., Brobeck J.R. Hypothalamic control of food intake in rats and cats. *Yale J. Biol. Med.* 24:123–146, 1951.

*Andersen A.E. *Practical Comprehensive Treatment of Anorexia Nervosa and Bulimia.* Baltimore, The Johns Hopkins University Press, 1985.

Andersen A.E., Hedblom J.E., Hubbard F.A. A multidisciplinary team-treatment program for patients with anorexia nervosa and their families: preliminary reports of long-term outcome. *Int. J. Eating Disorders* 2:181–192, 1983.

Babinski M.J. Tumeur du corps pituitaire sans acromégalie et avec le développement des organes génitaux. *Rev. Neurol.* 8:531–533, 1900.

Beutler B., Greenwald D., Hulmes J.D., et al. Identity of tumor necrosis factor and the macrophage secreted factor cachectin. *Nature* 316:552–554, 1985.

Bray G.A., Gallagher T.F. Jr. Manifestations of hypothalamic obesity in man. *Medicine* 54:301–330, 1975.

Brener W., Hendrix T.R., McHugh P.R. Regulation of the gastric emptying of glucose. *Gastroenterology* 85:76–82, 1983.

Cannon W.B., Washburn A.L. An explanation of hunger. *Am. J. Physiol.* 29:441–455, 1912.

Cantwell D.P., Sturzenberger S., Burroughs J., et al. Anorexia nervosa: an affective disorder? *Arch. Gen. Psychiatry* 34:1087–1093, 1977.

Cerami A., Ikeda Y., Le Trang N., et al. Weight loss associated with an endotoxin-induced mediator from peritoneal macrophages: the role of cachectin (tumor necrosis factor). *Immunol. Lett.* 11:173–177, 1985.

Erdheim J. Uber einen neven Fall von Hypophysengangeschwulst. *Zentralbl. Allg. Pathol.* 17:209–215, 1906.

Fomon S.J., Filer L.J., Thomas, et al. Relationship between formula concentration and rate of growth of normal children. *J. Nutr.* 198:241–251, 1969.

Fong, Y., Moldower L.L., Marano M., et al. Cachectin/TNF or IL-la induces cachexia with redistribution of body proteins. *Am. J. Physiol.* 256:R659–R665, 1989.

Fröhlich A. Ein Fall von Tumor der Hypophysis cerebrei ohne Akromegalie. *Wein. Klin. Rosch.* 15:883–886, 1901.

Garfinkel P.E., Garner D.M., eds. *The Role of Drug Treatments for Eating Disorders.* New York, Brunner/Mazel, 1987.

Garfinkel P.E., Moldofsky H., Garner D.M. The heterogeneity of anorexia nervosa. *Arch. Gen. Psychiatry* 37:1036–1040, 1980.

Garn S.M., Clark D.C. Trends in fatness and the origins of obesity. *Pediatrics* 57:443–456, 1976.

Garner D.M., Garfinkel P.E. Socio-cultural factors in the development of anorexia nervosa. *Psychol. Med.* 10:647–656, 1980.

*Garrow J.S. The regulation of energy expenditure in man. In Bray G., ed. *Recent Advances in Obesity Research.* Vol. II. London, Newman Publishing, pp. 200–210, 1978.

Gibbs J., Young R.C., Smith G.P. Cholecystokinin decreases food intake in rats. *J. Comp. Physiol. Psychol.* 84:488–495, 1973.

Gibbs J., Falasco J.D., McHugh P.R. CCK decreased food intake in Rhesus monkeys. *Am. J. Physiol.* 230:15–18, 1976.

Goldblatt P.B., Moore M.E., Stunkard A.J. Social factors in obesity. *J.A.M.A.* 192:1039–1042, 1965.

Gordon T., Kannel W.B. The effects of overweight on cardiovascular diseases. *Geriatrics* 28:80–90, 1973.

Halmi K.A., Eckert E., LaDu T.J., et al. Anorexia nervosa. Treatment efficacy of cyproheptadine and amitriptyline. *Arch. Gen. Psychiatry* 43:177–181, 1986.

Hetherington A.W., Ranson S.W. Hypothalamic lesions and adiposity in the rat. *Anat. Rec.* 76:149–172, 1940.

*Hirsch J., Knittle J.C. Cellularity of obese and non obese adipose tissue. *Fed. Proc.* 29:1516–1521, 1970.

Hunt J.N., Stubbs D.F. The volume and energy content of meals as determinants of gastric emptying. *J. Physiol. (Lond.)* 245:209–225, 1975.

Ingalls A.M., Dickie M.M., Snell G.D. Obesity, a mutation in the mouse. *J. Hered.* 41:317–318, 1950.

James W.P.T. *DHSSMRC Report on Research on Obesity.* London, Her Majesty's Stationery Office, 1976.

Kissileff H.R., Pi-Sunyer F.X., Thornton J., et al. C-terminal octapeptide of cholecystokinin decreases food intake in man. *Am. J. Clin. Nutr.* 34:154–160, 1981.

*Kral J. Surgical therapy for obesity. In Greenwood M.R.C., ed. *Obesity.* New York, Churchill Livingstone, 1983.

Krotkiewski M., Sjostrom L., Bjortorp P. Adipose tissue cellularity in relation to prognosis for weight reduction. *Int. J. Obes.* 1:395–416, 1977.

Mayer J., Marshall N.B., Vitale J.J., et al. Exercise, food intake and body weight in normal rats and genetically obese adult mice. *Am. J. Physiol.* 177:544–548, 1954.

*McHugh P.R. Aspects of the control of feeding: Application of quantitation in psychobiology. *Johns Hopkins Med. J.* 144:147–155, 1979.

McHugh P.R., Moran T.H. Accuracy of the regulation of caloric ingestion in the monkey. *Am. J. Physiol.* 235:R29–R34, 1978.

McHugh P.R., Gibbs J., Falasco J.D., et al. Inhibitions on feeding examined in rhesus monkeys with hypothalamic disconnexions. *Brain* 98:441–454, 1975.

McHugh P.R., Moran T.H., Killilea M. The approaches to the study of human disorders in food ingestion and body weight maintenance. *N. Y. Acad. Sci.* 575:1–12, 1989.

Moran T.H., McHugh P.R. Cholecystokinin suppresses food intake by inhibiting gastric emptying. *Am. J. Physiol* 242:R491–R497, 1982.

Moran T.H., Robinson P.H., Goldrich M.S., et al. Two brain cholecystokinin receptors: implications for behavioral actions. *Brain Res.* 362:175–179, 1986.

Oliff A. The role of tumor necrosis factor (cachectin) in cachexia. *Cell* 54:141–142, 1988.

Reeves A.G., Plum F. Hyperphagia, rage and dementia accompanying a ventromedial hypothalamic neoplasm. *Arch. Neurol.* 20:616–624, 1969.

Sclafani A., Springer D. Dietary obesity in adult rats, similarity to hypothalamic and human obesity syndromes. *Physiol. Behav.* 17:461–470, 1976.

Silverstone T. Psychosocial aspects of obesity. *Proc. R. Soc. Med.* 61:371–375, 1968.

Smith G.P., Jerome C., Cushin B., et al. Abdominal vagotomy blocks the satiety effect of cholecystokinin in the rat. *Science* 213:1036–1037, 1981.

*Smith G.T., Moran T.H., Coyle J.T., et al. Anatomic localization of cholecystokinin receptors to the pyloric sphincter. *Am. J. Physiol.* 246:R127–R130, 1984.

Stellar E. The physiology of motivation. *Psychol. Rev.* 61:5–22, 1954.

Stunkard A.J., Brownell K.D. Behavior therapy and self help programs for obesity. In Munro J.F., ed. *Treatment of Obesity.* London, MTP Press, 1979.

Stunkard A.J., Penick S.B. Behavior modification in the treatment of obesity. *Arch. Gen. Psychiatry* 36:801–806, 1979.

Stunkard A.J., Foch T.T., Hrubec Z. A twin study of human obesity. *J.A.M.A.* 256:51–54, 1986a.

Stunkard A.J., Sorenson T.R., Hanis C., et al. An adoption study of human obesity. *N. Engl. J. Med.* 314:193–195, 1986b.

Tepperman J., Brobeck J.R., Long C.N.H. The effects of hypothalamic hyperphagia and of alterations in feeding habits on the metabolism of the albino rat. *Yale J. Biol. Med.* 15:855–870, 1943.

38

Pathophysiology of Respiratory Dysfunction

Roger P. Simon

Respiration requires a combination of the mechanical aspects of ventilation with the physical and chemical events of alveolar gas exchange at the pulmonary capillary. The nervous system affects both processes, although much more is known about the mechanics of ventilation. (See also Chapter 108.)

NEURONAL CONTROL OF VENTILATION

Peripheral Receptor Systems

The carotid bodies of the carotid bifurcation and the aortic bodies of the anterior and posterior portions of the ascending aorta mediate increased central ventilatory drive in response to decreased P_{O_2} or an increase in P_{CO_2}; the carotid bodies respond to a fall in arterial pH as well. Receptor firing is also increased by a decrease in receptor blood flow, which may be caused either by a fall in systemic blood pressure or by an increase in sympathetic activity that reduces receptor blood flow by vasoconstriction. A rapid increase in chemoreceptor activity occurs as P_{O_2} falls from 100 to 30 torr. In laboratory experiments, the system is able to respond to changes in P_{O_2} values up to 500 torr. The response to P_{CO_2} and pH is linear over the physiologic range (20–60 torr; 7.2–7.7, respectively).

A number of neurotransmitters are found in the carotid body; the most prominent, dopamine, may act to inhibit impulses at the afferent nerve terminal in response to excitatory neurotransmitter release. Afferent nerve endings serve as the chemoreceptor (Mitchell et al., 1972).

Receptors sensitive to mechanical stimulation are found throughout the upper airway from the nasal mucosa to the trachea (Table 38–1). Activation of these receptors affects respiratory neurons in the medulla, producing apnea, coughing, or sniffing. The proximity of the medullary respiratory centers to cardiovascular control centers may explain the hypertension that accompanies these respiratory reflexes.

Within the lung tissue, three groups of receptors have been described (Table 38–2), each with vagal afferents projecting to the caudal medulla. The best characterized are the pulmonary stretch receptors of airway smooth muscle. Lung inflation produces activation of these receptors, which continues as long as lung distention is maintained, resulting in the Hering-Breuer reflex (a slowing of respiratory rate produced by an increase in expiratory time) (Hering, 1867). The reflex is centrally modulated and species dependent and is of greater significance in the respiratory regulation of animals than in that of humans (Guz et al., 1970). Thus, during normal breathing vagal blockade does not alter respiratory frequency or tidal volume in humans.

The role of the irritant receptors and the J receptors is less clear. These receptors are believed to detect airway irritants and pulmonary congestion, respectively, but the mechanism by which they produce this effect is uncertain. Nadel (1973) reported that irritant receptors in asthmatics are stimulated by histamine, with a resulting bronchoconstriction that does not occur by the direct application of histamine to the airway smooth muscle. Because these receptors have their afferent fibers in the vagus, a central nervous system (CNS) role in this reflex is possible.

Central Ventilatory Control

The brain stem transection experiments of Lumsden (1923) established the concept of respiratory

Table 38–1. UPPER AIRWAY RECEPTORS

Structure	Afferent Path	Efferent Respiratory Reflex	Other Effects
Nose	Trigeminal nerve	Apnea, sneezing	Bradycardia
Epipharynx	Glossopharyngeal nerve (pharyngeal branch)	Sharp inspiration (sniffling reflex)	Bronchodilation hypertension
Larynx	Superior laryngeal nerve (internal branch)	Cough, apnea, slow deep breathing	Bronchoconstriction hypertension
Trachea	Vagus	Coughing	Bronchoconstriction hypertension

centers in the hindbrain (Fig. 38–1). Transection of the brain stem at the level of the inferior colliculus does not alter the ventilatory pattern. If the vagi are cut as well, ventilation slows and deepens as it does after vagotomy in the absence of brain stem transection. Transection at the upper border of the cerebellar peduncles produces slow deep breathing. With the vagi cut, in addition, apneusis (markedly prolonged end-inspiratory time) occurs. The pneumotaxic center is found between these levels, and the apneustic center is below the level of the caudal transection. Transection at the pontomedullary junction produces rhythmic breathing with a gasping quality; this pattern is unchanged by vagal transection. Finally, brain stem transection at the medullary-cervical junction ablates all respiration. These ventilatory patterns are illustrated in Figure 38–2.

Pneumotaxic Center

The pneumotaxic center is localized by modern techniques to the area of the nucleus parabrachialis–Kölliker-Fuse complex (Kalia, 1977). The major role of this neuronal region is inspiratory "off switching," which is modified at least in part by the Hering-Breuer (and possibly other) afferents carried in the vagus (Gautier and Bertrand, 1975).

Apneustic "Center"

Although vagotomy combined with brain stem transection below the nucleus parabrachialis produces the phenomenon of the prolonged inspiratory state termed *apneusis*, no single neuronal pool producing this event has been identified. The apneustic

phenomenon is a respiratory state that is the end result of any one of several lesions or pharmacologic manipulations (Sears, 1977). Medullary stimulation in the reticular formation near the obex produces tonic diaphragmatic and external intercostal contraction (Andersen and Sears, 1970). Apneusis also follows lesioning of afferent pathways in ventrolateral cervical cord in animals previously vagotomized or prepared with lesions of the pneumotaxic center (Krieger et al., 1972). Apneusis occurs in vagotomized cats on the institution of anesthesia (Gautier and Bertrand, 1975). Apneustic breaths can be stopped by stimulation of intercostal afferents (Remmers and Marttila, 1975).

Thus, the phenomenon of apneusis results from the failure of one or more neural projection systems to produce inspiratory off switching. Berger et al. (1977) suggested that the state of sustained inspiration results from sustained firing of primary respiratory medullary inspiratory neurons.

Medullary Center

Two neuronal pools, the dorsal respiratory group (DRG) and the ventral respiratory group (VRG), constitute the medullary center (Fig. 38–3). A rhythmic but not normal ventilatory pattern is produced from these centers. The DRG is in the ventrolateral portion of the nucleus of the tractus solitarius, and the VRG is located in the nucleus ambiguus and the nucleus retroambiguus. The nucleus of the tractus solitarius receives all primary afferents from cranial nerves IX and X (Cottle, 1964), thus supplying the afferent projections from the pulmonary receptors and baroreceptors. The DRG is composed of

Table 38–2. INTRAPULMONARY RECEPTORS

Type of Receptor	Site	Excitation Stimulus	Afferent Pathway	Respiratory Effect	Other Effects
Pulmonary stretch receptors	Airway smooth muscle	Lung distention	Vagus—large myelinated fibers	Increased expiratory time resulting in decreased ventilatory rate (Hering-Breuer reflex)	Bronchoconstriction, increased heart rate
Irritant receptors	Airway epithelial cells	Chemical and particulate irritants	Vagus—large myelinated fibers	Hyperpnea	Bronchoconstriction
J receptors (juxtapulmonary capillary)	Pulmonary capillary wall	Increased interstitial fluid volume	Vagus—unmyelinated fibers	Apnea	Decreased heart rate and blood pressure

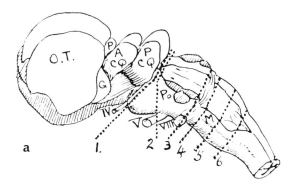

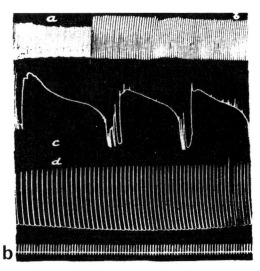

Figure 38–1. *(a)* The original illustration from Lumsden (1923), showing the level of critical sections in cats. *(b)* Respiratory tracings from Lumsden (1923): a, normal animal; b, after vagotomy; c, apneusis (transection 2, in *a*); d, gasping (after transection 4, in *a*). Transection between lines 5 and 6 produces cessation of all ventilatory movements. (From Lumsden T. Observations on the respiratory centres in the cat. *J. Physiol. [Lond.]* 57:153, 1923.)

primary inspiratory neurons that rhythmically drive the VRG and project to the contralateral cord to innervate phrenic motor neurons (Bystrzycka et al., 1975). The VRG contains both inspiratory and expiratory cells, the former projecting to the contralateral cord and innervating intercostal and some phrenic motor neurons. The latter cells project to the contralateral thoracic and high lumbar cord to innervate intercostal and abdominal respiratory musculature (Merrill, 1974). The neurotransmitters of these bulbospinal neurons innervating spinal respiratory motor neurons are excitatory amino acids (McCrimmon et al., 1989).

Transection at the medullary cervical junction ablates all respiratory movement; thus, the respiratory rhythm generator lies above this level. The site of the origin of normal respiratory rhythm generation, however, is not certain. Berger et al. (1977) stated that a site in or near the DRG is likely.

Forebrain Respiratory Influences

Plum (1970) reviewed the role of prepontine structures in ventilatory function. He described 15 elderly

patients with apraxia of volitional breathing. Each patient was unable to take a deep breath or to hold his or her breath on command. Evidence of diffuse CNS dysfunction was present in that the patients were easily confused in the hospital setting; however, none was felt to be incapacitated. Mild frontal release signs were present; some patients had difficulty in volitional swallowing. No other evidence of apraxia or corticobulbar dysfunction was present, and no patient had Cheyne-Stokes (CS) respiration. Although diffuse hemispheric disease may have been responsible for respiratory apraxia in these patients, an extrapyramidal cause, as well, is supported by the prominent inability of breath holding in postencephalitic Parkinson's disease (Kim, 1968).

Stimulation in the motor and premotor areas of the cortex may modestly increase ventilation; however, the major effect of cortical stimulation on respiration is that of inhibition (Plum, 1970; Plum and Leigh, 1981). Evidence for hemispheric inhibition comes from stimulation studies with animals (Kaada, 1960) (Fig. 38–4) and humans (Kaada and Jasper, 1952). Areas producing such inhibition (uncus, fornix, amygdala, anterior cingulate gyrus, anterior insular cortex, inferior medial temporal cortex, and posterior lateral frontal cortex) mainly form the limbic system (D.A. Nelson and Ray, 1968). Arrest of ventilation for 56 seconds has occurred after cortical stimulation in humans (Kaada and Jasper, 1952), and prolonged apnea and hypoventilation to the point of asphyxia have been demonstrated during cortical stimulation in animals (Reis and McHugh, 1968). Spontaneous seizures from limbic structures in humans have also produced apnea as an ictal event (Plum, 1970). In an additional patient reported by D.A. Nelson and Ray (1968), nine such episodes occurred; one that occurred during ictal monitoring via electroencephalography required mechanical ventilation for 30 hours.

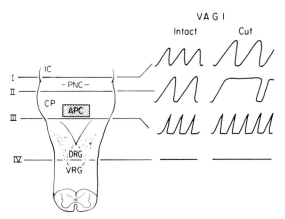

Figure 38–2. Effects of brain stem and vagal transections on the ventilatory pattern in an anesthetized animal. Tracings on the right represent the tidal volume with inspiration upward. APC = apneustic center; CP = cerebellar peduncle; DRG = dorsal respiratory group; IC = inferior colliculus; PNC = pneumotaxic center; VRG = ventral respiratory group. (From Berger A.J., Mitchell R.A., Severinghaus J.W. Regulation of respiration. *N. Engl. J. Med.* 297:138–143, 1977.)

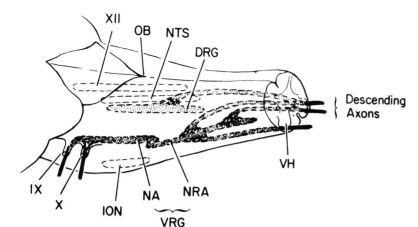

Figure 38-3. Schematic representation of the dorsal (DRG) and ventral (VRG) respiratory groups with their efferent projections in cat brain stem. ION = inferior olivary nucleus; NA = nucleus ambiguus; NRA = nucleus retroambiguus; NTS = nucleus tractus solitarius; OB = obex; VH = ventral horn; XII = hypoglossal nucleus. (From Mitchell R.A., Berger A. Neural regulation of respiration. *Am. Rev. Respir. Dis.* 111:206–224, 1975.)

Cortical structures also affect ventilation, although no specific anatomic region has been identified in this regard (Brown and Plum, 1961). This observation is based on increased ventilatory responses to CO_2 in patients with bilateral cortical infarctions who were compared with age-matched normal control subjects and patients with brain stem lesions. Heyman et al. (1958) noted hypocapnea at rest in such patients as well.

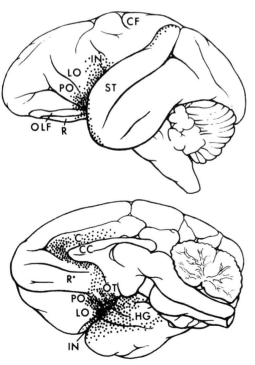

Figure 38-4. Points on the anterolateral *(upper)* and ventromedial *(lower)* cerebral cortex of *Macaca mulatta* at which electrical stimulation elicited inhibition of respiration. C = cingulate gyrus; HG = hippocampal gyrus; IN = insula; LO = lateral orbital gyrus; PO = posterior orbital gyrus; R = gyrus rectus; ST = superior temporal gyrus. (From Kaada B.R. Somato-motor, autonomic and electrocorticographic responses to electrical stimulation of "rhinencephalic" and other structures in primates, cat and dog. *Acta Physiol. Scand.* 24:1–285, 1951.)

Extrapyramidal Disorders

Disorders of respiratory rhythm were prominent features of postencephalitic parkinsonism (Turner and Critchley, 1925). Tachypnea to 100 breaths per minute was described, and respiratory tics were common. In the chronic phase of this disease, a fixed tachypnea occurred and the normal variation in respiratory amplitude was attenuated. The inability to alter the pattern of automatic respiration for speaking or breath holding was striking (Kim, 1968).

A syndrome of respiratory dyskinesias has been described in patients with tardive or levodopa-induced dyskinesia (Weiner et al., 1978; Zupnick et al., 1990). Tests of cardiopulmonary function are normal, but the patients' complaints are of true dyspnea. The apparent cause of this air hunger is dyskinesia of ventilatory muscles that produces respiratory irregularity resulting in the sensation of shortness of breath and chest discomfort. Upper airway muscles may be involved in extrapyramidal disorders as well. In 27 parkinsonian patients studied by Vincken et al. (1984), abnormal airflow was found in 24. This resulted from oscillation of flow related to rhythmic (4–8/second) contractions of glottic and supraglottic upper airway muscles. Upper airway obstruction was demonstrated in 10 patients, 4 of whom were symptomatic. Increased airway symptoms coincided with a marked increase in peripheral tremor in these patients.

Posthyperventilation Apnea

The observation that brief periods of apnea follow hyperventilation in anesthetized animals was made by Haring in 1867. Plum et al. (1962) studied respirations in patients, following five deep breaths on command, in whom arterial P_{CO_2} fell 8–14 torr. In normal subjects or patients without CNS disease, no posthyperventilation apnea (PHA) occurred in 83% and in only 2% of the control subjects did apnea persist for longer than 12 seconds ($n = 137$). The results were independent of age groupings of patients over or under 50 years old. In patients with bilateral disease of the CNS, PHA was absent in 6% and occurred for longer than 12 seconds in 78% ($n = 70$). Again, the results were independent of age. The authors concluded that prolonged (greater than 12 seconds) PHA suggested bilateral CNS disease.

Some different conclusions were drawn by Jennett et al. (1974), who compared PHA in 50 patients on a neurosurgical ward with 50 control subjects. Apnea in control subjects never exceeded 5–10 seconds. PHA occurred in 68% of the neurosurgical patients. However, PHA was as frequent (67%) in neurosurgical patients with unilateral damage as in those with bilateral (70%) damage. There was no correlation between a fall in end-tidal CO_2 and the occurrence of apnea, thus suggesting that hypocapnea may not be the cause of PHA. Patients who could not lower their end-tidal CO_2 were excluded from Plum's study. The most important factor in Jennett's patients was the level of consciousness: 95% of the drowsy neurosurgical patients demonstrated PHA as opposed to only 48% of those who were alert during the study. PHA, then, is an indication of CNS dysfunction, but the anatomic localization of such dysfunction is uncertain.

Cheyne-Stokes Breathing

CS breathing is a respiratory pattern in which escalating hyperventilation alternates with decremental hypoventilation ending in apnea. The cycle length in humans is approximately 40–100 seconds (R.I. Lange and Hecht, 1962) (Fig. 38–5). Arterial blood gases show a pattern of respiratory alkalosis (increased pH, decreased PCO_2), maximal at the apnea point and never returning to the normal range. PO_2 varies inversely with the respiratory frequency, with its nadir occurring at the apnea point (Fig. 38–6). Ventilatory periodicity is suppressed by breathing oxygen. The ventilatory cycles may be associated with cyclic variations in neurologic signs: diminished

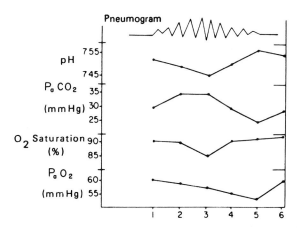

Figure 38–6. Relationship of blood gases to respiratory cycle in CS breathing. (From Brown W.H., Plum F. The neurologic basis of Cheyne-Stokes respiration. *Am. J. Med.* 30:849–860, 1961.)

consciousness, decreased muscle tone, miosis, and bradycardia. Cerebrovascular responsiveness to CO_2 produces alterations in cerebral blood flow during the ventilatory cycles and thus intracranial pressure varies (secondary to changes in the volume of the intravascular compartment) (Karp et al., 1961).

Although CS breathing may be a normal pattern during sleep and at altitude (Cherniack, 1981), its occurrence in CNS disease is well recognized. Its pathogenesis concerning circulatory versus neural factors continues to be a matter of debate, however, as discussed later.

In 1961 Brown and Plum studied 28 patients on a medical service who had waxing and waning ventilatory patterns. All had bilateral pyramidal signs, and five of these patients had no cardiac abnormalities. All had a fixed respiratory alkalosis, with a maximal PCO_2 at the peak of the ventilatory phase and a minimal PCO_2 at the onset of apnea. A rise in arterial pH mirrored the falling PCO_2. Although all patients had a circulation time greater than normal, many values were only modestly elevated and not greater than those in the elderly control patients. Patients with congestive heart failure but without CS ventilation had circulation times slightly greater than the CS patients under study. Brown and Plum hypothesized that this respiratory pattern resulted from an increased respiratory drive to CO_2, as previously described in patients with bilateral CNS disease (Heyman et al., 1958). Oxygen suppresses the respiratory periodicity by eliminating the hypoxic drive to respiration during the nadir of the PCO_2 levels.

The issue of abnormal feedback control to the CNS in the generation of respiratory oscillation has been studied by Cherniack et al. (1979). By using the phrenic nerve stimulus of an experimental animal to trigger a mechanical ventilator, the gain of which could be varied to amplify or retard the tidal volume produced by each such phrenic stimulus, it was found that periodic respirations were produced by an increased gain. This effect was eliminated by destruction of peripheral chemoreceptors but was

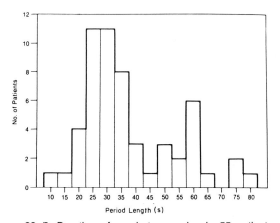

Figure 38–5. Duration of respiratory cycles in 55 patients with periodic breathing. (From North J.B., Jennett S. Abnormal breathing patterns associated with acute brain damage. *Arch. Neurol.* 31:338–344, 1974. Copyright 1974, American Medical Association.)

unaltered by vagotomy. The oscillation was enhanced by hypoxia and by depression (via local cooling) of the medullary CO_2 receptor areas. The breathing of 100% O_2 or of CO_2-enriched air also eliminated the oscillatory response. All animals with periodic respiration had respiratory alkalosis, as occurs in humans with CS breathing.

The issue of circulation time in the production of CS respirations stemmed from the observations by Guyton et al. (1956) that marked prolongation (2 minutes or more) of the transit time for blood from carotid artery to central receptors in brain resulted in respiratory oscillation. Guyton and colleagues suggested that a feedback delay to central receptors was responsible. R.I. Lange and Hecht (1962) studied nine patients with prolonged circulation times (lung to artery) related to congestive heart failure; each patient demonstrated CS breathing. There were no CNS abnormalities in five of the patients, and in two patients this was verified at postmortem examination. Thus, in this patient group, increased circulation time alone appeared to produce CS breathing. From plots of P_{CO_2} and ventilatory rates of these patients, the authors argued that the persistent respiratory alkalosis characteristic of CS breathing is explained by the ventilatory oscillations alone without invoking central hypersensitivity to P_{CO_2}.

Another study suggested that respiratory oscillations may be generated from the CNS itself. A central oscillatory drive to ventilation was described in experiments by Preiss et al. (1975) in a model of brain stem ischemia. The respiratory oscillations in this model persisted after elimination of afferent responses from chemoreceptors and baroreceptors, thus supporting a central origin.

Central Hyperventilation

This pattern of rapid regular ventilation is of prognostic but not localizing value (Leigh and Shaw, 1976; North and Jennett, 1974). In 1959, Plum and Swanson reported the phenomenon of "central neurogenic hyperventilation" in a patient with a brain stem tumor and suggested an association between this respiratory pattern and the patient's lesion site in the medial mesencephalic reticular formation. Later, McNealy and Plum (1962) included this ventilatory pattern as a localizing sign of midbrain compression during transtentorial herniation. Plum (1970) subsequently reported the inability to reproduce this respiratory pattern by mesencephalic and pontine lesions in experimental animals and noted that pulmonary congestion probably explained the hyperventilation in such patients. Such pulmonary congestion might be due to neurogenic pulmonary edema (Plum, 1972), with the stimulation of pulmonary afferents that responded to lung congestion producing the observed tachypnea (Plum, 1982). Experimental support for pulmonary edema in such patients awaits confirmation. Although an elevation in pulmonary transcapillary fluid flux has been demonstrated, frank pulmonary edema has not been reproduced from any focal CNS lesion in an animal model in which the permeability characteristics of the pulmonary capillary bed can be assessed (Simon and Bayne, 1984). At the San Francisco General Hospital, the author saw three patients who fulfilled the clinical requirements of central neurogenic hyperventilation after stroke. Their in vivo lung water was measured with a double-indicator dilution technique (Frank Lewis, Department of Surgery, personal communication). In each patient, the values were normal.

The localizing value of this respiratory pattern for midbrain lesions (Plum and Swanson, 1959) has not been confirmed. In the 227 neurosurgical patients studied by North and Jennett (1974), tachypnea was not associated with lesion site (from the hemisphere to medulla), and the site of the lesion (except medullary lesions) did not predict normal versus abnormal ventilatory patterns (Table 38–3). In addition, no localizing value of rapid regular ventilation was found in comatose patients studied by Leigh and Shaw (1976).

Studies such as these are open to criticism regarding mass effect, intracranial blood, and coexisting metabolic factors. Three cases of localized brain stem tumors in patients with central hyperventilation have been reported with postmortem data, thus permitting uncompromised pathophysiologic correlations. In two cases, the tumor involved the medulla and lower pons (Goulon et al., 1969; Rodriguez et al., 1982); in the third, the midbrain and pons were involved but the medulla was spared (L.S. Lange and Laszlo, 1965). Thus, a midbrain localization for lesions producing this ventilatory state is no longer tenable. Plum (1982) suggested that local lactate production from such tumors may produce stimulation of medullary chemoreceptors (Mitchell et al., 1963), thereby explaining the lack of correlation between anatomic site and ventilatory pattern in tumor patients.

Apneusis

The prominent, prolonged, end-inspiratory pause produced by pontine transection in vagotomized

Table 38–3. INCIDENCE OF EACH ABNORMAL VENTILATORY PATTERN IN ASSOCIATION WITH EACH SITE OF DAMAGE

Site	Periodic Pattern	Irregular Pattern	Tachypnea
Bilateral hemisphere	17	21	20
Unilateral hemisphere	30	21	27
Suprasellar	4	3	1
Midbrain	5	5	4
Pons	3	9*	5
Medulla	1	8†	4
Cerebellum	6	8	6

*Significant, $P = .01–.05$.
†Highly significant, $P < .01$.

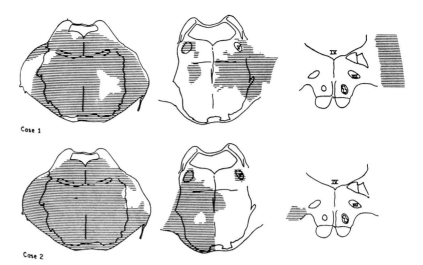

Figure 38–7. Areas of brain stem infarction in two patients with apneustic breathing. (From Plum F., Alvord E.C. Jr. Apneustic breathing in man. *Arch. Neurol.* 10:101–112, 1964. Copyright 1964, American Medical Association.)

Case 1

Case 2

animals (Lumsden, 1923; Sears, 1977) is rare in humans. This respiratory pattern was not seen in 23 patients with brain stem infarction who were being observed specifically for respiratory rate and pattern (Lee et al., 1976). The single clinical report of two human cases is of note, however, because the anatomic lesion (Fig. 38–7) caused by the basilar thrombosis in these patients corresponds closely to lesions producing apneusis in experimental animals (Plum and Alvord, 1964). Both patients had complete brain stem transection just rostral to the trigeminal motor nuclei and the nucleus parabrachialis. As opposed to the animal lesions producing apneusis, however, the vagi and their afferent connections were anatomically and clinically intact in these patients.

Ataxic Breathing

Marked irregularity of respiratory rhythm was most conspicuous in patients with bulbar poliomyelitis (Plum and Swanson, 1958) and has been reported with brain stem encephalitis (North and Jennett, 1974). Irregular ventilation occurred in 52 of 257 neurosurgical patients of North and Jennett (1974). Medullary lesions were most likely to produce this respiratory pattern, and each of the 12 patients with medullary involvement demonstrated an abnormal respiratory pattern (see Table 38–3). Medullary compression probably explains the irregular respiration seen in cerebellar hemorrhage (Fisher et al., 1965), as well.

Impaired Automatic Ventilation

Pathways from cortex subserving voluntary respiration and those from primary respiratory neuronal pools of the medulla descend to innervate spinal, phrenic, intercostal, and diaphragmatic respiratory motor neurons via separate pathways within the neuroaxis (Fig. 38–8). Thus, selective impairment of automatic or voluntary breathing is possible. Exper-

iments with animals (Aminoff and Sears, 1971) and observations in humans (Newsom-Davis, 1974) place the descending pathways that are under voluntary control within the dorsolateral cord in the region of the corticospinal tract. Pathways from primary medullary respiratory centers, providing the automatic respiratory drive, travel in the ventrolateral cord, with anatomic separation of inspiratory and expiratory pathways (Newsom-Davis and Plum, 1972).

Involvement of the lateral spinal cord with sparing of the ventral cord in a patient with transverse myelitis produced upper extremity and trunk paralysis but permitted automatic breathing that could not be voluntarily altered (Newsom-Davis, 1974). A patient with the converse situation, preserved voluntary but impaired automatic breathing, risks apnea during sleep (Cherniack, 1981). This symptom com-

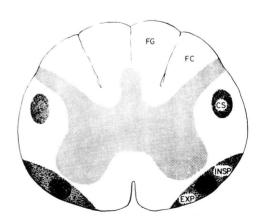

Figure 38–8. Location of the descending respiratory pathways in the cervical cord of cat. Voluntary control is in corticospinal tracts (CS). Involuntary pathways, both rhythmic and nonrhythmic, lie in the ventral and lateral columns *(cross-hatched regions)*. EXP = descending expiratory axons; INSP = inspiratory axons; FG = funiculus gracilis; FC = funiculus cuneatus. (From Mitchell R.A., Berger A. Neural regulation of respiration. *Am. Rev. Respir. Dis.* 111:206–224, 1975.)

plex has been termed *Ondine's curse* (Severinghaus and Mitchell, 1962), with reference to Jean Giraudoux's (translated 1956) interpretation of the mode of death of the Knight Hans, a German mythologic figure. Because of his infidelity to the sea nymph Ondine, Hans was cursed to require voluntary control over automatic functions: "He died, they will say, because it was a nuisance to breathe." This syndrome may be produced by lesions ranging from the area of the primary respiratory neurons of the medulla to the descending pathways in the cervical cord. Primary medullary lesions were responsible in bulbar poliomyelitis (Plum and Swanson, 1958). Both unilateral (Askenasy and Goldhammer, 1988; Levin and Margolis, 1977) and bilateral (Devereaux et al., 1973) medullary tegmental infarcts have produced the syndrome (Fig. 38–9). High cervical cord lesions are responsible after cervical cordotomy for pain or operative procedures in the region of the anterior cord (Krieger and Rosomoff, 1974; Tranmer et al., 1987). Idiopathic cases are referred to as idiopathic primary alveolar hypoventilation (Mellins et al., 1970); other abnormalities of autonomic function may be associated (Haddad et al., 1978).

Mechanical obstruction of the upper airway during sleep produces another group of sleep apneas (Onal et al., 1982), some of which have a neuropathic ideology, such as oropharyngeal weakness in syringobulbia (Haponik et al., 1983), olivopontocerebellar degeneration (Adelman et al., 1984), multiple system atrophy with autonomic failure (Munschauer et al., 1990), brain stem compression in achondroplasia (F.W. Nelson et al., 1988), and the lateral medullary syndrome (Chaudhary et al., 1982). Central and obstructive sleep apnea may coexist, as well (Guilleminault et al., 1976; Kales et al., 1987; Snyderman et al., 1982).

IMPAIRED PULMONARY GAS EXCHANGE

Regulation of the Starling Forces at the Pulmonary Capillary

Oxygen transport in the lung requires the mechanical action of ventilation combined with gas transport at the pulmonary capillary. A number of neurologic disorders may primarily affect capillary gas exchange in the lung; pulmonary edema of neurogenic origin is the most dramatic result (Simon, 1984).

The major effect of CNS disorders on pulmonary gas exchange is that of a neurally induced increase in fluid flux out of the pulmonary capillary bed into the interstitium and then into the alveolar air space. The variables for regulation of fluid flux from any capillary bed are dependent on the Starling equation:

$$\dot{Q}_f = K_f \left[(P_{mv} - P_{pmv}) - \sigma(II_{mv} - II_{pmv}) \right]$$

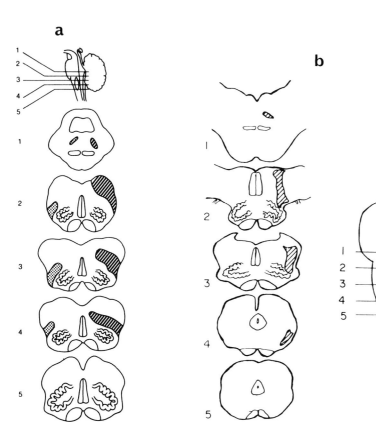

a

b

Figure 38–9. *(a)* Location of bilateral brain stem infarcts in a patient with automatic respiratory failure. *(b)* Brain stem sections showing a unilateral lesion that resulted in failure of automatic respiration. (*a* from Devereaux M.W., Keane J.R., Davis R.L. Autonomic respiratory failure associated with infarction of the medulla. *Arch. Neurol.* 29:46–52, 1973. Copyright 1973, American Medical Association. *b* from Levin B.E., Margolis G. Acute failure of autonomic respirations secondary to a unilateral brain stem infarct. Reprinted with permission from *Annals of Neurology*, volume 1, pages 583–586, 1977.)

where pmv = perimicrovascular; mv = microvascular. (Microvascular refers to the portion of the pulmonary capillary bed at which fluid exchange occurs.) Net fluid flux (Q_f) is the sum of the forces driving fluid out of the vascular lumen (intravascular pressure [P_{mv}] and oncotic forces outside the capillary lumen [II_{pmv}]) combined with the opposing forces driving the fluid into the vascular lumen (oncotic forces of intravascular proteins [II_{mv}] and the extravascular pressure [P_{pmv}]).

Whether pulmonary capillary permeability in the lung can be directly influenced by neuronal mechanisms remains uncertain (Rosell, 1980), but it is clear that there is a CNS effect on pulmonary intravascular pressure, the major factor in the outward movement of fluid from the pulmonary capillary bed (Minnear and Malik, 1982). Of these neural factors, generalized seizures and intracranial pressure elevation are the best studied.

Generalized seizures produce systemic and pulmonary vascular hypertension. The pulmonary vascular pressure, but not the systemic pressure, increases with the number and duration of seizures (Fig. 38–10). The pulmonary vascular pressures produced are well above the level of plasma oncotic pressures (Bayne and Simon, 1981) and result in a doubling of fluid flux out of the capillary bed into the interstitial space, which persists for at least 3 hours after the seizures (Simon et al., 1982) (Fig. 38–11). Such a sequence of events probably explains postictal pulmonary edema in humans (Darnell and Jay, 1982; Terrance et al., 1981).

Intracranial pressure elevation is frequently cited as the major cause of pulmonary edema from CNS injury (Bloch, 1967; Ducker et al., 1968). There is no effect of intracranial pressure elevation on pulmonary transcapillary fluid flux, however, until intracranial pressure approaches systemic pressure and the Cushing response of systemic hypertension occurs. Pulmonary vascular pressures rise as well, producing a doubling of pulmonary transcapillary fluid flux as a consequence of the increased pulmonary vascular pressure (Simon and Bayne, 1984). In humans, the major predictor of survival from head injury is this elevation in pulmonary vascular pressure and not the degree of increased intracranial pressure (Popp et al., 1982). In some animal studies, a change in pulmonary vascular permeability to protein has been described after increased intracranial pressure in the absence of prominent elevations of pulmonary vascular pressure (McClellan et al., 1989). Other studies with veratrine injection into the fourth ventricle identified pulmonary vascular hypertension as the major factor in neurogenic pulmonary edema (Maron, 1985, 1987).

Clinical studies suggest that brain stem lesions are the most likely focal areas of brain injury to result in frank pulmonary edema of CNS origin (Baker, 1957; Harari et al., 1976; Schlesinger, 1945; Yamour et al., 1980). Darragh and Simon (1985) lesioned central termini of pulmonary afferent and carotid baroreceptors in the nucleus tractus solitarius within the caudal

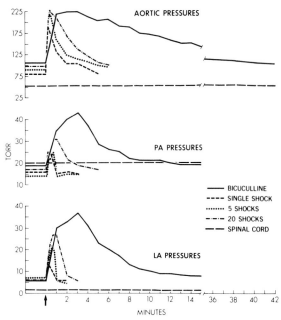

Figure 38–10. Time course of vascular pressure elevations during seizures. Arrow indicates seizure induction. Data are mean values at 10-second intervals. Spinal cord refers to animals with cervical cord transection before seizures. PA = pulmonary artery; LA = left atrium. (From Bayne L., Simon R.P. Systemic and pulmonary vascular pressures during generalized seizures in sheep. Reprinted with permission from *Annals of Neurology*, volume 10, pages 566–569, 1981.)

medulla. These lesions produced a pattern of elevated pulmonary arterial pressure and pulmonary transcapillary fluid flux without changing systemic or left atrial pressure. This pattern is similar to that reported with neurogenic pulmonary edema in humans by Popp (1982) and Harari et al. (1976). This lesion site has been implicated in acute pulmonary edema in patients with multiple sclerosis (Giroud et al., 1988).

RESPIRATION REFLEXES

Hiccup

Persistent hiccup has multiple causes (Samuels, 1952), including central (e.g., brain stem neoplasm [Stotka et al., 1962] and multiple sclerosis [McFarling and Susac, 1979]) and peripheral (thoracic zoster [Efrati, 1956]) nervous system disorders. This reflex seems to be modified by gastrointestinal (Newsom-Davis, 1970) or metabolic events (Gibbs, 1963). Males seem especially susceptible and constituted 181 of the 220 patients studied for intractable hiccup at the Mayo Clinic (Souadjian and Cain, 1968). Electromyographic studies of three patients by Newsom-Davis (1970) during persistent hiccup demonstrated synchronous inspiratory muscle activity in the diaphragmatic and inspiratory (external) intercostal muscle

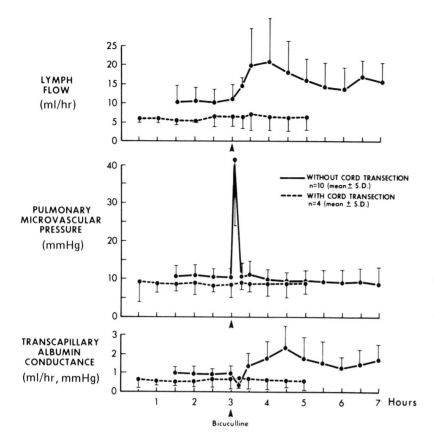

Figure 38–11. Pulmonary transcapillary fluid flux (lymph flow); calculated pulmonary microvascular pressure (microvascular pressure = left atrial pressure + 0.4 [pulmonary artery pressure − left atrial pressure]); and calculated transcapillary albumin conductance (cond = lung lymph flow × lymph albumin concentration/pulmonary microvascular pressure × plasma albumin concentration) before and during bicuculline-induced status epilepticus in nine paralyzed halothane-anesthetized sheep *(solid line)* and four sheep with cervical spinal cord transection *(dashed line).* (From Simon R.P. Bayne L.L., Tranbaugh R.F. Elevated pulmonary lymph flow and protein content during status epilepticus in sheep. *J. Appl. Physiol. Respir. Environ. Exercise Physiol.* 52:91–95, 1982.)

groups. Coincidental inhibition of expiratory intercostal muscles occurs, and glottal closure follows in 35 ms (Newsom-Davis, 1970); thus, air exchange is minimal. In a patient with a tracheostomy (by-passing glottal closure), hiccups produced a hyperventilation resulting in a respiratory alkalosis (pH = 7.58, P_{CO_2} = 28 mm Hg) (Newsom-Davis, 1970). In such cases, the decreased P_{CO_2} may perpetrate hiccup. Hiccups are most likely to occur during the period of maximal inspiration because lung inflation inhibits vagal mucosal and laryngotracheal afferents, which are known to inhibit hiccups (Salem et al., 1967).

In the study by Newsom-Davis (1970), patients' breath holding (increasing P_{CO_2}) had no effect on hiccup amplitude but markedly decreased hiccup frequency (confirming one common remedy). Decreasing P_{CO_2} increased hiccup amplitude, but hiccup frequency was unchanged. The inhibitory response of CO_2 to an inspiratory reflex is strong evidence against the origin of hiccups in the primary respiratory neuronal nuclei of the medulla, where P_{CO_2} has a major excitatory influence on the inspiratory neurons of the DRG. Thus, hiccup appears to be mediated through supraspinal mechanisms affecting primarily respiratory pathways at a spinal level similar to that for coughing, described next.

Coughing

Efferent pathways mediating coughing descend in the ventral columns of the spinal cord lateral to the ventral horn but are medial and distinct from pathways subserving automatic breathing. Thus, interruption of respiration could occur with preserved diaphragmatic innervation for coughing. Such a patient is described after high cervical cordotomy. The patient's maximal tidal volume during voluntary breathing was reduced to 200 ml, but tracheal stimulation resulted in coughing that produced tidal volumes of 1500 ml (Newsom-Davis and Plum, 1972).

Sneezing

Sneezing is rarely a manifestation of CNS disease (Co, 1979), although a patient described by Penfield and Jasper (1954) sneezed (and had chewing movements) during stimulation of the temporal lobe. A curious, common reflex is sneezing that occurs on an individual's sudden exposure to bright light. This phenomenon was found in nearly 30% of male medical students, was 50% as frequent in women, and was described in 80% of families of those with such photic-induced sneezing (Everett, 1964). The central mechanisms have not been studied.

Yawning

Although cortical factors, such as boredom, may modify or induce yawning, structures above the midbrain are not necessary for its production. Normal yawning has been described in an anencephalic newborn (Gamper, 1926). Although somnolence cannot be excluded as a factor, Penfield and Jasper (1954) described yawning (and hiccup) in the context of a seizure beginning within the temporal lobe. With the same proviso regarding somnolence, yawning often punctuates the progressive somnolence of an expanding intracranial mass (Fisher, 1969).

References

(Key references are designated with an asterisk.)

Adelman S., Dinner D.S., Goren H., et al. Obstructive sleep apnea in association with posterior fossa neurologic disease. *Arch. Neurol.* 41:509–510, 1984.

Aminoff M.J., Sears T.A. Spinal integration of segmental cortical breathing inputs to thoracic respiratory motoneurons. *J. Physiol. (Lond.)* 215:557–575, 1971.

Andersen P., Sears T.A. Medullary activation of intercostal fusimotor and alpha motoneurons. *J. Physiol. (Lond.)* 209:739–756, 1970.

Askenasy J.J.M., Goldhammer I. Sleep apnea as a feature of bulbar stroke. *Stroke* 19:637–639, 1988.

Baker A.B. A study of pulmonary edema. *Neurology* 7:743–751, 1957.

Bayne L., Simon R.P. Systemic and pulmonary vascular pressures during generalized seizures in sheep. *Ann. Neurol.* 10:566–569, 1981.

*Berger A.J., Mitchell R.A., Severinghaus J.W. Regulation of respiration. *N. Engl. J. Med.* 297:92–97, 138–143, 194–201, 1977.

Bloch M. Cerebral effects of rewarming following prolonged hypothermia: significance for the management of severe cranio-cerebral injury and acute pyrexia. *Brain* 90:769–784, 1967.

Brown H.W., Plum F. The neurologic basis of Cheyne-Stokes respiration. *Am. J. Med.* 30:849–860, 1961.

Bystrzycka E., Nail B.S., Purves M.J. Afferent neurones in the central pathway of the Hering-Breuer reflex. *J. Physiol. (Lond.)* 245:107–108, 1975.

Chaudhary B.A., Elguindi A.S., King D.W. Obstructive sleep apnea after lateral medullary syndrome. *South. Med. J.* 75:65–67, 1982.

Cherniack N.S. Respiratory dysrhythmias during sleep. *N. Engl. J. Med.* 305:325–330, 1981.

Cherniack N.S., von Euler C., Homma I., et al. Experimentally induced Cheyne-Stokes breathing. *Respir. Physiol.* 37:185–200, 1979.

Co S. Intractable sneezing: case report and literature review. *Arch. Neurol.* 36:111–112, 1979.

Cottle M.K. Degeneration studies of primary afferents of IXth and Xth cranial nerves in the cat. *J. Comp. Neurol.* 122:329–342, 1964.

Darnell J.C., Jay S.J. Recurrent postictal pulmonary edema: a case report and review of the literature. *Epilepsia* 23:71–83, 1982.

Darragh T.M., Simon R.P. Nucleus tractus solitarius lesions elevate pulmonary arterial pressure and lymph flow. *Ann. Neurol.* 17:565–569, 1985.

Devereaux M.W., Keane J.R., Davis R.L. Autonomic respiratory failure associated with infarction of the medulla. *Arch. Neurol.* 29:46–52, 1973.

Ducker T.B., Simons R.L., Anderson, R.W. Increased intracranial pressure and pulmonary edema. III. The effect of increased intracranial pressure on the cardiovascular hemodynamics of chimpanzees. *J. Neurosurg.* 29:475–483, 1968.

Efrati P. Obstinate hiccup as a prodromal symptom in thoracic herpes zoster. *Neurology* 6:601–602, 1956.

Everett H.C. Sneezing in response to light. *Neurology (Minneap.)* 14:483–490, 1964.

Fisher C.M. The neurological examination of the comatose patient. *Acta Neurol. Scand. Suppl.* 4–56, 1969.

Fisher C.M., Picard E.H., Polak, A. Acute hypertensive cerebellar hemorrhage diagnosis and surgical treatment. *J. Nerv. Ment. Dis.* 140:38–57, 1965.

Gamper E. Bau und Leistungen eines menschlichen Mittelhirnwesens (Arhinencephalie mit Encephalocele). *Z. Gesamte Neurol. Psychiatr.* 102:154–235, 1926.

Gautier H., Bertrand F. Respiratory effects of pneumotoxic center lesions and subsequent vagotomy in chronic cats. *Respir. Physiol.* 23:71–85, 1975.

Gibbs A.E. Two cases of persistent hiccup treated with orphenadrine. *Practitioner* 191:646–648, 1963.

Giraudoux J. *Ondine, A Romantic Fantasy in Three Acts* (translated by M. Valency). New York, Samuel French, 1956.

Giroud M., Guard O., Dumas R. Anomalies cardio-respiratoires dans la sclérose en plaques. *Rev. Neurol. (Paris)* 144:284–288, 1988.

Goulon M., Escourolle R., Augustin P., et al. Hyperventilation primitive par gliome bulbo-protuberantiel. *Rev. Neurol. (Paris)* 121:636–639, 1969.

Guilleminault C., Tilkian A., Dement, W. The sleep apnea syndromes. *Annu. Rev. Med.* 27:465–484, 1976.

Guyton A.C., Crowell J.W., Moore J.W. Basic oscillating mechanism of Cheyne-Stokes breathing. *Am. J. Physiol.* 187:395–398, 1956.

Guz A., Noble M.I.M., Eisele J.H., et al. The role of vagal inflation reflexes in man and other animals. In Porter R., ed. *Breathing: Hering-Breuer Centenary Symposium.* London, Churchill Livingstone, pp. 17–40, 1970.

Haddad G.G., Mazza N.M., Defendini R., et al. Congenital failure of automatic control of ventilation gastrointestinal motility and heart rate. *Medicine* 57:517–526, 1978.

Haponik E.F., Givens D., Angelo J. Syringobulbia-myelia with obstructive sleep apnea. *Neurology (N.Y.)* 33:1046–1049, 1983.

Harari A., Rapin M., Regnier B., et al. Normal pulmonary-capillary pressures in the late phase of neurogenic pulmonary oedema (letter). *Lancet* 1:494, 1976.

Hering P. Zusammensetzung der Blutgase während der Apnoe. *Dis. Dorpat.* 1867.

Heyman A., Birchfield R.I., Sieker H.O. Effects of bilateral cerebral infarction on respiratory center sensitivity. *Neurology* 8:694–700, 1958.

Jennett S., Ashbridge K., North J.B. Post-hyperventilation apnoea in patients with brain damage. *J. Neurol. Neurosurg. Psychiatry* 37:288–296, 1974.

Kaada B.R. Cingulate, posterior orbital, anterior insular and temporal pole cortex. In Magoun H.W., ed. *Handbook of Physiology.* Section 1. *The Nervous System.* Vol. II. *Neurophysiology.* Washington, DC, American Physiological Society, pp. 1345–1372, 1960.

Kaada B.R., Jasper H. Respiratory responses to stimulation of temporal pole, insula and hippocampal and limbic gyri in man. *Arch. Neurol. Psychiatry* 68:609–619, 1952.

Kales A., Vela-Bueno A., Kales J.D. Sleep disorders: sleep apnea and narcolepsy. *Ann. Intern. Med.* 106:434–443, 1987.

Kalia M. Neuroanatomical organization of the respiratory centers. *Fed. Proc.* 36:2405–2411, 1977.

Karp H.R., Sieker H.O., Heyman, A. Cerebral circulation and function in Cheyne-Stokes respiration. *Am. J. Med.* 30:861–870, 1961.

Kim R. The chronic residual respiratory disorder in post-encephalitic Parkinsonism. *J. Neurol. Neurosurg. Psychiatry* 31:393–398, 1968.

Krieger A.J., Christensen H.D., Sapru H.N., et al. Changes in ventilatory patterns after ablation of various respiratory feedback mechanisms. *J. Appl. Physiol.* 33:431–435, 1972.

Krieger A.J., Rosomoff H.L. Sleep-induced apnea. 1. A respiratory and autonomic dysfunction syndrome following bilateral percutaneous cervical cordotomy. *J. Neurosurg.* 40:168–180, 1974.

Lange L.S., Laszlo G. Cerebral tumour presenting with hyperventilation. *J. Neurol. Neurosurg. Psychiatry* 28:317–319, 1965.

Lange R.I., Hecht H.H. The mechanism of Cheyne-Stokes respiration. *J. Clin. Invest.* 41:42–52, 1962.

Lee M.C., Klassen A.C., Heaney L.M., et al. Respiratory rate and pattern disturbances in acute brain stem infarction. *Stroke* 7:382–385, 1976.

Leigh R.J., Shaw D.A. Rapid regular respiration in unconscious patients. *Arch. Neurol.* 33:356–361, 1976.

Levin B.E., Margolis G. Acute failure of automatic respirations secondary to a unilateral brain stem infarct. *Ann. Neurol.* 1:583–586, 1977.

Lumsden T. Observations on the respiratory centres in the cat. *J. Physiol. (Lond.)* 57:153–160, 1923.

Maron M.B. A canine model of neurogenic pulmonary edema. *J. Appl. Physiol.* 59:1019–1025, 1985.

Maron M.B. Analysis of airway fluid protein concentration in neurogenic pulmonary edema. *J. Appl. Physiol.* 62:470–476, 1987.

McClellan M.D., Dauber I.M., Weil J.V. Elevated intracranial pressure increases pulmonary vascular permeability to protein. *J. Appl. Physiol.* 67:1185–1191, 1989.

McCrimmon D.R., Smith J.C., Feldman J.L. Involvement of excitatory amino acids in neurotransmission of inspiratory drive to spinal respiratory motoneurons. *J. Neurosci.* 9:1910–1921, 1989.

McFarling D.A., Susac J.O. Hoquet diabolique: intractable hiccups as a manifestation of multiple sclerosis. *Neurology (Minneap.)* 29:797–801, 1979.

McNealy D.E., Plum F. Brainstem dysfunction with supratentorial mass lesions. *Arch. Neurol.* 7:10–32, 1962.

Mellins R.B., Balfour H.H., Turino G.M., et al. Failure of automatic control of ventilation. *Medicine* 49:487–504, 1970.

Merrill E.G. Finding a respiratory function for the medullary respiratory neurons. In Bellairs R., Gray E.G., eds. *Essays on the Nervous System.* Oxford, Clarendon Press, pp. 451–486, 1974.

Minnear F.L., Malik A.B. Mechanisms of neurogenic pulmonary edema. *Ann. N. Y. Acad. Sci.* 384:169–190, 1982.

Mitchell R.A., Loeschcke H.H., Massion W.H., et al. Respiratory responses mediated through superficial chemosensitive areas on the medulla. *J. Appl. Physiol.* 18:523–533, 1963.

Mitchell R.A., Sinha A.K., McDonald D.M. Chemoreceptive properties of regenerated endings of the carotid sinus nerve. *Brain Res.* 43:681–685, 1972.

Munschauer F.E., Loh L., Bannister R., et al. Abnormal respiration and sudden death during sleep in multiple system atrophy with autonomic failure. *Neurology* 40:677–679, 1990.

Nadel J.A. Neurophysiologic aspects of asthma. In Austen K.F., Lichenstein L.M., eds. *Asthma.* New York, Academic Press, pp. 29–37, 1973.

Nelson D.A., Ray C.D. Respiratory arrest from seizure discharges in limbic system. *Arch. Neurol.* 19:199–207, 1968.

Nelson F.W., Hecht J.T., Horton W.A., et al. Neurologic basis of respiratory complications in achondroplasia. *Ann. Neurol.* 24:89–93, 1988.

Newsom-Davis J. An experimental study of hiccup. *Brain* 93:851–872, 1970.

Newsom-Davis J. Control of the muscles of breathing. In Widdicombe J.G., ed. *Respiratory Physiology: MTP International Review of Science.* Ser. 1. Vol. 2. London, Butterworth, pp. 221–246, 1974.

Newsom-Davis J., Plum, F. Separation of descending spinal pathways to respiratory motoneurons. *Exp. Neurol.* 34:78–94, 1972.

North J.B., Jennett S. Abnormal breathing patterns associated with acute brain damage. *Arch. Neurol.* 31:338–344, 1974.

Onal E., Lopata M., O'Connor T. Pathogenesis of apneas in

hypersomnia-sleep apnea syndrome. *Am. Rev. Respir. Dis.* 125:167–174, 1982.

Penfield W., Jasper H. *Epilepsy and the Functional Anatomy of the Human Brain.* Boston, Little, Brown, p. 453, 1954.

Plum F. Neurological integration of behavioral and metabolic control of breathing. In Porter R., ed. *Breathing: Hering-Breuer Centenary Symposium.* London, Churchill Livingstone, pp. 159–175, 1970.

Plum F. Hyperpnea, hyperventilation, and brain dysfunction. *Ann. Intern. Med.* 76:328, 1972.

Plum F. Mechanisms of "central" hyperventilation. *Ann. Neurol.* 11:636–637, 1982.

Plum F., Alvord E.C. Jr. Apneustic breathing in man. *Arch. Neurol.* 10:101–112, 1964.

*Plum F., Leigh R.J. Abnormalities of central mechanism. In Hornbein T.F., ed. *Regulation of Breathing.* Part II. New York, Marcel Dekker, pp. 989–1067, 1981.

Plum F., Swanson A.G. Abnormalities in central regulation of respiration in acute and convalescent poliomyelitis. *Arch. Neurol. Psychiatry* 80:267–285, 1958.

Plum F., Swanson A.G. Central neurogenic hyperventilation in man. *Arch. Neurol. Psychiatry* 81:535–549, 1959.

Plum F., Brown H.W., Snoep, E. Neurologic significance of posthyperventilation apnea. *J.A.M.A.* 181:1050–1055, 1962.

Popp J.A., Gottlieb M.E., Paloski W.H., et al. Cardiopulmonary hemodynamics in patients with serious head injury. *J. Surg. Res.* 32:416–421, 1982.

Preiss G., Iscoe S., Polosa C. Analysis of a periodic breathing pattern associated with Mayer waves. *Am. J. Physiol.* 228:768–774, 1975.

Reis D.J., McHugh P.R. Hypoxia as a cause of bradycardia during amygdala stimulation in monkey. *J. Appl. Physiol.* 214:601–610, 1968.

Remmers J.E., Marttila I. Action of intercostal muscle afferents on the respiratory rhythm of anesthetized cats. *Respir. Physiol.* 24:31–41, 1975.

Rodriguez M., Baele P.L., Marsh H.M., et al. Central neurogenic hyperventilation in an awake patient with brainstem astrocytoma. *Ann. Neurol.* 11:625–628, 1982.

Rosell S. Neuronal control of microvessels. *Annu. Rev. Physiol.* 42:359–371, 1980.

Salem M.R., Baraka A., Rattenborg C.C., et al. Treatment of hiccups by pharyngeal stimulation in anesthetized and conscious subjects. *J.A.M.A.* 202:32–36, 1967.

Samuels L. Hiccup: a ten year review of anatomy, etiology, and treatment. *Can. Med. Assoc. J.* 67:315–322, 1952.

Schlesinger B. Neurogenic pulmonary edema, due to puncture wound of the medulla oblongata. *J. Nerv. Ment. Dis.* 102:247–255, 1945.

Sears T.A. The respiratory motoneuron and apneusis. *Fed. Proc.* 36:2412–2420, 1977.

Severinghaus J.W., Mitchell R.A. Ondine's curse—failure of respiratory center automaticity while awake (abstract). *Clin. Res.* 10:122, 1962.

Simon R.P. Neurogenic pulmonary edema. *Semin. Neurol.* 4:490–496, 1984.

Simon R.P., Bayne L.L. Pulmonary lymphatic flow alterations during intracranial hypertension in sheep. *Ann. Neurol.* 15:188–194, 1984.

Simon R.P., Bayne L.L., Tranbaugh R.F. Elevated pulmonary lymph flow and protein content during status epilepticus in sheep. *J. Appl. Physiol. Respir. Environ. Exercise Physiol.* 52:91–95, 1982.

Snyderman N.L., Johnson J.T., Møller M., et al. Brainstem evoked potentials in adult sleep apnea. *Ann. Otol. Rhinol. Laryngol.* 91:597–598, 1982.

Souadjian J.V., Cain J.C. Intractable hiccups. *Postgrad. Med.* 43:72–77, 1968.

Stotka U.L., Barcay S.J., Bell H.S., et al. Intractable hiccoughs as the primary manifestation of brain stem tumor. *Am. J. Med.* 32:313–315, 1962.

Terrance C.F., Rao G.R., Perper J.A. Neurogenic pulmonary edema in unexpected, unexplained death of epileptic patients. *Ann. Neurol.* 9:458–464, 1981.

Tranmer B.I., Tucker W.S., Bilbao J.M. Sleep apnea following percutaneous cervical cordotomy. *Can. J. Neurol. Sci.* 14:262–267, 1987.

Turner W.A., Critchley M. Respiratory disorders in epidemic encephalitis. *Brain* 48:72–104, 1925.

Vincken W.G., Gauthier S.G., Dollfuss R.E., et al. Involvement of upper-airway muscles in extrapyramidal disorders: a cause of airflow limitation. *N. Engl. J. Med.* 311:428–442, 1984.

Weiner W.J., Goetz C.G., Nausieda P.A., et al. Respiratory dys-

kinesias: extrapyramidal dysfunction and dyspnea. *Ann. Intern. Med.* 88:327–331, 1978.

Yamour B.J., Sridharan M.R., Rice J.F. Electrocardiographic changes in cerebrovascular hemorrhage. *Am. Heart J.* 99:294–300, 1980.

Zupnick H.M., Brown L.K., Miller A., et al. Respiratory dysfunction due to L-dopa therapy parkinsonism: diagnosis using serial pulmonary function tests and respiratory inductive plethysmography. *Am. J. Med.* 89:109–112, 1990.

39

Autonomic Function and Dysfunction

Ralph H. Johnson
David G. Lambie

Autonomic nervous system function is a feature of all human activity; it maintains homeostasis as various stresses, such as change in posture, exercise, or temperature changes, are placed on the individual. Autonomic dysfunction, therefore, affects the way the body can withstand such demands. In this chapter, disorders are considered according to the disease process in the part of the autonomic nervous system that is affected: within the brain, spinal cord, or peripheral nerves. Increased or decreased autonomic activity may result from lesions in any of these regions. Causes of arterial hypertension are given in Table 39–1. More commonly, however, neurologic lesions result in reduced autonomic activity. For example, the reflex arc subserving blood pressure may be affected on the afferent side from baroreceptors, within the brain, or in efferent pathways within the spinal cord or peripheral nerves (Table 39–2). Similarly, failure of thermoregulation may occur owing to widely dispersed dysfunction (Table 39–3).

Disorders of the system have been reviewed by Johnson and Spalding (1974) and Appenzeller (1982), and some features were amplified by Bannister (1983, 1988). The cardiovascular effects of autonomic dysfunction have been summarized by Johnson et al. (1984). Lack of specific tests means that examination depends on detailed studies of physiologic function; this information is given in the relevant sections of this book (see Chapters 32–36).

PARASYMPATHETIC AND SYMPATHETIC SYSTEMS

The autonomic nervous system has two major components: the sympathetic (with thoracolumbar outflows) and the parasympathetic (with craniosacral outflows) (Fig. 39–1). Although both are *efferent* systems, afferent fibers, sometimes called autonomic afferents, accompany some autonomic nerves and are part of reflex pathways involving the efferent systems. Investigation of autonomic function may require study of afferent activity and also individual parts of the autonomic nervous system. The texts noted earlier describe these investigations. Some disorders may have both parasympathetic and sympathetic dysfunction, for example, diabetes mellitus. Others, such as alcoholism, show predominantly parasympathetic abnormalities, whereas others, such as paraplegia, lead to sympathetic dysfunction. The descriptions that follow, however, are based on the major anatomic region affected, whether brain, spinal cord, or peripheral nerve.

CENTRAL AND BRAIN STEM LESIONS

Blood Pressure Control

Control of blood pressure is mediated through the brain stem. Intrinsic and extrinsic lesions may interrupt this control and cause orthostatic hypotension. Orthostatic hypotension has been reported with posterior fossa tumors, after surgery to brain stem neoplasms, and with craniopharyngiomas. It may be the presenting feature.

Raised intracranial pressure may be accompanied by an increase in arterial pressure, with bradycardia and slow irregular respiration (Cushing, 1902). The response may occur with relatively small increases in intracranial pressure if there is an acute distortion of the lower brain stem (Thompson and Malina,

Table 39–1. ARTERIAL HYPERTENSION ATTRIBUTABLE TO SYMPATHETIC HYPERACTIVITY

Tumor
Pheochromocytoma

Secondary to Neurologic Disorders
Diencephalic epilepsy
Intracranial disease
Other neurologic disorders
   Tetanus
   Familial dysautonomia
   Polyneuropathies
   Cervical spinal cord transection

Secondary to Cardiovascular Disorders
Myocardial infarction
Paroxysmal ventricular tachycardia

Unexplained Causes
Essential hypertension

Drugs
Monoamine oxidase inhibitors
Alcohol

1959), which is particularly likely to occur with space-occupying lesions in the posterior fossa; these demand immediate treatment. Lesions of the posterior fossa in which paroxysmal hypertension has been reported include astrocytoma, cerebellar tumor, and basilar artery aneurysm. Posterior fossa lesions should be considered in any patient with paroxysmal hypertension in whom a pheochromocytoma cannot be found, and radiologic investigation should be carried out.

Temperature Control

Localized lesions in or near the hypothalamus may cause abnormal temperature regulation, usually hypothermia (see Table 39–3). Of 60 patients with hypothalamic disease proved by biopsy, abnormalities of body temperature were recorded in 13 and were the first manifestation in 4 patients (Bauer, 1954). Other abnormalities indicating hypothalamic dysfunction include precocious puberty or hypogonadism, diabetes insipidus, somnolence, and obesity. Neurologic signs depend on the extent of involvement of neighboring structures; pyramidal, sensory, ophthalmologic, and cerebellar signs may develop with expanding lesions. Rarely, thermoregulation alone is affected and, if episodic, may be part of the syndrome of diencephalic epilepsy (see the later section on this disorder). The most common pathology is neoplasia, particularly craniopharyngiomas and astrocytomas. Infants may have intracranial hemorrhage in this region.

In Wernicke's encephalopathy, small petechial hemorrhages occur in the hypothalamus and upper brain stem, including the mamillary body. One of Wernicke's original series (1881) developed hypothermia; although hypothermia has subsequently been reported in only a small number of patients, it is important because it may mask other signs of the

syndrome. The disorder responds dramatically to thiamine. Agenesis of the corpus callosum associated with recurrent attacks of hypothermia has been described (Mooradian et al., 1984). It is unlikely that hypothermia is directly related to the abnormality of the corpus callosum, as surgical section in animals and humans does not lead to defects in temperature regulation. A relationship with accompanying lesions of the hypothalamus is more likely.

Hypothermia is a common and serious phenomenon in the elderly. It is particularly frequent in the winter. Clinical disorders that dispose to hypothermia include hypothyroidism and hypopituitarism; diabetes; mental impairment; vascular collapse, especially related to myocardial infarction; severe infections, especially pneumonia; drugs; and alcohol. However, hypothermia may develop in some elderly patients without exposure to undue cold, and it is

Table 39–2. DISORDERS IN WHICH THE PATIENT MAY DEVELOP ORTHOSTATIC HYPOTENSION AND THE PARTS OF THE REFLEX PATHWAY AFFECTED

Afferent Pathway (IX or X Nerves)
Acute polyneuropathy (?)
Chronic polyneuropathy (?)
Chronic alcoholism (?)
Diabetes mellitus (?)
Adie's syndrome
Renal failure
Hemodialysis
Tabes dorsalis

Central (Brain Stem Integration)
Acute polyneuropathy (?)
Acute alcoholism
Brain stem lesions
Familial dysautonomia (?)
Anorexia nervosa (?)
Drugs

Efferent Pathway
Spinal cord
Trauma
Transverse myelitis
Syringomyelia
Intramedullary tumors
Extramedullary tumors
Intermediolateral column degeneration
   Idiopathic orthostatic hypotension
   Multiple system atrophy
   Parkinson's disease
Sympathetic chain and postganglionic nerves
Acute polyneuropathy
Pure autonomic neuropathy
Idiopathic orthostatic hypotension
Chronic polyneuropathy
   Chronic alcoholism
   Diabetes mellitus
   Tumors (nonmetastatic complication?)
   Rheumatoid arthritis (?)
   Acute intermittent porphyria
   Amyloidosis
   Pernicious anemia
Failure of catecholamine release
   Anorexia nervosa
   Dopamine β-hydroxylase deficiency
Drugs
Adrenoreceptors
Orthostatic hypotension in the elderly (?)

Table 39–3. CAUSES OF HYPOTHERMIA

Neurologic Disease
Cerebrovascular disease (in the elderly)
Corpus callosum agenesis
Hypothalamic lesions
    Tumor
    Vascular lesion
    Wernicke's encephalopathy
    Parkinson's disease
    Idiopathic lesion
Spinal cord lesions
    Tetraplegia
    Paraplegia

Other Causes
Cold exposure
Drugs, alcohol
Hypothyroidism, hypopituitarism

evident that they suffer from a defect of temperature regulation (Collins et al., 1977; Macmillan et al., 1967).

Bladder Control

Lesions of the anterior frontal lobe in about the coronal plane of the tip of the frontal horn (Fig. 39–2), the anterior part of the cingulate gyrus, or the hypothalamus are liable to cause severe urgency, frequency, and incontinence with impaired awareness of the state of the bladder (Andrew and Nathan, 1965). Removal of a space-occupying lesion may reverse the urinary disturbance. Lesions of the frontal lobe, including the more extensive types of leukotomy, may also cause incontinence because of loss of inhibition and inattention to the demands of society. Brain stem vascular accidents may lead to retention of urine, which can be the presenting symptom. This is particularly apt to occur in elderly men, in whom such a vascular accident may cause a compensated degree of prostatic obstruction to become decompensated.

Diencephalic Epilepsy

Penfield (1929) described a patient with paroxysmal hypertensive attacks, defined as "diencephalic autonomic epilepsy," characterized by restlessness, flushing, a sudden rise in blood pressure, lacrimation, salivation, sweating, dilatation or constriction of the pupils, tachycardia, and, as the attack wore off, periodic (Cheyne-Stokes) respiration. At autopsy the patient had a cholesteatoma in the choroid plexus of the third ventricle causing internal hydrocephalus. The hypertension and respiratory disturbance may not have been related to the hypothalamus. Edema in the medulla and pons may have caused lower brain stem disturbance.

There have been occasional descriptions, since Penfield's report, of patients with paroxysmal disor-

ders characterized by autonomic features that have been attributed to diencephalic epilepsy (Duff et al., 1961; Fox et al., 1973). Lesions are usually in the third ventricle, notably colloid cysts, but there has been no clear evidence of epileptic foci in the diencephalon. Autonomic symptoms may also be a feature of temporal lobe epilepsy (van Buren, 1958). Sudden death in patients with epilepsy may occasionally be due to cardiac dysrhythmias resulting from autonomic activity associated with seizures, but this remains to be established (S. Oppenheimer, 1990).

Familial Dysautonomia (Riley-Day Syndrome)

Familial dysautonomia was first described by Riley et al. (1949). Although the majority of patients have been Jews of Ashkenazi extraction, a small number of patients of other races have been described. The disease tends to occur in siblings rather than in

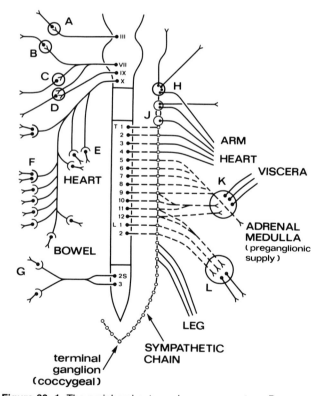

Figure 39–1. The peripheral autonomic nervous system. Parasympathetic system from cranial nerves III, VIII, IX, X and from sacral nerves 2 and 3: A = ciliary ganglion; B = sphenopalatine (pterygopalatine) ganglion; C = submandibular ganglion; D = otic ganglion; E = vagal ganglion cells in heart wall; F = vagal ganglion cells in bowel wall; G = pelvic ganglia. Sympathetic system from T-1 to L-2, preganglionic fibers (– – – –), postganglionic fibers (———): H = superior cervical ganglion; J = middle cervical ganglion and inferior cervical (stellate) ganglion including T-1 ganglion; K = celiac and other abdominal ganglia; L = lower abdominal sympathetic ganglia.

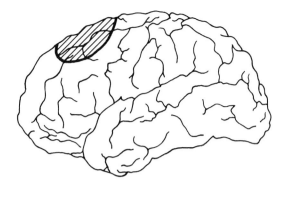

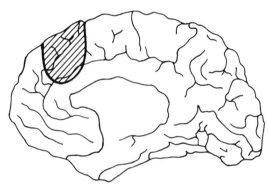

Figure 39–2. Lateral (*top*) and medial (*bottom*) views of the cerebral hemispheres, showing the region particularly important for the control of micturition and defecation. (Adapted from Andrew J., Nathan P.W., Spanos N.C. Disturbances of micturition and defaecation due to aneurysms of anterior communicating or anterior cerebral arteries. *J. Neurosurg.* 24:1–10, 1966.)

successive generations (Riley, 1957), thus suggesting that the disease is autosomal recessive. The molecular nature of the genetic defect may be related to nerve growth factor.

The patients are usually children and are liable to frequent infections. The autonomic disturbances are manifested by lability of the blood pressure, with both paroxysmal hypertension and orthostatic hypotension occurring. Other evidence of sympathetic failure may include blotching of the skin; erratic temperature control; alteration of sweating, which is usually increased; reduction of tear production; and diarrhea or constipation. Some patients show other neurologic involvement, including dysarthria, incoordination, vomiting attacks, insensitivity to pain, loss of tendon reflexes, and emotional instability.

The pathologic changes affecting the sympathetic and parasympathetic systems are by no means certain. Some workers have failed to demonstrate any relevant abnormality. Others have observed reduction in unmyelinated fibers in both peripheral nervous system and central tracts, with the sympathetic and parasympathetic systems being affected (Brown et al., 1964).

There is no specific treatment for the disease, and most children die of infection or hyperpyrexia. Some patients, however, survive into early adult life.

SPINAL CORD LESIONS

Lesions affecting the cervical spinal cord are particularly likely to produce symptoms related to autonomic dysfunction. Elegant correlation of clinical and subsequent neuropathologic studies showed that in the cervical cord, sympathetic pathways pass into the deeper white matter, close to and just posterior to the posterior angle of the anterior horn (Fig. 39–3). The sympathetic pathways to the head and neck are ipsilateral, whereas caudal to the head and neck sympathomotor fibers are supplied from both sides of the cord (Nathan and Smith, 1986, 1987). Cervical spondylosis may cause Horner's syndrome, and orthostatic hypotension may occur in syringomyelia. However, the most frequent cord disorder in which problems related to autonomic dysfunction occur is trauma.

Trauma

The various effects of traumatic lesions, including those affecting the autonomic nervous system, were reviewed by Guttmann (1976).

Orthostatic Hypotension

In a complete spinal cord lesion, the brain can no longer control the sympathetic outflow below the level of the lesion, although vascular reflexes may occur through the isolated spinal cord. If cord transection occurs above the sixth thoracic segment, orthostatic hypotension is the rule, particularly in

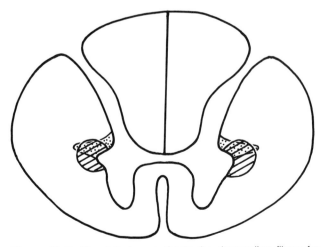

Figure 39–3. The dotted area shows the descending fibers for vasomotor control and the hatched area shows the descending fibers for sudomotor control. The oculomotor fibers lie in the same region. (From Nathan P.W., Smith M.C. The location of descending fibers to sympathetic preganglionic vasomotor and sudomotor neurons in man. *J. Neurol. Neurosurg. Psychiatry* 50:1253–1262, 1987.)

the acute stage. Hypotension may be severe, and great care must be taken to avoid raising the head above the horizontal in the recently injured patient, for example, in removing the patient from the scene of an accident. Any fall in blood pressure is more serious, because in the first few months after injury autoregulation of cerebral blood flow is impaired (Yamamoto et al., 1980). A patient with a high spinal cord lesion may need artificial respiration, and it is important not to embarrass the circulation while providing it. The ventilator must permit complete expiration to avoid impairing venous return by raising intrathoracic pressure. When secretions are aspirated from the trachea, the heart rate may slow dramatically because of unopposed action of the vagus. If this is suspected, care should be taken that the patient is fully oxygenated, and bradycardia can be prevented by atropine (Welply et al., 1975).

After several weeks or months, the orthostatic hypotension becomes less severe, so that patients are able to sit without the occurrence of symptoms for as long as they wish. Readjustment is assisted if the patient is exposed to a gradually increasing head-up position for longer periods each day or has the head of the bed progressively elevated. The mechanism of improvement is not clear. It is not accompanied by significant recovery of plasma catecholamine responses to tilting (Mathias et al., 1975). Patients with chronic high cord transections have high resting plasma renin activity and increased responses of renin to postural change; this may play a part in limiting hypotension (Johnson and Park, 1973). Sympathetic spinal reflexes may still be intact after cord transection, and these reflexes may also play a part in limiting orthostatic hypotension by causing vasoconstriction in the limbs. A local venoarteriolar reflex may act to reduce blood flow in subcutaneous tissues (Skagen et al., 1982).

Arterial hypotension, particularly orthostatic hypotension, may be exacerbated after meals (postprandial hypotension). It may occur in patients with autonomic failure and in elderly patients in whom there is no evidence of autonomic failure. It is likely to be due in part to redistribution of blood to the splanchnic and hepatic beds. It may also be due to the vasodilatory effect of insulin, mimicking the hypotension that may develop in diabetes mellitus after insulin injection, but other hormones, such as neurotensin and/or vasoactive intestinal polypeptide, may be involved.

Hypertension

Hypertension can occur because autonomic reflexes can develop through the isolated spinal cord and may be excessive if the lesion is above T-6; 50% of patients develop autonomic hyperreflexia at some stage after injury (Lindan et al., 1980). Prevalence is greater in patients with cervical lesions (60%) than in those with thoracic lesions (20%). Acute hypertension is usually first manifested during the first few months after injury, but occasionally the first attack does not occur until several years after injury. The increase in blood pressure may be severe and prolonged. Associated autonomic signs may include profuse sweating and piloerection below the level of the lesion. Headache is a characteristic symptom.

Various stimuli below the level of the lesion can raise blood pressure. They include reflex skeletal muscle activity (Corbett et al., 1971) and bladder contraction induced in any way (Cunningham et al., 1953).

Temperature Control

Spinal cord transection at the cervical level causes marked disturbance of temperature control (Johnson, 1976). This is due to interruption of sympathetic pathways controlling sweating and vasomotion and of motor pathways producing shivering. Spontaneous hypothermia is likely to occur in temperate climates, but hyperthermia may also occur, especially in warm climates. Patients with spinal cord lesions below the cervical level retain sympathetic activity subserving sweat glands and blood vessels in normally innervated regions and are therefore much less at risk.

Severe hypothermia is particularly likely to develop soon after acute spinal cord transection. This may happen because, in the acute stage, cutaneous vasodilatation and consequent loss of heat occur. Subsequently, tone returns to the vessels, and blood flow and heat loss are reduced. Shivering in response to a low central temperature can occur in muscles innervated from above the level of the lesion. In some patients with cervical cord lesions, such shivering may increase metabolism 50% above the resting level, but in others there is no detectable increase.

In spinal cord transection some thermoregulatory changes, vasomotor and sudomotor, apparently can occur in skin in which the sympathetic supply comes from below the level of the lesion. It is unproved whether this is due to spinal cord reflexes or to a direct effect on vessels and sweat glands. These mechanisms are inefficient, so that patients with cervical cord transection withstand heat and cold stress poorly.

Bladder Control

The conus medullaris contains the spinal integrating reflex center for micturition. If the spinal cord is damaged but the conus medullaris and its roots are intact, the reflexes through the pelvic (parasympathetic and sensory) and pudendal (somatic) nerves are intact. Activity of reflexes by way of the pudendal nerves is shown by examination of anal sphincter tone and the anocutaneous and bulbocavernous reflexes. When spinal shock after the acute lesion has subsided and if overdistention and infection of the bladder have been avoided, the bladder of a patient with a severe spinal cord lesion above the conus usually empties spontaneously or in response to abdominal pressure, tapping the suprapubic area, pulling the pubic hair, hitting the thighs, or stimulating the external rectal sphincter digitally. Once it starts to empty, it continues to do so.

As just described, if the lesion is above the mid-dorsal region a full bladder may cause sympathetic overactivity, including sweating and piloerection in the areas receiving sympathetic innervation from the isolated part of the spinal cord. These symptoms and the headache associated with hypertension may enable a patient to know when the bladder is full. Such direct "bladder sensation" is not evidence that a spinal cord lesion is incomplete. Chapter 36 also deals with bladder function.

Disturbances of Sexual Function

Priapism, continuous erection that normally resolves in days, occurs in patients with acute spinal cord transection, as well as in those with other spinal cord lesions, particularly when acute, including multiple sclerosis. It may also occur in those with tabes dorsalis, encephalitis, and epilepsy (Becker and Mitchell, 1965). Local lesions may cause penile erection as a symptom of spinal cord stenosis. It may occur during walking in affected patients, and symptoms may resolve after appropriate surgery (Hopkins et al., 1987).

A patient with a chronic complete bilateral upper motor neuron lesion resulting, for example, from trauma, may have a reflex erection (Guttmann, 1964). This is caused by manipulation of the genitalia, and the reflex arc passes through the isolated section of the spinal cord. A patient with a complete lower motor neuron lesion may have a psychogenic but not a reflex erection (Bors and Turner, 1967), even though the pelvic (parasympathetic) nerves are interrupted in such a lesion. It is suggested that erection results from impulses originating in the brain that reach the genitalia by the sympathetic nervous system (Bors and Turner, 1967). However, a substantial proportion of patients with lower motor neuron lesions do not have an erection.

Impotence (failure of erection) may result from any disorder that affects the sacral parasympathetic supply, including multisystem disease, chronic polyneuropathy, and multiple sclerosis.

Expulsion of semen into the urethra is dependent on the sympathetic nerve supply. Failure of sympathetic supply also causes failure of the internal urethral sphincter, and some patients may suffer retrograde ejaculation into the bladder if orgasm occurs. Ejaculation can occur, although uncommonly, in patients with complete upper motor neuron lesions as a reflex through the isolated spinal cord (Guttmann, 1964). It is less uncommon among patients with complete lower motor neuron lesions who have erections, for in these patients the sympathetic nerve supply is preserved (Bors and Turner, 1967). Semen is ejected from the urethra by rhythmic contraction

of the bulbocavernous and ischiocavernous muscles, which are supplied by the pudendal (somatic) nerves. Ejaculation does not therefore occur in patients with lower motor neuron lesions affecting these nerves and their roots, although the semen may dribble out. Various pharmacologic and other techniques to cause ejaculation have been reported. However, successful pregnancies are few, as spermatogenesis is considerably reduced in paraplegics. Neither male nor female patients with a complete spinal cord lesion experience orgasm. Patients with lower motor neuron lesions who have erections may experience all variations in degree of orgasm or have no orgasm. They may sometimes have painful sensations. The extent of sensory loss may be important, and orgasm is lost after bilateral and occasionally after unilateral cordotomy (Bors and Turner, 1967). Orgasm is possible even when ejaculation is absent. Chapter 35 also deals with sexual function.

Idiopathic Orthostatic Hypotension and Multiple System Atrophy

Bradbury and Eggleston (1925) first described idiopathic orthostatic hypotension. Their patients had orthostatic hypotension with fixed heart rate, anhidrosis, and lowered basal metabolic rate related to progressive autonomic failure (Bannister, 1983). Later studies have shown that some patients with these defects also have progressive degeneration elsewhere in the nervous system, first clearly described by Shy and Drager (1960) and often called the *Shy-Drager syndrome*, or multiple system atrophy. Some patients, however, have only autonomic dysfunction and apparently never develop evidence of other neurologic deficits. Some of these patients have evidence of peripheral failure of autonomic function, but the majority have similar changes in the cord affecting autonomic pathways such as those in the patients with Shy-Drager syndrome. Patients usually survive for several years; they frequently die from misadventure related to an episode of hypotension.

In both idiopathic orthostatic hypotension and multiple system atrophy, the autonomic nervous system progressively fails. The patients are usually middle-aged men, and the autonomic nervous system may fail as a whole over years or decades, the symptoms progressing through loss of sweating, impotence, sphincter disturbances, and orthostatic hypotension; the most incapacitating feature is the orthostatic hypotension. Other degenerative disorders may be closely related, as described later. All patients with idiopathic orthostatic hypotension or multiple system atrophy exhibit drops in blood pressure on standing. The supine blood pressure may be low, normal, or high. Some patients may show marked spontaneous fluctuations in blood pressure that are related to variations in peripheral resistance.

The most characteristic pathologic lesion in these patients is marked cell loss in the intermediolateral columns, the site of sympathetic preganglionic cell bodies (Fig. 39–4) (Bannister and Oppenheimer, 1972; Johnson et al., 1966). The lesion is close to the descending sympathetic pathways for vasomotor control already noted (see Fig. 39–3). In patients with multiple system atrophy, lesions in structures other than the intermediolateral columns may also contribute to autonomic failure: there may be degeneration in the locus ceruleus, nucleus tractus solitarius, or preganglionic vagal neurons (Bannister and Oppenheimer, 1972) and norepinephrine and dopamine depletion in the hypothalamus (Spokes et al., 1979). Patients with multiple system atrophy may also have

olivopontocerebellar atrophy and degeneration of corticobulbar, extrapyramidal, and cerebellar tracts. The clinical disorders that may be associated with autonomic failure are shown in Figure 39–5. The pathologic features have been reviewed (D.R. Oppenheimer, 1983). A genetic basis for progressive autonomic failure was suggested by a significant association between the disease and the frequency of human leukocyte antigen (HLA) antigen Aw32 (Bannister et al., 1983). It was suggested that progressive autonomic failure might indicate a lesion in a gene in the HLA region that is used in governing catecholamine metabolism.

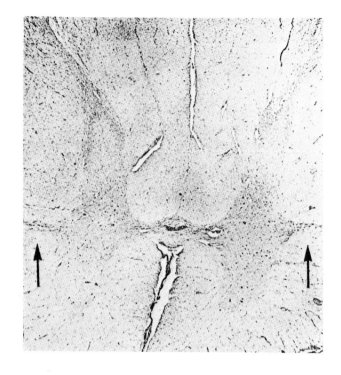

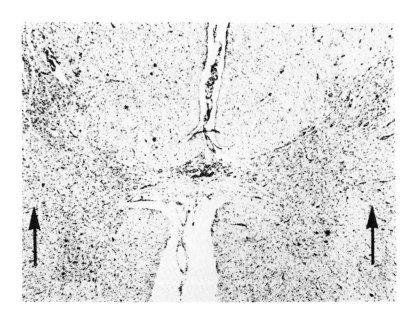

Figure 39–4. Sections of spinal cord at T-3 level in a normal subject (*top*) and in a patient with idiopathic hypotension (*bottom*). Arrows point to the intermediolateral cell columns, the site of sympathetic preganglionic cell bodies. In the patient, the cell population was much reduced. (From Johnson, R.H., Lee G. de J., Oppenheimer D.R., et al. Autonomic failure with orthostatic hypotension due to intermediolateral column degeneration. *Q. J. Med.* 35:276–292, 1966, by permission of Oxford University Press.)

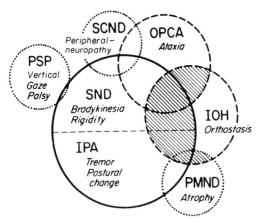

Figure 39–5. Relationships between idiopathic orthostatic hypotension and other neurologic degenerative disorders. The central solid circle represents the parkinsonism syndrome. The shaded area indicates the clinical findings in multiple system atrophy (Shy-Drager syndrome), in which there may be considerable variability in the neurologic findings in association with orthostatic hypotension. IPA = idiopathic Parkinson's disease; SND = striatonigral degeneration; PSP = progressive supranuclear palsy; IOH = idiopathic orthostatic hypotension; OPCA = olivopontocerebellar atrophy; PMND = parkinsonism with motor neuron disease; SCND = spinocerebellar-nigral degeneration. (Adapted from Ropper A.H., Hedley-White E.T. Parkinsonism associated with other neurologic manifestations. Reprinted, by permission of the *New England Journal of Medicine*, 308; 1406–1414, 1983.)

Patients with idiopathic orthostatic hypotension generally have low basal norepinephrine levels when supine, whereas patients with multiple system atrophy may have normal basal norepinephrine levels (Johnson, 1983a). In both idiopathic orthostatic hypotension and multiple system atrophy, the abnormality of sympathetic function produces depressed circulating norepinephrine responses to standing and exertion.

In both idiopathic orthostatic hypotension and multiple system atrophy, there is generally catecholamine depletion in sympathetic nerve endings around blood vessels (Bannister et al., 1981). However, catecholamine-specific fluorescence may be normal and there may be failure of norepinephrine release (Nanda et al., 1977).

An inherited syndrome of familial orthostatic hypotension has been described that resembles the multiple system degeneration syndrome of Shy and Drager (Lewis, 1964). In addition to orthostatic hypotension, symptoms include muscle wasting, ataxia, rigidity and tremor, and sphincter involvement. Symptoms appear in middle life, and the disease progresses slowly and without impairment of the intellect. The condition is probably autosomal dominant.

Parkinsonism and Idiopathic Paralysis Agitans

In patients with orthostatic hypotension associated with multiple system atrophy, parkinsonian features

are a frequent finding (Bannister and Oppenheimer, 1972). Occasionally, parkinsonism may precede the dysautonomia and lead to an erroneous diagnosis of idiopathic paralysis agitans. Some patients with autonomic failure, but without the widespread neurologic features of multiple system atrophy, may develop parkinsonism. These patients, unlike the majority of patients with multiple system atrophy, show Lewy-type inclusion bodies in the pigmented nuclei of the brain stem and in autonomic ganglia (D.R. Oppenheimer, 1983); this may represent an association of autonomic failure with idiopathic paralysis agitans.

Symptomatic orthostatic hypotension is rare in untreated patients with idiopathic paralysis agitans, although even in patients with mild paralysis agitans the postural fall in blood pressure is greater than in normal subjects (Gross et al., 1972). Circulatory reflexes are generally intact, but there may be some moderate reduction in sympathetic activity. Other autonomic symptoms may include impairment of thermoregulation and abnormal bladder function. The incidence of hypothermia is increased in patients with Parkinson's disease (Gubbay and Barwick, 1966) and is probably related to autonomic disturbances causing skin vasodilatation and excessive sweating.

Patients with parkinsonism who are treated with levodopa may develop hypotension in the horizontal position, and they may also develop orthostatic hypotension, which may be symptomatic in approximately 10% of patients (Marsden et al., 1973). An extracerebral dopa decarboxylase inhibitor only slightly improves orthostatic hypotension caused by levodopa, which suggests that orthostatic hypotension is principally related to a central, rather than a peripheral, effect of levodopa.

Infection with the Human Immunodeficiency Virus

The range of dysfunction that may occur with human immunodeficiency virus (HIV) infection has been shown to involve every system of the body. Neurologic complications include encephalopathy, myelopathy, and neuropathies, and autonomic dysfunction could be an early indication of HIV-related tissue damage. There have been few systematic studies of autonomic function, but a large number of case reports have now appeared and show that generalized autonomic insufficiency may be common. One of the first descriptions was of a patient who presented with syncopal episodes and was shown to have wide-ranging autonomic problems, including orthostatic hypotension, impotence, urinary urgency, extensive anhidrosis, and lack of response to the Valsalva maneuver (Lin-Greenberg and Taneja-Uppal, 1987). He had low supine norepinephrine levels, which suggested a peripheral postganglionic deficit (Polinsky et al., 1981).

Patients have been reported who developed syncopal reactions to fine-needle aspiration from the lung. Bradycardia and hypotension occurred immediately after the aspiration and progressed, in one instance, to death; the rapidity suggests a reflex neurologic mechanism, and autonomic abnormalities were found (Craddock et al., 1987).

Autonomic neuropathy has been found in association with parkinsonism and dementia (Miller and Semple, 1987), reminiscent of the Shy-Drager syndrome, and multiple system atrophy may be added to the list of neurologic manifestations of acquired immunodeficiency syndrome (AIDS). Patients have been studied to examine the possibility that autonomic dysfunction might occur before the development of other abnormalities. Abnormal autonomic function may occur in up to 30% of cases, often before other signs (Mulhall and Jennens, 1987). These observations suggest that dysautonomia may lead to complications over management, for example, with needle aspiration, or to modes of presentation, such as syncope related to orthostatic hypotension. It has been recommended that simple tests of heart rate should be carried out before invasive procedures on patients who are HIV positive (Villa et al., 1987), but false-positive results may occur because of weight loss, hypovolemia, or inactivity (Lohmöller et al., 1987).

PERIPHERAL NERVE LESIONS

Acute Polyneuropathy (Guillain-Barré Syndrome)

Autonomic dysfunction can be a feature of the acute polyneuropathy of the Guillain-Barré syndrome. The degree of autonomic failure is variable and only loosely related to the degree of muscle paralysis or sensory involvement. The mechanism of autonomic dysfunction has not been clearly established, but pathologic changes have been observed in the brain stem, the intermediolateral columns of the spinal cord, the sympathetic ganglia, and the vagi. Altered activity of sympathetic or parasympathetic nerves may cause electrocardiographic abnormalities. These include flat or inverted T waves, ST segment flattening, QT interval prolongation, and bursts of tachycardia or bradycardia. Autonomic dysfunction is associated with a poor prognosis in the Guillain-Barré syndrome, and cardiac arrhythmias may occasionally be a direct cause of death (Hodson et al., 1984).

Patients who have lost their circulatory reflexes are unable to maintain an adequate right-sided heart filling pressure when venous return is impeded by raised intrathoracic pressure (Watson et al., 1962). In patients with acute polyneuropathy requiring artificial ventilation, it is important to use a ventilator that does not raise the mean intrathoracic pressure unduly, for example, by obstructing expiration.

Hypertension may occur and may be severe enough to cause papilledema, retinal hemorrhages, and exudates (Hewer et al., 1966). In most patients, hypertension probably results from lesions in the afferent limb of the baroreflex arc (Fagius and Wallin, 1983), but there may also be a disturbance of central control of blood pressure caused by lesions in the brain stem (Appenzeller and Marshall, 1963). Severe hypertension should be treated, but special care is required because these patients do not have normal nervous control of their circulation.

Pure Autonomic Polyneuropathy

A small number of patients have been reported with isolated dysfunction of the peripheral autonomic nervous system of acute onset. The first patient was reported in 1969 (Young et al.), and a more extensive follow-up report appeared in 1975. Patients may present with involvement of any part of the autonomic nervous system, including abnormalities of lacrimation, loss of pupillary reflexes and accommodation, diarrhea or constipation, orthostatic hypotension, loss of sweating, and bladder paralysis. Both adrenergic and cholinergic fibers may be affected. In several patients, the condition has been self-limiting, with recovery over a period of months or many years. Sensory and motor systems have been generally normal apart from slight depression of tendon reflexes in some cases. Investigations have confirmed autonomic failure affecting either preganglionic or postganglionic (efferent) neurons (Okada et al., 1975). The condition may be a variant of acute idiopathic polyneuropathy because protein, but not cells, in cerebrospinal fluid has been raised in some cases. It may be preceded by infectious mononucleosis (Yahr and Frontera, 1975) or herpes simplex (Neville and Sladen, 1984). Pure autonomic polyneuropathy has also been reported as a stocking-glove sensorimotor loss occurring familially (Robinson et al., 1989).

An acute, self-limited condition characterized by hypertension and painful dysesthesias was described in children and suggested to be secondary to autonomic neuropathy (Nass and Chutorian, 1982). These subjects differed from other cases of acute dysautonomia in the prominent sensory symptoms and the presence of sustained hypertension, rather than orthostatic hypotension.

Dopamine β-Hydroxylase Deficiency

Orthostatic hypotension may result from congenital dopamine β-hydroxylase deficiency, in which there is a failure to β-hydroxylate dopamine into norepinephrine (Man in't Veld et al., 1987a; Robertson et al., 1986). Total absence of dopamine β-hydroxylase is rare, although low amounts are found in 3–4% of the population, and this trait, in apparently healthy individuals, is inherited as an autosomal recessive (Dunnette and Weinshilboum, 1977).

In clinically affected individuals, norepinephrine is absent from, or greatly reduced, in plasma, urine, and cerebrospinal fluid, and dopamine accumulates in plasma and cerebrospinal fluid. The condition is lifelong, and orthostatic hypotension, ptosis, and other symptoms of sympathetic failure, such as nasal stuffiness, are present. Impotence is present in males. Normal changes in heart rate to various tests imply normal baroreflex afferents and parasympathetic fibers. There is marked sensitivity to β adrenoreceptor and $α_1$ adrenoreceptor agonists. Tyramine fails to affect blood pressure, thus confirming the absence of norepinephrine. The absence of changes in norepinephrine and epinephrine in plasma on standing, together with rises in dopamine and the various metabolites of catecholamines, reflects the absence of the normal metabolism of dopamine to norepinephrine (Fig. 39–6), and plasma dopamine β-hydroxylase activity is depressed. Plasma dopamine concentrations could vary, implying that central preganglionic and postganglionic modulation of sympathetic activity is intact.

Patients may present in infancy with hypotonia and episodes of vomiting, coma, hypothermia, and hypoglycemia, together with hyperflexible joints. Because dopamine β-hydroxylase requires copper as a cofactor, it has been suggested that the syndrome could result from a disturbance of cellular handling of copper ions, as may occur in Minke's syndrome,

in which such abnormalities may be present, but this has not been confirmed. Treatment of this condition is described in the last section of this chapter.

Diabetes Mellitus

Patients with diabetes mellitus are liable to develop autonomic neuropathy. This occurs particularly in insulin-dependent diabetics; it is most common when the disease has lasted 20 years or more and if control has been poor. Pathologic changes in the autonomic nervous system include neuronal loss in the intermediolateral columns of the spinal cord, histologic changes in sympathetic ganglia, and loss of myelinated fibers in the vagus (Duchen, 1983).

Autonomic neuropathy may be manifested by impotence, bladder atony, nocturnal diarrhea, or orthostatic hypotension. Impotence and nocturnal diarrhea, however, cannot on their own be relied on as evidence of autonomic neuropathy. Patients with diabetes mellitus may show high resting heart rates, and these appear to be related to vagal neuropathy, which may accompany the disease (Ewing et al., 1981).

In a study of unselected nonketotic diabetics, two-thirds of whom were insulin dependent, one-fourth of the patients had orthostatic hypotension (Cryer et al., 1978). In a few patients, there was a reduced plasma norepinephrine response to standing, presumably related to sympathetic neuropathy, but in

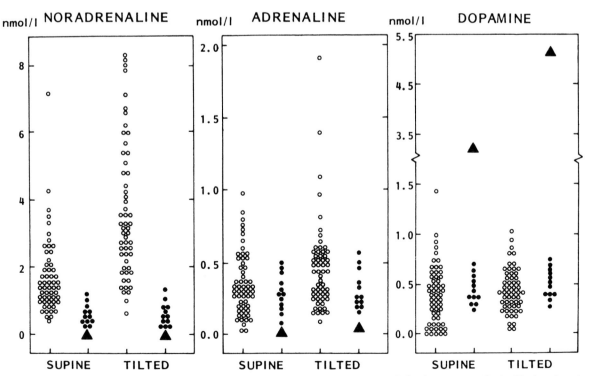

Figure 39–6. Basal and stimulated (5 min 60° head-up tilt) concentrations of plasma catecholamines: ● = patient with chronic autonomic failure; ○ = age- and sex-matched control; ▲ = patient with dopamine β-hydroxylase deficiency, in whom dopamine was released instead of norepinephrine and epinephrine, as normally occurs. (From Man in't Veld A.J., Boomsma F., Moleman P., et al. Congenital dopamine-beta-hydroxylase deficiency. *Lancet* 1:183–188, 1987.)

the remainder plasma norepinephrine responses to standing were either normal or exaggerated. Orthostatic hypotension in this latter group could be due to diminished response of blood vessels to norepinephrine, but this has not been confirmed (Tohmeh et al., 1979). Another possible cause of the orthostatic hypotension is reduced blood volume.

Intravenous injection of insulin may provoke orthostatic hypotension in diabetic patients with autonomic neuropathy but not in normal subjects or diabetics without neuropathy (Page and Watkins, 1976). Because orthostatic hypotension tends to be worse during the early morning, the effect of insulin may be lessened by delaying the morning dose of insulin for some hours after rising (Palmer et al., 1977).

Autonomic neuropathy in diabetics may be a contributing factor in the development of foot ulceration (Deanfield et al., 1980). The hypersensitivity to cold of denervated blood vessels in the foot might dispose to ischemia. Also, cracking of the dry skin of the foot with absent sweating related to sympathetic denervation might make it vulnerable to infection. Distal anhidrosis is common in diabetic patients with peripheral neuropathy (Fealey et al., 1989).

Diabetics may be impotent from autonomic neuropathy (Ewing et al., 1973). Vascular pathology and psychologic factors, however, may be more common causes.

Gustatory sweating can occur in diabetics. This may result from autonomic neuropathy followed by vagal regeneration of sympathetic sudomotor pathways (Watkins, 1973). However, Stuart (1981) considered that this does not satisfactorily explain the symmetry of the excessive sweating on both sides of the face seen in some patients and suggested that it is due to diabetic neuropathy causing impairment of a tonic suppressive influence on sweating.

Autonomic neuropathy in diabetics has a poor prognosis. Patients with symptomatic autonomic neuropathy showed a mortality after 2½ years of 44% and after 5 years of 56% (Fig. 39–7) (Ewing et al., 1980). Half of the deaths were due to renal failure, but some were "sudden" deaths. Sudden death in diabetics with autonomic neuropathy probably results from cardiorespiratory arrest (Page and Watkins, 1978), and the use of respiratory depressant drugs and anesthesia in such patients should be carefully monitored.

Alcoholism

Alcoholic subjects, while withdrawing from alcohol, may have orthostatic hypotension because of altered sympathetic nerve activity. Dehydration during the withdrawal period might also be a factor. Orthostatic hypotension may also occur, more rarely, as a chronic feature of sympathetic neuropathy in alcoholic patients (Birchfield, 1964; Eisenhofer et al., 1985).

Although sympathetic neuropathy and associated orthostatic hypotension are rare in alcoholic patients, abnormalities of parasympathetic nerves are rela-

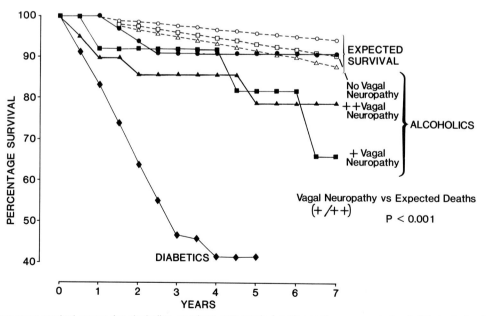

Figure 39–7. Seven-year survival curves for alcoholics on whom autonomic function tests were carried out: 32 alcoholics had no evidence of parasympathetic neuropathy (●), 25 alcoholics had only one abnormal test (■), and 22 alcoholics had two or more abnormal tests (▲). Expected survival curves for the general New Zealand population are shown by broken lines with age matching for each group (open symbols). Survival curve for a diabetic population with autonomic neuropathy is also shown (♦) (taken from Ewing D.J., Campbell I.W., Clarke B.F., The natural history of diabetic autonomic neuropathy. *Q. J. Med.* 49:95–108, 1980). The survival rate of alcoholics who had evidence of parasympathetic neuropathy was significantly decreased ($P < .001$). (From Johnson R.H., Robinson B.J. Mortality in alcoholics with autonomic neuropathy. *J. Neurol. Neurosurg. Psychiatry* 51:476–480, 1988.)

tively common (Johnson, 1988). A study of alcoholics with peripheral neuropathy found reduced esophageal mobility that probably resulted from vagal dysfunction (Winship et al., 1968). Novak and Victor (1974) described alcoholic patients with severe nervous system damage in whom dysphagia and hoarseness were prominent symptoms; postmortem examinations revealed extensive degeneration of the vagus nerves. Evidence of vagal neuropathy affecting the heart has been obtained (Duncan et al., 1980). Parasympathetic involvement may also affect fibers to the pupils (Tan et al., 1984c), and autonomic neuropathy occasionally may be a factor in alcoholic impotence (Tan et al., 1984b). Vagal abnormalities as a result of chronic alcoholism may show reversal after several months of abstinence and improved nutrition (Tan et al., 1984a). Autonomic neuropathy in chronic alcoholics may be associated with a significantly higher mortality than in the general population, and deaths caused by cardiovascular disease are a major cause (Johnson and Robinson, 1988; Thuluvath and Trigger, 1989; Villalta et al., 1989) (see Fig. 39–7).

Amyloidosis

The clinical manifestations of primary amyloidosis may include nervous system involvement, particularly a symmetric progressive sensorimotor neuropathy but also, commonly, autonomic disturbances (Rubenstein et al., 1983). Orthostatic hypotension may be the presenting symptom, and it may be severe (Kyle et al., 1966). It is probably due to abnormalities in efferent sympathetic fibers. Amyloid infiltration has been observed in autonomic ganglia of patients with amyloidosis at autopsy (Munsat and Poussaint, 1962), and catecholamine depletion has been observed in perivascular nerve endings (Rubenstein et al., 1978). Other autonomic symptoms occurring in amyloidosis include gastrointestinal disturbances, anhidrosis, bladder dysfunction, and impotence.

Renal Failure

Patients with chronic renal failure generally show evidence of peripheral neuropathy, and autonomic nerves may also be affected, causing sweating loss (Hennessy and Siemsen, 1968) and disorders of cardiovascular reflexes (Bach et al., 1979). Severe hypotension is a frequent complication of hemodialysis and results, in part, from autonomic neuropathy (Kersh et al., 1974). Hypovolemia appeared to be solely responsible for hypotension in patients with normal autonomic function. In these patients, but not the others, blood pressure returned to normal during volume expansion. Autonomic dysfunction may be due to lesions in afferent pathways to the baroreceptors (Lilley et al., 1976).

Acute Intermittent Porphyria

In porphyria, autonomic neuropathy has been held responsible for the tachycardia and hypertension that may be common and early features of a relapse (Ridley et al., 1968). Another feature of a relapse is severe colic. Acute demyelination in the vagus nerves and sympathetic chain and chromatolysis in the dorsal vagal nucleus of the medulla have been observed in patients dying of fatal episodes of porphyria (Gibson and Goldberg, 1965), and lesions in the central nervous system, including the hypothalamus, have also been reported (Perloth et al., 1966). Orthostatic hypotension may be accompanied by patchy loss of sweating and loss of sphincter control, which suggest that disturbance is due to efferent autonomic lesions.

Neurologic disturbances can be fatal and have apparently been precipitated by a large variety of drugs (Eales and Dowdle, 1968). Any patient suspected of having this disease should use only essential drugs until the diagnosis has been excluded.

Adie's Syndrome

The Adie or Holmes-Adie syndrome consists of a tonic pupil together with absent stretch reflexes. The pupillary abnormality, which is due to parasympathetic failure, is described in detail in Chapter 34. The discussion here is centered on the association with other, more widespread symptoms of autonomic dysfunction.

Orthostatic hypotension, segmental hypohidrosis, and diarrhea in the absence of structural bowel disease are occasional findings. There is no clear pattern of autonomic involvement. Those patients in whom segmental sudomotor dysfunction has been reported almost certainly had efferent sympathetic involvement, and generalized autonomic degeneration could be explained by postganglionic efferent lesions. In patients with orthostatic hypotension, the autonomic pathways may be blocked on the afferent side of the reflex or its connections (Johnson et al., 1971; Rubenstein et al., 1980). The association of the Adie syndrome with other symptoms of autonomic failure was reviewed in detail by Johnson (1983b).

Chagas' Disease

Infection with *Trypanosoma cruzi* (Chagas' disease) is common in certain rural areas of South America and in southern Mexico. The chronic form occurs both in children and in adults; dilatation of hollow organs, including the gastrointestinal and urinary tracts, as well as the heart, may occur. Patients with cardiomegaly from Chagas' disease are liable to sudden death, which may be at least partly related to destruction of the autonomic nerves to the heart. Degeneration of intracardiac ganglionic cells and cardiac nerves occurs, and there may be physiologic evidence of vagal dysfunction. Bradycardia is a feature of chronic Chagas' disease (Palmero et al., 1981) and is possibly due to sympathetic nervous dysfunction, but intrinsic dysfunction of the sinus node appears a more likely explanation.

In the esophagus, there is degeneration of considerable numbers of ganglion cells, and this degeneration probably prevents normal peristalsis (Long, 1983). The clinical picture of megaesophagus resembles that of achalasia of the cardia. The esophagus dilates, and stagnation of food causes esophagitis, ulcers, and hemorrhage. Diverticula and fistulas may develop. The possibility of both the colon and the esophagus being affected is considerable; about 50% of patients with megaesophagus have megacolon, and 27% of patients with megacolon have megaesophagus. The organisms multiply in the walls of the colon, destroy the intramural ganglion cells, and may eventually affect ganglion cells of the entire colon. Before this stage, the patient presents with constipation.

Orthostatic Hypotension in the Elderly

Up to one-sixth of elderly patients have minor falls of blood pressure on standing, with occasional dizziness and transient loss of consciousness (Caird et al., 1973; Johnson et al., 1965). The degree of the blood pressure fall may vary considerably over the course of the day and be more pronounced, in particular, after meals (Macrae and Bulpitt, 1989). In some elderly patients with orthostatic hypotension, the site of the block may be in the baroreceptors, their afferent nerves or the brain stem, but, in the majority of patients, plasma catecholamine responses to standing are normal (Robinson et al., 1983). Changes in adrenoreceptors may have a role in orthostatic hypotension in the elderly, and depression of α_2 adrenoreceptor sites measured on platelets has been observed, whereas an increase would be expected in autonomic failure (Robinson et al., 1990). Alteration in structure of the blood vessels may be the most important cause of orthostatic hypotension (MacLennan et al., 1980; Smith and Fasler, 1983), and the loss of baroreflex sensitivity that occurs with aging could be explained by arterial rigidity (Gribbin et al., 1971; Winson et al., 1974). Some patients with a minor degree of orthostatic hypotension have hyponatremia or hypokalemia, either of which responds to treatment.

Frequently, orthostatic hypotension in the elderly is multifactorial (Caird et al., 1973). Failure of cerebral autoregulation may contribute to symptoms of orthostatic hypotension in the elderly, as some symptomatic patients show bilateral or unilateral failure of cerebral autoregulation (Wollner et al., 1979). The pathophysiology of the condition is still debated (Johnson, 1991).

TREATMENT OF NEUROGENIC ORTHOSTATIC HYPOTENSION
(Table 39–4)

Many patients benefit from mechanical means to prevent blood pooling. Most effective are trousers that have inflatable components to compress the legs and abdomen; these are available from manufacturers of equipment for pilots. Elastic stockings are generally not effective alone but may be in combination with an elastic abdominal support, provided that the stockings are full length and the abdominal support is firm. Patients may also benefit from having the head of the bed raised at night. This probably works by reducing renal arterial pressure, promoting renin release, and increasing blood volume.

The most widely used pharmacologic agent in orthostatic hypotension is 9α-fluorohydrocortisone (fludrocortisone), which increases blood volume and maintains venous return to the heart. However, some patients who show benefit with the drug have only small increases in blood volume (Schatz et al., 1976). Fludrocortisone may also increase blood pressure by enhancing the sensitivity of vascular receptors to circulating norepinephrine (Davies et al., 1979). Chronic treatment with fludrocortisone may produce supine hypertension, and the risk of associated complications should be considered in evaluation of clinical benefit. Combined therapy with the vasodilator hydralazine has been suggested to be beneficial in improving control of orthostatic hypotension, with

Table 39–4. TREATMENT OF NEUROGENIC ORTHOSTATIC HYPOTENSION*

1. **Mechanical supports**
   Elastic stockings, abdominal binding, inflation suit
2. **Blood volume expansion**
   Response to raising head of bed
   9-α-Fluorohydrocortisone (fludrocortisone)
3. **Vasoconstrictors**
   Phenylephrine
   Ephedrine
   Midodrine
   Norepinephrine
   Tyramine with monoamine oxidase inhibition
   Dihydroergotamine
   Ergotamine
   Yohimbine
4. **Inhibition of prostaglandins**
   Indomethacin
   Flubiprofen
   Clonidine
5. **β₁ agonist**
   Prenalterol
6. **β blockers (inhibiting vasodilatation, reducing tachycardia during orthostatic hypotension)**
   Pindolol
   Propranolol
7. **DL-Dihydroxyphenylserine (for dopamine β-hydroxylase deficiency)**
8. **Atrial pacemaker**

*Treatments 1 and 2 are used together. If they are inadequate, treatments 3, 4, and 5 may be tried successively (see text). The importance of treatment 6 remains to be established by further use.

less supine hypertension (Jones and Reid, 1980), but this remains to be confirmed.

A variety of sympathomimetic substances have been used as vasoconstrictor agents in the treatment of orthostatic hypotension, including phenylephrine, ephedrine, and tyramine with a monoamine oxidase inhibitor. With all these agents, however, the side effect of supine hypertension may be a problem.

Ergotamine and its derivatives have vasoconstrictor actions that are mainly confined to the capacitance vessels. Dihydroergotamine (4–10 mg by mouth) has been used with some success in patients with orthostatic hypotension (Nordenfelt and Mellander, 1972), but it is not always effective. There may be a problem with bioavailability of oral dihydroergotamine (Olver et al., 1980), and ergotamine tartrate may be more useful for oral administration.

β receptor inhibition can reduce vasodilatation. The β blocker pindolol, which has intrinsic sympathomimetic activity, was reported to be effective in orthostatic hypotension associated with autonomic failure (Man in't Veld and Schalekamp, 1981). However, in patients with multiple system atrophy, pindolol was ineffective in all patients and may cause cardiac failure (Davies et al., 1981); pindolol should probably be restricted to patients with a postganglionic lesion.

Treatment of orthostatic hypotension related to dopamine β-hydroxylase deficiency is possible with the artificial norepinephrine precursor DL-dihydroxyphenylserine, which has a different metabolic pathway to norepinephrine compared with that via dopamine (Biaggioni and Robertson, 1987) (Fig. 39–8). Dose-dependent increases in blood pressure were obtained over the range of 150–600 mg, and the increases were closely correlated with increases in plasma norepinephrine. The treatment has been given for several months, during which freedom of symptoms occurred and a normal life could be lived (Man in't Veld et al., 1987b). This successful form of treatment helps to confirm that in this disorder the sympathetic neuron is intact but that dopamine, rather than norepinephrine, is released be-

cause of the congenital dopamine β-hydroxylase deficiency.

References

(Key references are designated with an asterisk.)

Andrew J., Nathan P.W. The cerebral control of micturition. *Proc. R. Soc. Med.* 58:553–555, 1965.

Andrew J., Nathan P.W., Spanos N.C. Disturbance of micturition and defaecation due to aneurysms of anterior communicating or anterior cerebral arteries. *J. Neurosurg.* 24:1–10, 1966.

*Appenzeller O. *The Autonomic Nervous System.* 3rd ed. Amsterdam, Elsevier North Holland Biomedical Press, 1982.

Appenzeller O., Marshall J. Vasomotor disturbance in the Landry-Guillain-Barré syndrome. *Arch. Neurol.* 9:368–372, 1963.

Bach C., Iaina A., Eliahou H.E. Autonomic nervous system disturbances in patients on chronic hemodialysis. *Isr. J. Med. Sci.* 15:761–764, 1979.

*Bannister R., ed. *Autonomic Failure: A Textbook of Clinical Disorders of the Autonomic Nervous System.* New York, Oxford University Press, 1983.

*Bannister R., ed. *Autonomic Failure: A Textbook of Clinical Disorders of the Autonomic Nervous System.* 2nd ed. New York, Oxford University Press, 1988.

Bannister R., Oppenheimer D.R. Degenerative diseases of the nervous system associated with autonomic failure. *Brain* 95:457–474, 1972.

Bannister R., Crowe R., Eames R., et al. Adrenergic innervation in autonomic failure. *Neurology (N.Y.)* 31:1501–1506, 1981.

Bannister R., Mowbray J., Sidgwick A. Genetic control of progressive autonomic failure: evidence for an association with an HLA antigen. *Lancet* 1:1017, 1983.

Bauer H.G. Endocrine and other clinical manifestations of hypothalamic disease: a survey of 60 cases with autopsies. *J. Clin. Endocrinol.* 14:13–31, 1954.

Becker L.E., Mitchell A.D. Priapism. *Surg. Clin. North Am.* 45:1523–1534, 1965.

Biaggioni I., Robertson D. Endogenous restoration of noradrenaline by precursor therapy in dopamine-beta-hydroxylase deficiency. *Lancet* 2:1170–1172, 1987.

Birchfield R. I. Postural hypotension in Wernicke's disease. *Am. J. Med.* 36:404–414, 1964.

Bors E., Turner R.D. History and physical examination in neurologic urology. In Boyarsky S., ed. *The Neurogenic Bladder.* Baltimore, Williams & Wilkins, 1967.

Bradbury S., Eggleston C. Postural hypotension. A report of 3 cases. *Am. Heart J.* 1:73–86, 1925.

Brown W.J., Beauchemin J.A., Linde L.M. A neuropathological study of familial dysautonomia (Riley-Day syndrome) in siblings. *J. Neurol. Neurosurg. Psychiatry* 27:131–139, 1964.

Caird F.I., Andrews G.R., Kennedy R.D. Effect of posture on blood pressure in the elderly. *Br. Heart J.* 35:525–530, 1973.

Collins K.J., Dore C., Exton-Smith A.N., et al. Accidental hypothermia and impaired temperature homeostasis in the elderly. *Br. Med. J.* 1:353–356, 1977.

Corbett J.L., Frankel H.L., Harris P.J. Cardiovascular changes associated with skeletal muscle spasm in tetraplegic man. *J. Physiol. (Lond.)* 215:381–393, 1971.

Craddock C., Pasvol G., Bull R., et al. Cardiopulmonary arrest and autonomic neuropathy in AIDS. *Lancet* 2:16–18, 1987.

Cryer P.E., Silverberg A.B., Santiago J.V., et al. Plasma catecholamines in diabetes. *Am. J. Med.* 64:407–416, 1978.

Cunningham D.J.C., Guttmann L., Whitteridge D., et al. Cardiovascular responses to bladder distension in paraplegic patients. *J. Physiol. (Lond.)* 121:581–592, 1953.

Cushing H. Some experimental and clinical observations concerning states of increased intracranial tension. *Am. J. Med. Sci.* 124:375–400, 1902.

Davies B., Bannister R., Sever P., et al. The pressor actions of noradrenaline, angiotensin II and saralasin in chronic autonomic

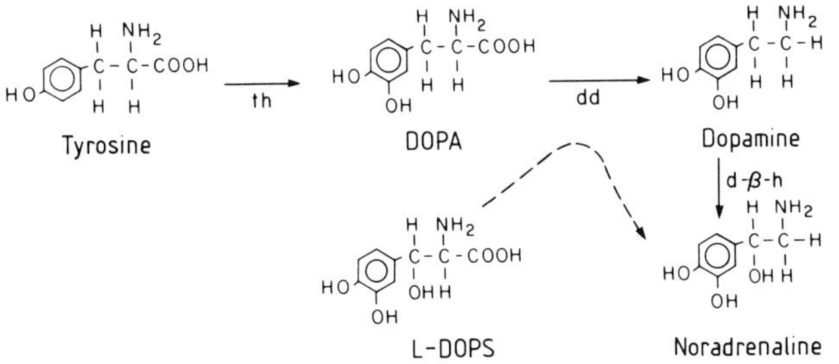

Figure 39–8. Primary biosynthetic pathway of catecholamines (*solid arrows*) and alternative formation of norepinephrine (*dashed arrow*) from DL-dihydroxyphenylserine (L-DOPS). th = tyrosine hydroxylase; dd = dopa decarboxylase; d-β-h = dopamine-β-hydroxylase. (From Biaggioni I., Robertson D. Endogenous restoration of noradrenaline by precursor therapy in dopamine-beta-hydroxylase deficiency. *Lancet* 2:1170–1172, 1987.)

failure treated with fludrocortisone. *Br. J. Clin. Pharmacol.* 8:253–260, 1979.

Davies B., Bannister R., Mathias C., et al. Pindolol in postural hypotension: the case for caution. *Lancet* 2:982–983, 1981.

Deanfield J.E., Daggett P.R., Harrison M.J.G. The role of autonomic neuropathy in diabetic foot ulceration. *J. Neurol. Sci.* 47:203–210, 1980.

Duchen L.W. Neuropathology of the autonomic nervous system in diabetics. In Bannister R., ed. *Autonomic Failure: A Textbook of Clinical Disorders of the Autonomic Nervous System.* New York, Oxford University Press, 1983.

Duff R.S., Ferrant P.C., Leveaux V.M., et al. Spontaneous periodic hypothermia. *Q. J. Med.* 30:329–338, 1961.

Duncan G., Johnson R.H., Lambie D.G., et al. Evidence of vagal neuropathy in chronic alcoholics. *Lancet* 2:1053–1057, 1980.

Dunnette J., Weinshilboum R.M. Inheritance of low immunoreactive human plasma dopamine hydroxylase. *J. Clin. Invest.* 60:1080–1087, 1977.

Eales L., Dowdle E.B. Clinical aspects of importance in the porphyrias. *Br. J. Clin. Pract.* 22:505–515, 1968.

Eisenhofer G.E., Whiteside E.A., Johnson R. H. Plasma catecholamine responses to change of posture in alcoholics during withdrawal and after continued abstinence from alcohol. *Clin. Sci.* 68:71–78, 1985.

Ewing D.J., Campbell I.W., Burt A.A., et al. Vascular reflexes in diabetic autonomic neuropathy. *Lancet* 2:1354–1356, 1973.

Ewing D.J., Campbell I.W., Clarke B.F. The natural history of diabetic autonomic neuropathy. *Q. J. Med.* 49:95–108, 1980.

Ewing D.J., Campbell I.W., Clarke B.F. Heart rate changes in diabetes mellitus. *Lancet* 1:183–186, 1981.

Fagius J., Wallin B.G. Microneurographic evidence of excessive sympathetic outflow in Guillain-Barré syndrome. *Brain* 106:589–600, 1983.

Fealey R.D., Low P.A., Thomas J.E. Thermoregulatory sweating abnormalities in diabetes mellitus. *Mayo Clin. Proc.* 64:617–628, 1989.

Fox R.H., Wilkins D.C., Bell J.A., et al. Spontaneous periodic hypothermia: diencephalic epilepsy. *Br. Med. J.* 2:693–695, 1973.

Gibson J.B., Goldberg A. The neuropathy of acute porphyria. *J. Pathol. Bacteriol.* 71:495–509, 1965.

Gribbin B., Pickering T.G., Sleight P., et al. Effect of age and high blood pressure on baroreflex sensitivity in man. *Circ. Res.* 29:424–431, 1971.

Gross M., Bannister R., Godwin-Austen R. Orthostatic hypotension in Parkinson's disease. *Lancet* 2:174–176, 1972.

Gubbay S.S., Barwick D.D. Two cases of accidental hypothermia in Parkinson's disease with unusual EEG findings. *J. Neurol. Neurosurg. Psychiatry* 29:459–466, 1966.

Guttmann L. The married life of paraplegics and tetraplegics. *Paraplegia* 2:182–188, 1964.

Guttmann L. *Spinal Cord Injuries: Comprehensive Management and Research.* 2nd ed. Oxford, Blackwell Scientific Publications, 1976.

Hennessy W. J., Siemsen A.W. Autonomic neuropathy in chronic renal failure. *Clin. Res.* 16:385, 1968.

Hewer R.L., Hilton P.J., Smith A.C., et al. Acute polyneuritis requiring artificial respiration. *Q. J. Med.* 37:479–491, 1966.

Hodson A.K., Horwitz B.J., Albrecht R. Dysautonomia in Guillain-Barré syndrome with dorsal root ganglioneuropathy, wallerian degeneration, and fatal myocarditis. *Ann. Neurol.* 15:88–95, 1984.

Hopkins A., Clarke C., Brindley G. Erections on walking as a symptom of spinal canal stenosis. *J. Neurol. Neurosurg. Psychiatry* 50:1371–1374, 1987.

Johnson R.H. Temperature regulation. In Vinken P.J., Bruyn G.W., eds. *Handbook of Clinical Neurology.* Vol. 26. *Injuries of the Spinal Cord.* Amsterdam, Elsevier North Holland Biomedical Press, pp. 355–376, 1976.

Johnson R.H. Autonomic dysfunction in clinical disorders with particular reference to catecholamine release. *J. Auton. Nerv. Syst.* 7:219–232, 1983a.

Johnson R.H. Autonomic failure and the eyes. In Bannister R., ed. *Autonomic Failure: A Textbook of Clinical Disorders of the Autonomic Nervous System.* New York, Oxford University Press, pp. 508–542, 1983b.

Johnson R.H. Autonomic failure in alcoholics. In Bannister R., ed. *Autonomic Failure: A Textbook of Clinical Disorders of the Nervous System.* 2nd ed. New York, Oxford University Press, pp. 690–714, 1988.

Johnson R.H. Orthostatic hypotension in the elderly. In Evans J.G., Williams T.F., eds. *Oxford Textbook of Geriatric Medicine.* New York, Oxford University Press, in press.

Johnson R.H., Park D.M. Effect of change of posture on blood pressure and renin-concentration in men with spinal transections. *Clin. Sci.* 44:539–546, 1973.

Johnson R.H., Robinson B.J. Mortality in alcoholics with autonomic neuropathy. *J. Neurol. Neurosurg. Psychiatry* 51:476–480, 1988.

*Johnson R.H., Spalding J.M.K. *Disorders of the Autonomic Nervous System.* Oxford, Blackwell, 1974.

Johnson R.H., Smith A.C., Spalding J.M.K., et al. Effect of posture on blood-pressure in elderly patients. *Lancet* 1:731–733, 1965.

Johnson R.H., Lee G. de J., Oppenheimer D.R., et al. Autonomic failure with orthostatic hypotension due to intermediolateral column degeneration. *Q. J. Med.* 35:276–292, 1966.

Johnson R.H., McLellan D.L., Love D.R. Orthostatic hypotension and the Holmes-Adie syndrome: a study of two patients with afferent baroreceptor block. *J. Neurol. Neurosurg. Psychiatry* 34:562–570, 1971.

*Johnson R.H., Lambie D.G., Spalding J.M.K. *Neurocardiology: The Interrelationship Between Dysfunction in the Nervous and Cardiovascular Systems.* London, Saunders, 1984.

Jones D.H., Reid J.L. Volume expansion and vasodilators in the treatment of idiopathic orthostatic hypotension. *Postgrad. Med. J.* 56:234–235, 1980.

Kersh E.S., Kronfield J., Unger A., et al. Autonomic insufficency in uremia as a cause of hemodialysis-induced hypotension. *N. Engl. J. Med.* 290:650–653, 1974.

Kyle R.A., Kottke B.A., Schirger A. Orthostatic hypotension as a clue to primary systemic amyloidosis. *Circulation* 34:883–888, 1966.

Lewis P. Familial orthostatic hypotension. *Brain* 87:719–728, 1964.

Lilley J.J., Golden J., Stone R.A. Adrenergic regulation of blood pressure in chronic renal failure. *J. Clin. Invest.* 57:1190–1200, 1976.

Lindan R., Joiner E., Freehafer A.A., et al. Incidence and clinical features of autonomic dysreflexia in patients with spinal cord injury. *Paraplegia* 18:285–292, 1980.

Lin-Greenberg A., Taneja-Uppal N. Dysautonomia and infection with the human Immunodeficiency virus. *Ann. Intern. Med.* 106:167, 1987.

Lohmöller G., Matuschke A., Goebel F.D. Testing for neurological involvement in HIV infection. *Lancet* 2:1532, 1987.

Long R.G. Chagas' disease. In Bannister R., ed. *Autonomic Failure: A Textbook of Clinical Disorders of the Autonomic Nervous System.* New York, Oxford University Press, 1983.

MacLennan W.J., Hall M.R.P., Timothy J.I. Postural hypotension in old age: is it a disorder of the nervous system or of blood vessels? *Age Ageing* 9:25–32, 1980.

Macmillan A.L., Corbett J.L., Johnson R.H., et al. Temperature regulation in survivors of accidental hypothermia of the elderly. *Lancet* 2:165–169, 1967.

Macrae A.D., Bulpitt C.J. Assessment of postural hypotension in elderly patients. *Age Ageing* 18:110–112, 1989.

Man in't Veld A.J., Schalekamp M.A.D.H. Pindolol acts as beta-adrenoceptor agonist in orthostatic hypotension: therapeutic implications. *Br. Med. J.* 282:929–931, 1981.

Man in't Veld A.J., Boomsma F., Moleman P., et al. Congenital dopamine-beta-hydroxylase deficiency. *Lancet* 1:183–188, 1987a.

Man in't Veld A.J., Boomsma F., Meiracker A.H., et al. Effect of unnatural noradrenaline precursor on sympathetic control and orthostatic hypotension in dopamine-beta-hydroxylase deficiency. *Lancet* 2:1172–1175, 1987b.

Marsden C.D., Parkes J.D., Rees J.E. A year's comparison of

treatment of patients with Parkinson's disease with levodopa combined with carbidopa versus treatment with levodopa alone. *Lancet* 2:1459–1462, 1973.

Mathias C.J., Christensen N.J., Corbett J.L., et al. Plasma catecholamines, plasma renin activity and plasma aldosterone in tetraplegic man, horizontal and tilted. *Clin. Sci.* 49:291–299, 1975.

Miller R.F., Semple S.J.G. Autonomic neuropathy in AIDS. *Lancet* 2:243–244, 1987.

Mooradian A.D., Morley G.K., McGeachie R., et al. Spontaneous periodic hypothermia. *Neurology (N.Y.)* 34:79–82, 1984.

Mulhall B.P., Jennens I. Testing for neurological involvement in HIV infection. *Lancet* 2:1531–1532, 1987.

Munsat T.L., Poussaint A.F. Clinical manifestations and diagnosis of amyloid polyneuropathy. Report of three cases. *Neurology (Minneap.)* 12:413–422, 1962.

Nanda R.N., Boyle F.C., Gillespie J.S., et al. Idiopathic orthostatic hypotension from failure of noradrenaline release in a patient with vasomotor innervation. *J. Neurol. Neurosurg. Psychiatry* 40:11–19, 1977.

Nass R., Chutorian A. Dysaesthesias and dysautonomia: a self-limited syndrome of painful dysaesthesias and autonomic dysfunction in childhood. *J. Neurol. Neurosurg. Psychiatry* 45:162–165, 1982.

Nathan P.W., Smith M.C. The location of descending fibres to sympathetic neurons supplying the eye and sudomotor neurons supplying the head and neck. *J. Neurol. Neurosurg. Psychiatry* 49:187–194, 1986.

Nathan P.W., Smith M.C. The location of descending fibres to sympathetic preganglionic vasomotor and sudomotor neurons in man. *J. Neurol. Neurosurg. Psychiatry* 50:1253–1262, 1987.

Neville B.G.R., Sladen G.E. Acute autonomic neuropathy following primary herpes simplex infection. *J. Neurol. Neurosurg. Psychiatry* 47:648–650, 1984.

Nordenfelt I., Mellander S. Central haemodynamic effects of dihydroergotamine in patients with orthostatic hypotension. *Acta Med. Scand.* 191:115–120, 1972.

Novak D.J., Victor M. The vagus and sympathetic nerves in alcoholic neuropathy. *Arch. Neurol.* 30:273–284, 1974.

Okada F., Yamashita I., Suwa N. Two cases of acute pandysautonomia. *Arch. Neurol.* 32:146–151, 1975.

Olver I.N., Jennings G.L., Bobik A., et al. Low bioavailability as a cause of apparent failure of dihydroergotamine in orthostatic hypotension. *Br. Med. J.* 281:275–276, 1980.

Oppenheimer D.R. Neuropathy of progressive autonomic failure. In Bannister R., ed. *Autonomic Failure: A Textbook of Clinical Disorders of the Autonomic Nervous System.* New York, Oxford University Press, 1983.

Oppenheimer S. Cardiac dysfunction during seizures and the sudden epileptic death syndrome. *J. R. Soc. Med.* 83:134–136, 1990.

Page M.M., Watkins P.J. Provocation of postural hypotension by insulin in diabetic autonomic neuropathy. *Diabetes* 25:90–95, 1976.

Page M.M., Watkins P.J. Cardiorespiratory arrest and diabetic autonomic neuropathy. *Lancet* 1:14–16, 1978.

Palmer K.T., Perkins C.J., Smith R.B.W. Insulin aggravated postural hypotension. *Aust. N. Z. J. Med.* 7:161–162, 1977.

Palmero H.A., Caeiro T.F., Iosa D. Prevalence of slow heart rates in chronic Chagas' disease. *Am. J. Trop. Med. Hyg.* 30:1179–1182, 1981.

Penfield W. Diencephalic autonomic epilepsy. *Arch. Neurol. Psychiatry* 22:358–374, 1929.

Perloth M.G., Tschudy D.P., Marver H.S., et al. Acute intermittent porphyria: new morphologic and biochemical findings. *Am. J. Med.* 41:149–162, 1966.

Polinsky R.J., Kopin I.J., Ebert M.H., et al. Pharmacologic distinction of different orthostatic hypotension syndromes. *Neurology (N.Y.)* 31:1–7, 1981.

Ridley A., Hierons R., Cavanagh J.B. Tachycardia and the neuropathy of porphyria. *Lancet* 1:708–710, 1968.

Riley C.M. Familial dysautonomia. *Adv. Pediatr.* 9:157–190, 1957.

Riley C.M., Day R.L., Greeley D.M., et al. Central autonomic dysfunction with defective lacrimation: report of 5 cases. *Pediatrics* 3:468–478, 1949.

Robertson D., Goldberg H.R., Onrot J., et al. Isolated failure of autonomic noradrenergic neurotransmission. Evidence for impaired β hydroxylation of dopamine. *N. Engl. J. Med.* 314:1494–1497, 1986.

Robinson B., Johnson R.H., Abernethy D., et al. Familial distal dysautonomia. *J. Neurol. Neurosurg. Psychiatry* 52:1281–1285, 1989.

Robinson B.J., Johnson R.H., Lambie D.G., et al. Do elderly patients with an excessive fall in blood pressure on standing have evidence of autonomic failure? *Clin. Sci.* 64:587–591, 1983.

Robinson B.J., Stowell L.I., Johnson R.H. Is orthostatic hypotension in the elderly due to autonomic failure? *Age Ageing* 19:288–296, 1990.

Ropper A.H., Hedley-White E.T. Parkinsonism associated with other neurologic manifestations. *N. Engl. J. Med.* 308:1406–1414, 1983.

Rubenstein A.E., Yahr M.D., Mytilineou C. Peripheral catecholamine depletion in amyloid autonomic neuropathy. *Mt. Sinai J. Med.* 45:57–61, 1978.

Rubenstein A.E., Yahr M.D., Mytilineou C., et al. Orthostatic hypotension in the Holmes-Adie syndrome. *Mt. Sinai J. Med.* 47:57–61, 1980.

Rubenstein A.E., Rudansky M.C., Yahr M.D. Autonomic failure due to amyloid. In Bannister R., ed. *Autonomic Failure: A Textbook of Clinical Disorders of the Autonomic Nervous System.* New York, Oxford University Press, 1983.

Schatz I.J., Miller M.J., Frame B. Corticosteroids in the management of orthostatic hypotension. *Cardiology* 61(Suppl. 1):280–289, 1976.

Shy G.M., Drager G.A. A neurological syndrome associated with orthostatic hypotension. *Arch. Neurol.* 2:511–527, 1960.

Skagen K., Jensen O., Henriksen O., et al. Sympathetic reflex control of subcutaneous blood flow in tetraplegic man during postural changes. *Clin. Sci.* 62:605–609, 1982.

Smith S.A., Fasler J.J. Age-related changes in autonomic function: relationship with postural hypotension. *Age Ageing* 12:206–210, 1983.

Spokes E.G.S., Bannister R., Oppenheimer D.R. Multiple system atrophy with autonomic failure. *J. Neurol. Sci.* 43:59–82, 1979.

Stuart D.D. Diabetic gustatory sweating. *Ann. Intern. Med.* 89:223–224, 1981.

Tan E.T.H., Johnson R.H., Lambie D.G., et al. Alcoholic vagal neuropathy: recovery following prolonged abstinence. *J. Neurol. Neurosurg. Psychiatry* 47:1335–1337, 1984a.

Tan E.T.H., Johnson R.H., Lambie D.G., et al. Erectile impotence in chronic alcoholics. *Alcoholism* 8:297–301, 1984b.

Tan E.T.H., Lambie D.G., Johnson R.H., et al. Parasympathetic denervation of the iris in alcoholics with vagal neuropathy. *J. Neurol. Neurosurg. Psychiatry* 47:61–64, 1984c.

Thompson R.K., Malina S. Dynamic axial brain-stem distortion as a mechanism explaining the cardio-respiratory change in increased intracranial pressure. *J. Neurosurg.* 16:664–675, 1959.

Thuluvath P.J., Trigger D.R. Autonomic neuropathy in chronic liver disease. *Q. J. Med.* 72:737–747, 1989.

Tohmeh J.F., Shah S.D., Cryer P.E. Pathogenesis of hyperadrenergic postural hypotension in diabetic patients. *Am. J. Med.* 67:772–778, 1979.

van Buren J.M. Some autonomic concomitants of ictal automatism. A study of temporal lobe attacks. *Brain* 81:505–528, 1958.

Villa A., Foresti V., Confalonieri F. Autonomic neuropathy and HIV infection. *Lancet* 2:915, 1987.

Villalta J., Estruch R., Antunez E., et al. Vagal neuropathy in chronic alcoholics: relation to ethanol consumption. *Alcohol Alcohol.* 24:412–428, 1989.

Watkins P.J. Facial sweating after food: a new sign of diabetic autonomic neuropathy. *Br. Med. J.* 1:583–587, 1973.

Watson W.E., Smith A.C., Spalding J.M.K. Transmural central venous pressure during intermittent positive pressure respiration. *Br. J. Anaesth.* 34:278–286, 1962.

Welply N.C., Mathias C.J., Frankel H.L. Circulatory reflexes in tetraplegics during artificial ventilation and general anaesthesia. *Paraplegia* 13:172–182, 1975.

Wernicke C. *Lehrbuch der Gehirnkrankheiten fur Aertze und Studierende*. Vol. 2. Berlin, Fischer, p. 229, 1881–1883.

Winship D.H., Caflisch C.R., Zboralske F.F., et al. Deterioration of esophageal peristalsis in patients with alcoholic neuropathy. *Gastroenterology* 55:173–178, 1968.

Winson M., Heath D., Smith P. Extensibility of the human carotid sinus. *Cardiovasc. Res.* 8:58–64, 1974.

Wollner L., McCarthy S.T., Soper N.D.W., et al. Failure of cerebral autoregulation as a cause of brain dysfunction in the elderly. *Br. Med. J.* 1:1117–1118, 1979.

Yahr M.D., Frontera A.T. Acute autonomic neuropathy. *Arch. Neurol.* 32:132–133, 1975.

Yamamoto M., Meyer J.S., Sakai F., et al. Effect of differential spinal cord transection on human cerebral blood flow. *J. Neurol. Sci.* 47:395–406, 1980.

Young R.R., Asbury A.K., Adams R.D. Pure pan-dysautonomia with recovery. *Trans. Am. Neurol. Assoc.* 94:355–357, 1969.

Young R.R., Asbury A.K., Corbett J.L., et al. Pure pan-dysautonomia with recovery. *Brain* 98:613–636, 1975.

40

Hypothalamic-Pituitary Function and Dysfunction

Paul E. Cooper
Joseph B. Martin

REGULATION OF ANTERIOR PITUITARY HORMONE SECRETION

Since the turn of this century, the observation by clinicians and scientists alike that disorders of the hypothalamus could cause symptoms of pituitary insufficiency had suggested that an important interface existed between the nervous and endocrine systems at this site. It was not until the early 1960s, however, that experiments involving pituitary transplantation showed that the hypothalamus had certain tropic influences on the anterior pituitary that were essential for its normal function.

Pituitary-Portal Circulation

The pituitary is supplied by two arteries: the superior and inferior hypophysial (Fig. 40–1). The superior hypophysial artery, a direct branch of the internal carotid, forms a capillary plexus in the hypothalamus and infundibulum that then drains into the hypophysial-portal system. Thus, most of the anterior pituitary is supplied by venous blood from the hypothalamus. The posterior pituitary, in contrast, receives a direct arterial blood supply from the inferior hypophysial artery.

Geoffrey Harris (see Martin and Reichlin, 1987) noted this special vascular relationship between the hypothalamus and anterior pituitary and postulated that the hypothalamus manufactured and released certain "hypophysiotropic" compounds that were carried to the anterior pituitary by the portal system to regulate function. A wide variety of experimental and clinical data now support this hypothesis. A closer examination of the venous drainage of the anterior pituitary, however, has led to the conclusion that, in addition to blood flow from the hypothalamus to the pituitary, it is possible for blood to flow retrogradely up the infundibular stem to the median eminence and thereby provide a route for pituitary hormones to control their own release by positive and negative feedback mechanisms (Page and Bergland, 1977).

The pituitary gland synthesizes and secretes at least six hormones, and each of these is under some type of hypothalamic control (Table 40–1). This control is achieved not only through the influence of the hypophysiotropic hormones (releasing or inhibiting factors) but also through other hypothalamic peptides and classic neurotransmitters and interactions among all three.

The hypophysiotropic hormones are synthesized and released from hypothalamic neurons into the portal vessels in the median eminence (Figs. 40–2 and 40–3). Although a particular hypothalamic factor may influence pituitary hormone release under one circumstance, it may not necessarily be the factor that causes release under all circumstances.

Regulation of Thyroid-Stimulating Hormone Secretion

Thyroid-stimulating hormone (TSH or thyrotropin) is a glycoprotein that is essential for thyroid homeostasis. It has a molecular weight of 28,000 and is formed by two non–covalently linked chains, the α and β subunits.

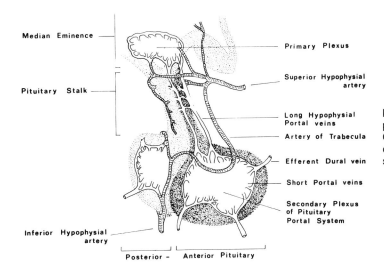

Median Eminence

Pituitary Stalk

Inferior Hypophysial
artery

Primary Plexus

Superior Hypophysial
artery

Long Hypophysial
Portal veins

Artery of Trabecula

Efferent Dural vein

Short Portal veins

Secondary Plexus
of Pituitary
Portal System

Posterior – Anterior Pituitary

Figure 40–1. The circulation of the median eminence and pituitary gland. (Reprinted, with permission, from Martin J.B., Cooper P.E. Neuroendocrine diseases. In Rosenberg R.N., ed. *The Clinical Neurosciences.* New York, Churchill Livingstone, 1983.)

Triiodothyronine (T_3) appears to be the most important factor regulating TSH secretion. It inhibits TSH release, primarily at the pituitary, although it does have some effect at the hypothalamus as well. At the pituitary, most of the T_3 is derived from the action of type II thyroxine 5-deiodinase on L-thyroxine (T_4). T_3 is likely the most important factor in the regulation of TSH homeostasis, but the neuropeptides neurotensin, cholecystokinin, opioid peptides, somatostatin, and thyrotropin-releasing hormone (TRH) have also been shown to influence its secretion. Neurotensin and cholecystokinin inhibit TSH release, whereas opioid peptides are stimulatory. Their physiologic role remains uncertain. The peptide with the best-characterized role in TSH physiology is TRH. A tripeptide, TRH was first isolated and characterized in 1969 (Guillemin, 1978; Schally, 1978). It is widely distributed in the nervous system, with especially rich concentrations being found in the median eminence. Its structure is

$$\overset{1}{\text{L-pyro-Glu}}\text{-}\overset{2}{\text{His}}\text{-}\overset{3}{\text{Pro}}\text{-amide}$$

Administered intravenously to humans, it causes a dose-related increase in TSH secretion and an increase in TSH synthesis. Somatostatin may play a role in control of TSH secretion. It can abolish the TSH response to TRH and will lower TSH levels in primary hypothyroidism. Norepinephrine (α receptor mediated) stimulates TSH release, as does serotonin. Dopamine directly inhibits TSH release at the level of the pituitary.

The failure of TSH to respond to synthetic TRH is one of the most sensitive clinical tests for hyperthyroidism, and TRH can also be used to assess TSH reserve in patients with pituitary disease.

Regulation of Luteinizing Hormone and Follicle-Stimulating Hormone Secretion

Luteinizing hormone (LH) and follicle-stimulating hormone (FSH) play essential roles in the regulation of gonadal function. Like TSH, they are glycoproteins composed of α and β subunits. The α subunits of LH, FSH, TSH, and the placental peptide human chorionic gonadotropin are virtually identical. Immunologic specificity of the intact hormone depends on the β subunit, and biologic activity depends on association of the α and β subunits. In 1971, gonadotropin-releasing hormone (GnRH) was isolated from the hypothalamus (Schally et al., 1971). Its structure is

$$\overset{1}{\text{pyro-Glu}}\text{-}\overset{2}{\text{His}}\text{-}\overset{3}{\text{Trp}}\text{-}\overset{4}{\text{Ser}}\text{-}\overset{5}{\text{Tyr}}\text{-}\overset{6}{\text{Gly}}\text{-}\overset{7}{\text{Leu}}\text{-}\overset{8}{\text{Arg}}\text{-}\overset{9}{\text{Pro}}\text{-}\overset{10}{\text{Gly}}\text{-NH}_2$$

This decapeptide stimulates the release of both LH and FSH. Norepinephrine is thought to be an im-

Table 40–1. ANTERIOR PITUITARY AND HYPOPHYSIOTROPIC HORMONES

Pituitary Hormones	Hypophysiotropic Hormones	
	Name	*Structure*
Growth hormone (GH)	Growth hormone–releasing hormone (GHRH)	44 amino acids
	Growth hormone release–inhibiting hormone (somatostatin)	14 amino acids
Prolactin (PRL)	Prolactin-releasing factor (PRF)	Unknown
	Prolactin release–inhibiting factor (PIF)	Dopamine 56 amino acids of the GnRH precursor
Thyrotropin (TSH)	Thyrotropin-releasing hormone (TRH)	3 amino acids
Proopiomelanocortin (POMC)	Corticotropin-releasing hormone (CRH)	41 amino acids
Luteinizing hormone (LH)	Gonadotropin-releasing hormone (GnRH)	10 amino acids
	Luteinizing hormone release–inhibiting factor	12-kd peptide
Follicle-stimulating hormone (FSH)	Gonadotropin-releasing hormone	10 amino acids

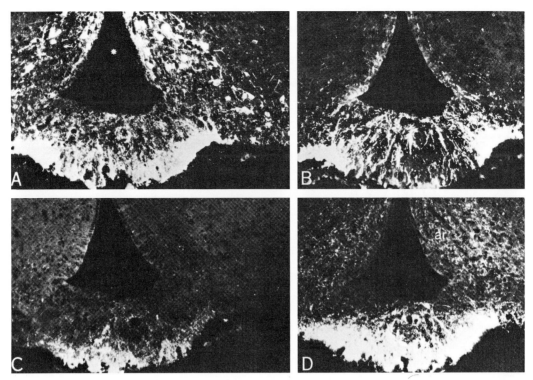

Figure 40–2. Immunofluorescence micrographs of consecutive sections of the basal hypothalamus including the median eminence after incubation with antiserum to tyrosine hydroxylase (*A*), luteinizing hormone–releasing hormone (*B*), thyrotropin-releasing hormone (*C*), and somatostatin (*D*). Luteinizing hormone–releasing hormone (*B*), thyrotropin-releasing hormone (*C*), and somatostatin (*D*) nerve endings are present in the median eminence but in different concentrations and with different distributions. Nerve endings positive for luteinizing hormone–releasing hormone are mainly present in the lateral parts, nerve endings positive for thyrotropin-releasing hormone are in the medial parts, and nerve endings positive for somatostatin are all over the median eminence, as well as also in the arcuate nucleus. In this area, there are also numerous basal hypothalamus–TH-positive cell bodies and nerve endings mainly representing dopamine neurons (*A*). Immunofluorescent cell bodies are not present after incubation with any of the antisera to the three peptides. Asterisk indicates the third ventricle. × 64. (From Hökfelt T., Elde R., Fuxe K., et al. Aminergic and peptidergic pathways in the nervous system with special reference to the hypothalamus. In Reichlin S., Baldessarini R.J., Martin J.B., eds. *The Hypothalamus.* New York, Raven Press, pp. 69–138, 1978.)

portant neurotransmitter in the pulsatile release of GnRH by the hypothalamus. Dopamine, depending on the circumstances, can have either a stimulatory or an inhibitory role. The presence of GnRH is necessary to "prime" the pituitary, but the feedback of gonadal steroids on the pituitary determines the actual pattern of LH and FSH release. The pituitary hormone prolactin (PRL) can inhibit the release of LH and FSH directly at the gonadotrophs in the pituitary.

A 105-amino-acid peptide has been isolated from rat hypothalamus (Hwan and Freeman, 1987) that blocks the release of LH from GnRH-stimulated pituitary cells in vitro. This peptide's physiologic role in LH secretion remains to be determined, as well as whether the entire peptide sequence is necessary for biologic activity or merely a fragment.

Regulation of Adrenocorticotropin Secretion

Adrenocorticotropin (ACTH) is synthesized in the pituitary as part of a larger precursor molecule—proopiomelanocortin (POMC) (Fig. 40–4). POMC is a 265-amino-acid peptide that contains within it the sequence of ACTH and β-lipotropin (β-LPH). ACTH, β-LPH, and the NH_2-terminal fragment of POMC (N-POMC) are secreted in equimolar amounts under a variety of circumstances. The endocrine role of ACTH has been studied extensively and is well understood, but the roles of β-LPH and N-POMC in endocrine regulation are uncertain.

ACTH increases corticosteroid production in the adrenal gland and also causes the gland to hypertrophy. The roles of N-POMC and β-LPH in adrenal physiology remain unclear. N-POMC potentiates ACTH-induced steroidogenesis, whereas β-LPH, particularly the β-melanocyte-stimulating hormone fragment, stimulates aldosterone secretion.

ACTH secretion has a circadian periodicity, with the highest levels occurring in the early morning before awakening and preceding the early-morning rise in cortisol. This rhythm persists even in the absence of the adrenal glands. Stress is an important stimulant for ACTH release.

The search for hypophysiotropic hormones began with a search for corticotropin-releasing factor; however, it was not until 1981 that Vale and colleagues isolated and characterized a 41-amino-acid peptide

HYPOTHALAMIC-NEUROHYPOPHYSIAL
SYSTEM

HYPOTHALAMIC-ADENOHYPOPHYSIAL
SYSTEM

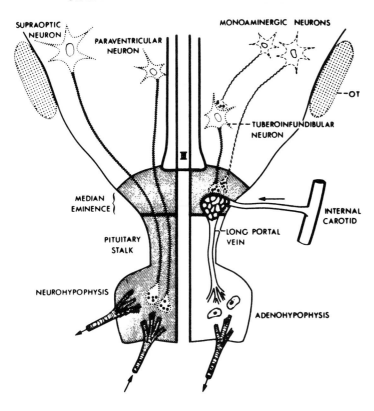

Figure 40–3. Diagram of the hypothalamic-pituitary axis in coronal section. (*Left*) The hypothalamic-neurohypophysial system. Supraoptic and paraventricular axons terminate on blood vessels in the posterior pituitary (neurohypophysis). (*Right*) The hypothalamic-adenohypophysial system. Tuberoinfundibular neurons, believed to be the source of the hypothalamic regulatory hormones, terminate on the capillary plexus in the median eminence. The pituitary-portal system is derived from branches of the internal carotid, which forms a primary capillary bed in the median eminence. The long portal veins drain the capillary plexus into the sinusoids of the anterior pituitary (adenohypophysis). Supraoptic, paraventricular, and tuberoinfundibular neurons are all classed as neurosecretory cells. The activity of tuberoinfundibular neurons is influenced by monoaminergic cells. (From Martin J.B., Reichlin S., Brown G.M. *Clinical Neuroendocrinology.* Philadelphia, Davis, p. 22, 1977.)

from sheep hypothalamus that caused ACTH release (Vale et al., 1981). Since then, corticotropin-releasing hormone (CRH) has been sequenced in the human (Shibahara et al., 1983) and shown to have the following primary structure:

$$\begin{array}{ccccccccccc} 1 & 2 & 3 & 4 & 5 & 6 & 7 & 8 & 9 & 10 & 11 \\ \text{H-Ser-Glu-Glu-Pro-Pro-Ile-Ser-Leu-Asp-Leu-Thr-} \end{array}$$

$$\begin{array}{ccccccccccc} 12 & 13 & 14 & 15 & 16 & 17 & 18 & 19 & 20 & 21 & 22 \\ \text{Phe-His-Leu-Leu-Arg-Glu-Val-Leu-Glu-Met-Ala-} \end{array}$$

$$\begin{array}{ccccccccccc} 23 & 24 & 25 & 26 & 27 & 28 & 29 & 30 & 31 & 32 & 33 \\ \text{Arg-Ala-Glu-Gln-Leu-Ala-Gln-Gln-Ala-His-Ser-} \end{array}$$

$$\begin{array}{ccccccc} 34 & 35 & 36 & 37 & 38 & 39 & 40 & 41 \\ \text{Asn-Arg-Lys-Leu-Met-Glu-Ile-Ile-NH}_2 \end{array}$$

At the level of the pituitary, CRH stimulates ACTH release directly. At the level of the hypothalamus, it enhances ACTH release induced by stress. The posterior pituitary hormone vasopressin (AVP) acts on pituitary corticotrophs to directly stimulate ACTH release and potentiate the action of CRH (C. Rivier et al., 1984).

Norepinephrine inhibits the release of CRH, whereas serotonin stimulates it. γ-Aminobutyric acid also appears to be inhibitory for CRH release. The opiate antagonist naloxone causes a rise in serum cortisol, possibly through inhibition of ACTH release. Angiotensin II, another neuropeptide, causes a rise in ACTH when administered intracerebroventricu-

larly. The mechanism for this is not known but may be due to release of AVP.

Regulation of Growth Hormone Secretion

Growth hormone (GH), initially isolated by Li in 1944, was not fully characterized until 1971 (Li and Dixon, 1971). It is a peptide with a molecular weight of 21,500. Hypothalamic control of GH secretion involves at least two peptides: growth hormone release–inhibiting hormone (somatostatin) and growth hormone–releasing hormone (GHRH).

Somatostatin was isolated from sheep hypothalamus by Guillemin's group in 1973 (Brazeau et al., 1973). This 14-amino-acid peptide is present in the hypothalamus, as well as being distributed widely throughout the human central nervous system (Cooper et al., 1981). Its structure is

$$\begin{array}{cc} 1 & 2 \\ \text{H}_2\text{N-Ala-Gly-} \end{array}$$

$$\begin{array}{cccccccccccc} 3 & 4 & 5 & 6 & 7 & 8 & 9 & 10 & 11 & 12 & 13 & 14 \\ \text{Cys-Lys-Asn-Phe-Phe-Trp-Lys-Thr-Phe-Thr-Ser-Cys-COOH} \end{array}$$

It blocks the release of GH induced by exercise, amino acids, and hypoglycemia; it is also effective in reducing the elevated GH levels in acromegaly. Somatostatin appears to be responsible for determining the basal levels of GH secretion because reduction of

Figure 40–4. The opiocortins are a family of peptides sharing a common, high-molecular-mass precursor: proopiocortin or POMC. The signal peptide and 16,000-dalton (16 K) fragment are sometimes referred to as N-POMC. N-POMC, ACTH, and β-LPH are released in equimolar amounts under physiological conditions. Note the recurring melanocyte-stimulating hormone (MSH) sequence (hatched areas). Although the sequence of met-enkephalin is contained within the sequence of β-endorphin (an opioid peptide, ■), present evidence indicates that met-enkephalin arises from a separate precursor molecule. (From Cooper P.E., Martin J.B. Neuroendocrinology and brain peptides. *Ann. Neurol.* 8:551–557, 1980.)

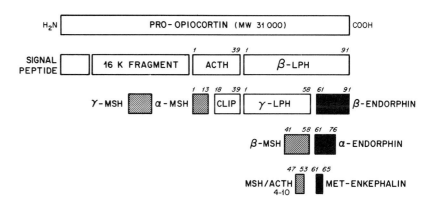

endogenous somatostatin secretion does not block the pulsatile release of GH.

GHRH was isolated in 1982 by two separate groups. Vale's group isolated a 40-amino-acid peptide (J. Rivier et al., 1982), and Guillemin and colleagues (1982) isolated an essentially identical peptide with four more amino acids. Both of these peptides were isolated from pancreatic tumors in patients with acromegaly. In 1984, an identical 44-amino-acid peptide was isolated from human hypothalamus (Ling et al., 1984); its structure is

$$\begin{array}{ccccccccccc} 1 & 2 & 3 & 4 & 5 & 6 & 7 & 8 & 9 & 10 & 11 \end{array}$$
Tyr-Ala-Asp-Ala-Ile-Phe-Thr-Asn-Ser-Tyr-Arg-

$$\begin{array}{ccccccccccc} 12 & 13 & 14 & 15 & 16 & 17 & 18 & 19 & 20 & 21 & 22 \end{array}$$
Lys-Val-Leu-Gly-Gln-Leu-Ser-Ala-Arg-Lys-Leu-

$$\begin{array}{ccccccccccc} 23 & 24 & 25 & 26 & 27 & 28 & 29 & 30 & 31 & 32 & 33 \end{array}$$
Leu-Gln-Asp-Ile-Met-Ser-Arg-Gln-Gln-Gly-Glu-

$$\begin{array}{ccccccccccc} 34 & 35 & 36 & 37 & 38 & 39 & 40 & 41 & 42 & 43 & 44 \end{array}$$
Ser-Asn-Gln-Glu-Arg-Gly-Ala-Arg-Ala-Arg-Leu-NH$_2$

GHRH-containing cells are found in the arcuate and ventromedial nuclei of the hypothalamus, and GHRH-rich bundles of fibers travel from the arcuate region to the median eminence. GHRH stimulates GH release both in vivo and in vitro.

GH can inhibit its own release by feedback effects on somatostatin. α-Adrenergic activity stimulates GH secretion; β-adrenergic activity is inhibitory. Dopamine, in normal humans, stimulates GH release, as does serotonin. In patients with acromegaly, dopamine inhibits GH release, probably by a direct action at the level of the pituitary. Stress is accompanied by GH release, as are exercise and slow-wave sleep. Various dietary factors affect GH release: glucose tends to suppress it, whereas certain amino acids stimulate it.

Regulation of Prolactin Secretion

PRL, in humans, was not known to be a distinct hormone until 1970, because human GH has marked PRL-like activity, which makes it difficult to distinguish between the two by bioassay alone. PRL has a molecular weight of 22,000 and, in contrast to all other pituitary hormones, is primarily under inhibitory hypothalamic control.

PRL, through feedback at the hypothalamus, can decrease its own release. Hypothalamic extracts with the most potent PRL-inhibitory effect do not contain peptides; however, they do contain dopamine, which has been shown by Hökfelt and Fuxe (1972) to be located in nerve terminals abutting directly on the pituitary portal capillaries. Several lines of experimental and clinical data suggest that dopamine is the principal physiologic PRL-inhibitory factor. The precursor of GnRH contains within it a 56-amino-acid sequence that strongly inhibits the release of PRL from cultured pituitary cells (Nikolics et al., 1985). Presumably, this peptide is coliberated with GnRH and may serve to reduce PRL levels, thereby enhancing the GnRH-induced release of LH and FSH.

TRH, a potent stimulator of PRL release, is probably not the physiologic PRL-releasing factor; evidence against this function arises from circumstances in which PRL release occurs without TSH secretion.

Serotonin may be important in stimulating the PRL rise induced by suckling, sleep, stress, and exercise. Opiates stimulate PRL secretion, as do a variety of peptides: cholecystokinin, vasoactive intestinal polypeptide, neurotensin, and substance P; however, the physiologic significance of these effects remains uncertain.

Estrogen is a potent modulator of PRL secretion. It appears to act on the hypothalamus to influence dopamine turnover and also at the level of the pituitary to desensitize PRL cells to the inhibitory action of dopamine. Testosterone stimulates PRL secretion, possibly through conversion to estrogen, whereas progesterone has an inhibitory effect on PRL secretion.

For a more detailed review of hypothalamic factors, readers are referred to Müller et al., 1989.

ABNORMALITIES OF PITUITARY SECRETION

Hypofunction

Dwarfism and Growth Failure

Growth failure may result from a number of conditions (Table 40–2).

Table 40–2. CAUSES OF GROWTH FAILURE

Familial causes
  Constitutional short stature
  Delayed adolescence

Environmental causes
  Emotional deprivation
  Inadequate nutrition

Endocrine and metabolic causes
  Chondrodystrophy
  Osteogenesis imperfecta
  Vitamin D–resistant rickets
  Hypoparathyroidism
  Pseudohypoparathyroidism
  Hypothyroidism
  Cushing's syndrome
  Hypopituitarism
  Adrenogenital syndrome
  Inborn errors of metabolism
  Primary growth hormone deficiency, resistance, or inactivity
  Precocious puberty

Inherited causes
  Turner's syndrome
  Down's syndrome

Associated with other organic disease
  Chronic infection
  Congenital and acquired heart disease
  Renal failure
  Hepatic failure
  Chronic lung disease
  Malabsorption syndromes
  Chronic anemia

In vivo, GH is essential for normal growth. The effects of GH are mediated by at least two growth factors in the human: (1) insulin-like growth factor I (IGF I), which is GH dependent and is now known to be identical with somatomedin-C; and (2) insulin-like growth factor II (IGF II), which is less GH dependent than IGF I. Administration of IGF I suppresses endogenous secretion of GH in the rat and also increases somatostatin content in the hypothalamus.

True GH deficiency is a rare condition with many causes, some of which have been demonstrated to be due to deletion or mutation of the GH gene. GH deficiency may occur as a monohormonal deficiency or as part of other anterior pituitary hormone deficiencies (e.g., of TSH and/or ACTH). Children with GH deficiency from any cause have round, doll-like facies with pudgy features. Some of these cases may be due to isolated deficiency of GHRH. Laron dwarfs have clinical features similar to those of GH-deficient individuals but have elevated GH levels by radioimmunoassay. Some of these individuals may have abnormal GH receptors, whereas others may produce a form of GH that is biologically inactive. The African Pygmy does not have the doll-like face seen in GH deficiency. Before puberty, Pygmy children have normal levels of IGF I and II; after puberty, the IGF I levels are low. One study showed that Pygmies have low levels of GH-binding protein in the plasma (Baumann et al., 1989). This suggests that their growth failure may be due to reductions in the number or function of GH receptors.

Delayed Puberty

Puberty is a complex physiologic process that requires normal function of the gonads, pituitary, and hypothalamus, as well as normal integration of their functions. In addition, chronic disease, a variety of other endocrine abnormalities, and even stress can interfere with the process.

Puberty is considered to be delayed in girls if breast or sexual hair development has not occurred by age 14 and in boys if testicular enlargement or sexual hair growth has not occurred by age 15. Delayed puberty can be due to a variety of causes (Table 40–3). At the level of the hypothalamus, GnRH is essential for the development of normal puberty. One of the first signs of the onset of puberty is the development of nocturnal pulses of LH secretion, which is dependent on hypothalamic GnRH release. Patients with GnRH deficiency are of normal to tall height. They may have some pubic and axillary hair growth (produced by adrenal androgens). Many such individuals show LH and FSH responses to the repeated administration of GnRH. If the syndrome is associated with hyposmia or anosmia, it is called Kallmann's syndrome. The condition of the so-called fertile eunuch is due to a deficiency of LH that leads to hypogonadal features clinically, but sperm formation occurs because of preserved FSH function. In cases of hypogonadotropic hypogonadism in which the pituitary responds to GnRH administration, the repeated administration of the synthetic peptide can be used to induce normal puberty. The peptide must be administered in a pulsatile fashion, however, as a continuous infusion causes tachyphylaxis and a progressive decline in LH and FSH release.

Table 40–3. CAUSES OF DELAYED PUBERTY

Idiopathic (constitutional)

Associated with chronic malnutrition or systemic disease

Gonadal insufficiency

  Primary (hypergonadotropic)

Girls	Boys
Turner's syndrome	Kleinfelter's syndrome
Gonadal dysgenesis	Anorchia
Syndrome of ovarian	Mumps orchitis
resistance	Noonan's syndrome
Androgen insensitivity	
(end organ)	
Autoimmune oophoritis	
Others	

  Secondary (hypogonadotropic)
    Panhypopituitarism (congenital or acquired)
    Isolated GnRH deficiency
    Kallmann's syndrome
    Prader-Willi syndrome
    Laurence-Moon-Biedl syndrome
    Holoprosencephaly
    Others

Table 40–4. CAUSES OF PITUITARY INSUFFICIENCY

Congenital
  Aplasia
  Familial hypopituitarism

Acquired
  After surgery
  After trauma
  After radiotherapy
  Pituitary apoplexy
  Infection
  Cysts and tumors
  Granulomatous disease
  Autoimmune disease
  Secondary to hypothalamic disease

Hypopituitarism

Many disorders can cause pituitary insufficiency (Table 40–4). Compressive lesions often produce slow pituitary failure, with hormonal loss occurring in the following sequence: GH, ACTH, TSH, and AVP. Exceptions to this sequence are not infrequent.

Panhypopituitarism is sometimes referred to as Simmonds' disease. Postpartum pituitary insufficiency that results from pituitary infarction is called Sheehan's syndrome. Hemorrhage into the pituitary gland, also known as pituitary apoplexy, may occur in up to one-fifth of all pituitary adenomas. It has been associated with a variety of underlying conditions: hypovolemia, diabetes mellitus, arterial hypertension, hypoparathyroidism, tuberculosis, tetanus, cardiac failure, hemolytic crises, meningitis, temporal arteritis, and intracranial hypertension. Signs and symptoms of pituitary apoplexy depend on the severity of the hemorrhage, the direction in which the gland enlarges, and whether the hemorrhage ruptures into the subarachnoid space. Severe cases may be clinically indistinguishable from subarachnoid hemorrhage manifested by headache, nuchal rigidity, third cranial nerve palsy, and blood-stained cerebrospinal fluid on lumbar puncture. Upward enlargement of the gland is associated with visual field defects and impairment of visual acuity, whereas lateral enlargement may cause cranial nerve palsies, especially of cranial nerves III and VI. Accompanying posterior pituitary dysfunction may occur, but it is rare.

The signs and symptoms of hypopituitarism depend on the hormones that are deficient (Table 40–5).

Hyperfunction

Precocious Puberty

In true precocious puberty there is activation of the hypothalamic-pituitary axis. Pseudoprecocious puberty is due to stimulation by gonadotropin-like hormone or by sex steroids themselves.

A familial form of precocious puberty exists that may be either autosomal recessive or dominant (Ro-

senfeld et al., 1980). Precocious puberty has also been described with a number of hypothalamic lesions. Most of these affect the posterior hypothalamus. Many different tumors can cause precocious puberty, but hamartoma, teratoma, and ependymoma are the most common. Other types of tumors that may affect the hypothalamus include optic nerve glioma, astrocytoma, chorioepithelioma, and neurofibroma (as part of von Recklinghausen's syndrome). Some of these tumors are thought to produce an irritant effect on the hypothalamus that causes GnRH release; however, this is not always the case. Judge et al. (1977) described precocious puberty in a patient with a hypothalamic hamartoma that contained GnRH; a pineal germinoma has been described that contained biologically active human chorionic gonadotropin (a placental peptide with LH- and FSH-like activity) (Wass et al., 1982).

The role of the putative pineal hormone melatonin in the control of human puberty and in the production of precocious puberty remains controversial.

The McCune-Albright syndrome occurs in females. It is characterized by irregular pigmented areas on the trunk and polyostotic fibrous dysplasia of bone. The syndrome may be complicated by the appearance of precocious puberty; however, there is no evidence that this is due to hypersecretion of hypothalamic GnRH.

The tachyphylaxis that develops in pituitary gonadotrophs with prolonged GnRH administration can be exploited to treat precocious puberty. The administration of long-acting GnRH analogues to patients with true precocious puberty, after an initial stimulation of LH and FSH, is associated with inhibition of gonadotropin secretion and a return of LH and FSH to prepubertal levels. This form of therapy has the advantage of not causing other pituitary dysfunction, and it prevents premature closure of the epiphyses (leading to short stature) that can be caused by the gonadal steroids.

Table 40–5. CLINICAL FEATURES OF ANTERIOR
PITUITARY HORMONAL DYSFUNCTION

Hormone	Clinical Features	
	Excess	*Deficiency*
GH	Gigantism or acromegaly	Growth failure Hypoglycemia
PRL	Amenorrhea, impotence, galactorrhea, infertility, or delayed puberty	Inability to breast-feed, ?infertility
LH and FSH	Precocious puberty Polycystic ovary syndrome	Amenorrhea, impotence, infertility, delayed puberty
TSH	Hyperthyroidism	Hypothyroidism
ACTH	Cushing's disease Nelson's syndrome	Addison's disease without mineralocorticoid deficiency

Table 40–6. CAUSES OF HYPERPROLACTINEMIA

Drugs
    Phenothiazines
    Reserpine
    Metoclopramide
    α-Methyldopa
    Tricyclic antidepressants (idiosyncratic)
    Benzodiazepines (idiosyncratic)

Hormones
    Estrogens (endogenous or exogenous)
    TRH (as in primary hypothyroidism)

PRL-producing pituitary adenoma

Disorders of hypothalamic inhibition of PRL secretion
    Pituitary tumor large enough to interfere with pituitary stalk
        and flow of prolactin-inhibitory factor
    Granulomatous disease
        Sarcoidosis
        Histiocytosis X
        Tuberculosis
    Craniopharyngioma
    Dermoid and epidermoid

After irradiation

Chest wall disease (chronic)

Chronic renal failure

Ectopic production

Idiopathic ("functional")

Hyperprolactinemia

In normal men and women, PRL secretion is episodic, with daytime levels less than 15 ng/ml.

Hyperprolactinemia is probably the most common pituitary disorder seen in most clinical practices. Its causes are outlined in Table 40–6.

In women, hyperprolactinemia may cause amenorrhea, irregular menses, or infertility. Decreased libido and galactorrhea are common, as is vaginal dryness because of estrogen deficiency. In men, hyperprolactinemia causes impotence, decreased libido, and, occasionally, galactorrhea. If the hyperprolactinemia occurs early in life, it may cause delayed or arrested puberty.

The single most important cause of hyperprolactinemia is pituitary adenoma. PRL levels higher than 200 ng/ml are almost always associated with adenoma; levels below that may be due to early adenoma or other causes. Primary hypothyroidism is associated with modest elevations of PRL because the increased TRH release also causes PRL release.

Dopaminergic blocking drugs cause hyperprolactinemia by interfering with the action of endogenous dopamine on the pituitary. Rarely do drugs of this type cause PRL levels to rise above 100 ng/ml. Although a history of oral contraceptive use is common in patients with PRL-secreting adenoma, the best evidence to date would suggest that the birth control pill does not induce adenoma formation (Franks et al., 1984). Long-standing hyperprolactinemia may cause osteoporosis in both males and females.

Acromegaly and Gigantism

Excessive GH secretion results in the clinical syndrome of acromegaly when it occurs after the epiphyses have fused and in gigantism if the GH hypersecretion occurs before epiphyseal closure. The common clinical features of acromegaly are summarized in Table 40–7.

Most patients with acromegaly have been found to have a GH-secreting pituitary adenoma; however, ectopic GH-secreting tumors have also been described. Thorner and colleagues (1982) described the details of a case of acromegaly that was due to somatotroph hyperplasia resulting from GHRH production by a pancreatic tumor. Hypothalamic tumors secreting a GHRH-like substance have been associated with adenoma formation in the pituitary. To date, somatostatin deficiency has not been described as a cause of acromegaly or gigantism.

Cushing's Disease and Nelson's Syndrome

Cushing's syndrome is a constellation of clinical signs and symptoms caused by prolonged elevation of plasma corticosteroids (Table 40–8). It can result from a variety of causes (Table 40–9). If the condition is due to pituitary-dependent hyperplasia of the adrenal glands, it is referred to as Cushing's disease; the majority of affected patients have an ACTH-secreting microadenoma of the pituitary. If patients with Cushing's disease are treated with bilateral adrenalectomy, a small percentage (about 10–15%) will develop increasing elevation of plasma ACTH, which causes hyperpigmentation of the skin. In addition, the pituitary adenoma may increase in size, cause local compressive symptoms, and invade bone locally. This condition is referred to as Nelson's syndrome.

When cases of steroid administration are excluded, about 80% of patients with Cushing's syndrome are found to have a pituitary microadenoma. In patients with Cushing's disease, serum ACTH levels are either normal or elevated; they will usually increase further if cortisol production is blocked by the administration of metyrapone (an inhibitor of adrenal 11β-hydroxylase) or if stimulated by insulin-induced

Table 40–7. COMMON CLINICAL FEATURES OF ACROMEGALY

Headache—frontal/retro-orbital
Hypermetabolism
Impaired glucose tolerance or overt diabetes mellitus
Acral growth and prognathism
Hypertension
Arthritic complaints
Menstrual irregularities
Soft tissue growth (may cause carpal tunnel syndrome)
    and thick skin
Visceromegaly
Proximal muscle weakness
Hyperhidrosis
Hypertrichosis

Table 40–8. COMMON CLINICAL FEATURES OF
HYPERCORTISOLISM

Obesity—centripetal (especially preauricular and supraclavicular
  fat pads)
Hypertension
Impaired glucose tolerance or diabetes mellitus
Menstrual irregularities or amenorrhea; sexual dysfunction
Hirsutism and acne
Striae
Proximal muscle weakness
Osteoporosis
Easy bruisability
Psychiatric disturbance

hypoglycemia or the administration of CRH. In patients with adrenal adenoma or carcinoma, the levels of ACTH are undetectable and usually do not respond to stimulation. In patients with ectopic ACTH production, ACTH levels are usually extremely elevated and unresponsive to stimuli. The exception to this is in cases of well-differentiated carcinoid tumors: the patterns of ACTH secretion and the responses to stimulation may be indistinguishable from those of pituitary adenoma (Carpenter, 1988). Apparent Cushing's disease has also been reported to occur because of excessive stimulation of the pituitary by CRH (Asa et al., 1984; Carey et al., 1984) or a CRH-like substance (Howlett et al., 1985).

The pathophysiology of Cushing's disease remains incompletely understood. Gross enlargement of the pituitary gland is rare, occurring in less than 10% of cases. Some patients with apparent Cushing's disease show no evidence of adenoma formation but have corticotroph hyperplasia. This, plus the observation that the serotonin antagonist cyproheptadine can restore normal circadian periodicity in at least some patients with Cushing's disease, suggests that Cushing's disease is probably not a single entity but may be due to different types of adenoma in some instances and excessive CRH secretion in others.

Serum levels of POMC, ACTH, and β-endorphin are elevated in cases of Cushing's disease, although the ratio of the three compounds may differ from that in normal individuals (Chan et al., 1983).

A single case of a β-endorphin–secreting tumor

Table 40–9. CAUSES OF CUSHING'S SYNDROME

ACTH dependent
  Administration of exogenous ACTH
  ACTH-producing pituitary adenoma
  Corticotroph cell hyperplasia
    Idiopathic
    Secondary to production of CRH
  Ectopic ACTH production

ACTH independent
  Administration of glucocorticoids
  Associated with alcoholism
  Adrenal
    Benign adenoma
    Adrenal carcinoma
    Hyperplasia—non–ACTH induced (rare)

has been reported (Trouillas et al., 1984). This patient presented with impotence, testicular atrophy, and an enlarged sella turcica but no evidence of glucocorticoid hypersecretion.

Inappropriate Secretion of Thyroid-Stimulating Hormone

Like all pituitary hormones, TSH shows a circadian variation. Its highest levels occur at 11 PM and the lowest 12 hours later.

One of the causes of inappropriate TSH secretion is TSH production by a pituitary adenoma. Such tumors are exceedingly rare. They are usually discovered in the investigation of patients with hyperthyroidism. Kourides et al. (1977) examined six hyperthyroid patients with inappropriate TSH elevation. In three patients with adenoma formation, there were marked elevations in the α subunit of TSH and undetectable levels of the β subunit. In addition, tumor patients showed little increase in TSH after the administration of TRH and little decrease with the administration of T_4 or T_3. Failure of TSH to suppress after administration of dexamethasone or dopamine is a common, but not universal, finding in patients with TSH-secreting tumors.

Ectopic TSH production has not been described to date. Two other conditions are associated with inappropriate TSH secretion. In the first, there is a peripheral resistance to T_4 and T_3. Such patients have elevated TSH levels and may be either euthyroid or hyperthyroid. In the second condition, the same type of resistance may be confined to the pituitary gland. In these cases, the patients have high TSH levels associated with peripheral signs and symptoms of hyperthyroidism.

Tumors Secreting Luteinizing Hormone and Follicle-Stimulating Hormone

Although gonadotropin-secreting tumors are rare, tumors that secrete the subunits α or β are relatively common. Most gonadotropin-secreting tumors secrete FSH, with approximately 90% of these being reported in males. FSH levels are markedly elevated, and LH levels may be normal or slightly high. Excessive secretion of the β or α subunits of FSH may occur. Patients usually have symptoms of mild hypogonadism. LH-secreting tumors are extremely rare and have occurred only in males. Gonadal dysfunction is not a symptom, although some features of partial hypopituitarism are common. The FSH level may be elevated, normal, or decreased, and the testosterone level is usually normal or increased. This subject has been reviewed by Snyder (1987).

Pituitary Pathology

Pituitary pathology may be classified morphologically, as outlined in Table 40–10.

Pituitary Tumors

Primary pituitary tumors account for 15% of all intracranial neoplasms. These tumors have been classified by Asa and Kovacs into seven groups (1983) (Table 40–11).

GH cell adenomas appear to arise from GH-secreting pituitary cells. They are associated with symptoms of either acromegaly or gigantism, and classic staining techniques show these tumors to be either chromophobic or acidophilic (Klibanski and Zervas, 1991). The chromophobic tumors have few secretory granules; the tumors that stain with acidophilic dyes are densely granulated. Similarly, PRL cell adenomas are densely and sparsely granulated, although the densely granulated form of the tumor is rare. This suggests that many of the chromophobic tumors in old series of pituitary tumors were actually prolactinomas. There are two types of corticotroph cell adenoma. One type is biologically active and associated with either Cushing's disease or Nelson's syndrome. These tumors are usually basophilic, and immunochemical staining reveals the presence of ACTH, β-LPH, and endorphins. A second type of corticotroph cell adenoma is clinically unassociated with any symptoms of hormone excess. Immunochemically, these tumors contain ACTH and fragments of POMC. TSH-secreting adenomas are usually chromophobic by classic staining. They may be associated with clinical symptoms of hyperthyroidism or can be seen in association with long-standing primary hypothyroidism. Gonadotroph cell adenomas are also chromophobic by classic staining. Immunochemically, they contain FSH, LH, and/or α or β subunits.

Table 40–10. MORPHOLOGIC CLASSIFICATION OF PITUITARY DISEASES

Developmental anomalies

Functional changes
 Crooke's hyaline change
 Hypertrophy
 Hyperplasia
 Atrophy or involution

Neoplasia
 Adenomas
 Carcinomas
 Craniopharyngiomas
 Other primary tumors
 Metastatic malignancies

Inflammatory lesions
 Acute
 Chronic
 Granulomatous

Vascular lesions
 Hemorrhage
 Infarction

Miscellaneous
 Amyloidosis
 Hemochromatosis or hemosiderosis
 Mucopolysaccharidoses
 Autoimmune

Table 40–11. PITUITARY ADENOMAS AND THEIR RELATIVE INCIDENCE IN SURGICAL MATERIAL

Tumor	Number	%
GH cell adenomas		
Densely granulated	47	7.0
Sparsely granulated	57	8.5
PRL cell adenomas		
Densely granulated	2	0.3
Sparsely granulated	191	28.3
Corticotroph cell adenomas		
Functioning	55	8.2
Silent	41	6.1
Thyrotroph cell adenomas	4	0.6
Gonadotroph cell adenomas	24	3.6
Null cell adenomas		
Nononcocytic type	127	18.8
Oncocytic type (oncocytoma)	46	6.8
Plurihormonal adenomas		
Mixed GH-PRL cell adenomas	31	4.6
Acidophilic stem cell adenomas	21	3.1
Mammosomatotroph cell adenomas	9	1.3
Unclassified plurihormonal adenomas	19	2.8
Total	674	100.0

From Asa S.L., Kovacs K. Histological classification of pituitary disease. *Clin. Endocrinol. Metab.* 12:567–596, 1983, © by The Endocrine Society.

Some tumors are associated with the production of more than one hormone. They may be composed of one cell type (monomorphous), in which each cell produces two or more hormones, or they may contain two or more cell types (plurimorphous). Mixed GH cell–PRL cell adenoma is one of the more common plurimorphous types. Clinically, it is associated with elevated GH levels. Acidophilic stem cell adenoma is a monomorphous tumor that produces both GH and PRL. Patients with this type of tumor have moderate hyperprolactinemia and acromegalic features without elevated GH levels. The mammosomatotroph cell adenoma is a more mature counterpart of the acidophilic stem cell tumor. Patients with this type have clinical features of acromegaly with elevated GH levels and modest elevation of serum PRL. Several other plurihormonal tumors have been described by Kovacs (see Martin and Reichlin, 1987) that contain various hormonal combinations: GH and TSH; PRL and TSH; GH, PRL, and ACTH; GH, ACTH, and α subunit of the gonadotropin or TSH.

It is difficult to decide whether a pituitary tumor is malignant or benign on morphologic grounds alone. Malignant pituitary tumors or primary pituitary carcinomas are most often ACTH secreting. Although histologic appearance may suggest malignancy, a tumor is judged to be malignant only after distant metastases have occurred. Histologically, benign-appearing tumors may behave in a malignant fashion, with local invasion and destruction of bone.

Pituitary Hyperplasia and Hypertrophy

Gonadotropin production by carcinoid, pancreatic, or hypothalamic tumors produces GH cell hyperplasia. PRL cell hyperplasia is seen most commonly during pregnancy and lactation but can also occur in infants as a response to maternal estrogen and in women given exogenous estrogen. Corticotroph hyperplasia occurs in primary hypoadrenalism that is incompletely treated with corticosteroids, and it may also occur with ectopic CRH production. Thyrotroph cell hyperplasia is seen with long-standing hypothyroidism, just as gonadotroph cell hyperplasia is seen in long-standing primary hypogonadism.

Inflammatory and Infiltrative Conditions

Now, in the antibiotic era, infective hypophysitis is a rare cause of hypopituitarism. Tuberculosis, syphilis, sarcoidosis, and giant cell granuloma can all cause hypopituitarism. Lymphocytic hypophysitis is a rare condition presumed autoimmune in which the pituitary gland is infiltrated by lymphocytes and enlarged. It may represent the pituitary equivalent of Hashimoto's thyroiditis. Clinically, it is associated with signs and symptoms of hypopituitarism and hyperprolactinemia. Infiltration of the pituitary with iron in hemochromatosis may also cause hypopituitarism, particularly hypogonadotropic hypogonadism.

Other Tumors

Null cell adenomas are chromophobic tumors composed of small cells that are nonsecretory and produce symptoms only by compression. Oncocytomas are chromophobic or acidophilic tumors that appear to arise through oncocytic transformation of null cell adenomas. They are characterized by the presence of numerous mitochondria. There is a tendency for both of these tumors to recur after surgical removal.

Craniopharyngiomas account for 3–5% of all intracranial tumors. These tumors are histologically benign and produce no hormones. They probably arise from squamous cell rests in the pars tuberalis. Histologically, they may be solid, cystic, or a mixture of the two types. Calcification is common and may be seen in the suprasellar region on a plain skull x-ray film. Despite being benign, they are often difficult to remove completely and tend to recur postoperatively if residual tumor remains. Symptoms arise from compression of local structures; GH deficiency and posterior pituitary dysfunction are particularly common.

A variety of other primary neoplasms may occur in the region of the pituitary: neurofibroma, angioma, glioma, meningioma, paraganglioma, cholesteatoma, chordoma, teratoma, dermoid, and epidermoid. Pituitary metastases are seen in 3–4% of patients with widespread metastatic cancer. Histiocytosis X, leukemia, and lymphoma may also affect the pituitary, particularly the secretion of the posterior lobe, which gives rise to diabetes insipidus (DI).

Empty Sella Syndrome

Radiologists coined this term to describe the sella turcica that is partly or completely filled with air during pneumoencephalography. The apparent cause, in the absence of pituitary tumor that has undergone infarction or necrosis, is an underdevelopment of the diaphragma sellae that allows herniation of the cerebrospinal fluid space into the sella turcica, thus resulting in the compression of the gland into a thin rim of tissue, but current evidence suggests that it occurs as a result of an autoimmune hypophysitis. Sellar enlargement may also result from this compression. This condition is seen most commonly in obese, middle-aged females with a history of chronic headache and documented pseudotumor cerebri (benign intracranial hypertension). Mild endocrine disturbances, such as hirsutism and irregular menses, are common in these women but do not appear to be related to significant disturbances of pituitary function. The diagnosis can be made fairly confidently by computed tomographic (CT) or magnetic resonance scanning, and metrizamide cisternography can be used to confirm the diagnosis in doubtful cases.

Pituitary microadenoma can occur in the pituitary tissue in the wall of the empty sella and, in the case of incomplete infarction of a macroadenoma, residual tissue may still give rise to signs and symptoms of hormonal hypersecretion. Rarely, the optic chiasm can herniate into the empty sella and cause visual field defects.

REGULATION OF POSTERIOR PITUITARY HORMONE SECRETION

Vasopressin

AVP is a nine-amino-acid peptide that is synthesized in the neurons of the supraoptic (SO) and paraventricular nuclei of the hypothalamus. In humans, the majority of cells in the SO nucleus and many of the cells in the paraventricular nucleus contain AVP.

Oxytocin

Oxytocin is a nine-amino-acid peptide with a physiologic role in humans that is far from clear. In the postpartum female, it is released in response to suckling or hearing an infant cry. It does not appear to initiate parturition, and its role in labor is uncertain. Vaginal distention and coitus induce its release, and it is postulated that it may play some role in aiding sperm transport. Oxytocin physiology in the male is even less clear. Chemically, its structure is similar to that of AVP.

Both AVP and oxytocin are derived from larger precursor molecules and are synthesized in association with a substance (separate for each hormone), called neurophysin, that acts as a carrier.

The structures of AVP and oxytocin are as follows:

Arginine Vasopressin

1 2 3 4 5 6 7 8 9
Cys-Tyr-Phe-Glu-Asp-Cys-Pro-Arg-Gly

Oxytocin

1 2 3 4 5 6 7 8 9
Cys-Tyr-Ile-Glu-Asp-Cys-Pro-Leu-Gly

A potent synthetic analogue of AVP is 1-desamino-D-8-arginine vasopressin (DDAVP):

Cys-Tyr-Phe-Glu-Asp-Cys-Pro-Arg-Gly

Physiology of Vasopressin Secretion

The magnocellular neurons of the SO nucleus or other neurons in the immediate vicinity are sensitive to osmotic changes in plasma. By controlling the release of AVP they maintain serum osmolality within narrow limits. Plasma levels of AVP of less than 1 pg/ml are associated with no antidiuretic effect, whereas levels of 5 pg/ml produce maximal antidiuresis. In severe dehydration, AVP alone is incapable of maintaining homeostasis because of the nonrenal losses of water. Therefore, thirst must stimulate an animal to drink enough water to maintain serum osmolality in the range at which AVP will be effective in fine-tuning the system. This seems to occur at a serum osmolality range of 296–280 mmol/kg. Normally, if the serum osmolality falls below 280 mmol/kg, AVP release is completely inhibited.

Volume receptors have been found in the arch of the aorta, the carotid arteries, the atria, and the major thoracic veins. If blood pressure falls by 15% or more, a maximal stimulation of AVP release occurs. With severe hypotension, baroregulation will override osmoregulation and AVP release will continue despite a low serum osmolality.

Nausea and vomiting are also potent releasers of AVP, and ethanol is a potent inhibitor of its release.

Hypothalamic Regulation of Drinking and Thirst

A "drinking center" has been postulated to exist in the far lateral hypothalamus at the level of the hypophysial stalk, just anterior to the "feeding center." It appears to play a dominant role in the hypothalamic control of fluid intake, whereas limbic centers play an important role in the motivation of drinking and the behavioral activities associated with a search for water.

The neuropeptide angiotensin has the ability to stimulate drinking behavior in animals and humans, an effect that appears to be mediated through the subfornical organ and the preoptic area. Excessive angiotensin release from the kidney in shock and in chronic renal failure may produce the severe thirst that occurs in these conditions.

Elderly persons are particularly prone to dehydration. This appears to result from at least two factors: (1) they have a defect in thirst perception that is probably central, and (2) their reduced renal function leads to an impaired response to normal or even high AVP levels.

Regulation of Sodium

The kidney plays a key role in the regulation of the body's sodium content. The need for sodium is primarily triggered by low blood volume, whereas osmolality appears to have a much lesser effect. The adrenal mineralocorticoid aldosterone is probably the single most important factor controlling sodium balance. Aldosterone levels are not particularly influenced by changes in ACTH (unless ACTH levels are excessive, as in Cushing's disease). β-LPH or a portion of it may stimulate aldosterone release under physiologic circumstances. A potent stimulator of aldosterone is angiotensin II. Angiotensin II is produced in the lung from angiotensin I, which, in turn, is produced by the action of renin from the kidney on angiotensinogen in plasma.

For many years, renal physiologists have postulated the existence of a third factor that controls urinary sodium excretion. de Bold and colleagues (1981) found a family of polypeptides in the rat atrium that produces natriuresis. Atrial natriuretic factor is a 28-amino-acid peptide that increases renal sodium excretion, relaxes smooth muscle in blood vessels, and inhibits renin and aldosterone secretion. It is also found in the hypothalamus (Tanaka et al., 1984), thus giving rise to the possibility that it plays a role in the central regulation of sodium homeostasis and water balance.

Diabetes Insipidus

A condition caused by a deficiency of AVP, DI is characterized by thirst, polyuria, and polydipsia. The amount of urine passed per day averages 8–10 L.

Etiology

The principal causes of DI are listed in Table 40–12. Forty percent of cases of DI are idiopathic. In some cases of heredofamilial DI there is a deficiency of AVP (central DI), whereas in others there is a failure of renal cyclic AMP to respond to AVP (nephrogenic DI). Most of the remaining cases of DI are due to dysfunction of the SO-hypophysial pathway. To cause permanent DI, at least 80% of the cells in the SO nucleus must be destroyed. This may occur by direct destruction or be secondary to interruption of efferent axons in the median eminence. Lesions of the pituitary stalk, without damage to the median eminence, rarely cause permanent DI.

Hypercalcemia or hypokalemia may make the renal tubule relatively insensitive to AVP and give rise to a clinical picture of nephrogenic DI. A similar condition can occur in patients treated with the drug lithium carbonate.

Shucart and Jackson (1976) divide postoperative and post-traumatic DI into four clinical syndromes:

1. Onset of polyuria within 24–72 hours and lasting 1–7 days. This form is the most common and is thought to be due to hypothalamic dysfunction associated with the onset and resolution of cerebral and hypothalamic edema.
2. Onset of polyuria within 24–48 hours and lasting 1–7 days, followed by normal urine output for 1 to several days, followed by permanent DI. This is postulated to be due to pituitary stalk damage that causes the initial failure of AVP release. As neuronal degeneration occurs and AVP is released, the DI then remits, only to be followed by permanent DI when degeneration is complete.
3. Onset of polyuria within 24–72 hours, followed by permanent partial DI.
4. Onset of persistent polyuria within 24–72 hours of surgery.

Table 40–12. CAUSES OF DIABETES INSIPIDUS

Idiopathic

Congenital

Post-traumatic
  Basilar skull fracture
  Damage to pituitary stalk
  After neurosurgery

Neoplastic
  Parasellar neoplasms (especially craniopharyngioma)
  Leukemia and lymphoma
  Secondary neoplasms

Granulomatous disease
  Histiocytosis X
  Sarcoidosis
  Tuberculosis
  Syphilis

Vascular disease
  Aneurysm with or without subarachnoid hemorrhage
  Pituitary apoplexy

Infections

Diagnosis

The water deprivation test is the single most useful procedure in the diagnosis of patients with polyuria. First, metabolic disturbances, drug use, and osmotic diuresis (e.g., diabetes mellitus) must be excluded. Then the patient undergoes a period of fluid deprivation until dehydration occurs (as evidenced by a rise in serum osmolality). This is then followed by the administration of exogenous vasopressin. At the end of water deprivation, a urine osmolality value of more than 750 mmol/kg excludes DI. An osmolality value of less than 300 mmol/kg suggests central or nephrogenic DI. The latter is diagnosed by the failure to respond to exogenous vasopressin.

Problems arise when there is a partial response. This can occur after a prolonged diuresis in a patient, because the loss of intrarenal electrolytes leads to a form of partial nephrogenic DI. If AVP levels cannot be measured, control of polyuria and regulation of fluid intake for several days, followed by repeat testing, are probably the best way to sort out difficult cases.

Management (Table 40–13)

Acute Diabetes Insipidus

In patients scheduled for neurosurgical procedures, in which the postoperative development of DI is a possibility, or in patients with head trauma, one should measure body weight, serum and urine osmolality, and serum electrolyte, glucose, urea, creatinine, calcium, and albumin levels preoperatively or immediately after the trauma, respectively. Every twelve hours thereafter, measurement of body weight, serum electrolyte levels, and serum and urine osmolality should be repeated. Accurate records of intake and output are essential to the diagnosis of acute DI and its management.

If polyuria appears, one must be certain that it is not due to excessive fluid administration or osmotic diuresis caused by diabetes mellitus or the administration of mannitol.

In the alert patient with normal osmoreceptor and thirst mechanisms, fluid balance is best maintained by oral intake. If urine output rises to 7 L/day or higher, most patients have difficulty maintaining this balance orally. In such cases, intravenous fluid replacement is made suboptimally so that the patient can still fine-tune the regulation with oral intake.

In the lethargic or unconscious patient, in the patient unable to drink, or in the patient in whom the administration of large volumes of fluid would be dangerous, exogenous vasopressin is administered.

In the afebrile patient, insensible fluid losses amount to approximately 1 L/24 hours. Electrolyte requirements are approximately 1 L of 0.9% sodium chloride solution and 60 mmol (mEq) of potassium during the same period. The remainder of the urinary losses are primarily water and are replaced with 5%

Table 40–13. THERAPY OF DIABETES INSIPIDUS

Compound	Dose	Duration of Action (h)	Comments
Aqueous vasopressin	2–20 IU IM q 4–6 h	4–6	Its brief duration of action makes it useful in the treatment of the unstable patient for whom long-acting compounds are less desirable.
1-Desamino-D-8 arginine vasopressin (DDAVP)	10–20 μg intranasally q 12 h	12–24	Treatment of choice for chronic DI. May be given intranasally, subcutaneously, intramuscularly, or intravenously. Individual requirements may vary considerably. The intranasal route is not used for the first 3 mo after transsphenoidal surgery.
Chlorpropramide*	50–250 mg/d	>24	Potentiates the effect of vasopressin on the kidney and is therefore effective only in partial DI. Hypoglycemia may be a troublesome side effect.
Hydrochlorothiazide*	50–100 mg b.i.d.	24	Contracts the extracellular fluid volume and reduces the amount of water presented to the kidney. May have a synergistic effect with chlorpropramide. Diabetogenic effect may counteract the tendency for chlorpropramide to cause hypoglycemia. Effective in nephrogenic DI.
Carbamazepine*	200 mg t.i.d.	>24	May potentiate the action of chlorpropramide as well as stimulate vasopressin release centrally.
Clofibrate*	500 mg b.i.d.	>24	Mode of action is uncertain. It may stimulate the release of vasopressin centrally.

*Most useful, in combination, in patients with partial diabetes insipidus while awaiting recovery of posterior pituitary function after surgery, or in the interval after transsphenoidal surgery in which intranasal DDAVP cannot be used.

dextrose in water. The replacement of urinary loss with sodium-containing intravenous solutions would result in a large solute load, further aggravation of the situation, and severe electrolyte disturbances. In patients with persisting DI associated with large urine volumes, administration of vasopressin is indicated. If it is used, one must be careful to avoid overcorrection and hyponatremia.

Chronic Diabetes Insipidus

Patients with central DI and intact thirst mechanisms usually maintain adequate fluid intake. Prolonged polyuria can result in renal concentrating problems and has been associated with lower urinary tract abnormalities; therefore, it should be controlled. DDAVP is the treatment of choice and should be given in a dose titrated to avoid water intoxication.

In patients with absent or impaired thirst, a fixed dose of DDAVP, coupled with a fixed fluid intake, is the usual treatment, although it seldom prevents wide fluctuations in serum sodium concentration. In such cases, a sliding scale of water intake based on body weight may be helpful.

"Essential" Hypernatremia

Some patients with partial DI develop chronic hypernatremia associated with mild dehydration and hypovolemia. It has been suggested that these patients have either an altered set point for their osmoreceptors or a defect in the ability to secrete AVP in response to osmotic stimuli, or it may be that these patients have a combination of partial DI and failure of normal thirst. Most patients with this syndrome described recently have had demonstrable hypothalamic lesions on CT scan. It is asymptomatic in its mildest form; however, symptoms begin to occur if the serum sodium level rises to 160 mmol/L or higher. The symptoms usually consist of weakness and muscle cramp. When sodium levels reach or exceed 180 mmol/L, stupor and coma occur and death can result if appropriate treatment is not instituted. See also Chapter 111.

Syndrome of Inappropriate Vasopressin Secretion

Hyponatremia in hospitalized patients is common and may be due to sodium loss (depletional hyponatremia), hyperlipidemia, hyperproteinemia, or hyperglycemia, all of which interfere with the biochemical measurement of sodium (artifactual or "delusional" hyponatremia), and dilutional hyponatremia resulting from the administration of sodium-poor solutions.

Schwartz and Barter postulated in 1967 (see Martin and Reichlin, 1987) that some cases of dilutional hyponatremia could be caused by the syndrome of inappropriate antidiuretic hormone (SIADH). Because they were unable to measure AVP levels, they relied on five clinical criteria to make the diagnosis:

1. Hyponatremia and hyposmolality of serum and extracellular fluid
2. Continued renal excretion of sodium in the face of hyponatremia
3. Formation of urine less than maximally dilute and usually hyperosmolar to serum
4. Absence of dehydration on clinical examination: normal mucous membrane moisture; lack of postural fall in blood pressure; and absence of edema-forming states, such as congestive failure
5. Normal renal, adrenal, and thyroid function

Etiology

SIADH occurs under a variety of circumstances (Table 40–14). Dilutional hyponatremia may complicate the treatment of DI because of the administration of long-acting vasopressin analogues and excessive fluid intake.

Table 40–14. CAUSES OF THE SYNDROME OF
INAPPROPRIATE ANTIDIURETIC
HORMONE SECRETION

Associated with nonhypothalamic, central nervous system
  disease
  Cerebral infarction
  Subdural hematoma
  Infections
    Meningitis
    Encephalitis

Hypothalamic causes
  After trauma (including surgery)
  Metabolic encephalopathy (including acute intermittent
    porphyria)
  Guillain-Barré syndrome
  Myxedema
  Subarachnoid hemorrhage
  Other vascular lesions

Ectopic production of AVP
  Neoplastic (especially carcinoma of lung)
  Associated with pneumonia

Drugs
  Vincristine
  Vinblastine
  Chlorpropamide
  Thiazide diuretics
  Carbamazepine
  Clofibrate
  Cisplatin
  Chlorpromazine

Certain intracranial diseases are commonly associated with SIADH, especially encephalitis. Extracranial disease may influence the nervous system to release AVP inappropriately or may produce AVP-like peptides that cause the syndrome.

Pathophysiology

Zerbe and associates (1980) examined the osmotic control of AVP release in 79 patients with SIADH. One group of these patients showed AVP fluctuations that appeared to be unrelated to serum osmolality. This is the type of release pattern thought to be characteristic of AVP production by tumor or of AVP release caused by nonosmotic stimuli. Another group of patients had a resetting of the osmotic threshold of AVP release. A third group showed an inability to turn off AVP secretion at low osmolalities. The fourth group appeared to have normal AVP regulation but an inability to excrete a water load, possibly because of some AVP-like factor that does not cross-react in the AVP immunoassay.

Clinical Manifestations

The symptoms and signs of SIADH are nonspecific and are related solely to the disturbance of osmolality. The accompanying water intoxication may initially cause fatigue, anorexia, headache, nausea, and vomiting. As the electrolyte disturbance becomes more severe, varying degrees of confusion and obtundation emerge. Delirium and agitation may intervene and, finally, coma (associated with convulsions) and even death may occur.

The onset of symptoms relates to the rapidity with which the serum sodium falls. The more rapid the change, the more severe are the symptoms and the quicker their onset. If the serum sodium level falls below 120 mmol/L, severe signs and symptoms are common.

Management

Acute

Prevention is the ideal form of treatment but is seldom possible. In the elderly and in patients with conditions that predispose to the syndrome, serum electrolytes should be carefully monitored and administration of large volumes of sodium-poor fluid avoided. Treatment of the underlying cause, in the case of pneumonia, infection of the central nervous system, or underlying malignant disease, is important but usually requires days or weeks before the circumstances leading to hyponatremia are reversed.

In most patients, the underlying cause is not known and specific treatment is not possible. In such instances, fluid restriction is the mainstay of therapy. Initially, the fluid intake should be reduced to insensible losses (i.e., 500–1000 ml/24 hours).

For the patient in deep coma or the patient with seizures, simple fluid restriction may not provide sufficiently rapid correction of the serum sodium. In such cases, Schrier's method of treatment is recommended (Hantman et al., 1973); however, great care must be taken to raise the serum sodium level only slowly. There is controversy in the literature about the safety of the rate of change in serum sodium in patients with hyponatremia. Even when the rate of correction has not exceeded 2 mmol/L/hour, central pontine myelinolysis has occurred. Some authors recommend that the serum sodium level should not be allowed to rise more than 10 mmol/L during the first week (Norenberg et al., 1982). This would seem to be a reasonable approach for the majority of patients; however, in the patient with acute hyponatremia and complications such as seizures, a safe rate of rise remains to be determined. Certainly, under any circumstances, the rate of rise should not exceed 2 mmol/L/hour and that rate should be maintained only until the sodium is elevated above the danger point of 120 mmol/L. Thereafter, a slower correction is warranted.

Chronic

Prolonged fluid restriction is unpleasant and may be particularly difficult in children and confused elderly persons. In such cases, if treatment of the underlying condition is not possible, demeclocycline (usual adult dose, 300–600 mg twice daily) can be used to block the action of AVP at the kidney. It is better tolerated than lithium carbonate (600–1200 mg daily) and is more effective than phenytoin. Ethanol is a potent inhibitor of AVP release, but this does not occur at levels unassociated with intoxication.

References

(Key references are designated with an asterisk.)

Asa S.L., Kovacs K. Histological classification of pituitary disease. *Clin. Endocrinol. Metab.* 12:567–596, 1983.

Asa S.L., Kovacs K., Tindall G.T., et al. Cushing's disease associated with an intrasellar gangliocytoma producing corticotrophin-releasing factor. *Ann. Intern. Med.* 101:789–793, 1984.

*Barkan A.L., guest ed. Medical therapy of endocrine tumors. *Endocrinol. Metab. Clin. North Am.* 18:259–276, 1989.

Baumann G., Shaw M.A., Merimee T.J. Low levels of high-affinity growth hormone–binding protein in African pygmies. *N. Engl. J. Med.* 320:1705–1709, 1989.

Brazeau P., Vale W., Burgus R., et al. Hypothalamic polypeptide that inhibits the secretion of immunoreactive growth hormone. *Science* 179:77–79, 1973.

Carey R.M., Varma S.K., Drake C.R. Jr., et al. Ectopic secretion of corticotropin releasing factor as a cause of Cushing's syndrome. *N. Engl. J. Med.* 311:13–20, 1984.

Carpenter P.C. Diagnostic evaluation of Cushing's syndrome. *Endocrinol. Metab. Clin. North Am.* 17:445–472, 1988.

Chan J.S.D., Seidah N.G., Chretien M. Measurement of N-terminal 1–76 of human pro-opiomelanocortin in human plasma:

correlation with adrenocorticotropin (ACTH). *J. Clin. Endocrinol. Metab.* 56:791–796, 1983.

Cooper P., Fernstrom M.H., Rorstad O.P., et al. The regional distribution of somatostatin, substance P and neurotensin in the human brain. *Brain Res.* 218:219–232, 1981.

de Bold A.J., Borenstein H.B., Veress A.T., et al. A rapid and potent natriuretic response to intravenous injection of atrial myocardial extract in rats. *Life Sci.* 28:89–94, 1981.

Franks S., Jacobs H.S., Hull M.G.R. The oral contraceptive and hyperprolactinemic amenorrhea. In Molinatti G.M., Crosignano P.G., Müller E.E., eds. *Pituitary Hyperfunction.* New York, Raven Press, pp. 175–178, 1984.

Guillemin R. Peptides in the brain: the new endocrinology of the neuron. *Science* 202:390–402, 1978.

Guillemin R., Brazeau P., Bohen P., et al. Growth hormone–releasing factor from a human pancreatic tumor that caused acromegaly. *Science* 218:585–587, 1982.

Hantman D., Rossier B., Zohlman R., et al. Rapid correction of hyponatremia in the syndrome of inappropriate secretion of antidiuretic hormone. An alternative treatment to hypertonic saline. *Ann. Intern. Med.* 78:870–875, 1973.

Hökfelt T., Fuxe K. On the morphology and neuroendocrine role of the hypothalamic catecholamine neurons. In Knigge K.M., Scott D.E., Weindl A., eds. *Brain Endocrine Interaction: Structure and Function.* Basel, Karger, p. 181, 1972.

Howlett T.A., Price J., Hale A.C., et al. Pituitary ACTH dependent Cushing's syndrome due to ectopic production of a bombesin-like peptide by a medullary carcinoma of the thyroid. *Clin. Endocrinol.* 22:91–101, 1985.

Hwan J.-C., Freeman M.E. A physiological role for luteinizing hormone release–inhibiting factor of hypothalamic origin. *Endocrinology* 121:1099–1103, 1987.

Judge D.M., Kulin H.E., Page R., et al. Hypothalamic hamartoma. A source of luteinizing-hormone–releasing factor in precocious puberty. *N. Engl. J. Med.* 296:7–10, 1977.

Klibanski A., Zervas N.T. Diagnosis and management of hormone-secreting pituitary adenomas. *N. Engl. J. Med.* 324:822–831, 1991.

Kourides I.A., Ridgway E.C., Weintraub B.D., et al. Thyrotropin-induced hyperthyroidism: use of alpha and beta subunit levels to identify patients with pituitary tumors. *J. Clin. Endocrinol. Metab.* 45:534–543, 1977.

Li C.H., Dixon J.S. Human pituitary growth hormone. XXXII. The primary structure of the hormone: revision. *Arch. Biochem. Biophys.* 146:233–236, 1971.

Ling N., Esch F., Böhlen P., et al. Isolation, primary structure, and synthesis of human hypothalamic somatocrinin: growth hormone–releasing factor. *Proc. Natl. Acad. Sci. U.S.A.* 81:4302–4306, 1984.

*Martin J.B., Reichlin S. *Clinical Neuroendocrinology.* 2nd ed. Philadelphia, Davis, 1987.

*Müller E.E., Nisticò G. *Brain Messengers and the Pituitary.* New York, Academic Press, 1989.

Nikolics K., Mason A.J., Szonyi E., et al. A prolactin-inhibiting factor within the precursor for human gonadotropin-releasing hormone. *Nature* 316:511–517, 1985.

Norenberg M.D., Leslie K.O., Robertson A.S. Association between rise in serum sodium and central pontine myelinolysis. *Ann. Neurol.* 11:128–135, 1982.

Page R.B., Bergland R.M. The neurohypophyseal capillary capillary bed. Part I. Anatomy and arterial supply. *Am. J. Anat.* 148:345–347, 1977.

Rivier C., Rivier J., Mormede P., et al. Studies of the nature of the interaction between vasopressin and corticotropin-releasing factor on adrenocorticotropin release in the rat. *Endocrinology* 115:882–886, 1984.

Rivier J., Spiess J., Thorner M., et al. Characterization of growth hormone–releasing factor from a human pancreatic islet tumour. *Nature* 300:276–278, 1982.

Rosenfeld R.G., Reitz R.E., King A.B., et al. Familial precocious puberty associated with isolated elevation of luteinizing hormone. *N. Engl. J. Med.* 303:859–862, 1980.

Schally A.V. Aspects of hypothalamic regulation of the pituitary gland. Its implications for the control of reproductive processes. *Science* 202:18–28, 1978.

Schally A.V., Arimura A., Baba Y., et al. Isolation and properties of the FSH and LH releasing hormone. *Biochem. Biophys. Res. Commun.* 43:393–399, 1971.

Shibahara S., Morimoto Y., Furutani Y., et al. Isolation and sequence analysis of the human corticotropin-releasing factor precursor gene. *EMBO J.* 2:775–779, 1983.

Shucart W.A., Jackson I. Management of diabetes insipidus in neurosurgical patients. *J. Neurosurg.* 44:65–71, 1976.

Snyder P.J. Gonadotroph cell pituitary adenomas. *Endocrinol. Metab. Clin.* 16:755–792, 1987.

Tanaka I., Misono K.S., Inagami T. Atrial natriuretic factor in rat hypothalamus, atria and plasma: determination by specific radio-immunoassay. *Biochem. Biophys. Res. Commun.* 124:663–668, 1984.

Thorner M.O., Perryman R.L., Cronin M.J., et al. Somatotroph hyperplasia. Successful treatment of acromegaly by removal of a pancreatic islet tumor secreting growth hormone–releasing factor. *J. Clin. Invest.* 70:965–977, 1982.

Trouillas J., Girod C., Sassolas G., et al. A human β-endorphin pituitary adenoma. *J. Clin. Endocrinol. Metab.* 58:242–249, 1984.

Vale W., Spiess J., Rivier C., et al. Characterization of a 41-residue ovine hypothalamic peptide that stimulates secretion for corticotropin and beta-endorphin. *Science* 213:1394–1397, 1981.

Wass J.A.H., Jones A.E., Rees L.H., et al. hCGβ-producing pineal choriocarcinoma. *Clin. Endocrinol.* 17:423–432, 1982.

Zerbe R., Stropes L., Robertson G.L. Vasopressin function in the syndrome of inappropriate antidiuresis. *Annu. Rev. Med.* 31:315–327, 1980.

Disorders of Development

41

Perinatal Brain Injury

E. Osmund R. Reynolds
John S. Wyatt

The perinatal mortality rate (stillbirths and neonatal deaths in the first week of life) continues to fall rapidly in developed countries. This fall is substantially attributable to social factors, but developments in obstetrics and neonatal care have played significant parts, resulting in remarkable improvements in the chances of survival for vulnerable infants, such as those of very low birth weight (<1500 g), most of whom are born "very preterm" (<33 weeks of gestation). These developments, including the general availability of mechanical ventilation for infants with respiratory failure, total parenteral nutrition for those who are too immature or ill to tolerate oral feeding, and sophisticated monitoring of a wide range of physiologic functions, have led to the survival of about 50% of infants born as early as 24 and 25 weeks of gestation who are admitted to modern units. Survival is even being reported at 22 and 23 weeks.

Inevitably, and quite properly, concern has been expressed about the long-term neurodevelopmental outcome for very small infants, whose brains are at high risk of perinatal brain injury, and also for other infants who may survive after aggressive management in the perinatal period, such as infants who have suffered severe birth asphyxia.

The purpose of this chapter is to consider the two main causes of perinatal brain injury, periventricular hemorrhage (PVH) in preterm infants and hypoxic-ischemic injury. No attempt is made to be comprehensive, but the contribution of noninvasive methods of assessing brain structure and function to the understanding of the pathogenesis and prognostic significance of these types of injury will be highlighted. Particular attention is paid to the use of ultrasound imaging for the investigation of PVH and of magnetic resonance spectroscopy and near-infrared spectroscopy (NIRS) for the exploration of oxidative metabolism and hemodynamics.

Certain other types of perinatal injury that were relatively common in the past have become more clearly understood and are now reasonably straightforward to prevent or treat. For example, hyperbilirubinemia caused by blood group (mainly rhesus) incompatibility can be largely prevented by the administration of anti–D immunoglobulin to the mother and treated by intrauterine intravascular (or intraperitoneal) transfusion. Phototherapy and exchange transfusion are available to prevent serious jaundice postnatally in these and other infants, such as preterm ones with immature glucuronyl transferase systems in the liver. Hence, kernicterus leading to athetoid cerebral palsy is now becoming a rarity, although moderate levels of hyperbilirubinemia are still implicated in some lesser forms of neurodevelopmental impairment including deafness (de Vries et al., 1985b). Hypoglycemia, which in the past was a significant cause of brain damage, especially in infants who suffered intrauterine growth retardation or were born to diabetic mothers, has become easy to detect and treat, although some doubt remains about the lowest safe level for blood glucose in newborn infants (Koh et al., 1988).

Many other aspects of perinatal neurology, some related to perinatal brain injury, are dealt with in other chapters. For example, neuromuscular diseases are covered in Chapters 14, 15, and 19, metabolic illnesses in Chapter 47, viral and bacterial infection in Chapters 97 and 100, and the subtle manifestations of seizures in newborn infants in Chapters 69 and 72. Several texts are available that provide comprehensive surveys of the field (e.g., Levene et al., 1988; Volpe, 1987).

PERIVENTRICULAR HEMORRHAGE

Significant cerebral hemorrhage in infants born at term is relatively rare. When it does occur, it is often due to bleeding from the choroid plexus or into regions of brain infarcted by arterial obstruction, particularly of the middle cerebral artery. Subdural hematomas, which follow rupture of superior cerebral bridging veins or tentorial tears resulting from birth trauma, are now uncommon.

By contrast, PVH—bleeding into the germinal layer and ventricles—in very preterm infants is a major cause of death (Fig. 41–1) and can cause neurodevelopmental impairment in survivors. Very preterm infants constitute the major workload of all neonatal intensive care units. Elucidation of the pathogenesis and prognostic significance of PVH is therefore a major focus of investigation by neonatal pediatricians.

Prevalence and Mortality

PVH has for many years been a common finding at autopsy in very low birth weight infants. About 75% of such infants who die are affected, and hypoxic-ischemic lesions are present in about 35% (Pape and Wigglesworth, 1979). The advent of computed tomography led to the surprising finding that PVH is also common in survivors (Papile et al., 1978). Burstein et al. showed in 1978 that 44% of a consecutively studied cohort of 100 very low birth weight infants had PVH, and the prevalence in survivors was 34%. Computed tomography has the disadvantage of employing ionizing radiation and also involves transporting small ill infants to the scanner, so the discovery in 1978 that a good image of the brain could be obtained with portable ultrasound equipment was a major advance. The linear array apparatus initially used was soon superseded by sector scanners, and repeated ultrasound imaging, via the anterior fontanelle, of the brains of vulnerable infants is now routine in most neonatal intensive care units.

The ability to image the brain repeatedly and safely has provided a wealth of information about PVH. The prevalence of the condition in very low birth weight or very preterm infants is generally reported as about 40–50%. Physical signs are commonly lacking or equivocal, unless the hemorrhage is quite large. The mortality rate increases with the size of the hemorrhage (Table 41–1).

Timing

Ultrasound imaging has enabled the onset of PVH to be timed with reasonable precision, although some dispute remains about how soon bleeding becomes visible after it starts. Data from numerous studies give fairly consistent results. For example, in one large study the sensitivity and specificity of identification of autopsy-proven PVH were first shown to be 86 and 94%, respectively (Thorburn et al., 1982a). It was then found in a cohort of 182 very preterm infants that 83 (46%) developed PVH (Table 41–2) (Hope et al., 1982; Thorburn et al., 1982b). Of 74 infants in whom satisfactory timing of the hemorrhage was possible, 37 (50%) bled during the first day, but in only 15 (20%) of the infants was the PVH present on the first scan performed, and it was

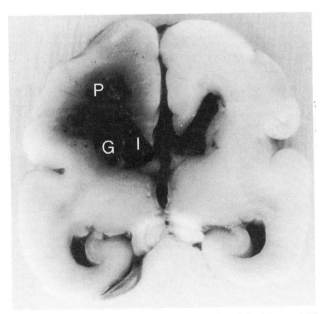

Figure 41–1. Coronal section of the brain of an infant born at 24 weeks of gestation who died at age 4 days. A large germinal layer hemorrhage (G) and an intraventricular hemorrhage (I) are present on the left, together with intraparenchymal hemorrhage (P) shown histologically to be due to venous infarction. Germinal layer and intraventricular hemorrhages are also present on the right. (From Gould S.J., Howard S., Hope P.L., et al. Periventricular intraparenchymal cerebral haemorrhage in the newborn: the role of venous infarction. *J. Pathol.* 151:197–202, 1987. Copyright 1987. Reprinted by permission of John Wiley & Sons, Ltd.)

Table 41–1. PERIVENTRICULAR HEMORRHAGE AND MORTALITY IN VERY PRETERM INFANTS ($n = 182$)

Ultrasound	Total Number	Died at <2 y ($n = 48$)
Normal	92 (51%)	8 (9%)
PVH grade*		
I	25	6 (24%)
II	29	14 (48%)
III	19	11 (58%)
IV	10	6 (60%)
All grades	83 (46%)†	37 (45%)
Other lesions (no PVH)	7 (4%)	3 (43%)

*The grading of PVH was as follows: I, PVH confined to the germinal layer and/or occupying less than half a lateral ventricle; II, PVH occupying more than half a lateral ventricle but not distending it; III, PVH distending a lateral ventricle; IV, PVH extending from the germinal layer into brain parenchyma.

†Eight infants had other lesions as well as PVH.

From Hope P.L., Thorburn R.J., Stewart A.L., et al. Timing and antecedents of periventricular haemorrhage in very preterm infants. In *Second Special Ross Laboratories Conference on Perinatal Intracranial Hemorrhage.* Columbus, OH, Ross Laboratories, pp. 78–101, 1982.

Table 41–2. GESTATIONAL AGE AND PREVALENCE OF PERIVENTRICULAR HEMORRHAGE IN VERY PRETERM INFANTS (n = 182)

Gestational Age	n	Number with PVH
23–24	8	7 (88%)
25–26	21	20 (95%)
27–28	39	22 (56%)
29–30	51	17 (33%)
31–32	63	17 (27%)

From Hope P.L., Thorburn R.J., Stewart A.L., et al. Timing and antecedents of periventricular haemorrhage in very preterm infants. In *Second Special Ross Laboratories Conference on Perinatal Intracranial Hemorrhage.* Columbus, OH, Ross Laboratories, pp. 78–101, 1982.

inferred that the PVH first became detectable toward the end of the first day of life. PVH was often progressive and reached its maximal extent on the third day. Only 6 (3%) of the 182 infants bled later than the fourth day. Many other studies have yielded similar results (reviewed by Martin, 1989), although some have concluded that PVH occasionally arises antenatally and others that a few hemorrhages may first develop as late as 1 month of age.

Pathogenesis

PVH arises in the germinal layer (or subependymal matrix), most commonly over the lower part of the head of the caudate nucleus opposite the foramen of Monro (Pape and Wigglesworth, 1979). The germinal layer largely involutes by about 35 weeks of gestation, so PVH is almost exclusively a problem of preterm infants. Early work suggested that thrombosis or rupture of the terminal (thalamostriate) vein draining the germinal layer might be important in the cause of PVH (Towbin, 1968). Defects of hemostasis (Gray et al., 1968) and hyaline membrane disease (Harrison et al., 1968) were also thought to be implicated. In 1974 Cole et al. showed that abnormal hemostasis was unlikely to be a major factor and postulated that hemodynamic influences were more relevant. Hambleton and Wigglesworth made the important observation in 1976 that PVH began as capillary bleeding in the vascular network of the germinal layer: they also showed that the layer had a substantial arterial supply (largely from Heubner artery, a branch of the middle cerebral artery), as well as a rich system of venous drainage to the terminal vein.

Work on an animal model demonstrated that PVH could be provoked in the germinal layer of the exteriorized preterm sheep fetus by a combination of impaired gas exchange with increased arterial or venous pressure or both (Reynolds et al., 1979), and Lou and colleagues (1979) showed that autoregulation of cerebral blood flow was often defective in small ill preterm infants, so that flow was pressure passive. The hypothesis emerged that PVH arose in the capillaries of the germinal layer largely because

of the hemodynamic consequences of impaired gas exchange associated with respiratory illnesses, which are extremely common in preterm infants. Ultrasound imaging has been an important means of testing this hypothesis.

Many studies have been performed with ultrasound imaging to compare variables in preterm infants who do and who do not develop PVH. The major aim has been to define apparently causal antecedents of the first detection of the hemorrhage. In the cohort study by Thorburn et al. (1982b) and Hope et al. (1982), the possible effects of a large number of antecedent social, obstetric, and neonatal events were explored. Univariate analysis provided no evidence for an effect of social background or of obstetric influences other than an apparently adverse effect of vaginal breech delivery. The prevalence of PVH increased sharply with decreasing gestation (see Table 41–2) and birth weight. Perhaps surprisingly, no indices of asphyxia around the time of birth reached significance as antecedents, although there was a trend in that direction. By contrast, the presence and severity of respiratory illnesses developing after birth were highly significant antecedents, especially hyaline membrane disease (caused by surfactant deficiency) necessitating mechanical ventilation. Pneumothorax was a particularly notable antecedent (Table 41–3). High arterial partial pressure of CO_2 ($PaCO_2$), low arterial partial pressure of O_2 (PaO_2), low pH, hypotension, and prolonged coagulation times were also significant antecedents. When these and other data were subjected to analysis of variance (multiple stepwise inclusion regression analysis), three factors—decreasing gestation (or birth weight), pneumothorax, and hyaline membrane disease—emerged as independent predictors of PVH. A number of other factors contributed to the variance—prolonged coagulation times, mechanical ventilation, breech delivery, abnormal blood gas tensions and pH values, hypotension, infusion of sodium bicarbonate, and administration of tolazoline (to dilate the pulmonary vasculature).

Other studies have yielded broadly similar results

Table 41–3. RESPIRATORY ILLNESS AND INCIDENCE OF PERIVENTRICULAR HEMORRHAGE IN VERY PRETERM INFANTS (n = 182)

Illness	n	Number with PVH
No respiratory illness	23	4 (17%)
Respiratory illness		
No mechanical ventilation	44	11 (25%)
Mechanical ventilation, no hyaline membrane disease	91	6 (25%)
Mechanical ventilation, hyaline membrane disease	67	40 (60%)
Pneumothorax during ventilation	15	13 (87%)

From Hope P.L., Thorburn R.J., Stewart A.L., et al. Timing and antecedents of periventricular haemorrhage in very preterm infants. In *Second Special Ross Laboratories Conference on Perinatal Intracranial Hemorrhage.* Columbus, OH, Ross Laboratories, pp. 78–101, 1982.

(e.g., Levene et al., 1982; Szymonowicz et al., 1984), and Perlman et al. (1985) have shown that fluctuations in cerebral arterial blood flow velocity may be particularly important in initiating PVH. Animal experimentation has provided further valuable information (reviewed by Goddard-Finegold, 1989). Of particular interest are studies showing that hypovolemic hypotension followed by reperfusion of the brain is a potent cause of bleeding in the germinal layer of the beagle puppy. These results, together with the findings that in the human infant hypotension (Hope et al., 1982) and an abnormal electroencephalogram (Connell et al., 1988) may precede PVH, suggest that in some infants the cerebral vasculature may be compromised by events occurring some time before the bleeding starts.

Synthesis. A reasonably plausible synthesis of the likely pathogenesis of PVH can be formulated from the available evidence. With decreasing gestation, the volume of the germinal layer with its vulnerable capillary bed becomes greater, and at the same time the likelihood of respiratory illnesses, particularly hyaline membrane disease, increases. In the smallest infants, fluctuations of blood gas tensions are common (because of immature control of breathing), even when no frank respiratory illness is present. With increasing severity of respiratory illnesses, abnormalities and fluctuations of PaO_2, $PaCO_2$, and blood pressure become more marked. Increased $PaCO_2$ causes cerebral blood flow to increase; low PaO_2 may also increase flow, as well as cause endothelial damage. Any acute worsening of gas exchange causes an abrupt increase in blood pressure, which, because of impaired autoregulation and the compliance of the preterm infant's skull, generates an increased distending pressure tending to rupture the fragile capillaries of the germinal layer. In addition to this sequence of events, when a tension pneumothorax develops, cerebral venous pressure rises, and this increase is also transmitted to the capillaries. If damage to these vessels has previously occurred, for example, because of birth asphyxia or hypotension, rupture is more likely; and if hemostasis is defective, bleeding will be more severe.

Prevention

It follows from the foregoing line of reasoning that PVH should be, at least theoretically, a preventable condition. The most efficient way to prevent it would be to prevent preterm birth, but so far methods for this are relatively ineffective. Avoidance of birth asphyxia and hypotension could have some effect in preventing PVH. Prevention or amelioration of hyaline membrane disease would probably lead to a considerable reduction in the incidence of PVH, and methods for achieving this are becoming available. Antenatal administration of glucocorticoid to the mother (to stimulate surfactant synthesis in the baby) has been shown to reduce the incidence of hyaline

membrane disease (Crowley et al., 1990), and intratracheal instillation of various forms of exogenous surfactant reduces its severity (Collaborative European Multicentre Study Group, 1988). Whether these treatments also reduce the likelihood of PVH remains to be established, although present evidence suggests trends in that direction for both glucocorticoids and exogenous surfactant. Pneumothorax, a particularly potent cause of PVH, is usually a complication of mechanical ventilation for hyaline membrane disease. Ventilator management should be designed to minimize this risk, and if pneumothorax occurs, diagnosis (by cold light) and drainage should be very swift.

Because abnormal cerebral hemodynamics particularly associated with deranged gas exchange are so clearly implicated in the pathogenesis of PVH, it is important to stabilize key variables controlling cerebral perfusion, notably $PaCO_2$, PaO_2, and blood pressure, at as normal levels as possible. This may be extremely difficult in ill preterm infants, especially because many medical and nursing procedures are needed to ensure other aspects of their well-being. There is some evidence that the incidence of PVH was lower when special attention was paid to controlling these variables than when customary management was applied (Szymonowicz et al., 1986). Also, Perlman et al. (1985) found that the use of muscle relaxation with pancuronium during mechanical ventilation reduced the incidence of PVH in infants selected for treatment because of fluctuating anterior cerebral arterial blood flow velocity. Other measures worthy of consideration are cesarean section for breech presentation (although this would seem likely to have only a small effect and could have other disadvantages) and possibly correction of abnormalities of hemostasis.

Various pharmacologic agents have been given to preterm infants in an attempt to prevent PVH. Pancuronium has already been mentioned. Claims for an effect of certain other drugs have been adduced, notably phenobarbital (Donn et al., 1981) and vitamin E (Sinha et al., 1987); for various reasons these have not found favor (de Vries et al., 1988). Ethamsylate is one agent for which convincing claims have been made (Benson et al., 1986; Morgan et al., 1981). This drug reduces prostaglandin synthesis and increases platelet adhesion. Its precise effects on the cerebral circulation are not yet known. Indomethacin, which is a powerful prostaglandin inhibitor, has also been found to reduce the incidence of PVH in experimental animals (Ment et al., 1983) as well as in preterm infants (Ment et al., 1985a). A study in which NIRS (see later) was used to test the effects on the cerebral circulation of this drug (given for closure of patent ductus arteriosus) showed marked reductions in cerebral blood flow, oxygen delivery, blood volume, and CO_2 reactivity (Edwards et al., 1990). In a minority of infants intracellular cytochrome aa_3 tended to become deoxidized (D.C. McCormick et al., 1990). Because hypoxic-ischemic injury to the brain is probably a more important cause than PVH of long-term neurodevelopmental impairment in preterm infants, great caution should be exercised when contemplating the use of this drug for prevention of PVH. Nevertheless, as NIRS and other methods become available for readily observing the cerebral effects of vasoactive agents in ill infants, it may become possible to use these agents to manipulate the cerebral circulation so that the risks of PVH and of hypoxic-ischemic injury are both minimized.

Posthemorrhagic Ventricular Dilatation and Hydrocephalus

Mild, usually reversible, dilatation of the ventricles with cerebrospinal fluid occurs in about 15% of infants with PVH and may be difficult or impossible to differentiate on ultrasound imaging from minor cerebral atrophy, especially that caused by periventricular leukomalacia (PVL) (see later).

Posthemorrhagic hydrocephalus is a serious complication of PVH. In a consecutive series of 125 very preterm infants who survived for more than 1 week studied by Lipscomb et al. (1982), 46 (37%) had PVH. Using the same definitions as in Table 41–1, the incidence of frank hydrocephalus in these infants was 4% (1 of 23) for infants with grade I PVH, 8% (1 of 13) for grade II, 40% (5 of 11) for grade III, and 57% (4 of 7) for grade IV; none of 77 infants without PVH developed hydrocephalus. Communicating hydrocephalus is more common than noncommunicating, and the site of the block appears usually to be at the base of the brain (because of obliterative arachnoiditis) or at the arachnoid granulations. Often, repeated lumbar punctures can be used to relieve the raised intracranial pressure. However, a multicenter controlled trial involving 157 infants with dilating ventricles showed no advantage for long-term outcome of intervening early by lumbar (or occasionally ventricular) puncture, when the width of the lateral ventricles had reached 4 mm above the 97th percentile for this dimension, rather than later, when the head circumference had increased by more than twice the normal rate over a period of 2 weeks (Ventriculomegaly Trial Group, 1990). Overall, 62% of survivors ultimately required ventricular shunts, and 73% had disabilities at 1 year of age. Secondary analysis showed some advantage of early intervention when parenchymal lesions were present at the time of entry to the trial.

Intraparenchymal Periventricular Hemorrhage

Hemorrhage apparently spreading superolaterally from the germinal layer into the brain parenchyma occurs in about 5–10% of infants with PVH. The hemorrhage is particularly likely to affect the caudate nucleus and the internal capsule (see Fig. 41–1). There has been some dispute about the mechanism of intraparenchymal hemorrhage. Initially, it was thought to be due to direct spread from bleeding vessels in the germinal layer into normal brain tissue. Later, evidence was acquired by positron emission tomography that the lesion was ischemic (Volpe et al., 1983) and histopathologic studies suggested that the hemorrhage represented spread of blood from the germinal layer into areas of PVL (Rushton et al., 1985). More recently, clear histologic evidence has been obtained that venous infarction is an important cause of intraparenchymal hemorrhage (see Fig. 41–1) (Gould et al., 1987). Large hemorrhages into the germinal layer and ventricles lead to distortion and obstruction of the terminal vein and initiate the infarction. Although more information about pathogenesis is needed, it is probable that most unilateral intraparenchymal hemorrhages are due to venous infarction, whereas large bilateral (and usually fatal) ones may often be caused by bleeding into tissue seriously damaged by arterial ischemia.

Infants with unilateral hemorrhages often survive. A porencephalic cyst develops at the site of the lesion within 6–8 weeks. Neurologic sequelae, particularly hemiparesis, are probably invariable, although these can be unexpectedly mild, presumably because of various aspects of brain plasticity (Dubowitz et al., 1985; McMenamin et al., 1984; Stewart et al., 1987).

Prognosis

Ultrasound imaging has been used extensively to investigate the prognostic significance of PVH and other lesions in surviving infants (e.g., Cooke, 1987; McMenamin et al., 1984). Some results from one large cohort study of 342 very preterm infants are given in Table 41–4 (Stewart et al., 1987). Useful prognostic information from the ultrasound scan alone could be obtained as early as the first week of life, and by the time the infants were discharged from the neonatal unit they could be assigned to one of three groups at low, intermediate, and high risk of neurodevelopmental impairment, detectable at 1 year of age. The largest group, 275 (80%) infants with normal scans or uncomplicated PVH, had low risk, with a 4% probability of a disabling impairment. In contrast, a small group of 26 (8%) infants with posthemorrhagic hydrocephalus or cerebral atrophy (any loss of brain tissue, including that following intraparenchymal PVH) were at high risk, with a probability of a disabling impairment of 58% (and of any impairment of 88%). Between the low- and high-risk groups lay the 41 (12%) infants with ventricular dilatation who were at intermediate risk, with a 27% probability of a disabling impairment. This group probably included infants with minor loss of brain tissue as a result of PVL as well as infants with partial obstruction to the flow of cerebrospinal fluid after intraventricular hemorrhage. The oldest 171 children from this cohort were re-examined at 4 years of age and the earlier conclusions were broadly confirmed,

Table 41–4. ULTRASOUND SCANS AT DISCHARGE IN 342 VERY PRETERM INFANTS AND NEURODEVELOPMENTAL IMPAIRMENTS AT 1 YEAR OF AGE

| Ultrasound | n | Impairments | | | Probability of Impairment (%) and 95% Confidence Internal | |
		Major (Disabling)	Minor	Total	Major	Total
Normal	174	6	6	12	4 (1–7)*	11 (8–17)*
Uncomplicated PVH†	101	4	15	19		
Ventricular dilatation with cerebrospinal fluid	41	11	3	14	27 (14–43)	34 (20–51)
Hydrocephalus	8	4	2	6	50 (16–84)	75 (35–97)
Cerebral atrophy‡						
Cysts	10§	8	2	10		
Generalized	8	3	4	7		
	18	11	6	17	61 (36–84)	94 (73–99)

*Infants with normal scans or uncomplicated PVH (unlike the other groups) were not statistically separable by logistical regression analysis and were analyzed together.

†Uncomplicated PVH refers to grade I–III periventricular hemorrhage not followed by ventricular dilatation with cerebrospinal fluid or hydrocephalus.

‡Cerebral atrophy means any loss of brain tissue.

§Four infants also had hydrocephalus and one had generalized atrophy.

From Stewart A.L., Reynolds E.O.R., Hamilton P.A., et al. Probability of neurodevelopmental disorders estimated from ultrasound appearance of brains of very preterm infants. *Dev. Med. Child Neurol.* 29:3–11, 1987.

although cognitive impairments (usually minor) that were not related to the ultrasound findings had by then emerged in a minority of the children (Costello et al., 1988). The pathogenesis of these cognitive impairments needs to be explored.

The most striking finding of this study was that PVH, although common and a major cause of death (see Table 41–1), was unlikely to lead to disability unless complicated by ventricular dilatation or frank hydrocephalus or by intraparenchymal bleeding. A further conclusion of this and other studies (de Vries et al., 1985a) was that hypoxic-ischemic injury leading to PVL is probably a more important cause than PVH of disability in surviving very preterm infants.

HYPOXIC-ISCHEMIC INJURY

The two main types of hypoxic-ischemic injury are birth asphyxia and PVL.

Birth Asphyxia

Birth asphyxia (interruption of gas exchange during labor) leading to hypoxic-ischemic encephalopathy can occur at any gestation but is much more readily recognized by clinical signs in term than preterm infants. Infants who are growing poorly in utero or who are post term are at increased risk of birth asphyxia because of inadequate placental function. Other common causes are preeclamptic toxemia, separation of the placenta, and prolapse of the umbilical cord.

In very acutely asphyxiated infants, the basal ganglia, which are highly metabolically active, are damaged. More commonly, asphyxia is less acute and complicated by hypotension, a situation that leads to injury in the parasagittal areas at the boundary zones between the territories of the anterior, middle, and posterior cerebral arteries. Both types of injury have

been modeled in newborn monkeys (Myers, 1972; Brann and Myers, 1975).

The clinical features depend on the severity of injury and bear a reasonably close relation to outcome. Several authors (Levene et al., 1988; Sarnat and Sarnat, 1976) have graded birth-asphyxiated infants as having mild, moderate, or severe encephalopathy. Infants with mild encephalopathy (minor disturbances of tone, hyperalertness, slight feeding difficulties lasting a few days) recovered completely. Those with moderate encephalopathy (lethargy, convulsions, poor feeding, signs of recovery by 1 week of age) had a 25% chance of death or survival with severe disabilities; and if severe encephalopathy was present (coma, profound hypotonia, inadequate ventilation), 75–100% of infants died or survived with severe disabilities.

Identification of fetuses at risk, intrapartum monitoring, and appropriate obstetric intervention will protect some infants from birth asphyxia, but in many infants problems are unforeseen. Current methods for the treatment of asphyxiated infants are unsatisfactory. Apart from rapid resuscitation, maintenance of oxygenation and cardiac output, and treatment of seizures, little can be done. No clear evidence exists that infusions of bicarbonate or glucose are more than occasionally indicated, and they can be dangerous. Neither is there current support for the use of various methods for reducing cerebral edema (which is often not marked), such as reducing $Paco_2$ below normal or administering steroids or osmotic agents such as mannitol. In the future the use of cerebroprotective drugs including N-methyl-D-aspartate (NMDA) blockers may find an important role (see later).

Periventricular Leukomalacia

This condition (Fig. 41–2) mainly affects infants born before 35 weeks of gestation and has a preva-

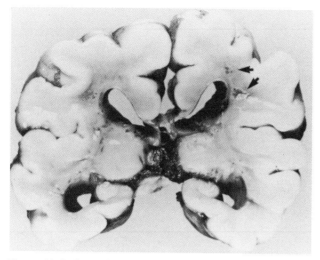

Figure 41–2. Coronal section of the brain of an infant born at 34 wk of gestation who died at age 11 d. Multiple small cavities caused by PVL can be seen *(arrows)*. (From Wigglesworth J.S. *Perinatal Pathology*. Philadelphia, Saunders, p. 274, 1984.)

lence of about 5–10% in survivors. It was first clearly recognized by Banker and Larroche (1962), and its pathology and likely pathogenesis have been amplified by de Reuek (1971), Armstrong and Norman (1974), Takashima and Tanaka (1978), and Pape and Wigglesworth (1979). These and many subsequent studies have shown that the condition principally affects the boundary zone between the centripetal and centrifugal arterial supplies of the developing brain, especially near the dorsolateral angle of the lateral ventricles at the point of junction of the corpus callosum and at the trigone of the lateral ventricle. In more mature infants a similar process may occur at the bases of the cortical sulci, causing subcortical leukomalacia (Takashima et al., 1978; Wigglesworth, 1989).

There is little doubt that PVL (and subcortical leukomalacia) is caused by hypoxemia and hypotension, which leads to necrosis in these zones (Ment et al., 1985b,c; Young et al., 1982) and may be followed by the development of cystic changes (see Fig. 41–2) or passive ventricular dilatation. Obtaining accurate information about the timing of the initiating insult is more difficult than for PVH, because the earliest changes of the lesion cannot be identified by ultrasound imaging (or any other currently available bedside technique). PVL may be suspected from persistently increased periventricular echo densities (Trounce et al., 1986), but for a certain diagnosis cystic changes, which occur from about 1 week to 1 month after the apparent time of the insult, should be awaited (Hope et al., 1988).

Strong evidence exists that in a proportion (of currently uncertain magnitude) of cases of PVL the insult occurs before the onset of labor, because characteristic cysts are seen in the first few days of life (Behar et al., 1988). In the remaining infants hypoxemia or hypotension during labor or associated with

a stormy neonatal course, particularly if prolonged mechanical ventilation is required, has been implicated (Sinha et al., 1985). As with PVH, abnormal clinical signs attributable to PVL are absent or equivocal in the neonatal period.

The long-term outcome for infants with PVL depends on the site and extent of the lesions. Because these are commonly symmetric and involve the motor fibers of the internal capsule, spastic diplegia or quadriplegia is a likely consequence (Dubowitz et al., 1985; Weindling et al., 1985).

Investigation of Cerebral Oxidative Metabolism

New methods have been introduced for investigating cerebral oxidative metabolism in infants suspected of hypoxic-ischemic brain injury. These methods, which include positron emission tomography, magnetic resonance spectroscopy, and NIRS, are proving valuable for defining the sequence of events that follows acute oxygen deprivation caused by, for example, birth asphyxia. They can also provide objective evidence about the effectiveness or otherwise of preventive strategies and treatment and about the prognosis of the infants.

The technique of positron emission tomography is dealt with in Chapter 121. It has been particularly employed by Volpe and co-workers to investigate regional cerebral blood flow in association with intraparenchymal PVH (see earlier) (Volpe et al., 1983) and birth asphyxia in term infants (Volpe et al., 1985).

The first studies of the human brain by the noninvasive technique of magnetic resonance spectroscopy were made in newborn infants, and a considerable amount of information about events in perinatal hypoxic-ischemic injury is now available (reviewed by Wyatt et al., 1989a). The technique is described in detail in Chapter 122. It is proving particularly valuable when used in conjunction with NIRS. These two methods provide complementary information about cerebral oxidative metabolism and hemodynamics, for reasons that are summarized in Figure 41–3. Electrons passing along the respiratory transport chain in the inner mitochondrial membrane initiate the synthesis of ATP from ADP and inorganic orthophosphate (P_i). The electrons then reduce cytochrome aa_3 (the terminal enzyme of the chain). Cytochrome aa_3 is reoxidized by molecular oxygen, a reaction that accounts for about 95% of the oxygen consumption of the body. Magnetic resonance spectroscopy allows noninvasive measurements in brain tissue of ATP and its "buffer," phosphocreatine (PCr). Intracellular pH (pH_i) can be derived from the difference in resonance frequency between PCr and P_i.

Near-Infrared Spectroscopy. This technique is used to measure, at the bedside, a wide range of indices related to oxygen delivery and utilization in

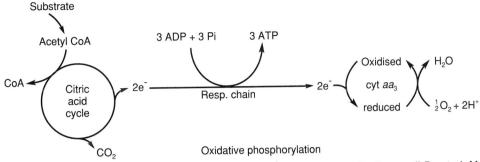

Figure 41–3. Simplified diagram of oxidative phosphorylation. (From Wyatt J.S., Edwards A.D., Azzopardi D., et al. Magnetic resonance and near infrared spectroscopy for investigation of perinatal hypoxic-ischaemic brain injury. *Arch. Dis. Child.* 64:953–963, 1989.)

the brain, including changes in the concentrations of oxyhemoglobin (HbO_2), deoxyhemoglobin, and oxidized cytochrome aa_3. Cerebral blood flow, oxygen delivery, and blood volume can also be measured, as can the reactivity of the cerebral circulation to carbon dioxide. Because NIRS has only recently been introduced into clinical investigation and shows promise of becoming useful for studies of older children and adults as well as newborn infants, a brief account of the technique is given here.

The principles of in vivo NIRS were first established by Jobsis (1977). They depend on the fact that light in the near-infrared (700–1000 nm) region of the spectrum penetrates tissue much more readily than does visible light. Technical developments have made possible the detection of light transmitted through the head of the newborn infant.

HbO_2, deoxyhemoglobin, and oxidized cytochrome aa_3 are pigmented compounds (chromophores) that absorb near-infrared light in predictable ways. The absorption characteristics of biologic tissue therefore give information about the presence of these compounds in the tissue. Brazy et al. (1985) were the first to obtain information about the brains of preterm infants. Subsequently, methods have been devised for quantitation of data for the brain (Wyatt et al., 1986, 1989a, 1990a).

Quantitation depends on the Beer-Lambert law describing optical absorption in a highly scattering medium, which may be expressed as absorption (OD) $= acLB + G$, where OD is optical density, a is the absorption coefficient of the chromophore (mM^{-1} cm^{-1}), c is the concentration of chromophore (mM), L is the distance between the points where light enters and leaves the tissue (the interoptode distance, cm), B is a path length factor that takes account of the scattering of light in the tissue (which causes the optical path length to be greater than L), and G is a factor related to the geometry of the tissue. If L, B, and G remain constant, changes in chromophore concentration can be derived from the expression $\Delta c = \Delta OD/aLB$. The absorption coefficients of HbO_2, deoxyhemoglobin, and oxidized cytochrome aa_3 are known (Wray et al., 1988), and a value for B of 4.4 has been obtained in preterm infants (Wyatt et al., 1990b). In practice, three to six wavelengths of light

are shone through the head, and an algorithm is used to obtain changes in chromophore concentration from changes in OD.

Processing of the changes in these indices that occur in response to alterations in arterial oxygen saturation (SaO_2) or $PaCO_2$ allows quantitation of a number of important hemodynamic variables. *Cerebral blood flow* (CBF) is measured by the Fick principle, using a small sudden change in arterial HbO_2 concentration (produced by altering the inspired oxygen concentration) as a tracer (Edwards et al., 1988). Cerebral blood flow can then be calculated from the expression:

$$CBF = k(\Delta[HbO_2](t)/tHb \int_0^t \Delta SaO_2)dt$$

where t is the time over which the observations are made, normally 6–8 seconds, less than the cerebral transit time; tHb is total large-vessel hemoglobin concentration; and k is 0.61, a constant that reflects the molecular weight of hemoglobin and tissue density. *Cerebral oxygen delivery* is calculated from the product of cerebral blood flow and arterial oxygen content.

Cerebral blood volume (CBV) can be measured from the observed effects of a small gradual change in SaO_2 on cerebral HbO_2 and deoxyhemoglobin (Wyatt et al., 1990a). As with measurement of cerebral blood flow, this method uses HbO_2 as a tracer molecule measured by NIRS, but the observations are made during a much slower change in SaO_2, over 5–10 minutes, so the tracer is at steady state and equilibrated throughout the brain. Changes in tracer concentration allow the calculation of cerebral blood volume from the equation

$$CBV = k \Delta([HbO_2] - [deoxyHb])/(2 \Delta SaO_2 tHb)$$

where deoxyHb is deoxyhemoglobin and k is 0.89, a constant reflecting the molecular weight of hemoglobin, tissue density, and the cerebral/large vessel hemoglobin ratio. Suitable calibration of the spectrometer then allows cerebral blood volume to be displayed continuously. The CO_2 reactivity of cerebral blood volume is tested by observing the effects of a small (~1 kPa) change in $PaCO_2$.

Data acquired with NIRS for normal infants are so far scant, but preliminary evidence suggests the following values for term infants: cerebral blood flow 20–40 ml/100 g/min; cerebral oxygen delivery, 2.5–5.0 ml/100 g/min; cerebral blood volume 2–3 ml/100 g; and CO_2 reactivity, 0.4–0.6 ml/100 g/kPa. In preterm infants CO_2 reactivity is reduced, but the other variables appear similar (Edwards et al., 1988; Wyatt et al., 1989a, 1990a).

Near-infrared light does not penetrate right through the adult head. However, NIRS can still be used to investigate regions of the brain, with the optodes placed 5–8 cm apart. As more information about the path length factor *(B)* is obtained, it will be possible to investigate the same hemodynamic variables described for newborn infants. Imaging of NIRS variables is a practical possibility for the future.

Abnormal Oxidative Metabolism

When the oxygen supply to tissue is critically reduced or the mitochondrial mechanisms for utilizing oxygen are damaged, the concentration of ATP tends to fall. This fall is initially extremely small because of the buffering effect of the creatine kinase reaction, which maintains the level of ATP. At the same time the concentration of PCr falls and an almost reciprocal rise takes place in P_i. Hence PCr/P_i falls. This ratio is related to the phosphorylation potential of the tissue and is often taken as an index of its energy state or reserve. Only when PCr/P_i falls to an extremely low level does the concentration of ATP fall appreciably (see Chapter 122).

Studies by phosphorus magnetic resonance spectroscopy of newborn experimental animals in which the oxygen supply to the brain was abruptly curtailed showed (as in adult animals) the expected changes in PCr/P_i and ATP levels (Hope et al., 1987). At the same time pH_i fell to an extremely low level, mainly because of the production of lactic acid. On reperfusion of the brain, recovery of the metabolite concentrations and pH_i was often rapid and could be complete in about an hour.

Studies of severely birth-asphyxiated babies have shown that PCr/P_i and pH_i (recorded from the temporoparietal cortex) were usually normal on the first day of life (Azzopardi et al., 1989; Hope et al., 1984). During the next few days, however, abnormalities developed (Figs. 41–4 and 41–5). In some infants with very low values, a fall in PCr/P_i took place together with a fall in the concentration of ATP. In the most affected infants PCr and ATP virtually disappeared as P_i continued to rise and death ensued. In less severely affected infants, the metabolite ratios returned to normal over about 2 weeks, but sometimes the total phosphorus signal remained low, indicating permanent loss of brain cells. This se-

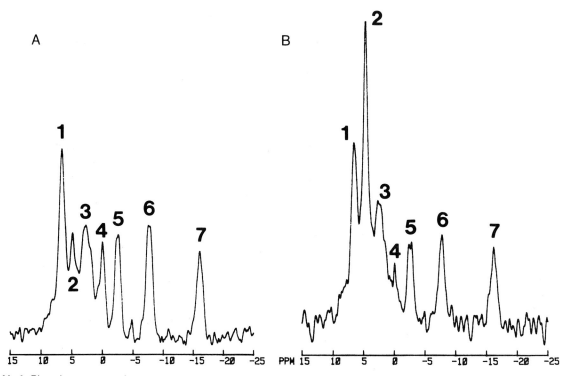

Figure 41–4. Phosphorus magnetic resonance spectra from the brains of two infants. *(a)* A normal infant born at 36 weeks of gestation who was studied at age 15 days. *(b)* An infant born at 36 weeks of gestation who had suffered severe birth asphyxia and was studied at age 2 days. The *x* axis is a frequency axis (chemical shift in parts per million [ppm] relative to PCr) and the *y* axis represents signal intensity; the area under the peaks is proportional to concentration. The seven labeled peaks are attributable to 1, phosphomonoesters; 2, P_i; 3, phosphodiesters; 4, PCr; and 5, 6, and 7, the γ, α, and β phosphorus nuclei of nucleotide triphosphates, mainly ATP. The spectrum from the infant in *a* is normal, $PCr/P_i = 1.15$. In the infant in *b*, PCr/P_i was grossly reduced, 0.08, and the concentration of ATP was also below normal; the infant subsequently died.

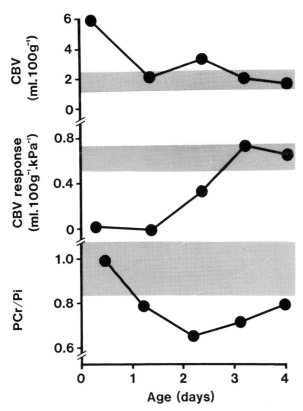

Figure 41–5. Cerebral blood volume, its response to changes in $Paco_2$, and PCr/P_i in a severely birth-asphyxiated baby born at 36 weeks of gestation; he died at age 7 weeks with evidence of cerebral atrophy. Normal ranges are shaded. (From Wyatt J.S., Edwards A.D., Azzopardi D., et al. Magnetic resonance and near infrared spectroscopy for investigation of perinatal hypoxic-ischaemic brain injury. *Arch. Dis. Child.* 64:953–963, 1989.)

quence of events (which evolved in spite of normal arterial blood pressure, blood gas and pH values, and glucose levels) may be called secondary energy failure to distinguish it from the events observed during acute oxygen deprivation, or primary energy failure, described earlier. Unlike the situation in primary energy failure, pH_i either remained normal or increased slightly in babies with secondary energy failure, indicating severe disruption of membrane function.

It can be presumed that severely birth-asphyxiated babies with normal magnetic resonance findings on the first day of life had gone through a phase of primary energy failure before delivery, at a time when they were inaccessible to study. The acute insult had, however, initiated a series of biochemical reactions and vicious circles that led to the secondary, damaging or lethal, phase.

If treatment designed to prevent secondary energy failure is to be put on a sound footing, more must be found out about the biochemical reactions set off by the acute insult. The likely candidates are dealt with in detail in Chapter 77 in the context of cerebroprotection. Synaptic release of excitatory neurotransmitters, particularly glutamate, in response to hypoxia is almost certainly of great importance, leading,

via stimulation of NMDA receptors, to both depolarization and massive entry of calcium ions to cells, which is one probable cause of mitochondrial damage and progression to secondary energy failure (Ikonomidou et al., 1989). Other reactions involving oxygen and hydroxyl free radicals during reperfusion are also likely to be damaging (see Chapter 77). These and other mechanisms cause energy failure by impairing the utilization of available oxygen. An additional factor may be inadequate oxygen delivery to tissue because of cerebral edema and damage to cerebral blood vessels and their control (Chapters 10 and 76).

The finding that the energy state of brain tissue was often normal shortly after delivery raises the intriguing possibility of intervening with cerebroprotective agents, such as NMDA receptor blockers and free radical scavengers. Accumulating evidence suggests that these agents are capable of preventing or ameliorating permanent damage to the brain (Olney et al., 1989; Thiringer et al., 1987). If this approach is to be tested in newborn infants, it will be important to identify, immediately after delivery, those who are destined to develop secondary energy failure. Preliminary evidence has been found by NIRS that before this failure is manifest, cerebral blood volume is increased and its reactivity to changes in $Paco_2$ is lost (Wyatt et al., 1989b) (see Fig. 41–5). If these abnormalities are confirmed, it will become possible to use them to select infants for enrollment in controlled trials of cerebroprotective agents such as NMDA receptor blockers and observe the effectiveness of these agents by NIRS, magnetic resonance spectroscopy, and other techniques.

Abnormal phosphorus spectra indicating impaired oxidative metabolism, and closely resembling those in babies with birth asphyxia, have been found in a variety of other conditions in which hypoxic-ischemic injury was suspected or known to have occurred, such as PVL, cerebral infarction, and intraparenchymal PVH (Wyatt et al., 1989a). Although systematic studies have not yet been done, the temporal progression of the spectral abnormalities in these conditions appears similar to that which follows birth asphyxia, implying that the initiating cerebral insult often occurred around the time of birth. A further implication (at least theoretically) is that, as in birth-asphyxiated infants, cerebroprotective agents may in the future find a role in preventing or ameliorating permanent ill effects.

Prognosis

After birth asphyxia, the neurologic state of the infants provides some guide to prognosis (see earlier), and data acquired by a number of other techniques, particularly computed tomography and Doppler velocimetry of the cerebral arteries, are useful (reviewed by Levene, 1988).

Magnetic resonance spectroscopy also provides

valuable prognostic information. Early studies suggested that low values for PCr/P$_i$ were predictive of the later loss of brain tissue (Hamilton et al., 1986). More recently, the prognostic significance of low values for PCr/P$_i$ and ATP concentration in the first days of life for survival and neurodevelopmental status at 1 year of age has been investigated in 61 infants born at 27–42 weeks of gestation (Azzopardi et al., 1989). They were studied because of evidence or suspicion of hypoxic-ischemic injury, and 40 had sustained birth asphyxia. Nineteen of the infants whose values for PCr/P$_i$ fell below 95% confidence limits for normal control infants died, and 7 of the 9 survivors developed multiple disabling impairments (sensitivity 74%, specificity 92%, positive predictive value for these outcomes 93%). Eleven of the 12 infants with similarly low values for ATP died, and the single survivor had severe multiple impairments (sensitivity 47%, specificity 97%, positive predictive value for death 91%). It was concluded that these data were secure enough to be taken into account when decisions were made about how far intensive care should be pursued in infants with hypoxic-ischemic injury.

This study also showed that the severity of adverse outcome was related to the minimal recorded value for PCr/P$_i$ (Fig. 41–6) and that the lower the value for PCr/P$_i$ the lower, in general, was the subsequent Griffiths general quotient. These findings demonstrate that the worse the impairment of oxidative metabolism in the first days of life, the worse the outcome, and are evidence for the existence of a continuum of reproductive casualty caused by hypoxic-ischemic brain injury arising in the perinatal period.

CONCLUSIONS

The two main causes of perinatal brain damage are PVH in very preterm infants and hypoxic-ischemic injury associated with birth asphyxia or causing PVL. Current epidemiologic evidence suggests that birth asphyxia accounts for about a quarter of all perinatal deaths in developed countries but no more than about 5% of the total number of disabled children at school age (Alberman, 1982). There has been much dispute about the latter figure and particularly about the contribution of birth asphyxia and other perinatal events (such as fetal hemodynamic derangements in late pregnancy) to the total number of children with cerebral palsy. Very low birth weight (<1500 g) infants account for roughly 50% of all perinatal deaths but only about 2% of disabled children, and there is abundant evidence that the widespread use of intensive care for these and other ill infants is associated with the increasing survival of normal children without significant salvage of disabled ones (e.g., M.C. McCormick, 1989).

The extent to which perinatal brain injury contributes to minor, as well as major, neurodevelopmental

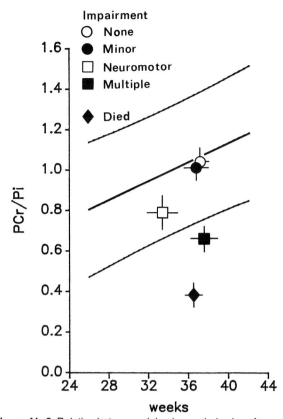

Figure 41–6. Relation between minimal recorded values for cerebral PCr/P$_i$ during the first 6 d of life and survival and neurodevelopmental outcome at age 1 year in 61 infants studied because of suspicion or evidence of hypoxic-ischemic brain injury. The regression line and 95% confidence limits for normal values versus gestational plus postnatal age are shown. Minor impairment refers to disorders of tone or reflexes not causing disability; neuromotor impairment, major neuromotor impairments causing disability; multiple impairments, more than one disabling impairment, including neuromotor, neurosensory (visual or hearing), neurobehavioral, and psychometric, often together with microcephaly. Mean values ± SEM are shown. (Data of Azzopardi D., Wyatt J.S., Cady E.B., et al. Prognosis of newborn infants with hypoxic-ischemic brain injury assessed by phosphorus magnetic resonance spectroscopy. *Pediatr. Res.* 25:445–451, 1989.)

impairments in childhood, or to neuropsychiatric illness in adult life, remains largely unresolved. Genetic factors clearly have the main influence and environmental factors are also extremely important. Nevertheless, clues exist that perinatal injury may be more prevalent than is currently appreciated. In particular, lesser degrees of hypoxic-ischemic injury often go unrecognized by currently available techniques (e.g., Hope et al., 1988), and some evidence has been presented that this form of injury may be involved in a variety of adverse outcomes including minor motor impairments (Marlow et al., 1989), cognitive and learning difficulties (Costello et al., 1988; Fuller et al., 1983; Lou et al., 1990; Njiokiktjien et al., 1988), and some cases of schizophrenia (Eagles et al., 1990; Owen et al., 1988).

A major focus of this chapter has been the ways in which noninvasive methods are providing new information about perinatal brain injury and its consequences. Ultrasound imaging has proved particularly valuable for the investigation of PVH, and magnetic resonance spectroscopy and NIRS give novel insights into the events that accompany hypoxic-ischemic injury. The introduction of these and many other methods for investigating the brain has been one of the most exciting developments in neonatal medicine, because it permits the prevalence and mechanisms of potentially brain-damaging influences to be explored, preventive measures and treatments to be tested, and the prognosis of small ill infants to be determined with reasonable confidence. In the future it will be possible to relate objective evidence of perinatal brain injury to a range of outcomes, including neuropsychiatric function in adult life. The ability to assign prognosis already has important implications for neonatal intensive care: parents of ill infants whose prognostic indicators are good can be reassured, early warning can be given if impairment can be foreseen, and, if it is plain that the prognosis is extremely bad, rational decisions can be made about how far to pursue treatment.

References

Alberman E.D. The epidemiology of congenital defects: a pragmatic approach. In Adinolfi M., Benson P., Gianelli F., et al., eds. *Paediatric Research: A Genetic Approach.* London, Heinemann, pp. 1–28, 1982.

Armstrong D., Norman M.G. Periventricular leukomalacia in neonates: complications and sequelae. *Arch. Dis. Child.* 49:367–375, 1974.

Azzopardi D., Wyatt J.S., Cady E.B., et al. Prognosis of newborn infants with hypoxic-ischemic brain injury assessed by phosphorus magnetic resonance spectroscopy. *Pediatr. Res.* 25:445–451, 1989.

Banker B., Larroche J.C. Periventricular leucomalacia of infancy: a form of neonatal anoxic encephalopathy. *Arch. Neurol.* 7:386–410, 1962.

Behar R., Wozniak P., Allard A., et al. Antenatal origin of neurologic damage in newborn infants. I. Preterm infants. *Am. J. Obstet. Gynecol.* 159:357–363, 1988.

Benson J.W.T., Drayton M.R., Hayward C., et al. Multicentre trial of ethamsylate for prevention of periventricular haemorrhage in very low birthweight infants. *Lancet* 2:1297–1299, 1986.

Brann A.W., Myers R.E. Central nervous system findings in the newborn monkey following severe in utero partial asphyxia. *Neurology (Minneap.)* 25:327–338, 1975.

Brazy J.E., Lewis D.V., Mitnick M.H., et al. Noninvasive monitoring of cerebral oxygenation in preterm infants: preliminary observations. *Pediatrics* 75:217–225, 1985.

Burstein J., Papile L.A., Burstein R. Intraventricular hemorrhage and hydrocephalus in premature newborns: a prospective study with CT. *A.J.R.* 132:631–635, 1979.

Cole V.A., Durbin G.M., Olaffson A., et al. Pathogenesis of intraventricular haemorrhage in newborn infants. *Arch. Dis. Child.* 49:722–728, 1974.

Collaborative European Multicentre Study Group. Surfactant replacement therapy for severe neonatal respiratory distress syndrome. *Pediatrics* 82:683–691, 1988.

Connell J., de Vries L., Oozeer R., et al. Predictive value of early continuous electroencephalogram monitoring in ventilated preterm infants with intraventricular hemorrhage. *Pediatrics* 812:337–343, 1988.

Cooke R.W.I. Early and late cranial ultrasonographic appearances and outcome in very low birthweight infants. *Arch. Dis. Child.* 62:931–937, 1987.

Costello A.M.de L., Hamilton P.A., Baudin J., et al. Prediction of neurodevelopmental impairment at four years from brain ultrasound appearance of very preterm infants. *Dev. Med. Child Neurol.* 30:711–722, 1988.

Crowley P., Chalmers I., Kierse M.J.N.C. The effects of corticosteroid administration before preterm delivery: an overview of the evidence from controlled trials. *Br. J. Obst. Gynaecol.* 97:11–25, 1990.

de Reuek J. The human periventricular arterial supply and the anatomy of cerebral infarctions. *Eur. Neurol.* 5:321–334, 1971.

de Vries L.S., Dubowitz L.M.S., Dubowitz V., et al. Predictive value of cranial ultrasound in the newborn baby: a reappraisal. *Lancet* 2:137–140, 1985a.

de Vries L.S., Lary S., Dubowitz L.M.S. Relationship of serum bilirubin levels to ototoxicity and deafness in high-risk low-birth-weight infants. *Pediatrics* 76:351–354, 1985b.

de Vries L.S., Larroche J.C., Levene M.I. Germinal matrix haemorrhage and intraventricular haemorrhage. In Levene M.I., Bennett M.J., Punt J., eds. *Fetal and Neonatal Neurology and Neurosurgery.* Edinburgh, Churchill Livingstone, pp. 319–322, 1988.

Donn S.M., Roloff D.W., Goldstein G.W. Prevention of intraventricular haemorrhage in preterm infants by phenobarbitone: a controlled trial. *Lancet* 2:215–217, 1981.

Dubowitz L.M.S., Bydder G.M. Nuclear magnetic resonance imaging in the diagnosis and follow-up of neonatal cerebral injury. *Clin. Perinatol.* 12:243–260, 1985.

Dubowitz L.M.S., Bydder G.M., Mushin J. Developmental sequence of periventricular leucomalacia. *Arch. Dis. Child.* 60:349–355, 1985.

Eagles J.M., Gibson I., Bremner M.H., et al. Obstetric complications in DSM-III schizophrenics and their siblings. *Lancet* 335:1139–1141, 1990.

Edwards A.D., Wyatt J.S., Richardson C., et al. Cotside measurement of cerebral blood flow in ill newborn infants by near infrared spectroscopy. *Lancet* 2:770–771, 1988.

Edwards A.D., Wyatt J.S., Potter A., et al. Effects of indomethacin on cerebral haemodynamics and oxygen delivery investigated by near infrared spectroscopy in very preterm infants. *Lancet* 335:1491–1495, 1990.

Fuller P.W., Guthrie R.D., Alvord E.C. A proposed neuropathological basis for learning difficulties in children born prematurely. *Dev. Med. Child Neurol.* 25:214–231, 1983.

Goddard-Finegold J. Experimental models of intraventricular hemorrhage. In Pape K.E., Wigglesworth J.S., eds. *Perinatal Brain Lesions.* Oxford, Blackwell Scientific Publications, pp. 115–134, 1989.

Gould S.J., Howard S., Hope P.L., et al. Periventricular intracerebral haemorrhage in the newborn: the role of venous infarction. *J. Pathol.* 151:197–202, 1987.

Gray O.P., Ackerman A., Fraser A.J. Intracranial haemorrhage and clotting defects in low birthweight infants. *Lancet* 1:545–547, 1968.

Hambleton G., Wigglesworth J.S. Origin of intraventricular haemorrhage in the preterm infant. *Arch. Dis. Child.* 51:651–659, 1976.

Hamilton P.A., Hope P.L., Cady E.B., et al. Impaired energy metabolism in brains of newborn infants with increased cerebral echodensities. *Lancet* 1:1242–1246, 1986.

Harrison V.C., Heese H.V. de, Klein M. Intracranial haemorrhage associated with hyaline membrane disease. *Arch. Dis. Child.* 43:116–120, 1968.

Hope P.L., Thorburn R.J., Stewart A.L., et al. Timing and antecedents of periventricular haemorrhage in very preterm infants. In *Second Special Ross Laboratories Conference on Perinatal Intracranial Hemorrhage.* Columbus, OH, Ross Laboratories, pp. 78–101, 1982.

Hope P.L., Costello A.M.de L., Cady E.B., et al. Cerebral energy metabolism studied with phosphorus NMR spectroscopy in normal and birth-asphyxiated infants. *Lancet* 2:366–370, 1984.

Hope P.L., Cady E.B., Chu A., et al. Brain metabolism and intracellular pH during ischaemia and hypoxia. An in vivo ^{31}P and ^{1}H nuclear magnetic resonance study in the lamb. *J. Neurochem.* 49:75–82, 1987.

Hope P.L., Gould S.J., Howard S., et al. Precision of ultrasound diagnosis of pathologically verified lesions in the brains of very preterm infants. *Dev. Med. Child Neurol.* 30:457–471, 1988.

Ikonomidou C., Price M.T., Mosinger J.L., et al. Hypobaric-ischemic conditions produce glutamate-like cytopathology in infant rat brain. *J. Neurosci.* 9:1693–1700, 1989.

Jobsis F.F. Noninvasive infrared monitoring of cerebral and myocardial oxygen sufficiency and circulatory parameters. *Science* 198:1264–1267, 1977.

Koh T.H.H.G., Aynsley-Green A., Tarbit M., et al. Neural dysfunction during hypoglycaemia. *Arch. Dis. Child.* 53:1353–1358, 1988.

Levene M.I. Management and outcome of birth asphyxia. In Levene M.I., Bennett M.J., Punt J., eds. *Fetal and Neonatal Neurology and Neurosurgery.* Edinburgh, Churchill Livingstone, pp. 383–392, 1988.

Levene M.I., Fawer C-L., Lamont R.F. Risk factors in the development of intraventricular haemorrhage in the premature neonate. *Arch. Dis. Child.* 57:410–417, 1982.

Levene M.I., Bennett M.J., Punt J. *Fetal and Neonatal Neurology and Neurosurgery.* Edinburgh, Churchill Livingstone, 1988.

Lipscomb A.P., Thorburn R.J., Stewart A.L., et al. Early intervention and outcome in very preterm infants with rapidly progressive post-haemorrhagic hydrocephalus. *Second Special Ross Laboratories Conference on Perinatal Intracranial Hemorrhage.* Columbus, OH, Ross Laboratories, pp. 840–881, 1982.

Lou H.C., Lassen N.A., Friis-Hansen B. Impaired autoregulation of cerebral blood flow in the distressed newborn infant. *J. Pediatr.* 94:118–121, 1979.

Lou H.C., Henriksen L., Bruhn P. Focal cerebral dysfunction in developmental learning disabilities. *Lancet* 1:8–11, 1990.

Marlow N., Roberts B.L., Cooke R.W.I. Motor skills in extremely low birthweight children at the age of 6 years. *Arch. Dis. Child.* 64:839–847, 1989.

Martin D.J. Cranial sonography in perinatology. In Pape K.E., Wigglesworth J.S., eds. *Perinatal Brain Lesions.* Oxford, Blackwell Scientific Publications, pp. 55–98, 1989.

McCormick D.C., Edwards A.D., Wyatt J.S., et al. Effect of indomethacin on cerebral oxidized cytochrome aa_3 in preterm infants. *Pediatr. Res.* 28:290, 1990.

McCormick M.C. Long-term follow-up of infants discharged from neonatal intensive care units. *J.A.M.A.* 261:1767–1772, 1989.

McMenamin J.B., Shakelford G.D., Volpe J.J. Outcome of neonatal intraventricular hemorrhage with periventricular echodense lesions. *Ann. Neurol.* 15:285–290, 1984.

Ment L.R., Stewart W.B., Scott D.T., et al. Beagle puppy model of intraventricular hemorrhage: randomised indomethacin prevention trial. *Neurology* 33:179–184, 1983.

Ment L.R., Duncan C.C., Ehrenkranz R.A., et al. Randomized indomethacin trial for prevention of intraventricular hemorrhage in very low birth weight infants. *J. Pediatr.* 207:937–943, 1985a.

Ment L.R., Stewart W.B., Duncan C.C., et al. Beagle puppy model of perinatal cerebral infarction: acute changes in cerebral blood flow and metabolism during hemorrhagic hypotension. *J. Neurosurg.* 63:441–447, 1985b.

Ment L.R., Stewart W.B., Duncan C.C., et al. Beagle puppy model of perinatal cerebral infarction: acute changes in cerebral prostaglandins during hemorrhagic hypotension. *J. Neurosurg.* 63:899–904, 1985c.

Morgan M.E.I., Benson J.W.T., Cooke R.W.I. Ethamyslate reduces the incidence of periventricular haemorrhage in very low birth-weight babies. *Lancet* 2:830–831, 1981.

Myers R.E. Two patterns of perinatal brain damage and their condition of occurrence. *Am. J. Obst. Gynecol.* 112:246–276, 1972.

Njiokiktjien C., Valk J., Ramaekers G. Malformation or damage of the corpus callosum? A clinical and MRI study. *Brain Dev.* 10:92–99, 1988.

Olney J.W., Ikonomidou C., Mosinger J.L., et al. MK-801 prevents hypobaric-ischemic neuronal degeneration in infant rat brain. *J. Neurosci.* 9:1701–1704, 1989.

Owen M.J., Lewis S.W., Murray R.M. Obstetric complications and schizophrenia: a computed tomographic study. *Psychol. Med.* 18:331–339, 1988.

Pape K.E., Wigglesworth J.S. *Haemorrhage, Ischaemia and the Perinatal Brain.* London, Heinemann, 1979.

Papile L.A., Burstein J., Burstein R., et al. Incidence and evolution of subependymal and intraventricular hemorrhage: a study of infants with birth weights less than 1500 gm. *J. Pediatr.* 92:529–534, 1978.

Perlman J.M., McMenamin J.B., Volpe J.J. Fluctuating cerebral blood flow velocity in respiratory distress syndrome: relation to the development of intraventricular hemorrhage. *N. Engl. J. Med.* 309:204–209, 1983.

Perlman J.M., Goodman S., Kreusser K.L., et al. Reduction in intraventricular hemorrhage by elimination of fluctuating cerebral blood flow in preterm infants with respiratory distress syndrome. *N. Engl. J. Med.* 312:1353–1357, 1985.

Reynolds M.L., Evans C.A.N., Reynolds E.O.R., et al. Intracranial haemorrhage in the preterm sheep fetus. *Early Hum. Dev.* 3:163–186, 1979.

Rushton D.I., Preston P.R., Durbin G.M. Structure and evolution of echodense lesions in the neonatal brain: a combined ultrasound and necropsy study. *Arch. Dis. Child.* 60:798–808, 1985.

Sarnat H.B., Sarnat M.S. Neonatal encephalopathy following fetal distress. *Arch. Neurol.* 33:696–705, 1976.

Sinha S., Davies J., Toner N., et al. Vitamin E supplementation reduces the incidence of periventricular haemorrhages in very preterm babies. *Lancet* 1:466–471, 1987.

Sinha S.K., Davies J.M., Sims D.G., et al. Relation between periventricular haemorrhage and ischaemic brain lesions diagnosed by ultrasound in very preterm infants. *Lancet* 2:1154–1156, 1985.

Stewart A.L., Reynolds E.O.R., Hamilton P.A., et al. Probability of neurodevelopmental disorders estimated from ultrasound appearance of brains of very preterm infants. *Dev. Med. Child Neurol.* 29:3–11, 1987.

Szymonowicz W., Yu V.Y.H., Wilson F.E. Antecedents of periventricular haemorrhage in infants weighing 1250 g or less at birth. *Arch. Dis. Child.* 59:13–17, 1984.

Szymonowicz W., Yu V.Y.H., Walker A., et al. Reduction in periventricular haemorrhages in preterm infants. *Arch. Dis. Child.* 61:661–665, 1986.

Takashima J., Tanaka K. Development of cerebral architecture and its relationship to periventricular leukomalacia. *Arch. Neurol.* 35:11–16, 1978.

Takashima J., Armstrong D., Becker L.E. Subcortical leukomalacia: relationship to the development of the cerebral sulcus and its vascular supply. *Arch. Neurol.* 35:470–472, 1978.

Thiringer K., Hrbek A., Karlson K., et al. Postasphyxial cerebral survival in newborn sheep after treatment with oxygen free radical scavengers and a calcium antagonist. *Pediatr. Res.* 22:62–66, 1987.

Thorburn R.J., Lipscomb A.P., Reynolds E.O.R., et al. Accuracy of imaging of the brains of newborn infants by linear-array real-time ultrasound. *Early Hum. Dev.* 6:31–46, 1982a.

Thorburn R.J., Lipscomb A.P., Stewart A.L., et al. Timing and antecedents of haemorrhage into the germinal layer and ventricles, and of cerebral atrophy in very preterm infants. *Early Hum. Dev.* 7:221–238, 1982b.

Towbin A. Cerebral intraventricular hemorrhage and subependymal matrix infarction in the fetus and premature newborn. *Am. J. Pathol.* 52:121–140, 1968.

Trounce J.Q., Fagan D., Levene M.I. Intraventricular haemorrhage and periventricular leucomalacia: ultrasound and autopsy correlation. *Arch. Dis. Child.* 61:1203–1207, 1986.

Ventriculomegaly Trial Group. Randomized trial of early tapping in neonatal posthaemorrhagic ventricular dilatation. *Arch. Dis. Child.* 65:3–10, 1990.

Volpe J.J. *Neurology of the Newborn.* 2nd ed. Philadelphia, Saunders, 1987.

Volpe J.J., Herscovitch P., Perlman J.M., et al. Positron emission tomography in the newborn: extensive impairment of regional blood flow with intraventricular hemorrhage and hemorrhagic intracerebral involvement. *Pediatrics* 72:589–601, 1983.

Volpe J.J., Herscovitch P., Perlman J.M., et al. Positron emission tomography in the asphyxiated term newborn: parasagittal impairment of cerebral blood flow. *Ann. Neurol.* 127:287–296, 1985.

Weindling A.M., Rochefort M.J., Calvert S.A., et al. Development of cerebral palsy after ultrasonographic detection of periventricular cysts in the newborn. *Dev. Med. Child Neurol.* 27:800–806, 1985.

Wigglesworth J.S. Current problems in brain pathology in the perinatal period. In Pape K.E., Wigglesworth J.S., eds. *Perinatal*

Brain Lesions. Oxford, Blackwell Scientific Publications, pp. 1–12, 1989.

Wray S., Cope M., Delpy D.T., et al. Characterisation of near infrared absorption spectra of cytochrome aa_3 and haemoglobin for the non-invasive monitoring of cerebral oxygenation. *Biochim. Biophys. Acta* 933:184–192, 1988.

Wyatt J.S., Cope M., Delpy D.T., et al. Quantitation of cerebral oxygenation and haemodyanamics in sick newborn infants by near infrared spectroscopy. *Lancet* 2:1063–1066, 1986.

Wyatt J.S., Edwards A.D., Azzopardi D., et al. Magnetic resonance and near infrared spectroscopy for investigation of perinatal hypoxic-ischaemic brain injury. *Arch. Dis. Child.* 64:953–963, 1989a.

Wyatt J.S., Edwards A.D., Azzopardi D., et al. Cerebral haemodynamics during failure of cerebral oxidative phosphorylation following birth asphyxia. *Pediatr. Res.* 26:510, 1989b.

Wyatt J.S., Cope M., Delpy D.T., et al. Quantitation of cerebral blood volume in human infants by near-infrared spectroscopy. *J. Appl. Physiol.* 68:1086–1091, 1990a.

Wyatt J.S., Cope M., Delpy D.T., et al. Measurement of optical path length for cerebral near-infrared spectroscopy in newborn infants. *Dev. Neurosci.* 12:140–144, 1990b.

Young R.S.K., Hernandez M.J., Yagel S.K. Selective reduction of blood flow to white matter during hypotension in newborn dogs: a possible mechanism of periventricular leukomalacia. *Ann. Neurol.* 12:445–448, 1982.

42

The Effects of Age: Normal Variation and Its Relation to Disease

Marilyn S. Albert
H. Harris Funkenstein

Many neurologic diseases have an increasing prevalence with age, particularly those that alter cognitive function, such as the primary progressive dementias and cerebrovascular disease. To understand these disease processes better, it is important to understand the age-related changes of cognition and neurologic function on which they are superimposed. This chapter presents a review of the cognitive and neurologic changes associated with age. The possible cause of these changes is discussed, as well as their potential impact on the presentation of disease.

DEMOGRAPHY

Although the demographic changes that have recently occurred in Western society are well known, it is useful to review them to gain a perspective on the problems facing the clinician dealing with a geriatric population. The gerontologic literature tells us that until the early 1800s the average life span of human beings was fairly constant, ranging from 30 to 40 years (Fig. 42–1). This began to change in the late 1800s. Death at age 30 was 10 times more likely to occur in 1820 than in 1975. During the 20th century, the average life expectancy of an American has increased by more than 25 years—from 47 years in 1900 to 75 years in 1980 (Kovar, 1977). In 1900, 4% of the population was over 65 (1 in 25). Today 11% are elderly (1 in 10). It is expected that by the beginning of the next century older individuals will account for about 17% of the population (1 in 5). In fact, more than half of the people who have lived

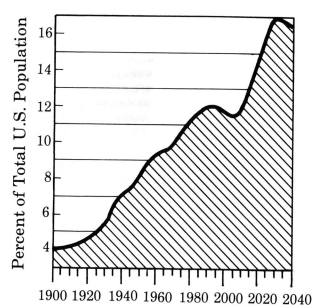

Figure 42–1. Percentage of the U.S. population aged 65 and over from 1900 to 2040. The estimates from 1980 to 2040 were projected by the U.S. Bureau of the Census. (From *Current Population Reports: Projections of the Population of the United States.* Washington, DC, U.S. Government Printing Office, 1975.)

past the age of 65 since the beginning of recorded history are alive today. Therefore, previously unimagined numbers of people are living to old age.

A number of factors are responsible for this demographic change. The first is the improvement in basic public health measures such as sanitation and sewage. Improved nutrition has also contributed to the dramatic reduction in death rate for infants and young adults. The development of antibiotics in the middle of this century further reduced the fatal diseases of the young. Most recently, there has been a rapid and significant fall in the death rate of the elderly, primarily because of a decrease in the incidence and fatality of cardiac and cerebrovascular disorders (Garraway et al., 1979). This decrease in fatality among the elderly is most pronounced among the "oldest old," those over 85, among whom deaths have dropped by more than 2% per year (Rosenwaike et al., 1980).

However, throughout this period of rapid demographic change there has been no alteration in the maximal attainable life span of human beings. The most long-lived individuals still do not exceed approximately 110 years of age (Comfort, 1979). The increase in the elderly population is therefore a reflection of the fact that more people are living to the normal human life span.

INCREASED PREVALENCE OF DISEASE

The extensions in the average life span have brought into sharp relief the fact that aging is also associated with an increased prevalence of disease. Various dementing disorders are strongly associated with age, as are cerebrovascular disorders that produce changes in mental function. Acute confusion, a syndrome of mental status change, is also more prevalent among older than younger individuals.

Dementia

Epidemiologic studies indicate that approximately 15% of the population older than 65 years of age suffer from some form of dementia (Katzman, 1976; Mortimer et al., 1981). On this basis, approximately 3.7 million people in the United States alone are affected. Results of autopsy (Tomlinson et al., 1970) and clinical (Mortimer, 1983) studies suggest that Alzheimer's disease, alone or in combination with other conditions, accounts for 50–70% of cases of dementia in the population over the age of 65. This means that, at present, more than 2 million individuals in the United States suffer from Alzheimer's disease.

The precise incidence of Alzheimer's disease has yet to be established. However, the best estimates at present suggest that less than 1 person in 1000 (0.1%) between the ages of 60 and 65 is at risk. The rate increases to 1.0% for individuals over 65 years of age and to more than 2.0% for individuals over 80 years of age (Hagnell et al., 1981, 1983). Thus, the probability of developing Alzheimer's disease increases with age. Figure 42–2 presents data on the prevalence of Alzheimer's disease in a community-dwelling population (Evans et al., 1989). It has been suggested that individuals who survive to their ninth decade

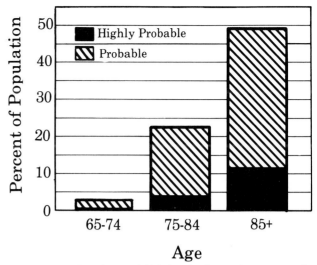

Figure 42–2. Prevalence of Alzheimer's disease in a community-dwelling population. Data were obtained for 3624 individuals, 65 years old and older, of whom 467 had detailed clinical assessments. (From Evans D., Funkenstein H., Albert M., et al. Prevalence of Alzheimer's disease in a community population of older persons. *J.A.M.A.* 262:2551–2556, 1989. Copyright 1989 by the American Medical Association.)

may show a decreased probability of developing the disease (Hagnell et al., 1981), but the numbers of individuals studied in this age range have been extremely limited.

Cerebrovascular Disease

Cerebrovascular disease occurs more commonly with age and may have substantial behavioral consequences. In particular, age is clearly a risk factor for most forms of stroke. With the exception of subarachnoid hemorrhage resulting from aneurysms and arteriovenous malformations, the incidence of most forms of stroke increases toward the end of life. This is most striking over the age of 70. Figure 42–3 illustrates this relationship (U.S. Department of Health, Education and Welfare, 1980). There is an almost eightfold increase in the incidence of stroke from age 60 to 80. Approximately 5% of individuals over age 65 have suffered at least one stroke.

The reasons for this strong relationship between age and stroke incidence are multiple. Hypertension, a major risk factor for stroke, is more prevalent in the older population. Systolic hypertension is particularly common. Data from the Framingham Heart Study indicate that both systolic and diastolic hypertensions are risk factors for stroke. Systolic blood pressure of 195 mm Hg is associated with a fivefold increase in the incidence of thrombotic stroke, whether one considers a population devoid of other risk factors for stroke or considers only those at high risk (Kannel and Wolf, 1983). Cardiac diseases—both coronary artery disease with consequent myocardial infarction and cardiac arrhythmias—are more com-

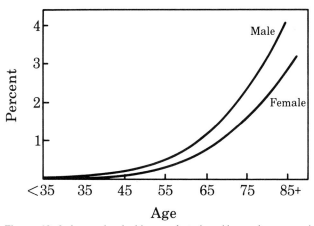

Figure 42–3. Increasing incidence of stroke with age in men and women living in the United States. (From U.S. Department of Health, Education and Welfare. *National Survey of Stroke.* Washington, DC, U.S. Public Health Service, NIH Publication No. 80–2069, 1980.)

mon in the elderly. The incidence of atherosclerosis, a major contributor to both thrombotic and embolic disease, increases with age, although the degree of vascular involvement may vary considerably depending on the individual constellation of risk factors for atherosclerosis, such as hypertension, hypercholesterolemia, smoking, and genetic predilection to vascular disease. In females, the menopause is accompanied by a fall in estrogen levels, which removes a hormonal factor that may protect women against the early appearance of atherosclerosis. Males are more frequently affected by stroke than females, by a ratio of 3:1 (Kurtzke, 1980).

Acute Confusion

An acute confusional state, also called a delirium, is a cognitive disorder of acute onset, usually of hours or days. Estimates of prevalence vary widely depending on the type of clinical facility from which patients are drawn (e.g., a psychiatric hospital, a geriatric unit, or a general medical ward) and on the cause of hospitalization. For the most common clinical setting, a general medical ward, there is surprising agreement. A British multicenter study found that about 26% of geriatric patients were acutely confused on admission (Hodkinson, 1973), and comparable estimates have been reported by others (Bergmann and Eastham, 1974; Seymour et al., 1980). Several studies have shown that 25–35% of hospitalized geriatric patients who are cognitively intact on admission develop acute confusion (Gillick et al., 1982; Hodkinson, 1973, 1981). Other estimates are higher but they derive from more specialized care settings, such as neurologic units (Bedford, 1959; Chisholm et al., 1982; Robinson, 1956; Warshaw et al., 1982).

There is less agreement concerning the incidence of confusion after surgical procedures. One study

found a 9.7% incidence of postoperative confusion in 258 elderly patients admitted to a general surgical unit (Seymour and Pringle, 1983). In this investigation there was no difference in incidence of acute confusion according to type of surgery (e.g., abdominal versus nonabdominal procedures), urgency of procedure, or preoperative activity level.

The association between confusion and advanced age has been demonstrated in several studies. They were significantly correlated in a retrospective survey of patients admitted to a general hospital (Warshaw et al., 1982). Two prospective studies also found a higher incidence of acute confusion in the elderly. One compared subjects under and over the age of 70 and reported incidences of 3.6 and 30%, respectively (Gillick et al., 1982). Another compared subjects with mean ages of 50 and 74 and found a greater degree of cognitive impairment after surgery in the older subjects, as measured by a neuropsychologic battery (Burrows et al., 1985). Furthermore, it is thought that the signs of acute confusion develop more insidiously, involve more severe behavioral symptoms (for comparable levels of underlying illness), and subside more slowly (Blass and Plum, 1983) in the elderly than in the young.

CHARACTERISTICS OF AGING

Whereas the phenomenon of aging, in the sense in which we have been discussing it, seems obvious, the study of aging is complex. There has even been considerable debate about the definition of aging. Most gerontologists agree that aging is an involuntary and irreversible process that occurs cumulatively with the passage of time and is revealed in different aspects of function. However, one gerontologist emphasized the losses associated with aging by saying that "senescence is a change in the behavior of the organism with age, which leads to a decreased power of survival and adjustment" (Comfort, 1956). Another stressed that both decremental and incremental changes occur over the adult life span and one might "regard the more constructive phenomena and the more degenerative ones as being mutually compensatory" (Bondareff, 1985). In either case, aging is a "process that begins or accelerates at maturity and results in an increasing number and/or range of deviations from the ideal state" (Gilchrest and Rowe, 1982).

Translating these definitions into the study of aging can be operationally difficult. Researchers are not interested in the passage of time per se but in the functions in which there is an accumulation of change over time. Chronologic age is merely an index of that accumulation of change. Investigators have, in fact, constructed a variable called functional age that might be used as a surrogate for chronologic age to predict function. However, a review of the data concerning functional age (Costa and McCrae, 1977) indicates that, to date, no single or multiple measure predicts performance on a physiologic or psychologic test better than chronologic age.

Aging Versus the Diseases of Older Age

The goal of identifying the changes that occur over time has led gerontologists to place great emphasis on distinguishing the effects of aging from the effects of the diseases that are more prevalent with age. This distinction is an important practical and theoretic one. If one evaluates all individuals, regardless of health status, one will obtain data regarding what is average for the population but will confound the effects of age with those of disease. For example, if one were studying cognitive changes with age and included in the population individuals with early Alzheimer's disease, the average scores would be substantially lower than if the subjects with disease were omitted. If one then developed test norms on the basis of these data, the norms would be inadequate to identify individuals with mild degrees of dysfunction because of the inclusion of individuals with disease in the original population. Similarly, if one were attempting to understand the mechanisms of age-related cognitive change by relating measures of cognition to other physiologic measures, important relationships might not be identified if individuals with disease were inappropriately included.

Because diseases in the elderly are superimposed on normal aging changes, any disease process will be understood better if the substrate on which it is based is well understood as well. Normal aging changes influence the presentation of illness, its response to treatment, and its potential complications.

For all of these reasons, gerontologists have begun to distinguish between primary (disease-free) aging and secondary (disease-related) aging. This is a relatively recent development, and most early studies of aging did not screen subjects carefully to discriminate between healthy subjects and those with disease. It is important to take this into account in reading their results. Today, most researchers either exclude subjects who do not meet their health criteria or describe the illnesses of their subjects in some detail. It is then up to the reader to determine whether the results apply to primary or secondary aging. Discrepancies in studies of aging that seem superficially similar can often be attributed to previously overlooked differences in subject selection.

At the same time, it is important to recognize that selecting only healthy subjects for a study may limit its generalizability. Thus, it may be necessary to evaluate optimally healthy individuals for an understanding of normal aging and then gather data for subjects with a range of common diseases to be able to generalize to the average individual. This may not be possible in all situations, but it is a goal worth striving for if we are to understand the aging process.

Variability in Aging

Although it might be supposed that by including only healthy individuals in studies of aging one would restrict the variability of the data, a striking characteristic of age-related change measured in this manner is its variability. In the same individual some functions change and others do not. This is true for both psychologic and physiologic data. An individual whose verbal IQ remains relatively stable into the eighth or ninth decade is likely to show a significant decline in performance IQ. Similarly, an individual whose nerve conduction velocity undergoes little significant change may well have considerable reductions in cardiac output.

Equally striking is the interindividual variability observed as people age. Although the mean value of a particular variable may decline substantially with age, many elderly subjects have scores that fall in the range for individuals 20 or 30 years younger than themselves.

Successful Aging

Because previous research on aging has focused primarily on general trends in the data and many functions (physiologic, behavioral, and cognitive) decline on the average with advancing age, gerontologists have tended to focus on whether declines in function occur and, if so, when. This focus on general trends has largely ignored the many older persons who show little cognitive, physiologic, or functional loss compared with their younger counterparts. More recently, these individuals have been said to represent "unusual" aging (Rowe and Kahn, 1987) because they have escaped the "usual" aging pattern. Such individuals might be considered to have aged "successfully," especially if they demonstrate little or no loss in several domains. This distinction between usual and successful aging has been applied to existing physiologic, sociologic, and cognitive data by Rowe and Kahn (1987), who pointed out that successful aging is likely to have at least two important dimensions. The first dimension pertains to a high level of basal function, that is, performance measured under relatively stable conditions. Examples are blood pressure measured when a person is sitting and the ability to remember a list of words when a subject is relaxed and unthreatened. The second dimension is related to response to perturbations in function, that is, performance measured after some type of stress or disturbance—for example, the time it takes blood pressure to return to normal after vigorous exercise or the ability to learn a list of words as quickly as possible while simultaneously trying to identify a repeating letter. An important question for gerontologists is what variables predict such successful aging.

It is unlikely that successful aging is merely the absence of physical illness, because even among such healthy individuals there is considerable variability in cognitive, physiologic, and functional status. One can therefore only hypothesize about what factors might contribute to the maintenance of high function with age. Are there hormonal responses to stress that predict who will recover from illness and regain functional independence? Are there psychosocial variables, such as a sense of self-efficacy, that predict who will recover from the death of a spouse? Are there intellectual abilities that predict who will be active and productive during retirement and who will not?

The study of successful aging is not merely the obverse of looking for age-related declines. The question is not just what is maintained with age and why, but also what factors enable some individuals to maintain high function when the average individual is showing declines. If it is found that the factors that contribute to successful aging are under external control, gerontologists may be able to help more people age successfully in future generations.

The present data base is, however, limited primarily to studies of general age-related trends. What follows, therefore, is a review of the cognitive and neurologic changes that are associated with increasing age.

AGE-RELATED COGNITIVE DIFFERENCES

Attention

The concept of attention is thought to encompass at least three interrelated aspects: sustained attention (vigilance), selective attention (the ability to extract relevant from irrelevant information), and attentional capacity (the total attentional resources available to an individual) (for reviews see Hasher and Zacks, 1979, and Parasuraman and Davies, 1984).

Tests that evaluate sustained attention assess an individual's ability to focus on a simple task and perform it without losing track of the object of the task. Memory demands are minimized in tests of sustained attention by limiting the information that must be remembered to material that falls within a person's immediate memory span (i.e., 7 ± 2). Digit span forward is the most commonly used test of attention and is included on both the Wechsler Adult Intelligence Scale (Wechsler, 1958) and the Wechsler Memory Scale (Wechsler, 1945). Visual and auditory continuous performance tasks that require the individual to identify a repeated letter (e.g., *A*) or a repeated letter sequence (e.g., *I* before *X*) are also commonly used to evaluate sustained attention (Mirsky, 1978).

Numerous studies have demonstrated that performance in tests of sustained attention is extremely good into old age. There is less than 1 SD of change between the ages of 20 and 80.

Selective attention is generally assessed by para-

digms that require the subject to ignore irrelevant information. For example, a subject may be asked to detect a target as the number of nontargets increases. Earlier studies indicated that older individuals have difficulty in performing tasks that require them to ignore irrelevant stimuli (Rabbitt, 1965), but more recent studies have shown that this is not the case (Nebes and Madden, 1983; Nissen and Corkin, 1985; Wright and Elias, 1979). It seems likely that previous results were related to the perceptual difficulties of older individuals in discriminating targets rather than attentional difficulties in ignoring irrelevant information.

Various procedures have been used to assess attentional capacity. These have typically used the dual-task methodology, in which two tasks must be performed simultaneously. The best known dual-task procedure is the dichotic listening paradigm of Broadbent (1958). In this task, two short series of digits, letters, or words are presented simultaneously through earphones, one series to each ear. The subject is asked to report both series. Results of dichotic listening tasks have typically shown large age differences, even among subjects in their early 60s (Braune and Wickens, 1985; Clark and Knowles, 1973; Wickens et al., 1987). However, it has been shown (Wickens et al., 1987) that performance in a dichotic listening paradigm, which was impaired with age, did not correlate with performance in other dual-task paradigms. These results suggest that not all performance in dual-task paradigms is impaired with age. It is important to determine why divided attention, as assessed by the dichotic listening task, is altered with age while other dual-task paradigms continue to be performed well. One possibility is that there are age-related decrements in dual-task paradigms that require the individual to deal with novel or complex material but not in paradigms involving familiar and well-practiced skills.

Language

Linguistic ability is thought to encompass at least four domains: phonologic, lexical, syntactic, and semantic. Until recently, it was assumed that all linguistic abilities are preserved into very old age, primarily because performance on the vocabulary subtest of the Wechsler Adult Intelligence Scale, the best general estimate of verbal intelligence, is well maintained until individuals are in their 80s (N.A. Owens, 1953). However, within the past decade a number of studies have shown that although most aspects of linguistic ability are preserved in the elderly, at least one aspect, semantic knowledge, declines with age.

Phonology refers to the use of the sounds of language and the rules for their combination. Phonologic capabilities are well preserved with age (Bayles and Kaszniak, 1987).

Lexical knowledge refers to both the lexical representation of a word (the name of an item) and its semantic representation (the meaning of a word). The lexicon of healthy older individuals appears to be intact, as are the semantic relationships of the lexicon (Bowles and Poon, 1985; Cerella and Fozard, 1984; Howard et al., 1981).

Syntactic knowledge refers to the ability to meaningfully combine words. A large number of studies have shown that age has little effect on syntax (DeRenzi, 1979; Noll and Randolf, 1978; Obler et al., 1985; Orgass and Poeck, 1966).

The one area of language function that appears to change significantly with age is semantic knowledge. One way of assessing the semantic aspects of word retrieval is by testing naming. In the most commonly used naming tests, the person is shown a picture of a common object and asked to produce the name. Several groups of investigators have reported that scores on naming tests such as these decrease with age (Borod et al., 1980; Goodglass, 1980; LaBarge et al., 1986). However, as shown in Figure 42–4, declines in naming ability do not become statistically significant until subjects are in their 70s (Albert et al., 1988).

Verbal fluency is also a measure of semantic ability. In a verbal fluency task a subject is asked to name as many examples of a category (e.g., animals or vegetables) or as many words beginning with a particular letter (e.g., *F*) as possible in a specified period (e.g., 1 minute). Several studies report a decline in verbal fluency with age (Albert et al., 1988; Obler and Albert, 1981; Spreen and Benton, 1969). These changes also occur relatively late in the life span (>70). Thus, semantic linguistic ability appears to change with advancing age, whereas other aspects of linguistic ability are relatively well preserved.

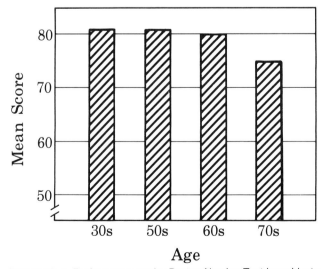

Figure 42–4. Performance on the Boston Naming Test by subjects aged 30–80 y. There is a significant decline in accuracy in subjects in their 70s. (Based on data in Albert M.S., Heller H.S., Milberg W. Changes in naming ability with age. *Psychol. Aging* 3:173–178, 1988.)

Memory

Memory is conceptualized as a series of specific yet interactive stores consisting of sensory memory, primary memory, and secondary memory (Tulving, 1972; Waugh and Norman, 1965). Sensory memory represents the earliest stage of information processing. It involves perceiving and attending to information and is modality specific (i.e., visual, auditory, haptic), highly unstable, and characterized by rapid decay.

A considerable amount of information indicates that changes in sensory memory are minimal with age (Cerella and Poon, 1981; Cerella et al., 1982). For example, the time necessary to identify a single letter does not change with age (Walsh et al., 1978).

Primary memory, once called short-term memory, pertains to the ability to retain a small amount of information over a brief period. Information must be actively rehearsed to be retained in primary memory. Numerous studies indicate that there are few, if any, losses of primary memory with age. For example, most studies have found no significant age differences in digit span forward (Drachman and Leavitt, 1972; Kriauciunas, 1968), no age differences in word span (Talland, 1965), and moderate differences in letter span (Botwinick and Storandt, 1974).

Secondary, or long-term, memory is viewed as a memory store that can contain an unlimited amount of information for an indefinite period of time (hours, days, years). In contrast to the minimal changes with age in sensory and primary memory, there are substantial changes in secondary memory. The degree of loss is related to the type of material to be remembered and the method of assessment. Large age differences are found in free recall (Erber, 1974; Gilbert and Levee, 1971; Schonfield and Robertson, 1966). When given a large amount of new information to retain over a relatively long period, individuals show declines in memory at a relatively early age. Figure 42–5 shows the performance of a group of optimally healthy subjects in delayed recall of two paragraphs from the Wechsler Memory Scale. Declines in memory are evident on this task by age 50 (Albert and Moss, 1988). Age decrements are, however, greater when subjects are asked to recall information than when they are asked to recognize which of several stimuli they were previously exposed to. This is true whether words, line drawings, or pictures are used (Harwood and Naylor, 1969).

Age-related changes in memory also appear to be related to initial intellectual ability, as well as socioeconomic status and personality characteristics. For example, Craik et al. (1987) and Arbuckle et al. (1986) found that the age at which declines in memory become significant is related to the amount of education and/or verbal intelligence of the subjects, with the better-educated subjects showing the least amount of change. Arbuckle et al. (1986) also found that personality characteristics, such as introversion, were related to performance on memory tests.

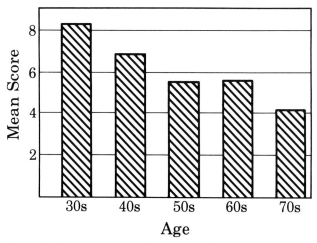

Figure 42–5. Delayed recall of the Logical Memory passages from the Wechsler Memory Scale by subjects 30–80 years old. There is a significant decline by age 50. (Based on data in Albert et al., Nonlinear changes in cognition with age and their neurophysiological correlates. *Can. J. Psychol.* 41:141–157, 1987.)

Visuospatial Ability

Visuospatial ability, the ability to perceive and function in the spatial domain, is generally assessed by both the production and recognition of figures. Performance of complex visual tasks, such as identifying incomplete figures (Danziger and Salthouse, 1978), recognizing embedded figures (Axelrod and Cohen, 1961), and arranging blocks into a design (Doppelt and Wallace, 1955; Klodin, 1975), declines in the elderly. Perhaps more important, the perception and production of relatively simple three-dimensional drawings are altered with age. For example, Plude et al. (1986) asked groups of young and old adults (mean ages 21 and 67) who were equated for static visual acuity to draw a cube to command. The drawings of the young adults were rated as significantly better than those of the old adults. In addition, the older subjects were less accurate in judging the adequacy of drawings of cubes that were distorted to varying degrees and in discriminating between distorted and undistorted cubes. Thus, the ability to perceive and to reproduce figures in three dimensions is altered with age.

Conceptualization

Conceptualization refers to the ability to form concepts, switch from one concept or category to another, generalize from a single instance, and apply rules or principles. Tests of conceptualization generally assess abstraction capacities and/or mental flexibility.

Many tests have been developed to examine conceptualization, including tests of proverb interpretation, reasoning, sorting, and set shifting. Some of these tasks make substantive memory demands and therefore show significant changes with age. How-

ever, conceptualization tasks that do not make substantive memory demands also demonstrate age differences. For example, series completion tasks that require the subject to examine a series of letters or numbers and determine the rule that governs the sequencing of the items show significant age-related change (Cornelius, 1984; Hooper et al., 1984; Lachman and Jelalian, 1984; Schaie, 1983). Investigators have developed specially constructed series completions problems to determine whether declines were related to the ability to appreciate abstract concepts or the ability to detect cyclic periodicity. They concluded that age-related alterations on series completion tasks were the result of progressive problems in abstraction and flexibility rather than inability to detect cyclic periodicity. Consistent with these findings are the results of proverb interpretation tasks, which also show substantial age-related change (Albert et al., 1990; Bromley, 1957). The greatest age differences appear among subjects in their 70s (Fig. 42–6).

General Intelligence

Although intelligence tests examine many of the abilities previously discussed, they do so in a complex way. Intelligence tests were designed to predict with a reasonable degree of certainty how a person would function in an academic environment; they were not designed to provide a complete assessment of cognitive function. Thus, intelligence tests do not assess all aspects of cognitive ability. For example, the Wechsler Adult Intelligence Scale does not include an evaluation of memory. In addition, IQ tests do not assess cognitive abilities in relative isolation from one another. Many of the tests require a com-

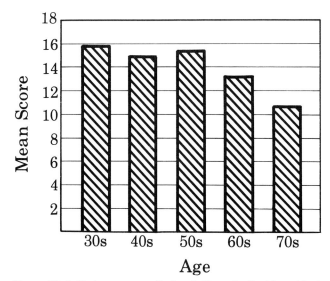

Figure 42–6. Performance on Gorham's Proverbs Test by subjects 30–80 years old. There is a significant decline in subjects in their 70s. (Based on data in Albert M., Wolfe J., Lafleche G. Differences in abstraction ability with age. *Psychol. Aging* 5:94–102, 1990.)

plex interaction of cognitive abilities and often depend on speed for an adequate level of performance. Nevertheless, intelligence testing has been one of the most widely explored topics in the field of the psychology of aging.

There is widespread agreement that there are changes in intelligence test performance with age. There has, however, been considerable debate about the point at which declines occur and the magnitude of the declines. The age at which decrements are observed appears to be determined by the methodology employed. There is some consensus that relatively little decline in performance occurs until people are about 50 (W.A. Owens, 1966; Schaie and Labouvie-Vief, 1974). After this age, results differ depending on whether cross-sectional or longitudinal methods were employed. The cross-sectional method shows declines of 1 SD or more beginning about age 60 (Doppelt and Wallace, 1955; Eisdorfer and Wilkie, 1973; Green, 1969; Schaie, 1958). Over the age of 70, scores drop sharply (Doppelt and Wallace, 1955). The longitudinal method shows declines beginning in the late 60s (Schaie and Parham, 1977). Both methodologies find substantial declines after individuals are in their mid-70s. Thus the major difference between the results of cross-sectional and longitudinal investigations is observed between subjects in their early 50s to late 60s. In this age range, the cross-sectional method shows greater age declines than the longitudinal method. Figure 42–7 shows the results of a cohort-sequential study of intelligence by Schaie (1983).

Summary: Age-Related Cognitive Differences

Several aspects of cognitive ability are altered with age. Cross-sectional studies indicate that the earliest

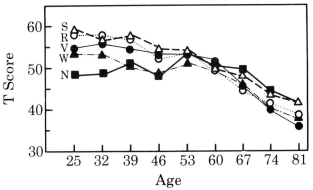

Figure 42–7. Factor score changes with age on the Primary Mental Abilities Test derived from a sequential design methodology. The within-subjects analysis showed significant age decrement on all subtests after approximately age 60. Factors in the Primary Mental Abilities Test: S = space; R = reasoning; V = verbal; W = word; N = number. (From Schaie K.W. The Seattle longitudinal study: a 21-year exploration of psychometric intelligence in adulthood. In Schaie K.W., ed. *Longitudinal Studies of Adult Psychological Development.* New York, Guilford Press, 1983. Copyright 1983 by the Guilford Press.)

change that occurs is in secondary memory function, the ability to retain relatively large amounts of information over long periods. In this respect, subjects in their mid-50s are significantly different from younger individuals. Proficiency at constructional tasks, divided-attention capabilities, and performance aspects of general intelligence are altered in the mid-60s. Abstraction and naming ability are significantly different when subjects are in their 70s. Results of longitudinal findings, where they exist, are comparable, although, as is generally the case with longitudinal studies, they show declines slightly later in the life span.

AGE-RELATED NEUROLOGIC DIFFERENCES

Most studies of change in neurologic function with age have evaluated older persons with no obvious neurologic abnormalities. However, some neurologic diseases that are increasingly common with age, such as Alzheimer's disease, produce subtle neurologic changes that can be confused with age-related change (Funkenstein et al., 1986).

We participated in a population study in East Boston, Massachusetts (Cornoni-Huntley et al., 1986) in which 467 individuals were systematically selected from a population of 3811 persons, aged 65 and older, and given a complete physical, neurologic, psychiatric, and neuropsychologic evaluation. Persons with cognitive impairments were identified; the prevalence of Alzheimer's disease and other dementing disorders in this population has been reported (Evans et al., 1989). One of the strengths of this study for the assessment of age-related neurologic change is that persons who were without evidence of neurologic, psychiatric, and neuropsychologic impairment could be identified. Because some dementing disorders common in the elderly do not produce striking medical or neurologic abnormalities early in their course, inclusion of a neuropsychologic evaluation is essential for establishing the normality of the population. To our knowledge, no other study of neurologic change with age has this characteristic. For the purposes of this chapter, the individuals with no evidence of cognitive impairment were identified. Neurologic differences across age strata (i.e., 65–69, 70–74, 75–79, 80–84, and 85+) were then examined by analysis of variance.

Oculomotor Function

The assessment of oculomotor function in the neurologic examination encompassed evaluations of eyelid elevation, pupillary constriction, and eye movements. These related functions depend on the integrity of cranial nerves III, IV, and VI (the oculomotor, trochlear, and abducens nerves).

Numerous investigators have reported that as people age there are decreases in pupillary size (Birren et al., 1950; Kumnick, 1954) and in the responsiveness of the pupil to light (Critchley, 1931; Howell, 1975; Kokmen et al., 1977). There is also evidence of diminished upward gaze with age (Critchley, 1956; Kokmen et al., 1977). Chamberlain (1971) reported an average decline in upward gaze from 37 to 16° between the ages of 15 and 75. Visual tracking is also altered, as reflected by an increase in the frequency of saccades (Jenkyn et al., 1985; Kokmen et al., 1977; Kuechenmeister et al., 1977; Sharpe and Sylvester, 1978; Spooner et al., 1985). Both pupillary size and pupillary reaction to light were decreased with age in the East Boston sample of older persons ($F(4, 146) = 4.31$, $P < .003$; $F(4, 146) = 7.23$, $P < .0001$) (Fig. 42–8).

Reflexes

Testing of deep tendon reflexes includes assessment of the biceps, triceps, knee, and ankle reflexes. Of the deep tendon reflexes, the ankle jerk has been most consistently reported to be lost with increasing age (Bhatia and Irvine, 1973; Carter, 1979; Critchley, 1956; Howell, 1975; Klawans et al., 1971; Skre, 1972). Most clinical studies indicate that 30–45% of elderly persons have lost their ankle reflex. Other deep tendon reflexes (e.g., knee and biceps) are less consistently abnormal with age. Ankle reflexes were not assessed in the East Boston study. No reflexes in the arms or the legs (other than the ankle reflex) were significantly different with age.

A set of reflexes collectively known as release signs includes the grasp reflex, the snout reflex, the suck reflex, the palmomental reflex, and the glabellar reflex. The palmomental, snout, and glabellar re-

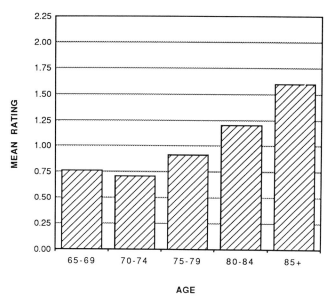

Figure 42–9. Snout reflex in subjects aged 65–85+. There is a significant increase in the prevalence of a snout reflex in subjects 75 years of age and older.

flexes have been reported to be increasingly present with age. The snout reflex is evident in 12–33% of elderly subjects (Jacobs and Gossman, 1980; Jenkyn et al., 1985; Klawans et al., 1971; Kokmen et al., 1977). The palmomental reflex reportedly appears in 10–37% of elderly subjects (Jacobs and Gossman, 1980; Kokmen et al., 1977) and the glabellar reflex in 6–29% (Jenkyn et al., 1985). In the East Boston study, the glabellar reflex was not evaluated. Of the four that were assessed (palmomental, snout, grasp, and suck), only the snout reflex was found to be increasingly prevalent with age ($F(4, 146) = 3.67$, $P < .007$) (Fig. 42–9).

Motor Function

An assessment of motor function includes an evaluation of muscle strength and tone. Several studies have found a 20% decline in strength in normal elderly persons (Potvin et al., 1980a,b; Welford, 1980). This decrease in muscle power is often accompanied by a loss of muscle bulk. There are, in particular, a number of reports of atrophy of the intrinsic muscle of the hand (Carter, 1979; Prakash and Stern, 1973). Increasing tone with age has also been reported (Jenkyn et al., 1985), although less consistently. In the East Boston study, increasing tone with age (marked by rigidity) was found in the legs ($F(4, 133) = 4.52$, $P < .002$) but not in the arms.

Sensory Functions

The sensory functions commonly evaluated during the neurologic examination are vibration sense, position sense, pain, and touch. Declines in vibratory

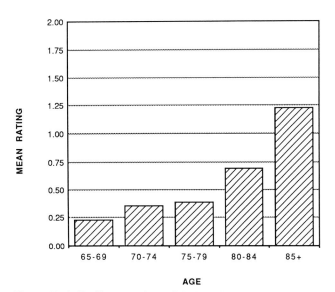

Figure 42–8. Pupillary reaction to light by subjects aged 65–85+. There is a significant decline in reactivity by subjects 80 years of age and older.

sense with age have been consistently reported, and inability to perceive a vibratory stimulus increases with age (Critchley, 1931; Howell, 1975; Kokmen et al., 1977). Where vibration thresholds have been quantitatively evaluated, a 2- to 10-fold increase has been reported (Perret and Regli; 1970; Potvin et al., 1980a,b). There is at least one report that the loss of vibration sense is greater in the upper than the lower extremities (Klawans et al., 1971). In the East Boston study, vibration sense was evaluated only in the toes and was found to be increasingly abnormal with increasing age (F(4, 146) = 7.26, $P < .0001$) (Fig. 42–10).

Abnormalities in joint position sense (Howell, 1975; Klawans et al., 1971) and light touch (Howell, 1975; Klawans et al., 1971; Potvin et al., 1980a,b) have not been consistently noted. They were not found to be increasingly abnormal with age in the East Boston study. Abnormalities in the sensation of light touch with age have also been inconsistently found (Howell, 1975; Kokmen et al., 1977; Potvin et al., 1980a,b).

Gait

An assessment of gait includes evaluations of posture, balance, arm swing, and step length. Gait is widely reported to change with age (Azar et al., 1964; Finley et al., 1969; Murray et al., 1969; Teravainen and Calne, 1984; Wolfson and Katzman, 1983). There is an alteration of posture (Murray et al., 1969), with older persons appearing more stooped. Diminished arm swing and shorter step length have also been reported (Murray et al., 1969). Difficulty in balance has also been noted (Potvin et al., 1980a,b). In the East Boston study, postural alterations were not

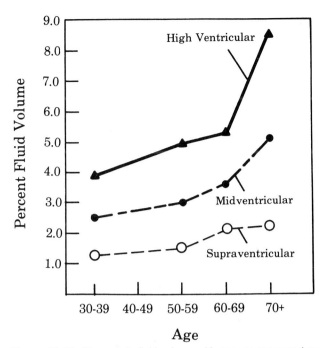

Figure 42–11. Changes in fluid volume with age, as measured on three computed tomographic slices. Computer programs were used to measure fluid volume. On ventricular slices, fluid volume measures primarily reflect ventricular size. (From Stafford J.L., Albert M.S., Naeser M.A., et al. Age-related differences in computed tomographic scan measurements. *Arch. Neurol.* 45:409–419, 1988. Copyright 1988 by the American Medical Association.)

evaluated, nor was balance. Of the aspects of gait that were evaluated (step length, arm swing, and timing), the only one found to be significantly altered with age was arm swing (F(4, 146) = 3.84, $P < .005$).

AGE-RELATED DIFFERENCES IN BRAIN STRUCTURE AND FUNCTION

There is evidence that at least some of the differences in cognitive and neurologic function observed as people age are related to structural and functional changes in the brain, even in optimally healthy individuals.

Computed tomographic studies indicate that the lateral ventricles increase in size with age, particularly after the age of 60 (Stafford et al., 1988; Zatz et al., 1982). Sulcal atrophy also increases with age, but this appears to occur more slowly than ventricular change (Stafford et al., 1988; Zatz et al., 1982) (Fig. 43–11). Electroencephalographic studies also show significant age-related change, primarily increased fast activity, in optimally healthy individuals (Duffy et al., 1984; Giaquinto and Nolfe, 1986). However, alpha activity remains little changed (i.e., 9.5 Hz), aside from diminished reactivity (Duffy et al., 1984; Giaquinto and Nolfe, 1986; Katz and Horowitz, 1982). Positron emission tomography has yielded conflicting results, with some studies showing declines of

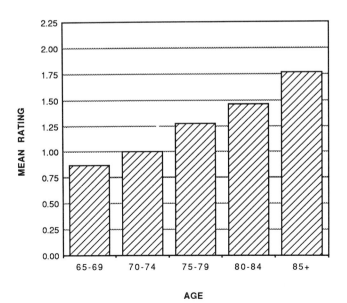

Figure 42–10. Vibration sense in the toes in subjects aged 65–85+. There is a significant decline in vibration sense in subjects 75 years of age and older.

about 20% (Kuhl et al., 1984), particularly in the inferior frontal lobe, and others showing no declines in either global or regional glucose metabolism (deLeon, 1983, 1984; Duara et al., 1983). With future technologic changes that make it possible to adjust for cerebral atrophy, this issue should be resolved.

A statistical analysis using linear structural relations modeling (LISREL) suggests that the cognitive differences among optimally healthy persons of different ages are causally related to measures of brain structure and function in these individuals. Using computed tomographic measures of brain structure, computerized electroencephalographic measures of brain function, and cognitive test scores, Jones et al. (1991) produced a LISREL model indicating that changes in brain structure and function significantly influence cognitive performance. The computed tomographic measures were associated with verbal and nonverbal memory and attention; the electroencephalographic measures were associated with verbal and nonverbal memory and speed. Some physiologic and psychosocial parameters also appeared to be related to cognitive performance, but the nature of these relationships has not yet been explored.

There are several specific hypotheses concerning the cause of the neurologic differences observed between younger and older persons. Many of the changes observed (increased rigidity, gait abnormalities, and the prevalence of release signs) have been attributed to alterations in the basal ganglia with age, which are well documented. There is a 50% loss of dopamine by age 60 (Hornykiewicz, 1988). Most of this decline with age has been attributed to loss of neurons in the substantia nigra, which decrease by 6% per decade (McGeer et al., 1977). Studies of dopamine D_1 and D_2 receptors indicate that there is a progressive decrease in the concentration of dopamine uptake sites with age (DeKeyser et al., 1990). Whether the concentration of the receptors themselves remains unchanged is controversial.

Alterations in the frontal lobes have also been cited as the cause of some of the neurologic changes with age (i.e., release signs and gait disturbances). Neuropathologic studies suggest that the atrophy seen with age is most marked in the frontal and temporal lobes (Kemper, 1984).

It has also been hypothesized that changes in the frontal lobe and basal ganglia are related to some of the alterations observed in cognitive function with age, in particular in abstraction, set shifting, and divided attention (Albert et al., 1990). Studies indicate that frontal lobe dysfunction leads to impairments of abstraction in general and of set shifting and set maintenance in particular (Cicerone and Lazar, 1983; Stuss and Benson, 1987).

Abnormalities in cognitive flexibility have also been attributed to loss of cells in the substantia nigra and decreases in dopamine levels, because patients with Parkinson's disease are particularly deficient in this cognitive domain (Taylor et al., 1987).

There are age-related changes in the prevalence of neurofibrillary tangles and neuritic plaques as well as decreases in choline acetyltransferase levels that are quantitatively greater than those seen in Alzheimer's disease (see Chapter 59). These changes have been cited as the likely cause of declines in naming and memory ability with age (Albert and Moss, 1988; Drachman and Leavitt, 1972). However, a more recent study suggests that the distribution of these changes is different in Alzheimer's disease, with greater concentrations in the temporal lobe in Alzheimer's disease and greater concentrations in frontal and anterior parietal regions in normal aging (Heilbroner and Kemper, 1990).

CONCLUSION

The cognitive and neurologic differences between younger and older persons have clear implications for the diagnosis of disease in older persons. Any abnormality found must be judged in terms of what is normal for age. Only changes beyond those associated with normal aging can be cited as a sign of disease. For example, whereas the presence of release signs would be considered a sign of disease in a young person, in the elderly they do not reliably differentiate normal individuals from patients with mild to moderate Alzheimer's disease (Galasko et al., 1990; Huff et al., 1987). Similarly, declines in abstraction do not consistently differentiate patients with mild Alzheimer's disease from controls (Albert et al., 1990). Further knowledge of age-related cognitive and neurologic changes should improve the diagnosis of disease in the elderly.

References

(Key references are designated with an asterisk.)
*Albert M., Moss M., eds. *Geriatric Neuropsychology*. New York, Guilford Press, 1988.
Albert M., Wolfe J., Lafleche G. Differences in abstraction ability with age. *Psychol. Aging* 5:94–102, 1990.
Albert M.S., Heller H.S., Milberg W. Changes in naming ability with age. *Psychol. Aging* 3:173–178, 1988.
Arbuckle T.Y., Gold D., Andres D. Cognitive function of older people in relation to social and personality variables. *Psychol. Aging* 1:55–62, 1986.
Axelrod S., Cohen L.D. Senescence and embedded-figure performance in vision and touch. *Percept. Mot. Skills* 12:283–288, 1961.
Bayles K.A., Kaszniak A.W. *Communication and Cognition in Normal Aging and Dementia*. Boston, Little, Brown, 1987.
Bedford P.D. General medical aspects of confusional states in elderly people. *Br. Med. J.* 2:185–188, 1959.
Bergmann K., Eastham E.J. Psychogeriatric ascertainment and assessment for treatment in an acute medical ward setting. *Age Ageing* 3:174–188, 1974.
Bhatia S.P., Irvine R.E. Electrical recording of the ankle jerk in old age. *Gerontol. Clin.* 15:357–360, 1973.
Birren J.E., Casperson R.C., Botwinick J. Age changes in pupil size. *J. Gerontol.* 5:216–221, 1950.
Blass J.P., Plum F. Metabolic encephalopathies in older adults. In Katzman R.J., Terry R.T., eds. *Neurology of Aging*. Philadelphia, Davis, pp. 189–220, 1983.
Bondareff W. The neural basis of aging. In Birren J.E., Schaie K.W., eds. *Handbook of the Psychology of Aging*. New York, Von Nostrand Reinhold, pp. 95–112, 1985.

Borod J., Goodglass H., Kaplan E. Normative data on the Boston Diagnostic Aphasia Examination, parietal lobe battery, and Boston Naming Test. *J. Clin. Neuropsychol.* 2:209–215, 1980.

Botwinick J., Storandt M. *Memory-Related Functions and Age.* Springfield, IL, Thomas, 1974.

Bowles N.L., Poon L.W. Aging and retrieval of words in semantic memory. *J. Gerontol.* 40:71–77, 1985.

Braune R., Wickens C.D. The functional age profile: an objective decision criterion for the assessment of pilot performance capacities and capabilities. *Hum. Factors* 27:549–554, 1985.

Broadbent D.E. *Perception and Communication.* New York, Pergamon, 1958.

Bromley D. Effects of age on intellectual output. *J. Gerontol.* 12:318–323, 1957.

Burrows J., Briggs R.S., Elkington A.R. Cataract extraction and confusion in elderly patients. *Clin. Exp. Gerontol.* 7:51–74, 1985.

Carter A.B. The neurologic aspects of aging. In Rossman I., ed. *Clinical Geriatrics.* Philadelphia, Lippincott, p. 292, 1979.

Cerella J., Fozard J.L. Lexical access and age. *Dev. Psychol.* 20:235–243, 1984.

Cerella J., Poon L.W. Age and parafoveal sensitivity (abstract). *Gerontologist* 76, 1981.

Cerella J., Poon L.W., Fozard J.L. Age and iconic read-out. *J. Gerontol.* 37:197–202, 1982.

Chamberlain W. Restriction in upward gaze with advancing age. *Trans. Am. Ophthalmol. Soc.* 68:234–244, 1970.

Chisholm S.E., Deniston O.L., Igrisan R.M., et al. Prevalance of confusion in elderly hospitalized patients. *Gerontol. Nurs.* 8:87–96, 1982.

Cicerone K.A., Lazar R.M. Effects of frontal lobe lesions on hypothesis sampling during concept formation. *Neuropsychologia* 21:513–524, 1983.

Clark L., Knowles J. Age differences in dichotic listening performance. *J. Gerontol.* 28:173–178, 1973.

Comfort A. *The Biology of Senescence.* London, Routledge & Kegan Paul, 1956.

Comfort A. *The Biology of Senescence.* New York, Elsevier, 1979.

Cornelius S.W. Classic pattern of intellectual aging: test familiarity, difficulty and performance. *J. Gerontol.* 39:201–206, 1984.

Cornoni-Huntley J., Ostfeld A., Taylor J., et al. *Established Populations for Epidemiologic Studies of the Elderly.* Washington, DC, U.S. Public Health Service, NIH Publication No. 86-2443, 1986.

Costa P.T., McCrae R.R. Functional age: a conceptual and empirical critique. In Haynes S.G., Feinleib M., eds. *Second Conference on the Epidemiology of Aging.* Washington, DC, U.S. Public Health Service, National Institutes of Health, p. 230, 1977.

Craik F.I.M., Byrd M., Swanson J.M. Patterns of memory loss in three elderly samples. *Psychol. Aging* 2:79–86, 1987.

Critchley M. The neurology of old age. *Lancet* 2:1119–1127, 1222–1230, 1931.

Danziger W.L., Salthouse T.A. Age and the perception of incomplete figures. *Exp. Aging Res.* 4:67–80, 1978.

DeKeyser J., Ebinger, G., Vauguelin G. Age-related changes in the human nigrostriatal dopaminergic system. *Ann. Neurol.* 27:157–161, 1990.

de Leon M.J., Ferris S.H., George A.E., et al. Positron emission tomography studies of aging and Alzheimer's disease. *Am. J. Neuroradiol.* 4:568–571, 1983.

de Leon M.J., Goege A.E., Ferris S.H., et al. Positron emission tomography and computed tomography. Assessments of the aging human brain. *J. Comput. Assist. Tomogr.* 8:88–94, 1984.

DeRenzi E. A shortened version of the Token Test. In Boller F., Dennis M., eds. *Auditory Comprehension: Clinical and Experimental Studies with the Token Test.* New York, Academic Press, pp. 33–44, 1979.

Doppelt J.E., Wallace W.L. Standardization of the Wechsler Adult Intelligence Scale for older persons. *J. Abnorm. Soc. Psychol.* 51:312–330, 1955.

Drachman D.A., Leavitt J. Memory impairment in the aged: storage versus retrieval deficit. *J. Exp. Psychol.* 93:302–308, 1972.

Duara R., Margolin R.A., Robertson-Tchabo E.A., et al. Cerebral glucose utilization as measured with positron emission tomography in 21 healthy men between the ages of 21 and 83 years. *Brain* 106:761–775, 1983.

Duffy F.H., Albert M.S., McAnulty G., et al. Age-related differences in brain electrical activity of healthy subjects. *Ann. Neurol.* 16:430–438, 1984.

Eisdorfer C., Wilkie F. Intellectual changes with advancing age. In Jarvik L.F., Eisdorfer C., Blum J.E., eds. *Intellectual Functioning in Adults.* New York, Springer-Verlag, pp. 21–29, 1973.

Ellenberg M. The deep reflexes in old age. *J.A.M.A.* 174:468–469, 1960.

Erber J.T. Age differences in recognition memory. *J. Gerontol.* 29:177–181, 1974.

Evans D., Funkenstein H., Albert M., et al. Prevalence of Alzheimer's disease in a community population of older persons. *J.A.M.A.* 262:2551–2556, 1989.

Finley F.R., Cody K.A., Finizie R.V. Locomotion patterns in elderly women. *Arch. Phys. Med. Rehabil.* 50:140–146, 1969.

Funkenstein H., Albert M., Cook N., et al. Relationship of neurological examination findings to diagnosis of SDAT in a defined community population (abstract). *Neurology* 36:267, 1986.

Galasko D., Kwo-on-Yuen P., Klauber M., et al. Neurological findings in Alzheimer's disease and normal aging. *Arch. Neurol.* 47:625–627, 1990.

Garraway W.M., Whisnant J.P., Furlan A.J., et al. The declining incidence of stroke. *N. Engl. J. Med.* 300:449–452, 1979.

Giaquinto S., Nolfe G. The EEG in the normal elderly: a contribution to the interpretation of aging and dementia. *Electroencephalogr. Clin. Neurophysiol.* 63:540–546, 1986.

Gilbert J.G., Levee R.F. Patterns of declining memory. *J. Gerontol.* 26:70–75, 1971.

Gilchrest B., Rowe J.W. The biology of aging. In Rowe J.W., Besdine R.W., eds. *Health and Disease in Old Age.* Boston, Little, Brown, pp. 15–24, 1982.

Gillick M.R., Serrell N.A., Gillick L.S. Adverse consequences of hospitalization in the elderly. *Soc. Sci. Med.* 16:1033–1038, 1982.

Goodglass H. Naming disorders in aphasia and aging. In Obler L.K., Albert M.L., eds. *Language and Communication in the Elderly: Clinical, Therapeutic and Experimental Issues.* Lexington, MA, Lexington Books, pp. 37–45, 1980.

Green R.F. Age-intelligence relationship between ages sixteen and sixty-four: a rising trend. *Dev. Psychol.* 1:618–627, 1969.

Hagnell O., Lanke J., Rorsman B., et al. Does the incidence of age psychosis decrease? A prospective, longitudinal study of a complete population investigated during the 25 year period 1947–1972: the Lundby study. *Neuropsychobiology* 7:201–211, 1981.

Hagnell O., Lanke J., Rorsman B., et al. Current trends in the incidence of senile and multi-infarct dementia. A prospective study of a total population followed over 25 years: the Lundby study. *Arch. Psychiatr. Nervenkr.* 233:423–438, 1983.

Harwood E., Naylor G.F.K. Recall and recognition in elderly and young subjects. *Aust. J. Psychol.* 21:251–257, 1969.

Hasher L., Zacks R.T. Automatic and effortful processes in memory. *J. Exp. Psychol.* 108:356–388, 1979.

Heilbroner P.L., Kemper T. Cytoarchitectonic distribution of senile plaques in three aged monkeys. *Acta Neuropathol.* 81:60–65, 1990.

Hodkinson H.M. Mental impairment in the elderly. *J. R. Coll. Physicians Lond.* 7:305–307, 1973.

Hodkinson H.M. Mental impairment in the elderly. *J. R. Coll. Physicians Lond.* 15:151–167, 1981.

Hooper F.H., Hooper J.O., Colbert K.C. *Personality and Memory Correlates of Intellectual Functioning: Young Adulthood to Old Age.* Basel, Karger, 1984.

Hornykiewicz O. Neurochemical pathology and the etiology of Parkinson's disease. *Mt. Sinai J. Med.* 55:11–20, 1988.

Howard D.V., McAndrews M.P., Lasaga M.I. Semantic priming of lexical designs in young and old adults. *J. Gerontol.* 36:707–714, 1981.

Howell T.H. Neurological problems of the elderly. In *Old Age.* London, Lewis, pp. 33–47, 1975.

Huff F.J., Boller F., Luchelli F., et al. The neurologic examination in patients with probable Alzheimer's disease. *Arch. Neurol.* 44:929–932, 1987.

Jacobs L., Gossman M.D. Three primitive reflexes in normal adults. *Neurology (N.Y.)* 30:184–188, 1980.

Jenkyn L.R., Reeves A.G., Warren T., et al. Neurologic signs in senescence. *Arch. Neurol.* 42:1154–1157, 1985.

Jones K.J., Albert M.S., Duffy F.H., et al. Modeling age using cognitive psychosocial, and physiological variables. *Exp. Aging Res.* (in press).

Kannel W.B., Wolf P.A. Epidemiology of cerebrovascular disease. In Ross Russell R.W., ed. *Vascular Disease of the Central Nervous System.* 2nd ed. Edinburgh, Churchill Livingstone, pp. 1–24, 1983.

Katz R., Horowitz G.R. Electroencephalogram in the septuagenarian: studies in a normal geriatric population. *J. Am. Geriat. Soc.* 3:273–275, 1982.

Katzman R. The prevalence and malignancy of Alzheimer disease. *Arch. Neurol.* 33:217–218, 1976.

Kemper T. Neuroanatomical and neuropathological changes in normal aging and in dementia. In Albert M.L., ed. *Clinical Neurology of Aging.* New York, Oxford University Press, pp. 9–52, 1984.

Klawans H.L., Tufo H.M., Ostfeld A.M., et al. Neurologic examination in an elderly population. *Dis. Nerv. Syst.* 32:274–279, 1971.

Klodin V.M. *Verbal Facilitation of Perceptual-Integrative Performance in Relation to Age.* Ph.D. thesis. Washington University, St. Louis, 1975.

Kokmen E., Bossemeyer R.W., Barney J., et al. Neurological manifestations of aging. *J. Gerontol.* 32:411–419, 1977.

Kovar M.G. *Elderly People: The Population 65 Years and Over.* Washington, DC, Department of Health, Education and Welfare, DHEW Publication No. (HRA) 77-1232, 1977.

Kriauciunas R. The relationship of age and retention interval activity in short term memory. *J. Gerontol.* 23:169–173, 1968.

Kuechenmeister C.A., Linton P.H., Mueller T.V., et al. Eye tracking in relation to age sex and illness. *Arch. Gen. Psychiatry* 34:578–579, 1977.

Kuhl D.E., Metter E.J., Riege W.H., et al. The effect of normal aging on patterns of local cerebral utilization. *Ann. Neurol.* 15(Suppl):133–137, 1984.

Kumnick L.S. Pupillary psychosensory restitution and aging. *J. Opt. Soc. Am.* 44:735–741, 1954.

Kurtzke J.F. Epidemiology of cerebrovascular disease. In Siekert R.G., ed. *Cerebrovascular Survey Report.* Bethesda, National Institute of Neurology and Communicative Disorders and Stroke, 1980.

LaBarge E., Edwards D., Knesevich J.W. Performance of normal elderly on the Boston Naming Test. *Brain Lang.* 27:380–384, 1986.

Lachman M.E., Jelalian E. Self-efficacy and attributions of intellectual performance in young and elderly adults. *J. Gerontol.* 39:557–582, 1984.

McGeer P.L., McGeer E.G., Suzuki J.S. Aging and extrapyramidal function. *Arch. Neurol.* 34:33–35, 1977.

Mirsky A. Attention: a neuropsychological perspective. In Chall J., Mirsky A., eds. *Education and the Brain: Seventy-Seventh Yearbook.* Part II. Chicago, University of Chicago Press, 1978.

Mortimer J.A. Alzheimer's disease and senile dementia; prevalence and incidence. In Reisberg B., ed. *Alzheimer's Disease.* New York, Free Press, pp. 141–148, 1983.

Mortimer J.A., Schuman L.M., French L.R. Epidemiology of dementing illness. In Mortimer J.A., Schuman L.M., eds. *The Epidemiology of Dementing Disorders.* New York, Oxford University Press, pp. 3–23, 1981.

Murray M.P., Kory R.C., Clarkson B.H. Walking patterns in healthy old men. *J. Gerontol.* 24:169–178, 1969.

Nebes R.D., Madden D.J. The use of focused attention in visual search by young and old adults. *Exp. Aging Res.* 9:139–143, 1983.

Nissen M.J., Corkin S. Effectiveness of attentional cueing in older and younger adults. *J. Gerontol.* 40:185–190, 1985.

Noll J.D., Randolph S.R. Auditory semantic, syntactic, and retention errors made by aphasic subjects on the Token Test. *J. Commun. Disord.* 11:543–553, 1978.

Obler L.K., Albert M.L. Language and aging: a neurobehavioral analysis. In Beasley D.S., Davis G.A., eds. *Aging: Communication Processes and Disorders.* New York, Grune & Stratton, pp. 107–121, 1981.

Obler L.K., NIcholas M., Albert M.L., et al. On comprehension across the adult life span. *Cortex* 21:273–280, 1985.

Orgass B., Poeck K. Clinical validation of a new test for aphasia: an experimental study of the Token Test. *Cortex* 2:222–243, 1966.

Owens N.A. Age and mental abilities: a longitudinal study. *Genet. Psychol. Monogr.* 48:3–54, 1953.

Owens W.A. Age and mental abilities: a second adult follow-up. *J. Educ. Psychol.* 57:311–325, 1966.

Parasuraman R., Davies R. *Varieties of Attention.* New York, Academic Press, 1984.

Perret E., Regli F. Age and the perceptual threshold for vibratory stimuli. *Eur. Neurol.* 4:65–76, 1970.

Plude D.J., Milberg W.P., Cerella J. Age differences in depicting and perceiving tridimensionality in simple line drawings. *Exp. Aging Res.* 12:221–225, 1986.

Potvin A.R., Syndulko K., Touretellotte W.W., et al. Human neurologic function and the aging process. *J. Am. Geriatr. Soc.* 28:1–9, 1980a.

Potvin A.R., Syndulko K., Tourtellotte W.W., et al. Human neurologic function and the aging process. *J. Am. Geriatr. Soc.* 1:1–9, 1980b.

Prakash C., Stern G. Neurological signs in the elderly. *Age Ageing* 2:24–27, 1973.

Rabbitt P.M.A. An age decrement in the ability to ignore irrelevant information. *J. Gerontol.* 20:233–238, 1965.

Robinson G.W. The toxic delirious reactions of old age. In Kaplan O., ed. *Mental Disorders in Late Life.* Stanford, CA, Stanford University Press, pp. 332–349, 1956.

Rosenwaike I., Yaffe N., Sagi P.C. The recent decline in mortality of the extreme aged: an analysis of statistical data. *Am. J. Public Health* 70:1074–1080, 1980.

Rowe J.W., Kahn R. Human aging: usual versus successful. *Science* 237:143–149, 1987.

Schaie K.W. Rigidity-flexibility and intelligence: a cross-sectional study of the adult life span from 20 to 70. *Psychol. Monogr.* pp. 72–462, 1958.

Schaie K.W. The Seattle longitudinal study: a 21-year exploration of psychometric intelligence in adulthood. In Schaie K.W., ed. *Longitudinal Studies of Adult Psychological Development.* New York, Guilford Press, pp. 64–135, 1983.

Schaie K.W., Labouvie-Vief G. Generational versus ontogenetic components of changes in adult cognitive behavior: a fourteen year cross-sequential study. *Dev. Psychol.* 10:305–320, 1974.

Schaie K.W., Parham I. A cohort-sequential analysis of adult intellectual development. *Dev. Psychol.* 13:649–653, 1977.

Schonfield D., Robertson B.A. Memory storage and aging. *Can. J. Psychol.* 20:228–236, 1966.

Seymour D.G., Pringle R. Post-operative complications in the elderly surgical patient. *Gerontologist* 29:262–270, 1983.

Sharpe J.A., Sylvester T.O. Effect of aging on horizontal smooth pursuit. *Invest. Ophthamol. Vis. Sci.* 17:465–468, 1978.

Skre H. Neurological signs in a normal population. *Acta Neurol. Scand.* 48:575–606, 1972.

Spooner J.W., Sakala S.M., Baloh R.W. Effect of aging on eye tracking. *Arch. Neurol.* 37:575–576, 1980.

Spreen O., Benton A. *Neurosensory Center Comprehensive Examination for Aphasia.* Victoria, B.C., Neuropsychology Laboratory, Department of Psychology, University of Victoria, 1969.

Stafford J.L., Albert M.S., Naeser M.A., et al. Age-related differences in computed tomographic scan measurements. *Arch. Neurol.* 45:409–419, 1988.

Stuss D.T., Benson D.F. *The Frontal Lobes.* New York, Raven Press, 1987.

Talland G.A. Three estimates of the word span and their stability over the adult years. *Q. J. Exp. Psychol.* 17:301–307, 1965.

Taylor A.E., Saint-Cyr J.A., Lange A.E. Parkinson's disease: cognitive changes in relation to treatment response. *Brain* 110:35–51, 1987.

Teravainen H., Calne D.B. Motor system in normal aging and Parkinson's disease. In Katzman R., Terry R.D., eds. *Neurology of Aging.* Philadelphia, Davis, pp. 85–109, 1984.

Tomlinson B.E., Blessed G., Roth M. Observations on the brains of demented old people. *J. Neurol. Sci.* 11:205–242, 1970.

Tulving E. Episodic and semantic memory. In Tulving E., Donaldson W., eds. *Organization of Memory.* New York, Academic Press, pp. 381–403, 1972.

U.S. Department of Health, Education and Welfare. *National Survey of Stroke.* Washington, DC, U.S. Public Health Service, NIH Publication No. 90-2069, 1980.

Walsh D.A., Till R.E., Williams M.V. Age differences in peripheral perceptual processing: a monoptic backward masking investigation. *J. Exp. Psychol. [Hum. Percept.]* 4:232–243, 1978.

Warshaw G.A., Moore J.T., Friedman S.W., et al. Functional disability in the hospitalized elderly. *J.A.M.A.* 248:847–850, 1982.

Waugh N.C., Norman D.A. Primary memory. *Psychol. Rev.,* 72:89–104, 1965.

Wechsler D. A standardized memory scale for clinical use. *J. Psychol.* 19:87–95, 1945.

Wechsler D. *The Assessment and Appraisal of Adult Intelligence.* Baltimore, Williams & Wilkins, 1958.

Welford A.T. Sensory, perceptual, and motor processes in older adults. In Birren J.E., Sloane R.B., eds. *Handbook of Mental Health and Aging.* Englewood Cliffs, NJ, Prentice-Hall, p. 192, 1980.

Wickens C.D., Braune R., Stokes A. Age differences in the speed and capacity of information processing. 1. A dual-task approach. *Psychol. Aging* 2:70–78, 1987.

*Wolfson L.I., Katzman R. The neurologic consultation at age 80. In Katzman R.O., Terry R.D., eds. *The Neurology of Aging.* Philadelphia, Davis, pp. 221–244, 1983.

Wright L.L., Elias J.W. Age differences in the effects of perceptual noise. *J. Gerontol.* 34:704–708, 1979.

Zatz L.M., Jernigan T.L., Ahumada A.J. Changes in computed cranial tomography with aging: intracranial fluid volume. *Am. J. Neuroradiol.* 3:1–11, 1982.

43

Mental Retardation

Arthur L. Prensky

Mental retardation is a symptom. As such, it is important to define its nature and its severity; to understand its anatomic basis, and to recognize its diverse etiologies. Because retardation is more of an expression of the overall function of the entire neocortex rather than any specific area, the pathophysiology of the disorder is not well described. There is not a specific cause that results in a unique pathology that can be associated with the severity of the intellectual disorder or with a failure to develop specific aspects of thought or reasoning in the affected individual. However, our understanding of the causes of retardation is rapidly expanding because of advances in three areas: (1) the neurophysiologic basis of animal cognition, (2) magnetic resonance imaging (MRI), and (3) application of the techniques of molecular genetics to the study of retarded populations.

The American Association of Mental Deficiency (AAMD) has stated: "Mental retardation refers to significantly sub-average intellectual functioning which manifests itself during the developmental period and is characterized by inadequacy in adaptive behavior" (Kidd, 1964).

Intellectual functioning is usually measured by one or more intelligence tests, the reliability and validity of which have been standardized on large populations. Reliability means that a child obtains approximately the same score on the test instrument at different ages with different examiners. Validity means that enough aspects of the child's behavior are measured to be able to estimate the concept of "intelligence." Many built-in hypotheses are accepted when measuring intelligence by such tests. The two most important of these are (1) intelligence is the sum of a series of the selected abilities that are being tested; and (2) intelligence can be described in comparative terms, that is, the performance of one child can be measured against that of a group of children of the same age taken from the general population. It is also agreed that the intelligence test measures only demonstrated abilities—skills and attainments that are evident during the test situation (Prensky and Palkes, 1982). The derived IQ has a predictive value if the test has been adequately standardized and other children's performances have been followed relative to their test scores over a long period of time. The most commonly used intelligence tests have been designed to predict school performance (i.e., the Stanford-Binet and the Wechsler Intelligence Scale for Children, Revised).

Because it is the practice to define intelligence by an IQ measured by tests, the exact nature of intelligence (and thus the exact nature of low intelligence) remains elusive. Such tests have often been standardized on white, middle-class populations. It has been said, therefore, that the tests have social, cultural, and economic biases built into them. Prevalence may vary by 10-fold. Investigations suggest a prevalence of 7–10 per 1000 in Scandinavia compared with 20–30 per 1000 in the United States. Much of this variation has to do with the way in which retardation is defined and with changing social conditions that influence reporting of the condition (Richardson, 1989). It has also been stated, with some truth, that school performance may not reflect later social adjustment. Cognition is a measure of adaptive behavior and can differ from intelligence as measured by tests (Escalona, 1974; Tarjan et al., 1972). For this reason, the AAMD added the phrase "deficits in adaptive behavior" to better define mental retardation. The addition of this clause has resulted in mental retardation's being considered a dynamic, rather than a static, condition. Tarjan et al. (1973) estimated that approximately 3% of all children born in the United States would be defined as mentally retarded at some time in their lives. Of these, nearly 90% would be in the mildly retarded group with an IQ of over 50. However, these authors noted that the prevalence of mild retardation varied with age, being approximately 0.25% in the 0- to 5-year-old group, 3% in the 9- to 16-year-old group, 0.4% in the 20- to 25-year-old group, and 0.2% over the age of 25. Dupont (1989) also noted that the peak prevalence of retardation in Danish population studies is in the 10- to 14-year-old group.

It would appear that sufficient numbers of mildly retarded children, as defined by IQ tests given during school years, are able to make suitable social adjustments, with a resulting drop in the prevalence of mental retardation in adult life to almost one-tenth of that seen during school years. Hagberg and Kyllerman (1983) found the incidence of severe mental retardation (IQ < 50) in Sweden to be 0.3% in school-age children, whereas mild retardation was 0.4%. A similar incidence was found in the city of Göteborg, where the overall incidence of the mentally retarded in the population was approximately 1% (Gillberg et al., 1983). Richardson (1989) is of the opinion that Scandinavian studies tend to underestimate the incidence of mild retardation in the population.

The AAMD has also set standards for the classification of mental retardation by severity (Covert, 1964). These are based entirely on IQ test performance. By the Wechsler Intelligence Test, a score of 55 to 69 is considered mildly retarded; 40 to 54, moderately retarded; 25 to 39, severely retarded; and 24 or below, profoundly retarded. Other investigators have chosen an IQ level of 50 to distinguish between the mildly retarded and the moderately and severely retarded.

Several observations about mental retardation are common to most population surveys. The mildly retarded make up about 60–70% of the total population of retarded children at school age (Drillien et al., 1966; Hagberg and Kyllerman, 1983; Mulcahy et al., 1983). Males are overrepresented in this population by a factor of at least 1.3 to 1 (Gillberg et al., 1983). A substantial number of the severe and profoundly retarded have gross anatomic defects of the nervous system; the mildly retarded often have no discernible anatomic abnormalities (Crome and Stern, 1973; Matti, 1974). A greater proportion of patients with IQ values below 40 have presumed etiologies for their deficits. Many investigators feel

that social and cultural factors are of great importance in the performance of the mildly retarded relative to anatomic insults. Mild retardation is more likely to occur in families of lower socioeconomic status and in those in which there are first-degree relatives who are also retarded (Barlow, 1978; Escalona, 1982; Lamont, 1988). However, Scandinavian studies indicate that a significant proportion of those considered mildly retarded have additional somatic handicaps (Akesson, 1987). Hagberg (1987) stresses the importance of the fetal alcohol syndrome and perinatal problems in mildly retarded children.

The causes of mental retardation can be placed into six broad categories:

1. *Genetic*: chromosomal defects that are acquired or inherited; diseases or syndromes that are usually inherited but without a known metabolic cause, such as neuroectodermal disorders; and inherited metabolic or degenerative diseases
2. *Developmental*: noninherited syndromes with specific physical features that suggest an insult early in development; malformations of the central nervous system (CNS) without consistent abnormalities in other organs but compatible with intrauterine insult; and destructive lesions related to acquired injuries of brain in utero before the perinatal period
3. *Perinatal*: acquired injuries that occur within the last several weeks of intrauterine life, during labor and delivery, or in the immediate postnatal period
4. *Postnatal*: exogenous insults that injure the brain after the perinatal period
5. *Environmental, social, or cultural*: retardation that may be said to result from inadequate stimulation to the maturing CNS during early postnatal life
6. *Unknown or unclassified*: no known cause

Many investigations of the causes of mental retardation combine genetic and developmental etiologies under the term *prenatal*. Table 43–1 reviews 12 series reported from 1966 to 1989 that classify the causes of mental retardation into these broad categories.

Table 43–1. TIMING OF INSULTS LEADING TO MENTAL RETARDATION

Author	IQ	Genetic	Genetic and/or Developmental	Developmental	Perinatal	Postnatal	Unclassified or Unknown	Socioeconomic
Drillien et al., 1966	<55	36		19.9	12.8	9	22.3	—
	>55	6.1		26.1	10.6	3.3	53.9	—
Moser and Wolf, 1971	<70	28.8		6.9	20.1	6.3	39.3	—
Kaveggia et al., 1973	<70	49		18	(15)	10	4.5	—
Gustavson et al., 1977	<55		73		10	3	14	—
Barlow, 1978	<70		37		12	4	28	19
Fryers and Mackay, 1979	<70		55		20	10	12	—
Bersena, 1980	<55		54		21	14	11.7	—
Van den Berghe et al., 1980	<55		37.8		13.7	8.3	40.2	—
Hagberg et al., 1981	>55	35		20	15	11	19	—
Chaney and Eyman, 1982	<70		45.3		13.9	11.6	29.2	—
Jaffe et al., 1984	<70		43.0		12	17	28	—
Krishman et al., 1989	<70	17	17		11.2	1.8	53	—

Clearly, most retarded children in these series have been believed to be the victims of prenatal disease, either because of associated physical findings or laboratory abnormalities or because of abnormalities in the structure of the nervous system. The incidence is probably higher than the table indicates; the possibility of genetic influences in the less severely retarded has been excluded because such influences cannot be determined by proof of chromosomal defects or known inherited metabolic disorders (Costeff et al., 1983). In most of these studies, only 10–12% of children are thought to be retarded as a result of neurologic disease in the perinatal period. This is true whether the patients are mildly or severely retarded. However, children who are damaged in the perinatal period have a higher incidence of associated motor deficits and of epilepsy. Most studies of the mentally retarded, whether in institutions or in the community, classify a large portion of these individuals into a group where the cause is indicated as unknown or undetermined.

The pathology of mental retardation has been reviewed by Crome and Stern (1973), Matti (1974), Friede (1975), Gilles et al. (1983), and Shaw (1987). Gross and microscopic aberrations in the development of the CNS, regressive changes in neurons, cell loss, demyelination, and vascular lesions have all been described in autopsies of retarded children and adults. The pathology of mental retardation is also subject to a number of generalizations. The profound and severely retarded are much more likely to have anatomic pathology than are the mildly retarded. Most patients who are severely retarded have evidence of morphologic alterations in the structure of the nervous system. According to Crome (1972), however, only about one-third of those patients have abnormalities that fall into the realm of recognizable syndromes. The majority of lesions noted appear to have developed prenatally, thus confirming the clinical impression that mental retardation is a symptom of insults that are predominantly genetic or developmental and expressed early in intrauterine life. As Matti (1974) noted in his review of the pathology of institutionalized patients with mental retardation, birth injuries are overdiagnosed. Crome (1972) also observed that the pathology of cases that have been placed clinically into an unclassified group with respect to etiology is in general similar to those cases with known cause (i.e., defects in structure that are gross or microscopic, cell loss, or vascular disease). The pathology of mental retardation seems to be more related to the time of the insult and its duration than to the specific etiology. Interestingly, even at the autopsy table, Shaw (1987) noted that fully 25% of the retarded individuals whose disorder was severe enough to require institutionalization had no significant morphologic abnormalities of the nervous system. A pathologic correlation may exist at a microscopic or submicroscopic level that could be defined only by quantitative studies in which the linkages among the billions of cells that make up the human brain are analyzed.

There is increasing evidence from animal studies that cognitive functions are localized in the brain and are as highly structured, anatomically and physiologically, as the neurons of the primary sensory-motor cortex. The anatomy of one aspect of cognition is beautifully summarized by Goldman-Rakic (1987a,b). She outlined the relation between structure and function of area 46 of the monkey prefrontal cortex, as well as its connections with parietal association areas, the neostriatum, the thalamus, and the brain stem. This particular area appears to control delayed responses over the short term to visual problems. Its linkage to the parietal cortex, as mapped by the firing patterns of single neurons, provides a visual map of space. Area 46 appears to provide an access to the stored memory of spatial organization that will help to resolve an immediate problem. Studies by Thompson et al. (1986, 1987) in the white rat also suggest that intelligence may be more localized than previously believed. Retardation was defined as a generalized learning impairment characterized by the inability to perform appropriately in any of six specific tasks thought to involve different aspects of cognition. Rats, which otherwise appeared to have normal sensory and motor functions, met this criterion when focal lesions were placed in the parietal cortex, globus pallidus, substantia nigra, ventrolateral thalamus, or median raphe of the pontine reticular system. Later, Thompson et al. (1987) added the superior colliculus and the dorsal lateral aspect of the neostriatum.

If those aspects of cognition that define mental retardation are indeed organized into several discrete areas of brain and are dependent on reciprocal circuits among those areas being intact, it may be extremely difficult to uncover the pathologic basis of mental retardation in many individuals not otherwise handicapped unless a great deal more is known about the anatomy of learned behaviors (Berenberg, 1977).

It is increasingly clear that the nervous system is not randomly organized at any level (Lund, 1978; Rabinowicz et al., 1977). In the normal nervous system, cells migrate at appropriate times to appropriate positions in the cortex. They are oriented correctly with regard to each other and the surface of the cortex; they grow to a predetermined size. Basilar and apical dendrites proliferate; the spines on these dendrites differentiate, and contact is made with appropriate axon terminals. This is a continuing process in which cells, parts of cells, and dendritic spines are lost. The dendritic field of a single cell is constantly remolded (Cotman and Nieto-Sampedro, 1984). The cells or parts of cells that are preferentially lost are frequently those that have formed incorrect connections with neurons during development to which they are usually not linked (Cowan et al., 1984).

The complexity of the process is perhaps best summarized by Lund (1978). Neurons must leave the cell cycle at a given time. They must migrate to an appropriate region. The neurons must develop a special identity relative to their neighbors. Dendrites must have a specific orientation. Axons must migrate appropriately. The axon must direct its branches appropriately. The terminal field of the axon must be ordered in a particular way in the region of termination. Axon terminals can end only on certain types of cells in an area and on certain parts of those cells. There must be a proper relationship among the number of synapses on the soma of the cell, proximal dendrites, and distal branches of the dendrites. Axons from appropriate cells must terminate at each of these. A neuron must select from a wide variety of connections and maintain this set of selections beyond a critical period to become physiologically stable and able to fulfill its potential functions. Aberrations in any of these events can lead to retardation.

The control of the number of neurons in the brain, their spatial organization, their synaptic connections, and the time of their death is genetic. The basic rules that govern the development of the nervous system are encoded in the genetic material of the organism. However, the number of possible interactions between neurons far exceeds the number of genes that a human being possesses (Gierer, 1988). The ultimate organization of the normal, as well as the abnormal, brain must depend on environmental influences that help to regulate the organization of neurons within a genetically determined envelope (Barth, 1987; Herschkowitz, 1988; Williams and Herrup, 1988).

With this in mind, it is probably best to approach what little is known about the etiology and pathophysiology of mental retardation by discussing discrete categories of insults (Table 43–2).

Here, too, several generalizations can be made. Insults that take place late in development and have severe consequences are more likely to be associated with destruction of neurons within the CNS than with aberrations in their organization and development. More sustained, milder lesions affect the growth of the neuropil. The effect of insults on the function of the nervous system is not always discernible immediately after the insults have taken place. The limitations that they produce may become more apparent as the organism is required to perform more complex functions in later stages of development. Alternatively, the limitations become clinically apparent when other parts of the nervous system that have been left relatively untouched mature normally but cannot interact with the neurons that have been damaged or destroyed.

GENETICALLY DETERMINED MENTAL RETARDATION OF KNOWN CAUSE

Chromosomal Disorders

Not all chromosomal abnormalities are associated with mental retardation, although the symptom occurs in the majority of cases in which genetic material is added to or subtracted from the cell. In one large study (Elejald and Opitz, 1978), the most common abnormality was a balanced translocation that occurred in 1 in 549 patients. Such individuals frequently have normal intelligence. Unbalanced translocations occurred in 1 in 2500 patients. The most common trisomies involved the sex chromosomes and occurred in about 1 in 1000 live births (47,XXY or 47,XYY). Trisomy 21 also occurred in approximately 1 in 1000 live births; trisomy 18, considerably more rare, occurred in 1 in 7500 live births; and trisomy 13 occurred in 1 in 15,000 live births. 45,X occurred in 1 in 10,000 live births. The figures are quite different for institutionally retarded populations, in which patients with Down's syndrome generally make up 75–80% of those children who have chromosomal abnormalities (Jacobs et al., 1978; Schreppers-Tijdink et al., 1988). Although some chromosomal abnormalities are inherited, most appear to be sporadic and the occurrence rates increase with maternal age at the time of pregnancy. While performing amniocentesis, Hook (1983) found that the incidence of chromosomal abnormalities was 5 in 1000 at age 35, 15 in 1000 at age 40, and 50 in 1000 at age 45. At age 33, the incidence of trisomy 21 was 1.6 in 1000; at age 49, it was 93.3 in 1000.

The higher incidence of retarded males relative to females is in part accounted for by a defect in the X chromosome. A constriction near the end of one long arm of the X chromosome is brought out when cells are grown in folate-deficient medium and is not seen in the folate-rich medium that is usually used to grow cells for chromosomal studies. Retardation is much more likely to occur in males who have a fragile X chromosome than in females, but heterozygous expression is seen. Turner et al. (1980) indicated the overall prevalence in females of school age to be 4 per 10,000. The frequency of the fragile X chromosome in noninstitutionalized subnormal children in Scandinavia varied from 0.8 to 2.8% (Gustavson et al., 1987; Kahkonen et al., 1986). Schreppers-Tijdink et al. (1988) found the chromosomal defect in 1.8% of the population in an institution for the mentally handicapped. Sutherland (1983) noted that no specific physical features separate males who have a fragile X chromosome from other mildly retarded men or boys. Furthermore, some individuals with

Table 43–2. CAUSES OF MENTAL RETARDATION

Genetic
    Chromosomal abnormalities
    Inherited metabolic disorders
    Inherited syndromes of unknown cause
    Degenerative diseases
Intrauterine developmental disorders
    Dorsal or ventral induction
    Neuronal multiplication
    Neuronal migration
    Cortical organization and synaptogenesis
    Myelination
Destructive disorders manifested in utero
Perinatal disorders
Postnatal disorders
Undetermined or unclassified

the fragile X chromosome have normal intelligence, which indicates that a great many factors (as in trisomy 21) can modify the effects of a structural anomaly of one or more chromosomes on intelligence.

The prevalence of chromosomal deficits in the entire population and in that subfraction who are mentally subnormal has probably been underestimated. Microdeletions within the chromosome, inversions of chromosomal material, and partially unbalanced translocations may not be identified by routine chromosomal studies, whereas many become apparent when chromosomes are studied in prometaphase by high-resolution banding techniques that use a variety of stains (Tengstrom and Autio, 1987). Many chromosomal aberrations have been shown to occur in individuals who have no significant somatic deformities by these techniques (Kikkawa et al., 1989).

Still other abnormalities can be defined by techniques employed in molecular genetics that use both linkage studies and specific probes to identify missing or altered sections of a chromosome. Until now, these techniques have been most effective in defining multiple sites on the X chromosome associated with familial retardation (Arveiler et al., 1988; Ballabio et al., 1989; Giannelli et al., 1987). The use of specific probes to define aberrancies in the long or short arm of the X chromosome (and eventually other chromosomes, as well) should improve the identification of carriers of submicroscopic chromosomal abnormalities associated with mental retardation and the diagnosis of their progeny early in intrauterine life (Goonewardena et al., 1987; Mulley et al., 1987; Oberlie et al., 1986). These techniques have also been used to localize the site on the chromosome responsible for several important neurologic disorders sometimes associated with retardation, such as Duchenne's dystrophy, neurofibromatosis, and Huntington's chorea (Rosenberg, 1990), and to clarify the molecular basis for highly disparate phenotypic syndromes that share the same chromosomal deletion— Angelman's syndrome and Prader-Willi syndrome. Both of these disorders share the same deletion site on chromosome 15, but in the first instance it is derived from the mother and in the second, from the father (Knoll et al., 1989).

Lejeune (1977) noted that the relationship of the symptom of mental retardation to any chromosomal abnormality is elusive. There is no specific pathology that links the chromosomal abnormalities to this symptom. Even the major trisomies have quite different brain lesions. There are no gross malformations in trisomy 21, although the superior temporal gyrus is increased in size and the frontal lobes diminished in size and weight, as is the cerebellum. Cortical laminae are irregularly formed, and the dendritic connections of pyramidal cells are decreased. There is reduced deposition of myelin (Banik et al., 1975). However, the most interesting change that has been described during the past 2 decades is the premature appearance of neurofibrillary tangles and

senile plaques (Schochet et al., 1973). In this disorder, there is a reduplication of chromosomal material that frequently results in severely retarded children, but the pathologic anatomy suggests that the process is not a static one. The disorder begins in the first months of intrauterine life and continues to develop after birth and into adulthood.

This picture is quite different from that of trisomy 13, in which approximately 80% of patients have arrhinencephaly or in which there may be a single ventricle with fusion of the frontal lobes. Patients who lack these major abnormalities still have extensive heterotopias in the cerebrum, anomalies of cerebellar development, and partial or complete agenesis of the corpus callosum. All of these are static defects and occur early in intrauterine life. They are incompatible with normal intelligence and are generally accompanied by abnormalities in other organ systems that end life between 1 and 3 years of age. Gross anomalies of neurologic development are also found in at least one-half of patients with trisomy 18. These include major defects, such as holoprosencephaly, severe hydrocephalus, and anencephaly, as well as less dramatic problems involving migration of cells with heterotopias in the cerebrum and cerebellum (Terplan et al., 1970) and abnormal layering of cells in the cerebellum.

In general, chromosomal disorders in which the brain exhibits the most significant developmental aberrations within the nervous system are associated with the greatest degree of retardation, although there is not a one-to-one correspondence. For example, patients with Klinefelter's or Turner's syndrome often have few gross or microscopic pathologic changes, but a higher percentage of this group suffers from microcephaly (perhaps the result of decreased cell proliferation). Although the incidence of mental retardation in this group of children is higher than that in the normal population, many of them have normal or borderline intelligence.

Mental retardation is a frequent symptom of chromosomal disorders, and, at least in the case of this class of diseases, the severity of that symptom is usualy related to the degree to which the organization of the brain within and between specific nuclear masses is altered.

Genetically Determined Developmental Diseases

Many autosomal dominant disorders have now been localized to defects in specific chromosomes. They are not, as far as we know, the result of disruption of catabolic pathways caused by a single enzyme defect. Tuberous sclerosis and neurofibromatosis are the classic examples of genetically determined developmental disorders. The gene for tuberous sclerosis appears to be on the long arm of chromosome 9, whereas the peripheral form of neurofibromatosis is at 7q11.2 and the central form at 22q11.1-13.0 (Rosenberg, 1990).

These diseases invariably affect both the skin and the CNS but also may affect visceral organs. Central to each of these disorders is disrupted growth. In prenatal life, this is expressed in the CNS of tuberous sclerosis patients by abnormal migration of cells with heterotopias, cortical dysplasias, abnormal cortical layering, and the presence of tubers that are sclerotic areas with an increased number of astrocytic nuclei and some neurons, many of which are 10 times larger than normal size and contain multiple nuclei (Bender and Yunis, 1982). They are usually surrounded by excessive numbers of fibrillary astrocytes. In less involved areas of cortex, neurons exhibit distortions in their apical dendrites that often contact glia rather than axons of other nerve cells (Machado-Salas, 1984). Megaspines are frequently seen, and there are excessive numbers of short thin spines, especially on the distal portions of the apical dendrites. In other areas, dendrites may be totally absent, thus distorting the normal architecture of the cortex. Tubers are actually more common in the subependymal zone where they are easily observed by computed tomographic (CT) scan. However, the cortical changes seem best related to retardation. Other abnormalities of growth also occur. Megalencephaly is found more often in patients with tuberous sclerosis and neurofibromatosis than in the general population. Some patients have enlargement of only one cerebral hemisphere. In postnatal life, growth abnormalities are expressed by an increased incidence of glial tumors of all varieties.

In neurofibromatosis, disturbances in both epidermal and nerve growth factors have been reported, but the relationship between these abnormalities and the pathogenesis of the disease is not clear (Riccardi and Mulvhill, 1981). The cortical architecture is less often distorted, and the degree of mental retardation is also less. Approximately 20% of patients with neurofibromatosis are retarded, whereas at least 60% of patients with tuberous sclerosis have intelligence that measures below the normal range.

The biochemical disturbances in these disorders may be analagous to that of Duchenne's dystrophy, in which a structural protein, dystrophin, is not synthesized because of a mutant gene at Xp211. What is not clear is how the failure to synthesize a single structural protein results in widespread defects involving several organ systems that become apparent throughout life. What is the common denominator, and why is neurologic involvement so variable?

Inherited Metabolic Disorders

Diseases with No Storage in Neurons

These disorders include most of the inherited diseases of amino and organic acid metabolism (Adams and Lyon, 1982). The most common is phenylketo-

nuria; it occurs in 1 in 7400 to 1 in 14,000 live births (Bickel et al., 1981; Levy, 1973). It is also the most thoroughly studied of these disorders, because it has been possible to simulate the effects of the disease on the CNS by administering phenylalanine to rodents in the perinatal period. Initially, examination of pathologic tissue from humans and from animal models suggested that the pathologic basis of the symptoms in phenylketonuria was hypomyelination (Prensky et al., 1968, 1971). Because untreated phenylketonurics are generally moderately to severely retarded and frequently without significant motor defects, the fact that the disease would preferentially attack this one membrane is rather simplistic, despite the fact that myelin is actively synthesized after birth in both humans and rodents (Davison and Dobbing, 1966). In later investigations, many aspects of brain development were found to be affected when severely retarded patients with phenylketonuria or animals made hyperphenylalaninemic were studied carefully (Cordero et al., 1983; Lacey, 1984). The width of the cortical plate is decreased; there is an increase in the density of cells; neuronal cell size and dendritic arborization decrease; and the number of dendritic spines and the amount of Nissl substance within the cells decrease. Cortical lamination is less distinct. It is much more likely that these abnormalities are the source of the patient's retardation. Similar and even more striking abnormalities in cortical architecture are reported in the offspring of female rats made hyperphenylalaninemic in pregnancy (Levy and Waisbren, 1983).

The enzyme defect that causes phenylketonuria is known. In most patients, the activity of phenylalanine hydroxylase, which converts phenylalanine to tyrosine, is virtually absent. Mental retardation is definitely related to blood levels of phenylalanine and/or alternative metabolites in utero (Mabry et al., 1963) or in the first years of postnatal life. However, the mechanisms by which high levels of this amino acid produce mental retardation are still unknown. Suppositions include interference with glycolysis or with oxidative metabolism in brain, decreased production of one or more neurotransmitters, and interference with protein synthesis by altering the transport of other neutral amino acids (Patel and Arinze, 1975). Similar mechanisms have been proposed for other aminoacidurias (Cremer et al., 1982; Pajari and Oja, 1983).

The degree of retardation depends not only on the severity of this type of metabolic insult but also its duration (Bickel, 1969; Msall et al., 1984). Thus, often it is possible to avoid or minimize the psychomotor retardation that accompanies these diseases by prompt reduction of the offending substrate in the blood and tissues. By inference, it is also possible to influence myelination and the cortical architecture by counteracting the chemical effects of these genetic insults. However, there is no indication in humans or experimental animals that the postnatal control of a metabolic deficit that has damaged the brain in utero results in more normal cytoarchitecture and function. The plasticity that is apparent in the human nervous system's response to disease appears to be limited to restructuring those processes that can take place when the insult is corrected.

Other more acute inherited metabolic disorders of amino and organic acid metabolism may be sufficiently severe to result in intracellular hypoxia, acidosis, and cell death, either directly or indirectly, through the production of cerebral edema, ischemia, or hypoglycemia (Naughten et al., 1982). Because some children can survive attacks of this type and are thereafter neurologically normal with no evidence of retardation, one must assume that the nervous system is capable of losing some cells without intelligence being significantly affected. What proportion of its cells can be lost and whether they must be limited to specific areas of brain have not been established.

Two new groups of biochemical diseases involving the CNS have become better characterized: the peroxisomal disorders (Moser, 1989; Moser et al., 1989) and the mitochondrial encephalomyopathies (DiMauro et al., 1990). Both categories of metabolic disease have multiple causes and multiple phenotypes. The causes vary from defects in the structure of, or even absence of, the organelle in cells of the nervous system to defects in the membrane of the organelle limiting transport or to defects of single enzymes located within the mitochondrion or the peroxisome. In peroxisomal disorders, there are reduced tissue levels of plasmalogens and accumulation of very long chain (C_{24} or greater) fatty acids. In the mitochondrial disorders, there is an increase in serum and often cerebrospinal fluid lactate, which is presumably the result of defective oxidation of glucose. Again, it is not known how these chemical disturbances affect cell function and the organization of brain neurons to result in retardation or progressive loss of mental function.

Diseases with Storage in Neurons

Lipid and carbohydrate storage disorders usually occur because of catabolic defects caused by the deficiency of a lysosomal enzyme that results in extensive intracellular accumulation of metabolites that cannot be degraded further. Initially, these metabolites are stored in a variety of membrane-bound inclusion bodies that probably were lysosomes. They markedly distend the cell soma. Eventually, the cell dies. The mechanism of death is not well understood. However, the degree of neurologic deterioration that occurs in these children and the severity of their retardation often far exceed the loss of cells. Purpura and Suzuki (1976) found a marked increase in the surface area of dendrites in these cells in the formation of massive dendritic-like structures, called meganeurites, which lie between the cell body and the axon hillock of the pyramidal neuron. They are often covered with spines and develop synapses that abut each other, the axons of other cells, or glial

cells. It would appear that this marked expansion of the dendritic surface with aberrant connections seriously compromises the function of the cell. One may also speculate that this significant alteration in the cell surface may play a part in shortening the life of the cell. Storage disorders are usually recessive diseases, but the genetic defects in several, such as Tay-Sachs disease, have been partially characterized (Galjaard and Reuser, 1989). In diseases in which there is accumulation of enormous amounts of substrate, localization of a DNA mutation may not aid in diagnosis, but it is hoped that such a determination will lead to improved treatment.

Inherited Disorders Characterized by Cell Death

Cell death is a part of the normal development of the nervous system (Cowan et al., 1984). After the middle third of intrauterine life and in postnatal life, however, the number of neurons in the cortex is stable or slowly decreases with age. Rapid destruction of neurons in childhood as part of an inherited degenerative disorder results in retardation as defined by the AAMD, although, in fact, it would be better characterized as a dementia. The severity and the form taken by this decrease in mental function relate to how many neurons in the cerebral cortex are lost and to the areas most severely affected. Dementia also occurs if neurons can no longer properly interact with one another because of destruction of elements in the cerebral white matter.

The accumulation of ceroid, probably made up of peroxidized lipid and protein, has led to the hypothesis that in some degenerative diseases free radicals peroxidize membrane lipids and so block normal degradation of intracellular organelles and their resynthesis, thus shortening the life of the cell. An alternative hypothesis is that many catabolic defects within the lysosome can result in accumulation of stored products that can be peroxidized, polymerized, and stored in the cell, thus leading to its death (Ivy et al., 1984). However, most disorders in which there is early neuronal death do not evidence production of excess lipofuscin, nor is there evidence of degeneration of neurotubes or filaments—all signs of premature aging of neurons. The mechanisms by which large numbers of cells are programmed to degenerate early in life are still not known. These disorders have been classified by Dyken and Krawiecki (1983).

INTRAUTERINE INSULTS ASSOCIATED WITH MENTAL RETARDATION

Developmental Malformations

Developmental malformations are defined as gross malformations of the nervous system that are present in intrauterine life and are associated with mental retardation. They sometimes occur with malformations of other organ systems that are specific enough to define a syndrome. Developmental malformations can be inherited, but they are usually the result of exogenous insults to the nervous system in intrauterine life. The malformations primarily reflect the time of the insult rather than the etiology.

The formation of the neural tube occurs during the third and fourth weeks of gestation. The tube begins as a plate of tissue differentiating in the middle of the ectoderm. Under the influence of the chordal mesoderm, closure begins anteriorly and proceeds caudally. During the fifth and sixth weeks of gestation, the prechordal mesoderm organizes the development of the face and forebrain rostrally. When these events are completed during the first 2 months of intrauterine life, they basically account for the major outline of the forebrain, hindbrain, and spinal cord. Thereafter, neurons proliferate and migrate. This process is usually completed by the fifth month of gestation; however, the migration of the glial cells that form satellite cells in the cortex and the oligodendroglial cells of the white matter continues until some months after birth, as does formation of the cerebellar cortex. As noted previously, the shaping of cortical architecture continues long after birth, as does myelination. Abnormalities in this sequence of events are reviewed by Volpe (1977).

Defects that occur early in embryogenesis are likely to be associated with severe retardation. Failure of the anterior neural tube to close results in anencephaly, in which the forebrain and parts of the upper brain stem fail to develop. The incidence in the United States is about 1 in 1000 live births (Volpe, 1977). If the lesion is somewhat more restricted, an encephalocele may develop, in which part of the brain and its coverings protrude in the midline. About four-fifths of these lesions are occipital, and most of the remainder are frontal or nasal. The protrusion of brain tissue itself is not the cause of retardation. However, it is often associated with extensive abnormalities of neural migration, resulting in abnormally organized cortex that usually extends to areas of brain remaining within the cranial cavity. About 60% of children with occipital encephaloceles are retarded (Guthkelch, 1970). Small encephaloceles, particularly nasal lesions, are often not associated with retardation (Mealey et al., 1970). The incidence is about 1–5 per 1000 live births. The highest incidence is in Ireland and parts of Britain during epidemic periods, which suggests an environmental cause for these insults. However, genetic determinants are also operative; the recurrence rate is increased in sibs, and there is also an increased incidence of anencephaly, spina bifida, and myelomeningocele (Warkany, 1971). About 50–70% of children born with congenital hydrocephalus, regardless of cause, are moderately to severely retarded (Noetzel, 1989).

Disturbances of ventral induction also result in major malformations; one group consists of the holoprosencephalies. The telencephalon remains as a single sphere, and, depending on the degree of the holoprosencephaly, the diencephalon is variably affected. The supralimbic cortex fails to develop. The child is usually severely retarded. Many of these fetuses die in utero; when they do survive, holoprosencephalies can be linked to chromosomal aberrations or the effect of teratogens. The subject is reviewed by Cohen (1989).

Disorders of neuronal proliferation with reduced numbers of neurons result in micrencephaly. In micrencephaly vera, there is no evidence of an intrauterine destructive disease. The brain is normal in shape but small. These children often have normal motor development during the first 18 months of life, but intellectual development is severely retarded. Cases can be sporadic or inherited as autosomal or X-linked recessive disorders in families (Volpe, 1977). Sporadic cases may be produced by external insults, such as irradiation; drugs, such as alcohol; or maternal hyperphenylalaninemia. Many cases have no known cause.

Failures of neuronal migration in their most severe form result in a complete agenesis of a portion of the cerebral wall that leaves bilateral clefts (schizencephaly). The walls of these clefts are abnormal. Polymicrogyria is usually present, as are neuronal heterotopias. Again, they may affect the cortex beyond the area of the cleft (Yakovlev and Wadsworth, 1946). In lissencephaly, the brain has few or no gyri and the surface is smooth. In type I lissencephaly, the cerebrum has four layers: (1) an outermost acellular layer (as it would be in the first trimester of gestation), (2) an outer cellular layer composed of normally migrating neurons, (3) a layer with sparse cells, and (4) a deep cellular layer with no organization that suggests the migration of these neurons was halted prematurely (Dobyns, 1989). In type II lissencephaly, there is a thickened, totally disorganized cortex of three layers (Dambska et al., 1983). Initially, lissencephaly was thought to result from insults occurring in the early part of the second trimester, but at least one form is genetic and associated with a deletion in the short arm of chromosome 17.

Lesser anomalies include excessively large or small gyri. Pachygyria is a condition in which the gyri are large and few with a thick cortical plate that is poorly developed. The neurons are not methodically arranged in columns. Pyramidal cells are abnormally oriented. Heterotopias are common, and there is abnormal dendritic branching (Fabregues et al., 1984). This disturbance probably occurs early in the second trimester. Large numbers of extremely small gyri (polymicrogyria) also contain cortex that is abnormally organized and are associated with neuronal heterotopias.

The development of high-resolution neuroimaging techniques, particularly MRI, has made it possible to diagnose many congenital brain anomalies during life. Migrational disorders, which are often unassociated with somatic malformations, can often be recognized easily by this radiologic technique (Byrd and Naidich, 1988; Dunn et al., 1986; Marchal et al.,

1989). In many instances, affected children have moderate to severe retardation associated with significant motor deficits. Until the patients have been scanned, their deficits are often incorrectly attributed to secondary problems occurring in the perinatal period. Unfortunately, no studies have yet screened an unselected population of retarded children to establish the incidence of these brain anomalies.

It is also possible to use neurosonography to diagnose major intracranial anomalies in utero. Some, such as encephaloceles, hydranencephaly, and alobar holoprosencephaly, can often be diagnosed early enough in the pregnancy to offer the option of abortion. Others, such as hydrocephalus, can be treated during gestation if the problem becomes severe (Fadel, 1989).

The cause of most of these intrauterine defects is not known. In experimental animals, deficiencies in vitamin A, riboflavin, folic acid, and vitamin B_{12} result in hydrocephalus (Kalter and Warkany, 1983). Deficiencies of pyridoxine can result in exencephaly. Deficiencies of either zinc or copper can result in small brains. Zinc, in particular, has the ability to produce in rats such major anomalies as anencephaly, hydranencephaly, exencephaly, and hydrocephalus. Alcohol and drugs, such as diphenylhydantoin, may produce a microcephaly (Hurley, 1976; Warkany and Petering, 1973). Viral infections are certainly known to produce major cerebral anomalies associated with abnormal brain function in animals and probably can do so in humans (Johnson, 1978). Severe restriction of protein or calories during pregnancy results in intrauterine growth retardation and a smaller than normal brain (Dodge et al., 1975). However, the insult primarily affects the development of the cortex, particularly dendritic arborization, synapse formation, and myelination, and thus its effects are most severe when continued after birth (Winick, 1976). In animals, it is possible to show that a variety of insults near the termination of development fail to produce qualitative changes in brain structure but result in a reduction in the total number of small neurons in the brain (Altman, 1987).

Drug ingestion during pregnancy has also proved to be harmful to fetal growth and resulted in a higher incidence of mental retardation than expected. The two types of drugs receiving the most attention have been anticonvulsants (Hanson et al., 1976) and alcohol (Hanson et al., 1978). It is estimated that 30–40% of children of alcoholic mothers have growth retardation and that a significant proportion are also mentally retarded. In one child, who died in infancy, dendritic spines were reduced in number and abnormally placed in the nerve cell (Ferrer and Galofre, 1987). The incidence of retardation is increased even in the absence of somatic abnormalities. Ingestion of excessive amounts of vitamin A and the use of oral anticoagulants are other exogenous insults associated with congenital anomalies of the fetus. However, Kalter and Warkany (1983) thought that *all* drugs accounted for only 1.3% of the malformations found in the population they studied.

Normal brain development, including cell differentiation, cell growth, and cell death, depends on a large number of endogenously produced chemicals. Hormones exert trophic, as well as metabolic, effects during intrauterine life (Goldstein, 1986). Neurotrophic compounds that are either produced within the nervous system or transferred to it also exert a profound effect on developmental events (Snider and Johnson, 1989). Except in thyroid disease, no hormonal imbalance has been shown to be associated with a specific defect in the brain or a specific chemical syndrome in which retardation plays a major role. It is likely, however, that many teratogens influence brain development by mechanisms that are similar to those by which hormones and neurotrophic factors operate. Preliminary information indicates that they may alter the balance of neurotransmitters in the CNS (Grimm, 1987; Lauder and Krebs, 1984).

The presence of endocrine disorders during pregnancy has a definite effect on the development of the CNS and intellectual function. Children of diabetic mothers have two to six times the chance of being born with a congenital anomaly of the nervous system than infants in the general population. The caudal dysplasia syndrome is most common, but anencephaly and microcephaly have been described as occurring with an increased incidence (Prensky and Dodson, 1978). However, the increased incidence of mental retardation in infants of diabetic mothers is not related only to malformations in utero. Many of these infants are small for gestational age and have postnatal hypoglycemia. They may also be large infants, and the resulting traumatic deliveries increase the risk for brain injury.

Fetal hypothyroidism, or iodine deficiency, is a major public health problem. It is important to distinguish between endemic and sporadic cretins. Sporadic cretinism is associated with the signs of neonatal hypothyroidism, including a hoarse cry and poor feeding habits. These children may often partially recover if treated early in postnatal life. If left untreated, they are almost always retarded. Endemic cretins are deaf, mute, and frequently have signs of spasticity and ataxia. They are invariably retarded. Postnatal administration of thyroid hormone is not effective in the great majority of endemic cretins, who do not themselves have evidence of thyroid deficiency (Raiti and Newns, 1971). Animal experiments suggest that a decrease in thyroid hormone retards cell division. Neurons are smaller and fewer, the development of the neuropil is poor, synaptogenesis is decreased in the cerebellum, and myelination is retarded (Balazs, 1972). A large number of experimental studies summarized by Nunez (1984) indicate that thyroid hormones affect neuronal growth to a greater degree than cell division. Thyroid hormones appear to be necessary for the assembly of microtubules, which are required for the cell to grow and function normally.

Steroids appear to decrease DNA synthesis in rat models (Balazs, 1972), but there is no indication that they have a similar effect in humans.

Many cases of multiple somatic anomalies are associated with idiopathic retardation (Smith and Bostian, 1964). The patients have no chromosomal abnormalities, no evidence of a metabolic disorder, and no history of toxic exposure. The nervous system appears to be normally formed, according to clinical and radiographic evaluation. The nature of the somatic abnormalities may help to date the time of the insult relative to gestation or, if sufficiently striking, may define a syndrome that will help the physician to give a prognosis for the child and advise the family about the chances of the disorder recurring (Opitz, 1982). The cause of mental retardation in these children and adults is not known.

It is characteristic of CNS development that the anatomic changes resulting from an insult set off a cascade of consequences that can continue after the insult ends. Thus, the failure of neurons to migrate to their proper places can result in profound effects on dendritic arborization, synaptogenesis, and neuronal growth that continue into postnatal life (Spero and Yu, 1983; Stoltenburg-Didinger and Spohr, 1983). The developing nervous system is restricted in its ability to compensate for major structural abnormalities.

Destructive Lesions of the Central Nervous System in Utero

Prenatal insults need not just impair normal growth; they also can destroy nervous tissue. Vascular disease can occur in utero, as can severe hypoxia. Depending on the nature of the involvement, destruction of tissue may occur in the area of a single major cortical vessel and produce a porencephalic cyst or more widespread neuronal destruction, particularly in the cortex where small, shriveled gyri (ulegyria) result.

Severe viral infections may produce cytolysis, focal necrosis, cerebral atrophy, and microcephaly (Stagno et al., 1981; Wolfe and Cowen, 1959). Intracranial calcifications may be present. The rubella virus can affect the process of cell division, but it also produces a severe vasculitis and may cause multiple areas of infarction in the brain (Rorke, 1973).

It is doubtful that many drugs that are not themselves toxins or that are not taken in toxic doses destroy fetal brain tissue.

PERINATAL BRAIN DAMAGE

Perinatal disorders usually produce mental retardation by the destruction of neural tissue and, less frequently, by interrupting the development of myelin or the neuropil (Gilles, 1985). By far, the most common cause of perinatal brain damage is hypoxic-ischemic disease (so called because poor oxygenation must be accompanied, in almost all cases, by hypotension and decreased cerebral blood flow to produce

serious brain damage). As outlined by Volpe (1987), this type of insult has five prominent forms: (1) selective neuronal necrosis involving neurons within the cortex; (2) status marmoratus involving cells in the basal ganglia; (3) parasagittal cerebral injury (watershed infarcts); (4) periventricular leukomalacia; and (5) focal or multifocal ischemic brain necrosis, including porencephaly, hydranencephaly, and multicystic encephalomalacia.

Intraventricular hemorrhage and periventricular hemorrhage are more likely to be related to changes in blood pressure and blood flow in the brain of the premature infant than in that of the term infant (Lou et al., 1979; Tarby and Volpe, 1982); However, they also have a strong association with hypoxia (Towbin, 1970). The damage caused by intraventricular hemorrhage depends in part on the severity of the hemorrhage (i.e., how much brain tissue is affected). The incidence of mental retardation also depends on associated insults that affect the brain before or at the time of the hemorrhage, such as the severity of associated hypoxic-ischemic disease, elevated intracranial pressure, and focal ischemia.

A frequent sequel to intraventricular hemorrhage, even when it does not severely damage the cells of the germinal matrix, is hydrocephalus. If this progresses without treatment, it can result in destruction of cerebral white matter and later of cortical tissue and produce retardation. However, even a thin rim of brain, 2–3 cm in thickness, often contains sufficient cells and axons to allow for normal or borderline mental function later in life if intracranial pressure is relieved by a shunt (Burstein et al., 1979).

Several studies show that it is not possible to relate hypoxic-ischemic disease in the neonate to any single factor occurring during labor or delivery (Chaney et al., 1986; Freeman, 1985; Holst et al., 1989; Niswander et al., 1984). Infants who are asphyxic at birth are often abnormal in utero (Garik et al., 1979; Susser et al., 1985). Most children with asphyxia at birth are normal later in life (Paneth and Stark, 1983). Only when multiple factors in the perinatal period are considered is there a relationship between hypoxic-ischemic disease and ultimate outcome (Rosen, 1985). Apgar scores are notoriously unreliable, particularly at 1 and 5 minutes, if unassociated with any other signs or symptoms of hypoxic-ischemic brain disease. Low Apgar scores at 10–15 minutes are much more reliable, but they are rarely recorded. The majority of babies with Apgar scores in the 0–3 range at 1 minute are normal by the time they are of school age (Nelson and Ellenberg, 1981). The association of low Apgar scores with repeated seizures, severe lethargy, hypotonia, and poor feeding markedly increases the possibility of subsequent mental retardation and/or motor difficulties as a consequence of a perinatal insult (Finer et al., 1981).

Because many hypoxic-ischemic lesions that occur in the perinatal period involve motor neurons or their axons, this particular type of insult has often been indicated to have a much higher incidence of association with cerebral palsy. Indeed, the incidence of such an association is quite high. Approximately 70% of severely or profoundly retarded children who have had definite perinatal injuries do have disease of the motor system with a spastic, athetoid, or ataxic motor deficit, or a combined form. A high percentage of these children also have epilepsy. However, epilepsy and static deficits of motor control also occur in many children who have developmental or destructive lesions in utero and in some children with genetic disorders. Therefore, the presence of these complications in a retarded child does not automatically point to hypoxic-ischemic disease in perinatal or postnatal periods of development.

Nelson and Browman (1977) demonstrated that low socioeconomic status, poor nutrition, smoking, and excessive alcohol ingestion during pregnancy lowered the IQ of the population of children they studied, but these insults failed to distinguish between severely retarded children and controls. A common denominator among these and many other less well-defined prenatal insults is low birth weight. Premature infants with birth weights of less than 1500 g have an increased incidence of hypoxic-ischemic disease and of intraventricular or periventricular hemorrhage with subsequent retardation. They are also more susceptible to effects on the brain of severe hypoglycemia and of hyperbilirubinemia (Brann, 1985). Infants who are small for gestational age usually have been subject to a disease, such as rubella, or had insufficient nutrition in utero as a result of maternal disease, poor maternal nutrition, or placental dysfunction. There is a significantly increased incidence of retardation in this group of children (Brann, 1985; Drillien, 1974).

POSTNATAL BRAIN DAMAGE

Postnatal brain damage, like perinatal brain damage, usually produces major symptoms by destruction of tissue. The many causes include infection; trauma; toxins, such as lead; acquired metabolic disorders; vascular disease; and hypoxia. It has been suggested that, in young children, the degree of intellectual dysfunction that is produced is related more to the amount of tissue destroyed than to the area of brain that is damaged (Chadwick et al., 1981). Damage is likely to be greater during the period of rapid growth (Rutter et al., 1983).

A controversial issue concerns the ability of environmental stimuli to modify the developing brain. Those who accept the idea of a sociocultural basis for mild retardation in many families with poor socioeconomic backgrounds point to animal studies in which overcrowding produced greater cell packing and less neuropil in the cortex than in the cortex of controls raised with smaller numbers of animals in each cage. Environmental stimuli in early life can influence the development of dendrites, the number of synapses in the cortex, and synaptic connections, and they may provide an anatomic basis for retar-

dation secondary to sociocultural deprivation. Certainly, children who undergo extreme deprivation are frequently backward in verbal skills, social interactions, and motor control (Avery, 1985; Werner et al., 1967). Many children who have lived in a deprived environment for long periods have damage that is not reversible. Extreme sociocultural deprivation is usually associated with nutritional deprivation and failure to thrive (Dodge et al., 1975). Thus, multiple variables influence brain development, and their effects often cannot be isolated from one another.

The association of a postnatal insult with a prenatal insult often has a devastating effect on mental development. This is clearly brought out in rodents in which the most serious consequences to brain development come from combining prenatal and postnatal undernutrition. The whole is frequently greater than the sum of each part.

IDIOPATHIC MENTAL RETARDATION

Idiopathic mental retardation usually affects children who have IQ values above 50. Pathology in this group is not well described. In profoundly or severely retarded children who have no known cause for the disability, studies have shown that there can be an abnormality in dendritic growth and organization. Huttenlocher (1974) noted that horizontal and tangential branches of apical dendrites are decreased in number and in length. There is also a decrease in the number of basal dendrites and their secondary branches, especially those arising directly from the perikaryon. He could find no changes in children with relatively mild mental retardation. Purpura (1974a,b) found similar dendritic abnormalities in children with profound mental retardation and believed that the more severe the intellectual deficit, the more prominent the abnormalities in cortical organization.

At the present time, there is too little quantitative information about brain structure and mental dysfunction to propose a relationship that includes children who are mildly retarded. It is not known how many cells or how many synapses on a cell need to be present for the brain to function properly or how many cells need to interact with one neuron to elicit proper responses. These subtle changes in structure probably define the limits of idiopathic retardation.

TREATMENT

The treatment of mental retardation is based directly on our limited understanding of pathophysiology. Generally, the treatment is prevention because destroyed brain cannot be restored. Many disorders that produce mental retardation, whether they are chromosomal, metabolic, structural, or destructive, can be diagnosed in utero and, if the family so desires, prevented by an abortion. In other instances, the chances of recurrence of the defect can be calculated and the family can decide whether to have more children. Certain metabolic and endocrine disorders can be prevented or ameliorated by dietary control or hormonal replacement early in the perinatal period. Infants at high risk for hypoxic damage or trauma at time of birth may have that risk lowered if they are delivered by cesarean section.

A major question still vexes neurologists and those in associated disciplines. Can the ultimate level of intellectual functioning be modified by early infant and childhood stimulation programs? The most objective answer would appear to be no, despite the animal literature cited earlier, suggesting that early stimulation should result in the modification of the dendritic architecture of the cortex. The subject is critically reviewed by Arendt et al. (1988). Apparently, these modifications are not sufficient to have a lasting effect on intelligence. However, such programs may have a permanent effect on behavior by giving the child from a deprived social background enough information and sufficient interest to function in a regular class.

References

(Key references are designated with an asterisk.)

*Adams R.D., Lyon G. *Neurology of Hereditary Metabolic Diseases of Children.* New York, McGraw-Hill, 1982.

Akesson H.O. Traditional views and new perspectives on the genetics of mild mental retardation. *Ups. J. Med. Sci. Suppl.* 44:30–33, 1987.

Altman, J. Morphological and behavioral markers of environmentally induced retardation of brain development: an animal model. *Environ. Health Perspect.* 74:153–168, 1987.

*Arendt R.E., MacLean W.E. Jr., Baumeister A.A. Critique of sensory integration therapy and its application in mental retardation. *Am. J. Ment. Retard.* 92:401–429, 1988.

Arveiler D., Alembik Y., Hanauer A., et al. Linkage analysis suggests at least two loci for X linked nonspecific mental retardation. *Am. J. Med. Genet.* 30:473–483, 1988.

Avery G. Effects of social, cultural and economic factors on brain development. In Freeman J.M., ed. *Prenatal and Perinatal Factors Associated with Brain Disorders.* Washington, DC, U.S. Public Health Service, NIH Publication No. 85–1149, pp. 163–176, 1985.

Balazs R. Hormonal aspects of brain development. In Cavanaugh J.B., ed. *The Brain: In Unclassified Mental Retardation.* Baltimore, Williams & Wilkins, pp. 61–72, 1972.

Ballabio, A., Bardoni, B., Carrozzo R., et al. Contiguous gene syndromes due to deletions in the distal short arm of the human X chromosome. *Proc. Natl. Acad. Sci. U.S.A.* 86:10001–10005, 1989.

Banik N.L., Davison, W.N., Palo J., et al. Biochemical studies on myelin isolated from brains of patients with Down's syndrome. *Brain* 98:213–218, 1975.

Barlow C.F. *Mental Retardation and Related Disorders.* Philadelphia, Davis, 1978.

Barth P.G. Disorders of neuronal migration. *Can. J. Neurol. Sci.* 14:1–16, 1987.

Bender B.L., Yunis E.J. The pathology of tuberous sclerosis. *Pathol. Annu.* 17(Part I):339–382, 1982.

*Berenberg S.R., ed. *Brain, Fetal and Infant: Current Research on Normal and Abnormal Development.* The Hague, Martinus Nijhoff, 1977.

Bersena N.H. Severe mental retardation among children in a Danish urban area: assessment and etiology. In Miller P., ed.

Frontiers of Knowledge of Mental Retardation. Vol. 2. *Biomedical Aspects.* Baltimore, University Park Press, pp. 53–61, 1980.

Bickel H. Recent advances in the early detection and treatment of inborn errors with brain damage. *Neuropaediatrie* 1:1–11, 1969.

Bickel H., Bachmann C., Beckers R., et al. Neonatal mass screening for metabolic disorders. *Eur. J. Pediatr.* 137:133–139, 1981.

Brann A.W. Jr. Factors during neonatal life that influence brain disorders. In Freeman J.M., ed. *Prenatal and Perinatal Factors Associated with Brain Disorders.* Washington, DC, U.S. Public Health Service, NIH Publication No. 85–1149, pp. 263–357, 1985.

Burstein J., Papile L.A., Burstein R. Intraventricular hemorrhage and hydrocephalus in premature infants: a prospective study with CT. *Am. J. Radiol.* 132:631–635, 1979.

Byrd S.E., Naidich T.P. Common congenital brain anomalies. *Radiol. Clin. North Am.* 26:755–772, 1988.

Chadwick O., Rutter M., Thompson J., et al. Intellectual performance and reading skills after localized head injury in childhood. *J. Child Psychol. Psychiatry* 22:117–139, 1981.

Chaney R.H., Eyman R.K. Etiology of mental retardation: clinical vs. neuroanatomic diagnosis. *Ment. Retard.* 20:123–127, 1982.

Chaney R.H., Givens C.A., Watkins G.P., et al. Birth injury as the cause of mental retardation. *Obstet. Gynecol.* 67:771–775, 1986.

Cohen M.M. Jr. Perspectives on holoprosencephaly. Part I. Epidemiology, genetics and syndromology. *Teratology* 40:211–235, 1989.

Cordero M.E., Trejo M., Colombo M., et al. Histological maturation of the neocortex in phenylketonuric rats. *Early Hum. Dev.* 8:157–173, 1983.

Costeff H., Cohen B.E., Weller L.E. Biological factors in mild mental retardation. *Dev. Med. Child Neurol.* 25:580–587, 1983.

Cotman C.W., Nieto-Sampedro M. Cell biology of synaptic plasticity. *Science* 225:1287–1294, 1984.

Covert C. *Mental Retardation: A Handbook for the Primary Physician: Report of the American Medical Association Conference on Mental Retardation, April 1964.* Chicago, American Medical Association, 1964.

Cowan W.M., Fawcett J.W., O'Leary D.D.M., et al. Regressive events in neurogenesis. *Science* 225:1258–1265, 1984.

Cremer J.E., Teal H.M., Cunningham V.J. Inhibition by 2-oxoacids that accumulate in maple-syrup-urine disease of lactate, pyruvate and 3-hydroxybutyrate transport across the blood-brain barrier. *J. Neurochem.* 39:674–677, 1982.

Crome L. Non-specific developmental abnormalities in unclassified mental retardation. In Cavanaugh J.B., ed. *The Brain: In Unclassified Mental Retardation.* Baltimore, Williams & Wilkins, pp. 283–289, 1972.

Crome L., Stern J. *The Pathology of Mental Retardation.* London, Churchill Livingstone, 1973.

Dambska M., Wisniewski K., Sher J.H. Lissencephaly: two distinct clinicopathological types. *Brain Dev.* 5:302–310, 1983.

Davison A.N., Dobbing J. Myelination as a vulnerable period in brain development. *Br. Med. Bull.* 22:40–44, 1966.

DiMauro S., Bonilla E., Lombes A., et al. Mitochondrial encephalomyopathies. *Neurol. Clin.* 8:483–506, 1990.

Dobyns W.B. The neurogenetics of lissencephaly. *Neurol. Clin.* 7:89–105, 1989.

*Dodge P.R., Prensky A.L., Feigin R.D. *Nutrition and the Developing Nervous System.* St. Louis, Mosby, 1975.

Drillien C.M. Prenatal and perinatal factors in etiology and outcome of low birth weight. *Clin. Perinatol.* 1:197–211, 1974.

Drillien C.M., Jameson S., Wilkinson E.M. Studies in mental handicap. Part I. Prevalence and distribution by clinical type and severity of defect. *Arch. Dis. Child.* 41:528–538, 1966.

Dunn V., Mock T., Bell W.E., et al. Detection of heterotopic gray matter in children by magnetic resonance imaging. *Magn. Reson. Imaging* 4:33–39, 1986.

Dupont A. 140 years of Danish studies on the prevalence of mental retardation. *Acta Psychiatr. Scand. Suppl.* 348:105–112, 167–178, 1989.

Dyken P., Krawiecki N. Neurodegenerative diseases of infancy and childhood. *Ann. Neurol.* 13:351–364, 1983.

Elejald B.R., Opitz J.M. Clinical cytogenetics. Part 2. *Postgrad. Med.* 63:207–209, 212–214, 1978.

Escalona S.K. The present state of knowledge and available

techniques in the area of cognition. In Purpura D.P., Reaser G.P., eds. *Methodological Approaches to the Study of Brain Maturation and Its Abnormalities*. Baltimore, University Park Press, pp. 135–140, 1974.

Escalona S.K. Babies at double hazard: early development of infants at biologic and social risk. *Pediatrics* 70:670–676, 1982.

Fabregues I., Ferrer I., Cusi M.V., et al. Fine structure based on the Golgi method of the abnormal cortex and heterotopic nodules in pachygyria. *Brain Dev.* 6:317–322, 1984.

Fadel H.E. Antenatal diagnosis of fetal intracranial anomalies. *J. Child Neurol.* 4(Suppl.):107–112, 1989.

Ferrer I., Galofre E. Dendritic spine anomalies in fetal alcohol syndrome. *Neuropediatrics* 18:161–163, 1987.

Finer N.N., Robertson C.M., Richards R.T., et al. Hypoxic-ischemic encephalopathy in term neonates: perinatal factors and outcomes. *J. Pediatr.* 98:112–117, 1981.

*Freeman J.M., ed. *Prenatal and Perinatal Factors Associated with Brain Disorders*. Washington, DC, U.S. Public Health Service, NIH Publication No. 85–1149, April 1985.

*Friede R.L. *Developmental Neuropathology*. New York, Springer-Verlag, 1975.

Fryers T., Mackay R.I. The epidemiology of severe mental handicap. *Early Hum. Dev.* 3:277–294, 1979.

Galjaard H., Reuser A.J.J. Genetic storage disorders. *Curr. Opin. Pediatr.* 1:428–435, 1989.

Garik T.J., Linzey E.M., Freeman R.K., et al. Fetal heart rate patterns and fetal distress in fetuses with congenital anomalies. *Obstet. Gynecol.* 53:716–720, 1979.

Giannelli F., Morris A.H., Garrett C., et al. Genetic heterogeneity of X-linked mental retardation with fragile X. Association of tight linkage to factor IX and incomplete penetrance in males. *Ann. Hum. Genet.* 51:107–124, 1987.

*Gierer A. Spatial organization and genetic information in brain development. *Biol. Cybern.* 59:13–21, 1988.

Gillberg C., Svenson B., Carlstrom G., et al. Mental retardation in Swedish urban children: some epidemiological considerations. *Appl. Res. Ment. Retard.* 4:207–218, 1983.

Gilles F.H. Neuropathological indicators of abnormal development. In Freeman J.M., ed. *Prenatal and Perinatal Factors Associated with Brain Disorders*. Washington, DC, U.S. Public Health Service, NIH Publication No. 85–1149, pp. 53–107, 1985.

*Gilles F.H., Leviton A., Dooling E.C. *The Developing Human Brain: Growth and Epidemiologic Neuropathology*. Boston, John Wright, 1983.

Goldman-Rakic P.S. Circuitry of the primate prefrontal cortex and the regulation of behavior by representational knowledge. In Mountcastle V., Plum K.F., eds. *Handbook of Physiology*. Section 1. *The Nervous System*. Vol. V. *Higher Functions of the Brain*. Bethesda, American Physiological Society, pp. 373–417, 1987a.

*Goldman-Rakic P.S. Development of cortical circuitry and cognitive function. *Child Dev.* 58:601–622, 1987b.

Goldstein R. Humoral mediation of the development of the mammalian nervous system. *Endocrinologie* 24:237–243, 1986.

Goonewardena P., Dahl N., Gustavson K.H., et al. DNA studies of X-linked mental retardation associated with a fragile site at Xq27.3. *Ups. J. Med. Sci. Suppl.* 44:155–164, 1987.

Grimm V.E. Effect of teratogenic exposure on the developing brain: research strategies and possible mechanisms. *Dev. Pharmacol. Ther.* 10:328–345, 1987.

Gustavson K.-H., Hagberg B., Hagberg G., et al. Severe mental retardation in a Swedish county. II. Etiologic and pathogenetic aspects of children born 1959–1970. *Neuropaediatrie* 8:293–304, 1977.

Gustavson K.-H., Holmgren G., Blomquist H.K. Chromosomal aberrations in mildly mentally retarded children in a northern Swedish county. *Ups. J. Med. Sci. Suppl.* 44:165–168, 1987.

Guthkelch A.N. Occipital cranium bifidum. *Arch. Dis. Child.* 45:104–109, 1970.

Hagberg B. Pre- and perinatal environmental origin in mild mental retardation. *Ups. J. Med. Sci. Suppl.* 44:178–182, 1987.

Hagberg B., Kyllerman M. Epidemiology of mental retardation—a Swedish survey. *Brain Dev.* 5:441–449, 1983.

Hagberg B., Hagberg G., Lewerth A., et al. Mild mental retardation in Swedish school children. *Acta Paediatr. Scand.* 70:441–452, 1981.

Hanson J.W., Myrianthopoulos N.C., Harvey M.A.S., et al. Risks to the offspring of women treated with hydantoin anticonvulsants, with emphasis on the fetal hydantoin syndrome. *J. Pediatr.* 89:662–668, 1976.

Hanson J.W., Streissguth A.P., Smith D.W. The effects of moderate alcohol consumption during pregnancy on fetal growth and morphogenesis. *J. Pediatr.* 92:457–460, 1978.

Herschkowitz N. Brain development in the fetus, neonate and infant. *Biol. Neonate* 54:1–19, 1988.

Holst K., Andersen E., Philip J., et al. Antenatal and perinatal conditions correlated to handicap among 4-year-old children. *Am. J. Perinatol.* 6:258–267, 1989.

Hook E.B. Chromosomal abnormality rate at amniocentesis and in live-born infants. *J.A.M.A.* 249:2034–2038, 1983.

Hurley L.S. Trace elements and teratogenesis. *Med. Clin. North Am.* 60:771–778, 1976.

Huttenlocher P.R. Dendritic development in neocortex of children with mental defect and infantile spasms. *Neurology (Minneap.)* 24:203–210, 1974.

Ivy G.O., Schottler F., Wenzel J., et al. Inhibitors of lysosomal enzymes: accumulation of lipofuscin-like dense bodies in the brain. *Science* 226:985–987, 1984.

Jacobs P.A., Matsumura J.S., Mayer M., et al. A cytogenetic survey of an institution for the mentally retarded: 1. Chromosome abnormalities. *Clin. Genet.* 13:37–60, 1978.

Jaffe M., Borochowitz Z., Dar H. Diagnostic approach to the etiology of mental retardation. *Isr. J. Med. Sci.* 20:136–140, 1984.

Johnson R.T. Teratogenic effects of viruses. In Vinken P.J., Bruyn G.W., eds. *Handbook of Clinical Neurology*. Vol. 34. Amsterdam, North Holland, pp. 369–389, 1978.

Kahkonen M., Leisti J., Thoden C.J., et al. Frequency of rare fragile sites among mentally subnormal school children. *Clin. Genet.* 30:234–238, 1986.

Kalter H., Warkany J. Congenital malformations. Etologic factors and their role in prevention. *N. Engl. J. Med.* 308:424–431, 491–497, 1983.

Kaveggia E.G., Durkin M.V., Pendleton E., et al. Diagnostic genetic studies on 1,224 patients with severe mental retardation. *Proceedings of the Congress of the International Association for Scientific Study of Mental Deficiency*. The Hague, Holland, September 4–12, 1973. Warsaw, Polish Medical Publishers, 1973.

Kidd J.W. Toward a more precise definition of mental retardation. *Ment. Retard.* 2:209–212, 1964.

Kikkawa K., Narahara K., Kimoto H. A cytogenetic study of nonpolymalformed patients with mental retardation of clinically undefined etiology: application of a high resolution banding technique. *Acta Med. Okayama* 43:105–114, 1989.

Knoll J.H., Nicholls R.D., Magenis R.E., et al. Angelman and Prader-Willi syndromes share a common chromosome 15 deletion but differ in parental origin of the deletion. *Am. J. Med. Genet.* 32:285–290, 1989.

Krishnan B.R., Ramesh A., Kumari M.P., et al. Genetic analysis of a group of mentally retarded children. *Indian J. Pediatr.* 56:240–250, 1989.

Lacey D.J. Hippocampal dendritic abnormalities in a rat model of phenylketonuria. *Ann. Neurol.* 16:577–580, 1984.

Lamont M.A. The socio-familial background and prevalence of medical aetiological factors in children attending ESN/M schools. *J. Ment. Defic. Res.* 32:221–232, 1988.

*Lauder J.M., Krebs H. Humoral influences on brain development. *Adv. Cell. Neurobiol.* 5:3–51, 1984.

Lejeune J. On the mechanism of mental deficiency in chromosomal diseases. *Hereditas* 86:9–14, 1977.

Levy H.L. Genetic screening. *Adv. Hum. Genet.* 4:1–104, 1973.

Levy H.L., Waisbren S.E. Effects of untreated maternal phenylketonuria and hyperphenylalaninemia on the fetus. *N. Engl. J. Med.* 309:1269–1274, 1983.

Lou H.C., Lassen N.A., Friis-Hansen B. Impaired autoregulation of cerebral blood flow in the distressed newborn. *J. Pediatr.* 94:118–121, 1979.

*Lund R.D. *Development and Plasticity of the Brain: An Introduction*. New York, Oxford University Press, 1978.

Mabry C.C., Denniston J.C., Nelson T.L., et al. Maternal phenylketonuria. A cause of mental retardation in children without the metabolic defect. *N. Engl. J. Med.* 269:1404–1408, 1963.

Machado-Salas J.P. Abnormal dendritic patterns and aberrant spine development in Bourneville's disease—a Golgi survey. *Clin. Neuropathol.* 3:52–58, 1984.

Marchal G., Andermann F., Tampieri D., et al. Generalized cortical dysplasia manifested by diffusely thick cerebral cortex. *Arch. Neurol.* 46:480–484, 1989.

Matti I., ed. *Study on the Origins of Mental Retardation. Clinics in Developmental Medicine.* Vol. 51. Spastics International Publications. London, Heinemann, 1974.

Mealey J. Jr., Dzenitis A.J., Hockey A.A. The prognosis of encephaloceles. *J. Neurosurg.* 32:209–218, 1970.

*Moser, H.W. Peroxisomal disorders. *Curr. Opin. Pediatr.* 1:284–289, 1989.

Moser H.W., Wolf P.A. The nosology of mental retardation: including the report of a survey of 1378 mentally retarded individuals at the Walter E. Fernald State School. *Birth Defects* 7:117–134, 1971.

Moser H.W., Mihalik S.J., Watkins P.A. Adrenoleukodystrophy and other peroxisomal disorders that affect the nervous system, including new observations on L-pipecolic acid oxidase in primates. *Brain Dev.* 11:80–90, 1989.

Msall M., Batshaw M.L., Suss R., et al. Neurologic outcome in children with inborn errors of urea synthesis: outcome of urea cycle enzymopathies. *N. Engl. J. Med.* 310:1500–1505, 1984.

Mulcahy M., O'Connor S., Reynolds A. Census of the mentally handicapped in the Republic of Ireland, 1981. *Ir. Med. J.* 76:71–75, 1983.

Mulley J.C., Gedeon A.K., Thorn K.A., et al. Linkage and genetic counselling for the fragile X using DNA probes 52A, F9, DX13 and ST14. *Am. J. Med. Genet.* 27:435–440, 1987.

Naughten E.R., Jenkins J., Francis D.E., et al. Outcome of maple syrup urine disease. *Arch. Dis. Child.* 57:918–921, 1982.

Nelson K.B., Browman S.H. Perinatal risk factors in children with serious motor and mental handicaps. *Ann. Neurol.* 2:371–377, 1977.

Nelson K.B., Ellenberg J.H. Apgar scores as predictors of chronic neurologic disability. *Pediatrics* 68:36–44, 1981.

Niswander K., Elbourne D., Redman C., et al. Adverse outcome of pregnancy and the quality of obstetric care. *Lancet* 1:827–830, 1984.

Noetzel M.J. Neural tube defects and other congenital and genetic disorders. *Curr. Opin. Pediatr.* 1:308–311, 1989.

Nunez J. Effects of thyroid hormones during brain differentiation. *Mol. Cell. Endocrinol.* 37:125–132, 1984.

Oberlie I., Heilig R., Moisan J.P., et al. Genetic analysis of the fragile X mental retardation syndrome with two flanking polymorphic DNA markers. *Proc. Natl. Acad. Sci. U.S.A.* 83:1016–1020, 1986.

Opitz J.M. The developmental field concept in clinical genetics. *J. Pediatr.* 101:805–809, 1982.

Pajari M., Oja S.S. Mutual inhibition of incorporation into protein of branched-chain amino acids in brain homogenates of developing and adult rats. *Neurochem. Int.* 5:213–220, 1983.

Paneth N., Stark R.I. Cerebral palsy and mental retardation in relation to indicators of perinatal asphyxia. *Am. J. Obstet. Gynecol.* 147:960–966, 1983.

Patel M., Arinze I.J. Phenylketonuria: metabolic alterations induced by phenylalanine and phenylpyruvate. *Am. J. Clin. Nutr.* 28:183–188, 1975.

Prensky A.L., Dodson W.E. Prenatal factors affecting future development. In Thompson R.A., Green J.R., eds. *Pediatric Neurology and Neurosurgery.* New York, SP Medical and Scientific Books, pp. 1–57, 1978.

Prensky A., Palkes H.S. *Care of the Neurologically Handicapped Child.* New York, Oxford University Press, 1982.

Prensky A.L., Carr S., Moser H.W. Development of myelin in inherited disorders of amino acid metabolism: a biochemical investigation. *Arch. Neurol.* 19:552–558, 1968.

Prensky A.L., Fishman M.A., Daftari B. Differential effects of hyperphenylalaninemia on the development of the brain of the rat. *Brain Res.* 33:181–191, 1971.

Purpura D.P. Morphological studies of brain maturation: approaches, advantages and limitations. In Purpura D.P., Reaser G.P., eds. *Methodological Approaches to the Study of Brain Maturation and Its Abnormalities.* Baltimore, University Park Press, pp. 75–84, 1974a.

*Purpura D.P. Dendritic spine dysgenesis and mental retardation. *Science* 186:1126–1128, 1974b.

Purpura D.P., Suzuki K. Distortion of neuronal geometry and formation of aberrant synapses in neuronal storage disease. *Brain Res.* 116:1–21, 1976.

Rabinowicz T., Leuba G., Heumann D. Morphologic maturation of the brain: a quantitative study. In Berenberg S.R., ed. *Brain, Fetal and Infant: Current Research on Normal and Abnormal Development.* The Hague, Martinus Nijhoff, pp. 28–53, 1977.

Raiti S., Newns G.H. Cretinism: early diagnosis and its relation to mental prognosis. *Arch. Dis. Child.* 46:692–694, 1971.

Riccardi V.M., Mulvhill J.J., eds. *Neurofibromatosis (von Recklinghausen Disease): Genetics, Cell Biology and Biochemistry. Advances in Neurology.* Vol. 29. New York, Raven Press, 1981.

Richardson S.A. Issues in the definition of mental retardation and the representativeness of studies. *Res. Dev. Disabil.* 10:285–294, 1989.

Rorke L.B. Nervous system lesions in the congenital rubella syndrome. *Arch. Otolaryngol.* 98:249–251, 1973.

Rosen M.G. Factors during labor and delivery that influence brain disorders. In Freeman J.M., ed. *Prenatal and Perinatal Factors Associated with Brain Disorders.* Washington, DC, U.S. Public Health Service, NIH Publication No. 85–1149, p. 237–261, 1985.

Rosenberg R.N. The triumph of linkage analysis (editorial). *Ann. Neurol.* 27:111–112, 1990.

Rutter M., Chadwick O., Shaffer D. Head injury. In Rutter M., ed. *Developmental Neuropsychiatry.* New York, Guilford Press, pp. 83–111, 1983.

Schochet S.S., Jr., Lampert P.W., McCormick W.F. Neurofibrillary tangles in patients with Down's syndrome: a light and electron-microscopic study. *Acta Neuropathol.* 23:342–346, 1973.

*Schreppers-Tijdink G.A., Curfs L.M., Wiegers A., et al. A systematic cytogenetic study of a population of 1170 mentally retarded and/or behaviorally disturbed patients including fragile X screening. The Hondsberg experience. *J. Genet. Hum.* 36:425–440, 1988.

Shaw C.M. Correlates of mental retardation and structural changes of the brain. *Brain Dev.* 9:1–8, 1987.

Smith D.W., Bostian K.E. Congenital anomalies associated with idiopathic mental retardation. *J. Pediatr.* 65:189–197, 1964.

*Snider W.D., Johnson E.M. Jr. Neurotrophic molecules. *Ann. Neurol.* 26:489–506, 1989.

Spero D.A., Yu M.C. Effects of maternal hyperphenylalaninemia on fetal brain development: a morphological study. *Exp. Neurol.* 79:655–665, 1983.

Stagno S., Pass R.F., Alford C.A. Perinatal infections and maldevelopment. *Birth Defects* 17:31–50, 1981.

Stoltenburg-Didinger G., Spohr H.L. Fetal alcohol syndrome and mental retardation: spine distribution of pyramidal cells in prenatal alcohol-exposed rat cerebral cortex: a Golgi study. *Dev. Brain Res.* 11:119–123, 1983.

Susser M., Hauser W.A., Kiely J.L., et al. Quantitative estimates of prenatal and perinatal risk factors for perinatal mortality, cerebral palsy, mental retardation and epilepsy. In Freeman J.M., ed. *Prenatal and Perinatal Factors Associated with Brain Disorders.* Washington, DC, U.S. Public Health Service, NIH Publication No. 85–1149, pp. 359–439, 1985.

Sutherland G.R. The fragile X chromosome. *Int. Rev. Cytol.* 81:107–143, 1983.

Tarby T.J., Volpe J.J. Intraventricular hemorrhage in the premature infant. *Pediatr. Clin. North Am.* 29:1077–1104, 1982.

Tarjan G., Tizard J., Rutter M., et al. Classification and mental retardation: issues arising in the fifth WHO seminar on psychiatric diagnosis, classification and statistics. *Am. J. Psychiatry* 128(Suppl.):34–45, 1972.

Tarjan G., Wright S.W., Eyman R.K., et al. Natural history of mental retardation: some aspects of epidemiology. *Am. J. Ment. Defic.* 77:369–379, 1973.

Tengstrom C., Autio S. Chromosomal aberrations in 85 mentally retarded patients examined by high resolution banding. *Clin. Genet.* 31:53–60, 1987.

Terplan K.L., Lopez E.C., Robinson H.B. Histologic and structural anomalies of the brain of the trisomy 18 syndrome. *Am. J. Dis. Child.* 119:228–235, 1970.

Thompson R., Huestis P.W., Crinella F.M., et al. The neuroanatomy of mental retardation in the white rat. *Neurosci. Biobehav. Rev.* 10:317–338, 1986.

Thompson R., Huestis P.W., Crinella F.M., et al. Further lesion studies on the neuroanatomy of mental retardation in the white rat. *Neurosci. Biobehav. Rev.* 11:415–440, 1987.

Towbin A. Central nervous system damage in the human fetus and newborn infant: mechanical and hypoxic injury incurred in the fetal-neonatal period. *Am. J. Dis. Child.* 119:529–542, 1970.

Turner G., Brookwell R., Daniel A., et al. Heterozygous expression of X-linked mental retardation and X-chromosome marker fra(X) (q27). *N. Engl. J. Med.* 303:662–664, 1980.

Van den Berghe H., Fryns J.-P., Parloir C., et al. Genetic causes of severe mental handicap: preliminary data from a University of Louvain study. In Miller P., ed. *Frontiers of Knowledge of Mental Retardation.* Vol. 2. *Biomedical Aspects.* Baltimore, University Park Press, pp. 71–79, 1980.

Volpe J.J. Normal and abnormal human brain development. *Clin. Perinatol.* 4:3–30, 1977.

*Volpe J.J. *Neurology of the Newborn.* Philadelphia, Saunders, 1987.

Warkany J. *Congenital Malformation.* Chicago, Year Book Medical Publishers, 1971.

Warkany J., Petering H.C. Congenital malformations of the brain produced by short zinc deficiencies in rats. *Am. J. Ment. Defic.* 77:645–653, 1973.

Werner E., Simonian K., Bierman J.M., et al. Cumulative effect of perinatal complications and deprived environment on physical, intellectual and social development of preschool children. *Pediatrics* 39:490–505, 1967.

Williams R.W., Herrup K. The control of neuron number. *Annu. Rev. Neurosci.* 11:423–453, 1988.

Winick M. *Malnutrition and Brain Development.* New York, Oxford University Press, 1976.

Wolfe A., Cowen D. Perinatal infections of the central nervous system. *J. Neuropathol. Exp. Neurol.* 18:191–243, 1959.

Yakovlev P.I., Wadsworth R.C. Schizencephalies. A study of congenital clefts in the cerebral mantle. I. Clefts with fused lips. II. Clefts with hydrocephalus and lips separated. *J. Neuropathol. Exp. Neurol.* 5:169–206, 1946.

44

The Normal and Abnormal Acquisition of Language

Trevor J. Resnick
Isabelle Rapin

STRUCTURE OF LANGUAGE AND LINGUISTIC OPERATIONS

Language is a socially derived, rule-governed symbolic system of communication used to convey ideas and wants, give orders, make comments, obtain information, and name people, objects, and events. It plays an essential role in social interaction and in thought. Speakers of a common language can engage in meaningful dialogue because they share a common set of word meanings and rules for communication.

Language processing has a number of stages in the brain. Language is encoded at several levels, each of which is rule governed. Although the details of the rules vary considerably from language to language, these linguistic levels are universal across languages.

Levels of Language

Phonology is language at the level of sound. *Phonemes* are the sound units of language. Phonology refers not only to the rules for producing speech sounds that make up words but also to intonation, rhythm, and pauses in speech *(prosody)*.

Morphology refers to the rules for the formation of words and their inflectional endings. *Morphemes* are the smallest linguistic units that have meaning. For example, "books" (book + s) has two morphemes.

This work was supported in part by an epilepsy fellowship from Montefiore Hospital and Medical Center (T.J.R.), by program project grant NS 20489 from the National Institute of Neurologic Diseases and Stroke, and by grants from the Rapaport Foundation and Peggy O'Malley Fund (I.R.). D.A. Allen reviewed the manuscript, which was ably prepared by H. Manigault.

Syntax (grammar) is a set of rules governing the way in which words are combined into well-formed sentences.

Semantics refers to the rules for generating meaningful verbal messages. Speakers of a language carry in their brains a learned repository of word meanings *(lexicon)*. Words may have different meanings in different sentences, as in "this is a telephone" versus "she telephoned me last week."

Pragmatics refers to the rules for using language communicatively. It encompasses verbal features, such as prosody, maintenance of topic, and turn taking, as well as nonverbal elements, such as posture, facial expression, and gesture. These features convey information regarding the intent of the utterance (e.g. criticism, joking, or questioning). Although pragmatics is often referred to as a nonlinguistic aspect of language, it is an integral and vital part of verbal communication.

Operational Stages of Linguistic Processing

Language processing proceeds through a series of operational stages. These take place both sequentially and in parallel, with numerous feedback loops and with interconnections between the processing of each of the language levels. Language can use several media for input (audition, vision, somatesthesia) and output (speech, signs, writing, and braille, as well as the facial and body movements that transmit the speaker's intent). All of these input-output channels are connected to common central language processing systems in the brain.

Sensation refers to the appreciation of the intensity and pitch of sound and to the localization of its source. Impairment of the cochlea or the auditory pathway degrades acoustic sensation. *Auditory perception* presupposes the ability to attend to stimuli, to discriminate speech from nonspeech sounds, and to store them in sequence at different rates and clarity of presentation to compare them with previously stored signals. One or more aspects of auditory perception may be deficient in some children with developmental language disorders (Frumkin and Rapin, 1980; Tallal and Stark, 1981). Whether these auditory perceptual deficits are necessary and sufficient causes of the child's language dysfunction or but one feature of a more complex disorder is debated (Rees, 1973).

Phonologic decoding of speech sounds is complex because discussed phonemes are coencoded rather than each being represented by one discrete sound (see later). The sound signal for a particular phoneme may also vary depending on the context in which it is produced (i.e., on the phonemes that precede or follow it).

Comprehension of a linguistic message involves recognition of its words with reference to words stored in the lexicon. It is also a function of the relationship of words in the sentence or even in several preceding sentences. Comprehension entails decoding at both the semantic and syntactic levels, as well as at the level of pragmatics. Pragmatic decoding necessitates correct assessment of the requirements of communicative context and of the intentions of the speaker, which are signaled by tone of voice, gestures, and facial expression as much as by words.

The *decision* whether and how to respond involves many nonlinguistic functions such as assessment of current needs, value judgment, and prior experience. *Formulation* entails selection and retrieval of words from the lexicon and their organization into a grammatically correct form, transforming thoughts and intentions into formulated language. This formulated language is encoded (i.e., *programmed*) into phonetic sequences that transmit the motor commands for speech production. *Production* engages upper and lower motor neurons to execute the coordinated movements of the oral, facial, and respiratory organs for the production of speech.

SOME BIOLOGIC CORRELATES OF LANGUAGE

Phonemes are coded by brief acoustic signals that comprise at least three bands of acoustic energy at different frequencies. *Formants* have a steady-state portion, lasting 200–300 ms, that carries the acoustic cues for vowels. They also have brief (<50 ms) formant transitions consisting of rapid shifts in frequency at the start or end of steady-state formants that code for consonants (Liberman et al., 1967).

Artificially produced in isolation, formant transitions do not sound like consonants; they do so only when they precede or follow steady-state formants. In short, consonants are coarticulated with vowels into syllables. In contrast, vowel sounds can be produced and perceived in isolation.

Categorical perception is another feature that distinguishes consonants from vowels. So-called stop consonants have well-defined acoustic boundaries. They do not blend into one another as their acoustic properties are changed artificially by computer; one hears either *b* or *p*, *g* or *k*, and *d* or *t*, even if the sound features that differentiate these stop consonants are changed gradually. The time that elapses between the plosive opening of the vocal tract and the onset of the vibration of the vocal cords (voice-onset time) determines which consonant of these pairs is heard. For example, one hears *da* if voice-onset time is less than 25 ms and *ta* if it is more than 45 ms, with an abrupt change centering on 35 ms. Stop consonants also differ by the place within the mouth where they are articulated: *b* and *p* on the lips, *d* and *t* on the alveolar ridge, and *g* and *k* on the soft palate. The place of articulation is coded by differences in the second formant transition and is also perceived categorically. Unlike consonants, vowels are not perceived categorically: one vowel changes gradually into another as the frequency of steady-state formants is changed gradually. This phenomenon is termed *continuous perception*.

Speech perception entails parallel processing and is context bound. The same phoneme (e.g., *d*) is coded by different formant transitions depending on which vowel follows it. Overlapping acoustic cues code several phonemes simultaneously (Liberman, 1970). This multilevel encoding accounts for one's ability to discriminate up to 30 phonemes/second, which would not be possible if phonemes were produced linearly. Consonants are more important than vowels for speech perception. This may be exemplified visually by the following example: *cnsnnts crr mr f th lngstc mssg* versus *ooa ay oe o e iuii eae* (consonants carry more of the linguistic message).

Infants have innate abilities to perceive and discriminate speech sounds. Behavioral studies indicate that, virtually from birth, infants are able to discriminate consonants, vowels, and differences in accent and pitch contour (Morse, 1977). They too perceive consonants categorically (Eimas, 1974; Eimas and Miller, 1980; Eimas et al., 1971). Different acoustic contrasts are linguistically relevant in different languages. Infants can perceive more acoustic contrasts than adults can. If a language does not rely on a particular contrast, a native speaker of the language loses the ability to discriminate this contrast, which has no relevance for her or him. This loss appears to occur as early as the end of the first year (Werker and Tees, 1984).

Hemispheric Specialization

In most persons, the planum temporale, which encompasses the auditory association cortex, has a considerably greater surface area in the left hemisphere than in the right (Geschwind and Levitsky, 1968). Asymmetry of the planum temporale has been noted in the 29-week-old fetus (Chi et al., 1977), suggesting that the asymmetry is genetic. The left hemisphere is more adept than the right at processing brief acoustic signals, including formant transitions. This is shown by dichotic listening tasks, in which competing sounds are presented simultaneously to each of the two ears. Right ear (left hemisphere) advantage exists for consonants, as opposed to vowels, which show no significant ear advantage (Studdert-Kennedy and Shankweiler, 1970).

The dichotic technique has been used to show right ear advantage for verbal stimuli and left ear advantage for music in 3- to 4-month-old infants (Glanville et al., 1977), as well as older children (Kimura, 1963). Even neonates are reported to show evoked potential asymmetry for speech and nonspeech sounds (Molfese, 1983), with greater amplitude over the left hemisphere for speech sounds and over the right for piano chords. Electroencephalographic studies in 6-month-old infants revealed greater desynchronization and suppression of alpha activity over the right hemisphere in response to music and over the left hemisphere in response to speech (Gardiner and Walter, 1977). Although the robustness of some of these behavioral and neurophysiologic findings has been questioned because differences are small and have not been replicated consistently in individual infants and in all studies (Colbourn, 1981), the convergence of findings is persuasive and seems to indicate that cerebral lateralization is present from infancy rather than developing with maturation.

The clinical observation that, in children as in adults, left-sided lesions are much more likely to produce acquired aphasia than right-sided ones (Satz and Bullard-Bates, 1981) is another facet of early hemispheric specialization for language. This commitment seems less absolute in young children than in adults, inasmuch as either hemisphere is able to sustain language acquisition: children with either left or right hemispherectomy carried out in infancy (Dennis and Kohn, 1975), as well as those with right or left infantile hemiparesis (Annett, 1973), typically learn to speak well. Yet there are subtle but definite differences between the effects of left- and right-sided damage: left-sided lesions produce deficits of the more complex syntactic aspects of language. Dichotic listening tasks and hemifield visual stimulation in adults who have undergone commissurotomies for intractable epilepsy show that the isolated right hemisphere comprehends words and short sentences but is unable to process more complex sentences (Zaidel, 1978). The right hemisphere is also inferior for tasks requiring fine-grained phonetic analysis. Not all linguistic functions are lateralized to the left hemisphere, however, in as much as the processing of prosody and of pragmatics takes place preferentially in the right hemisphere (Heilman et al., 1984; Weintraub and Mesulam, 1983).

LANGUAGE ACQUISITION

From birth, the infant starts to develop a communication system with other significant persons in his or her environment. The neonate, whose hearing is essentially mature, has an innate ability to attend to and discriminate speech-like sounds. The infant soon learns to recognize her or his mother's face and its various expressions. The infant smiles and coos responsively, thus giving positive feedback to the caretaker (Beebe et al., 1979; Brazelton et al., 1974). By 6 months, a complex system of communication has evolved between the infant and the caretakers. Taking turns in vocalizations is an example of the infant's early interactions. These nonlinguistic aspects of communication function as the precursors of pragmatics.

During the first year, the infant's vocal activities proceed through a number of stages (Martin, 1981; Stark, 1980). The first is cooing, which is well developed by 3 months and comprises both vowel- and consonant-like sounds. The infant coos playfully when he or she is alone, comfortable, and content; he or she also coos responsively while interacting with a caretaker. Babbling (repetitive consonant-vowel syllables) regularly begins in the latter half of the first year of life. At first, the sounds do not have referents; they appear to represent a child's joyous practicing of various articulated sounds. The child produces a wide range of sound sequences. These increasingly include the rhythms, pauses, intonations, and inflections of the language to which the child is exposed: sounds that do not occur in this language tend to drop out progressively.

Imitation plays an important role in the development of a child's vocalizations. By 9 months of age, the child can actively mimic a sound or action immediately after it has occurred. At a later stage of development, imitation can be delayed; the child can store the memory of an event or sound and is capable of reproducing it at a later time (Piaget, 1962). This internal representation is vital for the development of language, which entails the ability to retain, interpret, and reproduce symbolic information—to attach meaning to word or word to meaning.

With the foundations of pragmatics (interactive communication), practice with articulatory mechanisms (babbling), and the capacity for internal representation, the groundwork is laid for speaking; at about 1 year, the child starts to produce meaningful single-word utterances. The child points to a desired object, which indicates that she or he has discovered the power of symbolic communication over others' behavior. By 18 months or so, he or she has acquired a vocabulary of perhaps 10–50 single words. When the vocabulary has increased to several dozen content words, the child begins to appose them in ordered two-word utterances. At about 2 years of age, he or she progresses to three-word utterances governed by syntactic rules and, by 3 years, is usually producing the unstressed small words (*functors*) and word endings that supplement word order to indicate meaning more precisely (Bates et al., 1988; Brown, 1973; Menyuk, 1969).

Adults addressing toddlers tend to scale down their speech (caretaker speech, or "motherese") (Moskowitz, 1978). They speak slowly and clearly, exaggerate stress, and use a limited vocabulary of concrete referents and short simplified sentences. Yet early language is no mere imitation of adult models. Language acquisition is an active process (Brown, 1973): the child must discover how to segment the stream of speech into words and phrases, what words mean, and how to order words into meaningful sentences. In other words, the native speaker of a language must learn the syntactic rules that enable him or her to utter correct sentences that he or she may never have heard (Chomsky, 1957). How little children accomplish this monumental task easily and universally is not yet understood. In addition to their having an innate capacity for making relevant phonologic discriminations (Eimas et al., 1971), they are sensitive to stress and other prosodic features and to the order of sounds and words (Gleitman and Wanner, 1984). They have the ability to perceive salient features and to make some sense of the world about them. Whether they also have an innate ability for discovering and generating syntactic relations, as proposed by Chomsky (1957), is still debated.

A study of children's errors indicates that, from the start, children's utterances are lawful even when they do not match adult models. The tot's first rules tend to be overgeneralized, until new exemplars force him or her to apply new, more specific rules. For example, at the level of semantics, all men may be called "daddy," and all round objects, "ball." At the level of phonology, children may produce a single sound, *f*, for *f*, *s*, and *th*, or *w* for *w*, *l*, and *r*. There is usually a considerable lag between the child's ability to discriminate phonetic contrasts and her or his ability to produce the corresponding phonemes accurately.

Overextension also applies to syntax: for example, "no" is initially attached to the beginning of the sentence to connote all negative statements. Later, "no go" and "no Jimmy sleep," for example, are replaced by "don't go Mommy" and "Jimmy no sleep" and, much later, by "Jimmy doesn't want to sleep," or "I'm not sleepy." The toddler cannot benefit from correction, because he or she is able to say only what conforms to the rules he or she has internalized (Menyuk, 1969). For example, a child may say "bad boy" consistently when asked to repeat "he isn't a good boy"; this error indicates that the child understands the sentence but has not yet learned the rules for producing negative sentences.

Practice in conversational interaction plays a most important role in language development. Despite the child's seemingly innate capacity to acquire language without special instruction, he or she must hear language to acquire speech. Deaf infants, although they may begin to coo and vocalize like normal infants, decrease their verbal output after a few months, when acoustic feedback becomes increasingly important for language learning. If deaf children are provided with an adequate language model through the visual channel (sign language), they acquire a visual-manual language system in much the same way as hearing children learn to speak (Bonvillian et al., 1983; Klima and Bellugi, 1979).

Children master most of the basic rules of the language to which they are exposed within the first 5 years of life. Essentially, language learning is complete, even though vocabulary continues to increase throughout life, phonologic production may not be perfect for all speech sounds until the early school years, and the sophistication of grammatically complex sentences may not be acquired until the teenage years. Tots are capable of acquiring several languages apparently effortlessly and of learning to speak each of them idiomatically and without a foreign accent. These abilities are markedly curtailed in most older children and adults, in whom cerebral maturation is further advanced or essentially complete.

DYSPHASIC SYNDROMES

Developmental language disability, or dysphasia, refers to deviant or delayed language acquisition in the absence of hearing loss, motor or structural deficit of the oropharynx, or mental deficiency (Tallal, 1988). Emotional deficit almost never offers an adequate explanation of lack of language development but is its frequent concomitant or consequence (Baker et al., 1980). Except in the case of total isolation (Curtis, 1977), normal children learn language even if they are exposed to marginal models, so that purely environmental causes of dysphasia are exceptional (Skuse, 1988). Nonetheless, environment clearly plays a critical part in determining a child's level of cognitive and linguistic competence (Blank and Allen, 1976).

Language and its acquisition call into play such complex operations that it is surprising that it took so long for investigators to identify several different syndromes among dysphasic children. A number of classifications have been proposed (e.g., Aram and Nation, 1982). The nosology proposed by Rapin and Allen (1983, 1986) and Resnick et al. (1984) and described here groups patients according to the language-processing operations and language levels most severely affected. Receptive disorders are considered first, followed by disorders of processing, and finally disorders of expression.

Verbal Auditory Agnosia (Word Deafness)

Children with verbal auditory agnosia are unable to decode the phonologic aspects of language, despite adequate hearing. In very young children, this disorder forestalls comprehension and language development. Consequently, speech is dysfluent, with distorted phonology; children with severe impairment are mute. An older child who acquires the syndrome at an age when language is well developed may insist that he or she cannot hear, even though nonspeech sounds are discriminated; or he or she may complain that he or she hears sounds but is unable to understand what is being said. The child is word deaf, not cortically deaf (Rapin et al., 1977).

The children's visual skills are intact, as are nonverbal pragmatics; as a result, play is often age appropriate and the children communicate by gesture. They should be taught language by supplementing the auditory channel with the visual, using total communication, which encompasses speech and signs produced together, and reading, using a whole-word approach. Even with aggressive educational measures, these children are at high risk for learning disabilities because of inadequate language skills. Onset at a very young age carries a more guarded prognosis for the acquisition of good speech than onset after language skills are well developed (Dulac et al., 1983; Mantovani and Landau, 1980).

Word deafness may be associated with significant behavior problems. Many word deaf children are also autistic; their language disorder is but one feature of a more pervasive brain disorder that impairs socialization, cognitive skills, and affect, as well as language. Word deaf autistic children may remain mute and uncomprehending of speech, despite adequate visual-manual skills that rule out overall mental deficiency.

In some children, word deafness is present from infancy (Worster-Drought and Allen, 1930). In one child, it was associated with old bilateral temporal lobe infarcts encompassing primary and secondary auditory cortex (Landau et al., 1960). The syndrome replicates word deafness in adults with bilateral temporal pathologic alteration, with the crucial difference that the adults remain capable of verbal expression despite their lack of comprehension (Coslett et al., 1984). Adults whose routine language is well established do not depend on feedback to speak, in contrast to young children in whom either acquired deafness or acquired word deafness impairs speech ability promptly and severely.

The syndrome occurs frequently in the context of acquired epileptic aphasia; this is because loss of language may appear concurrently with absence or other seizure types in children whose language development was previously apparently normal or near-normal (Landau and Kleffner, 1957). The children's electroencephalograms typically show bilateral or left temporoparietal spike discharges. These paroxysmal abnormalities may be present only during sleep (Dulac et al., 1983).

Word deafness and epileptic aphasia are not interchangeable terms. Both the paroxysmal discharges and the language deficit may reflect temporal lobe damage or dysfunction; however, the paroxysmal disorder may not cause the phonologic decoding deficit: (1) not all children with word deafness have abnormal electroencephalograms or clinical seizures, (2) seizure control rarely improves language skills dramatically, and (3) there is often a poor correlation between the severity of the electroencephalographic discharges and the language deficit. Furthermore, occasional children with so-called acquired epileptic aphasia have predominantly expressive deficits (Sato and Dreifuss, 1973) and therefore should not be grouped with those with verbal auditory agnosia. A report (Morell et al., 1989) of improvement of the language disorder by surgical means requires confirmation.

Semantic-Pragmatic Syndrome

The semantic-pragmatic syndrome reflects problems with higher-order language processing (Rapin and Allen, 1983). It may not be modality specific, although some children's visual-manual skills are much superior to their auditory-verbal ones. Children comprehend discourse (connected language) inadequately and may respond to single words rather than to entire utterances, which gives their speech a tangential quality. Difficulty with pragmatics makes meaningful communication even more problematic. A characteristic feature is verbosity, with the child speaking aloud on favorite topics without the need for a conversational partner.

The children's comprehension deficit for the more abstract and complex aspects of language, such as drawing inferences, is exemplified by their problems with answering questions, notably "why," "when," and "how" questions. The child may know the answer to a question yet be unable to answer because he or she fails to understand it. For example: "How did you come to the office today?" No answer. "Did you come by bus?" "No." "By train?" "No." "By car?" "Yes." Or: "What is your sister's name?" "I don't know." "Your sister's name is . . . ." "Alissa." This child, who could not process a "how" or "what" question, was able to process the syntactically simpler question requiring a yes or no answer and to fill in the blanks of a declarative sentence with the correct answer. The comprehension deficit of these children is regularly underestimated; this often leads to behavior problems because the child is thought to be stubborn when in fact she or he does not know what is wanted of her or him.

The diagnosis is frequently missed because of the children's well-developed phonologic and syntactic skills. They speak in fluent, well-formed sentences, even though, by history, they often spoke late. Their prosody commonly remains aberrant; it may be singsong or overprecise and wooden. The content of their speech may be sadly lacking and has been compared with cocktail party chatter: they speak to maintain social contact rather than to convey a message.

Some of these children have a superior verbal

memory and repeat verbatim long and complex utterances *(immediate echolalia)*, including some utterances that they could not possibly have understood. They may perseverate and recite overlearned ditties, television commercials, and clichés *(delayed echolalia)*. Confrontation naming is usually intact, yet, paradoxically, the children often have significant word-finding difficulties *(anomia)* in discourse. Anomia in discourse may lead to verbal paraphasic errors or to the use of overlearned utterances as fillers. Perseverative return to favorite topics is often prominent.

The syndrome was originally described in hydrocephalic children (e.g., Swisher and Pinsker, 1971). Although it is characteristic of hyperverbal autistic children, it also occurs in nonautistic children. The semantic-pragmatic syndrome has features that are reminiscent of transcortical sensory aphasia as well as Wernicke's aphasia in adults (Rapin and Allen, 1988) (see Chapter 53).

Semantic Retrieval-Organization Syndrome

Semantic retrieval-organization syndrome is another higher-order processing disorder, also referred to as the lexical-syntactic syndrome, which does not affect pragmatics or phonology (Rapin and Allen, 1986). The children are dysfluent because of word retrieval problems and syntactic difficulties. Like the children with the semantic-pragmatic syndrome, they may have no difficulty naming to confrontation yet have such a severe anomia in discourse as to give the impression of stuttering when they are blocked in retrieving a word. They too make verbal paraphasic errors.

Their expressive syntax is immature and simplified. Typically, their spontaneous speech is superior to their elicited speech, and their sentence repetition is superior to their spontaneous speech. They have great difficulty formulating language, especially when they cannot choose their topic or are constrained by the demands of a conversation or a question. Comprehension of discourse and abstract questions is impaired.

This syndrome is reminiscent of some cases of transcortical motor aphasia in adults (Freedman et al., 1984) (see Chapter 53). It is common in both autistic and nonautistic children and is regularly the prelude to deficits in reading comprehension.

Mixed Expressive-Receptive Disorder (Phonologic Syntactic Syndrome)

Mixed expressive-receptive disorder is the most common dysphasic syndrome and resembles Broca's aphasia in adults (see Chapter 53). Speech is dysfluent, with faulty articulation and simplified, deviant syntax. Discourse has a telegraphic quality, lacking little *(closed class* or *function)* words such as

auxiliaries, prepositions, pronouns, and articles. Word inflection (morphology) is also defective. Comprehension is variably affected but equal to or superior to production, a distinguishing feature from verbal auditory agnosia. Comprehension of function words may be selectively impaired; for example, when asked "Where do you wear your mittens?" a child responded "When it snows."

Speech is used communicatively and is often augmented with gestures and signs. Many of the children have associated motor deficits, such as clumsiness and late walking, as well as oromotor problems that are not severe enough to account for their dysfluency. All but the most seriously affected children learn to express themselves verbally by school age. Prognosis is most closely related to the extent of the comprehension deficit. Most children are at risk for later learning disabilities and dyslexia (Rapin, 1982a,b).

Expressive Syndromes

Expressive deficit syndromes are confined almost entirely to the production of language. The children's ability to formulate speech sounds is defective. Comprehension and pragmatics are typically unaffected or affected to a much lesser degree than in the other dysphasic syndromes.

There are two types of expressive syndrome. In one, the children have minimal, highly dysfluent speech or are nonverbal. Comprehension is intact and gestures are used to communicate. Semantics and expressive syntax cannot be assessed because speech is so sparse. Oromotor problems such as drooling, pseudobulbar paresis, and oromotor dyspraxia may be associated but, when present, are not sufficiently severe to account for the child's inability to speak. The children are often able to imitate speech sounds in isolation but not in connected speech. Their production problems may be context bound, in that they are able to utter certain sounds in some speech contexts but not in others. This syndrome has been called *verbal* (not oromotor) *dyspraxia* (Ferry et al., 1975).

It is essential to provide these children with a channel for expression to lessen their frustration and attendant behavior problems. This is especially important because the prognosis for the development of fluent speech is guarded. Children with this syndrome can make excellent use of communication boards. Some are able to learn to read and write. Those who do not have a severe manual dyspraxia can acquire signs; few become proficient signers, but few have had adequate exposure to fluent signing. Some children learn to say their first words only after they have acquired them through signed or written language. Children with this syndrome resemble adults with aphemia who cannot speak but remain able to read and write (Schiff et al., 1983), rather than patients with Broca's aphasia who make the same errors in their written as in their oral speech.

A second group of children with a relatively isolated expressive deficit are quite fluent but largely unintelligible. They speak in long sentences. Speech sounds are distorted; there are sequencing errors and omissions. Syntax may be difficult to assess; if affected, it is simplified rather than deviant. Pragmatics and comprehension are intact. Children with this form of expressive syndrome, called the *speech-programming deficit syndrome*, usually persevere in their efforts to communicate and are not as frustrated as those with the nonverbal form of expressive disorder. Prognosis is usually quite good.

PATHOPHYSIOLOGIC CORRELATES OF DYSPHASIA

Although the receptive-expressive model of adult aphasia also pertains to the disorders of language acquisition, comparisons between disorders of developing and fully developed language remain tentative (Caramazza and Zurif, 1978; Rapin and Allen, 1988). Adult aphasics have sustained focal brain lesions, whereas computed tomography rarely discloses them in dysphasic children, notwithstanding the child with bilateral lobe porencephalies (Landau et al., 1960). Of course, a normal computed tomographic scan does not rule out microscopic developmental anomalies of the type described in a patient with dyslexia (Galaburda and Kemper, 1978). Unusual patterns of hemispheric asymmetry have been reported both in dysphasic, dyslexic children (Hynd and Semrud-Clikeman, 1989; Jernigan et al., 1991) and in autistic children (Damasio et al., 1980), but their relevance to these disorders is uncertain. Such findings are not helpful in an individual child, because they are inconstant and may be found in normal persons.

Dysphasia is not a single condition with a single cause (Tallal, 1988). Identifying the cause of the brain dysfunction responsible for a particular dysphasic syndrome is not as critical for understanding its pathophysiology as is determining what part of the language processing system is dysfunctional. Some investigators suggest that developmental language disorder is more often the result of a maturational lag than of brain pathologic change; even if this view is correct, it is a lag in the maturation of a particular brain system, so that questions concerning the identity of this system are still relevant.

The marked preponderance of boys over girls among dysphasics, a preponderance that also exists among autistic and dyslexic children, argues for a genetic cause in some of them. A common genetic cause can be expected to result in a behaviorally homogeneous dysphasic syndrome, as has been found to be the case in a familial dyslexia linked to the short arm of chromosome 15 (Smith et al., 1983). For example, children with Prader-Willi syndrome, half of whom have a deletion in the long arm of chromosome 15, often have a severe expressive language disability (Holm et al., 1981). The study of genetically and clinically homogeneous syndromes can be informative about the genetic programs that control language development.

Because brain pathologic alteration is rarely selective (unless it is a biochemical lesion restricted to a particular neurotransmitter or cell type), obvious or subtle nonlinguistic dysfunctions are often encountered in dysphasic children. Well-controlled and well-executed topographic studies of event-related potentials, power spectrum of the electroencephalogram, and cerebral blood flow and metabolism, which are carried out in children with homogeneous language syndromes while they are performing language-related tasks, hold the promise of providing more direct evidence regarding localization of brain dysfunction than do the associated sensorimotor and cognitive neuropsychologic deficits.

Children with expressive deficits are more likely than those with receptive ones to have motor signs suggesting frontal involvement. ^{133}Xe inhalation tomography carried out in three children with verbal dyspraxia and normal computed tomographic scans revealed bilateral frontal and, in one case, left perisylvian hypoperfusion; naming did not increase perfusion in Broca area. Three children with the phonologic-syntactic syndrome had both perisylvian hypoperfusion and lack of activation of the Broca area (Lou et al., 1984).

Autistic children do not have selective impairment of expressive language. Their comprehension is always impaired at some level, ranging from phonology to discourse. Their language deficits can take the form of all of the dysphasic syndromes described above, except for the two purely expressive ones. Autistic children are autistic *and* dysphasic, at least in the preschool years (Allen, 1988). Even hyperverbal autistic children with the semantic-pragmatic syndrome tend to acquire language late. Hydrocephalic children, in whom the white matter of the posterior part of the hemispheres is most severely affected, may also have the semantic-pragmatic syndrome but usually without autistic behaviors. This syndrome, like transcortical sensory aphasia, may reflect intracortical or corticosubcortical disconnection of the language areas.

Phonologic decoding is presumed to take place in the auditory association cortex, which is often the site of epileptic discharges in word deafness. A child with word deafness had hypoperfusion of both temporal lobes and lack of activation of either Wernicke or Broca areas during attempts at word naming (Lou et al., 1984). Five adults with partial or complete recovery from childhood verbal auditory agnosia had persistent deficits in phonologic discrimination tasks associated with deviant electrophysiologic activity over auditory association areas during the performance of these tasks (Klein et al., unpublished observations).

Brain stem auditory evoked potentials are unaffected in most if not all dysphasic and autistic children (Klin, 1991). Reports of abnormalities (e.g., Mason and Mellor, 1984; Piggot and Anderson, 1983) should be viewed cautiously. Brain stem auditory evoked potentials, together with reliable behavioral audiometry, are a first step in the evaluation of all young children with delayed or inadequate language definition, so as to avoid missing an unsuspected hearing loss.

A number of behavioral studies demonstrate auditory processing deficits in language-disordered children. For example, dysphasic children, as a group, had difficulty discriminating and ordering nonverbal stimuli, compared with age-matched controls, but had no deficit when rate of presentation was slowed or when the stimuli were visual. These same children had trouble discriminating between consonants but not vowels. Their ability to discriminate consonants improved dramatically when the short formant transitions that characterize different consonants were artificially lengthened (Tallal and Stark, 1981). This finding was replicated in seven children with language disorders whose phonology was defective, but not in nine who had normal articulation; these nine children had no difficulty with consonants but did with the order of stimuli. Four children with word deafness were quite unable to discriminate consonants, only one of them improving when the formant transitions were stretched (Frumkin and Rapin, 1980). These differences among groups of dysphasic children once again underline the importance of grouping children according to homogeneous syndromes when one is attempting to delineate the fundamental deficit that underlies their language disorder.

References

(Key references are designated with an asterisk.)

Allen D.A. Autistic spectrum disorders: clinical presentation in preschool children. *J. Child Neurol.* 3(Suppl.):S48–S56, 1988.

Annett M. Laterality of childhood hemiplegia and the growth of speech and intelligence. *Cortex* 9:4–33, 1973.

Aram D.M., Nation E. *Child Language Disorders*. St. Louis, Mosby, 1982.

Baker L., Dennis P.C., Mattison R.E. Behavior problems in children with pure speech disorders and in children with combined speech and language disorders. *J. Abnorm. Child Psychol.* 8:245–256, 1980.

Bates E., Bretherton I., Snyder L. *From First Words to Grammar: Individual Differences and Dissociable Mechanisms*. New York, Cambridge University Press, 1988.

Beebe B., Stern D., Jaffe J. The kinesic rhythm of mother-infant interactions. In Siegman A.W., Feldstein S., eds. *Of Speech and Time: Temporal Patterns in Interpersonal Contexts*. Hillsdale, NJ, Erlbaum Associates, pp. 23–34, 1979.

Blank M., Allen D. Understanding why: its significance in early intelligence. In Lewis M., ed. *Origins of Intelligence: Infancy and Early Childhood*. New York, Plenum Publishing, pp. 259–278, 1976.

Bonvillian J.D., Orlansky M.D., Novack L.L. Developmental milestones: sign language acquisition and motor development. *Child Dev.* 54:1435–1445, 1983.

Brazelton T.B., Koslowski B., Main M. The origins of reciprocity: the early mother-infant interaction. In Lewis M., Rosenblum L.A., eds. *The Effect of the Infant on its Caregiver*. New York, Wiley, pp. 49–76, 1974.

Brown R. *A First Language: The First Stages*. Cambridge, MA, Harvard University Press, 1973.

Caramazza A., Zurif E.B., eds. *Language Acquisition and Language Breakdown: Parallels and Divergencies*. Baltimore, Johns Hopkins University Press, 1978.

Chi J.G., Dooling E.C., Gilles F.H. Left-right asymmetries of the temporal speech areas of the human fetus. *Arch. Neurol.* 34:346–348, 1977.

Chomsky N. *Syntactic Structures*. The Hague, Mouton, 1957.

Colbourn C. What can laterality measures tell us about hemispheric functions during child development? In Lebrun Y., Zangwill O., eds. *Lateralization of Language in the Child*. Lisse, Swets and Zeitlinger, pp. 92–102, 1981.

Coslett H.B., Brashear H.R., Heilman K.M. Pure word deafness after bilateral primary auditory cortex infarcts. *Neurology (N.Y.)* 34:247–252, 1984.

Curtis S. *Genie: A Psycholinguistic Study of a Modern Day Wild Child*. New York, Academic Press, 1977.

Damasio H., Maurer R.G., Damasio A.R., et al. Computerized tomographic scan findings in patients with autistic behavior. *Arch. Neurol.* 37:504–510, 1980.

Dennis M., Kohn B. Comprehension of syntax in infantile hemiplegics after cerebral hemidecortication: left hemisphere superiority. *Brain Lang.* 2:472–486, 1975.

Dulac O., Billard C., Arthuis M. Aspects électro-cliniques et évolutifs de l'épilepsie dans le syndrome aphasie-épilepsie. *Arch. Fr. Pediatr.* 40:299–308, 1983.

Eimas P.D. Auditory and linguistic processing of cues for place of articulation by infants. *Percep. Psychophys.* 16:513–521, 1974.

Eimas P.D., Miller J.L. Contextual effects in infant speech perception. *Science* 209:1140–1141, 1980.

Eimas P.D., Siqueland E.R., Jusczyk P., et al. Speech perception in infants. *Science* 171:303–306, 1971.

Ferry P.C., Hall S.M., Hicks J.L. Dilapidated speech: developmental verbal dyspraxia. *Dev. Med. Child Neurol.* 17:749–756, 1975.

Freedman M., Alexander M.P., Naeser M.A. Anatomic basis of transcortical motor aphasia. *Neurology (N.Y.)* 34:409–417, 1984.

Frumkin B.A., Rapin I. Perception of vowels and consonant-vowels of varying duration in language impaired children. *Neuropsychologia* 18:443–454, 1980.

Galaburda A.M., Kemper T.L. Cytoarchitectonic abnormalities in developmental dyslexia: a case study. *Ann. Neurol.* 6:94–100, 1978.

Gardiner M.F., Walter D.O. Evidence of hemispheric specialization from infant EEG. In Harnad S., Doty R.W., Goldstein L., et al., eds. *Lateralization in the Nervous System*. New York, Academic Press, pp. 481–500, 1977.

Geschwind N., Levitsky W. Left/right asymmetries in temporal speech region. *Science* 161:186–187, 1968.

Glanville B., Best C., Levenson R. A cardiac measure of cerebral asymmetry in infant auditory perception. *Dev. Psychol.* 13:54–59, 1977.

Gleitman L.R., Wanner E. Current issues in language learning. In Bornstein M., ed. *Developmental Psychology*. Hillsdale, NJ, Erlbaum Associates, pp. 181–242, 1984.

Heilman K.M., Bower D., Speedie L., et al. Comprehension of affective and non-affective prosody. *Neurology (N.Y.)* 34:917–921, 1984.

Holm V.A., Sulzbacher S.J., Pipes P.L., eds. *Prader-Willi Syndrome*. Baltimore, University Park Press, 1981.

Hynd G.W., Semrud-Clikeman M. Dyslexia and brain morphology. *Psychol. Bull.* 106:447–482, 1989.

Jernigan T.L., Hesselink J.R., Sowell E., et al. Cerebral structure on magnetic resonance imaging in language- and learning-impaired children. *Arch. Neurol.* 48:539–545, 1991.

Kimura D. Speech lateralization in young children as determined by an auditory test. *J. Comp. Physiol. Psychol.* 56:899–902, 1963.

Klima E.S., Bellugi U. *The Signs of Language*. Cambridge, MA, Harvard University Press, 1979.

Klin A. Auditory brain stem response in autism: brain stem dysfunction or peripheral hearing loss? *J. Autism Dev. Disord.* (in press).

Landau W.M., Kleffner F.R. Syndrome of acquired aphasia with convulsive disorder in children. *Neurology (Minneap.)* 7:523–530, 1957.

Landau W.M., Goldstein R., Kleffner F.R. Congenital aphasia: a clinicopathological study. *Neurology (Minneap.)* 10:915–921, 1960.

*Liberman A.M., Cooper F.S., Shankweiler D.P., et al. Perception of the speech code. *Psychol. Rev.* 74:431–461, 1967.

Liberman A.M. The grammars of speech and language. *Cogn. Psychol.* 1:301–323, 1970.

Lou H.C., Henriksen L., Brunn P. Focal cerebral perfusion in children with dysphasia and/or attention deficit disorder. *Arch. Neurol.* 41:825–829, 1984.

Mantovani J.F., Landau W.M. Acquired aphasia with convulsive disorder: course and prognosis. *Neurology (N.Y.)* 30:524–529, 1980.

Martin J.A.M. *Voice, Speech, and Language in the Child: Development and Disorder.* New York, Springer-Verlag, 1981.

Mason S.M., Mellor D.H. Brain stem, middle latency and late cortical evoked potentials in children with speech and language disorders. *Electroencephalogr. Clin. Neurophysiol.* 59:297–309, 1984.

Menyuk P. *Sentences Children Use.* Cambridge, MA, M.I.T. Press, 1969.

Molfese D.L. Neural mechanisms underlying the processing of speech information in infants and adults: suggestion of differences in development and structure from electrophysiological research. In Kirk U., ed. *Neuropsychology of Language, Reading, and Spelling.* New York, Academic Press, pp. 109–128, 1983.

Morrell F., Whisler W.W., Smith M.C., et al. Landau-Kleffner syndrome: treatment with multiple subpial transections. *Epilepsia* 30:693, 1989.

*Morse P.A. Infant speech perception. In Sanders D.A., ed. *Auditory Perception of Speech.* New York, Prentice Hall, pp. 161–176, 1977.

Moskowitz B.A. The acquisition of language. *Sci. Am.* 239(5):92–108, 1978.

Piaget J. *Play, Dreams and Imitation in Childhood.* New York, Norton, 1962.

Piggot L.R., Anderson T. Brainstem auditory evoked responses in children with central language disturbance. *J. Am. Acad. Child Psychiatry* 22:535–540, 1983.

Rapin I. *Children with Brain Dysfunction: Neurology, Cognition, Language, and Behavior.* New York, Raven Press, 1982a.

Rapin I. Developmental language disorders and brain dysfunction as precursors of reading disability. In Wise G.A., Blaw M.E., Procopis P.G., eds. *Topics in Child Neurology.* Vol. 2. New York, Spectrum Publications, pp. 177–193, 1982b.

*Rapin I., Allen D.A. Developmental language disorders: nosologic considerations. In Kirk U., ed. *Neuropsychology of Language, Reading, and Spelling.* New York, Academic Press, pp. 155–184, 1983.

Rapin I., Allen D.A. The physician's assessment and management of young children with developmental language disorders. *Pädiat. Fortbildk. Praxis* 60:1–12, 1986.

Rapin I., Allen D.A. Syndromes in developmental dysphasia and adult aphasia. In Plum F., ed. *Language, Communication, and the Brain.* New York, Raven Press, pp. 57–75, 1988.

*Rapin I., Mattis S., Rowan A.J., et al. Verbal auditory agnosia in children. *Dev. Med. Child Neurol.* 19:192–207, 1977.

Rees N.S. Auditory processing factors in language disorders. The view from Procrustes' bed. *J. Speech Hear. Disord.* 38:304–315, 1973.

Resnick T.J., Allen D.A., Rapin I. Disorders of language development: diagnosis and intervention. *Pediatr. Rev.* 6:85–92, 1984.

Sato S., Dreifuss F.E. Electroencephalographic findings in a patient with developmental expressive aphasia. *Neurology (Minneap.)* 23:181–185, 1973.

Satz P., Bullard-Bates C. Acquired aphasia in children. In Sarno H.T., ed. *Acquired Aphasia.* New York, Academic Press, pp. 399–426, 1981.

Schiff H.B., Alexander M.P., Naesser M.A., et al. Aphemia: clinical-anatomic correlations. *Arch. Neurol.* 40:720–727, 1983.

Skuse D.H. Extreme deprivation in early childhood. In Bishop D., Mogford K., eds. *Language Development in Exceptional Circumstances.* Edinburgh, Churchill Livingstone, pp. 29–46, 1988.

Smith S.D., Kimberling W.J., Pennington B.F., et al. Specific reading disability: identification of an inherited form through linkage analysis. *Science* 219:1345–1347, 1983.

Stark R.E. Stages of speech development in the first year of life. In Yeni-Komshian G.H., Kavanagh J.F., Ferguson C.A., eds. *Child Phonology.* Vol. 1. *Production.* New York, Academic Press, pp. 73–92, 1980.

Studdert-Kennedy M., Shankweiler D. Hemispheric specialization for speech perception. *J. Acoust. Soc. Am.* 48:579–597, 1970.

Swisher L.P., Pinsker E.J. The language characteristics of hyperverbal hydrocephalic children. *Dev. Med. Child Neurol.* 13:746–755, 1971.

Tallal P. Developmental language disorders. In Kavanagh J.F., Truss T.J. Jr., eds. *Learning Disabilities: Proceedings of the National Conference.* Parkton, MD, York Press, pp. 181–272, 1988.

Tallal P., Stark R.E. A reexamination of some non-verbal perceptual abilities of language-impaired and normal children as a function of age and sensory modality. *J. Speech Hear. Res.* 24:351–357, 1981.

Weintraub S., Mesulam M.-M. Developmental learning disability of the right hemisphere: emotional interpersonal, and cognitive components. *Arch. Neurol.* 40:463–468, 1983.

Werker J.F., Tees R.C. Cross-language speech perception: evidence for perceptual reorganization during the first year of life. *Infant Behav. Dev.* 7:49–63, 1984.

Worster-Drought C., Allen I.M. Congenital auditory imperception (congenital word-deafness): and its relation to idioglossia and other speech defects. *J. Neurol. Psychopathol.* 10:193–236, 1930.

Zaidel E. Lexical organization in the right hemisphere. In Buser P.A., Rougeul-Buser A., eds. *Cerebral Correlates of Conscious Experience.* New York, Elsevier North Holland Biomedical Press, pp. 263–284, 1978.

45

Developmental Dyslexia

Martha Bridge Denckla
Judith M. Rumsey

DEFINITION

Developmental dyslexia is defined as a chronic constitutional condition characterized by difficulty with using written language (acquisition of reading skill being the index in childhood) that cannot be attributed to sensory impairment, limited intellect, emotional disturbance, educational deprivation, or *acquired* neurologic disorder. Despite all these exclusions, the constitutional element is presumed to be of central nervous system origin, although the definition (simply put) states only reading failure unexpected on the basis of intelligence level. Historically, developmental dyslexia has strong neurologic connections and continues to be the developmental disability that has been most intensively investigated by the neurosciences community.

One diagnostic point is a certainty: dyslexia should never be confused with the more inclusive plural-member diagnostic category learning disabilities. Dyslexia is only one, albeit the best known, of the several learning disabilities.

HISTORY

The first report of congenital word blindness (Morgan, 1896) made an overt analogy to then-recent concepts of acquired alexia, reflected not only in Morgan's choice of diagnostic label but also in the focus on the left angular gyrus.

Hinshelwood (1917) summarized 14 case reports of congenital word blindness resembling acquired left angular gyrus lesion cases in the "purity of symptoms . . . and the gravity of the defect." Gradually, the term *dyslexia* came to be preferred, and the term *word blindness* has been rarely used since the 1917 monograph.

The connection between research concerning dyslexia and neurologic concepts of alexia (Déjèrine, 1891) led to tacit acceptance of a brain basis for dyslexia in most special education literature and inspired much research on a neuropsychologic level. By 1937, another neurologist, Orton, formulated a theory of dyslexia that had two elements: (1) that reading disability was but the most visible and quantifiable aspect of a more generalized disorder of language and (2) that lack of clear and customary cerebral dominance, with consequent confusion about directional issues (e.g., *b* versus *d* and left versus right), characterized and underlaid dyslexia. The phenomenology of the second point, called descriptively *strephosymbolia* (meaning twisted symbols), so captured the public imagination that it overshadowed the great insights of Orton that related language inefficiency to anomalous cerebral dominance. Orton (1937) accepted the earlier interpretation that the angular gyrus was the critical region to be scrutinized but stressed that "deviation in the process of establishing unilateral brain superiority in individual areas" such as the angular gyrus, rather than maldevelopment of the left angular gyrus per se, might be due to "hereditary facts." Orton identified a spectrum of non–retarded developmental disabilities other than dyslexia, including developmental agraphia, dyscalculia, dyspraxia, and combinations of these. Orton's influence has persisted in special education and has been rehabilitated by Geschwind (Geschwind and Galaburda, 1987).

Epidemiologic studies (Spreen, 1989) provide confirmation of the probability that some neurologic explanation for dyslexia must be reasonable to seek, because there is an excess of cases of specific reading retardation beyond what a normal distribution curve for any specific ability predicts; there is a pathologic excess of unexpectedly poor readers.

CONCEPTS OF DEVELOPMENTAL DYSLEXIA

The neurologic dysfunction hypothesis regarding dyslexia has been aided by the renaissance of behavioral neurologic models (Geschwind and Behan, 1982; Geschwind and Galaburda, 1985, 1987), neuropsychologic approaches to the reading process, and more recently, application of studies involving in vivo anatomy (computed tomography, magnetic resonance imaging [MRI]) and neurophysiology (brain electrical mapping, ^{133}Xe regional cerebral blood flow measurement, and positron emission tomography) to the behavioral analyses. Persistent language inefficiencies (as a behavioral basis) and a left hemispheric lesion (as a neuroanatomic and neurophysiologic substrate) have most often, and with remarkable consensus, been the focus of neurologic thinking about dyslexia. Perhaps most influential of all thinking about dyslexia, among behavioral neurologists, was Geschwind's interest in a theory of how dyslexia is a consequence of a developmental anomaly or the almost incidental by-product of a different type of brain architecture. Briefly, Geschwind put together the phenomena related to dyslexia in terms of male preponderance, nonverbal giftedness, and a familial (not necessarily intraindividual) associated context of non–right-handedness and disorders of the immune system; he then synthesized an epigenetic theory of dyslexia, such that *immune* and *endocrine* factors operating during fetal life act on neuronal populations to "sculpt" diverse brains, conceptualized in the case of dyslexia as "specialized" toward more right hemisphere–mediated, nonverbal talents (Geschwind and Galaburda, 1985).

Through further histopathologic research, in animals as well as in accumulated human postmortem specimens, Galaburda refined and elucidated Geschwind's hypothetic formulation of the neurodevelopmental basis of dyslexia (Galaburda et al., 1986, 1987). It is of note that Geschwind's concept of the relevant genetics was a systemic, not a specifically brain-restricted view (i.e., that genetic variations of hormonal and immune systems affected the intrauterine environment in which brain development takes place) (see under Genetics). According to this theory, dyslexia is only one among several developmental disabilities that, perhaps on the basis of time periods (windows) of exposure to similar hormones or immune factors, could be produced even within the same sibship!

DIAGNOSIS

Although it appears simple enough to state that developmental dyslexia means unexpected reading failure, in practice (clinically or in research endeavors) it is no easy matter to decide whom to call dyslexic (Felton and Wood, 1989; Pennington, 1991;

Shaywitz et al., 1990; Vellutino and Denckla, 1991). It is uncomfortable for medically trained diagnosticians to depend on tests such as IQ and reading achievement measurement, such laboratory data being outside the usual medical education; thus, in *International Classification of Diseases*, Ninth Revision, Clinical Modification (ICD-9-CM) or *Diagnostic and Statistical Manual of Mental Disorders*, Third Edition, Revised (DSM-III-R), diagnostic codes for specific reading disability (the nearest one can come to dyslexia in a clinical practice manual), discrepancy between measures of intelligence and academic achievement is essentially the diagnostic approach. Little or nothing is said about personal or family history, the contexts of the measures, the problematic nature of the measures of intelligence and reading, as variables that change in their significance during the developmental and experiential life span, is not acknowledged. This decontextualization of laboratory data that are inherently rather mystifying to the medical clinician makes the diagnosis of dyslexia difficult and controversial.

Each research paper, likewise, must be read with consideration of the precise set of measurements (IQ, reading level) employed, the age and sex distribution and the educational experience of the subjects, and the criteria used to exclude, or filter, overlapping conditions. At the least, IQ must be viewed as a rough and potentially misleading index, not a constant value; and the range of tasks that may be described as reading must be appreciated as being diverse in demands. Both IQ and reading measures are environmentally influenced outcome measures, far removed from neurobiologic factors.

Issues of Overlap

Even after settling issues of measurement discrepancy (referable to establishing that reading achievement is significantly and unexpectedly lower than that predicted from intelligence) and factoring in personal (speech and language delay) and familial (speech, language, reading, spelling, and foreign language) underachievement as convergent confirmatory evidence, there remain issues of overlap and heterogeneity (see Denckla, 1985) in the diagnosis. The latter (heterogeneity) is discussed under Neuropsychology of Developmental Dyslexia. The issue of overlap remains a significant and serious one both in research and in clinical practice. The overlap is with the cognitive aspect of the DSM-III-R diagnostic category attention-deficit hyperactivity disorder (ADHD) and exemplifies current controversy about whether, or to what extent, ADHD is a learning disability or is a comorbid condition. Silver (1990) unequivocally separated ADHD as a comorbid condition because, in his view, it does not represent "one of the psychological processes necessary for learning."

Processes, however, are not synonymous with

processing; the latter term, *processing*, is commonly used by nonmedical professionals to refer to content domains (language and perception, auditory or visual) handled, or processed, presumably by the central nervous system. The term *processes* (whether preceded by the adjective psychologic, neuropsychologic, or cognitive) is commonly used in a broader sense that generally includes attention, intention, integration, and motor processes. In this sense, the opposing view to that of Silver (1990) would use the word processes to point out that *attention deficit* represents a zone of impaired cognitive process that extends into learning disability.

Multiple researchers have confronted this zone of overlap with respect to dyslexia. Hughes and Denckla (1978) suggested that *dyslexia-pure* should be distinguished by ADHD exclusion from *dyslexia-plus*; many researchers have employed this filtering approach and terminology. Significantly, the concern with overlap of attention deficit and dyslexia has come from many researchers who independently discovered the problem within their own data sets (Felton and Wood, 1989; Shaywitz et al., 1990).

Gender Ratio

Shaywitz et al. (1990) reported that school-identified samples of children with reading disability "are almost unavoidably subject to a referral bias" such that boys, because of "an excess of activity and behavior problems," are more often included. By contrast, research-identified samples reveal no significant differences in male and female prevalences of reading disability. This study is important because it reveals that the overlap of hyperactive characteristics and dyslexia, or dyslexia-plus, affects the sex ratio issue, which in turn influences conceptualization about the cause of the disorder. Pragmatically, this study suggests underserving of girls with reading disability but exemplary outward appearance of attentiveness and physical self-control; it does not, however, resolve the research question about cognitive aspects that may be shared by dyslexic boys and girls (i.e., disorders of self-regulation [attention, inhibition] and of executive function [planning, organization]).

Attentional and Inhibitory Inefficiencies Coexisting with Language Deficit (Dyslexia-Plus)

Whenever any aspect of ADHD is diagnosed in a child with a school-identified problem, the clinician is inevitably faced with the issue of stimulant medication. This situation arises daily in a clinic devoted to the evaluation of school problems.

Patients have report cards showing poor reading and spelling from the start of formal schooling and complaints that they get little out of reading, take inordinate amounts of time to read what is required, and/or "hate reading." They may or may not have test data yielding a discrepancy-based diagnosis of dyslexia (this is more often absent if patients are brighter or older); the direct cognitive assessment often yields significant attentional and organizational deficits (Denckla, 1989) without necessarily meeting the full-blown ADHD criteria threshold. The clinician attempts to understand the yearly changes in severity and the fundamental mechanisms whereby patients experience symptomatic distress in the acquisition and use of written language. In the authors' experience, the most common ingredients in dyslexia, in varying proportions, are language deficit and attentional inefficiency. That is, dyslexia-plus is far more common than dyslexia-pure, especially if *assessed* inattention is a component.

This is not an original observation, only a refinement of what led, in 1962, to the term *minimal brain dysfunctions* (later, minimal brain dysfunction, and now no longer used). The hyperactive component became overidentified with the advent of stimulant treatment (Wender, 1971). In 1962, however, minimal brain dysfunctions included the large group of dyslexia-plus disorders (i.e., dyslexia and hyperactivity) (Clemens and Peters, 1962). The more subtle cognitive element (as in Felton and Wood, 1989) applies to that group of patients who do not necessarily meet DSM-III-R diagnostic criteria for hyperactive.

Developmental dyslexia is now almost universally conceptualized as a subtle language-processing deficit syndrome. This is the basis for and outcome of the family studies undertaken by geneticists and genetic epidemiologists. This has long been the clinical rationale for inquiry into familial language achievements, ranging from delays in talking to failure in foreign language study. Unestablished, however, to date, is the threshold value at which subtle no longer describes the individual's language status, so that a spoken language disorder (whether expressive, receptive, or mixed) is the requisite diagnosis and dyslexia is only a symptom of that disorder. In other words, how normal must spoken language capabilities be to highlight written language as the deficient domain?

At first glance, this seems like an easy enough issue to resolve: simply set a basal level requirement for verbal IQ. Yet verbal IQ is not what it appears to be, especially in developmental disability related to elements of language. Astoundingly, youngsters routinely attain respectably average verbal IQ scores but, when assessed by language tests, score as much as 5 years below age expectation on one or more of these basic elements of language (phonology, semantics, syntax, and pragmatics). In developmental assessments, one often sees a whole that *is* more than the sum of its parts, a verbal intelligence score surpassing specific constituent spoken language competencies. Which of these spoken language competencies must be intact to preserve the notion of non–language-disordered but dyslexic diagnosis is not explicitly addressed in current literature, as few studies of dyslexic persons include a spoken language assessment per se, other than spoken language measures that are the foci of the research as dependent variables. So, although past speech and language delays in a dyslexic individual are respected as historical convergent data, a concurrent spoken language disorder as a disqualifying or overlapping (comorbid) diagnosis is not an explicit concern of research or clinical practice. Yet the educational prognosis for those with dyslexia may be powerfully influenced by the coexistence of spoken language deficiencies.

Diagnostic Guidelines: Summary

1. The acquisition and use of written language should stand out as *the* overriding and lifelong concern, even if other academic areas are somewhat problematic (but less so).

2. Personal history of preschool language inefficiency and family history of disorders of language acquisition and achievement should be solicited as convergent evidence of a biobehavioral at-risk status.

3. Assessments that document certain language deficits and inefficiencies and that may additionally document attentional or organizational dysfunctions should be ordered to provide laboratory data. Suggested neuropsychologic or cognitive assessment components (as constructs, not specific instruments) are reviewed later.

NEUROPSYCHOLOGY OF DEVELOPMENTAL DYSLEXIA: WHAT IS THE DOMAIN OF COGNITIVE DEFICIT?

For a thorough review of neuropsychologic issues, the reader is referred to Vellutino and Denckla (1991). In summary thereof, it may be stated that the cognitive psychology of reading is among the best developed in the field, far ahead of what is the state of the art with respect to any other learning disorder. In the past 2 decades, a convergent consensus has established that dyslexia (which means difficulty with words, after all) is basically a subtle language disorder; importantly—and despite lingering popular emphasis on reversals (such as *b* versus *d*) that on the surface appear visual in nature—dyslexia is *not* a disorder of visual and certainly not of visual-*spatial* processing. Other neurologic and cognitive explanations in the literature on dyslexia range from faulty eye movements to faulty general rule learning, running the gamut from motor to conceptual levels as the domains of neuropsychologic deficit.

Part of the reason for the many types and levels of deficits brought forth as explanations for dyslexia is related to the diagnostic and definitional issues discussed earlier. Insensitivity to such "fuzzy borders," indicated by lack of acknowledgment thereof in the literature on dyslexia, remains a serious source of confusion. This confusion not only hampers etiologically oriented research but also has an impact on therapeutic trials (see under Treatment). The major point is that none of the other explanations of dyslexia can claim the convergent, replicable empirical evidence available for a role of language deficit. Furthermore, the common core *within* linguistic explanations appears to be phonologic (speech sound) processing skills (Pennington, 1991). Although reading as a complex processing-of-information system involves oculovisuomotor directional consistency, visual perception (discrimination between symbols and words), visual memory, and the ability to detect and represent the visual-structural conventions of written language, these aspects (even if somewhat impaired) appear to present relatively minor, and transient obstacles to the acquisition of reading skill. Adequate development in both semantic (meaningful) and phonologic aspects of language appears from current evidence to be of most lasting import for reading skill. Of lesser, but possibly of contributory, compensatory, and ancillary importance *when* speech sound awareness or analysis is shaky, are speech-motor and visuographomotor abilities involved in, respectively, enunciating and writing words.

Word identification, or word recognition, the basic association of a visual symbol with a spoken sound, lies at the heart of reading. Skill in written word identification essentially entails retrieval either of spoken words (collections of speech sounds) or word meanings (referents that are directly imaged). The former is a surface operation, possible even for contrived nonsense words or foreign language words pronounceable by virtue of shared symbol-sound relationships. The latter is a deep association among a set of visual characters, a structural pattern, and an external referent. The problem with deep reading is that the little functor words (e.g., "the," "and," and "in") lack imageable external referents. Functor words exist largely within spoken language; some research suggests that the skilled grammarian (i.e., a person with solid linguistic skill at the syntactic level) may compensate by sentence completion for lack of direct surface symbol-sound decoding of "if's, and's, or but's" (Vellutino and Denckla, 1991). As with speech-motor and visuographomotor contributions to total reading success, competence with grammar may be more important in terms of available compensatory mechanisms than in terms of the common core of dyslexic deficit.

Poor readers as a group tend to be inefficient or inept with respect to phonologic processing of printed words, and convergent evidence that phonologic deficits directly cause poor reading is powerful. Even if adults with dyslexic past histories have adequate compensatory mechanisms, they often evidence poor word attack when meaning is removed from the printed words and phonologic processing (speech sound awareness and analysis) is paramount. Poor readers are more likely to detect similarities in visual configuration and in meaning of printed words than to detect common characteristics in phonologic attributes of printed words.

Theories about (and evidence appearing to support) deficiencies in more sweeping foundational processes (rule learning, associative learning, and intersensory learning) in dyslexia are suspected to be tainted by an overlap of ADHD and dyslexia. The most articulate of the groups investigating this overlap has been the North Carolina research effort led by Wood. Briefly, this group has shown that, within the verbal domain, dyslexia-pure is characterized by poor word retrieval, whereas ADHD and dyslexia-plus (the combination) are characterized by poor multitrial memorization of word lists, the overserved on-line new acquisition of verbal lists (Felton and Wood, 1989). Memorization, rule learning, associative learning, and the like are heavily identified with the domain that neuropsychologists call *executive function*, an anterior brain–based domain that includes sustained attention, selective attention, inhibition, set maintenance, and organization (Denckla, 1989; Pennington, 1991). This domain of executive function, which is broader than that of attention, may be a codeterminant of poor reading because effective compensatory strategies may exist if criteria for full-blown hyperactive disorders or ADHD are not met. Again, the language deficit and attentional inefficiency aspects of dyslexia-plus must be considered, both causally and therapeutically.

The core locus of deficit in dyslexia-pure is in word recognition by the surface route of phonologic coding. Even if there is a direct deep route to word recognition (and this has been questioned, especially developmentally, as opposed to postlesion circumstances in adults), it is probably a slow route. If spoken equivalence of printed letter strings, or the alphabet as a code for speech sounds, is not automatically and transparently available, reading is perforce slower (compensations use up time), and comprehension may be impeded. Spelling is even more vulnerable because the starting point is on the weak (speech sound) side of the association; poor spelling relative to verbal intelligence, or even relative to adult-acquired reading skill, indicates clinically the type of brain that is dyslexic. The most attenuated end of the spectrum of dyslexia is difficulty in acquiring speaking (not necessarily reading) competence in a foreign language.

How specific, restricted, or modular a domain, cognitively speaking, underlies the concept of dyslexia? Herein is the unsolved dispute about borders (other than the border between ADHD and executive function) regarding spoken language symptoms and syndromes. Clinical and research evidence points to the higher prevalence of spoken language problems in persons with dyslexia; symptoms occur in spontaneous speech and in daily life memory for meaningless sequences (months of year, telephone numbers, and proper names) and are not restricted to encounters with the printed word. These spoken language symptoms surrounding dyslexia are consistent with the construct that the core of the disorder is at the speech sound level rather than at visual, motor, or foundational levels. Problematic, however, is the allowable severity of the spoken language symptoms, the threshold level at which the diagnosis escalates from reading disorder to language disorder. This is not an esoteric concern when considering appropriate educational options.

STUDIES OF DYSLEXIA

Postmortem Studies

Postmortem studies of eight brains from dyslexic patients (six male, two female) by Galaburda (1989) and colleagues yielded two consistent findings. On a macroscopic level, all cases showed symmetry in the language-relevant, usually asymmetric planum temporale. Although not a pathologic finding, this represents a significant increase from the expected frequency (15–25%) in ordinary autopsy studies. Comparing symmetric and asymmetric plana temporale, Galaburda and colleagues (1987) found symmetric to be consistently larger than asymmetric plana, so that an enlarged right planum likely accounts for the symmetry of this structure in dyslexia (Galaburda and Kemper, 1979; Galaburda et al., 1985, 1987; Humphreys et al., 1990).

At a microanatomic level, all specimens showed disorganization of the cortical plate, generally consisting of nests of ectopic neurons in layer I and frequently associated with focally disordered underlying cytoarchitecture. Although these types of anomalies are found in other disorders (epilepsy, mental retardation), ectopic neurons in layer I are infrequent in routine autopsy studies (Galaburda, 1989; Kaufmann and Galaburda, 1989). Although distributions have been widespread, bilateral, and variable across brains, the left perisylvian cortex shows the greatest number of these developmental anomalies in the dyslexic brains.

Focal ectopias in layer I of the cortex and focal cytoarchitectonic abnormalities occur spontaneously in 20–30% of certain immunodefective mice (Sherman et al., 1985, 1987), and therefore, these mice may provide a model for the neuropathologic changes in dyslexic brains. Ectopias in these mice contain both neurons and glia, with some neurons showing abnormal morphologic features. Such ectopias in rat visual cortex reflect reduced cell death and differentiation, rather than simply disordered neuronal migration, and suggest the possibility of a similar mechanism (i.e., reduced cell death) underlying findings of increased planum size without differences in neuronal size or density in dyslexia (Galaburda et al., 1986).

If these focal dysgeneses contain abnormal axonal connections, focal abnormalities of cytoarchitecture may have widespread effects on cortical connectivity. Immunologic mechanisms may be etiologic (Geschwind and Behan, 1982; Pennington et al., 1987).

In addition, two female dyslexic brains and, to a lesser degree, one male brain had myelinated scars within the cortical plate, suggesting injury between the last prenatal trimester and third postnatal year. These scars were restricted to the left hemisphere in one female brain and were located in watershed areas of the three main cerebral arteries, suggesting a vascular mechanism, in the other female brain. One female brain also showed an oligodendroglioma involving the left hippocampus and an arteriovenous malformation (Galaburda, 1989).

Neuroanatomic Imaging

Neuroanatomic imaging in dyslexia began in the 1980s using computed tomographic scanning to examine hemispheric asymmetries, which are hypothesized to differ in dyslexia. Of the studies that examined parieto-occipital asymmetries (Denckla et al., 1985; Haslam et al., 1981; Hier et al., 1978; Leisman and Ashkenazi, 1980; Rosenberger and Hier, 1980), all reported increased incidence of either reversal of the usual left-predominant asymmetry seen most frequently in normal persons or symmetry in this region. Studies reporting reversed asymmetry found that this was related to a history of language delay and low verbal IQ compared with norms of the general population (Hier et al., 1978; Rosenberger and Hier, 1980). Inconsistencies in the studies possibly were due to failures to control for head tilt, bone artifact, and the use of different cutoff points for defining asymmetry. No differences in frontal asymmetry were found in the one computed tomographic study that examined this (Haslam et al., 1981).

Because bone artifact can easily distort or obscure true asymmetries on computed tomographic scans, MRI, which is free of such artifact, is a superior technique for in vivo anatomic studies. Other advantages of MRI include flexibility with respect to imaging planes, the ability to enhance contrast between structures through choice of pulsing sequences, increased resolution, and increased safety (lack of radiation).

The first MRI study of dyslexia (Rumsey et al., 1986) found a high incidence of symmetry of temporal lobe volumes and mild reversals of the usual left-predominant ventricular asymmetry on the basis of evaluations by two radiologists. This study examined healthy but severely dyslexic men without histories of developmental language disorder.

Two controlled, quantitative MRI studies reported unusual asymmetries, as well as other findings, in dyslexia. Duara et al. (1991) reported more rightward asymmetry of midposterior areas in the region of the angular gyrus and increased area of the splenium of the corpus callosum on MRI scans of 29 dyslexic individuals, relative to controls. Hynd and colleagues (1990) reported unusually symmetric anterior brain widths, bilaterally shorter insular regions, and a

shorter left planum temporale in 10 dyslexic children, relative to controls.

Like the dyslexics, 10 children with ADHD showed symmetric anterior brain widths. This finding was due to a reduction on the right side in both dyslexic and hyperactive children. Dyslexic and hyperactive children were distinguished by measures of insular or planar length, however. Nine of 10 dyslexics showed either symmetry or reversed asymmetry of planum length, whereas 70% of both hyperactive and normal children showed a left-predominant asymmetry. Neither dyslexic nor hyperactive children showed unusual posterior asymmetries (of posterior areas or widths) (Hynd et al., 1990).

Limitations include the failure to control for handedness and reliance on a single MRI image without control for head tilt. Three dyslexics were left-handed, whereas all control and hyperactive children were right-handed. Nonetheless, these findings suggest that the application of MRI methods to the study of brain morphologic features in dyslexia holds considerable promise.

Electrophysiology

Electroencephalographic (EEG) abnormalities in dyslexia are most frequently of questionable clinical significance. In a review of electrophysiologic studies of dyslexia, Hughes (1985) reported a 45% mean incidence of EEG abnormalities in dyslexia across 10 studies involving 530 patients. Reported abnormalities include 6–7/second and 14/second positive spikes and excessive occipital slow waves; these patterns may represent normal variants or nonspecific abnormalities. Epileptiform activity is rare. Results of visual and auditory evoked potential studies, also reviewed by Hughes (1985), are variable and inconsistent.

Approaches to identifying electrophysiologic abnormalities in dyslexia include (1) the use of computer-assisted techniques to quantify and topographically map the complex signals contained in multichannel EEG recordings and (2) the use of event-related potentials to study attention and information processing in dyslexia. The former approach breaks the EEG signal into classic frequency bands (spectrum analysis) and evaluates their scalp distribution. The latter focuses on late responses reflecting attention and cognitive processing.

Initial studies of EEG spectra in dyslexic boys (Duffy et al., 1980a,b) reported increased alpha and theta activity, suggesting relative cortical inactivation, in dyslexic boys without attention-deficit disorder, with a widespread distribution of these differences over the medial frontal and left frontal and posterior cortices. Although differences were seen at rest, a variety of activation tasks increased the differences.

More recent studies have shown fewer differences between dyslexics and controls. Studies of resting, nonhyperactive, severely dyslexic boys (Fein et al.,

1986; Yingling et al., 1986) reported lower power across right and left temporal, central, and parietal sites only in the high beta band, with no differences in alpha, theta, or delta. Although the significance of the difference in beta is unclear, the investigators speculated that this may have reflected a lesser capacity for maintaining a quiet, attentive state in the dyslexics. Two cohorts of dyslexic boys studied during narrative speaking and while performing a block design task showed normal patterns of EEG changes, including normal task-dependent asymmetries (Galin et al., 1988). Men with persistent, severe dyslexia studied at rest and during word- and design-recognition tasks showed minimal differences involving increased frontocentral theta and decreased posterior theta (a more activated state) on the more difficult design-recognition task (Rumsey et al., 1989). Because performance did not differ, this result was interpreted as compensatory for less efficient information processing. The word-recognition task elicited even fewer differences between dyslexics and controls.

The degree of cytoarchitectonic disorganization needed to disrupt the normal amplitude and spectrum of the EEG is unknown. EEG spectra reflect the participation of local brain regions but not their competence. Therefore, negative results argue against anomalous patterns of engagement but do not rule out the possibility of a local defect (Galin et al., 1988).

Event-related potential studies also failed to yield consistent findings. Variations in sample and task selection, behavioral performance, data analysis, and other technical aspects make this growing body of literature difficult to reconcile and interpret. Small samples and numerous statistical comparisons increase the likelihood of nonreplicable results. Paradigms yielding replicable results and an understanding of normal developmental effects are needed as a basis for hypothesis testing in dyslexia and other developmental and childhood disorders.

Nonetheless, studies using event-related potentials to compare dyslexic children and those with attention-deficit disorders consistently support the independence of dyslexia and attention-deficit disorder, although not reaching a consensus on the specific nature of the deficits (Harter et al., 1988a,b, 1989; Holcomb et al., 1985, 1986). Both groups show lower amplitude P300s, a nonspecific finding that is characteristic of many clinical syndromes and is thought to index context updating, whereby the subject keeps track of the sequential and probability structure of a series of stimuli (Donchin, 1981). Distinctive effects associated with reading disorder involve reduced P300s to unpronounceable letter strings when compared with nonmeaningful symbols, suggesting a specific deficit in processing word-relevant information. Specific to attention-deficit disorder are stimulus relevance effects, operationalized by comparing responses to target (relevant) stimuli with those to nontarget (irrelevant) stimuli.

Differences between relevant and irrelevant stimuli have been both decreased (Holcomb et al., 1985, 1986) and increased (Harter et al., 1988b) in hyperactive children relative to normal children. Harter et al. (1988b) suggested that this apparent contradiction may be attributable to differences in performance across studies, with decreased responses, accompanied by poorer performance, reflecting deficits and with enhanced responses, accompanied by good performance, reflecting compensatory processing.

Genetics

Considerable progress has been made during the past 10 years or so in defining the genetics and the behavioral phenotype of dyslexia. Studies of familial risk have reported estimates of 35–45% for males and 17–18% for females (Finucci et al., 1976; Vogler et al., 1985; Zahalkova et al., 1972). Both represent clinically significant increases for children with an affected parent when compared with a 5–10% risk for the general population. Within familial samples, the sex ratio (male/female) is approximately 2:1 (DeFries, 1989), considerably lower than the generally accepted 4:1 ratio for the population at large.

Twin studies suggest genetic influences on reading and/or spelling, which frequently remains impaired and dysphonetic in older dyslexics with improved reading (LaBuda et al., 1986; Pennington et al., 1986; Stevenson et al., 1986). Using a statistical technique (multiple regression) for testing genetic and environmental influences on continuous variables (in this case, test scores), DeFries et al. (1987) reported significant heritability for single-word reading recognition, spelling, and digit span, with an estimated heritability of about 30% for this cluster of skills, but a lack of heritability for reading comprehension and perceptual and motor speed, believed to be less affected in dyslexia. Other work (Olson et al., 1989) suggested significant heritability for phonologic coding (measured by nonword reading, which forces a reliance on phonologic rules) and phoneme awareness, but not for orthographic coding (i.e., knowledge of visual-structural conventions of written language, what letters can go together). Thus, what is inherited appears to be a deficit in single-word decoding, attributable to deficient phonologic coding and awareness.

Other work suggested the possibility of linkage to chromosome 15 heteromorphisms in a minority (about 20%) of families with apparent autosomal dominant transmission (Smith et al., 1983), as well as genetic heterogeneity (Smith et al., 1990). Patients whose dyslexia was linked and those whose dyslexia was unlinked to chromosome 15 have been found deficient in phonologic coding for reading and spelling, suggesting a common neuropsychologic pathway to dyslexia despite genetic heterogeneity. Because of associations of dyslexia with immune disorders (Geschwind and Behan, 1982; Pennington et al., 1987), Pennington (1991) is examining a locus near the HLA region on chromosome 6 as a possible second locus.

In summary, at least some dyslexia appears to be genetically based, but variable in mode of transmission, with evidence for major gene effects. The heterogeneity in genotype does not, however, appear to be accompanied by heterogeneity in neuropsychologic or behavioral phenotype. Instead, a common linguistic phenotype involving phonologic coding appears to be the case.

TREATMENT

For the clinician who makes the diagnosis, especially one based in a medical institution, it is frustrating that most of the means of treatment of dyslexic persons of any age are not in the hands of that clinician or under his or her control. The clinician is empowered to do the following, however: (1) establish the comorbidity of ADHD (or other related diagnoses) that may have therapeutic significance; (2) guide patients away from unproven, irrelevant treatments; (3) explain and interpret what dyslexia implies for the person and his or her family (past, present, and future) educationally, genetically, vocationally, psychodynamically, and philosophically; and (4) encourage the patient to act as an educated consumer of educational programs or, when possible, make educational suggestions.

If there is evidence of dyslexia-plus, whether the association is with full-blown ADHD or with executive dysfunction, recommendations referable to (1) stimulant medication, (2) home and school behavioral interventions (provision of support, supervision, or structure), and (3) a form of therapy that addresses organizational or metacognitive skills should be mapped out for the patient. If spoken language difficulty is ascertained to exceed the difficulty with the printed word, particularly in the older student who does not *understand* the instructional spoken language of the academic classroom, major efforts in language therapy and classroom accommodations (alterations in the rate and complexity of presentation, recapitulation) may supersede any reading instructional needs.

The use of nonstimulant medications (such as piracetam, which was tried in the *absence* of sufficient diagnostic sophistication in the 1970s) in dyslexia deserves reevaluation in the light of current conceptual advances in understanding both linguistic and other neuropsychologic factors, and advances in genetics and neuroanatomy.

Many treatments of undocumented efficacy and little or no scientific rationale continue to be popularized. Visual therapies (the use of convergence training, reading glasses that magnify print, eye movement exercises, peripheral field–reading devices, and colored lenses) are unsubstantiated and may be costly in time if not in money. The alleged effects of medications influencing the vestibular system, megavitamin administration, and special diets are similarly unsubstantiated (and often are supported by anecdotes that vaguely confound and conflate all manner of related diagnoses, barely touching on dyslexia). Because childhood is brief and therefore the time is precious, wasting of time in childhood cannot be dismissed as harmless. Medications and diets are even more deserving of scrutiny for physical risk than are exercise or training programs, but all share what is rarely mentioned, psychologic adverse effects, by delivering to those treated false messages about the nature of their problem. The quick, easy answers, implicit or explicit, in many of the noneducational treatments, run counter to the healthy self-knowledge that the dyslexic person needs to absorb.

Explanation and interpretation, not once but periodically (and in some instances, through psychotherapy, regularly and repeatedly) are essentially the delivery of the message, "You are not stupid!" Beyond that, the clinician educates the dyslexic patient as to the familial antecedents, the genetic probabilities for his or her offspring, and the neuropsychologic context. "You are not stupid" expands to "You have a differently built brain; you are specialized in dimensions of intelligence other than phonologic (speech sound) processing!" The balanced homology of the temporal lobes (left, phonologic; right, musical) affords an approach whereby the clinician may point out that, were schools to require the singing in tune of a certain curriculum of melodies, a different condition, "dysmusia," would replace dyslexia in importance. The helpful notion that phonologic processing is no more biologically valuable, no closer to the heart of what is meant by adaptive intelligence, than is processing of musical pitch, is followed by commiseration with what is, after all, the bad luck of a sociologic mismatch. Hence, good news (a different, not a damaged, brain; a different, not an inferior, intellect) is followed by bad news (the person with dyslexia is *un*talented in a skill that society demands). The clinician helps the dyslexic person begin to acquire and accept a philosophy of optimistic fatalism, meaning that he or she must remain confident and cheerful about life prospects in general while downscaling academic expectations in specific subjects. Such explanations and interpretations constitute major therapeutic interventions during the life span of the dyslexic individual.

Direct educational intervention of some sort, preferably one-on-one tutoring to some extent, is unavoidable as a prescription for dyslexia. How much (per session), how often (per week), how long (in duration of years), and the exact content of this educational intervention are decisions usually made within and by the educational establishment, although on some occasions the clinician is consulted for critical reappraisal of a program that is not working. The content of intervention is *not* universally agreed on, even when the core phonologic processing deficit *is* agreed on. Basically, there is the teach *to* the deficit approach (phonics approach), which uses explicit teaching, in a structured stepwise fashion, of symbol-sound associations, phonologic analysis, and synthesis. Phoneme awareness skills teaching, which was effective in treatment studies, may precede formal reading instruction in young, at-risk children and may continue to accompany symbol-sound instructional approaches. This head-on remediate-the-deficit cluster of phonologically explicit programs was well reviewed by Pennington (1991), who discussed its opposite, teaching to strength. Pennington represents the position of those who believe that phonologic coding cannot be by-passed, that reading as a "psycholinguistic guessing game" does not work often (only 20% accuracy is cited).

On the other hand, although total circumvention of phonologic coding (avoiding the deficit and teaching to the strength) is unlikely to work, other investigators are more eclectic in their conclusions about instructional strategies. A balanced approach to instruction, one that makes complementary and generous use of both "holistic/meaning-based and analytic/synthetic or code-oriented methods of teaching word identification" was proposed by Vellutino and Denckla (1991). They noted that meaning-based strategies may activate awareness of visual-orthographic attributes simultaneously with spoken equivalents. Use of context is important with respect to the many English words that fail to conform to coding regularities, words as simple and frequent as "of" and "have." Further, Vellutino and Denckla (1991) cautioned that the analytic and synthetic phonologic code approach in isolation may freeze into place an excessively part-oriented approach that detracts from integrated apperception of the words and may slow the reader down too much for efficient comprehension of meaning.

Vellutino and Denckla's (1991) instructional advice is a counsel of balance and moderation, advocating a diverse set of strategies for word identification, allowing for maximal flexibility. In addition, they exhorted instructors to buttress reading instruction with auditory training not only in phonemic awareness but also in general spoken language (vocabulary and syntactic) enrichment. Thus, both within and without books of printed words, multilevel linguistic remediation is their prescription for dyslexia (Vellutino and Denckla, 1991).

In summary, although fine-tuning of remedial instruction research is on the agenda for the next decade, a consensus exists that there is more than enough to remediate within the linguistic domain; that broader spoken language issues in academic or instructional language need special education expansion in future; and that disorders of self-regulatory and executive functions are in need of coexisting recognition and treatment in the many cases (the majority in clinical populations) of dyslexia-plus.

References

(Key references are designated with an asterisk.)

Clemens S.D., Peters J.E. Minimal brain dysfunction in the school-age child. *Arch. Gen. Psychiatry* 6:185–197, 1962.

DeFries J.C. Gender ratios in reading-disabled children and their affected relatives: a commentary. *J. Learn. Disabil.* 22:544–545, 1989.

DeFries J.C., Fulker D.W., LaBuda M.C. Reading disability in twins: evidence for a genetic etiology. *Nature* 329:537–539, 1987.

Déjèrine J. Sur un cas de cécité verbal avec agraphie, suivi d'autopsie. *Mem. Soc. Biol.* 3:197–201, 1891.

Denckla M.B. Dyslexia: issues of overlap and hetero-geneity. In Gray D., Kavanaugh J., eds. *Biobehavioral Measures of Dyslexia.* Parkton, MD, York Press, 1985.

Denckla M.B. Executive function, the overlap zone between attention deficit hyperactivity disorder and learning disabilities. *Int. Pediatr.* 4:155–160, 1989.

Denckla M.B., LeMay M., Chapman C.A. Few CT scan abnormalities found even in neurologically impaired learning disabled children. *J. Learn. Disabil.* 18:132–135, 1985.

Donchin E. Surprise! . . . Surprise? *Psychophysiology* 18:493–513, 1981.

Duara R., Kushch A., Gross-Glenn K., et al. Neuroanatomical differences between dyslexic and normal readers on MRI scans. *Arch. Neurol.* 48:410–416, 1991.

Duffy F.H., Denckla M.B., Bartels P.H., et al. Dyslexia: automated diagnosis by computerized classification of brain electrical activity. *Ann. Neurol.* 7:421–428, 1980a.

Duffy F.H., Denckla M.B., Bartels P.H., et al. Dyslexia: regional differences in brain electrical activity by topographic mapping. *Ann. Neurol.* 7:412–420, 1980b.

Fein G., Galin D., Yingling C.D., et al. EEG spectra in dyslexic and control boys during resting conditions. *Electroencephalogr. Clin. Neurophysiol.* 63:87–97, 1986.

*Felton R.H., Wood F.B. Cognitive deficits in reading disability and attention deficit disorder. *J. Learn. Disabil.* 22:3–22, 1989.

Finucci J.M., Guthrie J.T., Childs A.L., et al. The genetics of specific reading disability. *Ann. Rev. Hum. Genet.* 40:1–23, 1976.

*Galaburda A.M. Ordinary and extraordinary brain development: anatomical variation in developmental dyslexia. *Ann. Dyslexia* 39:67–80, 1989.

Galaburda A.M. The testosterone hypothesis: assessment since Geschwind and Behan (1982). *Ann. Dyslexia* (in press).

Galaburda A.M., Kemper T.L. Cytoarchitectonic abnormalities in developmental dyslexia: a case study. *Ann. Neurol.* 6:94–100, 1979.

Galaburda A.M., Sanides F. Cytoarchitectonic organization of the human auditory cortex. *J. Comp. Neurol.* 190:597–610, 1980.

*Galaburda A.M., Sherman G.F., Rosen G.D., et al. Developmental dyslexia: four consecutive patients with cortical anomalies. *Ann. Neurol.* 18:222–233, 1985.

Galaburda A.M., Aboitiz F., Rosen G.D., et al. Histological asymmetry in the primary visual cortex of the rat: implications for mechanisms of cerebral asymmetry. *Cortex* 22:151–160, 1986.

Galaburda A.M., Corsiglia J., Rosen G.D., et al. Planum temporale asymmetry, reappraisal since Geschwind and Levitsky. *Neuropsychologia* 25:853–868, 1987.

Galin D., Fein G., Yingling D.D., et al. EEG spectra during oral and silent reading in dyslexics. *J. Clin. Exp. Neuropsychol.* 9:50, 1987.

Galin D., Herron J., Johnstone J., et al. EEG alpha asymmetry in dyslexics during speaking and block design tasks. *Brain Lang.* 35:241–253, 1988.

Geschwind N., Behan P. Left-handedness: association with immune disease, migraine and developmental learning disorder *Proc. Natl. Acad. Sci. U.S.A.* 79:5097–5100, 1982.

*Geschwind N., Galaburda A.M. Cerebral lateralization: biological mechanisms, associations, and pathology. *Arch. Neurol.* 42:428–459, 521–552, 634–654, 1985.

Geschwind N., Galaburda A.M. *Cerebral Lateralization: Biological Mechanisms, Associations and Pathology.* Cambridge, MA, M.I.T. Press, 1987.

Geschwind N., Levitsky W. Human brain: left-right asymmetries in temporal speech region. *Science* 161:186–187, 1968.

Harter M.R., Anllo-Vento L., Wood F.B., et al. II. Separate brain potential characteristics in children with reading disability and attention deficit disorder: color and letter relevance effects. *Brain Cogn.* 7:115–140, 1988a.

Harter M.R., Diering S., Wood F.B. I. Separate brain potential characteristics in children with reading disability and attention deficit disorder: relevance-independent effects. *Brain Cogn.* 7:54–86, 1988b.

*Harter M.R., Anllo-Vento L., Wood F.B. Event-related potentials spatial orienting, and reading disabilities. *Psychophysiology* 26:404–421, 1989.

Haslam R.H.A., Dalby J.T., Johns R.D., et al. Cerebral asymmetry in developmental dyslexia. *Arch. Neurol.* 38:679–682, 1981.

Hier D.B., LeMay M., Rosenberger P.B., et al. Developmental dyslexia: evidence for a subgroup with a reversed cerebral asymmetry. *Arch. Neurol.* 35:90–92, 1978.

Hinshelwood J. *Congenital Word-Blindness.* London, Lewis, 1917.

Holcomb P.J., Ackerman P.T., Dykman R.A. Cognitive event-related brain potentials in children with attention and reading deficits. *Psychophysiology* 22:656–667, 1985.

Holcomb P.J., Ackerman P.T., Dykman R.A. Auditory event-related potentials in attention and reading disabled boys. *Int. J. Psychophysiol.* 3:263–273, 1986.

Hughes J.R. Evaluation of electrophysiological studies on dyslexia. In Gray D.B., Kavanagh J.F., eds. *Biobehavioral Measures of Dyslexia.* Parkton, MD, York Press, pp. 71–86, 1985.

Hughes J.R., Denckla M.B. Outline of a pilot study of electroencephalographic correlates of dyslexia. Benton A.L., Pearl D., eds. *Dyslexia: An Appraisal of Current Knowledge.* New York, Oxford University Press, pp. 112–122, 1978.

Humphreys P., Kaufmann W.E., Galaburda A.M. Developmental dyslexia in women: neuropathological findings in three patients. *Ann. Neurol.* 28:727–738, 1990.

Hynd G.W., Semrud-Clikeman M., Lorys A.R., et al. Brain morphology in developmental dyslexia and attention deficit disorder/hyperactivity. *Arch. Neurol.* 47:919–926, 1990.

Kaufmann W.E., Galaburda A.M. Cerebrocortical microdysgenesis in neurologically normal subjects: a histopathologic study. *Neurology* 39:238–244, 1989.

LaBuda M.C., DeFries J.C., Fulker D.W. Multiple regression analysis of twin data obtained from selected samples. *Genet. Epidemiol.* 3:425–433, 1986.

Leisman G., Ashkenazi M. Aetiological factors in cerebral asymmetry in developmental dyslexia. *Arch. Neurol.* 38:679–682, 1980.

*Morgan W.P. A case of congenital word-blindness. *Br. Med. J.* 2:1378, 1896.

Olson R., Wise B., Conners F., et al. Specific deficits in component reading and language skills: genetic and environmental influences. *J. Learn. Disabil.* 22:339–348, 1989.

*Orton S.T. *Reading, Writing and Speech Problems in Children.* New York, Norton, 1937.

Pennington B.F. Dyslexia. In *Differential Diagnosis of Learning Disorders in Children.* New York, Guilford Press, 1991.

Pennington B.F., McCabe L.L., Smith S.D., et al. Spelling errors in adults with a form of familial dyslexia. *Child Dev.* 57:1001–1013, 1986.

Pennington B.F., Smith S.R., Kimberling W., et al. Left-handedness and immune disorders in familial dyslexics. *Arch. Neurol.* 44:634–639, 1987.

Rosenberger P.B., Hier D.B. Cerebral asymmetry and verbal intellectual deficits. *Ann. Neurol.* 8:300–304, 1980.

Rumsey J.M., Dorwart R., Vermess R., et al. Magnetic resonance imaging of brain anatomy in severe developmental dyslexia. *Arch. Neurol.* 43:1045–1046, 1986.

Rumsey J.M., Coppola R., Denckla M.B., et al. EEG spectra in severely dyslexic men: rest and word and design recognition. *Electroencephalog. Clin. Neurophysiol.* 73:30–40, 1989.

Shaywitz S.E., Shaywitz B.A., Fletcher J.M., et al. Prevalence of reading disability in boys and girls. *J.A.M.A.* 264:998–1002, 1990.

Sherman G.F., Galaburda A.M., Geschwind N. Cortical anomalies in brains of New Zealand mice: a neuropathologic model of dyslexia? *Proc. Natl. Acad. Sci. U.S.A.* 82:8072–8074, 1985.

Sherman G.F., Galaburda A.M., Behan P.O., et al. Neuroanatomical anomalies in autoimmune mice. *Acta Neuropathol.* 74:239–242, 1987.

Silver L.B. Attention deficit hyperactivity disorder: is it a learning disability or a related disorder? *J. Learn. Disabil.* 23:394–397, 1990.

Smith S.D., Kimberling W.J., Pennington B.F., et al. Specific reading disability: identification of an inherited form through linkage and analysis. *Science* 219:1345–1347, 1983.

*Smith S.D., Pennington B.F., Kimberling W.F., et al. Familial dyslexia: use of genetic linkage data to define subtypes. *J. Am. Acad. Child Adolesc. Psychiatry* 29:204–213, 1990.

Spreen O. Learning disability, neurology, and long-term outcome: some implications for the individual and for society. *J. Clin. Exp. Neuropsychol.* 11:389–408, 1989.

Stevenson J., Graham P., Fredman G., et al. A twin study of genetic influences on reading and spelling ability and disability. *J. Child Psychol. Psychiatry* 28:231–247, 1986.

*Vellutino F.R., Denckla M.B. Cognitive and neuropsychological foundations of word identification in poor and normally developing readers. In Barr R., Kamil M.L., Mosenthal P.B., et al., eds. *Handbook of Reading Research.* Vol. II. New York, Longman, pp. 571–608, 1991.

Vogler G.P., DeFries J.C., Decker S.N. Family history as an indicator of risk for reading disability. *J. Learn. Disabil.* 18:419–421, 1985.

Wender P.H. *Minimal Brain Dysfunction in Children.* New York, Wiley, 1971.

Yingling C.D., Galin D., Fein G., et al. Neurometrics does not detect "pure" dyslexics. *Electroencephalogr. Clin. Neurophysiol.* 63:426–430, 1985.

Zahalkova M., Vrzal V., Klobouková E. Genetic investigations in dyslexia. *J. Med. Genet.* 9:48–52, 1972.

Genetic and Metabolic Diseases

46

Molecular Genetic Techniques and Their Applications to Clinical Neurology

A.E. Harding

Advances in molecular genetics have made a major impact in neuroscience and have many applications in the practice of clinical neurology. This chapter aims to provide an introduction to molecular genetic techniques and how they may be used in solving scientific and clinical problems related to diseases of the nervous system.

MENDELIAN INHERITANCE

An understanding of mendelian inheritance is an essential prerequisite for understanding genetics at a submicroscopic level. Every human cell contains a pair of each of 22 chromosomes, which are called the *autosomes*, and either two X chromosomes or one X and one Y chromosome, depending on the sex of the individual. During cell division, the process of mitosis results in two *daughter cells*, which are diploid (i.e., each contains an identical chromosomal complement to the parent cell). Gametogenesis involves the more complex process of meiosis, during which each pair of chromosomes exchanges genetic material, resulting in *gametes*, which are haploid (i.e., they contain half the number of chromosomes of the parent cell).

Mutant genes on the autosomes (chromosomes 1–22) may be inherited as dominant or recessive traits. An individual affected by an autosomal dominant disease has a 50% chance of transmitting it to each child. Thus, a heterozygous gene carrier manifests the disease, despite the presence of a normal corresponding gene (allele) on the other half of the chromosome pair. This is not so in autosomal recessive inheritance, in which it is necessary for both alleles to be abnormal for the disease to be expressed (i.e., the affected individual is homozygous). If two heterozygotes for the same autosomal recessive gene mate, on average one in four of their children will be affected, two of four will be carriers, and one in four will not carry the gene. Defective genes on the X chromosome show a distinctive pattern of inheritance in which males are most severely affected and females carrying the gene may be moderately or mildly affected or clinically normal. An important feature of X-linked inheritance is that male-to-male transmission never occurs, but all the female offspring of affected males inherit the abnormal gene. The variation in expression of an X-linked disorder in females is due to the process of lyonization, in which the expression of one X chromosome is suppressed randomly in each cell. The distinction between X-linked recessive and X-linked dominant disorders is rather loose, although these terms are often used.

NUCLEIC ACIDS

Both DNA and RNA consist of a string of nucleotides, each containing a nitrogenous base, a pentose sugar, and a phosphate group. Bases are either pyrimidines (uracil, cytosine, and thymine) or purines (adenine and guanine). DNA contains adenine (A), guanine (G), thymine (T), and cytosine (C). In RNA, uracil (U) replaces thymine. RNA is generally single stranded, but DNA is usually double stranded, forming an antiparallel double helix. A and T always pair together by means of hydrogen bonds and the same applies to G and C. Compact mammalian chromosomal DNA is supercoiled around proteins called histones. The human nuclear genome (i.e., all the chromosomal DNA) consists of about 3×10^9 base pairs of DNA.

Only about 1% of genomic DNA forms single-copy sequences (structural genes consisting of unique sequences). Nearly half of human DNA is composed of short repetitive sequences, which are either not transcribed or, less commonly, encode for small, high-abundance proteins such as histones. The function of the remaining 50% is not well understood. Some of it codes for *introns*, the noncoding parts of genes; the coding parts are called *exons*. There are also DNA sequences that initiate or stop *transcription*, the synthesis of mRNA complementary to single-stranded DNA sequences catalyzed by the enzyme RNA polymerase. The enzyme synthesizes RNA starting at its 5' end, traversing the DNA template strand from the 3' to the 5' end. A specific DNA sequence upstream from the coding region, the *promotor*, signals where RNA synthesis is to begin. When RNA polymerase reaches the termination signal (another specific sequence), it dissociates from the DNA and releases the RNA chain. A tail of up to 200 adenylic acids may be added to the 3' end of this chain, and it is capped with methylated guanosine residues at the 5' end.

In eukaryotes (higher organisms containing nuclei), most primary RNA transcripts contain introns that are spliced out, leaving a molecule consisting predominantly of exons. mRNA then moves from the nucleus to ribosomes in the cytoplasm. The genetic code dictates that each amino acid is encoded by a triplet of nucleotide bases (a *codon*) (e.g., AUG for methionine). Most amino acids are encoded by more than one codon (e.g., GAA or GAG for glutamine). tRNAs, each containing a complementary anticodon, successively pair with the mRNA and add amino acids to form a polypeptide chain. This process is known as *translation*. The ribosomes associated with one molecule of mRNA are referred to as a *polysome* (Alberts et al., 1989).

In addition to the nuclear genome, there exists an additional, much smaller, genome in mitochondria that is relevant to neurologic disease (Harding, 1991). Mammalian mitochondria contain 5–10 circular DNA (mtDNA) molecules, which are double stranded and about 16.6 kb in length, contributing about 1% of total cellular DNA. mtDNA encodes for 13 of the 67 or so subunits of the mitochondrial respiratory chain and oxidative phosphorylation system. It differs from nuclear DNA to some extent in its genetic code and because it contains little noncoding sequence; it also shows a different pattern of transmission from one generation to the next. A few paternal mitochondria may penetrate the ovum at the time of fertilization, but these appear to degenerate subsequently, and mtDNA has been shown to be exclusively maternally transmitted in many species, including humans.

GENE CLONING, GENE LIBRARIES, AND GENE PROBES

One of the most critical developments in molecular genetics was the discovery of *restriction endonucleases*. These enzymes occur in microorganisms and recognize specific sequences of the DNA molecule and cleave it at these sites and nowhere else (Fig. 46–1). They allow investigators to cut DNA into fragments and to insert the fragments into prokaryote vectors such as *bacteriophage* (often called *phage*, a virus that infects bacteria), *cosmids* (plasmid DNA packaged into phage), or *plasmids*. Plasmids are small circular DNA molecules that are found in the cytoplasm of bacteria and replicate independently of the host chromosomal DNA. Foreign DNA (e.g., a DNA fragment containing a human gene sequence) can be inserted into plasmids cleaved by restriction endonucleases using the enzyme DNA ligase. This hybrid DNA molecule is called recombinant DNA, and it is replicated on a large scale by transfecting bacteria (usually *Escherichia coli*) and culture, allowing the production of multiple copies of the inserted DNA fragment. This procedure is known as *DNA cloning*.

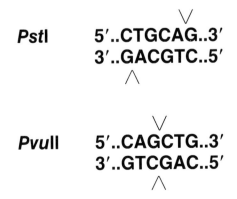

Figure 46–1. Restriction sites for the restriction endonucleases *Pst*I and *Pvu*II (arrowheads indicate cleavage sites). The former produces "sticky-ended" fragments, and the latter, blunt-ended fragments.

A human *genomic library* is produced when sequences from the entire human genome are cloned in a given vector, usually phage or cosmid. Genomic libraries can be enriched for sequences from a single chromosome, isolated by flow sorting; this is particularly useful if probes are needed for linkage studies (see later). It is often useful to construct libraries containing the DNA sequences complementary to mRNA transcribed in different tissues, such as muscle or brain. mRNA is extracted from the tissue, and cDNA to the mRNA sequences is synthesized using the enzyme reverse transcriptase. The cDNAs are then cloned into a vector, producing a cDNA library; this contains only sequences of DNA that are transcribed in the tissue studied.

A *gene probe* is a fragment of DNA that detects complementary sequences. Probes may be produced synthetically, and the nucleotide sequence can be inferred from the amino acid composition of the gene product if this is known. They are more frequently isolated from genomic or cDNA libraries (Emery, 1984; Rosenberg and Harding, 1988).

THE MOLECULAR BASIS OF GENETIC VARIATION

Nuclear DNA replication starts with separation of the two strands of the double helix; each strand then acts as a template for the formation of complementary sequences catalyzed by DNA polymerase. This enzyme adds complementary nucleotides to the growing chain and can also read and correct errors, allowing a high degree of precision in replication. When this mechanism fails, mutation occurs, either by substituting a single incorrect nucleotide *(point mutation)* or by skipping or adding a number of bases *(deletion* or *insertion,* respectively). Point mutations may lead to an amino acid substitution in a protein, such as the change from AGU (serine) to AGA (arginine), or premature termination of transcription if, for example, UAC (tyrosine) changes to UAG (stop codon). Deletions of one or more bases (but not three or multiples thereof) may result in a frameshift mutation, with misreading of the genetic code downstream from that site.

Genetic variation may be abnormal and result in disease. Yet much of the variation that occurs among normal humans is caused by changes in DNA sequences, and these molecular variations *(polymorphisms)* are inherited. This normal polymorphism may be externally apparent, such as differences in hair or eye color, or only evident subclinically, for example, in the different blood group systems and enzyme polymorphism. However, many DNA polymorphisms have no effect on the phenotype, as, on statistical grounds, these are more likely to occur in noncoding regions of the genome. DNA polymorphism can be detected by restriction endonucleases. One base change may lead to loss or gain of a specific recognition site for these enzymes. Thus, cleavage of

genomic DNA with any restriction endonuclease results in fragments that vary in length between individuals. These can be detected by hybridization with a labeled DNA probe. These polymorphisms are inherited and are known as *restriction fragment length polymorphisms* (RFLPs) (Davies and Read, 1988; Emery, 1984).

RESTRICTION FRAGMENT LENGTH POLYMORPHISM ANALYSIS

RFLPs are extremely useful as genetic markers in genetic linkage studies. The techniques used for detecting them are outlined in Figure 46–2. DNA is extracted from leukocytes and incubated with a restriction endonuclease to produce about 1 million DNA fragments up to 20 kb in length. These are separated by size using agarose gel electrophoresis. The DNA on the gel is then made single stranded (denatured) by alkaline treatment so that a complementary probe can hybridize to it later. The DNA fragments are then transferred to nitrocellulose or nylon membrane filters by a procedure known as Southern blotting. After blotting, they are permanently bound to the filter by baking or ultraviolet light (Davies and Read, 1988; Old, 1986).

DNA bound to filters can be stored virtually indefinitely. When required, the filter is placed in a hybridization solution containing the denatured labeled DNA probe complementary to the sequence of interest. The probe is usually labeled with ^{32}P, although nonradioactive labeling of probes is also possible. The location of the hybridized fragments is detected by autoradiography.

GENE MAPPING, GENE TRACKING, AND NEUROLOGIC DISEASE

The approach of reverse genetics (i.e., localizing a disease gene locus to a chromosomal region with the aim of identifying the abnormal gene product) has been applied to many neurologic disorders (Table 46–1) and is particularly useful in autosomal dominant disorders in which there are rarely identifiable metabolic markers. Genetic linkage analysis (gene tracking) has two major requirements: sufficient family material for the disease in question and sufficient variable DNA markers scattered throughout the genome at close intervals.

If two independent genes are located close together on the same chromosome, they are said to be linked. If they are very close together, they are tightly linked, and it is unlikely that they will be separated as a result of the exchange of genetic material that occurs between homologous chromosomes during meiosis (crossover). Early linkage studies used markers such as blood group antigens or serum proteins, but these are limited in number and are not as useful as RFLPs, which now almost saturate the genome. The likeli-

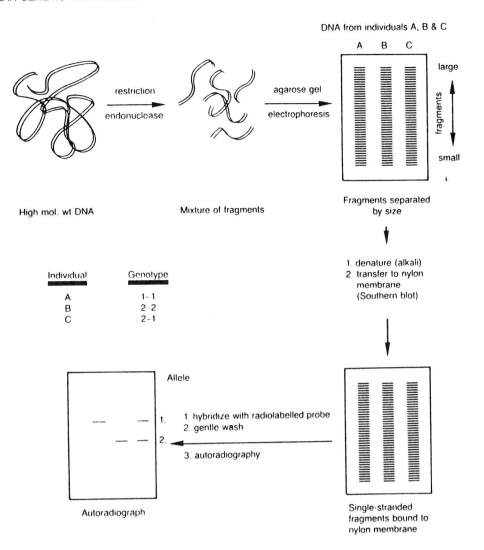

Figure 46–2. A diagrammatic summary of the techniques used for analyzing restriction fragment length polymorphisms. DNA is extracted from peripheral blood leukocytes and digested with a given restriction endonuclease. The genomic DNA fragments (about 10^6) are separated by agarose gel electrophoresis, shorter fragments migrating faster than long ones. They are then denatured with alkali and transferred to a nitrocellulose filter by Southern blotting. After baking or exposure to ultraviolet light, the DNA is permanently bound to the filter. A DNA probe, complementary to the genomic sequence of interest, is labeled with radioactive phosphorus and hybridized to the DNA on the filter. After autoradiography, the position of the fragments can easily be visualized; individual A is homozygous for the upper fragment (called 1), B is homozygous for the lower fragment (2), and C is heterozygous (1-2). (From Davies K.E., Read A.P. *Molecular Basis of Inherited Disease.* Oxford, IRL Press, p. 8, 1988, by permission of Oxford University Press.)

hood of linkage between two genetic loci is assessed statistically by using lod scores (Ott, 1986). *Lod* stands for the log of the odds; linkage between two loci at a given distance is usually considered to be proved or excluded if the lod score is greater than $+3$ or -2, respectively. A lod score of $+3$ means that the odds in favor of linkage are 1000 to 1, although because of the low prior probability of the linkage of two loci, the overall probability of linkage with a lod score of $+3$ is 95% (Davies and Read, 1988).

Lod scores are calculated using computer programs such as LIPED for a number of theoretic genetic distances (recombination fractions) between the marker and disease loci. If two loci are far apart, they should be transmitted together or separately in roughly equal proportions. The highest lod score would therefore be observed at a recombination fraction of 0.5. If the maximal lod score is $+3$ or greater at, for example, a recombination fraction of 0.05, the two loci are linked and recombination occurs, on average, during 1 of 20 meioses.

Often, during linkage studies, segregation of a disease locus is investigated in relation to a number

of markers in the same chromosomal region. The results can be analyzed by multilocus (or multipoint) analysis, and this technique is much more powerful than two-point lod scores, as individuals in the same pedigree who are informative for different markers contribute more information. Multipoint analysis also allows ordering of different loci in relation to each other (Davies and Read, 1988).

The distance between two loci is defined genetically in terms of potential recombination and is measured in centimorgans (cM). Crossing over between two loci 10 cM apart occurs in 10% of meioses. Genetic distance is not identical to physical distance; some parts of the genome appear to be more prone to recombination than others, but a distance of 1 cM approximates to 1 million base pairs.

One vital requirement for linkage analysis is that key individuals in the pedigree are informative for the marker studied (i.e., heterozygous). Thus, the best genetic markers for linkage studies are highly polymorphic. Many RFLPs have the disadvantage of only having two possible alleles, and even if the gene frequency for each allele is 50%, the chance

Table 46–1. NEUROLOGIC DISEASE GENES MAPPED BY LINKAGE ANALYSIS*

Disease	Chromosome/Location
HMSN type I (some families)	1q2
von Hippel–Lindau disease	3p
Huntington's disease†	4p16.3
Acute and chronic childhood SMA	5q11.2-q13.3
Juvenile myoclonic epilepsy	6p
Dominant ataxia (some families)	6p21.2-q12
Friedreich's ataxia†	9q13-q21
Tuberous sclerosis (some families)	9q
Torsion dystonia (some families)	9q34
Tuberous sclerosis (some families)	11q
Ataxia-telangiectasia	11q22-q23
Wilson's disease†	13q14
Batten's disease	16
HMSN type I (most families)†	17p11.2
von Recklinghausen's NF (NF 1)†	17q11.2
Myotonic dystrophy†	19p13.2-q12
Benign neonatal convulsions	20q
Early-onset Alzheimer's disease†	21pter-q21
Bilateral acoustic NF (NF 2)†	22q11-q13.1
Duchenne's and Becker's dystrophies†	Xp21.2
X-linked HMSN†	Xq13-q21
Bulbospinal neuronopathy†	Xq21.3-q22
Fabry's disease†	Xq22
Emery-Dreifuss muscular dystrophy†	Xq27.3-q28
Centronuclear myopathy†	Xq27-q28
Adrenoleukodystrophy†	Xq28

*HMSN = hereditary motor-sensory neuropathy; SMA = spinal muscular atrophy; NF = neurofibromatosis; p = short arm; q = long arm; ter = end of short or long arm. Examples: 1q2 = band 2 on the long arm of chromosome 1 (band numbers increase moving in either direction away from the centromere); 16 = localized to chromosome 16, but not to any specific region.

†Prenatal or presymptomatic diagnosis is possible or potentially possible.
From Human Gene Mapping 10: Tenth International Workshop on Human Gene Mapping. *Cytogenet. Cell Genet.* 51:1–1148, 1989, and/or references cited in text.

that any individual transmitting the disease locus is homozygous for the RFLP, and thus uninformative, is 50%.

The most useful polymorphic markers are derived from tandemly repeated sequences whose copy number varies between individuals because of unequal recombination (variable number of tandem repeats, or VNTR). A restriction fragment containing the whole block of tandem repeats varies in size considerably between different people, and the number of possible alleles makes these hypervariable loci useful in linkage analysis (Nakamura et al., 1987). Smaller sequences that share the characteristics of variable number tandem repeats are often referred to as *minisatellites*, and they are used in genetic fingerprinting. A further refinement in the development of hypervariable loci is the identification of microsatellites (extremely short sequences that contain a variable number of repeated dinucleotides, usually AC repeats). These occur frequently throughout the genome and have great potential for use in gene mapping (Weber and May, 1989). They are analyzed by high-resolution electrophoresis after amplification of the relevant DNA sequence (see later).

Linkage analysis in autosomal dominant neuro-

logic disorders is often limited by the availability of family material. This particularly applies in rare diseases or those with late onset and/or reduced life expectancy. Ideally, large multigeneration families are required, such as the Venezuelan pedigree studied to map the Huntington's disease gene (Gilliam and Gusella, 1988). It is possible to combine data from more than one family for the purposes of calculating lod scores, but this approach assumes that there is no question of genetic heterogeneity, which is rarely the case.

Anonymous RFLPs from gene libraries are mapped to specific chromosomal regions by using a number of methods. The anonymous DNA sequence can be hybridized to a fixed chromosomal preparation on glass slides (in situ hybridization [Buckle and Craig, 1986]). More frequently, the sequence is hybridized to DNA from somatic cell hybrids containing both human and, for example, hamster chromosomes, in which the human chromosomal content is randomly lost. It can then be mapped to a chromosome or a chromosomal region by a process of elimination, assuming that the human chromosomal content of the hybrids is known (Gilliam and Gusella, 1988). Alternatively, linkage studies between the new marker and other loci known to be in the relevant chromosomal region can be performed in large reference families (to establish the genetic distances between them).

Adult-onset neurologic disorders that have been localized to different chromosomal regions by means of linkage analysis are listed in Table 46–1. Most are autosomal dominant. Linkage analysis is more difficult in autosomal recessive disorders because affected individuals are usually confined to a single sibship, and families containing three or more affected persons are unusual. Nevertheless, this has been achieved by using random screening of the genome in Friedreich's ataxia (S. Chamberlain et al., 1988) and childhood spinal muscular atrophy (Gilliam et al., 1990).

Random genome searching is extremely time-consuming and labor intensive, and attempts are often made to accelerate gene mapping by initially studying candidate genes or chromosomal regions. For example, the long arm of chromosome 21 was suggested as a candidate region for the familial Alzheimer's disease locus because of the association between trisomy 21 and Alzheimer's disease. Linkage studies using RFLPs indicate that this hypothesis was correct, at least in early-onset familial Alzheimer's disease (St. George-Hyslop et al., 1987). This finding was of particular interest because the gene encoding the βA4 amyloid precursor protein maps to this region. However, it was subsequently suggested that amyloid precursor protein is not the gene causing familial Alzheimer's disease, as crossovers occur between the two loci (van Broeckhoven et al., 1987). A mutation in the amyloid precursor protein gene has since been demonstrated in an entirely different disorder, Dutch hereditary cerebral hemorrhage (Levy et al., 1990).

Candidate genes have led investigators to the right place, but the wrong gene, on a number of occasions. For example, linkage was established between the locus for von Recklinghausen's neurofibromatosis (neurofibromatosis type 1) and that encoding the nerve growth factor receptor, but again, several crossovers between the two loci disproved the candidate gene hypothesis (Seizinger et al., 1987).

In inherited tumor syndromes, molecular analysis of tumor tissue may provide clues for gene localization. This is because some inherited tumors are thought to arise as a result of loss of tumor suppressor genes, one copy of which bears an inherited mutation in affected family members. Seizinger et al. (1986) showed that there is loss of chromosome 22 in acoustic neuromas, and this provided a correct candidate chromosomal region for the gene giving rise to bilateral acoustic neurofibromatosis (type 2) (Rouleau et al., 1987). The same applies to loss of chromosome 3 in renal cell carcinoma in relation to von Hippel–Lindau disease (Seizinger et al., 1988).

FROM GENETIC LINKAGE TO GENE ISOLATION

One aim of genetic linkage studies is to isolate the defective gene itself, and then to study its abnormal product, to understand the disease pathophysiology and possibly develop a rational approach to therapy. Progressing from the establishment of genetic linkage to isolating the mutant gene is a formidable task. Even closely linked RFLPs are usually more than a 1 million base pairs away from the disease gene. The inherent difficulties in achieving the ultimate objective of reverse genetics are illustrated by the fact that the Huntington's disease gene was localized to the short arm of chromosome 4 in 1983, but it has not yet been isolated. This is probably largely due to the position of the gene, at the tip of chromosome 4 (the telomere), which means that no linked markers known to be on the other side of the gene from those originally described (flanking markers) have been identified (Bates et al., 1990).

A useful approach to disease gene cloning is provided by patients who have a chromosomal translocation associated with the disease of interest. The assumption is that the translocation disrupts the gene and that cloning the breakpoint identifies at least part of the gene itself. This approach proved useful in isolating sequences from the Duchenne muscular dystrophy gene (Davies and Read, 1988) and the neurofibromatosis type 1 gene (Ponder, 1990). If this approach is not possible, it is necessary to move from flanking linked DNA markers identified by linkage analysis toward the disease locus. This involves constructing a detailed physical map of the region using pulsed field gel electrophoresis, a technique that allows resolution of DNA fragments up to 2000 kb in length. These are produced by using restriction enzymes that cleave human DNA infre-

quently (van Ommen and Verkerk, 1986) and are also used to construct "jumping" and "linking" libraries, which allow fairly rapid honing in on a disease gene region from linked markers (Davies and Read, 1988). Gene isolation has been hampered by the limitations of cloning techniques with vectors that have a limited capacity for incorporating exogenous DNA, only up to about 50 kb. Fragments of DNA up to several hundred kilobases in length have been cloned into yeast and propagated as linear yeast artificial chromosomes. This system, together with pulsed field gel electrophoresis, addresses a major gap (between the resolution of the lower limits of cytogenetics and the upper limits of standard cloning techniques) in experimental methods for analyzing complex DNA sources (Burke et al., 1987). This approach is promising in relation to isolating the Huntington's disease gene, as the short arm telomere of chromosome 4 has been identified in a yeast artificial chromosome clone (Bates et al., 1990).

How is a gene recognized after the relevant sequence has been cloned? The following approaches, among others, may be used: (1) identifying *Hpa*II tiny fragment islands (recognized by rare cutting restriction enzymes), which are often associated with the 5' end of genes; (2) for a sequence of interest, searching for conservation by hybridizing it to Southern blots containing DNA from different species (zoo blots); and (3) examining affected and unaffected tissues for expression of the given sequence by screening cDNA libraries and Northern blotting (hybridizing to RNA on filters). Proof that the cloned gene is the disease gene requires demonstration of altered protein coding function—by mutation, deletion, or insertion—in affected individuals. Deletions or insertions are often detectable as alterations in DNA fragment size, analyzed by using Southern blotting or pulsed field gel electrophoresis. It is possible to screen rapidly for more discrete nucleotide changes, including point mutations, using single-strand conformation polymorphism analysis (Orita et al., 1989). Gene segments (usually from exons) of 100–400 base pairs in length are amplified by the polymerase chain reaction (see later), are heat denatured, and undergo electrophoresis on high-resolution polyacrylamide gels. Each single-stranded DNA fragment assumes a secondary structure determined partly by its nucleotide sequence under these conditions, and single base changes can alter electrophoretic mobility. The use of the various techniques mentioned earlier in isolating the neurofibromatosis type 1 gene is summarized in Table 46–2.

After a candidate gene has been cloned, its sequence can be determined in detail by a number of different methods, the most frequently used being the dideoxy method of Sanger et al. (1977). This involves using single-stranded DNA as a template to synthesize a complementary strand, incorporating dideoxynucleotides in place of normal nucleotides. The former lack the 3' hydroxy groups, and chain synthesis is terminated when they are incorporated. Four reactions containing template, DNA polymer-

Table 46–2. ISOLATION OF THE NEUROFIBROMATOSIS TYPE 1 GENE 1987–1990

1. Gene mapped to long arm of chromosome 17 by means of linkage analysis with restriction fragment length polymorphisms
2. Detailed genetic map of region obtained in collaborative effort analyzing 142 families
3. Two patients with translocations involving chromosome 17 (1;17 and 17;22) identified
4. Translocation breakpoints shown to lie about 60 kb apart by pulsed field gel electrophoresis
5. Conserved sequences in vicinity of translocated region identified by hybridization to zoo blots of sequence obtained by
   a. Chromosome jumping
   b. Cloning the translocation region in a yeast artificial chromosome
   c. Analyzing germline deletions in translocated region, found in 3 of 11 patients with neurofibromatosis type 1
6. Conserved sequences used to screen cDNA libraries (from peripheral nerve, fetal brain, and non-neurologic tissues)
7. Six exons spanning at least 33 kb of genomic DNA identified by Michigan group, and nine exons of more than 100 kb, by Salt Lake City group
8. Studies of patients with neurofibromatosis type 1 showed
   a. Transcript of gene interrupted by 17;22 translocation
   b. 500-bp insert in or close to one exon found in a new mutation
   c. 6 of 72 patients with neurofibromatosis type 1 had variant alleles in exons 4–9, detected by single-strand conformation polymorphism after DNA amplification
9. A 2485-amino-acid neurofibromatosis type 1 peptide predicted from reading frame sequence; a 360-residue region showed homology to both human and bovine guanosine triphosphatase–activating protein, an intermediate in the cellular transduction of extracellular signals, which is involved in the regulation of cell growth

From Ponder B. Neurofibromatosis gene cloned. Reprinted by permission from *Nature*, vol. 346, pp. 703–704. Copyright © 1990 Macmillan Magazines Ltd.

ase, the four normal nucleotides (one of which is radioactively labeled), and one of the four dideoxynucleotides are set up and then each is subjected to gel electrophoresis and autoradiography. The chains in all four reactions will end with one of the chain-terminating dideoxynucleotides, so the sequence of the DNA can be read directly from the autoradiograph. Short stretches of sequence can be compared with known genes and proteins by using established data bases, and the protein product of any unknown gene can be predicted from its sequence. Antibodies to corresponding synthetic peptides may then be used to study the distribution of the gene product in normal and affected tissues. Perhaps the most elegant way of demonstrating the effects of a mutant gene, and eventually investigating pathogenesis of the disease in question, is by producing transgenic animal models of the human condition by microinjecting the gene into the fertilized ova of mice. This has been achieved in one form of inherited spongiform encephalopathy, or prion disease (Gerstmann-Straussler syndrome), in which there is a mutation of codon 102 in the prion protein gene (Hsiao et al., 1990).

CLINICAL APPLICATION OF LINKED DNA MARKERS

The identification of a genetic marker linked to a disease locus has important clinical applications in presymptomatic and prenatal detection of gene carriers. After linkage has been established, it is often relatively easy to generate more closely linked DNA markers, thus enhancing the accuracy of gene tracking that is so important in genetic counseling. The diagnosis of genetic diseases using linked RFLPs is obviously an indirect method and has a number of disadvantages, not the least of which is the inaccuracy generated by the possibility of recombination during meiosis. It also necessitates studying several family members to establish how the genetic marker is segregating with the disease locus, and these individuals are not always available for study, particularly in a late-onset life-limiting disorder such as Huntington's disease (Harper and Sarfarazi, 1985). Nevertheless, the use of linked markers is well established in clinical practice in Huntington's disease, von Recklinghausen's neurofibromatosis, myotonic dystrophy, and a number of X-linked disorders, particularly Duchenne's and Becker's dystrophies, and is potentially possible in other neurologic disorders (see Table 46–1).

DIRECT TESTS FOR NEUROLOGIC DISEASE GENES

In some diseases, direct detection of a gene defect is possible by using DNA analysis (Table 46–3). This

Table 46–3. INHERITED NEUROLOGIC DISEASES IN WHICH GENE DEFECTS HAVE BEEN IDENTIFIED

Disease*	Genetic Defect
Nuclear Gene Defects	
Amyloid neuropathies	
Transthyretin related (5 types)	Point mutations
Apolipoprotein AII related	Point mutation
Dutch cerebral hemorrhage	Point mutation
Neurofibromatosis type 1	Insertion, deletions, point mutations
Hexosaminidase deficiencies	Deletions, insertion, point mutations
Prion diseases	Insertions, point mutations
Duchenne's and Becker's dystrophies	Deletions (70%), duplications
mtDNA Defects	
Leber's hereditary optic neuropathy	Point mutations
MERRF	Point mutation
MELAS	Point mutation
Ataxia, RP, neuropathy	Point mutation
Mitochondrial myopathy (PEO, KSS)	Deletions, duplications

*MERRF = myoclonic epilepsy with ragged red fibers; RP = retinitis pigmentosa; PEO = progressive external ophthalmoplegia; KSS = Kearns-Sayre syndrome; MELAS = mitochondrial encephalopathy, lactic acidosis, and stroke.

may be because the disease mutation alters a restriction site, as in the Portuguese type (and other types) of familial amyloid polyneuropathy. In this autosomal dominant disorder, the amyloid deposits are derived from an abnormal prealbumin, or transthyretin, in which there is a substitution of methionine for valine at position 30. This corresponds to a single base change in the gene for transthyretin, changing the codon GUG to AUG. This results in a new restriction site for the restriction endonuclease *Nsi*I, which can be detected by using a cDNA probe for the transthyretin gene (Fig. 46–3), making it possible to diagnose familial amyloid polyneuropathy presymptomatically and prenatally with a blood or tissue sample from a single individual (Holt et al., 1989a).

The mutation of mtDNA associated with about 50% of cases of Leber's hereditary optic neuropathy causes loss of a restriction site for the enzyme *Sfa*NI (Holt et al., 1989b), and this is a useful confirmatory test, particularly in patients who do not have affected relatives. Direct detection of mutations or insertions of the prion protein gene in inherited prion diseases is possible by using restriction endonuclease analysis or gene amplification (Westaway et al., 1989) (see later).

Direct mutation detection may be possible, even if the mutation does not result in a restriction site change. If the exact sequences of the normal and mutant genes are known, it is possible to synthesize complementary oligonucleotides to the mutated region, usually about 20 bases in length. If these are labeled and exposed to human DNA samples under strict conditions, only the perfectly matched sequences hybridize (Thein and Wallace, 1986). This technique has been applied in detecting the mtDNA mutation reported in myoclonic epilepsy with ragged red fibers (Shoffner et al., 1990).

Perhaps the most widespread use of direct detection of a gene defect in neurologic disease is the identification of deletions of the dystrophin gene in Duchenne's and Becker's muscular dystrophies. Deletions are identifiable in about 70% of cases (Davies and Read, 1988; Forrest et al., 1987). These are detected by hybridization with DNA probes complementary to various parts of the normal gene sequence. If a deletion is present, some restriction fragments are absent, or these may be of different lengths compared with the normal pattern. Deletions of the dystrophin gene may also be analyzed by using the polymerase chain reaction (PCR) (see later).

GENE AMPLIFICATION

Both research and clinical applications of molecular genetics to neurologic disease have been enhanced substantially by the technique of amplifying specific segments of DNA using the PCR. The sequence amplified is usually 1 kb or less in size. It is necessary to know the exact sequence of short sections of DNA flanking the region to be amplified (the template) so that two oligonucleotide primers (usually 20 nucleotides in length) can be synthesized, which hybridize to opposite strands of the template DNA at either end. The template, the primers, the nucleotides, a suitable buffer, and an enzyme called thermostable *Taq* polymerase are repetitively heated and cooled in a series of cycles until the desired amount of amplification is achieved (Eisenstein, 1990; Saiki et al., 1988; White et al., 1989) (Fig. 46–4).

In a standard PCR, the template DNA is denatured at 94°C, and then the single-stranded template anneals to the primers at 55°C. In the third part of the reaction (extension), the polymerase synthesizes cDNA on each strand of the template, starting from the 5' end of the oligonucleotide primers, at 72°C. Because the extension products are capable of hybridizing to the primers (which are present in excess), successive cycles of the PCR double the amount of DNA synthesized in the previous cycle. The result is exponential amplification of the target sequence, approximately 2^n, where n is the number of cycles. Most amplifications are performed using 20–30 cycles. The time for each part of the reaction varies with the length of the target sequence, the nucleotide composition of the primers, and the machine used for automating the reaction, but a typical cycle is shorter than 5 minutes. The exact temperatures used are also somewhat variable, depending on, for example, the GC content of the primers. The products of the PCR can be visualized and sized approximately

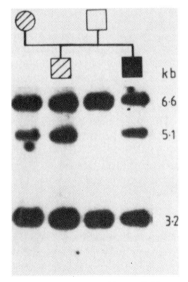

Figure 46–3. A 28-year-old man with amyloid neuropathy (*black square*) has a 5.1-kb DNA fragment (shown below after digestion with *Nsi*I, Southern blotting, and hybridization to a transthyretin cDNA probe) in addition to the normal 6.6- and 3.2-kb bands. The mutation for the Portuguese type of familial amyloid polyneuropathy results in a new restriction site for *Nsi*I, which cleaves one of the two homologous 6.6-kb fragments into two, 5.1 and 1.5 kb in length (latter not shown). The restriction fragment pattern from the patient's father (*open square*) is normal, but his clinically normal brother and mother (*hatched symbols*), aged 31 and 56 years, are carriers. (From Holt I.J., Harding A.E., Middleton L., et al. Molecular genetics of amyloid neuropathy in Europe. *Lancet* 1:524–526, 1989.)

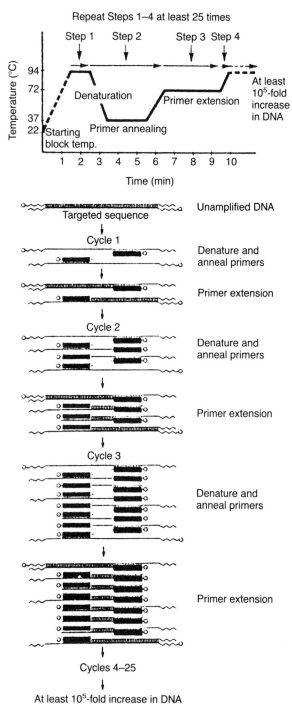

Figure 46–4. The polymerase chain reaction for amplifying DNA; see text for details. (From Anderson M. Perfecting the polymerase chain reaction. *Lab. Equip. Digest*, p. 30, January 1990.)

by running them on a small agarose gel and visualizing them under ultraviolet light after staining with ethidium bromide. More accurate size estimation, needed, for example, for detecting the length of fragments containing CA repeats referred to earlier, requires polyacrylamide gel electrophoresis and silver staining or radiolabeled hybridization.

The success of the PCR is largely determined by the selection of primers. These should have a random base distribution, with a GC content close to 50%; they should not have a significant secondary structure or be substantially complementary to each other. The major problems with the PCR are that it sometimes does not work for no obvious reason and contamination. Contamination with DNA other than the template can cause major difficulties, particularly in diagnostic work, in view of the exponential DNA amplification produced by the PCR. This problem can largely be avoided by obsessive attention to laboratory technique, particularly care in pipetting and keeping PCR equipment separate from general laboratory ware. Blank control samples (i.e., not containing template DNA) should always be used. Limiting the number of cycles also reduces the effects of contamination and the possibility of yielding a nonspecific product.

One major advantage of DNA amplification with the PCR is that PCR is a rapid alternative to cloning, and DNA can be sequenced directly from the PCR product using a modification of the dideoxy method referred to earlier (Schon et al., 1989). In diagnostic and research work, DNA amplification allows (1) detection of known point mutations by specific oligonucleotide hybridization or restriction endonuclease digestion of the product (e.g., the mtDNA mutation described in myoclonic epilepsy with ragged red fibers [Shoffner et al., 1990]); (2) detection of disease gene mutations by single-strand conformation polymorphism analysis or direct sequencing of the product, as has been achieved in neurofibromatosis type 1 (Cawthon et al., 1990) and a number of types of familial amyloid polyneuropathy (Mendell et al., 1990); (3) detection of suspected deletions by altered size or absence of the product (e.g., in Duchenne's and Becker's muscular dystrophies [J.S. Chamberlain et al., 1988]); and (4) detection of known or unknown RFLPs in the product for use in linkage analysis or the application of linked markers in clinical practice. The last has been used for rapid prenatal exclusion testing for Huntington's disease (McIntosh et al., 1989). Allele-specific PCR, using one primer with a 3' end complementary to a known mutation, has been employed to detect one of the types of familial amyloid polyneuropathy; amplification only occurs in the presence of the mutation (Mendell et al., 1990).

The major advantages of the PCR in clinical use are that it is extremely rapid compared with Southern blotting techniques (hours instead of days) and the amount of template DNA required is much less. For example, DNA from buccal epithelium cells isolated from saliva, a few hair roots, or a Guthrie spot can be used to detect cystic fibrosis carrier status (Williams et al., 1988). It is also theoretically possible to use template DNA obtained from archival material, such as paraffin-embedded sections of brain, which could be useful in gene tracking in families with limited pedigree structure (e.g., in Huntington's disease).

References

(Key references are designated with an asterisk.)

*Alberts B., Bray D., Lewis J., et al., eds. *Molecular Biology of the Cell*. 2nd ed. New York, Garland, 1989.

Bates G.P., MacDonald M.E., Baxendale S., et al. A yeast artificial chromosome telomere clone spanning a possible location of the Huntington disease gene. *Am. J. Hum. Genet.* 46:762–775, 1990.

Buckle V.J., Craig I.W. In situ hybridization. In Davies K.E., ed. *Human Genetic Diseases: A Practical Approach*. Oxford, IRL Press, pp. 85–100, 1986.

*Burke D.T., Carle G.F., Olson M.V. Cloning of large segments of exogenous DNA into yeast by means of artificial chromosome vectors. *Science* 236:806–812, 1987.

Cawthon R.M., Weiss R., Xu G., et al. A major segment of the neurofibromatosis type 1 gene: cDNA sequence, genomic structure, and point mutations. *Cell* 62:193–201, 1990.

Chamberlain J.S., Gibbs R.A., Ranier J.E., et al. Deletion screening of the Duchenne muscular dystrophy locus via multiplex DNA amplification. *Nucleic Acids Res.* 16:11141–11156, 1988.

Chamberlain S., Shaw J., Rowland A., et al. Mapping of mutation causing Friedreich's ataxia to human chromosome 9. *Nature* 334:248–250, 1988.

*Davies K.E., Read A.P. *Molecular Basis of Inherited Disease*. Oxford, IRL Press, 1988.

*Eisenstein B.I. The polymerase chain reaction. A new method of using molecular genetics for medical diagnosis. *N. Engl. J. Med.* 322:178–183, 1990.

Emery A.E.H. *An Introduction to Recombinant DNA*. Chichester, Wiley, 1984.

Forrest S.M., Smith T.J., Cross G.S., et al. Effective strategy for prenatal prediction of Duchenne and Becker musclar dystrophy. *Lancet* 2:1294–1297, 1987.

Gilliam T.C., Gusella J.F. Huntington's disease. In Rosenberg R.N., Harding A.E., eds. *The Molecular Biology of Neurological Disease*. London, Butterworth, 1988.

Gilliam T.C., Brzustowicz L.M., Castilla L.H., et al. Genetic homogeneity between acute and chronic forms of spinal muscular atrophy. *Nature* 345:823–825, 1990.

*Harding A.E. Neurological disease and mitochondrial genes. *Trends Neurosci.* 4:132–138, 1991.

Harper P.S., Sarfarazi M. Genetic prediction and family structure in Huntington's chorea. *Br. Med. J.* 290:1929–1931, 1985.

Holt I.J., Harding A.E., Middleton L., et al. Molecular genetic studies of amyloid neuropathy in Europe. *Lancet* 1:524–526, 1989a.

Holt I.J., Miller D.H., Harding A.E. Genetic heterogeneity and mitochondrial DNA heteroplasmy in Leber's hereditary optic neuropathy. *J. Med. Genet.* 26:739–743, 1989b.

Hsiao K.K., Scott M., Foster D., et al. Spontaneous neurodegeneration in transgenic mice with mutant prion protein. *Science* 250:1587–1590, 1990.

*Human Gene Mapping 10: Tenth International Workshop on Human Gene Mapping. *Cytogenet. Cell Genet.* 51:1–1148, 1989.

Levy E., Carman M.D., Fernandez-Madrid I.J., et al. Mutation of the Alzheimer's disease amyloid gene in hereditary cerebral hemorrhage, Dutch type. *Science* 248:1124–1126, 1990.

McIntosh I., Curtis A., Millan F.A., et al. Prenatal exclusion testing for Huntington disease using the polymerase chain reaction. *Am. J. Med. Genet.* 32:274–276, 1989.

Mendell J.R., Jiang X-S., Warmolt J.R., et al. Diagnosis of Maryland/German familial amyloidotic polyneuropathy using allele-specific, enzymatically amplified, genomic DNA. *Ann. Neurol.* 27:553–557, 1990.

*Nakamura Y., Leppert M., O'Connell P., et al. Variable number of tandem repeat (VNTR) markers for human gene mapping. *Science* 235:1616–1622, 1987.

Old J.M. Fetal DNA analysis. In Davies K.E., ed. *Human Genetic Diseases: A Practical Approach*. Oxford, IRL Press, pp. 1–17, 1986.

Orita M., Suzuki Y., Sekiya T., et al. Rapid and sensitive detection of point mutations and DNA polymorphisms using the polymerase chain reaction. *Genomics* 5:874–879, 1989.

Ott J. A short guide to linkage analysis. In Davies K.E., ed. *Human Genetic Diseases: A Practical Approach*. Oxford, IRL Press, pp. 19–32, 1986.

*Ponder B. Neurofibromatosis gene cloned. *Nature* 346:703–704, 1990.

Rosenberg R.N., Harding A.E., eds. *The Molecular Biology of Neurological Disease*. London, Butterworth, 1988.

Rouleau G.A., Wertelecki W., Haines J.L., et al. Genetic linkage of bilateral acoustic neurofibromatosis to a DNA marker on chromosome 22. *Nature* 329:246–248, 1987.

Saiki R.K., Gyllensten U.B., Erlich H.A. The polymerase chain reaction. In Davies K.E., ed. *Genome Analysis: A Practical Approach*. Oxford, IRL Press, pp. 141–152, 1988.

Sanger F., Nicklen S., Coulson A.R. DNA sequencing with chain-terminating inhibitors. *Proc. Natl. Acad. Sci. U.S.A.* 74:5463–5467, 1977.

Schon E.A., Rizzuto R., Moraes C.T., et al. A direct repeat is a hotspot for large-scale deletion of human mitochondrial DNA. *Science* 244:346–349, 1989.

Seizinger B., Martuza R.L., Gusella J.F. Loss of genes on chromosome 22 in tumorigenesis of human acoustic neuroma. *Nature* 322:644–647, 1986.

Seizinger B.R., Rouleau G.A., Ozelius L.J., et al. Genetic linkage of von Recklinghausen neurofibromatosis to the nerve growth factor receptor gene. *Cell* 49:589–594, 1987.

Seizinger B.R., Rouleau G.A., Ozelius L.J., et al. von Hippel-Lindau disease maps to the region of chromosome 3 associated with renal cell carcinoma. *Nature* 32:268–269, 1988.

Shoffner J.M., Lott M.T., Lezza A.M.S., et al. Myoclonic epilepsy and ragged-red fiber disease (MERRF) is associated with a mitochondrial DNA tRNA^{Lys} mutation. *Cell* 61:931–937, 1990.

St. George-Hyslop P.H., Tanzi R.E., Polinsky R.J., et al. The genetic defect causing familial Alzheimer's disease maps on chromosome 21. *Science* 235:885–890, 1987.

Thein S.L., Wallace R.B. The use of synthetic oligonucleotides as specific hybridization probes in the diagnosis of genetic disorders. In Davies K.E., ed. *Human Genetic Diseases: A Practical Approach*. Oxford, IRL Press, pp. 33–50, 1986.

van Broeckhoven C., Genthe A.M., Vandenberghe A., et al. Failure of familial Alzheimer's disease to segregate with the A4-amyloid gene in several European families. *Nature* 329:153–155, 1987.

van Ommen G.J.B., Verkerk J.M.H. Restriction analysis of chromosomal DNA in a size range up to two million base pairs by pulsed field gradient electrophoresis. In Davies K.E., ed. *Human Genetic Diseases: A Practical Approach*. Oxford, IRL Press, pp. 113–133, 1986.

*Weber J.L., May P.E. Abundant class of human DNA polymorphism which can be typed using the polymerase chain reaction. *Am. J. Hum. Genet.* 44:388–396, 1989.

*Westaway D., Carlson G.A., Prusiner S.B. Unravelling prion diseases through molecular genetics. *Trends Neurosci.* 12:221–227, 1989.

White T.J., Arnheim N., Erlich H.A. The polymerase chain reaction. *Trends Genet.* 5:185–189, 1989.

Williams C., Weber L., Williamson R., et al. Guthrie spots for DNA-based carrier testing in cystic fibrosis (letter). *Lancet* 2:693, 1988.

47

Heritable Disorders of the Nervous System

Orest Hurko

In the past decade there has been a greater appreciation and application of the methods of genetics and of molecular biology to the study and management of diseases of the nervous system (Antonarakis, 1989; Baraitser, 1990; Rosenberg and Harding, 1988). The theoretic framework and practical methods of these disciplines have proved powerful additions to the traditional approach of clinical neurologists, whose interest is in diagnosing, classifying and understanding the pathophysiology of disease, and neuroscientists, who are interested in the assembly and function of the nervous system (Greenspan, 1990).

GENETICS

It is important to recognize that genetics and molecular biology are separate, but unquestionably complementary, disciplines. Genetics is the study of biologic variation and its transmission (Sturtevant and Beadle, 1940). The theoretic framework of current genetics was established in the mid-1800s in the work of Gregor Mendel, an Austrian monk who studied the transmission of variation in domesticated plants. By crossing plants with different characteristics and carefully recording the appearance and numbers of their progeny, he enunciated principles that remain the cornerstone of genetics. He postulated that the characteristics of living organisms were encoded in immutable repositories of information that are now called genes. He further postulated that these genes occur in allelic pairs, and that only one allele of each pair is transmitted, at random, by an individual to its offspring. This recognition of randomness casts genetics as the first scientific discipline that is intrinsically probabilistic rather that determin-

istic—a major conceptual breakthrough (Murphy, 1979). Further, Mendel observed that an individual could be either homozygous (having two identical copies in a gene pair) or heterozygous (with two different copies, one dominant and the other recessive) for any gene pair.

In his first law, Mendel postulated segregation of alleles. Although alleles interact within an individual to give rise to the phenotype, this interaction in no way affects the alleles (the genotype) themselves, which are transmitted unchanged to the following generation. For example, in a species with two co-dominant alleles for flower color—red and white—a heterozygote would be pink. Crossing two such pink individuals would give rise to pink heterozygotes as well as pure white and pure red homozygotes in a characteristic mendelian ratio of 2:1:1. The red progeny is as red as any purebred red strain; the red allele is in no way diluted by its coexistence with a white allele in the previous generation. In his second law, Mendel postulated independent assortment of genes. Genes encoding distinct traits are transmitted independently of one another: crossing a wrinkled green pea with a smooth yellow variety would be as likely to produce offspring of the parental, nonrecombinant combination of traits (green and wrinkled, or yellow and smooth) as recombinant phenotypes (green and smooth, or yellow and wrinkled).

Subsequently, exceptions have been found to mendelism, the most important of which are two. First, not all genes are represented in individuals as allelic pairs. In the early 20th century, it was realized that certain genes are present in one copy in males, who are called hemizygous for those genes, but present in two copies or not at all in females. These genes are now known to be present on the sex chromosomes: X in the former case, Y in the latter. The majority of the genes, represented on the autosomes,

656

are present as allelic pairs. More recently mitochondrial genes have been discovered present in thousands of copies per cell. An individual whose mitochondrial genes are identical is homoplasmic, and one who has more than one type of mitochondrial genome, heteroplasmic (Rand and Harrison, 1989).

Second, not all genes segregate independently. In crosses of individuals heterozygous for several different genes, it was observed that some nonrecombinant phenotypes were more common than recombinant ones. Such genes are said to be linked (Smith, 1953). Tracking multiple pairs of such linked genes revealed that their segregation could be predicted by assuming that they were arranged as if they were beads on a string, the location of an allele being a fixed locus in this linear array. The farther apart any two loci are, the more likely they are to recombine, permitting construction of a genetic map. If recombinants for two traits are never observed (i.e., the recombination fraction is zero), the inference is that the two traits are encoded by exactly the same locus. If recombination does occur, the traits are encoded by different loci. Further, the relative frequency of recombinant and nonrecombinant progeny is a measure of the genetic distance between their loci. The maximal recombination fraction is 0.5 (50% of offspring are recombinant, and 50%, nonrecombinant), indicating that the genes are unlinked, segregating independently. A recombination fraction of less than 0.5 indicates linkage—the smaller the recombination fraction, the closer the loci. This behavior is based on the arrangement of genes on linear chromosomes. The locus for each gene occupies a characteristic location on a particular chromosome. Independent assortment implies that the genes in question are either on separate chromosomes, or are far enough apart on a given chromosome that a crossover (strictly, an *odd* number of crossovers) between their loci is as likely to occur as not. Such crossovers are most frequently observed during meiosis (the production of haploid sperm or egg cells) and are much less frequent during mitosis (the process by which one diploid somatic cell gives rise to two diploid daughter cells).

It is important to underscore that genetics need make no reference to the underlying physical nature of the gene, which is useful nevertheless as a theoretic construct, or for that matter, to chromosomes or crossovers. The mainstay of the geneticist is the breeding experiment. By analyzing the phenotypes of the parents and the offspring in a cross, the geneticist then makes inferences about their genotypes. The tools of the geneticist are probability algebra and statistics, not biochemistry. Unlike the neurologist or the neuroscientist, whose focus is the individual, the geneticist studies families.

MOLECULAR BIOLOGY

The origins of molecular biology were in the 1940s when investigators of bacteria and the viruses that infect them (bacteriophages) discovered the physical basis of the gene to be DNA. The focus of molecular biology is, as the name implies, not the family, but the structure of this macromolecule and its associated RNAs and proteins (Lewin, 1990). Unlike genetics, molecular biology is a deterministic rather than probabilistic discipline. A fundamental principle of molecular biology is the recognition that genetic information is based on the linear order of four bases—two purines, adenine (A) and guanosine (G); and two pyrimidines, thymidine (T) and cytosine (C). The faithful replication of DNA, as well as the formation of working blueprints as mRNA molecules, is based on the complementation of one purine with one pyrimidine: A with T, G with C. Proteins are assembled according to this blueprint by virtue of decoding by tRNA intermediates: each triplet of nucleotides in the nucleic acid corresponding to one amino acid, or a signal to terminate elongation of the growing polypeptide chain.

Molecular biology has proved extremely powerful for both theoretic and experimental reasons. Although secondary and more complex structures are unquestionably important, most of the information present in nucleic acids is readily deciphered from their primary linear structure. This greatly facilitates their analysis. One need only compare advances in the understanding of nucleic acids with the relatively slow progress made with proteins, in which most useful information is found in tertiary structure. Furthermore, the central dogma of molecular biology—unidirectional flow of information from DNA to RNA to protein and thence to other biochemical reactions—is a much more tractable paradigm, even with its known exceptions, than are other biologic processes, which often have no clear beginning or end and often consist of many processes occurring in parallel, with complex feedback loops.

Molecular biology also offers a tractable experimental system (Sambrook et al., 1989). DNA is a stable molecule, which is highly tolerant of multiple cycles of denaturation and renaturation without loss of information. Furthermore, base pair complementarity provides two major experimental advantages. Single-stranded nucleic acid probes prove to be ideal reagents: complementary copies can be detected in solution; after electrophoresis of experimental specimens and transfer to nitrocellulose or nylon membranes (DNA-DNA, Southern blotting; DNA-RNA, Northern blotting); on whole mounts of chromosomes, to determine the approximate locus of a particular sequence; and in in situ hybridization on histologic preparations, to determine the tissue and cellular distribution of transcripts from a particular gene.

Second, the principle of base pair complementarity allows generation of an unlimited number of copies of a nucleic acid sequence of interest, facilitating analysis and allowing ready modification. Unlike the protein chemist who has to husband microgram quantities of purified protein to perform analyses, the molecular biologist can readily make an indefinite number of replicates after a gene has been isolated. With the recognition of the similarity of nucleic acids and their processing enzymes in eukaryotes and prokaryotes, such replication was accomplished by cloning in bacteria: excising nucleic acid sequences from the genome of interest with restriction endonucleases, inserting these fragments individually into replicating vectors (plasmids, cosmids, or bacteriophage), and then propagating these vectors and their nucleic acid inserts in bacteria. Such in vivo molecular cloning is being supplanted by the polymerase chain reaction (Mullis et al., 1986). If the nucleic acid sequence of a region of interest is known well enough to permit synthesis of complementary oligonucleotide primers at two sites within several thousand base pairs of each other, the polymerase chain reaction permits an exponential amplification of the intervening sequence. Within several hours, one can amplify microgram quantities of pure sequence, starting with minute quantities of a crude biologic preparation as a template.

With such procedures, much has been learned about the structure and expression of genetic material (Lewin, 1990). In eukaryotes, genes consist of coding regions—*exons*, which dictate the amino acid sequence of the protein or proteins that they encode—separated by larger noncoding regions—*introns*, whose nucleic acid sequence is transcribed only to be spliced out and discarded in the formation of a mature mRNA. Tissue-specific variations in splicing allow selective removal of certain exons, permitting generation of different transcripts from a single gene. The beginning of the coding region is marked by a *start signal*, and the end, by a *stop signal*. Upstream of the start signal is a *promoter* region, to which can bind RNA polymerase and various transcriptional regulatory factors. Downstream of the stop signal is commonly found a signal for polyadenylation, permitting addition of a string of repeated adenine nucleotides that is a common feature of many mature mRNA molecules. Either upstream or downstream—frequently at distances of thousands of bases—exist *enhancer* elements, to which binding of regulatory factors can effect the tissue-specific expression of many regulated genes. The existence of certain repeated sequence motifs allows the recognition of the starting and ending points of genes (the bracketed interval being an *open reading frame*), the presence of intron and exon boundaries, and the presence of promoter and enhancer regions, even when the nucleic sequence derives from a region not previously encountered. This permits deduction of the amino acid sequence of the encoded protein, and often, by consideration of areas of hydrophobicity or signal sequence, the cellular region to which the encoded protein is likely to be targeted. From considerations of other amino acid motifs (e.g., leucine zippers, helix-loop-helix, and zinc fingers), one can estimate the probable functional role of the encoded protein. Deduction of the primary amino acid sequence allows synthesis of the encoded peptide and production of complementary antibodies for more direct studies.

Finally, the use of nucleic acid hybridization to chromosome spreads or to panels of somatic cell hybrids with limited complements of human chromosomes permits mapping of any sequence by physical methods. Such molecular mapping is possible even if no variation is known and therefore transmission genetic analysis is not possible. To map a mendelian trait genetically, it is necessary to demonstrate that the trait in question does not segregate independently of a marker whose chromosomal location is known. Such an analysis is possible only if there are at least two allelic variants of the trait in question (e.g., neurofibromatosis and not neurofibromatosis) and of the chromosomal marker. Another great boon to genetics provided by molecular biology has been polymorphic chromosomal markers (Botstein et al., 1980). There is sufficient variability between the nucleic acid sequence of any two individuals in a species that polymorphic markers can be found readily. Originally, the polymorphisms most exploited for such studies were *restriction fragment length polymorphisms* (RFLPs), resulting from single base pair variations in sequences of four to eight nucleotides that are recognized by a cleaving *restriction endonuclease*, thus changing the length of the resulting nucleic acid fragment. Increasingly, investigators are exploiting other commonly occurring variations in nucleic acid sequence (such as *variable numbers of tandem repeats* [Jeffreys et al., 1985]) as markers for genetic studies.

THE HUMAN GENOME

The bulk of the human genome resides in the nuclear chromosomes, of which there are 22 autosomal pairs as well as two sex chromosomes: an X and a Y in males, two Xs in females. Most somatic cells contain a diploid set (two copies of each autosome as well as two sex chromosomes), although some (e.g., Purkinje cells in the cerebellum) are tetraploid, containing four copies of each autosome. Germ cells (spermatocytes and oocytes) contain a haploid set—one copy of each autosome, and only one sex chromosome. The nucleotide content of the haploid human genome is about 3 billion base pairs (Kornberg, 1980). The sex-averaged genetic size of the human genome, as estimated from scoring recombinations between linked markers is about 3400 centimorgans (cM), a genetic distance of 1 cM between two loci being defined as a 1% probability of recombination per meiosis. Therefore, as a first approximation, 1 cM represents about 1 million base pairs (megabase) separation. This is only a rough approximation for several reasons. First, although the physical size of the autosomal genome is the same in men and in women, women have a twofold higher rate of recombination in autosomes than do men (Donis-Keller et al., 1987). The genetic size of the female autosomal complement is therefore almost 90% greater than it is for men. Second, although there is a monotonic relationship between genetic distance and physical distance, the relationship is not linear. Rates of recombination per unit of physical length differ throughout the genome, varying between large and small chromosomes, telomeric (near the ends) and centromeric regions of a given chromosome, and perhaps clustered in recombinational "hot spots," as has been demonstrated in other organisms (Bodmer, 1986).

It is estimated that the haploid human genome contains 30,000–100,000 unique, single-copy genes (McKusick, 1986). At present, only a small percentage of them are known. Some encode familiar, well-characterized proteins with names and known structure and function. Other encoded proteins are known only as spots on two-dimensional protein electrophoretic gels. As of this writing, 1884 of these human genes have been mapped. Many of these genes can be grouped on the basis of sequence similarities into gene families and superfamilies. Sequence similarity within a gene family indicates duplication of a primordial gene followed by evolution through accumulation of independent mutations. Some members of a gene family encode proteins with similar functions but with differing patterns of tissue and developmental expression. For example, different genes encode myosin heavy chains for smooth, cardiac, and fast and slow skeletal muscle during embryonic, neonatal, and adult life (Buckingham et al., 1986). Other members of these gene families are pseudogenes, bearing sequence similarities to functional genes, but are themselves incapable of encoding proteins and are presumably vestiges of evolutionary experiments that went awry. Lesser degrees of sequence similarity link members of superfamilies, whose members have diverged through evolution to acquire distinct functional properties.

Although each human cell contains the full complement of the human genome, it is estimated that a typical cell expresses only about 15,000 genes: 10,000 of them "housekeeping" genes, common to all cells, and about 3000–6000 "luxury," or tissue-specific, genes (Lewin, 1990). As in other species, in humans, housekeeping and luxury genes can be distinguished by sequence difference in their associated regulatory regions. The pattern of expression of a given gene can be directly verified by hybridization of a gene-specific nucleic acid probe to RNA extracted from different tissue specimens and transferred to a nylon or nitrocellulose membrane (Northern blotting) or by in situ hybridization in histologic preparations.

Only a fraction of the 3 billion base pairs in the haploid human genome code for amino acids. Complexity analysis of the human genome reveals that only a portion of its sequence is present in single copy (e.g., genes encoding protein products [see earlier]). A large proportion of these single-copy genes consist of noncoding introns. In addition to single-copy genes, a significant proportion of the human genome consists of medium-repetitive DNA, which is present in 10–100,000 copies per haploid human genome. Some of these sequences encode

tRNAs, rRNAs, and histone proteins. A still more abundant class of DNAs are highly repetitive and are present in more than 100,000 copies per haploid genome. Although many of these highly repetitive elements have been characterized, the most abundant classes being the Alu (Schmid and Shen, 1985) and long interspersed repeated elements (Singer and Skowronski, 1985), their function remains unknown.

The structure and organization of the human genome are being determined in increasing detail. In addition to the 1884 mapped genes, 4859 DNA segments have been mapped. Only a small fraction of these mapped DNA segments reveal sufficient polymorphism to be usable as genetic markers. A major achievement has been the generation of a linkage map of the human genome using that subset of cloned DNA segments that detect highly polymorphic RFLPs as markers. At present, this linkage map consists of more than 550 RFLP markers, covering more than 95% of the human genome, at an average spacing of 5–10 million base pairs between markers (Donis-Keller et al., 1987). With achievement of this map, one is virtually assured of finding linkage for any mendelian trait, provided that there are sufficient numbers of informative (e.g., heterozygous for a marker and also for the disease allele) families segregating the trait in question available for study *and* that affected individuals can be distinguished reliably from those that are not affected.

In humans, linkage analysis offers only a limited degree of precision, a few centimorgans resolution at best. In theory, given sufficient iterations, linkage analysis should be sufficient to resolve differences at the level of a single nucleotide. Indeed, such resolution has been achieved in prokaryotes and viruses (Lewin, 1977). However, such precision necessitates many iterations. Because the human geneticist has only a few meioses available for examination, she or he determines not the true recombination frequency between loci, but a statistical estimate of the true genetic distance. Because this is a statistical method, each arithmetic increase in the accuracy of the estimate necessitates a geometric increase in the number of meioses examined (Murphy, 1982; Ott, 1985). For example, mapping a gene whose true distance is 10 cM from a marker locus with precision of about 5 cM typically necessitates a pedigree with several dozen individuals; to estimate genetic distance with resolution of tens of kilobases (for positive identification of a single gene), hundreds of thousands of individuals must be examined. Thus, in human genetics, linkage analysis provides a good way to estimate roughly the location of a particular gene but is insufficient to identify the gene itself.

A similar level of resolution is offered by *somatic cell genetics* (Ruddle and Creagan, 1975), in which a panel of human-rodent hybrid cells, each of which contains a full complement of rodent chromosomes but only one or a few human chromosomes or chromosome fragments. Such hybrid panels can be used to score either for gene products (e.g., a human enzyme whose electrophoretic mobility allows it to be distinguished from its rodent counterpart) or for hybridization with nucleic acid probes. Concordance between detection of the human gene product and the presence of a given human chromosome permits mapping of its gene to that chromosome. Genes present on the same chromosome (though not necessarily linked through meiosis) are said to be *syntenic*.

The ultimate level of resolution is offered by *sequence analysis*, in which each nucleotide in a region of interest is determined. Current methods allow sequence determination of regions of several hundred base pairs at a time, and automated methods under development will extend this to 10,000 base pairs at a time. Currently, only about 0.2% of the human genome has been sequenced. An international effort to sequence the entire human genome within the next 2 decades has been undertaken under the auspices of the Human Genome Organization. For this effort to be successful, methods have to be developed to bridge the resolution gap between the 5–10 million base pair resolution afforded by linkage analysis, the 1- to 10-kb resolution afforded by cloning in plasmids or cosmids followed by restriction analysis, and the single base pair resolution afforded by sequence analysis. Two of the most promising methods for analysis of DNA segments in the range of 100,000–1 million base pairs involve restriction of genomic DNA with so-called *rare cutters* (restriction endonucleases whose recognition sites are, on average, this widely spaced in the human genome) and their subsequent analysis by *pulsed field gel electrophoresis* (allowing passage of such large segments through suitable gels, thus separating them by size) (Lawrence et al., 1986) or after cloning in *yeast artificial chromosomes* (Burke et al., 1987), which will accommodate inserts of several hundred thousand base pairs.

The storage and analysis of the large amounts of data generated by such investigation pose significant problems in informatics. In the past 16 years, the consensus human gene map has been compiled by an international consortium of geneticists meeting roughly biannually to review current data and to assemble the map. Initially, the map was constructed on paper, but in more recent years, it has been recorded on computerized data base systems. The most ambitious of these, the Genome Database, went on-line in September 1990. In it, mapping data derived at the various levels of resolution described earlier are stored and correlated. Data in the Genome Database are cross-referenced with phenotypic descriptions in a compendium of more than 5000 mendelian human traits (McKusick et al., 1990) (itself available on-line from a central computer) and sequence information formerly housed in the Howard Hughes–Yale GenBank.

MAPPING OF HUMAN NEUROLOGIC DISEASES

Long before the era of molecular genetics, many neurologic disorders were known to be genetically determined because of their pattern of transmission in families. Mere clustering of a disorder within families is insufficient to prove heredity (Edwards, 1960), inasmuch as family members share environmental exposures as well as genes: diet (as in the case of transmission of the infectious agent of kuru through ritual cannibalism), sanitary and living conditions (exposure to infectious agents), and learned behaviors (as in the acquisition of language and other behavioral traits—q.v., the jumping Frenchmen of Maine [St. Hilaire et al., 1986]).

In addition to familial clustering, proof of the genetic basis of a disorder entails observation of transmission of the disease to offspring at frequencies predicted by mendelian principles. For those disorders that segregate as autosomal dominant traits, one expects to find the disorder in several generations, each affected parent transmitting the disorder to 50% of the offspring. Rare autosomal recessive disorders are present in only one generation, with 25% of offspring of unaffected heterozygous parents being affected. If the allele responsible for an autosomal recessive disorder is sufficiently rare in a given population, one observes an increased frequency of consanguinity in the parents of affected children, each parent having received one copy of the recessive allele from a common ancestor. The analysis of such inheritance patterns is formalized in statistical segregation analyses (Murphy and Chase, 1975), in which the likelihood of a particular mode of inheritance is compared with that of a spurious familial grouping of the disorder occurring by chance alone. Heritability of a disorder can sometimes be inferred reliably even in the absence of data from transmission genetics: determination of a primary sequence alteration in the responsible protein or correlation of a consistent chromosomal aberration, such as a gross deletion or translocation, with a given disordered phenotype has often been used to indicate the genetic nature of a disease. Indeed, because of small nuclear families and rare consanguinity, most autosomal recessive disorders appear sporadically, the family history being negative.

Before the advent of chromosomal markers, the only mendelian disorders that could be mapped to a particular chromosome were those that were X linked. The hallmark of X-linked recessive inheritance is the transmission of the disorder from unaffected carrier mothers to half of their sons. Affected sons transmit the carrier state to half of their daughters but never transmit the disorder to their sons. As this pattern has long been easily recognized, there are considerably more neurologic disorders that have been mapped to the X chromosome than to any of the autosomes (McKusick et al., 1990).

Before the advent of a complete RFLP linkage map, assignment of disorders to particular autosomes was a hit-or-miss proposition, depending largely on the availability of other phenotypic markers, the chromosomal position of whose encoding locus was known. In this era, myotonic dystrophy was linked to the secretor locus (Harper et al., 1972), later shown to be on chromosome 19; the Schut-Haymaker and the Menzel forms of olivopontocerebellar degeneration, to the HLA gene cluster (Morton et al., 1980) on chromosome 6; and one form of demyelinating hereditary motor-sensory neuropathy (HMSN) (Charcot-Marie-Tooth disease Ib) (Guiloff et al., 1982), to the Duffy locus (the first autosomal marker discovered in humans) on chromosome 1 (Donahue et al., 1968).

Since RFLP markers and other molecular techniques have become available, there has been an explosion in the rate of chromosomal mapping of neurologic and muscular disorders (Fig. 47–1), with 140 such disorders being given at least provisional chromosomal assignments (McKusick et al., 1990). To these can be added several neurologic disorders associated with mutations in the mitochondrial genome (see later). Mapping has been accomplished in several ways. Perhaps the most straightforward has been the mapping of the locus encoding the normal gene product, mutation of which had been implicated by nongenetic biochemical studies as being the underlying cause of the disorder (Table 47–1).

Of greater interest are those disorders whose primary gene product is still unknown, but whose map location has been deduced, either by linkage analysis, in the case of mendelian disorders, or because of association of somatic chromosomal abnormalities (deletions, translocations, reduction to homozygosity) in tumors affecting muscle or nerve (e.g., glioblastoma, meningioma, and rhabdomyosarcoma) (Table 47–2). Even when the disease gene has not yet been determined, demonstration of linkage has important practical and theoretic implications. First, demonstration of linkage confirms the mendelian nature of the disorder (Edwards, 1960). Such confirmation is particularly important in behavioral disorders for which segregation analyses are ambiguous and learned behaviors are strongly suspected to be etiologic (e.g., schizophrenia, manic-depressive illness [Byerley et al., 1989], alcoholism [Goodwin, 1976], the Tourette syndrome, and obsessive compulsive disorder [Robertson, 1989]). Similarly, such confirmation is useful for understanding tumors, in which toxic or infectious agents might be suspected to be the sole etiologic factors. Second, the availability of linked markers for mendelizing traits affords the opportunity for presymptomatic diagnosis. In a small handful of disorders, this raises the prospect of presymptomatic and possibly preventive treatment. However, at the present time, such presymptomatic intervention is usually limited to the provision of counseling regarding family planning and, if requested, the termination of pregnancy. Third, linkage provides an extra measure of diagnostic accuracy in those disorders, such as the genetically distinct forms of demyelinating HMSN (Chance et al., 1990; Fischbeck et al., 1986; Guiloff et al., 1982; Vance et al., 1989), that are currently indistinguishable phenotypically. Such diagnostic accuracy is likely to be of great importance in nongenetic biologic investi-

gations of these disorders, preventing unwitting comparison of entities of dissimilar types.

From these early studies, some useful generalizations can be drawn. First, these studies offer confirmation of the robustness of many clinical diagnoses. It is reassuring that every disorder that clinicians recognize as Huntington's disease maps to the p terminus of chromosome 4 (Folstein et al., 1985); what is strictly defined as Friedreich's ataxia, to the long arm of chromosome 9 (Chamberlain et al., 1988); and Duchenne's muscular dystrophy, to chromosomal band Xp21 (Murray et al., 1982). When one considers the vast variety of gene products necessary to give rise to a healthy caudate, cerebellum, or skeletal muscle, it is satisfying to know that there is a manageable level of concordance between genotype and neurologic phenotype (even though it was assumed tacitly before the initiation of mapping studies!).

Second, in certain instances, mutations at any of a number of loci can give rise to an identical phenotype. The most common form of demyelinating HMSN results from mutation on chromosome 17 (Chance et al., 1990; Vance et al., 1989); another, from mutation of a yet unknown gene on the X chromosome (Fischbeck et al., 1986); another, from a mutation on chromosome 1 (Guiloff et al., 1982); and still at least one other form, from mutation at a yet undertermined autosomal locus (Chance et al., 1990). Such genetic heterogeneity complicates the provision of genetic counseling on the basis of linkage analyses in such disorders: even the most careful analysis of chromosome 17 markers in a family segregating HMSN Ib (encoded on chromosome 1) is meaningless and potentially misleading.

Third, even mutations at the same locus can give rise to different clinical syndromes. For example, deletion mutations that disrupt the reading frame in the dystrophin locus give rise to the severe Duchenne phenotype, whereas in-frame deletions allow the generation of partially functioning protein and the milder Becker phenotype (Monaco et al., 1988). Although not yet proved, it appears likely that many of the autosomal recessive spinal muscular atrophies, ranging from acute Werdnig-Hoffmann disease to chronic, adult-onset spinal muscular atrophy, may turn out to be allelic disorders (Brzustowicz, 1990). It is further interesting that different mutations at the same locus can give rise to phenotypes that differ not only in their severity and age of onset but also in the pattern of neural involvement: a mutation completely disrupting function of hexosaminidase A gives rise to the well-known amaurotic familial idiocy (Tay-Sachs disease [Okada and O'Brien, 1969]), whereas apparently allelic, but less disruptive, mutations give rise to spinocerebellar degeneration (W.G. Johnson et al., 1982). In addition to allelic variation, different phenotypes can result from a mutation at the same locus because of variable mosaicism, resulting from either (1) lyonization of X-linked traits, as in carriers of Duchenne's muscular dystrophy (Richards et al., 1990) and heterozygotes

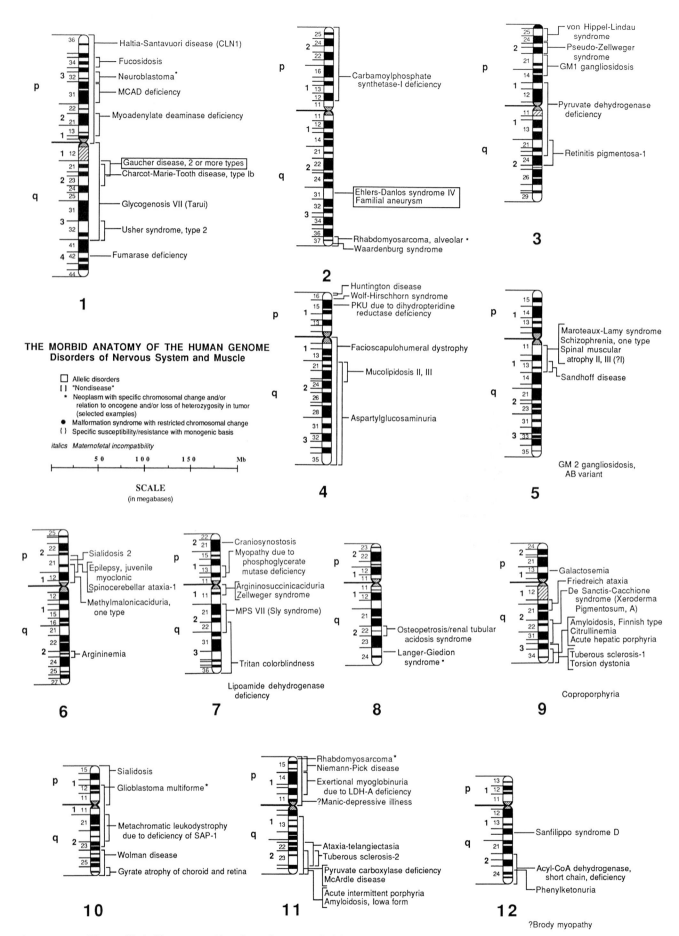

Figure 47–1. Chromosomal locations of genes underlying disorders of the nervous system or skeletal muscle.

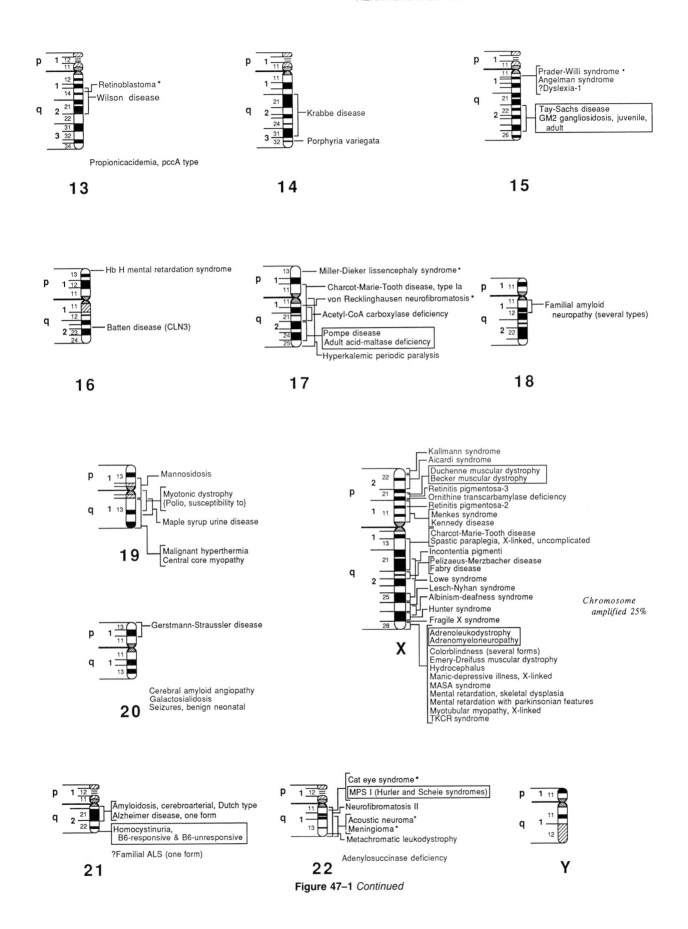

Figure 47–1 *Continued*

Table 47–1. HERITABLE NEUROLOGIC DISEASES: NORMAL GENE PRODUCT MAPPED

Map Position	Disease	Gene Product
1p21-p13	Myoadenylate deaminase deficiency	Myoadenylate deaminase
1p3	Fucosidosis	α-L-Fucosidase
1q	Glycogenosis VII (Tarui)	Phosphofructokinase M
1q21	Gaucher's disease 1, 2, and 3	Glucocerebrosidase
1q42.1	Fumarase deficiency	Fumarate hydratase
2p	Carbamoyl-phosphate synthetase deficiency	Carbamoyl-phosphate synthetase
3p13-q23	Pyruvate dehydrogenase deficiency	Pyruvate dehydrogenase E1α
3p21-p14.2	GM$_1$ gangliosidosis	β-Galactosidase 1
3p23-p22	Pseudo-Zellweger's syndrome	3-Oxo-acyl-CoA-thiolase
4p15.3	Phenylketonuria variant	Dihydropteridine reductase
4q21-q23	Mucolipidosis II	N-Acetylglucosamine-1-phosphotransferase
4q21-qter	Aspartylglucosaminuria	N-Aspartyl-β-glucosaminidase
5	GM$_2$ gangliosidosis AB variant	Hexosaminidase activator
5q13	Sandhoff's disease	β-Hexosaminidase
7	Pyruvate dehydrogenase deficiency	Pyruvate dehydrogenase E3
7cen-q11.2	Argininosuccinic aciduria	Arginosuccinate lyase
7p12.3-p13	Phosphoglycerate kinase	Phosphoglycerate mutase subunit M
7q22-qter	Tritan color blindness	Blue cone pigment
8q22	Osteopetrosis/renal tubular acidosis	Carbonic anhydrase II
9p13	Galactosemia	Galactose-1-phosphate uridyltransferase
9q33-34	Coproporphyria	Coproporphyroinogen oxidase
9q34	Acute hepatic porphyria	δ-Aminolevulinate dehydrase
9q34	Amyloidosis V (Finnish)	Prealbumin
9q34	Citrullinemia	Argininosuccinate synthetase
10p	Sialidosis	Neuraminidase
10q	Metachromatic leukodystrophy	Cerebroside sulfatase activator
10q24-q25	Wolman's disease	Lysosomal acid lipase
10q26	Gyrate atrophy	Ornithine aminotransferase
11p12-14	Myoglobinuria	Lactic dehydrogenase-A
11q	Pyruvate carboxylase deficiency	Pyruvate carboxylase
11q13	McArdle's disease	Muscle glycogen phosphorylase
11q23.2-ter	Acute intermittent porphyria	Porphobilinogen deaminase
12q14	Sanfillipo's syndrome D	N-Acetylglucosamine-6-sulfate sulfatase
12q22-qter	Lipid storage myopathy	Acyl CoA dehydrogenase
13	Propionic acidemia, type I	α-Propionyl-CoA carboxylase
14q21-q31	Krabbe's disease	Galactocerebrosidase
15q22-q25.1	Anterior horn disease (hexosaminidase A)	Hexosaminidase A
15q22-q25.1	GM$_2$ gangliosidosis, juvenile	Hexosaminidase A
15q22-q25.1	Tay-Sachs disease	α-1-Hexosaminidase
17	Niemann-Pick disease	Sphingomyelinase
17q	Acetyl coenzyme carboxylase deficiency	Acetyl-CoA carboxylase
17q23	Acid maltase deficiency	α-1,4-Glucosidase
19p13.2-q12	α-Mannosidosis	α-D-Mannosidase
19q13.1-q13.2	Maple syrup urine disease	Branched-chain α-keto acid dehydrogenase
20	Cerebral amyloid angiopathy	Cystatin C
20	Galactosialidosis	? 32-kd protein
21q21.3-q22.05	Cerebroarterial amyloidosis	β-A4 precursor protein
22	Adenylosuccinate lyase deficiency	Adenylosuccinate lyase
22ql	Mucopolysaccharidosis I	α-1-Iduronidase
22q13.31-qter	Metachromatic leukodystrophy	Arylsulfatase A
Xp	Pyruvate dehydrogenase deficiency	Pyruvate dehydrogenase E1β

Table 47–2. HERITABLE NEUROLOGIC DISEASES:
DISEASE MAPPED, GENE UNKNOWN

Map Position	Disease
1p	Haltia-Santavuori (neuronal ceroid lipofuscinosis, type 1)
1p32	Neuroblastoma
1q21.2-q23	Hereditary motor-sensory neuropathy, type Ib
1q32	Usher's syndrome, type II
2q37	Rhabdomyosarcoma, alveolar
3p25-p24	von Hippel–Lindau disease
4p16.3	Huntington's disease
4q31-qter	Facioscapulohumeral dystrophy
5q11-13	? Schizophrenia
5q11.2-13.3	Spinal muscular atrophy II and III
6p21	Juvenile myoclonic epilepsy
6p21.2-p11.3	Methylmalonic aciduria
6p21.3	Sialidosis 2 ?
6p21.3-p21.2	Olivopontocerebellar degeneration (one type)
6q2	Argininemia
7p12.3-p13	Craniosynostosis
7q11.23	Zellweger's syndrome
8q24.11-q24.13	Langer-Giedion
9q13-q21.1	Friedreich's ataxia
9q32-24	Torsion dystonia
9q33-q34	Tuberous sclerosis 1
10p12-q23.2	Glioblastoma multiforme ?
11p	? Manic-depressive illness
11pter-p15.5	Rhabdomyosarcoma
11q22-23	Ataxia-telangiectasia
11q23	Tuberous sclerosis 2
11q23-ter	Amyloidosis IV (Iowa)
13q14-21	Wilson's disease
13q14.1-q14.2	Retinoblastoma
14q32	Porphyria variegata
15	Xeroderma pigmentosum F
15q	Angelman's syndrome
15q11	Dyslexia ?-1
15q11	Prader-Willi syndrome
16pter-p13.3	Hemoglobin H mental retardation syndrome
16q	Batten's disease
17p11.2-q23	Hereditary motor-sensory neuropathy, type Ia
17p13.3	Miller-Dieker lissencephaly
17q	Hyperkalemic periodic paralysis
19q	Central core disease
19q13	Myotonic dystrophy
19q13.1-13.3	Malignant hyperthermia
20pter-p12	? Gerstmann-Straussler syndrome
21q11.2-q21	Familial Alzheimer's disease
21q22	Familial amyotrophic lateral sclerosis
22q11	Cat-eye syndrome
22q11-q13	Neurofibromatosis 2
22q12.3-qter	Meningioma
Xp	Kallmann's syndrome
Xp11	Incontinentia pigmenti
Xp11.3	Retinitis pigmentosa 2
Xp21	Retinitis pigmentosa 3
Xp222-223	Aicardi's syndrome
Xq12-13	Menkes' syndrome
Xq13	Hereditary motor-sensory neuropathy
Xq21-q22	Spastic paraplegia, uncomplicated
Xq21.3-q22	Kennedy's disease
Xq25	Lowe's oculocerebrorenal syndrome
Xq26.3-q27.1	Albinism-deafness syndrome
Xq27	? Manic-depressive illness
Xq27.3	Hunter's syndrome (mucopolysaccharidosis, II)
Xq28	Adrenoleukodystrophy
Xq28	Adrenomyeloneuropathy
Xq28	Emery-Dreifuss dystrophy
Xq28	Fragile X syndrome
Xq28	Myotubular myopathy
Xq28	Torticollis, keloids, cryptorchidism, and renal dysplasia syndrome

for ornithine transcarbamylase deficiency (Ricciuti et al., 1976), or (2) heteroplasmy for mtDNA mutations (Hurko et al., 1990) (see later).

Still the smallest group of mapped neurologic disorders are those in which the disorder itself was mapped by linkage methods and the normal gene product was either mapped independently, as was the case for one form of amyloidotic neuropathy (Tawara et al., 1983), or, as in the case of Duchenne's and Becker's muscular dystrophy (Kunkel, 1986; Monaco et al., 1986) and von Recklinghausen's neurofibromatosis (M.R. Wallace et al., 1990), in which the gene and its encoded product were determined largely on the basis of positional information provided by mapping experiments (Table 47–3).

FROM LINKAGE TO IDENTIFICATION OF A GENE

Perhaps the most interesting application of genetic and molecular techniques to the study of neurologic disorders is the isolation of the gene whose mutation underlies the disorder, when the primary defective gene product was not known. This approach, previously referred to as reverse genetics but perhaps more accurately termed *positional mapping*, has already proved successful in Duchenne's and Becker's muscular dystrophy (Kunkel, 1986; Monaco et al., 1986) and von Recklinghausen's neurofibromatosis (M.R. Wallace et al., 1990). As discussed earlier, owing to the inherent practical limitations of linkage analysis in humans, although genetic information can provide a useful first step to positive identification of a pathogenic gene, it is by no means sufficient. After linkage is established, any of a number of strategies can be employed to identify the pathogenic gene itself. These strategies can be laborious and far from straightforward. It is worthwhile to remember that the search for the Huntington disease gene still continues (MacDonald et al., 1989), even though

Table 47–3. HERITABLE NEUROLOGIC DISEASE: DISEASE AND DEFECTIVE GENE PRODUCT MAPPED

Map Position	Disease	Gene Product
12q24.1	Phenylketonuria	Phenylalanine hydroxylase
17q11.2	Neurofibromatosis 1	Antioncogene, ? adhesion molecule
18q11.2-q12.1	Amyloidotic neuropathy	Transthyretin
Xp21.1	Ornithine transcarbamylase deficiency	Ornithine transcarbamylase
Xp21.2	Becker's muscular dystrophy	Dystrophin
Xp21.2	Duchenne's muscular dystrophy	Dystrophin
Xq22	Fabry's disease	α-Galactosidase A
Xq22	Pelizaeus-Merzbacher disease	Proteolipid protein
Xq26-q27.2	Lesch-Nyhan syndrome	Hypoxanithine guanine phosphoribosyl transferase
Xq28	Color blindness	Green-red cone pigment

linkage to a 4p marker was established several years ago (Gusella et al., 1983).

The most conceptually straightforward of these approaches is the *candidate gene* approach. If there is biologic warrant to suspect a particular protein as the primary etiologic agent in a disorder, one can map the gene encoding the candidate protein to see if it is in the same location as the disease gene. The most powerful evidence resulting from such analysis is negative. Demonstration of a recombination between the candidate gene locus and the disease locus in a family heterozygous for each unequivocally proves that the candidate cannot be the primary etiologic agent for the disease. An example of such negative information came in the course of the initial mapping of the von Recklinghausen neurofibromatosis locus, with the demonstration of a crossover between the von Recklinghausen locus and that of the nerve growth factor receptor (Seizinger et al., 1987), a biologically attractive candidate known to map to chromosome 17. On the other hand, failure to demonstrate such a crossover in the limited number of meioses available in most investigations of human disease is corroboratory but not confirmatory. Several groups demonstrated tight linkage of the sodium channel and hyperkalemic periodic paralysis (Fontaine et al., 1990), other investigators, between the calcium release channel (the ryanodine receptor) and malignant hyperthermia (MacLennan et al., 1990). Confirmation of these genes as the primary etiologic factors in these two disorders awaits analysis of the candidate genes themselves in affected and normal individuals.

In the absence of viable candidates, considerable advantage can be gained from examination of those rare individuals who manifest the disease trait and also a gross chromosomal alteration, such as a deletion or a translocation, occurring in the vicinity of the disease gene locus (Kunkel, 1986; Kunkel et al., 1985). The assumption in such analyses is that the chromosomal alteration must disrupt the responsible gene itself. The object of the investigators is to identify, by molecular methods, the breakpoints of such a structural alteration and to determine which open reading frame was interrupted. When multiply affected individuals, each with slightly different chromosomal alterations, are available, the gene can be delimited by the common region of deletion. The inherent advantage of such gross structural alterations is that their locations are fixed and can therefore be determined directly, rather than by the intrinsically fuzzy statistical procedures inherent in strictly genetic analysis on limited samples. Such analyses were instrumental in the identification of the Duchenne and Becker gene and the von Recklinghausen neurofibromatosis gene.

If no patients with gross structural alterations in the region of interest can be found, genetic analysis continues in an effort to find additional, more closely linked markers. In addition to finding closer markers, it is especially useful to find bracketing markers (lying on either side of the disease locus). Bracketing markers not only improve the accuracy of presymptomatic diagnosis but also are useful in defining the limits within which the disease locus can be found. Such bracketing markers have been identified for myotonic dystrophy (Johnson et al., 1990; Schonk et al., 1990), raising hopes that the disease gene will be found. Determination of the order of closely spaced genes can be approached genetically, but at very close distances, physical maps, such as those afforded by pulsed field gel electrophoresis and yeast artificial chromosome cloning, are necessary. If the bracketing markers are separated by only a few hundred thousand kilobases, it is useful to determine a more detailed map of the bracketed interval, using overlapping cosmid, or λ, clones "contigs," each about 10–20 kb in length (Lawrence et al., 1986). Sequence analysis of a region completely covered with contigs may reveal several open reading frames, each of which becomes a candidate gene for the disorder.

Distinguishing between candidates can be far from straightforward and relies heavily on nongenetic, biologic information about the nature of the disease. One would select among the candidates the one whose developmental and tissue-specific pattern of expression matches that predicted by the known pathologic features of the disease. Nucleic acid probes generated from the candidate gene sequence can be hybridized to zoo blots (digests of genomic DNA from multiple species) on the assumption that a gene important enough that its disruption causes disease in humans must also be important enough to have been faithfully conserved through evolution. None of these analyses necessarily lead to incontrovertible proof, such as that which would obtain from transfer of the gene into another animal, rendering it transgenic. In a recessive disorder, transfer of the normal wild-type gene into an animal having the genetically identical disorder (itself no mean feat to establish!) should reverse the condition; in a dominant disorder, transfer of the candidate gene sequence into a healthy animal should induce the disorder.

EXCEPTIONS TO MENDELISM

Mitochondrial Disorders. To date, the majority of disorders associated with mutations of mtDNA have primarily displayed abnormalities in the nervous system or muscle, with variable involvement of other tissues. The common feature of these disorders has been impairment of the electron transport chain, a collection of some 70 proteins embedded in the inner mitochondrial membrane. The majority of these proteins are encoded by nuclear genes, mutations of which would segregate as mendelian disorders. However, 13 of the subunits of the electron transport chain are encoded by mtDNA, and their transmission is not expected to conform to mendelian principles: in humans, mtDNA is inherited exclusively from the mother and is present in thousands of copies per cell. Each of these copies is a separate genetic unit: a mutation affects itself and its progeny but not the other thousands of other mtDNAs within the same cell (D.C. Wallace, 1988).

Several different disorders have been associated with mutations in the mitochondrial genome. Some disorders, such as the original form of Leber's hereditary optic neuropathy for which the mutation has been mapped (D.C. Wallace et al., 1988), can be virtually homoplasmic in some individuals: every mitochondrion in the body bears the mutation. As might be expected, such mutations only disrupt the electron transport chain minimally. Curiously, the brunt of the pathologic phenotype is borne by the optic nerves and the cardiac conduction system, presumably reflecting special susceptibility of these tissues to minimal disruption of oxidative metabolism. Other mtDNA disorders result from large deletions of mtDNA (Holt et al., 1988), which delete entirely several genes encoding critical components of the electron transport chain as well as several tRNAs necessary for translation of all mitochondrially encoded proteins. Not surprisingly, such mutations have been observed only in the heteroplasmic state, the partially deleted mtDNA coexisting with variable numbers of normal species. There is no apparent correlation between the molecular site of the deletions and the clinical phenotype. Rather, the phenotype correlates most closely with the relative proportions of mutant and normal mtDNA present in a given organ (Hurko et al., 1990). These observations, plus the fact that mtDNA continues to replicate in postmitotic tissues such as the brain, suggest that mtDNA may be implicated in other neurodegenerative disorders.

Imprinting. According to mendelian theory, the phenotypic effects of a gene are the same whether it was inherited from the mother or the father. Several heritable disorders of the nervous system appear to violate that principle. The severe early-onset form of Huntington's disease (the Westphal variant) occurs only in children who inherit the Huntington gene from their father (Reik, 1988). Similarly, the severe early-onset form of myotonic dystrophy occurs only in those children who receive this autosomal gene from their mother (Harper and Dyken, 1972). Although imprinting (the reversible modification of genes during the formation of either male or female germ cells) has been proposed as an explanation for these curious phenomena, there is no proof of imprinting in either disorder, and these two examples admit to different explanations. Perhaps the most convincing example of the importance of the parental origin of genes is found in two clinically disparate mental retardation syndromes: the Angelman "happy puppet" syndrome (severe mental retardation, microcephaly, inappropriate laughter, and ataxia) and the Prader-Willi syndrome (mild-to-moderate mental retardation, obesity, short stature, and hypogonadism). The majority of cases of both syndromes are associated with similar, if not identical, deletions in the chromosomal region 15q11-q13 (Knoll

et al., 1989). In all informative cases of Angelman's syndrome associated with deletions, these deletions were found to be of maternal origin. Thus, affected children had only paternal genes in this region. In contrast, in Prader-Willi cases associated with deletions, these deletions were found to be of paternal origin. Furthermore, in studies of Prader-Willi patients with no grossly visible deletions, affected children were found to have maternal isodisomy for chromosome 15: two copies of the maternal chromosome, but no paternal copy (Nicholls et al., 1989). These studies strongly suggest that normal human development requires copies of genes from both parents.

Similar and more detailed observations of the parental origin of chromosomes in lower species further support the idea that certain genes may be modified differently during female and male gametogenesis. The mechanism underlying such differential processing (imprinting) is not known. However, a prevalent theory suggests that there may be different patterns of gene methylation imposed during gametogenesis in either sex. With the passage of genes through different sexes, they may again be modified, altering their pattern of expression in the somatic cells of the subsequent generation.

Multifactorial Inheritance. Many disorders of the nervous system appear to be inherited, but segregation analysis does not reveal simple mendelian ratios in affected families. Frequently, it is not known if familial clustering of these disorders results from genetic and/or shared environmental factors. Perhaps the most powerful method for sorting out the role of heredity in such disorders comes from studies of twins (Kinnunen et al., 1987), which are useful even if the mode of inheritance and relevant environmental factors are not known.

In some cases, expression of the disease phenotype requires not only the presence of a mutant allele but also exposure to a known environmental stressor. For example, malignant hyperthermia is expressed in an individual carrying a mutant autosomal gene only when that individual is exposed to halothane anesthesia. Segregation analyses that score only those individuals who have experienced a hyperthermic crisis as positive are confounded by those individuals who carry the mutant gene but who have not been exposed to general anesthetics. Ethical considerations preclude testing all family members with halothane. However, development of an in vitro halothane-caffeine contracture test on excised skeletal muscle has permitted ethical scoring of family members for malignant hyperthermia susceptibility and allowed the mapping of a gene responsible for susceptibility to this disorder to the long arm of chromosome 19 (MacLennan et al., 1990). In principle, such procedures could be applied to other multifactorial diseases in which exposure to environmental factors is important for expression of the disease phenotype. However, in many instances, suspected environmental triggers are not known or are not amenable to ethical testing.

Other disorders suspected of being heritable, but whose segregation does not conform to simple mendelian ratios may be *multilocal,* reflecting the summed contributions of alleles at several different loci. If the effect of each of the contributing genes is equal in magnitude, the inheritance pattern is said to be *multigenic;* if one gene has a considerably larger effect than do the others, the inheritance pattern is said to be *polymeric.* The distinction between unilocal (mendelian) inheritance and multilocal inheritance may be indistinct (Murphy and Bolling, 1967). One can model multilocal inheritance as a coin-tossing game, in which 10 pennies are tossed consecutively, the player winning any coin that comes up heads. It is obvious that, in this model, possible winnings range from nothing to 10 cents. However, it is impossible to tell from the final score which of the individual pennies were won. To model polymeric inheritance, the rules of the game stay the same, except that a silver dollar is substituted for one of the pennies. Again, the possible winnings vary, but the major effect of the dollar coin predominates, and loss or gain of that particular coin can be determined unequivocally. Intermediate inheritance patterns can be modeled by substituting a nickel, a dime, or a quarter for the dollar piece, or for one or several of the pennies.

Although such complex inheritance patterns have long been suspected in a number of neurologic disorders—autoimmune disorders such as multiple sclerosis (Haile, 1980) and myasthenia gravis (Kerzin-Storrar, 1988) known to be associated with certain HLA types; neuropsychiatric disorders such as schizophrenia and manic-depressive illness, in which segregation and linkage analyses have given contradictory results (Byerly et al., 1989); and disorders that contribute substantially to common neurologic dysfunction, such as atherosclerosis, hypertension, and diabetes—until recently, such models have been difficult to test. With the advent of a complete human gene map, permitting tracking of the human genome through multiple generations, as well as new mathematic paradigms for the analysis of such data (Ott, 1990), it may be possible to extend the impact of genetics on neurology far beyond those diseases currently recognized as mendelian disorders.

References

(Key references are designated with an asterisk.)

Antonarakis S.E.. Diagnosis of genetic disorders at the DNA level. *N. Engl. J. Med.* 320:153–163, 1989.

*Baraitser M. *The Genetics of Neurological Disorders.* 2nd ed. Oxford, Oxford University Press, 1990.

Bodmer W.F. Human genetics: the molecular challenge. *Cold Spring Harbor Symp. Quant. Biol.* 51:1–13, 1986.

Botstein D., White R.L., Scolnick M., et al. Construction of a genetic linkage map in man using restriction length polymorphisms. *Am. J. Hum. Genet.* 32:314–331, 1980.

Brzustowicz L.M., Lehner T., Castilla L.H., et al. Genetic mapping of chronic childhood spinal muscular atrophy to chromosome 5q11.2-13.3. *Nature* 344:540–541, 1990.

Buckingham M., Alonso S., Barton P., et al. Actin and myosin multigene families: their expression during the formation and maturation of striated muscle. *Am. J. Hum. Genet.* 25:623–634, 1986.

Burke D.T., Carle G.F., Olson M.V. Cloning of large segments of DNA into yeast by means of artificial chromosome vectors. *Science* 236:806–809, 1987.

Byerley W., Mellon C., O'Connell, P., et al. Mapping genes for manic-depression and schizophrenia with DNA markers. *Trends Neurosci.* 12:46–48, 1989.

Chamberlain S., Shaw J., Rowland A., et al. Mapping of a mutation causing Friedreich's ataxia to human chromosome 9. *Nature* 334:248–250, 1988.

Chance P.F., Bird T.D., O'Connell, P., et al. Genetic linkage and heterogeneity in type I Charcot-Marie-Tooth disease (hereditary motor and sensory neuropathy type I). *Am. J. Hum. Genet.* 47:915–925, 1990.

Donahue R.P., Bias W.B., Renwick J.H., et al. Probable assignment of the Duffy blood group locus to chromosome 1 in man. *Proc. Natl. Acad. Sci. U.S.A.* 61:949–955, 1968.

Donis-Keller H., Green P., Helms C., et al. A genetic linkage map of the human genome. *Cell* 51:319–337, 1987.

Edwards J.H. The simulation of mendelism. *Acta Genet.* 10:63–70, 1960.

Fischbeck K.H., ar-Rushdi N., Pericak-Vance M., et al. X-linked neuropathy: gene localization with DNA probes. *Ann. Neurol.* 20:527–532, 1986.

Folstein S.E., Phillips, J.A. III, Meyers D.A., et al. Huntington's disease: two families with differing clinical features show linkage to the G8 probe. *Science* 229:234–238, 1985.

Fontaine B., Khurana T.S., Bruns G.P., et al. Linkage analysis and periodic paralyses. *J. Neurol. Sci.* 98S:113, 1990.

Goodwin D. *Is Alcoholism Hereditary?* New York, Oxford University Press, 1976.

*Greenspan R.J. The emergence of neurogenetics. *Semin. Neurosci.* 2:145–157, 1990.

Guiloff R.J., Thomas P.K., Contreras M., et al. Evidence for linkage of type I hereditary motor and sensory neuropathy to the Duffy locus on chromosome 1. *Ann. Hum. Genet.* 46:25–27, 1982.

Gusella J.F., Wexler N.S., Conneally P.M., et al. A polymorphic DNA marker genetically linked to Huntington's disease. *Nature* 306:234–238, 1983.

Haile R.W. Genetic susceptibility to multiple sclerosis: a linkage analysis with age of onset corrections. *Clin. Genet.* 18:160–167, 1980.

Harper P.S., Dyken P.R. Early-onset dystrophia-myotonica: evidence supporting a maternal environmental factor. *Lancet* 2:53–55, 1972.

Harper P.S., Rivas M.L., Bias W.B., et al. Genetic linkage confirmed between the locus for myotonic dystrophy and the ABH-secretion and Lutheran blood group loci. *Am. J. Hum. Genet.* 24:310–316, 1972.

Holt I.J., Harding A.E., Morgan-Hughes J.A. Deletions of muscle mitochondrial DNA in patients with mitochondrial myopathies. *Nature* 331:717–719, 1988.

Hurko O., Johns D.R., Rutledge S.L., et al. Heteroplasmy in chronic progressive external ophthalmoplegia: clinical and molecular observations. *Pediatr. Res.* 28:542–548, 1990.

Jeffreys A., Wilson V., Thein S. Hypervariable "minisatellite" regions in human DNA. *Nature* 306:234–239, 1985.

Johnson K., Shelbourne P., Davies J., et al. A new probe that flanks myotonic dystrophy on the distal side. *J. Neurol. Sci.* 98S:38, 1990.

Johnson W.G., Wigger H.J., Karp H.R., et al. Juvenile spinal muscular atrophy: a new hexosaminidase deficiency phenotype. *Ann. Neurol.* 11:11–16, 1982.

Kerzin-Storrar, L. Genetic factors in myasthenia gravis. *Neurology* 38:38–42, 1988.

Kinnunen E., Koshenvuo M., Kapiro J. Multiple sclerosis in a nationwide study of twins. *Neurology* 37:1627–1629, 1987.

Knoll J.H.M., Nicholls R.D., Magenis R.E., et al. Angelman and Prader-Willi syndromes share a common chromosome 15 deletion but differ in parental origin. *Am. J. Hum. Genet.* 32:285–290, 1989.

Kornberg A. *DNA Replication.* San Francisco, Wiley, 1980.

Kunkel L.M. Analysis of deletions in DNA from patients with Becker and Duchenne muscular dystrophy. *Nature* 322:73–77, 1986.

Kunkel L.M., Monaco A.P., Middlesworth W., et al. Specific cloning of DNA fragments absent from the DNA of a male patient with an X chromosome deletion. *Proc. Natl. Acad. Sci. U.S.A.* 82:4778–4782, 1985.

Lawrence S.K., Srivastava R., Rigas B., et al. Molecular approaches to the characterization of megabase regions of DNA: applications to the human major histocompatibility complex. *Cold Spring Harbor Symp. Quant. Biol.* 51:123–130, 1986.

Lewin B. *Gene Expression. 3. Plasmids and Phages.* New York, Wiley, 1977.

*Lewin B. *Genes IV.* Chichester, Wiley, 1990.

MacDonald M.E., Haines J.L., Zimmer M., et al. Recombination events suggest potential sites for the Huntington's disease gene. *Neuron* 3:183–190, 1989.

MacLennan D.H., Duff C., Zorzato F., et al. Ryanodine receptor gene is a candidate for predisposition to malignant hyperthermia. *Nature* 343:559–561, 1990.

McKusick V.A. The gene map of *Homo sapiens*: status and prospectus. *Cold Spring Harbor Symp. Quant. Biol.* 51:15–27, 1986.

*McKusick V.A., Francomano C.A., Antonarakis S.E. *Mendelian Inheritance in Man: Catalogs of Autosomal Dominant, Autosomal Recessive, and X-Linked Phenotypes.* 9th ed. Baltimore, Johns Hopkins University Press, 1990.

Monaco A.P., Neve R.L., Colletti-Feener C., et al. Isolation of candidate cDNA's for portions of the Duchenne muscular dystrophy gene. *Nature* 323:646–650, 1986.

Monaco A.P., Bertelson C.J., Liechti-Gallati S, et al. An explanation for the phenotypic differences between patients bearing partial deletions of the DMD locus. *Genomics* 2:90–95, 1988.

Morton N.E., Lalouel J.-M., Jackson J.F. Linkage studies in spinocerebellar ataxia. *Am. J. Hum. Genet.* 6:251–257, 1980.

Mullis K., Faloona F., Scharf S. Specific enzymatic amplification of DNA in vitro: the polymerase chain reaction. *Cold Spring Harbor Symp. Quant. Biol.* 51:263–273, 1986.

Murphy E.A. *Probability in Medicine.* Baltimore, Johns Hopkins University Press, 1979.

Murphy E.A. *Biostatistics in Medicine.* Baltimore, Johns Hopkins University Press, 1982.

Murphy E.A., Bolling D.R. Testing of single-locus hypotheses where there is incomplete separation of the phenotypes. *Am. J. Hum. Genet.* 19:322–329, 1967.

*Murphy E.A., Chase G.A. *Principles of Genetic Counselling.* Chicago, Year Book Medical Publishers, 1975.

Murray J.M., Davies K.E., Harper P.S., et al. Linkage analysis of a cloned DNA sequence on the short arm of the X chromosome to Duchenne muscular dystrophy. *Nature* 300:69–71, 1982.

Nicholls R.D., Knoll J.H.M., Butler M.G., et al. Genetic imprinting suggested by maternal heterodisomy in non-deletion Prader-Willi syndrome. *Nature* 342:281–285, 1989.

Okada S., O'Brien J.S. Tay-Sachs disease: generalized absence of beta-D-N-acetylhexosaminidase component. *Science* 165:698–700, 1969.

Ott J. *Analysis of Human Genetic Linkage.* Baltimore, Johns Hopkins University Press, 1985.

Ott J. Invited editorial: Cutting a Gordian knot in the linkage analysis of complex human traits. *Am. J. Hum. Genet.* 46:219–221, 1990.

Rand D.M., Harrison R.G. Molecular population genetics of mtDNA size variation in crickets. *Genetics* 121:551–559, 1989.

Reik W. Genomic imprinting: a possible mechanism for the parental origin effect in Huntington's chorea. *J. Med. Genet.* 25:805–808, 1988.

Ricciuti F.C., Geleherter T.D., Rosenberg L.E. X-chromosome inactivation in human liver: confirmation of X-linkage of ornithine transcarbamylase. *Am. J. Hum. Genet.* 28:332–338, 1976.

Richards C.S., Watkins S.C., Hoffman E.P., et al. Skewed X inactivation in a female MZ twin results in Duchenne muscular dystrophy. *Am. J. Hum. Genet.* 46:672–681, 1990.

Robertson M.M. The Gilles de la Tourette syndrome: the current status. *Br. J. Psychol.* 154:147–169, 1989.

Rosenberg R.N., Harding A.E. *The Molecular Biology of Neurological Disease.* London, Butterworth, 1988.

Ruddle F.H., Creagan R.P. Parasexual approaches to the genetics of man. *Annu. Rev. Genet.* 9:407–486, 1975.

Sambrook J., Fritsch E.F., Maniatis T. *Molecular Cloning: A Laboratory Manual.* 2nd ed. Cold Spring Harbor, NY, Cold Spring Harbor Laboratory, 1989.

Schmid C.W., Shen C.K.J. The evolution of interspersed repetitive DNA sequences in mammals and other vertebrates. In MacIntyre R.J., ed. *Molecular Evolutionary Genetics.* New York, Plenum Publishing, 1985.

Schonk D., Vanijk P., Riegmann P., et al. Assignment of 7 genes to distinct intervals on the midportion of human chromosome-19q surrounding the myotonic dystrophy gene region. *Cytogenet. Cell Genet.* 54:15–19, 1990.

Seizinger B.R., Rouleau G.A., Ozelius L.J., et al. Genetic linkage of von Recklinghausen neurofibromatosis to the nerve growth factor receptor gene. *Cell* 49:589–594, 1987.

Singer M.F., Skowronski J. Making sense out of LINES: long interspersed repeat sequences in mammalian genomes. *Trends Biochem. Sci.* 10:119–123, 1985.

Smith C.A. The detection of linkage in human genetics. *J. R. Stat. Soc. Ser. B* 15:153–192, 1953.

St. Hilaire M.-H., Saint-Hilaire J.-M., Granger L. Jumping Frenchmen of Maine. *Neurology* 36:1269–1271, 1986.

Sturtevant A.M., Beadle G.W. *An Introduction to Genetics.* Philadelphia, Saunders, 1940.

Tawara S., Nakazato M., Kangawa K., et al. Identification of amyloid prealbumin variant in familial amyloidotic polyneuropathy. *Biochem. Biophys. Res. Commun.* 116:880–888, 1983.

Vance J.M., Nicholson G., Yamaoka L.H., et al. Linkage of Charcot-Marie-Tooth neuropathy type Ia to chromosome 17. *Cytogenet. Cell Genet.* 51:1097–1098, 1989.

Wallace D.C. Maternal genes: mitochondrial· inheritance. In McKusick V.A., Roderick T.H., Mori J., et al., eds. *Medical and Experimental Mammalian Genetics: A Perspective.* New York, Liss, 1988.

Wallace D.C., Singh G., Lott M.T., et al. Mitochondrial DNA polymorphism in Leber's optic atrophy. *Science* 242:1427–1430, 1988.

*Wallace M.R., Marchuk D.A., Andersen L.B., et al. Identification of a large transcript disrupted in 3 NF1 patients. *Science* 249:181–186, 1990.

48

Genetic and Metabolic Diseases: Mechanisms and Potential for Therapy

Hugo W. Moser

Since the previous edition of this book, the range and power of therapies for metabolic-genetic disorders of the nervous system have increased. This chapter subdivides therapies into two major categories. Indirect therapies include nutritional and metabolic manipulations, pharmocologic agents, and the avoidance of precipitating factors. These approaches were and continue to be the mainstay and may be remarkably effective. Enzyme replacement, transplants, and gene therapy are direct therapies because they aim to correct the fundamental deficit. These approaches are only now emerging, but success has been documented in some instances.

How many of the metabolic-genetic disorders of the nervous system can be treated? Table 48–1 lists 65 conditions in which specific therapies have had some degree of success. Indirect approaches were used in 53, and direct, in 16, with both approaches being used in 4. The degree of success is variable, depending on the condition or its subtype. The likelihood of success is increased by early diagnosis, because prevention of nervous system damage is more efficacious than restoration of function.

The future for patients with metabolic-genetic disorders of the nervous system is encouraging for at least two reasons. No doubt the direct therapeutic approaches will become available for a larger number of conditions and will also become more effective. In addition, the sensitivity of specific noninvasive diagnostic techniques is increasing, and their cost is diminishing. This, together with the improved prospects for therapy, is leading to more intensive efforts to achieve early and specific diagnosis. This trend is to be encouraged. There is no shotgun therapy for mental retardation or neurologic deficits. All medical successes are the consequence of specific diagnosis and the success is greatest when diagnosis is achieved before symptoms occur or before they are severe.

INDIRECT THERAPIES

Indirect therapies include all of the approaches used to ameliorate the ill effects of a genetic disorder without replacement of the defective enzyme or gene. These approaches are cited in Table 48–1. They are varied and necessitate an understanding of pathogenesis, ingenuity, and a high degree of life-long cooperation from the patient. They can be remarkably effective. The indirect approaches include the measures discussed in the following sections.

Reduce Intake of Substances to Which the Patient is Genetically Vulnerable

This goal is achieved by modification of diet and is applied in the therapy of phenylketonuria, galactosemia, maple syrup urine disease, Refsum's disease, the urea cycle disorders, methylmalonic aciduria, and other conditions (see Table 48–1).

Therapy of phenylketonuria is a significant public health issue. More than 100 million newborn infants throughout the world have been screened for this disorder. With an incidence of disease in 1 per 11,000, more than 10,000 children are now under treatment. The success of this therapeutic approach is possible because phenylalanine is an essential amino acid

Table 48–1. THERAPIES FOR METABOLIC-GENETIC DISORDERS THAT AFFECT THE NERVOUS SYSTEM*

Disorder	Diet	Drugs	Other
Abetalipoproteinemia	Restrict long chain triglycerides	Vitamins A and E	
Acyl-CoA dehydrogenase deficiency, medium chain			Avoid fasting; glucose in emergency
Acyl-CoA dehydrogenase deficiency, long chain	? Medium chain triglyceride Frequent feeding	? Carnitine	Avoid fasting
Adenosine deaminase deficiency			Enzyme replacement BMT† Gene therapy
Adrenoleukodystrophy, X linked	Restrict very long fatty acids	Glycerol trierucate	? BMT
Arginase deficiency	Low protein	Sodium benzoate Sodium phenylactate	
Argininosuccinic lyase deficiency	Low protein	Sodium benzoate	Hemodialysis
Biotinidase deficiency		Biotin	
Carbamoylphosphate-synthase deficiency	Low protein	Sodium benzoate Sodium phenylacetate	Hemodialysis
Carnitine palmitoyltransferase deficiency	High carbohydrate Low fat		Avoid strenuous exercise
Cholesterol ester storage disease		Hydroxymethylglutaryl-CoA reductase inhibitors	Liver transplant
Cerebrotendinous xanthomatosis		Chenodeoxycholic acid	
Citrullinemia	Low protein	Sodium benzoate Sodium phenylactate	
Cystinosis		Cysteamine	Kidney transplant Cysteamine eye drops
Fabry's disease		Diphenylhydantoin for acroparesisthesia	Enzyme replacement Kidney transplant
Folate malabsorption, hereditary		Folic acid	
Fructose-1,6-bisphosphatase deficiency	Low fructose Low sucrose		Avoid fasting
Galactosemia	Low galactose		
Gaucher's disease types 1 and 3			BMT Enzyme replacement
Globoid leukodystrophy			? BMT
Glutaric aciduria type I	Low protein Low lysine Tryptophan	? Riboflavin ? Carnitine	Metabolic Stress management
Glutaric aciduria type II, mild	Low protein	Carnitine Riboflavin	Treat acidosis
Glutathione synthetase deficiency		Vitamin E ?	Avoid specified drugs
Glycerol kinase deficiency			Avoid excessive glycerol Treat adrenal insufficiency
Glycogenosis type I	Nocturnal glucose by nasogastric route Uncooked starch		
Glycogenosis type IV			Treat liver cirrhosis Liver transplant
Glycogenosis type V (McArdle's)			Avoid strenuous exercise
Gyrate atrophy of retina	Restrict arginine	Pyridoxine	
Hartnup's disorder		Nicotinic acid	
Holocarboxylase synthetase deficiency	Restrict betaine, and methionine	Pyridoxine	
Hunter's syndrome (mucopolysaccharidosis II)			BMT
Hurler's syndrome			BMT
3-Hydroxy-3-methylglutaric aciduria	Low protein Low leucine Fat restriction	? Carnitine	
Hyperornithinemia, hyperammonemia, hypercitrullinemia	Low protein	Ornithine supplement ?	
Hyperoxaluria type 1		Pyridoxine ?	Treat renal disease Kidney or liver transplant

(Table continued on following page)

Table 48–1. THERAPIES FOR METABOLIC-GENETIC DISORDERS THAT AFFECT
THE NERVOUS SYSTEM* *Continued*

Disorder	Diet	Drugs	Other
Hypobetalipoproteinemia, familial	Low fat	Vitamin E	
Hypothyroidism, congenital		Thyroid hormone	
Isovaleric acidemia	Low protein	Glycine, carnitine	
Maple syrup urine disease	Restrict branched chain amino acids		
Metachromatic leukodystrophy			? BMT
Methionine synthase deficiency		Vitamin B$_{12}$	
2-Methylacetoacetyl-CoA thiolase deficiency	Low protein		
3-Methylcrotonyl-CoA carboxylase deficiency	Low protein	Biotin ?	Manage acidosis
3-Methylgutaconic aciduria	Low protein		
Methylenetetrahydrofolate reductase deficiency		Folate Vitamin B$_{12}$ Betaine, carnitine	
Methylmalonic aciduria and homocystinuria		Vitamin B$_{12}$	
Methylmalonyl-CoA mutase deficiency	Low protein Low valine Low isoleucine Low methionine Low threonine	Vitamin B$_{12}$ Carnitine	
Mucopolysaccharidosis type VI (Maroteaux-Lamy)			BMT
Mucopolysaccharidosis type VII (Sly's)			BMT
Ornithine transacarbamylase deficiency	Low protein	Sodium benzoate Sodium phenylacetate	Hemodialysis
Orotic aciduria, hereditary (uridine monophosphate synthase deficiency)		Uridine	
Phenylketonuria caused by dihydropteridine reductase deficiency	Phenylalanine restriction	Folinic acid Levodopa-dopa 5-Hydroxytryptophan	
Phenylketonuria caused by phenylalanine hydroxylase deficiency	Phenylalanine restriction		
Porphyria, acute intermittent			Avoid specified drugs
Propionic acidemia	Low protein Low leucine, isoleucine, valine, threonine, methionine	Biotin ?	
Pseudohypoparathyroidism		Calcium Vitamin D Acetazolamide	
Pyridoxine dependency		Pyridoxine	
Pyruvate decarboxylase deficiency	Low carbohydrate High fat	Dichloroacetate ? Thiamine ?	
Refsum's disease	Restrict phytanic acid		Plasma exchange
Sanfilippo's syndrome (mucopolysaccharidosis type III)			BMT ?
Sjögren-Larsson syndrome	Low fat Medium chain triglyceride		
Tyrosinemia type I (fumarylacetoacetate hydrolase deficiency)	Restrict phenylalanine, tyrosine		Liver transplant
Tyrosinemia type II (tyrosine aminotransferase deficiency)	Restrict phenylalanine, tyrosine		
Tyrosinemia, neonatal	Low protein	Ascorbic acid ?	
Wilson's disease		Penicillamine Trientine Zinc	Plasmapheresis Peritoneal dialysis Liver transplant for acute crisis

*This is a listing of genetic disorders that affect the nervous system, have a metabolic defect that can be defined biochemically, and can be improved at least to some least extent by therapy. For details see the text or Scriver C.R., Beaudet A.L., Sly, W.S., et al., eds. *The Metabolic Basis of Inherited Disease.* 6th ed. New York, McGraw-Hill, pp. 1–3006, 1989.

†BMT = bone marrow transplant.

(i.e., it is not synthesized in the body), so that dietary intake is the only source of this substance. The patient with phenylketonuria requires the same amount of phenylalanine, 200–500 mg/day for the first 5 years of life, as does the normal person. Patients with phenylketonuria differ from normal persons in that they are unable to dispose of amounts of phenylalanine in excess of this requirement. The aim of therapy is to provide a diet that contains no more than the minimal daily requirement of phenylalanine and that nevertheless contains all other nutrients and is palatable (Scriver and Clow, 1980). If the diet is begun early, preferably within the first 60 days of life, the risk of severe mental retardation (which is 99% in untreated patients) is greatly decreased. Longer follow-up studies indicate that the previous practice of relaxing dietary restriction of phenylalanine at 6 years of age is not desirable.

As part of a collaborative study of children treated for phenylaketonuria, intellectual function and behavior were evaluated in 110 10-year-old children who had started dietary therapy before 65 days of age. Children who had discontinued the diet at 6–8 years of age had significantly lower IQ scores than those in whom dietary control was maintained, and the severity of the deficit correlated inversely with the age at which the diet was discontinued (Holtzman et al., 1986). It is now recommended that dietary restriction of phenylalanine (250–500 mg/day) be continued throughout childhood and adolescence, and probably throughout life, with the aim of holding the plasma phenylalanine concentration below 1 mM and above 0.25 mM.

Two important issues have arisen in respect to phenylketonuria: maternal phenylketonuria and malignant phenylketonuria. *Maternal phenylketonuria* refers to the damage incurred during fetal life to a child born to a phenylketonuric woman. The child in almost all instances is a heterozygote for phenylketonuria and would not be handicapped by this were it not for the ill effects during pregnancy. Mental retardation (an IQ of less than 75) was observed in 91% of children born to mothers with a plasma phenylalanine level in excess of 1.2 mM (Lenke and Levy, 1980). The risk of maternal phenylketonuria has been increased greatly by the success of therapy of the phenylketonuric child. In the past, the untreated profoundly retarded woman with phenylketonuria hardly ever became pregnant. As a result of successful therapy, a large number of women with phenylketonuria and normal intelligence are now considering marriage. Two collaborative studies lead to the encouraging conclusion that phenylketonuric women can have normal children, provided that plasma phenylalanine levels are maintained below 0.6 mM before conception and throughout the pregnancy (Drogari et al., 1987; Rohr et al., 1987).

Malignant phenylketonuria refers to a group of disorders in which blood phenylalanine levels are elevated, and thus are detected by mass screening of newborns, but in which dietary restriction of phenylalanine does not prevent mental retardation or neurologic deficit. These patients may have several different enzyme defects, some of which lead to a deficiency of tetrahydropterin, a cofactor required for the conversion of phenylalanine to tyrosine. Malignant phenylketonuria is estimated to be present in 2% of children with significant and persistent hyperphenylalaninemia. Early detection methods are being developed (Danks, 1980). Folinic acid therapy, combined with neurotransmitter precursor replacement and dietary restriction of phenylalanine, can ameliorate this condition and, if begun early in infancy, may prevent neurologic deficits (Irons, 1987).

Other disorders in which success has been achieved by limiting the intake of precursors that may undergo toxic accumulation are maple syrup disease (Snyderman et al., 1964), galactosemia (Komrower and Lee, 1970), and Refsum's disease (Refsum, 1981). Komrower's (1982) review of 30 years' experience with galactosemia indicates that eventual intellectual function may be subnormal even in patients who maintained dietary restriction of galactose. Nearly all female patients also have ovarian dysfunction (Levy et al., 1984). The therapy of maple syrup urine disease differs from that of phenylketonuria in that the achievement of dietary restriction of the amino acids leucine, isoleucine, and valine is more difficult than that of phenylalanine alone. Furthermore, the restriction must be maintained for life, and there may be intermittent periods of life-threatening acidosis. Nevertheless, the oldest patient, who was 15 years old at the latest report, has normal intellectual function, is performing at grade level in regular school, and has achieved normal growth and sexual maturation (Moser, 1977).

Varying degrees of success with dietary restriction of leucine, isoleucine, or other amino acids have also been achieved in isovaleric acidemia (Levy and Erickson, 1974), methylmalonic acidemia (Nyhan et al., 1973), and propionic acidemia (Brandt et al., 1974). These disorders may also respond dramatically to the administration of vitamin cofactors (see later).

Replace Missing Metabolite in Physiologic Amounts

Apart from insulin, which is not discussed here, thyroid hormone is the most important substance for physiologic replacement. It assumes ever greater significance because most states in the United States and many countries throughout the world screen all newborns for hypothyroidism, in combination with Guthrie spot tests for phenylketonuria. The incidence of congenital hypothyroidism is 1 per 4000, more than twice that of phenylketonuria. Follow-up studies indicate that the adverse effects of prenatal hypothyroidism are largely avoided if treatment is begun before the age of 6 weeks (Hulse, 1984; New England Congenital Hypothyroidism Collaborative, 1981).

Follow-up studies in the United Kingdom (Hulse,

1984), Sweden (Ilicki and Larson, 1988), and Canada (Glorieux et al., 1988) document that congenitally hypothyroid children whose thyroid replacement therapy is begun before 1 month of age usually achieve normal IQ scores at 4–9 years. However, a subgroup of children who were most severely hypothyroid before therapy, as judged by plasma thyroxine level of less than 2 µg/dl and severely retarded bone maturation, had slightly subaverage IQ scores (86–91) in spite of early therapy (Glorieux et al., 1988). Even with this limitation, these outcome results differ dramatically from what would have been predicted without early intervention, namely, a mean IQ of 61 and a score of less than 45 in 25% of patients (Gesell et al., 1936).

Remove Toxic Substances

Copper Chelation Therapy in Wilson's Disease

A striking and important example of chelation therapy is removal of the excessive copper that accumulates, for reasons that are still unknown, in the brain, the liver, and the kidney of patients with Wilson's disease. The highly successful oral penicillamine therapy for this disorder was introduced by Walshe in 1955. Walshe (1983) summarized his unique experience with this disorder, stating that "most patients will respond, whether showing mainly hepatic or neurological signs and symptoms, and that however advanced the stage of the illness, no patient should be despaired of, though obviously the less tissue damage done before therapy is started the better the prognosis. . . . The neurological deficit, however severe, will almost always respond to treatment and . . . most patients are able to resume a normal life—although this takes time, 6 months at least—and often 2 or more years in those patients with the most severe disabilities."

About 20% of patients with Wilson's disease experience side effects of penicillamine during the first month of therapy (Marsden, 1987). These include fever, rash and lymphadenopathy, and more seriously, granulocytopenia and thrombocytopenia. In addition, there may be early and transient worsening of the neurologic disability (Brewer et al., 1987). The early neurologic worsening may be reduced by administering low doses of penicillamine initially (Brewer et al., 1987). An important additional measure is the simultaneous administration of zinc sulfate, which mobilizes copper for urinary excretion. Zinc sulfate has been proposed as an alternative to penicillamine therapy, and favorable results have been reported in 27 patients (Hoogenraad et al., 1987). The chelating agent trientine can be used as a substitute in patients who have adverse reactions to penicillamine (Scheinberg et al., 1987). Orthotopic liver transplantation was successful in a 13-year-old patient with Wilson's disease who had fulminant and life-threatening hepatic failure (Sokol et al., 1985).

The dramatic success in the therapy of Wilson's disease leads to several conclusions of general interest to neuroscientists. First, because copper removal reverses even severe symptoms, this metal is the toxic agent. It is extremely encouraging that, provided one truly has the right approach, even severe neurologic symptoms can be reversed. This observation has important implications for those who in the past viewed neurology as a diagnostically rather than a therapeutically oriented discipline. Walshe (1983) deplored the number of patients with Wilson's disease who remain undiagnosed. The incidence is probably of the order of 3 per 100,000 rather than the 3 per 1 million that had been cited by Walshe.

Reduction of Hyperammonemia in Patients with Inborn Errors of Urea Synthesis

The five inborn errors of urea synthesis have a combined incidence of 1 per 30,000, and affected infants accumulate ammonia and other nitrogenous compounds. Various methods have been used to reduce the accumulation of ammonia. The most effective method combines nitrogen restriction and the stimulation of alternative pathways of waste nitrogen excretion. Particularly effective agents are sodium benzoate, which is conjugated with glycine and excreted as hippuric acid, and sodium phenylacetate. Acute hyperammonemia represents an emergency that is treated with avoidance of all protein intake; intravenous administration of glucose, sodium benzoate, and phenylacetate; and hemodialysis if the response to initial therapy is insufficient (Brusilow et al., 1984). This therapy led to a striking reduction in mortality; the 1-year survival rate was 92%, and gratifying reduction of hyperammonemia was achieved. However, most treated children who had at least one episode of hyperammonemia coma lasting for more than 3 days eventually functioned in the severely retarded range (mean IQ, 43) (Msall et al., 1984). The challenge is to establish diagnosis early and to prevent the occurrence or shorten the duration of hyperammonemic coma.

Avoid Circumstances, Activities, or Drugs That Are Harmful in Specific Disorders

Precise diagnosis and understanding of pathogenesis make it possible to avoid precipitating factors that may lead to severe and, at times, irreversible worsening in several disorders. Striking examples are medium chain acyl-CoA dehydrogenase deficiency (Taubman et al., 1987) and glutaric aciduria type I (Bergman et al., 1989). In both of these disorders, the precipitating events are circumstances or illnesses that limit caloric intake, such as a gastrointestinal disturbance, an intercurrent illness, or a prolonged fast. These circumstances then lead to utilization of body fats or proteins as the prime source of energy, and this in turn accentuates the effects of the primary genetic defect and leads to a cascade of metabolic disturbances that may cause death owing to a Reye's syndrome–like condition in the medium acyl-CoA dehydrogenase deficiency or permanent damage to basal ganglia in glutaric aciduria. It is possible to diagnose these conditions in asymptomatic children who are known to be at risk (Rinaldo et al., 1988) and to institute measures that prevent the devastating acute decompensation. These measures include the prompt therapy of intercurrent illnesses, the reduction of protein load and the provision of carbohydrate-derived calories, and the avoidance of prolonged fasts. Other examples of such preventive measures are listed in Tables 48–1 and 48–2.

Administer Large Doses of Vitamins or Cofactors Under Clearly Defined Circumstances

In a rare but interesting group of disorders (see Table 48–1), administration of unusually large quantities of specified vitamins or cofactors can return a severely disabled individual to normal function. Some general characteristics of these disorders are

1. Vitamin cofactor action is specific and can be related to cofactor requirements of deficient enzyme reaction.
2. Effective vitamin cofactor dosage may be far in excess of the normal daily requirement.
3. Most of the inborn errors that may be responsive to cofactor also have variants that are unresponsive.
4. In most instances, the responsive and the unresponsive forms can be distinguished only by therapeutic trial.

Note that these disorders are specific for a single substance and that the benefits of therapy are well documented.

Included in this general disease category are the various types of carnitine deficiency states, which may occur with muscle weakness, encephalopathy, heart failure, or metabolic acidosis. Response to carnitine may be dramatic and even lifesaving (DiDonato et al., 1984). Although the vitamin- or metabolite-dependent disorders are relatively rare, recognition is of utmost importance, because it may provide a simple means of reversing an apparently untreatable developmental or neurodegenerative disorder.

Clinical presentation may differ from what had been reported previously. For instance, the first report of methylmalonic aciduria with homocystinuria disorder described a patient with severe psychomotor retardation and seizures that began in the neonatal period (Levy et al., 1970). It came as a surprise, therefore, when Shinnar and Singer (1984) reported two sisters with the same biochemical abnormalities but with quite different clinical manifestations. The older sister had been an A student until age 13 years but then began to do poorly in school. She was apathetic and showed ataxia, increased deep tendon reflexes, and an IQ of 50. Laboratory studies showed methylmalonic aciduria and increased homocystine levels, resulting from a defect of vitamin B_{12} metabolism. Administration of large doses of hydroxycobalamin was followed by marked improvement. An asymptomatic 12-year-old sister was found to have the same defect.

Reduce Formation of a Toxic Metabolite

Cerebrotendinous xanthomatosis is a progressive disorder with autosomal recessive inheritance that is associated with cerebellar ataxia, pyramidal tract and extrapyramidal dysfunction, dementia, cataracts, and tendon xanthomata. The tendon xanthomata in this condition occur in the presence of normal blood cholesterol levels. A characteristic abnormality is the presence of abnormal amounts of cholestanol in plasma, brain, and tendons. Cholestanol (which is identical with cholesterol, except that it lacks the double bond in the sterol nucleus) produces xanthoma formation in brain and tendons, which is the cause of the severe and progressive neurologic disability. The pathogenesis of the cholestanol accumulation is complex. The basic defect is impaired formation of bile acids. This in turn interferes with the feedback control of cholesterol and cholestanol biosynthesis, causing these substances to be produced in excess.

Berginer et al. (1984) used these concepts to devise a successful therapy for this disease. They gave 750 mg of chenodeoxycholic acid per day for at least 1 year to 17 patients with cerebrotendinous xanthomatosis. Plasma cholestanol levels declined by threefold, there was undoubted neurologic improvement, and serial computed tomographic scans showed clearing of brain xanthomata. The chenodeoxycholic acid was shown to diminish excessive cholesterol and cholestanol synthesis. This ingenious therapeutic approach was the culmination of a long series of investigations by Salen et al. (1983).

DIRECT THERAPEUTIC APPROACHES

Enzyme Replacement

Until recently, the results of enzyme replacement therapy were inconsistent and disappointing (Brady, 1984; Desnick et al., 1976). Results in patients with Gaucher's diseases are encouraging and most likely are applicable to other disorders. Brady (1984) administered purified placental glucocerebrosidase to patients with Gaucher's disease and found that the major portion of the enzyme had been taken up by hepatocytes, a cell type that does not show glucocerebroside accumulation; there was no definitive clinical improvement.

It is now known that enzyme uptake is determined by specific carbohydrate recognition sites, such as the mannose 6-phosphate group required for uptake

Table 48–2. CHARACTERISTICS OF DISORDERS RESPONDING TO LARGE DOSES OF VITAMINS OR COFACTORS

Vitamin (U.S. RDA*)	Disorder	Enzyme Defect	Daily Treatment Dose
Thiamine (B_1) (0.3–1.5 mg)	Megaloblastic anemia	Unknown	20 mg
	Intermittent cerebellar ataxia	Pyruvate dehydrogenase (?)	5–20 mg
	Lactic acidosis	Pyruvate carboxylase	5–20 mg
	Maple syrup urine disease	Branched chain keto acid	5–20 mg
Pyridoxine (B_6) (0.3–2.2 mg)	Convulsive disorder	Glutamic acid decarboxylase	10–80 mg
	Cystathioninuria	Cystathioninase	100–500 mg
	Xanthurenic aciduria	Kynureninase	5–10 mg
	Homocystinuria	Cystathionine synthetase	200–1200 mg
	Hypochromic anemia	Aminolevulinic acid synthetase	>10 mg
	Hyperoxaluria	α-Ketoglutarate carboxylase	100–500 mg
	Gyrate atrophy of choroid and retina	Ornithinic transaminase	50 mg
Cobalamin (B_{12}) (0.5–3 μg)	Megaloblastic anemia	Intrinsic factor, transcobalamin II, or defective ileal transport	>5 μg
	Methylmalonic aciduria	5′-Deoxyadenocobalamin synthesis	>250 μg
	Methylmalonic aciduria and homocystinuria	5′-Deoxyadenocablamin and methylcobalamin synthesis	>500 μg
	Methylmalonic aciduria	Methylmalonyl-CoA mutase (responsive in vitro only)	2000 μg
Folate (0.03–0.4 mg)	Megaloblastic anemia	Intestinal folate absorption	≥0.05 mg
	Aplastic anemia with megaloblastic changes	Cellular 5-methyltetrahydrofolate uptake	20 mg
	Megaloblastic anemia	Dihydrofolate reductase	>5 mg
	Homocystinuria and hypomethioninemia	5,10-Methylenetetrahydrofolate reductase	>10 mg
	Glutamate formininotransferase deficiency	Glutamate formininotransferase	>5 mg
	Sarcosinuria	Sarcosine dehydrogenase	5–30 mg
Biopterin (?)	Malignant hyperphenylalaninemia	Dihydropteridine reductase (lowers serum phenylalanine, but progressive neurologic deterioration)	30–1000 mg
	Malignant hyperphenylalaninemia	Dihydropteridine synthetase (lowers serum phenylalanine, but progressive neurologic deterioration)	20–500 mg
Biotin (0.3 mg)	Propionic acidemia	Propionyl-CoA carboxylase	10 mg
	β-Methylcrotonylglycinuria	β-Methylcrotonyl-CoA carboxylase	10 mg
	Multiple carboxylase deficiency	Holocarboxylase synthetase	10–40 mg
	Multiple carboxylase deficiency	Defect in biotin transport or metabolism	10 mg (oral or IM)†
Niacin (8–20 mg)	Hartnup's disease	Intestinal and renal transport of tryptophan	>40 mg
Vitamin D (400 IU or 10 μg)	Vitamin D–dependent rickets	1,25-Dihydroxycholecalciferol	$4–40 \times 10^3$ IU 0.1–1 μg
	X-linked hypophastemic rickets	Renal transport protein	$2.5–10 \times 10^5$ IU (6.25–25 μg)

*Recommended daily allowance.
†IM = intramuscular.
From Wolf B. Vitamin dependent metabolic diseases. In Kelly V.C., ed. *Practice of Pediatrics.* New York, Harper & Row, pp. 1–9, 1982.

by lysosomes (Kaplan et al., 1977). An important and exciting finding is that administration of a carbohydrate site–modified glucocerebrosidase resulted in unequivocal clinical improvement (Barton et al., 1990). The modification was achieved by sequential deglycosylation, which resulted in a mannose-terminated preparation, which is targeted to a lectin on the macrophage surface (the cell type consistently involved in Gaucher's disease). Administration of this enzyme during a 26-week period led to an increase of hemoglobin levels from 6.9 to 10.2 g/dl and also to increased platelet levels, decreased spleen size, and improvement in bone radiographic findings. These results are encouraging for other disease states also.

Cloning techniques are elucidating the structure of many enzymes and will permit their synthesis through genetic engineering. Study of targeting sequences will then make it possible to target the enzyme to the most involved cell types, as has been demonstrated in Gaucher's disease. In general, intravenously administered enzymes do not reach the brain, because they do not cross the blood-brain barrier. In experimental animals, this can be overcome to some extent by prior injection of hyperosmolar solutions of arabinose or mannose into the carotid artery. However, only 0.5–1% of injected enzymes entered brain, and for this reason, the procedure has not been used in patients (Brady, 1984).

Organ Transplants

Bone Marrow Transplants

The first successful allogeneic bone marrow transplants for genetic diseases were accomplished in two patients with the Wiscott-Aldrich syndrome (Parkman et al., 1978). Interest in applying this technique to storage disease was sparked by Hobbs et al. (1981), who noted striking improvement in patients with the Hurler syndrome. A report (Hugh-Jones et al., 1984) updates the experience with the 18 children with mucopolysaccharidoses who received bone marrow transplants at the Westminister Children's Hospital in London. Results have been spectacular in some respects. Corneal clouding and liver and spleen enlargement disappeared within 3–8 months, and urinary mucopolysaccharide levels became normal. In contrast, bone abnormalities showed little change, and it is not yet possible to assess the effects on mental function. Highly encouraging results in respect to non-neurologic aspects have been obtained in patients with the Maroteaux-Lamy syndrome (Krivit et al., 1984) and the Norbottnian form of Gaucher's disease (Svennerholm et al., 1984).

Clearly, bone marrow transplantation can produce striking improvement in some or most of the visceral manifestations of mucopolysaccharide storage disease, far more so than anything that has been achieved so far with other forms of therapy. It is a difficult and dangerous procedure, and even with HLA-matched donors, overall mortality approaches 20%. Under most circumstances, white blood cells cross the blood-brain barrier to only a slight extent but do so in considerable number when there is an inflammatory response (Oehmichen, 1978).

There are two reports of bone marrow transplants in experimental animal models of human genetic disease. Favorable results were obtained in a feline model of Maroteaux-Lamy disease (Gasper et al., 1984). In the twitcher mouse, a model of globoid leukodystrophy, bone marrow transplantation prolonged survival and improved peripheral nerve function but failed to alter brain pathologic changes (Yeager et al., 1984). Study of these animal models is of particular value, because it may help to determine the conditions under which transplantation is most beneficial.

Particularly encouraging are the reports of bone marrow transplants in patients with metachromatic leukodystrophy (Krivit et al., 1990) and adrenoleukodystrophy (Aubourg et al., 1990). The patient with metachromatic leukodystrophy underwent transplantation at 5 years of age. Five years later, she had moderate neurologic deficits but was clearly less disabled than was her untreated sibling at the same age. The patient with adrenoleukodystrophy underwent transplantation at 7 years of age, when he had a 6-month history of behavioral changes, ataxia, and dystonia. He had hyperreflexia and an extensor plantar response on the right side and moderate deficits on psychologic testing; magnetic resonance imaging showed small white matter lesions in the internal capsule, globus pallidus, and pons. His unaffected nonidentical twin was the bone marrow donor. Eighteen months after the transplant, the neurologic abnormalities and magnetic resonance imaging changes had disappeared and cognitive function was again equal to that of his unaffected twin. There is

no precedent for this type of improvement in untreated cases.

Bone marrow transplantation has substantial morbidity and mortality, and patients who have undergone transplantation in the advanced stages of leukodystrophy have not improved (Moser et al., 1984). Prospective randomized studies and additional studies in animal models of human disease are clearly needed. Nevertheless, the reported improvement in nervous system function in the patients with leukodystrophy and mucopolysaccharide disease has important implications. It suggests that bone marrow–derived cells enter the nervous system and that they can provide a sufficient quantity of normal enzyme to have a favorable effect on nervous system function. An exciting corollary is that, with somatic gene therapy, it may soon be possible to introduce normal genes into the patients' own bone marrow–derived cells. Positive results with allogeneic bone marrow transplants thus may serve as harbingers of what can be achieved with gene therapy.

Liver Transplants

Liver transplantation is being performed with increasing frequency, and 12-month survival rates exceed 50%. It has been used with a high degree of success in Wilson's disease, glycogen storage disease type I (Malatack et al., 1983), and homozygous familial hypercholesterolemia. In each of these instances, patients returned to an essentially normal function. Liver transplantation cannot affect the nervous system directly but can influence its function significantly by restoring normal metabolic function. Its dramatic benefit in homozygous familial hypercholesterolemia or in type I glycogen storage disease cannot be doubted. Patients with Wilson's disease experience great clinical improvement with the use of chelating agents (see earlier). Liver transplantation in Wilson's disease should be reserved for individuals with severe cirrhosis of the liver or possibly for those who cannot tolerate chelating agents.

Kidney Transplants

Kidney transplants are indicated for patients with Fabry's disease who have severely impaired renal function. The procedure does not normalize glycolipid metabolism in other tissues.

Gene Therapy

Gene therapy has been approved by the National Institutes of Health review board for human use, and it has been applied to one genetically determined disorder, namely, adenosine deaminase deficiency (S.A. Rosenberg et al., 1990). Application to disorders of the nervous system cannot be far away.

Prospects for gene therapy were presented in a systematic fashion by Anderson (1984). The following discussion summarizes the points presented by Anderson and includes results obtained since that time. The major concerns are decisions about what human diseases are candidates for gene replacement therapy at the current state of knowledge, methods of gene delivery, safety, and ethical issues.

Disease Candidates for Gene Therapy

Anderson (1984) proposed that gene therapy should be considered for the replacement of defective or missing enzymes whose level does not need to be regulated exactly. Because of the highly experimental nature and concerns about safety, the procedure is reserved for disorders that would be fatal without the intervention. With these criteria, Anderson (1984) cited three prime gene candidates: that which controls formation of hypoxanthine guanine phosphoribosyltransferase, the absence of which results in Lesch-Nyhan disease; purine nucleoside phosphorylase, the absence of which results in a severe immunodeficiency disease; and adenosine deaminase, the absence of which results in severe combined immunodeficiency disease. These three enzymes have simple "always-on" regulation. The level of their activity probably does not need to be exactly controlled, and the availability of a relatively small proportion of normal enzyme will likely prove beneficial. The same considerations probably apply to lysosomal enzymes, such as cerebroside β-glucosidase, the deficiency of which results in Gaucher's disease.

The favorable results with bone marrow transplants in the mucopolysaccharidoses and certain leukodystrophies (see earlier) also make these disorders suitable candidates. It is important to re-emphasize that present knowledge does not permit control or modulation of the expression of the transferred gene. This prohibits gene transfer for the therapy of pituitary dwarfism, because it would not be possible to hook into the feedback mechanisms that regulate the expression of the growth hormone gene. The need for regulation of gene expression also introduces caution in respect to gene therapy of hemoglobin disorders. Thus the hemoglobin α and β chain levels are always maintained in a 1:1 ratio, even though the genes that encode them are located in different chromosomes. The mechanisms responsible for these regulations are not yet understood.

Gene Delivery

At present, only bone marrow and skin cells can be used for gene transfer, because no other cells can be taken from the body, manipulated, and reinjected. Most work has been done with marrow cells. The prime targets are the nucleated bone marrow stem cells, which make up 0.1–0.5% of marrow cells. The issues and limitations relating to the techniques of administration, proliferation, and transport of bone marrow–derived cells to the nervous system thus are analogous to those with bone marrow transplantation, with the important exception that the cells would be autologous, and the complex immunologic problems associated with allogeneic donors are avoided.

Breakefield and Geller (1987) reviewed the prospects of gene transfer in the nervous system. The use of virus vectors is a promising procedure, but a great deal more study in experimental animals is needed. Another approach, which has produced exciting results in experimental animals, is the grafting of genetically modified cells. M.B. Rosenberg et al. (1988) grafted fibroblasts that had been genetically modified to secrete nerve growth factor into the brain of rats that had surgical lesions of the fimbria fornix. They showed that the grafted cells protected the animals against degeneration of cholinergic neurons. Wolff et al. (1989) grafted fibroblasts genetically modified to produce levodopa (L-dopa) into the caudate nucleus of a rat model of Parkinson's disease and showed that this reversed symptoms. Gene transfer into muscle may be achievable by direct injection (Wolff et al., 1990).

Several techniques can be used to transfer clonal genes into cells. These include the use of viruses, chemical techniques such as calcium phosphate–mediated DNA transfer, fusion of DNA-loaded membranous vesicles, and microinjection or electroporation. Discussion here is confined to the use of RNA retroviruses, which at this time represents the most practical and promising technique. The sequences for the gene to be transferred are first introduced into an infected retrovirus (Miller et al., 1983). RNA retroviruses are composed of an RNA-protein core and a glycoprotein envelope. They enter the cell, where the RNA acts as a template for the reverse transcription of genetic information into a double strand of DNA. Retroviruses are particularly advantageous vectors for gene delivery because up to 100% of cells can be infected and express the integrated viral and exogenous genes. Infection and long-term harboring of the retroviral vector does not usually harm the host cell. A particularly attractive feature is that it has been possible to alter the retrovirus vector in such a way that it enters the host cell but loses its capacity to leave the cell and infect others (Mann et al., 1983). The modified particle can infect just once. It acts as an effective delivery system but is no longer an infectious agent. This type of delivery system has been used in mice, and the new genetic material persisted for at least 6 months (Williams et al., 1984) and, as already noted, achieved partial correction of the phenotypic defect in fibroblast cell lines from patients with the Lesch-Nyhan syndrome (Willis et al., 1984). Retrovirus vector–mediated gene transfer has also been shown to correct the metabolic defect in hematopoietic progenitor cells of patients with Gaucher's diseases (Fink et al., 1990), in adenosine deaminase–deficient cultured human T and B cells (Kantoff et al., 1986), and in retinal pigment epithelial and bone marrow cells from an animal model of mucopolysaccharidosis type VII (Wolfe et al., 1990).

These reports make it clear that gene replacement therapy is indeed feasible. However, safety and ethical issues must be considered with utmost care.

Safety Issues

Anderson (1984) summarized the main concern about safety, which is that retroviruses can rearrange their own structure and exchange sequences with other retroviruses. This poses the risk that a retroviral vector might recombine with an endogenous viral sequence to produce an infectious recombinant virus, with a major concern being the formation of unknown primate cancer retroviruses or human T cell leukemia virus. Procedures are available to assess this risk. Anderson (1984) recommended a three-stage safety protocol before any retrovirus vector gene transfer experiments are performed in humans. Each stage must be passed successfully before proceeding to the next and, of course, prior to human use. These stages are in vitro studies with human bone marrow cells, followed by in vivo studies in mice, and finally in vivo studies with primates. At each stage, search must be made to rule out the formation of infectious or pathogenetic virus particles and to ascertain that the desired gene correction was achieved.

Ethical Issues

The ethical issues concerning gene therapy have been the subject of lengthy discussion. Anderson (1984) noted that "essentially all . . . believe that it would be ethical to insert genetic material into a human being for the sole purpose of medically correcting a severe genetic defect in that patient—that is, somatic cell gene therapy. As noted, this form of therapy has now been approved. Attempts to correct germ cells (that is, to permit the new gene to be passed on to the patient's children) or to enhance or improve a 'normal' person by gene manipulation do not have societal acceptance at this time." The National Institutes of Health announced that any federally funded gene therapy experiment must be approved by the National Institutes of Health after review by the Recombinant DNA Advisory Committee (Federal Register, 1984).

References

(Key references are designated with an asterisk.)

*Anderson W.F. Prospects for human gene therapy. *Science* 226:401–409, 1984.

Aubourg P., Stephane B., Jambaque I., et al. Reversal of early neurologic and neuroradiologic manifestations of X-linked adrenoleukodystrophy by bone marrow transplantation. *N. Engl. J. Med.* 322:1860–1866, 1990.

Berginer V.M., Salen G., Shefer S. Long-term treatment of cerebrotendinous xanthomatosis with chenodeoxycholic acid. *N. Engl. J. Med.* 311:1649–1652, 1984.

Barton M.W., Furbish F.S., Murray G.J., et al. Therapeutic response to intravenous infusion of glucocerebrosidase in a patient with Gaucher disease. *Proc. Natl. Acad. Sci. U.S.A.* 87:1913, 1990.

Bergman I., Finegold D., Gartner J.C., et al. Acute profound dystonia in infants with glutaric acidemia. *Pediatrics* 83:228–234, 1989.

Brady R.O. Enzyme replacement in the sphingolipidoses. In Barranger J.A., Brady R.O., eds. *Molecular Basis of Lysosomal Storage Disorders.* Orlando, FL, Academic Press, pp. 461–478, 1984.

Brandt I.K., Hsia E., Clement D.H., et al. Propionicacidemia (ketotic hyperglycinemia): dietary treatment resulting in normal growth and development. *Pediatrics* 53:391–395, 1974.

Breakefield X.O., Geller A.I. Gene transfer into the nervous system. *Mol. Neurobiol.* 1:339–371, 1987.

Brewer G.J., Terry C.A., Aisen A.M., et al. Worsening of neurologic syndrome in patients with Wilson's disease with initial penicillamine therapy. *Arch. Neurol.* 44:490–493, 1987.

Brusilow S.W., Danney M., Waber L.J., et al. Treatment of episodic hyperammonemia in children with inborn errors of urea synthesis. *N. Engl. J. Med.* 310:1630–1634, 1984.

Danks, D. Early diagnosis of hyperphenylalanimenia due to tetrahydrobiopterin deficiency (malignant hyperphenylalaninema). *J. Pediatr.* 96:854–856, 1980.

*Desnick R.J., Thorpe S.R., Fiddler M.B. Toward enzyme therapy for lysosomal storage diseases. *Physiol. Rev.* 56:57–99, 1976.

DiDonato S., Pelucchetti D., Rimoldi M., et al. Systematic carnitine deficiency: clinical, biochemical, and morphological cure with L-carnitine. *Neurology (N.Y).* 34:157–162, 1984.

Drogari E., Smith I., Beasley M., et al. Timing of strict diet in relation to fetal damage in maternal phenylketonuria. An international collaborative study by the MRC/DHSS Phenylketonuria Register. *Lancet* 2:927–930, 1987.

Federal Register. 49:17846, April 25, 1984.

Fink J.K., Correll P.H., Perry L.K., et al. Correction of glucocerebrosidase deficiency after retroviral-mediated gene transfer into hematopoietic progenitor cells from patients with Gaucher disease. *Proc. Natl. Acad. Sci. U.S.A.* 87:2334–2338, 1990.

Gasper P.W., Thrall M.A., Wenger D.A., et al. Correction of feline arylsulphatase B deficiency (mucopolysaccharidosis VI) by bone marrow transplantation. *Nature* 312:467–469, 1984.

Gesell A., Amatuda C.S., Culotta C.S. Effects of thyroid therapy in mental retardation and physical growth in cretins. *Am. J. Dis. Child.* 52:1117–1138, 1936.

Glorieux J., Desjardins M., Letarte J., et al. Useful parameters to predict the eventual mental outcome of hypothyroid children. *Pediatr. Res.* 24:6–8, 1988.

*Hobbs J.R., Hugh-Jones K., Barrett A.J., et al. Reversal of clinical features of Hurler's disease and biochemical improvement after treatment by bone-marrow transplantation. *Lancet* 2:709–712, 1981.

Holtzman N.A., Kronmal R.A., van Doorninck W., et al. Effect of age at loss of dietary control on intellectual performance and behavior of children with phenylketonuria. *N. Engl. J. Med.* 314:593–598, 1986.

Hoogenraad T.U., van Hattun J., van den Hamer C.J.A. Management of Wilson's disease with zinc sulphate: experience in a series of 27 patients. *J. Neurol. Sci.* 77:137–146, 1987.

Hugh-Jones K., Hobbs J., Chambers D., et al. Bone marrow transplantation in mucopolysaccharidoses. In Barranger J.A., Brady R.O., eds. *Molecular Basis of Lysosomal Storage Disorders.* New York, Academic Press, pp. 412–428, 1984.

Hulse J.A. Outcome for congenital hypothyroidism. *Arch. Dis. Child.* 59:23–30, 1984.

Ilicki A., Larsson A. Psychomotor developmental of children with congenital hypothyroidism diagnosed by neonatal screening. *Acta Paediatr. Scand.* 77:142–147, 1988.

Irons M., Levy H.L., O'Flynn M.E., et al. Folinic acid therapy in treatment of dihydropteridine reductase deficiency. *J. Pediatr.* 110:61–67, 1987.

Kantoff P.W., Kohn D.B., Mitsuya H., et al. Correction of adenosine deaminase deficiency in cultured human T and B cells by retrovirus-mediated gene transfer. *Proc. Natl. Acad. Sci. U.S.A.* 83:6563–6567, 1986.

Kaplan A., Achron D.T., Sly W.S. Phosphohexosyl components of a lysosomal enzyme are recognized by pinocytosis receptors on human fibroblasts. *Proc. Natl. Acad. Sci. U.S.A.* 74:2026–2030, 1977.

Komrower G.M. Galactosemia—thirty years on the experience of a generation. *J. Inherit. Metab. Dis.* 5:96, 1982.

Komrower G.M., Lee D.H. Long-term follow-up of galactosemia. *Arch. Dis. Child.* 45:367–373, 1970.

*Krivit W., Pierpont M.E., Ayaz K., et al. Bone-marrow transplantation in the Maroteaux-Lamy syndrome (mucopolysaccharidosis type VI). *N. Engl. J. Med.* 311:1606–1611, 1984.

Krivit W., Shapiro E., Kennedy W., et al. Treatment of late infantile metachromatic leukodystrophy by bone marrow transplantation. *N. Engl. J. Med.* 322:28–32, 1990.

*Lenke R.R., Levy H.L. Maternal phenylketonuria and hyperphenylalaninemia. An international survey of the outcome of untreated and treated pregnancy. *N. Engl. J. Med.* 303:1202–1208, 1980.

Levy H.L., Erickson A.M. Isovaleric acidemia: In Nyhan W.L., ed. *Heritable Disorders of Amino Acid Metabolism.* New York, Wiley, pp. 81–97, 1974.

Levy H.L., Mudd S.H., Schulman J.D., et al. A derangement in B_{12} metabolism associated with homocystinemia, cystathioninemia, hypomethioninemia and methylmalonic aciduria. *Am. J. Med.* 48:390–397, 1970.

Levy H.L., Driscoll S.G., Forensky R.S., et al. Ovarian failure in galactosemia. *N. Engl. J. Med.* 310:50, 1984.

Malatack J.J., Finegold D.N., Iwatsuki S., et al. Liver transplantation for type I glycogen storage disease. *Lancet* 1:1073–1075, 1983.

Mann R., Mulligan R.C., Baltimore D. Construction of a retrovirus packaging mutant and its use to produce helper-free defective retrovirus. *Cell* 33:153–159, 1983.

Marsden C.D. Wilson's disease. *Q. J. Med.* 65:959–966, 1987.

Miller A.D., Jolly D.J., Friedmann T., et al. A transmissible retrovirus expressing human hypoxanthine phosphoribosyltransferase (HPRT) gene transfer into cells obtained from humans deficient in HPRT. *Proc. Natl. Acad. Sci. U.S.A.* 80:4709–4713, 1983.

Moser H.W. Maple syrup urine disease: In Vinken P., Bruyn G, eds. *Handbook of Clinical Neurology.* Vol. 29. *Metabolic and Deficiency Diseases of the Nervous System.* Amsterdam, North Holland, 1977.

Moser H.W., Tutschka P.J., Brown F.R., et al. Bone marrow transplant in adrenoleukodystrophy. *Neurology* 34:1410–1417, 1984.

Msall M., Batshaw M.L., Suss R., et al. Neurologic outcome in children with inborn errors of urea synthesis. Outcome of urea-cycle enzymopathies. *N. Engl. J. Med.* 310:1500–1505, 1984.

*New England Congenital Hypothyroidism Collaborative: Effects of neonatal screening for hypothyroidism: prevention of mental retardation by treatment before clinical manifestations. *Lancet* 2:1095–1098, 1981.

Nyhan W.L., Fawcett N., Anda T., et al. Response to dietary therapy in B-12 unresponsive methylmalonic acidemia. *Pediatrics* 51:539–548, 1973.

Oehmichen M. *Mononuclear Phagocytes in the Central Nervous System.* New York, Springer-Verlag, 1978.

Parkman R., Rappeport J., Geha R. Complete correction of the Wiscott-Aldrich syndrome by allogeneic bone marrow transplantation. *N. Engl. J. Med.* 298:921–927, 1978.

Refsum S. Heredopathia atactica polyneuritiformis: phytanic-acid storage disease, Refsum disease. A biochemically well-defined disease with a specific dietary treatment. *Arch. Neurol.* 38:605–606, 1981.

Rinaldo P., O'Shea J.J., Coates P.M., et al. Medium-chain acyl-CoA dehydrogenase deficiency. *N. Engl. J. Med.* 319:1308–1313, 1988.

Rohr F.J., Doherty L.B., Waisbren S.E., et al. New England Maternal PKU Project: prospective study of untreated and treated pregnancies and their outcomes. *J. Pediatr.* 110:391–398, 1987.

Rosenberg M.B., Friedmann R., Robertson R.C., et al. Grafting genetically modified cells to the damaged brain: restorative effects of NGF expression. *Science* 242:1575–1578, 1988.

Rosenberg S.A., Aebersold P., Cornetta K., et al. Gene transfer into humans—immunotherapy of patients with advanced melanoma, using tumor-infiltrating lymphocytes modified by retroviral gene transduction. *N. Engl. J. Med.* 323:570–578, 1990.

Salen G., Shefer S., Berginer V.M. Familial diseases with storage of sterols other than cholesterol: cerebrotendinous xanthomatosis and sitosterolemia with xanthomatosis. In Frederickson D.S., Goldstein S.L., Brown M.S., eds. *The Metabolic Basis of Inherited Disease.* 5th ed. New York, McGraw-Hill, pp. 713–730, 1983.

Scheinberg I.H., Jaffe M.E., Sternlieb I. The use of trientine in preventing the effects of interrupting penicillamine therapy in Wilson's disease. *N. Engl. J. Med.* 317:209–213, 1987.

Scriver C.R., Clow C.L. Phenylketonuria: epitome of human biochemical genetics. *N. Engl. J. Med.* 303:1336–1342, 1394–1400, 1980.

Scriver C.R., Beaudet A.L., Sly W.S., et al., eds. *The Metabolic Basis of Inherited Disease.* 6th ed. New York, McGraw-Hill, 1989.

Shinnar S., Singer H.S. Cobalamin C mutation (methylmalonic aciduria and homocystinuria) in adolescence. A treatable cause of dementia and myelopathy. *N. Engl. J. Med.* 311:451–454, 1984.

Snyderman S.E., Norton P., Roitman E., et al. Maple syrup urine disease, with particular reference to diet therapy. *Pediatrics* 34:454–472, 1964.

Sokol R.J., Francis P.D., Gold S.H., et al. Orthotopic liver transplantation for acute fulminant Wilson disease. *J. Pediatr.* 107:549–552, 1985.

Svennerholm L., Mansson J.E., Nilsson O., et al. Bone marrow transplantation in the Norbottnian form of Gaucher disease. In Barranger J.A., Brady R.O., eds. *Molecular Basis of Lysosomal Storage Disease.* New York, Academic Press, pp. 441–459, 1984.

Taubman B., Hale D.E., Kelley R.I. Familial Reye-like syndrome: a presentation of medium-chain acyl-coenzyme A dehydrogenase deficiency. *Pediatrics* 79:382–385, 1987.

*Walshe J.M. Hudson Memorial Lecture: Wilson's disease: genetics and biochemistry—their relevance to therapy. *J. Inherit. Metab. Dis.* 6(Suppl. 1):51–58, 1983.

Williams D.A., Lemischka I.R., Nathan D.G., et al. Introduction of new genetic material into pluripotent haematopoietic stem cells of the mouse. *Nature* 310:476–480, 1984.

*Willis R.C., Jolly D.J., Miller A.D., et al. Partial phenotypic correction of human Lesch-Nyhan (hypoxanthine-guanine phosphoribosyltransferase–deficient) lymphoblasts with a transmissible retroviral vector. *J. Biol. Chem.* 259:7842–7849, 1984.

Wolfe J.H., Schuchman E.H., Stramm L.E., et al. Restoration of normal lysosomal function in mucopolysaccharidosis type VII cells by retroviral vector–mediated gene transfer. *Proc. Natl. Acad. Sci. U.S.A.* 87:2877–2881, 1990.

Wolff J.A., Fisher L.J., Xu L., et al. Grafting fibroblasts genetically modified to produce L-dopa in a rat model of Parkinson disease. *Proc. Natl. Acad. Sci. U.S.A.* 86:9011–9014, 1989.

Wolff J.A., Malone R.W., Williams P., et al. Direct gene transfer into mouse muscle in vivo. *Science* 247:1465–1468, 1990.

Yeager A.M., Brennan S., Tiffany C., et al. Prolonged survival and remyelination after hematopoietic cell transplantation in the twitcher mouse. *Science* 225:1052–1054, 1984.

Disorders of Higher Cerebral Function

49

Psychophysics and Central Processing

Günter Baumgartner

Nothing is learned or understood that is not perceived before.

Aristotle

Truth can emerge sooner from error than from confusion.

F. Bacon

PSYCHOPHYSICS IN CLINICAL NEUROPSYCHOLOGY

Long before the statement became trivial that perception and cognition derive from neuronal processes within the brain, the intensity of a sensation was known to depend on stimulus strength. The first measurements of thresholds and threshold differences were done only in the last century, however. They led to the foundation of psychophysics, the "science of the functional relationship between body and mind" (Fechner, 1860). This study started lively discussions in philosophic, psychologic, and physiologic circles. It was soon shown that the stimulus variable alone does not suffice to describe sensation (Mach, 1918; Wundt, 1901). Attention, expectancy, and context also required consideration. Signal detection theory was therefore applied to account for the internal state of the subject by comparing the relationship between responses.

Psychophysics so defined still relied on subjective responses. Later, objective criteria were added by measuring stimulus-associated brain events, trying to circumvent subjective reponses. Both procedures should be seen as complementary. They are separated by the mysterious gap between sensation or perception and the biophysics of neuronal activity. The two have in common that they can deal with only the quantity but not the quality of sensation. Just the opposite occurs in clinical experience. Clinicians confronted with lesions of the hemispheres are faced with psychophysical problems that can only be described qualitatively. Thus, the term *psychophysics* in the strict sense is not applicable. Nevertheless, neurology has contributed to psychophysics by pointing out the psychophysical relevance and qualitative impact of different cortical regions. Simply using clinical experience and improving it by better examination techniques will therefore provide more information about the organization of brain function.

For instance, the actual content of conscious experience is always limited by motivation and by directed attention. Normally, the details of its potential content can be retrieved. In pathologic conditions, however, the awareness of self or mental activity can be restricted partially or in a general way. Such conditions may often go unnoticed by the patient (McGlynn and Schacter, 1989). Subjects may not spontaneously complain about cortical scotomas.

681

A patient may be strangely unaware of changes in more complex cortical functions. This is illustrated by the neglects or anosognosias and is demonstrated dramatically in the transitory negation of the complete blindness in acute bioccipital lesions. Therefore, not only do cortical lesions produce defects of perception, as peripheral lesions do, but also these defects are at least transiently undetected by the subjects. In more general terms, if there is no cortical neuronal substrate for a certain function, its loss goes unnoticed.

Defects differ widely depending on localization. Therefore, it must be supposed that cortical functions must be topographically different, as proposed by Broca, Wernicke, and many others. The cytoarchitectonic differences in cortical areas were taken to support the localistic concept that "certain functions have a circumscribed regional localization" (Brodmann, 1909). Clinical observations led Riddock (1917) to formulate a dissociation of visual function into "light, movement and colour" components. He was severely criticized by representatives of a holistic view of brain function, a proposal first made by Flourens (1824) as a reaction to Gall's phrenology and continued with modifications by von Monakow (1914), Lashley (1937), and Goldstein (1946). It is now known that the more complex a task is, the more holistic features are required, but that the activity of circumscribed populations of neurons serves specific aspects of perception or cognition.

There is increasing evidence that the functional modularity is far more specified than was previously thought (McCarthy and Warrington, 1988). This holds true not only after structural lesions. It has long been recognized that uncontrolled cortical activity, as in focal seizures or after electrical stimulation (Ferrier, 1876; Jackson, 1870; Penfield and Rasmussen, 1957), leads to distorted sensations, specific to particular locations. Bipolar stimulation during brain surgery under local anesthesia has localized language areas in several mosaics of 1–2 cm^2 in the frontal and temporoparietal lobes of the left hemisphere. The precise locations show considerable interindividual variability, and the mosaics are much smaller than the classic fields of Broca and Wernicke. Neuronal recordings during these procedures indicate the participation of neurons over a much larger area in language processing (Ojemann et al., 1988, 1989).

The structure of cognitive processes and their corresponding neuronal mechanisms are still unknown. Within one modality, different cognitive defects may occur, as the variety of visual agnosias indicates. This shows that even submodalities or different properties within one sensory channel are processed separately in cortical pathways. With this in mind, the long discussion about the concept of agnosia (Bay, 1954; Critchley, 1966) can be more readily understood. Whether agnosia is defined as a pure cognitive defect with complete integrity of the sensory afferents (Freud, 1891) or as a consequence of a partial impairment of afferent processing depends on where,

if anywhere, one places the boundary between perception and cognition. If one defines the boundaries as lying between primary and secondary areas, Freud's (1891) definition remains adequate. If one assumes that it lies somewhere within the secondary cortical processing lines, agnosias are defects of specific subfunctions of a sensory system.

It is also well known from the study of the primary sensory and motor areas (Ferrier, 1876; Förster, 1936; Holmes, 1945) that the higher the available resolution is within a motor or a sensory system, the more extended is its cortical representation. The number of neurons and the intricacy of their connections obviously increases with the complexity of a given task. Higher brain functions depend on the normal function of many neuronal subsystems and can therefore be disturbed by lesions at many different sites. For instance, a rose can be recognized by sight, by touch, or by smell. Any single sensory channel activates the whole set of its qualities in the different modalities and evokes the full neuronal construct equivalent of a rose. This interpretation assumes that the neuronal level for recognition requires multimodal convergence. However, the occurrence of an isolated loss of submodalities is not compatible with this concept.

If convergence is a necessary condition, any loss of submodalities should become apparent by its effects on the functioning of still intact convergent recognition areas. At least this may be concluded from the immediate awareness of subcortical defects when cortical structures are intact. This difference can be understood by assuming that submodalities are not only processed in specific channels but also take on perceptual equivalence in the activity of neuronal assemblies in functionally specific sites. The completeness of the neuronal construct for perception and recognition within one and different modalities then depends on the activity in spatially distributed areas, which cooperate in space and time via intercortical connections by translating the local neuron code into a more holistic brain code (Cook, 1986). Under these conditions, different forms of modality-specific agnosias must occur.

In such an organization, an impairment of function should be more persistent the nearer the lesion is to the input or output regions of a system. A hemianopia persists after a complete lesion of striate area 17 because the main retinal input to the cortex has been destroyed. On the other hand, the hemineglect after a prestriate lesion may improve considerably by compensation via other pathways. This can be derived from observing simpler networks when they are disturbed. The execution of saccades, for instance, can be disturbed by parieto-occipital, premotor (area 8), or tectal lesions. If only one region is impaired, compensation occurs within days. If several are affected or the premotor neurons in the paramedian pontine reticular formation are destroyed, the impairment is permanent.

OBJECTIVE CONTRIBUTIONS TO PSYCHOPHYSICS

Neuroanatomy, Regional Cerebral Blood Flow, Positron Emission Tomography, and Evoked Potentials

The clinical and experimental neuropsychologic evidence of topographic differentiation of cortical functions (see Luria, 1980; Mishkin, 1972; Mishkin et al., 1983) continues to receive support from neuroanatomic and physiologic data. Subtle serial and parallel connections of cortical representation areas with multiple rerepresentation of sensory and motor systems have been demonstrated and defined (Jones and Powell, 1970; van Essen, 1985) and functionally differentiated (Zeki and Shipp, 1988) (Fig. 49–1). Stainings for the mitochondrial enzyme cytochrome oxidase revealed a further parceling within cytoarchitectonically homogeneous areas.

Almost all intracortical connections are organized in a reciprocal manner, but the laminar pattern of the axonal termination is different. Upward projections derive mainly from layers II and III and terminate in layer IV, as thalamocortical fibers do. Downward projections come from superficial and deep layers and reach preferentially layers I and VI.

The columnar arrangement of specific neuronal properties discovered by Mountcastle (1957) has been supported by morphologic data (Jones, 1981). Again in agreement with physiologic and clinical findings, the old assumption that the parietal and frontal homotypic association cortices are somewhat homogeneous regions of polymodal convergence must be modified. It has been shown that these areas retain, to a large extent, modal specificity and are divided into many mosaics with different intercortical connections (Goldman-Rakic, 1988). Each section of the parietal cortex projects to different nonoverlapping sites of the prefrontal cortex. Double-labeling techniques have demonstrated common target areas for the posterior parietal and dorsolateral prefrontal cortex in the monkey (supplementary motor area, anterior and posterior cingulate area, presubiculum, and many others). The terminations are not identical but occur either in a spatially alternating pattern or in complementary layers of columns. Furthermore, it has been found that there is convergence of thalamocortical connections from several nuclei to the association cortex, as well as divergence to several association cortical areas from one thalamic nucleus. The patchy connections from prefrontal, precentral, and parietal cortex to the striatum and other parts of the basal ganglia (Goldman and Nauta, 1977; Künzle, 1975) may explain the reports of aphasias and cognitive defects attributable to lesions of the head of the caudate nucleus and the dorsal putamen and thalamus (Wallesch et al., 1983).

Also, the neocortex and the allocortex receive several parathalamic inputs in addition to those of the familiar reticulothalamic arousal system of Moruzzi and Magoun (1949). Immunocytochemical and histochemical marker and tracing techniques indicate at least four ascending systems (noradrenergic from the locus ceruleus, serotoninergic from the raphe nucleus, dopaminergic from the substantia nigra and ventral tegmental complex, and cholinergic from the nucleus basalis), and some evidence of histaminergic and γ-aminobutyric acid (GABA)–ergic contributions from the hypothalamus have been found (Bloom, 1988). These systems originate from only some 10^4 cells each, but their projections, although distributed across wide cortical areas, show regional and laminar differences. Their functions are still not understood

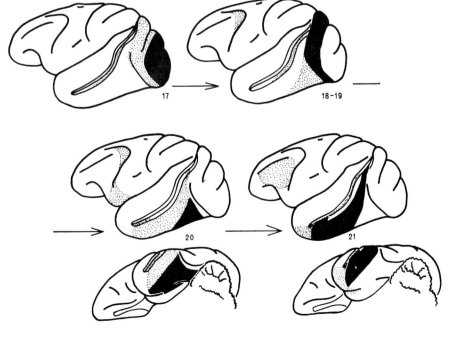

Figure 49–1. Schematic summary of Nauta-stained axonal degeneration (*stippled area*) after lesions (*black area*) in cortical visual areas to demonstrate the outward progression of corticocortical connections from the striate cortex (area 17). (From Jones E.G. The anatomy of extrageniculostriate visual mechanisms. In Schmitt F.O., Worden F.G., eds. *The Neurosciences*. Cambridge, MA, M.I.T. Press, pp. 215–222, 1974.)

and have been vaguely defined as modulation. However, they strongly influence behavior and are often discussed in the context of memory, learning, and plasticity. These deep nuclei are mentioned here because their normal functioning, as well as their interaction with the basal ganglia, is essential for normal cortical performance. Therefore, the concept of cortical function must be enlarged; here it is used with the implicit understanding of including subcortical contributions.

Measurements of *regional cerebral blood flow* during performance of defined tasks have shown a circumscribed increase, depending on language functions, audition, vision, and motor output and even on the intention of movement (Roland, 1984). Thus, during the verbal description of spatial scenery not only the motor speech area but also parts of the parietal region showed increased blood flow (Fig. 49–2). Comparable results were obtained by measuring the cortical metabolism with the glucose utilization method of Sokoloff in positron emission tomography (Ingvar, 1983; Phelps et al., 1986). Positron emission tomography has also shown that, after a cortical infarction, metabolic changes can be seen far away from the site of the lesion, which is a confirmation of von Monakow's (1914) concept of diaschisis.

The study of *evoked brain potentials* and *magnetoencephalography* provided evidence of pattern- and intention-dependent activity (Barber and Blum, 1987; Deecke and Weinberg, 1988; McCallum et al., 1987) and demonstrated changes of cortical potentials before the execution of a movement (Kornhuber and Deecke, 1965). Again, a topographic differentiation was observed. On the other hand, evoked potential mapping revealed certain similarities of topography and, thus, the location of neural generators during voluntary attention to, and automatic perception of, visual figures (Brandeis and Lehmann, 1989). Finally, measurements of field potentials showed source shifts over the cortex when potentials evoked by homophone verbs and nouns were analyzed. This indicates a topographic difference, even in the processing of words as a function of their syntactic category (Brown and Lehmann, 1979) (Fig. 49–3). Magnetoencephalography has proved to be another method for localizing functionally different regions (Deecke and Weinberg, 1989).

These methods have demonstrated psychophysical correspondences with the participating brain regions in humans. They provide an objective supplement to the classic approach of psychophysics and neuropsychology. However, because of their low spatial

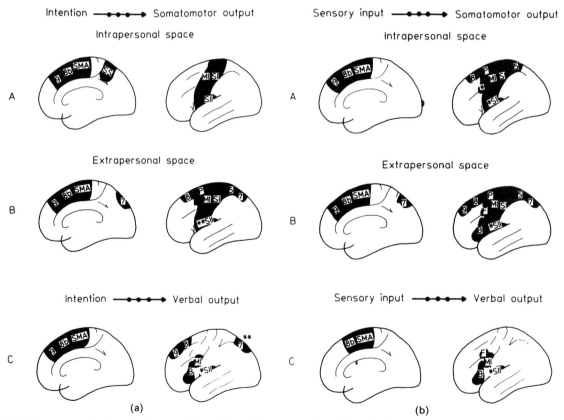

Figure 49–2. Measurements of regional cerebral blood flow during conversion of intention into voluntary motor output (*a*) and conversion of sensory input into voluntary motor output (*b*). Cortical areas for which regional cerebral blood flow increased more than 15% under a given condition are black. Areas that analyzed sensory information in *b* are not shown. (*A*) Movement of an extremity in intrapersonal space. (*B*) Movement of an extremity in extrapersonal space. (*C*) Conversion of internal language to speech. *Participation of this region possible but not verified. **Activated only on the right side when subjects reported from memory of extrapersonal space. (From Roland P.E. Organization of motor control by the normal human brain. *Hum. Neurobiol.* 2:205–216, 1984.)

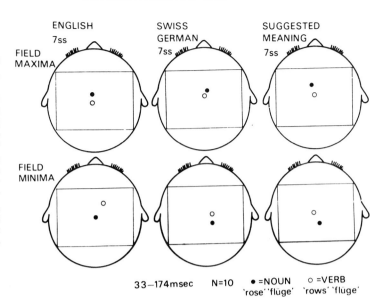

Figure 49–3. Characteristics of the scalp distribution of field potentials evoked by homophones of nouns and verbs in English, in Swiss German, and as suggested meaning. The distributions were defined by recording averaged evoked potentials from an array of 12 electrodes and determining the mean location of the maximal and minimal potentials during all analysis times between 33 and 174 ms after the onset of the homophone words. The mean of seven subjects (7ss) for each group was computed. It is shown that the field maxima (*black dots*) were in all groups significantly more anterior for nouns and more posterior for verbs; conversely, the field minima were more posterior for nouns and more anterior for verbs. (Data from Brown W.S., Lehmann D. Verb and noun meanings of homophone words activate different cortical generators: a topographic study of evoked potential fields. *Exp. Brain Res.* 2[Suppl.]:159–168, 1979.)

and (for the metabolic methods) temporal resolution, they allow no access to information regarding dynamic neuronal mechanisms. Moreover, predictions about the neuronal organization, as they were derived from old psychophysical data (Young-Helmholtz, three-color theory of color vision; Mach, contrast mechanisms; Hering, opponent color theory) are not possible. To be able to elucidate this level, neurophysiologic studies of neuronal activity and networks are necessary.

Entering the single-neuron level, one has to be aware that the main problem of central nervous function is far from being resolved: How is single neuron activity integrated to allow for adaptive conscious behavior (Sherrington, 1951)? How is the unification of neuronal activity (Griffith, 1968) performed? Conclusions regarding the neuronal basis of perception and behavior must therefore remain speculative at best, especially because until recently neurophysiologists were reluctant to use psychophysical evidence as guidance for designing experiments and to relate neuronal activity to perception (Baumgartner et al., 1987; Livingstone and Hubel, 1987b; Logothetis and Shall, 1989; Newsome et al., 1989).

Neuronal Physiology

Unimodal Processing

Every brain filters by its receptor surface the tiny fraction of available signals that fit the behavioral needs of the organism. For perception, this information must be classified. Therefore, elements of classification must be imposed at the single-neuron level as well. This is generally the case and has been recognized ever since J. Müller postulated the law of the specific sensory energies. Nevertheless, there are surprising similarities between the sensory systems. The numbers of cells and the proportion of pyramidal and stellate cells in an arbitrary cortical cylinder of 30-μm diameter were found to be constant (~110) in different areas and species of mammals, with the exception of the binocular parts of area 17 (V1) of primates, where the numbers are about twofold greater (Powell, 1981). The functional columnar arrangement in the somatosensory cortex (Mountcastle, 1957) is maintained in the visual, acoustic, and parietal cortices and seems to exist also in motor areas. In such columns with translaminar flow of information, the basic properties of neurons are the same (Edelman and Mountcastle, 1978; Hubel and Wiesel, 1977; Merzenich et al., 1979).

All systems perform serial and parallel processing in one area and in multiple rerepresented spatial maps. For the representation of somatic sensation, 8 areas are known, and for the visual field, 20 or so have been reported (Zeki and Shipp, 1988). The emphasis of these maps is on function, and somatotopic or retinotopic relations are therefore variable or even lost. The maps are repeated in a mirror-like fashion on the cortical surface. The vertical meridian in areas 17 (V1) borders on the vertical one in area 18 (V2). High/low frequency representation in one auditory area borders the high/low frequency zone of the next. Tonotopy (i.e., a spatially arranged acoustic map) is similar to the spatial representation in the visual system. Orthogonal to the tonotopic arrangement are binaural stripes with different input features from both ears reminiscent of the monocular dominance stripes of V1.

In higher-order areas, the size of receptive fields increases. Retinotopy, tonotopy, or somatotopy becomes therefore less precise, but the specificity of neuronal information increases.

In the best-known system, namely the visual system (for review, see Spillmann and Werner, 1990; von der Heydt, 1987), neurons in V1 having the same or overlapping receptive fields are combined in orientation-specific and ocular dominance columns. The functionally defined columnar organization has been confirmed by tracer studies, using the Sokoloff method, and by voltage-sensitive dyes (Blasdel and Salama, 1986). In general, only stimuli with a defined orientation, such as bars and edges, activate these cells, and one eye dominates the response in any column. Within a given column, although orientation and retinotopy remain the same, neurons with different functional properties are classified as simple, complex, or hypercomplex cells, depending on their receptive field characteristics. Each retinal receptive field area is represented by a complete set of orientation and ocular dominance columns extending over about 800 μm of the cortical surface. These sets, or hypercolumns, are repeated in cyclic fashion, forming a pattern of stripes. Intermingled with these stripes are dot-like patches (blobs) that can be seen in cytochrome oxidase stainings, mainly in layers II and III (Livingstone and Hubel, 1987a,b). Blob cells are not orientation selective but are often wavelength sensitive. Compared with the wavelength-sensitive cells of the parvocellular layers of the lateral geniculate body, they show double opponency (i.e., the color-opponent responses [for example, red—on; green—off] from the receptive field center are antagonized by stimuli in the surround). The parvocellular input is also fed via collaterals to the oriented cells outside the blobs, but color coding seems to be given up here in favor of orientation selectivity, so that a neuron can detect a bar in the appropriate orientation regardless of its color and independent of its brightness.

The information from the two non–wavelength-selective magnocellular layers of the lateral geniculate body terminates first in layer IV Cα. There is good evidence (Hubel and Livingstone, 1987; Livingstone and Hubel, 1984a,b, 1987a; Zeki, 1988) that the magnocellular and parvocellular systems are only partially overlapping in V1 but remain principally segregated and maintain this segregation in V2 and higher visual areas. In area V2, staining for cytochrome oxidase revealed an alternating pattern of thick and thin stripes separated by pale interstripes. The wavelength-selective blob cells project via the thin stripes to V4. The oriented cells of the interblob region project to the pale stripes and reach from there also to V3, V5 (also called middle temporal area), and other areas in the parietal and temporal cortex. The magnocellular input to V1 is connected via neurons of layer IVB directly with V3 and V5 and via the thick stripes of V2 again with V5 (Fig. 49–4).

Neurons of the parvocellular and magnocellular system have different properties and are therefore suited to transfer different visual information (Livingstone and Hubel, 1987b; Zeki and Shipp, 1988). The parvocellular blob system is thought to mediate color information via thin stripes of V2 to V4, where true color-coding neurons have been found (Zeki, 1985). The parvocellular connection to the interblob region via the pale stripes of V2 has been correlated with form perception owing to the higher resolution and the orientation of the receptive fields. The magnocellular input finally reaching V5 has been related to movement and stereopsis. This interpretation is supported by the predominance of disparity-selective cells in layer IVB of V1 (Poggio et al., 1985) and the thick stripes of V2, and by the finding of disparity and motion sensitivity of cells in V5. Cells that signal illusory contours (contours perceived in the absence of contrast edges) were found in the pale and the thick stripes of V2, but not in the thin stripes (Peterhans and von der Heydt, 1989; von der Heydt and Peterhans, 1989). These cells are obviously involved in form processing, supporting the assumption that form processing takes place in the pale stripes and not in the thin stripes. However, the thick stripes also seem to be involved. The combination of illusory contour perception with motion and disparity information in the thick stripes makes sense, because illusory figures are often seen in depth, and vivid contours are perceived also in random-dot stereograms and motion displays (Julesz, 1971).

The color-coded cells in V4 (Zeki, 1985) responded in a complex color scene, if their receptive area is seen in a defined color, independent of the wavelength reflected. Contrary to the case with wavelength-dependent cells in V1, they take into account the spectral reflectance of large areas and may explain color constancy. In the posterior bank of the superior temporal sulcus, neurons show considerably larger receptive field sizes (Zeki, 1978). Here and in the adjacent medial superior temporal area (Tanaka and Saito, 1989), neurons predominate that respond mostly to movement in a direction-specific way, often without shape or color preference. Disparity-tuned neurons in this area indicate the possibility of an analysis of the trajectories of moving objects (Maunsell and Newsome, 1987). Again, a columnar organization for the analysis of stimulus motion was found. Mikami et al. (1986a,b) demonstrated directional interactions over longer distances with stroboscopic motion stimuli.

In the inferior temporal cortex, cells have still larger receptive fields, often covering both visual hemifields (Gross, 1973), and are influenced by fixation and visual attention (Richmond et al., 1983). These neurons require specific trigger features just like neurons in the superior temporal sulcus, which respond to faces or even to a specific face independently of size, distance, color, or orientation (Perret et al., 1984). The reactions of these cells were diminished and the latency of response was larger when the recognition of the faces was made more difficult. Some neurons responded preferentially to an expression independently of the identity of the face. The neurons were also grouped in small clusters and again seem to be arranged in a columnar fashion.

These findings demonstrate trivially clear functional differences of higher-order visual areas. Together with the serial and parallel organization (see Fig. 49–4) of the visual areas, they are consistent with the notion that visual information from V1 is distributed to many channels, each subserving the processing of different visual qualities. A sufficient functional description of these areas is still not possible, because the studies are partially controversial and involve mostly limited regions of different areas.

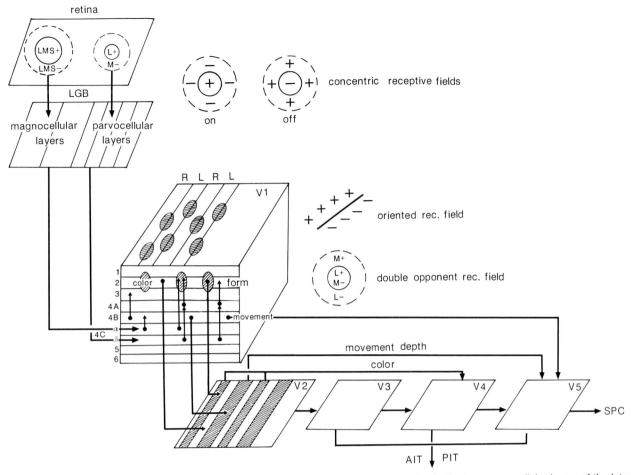

Figure 49–4. The visual pathway from large non–wavelength-selective retinal ganglion cells via the two magnocellular layers of the lateral geniculate body (LGB) to layer IVCα (4Cα) of V1. The smaller wavelength-selective ganglion cells of the retina project to the four parvocellular layers of LGB and terminate in layer IVCβ (4Cβ). The two pathways remain partially segregated. The magnocellular pathway reaches from IVβ directly and via the thick stripes of V2 to V5. A small part projects together with the parvocellular input to IVCβ (4Cβ) to the blobs in layers II (2) and III (3). Blob neurons reach the thin stripes of V2 and from there V4. Other cells from IVCβ remain in the interblob regions and project via layers II and III to the interstripes of V2 and to V3. Note the reorganization of receptive fields in V1 and the segregation of information for color, form, movement, and depth. LMS = long, medium, short wavelength; SPC = superior parietal cortex; AIT = anteroinferior temporal cortex; PIT = posteroinferior temporal cortex; blob = cytochromeoxidase–rich areas (see text); + = excitatory areas of the receptive field; − = inhibitory areas of the receptive field; R = right ocular dominance stripes; L = left ocular dominance stripe; M+ and M− = medium wavelength excitatory and inhibitory; L+ and L− = long wavelength excitatory and inhibitory.

The conclusion that the whole area is organized in the same fashion is therefore not justified. Furthermore, the back projections from V4 and V5 to V2 terminate not only at the forward projection sites of the thick stripes, but also, to a lesser degree, in the thin stripes and interstripes (Zeki, 1988). The significance of this back-propagation is not known. It may be necessary for perceptual coherence between functionally specific areas. Taken together, the physiologic evidence of highly specialized areas of visual processing is strong. It is therefore likely that different visual agnosias are due to defects within specific processing channels.

The distribution of function is, in a way, also proposed in the dual cortical pathways hypothesis of Mishkin et al. (1983): a parietal one for spatial vision probably related to reaching and tactile discrimination and an inferotemporal one for object vision. One should therefore expect different kinds of dysopsias (unformed phosphenes, chaotic form perceptions, and color dysopias, but also distortion of space and complex visual hallucinations) when neuronal activity is focally out of control, as in a focal seizure. The same considerations apply for other sensory channels that also reveal variable disorganized sensations related to circumscribed lesions.

Parietal Processing

The parietal cortex (areas 5 and 7) receives no direct input from primary sensory areas, but only preprocessed information from other cortical and thalamic sites: namely, somatosensory, prestriate, upper temporal, and frontal cingular cortex and callosal connections from homologous contralateral areas and pulvinar input. Neurons with convergent input (somatovisual, somatoauditory) have been found, but they account for only a small portion of the neuronal population (Lynch, 1980; Mountcastle et al., 1975). They do not readily explain the supposed function as an associative region for polymodal sensory integration. However, in the posterior parietal lobule, a higher-order processing of visual information exists, especially for the organization of space and the localization of objects, which is invariant for properties such as form and color (Robinson et al., 1978). Neuronal recordings (Mountcastle et al., 1975) revealed functionally different cells in a columnar arrangement, which were classified as eye fixation, eye tracking, saccade, or for arm and hand movements, reaching and manipulation neurons. In the posterior parietal lobule, neurons related to eye movements and, in the superior parietal lobule, neurons related to arm and hand movements were predominantly represented.

The activity of all neurons was strongly enhanced by stimuli of behavioral relevance, and they seemed not to be directly activated by sensory stimuli. Therefore, the unorthodox proposal was made that the posterior parietal cortex is not simply a sensory association area but is involved in the generation of action. This command system hypothesis was questioned by Robinson et al. (1978) after they found that all cells in their sample were visually responsive and that the response was behaviorally modifiable. Because this enhancement effect could be dissociated from movement, they saw it within the context of a process for stimulus selection (i.e., attention). They maintained, therefore, that the posterior parietal cortex is a sensory association area (see Lynch, 1980).

Hyvärinen (1982) questioned the validity of the dichotomy of sensory and motor functions in the association cortex and pointed to the integrational aspects between the two systems necessary for guiding movements in the surrounding space. It was then shown that those parietal neurons were correlated to sensory and motor responses as well. Cells related to reaching were activated more by tactile stimulation, and cells related to eye movements, by visual stimulation. The neurons seem indeed to act as sensorimotor synthesizers by using behaviorally dependent information from limbic regions to feed sensory signals into the beginning motor stream. Correspondingly, the functional properties, that is, their relation to sensory stimuli and motor behavior, were found to be increasingly diversified.

Motter et al. (1987) described cells in the inferior parietal lobule, where signals from visual areas, the superior colliculus and the pretectum, meet, with receptive fields varying with the behavioral state, the angle of gaze, and the variables of the stimuli. The cells responded to movement and direction, but less to speed. Within the often bilateral receptive fields, the direction sensitivity was antagonistic, resulting in responses to inward or outward movement of the stimulus. Steinmetz et al. (1987) proposed that these neurons are driven by the "apparent optic flow during self motion" and are part of the visual guidance system for projected movements. Another group of neurons depends on the retinal localization

of the stimulus and the position of the eyes. It was demonstrated that the retinotopy of such neurons is stable (i.e., the receptive fields move with the eyes), but the responsiveness is a function of the angle of gaze (Andersen et al., 1985). The interaction of these two variables tunes the neuronal response for the location of visual targets in head-centered space and theoretically could provide spatial constancy via body-centered coordinates (Andersen, 1988).

The understanding of the functions of the parietal cortex is just beginning, but research in anatomy (see Goldmann-Rakic, 1988) and physiology has revealed a parcellation not previously imagined. Hyvärinen (1982) proposed a functional differentiation as follows: area 5 subserves the somatosensory mechanisms for posture and movement, the anterior part of 7a contributes to visuospatial functions, and the lateral parts of 7a contribute to somatesthetic functions. He regarded the function of the posterior parietal cortex to be the combination of information for personal awareness of extrapersonal, mainly visuospatial, organization and the significance of external stimuli. The emphasis on the body image and its spatial relation to the immediate surround agrees with clinical knowledge concerning the defects after lesions of this area.

The extrapolation from animal experiments to humans, however, remains difficult owing to the large evolutionary increase of the parietal as well as the prefrontal homotypic cortex and the development of lateralization between the hemispheres from monkeys to humans. Nevertheless, the most common syndrome after lesions in the right parietal area (i.e., sensory and spatial neglect to the left [Mesulam, 1981]) can be related to the attention-dependent activity of these neurons if a left-sided dominance for attention in humans is assumed. The receptive fields of such neurons are frequently bilateral, and the weak hemi-inattention effects in monkeys after ablation of the parietal cortex could be due to the lack of lateralization. Split-brain patients do not show sensory or spatial neglects, possibly because of an inhibitory mechanism from the right to the left parietal cortex.

Prefrontal and Premotor Processing

The activity of the prefrontal cortex is less understood than that of the parietal cortex. Again, for evolutionary reasons, the relationship between animal data and human behavior is difficult to establish. The prefrontal cortex is reciprocally connected with the prestriate occipital, the temporal, and the parietal and cingular cortex. There is no area of convergence of the different sensory contributions. The prefrontal cortex seems to mark the end of preprocessed and parallel projected sensory and limbic information and the beginning of motor integration (Freund, 1987). How the necessary cooperation among its different parts and with its sites of projection is accomplished is not known. Considering its inputs, it is not astonishing that visual responses can be recorded not only from the frontal eye field, initially only during or after spontaneous saccades and later also in advance when the stimulus is of interest (Goldberg and Bushnell, 1981), but also from area 46. Goldberg and Bushnell (1981) also described an anticipatory activity before the appearance of the target, provided that several successive trials with the same target had preceded. The receptive fields are large, mostly contralateral, and not stimulus specific. In area 46 and in the frontal eye field, auditory responses have also been detected (Bruce and Goldberg, 1985; Ito, 1982). They have large receptive fields defined in space and not by sound composition. However, there have also been reports of neurons that respond best to species calls.

The impairment of delayed response tasks after prefrontal lesions led to neuronal studies with delayed response paradigms. It was shown that there is no common response. Some cells are activated by the cue; others respond with delay immediately before the behavioral response. Frontal eye field neurons related to ocular movement or visuomotor responses did respond often for seconds after a short target exposition; Bruce and Goldberg (1985) spoke of mnemonic activity. Again, in area 46, the same activity was detected (see Bruce, 1988).

It is still not possible to draw firm conclusions from these data. They indicate a higher-order function for motor behavior before the premotor areas. Rizzolatti and Gentilucci (1988) described, in the premotor cortex (area 6), a topographic arrangement for distal and proximal movements. Neurons for proximal movements are strongly activated by visual and tactile stimuli, with a visual receptive field around the body and in register with the tactile fields. The neurons for distal movement are activated during motor acts (e.g., tearing and grasping), no matter if the left or right hand or sometimes even the mouth is involved. Many neurons are specific for the type of object handling. Rizzolatti and Gentilucci (1988) proposed, therefore, that these neurons code for a motor vocabulary, which is thought to be a basis of cortical motor organization. One realizes that, just as one is confronted at the end of sensory processing with motor features, one is also confronted at the beginning of motor output with sensory information. This makes the separation of motor and sensory functions in the prefrontal and parietal cortex artificial.

The findings in the frontal eye field and area 6 may correspond to the deviation of gaze to the opposite side in focal seizures of the frontal eye field and the transitory deviation to the homolateral side after a lesion. By analogy, neglects after frontal lesions may be understood as defects in the motor programs for intentional visual and consequently manual exploration within extrapersonal space, as seen after ablation of frontal cortex in the monkey and also as recognized in humans (Mesulam, 1986).

NEURONAL ACTIVITY AND PERCEPTION

The following discussion concentrates on visual perception because it is by far the largest sensory input, constituting (with its cortical area) almost half of the macaque neocortex (see Spillmann and Werner, 1990). In addition, all anatomic and psychophysical evidence favors a comparable organization of the visual system in humans and monkeys. Neuronal responses recorded from monkeys have therefore been equated with the perceptive event by sensory physiologists (Jung, 1973). Such neuronal activity may correlate with human perceptive experience. At least this is assumed if, under comparable conditions, the neuronal activity parallels perception. Of course, such correlations cannot explain but indicates only the condition of how neuronal activity gives rise to conscious experience, with its wealth of qualities and emotional values.

Correlations between neuronal activity and perception are relatively easy to establish in the afferent pathways, but that is far from where it is assumed that perception arises. This derives trivially from the loss of sensation during still ongoing axonal activity distal to a nerve blockade. Relative brightness and darkness, simultaneous and successive contrast, color, flicker, and flicker fusion can be traced to the activity of neurons of the afferent visual system up to cells in layer IV of the striate cortex. Again, this activity is only a condition for, but not immediately related to, perception. Therefore, where within the system does neuronal activity become perceptive? Where does perception emerge? In other words, is there any evidence for separating detecting neurons (i.e., neurons depending reliably on the physical stimulus) from perceptive cells? The latter should be related to identical perception induced by a variety of different physical stimulus conditions.

A form-perceiving neuron so defined should indicate a bar no matter if it is real or illusory and its activity should fade with any change in the inducing stimulus that weakens the illusion. A movement-perceiving neuron should be activated by real or apparent movements, a depth-perceiving neuron should be driven by real depth cues or by stimuli that induce apparent depth, and the activation of a color-perceiving neuron should indicate the color of an object as long as it is seen in this color, regardless of the wavelength reflected. Even so, these conditions are certainly not sufficient to state that perception emerges simply from the activity of such neurons. This holds also for the implication that the term *perceptive neurons* stands always for an ensemble of functionally comparable neurons.

One can argue that the apparent-real relationship is still at a preprocessing mode or cannot contribute in isolation to perception proper. One has therefore to look for further evidence. In this context, several points are important:

1. The neuroanatomic data that demonstrate a parcellation of even cytoarchitectonically homogeneous areas and its segregation of connections to other visual areas.
2. The physiologic findings that relate segregated projections to different visual properties.

3. The psychophysical evidence that supports the segregation of function. Movement perception can be separated from form perception by stroboscopic stimulation or by variations of spatial frequency and contrast of moving gratings (Campbell and Maffei, 1981). Moreover, by eliminating luminance differences, color can be separated from form perception, at least partially (Koffka, 1935). Depth perception can be separated from pattern perception in random-dot stereograms (von der Heydt and Ben-Dov, 1990).

4. Brain injuries that lead to isolated loss of color and movement perception without impairment of form recognition, or to impairment of form recognition without or with only minor disturbances of other submodalities.

5. The specific code of neurons and its invariance for other properties. If a neuron is activated only by a face and is not affected by its size, location in space, movement, or color, these other properties must be defined somewhere else.

Taken together, these facts are fairly good evidence that vision is processed until the perceptual level in submodality-specific cortical pathways and areas. This implies that the different visual properties, such as form, color, depth, and movement, are compartmentalized. Thus, with regard to perceptive neurons, where within these channels does perception emerge? How to approach this problem can be illustrated by a simple example.

In the visual system, short-range border contrast can be found already in the distribution of neuronal activity around a contour in optic nerve cells or in neurons of the lateral geniculate body and in cells with concentric field organization in layer IV of V1 (Baumgartner and Hakas, 1962). This is the consequence of the reciprocal organization of neurons with concentric overlapping receptive on- and off-center fields, in which the receptive field center is always dominant. The on-center cells code for light increments, and the off-center cells, for decrements (Fiorentini et al., 1990). This organization gives rise to the illusion of a Hermann grid (Fig. 49–5); but this activity has to be processed further to reach awareness. This can be concluded from long-range area contrast, because there is no neuronal correlate to the perception of area contrast in the neurons of the afferent visual pathways. It must therefore be the product of exclusively cortical processing.

Possible candidates for the first step to build up area contrast are the cortical simple field neurons. Those neurons have a balanced excitatory and inhibitory input. They are therefore insensitive to diffuse illumination of their receptive fields. Neurons of this type signal only brightness gradients or contours of a target orientation if it fits the orientation of their receptive field axes. An area of equal brightness therefore activates only cells on its border. One may assume then that the brightness of the surface is approximated by the direction of the brightness gradient on its borders. Consequently, the brightness

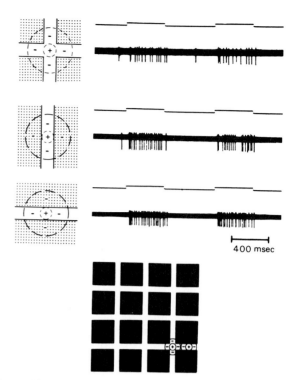

Figure 49–5. Hermann grid illusion and response of on-center neuron in the visual cortex (V1) of cat. Gray spots are seen at the bar intersection corresponding to the diminished neuronal response when the receptive field is centered on an intersection compared with the responses when the receptive field is centered within a vertical or horizontal bright bar. At reading distance, the gray spot disappears when fixated as a consequence of smaller receptive field size within the fovea. + = activating area of the receptive field; − = inhibiting area of the receptive field. The line above the neuronal response records the photo cell. When the line is up, the light is on.

should be neutralized by inverse gradients on the opposite side. This is indeed the case (Fig. 49–6). It is assumed that this is due to a long-range cooperation from border to border, which may be established first in V2 or some other prestriate area. This can be concluded because simple field neurons whose receptive fields lie within a uniform surface are not transferring any information under physiologic conditions. Their receptive area can be seen as brighter or darker. This means that the connected higher regions are not able to discriminate whether a lack of input from V1 is physiologic or is the consequence of a lesion. Cortical scotomata attributable to a lesion in V1 therefore should not be experienced, even with intact prestriate regions. They can, however, be made visible entoptically.

If one uses a stimulus that induces illusory contours, neurons of V1 respond only to the inducing features but do not indicate an illusory contour. However, in V2, some cells respond to both illusory and real contours. They are activated by the movement of a bright bar as well as by the movement of an illusory contour across their receptive field (Fig. 49–7). Their activity is diminished by any change in the stimulus configuration that reduces the illusion.

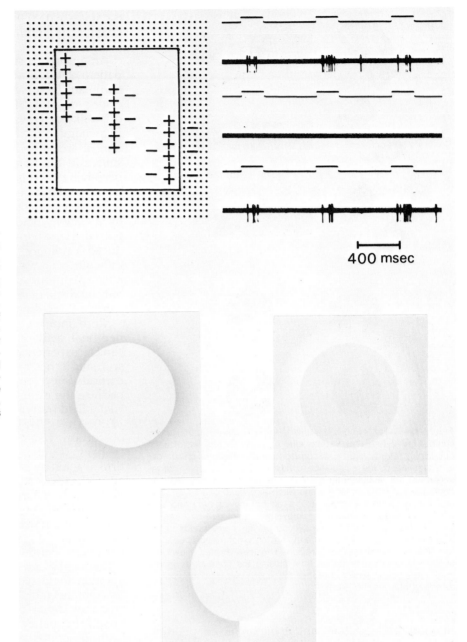

Figure 49–6. Area contrast (Craik-Cornsweet illusion) and the response of a simple field neuron of V1 of the cat. Although the discs are equal in diameter and luminance, the left is appearing larger and brighter. The neuron is activated only at the borders, because activating (+) and inhibiting (−) zones of the receptive field are balanced. Assuming that the area contrast is induced by the direction of the sudden step of luminance at the border, it should be reduced or neutralized when the gradients of luminance are reversed on the opposite side of an area, as it is shown below, where the apparent brightness appears as in between the two upper areas.

400 msec

Thus, border contrast could be considered a first-order contrast to enforce contours by amplifying intensity gradients. Area contrast can be thought of as a second-order contrast using only the enforced contours in generating surfaces to prepare form perception. The mechanisms underlying illusory contours may be a third-order contrast in generating form by abstracted features and using only a few widely separated picture elements.

Neurons responding to illusory contours were found in the pale interstripes, the termination site of the interblob neurons of V1, from which form processing is proposed to originate, and in the thick stripes of V2. In the thick stripes, there is an increased number of disparity-sensitive cells. This is in agreement with

the apparent depth frequently associated with illusory contours, which give the impression of an occlusion. Illusory contours have also been called cognitive contours and attributed to a top-down process. Their early occurrence in cortical processing does not exclude such an effect, but they are easier to explain by two inputs from V1 cells, which act as detecting and grouping mechanisms (Peterhans and von der Heydt, 1989).

Monkeys and cats can be trained to discriminate illusory contours. Therefore, a relationship between the activity of cells in V2 and the occurrence of illusory contours is assumed. Those cells are not mere detectors anymore but are rather organizers of visual information. One is still reluctant to call them perceptive neurons. They are not invariant for size,

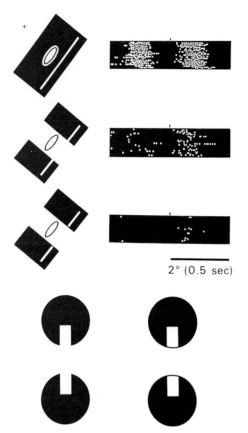

2° (0.5 sec)

Figure 49–7. Illusory contours and neuronal response to an illusory contour in V2 (area 18) of macaque monkey. On the left of each dot display (every bright spot corresponds to a neuronal discharge) is a scheme of the stimulation condition. The oval region corresponds to the receptive field and its orientation as measured with bright bars of different length and width at optimal orientation. The first display shows the response to a real bar moving back and forth above the receptive field with a movement amplitude of 2° and a cycle time of 0.5 second. The second display corresponds to the stimulation with an illusory figure by moving synchronously only the two notches within the black region. The third display shows the strongly diminished response after closing the notches as in the right figure below, which abolishes the illusory figure which is seen as a bright bar on the left.

rotation, and location, and a hierarchic cooperation along a channel of a specific function could make a strict definition entirely impossible.

Area contrast and illusory contours demonstrate the economy of the processing. The brain seems to rely on a minimum of neuronal activity. It modifies incoming information and builds up perception actively according to its intrinsic rules of organization.

The projection of the parvocellular blob system via the thin stripes in V2 to V4 reveals new features of color coding (see earlier). In V4, some cells code for color, as it is perceived, and not for the wavelength reflected. These cells become shape independent. The existence of these cells could explain why it is possible to see an object in a defined color under different conditions of illumination. After ablation of V4, monkeys are still able to discriminate light of different wavelengths. However, they are no longer able to make color discriminations in complex color

scenes when color constancy is required because of changes in illumination and reflectance (Wild et al., 1985).

An analogous situation was found in a color-blind patient. He too was still able to discriminate monochromatic light bands to a remarkable extent without color perception. He could not, however, copy Mondrian-like displays (Fries, personal communication). In analogy to the blindsight of patients with destruction of area 17 who are still able to point to a light source in the hemianopic field without consciously perceiving it, this patient could discriminate wavelength without perceiving color.

That the problem is still more complex is illustrated by a patient whom Wapner et al. (1978) have reported. He experienced a vascular accident that produced a homonymous hemianopia to the right and difficulties of visual recognition. He could not see illusory contours in a two-dimensional representation but could still detect them in random-dot stereograms using a three-dimensional display (Stevens, 1981).

More indirect support for the relation between neuronal activity and perception is derived from clinical experience. In area 17 (V1), the extent of a scotoma is not related to the geometric size of the cortical defect but to the localization of the lesion because the extent of cortical representation per unit visual field decreases toward the periphery (Holmes, 1919). This corresponds to the magnification factor of cortical visual representation measured in the monkey (Daniel and Whitteridge, 1961) and confirmed again by measurements of the phosphene size after electrical stimulation in humans (Cowey and Rolls, 1974). If a migrainous scotoma is indeed related to a spreading depression with a constant velocity of spread, one must expect the known accelerated expansion of the scotoma from central vision to the periphery (Baumgartner, 1977).

Interocular adaptation and therefore cortical adaptation for the discrimination of oriented patterns (Blakemore and Campbell, 1968) indicate the adaptation of defined channels for spatial frequencies. Spatial frequency–dependent cortical neurons have been described. The McCollough effect (1965) of pattern-related and therefore central color adaptation may be expected on the base of Zeki's (1985) neuronal data.

Neurons responding to movement in V5, where the magnocellular movement pathway terminates, were extensively studied and considered in relation to the principles of psychophysics. Such neurons respond to real motion in a certain direction and to apparent motion by stroboscopic stimuli, which show direction-dependent interaction over long distances (see Mikami et al., 1986a,b). The response is fairly independent of stimulus form and color. Some of the neurons are not related to the retinal stimulus, but to the "monkey's reported perception of motion direction" (Logothetis and Shall, 1989). Newsome et al. (1989) compared neuronal responses to a moving target with a direction discrimination task near the limits of performance. They found the sensitivity of the neurons to be as good or slightly better than the behavioral response. After ibotenic acid lesions in V5 (middle temporal area), eye movements (smooth pursuit movements and saccades) for following a moving target were impaired (Newsome and Wurtz, 1988). In the nearby medial superior temporal region, Tanaka and Saito (1989) found neurons responding to in-depth movements (i.e., to expansion or contraction) and to rotation of a stimulus. V5 and its neighborhood are obviously involved in the analysis of movement, and some V5 neurons may belong to the final perceptive movement assembly. Clinical support of such an interpretation derives from the patient of Zihl et al. (1983) who showed loss of movement perception after symmetric bilateral lesions in the lateral temporo-occipital cortex and white matter.

Of course, neuronal data alone cannot tell much about perception. They lead only to the trivial conclusion that detection and perception are processed in series and perception emerges somewhere at the end. The convergence of psychophysical and clinical experience with the spatially separated features of neuronal ensembles favors a rather direct relation between the activity of such neurons and perception. It still does not explain how this distributed activity is able to originate a coherent global percept. There are old proposals, such as that attention may occur via the reticular thalamic input and function as a search light for transiently combining selected neuronal groups (see Jung, 1967). It was found that neurons in a functional column of V1 do have synchronized oscillatory responses between 40–60 Hz after a proper stimulus. An analogue-synchronized oscillatory response to a light bar was then shown also in spatially separated columns with the same orientation preference in V1 and in V2 (Eckhorn et al., 1989). This led to the hypothesis that the stimulus-induced, spatially separated oscillations could reflect a transitory linkage of local features into a global percept. Time could therefore serve as the linking variable via intracortical and intercortical connections.

Advances in neurophysiology have led to some understanding of the importance of domain-specific contributions, allowing for the development of theories of processing, which can be tested by computer simulation, even with the implication of self-organization, and then applied to neural nets (Durbin and Mitchison, 1990; Eckhorn et al., 1989; Finkel and Edelman, 1989; Grossberg and Mignola, 1985; Haken, 1983; Marr, 1982; Rock, 1983; von der Marlsburg and Singer, 1988). All of these approaches modify thinking about the brain and its most wonderful creation, the mind, even if conclusions are still uncertain (Barlow, 1990) and the use of terms, such as modularity, is often inconsistent and contradictory (Fodor, 1983; Gazzaniga, 1988).

CONCLUSIONS

It is evident that the neocortex has a functional diversification that far exceeds the most speculative ideas and that is modifiable even in adults (Merzenich, 1987). It shows, however, some invariant features, such as the rerepresentation of sensory and motor systems, columnar organization, and the similarities of neuronal processing. It is inferred that the cortex is a rather uniformly organized matrix composed of modules with a shifting overlap (Creutzfeldt, 1976, 1983; Szentagothai, 1976)—each module containing the same number of neurons. This would be a logical consequence of handling complexity by grouping (Simon, 1962). The network of a module, no matter if it is considered to be a minicolumn (Hubel and Wiesel, 1977)or a macrocolumn composed of a set of minicolumns, could be similar, and differences in function depend on their connectivity and are reflected in differences in cytoarchitecture (Powell, 1981).

A cortical area is defined, then, morphologically and functionally strictly in relation to its input and output connections and is composed of columnar modules. Special intrinsic mechanisms may not be necessary, the processing in the different sets of modules being the same and therefore compatible. This seems not unlikely, considering the differences in function of a homogeneous structure such as the cerebellum.

In this view, the domain specificity does not depend on its circuitry but on the connectivity of input and output; the functional resolution derives from the number of modules per receptive or effective unit area. All the evidence shows that different properties of sensory information are processed repetitively in increasingly more dispersed and specialized pathways and remain domain specific, as must also be concluded from selective impairments after cortical injuries. The frequently encountered unawareness of such defects shows that global percepts are not based on a unitarian convergent principle but rather on a principle of cooperation. Distributed systems are bound together to establish new entities, whose functions cannot be predicted from knowing the activity of only one subsystem. If a part of this cooperation is injured, its respective contribution is lost. The patient may not see or recognize color anymore but has no difficulty in object or movement perception. This can be due to a disconnection between cooperating domains or to a lesion of a specific area. The clinical outcome may be similar (Geschwind, 1965), but the conditions are different. Although a lesion is always combined with disconnection too, the underlying difference becomes evident in results of studies in split-brain patients.

At first, sectioning of this largest commissure was reported to have no negative effect and, when tested with the usual neurologic and psychologic procedures, the patients were found free from symptoms. This changed dramatically after Sperry (1984) and collaborators entered the scene. With experience in animal split-brain research, Sperry applied the same test principles to humans. He made sure that sensory inputs reached always only one hemisphere and that motor responses were tested on the contralateral extremity. In these conditions, the patients acted as if they had two separated awareness systems or a double representation of consciousness. This was previously unheard of, and the finding was consequently widely criticized. The verbally dominant left hemisphere, which could easily express its conscious experiences, was previously considered a kind of unifier of the mind, and the mute right hemisphere, an unconscious automaton. Sperry and collaborators demonstrated convincingly, however, that split-brain patients live with two separated minds, each with different capacities and unaware of the other. The results of Levy et al. (1979) with chimeric faces and those of Gazzaniga et al. (1977) and Zaidel (1976) about the verbal functions of the right hemisphere and the superiority of the right hemisphere in some tasks involving logical reasoning could not be accounted for within the framework of an automaton scheme. This was further supported by the emotional expression of annoyance or satisfaction in response to certain visual inputs or at failure or completion of a motor task done with the right hemisphere.

Because it certainly cannot be assumed that an ape is unconscious because it cannot speak (Premack, 1988), the automaton conclusion was premature and indeed split-brain patients have two separated minds functioning at cognitive levels with different capacities. The conclusion that even the mind is compartmentalized seems unavoidable. What is lost after callosal section is the cooperation between the two hemispheres, which normally interact continuously and contribute with different weight in any processing to ensure the unity of behavior (Gazzaniga, 1988). Because intrahemispheric processing is unimpaired in split-brain conditions, the patients seem superficially intact in everyday life. Disconnection alone leaves domain-specific processing intact, but the cerebral hemispheres no longer have access to one another. If, in addition, a cortical injury occurs that involves not only disconnection or transfer of information but also information processing itself, defects in recognition or language result. This shows again that, as the mind can be split, a further parcellation of functions of the mind even within one hemisphere is possible.

So far, it can be said that neuronal processing applies rules that can contradict physical specifications of the input as shown by color-coded cells or neurons responding to illusory contours. The brain demonstrates here its intrinsic organization, which is designed to structure a wealth of information in a manageable manner. It organizes information so that the surroundings are not seen as they are, but in a way that makes an optimum of adaptive behavior possible. The plasticity of neuronal operations, including cortical maps, that does adjust for variations of input conditions and previous experiences means that the cortex cannot be described as a stable network but has its own ongoing dynamic, in which a downward flow of information must be of importance.

This may seem to be a rather reductionistic approach in true Gallic fashion, but it should not be understood so, because such an approach is certainly insufficient, and not only because of unanswered questions concerning the cooperation of distributed subsystems. A time-dependent linking feature concept with coincident covariation of activity (Philips et al., 1984) may perhaps explain finally the construction of global percepts. However, many findings (e.g., the patients of Bisiach [1988] with right parietal lesions, who described only the features of a familiar place located to the right of their imaginary line of sight, no matter if they were told to imagine the place first in one and then in the opposite view) show that there is still ample space and necessity for top-down approaches in addition. Lateralization must also be considered.

From the perspective of the present analyses of the sensory system, and on the basis of connectivity, one has to assume that the frontal lobes deal largely with integrated data preprocessed in the parietotemporo-occipital lobes and that their function is supported by information from the limbic system. Because the processing in these areas is not sufficiently understood, conclusions concerning frontal lobe functions are still more speculative. One could assume that the parietotemporal cortex establishes a continuously updated model of the world and the self. This may be used by the frontal cortex in conjunction with information of prior experiences as the basis for further abstractions, which allow planning or anticipating future events. For good reasons, the brain, especially the cortex, is considered the most sophisticated structure in the known universe. It may turn out that the miracle of its organization is its simplicity, hidden behind a complexity that is in essence the reason for the holistic-centralistic discussion. If Aristotle was right that it is not possible to understand what is not perceived before, what remains is the question of what is perceivable by the brain from the brain (i.e., a biologic paradox concerning the brain-mind problem).

References

(Key references are designated with an asterisk.)

*Andersen R.A. Visual and visual-motor functions of the posterior parietal cortex. In Rakic P., Singer W., eds. *Neurobiology of Neocortex.* Chichester, Wiley, pp. 285–295, 1988.

Andersen R.A., Essiek G.K., Siegel R.M. Encoding spatial location by posterior parietal neurons. *Science* 230:456–458, 1985.

Barber C., Blum T., eds. *Evoked Potentials III. The Third International Evoked Potential Symposium.* Stoneham, MA, Butterworth, 1987.

Barlow H. The mechanical mind. *Annu. Rev. Neurosci.* 13:15–24, 1990.

Baumgartner G. Neuronal mechanisms of the migrainous visual aura. In Clifford Rose F., ed. *Physiological Aspects of Clinical Neurology.* Oxford, Blackwell Scientific Publications, pp. 111–121, 1977.

Baumgartner G., Hakas P. Die Neurophysiologie des simultanen Helligkeitskontrastes. Reziproke Reaktionen antagonistischer Neuronengruppen des visuellen Systems. *Pfluegers Arch. Gesamte Physiol.* 274:489–500, 1962.

Baumgartner G., Peterhans E., von der Heydt R. Neuronal mechanisms of the first, second and third order contrast in the visual system. In Haken H., ed. *Computational Systems, Natural and Artificial.* New York, Springer-Verlag, pp. 35–43, 1987.

Bay E. Optische Faktoren bei den räumlichen Orientierungsstörungen. *Dtsch. Z. Nervenheilkde.* 171:454–459, 1954.

Bisiach E. Language without thought. In Weiskrantz L., ed. *Thought Without Language.* Oxford, Clarendon Press, pp. 464–484, 1988.

Blakemore C., Campbell F.W. Adaptation to spatial stimuli. *J. Physiol. (Lond.)* 200:11–13, 1968.

Blasdel G.G., Salama G. Voltage-sensitive dyes reveal a modular organization in monkey striate cortex. *Nature* 321:579–585, 1986.

*Bloom F.E. What is the role of general activating systems in cortical functions? In Rakic P., Singer W., eds. *Neurobiology of Neocortex.* Chichester, Wiley, pp. 407–421, 1988.

Brandeis D., Lehmann D. Segments of event-related potential map series reveal landscape changes with visual attention and subjective contours. *Electroencephalogr. Clin. Neurophysiol.* 73:507–518, 1989.

*Brodmann K. *Vergleichende Lokalisationslehre der Grosshirnrinde in ihren Prinzipien dargestellt auf Grund des Zellaufbaus.* Leipzig, Barth, 1909.

Brown W.S., Lehmann D. Verb and noun meanings of homophone words activate different cortical generators: a topographic study of evoked potential fields. *Exp. Brain Res.* 2(Suppl.):159–168, 1979.

Bruce C.J. Single neuron activity in the monkey's prefrontal cortex. In Rakic P., Singer W., eds. *Neurobiology of Neocortex.* Chichester, Wiley, pp. 297–329, 1988.

Bruce C.J., Goldberg M.E. Primate frontal eye fields. I. Single neurons discharging before saccades. *J. Neurophysiol.* 53:606–635, 1985.

Campbell F.W., Maffei L. The influence of spatial frequency and contrast on the perception of moving pattern. *Vision Res.* 21:713–721, 1981.

Cook N.D. *The Brain Code.* London, Methuen, 1986.

Cowey A., Rolls E.T. Cortical magnification factor and its relation to visual acuity. *Exp. Brain Res.* 21:447–454, 1974.

Creutzfeldt O. The brain as a functional entity. *Progr. Brain Res.* 45:451–462, 1976.

*Creutzfeldt O.D. *Cortex Cerebri.* Berlin, Springer, 1983.

*Critchley M. *The Parietal Lobes.* London, Arnold, 1966.

Daniel P.M., Whitteridge D. The representation of the visual field on the cerebral cortex of monkeys. *J. Physiol. (Lond.)* 159:203–221, 1961.

Deecke L., Weinberg H. Motor areas of the cerebral cortex as investigated by magnetoencephalography. In Erné S.N., Romani G.L., eds. *Advances in Biomagnetism, Functional Localization: A Challenge for Biomagnetism.* Singapore, World Scientific, pp. 256–264, 1989.

Durbin R., Mitchison G. A dimension reduction framework for understanding cortical maps. *Nature* 343:644–647, 1990.

Eckhorn R., Reitboeck H.J., Arndt M., et al. A neural network for feature linking via synchronous activity: results from cat visual cortex and from simulation. In Cotterill R.M.J., ed. *Models of Brain Function.* Cambridge, Cambridge University Press, pp. 225–272, 1989.

*Edelman G.M., Mountcastle V.B. *The Mindful Brain.* Cambridge, MA, M.I.T. Press, 1978.

Fechner G.T. (1860) Elemente der Psychophysik. In Boring E.G., Howes D.H., eds. *Elements of Psychophysics* (translated by H. Adler). New York, Holt, Rinehart & Winston, 1965.

Ferrier D. *The Function of the Brain.* London, Smith, Elder, 1876.

Finkel L.H., Edelman G.M. Integration of distributed cortical systems by reentry: a computer simulation of interactive functionally segregated visual areas. *J. Neurosci.* 9:3188–3208, 1989.

Fiorentini A., Baumgartner G., Magnussen S., et al. The perception of brightness and darkness. Relation to neuronal receptive fields. In Spillmann L., Werner J.S., eds. *Visual Perception. The Neurophysiological Foundations.* San Diego, Academic Press, pp. 129–161, 1990.

Flourens M.J.P. *Recherche Expérimentale sur les Propriétés et les Fonctions du Système Nerveux dans les Animaux Vertébrés.* Paris, Crevot, 1824.

*Fodor J.A. *The Modularity of Mind.* Cambridge, MA, M.I.T. Press, 1983.

Förster O. The motor cortex in man in the light of Hughlings Jackson's doctrine. *Brain* 59:135–159, 1936.

Freud S. *Zur Auffassung der Aphasien.* Leipzig, Deuticke, 1891.

*Freund H.J. Abnormalities of motor behaviour after cortical lesions in humans. In Plum F., ed. *Handbook of Physiology.* Section 1. *The Nervous System.* Vol. V. *Higher Functions of the Brain.* Part 2. Bethesda, American Physiological Society, pp. 763–810, 1987.

Gazzaniga M.S. The dynamic of cerebral specialization and molecular interaction. In Weiskrantz L., ed. *Thought Without Language.* Oxford, Clarendon Press, pp. 430–450, 1988.

Gazzaniga M.S., Le Doux J.E., Wilson D.H. Language, praxis and the right hemisphere: clues to mechanisms of consciousness. *Neurology* 27:1144–1147, 1977.

*Geschwind N. Disconnexion syndromes in animals and man. *Brain* 88:237–294, 585–644, 1965.

Goldberg M.E., Bushnell M.C. The role of the frontal eye fields in visually guided saccades. In Fuchs A.F., Becher W., eds. *Progress in Oculomotor Research.* Amsterdam, Elsevier North Holland Biomedical Press, 1981.

Goldmann P.G., Nauta W.J.H. An intricately patterned prefronto-caudate projection in the rhesus monkey. *J. Comp. Neurol.* 171:369–386, 1977.

*Goldman-Rakic P.S. Changing concepts of cortical connectivity. Parallel distributed cortical networks. In Rakic P., Singer W., eds. *Neurobiology of Neocortex.* Chichester, Wiley, pp. 177–202, 1988.

Goldstein K. Remarks on localization. *Confin. Neurol.* 7:25–34, 1946.

Griffith J.S. The unification of neural activity. *Proc. R. Soc. Lond. [Biol.]* 171:353–359, 1968.

Gross C. Visual function of intero-temporal cortex. In Jung R., ed. *Handbook of Sensory Physiology.* Vol. 7. Part 3B. Berlin, Springer, 1973.

Grossberg S., Mingola E. Neural dynamics of form perception: boundary completion, illusory figures, and neon color spreading. *Psychol. Rev.* 92:173–211, 1985.

*Haken H. Synopsis and introduction. In Basar E., Flohr H., Haken H., et al., eds. *Synergetics of the Brain.* Berlin, Springer-Verlag, pp. 3–25, 1983.

Holmes G. The cortical localisation of vision. *Br. Med. J.* 2:193–199, 1919.

Holmes G. The organization of visual cortex in man. *Proc. R. Soc. Lond. [Biol.]* 132:348–361, 1945.

Hubel D.H., Livingstone M.S. Segregation of form, colour and stereopsis in primate area 18. *J. Neurosci.* 7:3378–3415, 1987.

Hubel D., Wiesel T.N. Functional architecture of macaque monkey visual cortex. *Proc. R. Soc. Lond. [Biol.]* 198:1–59, 1977.

*Hyvärinen J. *The Parietal Cortex of Monkey and Man.* Berlin, Springer-Verlag, 1982.

Ingvar D.H., ed. Cognitive functions and cerebral metabolism. *Hum. Neurobiol.* 2:1–48, 1983.

Ito S. Prefrontal unit activity of macaque monkeys during auditory and visual reaction time task. *Brain Res.* 247:39–47, 1982.

Jackson J.H. (1870). A study of convulsions. London, Odell and Ives. Reprinted in Taylor J., ed. *Selected Writings of J.H. Jackson.* Vol. I. London, Hodder & Stoughton, pp. 8–36, 1931.

*Jones E.G. Anatomy of cerebral cortex: columnar input output organization. In Schmitt E.O., Worden A.G., Adelman G., et al., eds. *The Organization of Cerebral Cortex.* Cambridge, MA, M.I.T. Press, pp. 199–236, 1981.

Jones E.G., Powell T.P.S. An anatomical study of converging sensory pathways within the cerebral cortex of the monkey. *Brain* 93:793–820, 1970.

Julesz B. *Foundations of Cyclopean Perception.* Chicago, University of Chicago Press, 1971.

Jung R. Neurophysiologie und Psychiatrie. In Grühle H.W., Jung R., Mayer-Gross W., et al., eds. *Psychiatrie der Gegenwart.* Berlin, Springer-Verlag, pp. 325–928, 1967.

*Jung R. Visual perception and neurophysiology. In Jung R., ed. *Handbook of Sensory Physiology.* Vol. 7. Part 3A. Berlin, Springer-Verlag, 1973.

Koffka K. *Principle of Gestalt Psychology.* New York, Harcourt, Brace, 1935.

Kornhuber H.H., Deecke L. Hirnpotential-Aenderungen bei Willkürbewegungen des Menschen. Bereitschaftspotential und reafferente Potentiale. *Pfluegers Arch. Gesamte Physiol.* 184:1–17, 1965.

Künzle H. Bilateral projections from precentral motor cortex to the putamen and other parts of the basal ganglia. *Brain Res.* 88:195–209, 1975.

Lashley K.S. Functional determinants of cerebral localization. *Arch. Neurol. Psychiatry* 38:371–387, 1937.

Levy J., Trevarthen C., Sperry R.W. Perception of bilateral chimeric figures following hemispheric deconnexion. *Brain* 95:61–78, 1972.

Livingstone M.S., Hubel D.H. Anatomy and physiology of a colour system in the primate visual cortex. *J. Neurosci.* 4:309–356, 1984a.

Livingstone M.S., Hubel D.H. Specificity of intrinsic connections in primate primary visual cortex. *J. Neurosci.* 4:2830–2835, 1984b.

Livingstone M.S., Hubel D.H. Connections between layer 4B of area 17 and thick cytochrome oxidase stripes of area 18 in the squirrel monkey. *J. Neurosci.* 7:3371–3377, 1987a.

*Livingstone M.S., Hubel D.H. Psychological evidence for separated channels for the perception of form, colour, movement and depth. *J. Neurosci.* 7:3416–3468, 1987b.

Logothetis N., Shall J.D. Neuronal activity related to perception in the middle temporal (MT) area of the macaque. In Lam D.M.-K., Gilbert C.D., eds. *Neural Mechanisms of Visual Perception.* Woodlands, TX, Portfolio Publishing, pp. 199–222, 1989.

*Luria A.R. *Higher Cortical Function in Man.* 2nd ed. New York, Basic Books, 1980.

*Lynch J.C. The functional organization of posterior parietal cortex. *Behav. Brain Sci.* 3:485–534, 1980.

Mach E. *Die Analyse der Empfindungen.* 7th ed. Jena, Fischer, 1918.

*Marr D. *Vision.* San Francisco, Freeman, 1982.

Maunsell J.H.R., Newsome W.T. Visual processing in monkey extrastriate cortex. *Annu. Rev. Neurosci.* 10:363–401, 1987.

McCallum W.C., Zappoli R., Denoth F., eds. Cerebral psychophysiology: studies in event-related potentials. *Electroencephalogr. Clin. Neurophysiol. Suppl.* 38, 1986.

McCarthy R.A., Warrington E.K. Evidence for modality-specific meaning systems in the brain. *Nature* 334:428–430, 1988.

McCullough C. Colour adaptation of edge-detectors in the human visual system. *Science* 149:1115–1116, 1965.

McGlynn S.M., Schacter D.L. Unawareness deficits in neuropsychological syndromes. *J. Clin. Exp. Neuropsychol.* 11:143–205, 1989.

*Merzenich M.M. Dynamic neocortical processes and the origin of higher brain functions. In Changeux J.-P., Komiski M., eds. *The Neuronal and Molecular Bases of Learning.* Chichester, Wiley, pp. 337–358, 1987.

Merzenich M.M., Andersen R.A., Middlebrooks J.H. Functional organization of the auditory cortex. *Exp. Brain Res. Suppl. Ser.* 2:61–75, 1979.

Mesulam M.M. A cortical network for directed attention and unilateral neglect. *Ann. Neurol.* 10:309–325, 1981.

Mesulam M.M. Frontal cortex and behaviour. *Ann. Neurol.* 19:320–324, 1986.

Mikami A., Newsome W.T., Wurtz R.H. Motion selectivity in macaque visual cortex. I. Mechanisms of direction and speed selectivity in extrastrial area MT. *J. Neurophysiol.* 55:1308–1327, 1986a.

Mikami A., Newsome W.T., Wurtz R.H. Motion selectivity in macaque visual cortex. II. Spatio-temporal range of directional interaction in MT and V1. *J. Neurophysiol.* 55:1328–1339, 1986b.

Mishkin M. Cortical visual areas and their interaction. In Karczmar A.G., Eccles J.C., eds. *The Brain and Human Behaviour.* Berlin, Springer-Verlag, 1972.

Mishkin M., Ungerleider L.G., Macko K.A. Object vision and spatial vision: two cortical pathways. *Trends Neurosci.* 6:414–417, 1983.

Moruzzi G., Magoun H. Brain stem reticular formation and activation of the EEG. *Electroencephalogr. Clin. Neurophysiol.* 1:455–473, 1949.

Motter B.C., Steinmetz M.A., Duffy C.J., et al. Functional properties of parietal visual neurons: mechanisms of directionality along a single axis. *J. Neurosci.* 7:154–176, 1987.

*Mountcastle V.B. Modality and topographic properties of single neurons of cat's somatic sensory cortex. *J. Neurophysiol.* 20:408–434, 1957.

Mountcastle V.B., Lynch J.C., Georgopoulos A., et al. Posterior parietal association cortex of the monkey: command functions for operations within extrapersonal space. *J. Neurophysiol.* 38:871–908, 1975.

Newsome W.T., Wurtz R.H. Probing visual cortical functions with discrete chemical lesions. *Trends Neurosci.* 11:394–400, 1988.

Newsome W.T., Britten K.H., Morshon J.A., et al. Single neurons and the perception of visual motion. In Lam D.M.K., Gilbert C., eds. *Neural Mechanisms of Visual Perception. Proceedings of the Retina Research Foundation Symposium.* Vol. 2. Woodlands, TX, Portfolio Publishing, pp. 171–198, 1989.

Ojemann G.A., Creutzfeldt O., Lettich E., et al. Neuronal activity in human lateral temporal cortex related to short-term verbal memory, naming and reading. *Brain* 111:1383–1403, 1988.

Ojemann G.A., Ojemann J., Lettich E., et al. Cortical language localization in left, dominant hemisphere. *J. Neurosurg.* 71:316–326, 1989.

Penfield W., Rasmussen T. *The Cerebral Cortex of Man.* New York, Macmillan, 1957.

Perret D.I., Smith P.A.J., Potter D.D. Neurones responsive to faces in the temporal cortex: studies of functional organization, sensitivity to identity and relation to perception. *Hum. Neurobiol.* 3:197–208, 1984.

Peterhans E., von der Heydt R. Mechanisms of contour perceptive in monkey visual cortex. II. Contours bridging gaps. *J. Neurosci.* 9:1749–1763, 1989.

Phelps M.E., Maziotta J.C., Schelbert H.R., eds. *Positron Emission Tomography and Autoradiography. Principles and Applications for the Brain and Heart.* New York, Raven Press, 1986.

Phillips C.G., Zeki S., Barlow H.B. Localization of function in the cerebral cortex. Past, present, future. *Brain* 107:327–361, 1984.

Poggio G.F., Gonzalez F., Krause F. Stereoscopic mechanisms in monkey visual cortex: binocular correlation and disparity selectivity. *J. Neurosci.* 8:4531–4550, 1988.

*Powell T.P.S. Certain aspects of the intrinsic organization of the cerebral cortex. In Pompeiano O., Marsan C., eds. *Brain Mechanisms of Perceptual Awareness and Purposeful Behavior.* New York, Raven Press, pp. 1–19, 1981.

Premack D. Minds with and without language. In Weiskrantz L., ed. *Thought Without Language.* Oxford, Clarendon Press, pp. 46–65, 1988.

Richmond B.J., Wurtz R.H., Sato T. Visual responses of inferior temporal neurons in awake rhesus monkey. *J. Neurophysiol.* 50:1415–1432, 1983.

Riddock G. Dissociation of visual perception due to occipital injuries, with special reference to the appreciation of movement. *Brain* 40:15–57, 1917.

Rizzolatti G., Gentilucci M. Motor and visual-motor functions of the premotor cortex. In Rakic P., Singer W., eds. *Neurobiology of Neocortex.* Chichester, Wiley, pp. 269–284, 1988.

Robinson D.L., Goldberg M.E., Stanton G.R. Parietal association cortex in the primate cortex: sensory mechanisms and behavioural modulation. *J. Neurophysiol.* 41:910–932, 1978.

Rock J. *The Logic of Perception.* Cambridge, MA, M.I.T. Press, 1983.

Roland P.F. Organization of motor control by the normal human brain. *Hum. Neurobiol.* 2:205–216, 1984.

*Sherrington C.S. *Man on His Nature.* Cambridge, Cambridge University Press, 1951.

*Simon H.A. The architecture of complexity. *Proc. Am. Philos. Soc.* 106:467–482, 1962.

*Sperry R. Consciousness, personal identity and the divided brain. *Neuropsychologia* 22:661–673, 1984.

*Spillmann L., Werner J.S., eds. *Visual Perception. The Neurophysiological Foundations.* San Diego, Academic Press, 1990.

Steinmetz M.A., Motter B.C., Duffy C.J., et al. Functional properties of parietal visual neurons: radial organization of directionalities within the visual field. *J. Neurosci.* 7:177–191, 1987.

Stevens K.A. *Evidence Relating Subjective Contours and Interpretations Involving Occlusions.* Cambridge, MA, M.I.T. Artificial Intelligence Laboratory, A.I. Memo No. 637, 1981.

Szentagothai J. The "modul-concept" in cerebral cortex architecture. *Brain Res.* 95:475–496, 1976.

Tanaka K., Saito H.-A. Analysis of motion of the visual field by direction, expansion of contraction, and rotation cells clustered in the dorsal part of the medial superior temporal area of the macaque monkey. *J. Neurophysiol.* 62:626–641, 1989.

*van Essen D.C. Functional organization of primate visual cortex. In Peters A., Jones E.G., eds. *Cerebral Cortex*. Vol. 3. New York, Plenum Publishing, pp. 259–329, 1985.

*von der Heydt R. Approaches to visual cortical function. *Rev. Physiol. Biochem. Pharmacol.* 108:69–150, 1987.

von der Heydt R., Ben-Dov G. Stereopsis and metacontrast: pattern mashed, but depth perceived. *Invest. Ophthalmol. Vis. Sci.* 31:89, 1990.

von der Heydt R., Peterhans E. Mechanisms of contour perception in monkey visual cortex. I. Lines of pattern discontinuity. *J. Neurosci.* 9:1731–1748, 1989.

von der Malsburg C., Singer W. Principles of cortical network organization. In Rakic P., Singer W., eds. *Neurobiology of Neocortex*. Chichester, Wiley, pp. 69–99, 1988.

von Monakow K. *Die Lokalisation im Grosshirn*. Wiesbaden, Bergmann, 1914.

Wallesch C.M., Kornhuber H.H., Kunz T., et al. Neuropsychological deficits associated with small unilateral thalamic lesions. *Brain* 106:141–152, 1983.

Wapner W., Judd T., Gardner H. Visual agnosia in an artist. *Cortex* 14:343–364, 1978.

Wild H.M., Butter S.R., Carden D., et al. Primate cortical area V4 is important for colour constancy but not for wave length discrimination. *Nature* 313:133–135, 1985.

Wundt W. *Grundriss der Psychologie*. Leipzig, Engelmann, 1901.

Zaidel E. Auditory vocabulary of the right hemisphere following brain bisection or hemidecortication. *Cortex* 12:191–211, 1976.

Zeki S. Uniformity and diversity of structure and function in rhesus monkey prestriate visual cortex. *J. Physiol. (Lond.)* 277:273–290, 1978.

Zeki S. Colour pathways and hierarchies in the cerebral cortex. In Ottoson D., Zeki S., eds. *Central and Peripheral Mechanisms of Colour Vision*. Dobbs Ferry, NY, Sheridan Medical Books, pp. 19–44, 1985.

Zeki S. Anatomical guides to the functional organization of the visual cortex. In Rakic P., Singer W., eds. *Neurobiology of Neocortex*. Chichester, Wiley, pp. 241–251, 1988.

*Zeki S., Shipp S. The functional logic of cortical connections. *Nature* 335:311–317, 1988.

Zihl J., von Cramon D., Mai N. Selective disturbance of movement vision after bilateral brain damage. *Brain* 106:313–340, 1983.

50

Cortical Information Processing in the Normal Human Brain

Marcus E. Raichle

Substantial evidence supports the hypothesis that the human brain is structurally and functionally modular. One of the great challenges in neuroscience is to understand how this modularity is organized in support of mental activity. Such an understanding must at least accompany, if not precede, a knowledge of how specific components of a mental operation are implemented in individual modules (e.g., local ensembles of neurons). Modern imaging techniques substantially improve the ability to identify and study widely distributed component modules supporting specific mental operations. One approach is the measurement of local brain blood flow with positron emission tomography (PET). This technique is especially important because it permits an examination of these distributed modular relationships in the normal human brain. An understanding of the functional organization of the normal human brain is an essential step toward understanding the effect of injury and disease.

Examination of the functional organization of the normal human brain is based on the ability to measure neuronally induced changes in local blood flow in the brain. Interest in the relationship between brain blood flow and local functional activity has spanned nearly a century. The initial interest crystallized when Roy and Sherrington (1890) published a seminal paper in which they put forth the suggestion that there exists an "automatic mechanism" that provides for a local variation in blood supply in accordance with local differences in the functional activity of the brain. Subsequent experiments in laboratory animals and humans led to confirmation of these pioneering observations and to the establishment of PET as one of the most sensitive and accurate

means of studying the functional anatomy of the normal human brain in vivo (for review, see Raichle, 1987).

This chapter briefly outlines a strategy employing PET measurements of *changes* in local brain blood flow. These measurements are obtained by subtracting measurements made in a control state from those made in a functionally activated state in the same subject. These measurements are then averaged across subjects (and occasionally various measurements from a single subject are averaged) to improve the signal-to-noise properties of the resulting image. From such data emerges a map of the distributed modular brain organization underlying normal human cognition.

POSITRON EMISSION TOMOGRAPHY TECHNIQUE

Emission tomography produces an image of the distribution of a previously administered radionuclide in any desired section of the body. PET uses the unique properties of the annihilation radiation that is generated when positrons are absorbed in matter (Raichle, 1983) to provide an image that is a highly faithful representation of the spatial distribution of the radionuclide at a selected plane through the tissue. Such an image is effectively equivalent to a *quantitative tissue autoradiograph* obtained in laboratory animals. In standard tissue autoradiography, the animal is killed and the brain is removed after the systemic administration of a radiopharmaceutical. The brain is thinly sliced and layed on x-ray film to record the distribution of radioactivity in the brain.

PET can accomplish the measurement of regional brain radioactivity noninvasively; hence, studies are possible in living animals, including humans. PET has been used in humans to measure brain blood flow, blood volume, metabolism of glucose and oxygen, acid-base balance, receptor pharmacologic action, and transmitter metabolism (see Raichle, 1986).

The functional mapping of neuronal activity in the human brain with PET is composed of a number of important elements. These include the deliberate selection of blood flow measured with the PET adaptation of the Kety autoradiographic technique (Herscovitch et al., 1983, 1987; Raichle et al., 1983) or estimated from the radioactive counts accumulating in brain tissue during 40 seconds after the intravenous bolus administration of $H_2^{15}O$ (Fox et al., 1985) as the most accurate and flexible signal of changes in local neural activity that can be detected with PET (Fox et al., 1988a,b). Linearly scaled images of blood flow or radioactive counts in a control state are subtracted from images obtained during functional activation in each subject (i.e., paired image subtraction). The control state and the stimulated state are carefully chosen to isolate, as far as possible, a single mental operation (e.g., see Petersen et al., 1988). By subtracting blood flow measurements made in the control state from those for each task state, it is possible to identify those areas of the brain concerned with the mental operations unique to the task state. This employs a strategy first introduced to psychology by Donders (1868) in which reaction time was used to dissect out the components of mental operations. This process can now be accomplished for specific regions of the brain. These subtraction images form the basis of a data set that is composed of averaged responses across many individual subjects or across many runs in the same individual. Image averaging dramatically enhances the signal-to-noise properties of such data. This enables detection of even low-level responses associated with mental activity (Fox et al., 1988a; Mintun et al., 1989).

FUNCTIONAL MAPS OF SINGLE-WORD PROCESSING

Examination of the cortical anatomy of single-word processing (Petersen et al., 1988, 1989, 1990) is an initial step in the study of language processing. Because of the great complexity of language, restriction of initial efforts to an understanding of the processing of individual words seemed warranted. Furthermore, the design of tasks appropriate for such studies with PET was greatly aided by extant knowledge in cognitive psychology, linguistics, and clinical neurology (e.g., Coltheart, 1985; A.R. Damasio, 1984; LaBerge and Samuels, 1974).

Four behavioral conditions in each subject were used to form a three-level subtractive hierarchy in which each task state was intended to add a small number of mental operations to those of its subor-

dinate (control) state. The general results of this study are summarized in Figure 50–1; more detailed description follows.

In the first level of comparison, the visual presentation of single words without a lexical task was compared with visual fixation on small cross hairs on a television monitor without word presentation. Words were presented for 150 ms at the rate of 1/second on a television screen during the 40-second measurement of blood flow. No motor output or volitional lexical processing was required in this task; rather, simple sensory input and involuntary word form processing were targeted by this subtraction.

The areas of brain identified as active during the passive viewing of words appear to support two different computational levels, one of passive sensory processing in primary visual cortex and a second level of modality-specific word form processing in extrastriate areas. The main regions activated (see

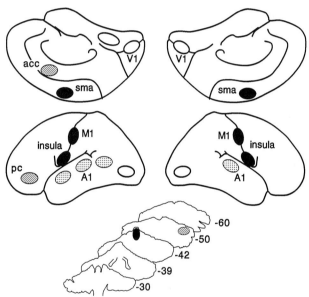

Figure 50–1. Functional anatomy of single-word processing. Location of averaged local blood flow changes in the brain during the processing of single words in normal adult subjects. Four different task states were studied in each subject (who were English speakers): passive presentation of visual words (open ovals), passive presentation of auditory words (stippled ovals), repetition of visual or auditory words (solid ovals), and generation of a verb for a presented noun (hatched ovals). The words, common English nouns, were presented at the rate of 1/second. The control state for the passive hearing or viewing of nouns was looking at a fixation point on a television monitor; the control state for repeating nouns was the passive presentation of the same nouns; the control state for generating verbs was repeating nouns. The right and left cerebral hemispheres are depicted on the right and left, respectively, with the medial surfaces above the lateral surfaces. Coronal sections through the cerebellum are shown below with distances (in millimeters) posterior to the midpoint between the anterior and posterior commissures shown to the right of each section (Talairach et al., 1967). V1 = primary visual cortex; A1 = primary auditory cortex; acc = anterior cingulate cortex; sma = supplementary motor area; M1 = primary motor cortex; insula, insular cortex; pc, prefrontal cortex. This figure summarizes results presented in greater detail elsewhere (Petersen et al., 1988, 1989, 1990).

Fig. 50–1, *open ovals*) were in the striate cortex bilaterally and extrastriate areas, several on the left and the right. The primary striate responses were similar to those produced by simple sensory stimuli, such as the checkerboard annuli used in earlier experiments (Fox et al., 1986, 1987). The regions in the extrastriate cortex were postulated to be a network of cortical modules that code for visual word form. Subsequent experiments (Petersen et al., 1990) demonstrated that the area located in the region of the left fusiform gyrus and the lingual gyrus (i.e., Brodmann areas 19 and 37; open oval anterior to V1 on the left in Fig. 50–1) was activated by words and nonwords obeying rules of English language and not by consonant letter strings or false fonts. Taken together, the several regions of the striate and extrastriate cortex activated by passive visual words appear to combine, functionally, to analyze visual symbols and to distinguish between those that behave according to rules of the English language and those that do not.

Words presented auditorily with subjects passively fixating on the visual cross hairs activated an entirely separate set of areas bilaterally in the temporal cortex (Petersen et al., 1988, 1989): the superior temporal gyrus and the supramarginalis gyrus (see Fig. 50–1, *stippled ovals*). Areas in left posterior temporal cortex (appropriate candidates for Wernicke area, which is thought to be involved in semantic processing) were clearly seen with auditory presentation but were conspicuously absent during the presentation of words visually. Only when subjects were asked to judge whether pairs of visual words rhymed were responses seen in these areas (Petersen et al., 1988, 1989), emphasizing the functionally flexible nature of these modular relationships.

In the second level of comparison, subjects were asked to repeat the words presented auditorily or visually. The control state for the PET blood flow subtraction was the passive presentation of auditory or visual words. Areas related to motor output and articulatory coding were activated (Petersen et al., 1988, 1989) (see Fig. 50–1, *solid ovals*). In general, similar regions were activated for visual and auditory presentation. Responses occurred in primary sensorimotor mouth cortex bilaterally, in the supplementary motor area, and in the insular cortex bilaterally. The left insular response is near Broca area, a region often viewed as specifically serving language output. Similar insular activation was also found when subjects were instructed to simply move their mouths and tongues (P.T. Fox, S.E. Petersen, C. Applegate, et al., unpublished), arguing against specialization of this region for speech output.

In the third and final level of comparison, subjects were asked to speak a verb for each noun presented, either auditorily or visually, again while monitoring a fixation point. Responses (see Fig. 50–1, *hatched ovals*) were identified in two areas of cerebral cortex as well as those areas identified for both auditory and visual word presentation: a region in left dorsolateral prefrontal cortex (Brodmann areas 45 and 46) and a second area in the anterior cingulate gyrus (Brodmann area 32). It is hypothesized that the responses in the anterior cingulate cortex are part of an anterior attentional system engaged in response selection. The localization of this function in the anterior cingulate cortex was suggested by the converging results of experiments (Pardo et al., 1990; Posner et al., 1988). The role of the left dorsolateral prefrontal cortex is less clear, but it may contribute short-term representational memory (Goldman-Rakic, 1987).

Responses in the cerebellum, especially in the right lateral cerebellar hemisphere, were also detected in this task. Because the motoric aspects of simply saying words were subtracted, this result strongly suggests that the cerebellum plays an important role in high-level information processing involving a novel task that engages the left prefrontal cortex. This is the first direct evidence in support of the hypothesis that the cerebellum plays an important role in high-level information processing in humans, as suggested by other investigators (Berntson and Torello, 1984; Bracke-Tolkmitt et al., 1989; Leiner et al., 1989). A study of an individual with an infarct confined to the right cerebellar hemisphere (Fiez et al., 1990) supports this hypothesis. At the time of examination, the subject had recovered from the motor signs of his lesions, and the results of a standard neurologic examination were normal. However, he was unable to perform the verb-generating task, producing significantly more errors than normal controls and showing no evidence of improvement with practice. This suggests that the cerebellum plays a significant role in response evaluation, even in high-level information-processing tasks.

Finally, one additional preliminary (M.E. Raichle, J. Fiez, S.E. Petersen, unpublished) observation may be of importance in understanding the information-processing role of the responses observed in this task. Specifically, the responses in the left prefrontal cortex, the anterior cingulate cortex, and the right cerebellar hemisphere were present only when subjects were first exposed to this task (i.e., when it was novel and required active attention). Practice generating verbs to a specific list of nouns resulted in the disappearance of the left inferior prefrontal, anterior cingulate, and right cerebellar hemisphere responses. These results suggest a role for these areas of cortex in the *acquisition* of a new skill, in this case linguistic. As such, they may represent part of a system responsible for the learning of habits or procedures (Mishkin, 1987).

What do such results suggest about the modular organization of the human brain for tasks associated with single-word processing? They indicate *flexible* modular organization consisting of multiple routes. For example, there is no activation in any of visual tasks near Wernicke area or the angular gyrus in the posterior temporal cortex unless a specific phonologic judgment must be made (e.g., rhyme judgment). Visual information from the occipital cortex appears to have access to output coding without undergoing phonologic recoding in these areas in posterior temporal cortex. Furthermore, tasks calling for semantic processing of single words activate frontal cortices (i.e., left prefrontal and anterior cingulate) and the cerebellum, rather than posterior temporal regions. Finally, sensory-specific information appears to have independent access to semantic and output codes; simple repetition of a presented word failed to activate the left frontal semantic areas.

The studies discussed earlier included mental operations devoid of any obvious emotional valence. It is clear, however, that the everyday cognitive activities are colored by feelings such as elation, sadness, and anxiety. Are these simply emergent properties of the brain or do they represent the coordinated activities of discrete regions of the brain? The limited data from studies in animals and lesion studies in humans argue that what are experienced as emotions are the result of specific systems within the brain (LeDoux, 1987). Until the advent of PET, however, no information was available on the normal human brain to test this hypothesis. Investigation of a disease identified as panic disorder in the *Diagnostic and Statistical Manual of Mental Disorders* (American Psychiatric Association, 1987; see also Reiman et al., 1984, 1986, 1989b) eventually led to studies of emotion in normal human subjects (Reiman et al., 1989a). From these studies, it is clear that a distinctive, distributed, modular, functional anatomic network also underlies the expression of emotion and its understanding can be approached in a manner similar to that used for the study of language.

CONCLUSIONS

Changes in neuronal activity are accompanied by rapid (<1 second) changes in local blood flow and metabolism in the brain. PET, a nuclear medicine brain-imaging technique, accurately and rapidly (<1 minute) measures changes in local blood flow. Assuming that all mental activity is accompanied by changes in local blood flow, PET is ideally suited to accomplish the task of relating changes in local neuronal activity to mental activity.

Using PET measurements of local blood flow and strategies for accurately localizing these changes in the normal human brain, the general topography of systems concerned with the analysis of words has been presented. These data demonstrate that a combination of cognitive and neurobiologic approaches to the study of normal human subjects, aided by modern imaging techniques such as PET, can give important information about the flexible, distributed, modular organization of cognition and emotion in the human brain.

Progress in the evolving understanding of the implementation of mental activities in the human brain will depend on an appreciation of the distributed nature of the processing. Inferences about the role of specific local neuronal ensembles in particular mental activities, heretofore inferred from the loss of function attributable to discrete lesions in humans, must now be guided by the knowledge that a region of the brain may be only a part of a distributed network in which local areas contribute highly specialized component functions. As this type of information accumulates on the normal functional anatomy of the human brain, it is likely that entirely new questions will be asked about neurologic disease. For example, it was only as a result of studies of normal language organization (Petersen et al., 1988, 1989, 1990) that the patient mentioned earlier with an injury to the right cerebellar hemisphere (Fiez et al., 1990) was evaluated for cognitive impairment and found to have a highly specific and profound deficit. It is expected that such examples will multiply rapidly in the future.

PET is not the only imaging technique likely to have an important impact on the understanding of the functional organization of the human brain. Magnetic resonance imaging provides superb gross anatomic images of the living brain and has been used with great success in delineating the anatomy of lesions in relation to specific behavioral deficits (H. Damasio and Damasio, 1989). It is likely that PET and magnetic resonance imaging will be used together to anatomically refine the interpretation of the PET blood flow responses. Neither PET nor magnetic resonance imaging provides insight into the temporal relationships among the several modules subserving a specific mental operation. Electrical measurements of brain activity from surface electrodes in the form of the electroencephalogram, event-related potentials (Hillyard and Picton, 1987), or electrically generated magnetic fields (magnetoencephalography) (Hillyard and Picton, 1987) provide excellent temporal information but variably have difficulty in localizing the source of the electrical signal.

In the future, PET and magnetic resonance imaging may interact with electroencephalography, event-related potentials, and magnetoencephalography, in which the former techniques will provide an accurate anatomic description of the functional anatomy of a system of modules underlying a particular mental operation and the latter techniques, using this information, will provide a description of the temporal relationships among the constituent modules. The prospect that new information will arise about the functional organization of the human brain from the *combined* use of these new imaging methods is quite exciting. I think there is hope that the insights gained from such work will provide a more rational basis for the understanding and treatment of some of the most devastating diseases of humans.

References

(Key references are designated with an asterisk.)
American Psychiatric Association. *Diagnostic and Statistical Manual of Mental Disorders.* 3rd ed., revised. Washington, DC, American Psychiatric Association, 1987.

Berntson G.G., Torello M.W. The paleocerebellum and the integration of behavioral function. *Physiol. Psych.* 10:2–12, 1984.

Bracke-Tolkmitt R., Linden A., Canavan A.G.M., et al. The cerebellum contributes to mental skills. *Behav. Neurosci.* 103:442–446, 1989.

Coltheart M. Cognitive neuropsychology and the study of reading. In Posner M.I., Marlin O.S.M., eds. *Attention and Performance XI.* Hillsdale, NJ, Erlbaum, pp. 3–37, 1985.

Damasio A.R. The neural basis of language. *Annu. Rev. Neurosci.* 7:127–147, 1984.

Damasio H., Damasio A.R. *Lesion Analysis in Neuropsychology.* New York, Oxford University Press, 1989.

Donders F.C. (1868) On the speed of mental processes. Reprinted in *Acta Psychol. (Amst.)* 30:412–431, 1969.

Fiez J., Petersen S.E., Raichle M.E. Impaired habit learning following cerebellar hemorrhage: a single-case study. *Soc. Neurosci. Abstr.* 16:287, 1990.

Fox P.T., Perlmutter J., Raichle M.E. A stereotactic method of anatomical localization for positron emission tomography. *J. Comput. Assist. Tomogr.* 9:141–153, 1985.

Fox P.T., Mintun M.A., Raichle M.E., et al. Mapping human visual cortex with positron emission tomography. *Nature* 323:806–809, 1986.

Fox P.T., Miezen F.M., Allman J.M., et al. Retinotopic organization of human visual cortex mapped with positron emission tomography. *J. Neurosci.* 7:913–922, 1987.

*Fox P.T., Mintun M.A., Reiman E.M., et al. Enhanced detection of focal brain responses using intersubject averaging and distribution analysis of subtracted PET images. *J. Cereb. Blood Flow Metab.* 8:642–653, 1988a.

Fox P.T., Raichle M.E., Mintun M.A., et al. Nonoxidative glucose consumption during focal physiologic neural activity. *Science* 241:462–464, 1988b.

Goldman-Rakic P.S. Circuitry of primate prefrontal cortex and regulation of behavior by representational memory. In Plum F., ed. *Handbook of Physiology.* Section 1. *The Nervous System.* Vol. V. *Higher Functions of the Brain.* Part 2. Bethesda, American Physiological Society, pp. 371–417, 1987.

Herscovitch P., Markham J., Raichle M.E. Brain blood flow measured with intravenous H$_2$^{15}O. I. Theory and error analysis. *J. Nucl. Med.* 24:782–789, 1983.

Herscovitch P., Raichle M.E., Kilbourn M.R., et al. Positron emission tomographic measurement of cerebral blood flow and permeability surface area product of water using ^{15}O-water and ^{11}C-butanol. *J. Cereb. Blood Flow Metab.* 7:527–542, 1987.

Hillyard S.A., Picton T.W. Electrophysiology of cognition. In Plum F., ed. *Handbook of Physiology.* Section 1. *The Nervous System.* Vol. V. *Higher Functions of the Brain.* Part 2. Bethesda, American Physiological Society, pp. 519–584, 1987.

LaBerge D., Samuels S.J. Toward a theory of automatic information processing in reading. *Cognitive Psychol.* 6:293–323, 1974.

LeDoux J.E. Emotion. In Plum F., ed. *Handbook of Physiology.* Section 1. *The Nervous System.* Vol. V. *Higher Functions of the*

Brain. Part 2. Bethesda, American Physiological Society, pp. 419–460, 1987.

Leiner H.C., Leiner A.L., Dow R.S. Reappraising the cerebellum: what does the hindbrain contribute to the forebrain? *Behav. Neurosci.* 103:998–1008, 1989.

Mesulam M.M. *Principles of Behavioral Neurology.* 2nd ed. Philadelphia, Davis, 1986.

Mishkin M., Appenzeller T. The anatomy of memory. *Sci. Am.* 256(6):80–89, 1987.

*Mintun M.A., Fox P.T., Raichle M.E. A highly accurate method of localizing regions of neuronal activation in the human brain with positron emission tomography. *J. Cereb. Blood Flow Metab.* 9:96–103, 1989.

Pardo J.V., Pardo P.J., Janer K.W., et al. The anterior cingulate cortex mediates processing selection in the Stroop attentional conflict paradigm. *Proc. Natl. Acad. Sci. U.S.A.* 87:256–259, 1990.

*Petersen S.E., Fox P.T., Posner M.I., et al. Positron emission tomographic studies of the cortical anatomy of single word processing. *Nature* 331:585–589, 1988.

Petersen S.E., Fox P.T., Posner M.I., et al. Positron emission tomographic studies of the processing of single words. *J. Cognitive Neurosci.* 1:153–170, 1989.

*Petersen S.E., Fox P.T., Snyder A.Z., et al. Activation of extrastriate and frontal cortical areas by visual words and word-like stimuli. *Science* 249:1041–1044, 1990.

*Posner M.I., Petersen S.E., Fox P.T., et al. Localization of cognitive functions in the human brain. *Science* 240:1627–1631, 1988.

Raichle M.E. Positron emission tomography. *Annu. Rev. Neurosci.* 6:249–268, 1983.

Raichle M.E., Martin W.R.W., Herscovitch P., et al. Brain blood flow measured with H$_2$^{15}O. II. Implementation and validation. *J. Nucl. Med.* 24:790–798, 1983.

Raichle M.E. Neuroimaging. *Trends Neurosci.* 9:525–529, 1986.

*Raichle M.E. Circulatory and metabolic correlates of brain function in normal humans. In Plum F., ed. *Handbook of Physiology.* Section 1. *The Nervous System.* Vol. V. *Higher Functions of the Brain.* Part 2. 1987. Bethesda, American Physiological Society, pp. 643–674, 1987.

*Reiman E.M., Raichle M.E., Butler F.K., et al. A focal brain abnormality in panic disorder, a severe form of anxiety. *Nature* 310:683–685, 1984.

Reiman E.M., Raichle M.E., Robins E., et al. The application of positron emission tomography to the study of panic disorder. *Am. J. Psychiatry* 143:469–477, 1986.

Reiman E.M., Fusselman M.J., Fox P.T., et al. Neuroanatomical correlates of anticipatory anxiety. *Science* 243:1071–1074, 1989a.

Reiman E.M., Raichle M.E., Robins E., et al. Neuroanatomical correlates of lactate-induced anxiety attack. *Arch. Gen. Psychiatry* 46:493–500, 1989b.

Roy C.S., Sherrington C.S. On the regulation of the blood supply of the brain. *J. Physiol. (Lond.)* 11:85–109, 1890.

Talairach J., Sxikla G., Tournoux P., et al. *Atlas d'Anatomie Stéréotaxique du Telencéphale.* Paris, Masson, 1967.

51

Memory Systems and Their Disorders

Barry Gordon

INTRODUCTION

Memory is an ambiguous term that has been used to refer to the entire series of processes involved in learning and remembering, to the act of learning alone, or just to the act of remembering itself. The memory disorders seen in clinical practice are an even more heterogeneous group, not all of which involve disorders of memory in the strict sense. It is also likely that there are some true memory disorders that are not yet appreciated in clinical practice. In addition, there is still no generally accepted way in which memory and its disorders can be described, nor are there as yet any proven connections between the memories of conscious experience and the synaptic and subsynaptic events that are generally assumed to underlie memory functions. Nonetheless, it is possible to sketch a working model of the processes that normally underlie memory, to identify some universal features of some of the recognized memory impairments within this working model, and to see the possible connections between behavioral expressions of memory and its disorders and underlying neuronal events. For more detailed discussions of normal memory and its pathologies, the reader is referred to reviews such as those of Baddeley (1990), Dudai (1989), and Squire (1987).

THE HUMAN AMNESTIC SYNDROME

The human amnestic syndrome (Milner et al., 1968; Squire, 1986) is the archetype of specific human

Preparation of this chapter was aided in part by National Institutes of Health grant 1 RO1 NS26553, by the Seaver Foundation, by the McDonnel-Pew Program in Cognitive Neurosciences, and by the Benjamin A. Miller Family Fund for Alzheimer's and Related Diseases.

memory impairments and undoubtedly an important component of the memory disorders that occur in common conditions such as Alzheimer's disease and the dementias, alcoholic Korsakoff's syndrome, postconcussive head injury, and postanoxic encephalopathy. In its idealized form, it is characterized by several features:

1. The patient's attention, concentration, general intellectual abilities, and language and other specific functions are intact.
2. Patients can retain information for short periods, so that abilities such as digit span and initial registration of materials to be remembered are intact.
3. Although they can register new information about explicit facts or events, patients have marked difficulty remembering it later (anterograde amnesia). In severe cases, the patients will not remember the physician's name if the physician leaves the room for a moment, nor do they remember much of anything that has happened to them since the onset of the memory impairment. This deficit in new learning does not extend to all types of material. In particular, new learning is normal for material that has been variously classified as implicit or procedural. Learning of skills such as those required for navigating a maze (Milner et al., 1968), problem solving (N.J. Cohen and Squire, 1980), or learning grammatical rules (Hirst, 1988) is normal in such patients, as is priming by previous experience. For example, amnesics show the normal benefit from prior exposure to words in reading or from prior exposure to words (such as "fragment") in identifying word fragments ("fr_g__nt").
4. Patients may have difficulty in remembering explicit facts or episodes that occurred before the

onset of their amnesia (retrograde amnesia). This retrograde amnesia may vary in temporal extent and in severity. The most common pattern in the purest cases of amnestic syndrome, in their chronic state, is one of no retrograde amnesia or of retrograde amnesia that extends back no more than weeks or months. However, it is possible for the retrograde amnesia to be more extensive, extending back months or years before the onset of the disease.

5. *Confabulation*—producing ridiculous stories or absurd scenarios in response to questions about memory—is not part of the pure amnestic syndrome. Rather, confabulation seems to require at least several types of problems in addition to memory deficits: deficits in self-monitoring and in inhibition of incorrect or inappropriate responses and a tendency to perseveration (Mercer et al., 1977; Shapiro et al., 1981), all of which are frequently associated with frontal lobe damage.

The most parsimonious account of the amnestic syndrome is that it represents a deficit in *consolidation*, the set of processes whereby information held in temporary, transient form is converted to more permanent storage. Nothing appears to be wrong with the amnesiac's ability to place information in temporary stores, nor is the information forgotten abnormally rapidly. A deficit in consolidation also accounts for the part of the retrograde amnesia that extends back no more than 1–2 years, because it is assumed that consolidative processes normally continue to fix memories into permanent form over this period (see Zola-Morgan and Squire, 1990). The more extensive retrograde amnesia that may occur, particularly acutely, probably represents a block in retrieval of existing memories, without damage to the memories themselves.

Only a few distinct sites of pathology have been responsible for almost all cases: the medial temporal lobes, in particular the amygdala and hippocampus; the mediodorsal nuclei of the thalamus; and their connections. It is likely that the amygdala, hippocampus, mediodorsal nuclei, and related structures are part of the circuits that determine which memories warrant saving and which do not and are therefore involved in the regulation of consolidative processes. When they are damaged, consolidation occurs much less reliably and efficiently. One important corollary of this newer view of the amnestic syndrome is that the memories themselves are not stored in the hippocampus and its associated structures. The storage sites are thought to be in the areas that are also involved in processing each type of information arriving in the brain. The hippocampus and its related systems instead regulate whether one aspect of the information that is constantly being processed in these sites, its explicit factual component, is committed to permanent storage. The hippocampal system apparently has no effects on the alterations of synaptic connectivity and strength that occur as part of the ongoing perceptual and motor experience in

these regions, which is why learning of skills and priming by prior exposure are unaffected in the amnestic syndrome.

The specific etiology of the structural damage in these critical sites does not appear to be important. Responsible etiologies have included bilateral medial temporal lobectomy (case H.M. of Milner et al., 1968), traumatic injury to the dorsomedial nuclei of the thalamus and other structures (case N.A. of Teuber et al., 1968), encephalitis with damage to the medial temporal lobes (Cermak, 1976; Cermak and O'Connor, 1983), and brief anoxia or ischemia causing damage restricted to the hippocampus, particularly its CA1 field (Press et al., 1989; Zola-Morgan et al., 1986). Nevertheless, the specific etiology of the amnestic syndrome helps determine how it presents and what other problems are associated with the core condition. For example, herpes is likely to manifest as an asymmetric encephalitis and often causes more extensive temporal and inferior frontal necrosis, which adds to the clinical picture.

In keeping with the hemispheric specialization of cerebral function, lesions of the left (dominant) hemisphere tend to affect verbal new learning and lesions of the right (nondominant) hemisphere to affect learning of nonverbal materials (e.g., visual patterns). When damage is unilateral, even the side-specific memory deficits tend to be milder than when the damage is bilateral. (Some investigators do not designate these more circumscribed problems as the amnestic syndrome, reserving that term for the more global and typically more dense impairments of bilateral disease.)

Other conditions sometimes involve elements of the pure amnestic syndrome, presumably because of pathology in the same regions. In Alzheimer's disease, for example, there is frequently disconnection of the hippocampal formation from the rest of the brain by focal degeneration (Hyman et al., 1990). The amnesia of closed head injury is sometimes circumscribed and perhaps then is due to diencephalic or medial temporal damage. The memory disorder that is a prominent part of alcoholic Korsakoff's syndrome frequently has features of a consolidative block (Shimamura et al., 1988) (although most of the apparent memory problems in many of these patients are due to impairments in initial information processing and in retrieval strategies; see later).

SYSTEMS INVOLVED IN HUMAN MEMORY

Data related to the human amnestic syndrome, other cases of pathologic memory, and normal and supranormal memory have suggested several features and processes of normal human memory (Fig. 51–1). These are discussed in the following subsections.

Units of Memory Storage. More than one and perhaps many basic units for memory processing

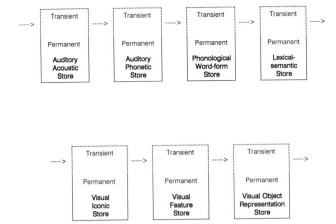

Figure 51–1. Outline of some of the processes involved in two memory systems, the verbal and the visual. Each system contains smaller subdivisions representing units of storage for different types of information. Verbal memory involves such components as the acoustic, auditory-phonetic, phonologic word form, and lexial-semantic memory stores. Visual memory involves stores such as those involved in processing and retaining iconic, visual featural, and visual object information. Each unit of information processing possesses a spectrum of capabilities for retaining information over short to long time intervals. Transient memory may be nearly identical to the actual processing of information in the stage or store. The various memory stores are interconnected through these transient processes. For clarity, the control processes that regulate the distribution of information around and from the various memory stores (informational codes) and the processes that regulate passage of information from the transient portions of the stores into more permanent form (consolidative processes) are not shown.

and storage exist in the human brain. Each basic unit of memory storage is concerned with a specific type or aspect of information, such as verbal or visual information. Where and how finely divisible these units are remain to be established. As a first approximation, it is reasonable to assume that the basic unit of information storage is part of the circuitry of the

cerebral cortex and that there are as many basic units as there are distinct cortical processing systems.

Each basic unit of information storage has the capacity to hold information temporarily or transiently. It also has the potential to store information in more permanent form (to consolidate information).

Encoding. Information coming in from the outside world must be distributed to the internal storage units before the units can learn the material. Therefore, the internal recoding and distribution of information have an important influence on what and how we learn. A subject who is given the word "red," for example, may encode only the sound internally (which is likely if the individual does not know the English language and has never heard the word before). However, it is also possible to extract from the stimulus not only the sound but also an appreciation of the meaning of red as a color, the image of redness, and perhaps associations with the word (the color of fire, the emotion of anger). All other things being equal, the more encodings, the better the memory for red is likely to be. In addition, memory will be better for encodings that are more permanent or more memorable than others. Whereas some encodings occur automatically, others are under conscious control. Either type depends on the prior experience of the individual; the varieties of conscious encodings are also a function of the individual's intelligence. These are therefore important influences on learning, independent of the process of information storage itself.

New Learning. The process of more permanent information storage (consolidation) within each memory unit appears to be regulated by a number of factors, including intent to remember and the interest or importance of the material. Some of these factors are unconscious, some are under conscious control. The mediodorsal nucleus, amygdala, and hippocampus (Fig. 51–2) play a role in weighing the

Figure 51–2. Structures in the human brain critical for regulating the storage and consolidation of new explicit knowledge. Mishkin (1990) proposed that two circuits are important in memory formation. One, indicated in light gray, includes the hippocampus (H), fornix (Fx), septal area (S), mamillary body (MB), anterior nuclei of the thalamus (Ant N of Th), and portions of the cingulate gyrus. The other, in medium gray, comprises the amygdala (A), ventral amygdalofugal pathway (VAP), stria terminalis (ST), bed nucleus of the stria terminalis (BNST), substantia innominata (SI), magnocellular portion of the mediodorsal nucleus (MDmc), and medial orbitofrontal cortex. A third region, the rhinal cortex (Rh, darkest gray) is part of both circuits. (Figure and modified caption reprinted by permission of the publisher from Vision, memory, and the temporal lobe: summary and perspective, by M. Mishkin, in E. Iwai and M. Mishkin, eds., *Vision, Memory, and the Temporal Lobe*, p. 432. Copyright 1990 by Elsevier Science Publishing Co., Inc.)

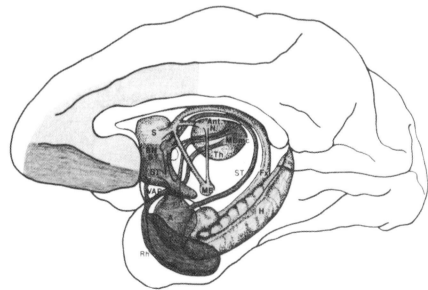

significance of information for the individual and accordingly regulating what information is consolidated in memory.

Forgetting. It may be intuitively thought that memories disappear, but this does not seem to be the case. Instead, it is more likely that the neural patterns for specific memories persist for an extremely long time but that new patterns, particularly those that are similar in some way to the existing patterns, overwrite the pre-existing patterns. This *interferes* with their storage, retention, or retrieval, so that memories do not vanish or become erased but instead become degraded or altered.

Retrieval. Retrieval of information may be straightforward, such as when the desired memory has been stored in the appropriate form and the retrieval question has the cue necessary to retrieve it (e.g., "Is your name X?"). In general, recognition of information is easier than recall, in large part because in recognition questions the basic material is given, whereas in recall questions it must be generated. Therefore, the ease of recall is strongly influenced by how easy it is to produce the item. Recognition questions that ask about a general sense of familiarity ("Have you seen me before?") are easier to answer than recognition questions that test a specific association or time tag ("Did you see me here yesterday?").

In real life, the information that is to be remembered is rarely so neatly packaged and explicitly defined as in the questions used for clinical memory testing. In real life also, what is in memory is often not exactly the information necessary to answer the question. Therefore, depending on the type of question and the way information relevant to it has been stored, retrieval of information from memory may be a very active process, strongly influenced by people's problem-solving skills and general intelligence in addition to their store of knowledge. For example, to answer the question "Who was your third grade teacher?" individuals may have to generate a series of questions for their memory, use the answers to those questions to generate more questions that might lead to the answer, or perhaps use external memory aids (e.g., find their third grade report card).

NORMAL AND PATHOLOGIC IMPAIRMENTS OF MEMORY

Individual Differences. Normal individuals differ in their ability to process various types of information; this has mostly been studied in the verbal-nonverbal dimension (e.g., Riding and Calvey, 1981; Woodhead and Baddeley, 1981). There may also be normal differences among individuals in ability to consolidate information within their memory store(s), although these have not been studied systematically. Most of the individual differences in memory capacity seem to be related to differences in the strategies used to encode information initially

and then retrieve it later. Popular mnemonic techniques are largely based on methods that force incoming information to be encoded in more ways than usual, make the encodings more distinctive (so that they suffer less interference from other memories), link them up with information that is already known (so that they can be retrieved more easily), and make them more interesting (more memorable), which may encourage consolidation.

Normal Memory. A number of characteristics of normal memory are often viewed as failings by anxious patients. Normal memory is far from perfect. People routinely forget where they have left their wallets or purses, the names and appearance of their acquaintances, and what they were supposed to get from the store (new memories). Normal people frequently fail to retrieve old information, including acquaintances' names, for example. For most people, information from several weeks ago seems harder to remember than events of many years back. Therefore, these kinds of problems are not necessarily causes for concern. Several inventories of memory abilities in everyday life, with tentative norms, have been developed (Crovitz and Daniel, 1984; Crovitz et al., 1984; B. Wilson et al., 1989).

Memory Disorders. These can be caused by impairments in any or all of the mechanisms subserving memory performance. For example, failure to attend to incoming information (because of depression or anxiety) leads to "forgetfulness," but nothing is intrinsically wrong with the underlying memory mechanisms. Similarly, in anxiety and depression, lack of the effort required to retrieve information is common. Such individuals may therefore appear to have very poor memories on tasks that require recall but perform much better (and often normally) on recognition tests, which require less effort.

Some disorders involve relatively specific effects on individual components or processes in human memory. Focal cortical lesions, although not commonly viewed as affecting memory, do destroy the basic substrate for memory storage. Because each specific type of information seems to be stored in essentially the same cortical region that is responsible for its processing, focal cortical lesions impair processing and memory together. Pure word deafness, for example, which is often due to a lesion of the left (dominant) superior temporal lobe, involves loss of stored information about the sounds of the individual's language, even though other aspects of auditory processing and verbal memory are intact. *Immediate memory* for auditory verbal material (e.g., digit span) is disrupted by lesions of the dominant posterior perisylvian region (Shallice and Warrington, 1977), presumably the region of early auditory processing. The consolidative deficit responsible for the *anterograde amnesia* in the amnestic syndrome has been noted. The strategies used for *initial encoding* of information and for its *recall* can be impaired separately from other memory functions, particularly by frontal disease.

Several different types of deficits in storage or

retrieval of previously learned material *(retrograde amnesias)* have been recognized (Fig. 51–3). Retrograde amnesia extending back weeks to at most 1–2 years (see Fig. 51–3, top) occurs in a number of the organic amnesias, such as those associated with medial temporal damage resulting from surgical resection (Marslen-Wilson and Teuber, 1975) or encephalitis (Cermak, 1976; Cermak and O'Connor, 1983) or with head trauma (Levin et al., 1985). This form of retrograde amnesia may represent a failure of complete consolidation of memory into the permanent stores (Zola-Morgan and Squire, 1990).

Retrograde amnesia that is more temporally extensive—that is, that encompasses many years or decades before the onset of illness—but still has a temporal gradient (older memories appear to be remembered better than more recent ones) (see Fig. 51–3, middle) is seen acutely with medial temporal damage and other forms of the classic human amnestic syndrome, with transient global amnesia, and with head injury. In the chronic state, it is more typical of alcoholic Korsakoff's disease and, less clearly, Alzheimer's disease. Acutely, the retrograde amnesia may extend back many decades but then shrinks in time to affect only more recent memories. The resolution or shrinkage in these cases shows that the older memories must have been present all along but were inaccessible during the acute phase of the illness.

In alcoholic Korsakoff's disease, the extensive retrograde amnesia may represent a combination of a consolidative impairment, a difficulty in learning new information that was present for a considerable time before the amnesia was formally recognized, and a retrieval deficit. The retrograde amnesia of Alzheimer's disease (Albert et al., 1981b; R.S. Wilson et al., 1981; but see Sagar et al., 1988) is probably, at least in part, an example of dissolution of the cerebral substrate for memory.

Temporally extensive retrograde amnesias, with little or no temporal gradient (the oldest memories are affected as severely as more recent ones; see Fig. 51–3, bottom), have been described in Huntington's chorea (Albert et al., 1981a) and in Alzheimer's disease (Albert et al., 1981b; R.S. Wilson et al., 1981; but see Sagar et al., 1988). Temporally extensive retrograde amnesias also occur in nonorganic contexts, in which they have somewhat different characteristics (see later).

"Recent" and "Remote" Memory in Memory Disorders. In the existing terminology there is confusion between the time course of the information in memory (was it recent or remote?) and the time course of the underlying processes responsible for memory (are they transient or permanent?). The clinical terms *recent memory* and *remote memory* are particularly ill-defined. The primary assessments that must be made for an etiologic understanding of memory disorders are how well new information can be learned and how well previously learned information can be retrieved. Depending on when the memory deficit developed in a patient and when the examiner tested

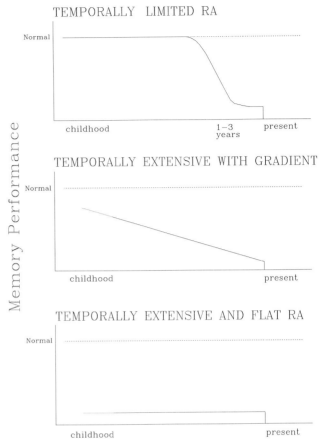

Figure 51–3. *(Top)* Retrograde amnesia (RA) extending back weeks to months. *(Middle)* Retrograde amnesia extending back many years, but with a temporal gradient. This retrograde amnesia follows the pattern described by Ribot (1881). *(Bottom)* Temporally extensive retrograde amnesia without a temporal gradient. This retrograde amnesia affects all memories learned before the "event" equally well.

the patient, material that is newly learned and material that was once known may fall into different time periods of recent or remote. In the frequent cases in which a deficit in new learning developed (or became obvious) relatively recently, the patient shows a greater deficit in recent memory (on direct testing of new learning and on testing of recently exposed material, such as new events) than in remote memory (where the problem is not with new learning, but with having full consolidation and retrieval). In this situation, the problems in trying to distinguish between recent and remote memory are not apparent. They will become evident if the consolidative deficit has been long-standing, so that even remote memories—that is, from times long before the period of examination, but which still represent a failure of new learning for the patient—are affected.

CLINICAL ASSESSMENT OF MEMORY AND ITS DISORDERS

Both the history and the examination provide information relevant to clinical assessment and diagnosis of memory disorders.

History. Although the patient's history is a necessary part of the evaluation of memory disorders, self-reported deficits are often not reliable guides to the presence of actual memory impairments, as might be expected (Larrabee and Levin, 1986; Shimamura and Squire, 1986; Sunderland et al., 1983). Self-perception of memory impairment is colored by expectations and by other deficits and biased by poor memory itself. Patients with depression or neurosis tend to overemphasize the severity of their problems (if any), patients with pure organic amnesia tend to be fairly accurate, and patients with global conditions such as Alzheimer's disease tend to minimize their memory problems. The inherent disadvantages of retrospective questioning can be somewhat reduced by having patients fill out diaries prospectively (Crovitz et al., 1984).

Other observers beside the affected patient are usually far more accurate raters of the presence and degree of memory impairment. The best clinical history may be obtained by having a daily diary of memory failures filled out by an observer such as a spouse or a therapist (Crovitz et al., 1984; B. Wilson et al., 1989).

Examination. The testing should assess attention, concentration, language, and visual perception, which are all important for proper memory performance, as well as intelligence and problem-solving ability. The basic memory functions to be tested are *registration* of information, *temporary* or *immediate* storage of information (e.g., digit span testing), *new learning* (consolidation) of information, and *retrieval* of information. Testing the retrieval of information that was once known (learned before the development of a memory deficit) is more reliable than testing the retrieval of newer information, which may not have been encoded or stored well in the first place. Retrieval of relatively recently learned information (e.g., knowledge of news events in the last several months) should be compared with retrieval of much more remotely learned information (news events of the patient's youth or information about family and personal identity).

Assessment of which of these processes involved in memory are intact and which are impaired allows an initial functional or neuroanatomic identification of the site(s) of pathology. Disturbances of registration or of immediate memory imply impaired attention or concentration or a specific processing deficit (an aphasia or visual perceptual deficit, for example). Disturbed new learning implicates the medial temporal structures or the mediodorsal nuclei of the thalamus. Retrograde amnesia that is temporally limited is consistent with a consolidative deficit and medial temporal or dorsomedial pathology. When acute, extensive retrograde amnesia can be due to medial temporal or dorsomedial pathology. When retrograde amnesia is so extensive or profound as to involve personal identity, it can signify a breakdown of the cerebral substrate for memory or a nonorganic amnesia.

The memory disorders of clinical practice are often

sufficiently severe that the standard mental status examination for memory—digit span, item recall, and recall of facts, including orientation—identifies them. The relationship between the questions on the standard mental status examination and some of the systems mediating verbal memories is outlined in Table 51–1.

However, the standard mental status examination has certain shortcomings. It is based primarily on verbal memory abilities, and it is too short and too uncontrolled for precise assessment of memory. For more sensitive, reliable, and reproducible testing, a number of memory tests are available. Objective tests widely used in clinical neuropsychologic testing include the Wechsler Memory Scale—Revised (Wechsler, 1989), with subtests for both verbal and visual memory; the Rey Auditory Verbal Learning Test (Rey, 1964), which measures recall and recognition of a list of 15 words; and the Warrington Recognition Memory Test (Warrington, 1984), which tests recognition memory for 50 words and 50 faces.

It is not easy to assess previous memories accurately. It is common clinical practice to ask patients about past events: what they had for breakfast in the morning, or where they were born and grew up. However, it is not fair to compare these types of memory, which differ in salience, strength, and likelihood of corruption by more recent information (the name of one's home town is likely to come up repeatedly in the course of a life, whereas what one was served for breakfast in the hospital may best be forgotten!). Research instruments for testing remote

Table 51–1. CORRELATES OF CLINICAL MEMORY TESTING ON STANDARD MENTAL STATUS TESTING

Task	Verbal Memory Store
Forward digit span	Immediate memory
582	
6439	
23157	
204781	
5604732	
48267039	
Immediate registration of three items "I want you to learn these three things. Repeat them after me: red, pencil, 35 Broadway"	
Three-item recall	New learning
Events of day	
Date (orientation)†	
Events of hospitalization	
Place (orientation)	
History of illness	
News items	Remote memory*
Presidents	(Retrieval of material learned before testing)
Towns/cities	(Most recent)
Family members	↓
Patient's name (orientation)	(Most remote)

*See text regarding the recent and remote memory distinction.
†In the hospital, many normal individuals lose track of the day and date.

memory use several methods to guarantee more balanced assessment. One common method tests for knowledge to which most people were only briefly exposed (Albert et al., 1981b; Sanders and Warrington, 1975; Warrington and McCarthy, 1988): events that were once prominent, but only briefly (e.g., the crash of an airplane into the Empire State Building in 1945); pictures of individuals who had only transient notoriety (Sanders and Warrington, 1975), or their voices (Meudell et al., 1980); or television programs that lasted only one or two seasons (Squire and Slater, 1978). All of these methods tap public knowledge only. Autobiographic knowledge can be ferreted out and then tested by systematic interviews and research (e.g., Treadway et al., 1991).

Additional tests that try to assess aspects of memory that are more relevant to real-life memory situations have been introduced. The most ambitious of these is the Rivermead Behavioural Memory Test (B. Wilson et al., 1985, 1989), which assesses memory for names, locations of personal items, appointments, newspaper articles, pictures and faces, routes, messages, and orientation. The test has good predictive utility for everyday memory problems and has four parallel forms for repeated administration. A test of everyday visual memory for misplaced objects has also been developed (Crook et al., 1990).

Relationship Between Symptoms and Signs. It is often difficult to relate patients' subjective complaints to test performance. There are at least two important reasons for this, in addition to the inherent problems of patients' self-reporting. First, memory testing may be too *insensitive* to the degree of deficit experienced by a patient. This is particularly true of bedside testing, which misses many problems of significance in everyday life, and this is another reason for using more standardized testing when sensitivity is an issue. Second, testing may not assess the *type* of memory that is causing difficulty for the patient. This is not usually a problem in clinical practice, because with most memory problems the effects are pervasive enough that testing will show something is wrong, even if it may not be able to pinpoint the basis for the specific complaints. However, if the patient has very circumscribed memory problems, they may not be detected by a given test.

CLINICAL SYNDROMES WITH MEMORY IMPAIRMENT

Amnesias Caused by Focal Lesions

Any disease affecting the structures critical for regulating memory storage—the amygdala, hippocampus, mediodorsal nuclei of the thalamus, and their interconnections and outflows—can cause an amnestic syndrome. The clinical presentation of the effects of lesions in these regions varies according to which modality is affected and how severely. Acutely, even with unilateral lesions, both verbal

and nonverbal memories seem to be equally affected. However, particularly with the passage of time, lesions of the left (dominant) hemisphere tend to affect verbal learning more than visual learning; the opposite is true for right (nondominant) lesions.

The degree of impairment in new learning varies widely. Some patients have mild deficits, which they may hardly notice and which may be clear only on formal testing. In severe cases, patients may be almost completely unable to learn explicitly anything new. The most severe amnesias are generally associated with bilateral lesions. Table 51–2 lists the principal anatomic sites and etiologies of amnestic syndromes, both partial and complete, caused by focal lesions.

Various degrees of pure amnesia are also observed in transient global amnesia and amnesia resulting from medial temporal lobe infarction.

Transient Global Amnesia. The prototypic presentation of transient global amnesia is the acute onset of a classic amnestic syndrome of anterograde and retrograde amnesia without alteration in consciousness or in most other neurologic functions. This amnesia persists for minutes to several hours and then disappears over the same time course. Patients who give detailed accounts of their experiences or who are examined during their episodes provide the

Table 51–2. PRINCIPAL ANATOMIC SITES AND ETIOLOGIES OF AMNESTIC SYNDROMES

Known or Presumed Anatomic Site	Etiology	Representative References
Amygdala/medial temporal lobe(s)	Surgical resection Herpes encephalitis Limbic (paraneoplastic) encephalitis Infarction (posterior cerebral artery territory) Transient ischemia (posterior cerebral artery territory)	Cermak, 1976; Cermak and O'Connor, 1983; Duyckaerts et al., 1985; Milner et al., 1968
	Anoxia/ischemia Seizure	Kritchevsky et al., 1988; Zola-Morgan et al., 1986
Mediodorsal nucleus of thalamus and adjacent regions	Infarction Tumors: craniopharyngioma, colloid cysts, pinealomas Penetrating injuries	Graff-Radford et al., 1990; Ignelzi and Squire, 1976; Markowitsch, 1988 Dusoir et al., 1990; Teuber et al., 1968
Connections between diencephalon and amygdala/ hippocampus	Fornix (variable; possibly caused by additional or synergistic lesions)	Grafman et al., 1985; Woolsey and Nelson, 1975 Kooistra and Heilman, 1988
Basal forebrain (e.g., septal nuclei)	Anterior communicating artery aneurysm and/or rupture	Damasio et al., 1985

most reliable and dramatic reports (e.g., Damasio et al., 1983; Gordon and Marin, 1979; Hodges and Ward, 1989; Kritchevsky and Squire, 1989; Kritchevsky et al., 1988). Many cases of less well documented transient impairments in new learning and retrieval have also been described (Hodges and Warlow, 1990). The etiology in most cases of the prototypic, well-described condition is likely to involve transient ischemic attacks in the vertebrobasilar system that affect the medial temporal regions bilaterally. The transient ischemia may be due to arteriosclerotic cerebrovascular disease or to migraine. Some episodes of transient global amnesia may be due to transient ischemia of the mediodorsal nuclei of the thalamus bilaterally. Seizures affecting the medial temporal lobes may arise as complications of the same ischemia that caused the amnesia or may themselves be the principal cause of the amnesia. It is not yet clear whether less severe or less pervasive cases of memory lapse have the same etiologic and pathologic significance as the more classic syndrome of transient global amnesia. The prognosis in classic transient global amnesia is generally benign (Hinge et al., 1986; Hodges and Ward, 1989; Miller et al., 1987), but some patients have persistent memory deficits (Hodges and Oxbury, 1990; Mazzucchi et al., 1980). In such patients decreased blood flow to the medial temporal lobe(s) may be shown by technetium 99m hexamethylpropyleneamine oxime (HM-PAO) single-photon emission computed tomography (SPECT) (B. Gordon et al., unpublished observations), or frank infarction in the area of the posterior cerebral artery may be revealed by computed tomography or magnetic resonance imaging.

Amnesia Resulting from Medial Temporal Lobe Infarction. Unilateral or bilateral medial temporal lobe infarction sometimes follows episodes of transient global amnesia or other warning signs of vertebrobasilar transient ischemic attack. The region involved is that supplied by the posterior cerebral artery or arteries (Benson et al., 1974; von Cramon et al., 1988). The resulting amnesia is a persistent one. It is often more marked for verbal memories if the infarction is on the left and for visual memories if the infarction is on the right. It is typically accompanied by a contralateral visual field deficit and by other concomitants of infarction in the distribution supplied by the posterior cerebral artery (Pessen et al., 1987). A model of posterior cerebral artery occlusion in the rhesus monkey has helped to confirm and extend many of the clinical observations of this condition (Bachevalier and Mishkin, 1989).

Amnesias Without Clearly Focal Etiologies, or Memory Impairments Occurring as Part of Other Conditions

Absent-Mindedness. This has several different definitions and several different causes (G. Cohen, 1989; Harris and Morris, 1984; Reason and Mycielska,

1982). Perhaps the most common manifestation is forgetfulness for both facts and intended actions. Information overload, stress, and rumination are frequent causes. Diagnosis is based on observation of the types of material that are forgotten, the situations under which forgetting (and remembering) occurs, introspection by the patient about likely causes, the observations of others, and the fluctuating course and generally good outcome.

Age-Associated Memory Impairment (Benign Senescent Forgetfulness). Age-associated memory impairment (Crook et al., 1986) describes middle-aged and older patients who report appreciable forgetfulness with otherwise intact functioning and self-insight. Formal neuropsychometric testing may show deficits in new learning, or the results may be normal. The patients who show mild deficits, either to other observers or on formal testing, are at appreciable risk (~ 35%) of developing Alzheimer's disease in a year's time (e.g., Berg et al., 1988). Many, if not most, however, have a stable or only slightly worsening memory deficit for years, without developing more florid disease. The condition that such patients have is unknown at present.

Alzheimer's Disease. Prototypically, Alzheimer's disease begins with a "memory" problem that usually includes difficulty in learning new declarative information and a variable degree of difficulty in retrieving old information, such as names (of people and things). An important feature of Alzheimer's disease is that the new learning disorder is coupled with other cognitive deficits, such as those of strategy or planning, even relatively early in the course. Therefore, the Alzheimer's patient is much more impaired by his or her memory problem than a patient with pure amnesia of an equivalent degree (Corkin, 1982). The pathology of Alzheimer's disease supports the idea of multiple deficits; there are lesions of the entorhinal cortex in a position to isolate the hippocampal formation (Hyman et al., 1990), as well as lesions of the parieto-occipital regions, the frontal lobes, and other regions (see Chapter 59).

Alcoholic Korsakoff's Disease. In its classic form, alcoholic Korsakoff's amnesia was the sequel of an acute episode of Wernicke's syndrome. This classic form is rarely seen now. More typically, a small subset of chronic alcoholics develop impairments gradually over the course of many years of drinking (and perhaps even for a period afterward).

The cognitive impairments in alcoholic Korsakoff's disease generally are not limited to memory functions. These patients have elements of a typical organic amnesia, with anterograde amnesia and a temporally extensive but gradated retrograde amnesia, as illustrated in Figure 51–4. In addition, however, they are frequently apathetic, have impairments of attention and concentration, are deficient in problem-solving and card-sorting tasks, and perform worse on free-recall testing of their memory than they do on recognition memory tests (Shimamura et al., 1988). These are the types of deficits seen in patients with frontal lobe damage, not in other cases

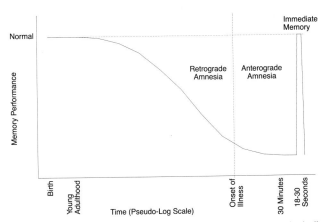

Figure 51–4. A typical organic amnestic condition (e.g., alcoholic Korsakoff's disease). Immediate memory is intact. There is an anterograde amnesia. Retrograde amnesia is extensive but with a marked temporal gradient (worse for more recently learned than for more remotely learned material). (Ribot's law [Ribot, 1881]; same pattern as illustrated in Fig. 51–3.)

of circumscribed organic amnesia. Also, confabulation, which occurs when patients have impaired self-monitoring and inability to inhibit responses (Mercer et al., 1977; Shapiro et al., 1981), is commonly associated with frontal-type deficits and is classic in alcoholic Korsakoff's disease.

Neuropathologic studies of patients with alcoholic Korsakoff's disease show two distinct areas of involvement that can explain their behavioral problems. The amnesia is reliably associated with lesions of the mediodorsal nuclei of the thalamus (Mair et al., 1979; Victor et al., 1989), a site where lesions routinely produce amnesia in animals (Aggleton and Mishkin, 1983; Zola-Morgan and Squire, 1985) and in humans (Graff-Radford et al., 1990) (see Table 51–2). Lesions also occur routinely in the mamillary bodies in these patients (Mair et al., 1979; Victor et al., 1989), but this site is probably not directly responsible for the amnesia (Zola-Morgan et al., 1989). The diencephalic damage can be appreciated on computed tomographic scans (Shimamura et al., 1988), and lesions of the mamillary bodies have been visualized with magnetic resonance imaging scans (M.E. Charness and DeLaPaz, 1987). These lesions appear to be caused by deficiency of riboflavin, vitamin B_2.

Frontal lobe–type deficits are correlated with frontal lobe atrophy, as seen on computed tomographic scans (Shimamura et al., 1988). This cortical damage may be caused by toxic effects of alcohol (Butters, 1985; Lishman et al., 1987).

The frontal-type dementia associated with alcoholic Korsakoff's disease helps explain why this condition has been such a misleading example of amnesia for so many generations of medical students and physicians. There is an amnestic component of Korsakoff's disease, but it is combined with a frontal lobe type of dementia that aggravates and alters the expression of the underlying memory deficits.

Closed Head Injury. Mild to moderately severe closed head injuries may result in classic examples of amnesia (Levin et al., 1982, 1989). Acutely, on regaining full alertness, these patients typically have an anterograde amnesia, an amnesia for the period of their unconsciousness (not surprisingly, but surprisingly often counted as part of their "anterograde amnesia"), and a variable degree of retrograde amnesia, which may be quite extensive (Fig. 51–5, top). The degree of anterograde amnesia (often called post-traumatic amnesia and clinically measured by the failure to remember events from day to day) has been used as a rough prognostic guide (Russell and Smith, 1961).

Most patients with mild head injury recover from the amnesia and other deficits (Levin et al., 1987). With recovery, an interval of total anterograde amnesia for the period of unconsciousness and the immediately subsequent period often remains, as well as a short period of dense retrograde amnesia (see Fig. 51–5, bottom). Presumably, the initial anterograde amnesia and the permanent hiatus in

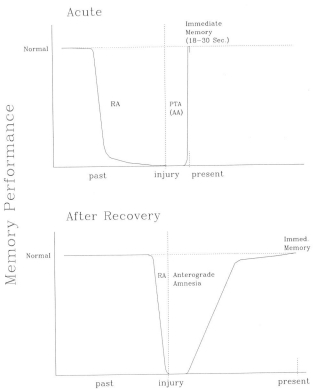

Figure 51–5. Examples of patterns of anterograde amnesia (AA) and retrograde amnesia (RA) frequently seen after mild to moderately severe closed head injuries. *(Top)* Acute pattern, with intact to mildly impaired immediate memory (attention and concentration, digit span), anterograde amnesia from time of injury (including period of unconsciousness), and marked retrograde amnesia with temporal gradient. *(Bottom)* Late pattern, after recovery, with intact immediate memory, amnesia for period of unconsciousness but no ongoing anterograde amnesia, and almost complete resolution of retrograde amnesia, with residual amnesia for periods of few seconds or minutes before the injury.

memory that results are due to failure to create long-term memories. The retrograde amnesia is resolved into two components by recovery. Its temporally extensive component is due to a temporary impairment in ability to retrieve old memories from more permanent storage. The component involving knowledge of the period just before the injury may never recover. This period of retrograde amnesia appears to result from interruption of processes of consolidation into longer-term memories.

Contusion of the medial temporal lobes and the orbitofrontal regions and perhaps twisting of the posterior diencephalon–upper midbrain are thought to be responsible for the amnesias of closed head injury (Adams et al., 1985; Povlishock et al., 1983). In most cases of mild head injury, these injuries cannot be detected by current magnetic resonance imaging or x-ray computed tomography scanning techniques. Whether regional metabolic impairments will be more reliably detected by SPECT or positron emission tomography has yet to be determined (see Humayan et al., 1989). Examinations shortly after the injury are more likely to reveal injuries than later ones.

Memory Impairments Associated with Depression. Depression is frequently accompanied by complaints of poor concentration and poor memory. Formal testing may yield normal results (Coughlan and Hollows, 1984), show only attention and concentration problems (Watts and Sharrock, 1985) with attendant impairment of registration (Sternberg and Jarvick, 1976), or show impaired new learning and remote recall as well. Typically, the patient complains of much worse impairment than is shown by formal testing (Squire and Zouzounis, 1988). Clues that the memory deficits are related to depression and not to organic illness (such as Alzheimer's disease) include a history of fluctuations over time, with periods of normal or near-normal memory; examination showing impaired attention and concentration; performance on memory tasks that require effort (such as recall) being disproportionately worse than performance on tasks that do not (such as recognition); and evidence of poor and variable effort on testing (Tancer et al., 1990). Patients with memory impairment associated with depression should have a good prognosis if the underlying depression can be treated, but there is some evidence that a significant proportion of patients with a severe, pseudodementia syndrome associated with depression develop Alzheimer's disease (Kral and Emery, 1989).

NONORGANIC AMNESIAS

Varieties of Nonorganic Amnesias

Various forms of memory loss that can occur without structural or biochemical pathology detectable by current techniques must be considered in the differential diagnosis of any memory loss. Such nonor-

ganic amnesias frequently have characteristic features that distinguish them from the organic amnesias.

Extensive Retrograde Amnesia. A dense, temporally extensive retrograde amnesia (Figs. 51–3 and 51–6) is a frequent presentation of a nonorganic amnesia. This amnesia typically affects even the oldest, most secure memories about the patient's personal identity, such as his or her name, birthplace, and other important items of the past history. In this respect, it differs from that seen in organic disease, where it is rarely so extensive unless combined with other deficits (as in dementia). Usually these patients cannot recall any event that triggered their amnesia. Nonetheless, they are alert, conscious, typically quite capable of taking in and using new information, and do not have anterograde amnesia. This extensive retrograde amnesia can result from either unconscious psychologic factors or conscious malingering.

Unconscious Retrograde Amnesia. A mild form of retrograde amnesia frequently occurs after emotional shocks. There is often relatively poor memory for the immediately preceding events (Loftus and Burns, 1982). Emotional shocks are also perhaps the most frequent precipitants of more marked forms of unconscious retrograde amnesia. These dramatic presentations are often reported in the newspaper: a young woman is found wandering about, not knowing who she is or how she got there; relatives then identify her from photographs; it turns out that a traumatic event had occurred; observers of the event may have noticed that the patient seemed to be in a detached state (a fugue state), from which she later emerged without memory. Usually, in these cases memory returns after a few hours or days, often when prompted, and frequently as a sudden rush of knowledge and awareness. The rare research studies of such individuals (Schacter et al., 1982; Treadway et al., 1991) have not yet provided a clear picture of the processes that are affected or of how this disorder fits into current theories of memory.

More rarely, unconcious retrograde amnesia occurs as part of the syndrome of multiple personality,

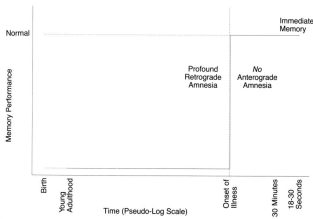

Figure 51–6. The pattern of extensive retrograde amnesia, without anterograde amnesia, frequently seen with nonorganic memory losses.

wherein the personas appear not to have access to each other's memories (Ludwig et al., 1972).

Feigned, Conscious, or Malingered Retrograde Amnesias. The inciting event is typically later found to be a crime or a financial problem. As in unconscious amnesia, the patients' knowledge of their identity and much or all of their prior life is apparently disrupted, without anterograde amnesia. In contrast to the unconscious retrograde amnesias, feigned amnesias are frequently maintained for weeks or months.

Anterograde Amnesias. Nonorganic amnesias also sometimes present as anterograde amnesias. Depression or lack of effort can lead to poor new learning and recall, as can simple malingering.

Amnesia in the Popular Imagination. Notably, the amnesia portrayed on television or in the movies usually resembles a nonorganic retrograde amnesia, although with some twists. For dramatic reasons, the inciting event is usually a blow to the head, which is often followed by a period of unconsciousness (presumably to convince the viewer of its severity), although the patient may sometimes merely be stunned. On awakening or recovering full consciousness, the individual has a marked retrograde amnesia for personal identity and prior life experiences, without any anterograde amnesia. This is, of course, quite different from the usual situation in closed head injury. Another characteristic feature of these cases is that the problem is cured by another blow to the head, or by the right clue. Again, this is unlike the situation in real closed head injury or other organic amnesias.

Differential Diagnosis

Retrograde amnesias are usually easier to diagnose than anterograde amnesias. Feigned deficits are usually easy to differentiate from organic and other nonorganic ones because the scope and depth of the "impairments" are more clearly nonphysiologic.

Clues to *malingered anterograde* amnesia (new learning impairment) include the following (see Brandt, 1988): internal inconsistencies in performance (frequently, recognition memory performance is worse than recall, the opposite of the expected pattern [Brandt et al., 1985]); consistent below-chance performance (Brandt et al., 1985); and much worse performance on formal testing than the patient's performance in everyday life would indicate (e.g., the patient gives no evidence of new learning on formal testing, yet has a normal ability to remember the testers, directions to the hospital or bathroom, and so forth).

A frequent clue to *feigned retrograde* amnesia is that it purportedly affects knowledge that is almost never altered in that fashion by organic disease. For example, a patient may claim loss of the ability to read or to understand the meaning of what has been read. Although some organic alexias do have these char-

acteristics (Friedman, 1988), patients with feigned amnesia do not have any other typical features. More blatantly, some patients will claim loss of knowledge of how to eat, use utensils, or drive. When such forms of knowledge are affected by organic disease, there are almost always more widespread problems (such as anterograde amnesia and/or dementia).

These features and the evolution of the disorder over time serve to differentiate most cases of nonorganic from organic memory loss. However, some complexities must be noted (Bernard, 1990; Brandt, 1988; Schacter, 1986; Wiggins and Brandt, 1988). Memory testing relies on reasonable effort; poor effort can give the appearance of a mild to moderately severe memory loss without any particular characteristics that clearly indicate its cause (Bernard, 1990). This is particularly vexing, because patients with true memory loss may exaggerate their deficits in an effort to be convincing.

More problematically, there are rare cases of organic memory problems in which many characteristics appear nonorganic by classic criteria. For example, relatively isolated, temporally extensive retrograde amnesias with little or no accompanying anterograde amnesia have been associated with structural disease (Andrews et al., 1982; Goldberg et al., 1981; Stuss and Guzman, 1988). As another example, patients with some of the apraxias may present with apparently bizarre loss of motor skills (e.g., inability to initiate gait). In addition, certain aspects of memory loss are not well measured, if they are measured at all, by current testing. For instance, forgetting an intended action (such as calling someone) is one of the most common examples of forgetting in everyday life, yet only one memory test (the Rivermead Behavioural Memory Test [B. Wilson et al., 1989]) tries to measure it directly. Therefore, one must be cautious in ascribing a nonorganic cause to a patient's complaints.

THE NEURONAL BASIS FOR HUMAN MEMORY AND ITS DISORDERS

How the memories of our conscious experience—the memory of what these words mean, for example—are represented at the neuronal level is becoming clearer, although the current understanding is far from definitive. It seems incontrovertible that such concepts are evoked as distinct patterns of neuronal and subneuronal activity, distributed over many neurons and neuronal processing elements and over time (tens to hundreds of milliseconds). In general, these representations are embodied in the orchestrated firing of many cells, rather than the activity of only one cell. It is important, therefore, to distinguish between the nature of the information that is stored at a single neuron (or single synaptic site) and the nature of the information stored in the *system* of neurons and their interconnections. What emerges from the system (or systems) of neurons is what we recognize as the memories of conscious experience, but these conscious memories are rooted in more elemental operations and storage processes.

Particular macroscopic patterns of activity arise because of the patterns of connectivity in cortical-cortical and cortical-subcortical neuronal networks. The term *patterns of connectivity* refers to both inter-neuronal connections and the strengths of those connections. One way in which memories can be formed is by making or breaking connections. This may be a particularly important mechanism in younger animals and in adults of some species. Most examples of flexible memory storage in the adult probably represent alterations in the strengths of existing synaptic connections. It is tempting to speculate that a form of neuronal immediate memory involves the transient activation of a neural circuit, whereas longer-term memory storage depends on altering the connectivity of the circuit so that it is more likely to fire the same way again. One particularly well-studied model system for long-term changes in neuronal connectivity is long-term potentiation, such as that seen in the hippocampal formation. A number of mechanisms through which synaptic strengths might be changed are known already, and new ones are constantly being discovered. For reviews, see Alkon and Rasmussen, 1988; Bear et al., 1987; Brown et al., 1988; Cotman and Lynch, 1989.

Most, if not all, of these possible synaptic mechanisms for memory are likely to be influenced by more or less specific neurotransmitter systems (see Bear and Singer, 1986). The cholinergic systems are known to be extremely important in human memory. Anticholinergic treatment can produce deficits in new learning for explicit material (Nissen et al., 1987). A cholinergic deficit associated with degeneration in the nucleus basalis of Meynert is one of the most frequent findings in Alzheimer's disease, although its etiologic significance is not clear (see Chapter 59). Neuropharmacologic manipulation of the mechanisms involved in memory storage and retrieval in humans is therefore just becoming a possibility.

METHODS FOR IMPROVING MEMORY PERFORMANCE

Normal Individuals

Mnemonic Strategies. Normal individuals can improve their memory performance through a number of strategies and techniques that have been known for at least 2000 years (Hirst, 1988; Morris, 1977). Having real interest in and *concentration* on the material to be learned probably helps to stimulate its transfer into longer-term forms and also to activate a wider net of connections to existing knowledge, which helps fix the new material in place. *Several learning sessions* spaced out result in better learning for the same amount of time spent than a single longer session (Dempster, 1988). *Organization* of the material into more meaningful or more connected patterns is a conscious strategy that clearly improves memory. *Distributed coding* of material—encoding it in more than one form, such as creating images to go with words—is another effective strategy. Most commonly, this takes the form of creating visual images to accompany or organize the material to be learned. Such distributed coding probably improves memory in several ways: through redundant encoding (information stored in two formats is more likely to be remembered than that stored in only one, all other things being equal); by taking advantage of the rapid learning and vast capacity of the visual system to supplement the abilities of the verbal system; and by giving additional organization to the material. Finally, more appropriate *retrieval cues* can be developed and learned. An ancient method for this is the *method of loci*. Material to be remembered is mentally "placed" in "locations" familiar to the individual, such as the rooms of a house. For retrieval, the rooms are entered in sequence and the material there is read out.

Diligent application of these mnemonic techniques can clearly improve memory performance, as professional mnemonists attest (Lorayne and Lucas, 1974). However, most individuals find that the effort to learn these methods is too great and the types of material that can be memorized best with these techniques differ from those that are most important for everyday life (Hirst, 1988). Also, most people prefer their memorization to be automatic, accomplished in the course of everyday events. Conscious memorization requires considerable effort and diminishes enjoyment of the experience itself.

External Memory Aids. Memory aids such as wrist alarms and notebooks have proved successful for many people and are much easier to apply than mnemonic strategies.

Drugs. There are no specific memory-enhancing agents or pharmacologic treatments. Nevertheless, stimulants such as caffeine, nicotine, ethyl alcohol, methylphenidate, and amphetamine are known to improve memory performance. Whether this is due to a specific improvement in memory storage ability or to less specific effects on concentration or mnemonic strategies is not known.

Amnesic Patients

Retraining and Mnemonic Techniques. Mnemonic retraining of memory-impaired patients has generally been disappointing (Cermak and O'Connor, 1988; Godfrey and Knight, 1987), for several instructive reasons. First, most clinical memory disorders are not pure but occur in the context of other cognitive deficits. The patients have impairments in attention, concentration, planning, sequencing, self-monitoring, and error recognition, so that the cognitive foundations necessary for use of mnemonic techniques are absent in these patients (Cermak and O'Connor, 1988). Second, the types of material that can best be learned with mnemonic techniques are, as noted, often irrelevant to the memory demands of everyday life. Third, the complex of skills required to learn any given task are often extremely specific and are difficult to generalize to other tasks. Last, for reasons that are far from clear, patients with memory impairments also find it hard to *learn how to learn*, that is, to remember that they have to apply mnemonic strategies (Schacter et al., 1985).

Successful retraining efforts have therefore generally focused on specific tasks that are important to the particular individual (e.g., being able to keep appointments) and have relied on several approaches to find those best suited for that individual and his or her environment (Cermak and O'Connor, 1988; N. Charness et al., 1988; Glisky and Schacter, 1987; B. Wilson, 1984; B.A. Wilson, 1987; B. Wilson and Moffat, 1984).

External Memory Aids. Memory aids such as an alarm that reminds the patient to consult an appointment book have been useful in some cases (Gouvier, 1982).

Drugs. Although there have been a few reports of drug therapy, usually cholinomimetic, improving some patients (e.g., Peters and Levin, 1977), no consistently useful results have been reported with the agents currently available. Newer cholinergic agonists that target more specific receptor subclasses, agents that act on other neurotransmitter systems, or drugs that seem to have more diffuse metabolic enhancement effects may prove to be more successful (Pepeu and Spognoli, 1989; Schindler, 1989).

Acknowledgments

I thank Drs. Guy McKhann, Pamela Talalay, and Arthur Asbury for their insightful and constructive comments on the manuscript.

References

(Key references are designated with an asterisk.)

Adams J.H., Graham D.I., Gennarelli T.A. Contemporary neuropathological considerations regarding brain damage in head injury. In Becker D.P., Povlishock J.T., eds. *Central Nervous System Trauma Status Report*. Washington, DC, National Institutes of Neurological and Communicative Disorders and Stroke, pp. 65–77, 1985.

Aggleton J.P., Mishkin M. Memory impairments following restricted medial thalamic lesions in monkeys. *Exp. Brain Res.* 52:199–209, 1983.

Albert M.S., Butters N., Brandt J. Development of remote memory loss in patients with Huntington's disease. *J. Clin. Neuropsychol.* 3:1–12, 1981a.

Albert M.S., Butters N., Brandt J. Patterns of remote memory in amnesic and demented patients. *Arch. Neurol.* 38:495–500, 1981b.

Alkon D.L., Rasmussen H. A spatial-temporal model of cell activation. *Science* 239:998–1005, 1988.

Andrews E., Poser C.M., Kessler M. Retrograde amnesia for forty years. *Cortex* 18:441–458, 1982.

Bachevalier J., Mishkin M. Mnemonic and neuropathological ef-

fects of occluding the posterior cerebral artery in *Macaca mulatta*. *Neuropsychologia* 27:83–106, 1989.

*Baddeley A. *Human Memory*. Hillsdale, NJ, Erlbaum, 1990.

Bear M.F., Singer W. Modulation of visual cortical plasticity by acetylcholine and noradrenaline. *Nature* 320:172–176, 1986.

Bear M.F., Cooper L.N., Ebner F.F. A physiological basis for a theory of synapse modification. *Science* 237:42–48, 1987.

Benson D.F., Marsden C.D., Meadows J.C. The amnestic syndrome of posterior cerebral artery occlusion. *Acta Neurol. Scand.* 50:133–145, 1974.

Berg L., Hughes C.P., Coben L.A., et al. Mild senile dementia of the Alzheimer type: 2. Longitudinal assessment. *Ann. Neurol.* 23:477–484, 1988.

Bernard L.C. Prospects for faking believable memory deficits on neuropsychological tests and the use of incentives in simulation research. *J. Clin. Exp. Neuropsychol.* 12:715–728, 1990.

Brandt J. Malingered amnesia. In Rogers R., ed. *Clinical Assessment of Malingering and Deception*. New York, Guilford Press, pp. 65–83, 1988.

Brandt J., Rubnisky E.W., Lassen G. Uncovering malingered amnesia. *Ann. N. Y. Acad. Sci.* 44:502–503, 1985.

Brown T.H., Chapman P.F., Kairiss E.W., et al. Long-term synaptic potentiation. *Science* 242:724–728, 1988.

Butters N. Alcoholic Korsakoff's syndrome: some unresolved issues concerning etiology, neuropathology, and cognitive deficits. *J. Clin. Exp. Neuropsychol.* 7:181–210, 1985.

Cermak L.S. The encoding capacity of a patient with amnesia due to encephalitis. *Neuropsychologia* 14:311–326, 1976.

Cermak L.S., O'Connor M. The anterograde and retrograde retrieval ability of a patient with amnesia due to encephalitis. *Neuropsychologia* 21:213–234, 1983.

Cermak L.S., O'Connor M. Mnemonic retraining of organic memory disorders. In Denes G., Semenza C., Bisiacchi P., eds. *Perspectives on Cognitive Neuropsychology*. Hillsdale, NJ, Erlbaum, pp. 313–324, 1988.

Charness M.E., DeLaPaz R.L. Mamillary body atrophy in Wernicke's encephalopathy: antemorten identification using magnetic resonance imaging. *Ann. Neurol.* 22:595–600, 1987.

Charness N., Milberg W., Alexander M.P. Teaching an amnesic a complex cognitive skill. *Brain Cogn.* 8:253–272, 1988.

Cohen G. *Memory in the Real World*. Hillsdale, NJ, Erlbaum, 1989.

Cohen N.J., Squire L.R. Preserved learning and retention of pattern-analyzing skill in amnesia: dissociation of knowing how and knowing that. *Science* 210:207–209, 1980.

Corkin S. Some relationships between global amnesias and the memory impairments in Alzheimer's disease. In Corkin S., Davis K.L., Growdon J.H., et al., eds. *Alzheimer's Disease: A Report of Progress in Research*. New York, Raven Press, pp. 149–164, 1982.

Cotman C.W., Lynch G.S. The neurobiology of learning and memory. *Cognition* 33:201–241, 1989.

Coughlan A.K., Hollows S.E. Use of memory tests in differentiating organic disorder from depression. *Br. J. Psychiatry* 145:164–167, 1984.

Crook T., Bartus S., Ferris S.H., et al. Age-associated memory impairment: proposed diagnostic criteria and measures of clinical change. *Dev. Neuropsychol.* 2:261–276, 1986.

Crook T.H. III, Youngjohn J.R., Larrabee G.J. The misplaced objects test: a measure of everyday visual memory. *J. Clin. Exp. Neuropsychol.* 12:819–833, 1990.

Crovitz H.F., Daniel W.F. Measurements of everyday memory: toward the prevention of forgetting. *Bull. Psychon. Soc.* 22:413–414, 1984.

Crovitz H.F., Cordoni C.N., Daniel W.F., et al. Everyday forgetting experiences: real-time investigations with implications for the study of memory management in brain-damaged patients. *Cortex* 20:349–359, 1984.

Damasio A.R., Graff-Radford N.R., Damasio H. Transient partial amnesia. *Arch. Neurol.* 40:656–657, 1983.

Damasio A.R., Eslinger P.J., Damasio H., et al. Multimodal amnesic syndrome following bilateral temporal and basal forebrain damage. *Arch. Neurol.* 42:252–259, 1985.

Dempster F.N. The spacing effect. *Am. Psychol.* 43:627–634, 1988.

*Dudai Y. *The Neurobiologic Systems of Memory*. Cambridge, Oxford University Press, 1989.

Dusoir H., Kapur N., Byrnes D.P., et al. The role of diencephalic pathology in human memory disorder: evidence from a penetrating paranasal brain injury. *Brain* 113:1695–1706, 1990.

Duyckaerts C., Durouesne C., Signoret J.L., et al. Bilateral and limited amygdalohippocampal lesions causing a pure amnesic syndrome. *Ann. Neurol.* 18:314–319, 1985.

Friedman R.B. Acquired alexia. In Boller F., Grafman J., eds. *Handbook of Neuropsychology*. Amsterdam, Elsevier, pp. 377–391, 1988.

Glisky E.L., Schacter D.L. Acquisition of domain-specific knowledge in organic amnesia: training for computer-related work. *Neuropsychologia* 25:893–906, 1987.

Godfrey H.P.D., Knight R.G. Interventions for amnesics: a review. *Br. J. Clin. Psychol.* 26:83–91, 1987.

Goldberg E., Antin S.P., Bilder R.M., et al. Retrograde amnesia: possible role of mesencephalic reticular activation in long-term memory. *Science* 213:1392–1394, 1981.

Gordon B., Marin O.S.M. Transient global amnesia: an extensive case report. *J. Neurol. Neurosurg. Psychiatry* 42:572–575, 1979.

Gouvier W. Using the digital alarm chronograph in memory retraining. *Behav. Eng.* 7:4–134, 1982.

Graff-Radford N.R., Damasio A.R., Hyman B.T., et al. Progressive aphasia in a patient with Pick's disease: a neuropsychological, radiologic, and anatomic study. *Neurology* 40:620–626, 1990.

Grafman J., Salazar A.M., Weingartner H., et al. Isolated impairment of memory following a penetrating lesion of the fornix cerebri. *Arch. Neurol.* 42:1162–1168, 1985.

Harris J.E., Morris P.E., eds. *Everyday Memory, Action and Absent-Mindedness*. Orlando, FL, Academic Press, 1984.

Hinge H.H., Jensen T.S., Kjaer M., et al. The prognosis of transient global amnesia: results of a multicenter study. *Arch. Neurol.* 43:673–676, 1986.

Hirst W. Improving memory. In Gazzaniga M.S., ed. *Perspectives in Memory Research*. Cambridge, MA, M.I.T. Press, pp. 219–244, 1988.

Hodges J.R., Oxbury S.M. Persistent memory impairment following transient global amnesia. *J. Clin. Exp. Neuropsychol.* 12:904–920, 1990.

Hodges J.R., Ward C.D. Observations during transient global amnesia: a behavioral and neuropsychological study of five cases. *Brain* 112:595–620, 1989.

Hodges J.R., Warlow C.P. The aetiology of transient global amnesia: a case-control study of 114 cases with prospective follow-up. *Brain* 113:639–657, 1990.

Humayan M.S., Presty S.K., LaFrance N.D., et al. Local cerebral glucose abnormalities in mild closed head injured patients with cognitive impairments. *Nucl. Med. Commun.* 10:335–344, 1989.

Hyman B.T., Van Hoesen G.W., Damasio A.R. Memory-related neural systems in Alzheimer's disease: an anatomic study. *Neurology* 40:1721–1730, 1990.

Ignelzi R.J., Squire L.R. Recovery from anterograde and retrograde amnesia after percutaneous drainage of a cystic craniopharyngioma. *J. Neurol. Neurosurg. Psychiatry* 39:1231–1235, 1976.

Kooistra C.A., Heilman K.M. Memory loss from a subcortical white matter infarct. *J. Neurol. Neurosurg. Psychiatry* 51:866–869, 1988.

Kral V.A., Emery O.B. Long-term follow-up of depressive pseudodementia of the aged. *Can. J. Psychol.* 34:445–446, 1989.

Kritchevsky M., Squire L.R. Transient global amnesia: evidence for extensive, temporally graded retrograde amnesia. *Neurology* 39:213–218, 1989.

Kritchevsky M., Squire L.R., Zouzounis J.A. Transient global amnesia: characterization of anterograde and retrograde amnesia. *Neurology* 38:213–219, 1988.

Larrabee G.J., Levin H.S. Memory self-ratings and objective test performance in a normal elderly sample. *J. Clin. Exp. Neuropsychol.* 8:275–284, 1986.

Levin H.S., Benton A.L., Grossman R.G. *Neurobehavioral Consequences of Head Injury*. New York, Oxford University Press, 1982.

Levin H.S., High W.M., Meyers C.A., et al. Impairment of remote memory after closed head injury. *J. Neurol. Neurosurg. Psychiatry* 48:556–563, 1985.

Levin H.S., Mattis S., Ruff R.M., et al. Neurobehavioral outcome following minor head injury: a three center study. *J. Neurosurg.* 66:234–243, 1987.

Levin H.S., Eisenberg M.M., Benton A.L., eds. *Mild Head Injury*. New York, Oxford University Press, 1989.

Lishman W.A., Jacobson R.R., Acker C. Brain damage in alcoholism: current concepts. *Acta Med. Scand.* 717:5–17, 1987.

Loftus E.F., Burns T.E. Mental shock can produce retrograde amnesia. *Memory Cogn.* 10:318–323, 1982.

Lorayne H., Lucas J. *The Memory Book*. New York, Stein & Day, 1974.

Ludwig A.M., Brandsma J.M., Wilbur C.B., et al. The objective study of a multiple personality: or, are four heads better than one? *Arch. Gen. Psychiatry* 26:298–310, 1972.

Mair W.G.P., Warrington E.K., Weiskrantz L. Memory disorder in Korsakoff's psychosis. *Brain* 102:749–783, 1979.

Markowitsch H.J. Diencephalic amnesia: a reorientation towards tracts. *Brain Res. Rev.* 13:351–370, 1988.

Marslen-Wilson W.D., Teuber H.L. Memory for remote events in anterograde amnesia: recognition of public figures from newsphotographs. *Neuropsychologia* 13:353–364, 1975.

Mazzucchi A., Moretti G., Caffarra P., et al. Neuropsychological functions in the follow-up of transient global amnesia. *Brain* 103:161–178, 1980.

Mercer B., Wapner W., Gardner H., et al. A study of confabulation. *Arch. Neurol.* 34:429–433, 1977.

Meudell P.R., Northen B., Snowden J.S., et al. Long term memory for famous voices in amnesic and normal subjects. *Neuropsychologia* 18:133–139, 1980.

Miller J.W., Peterson R.C., Metter E.J., et al. Transient global amnesia: clinical characteristics and prognosis. *Neurology* 37:733–737, 1987.

Milner B., Corkin S., Teuber H.L. A further analysis of the hippocampal amnesic syndrome: 14 year follow-up study of H.M. *Neuropsychology* 6:215–244, 1968.

Mishkin M. Vision, memory, and the temporal lobe: summary and perspective. In Iwai E., Mishkin M., eds. *Vision, Memory and the Temporal Lobe*. New York, Elsevier, pp. 427–436, 1990.

Morris P. Practical strategies for human learning and remembering. In Howe M.J.A., ed. *Adult Learning: Psychological Research and Applications*. New York, Wiley, 1977.

Nissen M.J., Knopman D.S., Schacter D.L. Neurochemical dissociation of memory systems. *Neurology* 37:789–794, 1987.

Pepeu G., Spignoli G. Nootropic drugs and brain cholinergic mechanisms. *Prog. Neuropsychopharm. Biol. Psychiatry* 13(Suppl.):S77–S88, 1989.

Pessen M.S., Lathi E.S., Cohen M.B., et al. Clinical features and mechanism of occipital infarction. *Ann. Neurol.* 21:290–299, 1987.

Peters B.H., Levin H.S. Memory enhancement after physostigmine in the amnesic syndrome. *Arch. Neurol.* 34:215–219, 1977.

Povlishock J.T., Becker D.P., Cheng C.L.Y., et al. Axonal change in minor head injury. *J. Neuropathol. Exp. Neurol.* 42:225–242, 1983.

Press G.A., Amaral D.G., Squire L.R. Hippocampal abnormalities in amnesic patients revealed by high-resolution magnetic resonance imaging. *Nature* 341:54–57, 1989.

Reason J., Mycielska K. *Absent-Minded? The Psychology of Mental Lapses and Everyday Errors*. Englewood Cliffs, NJ, Prentice-Hall, 1982.

Rey A. *L'Examen Clinique en Psychologie*. Paris, Presses Universitaires de France, 1964.

Ribot T. *Les Maladies de la Mémoire*. Paris, Germer Baillere, 1881. [English translation: *Diseases of Memory*. New York, Appleton-Century-Crofts, 1982.]

Riding R.J., Calvey I. The assessment of verbal-imagery learning styles and their effect on the recall of concrete and abstract prose passages by 11-year-old children. *Br. J. Psychol.* 72:59–64, 1981.

Russell W.R., Smith A. Post-traumatic amnesia in closed head injury. *Arch. Neurol.* 5:16–29, 1961.

Sagar H.J., Cohen N.J., Sullivan E.V., et al. Remote memory function in Alzheimer's disease and Parkinson's disease. *Brain* 111:185–206, 1988.

Sanders H.I., Warrington E.K. Retrograde amnesia in organic amnesic patients. *Cortex* 11:397–400, 1975.

Schacter D.L. Amnesia and crime: how much do we really know? *Am. Psychol.* 41:286–295, 1986.

Schacter D.L., Wang P.L., Tulving E., et al. Functional retrograde amnesia: a quantitative case study. *Neuropsychologia* 20:523–532, 1982.

Schacter D.L., Rich S.A., Stampp M.S. Remediation of memory disorders: experimental evaluation of the spaced-retrieval technique. *J. Clin. Exp. Neuropsychol.* 7:79–96, 1985.

Schindler U. Pre-clinical evaluation of cognition-enhancing drugs. *Prog. Neuropsychopharmacol. Biol. Psychiatry* 13(Suppl.):S99–S115, 1989.

Shallice T., Warrington E.K. Auditory-verbal short-term memory impairment and conduction aphasia. *Brain Lang.* 4:479–491, 1977.

Shapiro B.E., Alexander M.P., Gardner H. Mechanisms of confabulation. *Neurology* 31:1070–1076, 1981.

Shimamura A.P., Squire L.R. Memory and metamemory: a study of the feeling-of-knowing phenomenon in amnesia patients. *J. Exp. Psychol. [Learn. Mem. Cogn.]* 12:452–460, 1986.

Shimamura A.P., Jernigan T.L., Squire L.R. Korsakoff's syndrome: radiological (CT) findings and neuropsychological correlates. *J. Neurosci.* 8:4400–4410, 1988.

Squire L.R. Mechanisms of memory. *Science* 232:1612–1619, 1986.

*Squire L.R. *Memory and Brain*. New York, Oxford University Press, 1987.

Squire L.R., Slater P.C. Anterograde and retrograde memory impairment in chronic amnesia. *Neuropsychologia* 16:313–322, 1978.

Squire L.R., Zouzounis J.A. Self-ratings of memory dysfunction: different findings in depression and amnesia. *J. Clin. Exp. Neuropsychol.* 10:727–738, 1988.

Sternberg D.E., Jarvik M.E. Memory functions in depression: improvement with antidepressant medication. *Arch. Gen. Psychiatry* 33:219–224, 1976.

Stuss D.T., Guzman D.A. Severe remote memory loss with minimal anterograde amnesia: a clinical note. *Brain Cogn.* 8:21–30, 1988.

Sunderland A., Harris J.E., Baddeley A.D. Do laboratory tests predict everyday memory? A neuropsychological study. *J. Verb. Learn. Verb. Behav.* 22:341–357, 1983.

Tancer M.E., Brown T.M., Evans D.L., et al. Impaired effortful cognition in depression. *Psychiatry Res.* 31:161–168, 1990.

Teuber H.L., Milner B., Vaughan H.G. Jr. Persistent anterograde amnesia after stab wound of the basal brain. *Neuropsychologia* 6:267–282, 1968.

Treadway M., Cohen N.J., McCloskey M., et al. Landmark life events and the organization of memory: evidence from functional retrograde amnesia. In Christianson S.-A., ed. *Handbook of Emotion and Memory*. Hillsdale, NJ, Erlbaum, in press.

Victor M., Adams R.D., Collins G.H. *The Wernicke-Korsakoff Syndrome*. 2nd ed. Philadelphia, Davis, 1989.

von Cramon D.Y., Hebel N., Schuri U. Verbal memory and learning in unilateral posterior cerebral infarction: a report on 30 cases. *Brain* 111:1061–1077, 1988.

Warrington E.K. *Recognition Memory Test*. London, Nfer-Nelson, 1984.

Warrington E.K., McCarthy R.A. The fractionation of retrograde amnesia. *Brain Cog.* 7:184–200, 1988.

Watts F.N., Sharrock R. Description and measurement of concentration problems in depressed patients. *Psychol. Med.* 15:317–326, 1985.

Wechsler D. *WAIS-R Manual*. New York, Psychological Medicine, 1989.

Wiggins E.C., Brandt J. The detection of simulated amnesia. *Law Hum. Behav.* 12:57–78, 1988.

Wilson B. Memory therapy in practice. In Wilson B.A., Moffat N., eds. *Clinical Management of Memory Problems*. Rockville, MD, Aspen Systems, pp. 89–111, 1984.

Wilson B., Moffat N. Rehabilitation of memory for everyday life. In Harris J.E., Morris P.E., eds. *Everyday Memory, Actions, and Absent-Mindedness*. London, Academic Press, pp. 207–233, 1984.

Wilson B., Cockburn J., Baddeley A.D. *The Rivermead Behavioural Memory Test*. Titchfield, Thames Valley Test Co., 1985.

Wilson B., Cockburn J., Baddeley A. The development and validation of a test battery for detecting and monitoring everyday memory problems. *J. Clin. Exp. Neuropsychol.* 11:855–870, 1989.

Wilson B.A. *Rehabilitation of Memory*. New York, Guilford Press, 1987.

Wilson R.S., Kaszniak A.W., Fox J.H. Remote memory in senile dementia. *Cortex* 17:41–48, 1981.

Woodhead M.M., Baddeley A.D. Individual differences and memory for faces, pictures, and words. *Mem. Cogn.* 9:368–370, 1981.

Woolsey R.M., Nelson J.S. Asymptomatic destruction of the fornix in man. *Arch. Neurol.* 32:566–568, 1975.

Zola-Morgan S., Squire L.R. Amnesia in monkeys after lesions of the mediodorsal nucleus of the thalamus. *Ann. Neurol.* 17:558–564, 1985.

Zola-Morgan S., Squire L.R. The primate hippocampal formation: evidence for a time-limited role in memory storage. *Science* 250:288–290, 1990.

Zola-Morgan S., Squire L.R., Amaral D.G. Human amnesia and the medial temporal region: enduring memory impairment following a bilateral lesion limited to field CA1 of the hippocampus. *J. Neurosci.* 6:2950–2967, 1986.

Zola-Morgan S., Squire L.R., Amaral D.G. Lesions of the hippocampal formation but not lesions of the fornix or the mammillary nuclei produce long-lasting memory impairment in monkeys. *J. Neurosci.* 9:898–913, 1989.

52

Disorders of Memory

Elizabeth K. Warrington
Rosaleen A. McCarthy

The label *poor memory*, as used by both the patient and the clinician, encompasses a wide range of deficits such as the inability to retain short messages verbatim, the inability to recall names of objects, and forgetfulness or absentmindedness in everyday life. The patient complaining of poor memory may be referring to any of these difficulties. The selective impairment and selective preservation of different types of memory have frequently been documented in patients with cerebral lesions. This chapter presents an overview of the evidence for the fractionation of short-term memory, memory for facts (semantic memory), and memory for events. Evidence is drawn from single case studies and from the systematic investigation of groups of patients with well-localized cerebral lesions. The properties of each of these kinds of memory are described, and the importance of the types of test material and modality of presentation is considered. The evidence for the anatomic correlates of specific memory disorders is also discussed. The behavioral and neurologic evidence reviewed leads to the conclusion that there are multiple and mutually dissociable disorders of memory.

SHORT-TERM MEMORY

Experimental psychologists dating back to William James (1890) have identified a distinct short-term memory system. This system is held to be limited in terms of information load and has a duration that must be measured in *seconds*. These properties of short-term memory are evident in the normal person's ability to repeat a telephone number of about seven digits verbatim and equally in the inability to recall it after a few seconds unless it has been constantly rehearsed. The central representation in short-term memory is thus not only transient and labile, but also of strictly limited capacity.

The most commonly used measure of short-term memory is the individual's auditory digit span. Aphasic patients frequently have a reduced span for auditory verbal material; however, the relatively *selective* impairment of immediate memory span in the absence of other language impairments also occurs. Luria et al. (1967) described two patients whose major symptom was impairment in the repetition of strings of phonemes, words, and digits. They interpreted these observations in terms of a memory deficit and not as secondary to aphasia. Warrington and Shallice (1969) reported detailed investigations of a patient (KF) who had a profound inability to repeat spoken strings of digits, letters, and words. KF's performance on tests of auditory perception of the spoken word and on tests of single-word production was entirely normal. However, he had a digit, letter, and word span of only one or two items. His reduced verbal span was interpreted in terms of a selective impairment of auditory verbal short-term memory. In addition, KF forgot auditory verbal information abnormally quickly. Thus, for example, if rehearsal was prevented, his ability to recall even a single letter was significantly impaired and appeared to decay after only a few seconds (Fig. 52–1). The selective reduction in the capacity of auditory verbal span together with abnormal decay functions has been replicated frequently (Caramazza et al., 1981; Friedrich et al., 1984; McCarthy and Warrington, 1987; Saffran and Marin, 1975; Vallar and Baddeley, 1984; Warrington et al., 1971). The patients provide incontrovertible evidence for the selective impairment of auditory verbal short-term memory.

Patients with restricted digit and word spans may perform surprisingly well when repeating spoken sentences. Accurate repetition of sentences of up to seven words was recorded in two patients who had

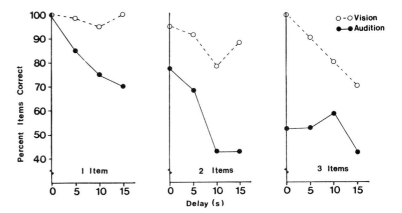

Figure 52–1. Short-term forgetting. KF's recall of visual and auditory letter stimuli after distraction.

a word span of only one item (McCarthy and Warrington, 1987). When errors are made, such patients typically produce a "paraphrase" of the sentence material (Saffran and Marin, 1975). The patients appear to be making use of the meaning of the sentence material in performing the task. In contrast, other patients may be particularly weak at recalling sentences as opposed to lists and make errors based on word sound rather than word meaning (McCarthy and Warrington, 1987). The double dissociation between sentence recall and list recall suggests that there are multiple verbal short-term memory systems, one of which is based on sound and another on meaning.

Modality Specificity

The evidence we have discussed so far has been confined exclusively to auditory verbal presentation. The questions arise as to whether a similar pattern of performance is observed with visual stimuli and whether short-term memory is similar in the two cases. There is, in fact, a significant double dissociation between the retention of auditory presented verbal stimuli and that of visually presented verbal stimuli. Thus, KF's performance on visually presented span tasks was superior to his performance with auditory presentation, and similarly, forgetting was much more rapid for auditory than for visual stimuli (the converse is the case for normal subjects) (Warrington and Shallice, 1972). KF's near-normal performance in the visual modality serves to underline the severity and selectivity of his auditory verbal short-term memory deficit. This superiority of the visual modality has been observed in a number of subsequent cases (McCarthy and Warrington, 1987; Vallar and Baddeley, 1984; Warrington et al., 1971).

If it is agreed that such evidence points to a modality-specific organization of short-term memory systems, it follows that selective impairments of *visual* short-term memory should also be observed. This is the case. Patients with a selective impairment in their visual span of apprehension have also been described. In the context of an investigation of si-

multaneous visual form perception, Kinsbourne and Warrington (1962) described four patients whose visual span was fewer than two items. Despite this deficit their auditory span was well within the normal range. This selective limitation in the visual span of apprehension was not material specific, because their recall after visual presentation was equally impaired for numbers, letters, and shapes (but not for spatial location). A systematic group study in which measures of both visual and auditory span were incorporated provided further evidence for the double dissociation of visual and auditory short-term memory systems (Warrington and Rabin, 1971). Patients with left hemisphere lesions were impaired on both auditory span and visual span of apprehension; however, performance on the two tasks was not significantly correlated.

Anatomic Considerations

The anatomic correlates of auditory and visual verbal short-term memory deficits appear to be relatively uncontroversial. First, consider auditory short-term memory (with the criterion of a selective reduction in auditory verbal span). The two cases of Luria et al. (1967) had damage in the left parietal region and the three cases of Warrington et al. (1971) also had a common area of damage in the inferior left parietal lobe. The locus of damage in the case reported by Saffran and Marin (1975) was similar. Benson et al. (1973) reviewed a series of cases in which there was a selective loss of auditory verbal "repetition" (which typically included a reduction in digit span). They concluded that the fasciculus arcuatus of the left hemisphere was the critical locus. Group studies of a consecutive series of patients with unilateral cerebral lesions consistently showed large and reliable left hemisphere impairments on a digit span task (e.g., McFie, 1975; Newcombe, 1969). A retrospective investigation, conducted in this department (in which the data from more than 650 patients were analyzed), confirmed the evidence of single case studies that the integrity of the left parietal lobe was necessary for normal auditory verbal short-term memory (Warrington et al., 1986).

The evidence concerning the anatomic correlates of impaired visual span is somewhat more sparse. The four patients with limited simultaneous form perception just discussed whose visual span was reliable for only one item all had a common area of damage in the posterior left hemisphere (Kinsbourne and Warrington, 1962). This location was corroborated and made more precise by one additional patient for whom there was autopsy evidence (Kinsbourne and Warrington, 1963). In this last patient there was a relatively small temporo-occipital infarction. The evidence from subsequent group studies is in good accord with that derived from single cases. Groups with left hemisphere damage were significantly impaired on all measures of visual span of apprehension both for verbal and for nonverbal stimuli. Furthermore, the groups with left posterior lesions were significantly more impaired than groups with left anterior lesions (e.g., Bisiach et al., 1979; Warrington and Rabin, 1971).

On the basis of the anatomic evidence, we suggest a provisional mapping of the lesion sites implicated by the two modality-specific short-term memory impairments that we described (Fig. 52–2).

MEMORY FOR FACTS

The distinction between memory for facts (or semantic memory) and memory for events has been recognized by neurologists for nearly a century, as evidenced by the distinction that is drawn between agnostic and amnestic syndromes. The term *memory for facts* is used to encompass that body of knowledge held in common by members of a culture or linguistic group. For example, vocabulary is probably the most extensive pool of verbal facts known by an individual. Thus, the average adult comprehends several thousand word meanings and in addition can retrieve them and utter them appropriately in the relevant context. There are many other classes of information

that can also be considered as factual: reading, writing, and arithmetic are such examples. It is appropriate to extend the concept of memory for facts to knowledge of the visual world. For people, visual knowledge is at least as important as verbal or symbolic knowledge. Objects, quite apart from having agreed names, have clearly defined attributes and/or functions. Knowledge of such visual facts is a sine qua non of normal existence.

Of all the impairments of verbal knowledge that are observed, the inability to retrieve words promptly and appropriately is perhaps the most common (nominal or amnestic aphasia). It has been the subject of extensive investigation and documentation. The importance of word frequency (how common the word is in the language), both for word retrieval and for word comprehension, cannot be overestimated. Rochford and Williams (1965), in a series of studies of naming skills, reported quantitative evidence for significant word frequency effects in groups of aphasic patients. It appeared as though the patients' naming vocabulary had contracted, the less common words being the more vulnerable. This robust effect has been replicated many times (e.g., McKenna and Warrington, 1980; Newcombe et al., 1965; Poeck et al., 1973).

Comparable effects of word frequency have been documented in studies of word comprehension. In testing a group of aphasic patients with a word-picture matching task, Schuell and Jenkins (1961) found a direct relationship between a word's frequency and the patient's ability to comprehend it. Massive word frequency effects were also observed in detailed studies of three patients who had particularly striking and relatively selective deficits in word comprehension (Warrington, 1975).

Poeck and colleagues argued that deficits in word retrieval and word comprehension can be completely specified in terms of word frequency (Poeck and Stachowiak, 1975; Poeck et al., 1973). Although there is no question of the importance of this variable, this view overlooks the growing body of evidence that impairments of verbal retrieval and verbal comprehension may be *category specific*. We would suggest that word frequency and word category are best considered as orthogonal dimensions.

Neurologists have long recognized that certain patients may have disproportionate impairments in the comprehension and the naming of certain categories of verbal information. In the case of body parts and colors, these deficits have been given the status of syndromes, namely, autotopagnosia and color agnosia. Goodglass et al. (1966) were the first to discuss such deficits in terms of the categorical organization of verbal knowledge systems. They documented retrieval and comprehension deficits for the categories color, concrete nouns, and action names in a group study of aphasic patients. They documented a high incidence of selective preservation and selective loss of each of these verbal categories. The patterns of deficit that they observed in the retrieval of words (naming to confrontation) were

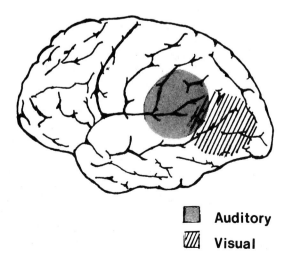

■ **Auditory**

▨ **Visual**

Figure 52–2. Provisional mapping of the lesion sites implicated by impaired auditory and visual short-term memory.

not identical with those observed for word comprehension (spoken word-picture matching).

Perhaps the most counterintuitive of their observations was the double dissociation of concrete nouns and action names. Some patients could comprehend and retrieve action verbs, such as drinking, running, and dripping, significantly better than they could matched concrete nouns, such as key, glove, and feather. For other patients the converse was the case: the concrete nouns presented less difficulty than the action verbs. The task demands (picture naming and picture recognition, respectively) would appear to be quite similar for these two categories. Miceli et al. (1984) reported a partial replication of this dissociation. They found that agrammatic aphasics had particular difficulty in naming pictures of actions. In a single case study, we demonstrated in an agrammatic patient a disproportionate impairment in the retrieval of verbs that was underpinned by a similar impairment at the level of comprehension. At the same time there was no evidence of impairment in the patient's retrieval or comprehension of common and proper nouns (McCarthy and Warrington, 1985). The fact that knowledge of proper nouns may be selectively impaired (McKenna and Warrington, 1980; Semenza and Zettin, 1988) or selectively preserved (McKenna and Warrington, 1978) provides a further example of a syntactically and/or semantically based division within verbal knowledge.

One of the major distinctions used to classify verbal knowledge in the experimental literature is the concrete-abstract dimension (e.g., Paivio et al., 1968). The more concrete the word is rated, the more likely it is to have a direct sensory referent (e.g., book, house, and car have high concrete ratings and luck, idea, and mind have low concrete ratings). This same concrete-abstract dimension has been shown to be relevant in patients with neurologic deficits. Knowledge of abstract words is frequently relatively more impaired than knowledge of concrete words. However, because of the problems of equating for task difficulty, this result can hardly provide compelling evidence for category specificity. The converse pattern, namely, a selective deficit affecting concrete words, is of considerable importance. Two well-documented patients (AB, SBY) had significant impairment in their definitions of concrete words (Warrington, 1975; Warrington and Shallice, 1984) (Table 52–1). It appeared that they had "forgotten" the

Table 52–1. WORD DEFINITIONS

Patient	% Correct	
	Concrete	*Abstract*
AB	24	85
SBY	47	94

Adapted from Warrington E.K. The selective impairment of semantic memory. *Q. J. Exp. Psychol.* 27:635–657, 1975; and Warrington E.K., Shallice T. Category specific semantic impairments. *Brain* 107:829–853, 1984, by permission of Oxford University Press.

Table 52–2. WORD DEFINITIONS

Patient	% Correct		
	Foods	*Living Things*	*Objects*
JBR	30	8	79
SBY	25	10	65

Adapted from Warrington E.K., Shallice T. Category specific semantic impairments. *Brain* 107:829–953, 1984, by permission of Oxford University Press.

meanings of all but the most common concrete words, words that were clearly well within their premorbid vocabulary. For example, they gave the following definitions of concrete words:

Garage: "Don't know."
Star: "It's a little creature, a little animal."
Frog: "Forgotten."
Harp: "Thing to measure things with."

These disastrous definitions serve to emphasize the patients' excellent ability to define abstract words.

Debate: "Argument."
Advantage: "Gain you get."
Indignation: "Not happy about something, to get angry about something."
Ratio: "Part of, percent of a thing."

Evidence for dissociations between subsets of the concrete word vocabulary has been documented. Warrington and Shallice (1984) reported on four patients who had relatively well-preserved knowledge of objects and their names but almost total loss of facts relating to foods and living things. Two of these patients were tested by use of a word definition task, and clear category effects were observed (Table 52–2). For example, the following definitions of foods and living things were given by two patients (JBR, SBY):

Brussels sprouts: "Area abroad."
Oak: "Animal."
Camel: "Animal, bird of some type."
Snake: "Animal, swims in the sea, eaten when caught."

By contrast some examples of their definitions of objects are as follows:

Helicopter: "Flying technique, vertical takeoff."
Screwdriver: "Device for fastening and unfastening screws."
Torch: "Device for showing the way in darkness."
Thermometer: "Device for registering temperature."

A similar pattern of deficit was observed in JBR and in two other patients in word-picture matching tests (Table 52–3).

A dissociation between these categories of factual knowledge could be arguably attributed to some artifact of task difficulty or item familiarity. The validity of this distinction would be supported by a

Table 52–3. WORD-PICTURE MATCHING

Patient	% Correct*		
	Foods	*Animals*	*Objects*
JBR	60	67	98
KB	55	45	85
ING	85	80	97
VER	88	86	58
YOT	93	85	63

*Chance score 20%.

Adapted from Warrington E. K., Shallice T. Category specific semantic impairments. *Brain* 107:829–853, 1984; and Warrington E. K., McCarthy R. Category specific access dysphasia. *Brain* 106:859–878, 1983, both by permission of Oxford University Press.

double dissociation. This double dissociation has now been documented (Warrington and McCarthy, 1983). VER, a patient who was severely aphasic after a left middle cerebral stroke, had no viable speech production, and thus word-picture matching techniques were used. She had a disproportionate difficulty in pointing to named pictures of objects compared with her ability to point to comparable stimuli depicting foods and living things. We also observed this dissociation in a second case (patient YOT) (Warrington and McCarthy, 1987).

Do these selective deficits in knowledge of certain facts reflect a fundamental division within the central representation of concrete words? It has been suggested that objects are differentiated primarily in terms of their functional properties (the physical or sensory attributes are frequently irrelevant or misleading, e.g., vase versus jug). In contrast, foods and living things are differentiated primarily in terms of their physical or sensory attributes, their functional properties being frequently irrelevant or insignificant, e.g., carrot versus parsnip (Warrington, 1981b). It now appears that although this typology is at least plausible, it may be an oversimplification and cannot account for all the dissociations that are observed within the concrete word vocabulary.

As long ago as 1946, Nielson claimed to have observed the selective *preservation* of knowledge of "flowers" in the context of widespread verbal impairments. Flower names are, of course, a subset of the living things vocabulary. A subset of the broad category of foods (subsumed within the more general category of things known by their physical or sensory attributes) may be selectively *impaired*. Hart et al. (1985) reported a single patient in whom it was claimed that there was a selective difficulty in retrieving the names of fruits and vegetables, other components of vocabulary being preserved.

Subsets of the category of objects can also be selectively impaired. Yamadori and Albert (1973) considered that their patient had more difficulty in the comprehension of indoor object names than outdoor object names. This indoor-outdoor dissociation was replicated and expanded in YOT. Her impairment in the knowledge of objects appeared to be greater for small manipulatable items than for large

outdoor objects. Thus she scored at the level of chance pointing to pictures of furniture and office objects but was significantly better with transport and types of accommodation. Such pointers toward a fine-grained organization of verbal knowledge systems will need to be incorporated in any future taxonomy of the systems subserving verbal facts.

Modality Specificity

There is no necessary parallel between impaired knowledge of verbal and visual facts. On the one hand, the selective impairment of either modality may be observed in isolation, the spared modality being normal or nearly so. On the other hand, there are instances in which there is impairment of both visual and verbal knowledge, and yet there is little concordance between the two modalities.

The selective impairment of verbal knowledge is the central component of the classic neurologic syndrome of transcortical sensory aphasia. These patients' comprehension deficits may be mainly or even entirely confined to the verbal domain. One such patient (EM) was unable to define an object name but had little difficulty in using the object or in describing its function (Warrington, 1975). By itself, this dissociation is perhaps not surprising. However, the converse material-specific dissociation, namely, selective impairment of visual semantic information, occurs in the classic neurologic syndrome of visual associative agnosia.

Convincingly documented cases of "pure" visual associative agnosia (that cannot be explained in terms of any simple disconnection syndrome) are rare. Hecaen et al. (1974), Pillon et al. (1981), and McCarthy and Warrington (1986) described individual patients in whom there was excellent evidence of a failure to recognize visually presented objects or demonstrate their use. In no case was there evidence of impaired verbal factual knowledge.

Selective impairment within the visual modality can also be category specific. A dissociation between visual representations of abstract and concrete concepts is on record (Warrington, 1981a). A patient (CAV) with unimpaired auditory verbal knowledge was unable to identify pictures with a concrete referent (e.g., hinge). However, his score on tasks requiring him to identify even uncommon abstract words pictorially presented was within normal limits (e.g., aptitude).

Of at least equal interest are patients with impairments in both verbal and visual modalities. The two patients described earlier (JBR and SBY) in whom clear category-specific effects were demonstrated for verbal knowledge had similar category-specific deficits for visual knowledge. Overall, JBR and SBY had equally marked impairments in their identification of pictorially presented living things and foods as in their comprehension of the spoken word. Similarly, their ability to identify pictures of objects was at a comparable level to their ability to define the object name. The concordance between visual and verbal deficits was considered for individual items, and there was little evidence of a direct mapping between the two modalities. Thus, specific items consistently lost to one modality were consistently known to the other and vice versa.

This lack of correspondence between the visual and verbal domains of knowledge is observed most dramatically in another patient (TOB) (McCarthy and Warrington, 1988) in whom there was a category-specific deficit in the verbal modality but not in the visual modality. TOB's verbal definitions of names of manufactured or constructed objects such as binoculars or a lighthouse were competent, whereas he had grave difficulties in defining names of living things. Yet his visual knowledge appeared to be intact and did not show this dissociation. He was equally competent in identifying pictures of living things and objects. Thus, his disorder was both category specific and modality specific (McCarthy and Warrington, 1988).

The evidence of selective visual and selective verbal impairments, together with a lack of correspondence between modalities, indicates that there are at least partially independent systems that subserve memory for verbal facts and memory for visual facts.

Anatomic Considerations

Impaired knowledge of verbal and visual facts typically involves damage to postrolandic regions of the left or language hemisphere. First, in the case of word retrieval: there is good evidence from group studies that patients with left temporal lobe lesions are more impaired in naming tasks than are patients with lesions in other sectors of the left hemisphere (Coughlan and Warrington, 1978; McKenna and Warrington, 1980). The single patient who had a selective impairment in naming proper nouns had a small lesion in the medial aspect of the left temporal lobe. Similar areas appear to be implicated in word comprehension deficits. In a group study, it was found that oral synonym judgments were particularly impaired in patients with left temporal lobe lesions (Coughlan and Warrington, 1978). A possible exception to this localization is that for verb retrieval and verb comprehension, for which, at present, the anatomic correlates are poorly defined.

Second, in the case of knowledge of visual facts there is a consensus that more posterior regions of the left hemisphere are implicated. In a large-scale group study, De Renzi et al. (1969) reported that patients with posterior left hemisphere lesions were particularly impaired on tasks of visual object knowledge. Using similar techniques testing functional knowledge of objects, Warrington and Taylor (1978) found that the group with posterior left hemisphere damage had significantly worse results than the other lesion groups tested. The evidence of single case studies also points to a fairly posterior left hemi-

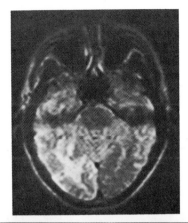
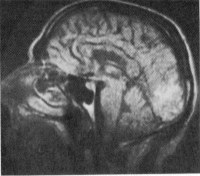

Figure 52–3. Magnetic resonance imaging scans of patient FRA showing the area of infarction in the territory of the left posterior cerebral artery.

sphere locus. A patient with a particularly pure case of visual associative agnosia underwent magnetic resonance imaging and was found to have a left hemisphere parieto-occipital boundary infarction with sparing of the splenium (McCarthy and Warrington, 1986) (Fig. 52–3). On the basis of anatomic evidence reviewed in this section, we suggest a provisional mapping of the lesion sites associated with modality-specific impairments in memory for facts (Fig. 52–4).

MEMORY FOR EVENTS

Memory for events is subserved by a system that provides a continually changing and updated record of autobiographic information unique to the individual. In this regard it is clearly different from memory for factual knowledge and poses different problems for the investigator. The most usual testing procedures involve the presentation of new information that is subsequently tested by recall or recognition. This approach rests on a long tradition in experimental psychology for investigating the parameters of verbal learning (e.g., Ebbinghaus, 1913).

The amnestic syndrome, known to neurologists since Korsakoff's (1889) classic description, exemplifies the global impairment of event memory. The amnesiac typically presents with an anterograde am-

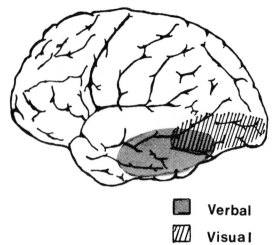

☐ **Verbal**
☒ **Visual**

Figure 52–4. Provisional mapping of the lesion sites implicated by impaired verbal and visual factual memory.

nesia and a retrograde amnesia, both of which can vary in degree of severity (Talland, 1965). In the extreme case the amnesiac appears to have an absolute deficit in accessing past events and in recalling new information (Butters and Cermak, 1986; Cermak and O'Connor, 1983; Sanders and Warrington, 1971; Warrington and McCarthy, 1988). Clinically it appears as though the patient's autobiographic record is impaired beyond a few minutes. At present, the relationship between the patient's incapacity to acquire new information and the rate at which such information is lost with the passage of time is unresolved.

Although the clinical impression may be that of a "total" amnesia, surprisingly there are certain types of learning and retention tasks that such patients perform normally or nearly so. These tasks include retention of a motor skill (Corkin, 1968; Milner, 1966), identification of stimuli on the basis of partial information (Warrington and Weiskrantz, 1970), and problem-solving techniques (Kinsbourne and Woods, 1975). One demonstration of preserved learning and retention has important implications for the rehabilitation of amnesic patients. Glisky and Schacter (1987) succeeded in training an amnesic patient in computer skills to a level that was viable in a "real world" environment. Whatever skills are required to perform such tasks, they are apparently independent of any phenomenologic autobiographic record and are unlikely to have an entry in event memory.

The global amnestic syndrome has been dealt with here summarily. To do anything like justice to this syndrome, a monograph would be required (for comprehensive reviews see Butters and Cermak, 1980; Mayes, 1983).

Modality and Material Specificity

For both short-term memory and memory for facts, there is good evidence of modality specificity. This does not appear to be the case for memory for events. No selective deficits in the recall of either auditory or visually presented words have been recorded (for review see Milner, 1971). The characteristics of the material to be remembered are of paramount importance. In a classic series of experiments Milner and colleagues demonstrated clear evidence for material-specific memory deficits. Patients after left temporal lobectomy were impaired in the learning and retention of verbal material. Conversely, patients after right temporal lobectomy were impaired in the recall and recognition of nonverbal pattern stimuli. The left hemisphere groups were relatively impaired in learning sentences, paired-associate learning tasks, and the like, whereas the right hemisphere groups had relatively more difficulty in recognizing tunes, faces, and complex patterns (e.g., Milner, 1958, 1965, 1971). This double dissociation appears to be robust. Comparable patterns of selective deficit are observed despite the fact that different testing procedures have been used for the assessment of verbal and nonverbal memory, and identical patterns of performance are obtained by using recognition memory tests in which task demands are equated for verbal and nonverbal material (Warrington, 1984).

Anatomic Considerations

In the early studies of learning and memory conducted by Milner and colleagues at Montreal, emphasis was placed on the importance of the temporal lobes in the etiology of memory loss (e.g., Kimura, 1963; Milner, 1958, 1965, 1966, 1971). Patients with right temporal lesions showed material-specific impairments in the retention of nonverbal material, whereas left temporal lobectomy resulted in impaired verbal retention. Furthermore, Milner and colleagues consistently reported that the greater the involvement of the hippocampus in temporal lobe ablations, the greater the severity of the material-specific memory deficit. However, their later studies were extended to the more detailed investigation of memory disorders in patients with frontal lobe lesions, and it is quite clear that certain aspects of memory function can be impaired after unilateral anterior cortical ablation (Milner, 1971, 1982; Petrides and Milner, 1982; Smith and Milner, 1984). Once again, material specificity related to laterality of the lesion has frequently been observed.

A study of patients assessed in the psychology department of the National Hospital in London has been reported (Warrington, 1984). Performance on a recognition memory test for words and faces was evaluated in a large group of patients (279) with well-localized unilateral lesions. There was a comparable incidence of visual memory deficit in all sectors of the right hemisphere and of verbal memory deficit in all sectors of the left hemisphere. Furthermore, in virtually all cases the memory deficit was disproportionately severe for words in the patients with left

Table 52–4. RECOGNITION MEMORY FOR WORDS AND FACES

	% of Cases			
Lesion Site	With Words Impaired	With Words Significantly Worse Than Faces	With Faces Impaired	With Faces Significantly Worse Than Words
Right frontal	11	7	23	19
Right temporal	4	4	36	40
Right parietal	10	5	35	35
Left frontal	37	15	20	5
Left temporal	42	35	19	5
Left parietal	34	31	15	2

Adapted from Warrington E. K. *Recognition Memory Test.* Windsor, England, NFER-Nelson Publishing, 1984.

hemisphere lesions and for faces in the patients with right hemisphere lesions. Once again, a significant incidence of material-specific deficits occurred in each cerebral sector (Table 52–4).

It is a matter of debate whether the frontal lobe deficit on a range of memory tests reflects a memory impairment per se or whether such effects are secondary to a higher-level cognitive dysfunction (e.g., Shallice, 1982). However, there is some evidence in the literature that there may be a qualitatively distinctive frontal lobe amnesia (Kapur and Coughlan, 1980; Logue et al., 1968; Volpe and Hirst, 1983). Analogously, it has been suggested that the memory deficit observed in patients with parietal lobe lesions is secondary to faulty processes at an input stage (De Renzi, 1968).

Although memory deficits observed in patients with diffuse brain disease are neutral with respect to the question of the localization of systems subserving memory for events, it is worth noting that material-specific deficits are not uncommon in such cases. In a retrospective series of 112 patients with proven cortical atrophy, 24% had a significant and selective verbal recognition memory deficit. A further 13% had an unequivocal and selective recognition memory impairment for faces (Warrington, 1984).

Paradoxically, no memory deficit is so severe or so global as that which can be observed in alcoholic patients with Korsakoff's syndrome, in whom there may be extremely small lesions. On the basis of evidence obtained at autopsy, the minimal lesion would appear to be in a restricted diencephalic area. Victor et al. (1971) reviewed a series of 26 cases and concluded that the dorsal medial nucleus of the thalamus was crucial in the etiology of the Korsakoff amnestic syndrome. Two other patients who were extensively investigated in life were reported to have lesions restricted to the mamillary bodies and in addition had a small area of degeneration in the thalamus, lying between the subependymal zone and the medial aspect of the medial dorsal nucleus (Mair et al., 1979). The problem of the relationship between the dense and often total memory deficit observed in the Korsakoff amnestic syndrome and the possibly less severe (but none the less important) memory impairments observed in patients with significantly

larger lesions remains to be resolved. From a more theoretic perspective, it seems likely that a more detailed investigation of the differences rather than similarities between lesion groups will lead to further refinement of the component processes involved in memory for events.

MULTIPLE MEMORY SYSTEMS

This chapter has reviewed the evidence that short-term memory, memory for facts, and memory for events are functionally and anatomically distinct systems. The evidence that they are systems independent of each other is reviewed here.

First, patients with auditory-verbal short-term memory disorders are considered. It is agreed that memory for verbal and visual facts (as tested by word definition or naming tasks) can be quite normal in these patients. However, perhaps more surprising, there is good evidence that memory for the same class of stimuli is impaired if recall is immediate (as in a span task) but entirely satisfactory if retention is tested outside the normal time scale of short-term memory (Shallice and Warrington, 1970). This is not to say that retention improves or that memory gets better with delay, but rather that normal subjects lose the benefit of the short-term memory component after 20–30 seconds. Their memory for events may thus be entirely normal.

Evidence such as this had led to the revision of the serial, or sequential, model of memory (e.g., Atkinson and Shiffrin, 1968; Broadbent, 1958), which viewed short-term memory systems as a gateway to long-term memory (which in our terms would be equivalent to retrieval from event memory). Current models favor a parallel organization of these systems (Baddeley, 1976; Morton, 1970).

Second, in the case of the relationship between impaired memory for facts (disorders of semantic memory) and the functioning of the other two memory systems, for many of the well-documented cases (e.g., those reviewed in this chapter) performance on short-term memory tasks can be entirely normal.

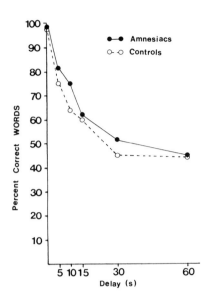

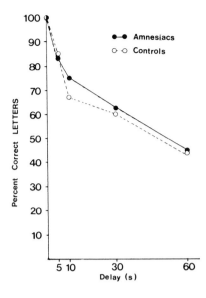

Figure 52–5. Short-term forgetting: amnesiacs and control subjects recall of printed words and letter stimuli after distraction.

Scores of several patients on conventional memory span tests were actually above the normal level. More problematic is the question of whether memory for facts is a system functionally independent of that subserving memory for events. In this case the evidence appears to favor serial rather than parallel organization. Clearly, the memory load imposed by a verbal learning task in which the meaningfulness of the test material was blunted or lost would be quite different from that for the patient with a normal memory for facts. In certain patients it has been shown that recall of categories of information that were spared in their factual knowledge was good. Furthermore, their personal orientation and their ability to recall current and past public events can be well preserved (Coughlan and Warrington, 1978; Warrington, 1975).

Finally, the amnesiac's performance on tests for factual memory and short-term memory must be considered. By definition, the pure amnesic syndrome is identified only when the patient can function at a normal level on tests of intelligence. Those in common use involve several measures of both verbal and visual factual knowledge. Reaction time measures have been used to obtain more accurate measures of retrieval of verbal facts in amnesic patients. No significant differences were observed between the experimental subjects and a matched group of control subjects in the ability to give word

opposites, word categories, and synonyms at speed (Meudell et al., 1981; Warrington and Weiskrantz, 1982). Evidence regarding short-term memory function in amnesic patients appears to be relatively clear. Not only can their performance on span tasks be normal, but, more dramatically, on short-term forgetting tasks (when rehearsal is prevented by a distracting task), their decay functions can be entirely normal. Thus, recall of letter stimuli and word stimuli tested at extremely short intervals after presentation can be normal (Fig. 52–5) (Baddeley and Warrington, 1970; Warrington, 1982). This is the task that is particularly impaired in patients with short-term memory deficits.

We described the dissociation between impaired short-term memory and intact memory for events. The converse pattern that is observed in amnesic patients provides compelling evidence for the mutual independence of the systems subserving short-term memory and memory for events.

When patients report poor memory, it is clear that they may be describing very distinct types of difficulty. A brief account was given here of the three major types of memory disorder that are frequently encountered in neurologic practice, as well as of these three major memory systems: short-term memory, memory for facts, and memory for events. An attempt was made to present an account of the principal characteristics of each system and to discuss

Table 52–5. SUMMARY OF THE PROPERTIES AND ANATOMIC CORRELATES OF SHORT-TERM MEMORY, MEMORY FOR FACTS, AND MEMORY FOR EVENTS

Types of Memory	Characteristics	Time Course	Modality Specific	Material Specific	Anatomy
Short-term	Labile and limited capacity	Short (seconds)	No	Yes	Left parietal
Factual	Static and large capacity	Long (years)	Yes	Yes	Left temporal
Event	Dynamic (capacity unknown)	Variable (>1 min)	Yes	No	Left and right hemispheres

each in terms of modality or material specificity; when possible, the anatomic correlates of each system were indicated (Table 52–5).

References

(Key references are designated with an asterisk.)

Atkinson R.C., Shiffrin R.M. Human memory: a proposed system and its control process. In Spence K., Spence R., eds. *The Psychology of Learning and Motivation.* Vol. 2. New York, Academic Press, pp. 90–195, 1968.

*Baddeley A.D. *The Psychology of Memory.* New York, Harper & Row, 1976.

Baddeley A.D., Warrington E.K. Amnesia and the distinction between long and short-term memory. *J. Verbal Learn. Verbal Behav.* 9:176–189, 1970.

Benson D.F., Sheremata W.A., Bouchard R., et al. Conduction aphasia: a clinicopathological study. *Arch. Neurol.* 28:339–346, 1973.

Bisiach E., Nichelli P., Sala C. Recognition of random shapes in unilateral brain damaged patients: a reappraisal. *Cortex* 15:491–500, 1979.

Broadbent D.E. *Perception and Communication.* London, Pergamon Press, 1958.

Butters N., Cermak L.S. *Alcoholic Korsakoff's Syndrome: An Information Processing Approach to Amnesia.* New York, Academic Press, 1980.

Butters N., Cermak L.S. A case study of the forgetting of autobiographical knowledge: implications for the study of retrograde amnesia. In Rubin D.C., ed. *Autobiographical Memory.* Cambridge, Cambridge University Press, pp. 253–272, 1986.

Caramazza A., Basili A.G., Koller J.J., et al. An investigation of repetition and language processing in a case of conduction aphasia. *Brain Lang.* 14:235–271, 1981.

Cermak L.S., O'Connor M. The retrieval capacity of a patient with amnesia due to encephalitis. *Neuropsychologia* 21:213–234, 1983.

Corkin S. Acquisition of motor skill after bilateral medical temporal lobe excision. *Neuropsychologia* 6:255–265, 1968.

Coughlan A.K., Warrington E.K. Word-comprehension and word-retrieval in patients with localised cerebral lesions. *Brain* 101:163–185, 1978.

De Renzi E. Non-verbal memory and hemispheric side of lesion. *Neuropsychologia* 6:181–189, 1968.

*De Renzi E., Scotti G., Spinnler H. Perceptual and associative disorders of visual recognition. Relationship to the site of the cerebral lesion. *Neurology (Minneap.)* 19:634–642, 1969.

Ebbinghaus H. *Memory: A Contribution to Experimental Psychology* (translated by Ruger H.A., Bussenius C.E.). New York, Dover Publications, 1913.

Friedrich F.J., Glenn C.G., Marin O.S.M. Interruption of phonological coding in conduction aphasia. *Brain Lang.* 22:266–291, 1984.

Glisky E.L., Schacter D.L. Acquisition of domain-specific knowledge in organic amnesia: training for computer-related work. *Neuropsychologia* 25:893–906, 1987.

Goodglass H., Klein B., Carey P., et al. Specific semantic word categories in aphasia. *Cortex* 2:74–89, 1966.

Hart J. Jr., Berndt R.S., Caramazza A. Category-specific naming deficit following cerebral infarction. *Nature* 316:439–440, 1985.

*Hécaen H., Goldblum M.C., Masure M.C., et al. Une nouvelle observation d'agnosie d'object. Deficit de l'association ou de la catégorization spécifique de la modalité visuelle? *Neuropsychologia* 12:447–464, 1974.

James W. *Principles of Psychology.* New York, Henry Holt, 1890.

Kapur N., Coughlan A.K. Confabulation and frontal lobe dysfunction. *J. Neurol. Neurosurg. Psychiatry* 43:461–463, 1980.

Kimura D. Right temporal lobe damage. *Arch. Neurol.* 8:264–271, 1963.

Kinsbourne M., Warrington E.K. A disorder of simultaneous form perception. *Brain* 85:461–486, 1962.

Kinsbourne M., Warrington E.K. The localising significance of limited simultaneous form perception. *Brain* 85:697–702, 1963.

*Kinsbourne M., Woods F. Shorter term memory processes and the amnesic syndrome. In Deutsch D., Deutsch J.A., eds. *Short Term Memory.* New York, Academic Press, 1975.

Korsakoff S.S. Étude médico-psychologique sur un forme de maladies de la mémoire. *Rev. Philos.* 28:501, 1889.

Logue V., Durwood M., Pratt R.T.C., et al. The quality of survival after rupture of an anterior cerebral aneurism. *Br. J. Psychiatry* 114:137–168, 1968.

Luria A.R., Sokolov E.N., Klimkowski M. Towards a neurodynamic analysis of memory disturbances with lesions of the temporal lobe. *Neuropsychologia* 5:1–10, 1967.

*Mair W.G.P., Warrington E.K., Weiskrantz L. Neuropathological and psychological examination of 2 patients with Korsakoff's psychosis. *Brain* 102:749–783, 1979.

*Mayes A.R. *Memory in Humans and Animals.* Wokingham, Van Nostrand Reinhold, 1983.

McCarthy R., Warrington E.K. Category specificity in an agrammatic patient: the relative impairment of verb retrieval and comprehension. *Neuropsychologia* 23:709–727, 1985.

McCarthy R.A., Warrington E.K. Visual associative agnosia: a clinicoanatomical study of a single case. *J. Neurol. Neurosurg. Psychiatry* 49:1233–1240, 1986.

McCarthy R.A., Warrington E.K. The double dissociation of short-term memory for lists and sentences. *Brain* 110:1545–1563, 1987.

McCarthy R.A., Warrington E.K. Evidence from modality specific meaning systems in the brain. *Nature* 334:428–430, 1988.

McFie J. *Assessment of Organic Intellectual Impairment.* London, Academic Press, 1975.

McKenna P., Warrington E.K. Category-specific naming preservation: a single case study. *J. Neurol. Neurosurg. Psychiatry* 41:571–574, 1978.

McKenna P., Warrington E.K. Testing for nominal dysphasia. *J. Neurol. Neurosurg. Psychiatry* 43:781–788, 1980.

Meudell P.R., Mayes A.R., Neary D. Amnesia is not caused by cognitive slowness. *Cortex* 16:413–419, 1981.

Miceli G., Silveri M.C., Villa G., et al. On the basis for the agrammatic's difficulty in producing main verbs. *Cortex* 20:207–220, 1984.

Milner B. Psychological defects produced by temporal lobe excisions. *Res. Publ. Assoc. Nerv. Ment. Dis.* 36:244–257, 1958.

Milner B. Visually-guided maze learning in man: effects of bilateral hippocampal bilateral frontal and unilateral cerebral lesions. *Neuropsychologia* 3:317–388, 1965.

Milner B. Amnesia following operation on the temporal lobes. In Whitty C.W.M., Zangwill O.L., eds. *Amnesia.* London, Butterworth, pp. 109–133, 1966.

*Milner B. Interhemispheric differences in the localisation of psychological processes in man. *Br. Med. Bull.* 27:272–277, 1971.

Milner B. Some cognitive effects of frontal-lobe lesions in man. *Philos. Trans. R. Soc. Lond [Biol.]* 298:3–13, 1982.

Morton J.A functional model for memory. In Norman D.A., ed. *Models of Human Memory.* New York, Academic Press, pp. 203–254, 1970.

Newcombe F. *Missile Wounds of the Brain.* London, Oxford University Press, 1969.

Newcombe F., Oldfield R.C., Wingfield A. Object naming by dysphasic patients. *Nature* 207:1217–1218, 1965.

Nielson J.M. *Agnosia, Apraxia, Aphasia: Their Value in Cerebral Localisation.* New York, Paul B. Hoeber, 1946.

Paivio A., Yuille J.C., Madigan J.A. Concreteness, imagery and meaningfulness values for 925 nouns. *J. Exp. Psychol. Monogr. Suppl.* 76:1–25, 1968.

Petrides M., Milner B. Deficits on subject ordered tasks after frontal and temporal lobe lesions in man. *Neuropsychologia* 20:249–262, 1982.

Pillon B., Signoret J-L., Lhermitte F. Agnosie visuelle associative. Rôle de l'hémisphère gauche dans la perception visuelle. *Rev. Neurol. (Paris)* 137:831–842, 1981.

Poeck K., Hartje W., Kerschensteiner M., et al. Sprachverstandnisstorung bie aphasischen und nichtaphasischen Hirnkranken. *Dtsch. Med. Wochenschr.* 98:139–147, 1973.

Poeck K., Stachowiak F-J. Farbenennungsstorungen bei aphasischen und nichtaphasischen Hirnkranken. *J. Neurol.* 209:95–102, 1975.

Rochford G., Williams M. Studies in the development and the

breakdown of the use of names. IV. The effects of word frequency. *J. Neurol. Neurosurg. Psychiatry* 28:407–413, 1965.

Saffran E.M., Marin O.S.M. Immediate memory for word lists and sentences in a patient with deficient auditory short-term memory. *Brain Lang.* 2:420–433, 1975.

Sanders H.I., Warrington E.K. Memory for remote events in amnesic patients. *Brain* 94:661–668, 1971.

Schuell H., Jenkins J.J. Reduction of vocabulary in aphasia. *Brain* 84:243–261, 1961.

Semenza C., Zettin M. Generating proper names: a case of selective inability. *Cognitive Neuropsychol* 5:711–721, 1988.

Shallice T. Specific impairments of planning. *Philos. Trans. R. Soc. Lond. [Biol.]* 298:199–210, 1982.

*Shallice T., Warrington E.K. The independence of the verbal memory stores: a neuropsychological study. *Q. J. Exp. Psychol.* 22:261–273, 1970.

Smith M.L., Milner B. Differential effects of frontal-lobe lesions on cognitive estimation and spatial memory. *Neuropsychologia* 22:697–705, 1984.

Talland G.A. *Deranged Memory. A Psychonomic Study of the Amnesic Syndrome.* New York, Academic Press, 1965.

Vallar G., Baddeley A.D. Fractionation of working memory: neuropsychological evidence for a phonological short-term memory store. *J. Verbal Learn. Verbal Behav.* 23:151–161, 1984.

Victor M., Adams R.D., Collins G.H. *The Wernicke-Korsakoff Syndrome.* Philadelphia, Davis, 1971.

Volpe B.J., Hirst W. Amnesia following the rupture and repair of an anterior communicating artery aneurism. *J. Neurol. Neurosurg. Psychiatry* 46:704–719, 1983.

*Warrington E.K. The selective impairment of semantic memory. *Q. J. Exp. Psychol.* 27:635–657, 1975.

Warrington E.K. Concrete word dyslexia. *Br. J. Psychol.* 72:175–196, 1981a.

Warrington E.K. Neuropsychological studies of verbal semantic systems. *Philos. Trans. R. Soc. Lond. [Biol.]* 295:411–423, 1981b.

Warrington E.K. The double dissociation of short- and long-term memory deficits. In Cermak L.S., ed. *Human Memory and Amnesia.* Hillsdale, NJ, Erlbaum, pp. 61–76, 1982.

Warrington E.K. *Recognition Memory Test.* Windsor, England, NFER-Nelson Publishing, 1984.

Warrington E.K., McCarthy R. Category specific access dysphasia. *Brain* 106:859–878, 1983.

Warrington E.K., McCarthy R.A. Categories of knowledge: further fractionations and an attempted integration. *Brain* 110:1273–1296, 1987.

Warrington E.K., McCarthy R.A. The fractionation of retrograde amnesia. *Brain Cogn.* 7:184–200, 1988.

Warrington E.K., Rabin P. Visual span of apprehension in patients with unilateral cerebral lesions. *Q. J. Exp. Psychol.* 23:423–431, 1971.

Warrington E.K., Shallice T. The selective impairment of auditory verbal short-term memory. *Brain* 92:885–896, 1969.

*Warrington E.K., Shallice T. Neuropsychological evidence of visual storage in short-term memory tasks. *Q. J. Exp. Psychol.* 24:30–40, 1972.

Warrington E.K., Shallice T. Category specific semantic impairments. *Brain* 107:829–853, 1984.

Warrington E.K., Taylor A.M. Two categorical stages of object recognition. *Perception* 7:695–705, 1978.

Warrington E.K., Weiskrantz L. Amnesic syndrome: consolidation or retrieval? *Nature* 228:628–630, 1970.

Warrington E.K., Weiskrantz L. Amnesia: a disconnection syndrome. *Neuropsychologia* 20:233–249, 1982.

Warrington E.K., Logue V., Pratt R.T.C. Anatomical localisation of selective impairment of auditory verbal short-term memory. *Neuropsychologia* 9:377–387, 1971.

Warrington E.K., James M., Maciejewski C. The WAIS as a lateralizing and localizing diagnostic instrument: a study of 656 patients with unilateral cerebral lesions. *Neuropsychologia* 24:223–239, 1986.

Yamadori A., Albert M.L. Word category aphasia. *Cortex* 9:112–125, 1973.

53

Acquired Language Disorders

J.P. Mohr

It is convenient to distinguish between disorders of speech and language. The former refers to brain, peripheral nerve, and muscle lesions that impair vocalization, writing or drawing, hearing, seeing, and searching the shapes and sounds used in interpersonal communication. The latter refers to less easily specified behaviors that permit individuals to communicate by using certain shapes and sounds individually or in groups according to rules acquired by experience and presumably improved by a certain degree of formal training.

The discussion in this chapter focuses on the neurology of aphasia, an emphasis that regrettably necessitates drastic condensations of the wide spectrum of the subject to more manageable topics and gives only passing reference to the larger subject of the theories of language, neurolinguistics, and cerebral organization, on which so much has been written during the past century and a half (Albert et al., 1981; Benson and Geschwind, 1976; Broca, 1861; Brown, 1972; Critchley, 1970; Dejerine and Mirallie, 1986; Foix, 1928; Geschwind, 1974; Head, 1926; Hecaen and Albert, 1978; Kleist, 1934; Lecours et al., 1983; Luria, 1966; Pick, 1905; Weisenberg and McBride, 1935; Wernicke, 1874; Wyllie, 1894).

GENERAL PRINCIPLES

The aphasias are most obvious from acute lesions in the sylvian region opposite the preferred hand, which for 95% of people is the left hemisphere. The farther from this zone and the smaller, deeper, and less acute the lesion, the less evident is the disturbance in speech and language.

These broad generalities underlie virtually all of the literature on the subject, but they have not proved enough in themselves to serve the needs of the clinician faced with aphasia as a diagnostic problem. Instead, more elaborate theoretic structures have been developed. For more than a century, the clinical findings in the aphasias have been explained by two somewhat incompatible views of cerebral function, one or both of which underlie the attitudes taken by clinician and researcher alike. In one, the syndromes of aphasia are interpreted as reflecting lesions of various origins involving relatively autonomous specialized cortical surface "centers" or white matter pathways, separately or in various combinations (Dejerine and Mirallie, 1986; Lichtheim, 1885; Wernicke, 1874). In terms less extreme, these concepts were resurrected in modern times in the theses of connectionism popularized by Geschwind (1965, 1974). In the second view, only one cerebral region, situated in the posterior portion of the sylvian fissure, is crucial for language behavior (Marie, 1906); other cerebral regions serve mainly as centripetal or centrifugal channels to this central zone. Syndrome analysis is directed toward discovering evidence of damage to the central language mechanism, regardless of the input or output channels involved in the behavior being tested. Damage to the former is aphasic in nature, whereas damage to the centrifugal or the centripetal pathways is not.

Although the issues raised by these theories have not yet been resolved, researchers have been distracted from them in recent years by other developments. The first was the emergence of the field of neurolinguistics; its adherents launched a major effort to study aphasic phenomena by the principles of this discipline, ably summarized by Lecours et al. (1983). This research has led to many reclassifications of the nature of the disturbed utterances by aphasics that now permit a more precise characterization of the deficits. Another development involved preliminary efforts by a small band of investigators who attempted to apply the principles of behavioral science (Sidman et al., 1971). Some initially encouraging results were obtained, but because of inadequate effort the power of this approach to aphasia has not been realized. However, it has had an impact on the design of tests to explore the behavior of aphasic patients (see the next section). Overshadowing these new methods has been the renewed interest in clinicoanatomic correlation by better imaging techniques, first with computed tomographic (CT) scanning and then by nuclear magnetic resonance scanning.

These techniques, which permit better estimates of the lesion in living individuals, have for the first time allowed researchers to focus their efforts on certain patients in a more efficient manner. Furthermore, regional cerebral blood flow studies and positron emission tomography have permitted inferences in cerebral regions activated in speech and language. Studies with regional cerebral blood flow have shown no difference between right and left hemisphere activation during humming, while vocal activation produced slightly more left-sided activation, with the sites of activation rather high over both convexities and the lowest site being about the middle rolandic region to the upper margin of the hemisphere (Ryding et al., 1987). These rather high sites are a bit above the regions usually considered to represent the face. Positron emission tomographic studies have challenged many of the assumptions of cerebral connectionism (Kempler et al., 1988).

These more focused studies have led to a revision of many of the traditional clinicopathologic correlations. Among them has been the demonstration that smaller, focal ischemic brain lesions that were once thought to produce the major syndromes of aphasia cause, at most, transient or minor abnormalities in production or comprehension of speech sounds and shapes; much larger lesions are necessary to produce major disruptions in language function (Mohr 1980; Mohr et al., 1978a). Lesions of deeper structures have increasingly been demonstrated to play important roles in disturbances of speech and language. Interruption of the medial subcallosal fasciculus, when inferior frontal infarcts extend deeply into the basal ganglia or affect the basal ganglia separately, has been postulated as the explanation for the severe nonfluency that occurs in some forms of aphasia (Naeser et al., 1989). Involvement of the thalamus from hemorrhage has been demonstrated not only clinically (Mohr et al., 1974) but also by regional cerebral blood flow studies in which changes this blood flow at the hemisphere surface have correlated with the nature of the errors found in thalamic hemorrhage occurring with syndromes of aphasia (Rousseaux et al., 1990) and in striatal infarcts (Viader et al., 1987). For other etiologies, such as neoplasms, some evidence suggests the exact lesion location is not a predictor of the occurrence of aphasia (Recht et al., 1989).

METHOD OF ANALYSIS

Physicians faced with the daily task of clinical management of aphasic patients generally agree on the importance of the following variables, in roughly descending order, in the diagnosis of aphasia: the methods used to delineate the syndrome; the site and size of the brain injury; the time after onset; the cause; and coexisting motor and sensory deficits. The importance of the first variable justifies a brief review of the main approaches.

Most major research centers tend to maintain and use their own methods of testing patients, and data from various centers are often not strictly comparable. Because ambiguities and differences in the observation of aphasic behavior constitute a paramount source of disagreement, a review of the major methods used to evaluate aphasic patients seems justified.

Tests to Corroborate Theories

A number of individual tests used and popularized by famous investigators were designed to demonstrate particular points concerning the nature of aphasia or to corroborate certain theories. An assumption underlying many of these individual tests was that failure to perform the test correctly would reflect a specific deficiency.

Many examples of such tests exist (Weigl, 1966). The most famous include the well-known three-paper test of Marie: The patient is presented with a piece of paper on which the examiner, in his or her own handwriting, has written an instruction to the effect that "When you have finished reading this page, tear the page into three parts. Give one to me. Throw a second on the floor. Put the third in your pocket." Another well-known set of tests was developed by Goldstein (1948) to assess impairment in "abstract attitude." In these tests, patients were asked to select from among a variety of stimuli the one that did not match the remainder of the group in terms of some functional principle or to name the overall categoric word that would best describe the functional class of which the demonstrated materials were members, for example, tools. Luria (1966) devised a special set of tests along pavlovian lines that were designed to pursue the ability of the patient to respond to increasingly complex demands, thus assuming that the failures represented higher-order disturbances.

Like many of the individual tests in the traditional test batteries, these theory-corroborating tests frequently are of greatest clinical value when the patient performs without errors. Confronted with a patient who is thought by others to have intact neurologic functioning, the consulting neurologist can often help to support this impression when the patient effortlessly responds to such tasks. But, when failures occur, so many variables are at work that one can conclude only that more work is required to settle the nature of the disturbances.

Test Batteries for Aphasic Syndromes

Another major approach to aphasic deficits involves the presentation of a wide variety of individual tests, each designed to assess a given aspect of behavior (Eisenson, 1954; Goodglass and Kaplan, 1972; Head, 1926; Kertesz and Poole, 1974; Porch, 1970; Weisenberg and McBride, 1935). Each test in the subgroups is constructed to stand alone with its own validity. The performance profile that results for a given patient is compared with that obtained in normal individuals and other aphasic patients.

These batteries appear to have arisen from the large variety of individual tests created by previous aphasiologists and have been steadily modified by experience. Credit is due to Weisenburg and McBride (1935) for the first systematic use of standard clinical psychologic tests, including IQ tests, in the evaluation of aphasia. Several other groups of investigators have also developed and validated their own batteries to an impressive level of complexity and reliability. In North America, the most popular have been the Boston Veterans Administration Diagnostic Test for Aphasia (Goodglass and Kaplan, 1972) and a somewhat shorter one derived from it, the Western Aphasia Battery (Kertesz and Poole, 1974).

These tests have the advantage of considerable use in the clinical characterization of aphasic patients and have been used for correlations with CT scan and autopsy data. In experienced hands, they have been useful in characterizing the syndrome in traditional eponymic terms, which has had some predictive value for lesion location and prognosis. Because they are time-consuming, they are often administered by specially trained speech pathologists, although fragments of the tests have become parts of the bedside tests used by many clinical neurologists.

The assumptions basic to use of the tests are that the patient's behavior is stable, he or she is motivated to a degree that success or failure will not significantly affect on performance, and the scores obtained fairly represent a best effort. The limitations on testing imposed by these assumptions make these batteries somewhat unsuitable for severely aphasic individuals, those easily dismayed by failure, or those with major disturbances in response constancy, hemineglect, or failure to grasp the principle of the tests. Although extensively validated, the tests suffer from a necessary limitation on the number of stimuli in each test group and rest on the assumption that some five or six items suffice to adequately sample the behavior. They also have only limited continuity of stimulus materials; for example, the items written from dictation are often different from those read aloud. Also, conduct of the testing does not take into account the effects of reinforcement across the spectrum of tests.

Behavioral Tests

In his monograph on aphasia more than a century ago, Wernicke (1874) noted a tendency for patients to seize upon any available cues to help themselves get a correct answer when they experienced difficulties with bedside tests. The fact that patients use cues, including those unrecognized or thought irrelevant by the examiner, is basic to all testing for aphasia; failure to take it into account is the usual explanation for a difference between examiners in their impression of the nature and severity of an individual aphasic syndrome.

Although all aphasia tests are behavioral, few investigators explicitly and systematically use the principles and techniques that stem from objective behavioral science (Sidman et al., 1971). With some oversimplification, three major variables may be said to govern a person's interaction with his or her environment. First, all behavior, including that exhibited in aphasia tests, is governed by its consequences. Rather than depend solely on a patient's presumed motivation to do well during tests, the author has found it useful to provide explicit positive reinforcement to encourage correct responses. Behavioral deficits, aphasic or other, may result when the expected control over behavior fails to be exerted by its consequences. Under such conditions, a patient shows no consistent behavior. Failure of consequences to govern the response may be referred to as motivational (reinforcement) deficits. There is little known about these states. In such circumstances, which are often met in severe aphasics and in those with deep lesions, attempts to construct a typical traditional eponymic syndrome based on a few observations usually proves untenable.

The second behavioral variable involves response to instructions. The task the patient is asked to perform involves a response to test stimuli, such as printed words, and the response called for is not just any response but one specific to the test procedure itself, such as reading aloud. A patient who is not sensitive to such instructions may show behavior that is unrelated to the purposes of the test. The author refers to such failures as instructional deficits. Like motivational deficits, instructional deficits invalidate any conclusions specific to aphasia. Because aphasia, by its nature, represents a communication disorder, instructional deficits in a variety of forms are often present and frequently prove difficult to circumvent during evaluation of the aphasia. Extra time and effort in overcoming the problem, sometimes by changing the reinforcers and at other times by slowing the rate of testing, may be rewarded by the observation of a far superior level of performance than that obtained by more casual testing. Instructional deficits seem especially common among patients with Wernicke's aphasia. Most aspects of instructional deficits, like motivational deficits, are incompletely understood, including clinical correlation, prognosis, and the extent to which they impact on performance to different tasks.

Assuming the first two variables are adequately accounted for, much of the testing of aphasia involves what can be called stimulus decontrol. Appropriate behavior occurs in response to stimuli that set the occasion for reinforcement, as determined by a person's behavioral history. When a particular stimulus occasions a response and its absence fails to do so, a controlling relation exists between stimulus and response. An example of the complexity involved in stimulus control is the relation between traffic lights and a driver's behavior. Many of the deficits labeled as aphasic represent breakdowns of stimulus control. Examples include the faulty naming of colors but intact ability to say these words when asked to read their printed names aloud. A huge literature exists on the details of stimulus control in normal animals and humans but has barely been developed for aphasic subjects (Leicester et al., 1971).

In approaching patients at the bedside and in the laboratory, the author has found it essential to build controls for reinforcement and instructional deficits into the test procedures, which are, themselves, oriented toward the analysis of stimulus-control deficits characteristic of aphasia. The sequence of tests is designed to reveal intact forms of stimulus control, thereby reducing the number of factors that must be considered to play a role in the patient's deficit. The tests themselves simply require the patient to name orally, write, or match (select from a number of alternatives) visual, auditory, or palpated test stimuli, such as single letters, three-letter picturable nouns and their pictures, color names and their colors, digit names and their digits, and manipulable objects. These tests demonstrate the control exerted by each stimulus (visual, auditory, or palpated) over each type of response (oral, naming, writing, and matching). The test battery yields a stimulus-control matrix in which stimulus (input) channels, response (output) channels, and controlling stimulus-response or stimulus-stimulus relations can be evaluated.

Other investigators have independently devised methods similar in principle, among them the well-validated Porch Index of Communicative Ability. The principle of using common manipulable object stimuli presented separately in visual, auditory, and palpated form for separate spoken and written naming responses began with Head's six objects (Head, 1926). It was popularized in the United States (Chesher, 1937) and was later increased to 20 objects (Weigl, 1966). It is found in modified form as a part of the Porch Index of Communicative Ability (Porch, 1970) and, in reduced form, is present as a subtest in many other aphasia test batteries. Extensive use has been made of the matching-to-sample paradigm as a means of "facilitating" correct responses on verbal tests requiring spoken or written responses in which errors appeared. Similar procedures have seen extensive use in production examinations of intermodality and intramodality performances in cases of surgical sections of the corpus callosum. Although time-consuming, tests of this sort can be easily used at the bedside and the stimulus materials readily carried in a small bag.

CONVERSATIONAL ASSESSMENT OF APHASIA

Most of the data on which a diagnosis of aphasia, its severity, and type is made are obtained by means of the conversational interaction during attempts at history taking. Yet even this limited exposure can yield useful data, if enough effort is made to ensure that the sample of behavior is guided to document the errors discussed in this section.

Error Patterns in Words

The structures grouped around the left sylvian fissure serve to discriminate, echo, and produce the phonologic stimuli used to convey language. When these systems are disturbed, the resulting abnormal activities are, in principle, failures in elemental afferent and efferent channels, such as the faulty oropharyngeal positionings from a weak tongue or oropharynx, the impaired discrimination of individual sounds or shapes from damaged pathways or primary sensory cortices, and the like. These disturbances are often referred to as *phonetic* errors in neurolinguistic parlance. The documentation of these disturbances is thought useful to separate them from disorders of higher function, which they often mimic and which are often difficult to study when phonetic errors predominate. If phonetic errors are gross enough, they may preclude further observations on other behaviors and require the examiner to try writing, drawing, or pointing responses for further testing.

Fiber pathways in the arcuate fasciculus, deep to the insula, may link the auditory and vocal motor regions to permit repeating aloud from dictation (Geschwind, 1965), although the role of this structure is still in dispute (see the later section on conduction aphasia). Damage to these connecting pathways produces substitutions of sounds, shapes, and sometimes whole syllables that share with the desired response a similarity of form or sound. In neurolinguistic terms, they are *phonemic*, not phonetic; in neurologic terms, dyspraxic, not paretic; and they are known traditionally as literal paraphasias. Like phonetic errors, they constitute an obstacle to the analysis of more complex language disturbances but are part of the usual picture of the communication disorder. A combination of phonetic and phonemic errors can make spoken responses all but incomprehensible, a state known as *jargon speech*. Although jargon speech often reflects serious disturbances in the language zone, in some cases it is not indicative of major language disturbance. To settle this point, tests involving selection of choices to dictated commands or manual responses to printed commands may help in the differentiation.

At a more complex level, that involving the organization and comprehension of conversational language, especially its semantic and syntactic aspects, the whole language zone has been thought to be involved, especially the posterior temporoparietal regions. Damage to these regions produces substitutions of whole words, sometimes whole phrases, for those intended; these errors are known as *verbal paraphasias* in all methods of classification. Erroneous responses consisting of words or phrases that bear some resemblance to the target responses in sound or shape, such as "through kink and keen" for "the king and queen," are known as *formal* verbal paraphasias. Those approximating the target word in meaning but not form, such as "the prince and duchess" for "the king and queen," are known as *semantic* verbal paraphasias. The occurrence of many such errors is the combination usually referred to as *Wernicke's aphasia*. Verbal paraphasias are a fairly reliable indication of aphasia from posterior hemispheral lesions. Because they rarely occur alone, they must be sought among the phonetic and phonemic errors that often accompany them. When the latter are plentiful, the task may not be an easy one. The analysis can be made more easily by emphasizing tests of repeating aloud, in which the examiner can at least be certain of the target words. Because such errors are common in normal individuals under stress, this assessment is sometimes best done by posing unusual questions to the patient—questions that might prompt a quizzical echoic response without arousing the patient's awareness that he or she is being specifically tested.

Errors in Conversation and Discourse

Lengthy responses permit observations on sentence structure and the sequence of utterances at paragraph length and longer. The disturbed coordination of breathing and speaking that occurs in small frontal lesions alters the rhythm of speech and results in a dysmelodic intonation of whole strings of words, an unsettling of the phrasing in parts of sentences, and even grossly inaccurate stress on syllables of longer words, a state known as *speech dyspraxia* or *dysprosody* (Alajouanine et al., 1939; Mohr, 1976).

In patients with larger lesions of the sylvian region, the utterances that are expected in full sentence form, usually accompanied by such filler words as "well," "you know," are dramatically condensed to the main predicative items and approach the simplified structure of a telegram. The terms *agrammatism* (Pick, 1913), *telegraphic speech* (Kleist, 1934), and *nonfluency* (Naeser et al., 1989) are in popular use to describe this finding. This latter term has previously suffered from its inherent ambiguity because it was not clear if the user meant the hesitancy, the dysmelodic flow of sounds, or the condensed grammar in the speech

of the patient. Each of the elements alone may reflect lesions other than those responsible for motor aphasia. However, the term, as currently defined, now encompasses all of the elements together: "effortful, dysmelodic speech, often with impaired articulation and impoverishment of grammatical form" (Knopman et al., 1983). With the current definition, the persistence of nonfluency correlates well with lesion size. Among the group of infarcts studied by Knopman et al. (1983), 10 of the 17 patients with persisting nonfluency had lesions with CT size measuring more than 100 cm^3; six lesions were larger than 25 cm^3, and only one was smaller. More recently, this nonfluency has been related to deeper lesions reaching the ventricular wall (Naeser et al., 1989).

Agrammatism, telegraphic speech, or dysfluency is part of a wider disorder in dealing with grammatical elements. The disturbance is also apparent when the patient is asked to point on command to single letters and small grammatical words, such as *c* and "are," to which errors occur more often than to "sea" and "ear." Even silent reading comprehension is disturbed if the materials emphasize grammatical elements, such as "give this to her, not to me."

In large lesions involving the posterior portions of the brain, the effects are almost the reverse of the insular-opercular syndromes: the structures of the sentences seem better preserved than the selection of words that give the sentences unique meaning, and speech flows more smoothly with most of the expected small grammatical words in place. However, with many of the predicative words either absent or substituted by verbal paraphasias, the otherwise adequately constructed utterances have little communicative value, a state known as *empty speech* (Benson, 1979). When such utterances contain many phonetic and phonemic errors, they may be completely incomprehensible. A similar disturbance affects attempts to understand the words heard or seen.

Little is known of the sites involved in the most complex, abstract levels of language activity, including such poorly understood activities referred to as preverbal thought (i.e., the formulation of the basic message to be conveyed) (Brown, 1972). Posterior and deep temporal lobe activity may underlie these processes. In the few patients analyzed in any detail, the discourse has approached that encountered in states of delirium. In some patients, the most remarkable feature has been the occurrence of grossly neologistic paraphasias in the place of the expected nouns, such as "that's a skert pladny," uttered with no hint of self-correction and easily written down on request to the astonishment of the examiner. For reasons not clear, this unusual syndrome seems to occur more commonly in patients with tumors and herpes simplex encephalitis but rarely in those with vascular disease. Thalamic activity appears important in maintaining a steady state in the cerebral structures involved in language, as some thalamic lesions mimic lesions in these areas. Most of the few patients documented with the syndrome have had small thalamic hemorrhages (Mohr et al., 1975), although some cases have been reported from infarction (Gorelick et al., 1984).

TRADITIONAL SYNDROMES

The following discussion is keyed to the syndromes that have eponyms or general descriptive terms, partly because of their common usage. Many studies of acquired language disorders have been made in patients with cerebrovascular disease. A convenient point from which to approach these syndromes is relating them to the usual site and size of stroke and emphasizing the differences with other etiologies as they apply. Fewer studies have been made of the syndromes of aphasia from other etiologies, but when such studies have been done surprising differences seem to exist in the syndromes associated with brain infarction and hemorrhage. Some differences are great enough to suggest that the insights into language function gleaned from the focal infarct model might be less general than has been thought.

In brain tumors, the syndromes of aphasia seem to feature more semantic and syntactic errors (Haas et al., 1982), more often found in the elderly, that are related to the histologic degree of malignancy but only slightly to lesion size and that are not well correlated with exact lesion location (Recht et al., 1989). After Mesulam's (1982) seminal work on a syndrome of progressive pure aphasia without dementia, which he ascribed to degenerative disease affecting the left perisylvian cortex, a flurry of reports on isolated aphasia as a presenting sign of various forms of disease appeared, including Alzheimer's disease (Pogacar and Williams, 1984), Pick's disease (Holland et al., 1985), Creutzfeldt-Jakob disease (Mandell et al., 1989), and a form of status spongiosis not further defined (Kirshner et al., 1987).

Wernicke's Aphasia

This syndrome is central to all writings on the aphasias. Damage to the putative Wernicke area is assumed to trigger not only the defective auditory comprehension but also the verbal and phonemic paraphasias and even, in some views, the disordered reading and writing. For some authors, this is the true aphasia, whereas Broca's aphasia is but a disturbance in motor function (Marie, 1906). Wernicke's aphasia has long been thought of as a unitary disorder (Benson and Geschwind, 1976) stemming from the locus of the lesion in the auditory zone, from which traditionalists inferred all language-related behavior arose (Wernicke, 1874). In support of this contention was the assumption that the same sort of phonemic and verbal paraphasias that contaminate speaking and writing were to be found in the disturbed comprehension of spoken and written language. Yet it has proved difficult to demonstrate the presumed disturbance in phonemic processing (Lecours et al., 1983); instead, the phonemes seem adequately discriminated but their linguistic significance seems poorly understood (Blumstein et al., 1977).

Furthermore, numerous cases have been found in which reading comprehension has proved superior to auditory comprehension and writing superior to oral naming (Hier and Mohr, 1977) and, in some instances, real words were read aloud when nonwords were not (Lytton and Brust, 1989). These findings are the reverse of the prediction that reading is subservient to auditory comprehension and that writing is dependent on speaking, and they suggest that different tasks utilize different pathways or behaviors. Evidence of this sort argues against a unitary nature of aphasia in general and the Wernicke aphasia syndrome in particular.

In the essential nature of Wernicke's aphasia, its pathoanatomic substrate is of special neurologic interest (Bogen and Bogen, 1976). For the school based on the notion of connectionism, it has been of some importance to show that the Wernicke area is a relatively small region from which fiber pathways project to other centers and is discrete enough to be disconnected from other regions of the brain. The postulation that the Wernicke area is contained in the posterosuperior temporal plane (Geschwind, 1969) fits both of these needs. Methods of lesion mapping almost always include at least this zone (Kertesz, 1983). Yet, the reason for the correlation may simply be that embolic occlusions of the lower division of the middle cerebral artery—the usual cause of Wernicke's aphasia—typically start at this point, where the lower division branches begin and spread varying distances distally.

Patients with Wernicke's aphasia with the lesion confined to the superior temporal plane are difficult to find (Mohr, 1980; Starr, 1889). Modern studies based on CT scanning show medium to large lesions (Mazzochi and Vignolo, 1979; Naeser, 1983). The autopsy literature is similarly unrewarding: In 1920, Henschen concluded that a superior temporal plane lesion did not cause the full picture of Wernicke's aphasia; he based his opinion on 35 cases with temporal lobe lesions and echoed the earlier work of Bastian. Mohr (1980) found that two of the three cases used to support the argument for a small lesion showed residue of an old subcortical (so-called slit) hemorrhage at autopsy years later; the hematomas presumably were large enough initially to trigger a picture of Wernicke's aphasia. Details on the third case (Kleist, 1934) were meager, but the patient was said to have had sensory aphasia for 2 months until another stroke altered the clinical picture.

Studies drawing on personally acquired case material seeking to document Wernicke's aphasia with small lesions have regularly found the lesions larger than the posterosuperior temporal plane. The four autopsied cases of Kertesz and Benson (1970) spread into the insula and supramarginal gyri, even into the angular gyri. Luria (1966) considered the superior temporal plane to be the Wernicke area, but his case material was of traumatic origin from World War II, a notoriously inadequate source material for precise localization. Benson and Geschwind (1976) claimed that severe alexia (part of the full Wernicke's aphasia syndrome) can arise from a lesion confined to the superior temporal plane and cited Nielsen's (1946) earlier report of 12 cases of Wernicke's aphasia in which the deficit included reading disturbances with lesions that spared the angular gyrus. Yet, three of these cases had been originally reported with no alexia; six others had large posterior sylvian lesions that included the superior temporal plane. Wernicke's original contribution (1874) left the issue of the size of the lesion in doubt.

Where documentation exists, the correlation is fairly high between the extent of the aphasia and the size of the lesion. Most patients showing the full syndrome of Wernicke's aphasia have a large infarct involving the posterior temporal, inferior parietal, and lateral temporo-occipital portions of the brain, or most of its posterior half (Mohr et al., 1978a, b). Naeser et al. (1987), in a study based on CT scanning, found that when the lesion affected half or less than half of the posterior temporal plane auditory comprehension was good within 6–13 months. Involvement of the parietal region did not add to the auditory comprehension disturbance.

Subcortical Sensory Aphasia: Pure Word Deafness

This rare disorder presumably represents the disruption of subcortical pathways from the ears to the main sensory language zone in the posterosuperior temporal plane. By classic disconnection criteria, the only deficit should be in auditory comprehension, but the clinical picture and the lesion site are not congruous. Schuster and Taterka's (1926) famous case was a disappointment: in the acute phase, paraphasic speaking existed for well over a month and when the patient was examined at 7 months, no tests of reading were performed. The autopsy revealed an old slit hemorrhage, somewhat disappointing material for precise correlation. Nielsen's (1946) case was reported with few clinical details, but the patient had a left superior temporal plane lesion. Eight well-known cases exist with a unilateral lesion confined to the superior temporal plane in the dominant hemisphere; in seven of the patients, paraphasic speaking was prominent. In many, however, the elements of paraphasic speech later cleared.

Many of the patients with bilateral lesions also experienced paraphasic speaking with poor comprehension during the acute phase of the stroke. In the famous case reported by Pick (1905), bilateral lesions, including a large left temporal plane lesion, left the patient paraphasic for 4 years. The deficit was only slight when she was examined by the author 10 years

later. Other cases of bilateral infarction described as pure word deafness (Coslett et al., 1984) have also shown paraphasic errors in spoken speech, often uncorrected, and in tests involving comprehension of printed words.

Transcortical Sensory Aphasia

This unusual syndrome was postulated in the early days of aphasiology as a consequence of disconnecting the sensory language zone from the centers of concepts, that is, other cortical regions that ordinarily receive projections from the sensory language zone to arouse associations that permit the appreciation of the meaning of sounds heard and perhaps also of words seen. Few examples have emerged over the years, and fewer still with documentation by autopsy or radiologic images. The clinical examples have often been patients with Alzheimer's disease, a state that comes closer to satisfying the anatomic requirements than most others; the lesions presumably have been of the cortical regions themselves, rather than of any putative transcortical pathways.

Kertesz et al. (1982) have risen to the challenge by using CT scans and the Western Aphasia Battery tests with patients satisfying criteria for the syndrome. The lesion was diagnosed by isotopic brain scan in 12 patients and by CT scan in 6. The lesions were rather large and involved the posterior half of the brain from the occipital pole forward on both the medial and lateral surfaces. In many of the patients, the lesions reached far forward along the mesial occipital lobe, but most were in the territory of the posterior cerebral artery. The high incidence of hemianopia, "visual agnosia," and sensory loss supports this location. Speech was described as fluent and circumlocutory, often semantic jargon. Strings of well-articulated and acceptable English words semantically not relevant to the questions or to the previous sentence were frequently observed. Comprehension was poor, and repetition was intact. This syndrome remains infrequently reported and its status is still unclear.

Alexia with Agraphia

Like many other classic syndromes, the clinical features and lesion sites of this disorder rarely agree with the predictions based on dogma. It is quite rare. Henschen (1920) uncovered a mere 5 pure cases; in more than 250 others, dyslexia and dysgraphia were part of a larger clinical syndrome, one often including paraphasia in speaking.

The disorder has been described (Benson and Geschwind, 1976) as a disturbance in reading comprehension and writing, with little or no disturbance in auditory comprehension or spontaneous speech. However, most patients have an aphasia that ranges from a minimal degree of word-finding difficulty to a more marked sensory aphasia with paraphasia and comprehension disturbance. In Dejerine's oft-quoted (1891) case, the patient suffered a lateral large parietal infarct that penetrated deep to the ventricle. Dejerine did not see the patient in the acute phase but found a striking disturbance in reading and writing that contrasted with the modest dysphasia in conversation. deMassary (1934) suggested that Dejerine himself considered this form of alexia as a form of the syndrome of sensory aphasia, which is more evident when the patient is seen in the early phase of the stroke. This frequently underemphasized point is worthy of note, because examples of isolated alexia with agraphia at any stage of the syndrome are all but nonexistent. When such patients are studied in detail over time, the alexia with agraphia is seen to be relative at best and emerges from an earlier picture of Wernicke's aphasia (Sidman et al., 1971).

Conduction Aphasia

The existence of this syndrome is fundamental to connectionism and shows a separation between sensory and motor zones for language. The syndrome is defined as poor repetition with normal auditory and visual comprehension of language, thus reflecting the basic disorder as a lesion in the pathway conveying instructions from the sensory language zone to the motor zone and involving the arcuate fasciculus (Benson and Geschwind, 1976; Benson et al., 1973). Yet, the available clinical and anatomic evidence does not support the prediction of a predominantly subcortical lesion. The documented lesions (Benson et al., 1973) have all been superficial infarcts, with considerable variation in their subcortical penetration. In some patients, the infarction was only superficial.

More than 20 cases with CT or autopsy correlation have been reported with this syndrome, and many patients show the lesion located in the same area usually attributed to Wernicke's aphasia. Naeser (1983) found no difference in the lesion size per slice in cases with conduction or Wernicke's aphasia, although the mean size of the left hemisphere lesion was larger in the patients with Wernicke's aphasia than in those with conduction aphasia. The theory has been rescued somewhat by H. Damasio and Damasio's (1983) postulates that two projecting systems may exist and may be susceptible to injury even by superficial lesions. Their cases were not pure, however; some degree of disturbance in auditory and reading comprehension was present. In a positron emission tomographic study of conduction aphasia, one-half of the patients failed to show the predicted hypometabolism in the inferior frontal region. The authors proposed a model whereby conduction aphasia is the result of damage to the perisylvian cortex and not primarily a disconnection syndrome (Kempler et al., 1988).

These unsettling clinical and anatomic findings

have done little to resolve the long-standing arguments on the fundamental nature of the syndrome, although fewer claims are now heard that the syndrome does not even exist. Wernicke (1874) first proposed it as a disconnection but was satisfied of its existence in only one case. Goldstein (1948) viewed the disorder as a sign of disruption of a brain region located between the major sensory and motor centers and emphasized the central, but not so much the conduction, aspects. Luria (1966) coined the term afferent motor aphasia to represent his view that it was a disturbance in kinesthetic feedback caused by a superficial lesion of the sylvian operculum posterior to the rolandic fissure, as has been demonstrated in at least one case documented by CT scan (Lhermitte et al., 1980). One of the early authors who was aware that the syndrome could result from an infarction of the posterosuperior temporal plane, Kleist (1934) speculated on mixed hemisphere dominance that could produce conduction aphasia instead of the expected Wernicke's aphasia.

In clinical studies, spontaneous speech is often contaminated by paraphasic utterances, and auditory and visual language comprehension is impaired at any stage of the disorder. The disturbance in repeating aloud, on which great stress has been laid, is not a useful distinguishing point from Wernicke's aphasia in the acute stage of the syndrome (Burns and Cantor, 1977), although conduction aphasics make a greater effort at self-correction (Benson, 1979). The syndrome is often diagnosed as Wernicke's aphasia initially and as conduction aphasia later. Many patients show some degree of decreased auditory comprehension when tested, but their ability to read aloud and to comprehend is so much superior that they do not easily qualify for the full syndrome of Wernicke's aphasia, as traditionally defined; however, they could easily be described as examples of the mild form of Wernicke's aphasia (Hier and Mohr, 1977).

Broca's Aphasia

If Wernicke's aphasia is a concept filled with contradictions and incomplete documentation for dogma, those applicable in Broca's aphasia are at least a bit better understood. Classically, the syndrome represents a defect in skills involving the act of speaking, together with a disturbance in the organization of language (agrammatism) attributed to a lesion confined to the third frontal gyrus (Broca area) (Broca, 1861). Each point has been well documented but, except in rare cases, not all three together. One patient, a 60-year-old man, was described by Van Gehuchten (1974). He experienced sudden total loss of speech with right upper limb paresis and a small amount of facial involvement. Although the weakness improved, the speech disturbance remained unchanged until his death 1 year later. The patient was incapable of speaking. He uttered only a few sounds and sometimes a word or two. However, he expressed himself adequately by gestures and wrote some letters and ordinary words from dictation, but he was unable to write spontaneously or from dictation under demanding circumstances. Van Gehuchten characterized the syndrome as "pure motor aphasia with agraphia with no word blindness or deafness." Autopsy revealed an infarct involving the inferior half of the middle frontal gyrus from the top to the bottom of what was described as the Broca area. The published photograph did not indicate the involvement or sparing of the insula or whether the lesion extended deep into the brain.

Such cases are decidedly rare. No other case known to the author has produced a lasting severe Broca's aphasia (Mohr, 1976). An infarction in the Broca area usually precipitates complete mutism, ideomotor buccofacial dyspraxia, and virtually normal auditory and visual comprehension; many patients can write properly with the unaffected left hand. Evidence of grammatical condensation and simplified sentence structure is rare. The mutism often fades within days, rarely weeks, and any language deficit evident by careful testing usually disappears quickly, along with the buccolinguofacial dyspraxia. Although contralateral hemiparesis may occur, some patients are completely spared (Bramwell, 1898; Masdeu and O'Hara, 1983). Others become fluent after a few months and appear abnormal only to those persons who are most familiar with their daily routines.

The disturbance in the small number of cases of infarction in the lower rolandic region has been similar but lacks any evidence of language disorder (Mohr et al., 1978a,b). However, one patient had persisting Broca's aphasia with infarction limited to the cortex and subcortical white matter of the precentral gyrus but sparing the deeper structures and largely sparing the adjacent third frontal convolution (Trojanowski et al., 1980). This case is important because it resurrects theories of a lower rolandic role in Broca's aphasia (Levine and Sweet, 1983). Another case, described as Broca's aphasia, mainly involved disturbance in speech praxis and dysgraphia, with no agrammatism or disturbance in comprehension of auditory or visual language comprehension (Mori et al., 1989), but the disturbance persisted for some 3 years until death. Using CT scanning for veterans of the Vietnam conflict, Ludlow et al. (1986) showed that subcortical penetration of the missile greatly added to the persistence of nonfluency and that the posterior extension of the lesion also added to the degree of language disturbance.

Alexander et al. (1990) have demonstrated several distinct and overlapping subtypes of speech disorder from infarcts confined to the frontal operculum, including the inferior rolandic region, but have also documented some degree of individual variability in the syndrome from a given small focal lesion. Although all modern studies argue against Broca's original claim that a small, focal opercular infarction causes the full syndrome of Broca's aphasia, each

study has shown enough variation in the minor syndromes to predict that the factor of individual variation will continue to plague efforts to force an exact and stable correlation between a given lesion site and syndrome.

Broca's aphasia usually results from a major infarction involving most of the insula, upper and lower opercula, and adjacent regions surrounding the sylvian fissure (Mohr et al., 1978a, b). The diagnosis is made easier by the accompanying disturbances in motor, sensory, and visual function, effects that are occasionally minimized when the lesion is confined to the insula and operculum alone. In these cases of large infarcts, the agrammatism is evident in tests of comprehension, as well as in speaking and writing. The disturbances are especially evident in responses to spoken or written material that feature small grammatical words, such as "the," "are," and "then," or involve spelling. Silent reading comprehension, which requires no overt vocalization, is disturbed, especially with material containing a particularly high density of such grammatical words, a condition termed *deep dyslexia* (Benson, 1977). Finally, Broca's aphasia is rarely an acute syndrome. With the typical lesion that produces the syndrome, the acute clinical picture features global aphasia, which yields to Broca's aphasia only after some weeks or months.

Subcortical Motor Aphasia

Classic formulations included the notion that a subcortical lesion or lesions could interrupt efferent pathways from the motor speech zone to the bulbar apparatus, thus producing mutism with paralysis of the face, oropharynx, and tongue. Among the famous cases was Bonhoeffer's (1914) patient, who had a large, deep infarct in the striatum and capsule and a second infarct in the cortical surface territory of the anterior cerebral. The patient spoke only a few poorly formed vowels. The syndrome was formulated as a double disconnection from the Broca area: the giant lacuna prevented innervation of the bulbar apparatus from ipsilateral pathways, and the anterior cerebral territory infarct cut off transcallosal projections.

A few cases have been described from unilateral lesion alone. Marie (1906) used the term anarthria for a patient with a putaminal hemorrhage but with no aphasic symptoms. In Kleist's (1934) case, the patient had a large, deep infarct involving the putamen, caudate, both limbs of the internal capsule, and much of the corona radiata and centrum semiovale. The patient showed severe dysarthria and rare paraphasias but little disturbance in comprehension. In Fisher's (1979) case of "modified PMH with 'motor aphasia'" the patient had a large infarct of the genu and anterior limb of the internal capsule that included the adjacent corona radiata. Dysarthria worsened to single syllables, unintelligible sounds, and finally mutism, but comprehension remained intact.

Apart from these cases, in which the syndrome can be formulated as severe pareses of the speech apparatus, a few others have been described in which a single deep infarct has produced enough disturbance in speech and language to warrant the term aphasia. Typical of the individual cases reported was that of Santamaria et al. (1983), described as an "expressive dysphasia" featuring "non-fluent conversational speech, naming and reading difficulties, dysgraphia, and normal auditory comprehension." A mixture of deficits in syntactic and semantic functions not typical for any of the classic syndromes of dysphasia, in addition to a remarkable dysprosody, at times accompanied by dysarthria, and with little or no dyspraxia of limbs on either side, was reported by A.R. Damasio et al. (1982) in six patients diagnosed by CT scan and in seven by Naeser et al. (1982). At least three of the latter had accompanying surface infarcts, a finding that may indicate the main language disturbance represents surface disease, not infarction in the depths. In the others patients, however, the CT findings were predominantly in the anterior limb of the internal capsule, putamen, and caudate. The meaning of these cases remains unclear at present, but they open the path to reconsideration of deep aphasias.

Mixed Transcortical Motor Aphasia

Claims have been made for a form of transcortical aphasia, which is mixed, that is, with combined motor and sensory components. The syndrome is said to be characterized by nonfluent spontaneous speech and poor naming and comprehension but with preserved repetition. Earlier called the syndrome of isolation of the speech area (Geschwind et al., 1968), its essence, to the extent it can be said to have one, is the preservation of repetition when the remainder of speech and language functions are deranged. There is little wonder that a wide variety of lesion locations have been described with this condition, most of which lie away from the sylvian area. Included are the distal field or watershed infarcts that occur in carotid occlusive disease (Bogousslavsky et al., 1988), multiple infarcts (Assal et al., 1983), and infarcts of the supplementary motor area after subarachnoid hemorrhage (Ross, 1980) and in the late stages after global aphasia. Unhappily, the preserved repeating aloud with poor speech and language function is also observed in states of intoxication and in dementia, to name but a few, and thus far the postulates of this syndrome seem more to represent an attempt to preserve the connectionist model for language disturbances than to provide help in differential diagnosis of the lesion location or clinical features of speech or language syndromes.

Amnestic Aphasia

This disorder, separate from the major syndromes of Wernicke's and Broca's aphasias, is characterized by a failure to recall the names of people, as well as many other individual nouns, when the stimuli are presented in visual or auditory form. Instead of paraphasic errors, however, the amnestic aphasic usually merely fails to respond, often falling silent or hesitating as if the name is about to be produced momentarily ("tip of the tongue" effect). Often, the patient indicates familiarity with the missing name by describing attributes of the item, engages in circumlocution, or, occasionally, offers lame excuses for failure, testimonials of prowess in other areas, or protestations that such testing is irrelevant. Although not invariable, it is a common finding that the correct name is accepted among choices offered. A surprising specificity of the errors may occur, with the names of same items repeatedly failing to occur, and other items in the same stimulus class (i.e., fruits) named without hesitation.

Amnestic aphasia is considered classically as a sign of deep temporal lobe involvement but has been reported from posterior cerebral artery territory infarction in the dominant hemisphere (Wyllie, 1894).

OUTCOME

Although the most common preoccupation of the harried clinician is to characterize the nature of the aphasic deficit quickly in the acute stage only for the purpose of diagnosis, other clinicians are equally preoccupied with the predictions of outcome. Because the initial clinical contact with the patient is often brief, the sample of behavior from which predictions are made may prove frustratingly small, especially when the physician is confronted by the family. Each family member usually has a special anecdote concerning the patient's behavior and requests the physician to comment on its significance. The following observations are noted in the hope of easing this burden on all participants.

When the disease has acutely erased interpersonal communication using words as sounds or sights and shuts off speech, the outlook for a good functional result is poor unless the cause is epilepsy and the state is immediately postictal. This grim outlook applies equally to those who have no interpersonal communication but can say a few words; verbal stereotypes, such as "hello," "yes," "home," are but another sign of the heavy damage to the language mechanism. Interpersonal communication using gestures or tone of voice with high emotional contact (e.g., threats, supplications), shoulder shrugs, nods, and pantomime often succeeds even in these circumstances but should not be taken as hopeful prognostic signs. They may merely provide misleadingly encouraging indications of functions of the nondominant hemisphere.

Regardless of the cause of the disorder, the less the evidence of language disturbance and the more the deficit can be found confined to disturbances at the phonetic level, in either speech comprehension or production, the smaller the lesion and the better the prognosis. In particular, isolated mutism from a small surface infarct, even in the Broca area, has an excellent functional prognosis, often apparent within days to weeks. When the lesion extends deep into the inferior frontal region, the prognosis for functional speech recovery is poor (Kleist, 1934; Naeser et al., 1989). For reasons still obscure, instances of Wernicke's aphasia with fairly small surface infarcts may undergo striking improvement within the same time frame. Hematomas of the thalamus, which produce such a striking aphasic delirium acutely, usually have little or no permanent residual deficit, although a period of many weeks may occur before improvement begins. There are some exceptions. When bilateral lesions occur in approximately the same location, the initial deficit, even if confined to a disorder at the phonetic level, often is slow to improve and may stabilize at a disappointingly low level. Some deficits, especially the cortical deafness from bilateral disease, may be permanent with little improvement from the start. When alexia occurs from an extensive posterior cerebral infarct in the hemisphere dominant for language, the effect is usually permanent. In these cases, the guide to the prognosis is whether the alexia is absolute. Even the slightest residual reading skill at the extremes of vision is a hopeful sign that the dyslexia is part of a temporary, albeit severe, hemineglect syndrome.

Therapy for impaired speech and language function is a good plan from the first day. At most, the patient may quickly reacquire the impaired skills and shorten the period of disability. In many, it serves to document the rate of improvement. In the worst case, although little benefits can be documented, the grieving family is aware that the clinical team is doing the most that can be done.

References

(Key references are designated with an asterisk.)

Alajouanine T., Ombredane A., Durand M. *Le Syndrome de Désintégration Phonetique dans L'Aphasie.* Paris, Masson, 1939.

Albert M.L., Goodglass H., Helm N.A., et al. *Clinical Aspects of Dysphasia.* New York, Springer-Verlag, 1981.

Alexander M.P., Naeser M.A., Palumbo C. Broca's area aphasias. Aphasia after lesions including the frontal operculum. *Neurology* 40:353, 1990.

Assal G., Regli F., Thuillard F., et al. Syndrome d'isolement de la zone du langage: étude neuropsychologique et pathologique. *Rev. Neurol. (Paris)* 139:417, 1983.

Benson D.F. The third alexia. *Arch. Neurol.* 36:317, 1977.

Benson D.F. *Aphasia, Alexia and Agraphia.* New York, Churchill Livingstone, 1979.

Benson D.F., Geschwind N. The aphasias and related disorders. In Baker A.B., Baker L.H., eds. *Clinical Neurology.* Vol. 1. Hagerstown, MD, Harper & Row, 1976.

Benson D.F., Sheremata W.A., Bouchard R., et al. Conduction aphasia. *Arch. Neurol.* 28:339, 1973.

Blumstein S.E., Baker E., Goodglass H. Phonological factors in auditory comprehension in aphasia. *Neuropsychologia* 15:19, 1977.

*Bogen J.E., Bogen G.M. Wernicke's region—where is it? *Ann. N. Y. Acad. Sci.* 280:834, 1976.

Bogousslavsky J., Regli F., Assal G. Acute transcortical aphasia. *Brain* 111:631, 1988.

Bonhoeffer K. Klinischer und anatomischer Befund zur Lehre von der Apraxie und der "Motorischen Sprachbahn." *Monatsschr. Psychiatr. Neurol.* 35:113, 1914.

Bramwell B. A remarkable case of aphasia. *Brain* 21:343, 1898.

*Broca P. Remarques sur le siège de la faculté du langage articulé, suivies d'une observation d'aphemie (père de la parole). *Bull. Soc. Anat. Paris* 6:330, 1861.

Brown J.W. *Aphasia, Apraxia, and Agnosia.* Springfield, IL, Thomas, 1972.

Burns M.S., Cantor C.J. Phonemic behavior of aphasic patients with posterior cerebral languages. *Brain Lang.* 4:492, 1977.

Chesher E.D. Aphasia. *Bull. Neurol. Inst.* 6:134, 1937.

Coslett H.B., Saffran E.M. Evidence for preserved reading in "pure alexia." *Brain* 112:327, 1989.

Critchley M. *Aphasiology and Other Aspects of Language.* London, Edward Arnold, 1970.

Damasio A.R., Damasio H., Rizzo M., et al. Aphasia with non-hemorrhagic lesions of the basal ganglia and the internal capsule. *Arch. Neurol.* 39:15, 1982.

Damasio H., Damasio A.R. Localization of lesions in conduction aphasia. In Kertesz A., ed. *Localization in Neuropsychology.* New York, Academic Press, 1983.

Dejerine J. Sur un cas de cécité verbale avec agraphie, suivi d'autopsie. *Mem. Soc. Biol.* 3:197, 1891.

Dejerine J., Mirallie C. *L'Aphasie Sensorielle.* Paris, Steinheil, 1896.

deMassary J. L'alexie. *Encephale* 27:134, 1934.

Eisenson J. *Examining for Aphasia.* New York, Psychological Corporation, 1954.

Fisher C.M. Capsular infarcts. *Arch. Neurol.* 36:65, 1979.

Foix C. Aphasies. In Roger G.H., Widal F., Teissier P.J., eds. *Nouveau Triete de Médicine.* Vol. 18. Paris, Masson et Cie, 1928.

Geschwind N. Disconnexion syndromes in animals and man. Parts 1 and 2. *Brain* 88:237, 585, 1965.

*Geschwind N. *Selected Papers on Language and the Brain.* Boston, Reidel, 1974.

Geschwind N., Quadfasel F.A., Segarra J.M. Isolation of the speech area. *Neuropsychologia* 6:327, 1968.

*Goldstein K. *Language and Language Disturbances.* New York, Grune & Stratton, 1948.

Goodglass H., Kaplan E. *The Assessment of Aphasia and Related Disorders.* Philadelphia, Lee & Febiger, 1972.

Gorelick P.B., Hier D.B., Beevento L., et al. Aphasia after left thalamic infarction. *Arch. Neurol.* 41:1296, 1984.

Haas J., Vogt G., Schiemann M., et al. Aphasia and non-verbal intelligence in brain tumour patients. *J. Neurol.* 227:209–218, 1982.

Head H. *Aphasia and Kindred Disorders of Speech.* London, Cambridge University Press, 1926.

Hecaen H., Albert M.L. *Human Neuropsychology.* New York, Wiley, 1978.

Henschen S.E. *Klinische und anatomische Beitrage zur Pathologie des Gehirns.* Stockholm, Nordiska Bokhandeln, 1920.

Hier D.B., Mohr J.P. Incongruous oral and written naming. Evidence for a subdivision of the syndrome of Wernicke's aphasia. *Brain Lang.* 4:115, 1977.

Holland A.L., McBurney D.H., Moossy J., et al. The dissolution of language in Pick's disease with neurofibrillary tangles: a case study. *Brain Lang.* 24:36, 1985.

Kempler D., Metter E.J., Jackson C.A., et al. Disconnection and cerebral metabolism. *Arch. Neurol.* 45:275, 1988.

Kertesz A. Localization of lesions in Wernicke's aphasia. In Kertesz A., ed. *Localization in Neuropsychology.* New York, Academic Press, 1983.

Kertesz A., Benson D.F. Neologistic jargon: a clinical pathological study. *Cortex* 6:362, 1970.

Kertesz A., Poole E. The aphasia quotient: the taxonomic approach to measurement of aphasic disability. *Can. J. Neurol. Sci.* 1:7, 1974.

Kertesz A., Sheppard A., MacKenzie R. Localization in transcortical sensory aphasia. *Arch. Neurol.* 39:475, 1982.

Kirshner H.S., Tanridag O., Thurman L., et al. Progressive aphasia without dementia: two cases with focal spongiform degeneration. *Ann. Neurol.* 22:527–532, 1987.

Kleist K. *Gehirnpathologie.* Leipzig, Barth, 1934.

Knopman D.S., Selnes O.A., Niccum N., et al. A longitudinal

study of speech fluency in aphasia: CT correlates of recovery and persistent nonfluency. *Neurology (N.Y.)* 33:1170, 1983.

*Lecours A.R., Lhermitte F., Bryans B. *Aphasiology*. London, Bailliere Tindall, 1983.

Leicester J., Sidman M., Stoddard L.T., et al. The nature of aphasic responses. *Neuropsychologia* 9:141, 1971.

Levine D.N., Sweet E. Localization in lesions in Broca's motor aphasia. In Kertesz A., ed. *Localization in Neuropsychology*. New York, Academic Press, 1983.

Lhermitte F., Desi M., Signoret J.L., et al. Aphasie kinesthetique associée à un syndrome pseudothalamique. *Rev. Neurol. (Paris)* 136:675, 1980.

Lichtheim L. On aphasia. *Brain* 7:433, 1885.

Ludlow C.L., Rosenberg J., Fair C., et al. Brain lesions associated with nonfluent aphasia fifteen years following penetrating head injury. *Brain* 109:55, 1986.

*Luria A.R. *Higher Cortical Functions in Man*. New York, Basic Books, 1966.

Lytton W.W., Brust J.C.M. Direct dyslexia. *Brain* 112:583, 1989.

Mandell A.M., Alexander M.P., Carpenter S. Creutzfeldt-Jakob disease presenting as isolated aphasia. *Neurology* 39:55–58, 1989.

Marie P. Revision de la question de l'aphasie. *Semin. Med.* 26:241, 493, 565, 1906.

Masdeu J.C., O'Hara R.J. Motor aphasia unaccompanied by faciobrachial weakness. *Neurology (N.Y.)* 33:519, 1983.

Mazzochi F., Vignolo L.A. Localisation of lesions in aphasia: clinical-CT scan correlations in stroke patients. *Cortex* 15:627, 1979.

Mesulam M.M. Slowly progressive aphasia without generalized dementia. *Ann. Neurol.* 11:592, 1982.

Mohr J.P. Broca's area and Broca's aphasia. In Whitaker H., ed. *Studies in Neurolinguistics*. New York, Academic Press, 1976.

Mohr J.P. The vascular basis of Wernicke aphasia. *Trans. Am. Neurol. Assoc.* 105:133, 1980.

Mohr J.P., Watters W.E., Duncan G.W. Thalamic hemorrhage and aphasia. *Brain Lang.* 2:3, 1975.

Mohr J.P., Pessin M.S., Finkelstein S., et al. Broca aphasia: pathologic and clinical aspects. *Neurology (N.Y.)* 28:311, 1978a.

Mohr J.P., Hier D.B., Kirshner H.S. Modality bias in Wernicke's aphasia (abstract). *Neurology (N.Y.)* 4:395, 1978b.

Mori E., Yamadori A., Furumoto M. Left precentral gyrus and Broca's aphasia. *Neurology* 39:51, 1989.

Naeser M.A. CT scan lesion size and lesion locus in cortical and subcortical aphasias. In Kertesz A., ed. *Localization in Neuropsychology*. New York, Academic Press, 1983.

Naeser M.A., Alexander M.P., Helm-Estabrooks N., et al. Aphasia with predominantly subcortical lesion sites: description of three capsular/putaminal aphasia syndromes. *Arch. Neurol.* 39:2–14, 1982.

*Naeser M.A., Helm-Estabrooks N., Haas G., et al. Relationship between lesion extent in "Wernicke's area" on computed to-

mographic scan and predicting recovery of comprehension in Wernicke's aphasia. *Arch. Neurol.* 44:73–82, 1987.

Naeser M.A., Palumbo C.L., Helm-Estabrooks N., et al. Severe nonfluency in aphasia. Role of the medial subcallosal fasciculus and other white matter pathways in recovery of spontaneous speech. *Brain* 112:1–38, 1989.

Nielsen J.M. *Agnosia, Apraxia, Aphasia*. New York, Hoeber, 1946.

Pick A. *Studien uber motorische Apraxie und ihre mahestehende Erscheinungen*. Liepzig, Deuticke, 1905.

Pogacar S., Williams R.S. Alzheimer's disease presenting as slowly progressive aphasia. *R. I. Med. J.* 67:181, 1984.

Porch B. *Porch Index of Communicative Abilities*. Palo Alto, CA, Consulting Psychologist Press, 1970.

Recht L.D., McCarthy K., O'Donnell B.F., et al. Tumor-associated aphasia in left hemisphere primary brain tumors: the importance of age and tumor grade. *Neurology* 39:48, 1989.

Ross E.D. Left medial parietal lobe and receptive language functions: mixed transcortical aphasia after left anterior cerebral artery territory infarction. *Neurology (N.Y.)* 30:144, 1980.

Rousseaux M., Steinling M., Griffie G., et al. Correlations de l'aphasie thalamique avec le débit sanguin cérébral. *Rev. Neurol. (Paris)* 146:345, 1990.

Ryding E., Bradvik B., Ingvar D.H. Changes in regional cerebral blood flow measured simultaneously in the right and left hemisphere during automatic speech and humming. *Brain* 110:1345, 1987.

Santamaria J., Graus F., Rubio F., et al. Cerebral infarction of the basal ganglia due to embolism from the heart. *Stroke* 14:911, 1983.

Schuster P., Taterka H. Beitrag zur Anatomie und Klinik der reinen Wourttaubheit. *Z. Neurol. Psychiatrie* 105:494, 1926.

Sidman M., Stoddard L.T., Mohr J.P., et al. Behavioral studies of aphasia: methods of investigations and analysis. *Neuropsychologia* 9:119, 1971.

Starr A. The pathology of sensory aphasia. *Brain* 12:82, 1889.

Trojanowski J.Q., Green R.C., Levine D.N. Crossed aphasia in a dextral: a clinical pathological study. *Neurology (N.Y.)* 30:709, 1980.

Van Gehuchten P. *The scientific work of Arthur Van Gehuchten*. Louvain, Francqui Fondation, 1974.

Viader F., Lechevalier B., Eustache F., et al. Un cas d'aphasie avec troubles du discours par infarctus des noyaux caudé et lenticulaire gauches. *Rev. Neurol. (Paris)* 143:814–822, 1987.

Weigl E. On the construction of standard psychological tests in cases of brain damage. *J. Neurol. Sci.* 3:123, 1966.

Weisenberg T., McBride K. *Aphasia: A Clinical and Psychological Study*. New York, Hafner, 1935.

Wernicke C. *Der aphasische Symptomcomplex*. Breslau, Cohn & Weigert, 1874.

Wyllie J. *The Disorders of Speech*. Edinburgh, Oliver & Boyd, 1894.

54

The Agnosias

Antonio R. Damasio
Daniel Tranel
Paul Eslinger

The mastering of the concept of agnosia and its application to diagnosis are complex but necessary tasks for neurologists and researchers in cognitive neuroscience. The appropriate detection of agnosia is essential for the understanding of many cerebral diseases, and the experimental study of agnosic syndromes is crucial to progress in the pathophysiology of higher nervous function.

The Greek-derived term *agnosia*, which signifies absence of knowledge, was introduced by Freud (1891) to designate impaired recognition of a stimulus, as distinct from the impaired naming that characterized aphasia. Since its inception (Lissauer, 1890), agnosia has been subdivided into two main forms: (1) *apperceptive*, referring to a recognition impairment that was caused by disturbed integration of otherwise normally perceived components of a stimulus; and (2) *associative*, referring to defective recognition of normally perceived and normally integrated percepts, and deemed a more pure recognition impairment. From a strict scientific perspective, this subdivision is not valid because it is based on the nonverifiable assumption that there is some point in the processing of a stimulus at which perception ends and recognition takes over. In practice, however, most agnosic patients can be reliably classified as apperceptive or associative, and the distinction appears to have consistent neural correlates.

The associative variety conforms to the modern definition of agnosia as articulated by Teuber (1968): "a normal percept that has somehow been stripped of its meaning." The authors' operational definition of associative agnosia is as follows: "a modality-specific impairment of the ability to recognize previously learned stimuli (or to recognize stimuli that would normally have been learned after adequate exposure) that cannot be attributed to disturbances of intellect, language, or perception and that results from acquired cerebral damage."

A reference to current models of learning and recognition can facilitate the understanding of this problem. The authors' account of the neural substrates of recognition is based on a systems-level model of learning and memory (A.R. Damasio, 1989a,b). Briefly, the model posits that: (1) the representations of the physical properties of entities at feature level are inscribed in anatomically separate regions of early sensory and motor cortices in fragmented fashion. The patterns of neural activity that correspond to different features of entities are thus recorded, in a distributed manner, in the same neural ensembles that were engaged during perception. (2) The integration of varied aspects of external and internal reality, in both perception and recall, depends on the time-locked activation of those geographically separate sites of neural activity. (3) Separate neural ensembles, called *convergence zones*, are used to record the combinatorial codes that hold the recipes for binding features into entities and entities into events (i.e., their spatial and temporal coincidences). (4) Feedforward and feedback projections are used to interconnect (a) the separate cortical regions that record featural fragments and (b) the convergence zones that record the combinatorial binding codes that correspond to their linkage in previous perceptual or recorded experiences. Convergence zones can trigger and synchronize neural activity in a way that attempts to replicate patterns that were associated in previous experience. *Local* convergence zones are located near early sensory and motor cortices and bind featural components of entities; *nonlocal* convergence zones are located in later sensory association cortices and in higher-order, multimodal association cortices and bind more complex entities and events.

Confronted with a previously known stimulus in a given modality, the agnosic patient fails to experience any familiarity i.e., he or she is unable to evoke relevant relationships of the stimulus both in nonverbal and in verbal terms and thus cannot arrive at its meaning. Recognition of the same stimulus occurs normally when the presentation is made in a nonaffected modality (e.g., the patient who fails to recognize the face of a friend rapidly recognizes the voice that belongs to that face), a fact that establishes the intactness of memories pertinent to the stimulus and that underscores the circumscribed nature of the defect. It should be clear, then, that agnosia is not limited to an inability to conjure the name of a stimulus or verbal associations of a stimulus, disturbances that should be classified under anomia. Agnosia is a pervasive defect of the evocation of extensive knowledge, verbal and nonverbal, related to a stimulus when the stimulus is presented in the affected modality.

The proper analysis of associative agnosia is based on the establishment that (1) the defect is not limited to an inability to name or describe verbally the stimulus in question and does correspond to a paucity of evocation of previous knowledge related to the stimulus; and (2) the impairment cannot be explained by a disturbance of the ability to perceive, or by a disorder of attention or problem solving.

It is necessary to confirm that the patient's language ability is normal. The ability to converse and give a verbal report of experience must be intact.

The integrity of perception in the affected modality is just as important to demonstrate. A large degree of perceptual impairment may not be compatible with normal recognition; in certain cases, this presentation conforms to apperceptive agnosia (see later). The observer must make sure that the patient perceives enough of a stimulus to permit recognition. Finally, attention to the task and the patient's intention to cooperate with the observer, as well as his or her problem-solving ability, must be intact for the patient to qualify as agnosic. Most patients with true agnosia have normal intellect, although many patients with dementia, for instance of the Alzheimer's type, develop agnosia. It should be noted that, even in those cases, the intellectual impairment does not explain the agnosia. The notion that agnosia results from a combination of perceptual and intellectual defects (see Bay, 1953; Bender and Feldman, 1972) is not tenable.

The principal means to assess the experience of recognition is the verbal report of that experience. In most instances, provided language abilities are intact, this means is reliable for obtaining an account of multimodal sensory activity accessible to consciousness. One of the few exceptions to take into consideration is that of patients with callosal section who might be unable to give a verbal account of activity occurring in the nondominant hemisphere for language. The authors, however, have never encountered a case of agnosia in a patient with complete callosal section and are not aware that such has been described. Nonetheless, recognition can be investigated by other means. A nonagnosic subject can match the recognized stimulus with other stimuli that are meaningfully related and can reject the matching of unrelated items. For instance, given the object "pipe" as a stimulus, the subject may be asked to decide which objects within an adjoining group are directly related to it; the group should contain two or three items that are directly or indirectly connected to pipe and several others that bear no possible logical relationship. Such tasks, which are commonly used in the experimental study of recognition, do reduce language participation in the elaboration of responses and may be used with advantage in agnosic patients.

For research purposes, the process of recognition can also be evaluated by using indices of processes for which there is no awareness (e.g., autonomic responses). It has now been shown that patients with agnosia for faces may indeed respond, at an autonomic level, to a previously familiar face they are consciously unable to recognize (Tranel and Damasio, 1988) or to correct face-name pairs (Bauer, 1984). The finding indicates that some steps of the complex process of recognition are still taking place, although the outcome of those levels of operation is not made available to consciousness (i.e., is not experienced) and thus cannot be reported verbally or investigated by nonverbal matching tasks. But it must be clear that patients who show some index of covert recognition of a stimulus should still be diagnosed as agnosic.

Theoretically, agnosia can occur in relation to any sensory modality, and numerous instances of visual, auditory, and tactile agnosia have been described. In practice, however, the most unequivocal examples occur in the visual and auditory realms. The presentation, physiopathology, and pathologic correlates of visual and auditory agnosia are discussed here.

VISUAL AGNOSIA

The authors' operational definition of visual agnosia is as follows: "a disorder of recognition confined to the visual realm, in which an alert, attentive, nonaphasic patient fails to arrive at the meaning of some or all categories of previously known nonverbal visual stimuli. When visual perception is normal or near normal, the condition may be further designated as *associative* visual agnosia." As indicated in the general definition of agnosia, all patients also have an anterograde learning defect. Stimuli that would normally have been learned but for which there is a learning impairment will be encompassed in the agnosia.

The patient's neuro-ophthalmologic status should be assessed in detail. Patients with prosopagnosia generally have some form-vision field defect, often a superior quadrantanopia or a hemianopia. In the authors' experience, however, at least one-half, but more often three-fourths, of central vision is intact. Testing of visual acuity, which should be normal, and of perimetry and contrast sensitivity should be carried out. The examiner should obtain a verbal account of what the patient sees in the intact portion of the visual field. A wide variety of stimuli should be used—objects, faces, colors, meaningful and meaningless geometric forms, and signs. Real objects, as well as graphic representations, should be used. Static as well as moving stimuli should be shown. Accurate description of general shape, number, and position of stimuli establishes that visual form perception is normal. A statement by the patient that vision is blurred or foggy excludes the diagnosis of visual associative agnosia. When it is clear that patients apprehend the entire shape of a stimulus and yet fail to recognize it, the traditional classification *associative visual agnosia* applies. However, if the patient can only apprehend the shapes of fragments and cannot grasp the whole stimulus, the term *apperceptive visual agnosia* is more appropriate. Drawing stimuli from copy or matching a stimulus with the appropriate drawing or photograph of a similar stimulus indicates the patient's ability to perceive normally. Visual perception can be judged with more demanding tasks, such as the test of facial discrimination (Benton et al., 1983). Patients affected by associative visual agnosia perform normally or near normally in such procedures.

Prosopagnosia

Clinical Presentation

The term *prosopagnosia* was introduced by Bodamer (1947). The word derives from the Greek *prosopon* (for face) and *gnosis* (for knowledge); although this is an entirely well-formed medical term, it has proved somewhat misleading by suggesting that the agnosia is confined to human faces. The erroneous notion has been perpetuated in textbooks and review articles, but the defect is of a far greater magnitude, as later noted.

Prosopagnosia is a form of visual agnosia hallmarked by an inability to recognize previously known human faces or equivalent stimuli (the retrograde defect) and to learn new ones (the anterograde defect). The onset is almost always sudden. The patient realizes that his or her own face in the mirror or the well-known face of a relative or friend can no longer be recognized visually and appears unfamiliar. The voice easily gives away the identity of the unrecognized face, as do such clues as attire, posture, or accessories of clothing. The possibility of recognition through alternate channels underscores the intactness of a vast pool of pertinent memories, as well as the preservation of the means to formulate intelligent analyses of the environment. But prosopagnosics also become entirely unable to recognize their own cars or clothes, and they can neither recognize nor learn new buildings, landscapes, or even rooms, to name just the most frequently affected items. (The loss of topographic memory that is invariably noted in prosopagnosia is a special instance of the defect, if only one considers facades of buildings, landscapes, or decoration details as specific "faces" that require specific recognition and that can trigger appropriate associated memories.) If patients' activities call for the frequent recognition of visually similar items, they are at a loss. For instance, a bird watcher will no longer identify different species of birds and a farmer will no longer be able to recognize individual cows in the herd. Needless to say, the lack of human face recognition remains the symptom that patients most complain about and explains why the impairment for other stimuli has often been overlooked.

The ability to read may be intact, a striking dissociation of abilities that supports the notion of diverse template systems for different categories of stimuli within each modality. The absence or presence of alexia is closely associated with the anatomic placement of the left hemisphere component of the lesions in these patients. When the lesion encompasses both the left occipitotemporal region *and* the left periventricular region (the white matter beside, beneath, and behind the occipital horn), alexia coexists with prosopagnosia (A.R. Damasio and Damasio, 1983).

Most prosopagnosics also have an impairment of color perception (achromatopsia). The association of the defects is fortuitous, caused by contiguity of visual association areas that are damaged by the lesion. The loss of color perception is not likely to play a role in the impairment of recognition (one can recognize the black and white Ingrid Bergman and Humphrey Bogart of *Casablanca* without any difficulty). But in the authors' experience, some of these patients also have a defect in the appreciation of the visual processing of texture, and it is conceivable that such a disturbance might contribute to agnosia.

The presence of achromatopsia appears related to the caudalward extension into the occipitotemporal region in such a way that it damages or disconnects the inferior visual association cortex closest to the macular representation, which is generally located about the occipital pole (A. Damasio et al., 1980).

Physiopathologic Mechanism

Patients with prosopagnosia fail to recognize any stimuli that, as faces, belong to a group containing numerous, visually "ambiguous" members. The authors define visually ambiguous stimuli operationally, as stimuli that share the same type of subcomponents, spatially arranged in a similar way, and that can be distinguished only by small differences of shape or of those subcomponents. Human faces form a group of visually ambiguous stimuli, with numerous members. The specific recognition of those members is a social necessity, more often than not, and the survival value of this deceivingly simple ability is obvious. Automobiles, some food ingredients, or articles of clothing constitute other prominent groups of visually ambiguous stimuli. The separation of each specific item in those groups also depends on small distinguishing features.

The recognition of such ambiguous stimuli presupposes the discrimination of each individual stimulus within the visual system and the subsequent activation, both within and beyond the visual system, of a host of pertinently associated memories. The activation of this broad matrix of contextual material appears never to take place in prosopagnosia.

Prosopagnosics can recognize most objects in the environment, provided the examiner does not require recognition of a specific object within the group. Patients are able to recognize a piece of furniture or a car as, respectively, furniture and a car. They are not able, however, to discover if such an item belongs to them or to indicate the specific make of a given car. Patients perform a *generic*, superordinate recognition that clearly testifies to their knowledge of the class to which a stimulus belongs. However, the identification of a specific member within the generic class eludes these patients, and the subordinate placement of an item is no longer possible. This dissociation is especially dramatic with human faces. Prosopagnosics are unable to recognize any previously known face, including their own. Yet, they do know that a face is a face, and they can point to or name the eyes, ears, or nose of the observer or examiner, a test which should assure the examiner that a patient's perception of both the whole and the parts of a facial stimulus is intact. Thus, prosopagnosia is a defect of visually triggered memory for unique information. It is of interest to note that most prosopagnosic patients can perform complex perceptual tasks, whereas most patients with severe disturbances of visuospatial performance (e.g., neglect, visual disorientation) do not have prosopagnosia (Meier and French, 1965; Newcombe and Russell, 1969).

From a cognitive standpoint, face recognition is a process of relating *some* face records specific to a face to a set of *some* non–face records specific to the entity behind the face. At the identity level, the process of face recognition is one of conjuring up meaning for a familiar face in the form of a unique set of coactivated memoranda (i.e., recognition is subsidiary to recall of a pertinent set of memories). But not all levels and types of face processing are aimed at the same cognitive demands. Recognizing a facial expression among a limited set of possible facial expressions, although of great relevance in social interactions, requires evocation of a specific but nonunique set of memoranda.

In the authors' model (A.R. Damasio et al., 1990b), recognition of identity from faces depends on (1) the establishment of face records (records of the physical characteristics of a unique face, apprehended by vision); (2) the establishment of linkages between face records and non–face records (non–face records inscribe other characteristics pertinent to the entity);

and (3) access to 1 and 2, leading to simultaneous reactivation (recall), at a conscious level, of a set of non–face records sufficient for unequivocal identification of the possessor of the face.

The process described in 1 is necessary because the separation of extremely similar face patterns requires detailed mapping of face features and configurational arrangements to render records distinctive (A.R. Damasio et al., 1990a,b). As mentioned, parallel sources of information (e.g., telltale appendages, movement, special environmental context) do assist with disambiguation. However, the information available in the face alone is often enough, and thus there is a clear advantage to record as much of it as possible for each individual face. In other words, even if it can be argued that recognizing the identity of a given person can be successfully achieved without recording or accessing *all* physical details of a face, a perceiver is likely to recognize more quickly and accurately if the details are actually recorded and accessible. Incidentally, such detailed records are indeed laid down for faces of significant individuals, or it would not be possible for normal perceivers to recall the extraordinary amount of physical structure features that they do and to inspect these features and ensembles with the mind's eye.

The process described in 2 is necessary because visual records of face structure do not contain information relative to other characteristics of the entity behind the face (A.R. Damasio et al., 1982). It is necessary to link face records to non–face records, first during learning and later during recognition. Non–face records are both nonverbal and verbal. They include visual records, such as body parts, typical attire, typical context, and characteristic motion, and verbal information, such as names, certain demographic information, and other characteristic lexical descriptors of the entity.

For face recognition, then, the critical ingredient is the partial reconstruction of previous experiences related to a target face, which in turn depends on the simultaneous reconstruction of key sensory and motor components of those experiences. Viewing a familiar face leads to the activation of face records learned during previous exposures to the face, including the shape of face components, face contour, face motion during facial expressions and face turning, scan paths (transition of fixations) used to perceive all of the above, texture, and color. In turn, based on those many sources, combined or in isolation, non–face records acquired during previous exposures and pertinently associated with the familiar face also become activated. The success of recognition depends on the activation of a sufficiently comprehensive set of non–face records and face records in synchronous fashion. In other words, within approximately the same time window, the perceiver must not only see aspects of the face but also have an internally recalled experience of information that pertains uniquely to that face.

In cognitive terms, face agnosia can be caused by a disturbance at any point in this multicomponent process. For instance, some perceptual defects may preclude the activation of some types of face records, or the process that mediates activation of non–face records may be defective and fail to evoke a sufficient amount of pertinent information relative to an otherwise normal percept. It is also possible that the process may generate activations that fail to reach a level commensurate with conscious experience and thus go unattended. Such activations would not produce *evocations* but rather *covert* activity sufficient to influence behavior in some experimental paradigms, although not enough to generate conscious mental contents. In traditional psychologic terminology, one might say that these activations do not produce true recall or that they produce only partial recall.

The authors' account of the neural substrates of facial recognition is based on the application of their systems-level model of learning and memory, as outlined at the beginning of this chapter (A.R. Damasio, 1989a,b).

Drawing on this framework, the authors propose the following:

1. Face records are made up of a variety of fragmentary representations of the physical structure of faces and of processes used by the brain during repeated perception of such physical structures. They include unique shapes of face contour and face components, linkage codes for their spatial assembly, their spatial transformations as viewing perspectives change, and scan paths (transition of fixations) used and modified by repeated exposure.

2. Face records are bound by local convergence zones located in association cortices near and directly downstream from the cortices where separate face components or scan paths are represented. Such convergence zones thus subsume sets of descriptive characteristics for different faces (i.e., they represent amodally a combinatorial arrangement of characteristics), although no single convergence zone is presumed to subsume *all* traits of one face. Local convergence zones interact with other local convergence zones and also with non–local convergence zones located downstream in the system. The latter bind events in which a specific face has participated. When signaled by feedforward projections, non–local convergence zones project back to a multiplicity of sensory cortices—visual and not visual, verbal and nonverbal—where the components of events pertinent to a face (non–face records) can be simultaneously coactivated.

3. Face records are contained in posterior visual association cortices bilaterally (in functional regions within cytoarchitectonic fields 18, 19, 39, and 7) but are not evenly or symmetrically distributed in those cortices. This is a consequence of a particular anatomic and physiologic arrangement of the visual cortices. The processing of visual properties, such as shape, texture, color, and motion, depends on varied cellular channels and cortical regions within the visually related cortices, and such a functional segregation imposes a separation of the corresponding face records (A.R. Damasio, 1985; Livingstone and Hubel, 1988; Van Essen and Maunsell, 1983).

The evidence suggests persuasively that shape-related face records are probably based on inferior visual association cortices (i.e., the records and the binding local convergence zones are preferentially located in the inferior visual cortices). This is in agreement with behavior lesion data in both humans (A.R. Damasio, 1985) and nonhuman primates (Ungerleider and Mishkin, 1982). There is also preliminary evidence that static records might be skewed toward the left sector of those cortices, whereas records in which shape would be recorded dynamically with transformations around vertical and anteroposterior axes would be recorded in the right sector of the system. The findings in the authors' patients with unilateral occipital lesions speak to this point and so do studies of face processing in normal subjects (Ellis, 1983; Gazzaniga and Smylie, 1984; Sergent and Bindra, 1981). The mappings of linkages among face components, as related to scan paths over a unique face, are likely to depend on superiorly located cortices in the right occipitoparietal region (fields 18 and 19, as well as field 39 and perhaps 7), in keeping with the clear role of such cortices in motion detection, motion learning, and eye movement control.

4. Non–local convergence zones, on the basis of which event level information can be reconstituted, are located bilaterally in temporal neocortices of fields 20, 21, 22, 35, 36, and 37; in paralimbic and limbic fields 28 and 38, hippocampus and amygdala; in insular cortices; and in prefrontal cortices.

Recognition of a familiar face thus starts as face perception, in multiple visual association cortices, and terminates as synchronized multimodal recall, in multiple discrete cortical regions. The process starts in early cortices and returns to early cortices, recurrently and iteratively. By holding the record to pertinent combinatorial arrangements, convergence zones at all levels, local and nonlocal in early-, intermediate-, and high-order cortices, guide the process of recurrence and iteration.

Pathologic Correlates

Analysis of postmortem studies of prosopagnosia, as well as analysis of modern neuroimaging studies, such as computed tomography, magnetic resonance imaging, and emission tomography, reveals that most patients with prosopagnosia, in whom the defect persists beyond the acute period, prove to have bilateral lesions (Arseni and Botez, 1965; Benson et al., 1974; Bornstein, 1965; Brazis et al., 1981; Cohn et al., 1977; A.R. Damasio et al., 1982; Gloning et al., 1970; Hecaen and Angelergues, 1962; Heidenhain, 1927; Lhermitte et al., 1972; Nardelli et al., 1982; Pevzner et al., 1962; Wilbrand, 1892). The lesions compromise either the inferior and mesial visual association cortices, in the lingual and fusiform gyri, or their subjacent white matter. From the functional point of view, the lesions are approximately symmetric (i.e., they involve equivalent portions of the central visual system in the left and right hemispheres) (A.R. Damasio et al., 1982; Meadows, 1974).

Although the inferiorly located lesions can extend into parts of the superior visual association cortex in some patients, instances of prosopagnosia with bilateral lesions located exclusively in the superior visual association cortices have never been reported. There is additional evidence that right hemisphere lesions alone are not likely to cause prosopagnosia (i.e., patients with right hemispherectomy recognize faces normally) (A.R. Damasio et al., 1975), and split-brain patients have no difficulty recognizing faces presented separately, by tachistoscope, to each hemisphere (Levy et al., 1972). The authors believe that the value of human facial recognition is such that the process is generally represented in both hemispheres, although they have postulated that the mechanisms for facial learning and recognition are, in all likelihood, different in each hemisphere (A.R. Damasio et al., 1982). There is no doubt that the right hemisphere is far more efficient at facial recognition than the left.

A few exceptional cases have been reported in which prosopagnosia was caused by a lesion confined to the right hemisphere (A.R. Damasio et al., 1990b; De Renzi, 1986; Landis et al., 1986; Sergent and Villemure, 1989). These patients have difficulty in perceiving all parts of a visual array simultaneously and in generating the image of a whole entity where given a part. A related defect is the inability to assemble parts of a model into a meaningful ensemble (e.g., the patient may be unable to assemble various face parts to form a spatially correct whole). Such patients are properly termed apperceptive agnosics; unlike the associative agnosics who often have bilateral lesions of the type described earlier, the apperceptive patients fail many standard neuropsychologic tests of visual perception. From evidence available thus far, it appears that combined superior *and* inferior damage in right posterior association cortices is a requisite for prosopagnosia of this type (A.R. Damasio et al., 1990b; Landis et al., 1988).

Most cases of prosopagnosia are caused by cerebrovascular accidents, generally embolic, resulting from occlusion of branches of the posterior cerebral arteries. The authors have noted that the lesions may occur on different occasions, in some instances separated by months or years. In such cases, a first stroke may cause a mere upper quadrantic visual field defect, hemiachromatopsia, or alexia on the basis of a unilateral occipitotemporal lesion. Some time later, another stroke leads to the development of a second contralateral lesion that renders the patient agnosic.

Rarely, prosopagnosia may be caused by cerebral tumors, especially by gliomas originating in one occipital lobe that traverse to the opposite hemisphere via the splenium of the corpus callosum. Paroxysmal prosopagnosia is rare and is generally caused by bilateral epileptic foci or by a unilateral focus with momentary spreading to the opposite hemisphere as described by Agnetti et al. (1978). The authors have also seen it, just as rarely, as a circumscribed form of the elusive syndrome of transient amnesia in the setting of classic migraine.

Prosopagnosia can also occur as a consequence of herpes simplex encephalitis, a process that generally causes extensive, bilateral damage to temporal and occasionally mesial occipital regions. In the authors' experience with that disease, however, prosopagnosia is generally part of an extensive syndrome of amnesia in which the evocation of contextual memories from visual modalities, as well as other sensory modalities, was affected (A.R. Damasio et al., 1989).

Visual Object Agnosia

Visual object agnosia is both less frequent and less stable than prosopagnosia. The pathologic causes and clinical presentations are quite different. Visual object agnosia has most often been seen in the setting of large bilateral strokes or tumors of the occipital lobes, advanced degenerative dementia, and carbon monoxide poisoning. In patients in whom the lesion stabilizes, the syndrome may be preceded by cortical blindness and ultimately evolve to prosopagnosia. In the rare instances in which the condition is stable, the patients are behaviorally and anatomically distinct from those with prosopagnosia and have a far more pervasive disturbance. In addition to prosopagnosia, they have an inability to recognize even the generic class to which an object belongs (i.e., the patients do not know that a face is a face). They may also have a defect of visual naming, which in the presence of intact auditory and tactile naming is known as *optic aphasia* (Freud's rarely used term, 1889). In the authors' experience, such patients are invariably alexic. Some patients with object agnosia may suddenly "unblock" their agnosia and describe the use of the object or even name it if the actual object is moved slowly in front of them. Because of the effect of movement on performance, this defect has been called *static visual agnosia* (Botez, 1975). Components of the Balint syndrome, such as visual disorientation and optic ataxia, are often present.

Some patients with visual object agnosia complain of unclear, blurred vision, and they possibly have selective defects of spatial frequency vision. These patients do not fit the diagnosis of visual agnosia in the associative sense. At best they may be classified as visual apperceptive agnosics.

Visual object agnosia is associated with comparable but more extensive damage than prosopagnosia. There are bilateral lesions in the ventral and mesial parts of occipitotemporal visual areas that often extend dorsally and laterally. Exceptionally, it can be seen with unilateral *left* visual system lesions (Hecaen and Ajuariaguerra, 1956).

AUDITORY AGNOSIA

Many of the comments made in regard to visual agnosia are applicable to the auditory variety. A parallel operational definition is as follows: "a disorder of recognition confined to the auditory realm, in which an alert, attentive, and intelligent patient with normal auditory perception fails to arrive at the meaning of previously known nonverbal auditory stimuli."

In contrast to the definition of visual agnosia, it should be noted that aphasia is not an exclusionary criterion. In fact, because most patients with auditory agnosia have bilateral lesions of auditory cortex, some degree of aphasia is inevitably present. Nonetheless, the patients must have some form of intact language channel available so that they can still give reliable verbal testimony of their experience. In most patients, that intact channel is visual and the patient should be tested by being asked to read the examiner's questions and to write the appropriate answers. In spite of the presence of aphasia, patients often remain capable of giving an entirely satisfactory oral account of nonverbal experiences. It should be clear that although many cases of auditory agnosia are accompanied by aphasia, generally of the Wernicke type, the term agnosia refers only to the impairment of nonverbal sound recognition and is so used in the literature (Albert et al., 1972; Rubens, 1979; Vignolo, 1969). Thus, auditory agnosia may coexist with Wernicke's aphasia (word deafness), or with pure word deafness (patients with pure word deafness fail to comprehend and repeat words but produce normal, nonparaphasic speech, as described by Liepmann [1898] and Liepmann and Storch [1902]), and is invariably accompanied by a sensory amusia.

As with visual agnosia, auditory agnosia may be limited to the recognition of specific subordinate stimuli within a large class (e.g., the recognition of the voice of a friend or relative, the detection of the distinctive timbre of an opera singer or actor) or encompass the larger universe of generic, supraordinate sounds in the environment (e.g., the sound of a train whistling, musical sounds, the roar of a jet aircraft, the cry of a baby). Unlike visual agnosia, however, the more pervasive defect occurs more frequently than the circumscribed defect. Furthermore, if the distinction between apperceptive and associative agnosia is controversial for the visual domain, it is even more so for the auditory realm, and it could be argued that separate designations of apperceptive auditory agnosia and associative auditory agnosia are simply not valid (Anderson et al., 1991).

The patency of the auditory channel may be tested in several ways. At the bedside by means of written notes, the examiner can instruct the patient to raise a hand when he or she hears a sound produced outside the field of vision (standing behind the patient, the examiner can snap fingers or clap hands). The examiner may also have the patient repeat a finger-tapping pattern on a tabletop, for instance, two short and three long taps given without visual or vibratory cues. Correct detection of sounds or correct finger-tapping certainly indicates that the patient is hearing, but this form of bedside testing should be complemented by pure-tone audiometry, formal tests for recognition of recorded environmental sounds, and auditory evoked potentials.

In most instances, the disorder starts acutely and is accompanied by a severe auditory defect (i.e., the patient is entirely or almost entirely deaf). Either orally or by writing, the patient complains of complete, or almost complete, lack of hearing. It is not uncommon for this acute auditory deprivation to be accompanied by anxiety, agitation, and even socially inappropriate behavior. The diagnosis of agnosia does not apply at that point; the term *cortical deafness* is appropriate at that time. Many patients with cortical deafness evolve rapidly, and within days or weeks they report being able to hear sounds and clearly respond to the presence of sounds when blindfolded. If the audiometric pattern becomes normal and if the patient is still unable to recognize sounds, the diagnosis of auditory agnosia applies.

The following is an example of a typical presentation:

K.J. is a 27-year-old left-handed woman who complained of sudden deafness on October 22, 1982. She was taken to the emergency room of a local hospital where she arrived in great distress, reiterating that she could hear neither speech nor other sounds. Vision and somatic sensation were normal. There was no paralysis and no gait abnormality. Two weeks later, after no improvement was noted, she was referred to our care.

K.J. had fluent, effortless, well-articulated speech, but produced frequent semantic paraphasias. She was composed but concerned about her condition. Her auditory comprehension was impaired but written language and gestures were quite effective to communicate with her. Audiometry revealed a 40–50 dB loss at 125 Hz pure-tone stimulation, and stable 60–80 dB loss in the 250–8000 Hz range. Her comprehension of conversational speech was limited to occasional single words. She made obvious attempts to lip-read to aid comprehension. During tests of dichotic listening, sound recognition, and rhythm detection without visual or vibratory cues, K.J. could localize and thus appeared to hear many sounds despite being unable to recognize them. For instance, on presentation of a single word to one or the other ear by headphones, she could correctly localize in which ear each word was presented but could not indicate what word it was. Recognition of nonverbal sounds was also extremely poor. In a formal test of nonverbal recognition of recorded environmental sounds, she performed randomly. Reading comprehension of words, phrases, and simple sentences was normal but comprehension of complex sentences and paragraphs was impaired. Visual naming and tactile naming, as well as writing with her preferred hand, were normal.

Constructional ability, gestural praxis, visuospatial judgment, visuoperceptive discrimination of unfamiliar faces, and right-left discrimination were all normal. Intellectual abilities, assessed by a written form of the Wechsler Adult Intelligence Scale–Revised subtests, were average on the nonverbal section (45th percentile) but low average on the verbal section (13th percentile). K.J. was fully oriented to time, place, and personal information.

The initial computed tomographic scan on the day of onset had revealed a hypodense region in the right posterior temporal region, thought to represent an area of old infarction. No lesion was seen on the left. Cerebrospinal fluid examination and angiography results were both normal. Another computed tomographic scan 7 days later revealed lucencies in both the right *and* the left posterior temporal region. Single-photon emission tomography confirmed the presence of bilateral areas of reduced cerebral flow in the auditory regions.

Analysis of these data suggests that the patient first developed cortical deafness that evolved into a combined picture of auditory agnosia and Wernicke's aphasia. The emotional disturbance that characterized the onset was typical. Not infrequently, these patients are considered to be hysterical or even psychotic. The auditory disorders were related to bilateral lesions of the auditory cortices caused by strokes. In retrospect, it appears that the patient sustained the first of these strokes 2 years previously. During one interview, she described several episodes of left-hand numbness and what she called a "flying hand" that had occurred approximately 2 years before. She had to hold on to her left hand to control it. She did not seek medical attention for this. In all likelihood, these were the only signs of her previous stroke. The event involved the right auditory association cortex. The second stroke occurred at the time deafness started.

The authors have often seen this presentation of cortical deafness on the basis of "staged lesions," and always in a setting of cerebrovascular disease.

The bilaterality of the lesions is practically a rule, especially when patients have both auditory agnosia and aphasia (for an example of typical lesions and review of the literature, see Oppenheimer and Newcombe, 1978). Most patients with single lesions of the left or right auditory cortex can recognize environmental sounds normally, in laboratory tests and in situ. But some patients with such single, unilateral lesions may have defective performance in tests of sound recognition. The significance of such findings and their relation to recognition in situ have not been properly ascertained. In one instance, auditory agnosia (without aphasia) has been correlated with a single, unilateral lesion of the right hemisphere damaging the auditory cortex and the adjoining parietal, frontal, and insular cortices (Spreen et al., 1965). The authors believe the precise anatomic endowment necessary to recognize sounds is a highly variable individual feature that probably covaries with the anatomic endowment for language.

OTHER FORMS OF AGNOSIA

As indicated previously, it is theoretically possible to develop agnosia for any of the sensory modalities. But in practice, agnosia for modalities other than vision or audition is difficult to establish with certainty. Few studies have demonstrated convincingly a disturbance of tactile recognition in the absence of somatosensory impairment, although a study by Caselli (1991) reported several cases that conform closely to the characterization of tactile agnosia (see Semmes, 1965, for another similar exception).

Other alleged forms of agnosia have a debatable status. For instance, the designation *color agnosia* has been variably applied to patients with a defect in color naming, and to patients who fail to perceive color. To avoid error, the former is best designated as *color naming disorder,* because the objective findings are failure to name colors and to point to colors when given their names (in some extreme cases, a complete dissociation between names of colors and color perception probably does compromise the experience of color and might thus be conceptualized as an agnosia).

The designation *simultanagnosia* is a useful but misleading term; it stands for the phenomenon of *visual disorientation,* a perceptually related component of Balint's syndrome. Patients fail to perceive more than a fragment of the visual field at any one time, and that fragment of clear vision may shift from region to region rather erratically. As noted earlier, most of these patients generally recognize objects and faces, provided their erratic scanning does bring a crucial fragment into the central vision. Clearly, they do not have an agnosia. The problems with the term *anosognosia,* which designates a lack of awareness of disease, are similar. The physiopathology of the phenomenon is different from that of the agnosias and corresponds to a defect in higher-level cognitive integration (see A.R. Damasio et al., 1990c, for a related discussion).

CONCLUSION

The importance of the agnosias, both for the clinician and for the researcher, is apparent. The appropriate diagnosis of visual or auditory agnosia generally indicates the presence of bilateral cerebral dysfunction, most often caused by cerebrovascular disease in the territories, respectively, of the posterior cerebral arteries or the middle cerebral arteries. It is important for the clinician to realize the bilaterality of the process at the bedside as early as possible, because even the most modern imaging techniques may fail to reveal any or both areas of dysfunction early after onset. The appropriate diagnosis of agnosia is also important to avoid dangerous errors of clinical judgment. Patients with visual agnosia may appear demented, or their complaints may seem so bizarre as to raise doubts about their true nature. Similarly, in the acute phase of auditory agnosia, patients may be considered psychotic and time precious for potential treatment may be wasted. Needless to say, the rehabilitation of such patients depends quite remarkably on the accuracy of the diagnostic formulation.

From a research standpoint, the agnosias often provide ideal experiments of nature, essential for understanding the organization of human memory. A consensus is developing that most agnosias are disorders of sensorily triggered memory and that, in fact, it is possible to conceptualize the global amnesia syndromes as multiple agnosias. The important issue here is the discovery of a relation between specific structures within large networks, cortical and subcortical, and specific steps of complex physiologic mechanisms. The lesion method, especially now that advances in neuroimaging technology have greatly enhanced the ability to study changes in vivo, remains a fundamental approach to experimental work in the agnosias in humans (H. Damasio and Damasio, 1989).

References

(Key references are designated with an asterisk.)

Agnetti V., Carreras M., Pinna L., et al. Ictal prosopagnosia and epileptogenic damage of the dominant hemisphere: a case history. *Cortex* 14:57, 1978.

Albert M.L., Sparks R., von Stockert T., et al. A case study of auditory agnosia: linguistic and non-linguistic processing. *Cortex* 8:427–443, 1972.

Anderson S.W., Damasio H., Robin D.A., et al. Perceptual impairments following bilateral lesions in auditory cortex. *J. Clin. Exp. Neuropsychol.* 13:94, 1991.

Arseni C., Botez M. Consideracions sobre un caso de agnosia de las fisonomias. *Rev. Neuropsiquiatr.* 3:157–160, 1965.

Bauer R.M. Autonomic recognition of names and faces in prosopagnosia. *Neuropsychologia* 22:457–469, 1984.

Bay E. Disturbances of visual perception and their examination. *Brain* 76:515–550, 1953.

Bender M.B., Feldman M. The so-called "visual agnosias." *Brain* 9:173–186, 1972.

Benson D.F., Segarra J., Albert M.L. Visual agnosia-prosopagnosia. *Arch. Neurol.* 30:307–310, 1974.

Benton A.L., Hamsher K., Varney N.R., et al. *Contributions to Neuropsychological Assessment.* New York, Oxford University Press, 1983.

Bodamer J. Die Prosop-Agnosie. *Arch. Psychiatr. Nervenkr.* 179:6–54, 1947.

Bornstein B. Prosopagnosia. *8th International Congress of Neurology Proceedings* 3:157–160, 1965.

Botez M.I. Two visual systems in clinical neurology: readaptive role of the primitive system in visual agnosic patients. *Eur. Neurol.* 13:101–122, 1975.

Brazis P.W., Biller J., Fine M. Central achromatopsia (letter). *Neurology (N.Y.)* 31:920–921, 1981.

Caselli R.J. Rediscovering tactile agnosia. *Mayo Clin. Proc.* 66:129–142, 1991.

Cohn R., Neumann M.S., Wood D.H. Prosopagnosia: a clinicopathological study. *Ann. Neurol.* 1:177–182, 1977.

Damasio A.R. Disorders of complex visual processing: agnosias, achromatopsia, Balint's syndrome, and related difficulties of orientation and construction. In Mesulam M-M., ed. *Principles of Behavioral Neurology.* Philadelphia, Davis, pp. 259–288, 1985.

Damasio A.R. The brain binds entities and events by multiregional activation from convergence zones. *Neural Comput.* 1:123–132, 1989a.

*Damasio A.R. Time-locked multiregional retroactivation: a systems level proposal for the neural substrates of recall and recognition. *Cognition* 33:25–62, 1989b.

*Damasio A.R., Damasio H. The anatomic basis of pure alexia. *Neurology (N.Y.)* 33:1573–1583, 1983.

Damasio A.R., Lima P.A., Damasio H. Nervous function after right hemispherectomy. *Neurology (Minneap.)* 25:89–93, 1975.

Damasio A., Yamada T., Damasio H., et al. Central achromatopsia: behavioral, anatomical and physiologic aspects. *Neurology (N.Y.)* 30:1064–1071, 1980.

*Damasio A.R., Damasio H., Van Hoesen G.W. Prosopagnosia: anatomic basis and behavioral mechanisms. *Neurology (N.Y.)* 32:331–341, 1982.

Damasio A.R., Tranel D., Damasio H. Amnesia caused by herpes simplex encephalitis, infarctions in basal forebrain, Alzheimer's disease, and anoxia. In Boller F., Grafman J., eds. *Handbook of Neuropsychology.* Vol. 3. Amsterdam, Elsevier, pp. 149–166, 1989.

Damasio A.R., Damasio H., Tranel D. Impairments of visual recognition as clues to the processes of memory. In Edelman G., Gall E., Cowan M., eds. *Signal and Sense: Local and Global Order in Perceptual Maps.* New York, Wiley-Liss, pp. 451–473, 1990a.

*Damasio A.R., Tranel D., Damasio H. Face agnosia and the neural substrates of memory. *Annu. Rev. Neurosci.* 13:89–109, 1990b.

*Damasio A.R., Tranel D., Damasio H. Individuals with sociopathic behavior caused by frontal damage fail to respond autonomically to social stimuli. *Behav. Brain Res.* 41:81–94, 1990c.

*Damasio H., Damasio A.R. *Lesion Analysis in Neuropsychology.* New York, Oxford University Press, 1989.

De Renzi E. Prosopagnosia in two patients with CT scan evidence of damage confined to the right hemisphere. *Neuropsychologia* 24:385–389, 1986.

Ellis H.D. The role of the right hemisphere in face perception. In Young A.W., ed. *Functions of the Right Cerebral Hemisphere.* London, Academic Press, 1983.

Freud S. Zur ueber optische Aphasie und Seelenblindheit. *Arch. Psychiatr. Nervenkr.* 20:276–297, 371–416, 1889.

Freud S. *Zur Auffasung der Aphasien. Einekritische Studie.* Leipzig, Deuticke, 1891.

Gazzaniga M.S., Smylie C.S. Facial recognition and brain asymmetries: clues to underlying mechanisms. *Ann. Neurol.* 13:537–540, 1984.

Gloning I., Gloning K., Jellinger K., et al. A case of "prosopagnosia" with necropsy findings. *Neuropsychologia* 8:199–204, 1970.

Hecaen H., Ajuariaguerra J. Agnosie visuelle pour les objets inanimés par lésion unilatérale gauche. *Rev. Neurol. (Paris)* 94:222–233, 1956.

Hecaen H., Angelergues R. Agnosia for faces (prosopagnosia). *Arch. Neurol.* 7:92–100, 1962.

Heidenhain A. Beitrag zur Kenntnis der Seelenblindheit. *Monatsschr. Psychiatr. Neurol.* 66:61–116, 1927.

Landis T., Cummings J.L., Christen L., et al. Are unilateral right posterior cerebral lesions sufficient to cause prosopagnosia? Clinical and radiological findings in six additional patients. *Cortex* 22:243–252, 1986.

Landis T., Regard M., Bliestle A., et al. Prosopagnosia and agnosia for noncanonical views. *Brain* 111:1287–1297, 1988.

*Levy J., Trevarthen C., Sperry R.W. Perception of bilateral chimeric figures following hemispheric disconnection. *Brain* 95:61–78, 1972.

Lhermitte J., Chain F., Escourolle R., et al. Etude anatomo-clinique d'un cas de prosopagnosie. *Rev. Neurol. (Paris)* 126:329–346, 1972.

Liepmann H. Ein Fall von reiner Sprachtaubheit. In *Psychiatrische Abhandlungen* 1. Breslau, Schletter, 1898.

Liepmann H., Storch E. Der mikroskopische Gehirnbefund bei dem Fall Gorstelle. *Monatsschr. Psychiatr. Neurol.* 11:115–120, 1902.

Lissauer H. Ein Fall von Seelenblindheit nebst einem Beitrag zur Theorie derselben. *Arch. Psychiatr. Nervenkr.* 21:22–70, 1890.

*Livingstone M.S., Hubel D.H. Segregation of form, color, movement, and depth: anatomy, physiology, and perception. *Science* 240:740–749, 1988.

*Meadows J.C. The anatomical basis of prosopagnosia. *J. Neurol. Neurosurg. Psychiatry* 37:489–501, 1974.

Meier M.J., French L.A. Lateralized deficits in complex visual discrimination and bilateral transfer of reminiscence following unilateral temporal lobectomy. *Neuropsychologia* 3:261–272, 1965.

Nardelli E., Buonanno F., Coccia G., et al. Prosopagnosia, report of four cases. *Eur. Neurol.* 21:289–297, 1982.

Newcombe F., Russell W.R. Dissociated visual perceptual and spatial deficits in focal lesions of the right hemisphere. *J. Neurol. Neurosurg. Psychiatry* 32:73–81, 1969.

*Oppenheimer D.R., Newcombe F. Clinical and anatomic findings in case of auditory agnosia. *Arch. Neurol.* 35:712–719, 1978.

Pevzner S., Bornstein B., Loewenthal M. Prosopagnosia. *J. Neurol. Neurosurg. Psychiatry* 25:336–338, 1962.

Rubens A.B. Agnosia. In Heilman K.M., Valenstein E., eds. *Clinical Neuropsychology.* New York, Oxford University Press, 1979.

Semmes J. A non-tactual factor in astereognosis. *Neuropsychologia* 3:295–315, 1965.

*Sergent J., Bindra D. Differential hemispheric processing of faces: methodological considerations and reinterpretation. *Psychol. Bull.* 89:541–554, 1981.

Sergent J., Villemure J-G. Prosopagnosia in a right hemispherectomized patient. *Brain* 112:975–995, 1989.

Spreen O., Benton A.L., Fincham R. Auditory agnosia without aphasia. *Arch. Neurol.* 16:84–92, 1965.

Teuber H.L. Alteration of perception and memory in man: reflections on methods. In Weiskrantz L., ed. *Analysis of Behavioral Change.* New York, Harper & Row, 1968.

*Tranel D., Damasio A. Knowledge without awareness: an autonomic index of facial recognition by prosopagnosics. *Science* 228:1453–1454, 1985.

Tranel D., Damasio A.R. Nonconscious face recognition in patients with face agnosia. *Behav. Brain Res.* 30:235–249, 1988.

Ungerleider L.G., Mishkin M. Two cortical visual systems. In Ingle D.J., Mansfield R.J.W., Goodale M.A., eds. *The Analysis of Visual Behavior.* Cambridge, MA, M.I.T. Press, pp. 549–586, 1982.

Van Essen D.C., Maunsell J.H.R. Hierarchical organization and functional streams in the visual cortex. *Trends Neurosci.* 6:370–375, 1983.

Vignolo L.A. Auditory agnosia: a review and report of recent evidence. In Benton A.L., ed. *Contributions to Clinical Neuropsychology.* Chicago, Aldine Publishing, 1969.

Wilbrand H. Ein Fall von Seelenblindheit und Hemianopsie mit Sectionsbefund. *Dtsch. Z. Nervenheilkd.* 2:361–387, 1892.

55

The Apraxias

Hans-Joachim Freund

The apraxias have been identified as higher-order motor disturbances that are not due to paresis, ataxia, aphasia, or dementia (Liepmann, 1900). They can affect almost any aspect of motor behavior. The intriguing complexity of the wide range of possible disturbances of higher-order motor behavior has led to various classifications, most of them based on clinical phenomena.

Many clinicians are frustrated by the vagueness of the definition of the apraxias and the changing views on terminology. In contrast to the situation for other neurologic disorders, the issue of the apraxias has not benefited from the progress in pathophysiology, identification of causes, or other medical research in the nondescriptive realm. According to Ettlinger (1969), there are no reports on apraxia in experimental animals. The progress that has been made in the understanding of motor control and sensorimotor interactions in nonhuman primates and the emergent views on their cortical organization has therefore had little impact on current concepts on the apraxias, whose study is still a domain of traditional neuropsychology. The analysis of lesions that became possible with the advent of the organ-imaging techniques is beginning to change this situation.

Liepmann (1900, 1908, 1920) proposed the original definition of the apraxias. Because the initial description had such clarity and influence and the classification into three types still underlies the most widely used present schemes of apractic disturbances, his classification provides the point of departure. (For more detailed accounts of subsequent modifications and special forms of apraxia, see Hecaen and Albert [1987].) A discussion of the issue of the apraxias on the basis of recent concepts about sensorimotor functions and of the anatomic and physiologic basis of higher-order motor disturbances follows.

CLINICAL SPECTRUM OF APRAXIAS

Liepmann's Classification

Liepmann (1908) described three types of apraxia. The common denominator was a disturbance of purposive movements that was not due to paresis, ataxia, aphasia, or dementia. The characteristic features were described as follows.

1. *Ideatorische Apraxie* (ideational apraxia) was differentiated by Liepmann from the frequently associated aphasia. Aphasia and apraxia had previously been confused, so that the apractic deficit was attributed to the lack of comprehension in sensory aphasia. This type of apraxia was allocated to lesions of the left temporoparieto-occipital area.
2. *Ideokinetische Apraxie* (ideokinetic apraxia) corresponds to what Liepmann had formerly called *motorische Apraxie*. In this condition the limb kinetics were maintained but were disconnected from the ideation of movement. (He therefore regarded a hyphen between ideo and kinetic as relevant.) This form of apraxia was attributed to a disconnection between the visual, tactile, or acoustical cortical areas, especially those of the left hemisphere, and the precentral gyrus. This form of apraxia is now frequently called *ideomotor apraxia*. For the sake of simplicity, ideational and ideokinetic apraxia are sometimes referred to as posterior apraxias, because the lesion site is most frequently posterior to the central sulcus.
3. *Gliedkinetische Apraxie* (limb-kinetic apraxia) was regarded as a loss of kinetic memories for the use of a limb, which is produced by lesions of the precentral gyrus and possibly also the cortex of its immediate neighborhood, either anterior or

751

posterior. Liepmann conceived three major steps in the genesis of movement:

a. *Die Bewegungsformel* (the movement formula)
b. The ability to transform this formula into a scheme of motor innervation
c. A kinetic memory for the storage of learned movements

Movement execution would thus depend on the interaction of these three components.

Clinical Picture and Examination

The three types of apraxia described by Liepmann (1908) have been further elaborated by subsequent studies so that the characteristic deficits can be summarized as follows.

Ideational apraxia is characterized by a deficit of the conception of the movement so that the patient does not know *what* to do or how to organize movement sequences. Such patients cannot perform a complex motor task on command, no matter whether ordered verbally or by the request to imitate it. Because imitation or spontaneous action is disturbed, the apraxia cannot be attributed to a lack of language comprehension. The patients may be unable to do anything at will or may confuse the sequence of the different movement components, although single actions are executed properly. The introduction of objects does not help but rather inhibits the performance of the movements (Brown, 1979). In contrast to ideokinetic apraxia, this movement disorder is experienced by the patients as a disability because it interferes with their everyday motor activities.

Ideational apraxia is less common than ideokinetic apraxia. About 90% of the patients have concomitant aphasia (De Renzi, 1986). The clinical examination aims to disclose the patients' inability to organize action sequences (e.g., making coffee). In contrast to the case with ideokinetic apraxia, video analysis of patients with ideational apraxia showed that manipulation of single objects is correct (Lehmkuhl et al., 1983). If the task does not involve the use of different objects in a complex sequence, the disturbance may not become apparent.

In *ideokinetic (ideomotor) apraxia*, the patient does not know *how* to perform a particular motor act. The introduction of objects facilitates the performance. The action is conceptually determined but faulty in the execution of its parts. Although the ideation necessary for complex gestures is preserved, the disorder typically becomes apparent during the performance of elementary single gestures. Therefore, complex acts can be executed properly, whereas their constituent elements may be disturbed. The response by imitation is frequently better than the response to verbal commands. The flawless execution of movements that cannot be performed at will during automatic motor behavior (voluntary-automatic dissociation) illustrates that it is not the movement pattern per se nor the kinetic memory that is disturbed but

the voluntary evocation. Various tests have been elaborated to examine patients with ideokinetic apraxia, including tests for facial, extremity, and trunk movements that consist partly of transitive and intransitive movements and of representational and nonrepresentational motor acts. Most patients do not recognize that their performance is in error (anosognosia), although they can distinguish appropriate from nonappropriate pantomime (Heilmann et al., 1982).

In practice, the differences between ideational and ideokinetic apraxia are not always clear. Different mixtures of apractic phenomena often make a clear grouping difficult. In addition, the test procedures and the terminology used vary. From the linguistic angle, apraxia is regarded as a disturbance of symbolic communication and representational movement, whereas most neurologists envisage it as a higher-order motor disorder. Because limb-kinetic, or frontal, apraxia is frequently not accepted as a true apraxia, ideational apraxia and ideomotor apraxia remain the most widely used terms.

Limb-kinetic apraxia has been described as a slowness, clumsiness, and awkwardness of movements with loss of the kinetic melody, temporal deordering, and decomposition of movement (Luria, 1966). Liepmann's (1908) original description of this type of apraxia was not based on his own observations but on a case by Westphal (1908). Westphal's patient showed a gross disturbance of the ability to assume certain positions or to perform certain movements with his right arm. There was also a loss of skill of the right hand with open eyes that differed from ataxia. It was in particular the inability to perform purposive movements. Liepmann assigned the disturbed security and positioning of movement to a loss of kinesthetic memories that usually would be a substantial part of the sensorimotor function. Kleist (1907) called this type of apraxia *innervatorische Apraxie* and regarded the loss of hand skill and facial and oral movements as well as the apraxia of standing and of gait as typical dysfunctions; he allocated the motor disorder to damage of area 6. For the hands, fine and composite movements such as sewing, playing the piano, and typing were particularly abnormal, but it was possible to recognize the type of movement that was intended.

De Renzi (1986) correctly emphasized the dearth of well-documented case reports of apraxia associated with frontal damage not extending behind the rolandic fissure. No more than seven such cases could be gleaned by Faglioni and Basso (1985) in a review of the literature. For these reasons, many neurologists refrain from accepting limb-kinetic apraxia as a true apraxia and consider it as clumsiness associated with paresis or prefer the use of other descriptive terms such as awkwardness of movement, loss of kinetic melody, and temporal decomposition of movement. The lack of voluntary-automatic dissociation is regarded as further evidence for such a view.

The premotor syndrome described by Freund and Hummelsheim (1985) illustrates the difficulty in the delineation of a limb-kinetic apraxia. Many of these patients had a mild or moderate proximal weakness of the limbs contralateral to the lesion, which usually resolved rapidly after the stroke and which would have been regarded as indicating concomitant damage of the precentral gyrus by many neurologists. Initially, the patients reported that their hand and arm did not function normally and that skilled hand activities such as writing were difficult. Closer analysis of the motor deficits in these patients showed that arm and hand activities were mainly disturbed by the deficient postural stability of the arm at the shoulder joint. What was apparent in all cases with symptomatic lesions of the premotor area was a limb-kinetic apraxia for coordinated movements between the two limbs of either side.

I have seen this deficit in more than 40 patients. None of the patients had ideomotor apraxia. In all cases, some of them without any proximal weakness, the limb-kinetic apraxia was not obvious for any arm-hand function but became apparent only when the activities of proximal muscles had to be adjusted between the two sides. The apraxia was not obvious when not specially tested and was not noticed by the patients themselves. Observing their spontaneous motor behavior did not help to disclose the apractic deficit. Patients were able to rotate one arm at the shoulder when asked to do so but had difficulties in rotating both arms simultaneously in the forward or backward direction. The dysfunction became most pronounced when the patient was asked to produce a windmill movement forward or backward with both arms in an alternating manner. The movement degraded and decomposed from the beginning, sometimes turning in the opposite direction. This difficulty could not be overcome by several weeks of exercise. Distal movements such as circling hands or fingers in the air could be performed correctly, as could bimanual aiming tasks or everyday activities requiring bimanual coordination (e.g., tying shoelaces). A similar disturbance appeared in the legs when the patients lay supine and attempted to make bicycling movements. Backward cycling movements in particular showed a disturbance similar to that described for the windmill movement of the arms. In contrast to the proximal weakness seen in some of these cases, these deficits remained permanently and did not improve with time or exercise in most cases.

DISTRIBUTION OF THE APRAXIAS IN DIFFERENT BODY PARTS

Apractic disturbances may be global or restricted to certain body parts. Because ideational apraxia represents a disturbance of the action plan, it interferes with the general organization and orderly sequencing of complex motor acts, irrespective of which body parts contribute to the performance. Ideomotor apraxia may affect both sides but can also be restricted to the side opposite to the lesion. Limb-kinetic apraxia affects mainly the limbs opposite to the damaged hemisphere. As illustrated by the cases with premotor lesions, the dysfunction may also affect temporal adjustment between limb movements on both sides.

The disturbances of whole-body movements in limb-kinetic apraxia were mentioned in the first reports by Liepmann (1900) and Sittig (1931). They described the patient's inability to perform whole-body movements such as lying down, rising, sitting, and rolling over, disturbances that have been referred to as truncopedal apraxia. These disturbances could not be attributed to paresis, hypokinesia, ataxia, or other causes on the executional side of movement. The so-called apraxia of gait, which has been distinguished as a separate form by Gerstmann and Schilder (1926), and other special types of apraxia such as dressing apraxia have also been isolated.

Liepmann (1920) emphasized similarities between the language disorders and the disorders of facial innervation. He considered disorders of verbal expression as an apraxia of the speech muscles and drew attention to the frequent association between the impairment of the facial and oral movements (later called buccofacial apraxia) and motor aphasia. Nathan (1947) and Bay (1957) used the term cortical anarthria, or apraxic dysarthria. Alajouanine and Lhermitte (1960) found buccofacial apraxia as a constant accompanying sign in the initial stages of anarthria. De Renzi (1986) reported a 90% incidence of buccofacial apraxia in patients with expressive (Broca's) aphasia. In spite of the similarities between limb-kinetic and buccofacial apraxia and the preferential damage of frontal areas in both groups, buccofacial apraxia has even been considered as part of ideomotor apraxia—an example of how widely classification varies.

Nielsen (1946) discussed the issue of axial versus distal apractic disturbances on anatomic grounds. He assumed three different levels of movement control: (1) purely unilateral voluntary control (e.g., of the fingers and hand) by the contralateral precentral gyrus; (2) bilateral control of centrally located musculature or paired muscles that always function as a unit, such as the diaphragm or the abdominal muscles; and (3) the coordination of large groups of muscles of mixed type, such as those used for writing, speaking, or musical performances. Impairment of the corresponding motor engrams located anterior to the precentral gyrus leads to a loss of the memory for the use of the hand only for these movements and not for other uses of the hand. According to Nielsen (1946), the plan for the coordination of periaxial musculature has a different cortical control mechanism from that laid down in the precentral gyrus and is further integrated in the brain stem reticular formation and spinal cord.

Although Poeck et al. (1982) did not observe a relative preservation of axial commands, Geschwind (1967) used illustrative cases to contrast the grace and elegance of whole-body movements with the awkwardness and clumsiness of apractic limb movements. Even severely apractic patients may be able to perform whole-body postures similar to those of a boxer or a fencer. Geschwind (1967) did not consider the preservation of the whole-body movements as indicating their greater simplicity but regarded it as reflecting the utilization of different anatomic arrangements from those involved in movements of individual limbs. With respect to the axial musculature, he therefore arrived at conclusions similar to those of Freund and Hummelsheim (1985), Howes (1988), and Nielsen (1946).

APRAXIA AND THE DOMINANT HEMISPHERE

The striking association between disorders of language and those of praxis has been subject of numerous studies. This association was revealed for motor aphasia and buccofacial apraxia and for sensory aphasia and ideational or ideomotor apraxia. The relationship between aphasia and apraxia raises two possibilities:

1. The two disorders are independent and their frequent association is due to the proximity of the cortical areas within which lesions produce these disturbances.
2. The two disorders are the expression of a common underlying deficit of communication affecting linguistic and gestural behavior in a general sense. This hypothesis dates to Liepmann's (1908) original definition of aphasia as an apraxia of the speech muscles and was re-emphasized by Ettlinger (1969).

Some reports describe posterior apraxia resulting from right hemisphere damage in left-handed persons. The evaluation of these reports is difficult in many cases because of the problems in defining handedness. Studies on large series of patients support the association between ideational or ideomotor apraxia and the speech-dominant hemisphere. In 415 cases of parietal, temporal, or occipital lesions, all patients with such apraxias had left hemisphere or bilateral damage (Hecaen, 1962). Similarly, De Renzi et al. (1968) found such apractic disturbances only in association with left-sided lesions in a study of 205 patients (45 right hemisphere and 160 left hemisphere lesions).

The dominance of the left hemisphere for language and motor programming in right-handed persons raises a number of questions. Studies on patients with commissurotomies make it clear that the right hemisphere possesses the full potential for programming and initiating skillful left hand motor acts. Sectioning of the corpus callosum produces apraxia of the left hand only when the response-eliciting stimulus is not available to the hemisphere contralateral to the acting limb. In all other conditions, the right hemisphere is fully capable of organizing even the most complex motor behavior of the left side of patients who undergo commissurotomy. Freeman (1984) called the ensuing difficulties in explaining the apraxias as disconnection syndromes the paradox of disease of the left hemisphere:

> If the left hand split-brain patient is fully capable of performing a wide variety of motor tasks without the participation of the (disconnected) left hemisphere and under circumstances in which the left hemisphere cannot "know" what instructions the right hemisphere has received, then why should a lesion of the left hemisphere disrupt the control by the right hemisphere of the motor behavior of the left hand, even though, as in the case of (nonverbal) imitation tasks and demonstration of use-tasks, the (intact) right hemisphere is fully informed about the task to be performed by the left hand?

To solve this problem, Freeman suggested that the principal function of the left hemisphere may be to exert a priority of motor control in situations appropriate to its action.

THE ISSUE OF DISCONNECTION SYNDROMES

Liepmann (1920) was the first to promote the concept that some apractic disturbances result from the disconnection between interacting cortical areas. This concept was further elaborated by Geschwind (1965a,b). Geschwind considered the disconnection of the speech areas from the motor regions as the simplest type of apraxia: callosal lesions disconnect the right hemisphere from any language processing. A patient described by Geschwind and Kaplan (1962) had a mild pyramidal disturbance of the right hand with a severe grasp reflex but could write properly with the right hand in spite of this impairment. The patient could not, however, write with the left hand, although it showed no other motor disturbance at all. It was further observed that verbal commands were carried out with the right hand but not with the left, which was consistent with an apraxia of the minor hand. The disturbance of writing with the left hand was, however, shown to be an aphasic deficit. This was demonstrated when the patient's writing movements were appropriate but the words written were incorrect. This was true for handwriting as well as for typing with the fingers of the left hand. The patient could recognize the errors produced but could not correct them with the left hand. The patient also could not execute left hand movements in response to verbal commands but could copy movements flawlessly. Geschwind and Kaplan (1962) assumed that this dysfunction was due to a disconnection of the right motor cortex from the left language center, a postulate supported by postmortem examination, which showed an extensive infarction of the corpus callosum. Movements in response to verbal commands involving symmetric bilateral muscle activities such as facial movements were intact.

Geschwind (1965a) used this case not only to disclose the nature of the apractic deficit as a disconnection syndrome but also to emphasize that the designation apractic would be inadequate unless the stimulus condition was specified: the left hand of this patient was apractic to verbal command but intact on imitation or during object handling. The right hand performed incorrectly when it was required to respond to somatesthetic stimuli applied to the left hand. Geschwind and Kaplan (1962) therefore recommended specifying apraxia as a disturbance of stimulus-response combinations and viewed the different forms of apraxia as modality-specific dysfunctions. They may also involve several modalities if the fiber systems connecting the different posterior sensory areas with the motor centers are damaged. The preservation of automatic movements in apraxia illustrates the specificity of the access of certain stimuli to the retrieval of motor patterns from the frontal cortical motor fields. On the basis of these observations, Geschwind and Kaplan proposed a distinction between aphasic and apractic agraphia. They regarded the concept of modality-specific disconnection syndromes as more relevant for understanding the pathophysiology and for the clinical analysis of such patients than the concept of classification into the three types as postulated by Liepmann.

Apraxia After Subcortical Lesions

Geschwind's (1965a,b) hypothesis that apraxias represent an ensemble of disconnection syndromes interrupting the information flow between sensory and motor areas or between speech and motor centers is attractive and in heuristic terms can explain the bewildering multiplicity of apractic phenomena. The issue of the disconnection syndromes, however, raises the question whether and, if so, how apractic phenomena attributable to fiber disconnection and those caused by cortical damage can be distinguished. It was noticed from the beginning of the lesion studies on brain function that damage of the immediately subcortical white matter would produce similar clinical deficits to those produced by cortical damage. Because all cortical lesions also affect underlying fibers, the relative contribution of the cortical and subcortical impairment to the resulting deficit often cannot be differentiated. The situation is different with purely subcortical lesions. As in the case of subcortical aphasias, the issue of subcortical apraxias has been advanced by the results of computed tomographic studies (Alexander, 1989). Damage to the deep superior paraventricular white matter produces lasting left limb apraxia or bilateral limb apraxia. This is attributed to the interruption of the intrahemispheric connections between the posterior parietal lobe and premotor areas, involving the intrahemispheric fibers and the ascending and descending fibers.

The study of aphasic syndromes with organ-imaging techniques during the past decade yielded new insights about the role of subcortical lesions in aphasia. Alexander (1989) concluded that the classic syndromes of aphasia are not the most useful independent variables for aphasia research. He pointed out that Broca's aphasia comprises nine separate aphasic signs, each of which probably having its own pathologic anatomic features. Regarding the role of aphasic phenomena produced by purely subcortical lesions, the clinicopathologic correlations show that damage to the paraventricular or periventricular white matter can interfere with different fiber systems relevant for specific parts of language or speech processing (Naeser et al., 1982). Reduced language output, dysarthria, hemiparesis, and left limb apraxia were observed after damage to the middle one-third of the superior paraventricular white matter (Alexander et al., 1987). Ideomotor apraxia of specific body parts has been described in cases with specified pathologic anatomic changes. More work will have to be done before clearer views about the pathologic anatomic features of various subcortical and cortical apractic phenomena become apparent. In this context, positron emission tomographic studies will play an important role, because they can elucidate the disturbance of cortical function ensuing from purely subcortical damage.

NEW APPROACHES TO THE UNDERSTANDING OF HIGHER-ORDER MOTOR DYSFUNCTIONS

Motor Dysfunctions After Damage of Unimodal Sensory Association Areas

Motor disturbances attributable to interference with sensory inputs have been analyzed in great detail. These studies showed that complete peripheral deafferentation interferes grossly with motor functions. The motor disturbances accompanying parietal lobe pathologic changes are similar to those that occur after interference with afferent input to the somatosensory cortex (Nathan et al., 1986). This situation becomes more complex in cases with lesions of the posterior parietal cortex (Pause et al., 1989). Such patients showed preferential impairment of complex somatosensory and motor functions interfering with stereognosis, recognition of textured surfaces, and the execution of purposive, exploratory, and manipulative finger movements.

Quantitative analysis of hand and finger movements in these patients revealed that the dynamics of digital palpation of objects was grossly disturbed. The breakdown of the finely tuned scanning process of the fingers prevents the sequential sampling of mechanoreceptor information. The essence of the motor disturbance of the hand in posterior parietal lobe disease lies in the disturbance of the conception and generation of the movement patterns necessary to bring those receptors into action that would normally provide the information required for the identification and manipulation of objects. The somatosensory association areas in the parietal lobe are involved not only in the elaboration and further processing of somatosensory information but also in the conception and generation of the motor programs required to collect this information. This illustrates an important aspect of sensorimotor integration: the dependence of feature extraction on purposive action. Lesions of the somatosensory association areas 5 and 7 on the superior parietal lobe therefore produce a deficit of purposive and skillful behavior of the hand. Although force production and rapid movement generation may be completely normal, there is a grossly disturbed motor behavior for a restricted range of activities that elaborate on the use of the hand as a sense organ. Even though the motor system is completely normal, patients with such lesions often consider their affected hand as completely useless. This deficit of active touch and manipulation represents a tactile apraxia (Delay, 1935; Pause et al., 1989).

Another unimodal higher-order motor disturbance that follows lesions of a sensory association area is known as visuomotor ataxia. This disorder of visually guided motor behavior in conditions in which the motor, cerebellar, somatosensory, and visual pathways function satisfactorily is seen after bilateral or sometimes unilateral parieto-occipital lesions (Balint, 1909; Gowers, 1887; Holmes, 1918; Holmes and Horrax, 1919; Rondot et al., 1977). A deficit similar to that caused by cutting the occipitofrontal connections of one hemisphere could be produced by a dorsal commissurotomy under conditions of hemifield stimulation. When the occipitofrontal fiber connections were severed in monkeys, visuomotor ataxia ensued. Haaxma and Kuypers (1975) regarded this as a disconnection syndrome in which the visual information did not reach the motor centers.

Many patients have an inability to orient the eyes, the head, and the body toward a peripheral stimulus, without regard to which modality is channeling the information. Imperfect perception of distances, disturbances of exploring extrapersonal space with the arms and the eyes, and inappropriate performance of the act of reaching or grasping is strikingly different from the disturbed motor behavior seen in adult patients with acute blindness. The analysis of movement trajectories (Jeannerod, 1988) showed grossly deranged trajectories of reaching, aiming, grasping, and exploring movements. Such patients are barely able to learn to reach for targets with locations in space cued by proprioceptive or acoustic input. The wrong conception of the trajectories is repeated again and again with little improvement by training. It is therefore likely that this disturbance represents an apractic deficit of cortical synthetic function rather than a pure visuomotor disconnection syndrome, in which the disturbances should resemble those in blind subjects.

Quantitative analysis of movement trajectories has shown that a dissociation between perceiving and grasping of visualized objects can occur. Goodale et al. (1991) described a patient with strikingly accurate guidance of hand and finger movements directed at the objects whose qualities she failed to perceive.

Conversely, the typical patient with visuomotor apraxia cannot reach accurately toward visualized targets that they perceive correctly. This dissociation suggests that the visual processing underlying conscious perceptual judgments operates separately from that underlying the visual guidance of limb movements. Because the adjustment of egocentric and allocentric maps as well as various coordinate transformations are required for sensorimotor functions in various modalities, quantitative movement analysis must show whether the unimodal apraxias after lesions of the superior parietal lobe exhibit additional space-specific deficits.

The impaired motor behavior in patients with unimodal sensory disturbances and consecutive motor deficits is usually described as atactic. This applies for limb ataxia seen after damage of the somatosensory part of the parietal lobe or after damage of the visual association areas. The term *atactic* is appropriate insofar as the deficient somatosensory or visual information cannot satisfy the demands for movement precision. In addition to having an atactic component, the performance of the movement is deranged, decomposed, and faulty in the execution of its parts. This fulfills the criteria for apractic movements. I have therefore proposed that these disturbances of higher-order motor behavior in relation to somatosensory or visual functions be considered tactile and visuomotor apraxia (Freund, 1987). These apraxias do not represent simple disconnection syndromes interrupting sensorimotor information flow but rather are a disturbance of cortical synthetic functions (the elaboration of the motor programs that are required for the explorative motor or oculomotor behavior that is necessary to collect, select, and shape the sensory input). This concept is in agreement with the hypothesis about the command function of the posterior parietal lobe for the exploration of extrapersonal space (Mountcastle et al., 1975). This integrative function of the posterior parietal lobe is obviously disturbed in patients with visuomotor and tactile apraxia. In contrast to the case in the polymodal ideational and ideomotor apraxias, there is no voluntary-automatic dissociation and the deficit does not depend on the side on which the lesion occurs.

Similar effects on motor function of damage to a sensory area can be seen after lesions of an auditory association area. Lesions of Wernicke posterior speech area not only compromise the perception and comprehension of language but also produce a severe motor language disturbance. Language production in such patients is typically increased but grossly deranged in its lexical, syntactic, and semantic context. The operational principle thus seems similar to that in the other unimodal motor apraxias: the production of adequate motor patterns is no longer possible for all motor behavior that is based on a particular modality.

Sign Language Aphasia and Apraxia in Deaf-Mute Patients

The relation between aphasic and apractic disturbances is further elucidated by studies of left or right hemisphere strokes in deaf-mute patients who use American Sign Language (ASL). Bellugi et al. (1989) described second- or third-generation deaf-mutes who learned ASL from their deaf-mute parents. ASL exhibits format structuring at the same levels as spoken languages, but the form of grammatic structuring is transmitted in a visual-manual language rather than in the auditory-vocal mode. ASL specifies relations among signs through the manipulation of sign forms in space, so that space itself bears linguistic meanings. The signing capacity of three patients with left hemisphere lesions and three patients with right hemisphere lesions was analyzed by means of three-dimensional computer graphics of movement. This was combined with a linguistic analysis to explore how the brain controls movement at different levels: linguistic, symbolic, spatial, and motor.

In the patients with left hemisphere damage, clear sign language aphasias were apparent in all cases as revealed by sign aphasia examination and on linguistic analysis of signing. One patient was agrammatic for ASL. Her lesion was typical of those that produce agrammatic aphasia for spoken language. Another patient produced the ASL equivalent of phonemic paraphasias and had severe and lasting sign comprehension loss. Remarkably, both major language-mediating areas for spoken language (Broca and Wernicke areas) were intact. The lesion was in the parietal area known to function in higher spatial analysis. The third patient produced grammatically inappropriate signs in the context of fluent sign output; he also showed errors of spatially organized syntax of ASL.

In contrast, the signers with right hemisphere damage were not aphasic. They showed fluent, grammatic, and virtually error-free signing in spite of the spatial nature of sign language. There was no impairment in the grammatic aspect of signing, including the spatially organized syntax. In remarkable contrast to their flawless performance on sign language tasks, the patients with right hemisphere damage showed classic visuospatial impairments, which were apparent in the range of tasks including drawing, spatial construction, spatial attention, judgment of line orientation, and spatial discrimination. As expected, these functions were normal in the patients with left hemisphere lesions. Bellugi and co-workers (1989) concluded that the right hemisphere in deaf signers can develop cerebral specialization for nonlanguage visuospatial functions but has little effect on the spatial organization of language. It was further concluded that the primary specialization of the left hemisphere does not rest on the form of the signal but rather on the linguistic function it subserves.

These remarkable data show that hearing and speech are not necessary for the development of hemispheric specialization. They show further that the left hemisphere is dominant for sign language, suggesting that the left hemisphere in humans has an innate predisposition for language, regardless of the modality. The human capacity for language is not linked to some privileged, cognitive-auditory connections. These studies also shed some light on the long-standing discussion of the nature of aphasic and apractic disorders.

Gesture and linguistic symbols are transmitted in the same modality in sign language. A series of apraxia tests in the signers with left hemisphere lesions, all of whom were aphasic for sign language, showed that the language deficits of these signers were related to specific linguistic components of sign language rather than to an underlying motor disorder for the capacity to express and comprehend symbols or for the production and imitation of representational and nonrepresentational movements. This reveals that, in aphasic and apractic disturbances, only specific functions are selectively disturbed. Nevertheless, the studies of lesions in deaf-mute signers demonstrate that sign language aphasia represents a special type of apraxia affecting the understanding and production of limb movements that convey linguistic information. This comes close to Liepmann's (1908) interpretation of the disorders of verbal expression as apraxia of the speech muscles.

Anatomic and Physiologic Basis of Unimodal Apraxias

The lesions underlying the unimodal apraxias are all located in the posterior parietal lobe or its junctional zones with the temporal and occipital lobes. Therefore, it appears useful to analyze the connectional pattern of the corresponding regions in nonhuman primates, because this was not studied in sufficient detail with modern anatomic and physiologic methods in the human brain.

Figure 55–1 shows the location and classifications of the sensory projection and association areas on the lateral and medial aspects of the rhesus monkey cerebral hemisphere. The classification is based on interareal differences in thalamocortical projections, long association fiber systems, and functional considerations. In contrast to the situation for the primary cortical projection areas, which receive their major thalamic input from strictly unimodal thalamic nuclei, the thalamic input to the somatosensory association areas originates predominantly in the lateral posterior, pulvinar, and intralaminar thalamic nuclei, which have been identified as targets of projections from different modalities (Jones and Burton, 1976). The somatosensory association areas SA_1–SA_3 lie caudal to the primary somatosensory cortex S1; the visual association areas VA_1–VA_3 are located rostral to the primary visual cortex V1 at the parieto-occipital transition zone and extend into the temporal lobe below the superior temporal sulcus. The auditory association areas AA_1–AA_3 are found above this sulcus and adjoin the primary auditory cortex A1, which is located on the dorsal surface of the superior temporal gyrus within the lateral fissure. Additionally, supplementary motor (M2) and somatosensory

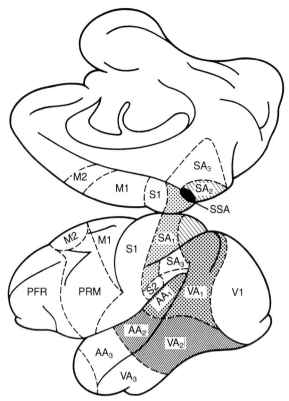

Figure 55–1. Lateral and medial surfaces of rhesus monkey cerebral hemisphere showing three major divisions of the association cortex: (1) parasensory association cortex: auditory association areas AA_1–AA_3, somatic sensory association areas SA_1–SA_3, and visual association areas VA_1–VA_3; (2) frontal association cortex: premotor (PRM) and prefrontal (PFR) areas; and (3) paralimbic association cortex: cingulate gyrus, parahippocampal gyrus, temporal pole, and orbitofrontal cortex. Additionally, the primary motor (M1), somatosensory (S1 and visual (V1) areas are shown together with the secondary and supplementary areas of the motor (M2) and somatosensory (S2 and SSA) cortices. (Adapted from Pandya D.N., Yeterian E.H. Cortico-thalamic connections of the posterior parietal cortex in rhesus monkeys. *Anat. Rev.* 202:211A, 1982, and modified by Zilles K. The cortex. In Paxinos G., ed. *The Human Nervous System*. San Diego, CA, Academic Press, pp. 757–802, 1990.)

(SSA and S2) areas are visible on the lateral and medial surfaces of the hemisphere. It appears that the posterior part of the lateral aspect of the monkey hemisphere is covered by unimodal association areas. The polymodal association areas, which are characterized by their widespread connections with visual, auditory, and somatosensory association areas, are buried in the sulci at the junctions between the unimodal association areas of the parietal, temporal, and occipital lobes.

The sensory association areas of the posterior lobes are connected with the prefrontal, premotor, and supplementary motor areas of the frontal lobe and with the cingulate and parahippocampal regions. The trunk and extremity representation areas in S1 project to the superior parietal lobule (SPL), whereas the face, head, and neck regions of S1 project to the inferior parietal lobule (IPL). In spite of the overall similarities in the connective scheme, there are quan-

titative differences. SA_1 is reciprocally connected with S1, S2, SSA, M2, and the caudal premotor region. The major connections of SA_2 are shifted more rostrally to the premotor and prefrontal cortices and to the cingulate and parahippocampal regions. This connectivity pattern suggests a more direct interaction between the motor and somatosensory projection areas on SA_1 than on SA_2 or SA_3 (Pandya and Yeterian, 1982).

As shown by the pioneering work of Hyvärinen (1982), Mountcastle et al. (1975), and Wurtz and Mohler (1976), neurons in the IPL play a critical role not only in the elaboration of higher-order sensory information but also in the sensory-to-motor transformation. The IPL is therefore considered to be part of an interface between sensory and motor systems for the achievement of sensory-guided motor behaviors. Characteristically, many classes of IPL neurons have both sensory and motor-related responses. The motor-related responses appear to represent efference copies of motor commands rather than actual motor commands, thus providing information about position or velocity. Efference copies may play an important role in the transformation of sensory coordinate frames to spatial coordinate frames as they are needed for the elaboration of motor programs.

The sensorimotor transformation processes of each modality are organized in submodal task groups. This is briefly outlined here only for the visual channel. The segregation of information channels subserving different visual functions such as form, color, depth, and motion is firmly established (Hubel and Livingstone, 1987; Ungerleider and Mishkin, 1982; Van Essen and Maunsell, 1983). The progression for visual processing can be traced from area V1 to middle temporal, medial superior temporal, lateral intraparietal, dorsal prelunate, and 7a areas (Fig. 55–2). The anatomic mapping of these subsequent stages in visuomotor processing shows that large aspects of these areas are buried in sulci (Fig. 55–3). Motion processing is accomplished by a pathway that begins in area V1 and passes through middle temporal and medial superior temporal areas to area 7a. This pathway represents the dorsolateral visual projection (the "where" system) as compared with the ventromedial "what" system that conveys form information from occipital to inferotemporal areas. The dorsolateral pathway and its cortical relay zones (middle temporal and medial superior temporal, and 7a areas) provide the source of strong corticopontine projections (Brodal, 1978; Glickstein et al., 1980, 1985). The target of the pontine projections, the cerebellum, plays a prominent role in smooth pursuit oculomotor functions. Dorsal prelunate and lateral intraparietal areas project to the dorsal and dorsolateral pons, whereas area 7a projects to three areas of the lateral margin of the pons: the ventral, lateral, and dorsolateral nuclei. In contrast, area 7b, involved in the elaboration of somatosensory information, projects to the same lateral areas but also sends fibers to ventromedial portions of the ventral peduncular and paramedian pontine nuclei.

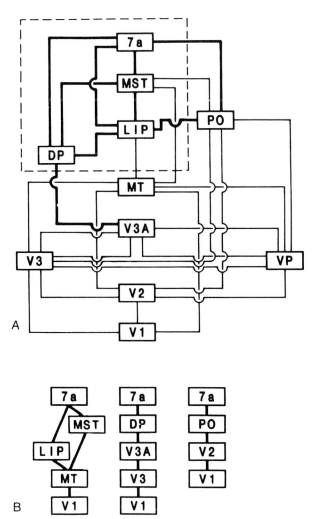

Figure 55–2. *(A)* Hierarchy of visual pathways from area V1 to the inferior parietal cortex determined by laminar patterns of sources and terminations of projections. Box outlined by dashed lines delineates cortical areas of the inferior parietal lobule and the dorsal aspect of the prelunate gyrus. *(B)* Three of shortest pathways for visual information travel from area V1 to area 7a. MST = medial superior temporal area; LIP = lateral intraparietal area; DP = dorsal prelunate area; VP = ventral posterior; MT = middle temporal area. (From Andersen R.A. Inferior parietal lobule function in spatial perception and visuomotor integration. In Plum F., ed. *Handbook of Physiology.* Section 1. *The Nervous System.* Vol. V. *Higher Functions of the Brain.* Part 2. Bethesda, American Physiological Society, pp. 483–518, 1987.)

Of all the regions, area 7a demonstrates the most extensive corticocortical connections with the frontal and temporal lobes and the cingulate gyrus as compared with other cortical fields in the IPL. It has strong projections to the prefrontal cortex in and around the principal sulcus (area 46 of Walker), but unlike the lateral intraparietal area, it connects only weakly to the frontal eye fields (Andersen, 1987; Barbas and Mesulam, 1981). This picture is at considerable variance with the customary neurologic schemes of visuomotor processing, in which the visual information was considered to reach the premotor areas via direct occipitofrontal projections, so that the interruption of this projection would cause

a visuomotor disconnection syndrome resulting in visuomotor ataxia (Geschwind, 1975). More recent findings elucidate why visuomotor dysfunctions have never been observed after more anterior lesions. The corticopontine projections funnel the visual signals that are relevant for motion perception and the generation of motor signals to the brain stem and cerebellum (Glickstein et al., 1985), where they are integrated with vestibular, oculomotor, and proprioceptive inputs from the neck and the body and from where they reach the frontal motor fields via the ventrolateral thalamus.

Supramodal Apraxias and the Problem of Comparative Anatomy

Ideational and ideomotor apraxias represent supramodal apraxias. Although the apractic disturbance may be differently expressed at imitation or verbal command, the disturbed motor behavior is not restricted to a particular modality but affects the ideation, and conception of the intended motor acts at a global level. These most complex forms of apraxia have been frequently attributed to lesions of the supramarginal or angular gyrus. In contrast to the unimodal apractic disturbances, they only occur after lesions of the language-dominant hemisphere. As illustrated in Figure 55–3, the polymodal sensory association areas in the monkey are buried in the sulci. In the human, the location of these functional areas is unclear. Figure 55–4 shows the differences in the cytoarchitectonic maps of the posterior parietal cortex in humans and monkeys. Brodmann (1909) identified area 5 in the SPL and area 7 in the IPL in monkeys (see Fig. 55–4*A*). In the comparable view of the human cortical map according to Brodmann (1909) (see Fig. 55–4*B*), it appears that area 5 represents a much smaller proportion of SPL, whereas the largest part of the SPL is covered by area 7.

The IPL in humans consists of the two areas 39 and 40. They correspond to the angular and the supramarginal gyrus. Brodmann (1909, p. 157) recognized this problem:

> Since the homology of area 5 is clear, the question arises, which area in the human cortex is comparable to area 7 of the monkey. Its position ventrally of the intraparietal sulcus argues for a homology with areas 39 and 40 of the human inferior parietal lobule. Because of comparative anatomical arguments, I believe, that area 7 in monkeys corresponds to the whole parietal region in humans and is, therefore, the undifferentiated primordial region for all human parietal areas (except area 5).

A different view was taken by Bailey and von Bonin (1951), who designated areas PG and PF as the homologue for area 7 in monkeys (see Fig. 55–4*C* and *D*). These authors regarded the areas PG and PF as homologous to von Economo's PG and PF in humans. It is therefore unclear whether homologies exist between the areas of the human inferior parietal cortex and those of the monkey brain.

According to Zilles (1990), the anatomic evidence

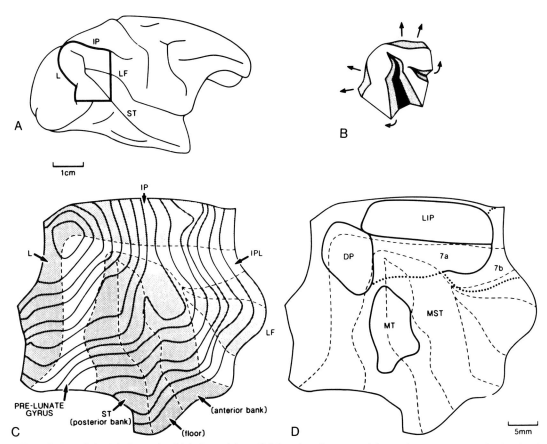

Figure 55–3. Parcellation of the inferior parietal lobule and the adjoining dorsal aspect of the prelunate gyrus on the basis of physiologic, connectional, myeloarchitectural, and cytoarchitectural criteria. Cortical areas are represented on flattened reconstructions of cortex. *(A)* Lateral view of monkey hemisphere. (Heavier lines outline flattened area.) *(B)* Same cortex isolated from the rest of the brain. Cortex buried in sulci *(shaded areas)*; floor of the superior temporal sulcus (ST) *blackened area;* movement of local cortical regions resulting from mechanical flattening *(arrows)*. *(C)* Completely flattened representation of same area. Cortical regions buried in sulci *(shaded areas)*; tracing of layer IV taken from frontal sections through this area *(contour-like lines)*. *(D)* Locations of several cortical areas. *Dotted lines* indicate borders of cortical fields not precisely determinable. DP = dorsal prelunate area; IP = intraparietal sulcus; IPL = inferior parietal lobule; L = lunate sulcus; LF = lateral fissure; LIP = lateral intraparietal area; MST = medial superior temporal area; MT = middle temporal area. (From Andersen R.A. Inferior parietal lobule function in spatial perception and visuomotor integration. In Plum F., ed. *Handbook of Physiology.* Section 1. *The Nervous System.* Vol. V. *Higher Functions of the Brain.* Part 2. Bethesda, American Physiological Society, pp. 483–518, 1987.)

makes it more likely that Brodmann's view is correct, so that areas 39 and 40 are not directly comparable with area 7 of the monkey brain but have been derived from a primordial region during human evolution, which is represented by that part of area 7 located in the IPL of monkeys. Areas 39 and 40 may thus be cortical convolutions representing higher-order polymodal association areas. Lesions of areas 39 and 40 in the language-dominant hemisphere of human subjects cause complex deficits of sophisticated, lateralized human functions, such as reading, writing, and calculating, and of the conception and organization of higher-order motor behavior. Future studies have to settle the question about the polymodal nature of these gyri on the basis of more precise morphologic (magnetic resonance imaging) and functional analysis (positron emission tomography, magnetoencephalography). It thus seems possible that, in contrast to the situation in the monkey brain, the polymodal sensory association

areas in humans have a large representation on the gyral surface of the hemisphere. The supramodal conceptual apraxias interfere grossly with human motor behavior, which is further evidence of the significance of the sensory association areas for movement.

Comparative Anatomy of the Frontal Motor Fields

Fulton (1935) originally delineated the human premotor areas as the frontal agranular cortex (PMC, area 6) rostral to the primary motor cortex (M1, area 4). PMC shows particular enlargement in humans, in whom it is five times larger than area 4 as compared with a 1:1 relationship in the macaque (Bailey and von Bonin, 1951). Figure 55–5 shows the distribution of Brodmann frontal agranular and dysgranular cytoarchitectonic areas 4, 6, 8, and 44 on the precentral

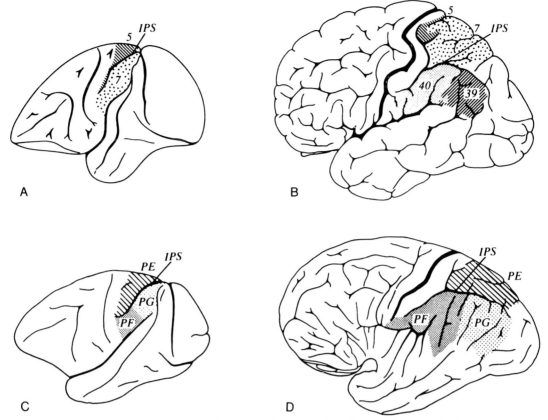

Figure 55–4. Lateral views of monkey and human cerebral hemispheres showing different cytoarchitectural parcellation schemes of the posterior parietal cortex. *(A)* Brodmann's subdivisions of monkey cortex *(Cercopithecus). (B)* von Bonin and Bailey's classification of monkey cortex *(Macaca mulatta). (C)* Brodmann's parcellation of human cortex. *(D)* von Economo's parcellation of human posterior parietal cortex. IPS = intraparietal sulcus. (From Andersen R.A. Inferior parietal lobule function in spatial perception and visumotor integration. In Plum F., ed. *Handbook of Physiology.* Section 1. *The Nervous System.* Vol. V. *Higher Functions of the Brain.* Part 2. Bethesda, American Physiological Society, pp. 483–518, 1987.)

and frontal gyri. When the human inferior precentral sulcus represents the homologue of the arcuate sulcus in monkeys, the ventral compartment of area 6 (PMC v in Fig. 55–5) covering the banks of the precentral sulcus and the anterior part of the precentral gyrus corresponds to the monkey arcuate premotor area. The largest part (the dorsal compartment [PMC d]) lies on the superior and middle frontal gyri. This area may correspond to PMd as outlined by Wise (1991) and by Humphrey and Tanji (1991). The human premotor lesions were located in this dorsal compartment of the PMC (Freund and Hummelsheim, 1985; Fulton, 1935). To my knowledge, there are no published records of lesions restricted to PMC v and not affecting area 4. In the human, the pyramidal syndrome represents a typical deficit after lesions confined to the precentral gyrus (PMC and PMC v). The part of area 6 that lies on the medial side of the hemisphere represents the supplementary motor area. In conjunction with the premotor areas that have been identified on the monkey's cingulate gyrus (Dum and Strick, 1991a,b), these motor areas seem relevant for the planning and initiation of motor behavior.

Higher-Order Motor Disturbances After Frontal Lobe Lesions

Faglioni and Basso (1985), in their review of the literature, found only seven cases that fit the criteria of a classic limb-kinetic apraxia. Special forms of executional apraxias, such as the apraxia of gait (Gerstmann and Schilder, 1926) and the disturbance of interlimb coordination (Freund and Hummelsheim, 1985), were described earlier. There is increasing evidence that the frontal motor fields are involved in the temporal organization of motor behavior and in motor learning. This is in accord with the concept (Fuster, 1989) that the frontal lobes are involved in the temporal organization of behavior, in planning, focusing attention, and evaluating behavioral goals in the context of limbic drive, present behavioral states, and long-term aspects of behavior that are related to the "memory of the future" (Ingvar, 1985).

The significance of the supplementary motor area in the preparation and initiation of movement has been elaborated on the basis of *Bereitschaftspotential* studies (Kristeva et al., 1979) and regional blood flow investigations (Orgogozo et al., 1979; Roland et al.,

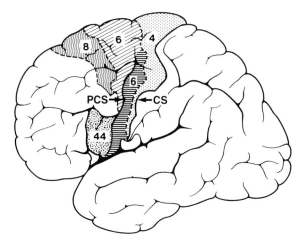

dorsal compartment of area 6 on superior and middle frontal gyrus (PMC d)

ventral compartment of area 6 on precentral gyrus (PMC v)

PCS precentral sulcus

CS central sulcus

Figure 55–5. Distribution of Brodmann agranular and dysgranular cytoarchitectonic areas 4, 6, 8, and 44 on the frontal gyri. Different labels designate the different cytoarchitectonic areas and subdivide area 6 into a ventral compartment that lies on the precentral gyrus (PMC v) and a dorsal part (PMC d) covering the superior and middle frontal gyri. (From Freund H.-J. What is the evidence for multiple motor areas in the human brain? In Humphrey D.R., Freund H.-J., eds. *Motor Control: Concepts and Issues.* Dahlem Konferenzen. New York, Wiley, 1991.)

1982). For the premotor area, the behavioral effects of ablation studies (Halsband and Passingham, 1985) and the results of single-unit recordings in monkeys suggested that PMC is concerned with the conditions for action (Godschalk et al., 1981; Wise et al., 1983). Petrides and Pandya (1984) found that periarcuate lesions caused a severe impairment in the learning of motor conditional tasks. Halsband and Passingham (1985) showed that monkeys with premotor ablations were impaired in relearning a task in which they had to select one of two movements as instructed by a visual cue. In contrast, these animals were not impaired in learning a nonmotor conditional task, in which the visual cues specified which object should be chosen.

These results were expanded by conducting similar experiments in humans. Halsband and Freund (1990) showed that patients with PMC lesions were impaired in their ability to learn an association task between six visual, tactile, or auditory stimuli and six different arm postures, which had been previously learned. This impairment was almost equally pronounced on the side ipsilateral and that contralateral to the lesion. The same patients were not impaired in learning an association between the same set of sensory stimuli and six spatial locations. This selective impairment in sensory conditional motor learning was not found in the comparative evaluation of patients with lesions of primary motor or parietal cortex. For the experiment conducted by Petrides

(1982) on patients with prefrontal lobe damage, no significant deficit of visual conditional motor learning could be detected. The significance of PMC for motor learning is further supported by results of Roland and Seitz (1989), who showed in consecutive experiments on the progress of motor learning that, during a complicated finger sequencing task or during tactile learning (Roland et al., 1989), there was a prominent activation of the contralateral primary motor and sensory hand area and bilaterally of the supplementary motor area and PMC.

Patients with premotor lesions have disturbances not only in motor learning paradigms but also in skilled motor behaviors that had been acquired before damage (Freund, 1989). When the lesion was located in the left hemisphere and affected the more lateral part of the premotor zone close to Broca area, severe agraphia was observed. Closer analysis of this disturbance showed that this was a purely apractic agraphia without a disturbance of the spatial, constructive abilities and without aphasic disturbances. Only the graph, the motor template for the hand-written word, was destroyed, so that the patient could not write without severe derangement and destruction of the written pattern, although the patient could faultlessly execute the letter sequence on a typewriter.

The same study showed that these patients were not disturbed in their capacity to carry out fractionated independent distal movements or in their ability to master tasks involving manual dexterity or tactile exploration, but they showed a pronounced impairment of rhythm production. This was again seen for both hands in patients with lesions of the left PMC but was mainly contralateral with right-sided PMC lesions. Although these patients evidenced a severe disturbance in rhythm production, they were able to discriminate the rhythm pattern without any difficulty, so that they achieved the same score on the Seashore Rhythm Discrimination Test as normal controls. The severe deficit in rhythm production illustrates that the PMC participates in the temporal organization of movement. The composition of muscle synergies and their temporal adjustment is an important component of movement preparation. The elaboration of a "vocabulary of motor acts" (Rizzolati et al., 1983) may represent a significant aspect of premotor function, particularly for the most cortical motor functions of spoken and written language.

Patients with Broca's aphasia have deficits not only in producing speech and writing but also in understanding language. Conversely, those with Wernicke's aphasia show, in addition to the deficits of the production of language and comprehension, pronounced speech dysfunctions. These clinical observations are complemented by stimulation studies on the human brain. The language disturbances elicited by stimulation of Wernicke area are similar to those produced by stimulation of Broca area (Lüders et al., 1989). In both cases, speech arrest was associated with impairment of language comprehension. Patients were unable to follow written or oral commands or to repeat words or sentences. Nonverbal tasks, such as producing complex block designs or copying figures from the Benton Visual Retention Test, could be flawlessly performed. Stimulation of Broca area in three patients elicited agraphia (Lesser et al., 1984). In these three cases, all frontal electrodes that elicited writing arrest also produced speech arrest and an inhibition of other voluntary movements of the contralateral right hand. These results illustrate the interdependence of the sensorimotor interactions involved in language processing.

In spite of the strong sensory projections to the frontal motor fields, there are, however, no reports of cases with unimodal or supramodal apraxias after frontal lobe lesions. From the human studies, it appears that these complex motor disturbances are only seen in the cases with posterior apraxias. The motor dysfunctions ensuing from frontal lesions are characterized by a disturbance of the fine temporal adjustment of motor acts, a disturbance of their kinetic melody, and a disturbance of the sensory cueing of movement and of motor learning.

The Problem of Localization of Apractic Deficits

The problem of localization of complex functions such as language or higher-order motor behavior has two aspects. At first, it seems impossible to draw conclusions from controversial results obtained on the basis of different terminologies, badly defined temporal relationships between damage and assessment, and vaguely described qualitative deficits. In addition, it is presently impossible to determine whether and to what extent a lesion as shown by computed tomography or magnetic resonance imaging is functionally relevant. In addition, the relative contributions of cortical and subcortical damage are difficult to assess. Similar to the results of studies on aphasia, findings regarding large perisylvian lesions of the left hemisphere involving long deep paraventricular subcortical white matter are most consistently associated with apractic deficits.

The second, more pertinent problem of functional localization is the issue of centers versus distributed networks. This controversy is, however, a semantic artifact rather than an issue that promotes the understanding of motor functions and their disturbances. Humans can be paralyzed by the destruction of a small strand of output neurons of the motor cortex to the spinal cord. This final common path of the motor system is the basic prerequisite for conveying all the earlier-mentioned facets of motor behavior to the muscles. The situation is similar to that of the sensory systems in which functional loss ensues when the receptors or their afferent projections are destroyed. It therefore seems equally inappropriate to discuss whether M1 is a motor center or area 17 is a visual center. The further one moves from these nodal points to those areas subserving

more complex aspects of sensorimotor functions, the more difficult is the precise delineation of the neural contributors. The most sophisticated aspects of motor behavior such as pantomime are associated with correspondingly complex neural interactions, so that a pantomime center would be a misnomer as awkward as an apraxia center.

Recovery from apraxia must also be considered in determining the significance of certain brain areas for producing apractic deficits. Basso et al. (1987) followed recovery in 26 patients with ideomotor apraxia and left hemisphere acute stroke lesions. Of these 26 patients who were apractic at the first examination between 15 and 30 days after stroke, 13 were still apractic at the second examination 5–23 months later, but only 5 remained apractic until tested the third time another 5 months later. It was found that "there is no one brain area, a lesion of which is sufficient to prevent recovery" (Basso et al., 1987). The patients with poor prognoses were those with damage to the posterior temporal area and the parieto-occipital junction. Six patients with bilateral damage improved as much as the patients with unilateral lesions. The type of aphasia associated with apraxia had no effect on recovery.

Are Different Lesion Sites Associated with Different Types of Apraxia?

Whether specific lesion sites are associated with certain types of apraxia is controversial. There seems to be some agreement that patients with nonfluent aphasia and buccofacial apraxia have more anterior lesions and patients with fluent aphasia and ideomotor apraxia have more posterior lesions. In some cases, however, the situation may be reversed (Basso et al., 1985). This situation is particularly confusing because buccofacial, or oral, apraxias are frequently included in the category of ideomotor apraxias. Such a classification contradicts previous definitions. Liepmann (1920) and Kleist (1934) clearly included buccofacial apraxia with the limb-kinetic forms. Kleist (1934, p. 467) used the term "limb-kinetic apraxia of the movements of the face, tongue and head." Of course, limb-kinetic is not the adequate term here, but limb-kinetic and facial-oral apraxias were regarded as the same type of disturbance. Transitional forms between limb-kinetic and ideomotor disturbance were also described.

This dilemma shows that the different types of apractic disturbances are obviously not always unambiguously discernible. As is expected from a wide range of different pathophysiologic changes, there ought to be an equally diverse group of apractic phenomena. A scheme with rigidly defined groups is therefore a difficult construction.

Computer graphic recordings may help to arrive at assessments that are based on better insights into the pathophysiology of apractic disturbances. Figure 55–6 shows an example of an arm movement record-

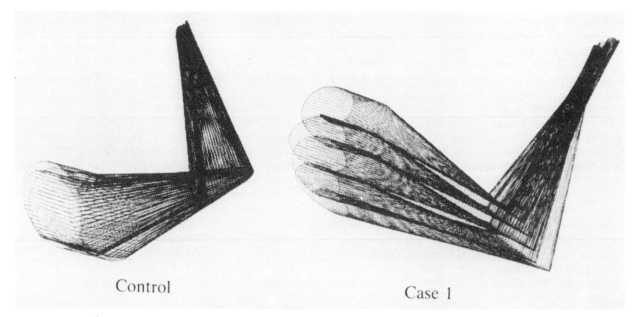

Figure 55–6. Three-dimensional reconstruction of motions of the hand and arm in a gesture simulating rolling up an automobile window for a normal subject *(left)* and a patient with ideomotor apraxia *(right)*. Note added downward movement axis on the right. (From Poizner H., Mack L., Verfaellie L.J., et al. Three-dimensional computergraphic analysis of apraxia. Neural representations of learned movement. *Brain* 113:85–101, 1990 by permission of Oxford University Press.)

ing by means of an optoelectronic camera system. The patient had an ideomotor apraxia and was asked to make a gesture such as to roll up an automobile window. Whereas the control subject performed a smooth circular movement repeated about a well-defined center point, the patient added a downward movement to the circular motions. Variability of movements and impairment in joint control and in the timing associated with loss of regularity and fluidity of the movement were prominent features in the patient (Poizner et al., 1990).

The pattern of disturbance of explorative finger movements in a patient with a unimodal, tactile apraxia attributable to a posterior parietal lesion is shown in Figure 55–7. The movement trajectories of the thumb and the forefinger are grossly deranged on the affected side and the temporal profile shows few irregular movements. The quasisinusoid performance with a preferred frequency of approximately 1 Hz that is typical for the normal hand is substituted by a chaotic pattern on the affected side.

The computer graphic recordings available reveal a substantial alteration of the spatial-temporal aspects of the movement pattern in all cases of apraxia. It remains an open question whether the systematic application of these techniques in examining patients with different types of apraxias will lead to a new taxonomy of the apraxias based on distinguishing features in the movement trajectories or temporal profiles.

CONCLUSIONS

The deep-rooted desire of many neurologists to abandon the term apraxia and to introduce a new

terminology that is based on closer insights into higher-order motor disturbances is now difficult to fulfill. The scheme shown in Table 55–1 attempts a linkage between the traditional concepts and other motor dysfunctions that can be designated as apractic on the basis of the disordered motor behavior and the underlying pathophysiologic changes of disturbed sensorimotor integration. What emerges from the observation of apractic motor behavior and the corresponding lesions is the prominent role of the unimodal and polymodal sensory association areas for motor control. These areas subserve the processing of sensory information not only for perceptive and congitive purposes but also for the elaboration of motor behavior that in turn selects and shapes sensory input. Lesions posterior to the central sulcus leaving the "motor system" intact can cause gross motor disabilities. This is a major contribution of clinical neurology to the field of motor control because this effect did not become apparent from studies on nonhuman primates. The surprisingly discrete sequelae of damage to the premotor areas are most likely due to their bilateral organization.

There is little hope that the present confusion about the phenomenology and terminology of the apraxias could be solved by consensus conferences. Rather, progress in the elucidation of different pathophysiologic and anatomic patterns will allow understanding of apractic disturbances in terms of mechanisms rather than at a descriptive level. The pathophysiology of the higher-order motor disturbances of the apractic type is beginning to emerge from computer graphic movement recordings. Higher-resolution magnetic resonance images have become available, so that precise studies on patients with small lesions

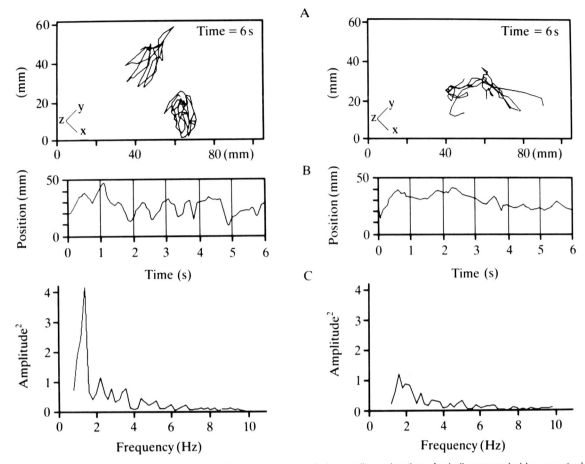

Figure 55–7. Spatial and temporal characteristics of finger movements during tactile exploration of a ball as revealed by an optoelectronic system. *(A)* The movement trajectories of the forefinger and the thumb are shown as viewed from the front, so that the vertical and horizontal movement components are displayed. On the left is the performance of the unaffected, and on the right, of the affected hand. The workspace of the scanning movements is smaller and more irregular for the affected hand, and the finger and the thumb are closer together because the patient had already lost the ball without noticing it. *(B)* The temporal profile of the vertical movement trajectories for the unaffected *(left)* and the affected hand *(right)*. *(C)* The corresponding power spectra show that the normal regular sinusoid movement, as reflected by a prominent peak, is decomposed for the affected hand. (From Pause M., Kunesch E., Binkofski F., et al. Sensorimotor disturbances in patients with lesions of the parietal cortex. *Brain* 112:1599–1625, 1989, by permission of Oxford University Press.)

restricted to cortical and subcortical areas relevant for higher-order motor functions can now be conducted (Damasio and Damasio, 1989). Functional methods such as positron emission tomography and magnetoencephalography, along with the quantitative analysis of motor and oculomotor behavior, hold promise for closer insights into the disordered control mechanisms underlying apractic behavior. It is thus likely that an exciting development in the understanding of the apraxias will occur about a century after Liepmann's ingenious analysis of the clinical picture of the apraxias.

Acknowledgment

I am indebted to Prof. K. Zilles for his advice on the anatomic aspects of this article and for his modification of Figure 55–1.

Table 55–1. THE APRAXIAS*

Posterior Apraxias		Frontal Apraxias
Unimodal Apraxias	*Supramodal Apraxias*	*Executional Apraxias*
Tactile apraxia	Ideational apraxia	Limb-kinetic apraxia
Visuomotor apraxia	Ideomotor apraxia	Disorders of motor
Apraxia of speech		learning and
		rhythm production
Lesion Site		
Unimodal sensory association areas	Polymodal association cortex	Premotor cortex

*Subcortical (disconnection) apraxias can produce any type of apraxia and disturbances of distinct stimulus-response relationships.

References

Alajouanine T., Lhermitte F. Les troubles des activités expressives du langage dans l'aphasie, leurs relations avec les apraxies. *Rev. Neurol. (Paris)* 102:604–629, 1960.

Alexander M.P. Clinical-anatomical correlations of aphasia following predominantly subcortical lesions. In Boller F., Grafman J., eds. *Handbook of Neuropsychology.* Vol. 2. Amsterdam, Elsevier, pp. 47–66, 1989.

Alexander M.P., Baker E., Naeser M.A., et al. The anatomical basis of ideomotor apraxia. *Neurology* 36(Suppl. 1):319, 1986.

Alexander M.P., Naeser M.A., Palumbo C.L. Correlations of subcortical CT lesion sites and aphasia profiles. *Brain* 110:961–991, 1987.

Andersen R.A. Inferior parietal lobule function in spatial perception and visuomotor integration. In Plum F., ed. *Handbook of Physiology*. Section 1. *The Nervous System*. Vol. V. *Higher Functions of the Brain*. Part 2. Bethesda, American Physiological Society, pp. 483–518, 1987.

Bailey P.A., von Bonin G. *The Isocortex of Man*. Urbana, IL University of Illinois Press, 1951.

Balint, R. Seelenlähmung des Schauens, optische Ataxie, räumliche Störung der Aufmerksamkeit. *Monatsschr. Psychiatr. Neurol.* 250:51–81, 1909.

Barbas H., Mesulam M.-M. Organization of afferent input to subdivisions of area 8 in the rhesus monkey. *J. Comp. Neurol.* 200:407–431, 1981.

Basso A., Lecours A.R., Moraschini S., et al. Anatomoclinical correlations of the aphasias as defined through computerized tomography: exceptions. *Brain Lang.* 26:201–229, 1985.

Basso A., Capitani E., Della Sala S., et al. Recovery from ideomotor apraxia: a study on acute stroke patients. *Brain* 110:747–760, 1987.

Bay E. Die corticale Dysarthrie und ihre Beziehungen zur sogenannten motorischen Aphasie. *Dtsch. Z. Nervenheilkd.* 176:553–594, 1957.

Bellugi U., Poizner H., Klima E.S. Language, modality and the brain. *Trends Neurosci.* 12:380–388, 1989.

Brodal P. Principles of organization of the monkey cortico-pontine projection. *Brain* 148:214–218, 1978.

Brodmann K. *Vergleichende Lokalisationslehre der Grosshirnrinde in ihren Prinzipien dargestellt auf Grund des Zellenbaus*. Leipzig, Barth, 1909.

Brown J.W. *Aphasia, Apraxia and Agnosia, Clinical and Theoretical Aspects*. Springfield, IL, Thomas, 1979.

Damasio A.R., Damasio H. *Lesion Analysis in Neuropsychology*. New York, Oxford University Press, 1989.

Delay J. *Les Astéréognosies. Pathologie du Toucher*. Paris, Masson & Cie, 1935.

De Renzi E. The apraxias. In Asbury A.K., McKhann G.M., McDonald W.I., eds. *Diseases of the Nervous System. Clinical Neurobiology*. Vol. II. London, Heinemann, pp. 848–854, 1986.

De Renzi E., Faglioni P., Scotti G. Tactile spatial impairment and unilateral cerebral damage. *J. Nerv. Ment. Dis.* 146:468–475, 1968.

Dum R.P., Strick P.L. Premotor areas: nodal points for parallel efferent systems involved in the central control of movement. In Humphrey D.R., Freund H.J., eds. *Motor Control: Concepts and Issues*. Dahlem Konferenzen. New York, Wiley, 1991a.

Dum R.P., Strick P.L. The origin of corticospinal projections from the premotor areas in the frontal lobe. *J. Neurosci.* 11:667–689, 1991b.

Ettlinger G. Apraxia considered as a disorder of movements that are language-dependent: evidence from cases of brain bisection. *Cortex* 5:285–289, 1969.

Faglioni P., Basso A. Historical perspectives on neuroanatomical correlates of limb apraxia. In Roy E.A., ed. *Neuropsychological Studies of Apraxia and Related Disorders*. Amsterdam, Elsevier, 1985.

Freeman R.B. Jr. The apraxias, purposeful motor behavior, and left-hemisphere function. In Prinz W., Saunders A.F., eds. *Cognition and Motor Processes*. New York, Springer-Verlag, pp. 29–50, 1984.

Freund H.-J. Abnormalities of motor behavior after cortical lesions in humans. In Plum F., ed. *Handbook of Physiology*. Section 1. *The Nervous System*. Vol. V. *Higher Functions of the Brain*. Part 2. Bethesda, American Physiological Society, pp. 763–810, 1987.

Freund H.-J. Motor dysfunctions in Parkinson's disease and premotor lesions. *Eur. Neurol.* 29(Suppl. 1):33–37, 1989.

Freund H.-J. What is the evidence for multiple motor areas in the human brain? In Humphrey D.R., Freund H.-J., eds. *Motor Control: Concepts and Issues*. Dahlem Konferenzen, New York, Wiley, 1991.

Freund H.-J., Hummelsheim H. Lesions of premotor cortex in man. *Brain* 108:697–733, 1985.

Fulton J.F. A note on the definition of the "motor" and "premotor" areas. *Brain* 58:311–316, 1935.

Fuster J.M. *The Prefrontal Cortex: Anatomy, Physiology, and Neuropsychology of the Frontal Lobe*. New York, Raven Press, 1989.

Gerstmann J., Schilder P. Über eine besondere Gangstörung bei Stirnhirnerkrankung. *Wien. Med. Wochenschr.* 76:97–102, 1926.

Geschwind N. Disconnexion syndromes in animals and man. I. *Brain* 88:237–294, 1965a.

Geschwind N. Disconnexion syndromes in animals and man. II. *Brain*. 88:585–644, 1965b.

Geschwind N. The apraxias. In Straus E.W., Griffith R.M., eds. *Phenomenology of Will and Action*. Pittsburgh, PA, Duquesne University Press, pp. 91–102, 1967.

Geschwind N. The apraxias: neural mechanisms of disorders of learned movements. *Am. Sci.* 63:188–195, 1975.

Geschwind N., Kaplan E. A human cerebral deconnection syndrome. *Neurology (Minneap.)* 12:675–685, 1962.

Glickstein M., Cohen J.L., Dixon B., et al. Corticopontine visual projections in macaque monkeys. *J. Comp. Neurol.* 190:209–229, 1980.

Glickstein M., May J., Mercer B. Cortico-pontine projection in the macaque: the distribution of labelled cortical cells after large injections of horseradish peroxidase in the pontine nuclei. *J. Comp. Neurol.* 235:343–359, 1985.

Godschalk M., Lemon R.N., Nijs H.G.T., et al. Behavior of neurones in monkey periarcuate and precentral cortex before and during visually guided arm and hand movements. *Exp. Brain Res.* 44:113–116, 1981.

Goodale M.A., Milner A.D., Jakobson L.S., et al. A neurological dissociation between perceiving objects and grasping them. *Nature* 349:154–156, 1991.

Gowers W. *Lectures on the Diagnosis of Diseases of the Brain*. London, Churchill, 1887.

Haaxma R., Kuypers H.G.J.M. Intrahemispheric cortical connections and visual guidance of hand and finger movements in the rhesus monkey. *Brain* 98:239–260, 1975.

Halsband U., Freund H.-J. Premotor cortex and conditional motor learning in man. *Brain* 113:207–222, 1990.

Halsband U., Passingham R. Premotor cortex and the conditions for movement in monkeys (*Macaca fascicularis*). *Behav. Brain Res.* 18:269–277, 1985.

Hecaen H. Clinical symptomatology in right and left hemisphere lesions. In Mountcastle V.B., ed. *Interhemispheric Relations and Cerebral Dominance*. Baltimore, Johns Hopkins University Press, pp. 215–243, 1962.

Hecaen H., Albert M.L. *Human Neuropsychology*. New York, Wiley, 1978.

Heilman K.M., Rothi L.J.G. Apraxia. In Heilman K.M., Valenstein E., eds. *Clinical Neuropsychology*. New York, Oxford University Press, pp. 131–150, 1985.

Heilman K.M., Rothi L., Valenstein E. Two forms of ideomotor apraxia. *Neurology (N.Y.)* 32:342–346, 1982.

Holmes G. Disturbance of visual orientation. *Br. J. Ophthalmol.* 2:440–468, 506–516, 1918.

Holmes G., Horrax G. Disturbances of spatial orientation and visual attention with loss of stereoscopic vision. *Arch. Neurol. Psychiatry* 1:385–407, 1919.

Howes D.H. Ideomotor apraxia: evidence for the preservation of axial commands. *J. Neurol. Neurosurg. Psychiatry* 51:593–593, 1988.

Hubel D.H., Livingstone M.S. Segregation of form, color, and stereopsis in primate area 18. *J. Neurosci.* 7:3378–3415, 1987.

Humphrey D.R., Tanji J. What features of motor control are encoded in the neuronal discharge in different cortical motor areas? In Humphrey D.R., Freund H.-J., eds. *Motor Control: Concepts and Issues*. Dahlem Konferenzen. New York, Wiley, 1991.

Hyvärinen J. *The Parietal Cortex of Monkey and Man*. New York, Springer-Verlag, 1982.

Ingvar D.H. Memory of the future. An essay on the temporal organization of conscious awareness. *Hum. Neurobiol.* 4:127–136, 1985.

Jeannerod M. *The Neural and Behavioural Organization of Goal-Directed Movements*. Oxford, Clarendon Press, 1988.

Jones E.G., Burton H. Areal differences in the laminar distribution of thalamic afferents in cortical fields of the insular, parietal and temporal regions of primates. *J. Comp. Neurol.* 168:197–248, 1976.

Kleist K. Kortikale (innervatorische) Apraxie. *Jahrb. Psychiatr. Neurol.* 28:46–112, 1907.

Kleist K. *Gehirnpathologie.* Leipzig, Barth, 1934.

Kristeva R., Keller E., Deecke L., et al. Cerebral potentials preceding unilateral and simultaneous bilateral finger movements. *Electroencephalogr. Clin. Neurophysiol.* 47:229–238, 1979.

Lehmkuhl G., Poeck K., Willmes K. Ideomotor apraxia and aphasia: an examination of types and manifestations of apraxic symptoms. *Neuropsychologia* 21:199–212, 1983.

Lesser R.P., Lüders H., Dinner D.S., et al. The location of speech and writing functions in frontal language area. *Brain* 107:275–291, 1984.

Liepmann H. Das Krankheitsbild der Apraxie ("motorische Asymbolie"), auf Grund eines Falles von einseitiger Apraxie. *Monatsschr. Psychiatr. Neurol.* 8:182–197, 1900.

Liepmann H. *Drei Aufsätze aus dem Apraxiegebiet.* Berlin, Karger, 1908.

Liepmann H. Apraxie. In *Brugsch's Ergebnisse der Gesamten Medizin.* Berlin, Urban & Schwarzenberg, pp. 518–543, 1920.

Lüders H., Lesser R.P., Dinner D.S., et al. Localization of cortical function: new information from extraoperative monitoring of patients with epilepsy. *Epilepsia* 29(Suppl. 2):56–65, 1989.

Luria A.R. *Higher Cortical Functions in Man.* New York, Basic Books, 1966.

Mountcastle V.B., Lynch J.C., Georgopolous A.P., et al. Posterior parietal association cortex of the monkey: command functions for operations within extrapersonal space. *J. Neurophysiol.* 38:871–908, 1975.

Naeser M.A., Alexander M.P., Helm-Estabrooks N., et al. Aphasia with predominantly subcortical lesion sites. *Arch. Neurol. (Chicago)* 39:2–14, 1982.

Nathan P.W. Facial apraxia and apraxic dysarthria. *Brain* 70:449–478, 1947.

Nathan P.W., Smith M.C., Cook A.W. Sensory effects in man of lesions of the posterior columns and of some other afferent pathways. *Brain* 109:1003–1041, 1986.

Nielsen J.M. *Agnosia, Apraxia, Aphasia: Their Value in Cerebral Localization.* 2nd ed. New York, Hoeber, 1946.

Orgogozo J.M., Larsen B., Roland P.E., et al. Activation de l'aire motrice supplémentaire au cours des mouvements volontaires chez l'homme. *Rev. Neurol. (Paris)* 135:705–717, 1979.

Pandya D.N., Seltzer B. Association areas of the cerebral cortex. *Trends Neurosci.* 5:386–390, 1982.

Pause M., Kunesch E., Binkofski F., et al. Sensorimotor disturbances in patients with lesions of the parietal cortex. *Brain* 112:1599–1625, 1989.

Petrides M. Deficits on conditional associative-learning tasks after frontal- and temporal-lobe lesions in man. *Neuropsychologia* 23:601–614, 1985.

Petrides M., Pandya D.N. Projections to the frontal cortex from the posterior parietal region in the rhesus monkey. *J. Comp. Neurol.* 228:105–116, 1984.

Poeck K., Lehmkuhl G. Das Syndrom der ideatorischen Apraxie und seine Lokalisation. *Nervenarzt* 51:217–225, 1980.

Poeck K., Lehmkuhl G., Wilmes K. Axial movements in ideomotor apraxia. *J. Neurol. Neurosurg. Psychiatry* 45:1125–1129, 1982.

Poizner H., Mack L., Verfaellie L.J., et al. Three-dimensional computergraphic analysis of apraxia. Neural representations of learned movement. *Brain* 113:85–101, 1990.

Rizzolatti G., Matelli M., Pavesi G. Deficits in attention and movement following the removal of postarcuate (area 6) and prearcuate (area 8) cortex in macaque monkeys. *Brain* 43:118–136, 1983.

Roland P.E., Seitz R.J. Mapping of learning and memory functions in the human brain. In Ottoson D., Rostene W., eds. *Visualization of Brain Functions.* New York, Macmillan, pp. 141–151, 1989.

Roland P.E., Meyer E., Shibasaki T., et al. Regional cerebral blood flow changes in cortex and basal ganglia during voluntary movements in normal human volunteers. *J. Neurophysiol.* 48:467–480, 1982.

Roland P.E., Eriksson L., Widen A. Changes in regional cerebral oxidative metabolism induced by tactile learning and recognition in man. *Eur. J. Neurosci.* 1:3–18, 1989.

Rondot P., de Recondo J., Ribadeau Dumas J.L. Visuomotor ataxia. *Brain* 100:355–376, 1977.

Sittig O. *Über Apraxie.* Berlin, Karger Verlag, 1931.

Ungerleider L.G., Mishkin M. Two cortical visual systems. In Ingle D.J., Goodale M.A., Mansfield R.J.W., eds. *Analysis of Visual Behavior.* Cambridge, MA, M.I.T. Press, pp. 549–586, 1982.

Van Essen D.C., Maunsell J.H.R. Hierarchical organization and functional streams in the visual cortex. *Trends Neurosci.* 6:370–375, 1983.

von Economo C., Koskinas G.N. *Die Cytoarchitektonik der Hirnrinde des erwachsenen Menschen.* Wien, Springer-Verlag, 1925.

Westphal S. Über einen Fall von "amnestischer Aphasie," Agraphie und Apraxie nebst eigenartigen Störungen des Erkennens und Vorstellens im Anschluss an eine eklamptische Psychose. *Dtsch. Med. Wochenschr.* 34:2326–2327, 1908.

Wise S.P. The primate premotor cortex: past, present, and preparatory. *Annu. Rev. Neurosci.* 8:1–19, 1985.

Wise S.P. What are the specific functions of the different motor areas? In Humphrey D.R., Freund H.-J., eds. *Motor Control: Concepts and Issues.* Dahlem Konferenzen. New York, Wiley, 1991.

Wise S.P., Weinrich M., Mauritz K.-H. Motor aspects of cue-related neuronal activity in premotor cortex of the rhesus monkey. *Brain Res.* 260:301–305, 1983.

Wurtz R.H., Mohler C.W. Enhancement of visual responses in monkeys striate cortex and frontal eyefields. *J. Neurophysiol.* 39:766–712, 1976.

Zilles K. The cortex. In Paxinos G., ed. *The Human Nervous System.* San Diego, CA, Academic Press, pp. 757–802, 1990.

56

Neglect

Kenneth M. Heilman
Edward Valenstein
Robert T. Watson

A patient with the neglect syndrome fails to report, or to respond or orient to, novel or meaningful stimuli presented to the side opposite a brain lesion (Heilman, 1979). If this failure can be attributed to either sensory or motor defects, the patient is not considered to have neglect.

The two basic mechanisms that are thought to be responsible for the failure to report, respond, or orient are defects in the systems that mediate sensory attention or motor intention. Whereas attentional defects may be associated with unawareness, intentional disorders may cause a failure to respond despite awareness of the stimulus. Attention and intention defects may occur in two domains: spatial and personal. Therefore, attentional failures may occur for stimuli presented in space or on the body. Similarly, intentional failures may be associated with failure to act in a part of space, in a particular direction, or with a specific body part. Patients with neglect can also have a spatial memory defect. This defect can be for new information or old memories (representational defects). Different manifestations of neglect may occur at different times, and in some patients some of these manifestations are never seen. This chapter describes tests that may be used to assess patients and behaviorally define these disorders and discusses the pathophysiology underlying them.

BEHAVIORAL TESTING FOR THE COMPONENTS OF NEGLECT

Tests for Inattention and Extinction

The attentional aspects of the neglect syndrome are detected by observing abnormal responses to sensory stimuli. Stimuli should be given in at least three modalities—somatesthetic, visual, and auditory—but other stimuli, such as gustatory and olfactory, may be used. Examiners often request immediate response; however, delaying the response and using distractor techniques may help amplify the symptoms.

When testing with somatesthetic stimuli, one may control the intensity of a tactile stimulus by using Von Frei's hairs. However, fingers or cotton applicators are more convenient. Other cutaneous stimuli, such as pins, may be used. For bedside auditory testing, we use sounds made by either rubbing the fingers together or snapping them. When possible, perimetric and tangent screen studies should be used for testing visual fields. However, for bedside testing the confrontational method may be used; the examiner's finger movement can be used as the stimulus. A modified Poppelreuter diagram or written sentences may also be used.

These somatesthetic, auditory, and visual stimuli should be presented to the abnormal (contralateral) side and to the normal side of the body in random order. If the patient responds normally to unilateral stimulation, simultaneous bilateral stimulation may be used. Unilateral stimuli should be randomly interspersed with simultaneous bilateral stimuli. Bender (1952) noted that normal subjects may show extinction to simultaneous stimulation when the stimuli are delivered to two different (asymmetric) parts of the body (simultaneous bilateral heterologous stimulation). For example, if the right side of the face and the left hand are stimulated simultaneously, normal subjects sometimes report only the stimulus on the face. Normal subjects do not extinguish symmetric simultaneous stimuli (simultaneous bilateral homologous stimulation). Simultaneous bilateral heterologous stimulation can sometimes be used to test for milder defects in patients with extinction. For example, when the right side of the face and the left hand are stimulated, patients with left-sided neglect do not report the stimulus on the left hand, but when the left side of the face and the right hand are stimulated, they report both stimuli.

The most frequent response by patients is verbal (i.e., right, left, or both). In addition, the patient may be instructed (verbally or nonverbally by gesture) to move the extremity or extremities the examiner has touched.

Patients may be considered to have hemi-inattention when they fail to orient, report, or respond to contralateral stimuli and when it can be demonstrated that the lesions does not interrupt afferent projections and does not destroy primary sensory cortex or sensory thalamic nuclei. However, unless the site of the lesion is known, it may be difficult to distinguish between hemianesthesia or hemianopia and severe somathesthetic and visual hemiattention. Occasionally, visual inattention may be distinguished from hemianopia by changing the hemispace of presentation. Kooistra and Heilman (1989) reported a patient who could not detect single stimuli presented in the left visual field when the eyes were directed straight ahead but could detect stimuli in the same retinotopic position when the eyes were directed toward right hemispace so that the left visual half-field was in the right hemispace.

Although hemianesthesia and hemianopia are fairly common manifestations of central nervous system lesions, unilateral hearing loss is almost always due to a disturbance in the peripheral hearing mechanisms or in the auditory nerve. Because the auditory pathways that ascend from the brain stem to the cortex are bilateral, each ear projects to both hemispheres. Thus, a unilateral central nervous system lesion will not produce unilateral hearing loss. Consequently, patients without peripheral hearing loss who fail to orient to, or report, unilateral auditory stimulation usually have hemi-inattention. Furthermore, because sound presented on one side of the body projects to both ears, patients with unilateral hearing loss caused by a peripheral lesion usually respond to unilateral auditory stimulation unless the stimulus is extremely close to the ear. Therefore, patients who neglect unilateral auditory stimuli most often have unilateral inattention.

Patients with unilateral neglect are most inattentive to stimuli contralateral to the lesion, but they are often inattentive to ipsilateral stimuli, although ipsilateral inattention is not so severe.

Tests for Personal Neglect

Whereas the failure to detect tactile stimuli described in the preceding section may be a sign of personal neglect, patients with flagrant personal inattention may deny that their own limbs belong to them. The examiner can demonstrate personal ne-

glect by asking patients to show a limb or by showing them their own limb and asking them who the limb belongs to. Patients with personal neglect may also fail to groom or dress half of their body. Although anosognosia of a left hemiplegia and alloesthesia (misplacing contralesional stimuli to the ipsilesional part of the body) are often associated with personal neglect, these three signs are often dissociable.

Tests for Spatial Neglect

Patients who are able to detect contralesional visual stimuli and who may not even have extinction may fail to act on contralesional stimuli presented in space. They may fail to act in left hemispace (egocentric hemispatial neglect), or they may fail to act on the left side of the stimulus (allocentric spatial neglect). The two most frequently used methods for testing spatial neglect are the line bisection and cancellation tasks. In the cancellation test, small lines are randomly drawn on a sheet of paper and the patient is asked to cross out all the lines. This can be made more difficult by using a task in which patients must either discriminate or focus their attention (Rapcsak et al., 1989). In the line bisection task an 8- to 10-inch line is presented to the patient, who is asked to bisect the line (find the middle of the line). This task can be made more difficult by using longer lines (Butter et al., 1988a) or by placing lines to the left of the midsagittal plane (Heilman and Valenstein, 1979). Last, one can test for spatial neglect by having a subject copy drawings. Because neglect is often associated with right hemisphere lesions, patients may have constructional apraxia. Therefore, simple drawings (flower, clock) should be used.

Although spatial neglect is most often described in the horizontal plane (left spatial neglect), vertical neglect (Rapcsak et al., 1988) and radial neglect (Shelton et al., 1990) have been reported. Vertical neglect and radial neglect can be assessed by orienting the line to be bisected in a radial or vertical direction.

Bisiach and Luzzatti (1978) asked patients to describe a familiar scene. Patients with left-sided neglect failed to recall the left side of the scene. Unfortunately, there is no simple bedside test for examining spatial representations. However, one can ask patients to describe the layout of their house, describe the sites on a famous street in their hometown going in a specific direction, or name the cities in the state in which they live. Failure to describe more items on one side than the other may suggest spatial representational neglect. Asking a patient to spell words from memory may also elicit spatial representational neglect but is an insensitive test. Finally, one could ask a patient who can copy drawings well to make the same drawings from memory to see if one side is neglected.

H.B. Coslett (personal communication) showed patients diagrams of the palmar or dorsal aspect of the right or left hand and asked them to tell if the picture showed a right or left hand. To perform this task, one has to image one's own right or left hand in either the prone or supine position. Coslett's patients were impaired when shown diagrams of the left hand but not the right hand, suggesting a defect in the left side of a personal representation.

Tests for Akinesia and Related Disorders: Motor Neglect

Akinesia is the inability to initiate a movement that cannot be attributed to a defect in the motor unit or corticospinal neurons. Milder forms of akinesia may be expressed as a delay in initiating a movement (hypokinesia) or decreased amplitude of movement (hypometria). Akinesia may affect one or more body parts (legs, limbs, eyes, head) and may be spatial or directional. It may be seen only with spontaneously evoked activities (endo-evoked akinesia) or only in response to stimuli (exo-evoked akinesia) or may be mixed. When akinesia is mixed, involves a limb, and is not spatially or directionally specific, it may be difficult to dissociate from a motor defect caused by corticospinal tract damage, and one may have to rely on imaging studies.

When examining a patient for akinesia one must make multiple observations, including watching spontaneous activity to see if the patient moves eyes, head, and limbs in all directions. After an acute insult to the right hemisphere, it is not unusual for the head and eyes to be deviated to the right and not to move toward the left either spontaneously or in response to stimuli or instructions. However, even in the absence of this florid manifestation, contralesional directional akinesia may be detected using a modification of the crossed response task (Watson et al., 1978). The examiner holds one hand in the patient's right visual half-field and the other in the left visual half-field. In the first series of trials, the index finger of the examiner's right or left hand is moved and the patient is instructed to look at the finger. A patient who fails to look at the contralesional stimulus may be hemianopic, have visual inattention, or have directional akinesia. These can be dissociated by instructing the patient to look to the side opposite that stimulated, so that when the examiner's right index finger is moved the patient looks at the left hand and vice versa. Failure to look at the contralesional finger indicates directional akinesia, and failure to look at the ipsilesional finger suggests inattention or hemianopia (Butter et al., 1988b). In less severe cases of directional akinesia, patients may move in a contralesional direction by making multiple hypometric saccades (Heilman et al., 1980).

A condition similar to eye deviation may be detected in the arm by asking blindfolded patients with neglect to point to their midsagittal plane (Heilman et al., 1983a). Patients may point toward the ipsilat-

eral hemispace. To detect directional akinesia of the limbs, a blindfolded patient may be placed before a table that has pennies randomly distributed over the top and be asked to pick up all the pennies. Patients with directional akinesia may fail to explore left hemispace. Patients may also have a directional hypokinesia of the limbs, so that movements toward the left are initiated more slowly than movements toward the right (Heilman et al., 1985). Patients may demonstrate hemispatial akinesia of the limbs such that when the limb is in contralateral hemispace it does not move or it moves less than when it is in ipsilateral hemispace (Meador et al., 1986).

Testing for Denial of Illness

Explicit verbal denial of illness is termed *anosognosia*. Patients with neglect often deny a left hemiplegia, and they may also be unaware of a left hemianopia. Verbally acknowledging a problem but failing to be concerned is called *anosodiaphoria*. Anosognosia and anosodiaphoria are best tested by asking patients why they came to the hospital. If they fail to describe their problems, more specific questions may be asked. If patients have hemispatial inattention, the hemiparetic limbs should be brought into ipsilesional hemispace and the patients should be asked to move the limb and then asked again if they are impaired.

Testing for Alloesthesia and Allokinesia

When stimulated on the side contralateral to a lesion, patients with alloesthesia misplace the location of the stimulus to the normal side. Patients with allokinesia respond with the wrong limb or move in the wrong direction. Alloesthesia and allokinesia should be distinguished from right-left confusion. Patients with right-left confusion do not make systematic directional errors, whereas patients with alloesthesia misattribute left side stimuli to the right but not vice versa.

PATHOPHYSIOLOGY OF THE COMPONENTS OF NEGLECT

Pathophysiology of Inattention

Unilateral inattention can be induced in humans by lesions in a variety of loci. Contralateral inattention may be induced by lesions in the temporoparietal occipital junction or inferior parietal lobe (Critchley, 1966; Heilman et al., 1983b). In humans, inferior parietal lobe lesions are probably most commonly associated with inattention, but lesions of the dorsolateral frontal lobe may also be associated with inattention (Damasio et al., 1980; Heilman and Valenstein, 1972). In humans and monkeys, lesions in the cingulate gyrus (Heilman and Valenstein, 1972; Watson et al., 1973) and subcortical lesions in such areas as the thalamus and mesencephalic reticular formation (Watson and Heilman, 1979; Watson et al., 1974) may also induce inattention.

Cerebral infarction is the most common cause of cortical lesions associated with neglect. Intracerebral hemorrhage is the cause of most subcortical lesions associated with inattention; however, other disease processes, including tumors, may induce inattention.

Inattention is probably caused by dysfunction in a corticolimbic reticular formation network (Heilman and Valenstein, 1972; Watson et al., 1974, 1981) (Fig. 56–1). A discussion of possible mechanisms requires some consideration of the phenomena of arousal, a physiologic state that prepares the organism for sensory and motor processing.

Stimulation of the mesencephalic reticular formation is associated with arousal and also with desynchronization of the electroencephalogram, a physiologic measure of arousal (Moruzzi and Magoun, 1949). Unilateral stimulation induces greater desynchronization of the electroencephalogram in the ipsilateral than in the contralateral hemisphere (Moruzzi and Magoun, 1949). Bilateral mesencephalic reticular formation lesions result in coma. Unilateral lesions result in contralateral inattention, which is probably due to unilateral hemispheric hypoarousal (Reeves and Hagamen, 1971; Watson et al., 1974). The mesencephalic reticular activating system probably projects to the cortex in a diffuse polysynaptic fashion (Schiebel and Schiebel, 1967). This projection may occur through the thalamus (Steriade and Glenn, 1982) or basal forebrain.

There is another way in which the mesencephalic reticular activating system can affect cortical process-ing of sensory stimuli. Sensory information that reaches the cortex is relayed through specific thalamic nuclei. The nucleus reticularis thalami, a thin reticular nucleus enveloping the thalamus, projects to the thalamic relay nuclei and appears to inhibit thalamic relay to the cortex (Schiebel and Schiebel, 1966). The mesencephalic reticular formation projects to the nucleus reticularis. Rapid stimulation of the mesencephalic reticular formation (or behavioral arousal) inhibits the nucleus reticularis and is thereby associated with enhanced thalamic sensory transmission to the cerebral cortex (Singer, 1977). Unilateral lesions of the mesencephalic reticular formation may induce neglect because in the absence of mesencephalic reticular formation–mediated arousal, the cortex is not prepared for processing sensory stimuli and the thalamic sensory relay nuclei are being inhibited by the nucleus reticularis thalami.

Modality-specific association areas may detect stimulus novelty (Sokolov, 1963). When a stimulus is neither novel nor significant, corticofugal projections to the nucleus reticularis thalami may allow habituation to occur by selectively influencing thalamic relay. When a stimulus is novel or significant, the corticofugal projections may inhibit the nucleus reticularis thalami and allow the thalamus to relay additional sensory input.

Unimodal association areas converge on polymodal association areas (see Fig. 56–1) in the prefrontal cortex and in the posterior superior portion of the temporal lobe and inferior parietal lobe (Pandya and Kuypers, 1969). Polymodal convergence areas may subserve cross-modal associations and polymodal sensory synthesis. Polymodal sensory synthesis may also be important in the detection of stimulus novelty (modeling) and significance. In contrast to the uni-

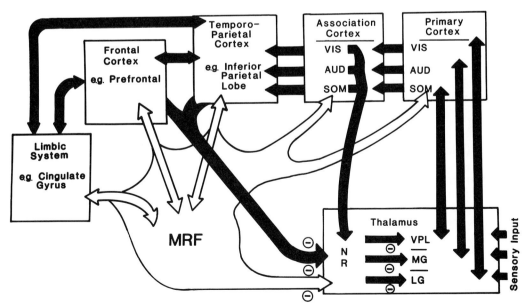

Figure 56–1. Schematic representation of systems important in attention and arousal (see text for details). NR = nucleus reticularis thalami; MRF = mesencephalic reticular formation; VPL = ventralis posterolateralis; MG = medial geniculate; LG = lateral geniculate; VIS = visual; AUD = auditory; SOM = somatosensory.

modal association cortex that projects to specific parts of the nucleus reticularis thalami and thereby gates sensory input in one modality, these multimodal convergence areas may have a more general inhibitory action on the nucleus reticularis thalami and provide further arousal after cortical analysis. These convergence areas also may project directly to the mesencephalic reticular formation, which may either induce a general state of arousal because of diffuse multisynaptic connections to the cortex or increase thalamic transmission through connections with the nucleus reticularis thalami, or both. Evidence that polymodal areas of the cortex, such as the prefrontal and inferior parietal lobe, are important in arousal comes from neurophysiologic studies showing that stimulation of these cortical sites induces a generalized arousal response (Segundo et al., 1955). When similar sites are ablated, there is electroencephalographic evidence of ipsilateral hypoarousal (Watson et al., 1977).

Although the sensory association cortex may mediate determination of stimulus novelty, stimulus significance is determined in part by the needs of the organism (motivational state). Limbic system input into the brain regions important for determining stimulus significance may provide information about biologic needs. The frontal lobes may provide input about needs related to goals that are neither dependent directly on the stimulus nor motivated by an immediate biologic need, because the frontal lobes have a critical role in goal-mediated behavior and in developing sets.

The inferior parietal lobe has prominent limbic (cingulate) and frontal connections (Baleydier and Mauguière, 1980; Pandya and Kuypers, 1969; Vogt et al., 1979) that may provide an anatomic substrate through which motivational states (for example, biologic needs, sets, and long-term goals) may influence stimulus processing (Heilman, 1979; Heilman and Valenstein, 1972; Watson et al., 1981).

Investigators have been able to study the physiologic function of specific areas of the nervous system by recording from single neurons in awake animals. In this experimental situation, the firing characteristics of individual neurons can be measured in relation to specific sensory stimulation or motor behavior. Investigators have thus defined the properties of neurons in the inferior parietal lobule (area 7) of the monkey (Lynch, 1980; Mountcastle et al., 1975). Unlike the activity of single cells in primary sensory cortex, the activity of many neurons in the inferior parietal lobule correlates best with stimuli or responses of importance to the animal, and similar stimuli or responses that are unimportant are associated with either no change or a lesser change in neuronal activity. These cells appear to be critical in directing attention.

The attentional model we have discussed is summarized in Figure 56–1. Unilateral inattention follows lesions of the unilateral mesencephalic reticular activating system because loss of inhibition of the ipsilateral nucleus reticularis by the mesencephalic

reticular activating system decreases thalamic transmission of sensory input to the cortex or because the mesencephalic reticular formation does not prepare the cortex for sensory processing, or both. Unilateral lesions of the primary or association cortices cause contralateral unimodal sensory loss or inability to synthesize contralateral unimodal sensory input. Corticothalamic collaterals from the association cortex to the nucleus reticularis may serve unimodal habituation and attention. Unilateral lesions of multimodal sensory convergence areas that project to mesencephalic reticular activating system and nucleus reticularis induce contralateral inattention because the subject cannot be aroused to, or process, multimodal contralateral stimuli. A lesion of the inferior parietal lobule, because of its reciprocal connections with polymodal areas and the limbic system, may impair the subject's ability to determine the significance of a stimulus.

EXTINCTION TO SIMULTANEOUS STIMULATION

Although patients may initially have hemi-inattention, most improve. Whereas at first they fail to detect stimuli presented to the side opposite the lesion, they eventually become able to report these stimuli. When given bilateral simultaneous stimulation, however, they often fail to report the stimulus presented to the side contralateral to the lesion (Anton, 1899; Bender, 1952; Loeb, 1885; Poppelreuter, 1949).

Extinction can be seen in normal subjects as well as in patients with central nervous system lesions (Benton and Levin, 1972; Kimura, 1967). The lesions causing extinction are often in the same areas as lesions that cause inattention. However, certain forms of extinction may also occur after lesions of the corpus callosum (Milner et al., 1968; Sparks and Geschwind, 1968), and left-sided extinction has even been reported after left hemisphere lesions (Schwartz et al., 1979).

The mechanisms underlying extinction in normal subjects and in patients with callosal lesions, sensory defects, or hemispheric lesions may differ and in general are poorly understood. Several investigators have suggested that extinction and perhaps obscuration in normal subjects and patients with sensory loss result from suppression or reciprocal inhibition. In the case of cerebral damage, the normal hemisphere inhibits the damaged hemisphere more than the damaged hemisphere inhibits the normal hemisphere. Consequently, stimuli contralateral to the damaged hemisphere are not perceived when the normal side is stimulated. The physiologic mechanisms that induce this reciprocal inhibition are unknown. However, as discussed earlier, the thalamic reticular nucleus can selectively inhibit various thalamic sensory nuclei. Each association cortex may not only project to the ipsilateral thalamic reticular nucleus but also influence the contralateral thalamic reticular nucleus. Unlike the ipsilateral connections, which are inhibitory, the contralateral projections may be facilitatory. Therefore, even under normal conditions, a stimulus on one side should induce an increase of threshold for stimuli on the other side. With a lesion of association cortex there should be less ipsilateral inhibition of nucleus reticularis thalami, which in turn should inhibit the thalamic sensory nuclei, thus making the thalamus less sensitive to contralateral stimuli. If the opposite side were simultaneously stimulated, activated attentional cells should further increase contralateral nucleus reticularis thalami activity, further inhibiting the thalamic sensory nuclei and thereby inducing extinction. The pathway by which one association cortex may influence the contralateral nucleus reticularis thalami is unknown.

Birch et al. (1967) proposed and provided support for the hypothesis that the damaged hemisphere processes information more slowly than does the intact hemisphere. Because of this inertia, the damaged side is more subject to interference from the normal side. When stimuli must be processed by a lateralized system, callosal lesions may induce extinction because the information cannot reach the processor or is delayed.

Another explanation for extinction, the limited attention theory, proposes that under normal circumstances bilateral simultaneous stimuli are processed simultaneously, each hemisphere processing the contralateral stimulus (Heilman, 1979). However, a damaged hemisphere may be unable to attend to contralateral stimuli, making the organism inattentive to those stimuli. As the organism recovers, it can attend to contralateral stimuli. This improvement may be mediated by the normal (ipsilateral) hemisphere. The normal hemisphere, however, may have a limited attentional capacity. Therefore, with bilateral simultaneous stimulation the normal hemisphere's attentional mechanism, occupied with the contralateral stimulus, may be unable to attend to the ipsilateral stimulus (Heilman, 1979).

These theories may not be mutually exclusive. Because extinction can be caused by lesions in a variety of anatomically and functionally different areas, the reciprocal inhibition, limited attention, and interference theories may each be correct, but for different lesions.

Pathophysiology of Akinesia

Attention and intention (preparation to make a movement) are closely linked, and lesions in many of the areas that induce inattention and extinction may also induce akinesia. For example, unilateral sensory neglect (inattention) has been reported to follow unilateral dorsolateral frontal lesions in monkeys (Bianchi, 1895; Kennard and Ectors, 1938; Welch and Stuteville, 1958) and humans (Heilman and Val-

enstein, 1972). In most testing paradigms the animal is required to respond to a stimulus contralateral to the lesion either by orienting to the stimulus or by moving the limbs on the side of the stimulus. These animals with frontal lobe lesions were not weak, so it was assumed that they had sensory neglect when they failed to make the appropriate response. Although this neglect was usually assumed to result from inattention to the sensory stimuli, we suggested that it could equally well be caused by unilateral akinesia (Watson et al., 1978). Therefore, we trained monkeys to use the left hand to respond to a tactile stimulus on the right leg and the right hand to respond to a tactile stimulus on the left. After a unilateral frontal arcuate lesion, the monkeys appeared to have contralateral neglect, but when stimulated on their neglected side, they responded normally with the limb on the side of the lesion. When stimulated on the side ipsilateral to the lesion, however, they often failed to respond (with the limb on the neglected side) or responded by moving the limb ipsilateral to the lesion. These results cannot be explained by sensory or perceptual hypotheses and are thought to reflect a defect in intention to make a correct response.

In considering the possible role of the dorsolateral frontal lobes in attention and intention related to multimodal sensory and limbic inputs, it is important to examine their connections. The dorsolateral frontal lobe has reciprocal connections with unimodal and polymodal posterior sensory association cortex (Chavis and Pandya, 1976) and is an area of sensory convergence (Bignall and Imbert, 1969). The dorsolateral frontal lobe has reciprocal connections with medial (nonspecific) thalamic nuclei. Projections to the mesencephalic reticular formation (Kuypers and Lawrence, 1967) and nonreciprocal projections to caudate also exist. Also, the dorsolateral frontal lobe receives input from the limbic system, primarily from the anterior cingulate gyrus (Baleydier and Mauguière, 1989).

Its connections with neocortical sensory association and sensory convergence areas may provide the frontal lobe with information about external stimuli that may call the organism to action. The limbic connections (anterior cingulate gyrus) may provide the frontal lobe with motivational information. Connections with the mesencephalic reticular formation may be important in arousal.

Because the dorsolateral frontal lobe has sensory association cortex and limbic and reticular formation connections, it seems to be ideal for mediating a response to a stimulus to which the subject is attending. Physiologic studies support this hypothesis (Goldberg and Bushnell, 1981).

Motor neglect or akinesia may also accompany lesions of the nonspecific intralaminar thalamic nuclei (Watson et al., 1978), which project to both the frontal lobe and the neostriatum. Akinesia may result from basal ganglia and ventral thalamic lesions (ventralis lateralis and ventralis anterior) (Velasco and Velasco, 1979). The basal ganglia project to the ventral thalamus, and this motor portion of the thalamus is also gated by nucleus reticularis thalami. The nucleus reticularis thalami may be inhibited by the mesencephalic reticular formation during an arousal or orienting response and be inhibited by the frontal lobes during a motor set.

Akinetic mute states are often induced by bilateral lesions of the frontal lobes, cingulate gyri, and medial thalamus. These lesions are usually caused by vascular disease (Segarra and Angelo, 1970). A cingulate gyrus lesion may be induced by an infarct in the distribution of the anterior cerebral artery, secondary to thrombosis, embolism, or aneurysm-induced spasm. Akinetic mutism of thalamic origin is most often the result of occlusion of the posterior thalamic-subthalamic paramedian arteries (Segarra and Angelo, 1970).

Degenerative diseases that affect the basal ganglia, limbic system, and frontal lobes may also induce akinesia. These include Parkinson's disease, progressive supranuclear palsy, striatonigral degeneration, olivopontocerebellar degeneration, and related diseases. Late in the course of several degenerative dementias, including Pick's disease and Alzheimer's disease, akinesia may be a prominent sign.

Lesions that disrupt the connections of the frontal lobes, limbic system, basal ganglia, and thalamus may also be associated with akinesia. Hydrocephalus, tumors (such as butterfly gliomas), lacunae, and Binswanger's disease are common causes of such lesions.

Pathophysiology of Spatial Neglect

Lesions associated with hemispatial neglect are similar to those associated with inattention and extinction. Although hemianopia may enhance the symptoms of hemispatial neglect, hemianopia alone cannot account for the deficit because some patients with hemispatial neglect are not hemianopic (McFie et al., 1950) and some hemianopic patients do not have spatial neglect.

The abnormal performance of patients in and toward contralateral space suggests that brain mechanisms related to the opposite hemispace have been disturbed. It also suggests that each hemisphere is responsible not only for receiving stimuli from the contralateral visual field and for controlling the contralateral limbs but also for attention and intention in and toward contralateral hemispace, independent of which visual field the stimulus enters or which hand is used (Bowers and Heilman, 1980; Heilman, 1979). The postulate that each hemisphere attends to and intends in and toward contralateral hemispace has been supported by studies of normal subjects (Bowers et al., 1981).

Hemispace can be defined according to the visual half-field (eye position), head position, or trunk position. With the eyes and head facing directly ahead, the hemispaces defined by the eyes, head, and body

are congruent. But if the eyes are directed to the far right, for example, the left visual field falls in large part in the right hemispace, as defined by the head and body midline. Similarly, if the head and eyes are turned far to the right, the left head and eye hemispaces can both be in the right hemispace of the body. There is evidence that head and body hemispaces are important in determining the symptoms of hemispatial neglect (Bowers and Heilman, 1980; Heilman and Valenstein, 1979). For example, when patients with left hemispatial neglect are asked to bisect a line, their performance is poorer in left body hemispace than in right body hemispace even when a strategy is used to ensure that the line is seen in the normal right body hemifield (Heilman and Valenstein, 1979). Similarly, independent of visual field and body hemispace, lines are more poorly bisected in left head hemispace than in right head hemispace (Coslett et al., 1985).

Several neuropsychologic mechanisms could account for the hemispatial defect associated with neglect. Patients with hemispatial neglect may have a hemispatial attentional deficit. Although the line is seen in the normal visual field, it is not attended and thus is not fully processed; the percept is therefore not consolidated and the stimulus does not affect the patient's behavior. The attentional defect may also be associated with a hemispatial memory defect (Heilman et al., 1974).

Patients with neglect may have an attentional bias such that their attention is drawn to the side of space ipsilateral to their lesion (Kinsbourne, 1970) and they are unable to draw their attention away from the ipsilateral part of space. Partial support for the attentional bias hypothesis comes from the observation that in a cancellation task, erasing lines is associated with better performance than canceling lines. When lines are erased they no longer draw attention (Mark et al., 1988).

Hemispatial neglect may be associated with a directional and hemispatial akinesia of the eyes and the arm. The former together with inattention would prevent patients from fully exploring the left side of space, and the latter would prevent patients with neglect from acting with their arms in the left side of space. As previously discussed, patients with neglect may have a directional akinesia of their eyes that is independent of their inattention (Butter et al., 1988b). In regard to the arm, Coslett et al. (1990) prevented patients from looking directly at their hand when performing a line bisection task; instead, a video camera projected the hand and the line to a video monitor. Using this technique, the hemispace where the action took place could be dissociated from the hemispace where visual feedback took place. Some patients did better when the monitor was in ipsilateral hemispace than in contralateral hemispace. Others were not affected by the position of the monitors but did better when the action took place in ipsilateral hemispace than they did when the action took place in contralateral hemispace. Coslett et al. (1990) suggested that patients with intentional neglect had more involvement of the frontal lobes than those with attentional spatial neglect who had involvement of the parietal lobes.

Pathophysiology of Representational Defects

Bisiach and Luzzatti (1978) asked two patients with right hemisphere damage to describe from memory a familiar scene in Milan from two different perspectives, one facing the cathedral and the other facing away. In both orientations, left-sided details were omitted. On the basis of these findings, the investigators postulated that the mental representation of the environment is structured topographically and is mapped across the brain so that it is split between the two hemispheres (like the projection of a real scene). With hemispheric damage there is a representational disorder for the contralateral half of this image. Brain (1941) proposed that the parietal lobes contain personal (body) and spatial schemata (representations). The two patients of Bisiach and Luzzatti (1978) and the three described by Meador and colleagues (1987) with hemispatial representational disorder all had right temporoparietal damage.

There are at least three explanations for the failure of Bisiach and Luzzatti's patients to envision one half of the mental image: (1) the representation may have been destroyed, as suggested by Bisiach and Luzzatti; (2) the representation may have been intact but could not be activated, so an image could not be formed; and (3) the image was formed, but it could not be fully explored or attended to (e.g., hemispatial inattention to an internal representation). If a representation is destroyed, attentional manipulation should not affect retrieval, but if patients with neglect have an activational or attentional deficit, attentional manipulation may affect retrieval. Meador et al. (1986) not only replicated Bisiach and Luzzatti's observations but also provided evidence that behavioral manipulations could affect performance. When normal subjects are asked to recall an object in space, they move their eyes to the position the object occupied in space (Kahneman, 1973). Moving one's eyes to a specific spatial location may aid recall. Having patients move their eyes toward neglected hemispace may aid recall because the eye movement induces hemispheric activation or helps direct attention. Meador et al. (1986) asked a patient with left hemispatial neglect and defective left hemispatial recall to move his eyes to either right or left hemispace while recalling a scene. The patient's recall of details on the left side was better when he was looking toward the left than toward the right. This finding provides evidence that hemispatial representational deficit may be induced by activation or an exploratory-attentional deficit.

Pathophysiology of Denial of Hemiplegia (Anosognosia)

Denial of hemiplegia is most often seen with right hemisphere lesions. The lesion usually includes both the frontal and parietal regions.

There have been many explanations of this dramatic behavioral aberration. Weinstein and Kahn (1955) studied the premorbid personalities of patients with anosognosia and found that before their strokes, they used denial mechanisms more frequently than did controls. However, Weinstein and Kahn's study cannot explain why denial of hemiplegia is more frequently associated with right hemisphere lesions. Denial of hemiplegia is often associated with neglect, and perhaps patients do not recognize that they are hemiplegic because they have personal neglect. However, Bisiach et al. (1986) demonstrated that personal neglect was not always associated with denial of hemiplegia. The disconnection hypothesis has also been used to explain denial of hemiplegia, postulating that the damaged right hemisphere is disconnected from other areas of the brain, including speech-language areas (Geschwind, 1965). It is well established that the left hemisphere speech areas in the absence of input often confabulate a response (Gazzaniga, 1970). Neither the disconnection hypothesis nor the neglect hypothesis can explain why patients still deny hemiplegia when the paretic hand is brought into right hemispace or into the right visual field, where it gains direct access to the left hemisphere.

Many theories of anosognosia are related to defective feedback. Even though these feedback theories may help explain failure to recognize a hemianopia or unawareness of hemiplegia, they cannot explain denial or hemiplegia when the arm is brought into a normal visual field. We propose a "feed-forward" or "intentional" theory of denial of hemiplegia, in which the previously discussed intentional system may be responsible not only for activating the motor systems but also for feeding information about motor expectations to comparator systems. When a patient without anosognosia attempts to move a paretic limb, the comparator notes a mismatch between expectations and performance. However, when the intentional system is impaired (independently or along with the motor systems), not only is there inability to activate the motor neurons but also expectations are not fed to the comparator. When the patient fails to move there is no mismatch and, therefore, no awareness of a deficit. Perhaps this is why patients who have denial of left hemiplegia, when asked why they are not moving their arm, call it "lazy" (Weinstein and Kahn, 1955). As discussed, intentional defects such as akinesia are more commonly associated with right than left hemisphere lesions. If denial of hemiplegia is related to intentional defects, it is not surprising that denial of hemiplegia is also more common with right hemisphere lesions.

HEMISPHERIC ASYMMETRIES AND THE NEGLECT SYNDROME

Many early investigators noted that inattention is more often associated with right than with left hemisphere lesions (Brain, 1941; Critchley, 1966; McFie et al., 1950). To account for hemispheric asymmetry of attention in humans, it has been postulated that temporoparietal regions of the human brain also have attentional or comparator neurons but that the neuronal networks in the right hemisphere are more likely to have bilateral receptive fields than those in the left hemisphere. Thus, the networks in the left hemisphere would be activated predominantly by novel or significant stimuli on the right, but the networks in the right hemisphere would be activated by novel or significant stimuli on either or both sides (Heilman and Van Den Abell, 1980). If this were the case, right hemisphere lesions would cause inattention more often than left hemisphere lesions. When the left hemisphere is damaged, the right can attend to ipsilateral stimuli, but the left hemisphere cannot attend to ipsilateral stimuli after right-sided damage. Support for this hypothesis has been provided by electrophysiologic (Heilman and Van Den Abell, 1980) and imaging (Prohovnik et al., 1981; Rosen et al., 1981) studies. Extinction has also been shown to be more frequent with right than left hemisphere dysfunction (Meador et al., 1988) and may also be related to the hemispheric asymmetries in attentional capacity.

Some patients with right hemisphere lesions are also inattentive to right-sided stimuli (Albert, 1973). Although damage to attentional or comparator networks in the right hemisphere may induce an ipsilateral defect, the cortical lesions may also induce an arousal defect. Using a galvanic skin response and electroencephalographic power spectrum recording, it has been shown that right hemisphere lesions reduce arousal to stimuli presented to the hand ipsilateral to the lesion (Heilman et al., 1978) as well as to the opposite hand.

Patients with right hemisphere lesions also have contralateral limb akinesia more often than do patients with left hemisphere lesions (Coslett and Heilman, 1989). Hypokinesia, however, is not always limited to the contralateral extremities. Howes and Boller (1975) found that patients with right hemisphere lesions had slower reaction times than did patients with left hemisphere lesions. In their patients, the right hemisphere lesions associated with this slowing were not larger than those on the left. Although the right parietal lobe lesions appeared to induce the most profound slowing, these investigators did not mention whether the patients with ipsilateral slowing had unilateral neglect. In monkeys, no hemispheric asymmetries in production of the neglect syndrome have been noted. However, monkeys with lesions inducing neglect had slower ipsilateral reaction times than did monkeys with equal-sized lesions that did not induce neglect (Valenstein et al., 1987).

Lansing and colleagues (1959) have shown that warning stimuli may prepare an organism for action and thereby reduce reaction times. Pribram and McGuinness (1975) used the term activation to define the physiologic readiness to respond to environmental stimuli. Because patients with right hemisphere lesions have reduced behavioral evidence of activation (Howes and Boller, 1975), it has been postulated that in humans the right hemisphere dominates in mediating the activation process (Heilman and Van Den Abell, 1979). That is, the left hemisphere prepares the right extremities for action, and the right prepares both. Therefore, with left-sided lesions, left-sided limb akinesia is minimal, but with right-sided lesions there is severe left limb akinesia. In addition, because the right hemisphere is more involved than the left hemisphere in activating the right extremities, there is more ipsilateral hypokinesia with right hemisphere lesions, than with left hemisphere lesions.

That the right hemisphere dominates mediation of activation or intention (physiologic readiness to respond) has been demonstrated in normal subjects. They show more activation (measured behaviorally by the reaction time) with warning stimuli delivered to the right hemisphere than to the left hemisphere. That is, warning stimuli projected to the right hemisphere reduced reaction times of the right hand more than stimuli projected to the left hemisphere reduced left-hand reaction times; warning stimuli projected to the right hemisphere reduced reaction times of the right hand even more than did warning stimuli projected directly to the left hemisphere. These results support the hypothesis that the right hemisphere dominates activation or intention (Heilman and Van Den Abell, 1979).

Physical therapists and occupational therapists have noted that it is more difficult to rehabilitate patients with right hemisphere damage than those with left hemisphere damage. Right hemisphere–damaged patients have a greater mortality (related to pulmonary emboli and pneumonia) immediately after stroke. Both the difficulties in rehabilitation and the greater mortality after stroke may be related to the akinesia induced by right hemisphere lesions.

Lesions in the right hemisphere more often induce hemispatial neglect than do those in the left hemisphere. The neglect induced by right hemisphere lesions is also more severe (Albert, 1973; Costa et al., 1969; Gainotti et al., 1972). Verbal stimuli might activate the left hemisphere and thereby further enhance attentional-intentional hemispatial asymmetry (Heilman and Watson, 1978). However, when paradigms that do not use verbal stimuli or verbal instructions are tested, right hemisphere lesions induce more severe hemispatial neglect than do those on the left (Albert, 1973). The mechanism of this asymmetry may be similar to mechanisms already discussed. The left hemisphere may be able to attend and intend only in and toward the right hemispatial field. Therefore, with left hemisphere lesions the right hemisphere will attend and intend in and toward ipsilateral (right) hemispace. However, with right hemisphere lesions, the left hemisphere attends and intends in and toward the right hemispace and the left hemispace is neglected.

RECOVERY OF FUNCTION AND TREATMENT

Hier et al. (1983) demonstrated that neglect improves in many patients. The mechanism underlying recovery is not completely understood. One hypothesis is that the undamaged hemisphere is involved in recovery.

Crowne et al. (1981) showed that neglect resulting from frontal ablations was worse when the corpus callosum was simultaneously transected than when the callosum was intact, and Watson et al. (1984) demonstrated that monkeys that had a frontal arcuate gyrus ablation several months after a corpus callosum transection had worse neglect than did animals with an intact callosum. Although callosal section worsened the severity of neglect, it did not influence the rate of recovery, suggesting that recovery is an intrahemispheric process.

Hughlings Jackson (Taylor, 1932) postulated that certain functions could be mediated at several levels of the nervous system. Lesions of higher areas (e.g., cortex) would release phylogenetically more primitive areas that might take over the function of the lesioned cortical areas. The superior colliculus receives not only optic but also somatesthetic projections (Sprague and Meikle, 1965) and fibers from the medial and lateral lemnisci and from the inferior colliculus (Truex and Carpenter, 1964). Sprague and Meikle thought that the colliculus is more than a reflex center controlling eye movements: it is a sensory integrative center. Tectoreticular fibers project to the mesencephalic reticular formation, and ipsilateral fibers are more abundant than contralateral fibers (Truex and Carpenter, 1964). Stimulation of the colliculus (like stimulation of the arcuate gyrus or the inferior parietal lobe) induces an arousal response (Jefferson, 1958). Unilateral lesions of the superior colliculus induce a multimodal unilateral neglect syndrome, and combined cortical-collicular lesions induce a more profound disturbance, regardless of the order of removal (Sprague and Meikle, 1965). On the basis of these observations, we suspect that much of the recovery seen after cortical lesions may be mediated by the colliculus.

Subcortical lesions of ascending dopamine projections in rats induce permanent neglect (Marshall, 1982). The severity and persistence of neglect induced by 6-hydroxydopamine injections into the ventral tegmental area of rats are correlated with the amount of striatal dopamine depletion: those with more than 95% loss of striatal dopamine have a permanent deficit. The extent of recovery of these animals is also directly related to the quantity of neostriatal dopamine present when the animal is killed. Nonrecovered rats show pronounced contralateral turning after injections of apomorphine, a dopamine receptor stimulant. Recovered rats given metyrosine (methyl-p-tyrosine), a catecholamine synthesis inhibitor, or spiroperidol, a dopamine receptor blocking agent, had their deficits reappear. These results suggest that restoration of dopaminergic activity in dopamine-depleted rats is sufficient to reinstate orientation (Marshall, 1979). Further investigation of these findings indicates that proliferation of dopamine receptors may contribute to pharmacologic supersensitivity and recovery of function (Neve et al., 1982). Implanting dopaminergic neurons from the ventral tegmental area of fetal rats adjacent to the striatum ipsilateral to the lesion induces recovery in rats with unilateral neglect resulting from a 6-hydroxydopamine lesion in the ascending dopamine tracts (Dunnett et al., 1981). This recovery is related to growth of dopamine-containing neurons into the partially denervated striatum.

Incorporation of ^{14}C-labeled 2-deoxy-D-glucose (2-DG) permits a measure of metabolic activity. In rats with 6-hydroxydopamine lesions of the ventral tegmental areas that had shown no recovery from neglect, the uptake of labeled 2-DG into the neostriatum, nucleus accumbens septi, olfactory tubercle, and central amygdaloid nucleus was significantly less on the denervated side than on the normal side. Rats that recovered by 6 weeks showed equivalent 2-DG uptake in the neostriatum and central amygdaloid nucleus on the two sides. Recovery is therefore associated with normalization of neostriatal metabolic activity (Kozlowski and Marshall, 1981).

Similar results have been obtained for monkeys recovering from frontal arcuate gyrus–induced neglect (Deuel et al., 1979). Animals with neglect showed depression of ^{14}C-labeled 2-DG in ipsilateral subcortical structures, including the thalamus and basal ganglia. Recovery from neglect occurred concomitantly with reappearance of symmetric metabolic activity.

Because alterations of the dopamine system may be partly responsbile for the symptoms of neglect and recovery from neglect, we decided to learn whether we could improve frontal lesion–induced neglect in rats by using the dopamine agonist apomorphine (Corwin et al., 1986). Because the animals showed dramatic improvement, we gave bromocriptine to patients with neglect. Patients improved with the medication and had a relapse after the medication was withdrawn. The results suggest that improvement may have been related to the medicine and not to the natural history of the disease (Fleet et al., 1987). Unfortunately, a double-blind study has not been done. Rubens (1985) observed improvements in humans with neglect when the labyrinth was stimulated. This finding suggests that stimulation of the labyrinth or brain stem may be useful in treating these patients. Also, several things can be done to manage the symptoms of the neglect syndrome. Patients with neglect should be placed so that their "good" side faces the area where interpersonal actions are most likely to take place. Fleet and Heilman (1986) have demonstrated that hemispatial neglect may become worse with repeated trials. However, knowledge of results (i.e., feedback to the patient) that induces increased arousal and effort may reverse this fatigue effect.

In addition, because patients with neglect remain inattentive to their left side and in general are poorly motivated, training and rehabilitation efforts are laborious and in many cases nonrewarding. Diller and Weinberg (1977) were able to train patients with neglect to look to their neglected side, but it has not been shown that the patients can fully generalize this training to nontask situations.

References

Albert M.L. A simple test of visual neglect. *Neurology (Minneap.)* 23:658–664, 1973.

Anton G. Über die Selbstwahrnehmung der Herderkrankungen des Gehirns durch den Kranken der Rindenblindheit und Rindentaubheit. *Arch. Psychiatr.* 32:86–127, 1899.

Baleydier C., Mauguière F. The duality of the cingulate gyrus in monkey—neuroanatomical study in functional hypothesis. *Brain* 103:525–554, 1980.

Bender M.B. *Disorders of Perception.* Springfield, IL, Thomas, 1952.

Benton A.L., Levin H.S. An experimental study of obscuration. *Neurology (Minneap.)* 22:1176–1181, 1972.

Bianchi L. The functions of the frontal lobes. *Brain* 18:497–522, 1895.

Bignall K.E., Imbert M. Polysensory and cortico-cortical projections to frontal lobe of squirrel and rhesus monkey. *Electroencephalogr. Clin. Neurophysiol.* 26:206–215, 1969.

Birch H.G., Belmont I., Karp E. Delayed information processing and extinction following cerebral damage. *Brain* 90:113–130, 1967.

Bisiach E., Luzzatti C. Unilateral neglect of representational space. *Cortex* 14:29–133, 1978.

Bisiach E., Valler G., Perani D., et al. Unawareness of disease following lesions of the right hemisphere: anosognosia for hemiplegia and anosognosia for hemianopsia. *Neuropsychologia* 24:471–482, 1986.

Bowers D., Heilman KmM. Pseudoneglect: effects of hemispace on tactile line bisection task. *Neuropsychologia* 18:491–498, 1980.

Bowers D., Heilman K.M., Van Den Abell T. Hemispace-VHF compatibility. *Neuropsychologia* 19:757–765, 1981.

Brain W.R. Visual disorientation with special reference to lesions of the right cerebral hemisphere. *Brain* 64:224–272, 1941.

Butter C.M., Mark V.W., Heilman K.M. As experimental analysis of factors underlying neglect in line bisection. *J. Neurol. Neurosurg. Psychiatry* 51:1581–1583, 1988a.

Butter C.M., Rapcsak S.Z., Watson R.T., et al. Changes in sensory attention, directional hypokinesia and release of the fixation reflex following a unilateral frontal lesion: a case report. *Neuropsychologia* 26:533–545, 1988b.

Chavis D.A., Pandya D.N. Further observations on cortico-frontal connections in the rhesus monkey. *Brain Res.* 117:369–386, 1976.

Corwin J.V., Kanter S., Watson R.T., et al. Apomorphine has a therapeutic effect on neglect produced by unilateral dorsomedial prefrontal cortex lesions in rats. *Exp. Neurol.* 36:683–698, 1986.

Coslett H.B., Heilman K.M. Hemihypokinesia after right hemisphere strokes. *Brain Cogn.* 9:267–278, 1989.

Coslett H.B., Bowers D., Heilman K.M. An analysis of the determinants of hemispatial performance. Presented at the Meeting of the International Neuropsychological Society, San Diego, February 1985.

Coslett H.B., Bowers D., Fitzpatrick E., et al. Hemispatial hypokinesia and hemisensory inattention in neglect. *Brain* 113:475–486, 1990.

Costa L.D., Vaughan H.G., Horwitz M., et al. Patterns of behavior deficit associated with visual spatial neglect. *Cortex* 5:242–263, 1969.

Critchley M. *The Parietal Lobes.* New York, Hafner Publishers, 1966.

Crowne D.P., Yeo C.H., Russell I.S. The effects of unilateral frontal eye field lesions in the monkey: visual-motor guidance and avoidance behavior. *Behav. Brain Res.* 2:165–185, 1981.

Damasio A.R., Damasio H., Chui H.G. Neglect following damage to frontal lobe or basal ganglia. *Neuropsychologia* 18:123–131, 1980.

Deuel R.K., Collins R.C., Dunlop N., et al. Recovery from unilateral neglect: behavioral and functional anatomic correlations in monkeys. *Soc. Neurosci. Abstr.* 5:624, 1979.

Diller L., Weinberg J. Hemi-inattention in rehabilitation: the evolution of a rational remediation program. *Adv. Neurol.* 18:63–82, 1977.

Dunnett S.B., Björklund A., Stenevi U., et al. Behavioral recovery following transplantation of substantia nigra in rats subjected to 6-OHDA lesions of the nigrostriatal pathway. I. Unilateral lesions. *Brain Res.* 215:147–161, 1981.

Fleet W.S., Heilman K.M. The fatigue effect in hemispatial neglect. *Neurology* 35(Suppl. 1):258, 1986.

Fleet W.S., Valenstein E., Watson R.T., et al. Dopamine agonist therapy for neglect in humans. *Neurology* 37:1765–1771, 1987.

Gainotti G., Messerli P., Tissot R. Qualitative analysis of unilateral spatial neglect in relation to laterality of cerebral lesions. *J. Neurol. Neurosurg. Psychiatry* 35:545–550, 1972.

Gazzaniga M.S. *The Bisected Brain.* New York, Appleton, 1970.

Geschwind N. Disconnexion syndromes in animals and man. *Brain* 88:237–294, 585–644, 1965.

Goldberg M.E., Bushnell M.C. Behavioral enhancement of visual responses in monkey cerebral cortex: II. Modulation in frontal eye fields specifically related to saccades. *J. Neurophysiol.* 46:773–787, 1981.

Heilman K.M. Neglect and related disorders. In Heilman K.M., Valenstein E., eds. *Clinical Neuropsychology.* New York, Oxford University Press, 1979.

Heilman K.M., Valenstein E. Frontal lobe neglect in man. *Neurology (Minneap.)* 22:660–664, 1972.

Heilman K.M., Valenstein E. Mechanisms underlying hemispatial neglect. *Ann. Neurol.* 5:166–170, 1979.

Heilman K.M., Van Den Abell T. Right hemispheric dominance for mediating cerebral activation. *Neuropsychologia* 17:315–321, 1979.

Heilman K.M., Van Den Abell T. Right hemisphere dominance for attention: the mechanisms underlying hemispheric asymmetries of inattention (neglect). *Neurology (N.Y.)* 30:327–330, 1980.

Heilman K.M., Watson R.T. Changes in the symptoms of neglect induced by changing task strategy. *Arch. Neurol.* 35:47–49, 1978.

Heilman K.M., Watson R.T., Schulman H. A unilateral memory defect. *J. Neurol. Neurosurg. Psychiatry* 37:790–793, 1974.

Heilman K.M., Schwartz H.B., Watson R.T. Hypoarousal in patients with the neglect syndrome and emotional indifference. *Neurology (N.Y.)* 28:229–232, 1978.

Heilman K.M., Watson R.T., Valenstein E. A unidirectional gaze deficit associated with hemispatial neglect (abstract). *Neurology (N.Y.)* 30:360, 1980.

Heilman K.M., Bowers D., Watson R.T. Performance on a hemispatial pointing task by patients with neglect syndrome. *Neurology (N.Y.)* 33:661–664, 1983a.

Heilman K.M., Valenstein E., Watson R.T. Locailzation of neglect. In Kertesz A., ed. *Localization in Neuropsychology.* New York, Academic Press, 1983b.

Heilman, K.M., Bowers D., Watson R.T. Pseudoneglect in a patient with partial callosal disconnection. *Brain* 107:519–532, 1984.

Heilman K.M., Bowers D., Coslett H.B., et al. Directional hypokinesia in neglect. *Neurology (Cleve.)* 35(Suppl. 2):855–860, 1985.

Hier D.B., Mondock J., Caplan L.R. Recovery of behavioral abnormalities after right hemisphere stroke. *Neurology (N.Y.)* 33:345–350, 1983.

Howes D., Boller F. Evidence for focal impairment from lesions of the right hemisphere. *Brain* 98:317–332, 1975.

Jefferson G. Substrates for integrative patterns in the reticular core. In Scheibel M.E., Scheibel A.B., eds. *Reticular Formation.* Boston, Little Brown, 1958.

Kahneman D. *Eye Movement Attention and Effort.* Englewood Cliffs, NJ, Prentice-Hall, 1973.

Kennard M.A., Ectors L. Forced circling movements in monkeys following lesions of the frontal lobes. *J. Neurophysiol.* 1:45–54, 1938.

Kimura D. Function asymmetry of the brain in dichotic listening. *Cortex* 3:163–178, 1967.

Kinsbourne M. A model for the mechanism of unilateral neglect of space. *Trans. Am. Neurol. Assoc.* 95:143, 1970.

Kooistra C.A., Heilman K.M. Hemispatial visual inattention masquerading as hemianopsia. *Neurology* 39:1125–1127, 1989.

Kozlowski M.R., Marshall J.F., Plasticity of neostriatal metabolic activity and behavioral recovery from nigrostriatal injury. *Exp. Neurol.* 74:313–323, 1981.

Kuypers H.G.J.M., Lawrence D.G. Cortical projections to the red nucleus and the brain stem in the rhesus monkey. *Brain Res.* 4:151–188, 1967.

Lansing R.W., Schwartz E., Lindsley D.B. Reaction time and EEG activation under alerted and nonalerted conditions. *J. Exp. Psychol.* 58:1and7, 1959.

Loeb J. Die elementaren Storüngen einfacher Functionen nach oberflächlicher umschriebener Verletzung des Grosshirns. *Pfluegers Arch.* 37:51–56, 1885.

Lynch J.C. The functional organization of posterior parietal association cortex. *Behav. Brain Sci.* 3:485–534, 1980.

Mark V.W., Kooistra C.A., Heilman K.M. Hemispatial neglect affected by non-neglected stimuli. *Neurology* 38:1207–1211, 1988.

Marshall J.F. Somatosensory recovery and pharmacological control. *Brain Res.* 177:311–324, 1979.

Marshall J.F. Neurochemistry of attention and attentional disorders. Annual course 214, Behavioral Neurology. Presented at the American Academy of Neurology, April 27, 1982.

McFie J., Piercy M.F., Zangwill O.L. Visual spatial agnosia associated with lesions of the right hemisphere. *Brain* 73:167–190, 1950.

Meador K., Watson R.T., Bowers D., et al. Hypometria with hemispatial and limb motor neglect. *Brain* 109:293–305, 1986.

Meador K.J., Loring D.W., Bowers D., et al. Remote memory and neglect syndrome. *Neurology* 37:522–526, 1987.

Meador K.J., Loring D.W., Lee G.P., et al. Right cerebral specialization for tactile attention as evidenced by intracarotid sodium amytal. *Neurology* 38:1763–1766, 1988.

Milner B., Taylor L., Sperry R.W. Lateralized suppression of dichotically presented digits after commissural section in man. *Science* 161:184–186, 1968.

Moruzzi G., Magoun H.W. Brainstem reticular formation and activation of the EEG. *Electroencephalogr. Clin. Neurophysiol.* 1:455–473, 1949.

Mountcastle V.B., Lynch J.C., Georgopoulos A., et al. Posterior parietal association cortex of the monkey: command function from operations within extrapersonal space. *J. Neurophysiol.* 38:871–908, 1975.

Neve K.A., Kozlowski M.R., Marshall J.F. Plasticity of neostriatal dopamine receptors after nigrostriatal injury: relationship to recovery of sensorimotor functions and behavioral supersensitivity. *Brain Res.* 244:33–44, 1982.

Pandya D.M., Kuypers H.G.J.M. Cortico-cortical connections in the rhesus monkey. *Brain Res.* 13:13–36, 1969.

Poppelreuter W.L. *Die psychischen Schädigungen durch Kopfshuss in Krieg 1914–1916: die Störungen der niederen und hoheren Leistungen durch Verletzungen des Okzipitalhirns.* Vol. 1. Leipzig, Leopold Voss, 1917. [Referred to by Critchley M. *Brain* 72:540, 1949.]

Pribram K.H., McGuinness D. Arousal, activation and effort in the control of attention. *Psychol. Rev.* 82:116–149, 1975.

Prohovnik I., Risberg J., Hagstadius S., et al. Cortical activity during unilateral tactile stimulation: a regional cerebral blood flow study. Presented at the meeting of the International Neuropsychological Society, Atlanta, February 1981.

Rapcsak S.Z., Cimino C.R., Heilman K.M. Altitudinal neglect. *Neurology* 38:277–281, 1988.

Rapcsak S.Z., Fleet W.S., Verfaellie M., et al. Selective attention in hemispatial neglect. *Arch. Neurol.* 46:178–182, 1989.

Reeves A.G., Hagamen W.D. Behavioral and EEG asymmetry following unilateral lesions of the forebrain and midbrain of cats. *Electroencephalogr. Clin. Neurophysiol.* 30:83–86, 1971.

Rosen A.D., Gur R.C., Reivich M., et al. Preliminary observation of stimulus-related arousal and glucose metabolism. Presented at the meeting of the International Neuropsychological Society, Atlanta, February 1981.

Rubens A. Caloric stimulation and unilateral visual neglect. *Neurology* 35:1019–1024, 1985.

Schiebel M.E., Schiebel A.B. The organization of the nucleus reticularis thalami: a golgi study. *Brain Res.* 1:43–62, 1966.

Schiebel M.E., Schiebel A.B. Structural organization of nonspecific thalamic nuclei and their projection toward cortex. *Brain* 6:60–94, 1967.

Schwartz A.S., Marchok P.L., Kreinich C.J., et al. The asymmetric lateralization of tactile extinction in patients with unilateral cerebral dysfunction. *Brain* 102:669–684, 1979.

Segarra J.M., Angelo J.N. Presentation I. In Benton A., ed. *Behavioral Change in Cerebrovascular Disease.* New York, Harper & Row, 1970.

Segundo J.P., Naguet R., Buser P. Effects of cortical stimulation on electrocortical activity in monkeys. *J. Neurophysiol.* 18:236–245, 1955.

Shelton P.A., Bowers D., Heilman K.M. Peripersonal and vertical neglect. *Brain* 113:191–205, 1990.

Singer W. Control of thalamic transmission by corticofugal and ascending reticular pathways in the visual system. *Physiol. Rev.* 57:386–420, 1977.

Sokolov Y.N. *Perception and the Conditioned Reflex.* Oxford, Pergamon Press, 1963.

Sparks R., Geschwind N. Dichotic listening in man after section of the neocortical commissures. *Cortex* 4:3–16, 1968.

Sprague J.M., Meikle T.H. The role of the superior colliculus in visually guided behavior. *Exp. Neurol.* 11:115–146, 1965.

Steriade M., Glenn L. Neocortical and caudate projections of intralaminar thalamic neurons and their synaptic excitation from the midbrain reticular core. *J. Neurophysiol.* 48:352–370, 1982.

Taylor J., ed. *Selected Writings of John Hughlings Jackson.* London, Hodder and Stoughton, 1932.

Truex R.C., Carpenter M.B. *Human Neuroanatomy.* Baltimore, Williams & Wilkins, 1964.

Valenstein E., Watson R.T., Van Den Abell T., et al. Response time in monkeys with unilateral neglect. *Arch. Neurol.* 44:517–520, 1987.

Velasco F., Velasco M. A reticulothalamic system mediating proprioceptive attention and tremor in man. *Neurosurgery* 4:30–36, 1979.

Vogt B.A., Rosene D.L., Pandya D.N. Thalamic and cortical afferents differentiate anterior from posterior cingulate cortex in the monkey. *Science* 204:205–207, 1979.

Watson R.T., Heilman K.M. Thalamic neglect. *Neurology (N.Y.)* 29:690–694, 1979.

Watson R.T., Heilman K.M., Cauthen J.C., et al. Neglect after cingulectomy. *Neurology (Minneap.)* 23:1003–1007, 1973.

Watson R.T., Heilman K.M., Miller B.D., et al. Neglect after mesencephalic reticular formation lesions. *Neurology (Minneap.)* 24:294–298, 1974.

Watson R.T., Andriola M., Heilman K.M. The EEG in neglect. *J. Neurol. Sci.* 34:343–348, 1977.

Watson R.T., Miller B.D., Heilman K.M. Nonsensory neglect. *Ann. Neurol.* 3:505–508, 1978.

Watson R.T., Valenstein E., Heilman K.M. Thalamic neglect; possible role of the medial thalamus and nucleus reticularis thalami in behavior. *Arch. Neurol.* 38:501–506, 1981.

Watson R.T., Valenstein E., Day A.L., et al. The effect of corpus callosum lesions on unilateral neglect in monkeys. *Neurology (N.Y.)* 34:812–815, 1984.

Weinstein E.A., Kahn R.L. *Denial of Illness.* Springfield, IL, Thomas, 1955.

Welch K., Stuteville P. Experimental production of neglect in monkeys. *Brain* 81:341–347, 1958.

57

Disorders of Sleep

David R. Fish

Sleep complaints are common in community-based surveys (Ford and Kamerow, 1989) and have become a significant part of neurologic practice. The principal symptoms relate to insomnia, excessive daytime sleepiness, and episodes of abnormal nocturnal behavior. In addition, clinically or diagnostically important changes in sleep may be found in certain neurologic disorders. For example, frequent nocturnal arousals and parasomnias are common in Gilles de la Tourette's syndrome (Glaze et al., 1983). Although simultaneous clinical and neurophysiologic monitoring has helped to define specific diagnostic entities and relate these to basic disease mechanisms, a careful sleep history remains paramount (A. Kales et al., 1980b).

NORMAL SLEEP PROCESSES

Normal sleep occupies about one-third of human life. The timing and duration of sleep are governed by internal clocks and environmental cues. Overnight sleep is organized into cycles lasting for 1–2 hours. Within these cycles, there is a clear distinction between non–rapid eye movement (NREM) and rapid eye movement (REM) sleep. The former predominates in the initial cycles, and the latter, in the later cycles. REM sleep is characterized by electroencephalographic desynchronization, muscle atonia, and REMs. NREM sleep may be subdivided on the basis of polysomnography into stage 1 (rolling eye movements, loss of alpha rhythm, and vertex sharp waves), stage 2 (sleep spindles, K complexes), stage 3 (20–50% slow waves), and stage 4 (>50% slow waves) (see Rechtschaffen and Kales, 1968). Although these subdivisions may be clinically useful, they are somewhat artificial (Fish et al., 1991) and do not necessarily reflect discrete stepwise changes in the mechanisms underlying sleep.

Theories of sleep mechanisms have changed substantially during the past decade, and yet much uncertainty remains about the basic processes (Parkes and Lock, 1989). Insights into human sleep are sometimes derived from patients with specific lesions and changes in sleep structure (e.g., Aldrich et al., 1989; Bremmer, 1977; Tinuper et al., 1989). However, sleep structure can be affected by many nonspecific factors. In the evaluation of new hypotheses, it is important to ascertain not only that lesions to a particular site or neurochemical process result in specific sleep changes but also that stimulation of these systems may induce opposite effects, that activition is seen during the relevant period of normal sleep, and that there is interaction between the different control processes.

The control of NREM sleep appears to involve a complex series of interactions among widely located brain structures rather than the action of a single center (for review, see Siegel, 1990). For example, wakefulness may be promoted by cells in the posterior hypothalamus (Lin et al., 1989), and NREM sleep, by activity in specific regions of the basal forebrain (Szymusiak and McGinty, 1989), the brain stem (Eguchi and Satoh, 1980), and the thalamus (Imeri et al., 1988; Lugaresi et al., 1986c). Detailed studies with animals and humans confirmed the importance of thalamocortical connections in sleep spindle generation (for reviews, see Jankel and Niedermyer, 1985; Steriade and Llinas, 1988).

Transection experiments in animals demonstrated that pontomedullary structures, particularly in the region of the locus cereleus, are crucially involved in the production of REM sleep phenomena (Jouvet, 1962; Jouvet and Delorme, 1965; Sastre et al., 1978; Siegel et al., 1983). Cholinergic stimulation of this region may induce REM sleep phenomena (Amatruda et al., 1975), and cells in this region are particularly active during stage REM sleep (Sakai et al., 1981). Nevertheless, interactions with other cerebral structures, such as the hypothalamus, undoubtedly influence the control of REM sleep (e.g., Jouvet, 1988).

The descending inhibitory pathway from the region of the locus ceruleus leading to the production of REM atonia probably involves the lateral tegmentoreticular tract (Webster et al., 1986); projections to the nucleus magnocellularis (Kanamoni et al., 1980) and then to the ventrolateral reticulospinal tract (Jankowska et al., 1968) leading to postsynaptic inhibition of α motor neurons (Morales and Chase, 1983). Ascending projections from the pons to the lateral geniculate body and onto the cortex are involved in the expression of pontogeniculo-occipital waves, which are seen during wakefulness and REM sleep and may be related to phasic REM events such as REMs and muscle twitches. Projections to the thalamus may mediate the desynchronization of cortical activity seen during REM sleep (Steriade and Llinas, 1988).

INSOMNIA

Temporary insomnia relating to acute environmental or personal events is common, and at least 10% of the population experience chronic insomnia (National Institute of Mental Health Catchment Area Study, Ford and Kamerow, 1989). A broad range of psychiatric conditions, particularly affective disorders, may be of etiologic significance. However, psychopathologic changes are absent in up to half of the cases (Ford and Kamerow, 1989), and many other factors may be involved alone or in combination (Gillin and Byerley, 1990). These factors may act directly to interfere with the cerebral structures controlling sleep or activate arousal mechanisms. They include obsessional thoughts and ruminations; environmental factors, such as shift work; alcohol or other drug abuse; chronic pain; the restless leg syndrome; and sleep apnea.

The restless leg syndrome accounts for about 4% of hospital referrals for insomnia (Coleman et al., 1982). It is characterized by an unpleasant creeping sensation, usually in both legs; it is sometimes asymmetric or may involve the upper limbs. This sensation is worse on lying or sitting in the evening and is associated with an urge to move. Most cases are of unknown cause, although associated factors include iron deficiency anemia and peripheral neuropathy or radiculopathy. A familial form with autosomal dominant inheritance commences in adolescence (Montplaisir et al., 1985), but most other cases begin in middle or old age. Polysomnography nearly always reveals additional periodic movements of sleep, sometimes with persistence into wakefulness, or additional dyskinesias such as fragmentary myoclonus (Hening et al., 1986).

Sleep apnea usually manifests as excessive daytime sleepiness but may cause difficulty in initiating or maintaining sleep because of either apneic arousals or overall disruption of the circadian sleep-wake cycle.

The cerebral structures responsible for initiating and maintaining sleep are widespread. Ischemic, degenerative, or expanding lesions in the forebrain, the hypothalamus, the thalamus, and the pontomedullary regions may affect the sleep-wake cycle (Parkes, 1987). Lugaresi et al. (1986c) described two families in whom selective degeneration of the anterior and dorsal medial thalamic nuclei was associated with dysautonomia and insomnia. The latter was characterized by progressive loss of REM, slow waves, and sleep spindles. Nocturnal sweating was profuse, and restless or even violent behavior was sometimes evident in sleep. Symptoms began in adult life and rapidly progressed through a vegetative state to death.

Rarely, the internal clock controlling the sleep-wake cycle is delayed. Subjects with this condition may retire in the early hours of the morning but then have a normal duration of sleep (Weitzman et al., 1981).

Insomnia may be an important problem in a variety of neurologic disorders. Any cause of chronic pain or immobility may lead to difficulties in initiating or maintaining sleep. In Parkinson's disease (Askenasy and Yahr, 1985) and even more so in progressive supranuclear palsy (Aldrich et al., 1989), insomnia may be more severe than would be expected from the degree of physical disability alone. In Gilles de la Tourette's syndrome, an excessive or disordered arousal may be the cause of frequent awakenings or difficulty in falling asleep (Glaze et al., 1983).

Insomnia may result from stimulant drugs such as amphetamines, which enhance arousal, or by direct interference with sleep mechanisms. For example, anticholinergic medication inhibits the output from the region of the locus ceruleus, which appears to be involved in the initiation and maintenance of REM sleep.

The treatment of chronic insomnia should initially be directed at the specific cause. If appropriate, improved sleep hygiene may be helpful (e.g., going to bed at regular times and avoiding stimulants such as caffeine in the evening). Benzodiazepines may increase the duration of stage 2 sleep but often reduce slow-wave and REM sleep. In addition, they may cause daytime drowsiness and, with longer-term use, tolerance, addiction, and rebound insomnia. The restless leg syndrome is often difficult to treat (Brodeur et al., 1988). Occasionally, patients benefit from benzodiazepines, codeine, or low doses of levodopa (L-dopa).

DAYTIME HYPERSOMNOLENCE

Although less frequent in the community than is insomnia (3% versus 10% [Ford and Kamerow, 1989]), daytime hypersomnolence is the most common sleep complaint in patients who are referred for polysomnography (Coleman et al., 1982). Sleep apnea and narcolepsy together account for about 75% of cases (Table 57–1), although psychologic factors are of greater significance in those who do not seek medical advice (Ford and Kamerow, 1989), possibly reflecting their less severe symptoms. Clinically, it is important to differentiate causes that relate to disturbed nocturnal sleep from disorders of the sleep-wake mechanisms themselves.

Narcolepsy

The reported prevalence of narcolepsy varies geographically, being only 0.2 per 10,000 persons in Israel, 5–7 per 10,000 in San Francisco, and 16 per 10,000 in Japan (Parkes and Lock, 1989). Both sexes are similarly affected. It is often familial and probably of autosomal dominant transmission with low penetrance. It is possible that environmental factors trigger the disorder in genetically susceptible individuals. Virtually all cases have HLA-DR2 and HLA-DQw1 genotypes, which are located on chromosome 6, although there are a few well-documented exceptions. These genotypes are present in about one-third of the population. Therefore, tissue typing can help to exclude, but not establish, the diagnosis. Unfortunately, there are no identified pathologic or neurochemical markers for the human disease.

The onset of symptoms is usually in adolescence or early adulthood. Daytime hypersomnolence is characterized by sudden episodes of an irresistible urge to sleep. Most affected patients report attacks in inappropriate circumstances, such as during meals or while standing up. These naps usually last less than 30 minutes. Initially, nocturnal sleep is unaffected, but this is progressively disrupted as the disease evolves. Cataplexy, presleep hallucinations, or sleep paralysis may occur in association with narcolepsy, although many cases are monosymptomatic. These associated features represent the inappropriate occurrence or persistence of fragmented REM sleep phenomena during wakefulness. Daytime automatisms, on the other hand, which also occur not infrequently, are nonspecific, being found with other causes of daytime hypersomnolence.

Narcolepsy remains a clinical diagnosis. However, most patients show episodes of REM sleep onset, provided that sufficient recordings are made. The Multiple Sleep Latency Test shows two or more episodes per seven trials of REM-onset daytime sleep in approximately 90% of narcoleptics (Baker et al., 1986). Unfortunately, REM-onset sleep is not specific to narcolepsy and may be seen with other causes of severely disturbed nocturnal sleep.

Relatively low doses of central nervous system (CNS) stimulants such as methylphenidate or *d*-amphetamine may relieve sleepiness but not the REM-related symptoms. The latter sometimes respond to tricyclic antidepressants such as clomipramine. Mazindol is useful in mild cases and occasionally benefits both types of symptoms.

Idiopathic Central Nervous System Hypersomnolence

CNS hypersomnolence accounts for about 5% of patients with excessive daytime somnolence who are referred for polysomnography. Although largely a diagnosis of exclusion, it appears to be a distinct clinical entity (Parkes, 1988) and probably reflects a disorder of NREM sleep mechanisms (Baker et al., 1986). A positive family history is reported in about one-third of cases. There is no definite association with HLA-DR2 or -DQw1 but some association with HLA-Cw2, -DR5, and -B27 (Poirier et al., 1986). Onset is usually in early adulthood.

Nocturnal sleep is largely unaffected, although some patients are difficult to arouse in the morning and then experience sleep drunkenness. Daytime sleep attacks usually occur when the patient is bored or relaxed. They are of gradual onset and often of longer duration than narcoleptic attacks. Daytime automatisms may occur, but cataplexy, sleep paralysis, and presleep hallucinations are not associated with idiopathic CNS hypersomnolence. Overnight polysomnography shows a normal REM latency and sleep structure. The disorder may become severely disabling and may necessitate the use of stimulant drugs, which are given in the morning or twice a day.

Sleep Apnea

The overwhelming proportion of cases of sleep apnea involve intermittent upper airway obstruction. Rarely, restrictive pulmonary disease or brain stem abnormalities are responsible.

Obstructive sleep apnea is much more common in men and usually presents in middle age. It is asso-

Table 57–1. CAUSES OF EXCESSIVE SLEEPINESS IN 1983 PATIENTS REFERRED FOR POLYSOMNOGRAPHY

Diagnosis*	%
Sleep apnea	43.2
Narcolepsy	25.0
Idiopathic CNS hypersomnia	8.8
No hypersomnia found	5.4
Other hypersomnia	5.0
Sleep-related myoclonus and RLS	3.5
Medical, toxic, or environmental factors	2.7
Drug and alcohol dependency	1.5
Psychophysiologic condition	1.1

*CNS = central nervous system; RLS = restless leg syndrome.
From Coleman R.M., Roffwarg H.P., Kennedy S.J., et al. Sleep-wake disorders based on a polysomnographic diagnosis. *J.A.M.A.* 247:997–1003, 1982. Copyright 1982, American Medical Association.

ciated with obesity, a short neck, a small pharynx, hyperglossia, micrognathia, and nasal septal deformities (Bradley and Phillipson, 1985; Kuna and Remmers, 1985). The airway obstruction is usually pharyngeal. A variety of predisposing factors may lead to narrowing of the pharyngeal lumen, which may then become occluded during a fall in intrapharyngeal pressure in sleep. There is usually a long history of excessive snoring. Apneic episodes are frequent and may last 10–180 seconds. During these episodes, chest and abdominal movements are prominent. Apneic episodes terminate with gasping or choking noises. Arousals and severe nocturnal restlessness are common. Patients often feel tired and complain of headaches in the morning.

Polysomnography with percutaneous oximetry and chest and abdominal movement detectors readily confirms the diagnosis. Advanced cases may show additional central-type apneic episodes, possibly resulting from the chronic effect of hypoxia or hypercarbia on brain stem structures. Respiratory problems are most severe in REM sleep, presumably because of the concomitant atonia. They may be associated with acute cardiovascular changes, particularly bradycardia, leading to a risk of sudden death, or chronic pulmonary hypertension.

Weight reduction and the avoidance of sedating medicines and evening alcohol ingestion may be helpful. Continuous positive airway pressure at 4–10 cm H_2O applied to the nares may maintain upper airway patency (Sullivan et al., 1981). Specific abnormalities of the oropharynx may be amenable to surgery. Uvulopharyngoplasty may benefit some patients with selected deformities leading to obstruction at the level of the soft palate. Occasional severe cases require tracheostomy.

Several neurologic disorders may cause apneic episodes during sleep or be associated with a nocturnal exacerbation of respiratory difficulties. These usually occur predominantly with restrictive respiration (e.g., in Guillain-Barré syndrome) (George and Kryger, 1987). Less commonly, the effect may be on brain stem respiratory centers, as in the Arnold-Chiari malformations (Balk et al., 1985). Overnight polysomnography should be considered in patients at high risk for such difficulties, particularly if surgical intervention for the primary CNS disorder is being considered.

Other Causes of Daytime Hypersomnolence

Any cause of chronic nocturnal sleep disruption may result in daytime hypersomnolence. Rarely, lesions of the CNS affecting sleep-wake mechanisms, such as posterior hypothalamic tumors, are responsible. Metabolic or other medical conditions, such as hepatic or renal failure, hypothyroidism, and hypoglycemia, should be excluded, and all drug con-

sumption should be reviewed. The time course of hypersomnolence in Kleine-Levin syndrome is quite different from that in the conditions cited earlier. Hypersomnolence, sometimes associated with hyperphagia and hypersexuality in adolescent males, occurs for weeks or months, interspersed with periods of more normal sleep-wake cycles (Critchley, 1962).

EPISODES OF ABNORMAL NOCTURNAL BEHAVIOR

Clinically, abnormal nocturnal behavior can be divided into simple brief movements and prolonged episodes of complex motor behavior.

Nocturnal Twitches

Whole-body jerks on falling asleep, or hypnic jerks (Oswald, 1959), and fragmentary twitches, particularly of the hands and the face (De Lisi, 1932), during stages 1, 2, and REM sleep are normal. Frequent fragmentary twitches that persist into stages 3 and 4 are associated with a variety of disorders causing sleep disruption (Broughton et al., 1985).

Periodic Movements of Sleep

Periodic movements of sleep occur in 5% of normal subjects between 30 and 50 years of age and in 29% of those older than 50 years of age (Lugaresi et al., 1986a). They have an increased prevalence in patients with pathologically disturbed sleep (e.g., narcolepsy and sleep apnea) and are nearly always present in the restless leg syndrome (Hening et al., 1986; Krueger, 1990). They involve dorsiflexion of the great toe and ankle, with flexion of the knee and sometimes the hip. Occasionally, there may be involvement of the upper limb. The movements last for 3–5 seconds and occur with a periodicity of 15–60 seconds. They are more common during light NREM sleep and rarely awaken the patient; however, in severe cases, they may occur in wakefulness. The underlying periodicity of the movements shows a similar time course to changes in pulse, blood pressure, and respiration, suggesting possible control by a brain stem pacemaker (Coleman et al., 1980).

Sleepwalking and Night Terrors

Sleepwalking and night terrors are NREM parasomnias that usually commence in childhood or adolescence and may be precipitated by emotional stress (A. Kales et al., 1980a; J.D. Kales et al., 1980). They occur during slow-wave sleep and therefore rarely happen after the first 3 hours of sleep. Both conditions are often familial and may be concomitant. They may represent an immaturity or abnormality of the arousal mechanisms (Broughton, 1968).

During somnambulism, complex tasks may be undertaken, sometimes with accidental self-injury. Spontaneous or responsive speech may occur during an attack but is often slow or monosyllabic. Sometimes, it is possible to lead patients back to bed without awakening them. Abortive attacks in which the patient sits up and makes small, semipurposeful movements such as fidgeting or shuffling leg movements are more common than full-blowm episodes. The latter rarely last longer than 5 minutes and occur too infrequently to be readily documented by polysomnography.

Night terrors may represent a more severe form of somnambulism. The patient usually sits up and looks terrified. Vocalizations are often loud. Autonomic changes such as sweating, tachycardia, and pupillary dilatation are marked. Patients may thrash about and get out of bed. They are difficult to arouse and have little recall, although they may report vaguely a frightening scene. Self-injury, as opposed to other-directed aggression, is not uncommon.

Enuresis may be associated with somnambulism or night terrors. Benzodiazepines may help NREM parasomnias acutely, probably by reducing slow-wave sleep, but are rarely of long-term benefit. Attention should be given to psychologic factors, and organic CNS lesions should be excluded in late-onset cases.

Rapid Eye Movement Sleep Behavior Disorder

Interruption of the descending inhibitory system responsible for REM atonia in cats leads to complex motor behavior, such as hunting, during REM sleep (Sastre and Jouvet, 1979). Similarly, in humans, a loss of REM atonia may cause the syndrome of chronic REM sleep behavior disorder (Schenk et al., 1987). This is more common in middle-age or elderly males and may be associated with depression, excessive alcohol ingestion, cerebrovascular disease, and degenerative or structural brain stem lesions. Complex, often violent or aggressive behavior occurs during REM sleep, frequently with shouting and screaming. These episodes may last from seconds to several minutes, and self-injury or injury to a partner may occur. If awakened, the patient may recount a dream that can be related to the clinical episodes.

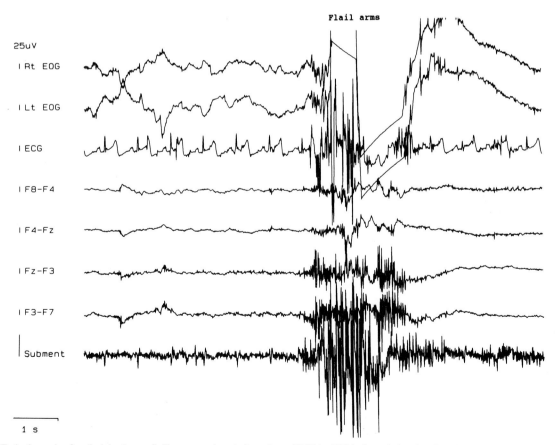

Figure 57–1. An episode of violent arm flailing occurring during stage REM in REM sleep behavior disorder. Note the burst of elevated submental electromyographic tone in association with the behavioral episode. Rt EOG = right electro-oculogram; Lt EOG = left electro-oculogram; ECG = electrocardiogram; Subment = submental EMG. Displayed ECG channels show a bipolar transfrontal chain.

Table 57–2. COMPARISON OF NON–RAPID EYE MOVEMENT AND RAPID EYE MOVEMENT PARASOMNIAS

Parameter	NREM Parasomnia	REM Parasomnia
Onset	Adolescence	Middle or old age
Sex	Male = female	Male > female
Positive family history	>80%	None
Timing	<2 AM	>2 AM
Duration	Usually <5 min	Brief or prolonged
Vocalization	Yes	Yes
Dream recall	Rare	Common
Aggression	Rare	Common
Responsiveness	Sometimes	Rarely
Electroencephalographic findings	Slow wave	REM
Benefit with benzodiazepines	Transient	May be persistent
Associated sleep problems	Enuresis common	Enuresis rare, marked increased in REM twitches
Associated diseases	Depression	Depression
	Anxiety	Alcoholism
		Brain stem lesions, other CNS lesions

Polysomnography shows a lack of sustained atonia during REM sleep, particularly during the sleep behavior disorder episodes (Fig. 57–1). Treatment with clonazepam or imipramine may be helpful. (Schenck et al., 1987). Differentiation from NREM parasomnias is usually possible on clinical grounds (Table 57–2) and has important therapeutic implications.

Nocturnal Seizures

Nocturnal seizures with tonic-clonic manifestations, or additional daytime attacks, rarely present diagnostic difficulties if a reliable witness is available. However, partial seizures restricted to sleep may be more troublesome, particularly if they are of frontal lobe origin. The latter may be brief (<1 minute), frequent, and sometimes only nocturnal. Posturing of one of more limbs, vocalization, and some retention of awareness may occur, particularly with lesions arising in the supplementary motor area. If present, automatisms such as bicycling leg movements may be diagnostically helpful. Interictal scalp electroencephalograms may fail to show epileptiform abnormalities, even with the use of supraorbital electrodes. Ictal scalp recordings are often obscured by muscle artifact. Partial seizures of temporal lobe origin more often show additional daytime seizures; a longer duration; automatisms such as chewing, swallowing, or fidgeting; and interictal scalp electroencephalographic abnormalities.

Lugeresi et al. (1986b) introduced the term *paroxysmal nocturnal dystonia* to describe certain attacks arising during NREM sleep. The characteristics of the attacks are similar to those of frontal lobe epilepsy in many of the cases described. Lugeresi et al. (1986b) reported 12 patients with frequent nocturnal attacks characterized by choreoathetoid, dystonic, or ballistic movements. In 10 patients, the attacks were short (<1 minute). They were frequent (up to 20 per night), stereotyped within an individual, and often accompanied by vocalization. There was no postictal confusion. In two cases, the attacks were much longer (up to 50 minutes). Most patients responded to anticonvulsants, and some had associated daytime seizures. The clinical features of the nocturnal attacks in patients labeled as having nocturnal paroxysmal dystonia are similar to those that may occur in patients with proven frontal lobe epilepsy (Meierkord et al., 1991). It remains to be established whether all of the patients with nocturnal dystonic attacks, of the type described by Lugaresi et al., have hidden frontal epileptic foci or whether there are other causes for this syndrome.

Most involuntary movement disorders are much reduced or virtually stopped by sleep. Spinal myoclonus, palatal myoclonus, and epilepsia partialis continua show a variable persistence. The dyskinesias of torsion dystonia, Huntington's chorea, Parkinson's disease, Gilles de la Tourette's syndrome, and several other movement disorders may occur occasionally during sleep, particularly in association with arousals (Fish et al., 1991; Glaze et al., 1983; Mano et al., 1982). Gilles de la Tourette's syndrome may be associated with slow-wave sleep parasomnias, characterized by confusion or combativeness (Glaze et al., 1983). Severe nocturnal myoclonic attacks affecting the whole body may be seen in patients receiving levodopa (L-dopa) (Klawans et al., 1975; Vardi et al., 1978). Bruxism may persist into, or even commence in, light sleep (Satoh and Haroda, 1973). Similarly, jactatio nocturna, characterized by rocking movements of the neck or the whole body associated with grunting or muttering, usually commences on retiring and is most prominent in stage 2 sleep (Drake, 1986). These movement disorders occur rarely and may persist into sleep, which is important in the interpretation of symptoms reported by the patient or spouse.

References

(Key references are designated with an asterisk.)

Aldrich M.S., Foster N.L., White R.F. Sleep abnormalities in progressive supranuclear palsy. *Ann. Neurol.* 25:577–581, 1989.

Amatruda T.T., III, Black D.A., McKenna T.M., et al. Sleep cycle control and cholinergic mechanisms: differential effects of carbachol at pontine brain stem sites. *Brain Res.* 98:501–515, 1975.

Askenasy J.J.M., Yahr M.D. Reversal of sleep disturbance in Parkinson's disease by antiparkinsonian therapy. *Neurology* 35:527–532, 1985.

Baker T.L., Guilleminault C., Nino-Muria G. et al. Comparitive polysomnographic study of narcolepsy and idiopathic central nervous system hypersomnia. *Sleep* 9:232–242, 1986.

Balk R.A., Hiller F.C., Lucas E.A., et al. Sleep apnea and the Arnold-Chiari malformation. *Am. Rev. Respir. Dis.* 132:929–930, 1985.

Bradley T.D., Phillipson E.A. Pathogenesis and pathophysiology of the obstructive sleep apnea syndrome. *Med. Clin. North Am.* 69:1169–1185, 1985.

Bremmer F. Cerebral hypnogenic centres. *Ann. Neurol.* 2:1–6, 1977.

Brodeur C., Montplaisir J., Godbout R., et al. Treatment of restless legs syndrome and periodic movements of sleep with L-dopa. *Neurology* 38:1845–1848, 1988.

*Broughton R. Sleep disorders: disorders of arousal. *Science* 159:1070–1078, 1968.

Broughton R., Tolentino M.A., Krelina M. Excessive fragmentary myoclonus in NREM sleep: a report of 38 cases. *Electroencephalogr. Clin. Neurophysiol.* 61:123–133, 1985.

Coleman R.M., Pollak C.P., Weitzman E.D. Periodic movements in sleep (nocturnal myoclonus): relation to sleep disorders. *Ann. Neurol.* 8:416–421, 1980.

Coleman R.M., Roffwarg H.P., Kennedy S.J., et al. Sleep-wake disorders based on polysomnographic diagnosis a national cooperative study. *J.A.M.A.* 247:997–1003, 1982.

Critchley M. Periodic hypersomnia and megaphagia in adolescent males. *Brain* 85:628–656, 1962.

De Lisi L. Si di un fenomeno motorio constante del somno normale: le myoclonie ipniche fisiologishe. *Rev. Patol. Nerv. Ment.* 39:481–496, 1932.

Drake M.E. Jactatio nocturna after head injury. *Neurology* 36:867–868, 1986.

Eguchi K., Satoh T. Convergence of sleep wakefulness subsystems onto single neurones in the region of cat's solitary tract. *Arch. Ital. Biol.* 118:331–345, 1980.

Fish D.R., Sawyers D., Blackie J.D. The effect of sleep on the dyskinesias of Parkinson's disease, Huntington's chorea, Gilles de la Tourette syndrome and torsion dystonia. *Arch. Neurol.* 48:210–214, 1991.

Ford D.E., Kamerow D.B. Epidemiologic study of sleep disturbances and psychiatric disorders. *J.A.M.A.* 262:1479–1484, 1989.

George C.F., Kryger M.H. Sleep in restrictive lung disease. *Sleep* 10:409–418, 1987.

*Gillin J.C., Byerley W.F. The diagnosis and management of insomnia. *N. Engl. J. Med.* 322:239–248, 1990.

Glaze D.G., Frost J.D., Jankovic J. Sleep in Gilles de la Tourette syndrome: disorder of arousal. *Neurology (N.Y.)* 33:586–592, 1983.

Hening W.A., Walters A., Kavey N., et al. Dyskinesia while awake and periodic movements in sleep in the restless leg syndrome: treatment with opioids. *Neurology* 36:1363–1366, 1986.

Imeri L., Moneta M.E., Mancia M. Changes in spontaneous activity of medialis dorsalis thalmic neurones during sleep and wakefulness. *Electroencephalogr. Clin. Neurophysiol.* 69:82–84, 1988.

*Jankel W.R., Niedermyer E. Sleep spindles. *J. Clin. Neurophysiol.* 2:1–35, 1985.

Jankowska E., Lund S., Lundberg A., et al. Inhibitory effects evoked through ventral reticulospinal pathways. *Arch. Ital. Biol.* 105:124–140, 1968.

Jouvet M. Recherches sur les structures nerveuses et les mécanismes responsables des différentes phases du sommeil physiologique. *Arch. Ital. Biol.* 100:125–206, 1962.

Jouvet M. Hypothalamic-hypophyseal interactions in REM sleep. *Acta Ital. Biol.* 126:259–274, 1988.

Jouvet M., Delorme F. Locus coereleus et sommeil paradoxal. *C.R. Soc. Biol. (Paris)* 159:895–899, 1965.

Kales A., Soldatos A.B., Caldwell A.B., et al. Somnambulism. Clinical characteristics and personality patterns. *Arch. Gen. Psychiatry* 37:1406–1410, 1980a.

Kales A., Soldatos C.R., Kales J.D. Taking a sleep history. *Am. Fam. Physician* 22:101–108, 1980b.

Kales J.D., Kales A., Soldatos C.R., et al. Night terrors. Clinical characteristics and personality patterns. *Arch. Gen. Psychiatry* 37:1413–1417, 1980.

Kanamoni N., Sakai K., Jouvet M. Neuronal activity specific to paradoxical sleep in the ventromedial medullary formation of unrestrained cats. *Brain Res.* 189:251–255, 1980.

Klawans H.L., Goetz C., Bergen D. Levodopa-induced myoclonus. *Arch. Neurol.* 32:331–334, 1975.

Krueger B.R. Restless legs and periodic movements of sleep. *Mayo Clin. Proc.* 65:999–1006, 1990.

Kuna S.T., Remmers J.E. Neural and anatomic factors related to upper airway obstruction. *Med. Clin. North Am.* 69:1221–1242, 1985.

Lin J.S., Sakai K., Vanni-Mercier G., et al. A critical role of the posterior hypothalamus in the mechanisms of wakefulness determined by microinjection of muscimol in freely moving cats. *Brain Res.* 479:225–240, 1989.

Lugaresi E., Cirignotta F., Coccagna G., et al. Nocturnal myoclonus and the restless legs syndrome. *Adv. Neurol.* 43:295–307, 1986a.

Lugaresi E., Cirignotta F., Montagna P. Nocturnal paroxysmal dystonia. *J. Neurol. Neurosurg. Psychiatry* 49:375–380, 1986b.

Lugaresi E., Medori R., Montagna P., et al. Fatal familial insomnia and dysautonomia with selective degeneration of thalamic nuclei. *N. Engl. J. Med.* 315:997–1003, 1986c.

Mano T., Shiozawa Z., Sobue I. Extrapyramidal involuntary movements during sleep. *Electroencephalogr. Clin. Neurophysiol.* 35S:431–441, 1982.

Meierkord H., Fish D.R., Smith S.J.M. Is nocturnal paroxysmal dystonia a form of frontal lobe epilepsy? *Mov. Disord.* (in press).

Montplaisir J., Godbout R., Boghen D., et al. Familial restless legs with periodic movements in sleep: electrophysiologic, biochemical, and pharmacologic study. *Neurology* 35:130–134, 1985.

Morales F.R., Chase M.H. Postsynaptic mechanisms responsible for motor inhibition during active sleep. In Weitzman E.D., Chase M.H., eds. *Sleep Disorders: Basic and Clinical Research.* New York, Spectrum Publications, pp. 71–93, 1983.

Oswald I. Sudden body jerks on falling asleep. *Brain* 82:93–103, 1959.

*Parkes J.D. Day-time drowsiness. *Lancet* 2:1213–1218, 1981.

*Parkes J.D. *Sleep and Its Disorders.* New York, Churchill Livingstone, 1987.

*Parkes J.D., Lock C.B. Genetic factors in sleep disorders. *J. Neurol. Neurosurg. Psychiatry* 52S:101–108, 1989.

Poirier G., Montplaisir J., Decary F., et al. HLA antigens in narcolepsy and idiopathic central nervous system hypersomnolence. *Sleep* 9:153–158, 1986.

*Rechtschaffen A., Kales A., eds. *A Manual of Standard Terminology, Techniques and Scoring System for Sleep Stages of Human Subjects.* Washington, DC, U.S. Public Health Service, U.S. Government Printing Office, 1968.

Sakai K., Sastre J.P., Kanamoni N., et al. State specific neurons in the pontomedullary reticular formation with special reference to the postural atonia during paradoxical sleep in the cat. In Pompeiano O., Ajmone-Marsan C., eds. *Brain Mechanisms and Perceptual Awareness.* New York, Raven Press, pp. 405–429, 1981.

Sastre J.P., Jouvet M. Le comportment onirique du chat. *Physiol. Behav.* 22:979–989, 1979.

Sastre J.P., Sakai K., Jouvet M. Bilateral lesions of the dorsolateral pontine tegmentum II. Effect upon muscle atonia. *Sleep Res.* 7:44, 1978.

Satoh Y., Haroda Y. Electrophysiological study on tooth grinding during sleep. *Electroencephalogr. Clin. Neurophysiol.* 35:267, 1973.

*Schenck C.H., Bundlie S.R., Patterson A.L., et al. Rapid eye movement sleep behavior disorder. A treatable parasomnia affecting older adults. *J.A.M.A.* 257:1786–1789, 1987.

*Siegel J.M. Mechanisms of sleep control. *J. Clin. Neurophysiol.* 7:49–65, 1990.

Siegel J.M., Nienhuis R., Tomaszewski K.S. Rostral brainstem contributes to medullary inhibitions of muscle tone. *Brain Res.* 268:344–348, 1983.

Steriade M., Llinas R.R. The function of the thalamus and associated neuronal interplay. *Physiol. Rev.* 68:649–742, 1988.

Sullivan C.E., Issa F.G., Berthan-Jones M., et al. Reversal of obstructive sleep apnoea by continuous positive airways pressure applied through the nares. *Lancet* 1:862–865, 1981.

Szymusiak R., McGinty D. Effects of basal forebrain stimulation on the waking discharge of neurones in the midbrain reticular formation of cats. *Brain Res.* 498:355–359, 1989.

Tinuper P., Montagna P., Medori R., et al. The thalamus participates in the regulation of the sleep waking cycle. A clinico-

pathological study in fatal familial thalamic degeneration. *Electroencephalogr. Clin. Neurophysiol.* 73:117–123, 1989.

Vardi J., Glaubman H., Rabey J.M., et al. Myoclonic attacks induced by L-dopa and bromocriptine in parkinsonian patients. A sleep EEG study. *J. Neurol.* 218:35–42, 1978.

Webster H.H., Friedman L., Jones B.E. Modification of paradoxical sleep following transection of the reticular formation at the pontomedullary junction. *Sleep* 9:1–23, 1986.

Weitzman E.D., Czeisler C., Coleman R., et al. Delayed sleep phase syndrome. A chronobiological disorder with sleep-onset insomnia. *Arch. Gen. Psychiatry* 38:737–746, 1981.

Disorders of Psychic Function

58

Dementia

M. Rossor

The term *dementia* is used to describe a state of cognitive impairment that involves multiple domains of function without impairment of consciousness. It is not a diagnosis in itself and merely reflects widespread dysfunction of the neural network of the cerebral cortex. The term is useful clinically but eludes precise definition; thus, it should be used with caution, especially because of its frequent association with irreversible degenerative processes. Dementia is particularly common in the elderly, with prevalence rates as high as 5% in the population above 65 years of age and rising to 20% in persons older than age 80 (Kay Beamish and Roth, 1964). With increasingly severe loss of cognition, the ability to function in society is impaired and there is a subsequent inability to perform the ordinary activities of daily living. The care of patients with dementia presents major social and financial burdens. Because life expectancy is usually significantly shortened by dementing diseases, they can be considered a leading cause of death (Katzman, 1976). With the general increase in life expectancy and a predicted substantial increase in the aged population by the end of this millennium, dementia, and more specifically Alzheimer's disease, may reach epidemic proportions (Plum, 1979).

Alzheimer's disease is the most common cause of dementia and in clinical and pathologic series constitutes 50–60% of cases. The second most frequent disorder is dementia resulting from cerebrovascular disease, which accounts for about 20% of cases. For many years, dementia, particularly in the elderly, was ascribed to cerebral arteriosclerosis with associated reduction in blood flow. Cerebral blood flow is indeed reduced in many patients with dementia, not only those who have vascular disease but also patients with degenerative dementia, such as Alzheimer's disease. However, the cerebral blood flow is coupled to metabolism and, in general, represents a concomitant fall rather than a causative factor.

Prospective neuropathologic studies during the 1960s (Tomlinson et al., 1970) established that the predominant cause of dementia in the elderly was an Alzheimer-type histopathologic change. Moreover, even dementia caused by cerebrovascular disease is now seen as constituting a variety of pathologic processes that include strategic large cortical infarcts, multiple small lacunar infarcts, and diffuse white matter ischemia; often these different processes coexist in the same patient. The causes of dementia are legion, and some of the many associated diseases are listed in Table 58–1. The most common causes vary with geographic location and with the age of the patient. Alzheimer's disease is less common in young patients in their 30s, in whom human immunodeficiency virus–related dementia is becoming increasingly prevalent. In Third World countries, infectious causes are proportionally more common.

PROBLEMS OF DEFINITION

The severely demented patient is easily recognized; the problem is to delineate the demented patient from a person with mild cognitive inefficiency. There are three essential features of the definition: (1) multiple domains of cognitive impairment should be apparent to distinguish the dementia patient from

Table 58-1. DISORDERS THAT MAY PRODUCE DEMENTIA

Alzheimer's disease*

Vascular dementia†
    Varieties: Multiple infarcts (called multi-infarct dementia)
          Lacunae
          Binswanger's disease
          Cortical microinfarction

Drug and toxins (including chronic alcoholic dementia)‡

Intracranial masses: tumors, subdural masses, brain abscesses‡

Anoxia

Trauma
    Head injury‡
    Dementia pugilistica (punch-drunk syndrome)

Normal-pressure hydrocephalus‡

Neurodegenerative disorders
    Parkinson's disease§
    Huntington's chorea§
    Progressive supranuclear palsy§
    Pick's disease§
    Amyotrophic lateral sclerosis
    Spinocerebellar degenerations
    Ophthalmoplegia plus
    Metachromatic leukodystrophy (adult form)
    Hallervorden-Spatz disease

Infections
    Creutzfeldt-Jakob disease*
    AIDS§
    Viral encephalitis
    Progressive multifocal leukoencephalopathy
    Behçet's syndrome
    Neurosyphilis
    Chronic bacterial meningitis
    Cryptococcal meningitis
    Other fungal meningitides

Nutritional disorders
    Wernicke-Korsakoff syndrome (thiamine deficiency)‡
    Vitamin B_{12} deficiency
    Folate deficiency
    Pellagra
    Marchiafava-Bignami disease
    ?Zinc deficiency

Metabolic disorders
    Dialysis dementia
    Hypo- and hyperthyroidism
    Renal insufficiency, severe
    Cushing's syndrome
    Hepatic insufficiency
    Parathyroid disease

Chronic inflammatory§
    Lupus and other collagen-vascular§ disorders with
        intracerebral vasculitis
    Multiple sclerosis
    Whipple's disease

---

*Accounts for 50–60% of cases.
†Accounts for 10–20% of cases.
‡Accounts for 1–5% of cases.
§Accounts for about 1% of cases; no symbol: less than 1% of cases.
Modified and updated from Haase G.R. Diseases presenting as dementia. In Wells C.E., ed. *Dementia.* 2nd ed. Philadelphia, Davis, pp. 27–67, 1977. This table includes disorders seen in the United States. Frequency of diseases estimated from Jellinger (1976), Wells (1977), and Katzman (1986).

the person with a focal neuropsychologic deficit, such as a dysphasia; (2) the patient should not have disturbance of consciousness; and (3) the cognitive impairment should be of sufficient severity to interfere with occupational or social function. These cri-

teria are formulated in the *Diagnostic and Statistical Manual of Mental Disorders* (DSM-III-R) (American Psychiatric Association, 1987).

The stipulation of a normal consciousness level serves to distinguish the patient with a confusional state, although this distinction may be more difficult in clinical practice than the definition implies because patients with dementia may have impairment of selective attention. People are often forgetful, make occasional dysphasic errors, and occasionally misinterpret visual and auditory stimuli. Such errors are more apparent during concurrent illness, with fatigue, and during the use of drugs, of which alcohol is the most common. Moreover, cognition, particularly the speed of cognition, declines with age. A distinction has been drawn between the forgetfulness of old age, which may have a benign course, and that of dementia. Kral (1962) introduced the term *benign senescent forgetfulness*. More recently, the term *age-associated memory impairment* (Crook et al., 1986) has been widely used in the United States and avoids the implication of a benign prognosis. These terms imply categorical differences in dementia that have yet to be established, and it may be quite difficult to decide when forgetfulness and cognitive inefficiency become sufficiently noticeable to justify the label of dementia. Although DSM-III-R criteria state that occupation and social function should be impaired, these are clearly variable and depend on premorbid intellect and occupation. Some patients with Alzheimer's disease preserve social skills until late in the disease, whereas the demands of a high-powered job may defeat the same patient at an early stage.

A number of bedside mental tests have been developed (Table 58-2) that are useful as brief clinical assessments of overall function; as such, they are suitable for patients who have diseases with the widespread cognitive disturbance that characterizes dementia. These tests also serve to assess in broad terms the areas of cognition affected but are quite crude for specific neuropsychologic deficits. With severe dementia, cognitive impairment is generalized. In general, however, the term *global impairment* is a misleading definition because dementias may start with characteristic patterns, such as the prominent early memory impairment with visuospatial dysfunction in Alzheimer's disease. Some diseases, such as primary progressive dysphasia, may begin with a strikingly focal deficit and only later develop more widespread impairment.

CLINICOPATHOLOGIC CORRELATES

Is there a common mechanism underlying the various diseases that produce dementia? At its simplest, dementia arises when there is widespread disruption of the cortical neural network, either from impairment of synaptic transmission or structural disintegration. Diffuse brain dysfunction, such as that occurring, for example, with drug intoxication,

Table 58–2. MENTAL STATUS TESTS

Orientation-Memory-Concentration Test	Mini-Mental State
Name	Year/season/date/day/month
Age	State/country/town/hospital/floor
When born	Remember three objects
Where born	Serial 7's
Place	Name pencil and watch
Street	Repeat "No ifs, ands, or buts"
How long	Follow three-stage command
City	Read and obey instruction
Today	Write a sentence
Month	Copy design
Year	
Day of week	
Part of day	
Time	
Season	
Name of mother	
School attended	
Work	
Head of state	
Prior head of state	
Date of World War I	
Date of World War II	
Months backwards	
Count 1–20	
Count 20–1	
Memory phase	

From Blessed et al. (1968), as modified by Katzman et al. (1983) and Folstein et al. (1975).

also normally causes impairment of consciousness resulting from involvement of the reticular activating system. As discussed earlier, however, a global impairment does not occur in early dementia, and the distinctive clinical patterns arise from the selectivity of the disease process. There are variations in regional vulnerability, but also within particular areas of the cerebral cortex only certain neurons may be disrupted to further define the topography of the dementia. In this regard, two extremes can be considered: anatomically focal damage involving all neurons, such as that occurring with an infarct, or diffuse involvement of only one type of cell. No pure example of the latter has been found, although Parkinson's disease and the cognitive impairment that may occur with the neurotoxin 1-methyl-4-phenyl-1,2,3,6-tetrahydropyridine (MPTP), which selectively destroys the substantia nigra, approach it (Stern et al., 1990).

The pattern of selective vulnerability determines the clinical features, but there is rarely sufficient correlation to allow precise diagnosis of the underlying disease from the clinical presentation (Chui, 1989). A broad clinical distinction has been drawn between cortical and subcortical dementias (Cummings, 1986; Cummings and Benson, 1983) (Table 58–3). Alzheimer's disease, the prototypic cortical dementia, is characterized by damage to the association cortices that results in dysphasia, agnosia, and dyspraxia, in addition to memory disturbance. Progressive supranuclear palsy, the prototypic subcortical dementia (Albert et al., 1974) is characterized by memory complaint, but an absence of dysphasia, agnosia, and dyspraxia; a striking slowness of cognition; and a frequent association with motor deficits. The distinction between cortical and subcortical dementias might be paraphrased as a contrast between speed and accuracy, with cortical dementias having normal speed but frequent errors.

The terms *cortical dementia* and *subcortical dementia* have come under criticism, particularly in view of the fact that the distribution of the neuropathology in the various diseases does not precisely segregate between cortical and subcortical structures. Thus, Alzheimer's disease includes damage to subcortical structures, such as the nucleus basalis of Meynert and the locus ceruleus. Subcortical dementias, such as Parkinson's disease and progressive supranuclear palsy, may also be associated with cortical biochemical changes in addition to the classic changes in subcortical nuclei. Positron emission tomography has also demonstrated that subcortical lesions, either in such degenerative processes as progressive supranuclear palsy (D'Antona et al., 1985) or with subcortical infarcts, can result in hypometabolism over the cortical projection area. The clinical deficit that arises from such subcortical lesions differs from that involving the cortical projection site per se, but the overall different patterns have not yet been reliably established.

Alzheimer's Disease

The characteristic features of Alzheimer's disease, namely senile plaques and neurofibrillary tangles, predominantly affect the association neocortices and

Table 58–3. CORTICAL AND SUBCORTICAL DEMENTIAS

Parameter	Subcortical Dementia	Cortical Dementia
Severity	Mild to moderate	Severe earlier in course
Speed of cognition	Slowed	Normal
Behavioral changes	Apathy, depression	Depression less common
Neuropsychologic deficits	Memory impairment (recall aided by cues)	Dysphasia, dyspraxia, agnosia, memory impairment
Motor abnormalities	Extrapyramidal	Uncommon Gegenhalten
Neuropathology	Major changes in striatum and thalamus	Major changes in cortical association areas

Data from Cummings J.L. Subcortical dementia. Neuropsychology, neuropsychiatry, and pathophysiology. *Br. J. Psychiatry* 149:682–697, 1986.

hippocampus in a symmetric pattern. This pattern of selective vulnerability determines the characteristic early features of memory and visuospatial impairment and language disturbance. The dysphasia is characterized by poor comprehension and empty speech resembling a transcortical sensory dysphasia. Plaques and tangles are also seen in large numbers in the amygdala and olfactory bulb; their presence has generated theories of a toxic agent that may gain access to the central nervous system via the nasal mucosa (Pearson et al., 1985). Disturbance of olfaction is often found if specifically looked for in Alzheimer's disease but is rarely a presenting complaint. Within these areas of selective vulnerability, there is also selectivity of neuronal damage; thus, pyramidal cells within the cortex are particularly vulnerable, as reflected in the reduced counts of large cortical neurons. Pyramidal cells are the origin of the cortico-cortical association fibers, and disruption of these association pathways further determines the disturbance of higher cortical function. In addition, the projection fibers from subcortical nuclei, such as nucleus basalis of Meynert and locus ceruleus, and the dorsal raphe nuclei are also involved.

After the success of neurotransmitter replacement in Parkinson's disease, much attention has been directed toward the neurotransmitter changes in neurodegenerative disease. The selectivity of neurotransmitter changes in Alzheimer's disease essentially reflects the loss of pyramidal cells, which utilize glutamate, and damage to the subcortical diffuse projections, which utilize acetylcholine, norepinephrine, and 5-hydroxytryptamine. The damage to the cholinergic system has attracted particular attention because of its role in memory. Scopolamine in young adults results in impaired recall that can be reversed with cholinergic drugs but not by stimulants, such as amphetamine (Drachman and Leavitt, 1974). However, the cognitive impairment arising from the experimental disruption of cholinergic transmission is not sufficiently similar or generalized to explain the dementia of Alzheimer's disease (Kopelman and Corn, 1988). Nevertheless, a diffuse cortical projection system may theoretically have profound effects over a wide area of cortical function, and thus disruption to such a system may be manifested as a dementia even though only a small number of neurons are involved.

The underlying cause of Alzheimer's disease is unknown, although deposition of amyloid both in the senile plaques and blood vessels is seen as an important and consistent feature. The brain amyloid of Alzheimer's disease (referred to as A4 or B amyloid) is distinct from systemic amyloidoses but shares the feature of a β-pleated structure that determines the characteristic staining. A4 amyloid is part of a much larger membrane-bound molecule, the amyloid precursor protein (APP), which is encoded on chromosome 21 (Kang et al., 1987). The precise role of this protein is still unknown, but with alternative splicing of the mRNA a protease inhibitor domain is variably expressed. Cell proliferation and differentia-

tion are known to involve surface-associated serine protease inhibitors, the protease nexins. Part of the APP molecule is homologous to protease nexin II (Van Nostrand et al., 1989). A4 amyloid has been found to enhance the survival of hippocampal neurons in vitro (Whitson et al., 1989); on the other hand, a fragment of the APP molecule has been shown to be neurotoxic (Yankner et al., 1989). This variable biologic activity raises intriguing possibilities for a pathophysiologic role of APP and A4 amyloid, both of which may initiate dystrophic neuritic outgrowth and have a neurotoxic action.

Young-onset familial Alzheimer's disease is linked to chromosome 21 (St. George-Hyslop et al., 1990), but the familial Alzheimer's disease gene appeared to be distinct from the APP gene. More recently, however, a small number of familial Alzheimer cases have been attributed to a point mutation in the APP gene (Goate et al., 1991). Hereditary cerebral hemorrhage with amyloidosis of the Dutch type that causes dementia with hemorrhages and deposition of parenchymal amyloid can be directly attributed to a defect in the APP gene (Levy et al., 1990; Van Broeckhoven et al., 1990).

Other Degenerative Diseases

As with the recognition that not all dementia is cerebrovascular disease, it is now clear that not all degenerative dementia is due to Alzheimer's disease. The features of Pick's disease have long been recognized, and the focal frontotemporal atrophy determines the prominent dysphasia and behavioral abnormalities. Patients have been described with mild memory impairment but with early dysphasia characterized by low speech output, apathy, and personality change. These patients do not have Alzheimer- or Pick-like changes but do show degenerative changes in the frontal lobe (Gustafsson, 1987; Neary et al., 1988). Primary progressive dysphasia (Mesulam, 1982) is another example of a focal atrophy, selectively involving the dominant perisylvian area. Patients ultimately develop dementia but may retain a striking selectivity with sparing of visuospatial function until late in the disease. Positron emission tomography reveals focal hypometabolism that spreads to contiguous areas with progression of the disease (Tyrrell et al., 1990).

Dementia occurring in the setting of extrapyramidal disease usually has characteristics of a subcortical dementia with slowness and frontal features that can be attributed to disruption of frontostriatal projections, and positron emission tomographic scanning in progressive supranuclear palsy confirms frontal hypometabolism (D'Antona et al., 1985). Nevertheless, cognitive impairment in extrapyramidal disease, such as Parkinson's, is more prevalent in the elderly, in whom an overlap with Alzheimer's disease may occur (Dubois et al., 1990).

Vascular Dementia

With the demonstration that vascular dementia was not due to a simple reduction in cerebral blood flow but rather to multiple infarcts, it was established that there was an overall association between the amount of tissue lost and the occurrence of dementia. Tomlinson et al. (1970) found that patients with more than 100 ml of cerebral cortical infarction were demented and a number of those with 50 to 100 ml of infarction were also demented. This observation was related to the experiments of Lashley (1963), who demonstrated that the impairment of learning in rats was proportional to the amount of cerebral cortex, other than primary motor and sensory areas, that was excised. This result is perhaps not surprising in a clinical syndrome that arises from widespread destruction of cerebral cortex. Nevertheless, strategic infarcts of certain association cortical areas, such as the angular gyrus (Benson and Cummings, 1982), may result in a dementia syndrome. Theoretically, lesions of the diffuse projection systems would likewise result in dementia and represent an exception to theories of critical mass effect. The search for vascular lesions selectively affecting the nucleus basalis in cases of multi-infarct dementia have been generally unrewarding, although bilateral forebrain infarcts can result in severe amnesia (Phillips et al., 1987). In addition to cortical infarcts, widespread subcortical lacunar or diffuse white matter ischemia (Binswanger's disease) may occur with motor disturbance and a subcortical dementia. These diffuse white matter changes can be seen on computed tomographic scans and more frequently on magnetic resonance imaging scans. White matter changes have also been reported in Alzheimer's disease, and it has been suggested that amyloid deposition in blood vessels may contribute to the pathophysiology of Alzheimer's disease.

As listed in Table 58–1, many diseases may result in dementia. It is not possible to review the clinicopathologic correlates of all of these diseases, but they share the feature of widespread disruption of cerebral cortex or subcorticocortical connections. The majority of metabolic, infective, and nutritional disorders present a picture of subcortical dementia. Normal-pressure hydrocephalus is also characterized by a striking slowing of cognition that is useful in predicting the outcome of shunting. The cognitive impairment associated with depressive illness is often referred to as depressive pseudodementia, which serves the useful purpose of reminding the clinician of the importance of depression as a cause of dementia but implies that the cognitive impairment is, in some sense, unreal or simulated. This is not the case, and the biochemical changes that underlie depression, such as those of the diffuse aminergic projections, may also contribute to the cognitive impairment.

ASSESSMENT OF PATIENTS WITH DEMENTIA

The diagnostic work-up of the patient with dementia includes careful history taking, mental status examination, neurologic and general physical examination, laboratory investigations, and neuroimaging (Cummings and Benson, 1983; Katzman and Terry, 1983). Many aspects of the history taken directly from the patient can be used to contribute to the mental state assessment. Thus, a short biographic history permits some simple assessment of memory in terms of knowledge of address, place, and family details. It also provides information of the previous occupation and level of functioning. Some idea of the current impairment and the length of history may be obtained, and it is important to assess the degree of insight. Nevertheless, many patients are unaware of their deficits or are prevented from providing a reliable history by the severity of the impairment. Interviewing a second informant, normally the spouse or close family member, is therefore essential to provide information on the onset and progression of the illness, the presence of personality and behavioral disturbances, and the presence of any depressive symptoms. An indication of the main areas of affected cognition, such as memory, language, and visuospatial function, can be obtained, and the physician can determine whether there are occupational problems if the patient is still working and whether the patient is coping with family affairs, still driving, and performing the functions of daily living. It is also important to determine what medications the patient is taking. The interview with the second informant may take place when the patient is preparing for the physical examination, or it may need to be obtained at the end of the consultation or at an entirely separate time to avoid causing distress.

On examination, the mental status assessment can be completed and any particular areas of cognitive impairment can be further explored. Physical examination may provide evidence of such additional features as motor abnormalities that may direct the physician toward diagnoses other than Alzheimer's disease, which tends to be associated with a paucity of neurologic signs. The general examination may provide evidence of systemic disturbances, hypertension, and generalized cardiovascular disease.

Formal neuropsychologic assessment provides more precise measures of impairment of specific functions that cannot be obtained with a simple bedside mental state assessment. Routine hematologic and biochemical assays should include thyroid function and vitamin B_{12} estimations and treponemal serology. A routine chest x-ray film and electrocardiogram exclude relevant cardiovascular disease. Neuroimaging with either computed tomography or magnetic resonance imaging can exclude structural lesions, such as tumors and hydrocephalus. Focal atrophy may also be apparent, but assessment of generalized cerebral atrophy is unreliable as a diagnostic marker. The electroencephalogram provides specific diagnostic information, as in Creutzfeldt-Jakob disease, or supplementary information, as in Alzheimer's disease, when early slow-wave changes occur in contrast to the normal electroencephalogram in Pick's disease and frontal lobe dementia. Examination of the cerebrospinal fluid excludes low-grade meningitic infections and allows measurement of the pressure. Many other tests may be necessary, such as screening for inherited metabolic disorders and human immunodeficiency virus status, but the detail of investigation depends much on the age of the patient because these disorders are more common in the young.

THERAPEUTIC APPROACHES

The definition of dementia does not imply that the cognitive impairment is irreversible; in most series, 5–15% of patients are treatable (Cummings et al., 1980; Marsden and Harrison, 1972). However, because there is no single cause of dementia, there is no simple treatment. In a number of cases, the underlying cause can be identified and treated, with resolution or arrest of the cognitive impairment. The most common reversible dementia in most series is that of depression. This finding underlines the importance of considering this diagnosis in patients with dementia. Drug intoxication is another important cause, as well as with benign tumors, in which significant or complete reversal can be anticipated. Treatment of vascular disease, vitamin B_{12} deficiency, and hypothyroidism may cause partial reversal but rarely complete resolution.

The majority of patients, however, have degenerative dementia, of which Alzheimer's disease is the most common. Most efforts have been directed at facilitating synaptic transmission at those sites preferentially affected in the disease. The cholinergic projection system has provided a basis for drugs, such as the anticholinesterases, physostigmine, and tetrahydroaminoacridine, for which limited effects have been claimed (Mayeux, 1990), although such treatment is only symptomatic. The current work on amyloid deposition and the elucidation of the molecular genetics of chromosome 21–linked familial Alzheimer's disease (St. George-Hyslop et al., 1990) can be anticipated to provide rational strategies based on underlying mechanisms. With the currently limited prospects of treatment, explanation to the family becomes even more important. The patient should avoid fatigue and drugs that may impair cognition, and systemic illness should be vigorously treated. An explanation of the prognosis, once the diagnosis is established, is important, particularly for the appropriate planning of long-term care, which remains one of the major problems of health care.

References

(Key references are designated with an asterisk.)

*Albert M.L., Feldman R.G., Willis A.L. The "subcortical dementia" of progressive supranuclear palsy. *J. Neurol. Neurosurg. Psychiatry* 37:121–130, 1974.

American Psychiatric Association. *Diagnostic and Statistical Manual of Mental Disorders.* 3rd ed. revised. Washington, DC, American Psychiatric Association, 1987.

Benson D.F., Cummings J.L. Angular gyrus syndrome simulating Alzheimers disease. *Arch. Neurol.* 39:616–620, 1982.

*Blessed G., Tomlinson B.E., Roth M. The association between quantitative measurements of dementia and of senile changes in the cerebral gray matter of elderly subjects. *Br. J. Psychiatry* 114:797–811, 1968.

Chui H.C. Dementia. A review emphasizing clinicopathologic correlation and brain-behavior relationships. *Arch. Neurol.* 46:806–814, 1989.

*Crook T., Bartus R.T., Ferris S.H., et al. Age-associated memory impairment. Proposed diagnostic criteria and measures of clinical change; report of a National Institute of Mental Health work group. *Dev. Neuropsychol.* 2:261–276, 1986.

Cummings J.L. Subcortical dementia. Neuropsychology, neuropsychiatry, and pathophysiology. *Br. J. Psychiatry* 149:682–697, 1986.

Cummings J.L., Benson D.F. *Dementia: A Clinical Approach.* London, Butterworth, 1983.

Cummings J.L., Benson D.F., Lo Verma S. Reversible dementia, illustrative cases, definition and review. *J.A.M.A.* 243:2434–2439, 1980.

D'Antona R., Baron J.C., Samson Y., et al. Frontal cortex hypometabolism detected by positron tomography in patients with progressive supranuclear palsy. *Brain* 108:785–799, 1985.

Drachman D.A., Leavitt J. Human memory and the cholinergic system: a relationship to aging? *Arch. Neurol.* 30:113–121, 1974.

Dubois B., Pillon B., Sternic N., et al. Age-induced cognitive disturbances in Parkinson's disease. *Neurology* 40:38–41, 1990.

*Folstein M., Folstein S., McHugh P.R. Mini-mental state: a practical method for grading the cognitive state of patients for the clinician. *J. Psychiatr. Res.* 12:189–198, 1975.

*Goate A., Chartier-Harlin M-C., Mullan M., et al. Segregation of a missense mutation in the amyloid precursor protein gene with familial Alzheimer's disease. *Nature* 349:704–706, 1991.

Gustafsson L. Frontal lobe degeneration of non-Alzheimer type. II. Clinical picture and differential diagnosis. *Arch. Gerontol. Geriatr.* 6:209–223, 1987.

Jellinger J. Neuropathological agents and dementia. *Acta Neurol. Belg.* 76:83–102, 1976.

*Kang J., Lemaire H.G., Unterbeck A., et al. The precursor of Alzheimer's disease amyloid A4 protein resembles a cell surface receptor. *Nature* 325:733–736, 1987.

Katzman R. The prevalence and malignancy of Alzheimer disease. *Arch. Neurol.* 33:217–218, 1976.

Katzman R., Terry R.D. *The Neurology of Aging.* Philadelphia, Davis, 1983.

Katzman R., Brown T., Fuld P., et al. Validation of a short orientation-memory-concentration test of cognitive impairment. *Am. J. Psychiatry* 140:734–739, 1983.

Kay D.W.K., Beamish P., Roth M. Old age mental disorders in Newcastle upon Tyne. Part 1. A study of prevalence. *Br. J. Psychiatry* 110:146–158, 1964.

Kopelman M.D., Corn T.H. Cholinergic "blockade" as a model for cholinergic depletion. A comparison of the memory deficits with those of Alzheimer-type dementia and the alcoholic Korsakoff syndrome. *Brain* 111:1079–1110, 1988.

Kral V.A. Senescent forgetfulness, benign and malignant. *Can. Med. Assoc. J.* 86:257–260, 1962.

Lashley K.S. *Brain Mechanisms and Intelligence: A Quantitative Study of Injury to the Brain.* New York, Hafner Publishers, 1963.

Levy E., Carman M.D., Fernandez-Madrid I.J., et al. Mutation of the Alzheimer's disease amyloid gene in hereditary cerebral hemorrhage, Dutch type. *Science* 248:1124–1126, 1990.

*Marsden C.D., Harrison M.J.G. Outcome of investigation of patients with presenile dementia. *Br. Med. J.* 2:249–252, 1972.

Mayeux R. Therapeutic strategies in Alzheimer's disease. *Neurology* 40:175–180, 1990.

*Mesulam M-M. Slowly progressive aphasia without generalized dementia. *Ann. Neurol.* 11:592–598, 1982.

Neary D., Snowden J.S., Northen B., et al. Dementia of frontal lobe type. *J. Neurol. Neurosurg. Psychiatry* 51:353–361, 1988.

Pearson R.C.A., Esiri M.M., Hiorns R.W., et al. Anatomical correlate of the distribution of the pathologic changes in the neocortex in Alzheimer's disease. *Proc. Natl. Acad. Sci. U.S.A.* 82:4531–4534, 1985.

Phillips S., Sangalang V., Sterns G. Basal forebrain infarction. A clinicopathologic correlation. *Arch. Neurol.* 44:1134–1138, 1987.

Plum F. Dementia: an approaching epidemic. *Nature* 279:372–373, 1979.

Stern Y., Tetrud J.W., Martin W.R.W., et al. Cognitive change following MPTP exposure. *Neurology* 40:261–264, 1990.

*St. George-Hyslop P.H., Haines J.L., Farrer L.A., et al. Genetic linkage studies suggest that Alzheimer's disease is not a single homogeneous disorder. *Nature* 347:194–197, 1990.

Tomlinson B.E., Blessed G., Roth M. Observations on the brains of demented old people. *J. Neurol. Sci.* 11:205–242, 1970.

Tyrrell P.J., Warrington E.K., Frackowiak R.S.J., et al. Heterogeneity in progressive aphasia due to focal cortical atrophy. A clinical and PET study. *Brain* 113:1321–1336, 1990.

Van Broeckhoven C., Haan J., Bakker E., et al. Amyloid B protein precursor gene and hereditary cerebral hemorrhage with amyloidosis (Dutch). *Science* 248:1120–1122, 1990.

Van Nostrand W.E., Wargner S.L., Suzuki M., et al. Protease nexin-2, a potent antichymotrypsin, shows identity to amyloid beta protein precursor. *Nature* 341:546–549, 1989.

Wells C.E., ed. *Dementia.* 2nd ed. Philadelphia, Davis, 1977.

Whitson J.S., Selkoe D.J., Cotman C.W. Amyloid B protein enhances the survival of hippocampus neurons in vitro. *Science* 243:1488–1490, 1989.

*Yankner B.A., Dawes L.R., Fisher S., et al. Neurotoxicity of a fragment of the amyloid precursor associated with Alzheimer's disease. *Science* 245:417–420, 1989.

59

Alzheimer's Disease

William R. Markesbery

Alzheimer's disease (AD) was initially described in 1907 in a 51-year-old woman with a 4½-year course of progressive dementia (Alzheimer, 1907). Clinical features included memory decline, paranoid delusions, auditory hallucinations, aphasia, apraxia, and agnosia. Autopsy of the patient showed the presence of masses of silver-positive fibers, or neurofibrillary tangles (NFTs), in many neurons in the cerebral cortex, in addition to a severe loss of cortical neurons. During the next 5 years, 12 cases of this new entity were described; several were referred to as AD (Beach, 1987), although there was considerable disagreement about whether AD and senile dementia were the same disorder. Early pathologists viewed atherosclerosis as a prominent disease mechanism, and many thought that cerebral atherosclerosis was the cause of dementia in the elderly. Not until the early 1960s did the modern era of knowledge about AD begin. In 1963, ultrastructural studies of the cerebral cortical lesions in AD were described. During the 1970s, specific neurotransmitter deficits were found in AD. The discovery raised the possibility that some symptoms of the disease could be ameliorated by pharmacologic intervention. More recently, molecular biologic approaches and other new technologies have offered better insight into molecular mechanisms in AD and have set the stage for potentially understanding the pathogenetic mechanisms in this disorder, with the ultimate goal of treatment or prevention.

CLINICAL FEATURES

Dementing diseases represent one of the major health problems facing society. The symptom complex of dementia can be caused by more than 70 different disorders (Katzman et al., 1988). Many of these disorders are treatable or reversible, including drug toxicity, depression, central nervous system infections, subdural hematomas, primary brain tumors, normal-pressure hydrocephalus, metallic and organic poisoning, nutritional disorders (vitamin B_{12}, vitamin B_6, thiamine, and folic acid deficiencies), and numerous metabolic disorders (especially thyroid and parathyroid disorders). AD is the most common form of adult-onset dementia. A community-based study suggested that approximately 4 million persons in the United States have AD (Evans et al., 1989), and it is said to be the fourth or fifth leading cause of death in the United States (Katzman, 1976).

Diagnostic Criteria

Criteria for the clinical diagnosis of AD have been established (McKhann et al., 1984) and validated by autopsy findings (Morris et al., 1988). Six primary criteria are (1) dementia established by the clinical examination and documented by neuropsychologic testing; (2) deficits in two or more areas of cognition; (3) progressive worsening of memory and other cognitive function, such as abstract thinking, judgment, problem solving, language, perception, praxis, and ability to learn new skills; (4) no disturbance of consciousness; (5) onset between ages 40 and 90; and (6) absence of systemic disorders or other brain diseases that could account for the progressive memory and cognitive changes.

Supportive criteria include progressive decline in specific functions, such as language, motor skills, and perception; impaired activities of daily living and altered behavior; family history of a similar disorder; plateaus in the course of the illness; and associated symptoms of depression, insomnia, incontinence, delusions, illusions, hallucinations, and verbal, emotional, or physical outbursts. Diagnostic accuracy for AD in the most recent series is approximately 90% (Katzman et al., 1988).

Clinical Picture

The typical clinical picture of AD is characterized by early decline in recent memory, often demonstrated by the inability to remember names and repeating oneself, misplacement of objects, and the inability to carry out simple tasks. The patient loses spontaneity and initiative, reacts more slowly, uses poor judgment, does not make decisions well, and prefers to remain in familiar surroundings. He or she is unable to reason clearly and especially shows deficits when confronted with new situations. Social judgment is usually maintained in the early and middle stages of the disease. With time, there are alterations in the ability to use words correctly and a loss of ability to do simple calculations. The patient becomes disoriented to time and place and often becomes lost in familiar surroundings. The memory loss gradually becomes much more severe, and only highly learned material is retained. Interests are quite restricted and poorly sustained. In the moderately impaired stages, assistance is required in dressing and personal hygiene. In the late stage of the disease, only fragments of recent and remote memory remain. The patient is oriented to person only; is apathetic, lethargic, and withdrawn; becomes easily lost; and has no judgment or ability to solve problems. Help is required with personal care, and the patient is often incontinent and bedridden. Generalized seizures occur in approximately 10% of patients (Hauser et al., 1986).

Behavior problems, such as agitation, wandering, hallucinations, and suspicion, frequently occur and rise significantly with increased cognitive impairment (Teri et al., 1988). Hostile, obstreperous, occasionally combative behavior is also frequently observed. The frequency and degree of depression in AD have varied considerably in several studies (reviewed in Merriam et al., 1988), but severe depression is not common.

Atypical clinical presentations of AD occur in approximately 10% of patients (Katzman, 1986). They include progressive aphasia, visual agnosia, pure memory loss, right parietal lobe syndrome of spatial disorientation, and personality changes (paranoid or bizarre behavior). Some patients may initially present with atypical features for several years, but all patients subsequently develop more generalized cognitive deterioration.

Neurologic Examination

The neurologic examination reveals a few subtle abnormalities. The cranial nerves are intact except for olfactory identification deficits in a few patients (Corwin et al., 1986). Primitive reflexes, such as the grasp, snout, suck, tonic-foot, and palmomental reflexes, are found frequently in middle and late stages of AD. Cummings et al. (1985) reported the presence of language abnormalities in 100% of AD patients.

The earliest abnormality is impaired word finding, followed by frank anomia and paraphasia. Subsequently, comprehension of spoken language is altered and a transcortical sensory fluent aphasia develops. The patient frequently repeats words spoken to him or her. Terminally, few spontaneous meaningful sounds are uttered. Varying degrees of apraxia, especially dressing and constructional apraxias, are found in middle stage AD patients. Visual agnosias are encountered in some patients. Myoclonic jerks are found in approximately 10% of patients (Mayeux et al., 1985).

The hallmark of AD is a steadily progressive deterioration of intellectual function, although the rate of progression is highly variable. Many patients have plateau periods in which there is an apparent arrest of progression. Remissions have never been reported. The mean survival time of AD patients in the United States is 8.1 years (Barclay et al., 1985); the range of survival is 1 to 20 years.

Laboratory and Diagnostic Tests

There are no definitive diagnostic laboratory studies for AD, but numerous laboratory studies are of value in excluding other dementing illnesses. A complete blood count; erythrocyte sedimentation rate; electrolyte assays; calcium, phosphorus, renal, liver, and thyroid function studies; vitamin B_{12} and folic acid levels; drug screen; and serologic tests exclude many of the treatable or reversible entities just mentioned. An electrocardiogram and chest x-ray film can yield useful information in a dementia evaluation. The electroencephalogram shows nonspecific progressive slowing as intellectual deterioration progresses. The electroencephalogram can be useful in a small number of patients who have cognitive impairment resulting from seizure activity or in patients with Creutzfeldt-Jakob disease (CJD) who may have a periodic rhythm. Computed tomography and magnetic resonance imaging are of value in excluding other lesions, such as brain tumors, abscesses, subdural hematomas, hydrocephalus, cerebral hemorrhages, and infarctions. Magnetic resonance imaging is especially useful in defining multi-infarct dementia.

Cerebral atrophy and ventricular enlargement are commonly found in the middle and late stages of AD, although some patients with AD do not show significant atrophy and these findings can occur in normal, nondemented elderly. Positron emission tomography has revealed a relatively characteristic pattern of symmetrically reduced regional cerebral blood flow and glucose and oxygen metabolism in the parietal and adjacent temporal lobes in AD (reviewed in Frackowiak, 1988). Similar changes are found in the frontal lobes to a lesser degree. The sensory-motor and visual cortex, cingulate gyri, basal ganglia, and cerebellum are normal. Single-photon emission computed tomography measures regional blood flow and defines similar changes.

Neuropsychologic assessment is important in confirming the presence of a dementing process, defining the kinds of impaired cognitive function, separating psychiatric illnesses from dementia, and following changes in cognition. Neuropsychologic testing does not give a definitive diagnosis. A simple, convenient screening battery consists of the Folstein Mini-Mental Status Examination, the Blessed Dementia Rating Scale, and the Alzheimer's Disease Assessment Scale.

Differential Diagnosis

It is occasionally difficult to differentiate AD from vascular dementia (multi-infarct dementia), Pick's disease, diffuse Lewy body disease (DLBD), and some cases of CJD.

The characteristics of vascular dementia are a history of clinical stroke and hypertension; abrupt onset; stepwise deterioration; relative preservation of the personality; and focal neurologic symptoms and signs, most frequently motor, reflex, sensory, and/or visual changes. These items and others are a part of the Hachinski Ischemic Score, an 18-point scale to identify dementia on a vascular basis (Hachinski et al., 1975). If a patient scores 7 or more, a vascular dementia is most likely, whereas a score of 4 or less makes a primary degenerative dementia more probable. In most instances, the ischemic score and magnetic resonance imaging of the brain are helpful in differentiating AD and vascular dementia. It should be remembered, however, that approximately 15% of patients have a combination of AD and vascular dementia.

Pick's disease is often difficult to differentiate from AD. The early stages of Pick's disease are often characterized by personality and behavior changes with relative preservation of visuospatial skills and memory, but most AD patients suffer early impaired memory and visuospatial disturbances (Cummings and Benson, 1983). Although both disorders include language disturbances, Pick's disease patients demonstrate early semantic anomia and circumlocution. Computed tomography and magnetic resonance imaging may show generalized cortical atrophy in AD and frontal and temporal atrophy in Pick's disease; the latter can also be found in AD patients.

The relationship between Parkinson's disease and AD is not clearly defined and can present diagnostic problems. A moderate number of AD patients show extrapyramidal signs, primarily rigidity and bradykinesia, and may represent a subgroup (Mayeux et al., 1985). A significant number of patients with Parkinson's disease have mild to severe dementia (Boller et al., 1980). The clinical picture is often complicated by psychotropic medication–induced extrapyramidal signs in some AD patients. In addition, patients with DLBD can be difficult to diagnose.

DLBD is a newly recognized entity with Lewy's bodies in the brain stem and other subcortical structures and Lewy-like bodies in the cerebral cortex (Burkhardt et al., 1988). In addition, many patients have numerous cortical senile plaques (SPs) and a decline in cholinergic markers, thus raising the question of whether DLBD is a variant of AD (Hansen et al., 1990). The brains of DLBD patients contain few NFTs and neuropil threads. Autopsy studies have suggested that it is the second most common cause of dementia in adults (R.H. Perry et al., 1989). Progressive dementia or psychosis is the most prominent early clinical feature. Parkinsonism signs are usually mild except for rigidity. Involuntary movements, myoclonus, orthostatic hypotension, and dysphagia have been described (Burkhardt et al., 1988; Hansen et al., 1990).

In general, typical cases of CJD with dementia, myoclonus, visual disturbances, pyramidal and extrapyramidal signs, sensory signs, ataxia, fasciculations, and periodic electroencephalographic activity are not difficult to differentiate from AD. However, it is difficult to distinguish slowly progressive CJD from AD. Five to 10% of CJD patients have a clinical course of 2 years or more, with the longest case of 13 years' duration (Brown et al., 1984). Slowly progressive CJD is more often familial; patients have a younger age of onset and a lower frequency of myoclonus and periodic electroencephalographic activity. These patients have a slowly progressive initial stage with intellectual decline or behavior abnormalities and a more rapidly progressive terminal stage.

NEUROPATHOLOGY

Although the clinical criteria for AD are relatively distinct, a definitive diagnosis cannot be made without neuropathologic confirmation. In considering the pathologic features of AD, the examiner must remember that most of the alterations observed are found to a lesser extent in the normal aged brain.

Grossly, the AD brain shows variable degrees of cerebral cortical atrophy, more in younger than in older patients. The atrophy is usually generalized but is most prominent in the frontal and temporal lobes. It should be underscored that some individuals with clinical and histologic features of AD show minimal atrophy. The centrum ovale white matter is diminished in size, and the lateral ventricles are variably enlarged.

The major microscopic alterations in AD are neuritic or SP formation, NFT formation, selective neuron loss and shrinkage, altered neuritic processes, and synapse loss. Specific diagnostic criteria for quantitation of SP and NFT in various age groups have been suggested (Khachaturian, 1985).

Senile Plaques. SPs are complex structures composed of dystrophic neuritic processes, extracellular amyloid, astrocytes and their processes, and microglia (Tomlinson and Corsellis, 1984). These structures are divided into (1) diffuse plaques (Yamaguchi et al., 1988) that contain nonfibrillar amyloid precursor protein; (2) primitive plaques composed of distended neuritic processes; (3) mature plaques composed of neurites, occasionally astrocytes, microglial cells, and a dense core of amyloid; and (4) burned-out plaques consisting primarily of a core of amyloid (Tomlinson and Corsellis, 1984). SPs are present in abundance in the association areas of the frontal, temporal, and parietal lobes; amygdala; hippocampus; and piriform cortex and in lesser numbers in primary motor, somatosensory, visual, and auditory cortex. A direct correlation of SP density, severity of dementia, and decline in cholinergic markers has been reported (E.K. Perry et al., 1978). Some AD patients have abundant SP formation and decreased cholinergic markers and somatostatin but insignificant numbers of NFTs (Terry et al., 1987). These findings suggest that the SP is the most important and consistent microscopic lesion in AD.

Most SPs contain amyloid, the subject of intense research in AD (reviewed in Selkoe, 1989a,b). The extracellular amyloid fibrils present in SPs are composed of a 4-kd peptide of 42 amino acids referred to as βA4 protein or β-amyloid protein (BAP). BAP is a fragment of a larger amyloid precursor protein (APP). Four different forms of APP have been identified to date. Three of these contain 714, 751, and 770 amino acids and have a serine protease inhibitor domain (Kang and Müller-Hill, 1990; Kitaguchi et al., 1988; Ponte et al., 1988). A fourth form contains 695 amino acids and does not have a protease inhibitor domain. The four forms of APP are encoded by four distinct mRNAs. The gene coding for APP maps to the long arm of chromosome 21 (Goldgaber et al., 1987; Tanzi et al., 1987). One fragment of the complex APP molecule has been shown to be toxic to cultured neurons (Yankner et al., 1989), whereas another has been found to prolong survival of cultured neurons (Whitson et al., 1989).

Amyloid, similar to that in SPs, is present in blood vessel walls in the brain and leptomeninges in almost all AD patients (Selkoe, 1989b). The exact site of BAP production in SPs and blood vessels is not known. BAP has been found in the skin, subcutaneous tissues, and intestines of patients with AD (Joachim et al., 1989). It has been hypothesized that in AD there is an age-related alteration in the brain's degradative processing of APP that leads to BAP fragment deposition and a subsequent cascade of pathologic changes culminating in SP and neuritic changes (Selkoe, 1989b).

Neurofibrillary Tangles. NFTs are neuronal cytoplasmic collections of tangled, silver-positive filaments (Tomlinson and Corsellis, 1984). They are present in the neocortex, hippocampus, amygdala, substantia nigra, locus ceruleus, dorsal raphe, and other scattered brain stem nuclei in AD. In the cortex, they occur most frequently in the outer and middle layers. In the hippocampus, they are present in greatest numbers in CA1 and the subiculum.

By electron microscopy, NFTs are composed of paired helical filaments (PHFs), 10 nm in diameter (Kidd, 1963). PHFs are highly insoluble, crossed-linked protein polymers of an uncertain origin. Available evidence reveals that PHFs contain a number of proteins, including tau, microtubule-associated protein, neurofilament protein, and ubiquitin (Kosik, 1989). Tau contains the entire or almost all of the parent protein and may be the major protein in PHF.

NFTs are also found in Down's syndrome, dementia pugilistica, Parkinson-dementia complex of Guam, postencephalitic Parkinson's disease, subacute sclerosing panencephalitis, Hallervorden-Spatz disease, and the brain of normal aging individuals. They probably represent a nonspecific response of neurons to a variety of cellular insults.

Neuron Loss. Perhaps the most important microscopic feature of AD is selective neuron loss (reviewed in Coleman and Flood, 1987). In the neocortex, the greatest loss has been found in pyramidal neurons of the temporal and frontal lobes. A consistent neuron loss is also found in the CA1 area and subiculum of the hippocampus and the basolateral amygdala. Neuronal loss is a feature of the cholinergic nucleus basalis of Meynert (Whitehouse et al., 1982) and septal nuclei in AD. Loss of neurons from the noradrenergic locus ceruleus in AD is present in the central region projecting to the temporal and parietal cortex but not in the region projecting to the basal ganglia, cerebellum, or spinal cord (reviewed in Hardy et al., 1986). Neuron loss from the serotoninergic dorsal raphe nucleus, superior central nucleus, and dorsal tegmental nucleus also has been reported in AD (Hardy et al., 1986).

Neuronal Changes. In addition to neuron loss, many surviving neurons undergo degenerative changes and shrinkage. It has been shown that the apical and basal dendritic spines undergo degeneration in AD more than in normal aging (Coleman and Flood, 1987). Dendritic plasticity is also reduced in AD. Some surviving neurons have been shown to have a decreased capacity for protein synthesis (Doebler et al., 1987). Surviving atrophic neurons may become the target of therapeutic efforts utilizing growth factors. Nerve growth factor has been shown to attenuate cholinergic neuron degeneration induced by experimental lesions in animals (reviewed by Hefti et al., 1989).

Dystrophic Neurites. Another important lesion in the AD cortex consists of copious numbers of dystrophic neurites referred to as neuropil threads, or curly fibers (Kosik, 1989). These tau-reactive neurites dominate the neuropil in the AD cortex and may be a factor in the clinical picture of cognitive decline.

Synapse Loss. Immunohistochemical studies using an antibody against the presynaptic terminal marker synaptophysin revealed approximately 50% synaptic loss in the AD neocortex (Masliah et al., 1989). Quantitative electron microscopic studies of AD frontal laminae III and V revealed a 29–42% decrease in synaptic number (Scheff et al., 1990). It has been suggested that synaptic loss correlates with cognitive decline and neuron loss and might be the anatomic substrate of dementia in AD, rather than SP or NFT formation.

NEUROCHEMISTRY

The most consistent neurotransmitter alteration found in the AD brain is a loss of the cholinergic markers choline acetyltransferase and acetylcholinesterase (reviewed in Bartus et al., 1982). Brain biopsy studies have shown that choline acetyltransferase is diminished early in the disease and that high-affinity choline uptake and acetylcholine synthesis are reduced in AD (reviewed in Bowen et al., 1988). These findings, the loss of neurons in the cholinergic nucleus basalis of Meynert, a correlation between the loss of choline acetyltransferase and decline in mental status scores (Wilcock et al., 1982), and scopolamine-induced memory loss in normal individuals have led to the cholinergic hypothesis in AD (Bartus et al., 1982), which has served as the basis for therapeutic trials.

It is now readily apparent that AD is a multineurotransmitter deficiency disease. Biopsy and postmortem studies have shown a presynaptic noradrenergic deficit in AD neocortex (Bowen et al., 1988). Concentrations of norepinephrine are decreased in pre- and postmortem specimens of AD cerebral cortex (Palmer et al., 1987b; Reinikainen et al., 1988). Levels of the norepinephrine metabolites 3-methoxy-4-hydroxyphenylglycol and dopamine β-hydroxylase are also reduced in the AD brain. Despite the loss of noradrenergic presynaptic markers, the density of adrenergic receptor–binding sites is not changed in AD (Rossor and Iverson, 1989). The marked loss of neurons in the dorsal part of the locus ceruleus, the major noradrenergic projection area to the cerebral cortex, appears to correlate with the cortical noradrenergic deficit in AD. The neuron loss in the locus ceruleus and substantia nigra has been hypothesized to correlate with the presence of depression in AD patients (Zubenko and Moossy, 1988).

Alterations in serotonin (5-hydroxytryptamine) have been described in both biopsy and autopsy material in AD (reviewed in Bowen et al., 1988). The concentrations of serotonin and the metabolite 5-hydroxyindoleacetic acid, serotonin uptake, and potassium-stimulated release of endogeneous serotonin are reduced in AD cerebral cortical biopsy specimens (Palmer et al., 1987a). Binding to serotonin type 1 and 2 receptors is consistently reduced in AD. It has been shown that serotonin, 5-hydroxyindoleacetic acid, and presynaptic receptor binding are reduced in the nucleus basalis of Meynert in AD (Sparks et al., 1986). Cortical serotoninergic changes correlate with neuron loss and NFT formation in the dorsal raphe nucleus, the major serotoninergic projection nucleus (Hardy et al., 1986).

The major change found in the neuropeptides of AD patients is a decline in somatostatin-like immu-noreactivity (Davies et al., 1980). Somatostatin-like immunoreactivity is reduced most severely in the temporal lobe and, to a lesser extent, in the parietal lobe of autopsy specimens. Cerebral biopsy specimens of patients in the early stage of AD showed no alteration in somatostatin-like immunoreactivity, thus suggesting that this is a late-stage change (Bowen et al., 1988). Corticotropin-releasing factor concentrations are markedly reduced in the frontal and temporal cortex and caudate nucleus in AD (Bissette et al., 1985). Concentrations of other neuropeptides, neuropeptide Y, vasoactive intestinal polypeptide, neurotensin, and thyrotropin-releasing hormone, are not altered in AD.

In several studies, γ-aminobutyric acid concentrations have been found to be normal, as has its biosynthetic enzyme glutamic acid decarboxylase, in postmortem and biopsied AD specimens (Bowen et al., 1988; Reinikainen et al., 1988). Cortical γ-aminobutyric acid receptors have been reported to be unchanged or reduced in AD (Chu et al., 1987).

GENETICS

Genetic factors are important in some patients with AD. Current data do not give a definitive answer regarding the proportion of familial AD cases, but estimates vary from 5 to 100% (reviewed in St. George-Hyslop et al., 1989). It is most likely that familial examples make up approximately 40% of cases (Fitch et al., 1988). In most large families with AD, an autosomal dominant inheritance pattern is present. This is especially true in families with early-onset AD, in which at-risk offspring have an estimated lifetime risk of 53% (Farrer et al., 1990). AD offspring in families with late-onset AD, however, have a lifetime risk of 86%, thus suggesting that some causes of late-onset cases may be autosomal dominant inheritance, genes that determine longevity, and environmental factors.

Comparison of the concordance rate of AD in twins reveals a 44% rate for monozygotic twins and a 40% rate for dizygotic twins (St. George-Hyslop et al., 1989). A striking difference in ages of expression of the concordant twins has been observed in some instances. These data support a genetic component in AD but also suggest that environmental factors may modify the expression of AD genes.

Genetic linkage studies using recombinant DNA techniques have shown that the proximal region of chromosome 21 contains a locus for susceptibility to familial early-onset AD in some pedigrees (Goate et al., 1989; St. George-Hyslop et al., 1987). This factor is of considerable interest because the defective gene in Down's syndrome and the gene coding APP are on chromosome 21. However, two other groups of investigators using autopsy-documented kindreds have not shown evidence for linkage between chromosome 21 and familial AD (Pericak-Vance et al., 1988; Schellenberg et al., 1988). More recent linkage studies have suggested the existence of a locus on chromosome 19 in late-onset familial AD (Roses et al., 1990). Thus, it seems most likely that familial AD is a heterogeneous disorder.

An additional feature of the genetic hypothesis of AD is the link with Down's syndrome (Karlinsky, 1986). Most individuals with Down's syndrome have an extra copy of chromosome 21. The patients who live into their 40s or longer develop SPs and NFTs and have a decline in brain cholinergic markers similar to that in AD. This suggests that Down's syndrome and AD may have common etiologic or pathogenetic mechanisms. Of added interest, studies have shown an increase in Down's syndrome in families with AD.

EPIDEMIOLOGY

Age is a strong risk factor for AD. A community-based study has shown that the overall prevalence of AD in the United States is 3% for persons 65–74 years old, 18.7% for those 75–84 years old, and 47.2% for those over age 85 (Evans et al., 1989). Demographic trends indicate that there will be a sizable increase in the number of AD patients over age 65 during the next few decades. In addition, the over-85 age group is the most rapidly growing segment of the U.S. population. It has been suggested that there could be 14 million individuals with AD by the year 2040.

Other risk factors for AD have been identified (reviewed in Henderson, 1986; Mortimer and Hutton, 1985). A family history of dementia or AD is a significant risk factor for AD, especially in cases with onset before age 70. Several studies have shown a significantly greater occurrence of concussive head trauma in AD patients. This is of interest in relation to the repeated head trauma experienced by boxers who develop dementia pugilistica, in which NFTs are prominent histopathologic findings. One case-control study revealed a higher frequency of prior thyroid disease in women AD patients than in control subjects (Heyman et al., 1984). Several reports have indicated that late maternal age is a risk factor for AD, but other reports have not supported this possibility. Other studies have not found a relationship between medication use, unusual food ingestion, surgical procedures, or occupational exposure and AD.

A possible link between cardiovascular disease and AD has been more recently postulated. AD patients have been reported to have a significant increase in myocardial infarction, atherosclerotic cardiovascular disease, left bundle branch block, and atrial fibrillation (Martins et al., 1990). Other investigators have shown that older females with a history of myocardial infarction are five times more prone to develop dementia than those without such a history (Aronson et al., 1990).

ETIOLOGY AND PATHOGENESIS

The etiology and pathogenesis of AD are not known. Any hypothesis about the etiology or pathogenesis must consider many factors, including genetic; known risk factors; environmental variables; variable clinical course; neuropathologic features, such as specific neuron loss and synapse loss; neuritic pathology and amyloid deposition; multiple neurotransmitter deficits; relationship to Down's syndrome; and the normal aging process.

The basic pathologic alteration in AD consists of neuronal degeneration and death in specific brain areas that leads to gradual decline in memory and other cognitive functions. The same process probably takes place at a lower rate in the brain in normal aging. One must also consider that the degenerative process in the brain has its onset many years before the onset of clinical symptoms, that is, neuron degeneration has progressed for many years before it reaches a critical threshold resulting in cognitive dysfunction.

The cellular and molecular events leading to degenerative changes and cell death in AD are beginning to be approached. Deficiency of growth factors or excess of excitatory amino acids could play a role in selective death of neurons. It is possible that cell degeneration can be correlated with increased intracellular calcium, altered general energy metabolism, formation of free radicals, or production of abnormal proteins, such as heat shock proteins or those accumulating in NFT-bearing cells (see the earlier section on neuropathology).

Many etiologic and pathogenetic hypotheses have been advanced for AD, including genetic defect, systemic metabolic defect, slow or latent virus disorders, environmental toxins, and endogenous toxins.

There is compelling evidence for the presence of a genetic influence in some AD patients, as reviewed earlier. Some investigators have suggested that all AD is inherited, although it is more likely that nongenetic factors are also involved. It is also possible that nongenetic, environmental factors may serve to trigger genetic factors.

The genetic hypothesis is complementary to the idea of a systemic molecular defect in AD. No precedent is known for genetic diseases in which the gene of interest is expressed only in the nervous system (Blass et al., 1990). Thus, it is possible that a gene or genes involved in AD are also expressed in extraneural tissues, although the functional alterations might be expressed only in the brain. Numerous studies (reviewed in Baker et al., 1988) have described alterations in AD erythrocytes, leukocytes, platelets, and fibroblasts.

Solid evidence for an infectious etiology of AD is lacking; however, it has been hypothesized that an unconventional slow infectious agent similar to agents that cause CJD, kuru, and Gerstmann-Straussler syndrome in humans and scrapie in animals may be present in AD. The evidence supporting this hypothesis includes characteristics that are similar in AD and unconventional slow virus infections: (1) clinical manifestations during a long and irrevocable course that ends in death, (2) no demonstrated specific immune response to a foreign protein by the host, (3) myoclonus (common in CJD and occasionally seen in AD), (4) amyloid plaques present in the central nervous system in AD patients and in some patients with unconventional slow virus diseases, (5) spongiform changes in unconventional slow virus diseases and some AD cases, and (6) a genetic susceptibility component in AD, CJD, and Gerstmann-Straussler syndrome.

The role of transmissible agents in AD received a boost when Manuelidis et al. (1988) reported that hamster brains injected with buffy coat specimens from 5 of 11 relatives of AD patients developed spongiform changes similar to experimental CJD. Material from three of the positive cases was serially transmitted in a second passage. Two of the subjects studied subsequently developed AD. Previous studies have shown that infectivity is found in buffy coats of CJD patients and in buffy coats of animals during preclinical phases of experimental CJD. This study raises the possibility of a transmissible CJD-like agent in some forms of AD.

Trace element neurotoxicity has been hypothesized to play a role in AD (reviewed in Markesbery and Ehmann, 1988). Several trace elements, including aluminum, silicon, mercury, and zinc, have been implicated in AD. Aluminum has received the most attention as a potential neurotoxin in AD, although there are conflicting reports about aluminum imbalances in bulk brain tissue (Crapper et al., 1976; Markesbery et al., 1981). Microprobe studies have shown an aluminum increase in NFT-bearing neurons compared with NFT-free neurons in AD and in NFTs in Guamanian parkinsonism-dementia complex (Perl and Brody, 1980). Other microprobe studies have not shown elevated aluminum in NFT-containing neurons. In addition, aluminum and silicon have been found in SPs by some investigators (Candy et al., 1985). Aluminum is a neurotoxin, and small amounts in neurons could lead to severe functional and morphologic alterations. It is not clear if the aluminum reported in NFTs and SPs represents an early, potentially causative event or a terminal event superimposed on the primary neuronal degenerative process.

Other studies have shown a consistent elevation of mercury in bulk brain specimens (Ehmann et al., 1986) and subcellular fractions (Wenstrup et al., 1990) of AD brains. Imbalances also have been found in bromine, chlorine, nitrogen, phosphorus, rubidium, and sodium in AD patients (Ehmann et al., 1986). Clearly, a number of brain elemental imbalances exist in AD, but their roles in the pathogenesis await further studies.

It has been suggested that excitatory amino acids, such as glutamate, may be involved in the pathogenesis of AD by virtue of their neurotoxic (excitotoxic)

properties (Greenamyre and Young, 1989). This factor could be related to depolarization through N-methyl-D-aspartate receptors that causes calcium influx, leading to disrupted cellular energy metabolism and delayed neuronal damage.

Most likely, this complex disorder has multiple causes. It is highly probable that there are genetic etiologies, one or several primary environmental etiologies, and other instances with strong interplay between genetic and environmental factors. A rational basis for therapy and/or prevention will not be available until the etiologies and pathogenesis of the disorder are determined. The understanding of AD has progressed rapidly during the past 10 years. Research, accelerating at an exciting pace, is the hope for eventual prevention or treatment of this most devastating of all disorders.

REFERENCES

Alzheimer A. Uber eine eigenartige Erkrankung der Hirnride. *Allg. Z. Psychiatr.* 64:146–148, 1907.

Aronson M.K., Ooi W.L., Morgenstern H., et al. Women, myocardial infarction and dementia in the very old. *Neurology* 40:1102–1106, 1990.

Baker A.C., Ko L., Blass J.P. Systemic aspects of Alzheimer's disease. *Age* 11:60–65, 1988.

Barclay J.L., Zemcov A., Blass J.P., et al. Factors associated with duration of survival in Alzheimer's disease. *Biol. Psychiatry* 20:86–93, 1985.

Bartus R.T., Dean R.L., Beer B., et al. The cholinergic hypothesis of geriatric memory dysfunction. *Science* 217:408–417, 1982.

Beach T.G. The history of Alzheimer's disease: three debates. *J. Hist. Med. Allied Sci.* 42:327–349, 1987.

Bissette G.O., Reynolds G.P., Kilts C.A., et al. Corticotropin-releasing factor-like immunoreactivity in senile dementia of the Alzheimer type. *J.A.M.A.* 254:3067–3069, 1985.

Blass J.P., Baker A.C., Ko L. Alzheimer's disease: inborn error of metabolism of late onset. *Adv. Neurol.* 51:199–200, 1990.

Boller F., Mizutani T., Roessmann U., et al. Parkinson disease, dementia, and Alzheimer's disease: clincopathological correlations. *Ann. Neurol.* 7:329–335, 1980.

Bowen D.M., Palmer A.M., Francis P.T., et al. Classical neurotransmitters in Alzheimer's disease. In Terry, R.D., ed. *Aging and the Brain.* New York, Raven Press, pp. 115–128, 1988.

Brown P., Rodgers-Johnson P., Cathala F., et al. Creutzfeldt-Jakob disease of long duration: clinicopathological characteristics, transmissibility and differential diagnosis. *Ann. Neurol.* 16:295–304, 1984.

Burkhardt C.R., Filley C.M., Kleinschmidt-DeMasters B.K., et al. Diffuse Lewy body disease and progressive dementia. *Neurology* 38:1520–1528, 1988.

Candy J.M., Edwardson J.A., Klinowski J., et al. Co-localization of aluminum and silicon in senile plaques: implications for the neurochemical pathology of Alzheimer's disease. In Traber J., Gispen W., eds. *Senile Dementia of Alzheimer Type.* Heidelberg, Springer-Verlag, pp. 183–197, 1985.

Chu D.C.M., Penny J.B., Young A.B. Cortical GABA$_B$ and GABA$_A$ receptors in Alzheimer's disease. *Neurology* 37:1454–1459, 1987.

Coleman P.D., Flood D.G. Neuron numbers and dendritic extent in normal aging and Alzheimer's disease. *Neurobiol. Aging* 8:521–545, 1987.

Corwin J., Serby M., Rotrosen J. Olfactory deficits in AD: what we know about the nose. *Neurobiol. Aging* 7:580–582, 1986.

Crapper D.R., Krishnan S.S., Quittkat S. Aluminum, neurofibrillary degeneration and Alzheimer's disease. *Brain* 102:67–80, 1976.

Cummings J.L., Benson F.D. *Dementia: A Clinical Approach.* Boston, Butterworth, pp. 57–72, 1983.

Cummings J.L., Benson F.D., Hill M.A., et al. Aphasia in dementia of the Alzheimer type. *Neurology* 35:394–397, 1985.

Davies P., Katzman R., Terry R.D. Reduced somatostatin-like immunoreactivity in cerebral cortex from cases of Alzheimer disease and Alzheimer senile dementia. *Nature* 288:279–280, 1980.

Doebler J.A., Markesbery W.R., Anthony A., et al. Neuronal RNA in relation to neuronal loss and neurofibrillary pathology in the hippocampus in Alzheimer's disease. *J. Neuropathol. Exp. Neurol.* 46:28–39, 1987.

Ehmann W.D., Markesbery W.R., Alauddin M., et al. Brain trace elements in Alzheimer's disease. *Neurotoxicology* 7:197–206, 1986.

Evans D.A., Funkenstein H.H., Albert M.S., et al. Prevalence of Alzheimer's disease in a community population of older persons. *J.A.M.A.* 262:2551–2556, 1989.

Farrer L.A., Myers R.H., Cupples P.H., et al. Transmission and age-at-onset patterns in familial Alzheimer's disease: evidence of heterogeneity. *Neurology* 40:395–403, 1990.

Fitch N., Becker R., Heller A. The inheritance of Alzheimer's disease: a new interpretation. *Ann. Neurol.* 23:14–19, 1988.

Frackowiak R.S.J. Cerebral imaging and function in the dementias. In Terry R.D., ed. *Aging and the Brain.* New York, Raven Press, pp. 89–107, 1988.

Goate A.M., Haynes A.R., Owen M.J., et al. Predisposing locus for Alzheimer's disease on chromosome 21. *Lancet* 1:352–355, 1989.

Goldgaber D., Lerman M.I., McBride O.W., et al. Characterization and chromosomal localization of a cDNA encoding brain amyloid of Alzheimer's disease. *Science* 235:877–880, 1987.

Greenamyre J.J., Young A.B. Excitatory amino acids and Alzheimer's disease. *Neurobiol. Aging* 10:593–602, 1989.

Hachinski V.C., Iliff L.D., Zilhka E., et al. Cerebral blood flow in dementia. *Arch. Neurol.* 32:632–637, 1975.

Hansen L., Salmon D., Galasko D., et al. The Lewy body variant of Alzheimer's disease: a clinical and pathologic entity. *Neurology* 40:1–8, 1990.

Hardy J.A., Mann D.M.A., Wester P., et al. An integrative hypothesis concerning the pathogenesis and progression of Alzheimer's disease. *Neurobiol. Aging* 7:489–502, 1986.

Hauser W.A., Morris M.L., Heston L.L., et al. Seizures and myoclonus in patients with Alzheimer's disease. *Neurology* 36:1226–1230, 1986.

Hefti F., Hartikka J., Knusel B. Function of neurotrophic factors in the adult and aging brain and their possible use in the treatment of neurodegenerative diseases. *Neurobiol. Aging* 10:515–533, 1989.

Henderson A.S. The epidemiology of Alzheimer's disease. *Br. Med. Bull.* 42:3–10, 1986.

Heyman A., Wilkinson W.E., Stafford J.A., et al. Alzheimer's disease: a study of epidemiological aspects. *Ann. Neurol.* 15:335–341, 1984.

Joachim C., Mori H., Selkoe D.J. Amyloid B-protein deposition in tissues other than brain in Alzheimer's disease. *Nature* 341:226–230, 1989.

Kang J., Müller-Hill B. Differential splicing of Alzheimer's disease amyloid A4 precursor RNA in rat tissues: PreA4$_{695}$ mRNA is predominantly produced in rat and human brain. *Biochem. Biophys. Res. Commun.* 166:1192–1200, 1990.

Karlinsky H. Alzheimer's disease in Down's syndrome. *J. Am. Geriatr. Soc.* 34:728–734, 1986.

Katzman, R. The prevalence and malignancy of Alzheimer's disease: a major killer. *Arch. Neurol.* 33:217–218, 1976.

Katzman R. Alzheimer's disease. *N. Engl. J. Med.* 314:964–987, 1986.

Katzman R., Lasker B., Bernstein N. Advances in the diagnosis of dementia: accuracy of diagnosis and consequence of misdiagnosis of disorders causing dementia. In Terry R.D., ed. *Aging and the Brain.* New York, Raven Press, pp. 17–62, 1988.

Khachaturian Z.S. Diagnosis of Alzheimer's disease. *Arch. Neurol.* 42:1097–1105, 1985.

Kidd M. Paired helical filaments in electron microscopy of Alzheimer's disease. *Nature* 197:192–193, 1963.

Kitaguchi N., Takahashi Y., Tokushima Y., et al. Novel precursor of Alzheimer's disease amyloid protein shows protease inhibitory activity. *Nature* 311:530–532, 1988.

Kosik K.S., Minireview: the molecular and cellular pathology of Alzheimer neurofibrillary lesions. *J. Gerontol.* 44:B55–B58, 1989.

Manuelidis E.E., de Figueiredo J.M., Kim J.H., et al. Transmission studies from blood of Alzheimer disease patients and healthy relatives. *Proc. Natl. Acad. Sci. U.S.A.* 85:4898–4901, 1988.

Markesbery W.R., Ehmann W.D. Trace elements in dementing disorders. In Morley J.E., Walsh J.H., Sterma M.B., eds. *Nutritional Modulation of Neural Function.* Orlando, FL, Academic Press, pp. 179–190, 1988.

Markesbery W.R., Ehmann W.D., Hossain T.I.M., et al. Instrumental neutron activation analysis of brain aluminum in Alzheimer's disease and aging. *Ann. Neurol.* 10:511–516, 1981.

Martins C., Gambert S.R., Gupta K.L., et al. Effect of age and dementia on the prevalence of cardiovascular disease. *Age* 13:9–11, 1990.

Masliah E., Terry R.D., DeTeresa R.M., et al. Immunohistochemical quantification of the synapse-related protein synaptophysin in Alzheimer's disease. *Neurosci. Lett.* 103:234–239, 1989.

Mayeux R., Stern Y., Spanton, S. Heterogeneity in dementia of the Alzheimer type: evidence of subgroups. *Neurology* 35:453–461, 1985.

McKhann G.D., Drachman D.A., Folstein M.F., et al. Clinical diagnosis of Alzheimer's disease: report of the NINCDS-ADRDA Work Group under the auspices of the Department of Health and Human Services Task Force on Alzheimer's Disease. *Neurology (N.Y.)* 34:939–944, 1984.

Merriam A.E., Aronson M.K., Gaston P., et al. The psychiatric symptoms of Alzheimer's disease. *J. Am. Geriatr. Soc.* 36:7–12, 1988.

Morris J.C., McKeel D.W., Fulling K., et al. Validation of clinical diagnostic criteria for Alzheimer's disease. *Ann. Neurol.* 24:17–22, 1988.

Mortimer J.A., Hutton J.T. Epidemiology and etiology of Alzheimer's disease. In Hutton J.T., Kenny A.D., eds. *Senile Dementia of the Alzheimer's Type.* New York, Liss, pp. 177–196, 1985.

Palmer A.M., Francis P.T., Benton J.S., et al. Presynaptic serotonergic dysfunction in patients with Alzheimer's disease. *J. Neurochem.* 48:8–15, 1987a.

Palmer A.M., Francis P.T., Bowen D.M., et al. Catecholaminergic neurons assessed ante-mortem in Alzheimer's disease. *Brain Res.* 414:365–375, 1987b.

Pericak-Vance M.A., Yamaoka L.H., Haynes C.S., et al. Genetic linkage studies in Alzheimer's disease families. *Exp. Neurol.* 102:271–279, 1988.

Perl D.P., Brody A.R. Alzheimer's disease: x-ray spectrometric evidence of aluminum accumulation in neurofibrillary tangle-bearing neurons. *Science* 208:297–299, 1980.

Perry E.K., Tomlinson B.E., Blessed G., et al. Correlation of cholinergic abnormalities with senile plaques and mental test scores in senile dementia. *Br. Med. J.* 2:1457–1459, 1978.

Perry R.H., Irving D., Blessed G., et al. Clinically and neuropathologically distinct form of dementia in the elderly. *Lancet* 1:166, 1989.

Ponte, P., Gonzale-DeWhitt P., Schilling J., et al. A new A4 amyloid mRNA contains a domain homologous to serine proteinase inhibitors. *Nature* 331:525–527, 1988.

Reinikainen K.J., Paljarvi L., Huuskonen M., et al. A post-mortem study of noradrenergic, serotonergic and GABAergic neurons in Alzheimer's disease. *J. Neurol. Sci.* 84:101–116, 1988.

Roses A.D., Bebout J., Yamaoka P.C., et al. Linkage studies in familial Alzheimer's disease (FAD): application of the affected pedigree member (APM) method. *Neurology* 40(Suppl. 1):275, 1990.

Rossor M., Iverson L.L. Non-cholinergic neurotransmitter abnormalities in Alzheimer's disease. *Br. Med. Bull.* 42:70–74, 1989.

Scheff S.W., DeKosky S.T., Price D.A. Quantitative assessment of cortical synaptic density in Alzheimer's disease. *Neurobiol. Aging* 11:29–38, 1990.

Schellenberg G.D., Bird T.D., Wijsman E.M., et al. Absence of linkage of chromosome 21q21 markers to familial Alzheimer's disease. *Science* 241:1507–1509, 1988.

Selkoe D.J. Biochemistry of altered brain proteins in Alzheimer's disease. *Annu. Rev. Neurosci.* 12:463–490, 1989a.

Selkoe D.J. Molecular pathology of amyloidogenic proteins and the role of vascular amyloidosis in Alzheimer's disease. *Neurobiol. Aging* 10:387–395, 1989b.

Sparks D.L., Markesbery W.R., Slevin J. Alzheimer's disease: monoamines and spiperone binding reduced in nucleus basalis. *Ann. Neurol.* 19:602–604, 1986.

St. George-Hyslop P.H., Tanzi R.E., Polinsky R.J., et al. The genetic defect causing familial Alzheimer's disease maps on chromosome 21. *Science* 235:885–890, 1987.

St. George-Hyslop P.H., Myers R.H., Hainer J.L., et al. Familial Alzheimer's disease: progress and problem. *Neurobiol. Aging* 10:417–425, 1989.

Tanzi R.E., Gusella J.F., Watkins P.C., et al. Amyloid B protein gene: cDNA, mRNA distribution, and genetic linkage near the Alzheimer locus. *Science* 235:880–884, 1987.

Teri L., Larson E.B., Reifler B.V. Behavioral disturbance in dementia of the Alzheimer's type. *J. Am. Geriatr. Soc.* 36:1–6, 1988.

Terry R.D., Hansen L.A., DeTeresa R., et al. Senile dementia of the Alzheimer's type without neocortical neurofibrillary tangles. *J. Neuropathol. Exp. Neurol.* 46:262–268, 1987.

Tomlinson B.E., Corsellis J.A.N. Ageing and the dementias. In Adams J.H., Corsellis J.A.N., Duchen L.W., eds. *Greenfields Neuropathology.* New York, Wiley, pp. 958–980, 1984.

Wenstrup D.E., Ehmann W.D., Markesbery W.R. Trace element imbalance in isolated subcellular fractions of Alzheimer's disease brains. *Brain Res.* 553:125–131, 1990.

Whitehouse P.J., Price D.L., Struble R.G., et al. Alzheimer's disease and senile dementia: loss of neurons in the basal forebrain. *Science* 215:1237–1239, 1982.

Whitson J.S., Selkoe D.J., Cotman D.W. Amyloid B protein enhances the survival of hippocampal neurons in vitro. *Science* 243:1488–1490, 1989.

Wilcock G.K., Esiri M.M., Bowen D.M., et al. Alzheimer's disease: correlation of cortical choline acetyltransferase activity with the severity of dementia and histological abnormalities. *J. Neurol. Sci.* 57:407–417, 1982.

Yamaguchi H., Hirai S., Morimatsu M., et al. Diffuse type of senile plaques in the brains of Alzheimer-type dementia. *Acta Neuropathol.* 77:113–119, 1988.

Yankner B.A., Dawes L.R., Fisher S., et al. Neurotoxicity of a fragment of the amyloid precursor associated with Alzheimer's disease. *Science* 245:417–420, 1989.

Zubenko G.S., Moossy J. Major depression in primary dementia. *Arch. Neurol.* 45:1182–1186, 1988.

60

Neurologic Aspects of Functional Disorders

Maria A. Ron

Patients with neurologic symptoms for which there is no organic explanation are familiar to neurologists and psychiatrists. The time-honored diagnosis of conversion hysteria serves a useful function and has survived, with some modifications, the changing fashions in diagnostic classification. It is discussed, together with the related syndrome of Briquet's hysteria, or somatization disorder. Panic and obsessive compulsive disorder (OCD), two of the most common anxiety disorders, whose biologic bases are becoming increasingly clear, are also included. Finally, the psychiatric abnormalities detected in those with neurologic disease are considered.

SOMATOFORM DISORDER

A variety of psychiatric disorders have symptoms that suggest the presence of physical illness but for which no organic explanation can be found. In the *Diagnostic and Statistical Manual of Mental Disorders,* Third Edition, Revised (DSM-III-R), these conditions are classified as somatoform disorders. Of interest here are those that have neurologic manifestations, as is the case in conversion disorder and somatization disorder (the two main variants of the previous diagnosis of hysteria).

In *conversion disorder,* the predominant disturbance is often an alteration of neurologic function. The presentations of conversion disorder are protean and have been comprehensively reviewed (Pincus, 1982; Weintraub, 1983). Pseudoepileptic seizures, motor and sensory disturbances, fugues, amnestic states, and blindness are among the most common manifestations. Pain of unexplained origin may also be present, but, in accordance with DSM-III-R, in isolation it is not sufficient to make the diagnosis of

conversion disorder. In most cases, the symptoms and signs fail to conform to well-established patterns of neurologic abnormality and cannot, after appropriate investigation, be attributed to a known disorder.

In making the diagnosis, it is important to determine whether the patient has previously experienced similar or related symptoms without organic explanation. In the DSM-III-R classification, the presence of relevant psychologic factors is also required to make the diagnosis, but this is an unreliable criterion open to subjective interpretation and it should not be given priority when making the diagnosis. Another difficulty in diagnosing conversion symptoms is the need to establish that they are not under voluntary control, which is extremely difficult to do, given that the patient's awareness is likely to fluctuate during the course of the illness. These two criteria, of little relevance in the management of these patients, are a legacy of the psychoanalytic concept of hysteria, and strong arguments have been put forward for omitting them in future diagnostic revisions (Cloninger, 1987; Miller, 1988). The symptom of la belle indifférence, an indicator of lack of concern that is inappropriate in the presence of considerable physical impairment, is also of limited diagnostic value, and psychophysiologic studies (Lader, 1982) have demonstrated that high arousal is often present in those with chronic conversion symptoms.

Somatization disorder (Briquet's syndrome) (Guze and Perley, 1963) is a narrowly defined, chronic syndrome that has recurrent and fluctuating symptoms in many organ systems, begins before the age of 30 years, is predominantly diagnosed in women, and is associated with psychiatric but not physical pathologic changes. Patients regularly come to medical and surgical attention, and neurologic symptoms, similar to those seen in conversion disorder, are often present.

The Validity of the Diagnosis

Doubts about the validity of these diagnoses originate from their low stability in early follow-up studies, in which brain disease and major psychiatric illness turned out to be the final diagnosis in many patients. In separating Briquet's syndrome from conversion disorder, the diagnostic validity of the former has become clearer, even if it can be argued that this is the result of the rigid diagnostic criteria that require chronicity, and therefore a well-established behavior pattern, before the diagnosis can be made (Kendell, 1982; Lipowski, 1988b). The early studies of Guze and Perley (1963) suggested that the clinical picture was consistent over time, and those findings have been confirmed in a follow-up study (Guze et al., 1986). Thus, 80% of the patients had the same diagnosis of conversion disorder 6 to 12 years later; however, the retrospective stability was much lower and only one-third of those who received the diagnosis at follow-up had the same initial diagnosis. Adoption studies (Cloninger et al., 1984) also identified a small group of women (5% of the adopted population) with a recurrent pattern of somatic complaints and frequent psychiatric disturbances, similar to those in Briquet's syndrome. No such studies have been performed more recently in conversion disorder, but it seems likely that the stability of the diagnosis would be much lower.

Other psychiatric conditions are often associated with conversion and somatization disorders. Depressive symptoms have been found in patients with conversion disorder as often as in those with a primary diagnosis of affective illness (Roy, 1980). Other studies reported a high frequency of other psychiatric diagnoses in those with Briquet's syndrome. Major depression was the most frequent, with prevalence rates between 94% (Liskow et al., 1986) and 52% (Zocolillo and Cloninger, 1986); agoraphobia, panic disorder, and obsessive compulsive disorder were also commonly associated with somatization disorder. However, these psychiatric symptoms were often overlooked by clinicians. The inability to communicate psychic distress and the lack of awareness of inner feelings and attitudes, known as alexithymia, may be crucial in determining the somatic presentation of psychiatric illness (Taylor, 1984).

Prevalence

Patients who have symptoms without adequate organic explanation are ubiquitous in all clinical settings. In an annual hospital survey that involved more than 300 American hospitals and 260,000 patients (Wallen et al., 1987), 5% of patients had symptoms and ill-defined conditions without a clear organic basis, most of them attributable to psychiatric

disturbance. Somatic presentations of psychiatric disorder are even more common in primary care settings. Bridges and Goldberg (1985) reported this to be the case in 30% of those seen by general practitioners in the United Kingdom.

The overlapping clinical findings in the different somatoform disorders make it difficult to determine their individual prevalences; in addition, the rates vary depending on the setting from which patients are selected. Schiffer (1983) in a cross-sectional study reported a prevalence of 17.5% of primary psychiatric illness initially manifesting with neurologic symptoms and signs. The rate was the same for inpatient and outpatient populations and encompassed patients with conversion, anxiety neurosis, and somatization disorder. In the United Kingdom, lower rates have been reported retrospectively. Perkin (1989) found a 3.8% prevalence of conversion symptoms, a frequency greater than that of multiple sclerosis (3.5%); and Stevens (1989) reported a frequency of 2.5%. In both studies, additional groups of patients were undiagnosed and were likely to contain many with conversion disorder.

Reports on the prevalence of Briquet's syndrome have to be interpreted cautiously. Farley et al. (1968), in one of the first studies of the syndrome, found a prevalence of 1–2% in a group of American women in the puerperium, but the small sample size and the presence of affective changes in the puerperium may have produced artificially inflated rates. Another American study (Weissman et al., 1984) reported a much lower prevalence (4 per 1000) in a household survey that also included men. In the United Kingdom, the prevalence for women aged 16 to 25 years from a general practice setting was even lower (2 per 1000) (Deighton and Nicol, 1985). Several reasons are likely to account for these transatlantic discrepancies. The variations between the two health care systems are perhaps the most important, followed by the use of different classification systems (DSM-III-R and *International Classification of Diseases*, Ninth Revision [ICD-9], which may result in the inclusion of U.K. patients with somatization disorder under other categories such as hypochondriasis.

Genetics

Genetic studies have contributed little to the understanding of hysteria. The increased risk reported in relatives, predominantly in women, of those with conversion disorder (Guze et al., 1986; Ljungberg, 1957) could be accounted for by shared environmental factors rather than by genetic inheritance. Higher concordance rates for monozygotic twins have also been reported (Torgersen, 1986), but the differences with dizygotic twins were not statistically significant and could be accounted for by the greater environmental similarity shared by monozygotic twins. Adoption (Cloninger et al., 1984; Sigvarsdsson et al., 1984) and twin studies (Torgersen, 1986) highlighted the increased prevalence of anxiety neurosis, alcohol abuse, and criminality in the relatives of those with somatoform disorder. Whether this is a specific link or whether it is also present in other neuroses remains uncertain.

Pathophysiologic Mechanisms

The pathophysiologic mechanisms of conversion symptoms are still unknown. The curious observation (Galin et al., 1977; Stern, 1977) that conversion symptoms are more common on the left side of the body, more significantly so in women and when sensory symptoms are involved, led to the suggestion that the nondominant hemisphere plays a role in their production. The parallel has also been drawn between this phenomenon and the unilateral unawareness and neglect found in patients with right-sided parietal lesions (Stern, 1977). In anosognosia, a related condition, the unawareness of disease is also more common in left limbs, and it is often accompanied by an inappropriately flat affect (anosodysphoria) reminiscent of la belle indifférence.

Psychophysiologic studies (Lader and Sartorius, 1968) reported high arousal levels with slow habituation in patients with chronic conversion disorders, in keeping with subjective high-anxiety ratings. Meares and Horvath (1972), although confirming these findings in chronic disorders, reported normal psychophysiologic arousal in those with acute conversion symptoms, suggesting different mechanisms in initiating and perpetuating symptoms. The gross delay in habituation in these patients, when compared with findings in normal controls (Horvath et al., 1980), led to the suggestion that an attention disorder may be relevant in the causation or maintenance of these symptoms. The study of evoked responses in conversion disorder was popular in the 1960s and 1970s, with largely normal results using somatosensory evoked responses (Halliday, 1968; Levy and Mushin, 1973) and cognitive evoked potentials P300 (Gordon et al., 1986). More recently, magnetic stimulation of the motor cortex (Schriefer et al., 1987) in a small group of patients with hysterical arm weakness demonstrated normal latency and amplitude of responses, contrary to the pattern encountered in patients with demonstrable brain disease such as multiple sclerosis (Hess et al., 1987).

Psychologic theories, although failing to clarify the final pathophysiologic mechanism, still provide the best explanation of the genesis of these disorders. These theories have been extensively reviewed (Lipowski, 1988b; Lloyd, 1986), and only a brief summary is given here. Many of the symptoms experienced by those with somatization disorder can be considered a magnification of normal sensations (Mayou, 1976) or physiologic symptoms such as those resulting from hyperventilation (Smith et al., 1986). In other cases, the process of morbid magnification may be triggered by the presence of genuine, usually mild, organic symptoms. The link between the stimulus that causes physiologic arousal and the ensuing physical symptoms is not recognized by the subject and the symptoms come to be seen as primary (Tyrer, 1973). Other mechanisms such as abnormal illness behavior (Parsons, 1951) and the adoption of the sick role (Mechanic, 1962), which can be seen as attempts to relinquish responsibilities and to gain help and attention, are more likely to play a role in chronic disorders.

The Prevalence of Organic Disease in Conversion Disorder

The precise prevalence of organic disease in conversion disorder is not known, although their coexistence is well documented. Marsden (1986), in looking at consecutive neurologic referrals, found that nearly half of those diagnosed with conversion symptoms had organic pathologic changes. Slater (1965), in a study of psychiatric referrals in a neurologic hospital, reported the presence of organic pathology in more than two-thirds of a group of patients who some years previously had received the diagnosis of hysteria. Major psychiatric illness was also apparent at follow-up in nearly half of those without organic pathologic findings. The high frequency of organic disease in these patients has been interpreted as evidence of a causal link between the two (Merskey and Buhrich, 1975). The prevalence of organic disease in conversion disorder appears to be considerably lower (3%) in patients admitted to psychiatric hospitals (Roy, 1979), highlighting the differences between these populations. Mistakes in the diagnosis are more likely to occur when the results of the investigations are inconclusive or when the symptoms are those of a condition that has only recently been identified as organic (e.g., torsion dystonia, spastic dysphonia, and stiff-man syndrome).

The presence of organic pathologic change may both predispose to and provide a model for conversion symptoms. This is commonly seen in epileptics who also experience pseudoepileptic seizures (between 5 and 25% of all epileptics (Merskey and Buhrich, 1975; Scott, 1982). Brain damage sustained during childhood, cognitive impairment, and anticonvulsant intoxication are found to operate more frequently in epileptic patients who also have pseudoepileptic seizures (Fenton, 1986). Even in these patients, factors other than brain damage are likely to play a significant role, as suggested by the high prevalence of coexisting psychiatric symptoms and a history of previous or family psychiatric illness (Roy, 1977). The clinical features that distinguish epileptic from psychogenic attacks are familiar to neurologists (Lishman, 1987). Suffice it to say that bizarre, changing seizure patterns that occur in stressful situations without reflex or pupillary changes and with retained awareness in the presence of generalized convulsions should suggest the diagnosis of hysteria. Unfortunately, the diagnostic difficulties are much greater in patients with complex partial seizures and the correct diagnosis may only be reached after careful observation and the use of telemetry.

Management

The treatment of somatoform disorders has been reviewed in detail (Bass and Murphy, 1990; Lipowski, 1988b), but several therapeutic principles are worth mentioning here. A comprehensive neurologic and psychiatric evaluation is always mandatory, as is a close collaboration among all the physicians dealing with the patient. When investigations have ruled out the presence of neurologic disease or revealed the extent of its contribution to the total clinical picture, the patient needs to be told of these results in clear and unequivocal terms and further medical investigations avoided. At this point, further psychiatric exploration may be necessary to assess the role of precipitating factors and the mechanisms that perpetuate the symptoms. In the cases in which a definite psychiatric diagnosis can be made, treatment should be instituted. Antidepressant medication may be used if depressive symptoms or panic disorder is prominent, and brief cognitive or behavior psychotherapy may also be useful. The use of analgesics and benzodiazepines should be restricted and carefully monitored, as drug abuse often occurs.

Patients with chronic conversion symptoms or Briquet's syndrome present far more complex therapeutic problems. In these patients, the aims of treatment are twofold: (1) to minimize the extent of the physical and mental disability and (2) to avoid further, unnecessary, and costly treatment. Bass and Murphy (1990) underlined the principles likely to be useful. They recommended that a specific physician, usually the psychiatrist or the general practitioner, be in overall charge of the treatment, avoiding multiple consultations. Patients should be seen at regular intervals rather than on an emergency basis; the latter tends to perpetuate the use of symptoms as a means of getting medical attention. In the consultations, psychologic problems should be explored and the patient helped to make links between them and the physical symptoms. Coexisting psychiatric problems such as depression and anxiety should be treated appropriately and unnecessary medications should be withdrawn.

In some cases, especially when severe conversion symptoms are present, inpatient treatment may be required to implement carefully designed behavior therapy programs (Lipowski, 1988a). The results of a much simpler approach limited to advising the referring physician about how to deal with the patients to minimize unnecessary consultations (Smith et al., 1986) have been encouraging in terms of reducing health care costs. Unfortunately, the significant savings were not necessarily accompanied by a reduction in symptoms and overall disability or by an increase in patients' satisfaction with treatment.

ANXIETY DISORDER

In DSM-III-R terminology, the main categories of psychiatric disorder subsumed under anxiety disorder are generalized anxiety, panic, phobic, and obsessive compulsive disorders. Diagnostic labels have been somewhat different in countries where the ICD-9 classification has been used, but the increasing acceptance of the American system makes it more appropriate to use DSM-III-R terminology here. The two cardinal features common to all anxiety disorders are anxiety symptoms and avoidance behavior. The principal psychologic symptom of anxiety is fearful anticipation. Recurrent worrying thoughts, irritability, restlessness, hypersensitivity to light or noise, and difficulty in concentration are also common. Physical symptoms are protean and are referred to many systems. Dizziness, muscle tension, headaches, restlessness, tremors, fatigability, initial insomnia, and intermittent waking are extremely common. Gastrointestinal symptoms include dry mouth, nausea, abdominal pain, and diarrhea. Cardiorespiratory symptoms include shortness of breath, palpitations, tachycardia, and chest discomfort. Genitourinary and gynecologic symptoms also occur.

Panic Disorder

In panic attacks, the physical and psychologic features of anxiety occur in discrete episodes of sudden onset, which are sometimes unrelated to exposure to anxiety-provoking situations. The attacks may also start during sleep stages 2 and 3. Before the diagnosis is established, the role of alcohol, caffeine, and drugs such as amphetamine needs to be ruled out and conditions such as hyperthyroidism, pheochromocytoma, and hypoglycemia excluded. Panic disorder is often associated with other anxiety disorders, particularly agoraphobia.

Markowitz et al. (1989), in a large epidemiologic study, reported a prevalence of 1.5% for panic disorder as compared with 4.2% for major depression. Panic disorder was three times more common in women, and it occurred in association with agoraphobia in a third of the patients and with major depression in an additional third. Somatic symptoms, excessive alcohol intake, and drug abuse were also overrepresented. Other epidemiologic (Reich, 1986; Robins et al., 1984) and family studies (Noyes et al., 1986) also reported an increase in the incidence of agoraphobia in the relatives of those with panic disorder.

Genetic factors appear to be relevant in panic and associated anxiety disorders. Crowe et al. (1983), in a large family study of panic disorder, found the risk in first-degree relatives to be 17.3%, compared with 1.8% for the relatives of normal controls. These findings were replicated by Noyes et al. (1986), who found secondary cases of panic disorder in two-thirds of the families. In the study of Crowe et al. (1983), panic disorder in isolation did not increase the risk of other psychiatric conditions in first-degree relatives (Crowe et al., 1983), but other studies (Leckman et al., 1983) reported that, when panic disorder coexists with major depression in the proband, the risks of depression, anxiety disorders, and alcoholism double in first-degree relatives. Family studies have put forward the hypothesis that some specific childhood disturbances could be the forerunners of adult panic and anxiety disorders. Weissman et al. (1984) found a threefold increase in the incidence of separation anxiety in children of parents with panic disorder, and Rosenbaum et al. (1988) found that these children were also more likely to show behavioral inhibition when confronted with novel objects or situations. Long-term follow-up studies are required test this hypothesis.

Twin studies also support the role of genetic factors. Torgersen (1983) found concordance rates for panic disorder with or without agoraphobia to be three times higher in monozygotic than in dizygotic twins (45 versus 15%), a difference similar to that for schizophrenia. In this study, depression was rare in the cotwins of both monozygotic and dizygotic probands. Similar results were reported much earlier by Slater and Shields (1969) for anxiety neurosis as a whole. In their study, the concordance rate for monozygotic twins was 41%, and for dizygotic twins, 4%. These rates contrasted sharply with the lack of concordance for minor depression in monozygotic and dizygotic twins (Slater and Shields, 1969).

Pathophysiology

The current interest in the study of panic disorder has been fueled by the possibility that panic attacks that occur without provocation may represent a key biologic symptom with a specific neurochemical cause from which other anxiety disorders (e.g., agoraphobia) would originate. This hypothesis has been criticized by Gelder (1989) on the grounds that the distinction between spontaneous and provoked attacks may be artifactual and that in most patients a combination of biologic and psychologic factors are likely to have a role.

On the other hand, the renewed interest in panic disorder has resulted in the search for biologic markers. This field has been reviewed by Szabadi and Bradshaw (1988). Increased plasma and urinary levels of epinephrine, norepinephrine, and their metabolites (Cameron et al., 1984; Nesse et al., 1984) were noted in panic disorder and less consistently in generalized anxiety. In panic disorder, the exaggerated response of the catecholamine system to anxiogenic (e.g., yohimbine) and anxiolytic drugs (e.g., clonidine) was interpreted as a defect in the regulatory mechanisms of the α_2-adrenergic receptors in the noradrenergic neurons in the locus ceruleus (Charney and Heninger, 1986). These responses do not appear to be related to the severity or the duration of symptoms, suggesting that they are trait rather than state related (Nutt, 1989). The same conclusion has been drawn from sleep studies performed between attacks (Mellman and Thomas, 1989), reporting longer sleep latencies, decreased total sleep time, fewer rapid eye movement periods, and less total rapid eye movement sleep in those with panic attacks compared with controls. Other abnormalities such as the low plasma levels of thyrotropin, the blunted response to thyrotropin-releasing hormone, and variable response to dexamethasone are less consistent and could be attributed to the presence of depression.

The observation that panic attacks can be provoked in susceptible subjects using a variety of stressors such as lactate infusion and carbon dioxide inhalation focused attention on the underlying pathophysiologic mechanisms. Hyperventilation, with the resulting hypocapnia and depression of the parasympathetic system, appears to be the common path leading to panic attacks (Bass et al., 1987). Lactate infusion, the more reliable of these triggers, increases cardiac output and causes hypernatremia and hypocalcemia. The partial pressure of carbon dioxide (P_{CO_2}) falls acutely, and this leads to hyperventilation and the clinical development of a panic attack. In the case of carbon dioxide inhalation, the increased respiratory rate that follows is probably due to hypersensitivity of the brain stem regulatory mechanisms, and they in turn lead to hypocapnia, respiratory alkalosis, and the clinical symptoms of anxiety (Gorman et al., 1988). Although there is little doubt that these stressors act preferentially in persons with panic attacks, there is no definite evidence that their biologic responses are different from those observed in controls (Gaffney et al., 1988; Liebowitz et al., 1985; Woods et al., 1988).

The greater vulnerability of persons who experience panic attacks to the effects of these triggers has been explained as resulting from dysfunction of the hypothalamic-pituitary-adrenal axis (Hollander et al., 1989). Some support for this accrues from positron emission tomographic studies in lactate-sensitive subjects. Reiman et al. (1986) described increased blood flow, increased blood volume, and heightened oxygen metabolism in the right parahippocampal region, on a background of generally increased brain metabolism. The parahippocampal region receives noradrenergic projections from the locus ceruleus and projects to the hypothalamus and in turn to the respiratory centers in the brain stem. Whatever the nature of the parahippocampal abnormalities (e.g., increased neuronal activity and breakdown of the blood-brain barrier, dysfunction in this area could be the key in explaining vulnerability to panic disorder.

The observation that different triggers are capable of producing panic attacks in normal persons and in those with depression, albeit less frequently than in those with panic disorder, suggests that the mechanisms involved are nonspecific and that it would be unwarranted to ignore the role of psychologic factors (Bass et al., 1987). The initial physical symptoms of the attack could be produced by one of the stressors mentioned earlier or less commonly by unrelated physical disease (e.g., dizziness attributable to vestibular or central neurologic disturbances). In predisposed subjects, a mechanism of interoceptive conditioning, determined by the experience of similar symptoms on previous occasions, may result in interpretation of the symptoms as serious physical disease; fearful thoughts and anxious mood follow, completing the picture of the panic attack.

Treatment

Imipramine administration and behavior therapy are the main approaches to the treatment of panic and related anxiety disorders. The value of imipramine was clearly shown in short-term double-blind studies (Mavissakalian and Perel, 1989) in patients who did not have symptoms of depression. Improvement was dose related, and nearly two-thirds of those taking standard doses showed significant gains. More modest effects were claimed with alprazolam, a benzodiazepine derivative (Ballenger et al., 1988), and less well controlled trials suggested that other tricyclic antidepressants and monoamine oxidase inhibitors may also be effective.

The principal component of behavior therapy that appears to be effective in panic disorder is exposure to the feared stimulus. Used alone, behavior therapy produces recovery in 20–30% of patients with panic disorder with or without agoraphobia and benefits an additional 30–40% (Swinson and Kuch, 1989). The use of behavior therapy in combination with psychotropic medication has steadily gained ground. A review of the subject (Mavissakalian and Jones, 1989) suggested that the combination of imipramine and exposure is superior to either used in isolation. There is also indication that the long-term use of imipramine continues to be beneficial, although long-term follow-up studies are needed to determine the optimal dosage and duration of treatment. In some patients, cognitive therapy can be a useful addition to this treatment.

Obsessive Compulsive Disorder

According to DSM-III-R, obsessions are recurrent and persistent thoughts or impulses experienced as intrusive and senseless. The person recognizes obsessions as originating in his or her mind and makes attempts to ignore or to neutralize them by means of competing thoughts or actions. Compulsions are repetitive, stereotyped, and purposeful actions performed to respond to obsessions or to avert a dreaded event or situation. These actions are only tenuously connected with the event they try to avert and their magnitude is out of proportion. Insight is preserved, but the symptoms cause distress and interfere with everyday life. Obsessions and compulsions do not always occur together. Karno et al. (1988), in a large epidemiologic study of five U.S. communities, found that approximately 50% of patients with OCD experienced only obsessions, and another 50%, only compulsions, whereas slightly more than 8% experienced both together.

OCD often starts during adolescence, and both sexes are affected in equal numbers. The disorder is probably much more common than previously thought. Rudin (1953) estimated a prevalence of 0.05% in the general population, but Karno et al. (1988) reported a lifetime prevalence of 1.9–3.3% using a broad definition of OCD. When Karno et al. (1988) excluded patients with concurrent psychiatric diagnoses, the prevalence rates (1.2–2.4%) were still considerably higher than those found by Rudin (1953), and a similar figure (1.9%) was reported in an unselected adolescent population (Flament et al., 1988).

The association of OCD with other psychiatric conditions, particularly depression and other anxiety disorders, is well known. In the study by Karno et al. (1988), phobias occurred in 46% of individuals with OCD, depression in 32%, panic disorder in 14%, and schizophrenia in 12%. A follow-up study of OCD with childhood onset (Flament et al., 1990) further illustrated this point. Thus, when the patients were seen at follow-up some years later, the diagnosis of OCD had held true, but nearly half of them had also experienced at least one episode of major depression, 11% were diagnosed as having anxiety disorder, and 7% were abusing alcohol.

Genetic factors appear to be relevant in the causation of OCD. Carey and Gottesman (1981) found the incidence of OCD to be increased in the parents and children (6% for both) and siblings (3%) of OCD probands compared with the rates found in the general population (1.2–2.4%). The same study reported a higher concordance rate in monozygotic than in dizygotic twins (33 and 7%, respectively), adding support to the relevance of inheritance in this disorder.

Organic Basis

Support for an association between brain pathologic change and OCD accrues because minor neurologic and radiologic abnormalities may occur in patients with OCD and obsessive compulsive symptoms are present in a variety of neurologic conditions. Hollander et al. (1990) investigated the presence of minor, or soft, neurologic signs in 41 adults with OCD and a group of normal controls. Difficulties in coordination, abnormal movements, and visuospatial difficulties were significantly more common in patients with OCD. Neurologic abnormalities tended to occur predominantly on the left side of the body. This, together with impaired performance on tests of visual memory (also a feature of the study) by patients with OCD, suggested that right hemisphere function may be preferentially impaired in OCD.

Ventricular enlargement on computed tomography has also been reported in a small group of adolescents with OCD (Behar et al., 1984). In this study, the normal scans of neurologic patients were used for comparison. Other studies, using normal volunteers (Luxemberg et al., 1988), failed to replicate these findings, which possibly resulted from the differences in the control populations. The cause of these putative abnormalities is uncertain, but the possible role of perinatal insults received some attention after Capstick and Seldrup (1977) reported greater frequency of birth trauma in a small group of patients with OCD compared with controls with a mixed group of psychiatric disorders. Nonspecific abnormalities have also been reported using magnetic resonance imaging. Garber et al. (1989) found increased relaxation time (T1 time) in the right orbital frontal white matter of a group of patients with OCD compared with controls. The differences in T1 relaxation times between the right and left sides of the frontal regions were positively correlated with the severity of symptoms. The significance of these findings, which await replication, remains uncertain.

Neuropsychologic deficits have also been described in some patients with OCD, but the results of these studies have often been contradictory. Flor-Henry et al. (1979) reported poor performance on tests of language and frontal lobe functions in 11 patients with OCD, and the findings of Behar et al. (1984), in another small group, suggested that frontal lobe functions may be impaired. However, other studies (Insel et al., 1983) failed to confirm these findings. In those patients in whom cognitive deficits have been detected, there is no evidence of progressive deterioration. Flament et al. (1990) re-examined the cohort of Behar et al. (1984) some years later and reported some improvement in those persons who were initially impaired. No clear relationship has been found in any of these studies between poor performance on psychometric tests and the severity or duration of the clinical symptoms, and more comprehensive studies are needed before the extent and significance of these mild cognitive abnormalities can be firmly established.

Electrophysiologic studies have so far not contributed significantly to the understanding of the pathophysiologic process of OCD. No abnormalities have been reported during routine electroencephalography (Flor-Henry et al., 1979), and sleep recordings in those with abnormal sleep patterns are not significantly different from patterns encountered in depressed patients (Insel et al., 1982). Ciesielski et al. (1981) reported shortened latencies and reduction in amplitude of the N200 component of the visual evoked responses in a small group of patients, but the significance of these findings remains uncertain.

Baxter et al. (1987) used positron emission tomography and described an abnormal pattern of glucose metabolism in a group of 14 patients with OCD when compared with normal persons and with patients with unipolar depression. The main difference between the groups was the increase in metabolism in the left orbital gyrus and caudate nuclei in patients with OCD. In those patients who responded to pharmacologic treatment, the metabolic rate in the caudate increased relative to the hemisphere metabolic rate, whereas the metabolism in the left orbital gyrus remained unchanged. The interpretation of these findings is complex. In symptomatic patients, the heightened metabolism in the orbital gyrus has been interpreted as reflecting dysfunction of attentional and integrative mechanisms subserved by this area. The gating of sensory information, normally mediated by the caudate, would in turn be unable to cope with the increased activity of the orbital gyrus, despite a concurrent increase in metabolic rate. With successful treatment, the caudate re-establishes its processing capacity through an increase in metabolic rate relative to those structures with which it interacts.

Further support for the role of the caudate in OCD comes from the study of Luxemberg et al. (1988) who found, using computed tomography, the volume of these nuclei significantly diminished in a small group of patients with OCD compared with normal control subjects. The beneficial effects of leukotomy in OCD also add support to the role of the limbic system in the genesis of the symptoms. Leukotomy lesions are placed in the lower medial quadrant of the frontal lobes, orbital convexity, and cingulate gyri, with the aim of disconnecting the frontal cortex from the limbic circuit (Kelly, 1973).

Increased serotoninergic activity has been postulated as playing a role in the genesis of OCD symptoms. The main support for this hypothesis accrues from the well-replicated finding that clomipramine and other serotonin reuptake blockers are effective in the treatment of this condition (Thoren et al., 1980). However, there is no direct and conclusive evidence of abnormal serotonin metabolism. Studies of 5-hydroxyindoleacetic acid in cerebrospinal fluid produced contradictory results (Insel et al., 1985; Thoren et al., 1980), and behavioral and biochemical responses to serotonin agonists (m-chlorophenylpiperazine) and precursors (tryptophan) were also inconclusive (Charney et al., 1988).

Stronger links between OCD and brain disease can be inferred from the presence of obsessive compulsive symptoms in well-characterized neurologic disease. Obsessive compulsive symptoms have been described in association with head injury, with epilepsy, and after lethargic encephalitis (Cummings and Frankel, 1985; Lishman, 1987). In many of these cases, the diffuseness of the brain pathologic changes makes it impossible to draw conclusions as to the specific brain structures responsible for the symptoms. Of greater interest is their association with movement disorders such as Parkinson's disease and Gilles de la Tourette's syndrome because of the pathophysiologic mechanisms that may be implicated.

Robertson (1989) reported a prevalence of 37% for obsessive compulsive symptoms in Gilles de la Tourette's syndrome. In her study, as in several other studies, obsessive compulsive symptoms were also a common feature in the relatives who did not have the tics or vocalizations typical of the syndrome. There are other similarities between the two conditions, such as the age at onset, the waxing-and-waning course, the occurrence after lethargic encephalitis, and the response to the same pharmacologic agents. The neuropathologic basis of Gilles de la Tourette's syndrome is still unknown, but it is widely regarded as a disease of the basal ganglia. By implication, it has been suggested that dysfunction of these structures may also be relevant in OCD (Cummings and Frankel, 1985), although different neurotransmitter systems may be implicated in the two conditions (dopaminergic in Gilles de la Tourette's syndrome and serotoninergic in OCD).

Treatment

Behavior therapy and the administration of serotonin reuptake blockers are the main treatments of OCD. Clomipramine and other nontricyclic drugs such as fluoxetine and fluvoxamine are effective short-term agents in children and adults with OCD (Thoren et al., 1980; Turner et al., 1985), and their action appears to be independent of antidepressant and anxiolytic properties. The long-term effect of these drugs is less well established, and relapses are common after drug withdrawal (Thoren et al., 1980).

The use of behavior therapy in OCD was reviewed by Cottraux (1989). Exposure in vivo appears to be effective in three-fourths of those who engage in treatment, and the benefits are more persistent than those of drug treatment (Marks et al., 1988). The combination of behavior therapy and clomipramine or fluvoxamine appears to be superior in the short term to either of these treatments used separately, but drug treatment does not appear to enhance the long-term outcome. Leukotomy is now rarely used in the treatment of OCD and should only be considered in the severe cases resistant to behavior and drug treatment. Beneficial effects have been reported after limbic leukotomy in some of these patients (Goktepe et al., 1975; Mitchell-Heggs et al., 1976), but the long-term benefits of the operation have not been clearly proved.

PSYCHIATRIC ILLNESS IN NEUROLOGIC DISEASE

Psychiatric illness is often present in patients with neurologic disease, and it may be responsible for a substantial part of their disability.

The prevalence of psychiatric disease in patients with neurologic disorders has been studied in a number of different settings. In the United States, DePaulo and Folstein (1978) reported a prevalence of 50% in a series of consecutive admissions to a hospital neurologic unit, whereas Schiffer (1983) reported a prevalence of 41%, for both inpatients and outpatients. Similar figures were reported in the United Kingdom for outpatient populations (Kirk and Saunders, 1979) and for consecutive admissions to a regional neurologic unit (Bridges and Goldberg, 1984). These figures are higher than those encountered by general physicians, reported to be approximately 15% by Feldman et al. (1987). Women with neurologic disease appear to have higher rates of psychiatric morbidity than men. Thus, Bridges and Goldberg (1984) reported a prevalence of 53% in women as compared with 27% in men, a finding similar to that of Feldman et al. (1987). An explanation of these discrepancies is not immediately forthcoming, but the factors that generally make women more vulnerable to primary psychiatric illness are also likely to be relevant.

There is broad agreement among the various studies as to the psychiatric symptoms more often seen in patients with neurologic disease: depression and anxiety, which often coexist, are by far the most common, followed by alcohol abuse. These diagnostic categories contrast sharply with those seen in patients in whom the neurologic symptoms are thought to be somatic manifestations of primary psychiatric disease. In the latter group, as discussed earlier, conversion and somatoform disorders are more common, even if symptoms of depression and anxiety are often present. Another important point to emerge from these studies is that psychiatric morbidity often remains undetected, and therefore untreated, in as many as three-fourths of patients with neurologic disorders on both sides of the Atlantic (Bridges and Goldberg, 1984; DePaulo and Folstein, 1978).

This apparent inability of neurologists to detect psychiatric disability may be due to the tendency to consider psychiatric and neurologic diagnoses as simple alternatives, to the work pressures that prevent physicians from spending more time with their patients, and to the reluctance of patients to discuss psychologic matters with physicians whom they consult for physical symptoms (Bridges and Goldberg, 1984). Shortcomings of the present diagnostic systems are also highlighted by these patients in whom, despite extensive investigations, disorders often remain undiagnosed because no neurologic or psychiatric label can be legitimately applied. In the study of Bridges and Goldberg (1984), this was the case in two-thirds of those in whom no definite neurologic diagnosis could be reached. A symptomatic approach to treatment and a careful follow-up are the only sound strategies.

Psychiatric abnormalities have been described in conjunction with most neurologic diseases. Schiffer (1983) found the greatest psychiatric morbidity in those with chronic pain or epilepsy, whereas DePaulo et al. (1980), in looking at consecutive admissions to a neurologic ward, found psychiatric symptoms to be most common in patients with myasthenia gravis (78%) and multiple sclerosis (68%), followed by Parkinson's disease and stroke (50% in both cases). Starkstein and Robinson (1989) also reported a prevalence of 30–50% for affective disorders in stroke patients.

The link between neurologic and psychiatric symptoms is complex. In some cases, psychiatric symptoms are an integral part of the manifestations of neurologic disease (Lishman, 1987), whereas in other cases, the presence of brain disease may act as an indirect etiologic factor by increasing the patient's vulnerability to environmental stress. This complex interaction is exemplified by the high prevalence of psychiatric symptoms in patients with multiple sclerosis (43%) compared with those with rheumatoid arthritis (4%) who were matched for disability (Ron and Logsdail, 1989). In these patients, depression and anxiety were more closely related to the severity of social stress subjectively experienced by the patients than to the degree of brain pathologic change detected by magnetic resonance imaging. The importance of nonorganic factors in the causation of psychiatric symptoms has been further highlighted by the low psychiatric morbidity in patients with clinically isolated syndromes of the type seen in multiple sclerosis (optic neuritis, cord and brain stem syndromes) (Logsdail et al., 1988). Two-thirds of these patients had widespread brain lesions detectable with magnetic resonance imaging, but their physical disability was minimal and nonspecific risk factors were no greater than in the control population. On the other hand, symptoms such as euphoria are more clearly linked to the presence and severity of brain damage and tend to occur only in those with advanced brain disease and severe cognitive impairment (Ron and Logsdail, 1989).

The relation between psychiatric symptoms and the site of the brain lesion is often unclear. Convincing evidence was advanced by Robinson et al. (1984), who linked the presence of depression with anterior left-sided lesions in stroke patients. The presence of mania in these patients was attributed to lesions in the limbic and related areas of the right hemisphere by the same authors (Starkstein and Robinson, 1989). However, no evidence of lesion lateralization was found in patients with multiple sclerosis with elevated mood (Ron and Logsdail, 1989) or in patients with different types of brain pathologic changes (Krauthammer and Klerman, 1978). Schizophrenia caused by brain disease also occurs in the presence of heterogeneous pathologic change in variable sites (Feinstein and Ron, 1990), but in epileptic patients, a closer association has been described with temporal lobe pathologic change, preferentially left sided (Perez et al., 1985), and temporal lobe lesions were also more common in patients with multiple sclerosis with delusions and thought disorder (Ron and Logsdail, 1989). Functional imaging studies able to detect the distant metabolic effects of localized lesions are bound to clarify these issues. Treatment of psychiatric illness in patients with neurologic conditions has proceeded empirically, but evidence is beginning to emerge suggesting that response to standard psychiatric treatments is likely to be rewarding in these patients.

REFERENCES

(Key references are designated with an asterisk.)

Ballenger J.C., Burrows G.D., DuPont R.L., et al. Alprazolam in panic disorder and agoraphobia: results from a multicenter trial. *Arch. Gen. Psychiatry* 45:413–422, 1988.

Bass C.M., Murphy M.R. Somatization disorder: critique of the concept and suggestions for future research. In Bass C.M., ed. *Somatization: Physical and Psychological Illness*. Oxford, Blackwell Scientific Publications, pp. 301–333, 1990.

Bass C., Kartsounis L., Lelliott P. Hyperventilation and its relationship to anxiety and panic. *Integrative Psychiatry* 5:274–291, 1987.

Baxter L.R., Phelps M.E., Mazziotta J.C., et al. Local cerebral glucose metabolic rates in obsessive-compulsive disorder. *Arch. Gen. Psychiatry* 44:211–218, 1987.

Behar D., Rapoport J.L., Berg C.J., et al. Computerized tomography and neuropsychological test measures in adolescents with obsessive-compulsive disorder. *Am. J. Psychiatry* 141:363–369, 1984.

Bridges K.W., Goldberg D.P. Psychiatric illness in patients with neurological disorders: patient's views on discussion of emotional problems. *Br. Med. J.* 289:656–658, 1984.

Bridges K.W., Goldberg D.P. Somatic presentation of DSM-III psychiatric disorders in primary care. *J. Psychosom. Res.* 29:563–569, 1985.

Cameron O.G., Smith C.B., Hollingsworth P.J., et al. Platelet alpha-2 adrenergic receptor binding and plasma catecholamines. *Arch. Gen. Psychiatry* 41:1144–1148, 1984.

Capstick N., Seldrup J. Obsessional states. A study in the relationship between abnormalities occurring at the time of birth and the subsequent development of obsessional symptoms. *Acta Psychiatr. Scand.* 56:427–431, 1977.

Carey G., Gottesman I.I. Twin and family studies of anxiety, phobic and obsessive disorders. In *Anxiety: New Research and Changing Concepts*. New York, Raven Press, pp. 117–135, 1981.

Charney D.S., Heninger G.R. Abnormal regulation of noradrenergic function in panic disorders. Effects of clonidine in healthy subjects and patients with agoraphobia and panic disorder. *Arch. Gen. Psychiatry* 43:1042–1054, 1986.

Charney D.S., Goodman W.K., Price L.H., et al. Serotonin function in obsessive-compulsive disorder. *Arch. Gen. Psychiatry* 45:177–185, 1988.

Ciesielski K.T., Beech H.R., Gordon P.K. Some electrophysiological observations in obsessional states. *Br. J. Psychiatry* 138:479–484, 1981.

Cloninger C.R. Diagnosis of somatoform disorders. A critique of DSM-III. In Tischler G.L., ed. *Diagnosis and Classification in Psychiatry. A Critical Appraisal of DSM-III*. New York, Cambridge University Press, pp. 243–259, 1987.

Cloninger C.R., Sigvardsson S., von Knorring A.L., et al. An adoption study of somatoform disorders, II: identification of two discrete somatoform disorders. *Arch. Gen. Psychiatry* 41:863–871, 1984.

Cottraux J. Behavioural psychotherapy for obsessional-compulsive disorder. *Int. Rev. Psychiatry* 1:227–234, 1989.

Crowe R.R., Noyes R., Pauls D.L., et al. A family study of panic disorder. *Arch. Gen. Psychiatry* 40:1065–1069, 1983.

Cummings J.L., Frankel M. Gilles de la Tourette syndrome and the neurological basis of obsessions and compulsions. *Biol. Psychiatry* 20:1117–1126, 1985.

Deighton C.M., Nicol A.R. Abnormal illness behaviour in young women in a primary care setting: is Briquet's syndrome a useful category? *Psychol. Med.* 15:515–520, 1985.

DePaulo J.R., Folstein M.F. Psychiatric disturbances in neurological patients: detection, recognition and hospital course. *Ann. Neurol.* 4:225–228, 1978.

DePaulo J.R., Folstein M.F., Gordon B. Psychiatric screening on a neurological ward. *Psychol. Med.* 10:125–132, 1980.

Farley J., Woodruff A., Guze S. The prevalence of hysteria and conversion symptoms. *Br. J. Psychiatry* 114:1121–1125, 1968.

Feinstein A., Ron M.A. Psychosis associated with demonstrable brain disease. *Psychol. Med.* 20:793–803, 1990.

Feldman E., Mayou R., Hawton K., et al. Psychiatric disorders in medical in-patients. *Q. J. Med.* 63:405–412, 1987.

Fenton G. Epilepsy and hysteria. *Br. J. Psychiatry* 149:28–37, 1986.

Flament M.F., Whitaker A., Rapoport J.L., et al. Obsessive compulsive disorder in adolescence: an epidemiological study. *J. Am. Acad. Child Adolesc. Psychiatry* 27:764–771, 1988.

Flament M.F., Koby E., Rapoport J.L., et al. Childhood obsessive-compulsive disorder: a prospective follow up study. *J. Child Psychol. Psychiatry* 31:363–380, 1990.

Flor-Henry P., Yeudall L.T., Koles Z.J., et al. Neuropsychological and power spectral EEG investigations of the obsessive-compulsive syndrome. *Biol. Psychiatry* 14:119–130, 1979.

Gaffney F.A., Fenton B.J., Lane L.D., et al. Hemodynamic, ventilatory and biochemical responses of panic patients and normal controls with sodium lactate infusion and spontaneous panic attacks. *Arch. Gen. Psychiatry* 45:53–60, 1988.

Galin D., Diamond R., Braff D. Lateralization of conversion symptoms: more frequent on the left. *Am. J. Psychiatry* 134:578–580, 1977.

Garber H.J., Ananth J.V., Chiu L.C., et al. Nuclear magnetic resonance study of obsessive-compulsive disorder. *Am. J. Psychiatry* 146:1001–1005, 1989.

Gelder M.G. Panic disorder: fact or fiction. *Psychol. Med.* 19:277–283, 1989.

Goktepe E.O., Young L.B., Bridges P.K. A further review of the results of stereotactic tractotomy. *Br. J. Psychiatry* 126:270–281, 1975.

Gordon E., Kraiuhin C., Kelly P., et al. A neurophysiological study of somatization disorder. *Compr. Psychiatry* 27:295–301, 1986.

Gorman J.M., Fyer M.R., Goetz R., et al. Ventilatory physiology of patients with panic disorder. *Arch. Gen. Psychiatry* 45:31–39, 1988.

Guze S.B., Perley M.J. Observations on the natural history of hysteria. *Am. J. Psychiatry* 119:960–965, 1963.

Guze S.B., Cloninger C.R., Martin R.L., et al. A follow up and family study of Briquet's syndrome. *Br. J. Psychiatry* 149:17–23, 1986.

Halliday A.M. Computing techniques in neurological diagnosis. *Br. Med. Bull.* 24:253–259, 1968.

Hess C.W., Mills K.R., Murray N.M.F., et al. Magnetic brain stimulation: central motor conduction studies in multiple sclerosis. *Ann. Neurol.* 22:744–752, 1987.

Hollander E., Liebowitz M.R., Gorman J.M., et al. Cortisol and sodium lactate induced panic. *Arch. Gen. Psychiatry* 46:135–140, 1989.

*Hollander E., Schiffman E., Cohen B., et al. Signs of central nervous system dysfunction in obsessive-compulsive disorder. *Arch. Gen. Psychiatry* 47:27–32, 1990.

Horvath T., Friedman J., Meares R. Attention in hysteria: a study of Janet's hypothesis by means of habituation and arousal measures. *Am. J. Psychiatry* 137:217–220, 1980.

Insel T.R., Gillin C., Moore A., et al. The sleep of patients with obsessive-compulsive disorder. *Arch. Gen. Psychiatry* 39:1372–1377, 1982.

Insel T.R., Donnelly E.F., Lalakea M.L., et al. Neurological and neuropsychological studies of patients with obsessive-compulsive disorder. *Biol. Psychiatry* 18:741–750, 1983.

Insel T.R., Mueller E., Alterman I., et al. Obsessive-compulsive disorder and serotonin: is there a connection? *Biol. Psychiatry* 20:1174–1188, 1985.

Karno M., Golding J.M., Sorenson S.B., et al. The epidemiology of obsessive-compulsive disorder in five US communities. *Arch. Gen. Psychiatry* 45:1094–1099, 1988.

Kelly D. Therapeutic outcome of limbic leucotomy in psychiatric patients. *Psychiatr. Neurol. Neurochir.* 76:353–363, 1973.

*Kendell R.E. A new look at hysteria. In Roy A., ed. *Hysteria.* New York, Wiley, pp. 27–36, 1982.

Kirk C.A., Saunders M. Psychiatric illness in a neurological out-patient department in North East England. *Acta Psychiatr. Scand.* 60:427–437, 1979.

Krauthammer C., Klerman G.L. Secondary mania. Manic syndromes associated with antecedent physical illness or drugs. *Arch. Gen. Psychiatry* 35:1333–1339, 1978.

Lader M. The psychophysiology of hysteria. In Roy A., ed. *Hysteria.* New York, Wiley, pp. 81–87, 1982.

Lader M.H., Sartorius N. Anxiety in patients with hysterical conversion symptoms. *J. Neurol. Neurosurg. Psychiatry* 31:490–497, 1968.

Leckman J.F., Weissman M.M., Merikangas K.R., et al. Panic disorder and major depression. *Arch. Gen. Psychiatry* 40:1055–1060, 1983.

Levy R., Mushin J. Somatosensory evoked responses in patients with hysterical anaesthesia. *J. Psychosom. Res.* 17:81–84, 1973.

Liebowitz M.R., Gorman J.M., Fyer A.J., et al. Lactate provocation of panic attacks. *Arch. Gen. Psychiatry* 42:709–719, 1985.

Lipowski Z.J. An in-patient programme for persistent somatizers. *Can. J. Psychiatry* 33:275–278, 1988a.

*Lipowski Z.J. Somatization: the concept and its clinical application. *Am. J. Psychiatry* 145:1358–1368, 1988b.

Lishman W.A. *Organic Psychiatry.* 2nd ed. Oxford, Blackwell Scientific Publications, 1987.

Liskow B., Penick E.C., Powell B.J., et al. In-patients with Briquet's syndrome: presence of additional psychiatric syndromes and MMPI results. *Compr. Psychiatry* 27:461–470, 1986.

Ljungberg L. Hysteria: a clinical, prognostic and genetic study. *Acta Psychiatr. Neur. Scand.* 32(Suppl. 112), 1957.

Lloyd G.G. Psychiatric symptoms with a somatic presentation. *J. Psychosom. Res.* 30:113–120, 1986.

Logsdail S.J., Callanan M.M., Ron M.A. Psychiatric morbidity in patients with clinically isolated lesions of the type seen in multiple sclerosis: a clinical and MRI study. *Psychol. Med.* 18:355–364, 1988.

Luxemberg J.S., Swedo S.E., Flament M.F., et al. Neuroanatomical abnormalities in obsessive-compulsive disorder detected with quantitative x-ray computed tomography. *Am. J. Psychiatry* 145:1089–1093, 1988.

Markowitz J.S., Weissman M.M., Ouellette R., et al. Quality of life in panic disorder. *Arch. Gen. Psychiatry* 46:984–992, 1989.

Marks I., Lelliott P., Basoglu M., et al. Clomipramine, self-exposure and therapist aided exposure in obsessive-compulsive ritualisers. *Br. J. Psychiatry* 152:522–534, 1988.

*Marsden C.D. Hysteria. A neurologist's view. *Psychol. Med.* 16:277–286, 1986.

Mavissakalian M.R., Jones B.A. Antidepressant drugs plus exposure treatment of agoraphobia/panic and obsessive-compulsive disorders. *Int. Rev. Psychiatry* 1:275–282, 1989.

Mavissakalian M.R., Perel J.M. Imipramine dose-response relationship in panic disorder with agoraphobia. *Arch. Gen. Psychiatry* 46:127–131, 1989.

Mayou R. The nature of bodily symptoms. *Br. Med. J.* 129:55–60, 1976.

Meares R., Horvath T. Acute and chronic hysteria. *Br. J. Psychiatry* 121:653–657, 1972.

Mechanic D. The concept of illness behaviour. *J. Chronic Dis.* 15:189–194, 1962.

Mellman T.A., Thomas W.U. Electroencephalographic sleep in panic disorder. *Arch. Gen. Psychiatry* 46:178–184, 1989.

Mersky H., Buhrich N.A. Hysteria and organic brain disease. *Br. J. Med. Psychol.* 48:359–366, 1975.

Miller E. Defining hysterical symptoms. *Psychol. Med.* 18:275–277, 1988.

Mitchell-Heggs N., Kelly D., Richardson A. Stereotactic limbic leucotomy: a follow up after 16 months. *Br. J. Psychiatry* 128:226–241, 1976.

Nesse R.M., Cameron O.G., Curtis G.C., et al. Adrenergic function in patients with panic anxiety. *Arch. Gen. Psychiatry* 41:771–776, 1984.

Noyes R., Crowe R.R., Harris E.L., et al. Relationship between panic disorder and agoraphobia. *Arch. Gen. Psychiatry* 43:227–233, 1986.

Nutt D.J. Altered central alpha-2 adrenoceptor sensitivity in panic disorder. *Arch. Gen. Psychiatry* 46:165–169, 1989.

Parsons T. *The Social System.* New York, Free Press, 1951.

Perez M.M., Trimble M.R., Murray N.N.F., et al. Epileptic psychosis: an evaluation of PSE profiles. *Br. J. Psychiatry* 146:155–163, 1985.

Perkin G.D. An analysis of 7836 successive new out-patient referrals. *J. Neurol. Neurosurg. Psychiatry* 52:447–448, 1989.

Pincus J. Hysteria presenting to the neurologist. In Roy A., ed. *Hysteria.* New York, Wiley, pp. 131–143, 1982.

Reich J. The epidemiology of anxiety. *J. Nerv. Ment. Dis.* 174:129–136, 1986.

Reiman E.M., Raichle M.E., Robins E., et al. The application of positron emission tomography to the study of panic disorder. *Am. J. Psychiatry* 143:469–477, 1986.

Robertson M.M. The Gilles de la Tourette syndrome: the current status. *Br. J. Psychiatry* 154:147–169, 1989.

Robins H., Helzer J.E., Weissman M.M., et al. Lifetime prevalence of specific psychiatric disorders in three sites. *Arch. Gen. Psychiatry* 41:949–958, 1984.

Robinson R.G., Kubos K.G., Starr L.B., et al. Mood disorders in stroke patients: importance of location of lesion. *Brain* 107:81–93, 1984.

Ron M.A., Logsdail S.J. Psychiatric morbidity in multiple sclerosis: a clinical and MRI study. *Psychol. Med.* 19:887–895, 1989.

Rosenbaum J.F., Biederman J., Gersten M., et al. Behavioural inhibition in children of parents with panic disorder and agoraphobia. *Arch. Gen. Psychiatry* 48:463–470, 1988.

Roy A. Hysterical fits previously diagnosed as epilepsy. *Psychol. Med.* 7:271–273, 1977.

Roy A. Hysteria: a case note study. *Can. J. Psychiatry* 24:157–160, 1979.

Roy A. Hysteria. *J. Psychosom. Res.* 24:53–56, 1980.

Rudin E. Beitrag zur Frage der Zwangskrankheit insbesondere iherere herediteren Beziechungen. *Arch. Psychiatr.* 191:14–54, 1953.

*Schiffer R.B. Psychiatric aspects of clinical neurology. *Am. J. Psychiatry* 140:205–207, 1983.

Schriefer T.N., Mills K.R., Murray N.M.F., et al. Magnetic brain stimulation in functional weakness. *Muscle Nerve* 10:643, 1987.

Scott D.F. Recognition and diagnostic aspects of non-epileptic seizures. In Riley T.L., Roy A., eds. *Pseudoseizures.* Baltimore, Williams & Wilkins, 1982.

Sigvarsdsson S., Knorring A.L., Bohman M., et al. Adoption study of somatoform disorders. I: the relationship of somatization to psychiatric disability. *Arch. Gen. Psychiatry* 41:853–859, 1984.

Slater E. Diagnosis of hysteria. *Br. Med. J.* 1:1395–1399, 1965.

Slater E., Shields J. Genetical aspects of anxiety. In Lader M.H., ed. *Studies of Anxiety.* Ashford, U.K., Headley Brothers, pp. 62–71, 1969.

Smith G.R., Monson R.A., Ray D.C. Patients with multiple unexplained symptoms. *Arch. Intern. Med.* 146:69–72, 1986.

Starkstein S.E., Robinson R.G. Affective disorders in cerebral vascular disease. *Br. J. Psychiatry* 154:170–182, 1989.

Stern D.B. Handedness and the lateral distribution of conversion reactions. *J. Nerv. Ment. Dis.* 164:122–128, 1977.

Stevens D.L. Neurology in Gloucestershire: the clinical workload of an English neurologist. *J. Neurol. Neurosurg. Psychiatry* 52:439–446, 1989.

Swinson R.P., Kuch K. Behavioural psychotherapy of agoraphobia/panic disorder. *Int. Rev. Psychiatry* 1:195–205, 1989.

*Szabadi E., Bradshaw C.M. Biological markers of anxiety states. In Granville-Grossman K., ed. *Recent Advances in Clinical Psychiatry.* New York, Churchill Livingstone, pp. 69–99, 1988.

Taylor G.J. Alexithymia: concept, measurement and implications for treatment. *Am. J. Psychiatry* 141:725–732, 1984.

Thoren P., Asberg M., Bertilsson L., et al. Clomipramine treatment of obsessive-compulsive disorder: biochemical aspects. *Arch. Gen. Psychiatry* 37:1289–1294, 1980.

Torgersen S. Genetic factors in anxiety disorders. *Arch. Gen. Psychiatry* 40:1085–1089, 1983.

Torgersen S. Genetics of somatoform disorders. *Arch. Gen. Psychiatry* 43:502–504, 1986.

Turner S.M., Jacob R.G., Beidel D.C., et al. Fluoxetine treatment of obsessive-compulsive disorder. *J. Clin. Psychopharmacol.* 5:207–212, 1985.

Tyrer P.J. Relevance of bodily feelings in emotion. *Lancet* 1:915–916, 1973.

Wallen J., Pincus H.A., Goldman H.H. Psychiatric consultation in short-term general hospitals. *Arch. Gen. Psychiatry* 44:163–168, 1987.

Weintraub M.I. *Hysterical Conversion Reaction: A Clinical Guide to Diagnosis and Treatment.* Jamaica, NY, S.P. Medical & Scientific Books, 1983.

Weissman M.M., Myers J.K., Harding P.S. Psychiatric disturbance in a US urban community: 1975–76. *Am. J. Psychiatry* 135:459–462, 1984.

Woods S.W., Charney D.S., Goodman W.K., et al. Carbon dioxide–induced anxiety. *Arch. Gen. Psychiatry* 45:43–52, 1988.

Zocolillo M., Cloninger C.R. Somatization disorder: psychological symptoms, social disability and diagnosis. *Compr. Psychiatry* 27:65–73, 1986.

61

Neurochemistry of Mood Disorders

David Healy
Eugene S. Paykel

This chapter reviews developments in the study of the neurochemistry of the affective disorders. The methodologic difficulties in establishing reliable correlates of central control of human mood are also considered.

The study of the neurobiologic bases of mood disorders is still beset by considerable difficulties, mainly because the direct localized study of functional disturbances in the intact human brain is not yet fully possible. Even the most recent techniques for functional imaging of central processes are still relatively coarse in their powers of localization. Given this fundamental difficulty, research has been dominated by attempts to establish the effects of antidepressants on a variety of peripheral processes, in the hope that inferences can be made to central mechanisms. Such a method is obviously open to the objection that drug treatments may act via compensatory mechanisms rather than directly on an illness process.

Currently, most studies therefore depend on indirect approaches, using peripheral markers such as platelets, which in themselves appear unlikely to reflect specific central nervous state changes. Alternatively, the neuroendocrine window on the brain is used, mainly in neuroendocrine challenge studies. This enables access to hypothalamic dysfunctions, but they are more likely to be secondary rather than primary and may not be accompanied by parallel changes in mood-regulatory systems. Furthermore, both of these approaches are compromised because depression produces profound secondary disturbances in food intake, weight, activity level, and sleep patterns, which it is difficult to control for satisfactorily. A further compromising factor is that most depressed patients entering a research study

have recently received a variety of psychotropic medications, and the duration of their effects on receptor plasticity remains unknown.

THE ORIGINAL AMINE HYPOTHESES

An association between monoamines and mental life has been recognized since Cannon (1929) demonstrated the involvement of the sympathetic nervous system in the peripheral manifestations of the emotions. However, the central neurochemical studies of the affective disorders have had a surprisingly brief history. In 1954, norepinephrine was identified in the brain. At the same time, it was noted that serotonin (5-hydroxytryptamine, 5-HT) and lysergic acid diethylamide were structurally similar and that breakdown products of 5-HT, such as dimethyltryptamine, had potent hallucinogenic properties (Carlsson, 1990).

As late as 1960, there was a general tendency to regard the central nervous system as functioning electrically in a manner that disregarded chemical neurotransmitters (Carlsson, 1990). This began to change only with the discovery of dopaminergic deficits in Parkinson's disease and after the development of effective drug therapies for psychiatric disorders. The introduction, in the late 1950s, of the tricyclic iminodibenzyls and the monoamine oxidase inhibitors gave neurobiologists their first specific tools to probe the cerebral substrates of the affective disorders (Kuhn, 1958; Loomer et al., 1958). Subsequent basic research suggested that the monoamine oxidase inhibitors increased synaptic norepinephrine concentrations (Spector et al., 1960) and brain catecholamine levels (Spector et al., 1963). The tricyclic antidepressants were found to inhibit amine reuptake (Axelrod and Inscoe, 1963; Axelrod et al., 1961), to potentiate the effect of amines postsynaptically (Sigg et al., 1963), and to protect against the depleting effects of reserpine (Sulser and Bickel, 1962; Sulser et al., 1964). These findings were complemented by reports that reserpine, used in the treatment of hypertension, could precipitate depression in up to 15% of those taking it (Frize, 1954; Harris, 1957). Brodie and co-workers showed that reserpine depleted 5-HT from the brain (see Carlsson, 1990), and Carlsson et al. demonstrated that it also depleted catecholamines (Carlsson et al., 1957a,b).

These findings set the scene for the first specific proposal concerning the neurochemistry of depression: that there was a consistent relationship between drug effects on catecholamines and mood, with agents causing depletion of norepinephrine leading to depression and antidepressant action being mediated through an increase in, or potentiation of, brain norepinephrine activity (Bunney and Davis, 1965; Schildkraut, 1965). Comparable hypotheses concerning the role of the indolamine 5-HT in the affective disorders were put forward by Coppen (1967) and Glassman (1969).

STUDIES OF MONOAMINES AND THEIR METABOLITES

A considerable amount of clinical research was undertaken to find evidence of a simple deficit of catecholamines or indolamines in depressed persons. Initially, the only available indicators of amine activity were urinary and cerebrospinal fluid (CSF) 3-methoxy-4-hydroxyphenylglycol (MHPG) and CSF 5-hydroxyindoleacetic acid (5-HIAA).

3-Methoxy-4-hydroxyphenylglycol

A number of early reports suggested that urinary or CSF MHPG levels might be largely central in origin and might be reduced in persons who were depressed (Maas, 1975; Maas et al., 1972; Schildkraut et al., 1978). In general, however, such findings have not been consistently borne out. The difficulties of research in this area have become increasingly apparent, as urinary MHPG measurement has been found to have a wide range of normal values (Hollister et al., 1978), to be affected by diet (Muscettola et al., 1977) and by physical activity (Ebert et al., 1972), and also to be influenced by weight, age, sex, urinary pH, and the consumption of alcohol or nicotine (Annitto and Shopsin, 1979). In addition, it appears that little of the MHPG found in urine is derived from central sources (P. Blumberg et al., 1980). This led to a consensus that urinary MHPG is too influenced by external factors to indicate reliably central noradrenergic function (Ridges, 1980). Much the same is true of CSF MHPG. Its levels appear to reflect

general activity level or the anxiety at the stress of lumbar sampling (Annitto and Shopsin, 1979; Zis and Goodwin, 1982).

3,4-Dihydroxyphenylethyleneglycol

More recently, the noradrenergic metabolite 3,4-dihydroxyphenylethyleneglycol has been a focus of interest, as it is specific to nerve and endocrine tissues and hence can be usefully measured in blood, unlike MHPG, which also derives from liver and other sources (Scatton et al., 1986). There was one report that its levels were lowered in depression (Scatton et al., 1986), but another study found no difference between depressed and control subjects (Healy et al., 1991c).

Norepinephrine

Catecholamine metabolites had until recently been the focus of research because norepinephrine and epinephrine are highly unstable in plasma and there have been technical difficulties in measuring them reliably (Barrand and Callingham, 1985). Initial reports suggested that norepinephrine levels were elevated in the plasma of depressed subjects (Lake et al., 1982; A. Roy et al., 1985). Later studies have not confirmed this (Healy et al., 1991c; Siever et al., 1986).

5-Hydroxyindoleacetic Acid

There has been a similar pattern of research on CSF 5-HIAA, one of the metabolites of 5-HT. A number of early reports suggested that its levels were lowered in depressed persons (Asberg et al., 1973, 1976; Ashcroft et al., 1966). Additional research indicated that its accumulation in the CSF, after egress has been blocked by probenecid, was also reduced (F.K. Goodwin and Post, 1974; van Praag et al., 1973). However, by 1979, there had been 14 studies of this metabolite, with the majority finding no abnormality in depression (Annitto and Shopsin, 1979).

Even if 5-HIAA levels were lowered, there would be grounds for caution in the interpretation of the findings because amine metabolites may reflect metabolism divorced from function (Green and Grahame-Smith, 1975). Furthermore, 5-HIAA passes directly into the bloodstream and therefore CSF levels may reflect altered hemodynamics rather than altered cerebral function (Post et al., 1973a). The results are also affected by physical activity (Meek and Neff, 1973). In addition, it has been argued that lumbar sampling may reveal no more than the metabolism in the lumbar cord (Bulat, 1984).

In contrast to the lack of findings regarding a consistent association with depressive disorder itself, evidence for an association between diminished CSF 5-HIAA levels and aggression or autoaggression has been strengthening. Starting with the early studies by Asberg et al. (1976), it appeared that depressed subjects with lowered CSF 5-HIAA levels were more likely to have attempted suicide during the course of the index illness, especially by violent means. A number of studies now support the possibility of a link between this variable and suicidal behavior, cutting across psychiatric diagnoses (Agren, 1980; Banki and Arató, 1983; Oreland et al., 1981; Träskman et al., 1981; van Praag, 1983), although some studies have not found this (P. Roy et al., 1984; Vestergaard et al., 1978). It has been suggested that diminished serotoninergic function, as reflected in 5-HIAA levels, may correlate with poor impulse control (van Praag, 1986) and that this leads to both aggressive and autoaggressive behavior. Lowered 5-HIAA levels also appear to predict future suicide attempts (Träskman et al., 1981; Träskman-Bendz et al., 1984).

However, it should be noted that alcohol can profoundly alter the metabolism of 5-HT. In particular, it biases its breakdown away from 5-HIAA and toward 5-hydroxytryptophol (V.E. Davis et al., 1966; Feldstein et al., 1967). Many mental states dominated by either suicidal or aggressive ideation are associated with alcohol consumption, either preceding a suicidal or violent act or on a long-term basis. This is a possible confounding factor that has not been properly addressed to date.

CATECHOLAMINE RECEPTORS

A number of problems with the classic monoamine hypotheses have become apparent. Measured levels of neurotransmitters and their metabolites vary rapidly and in response to a multitude of influences (see earlier). The basis for the relatively unvarying state of major depressive disorder is unlikely therefore to lie in the levels of any one neurotransmitter. There is also a logical consequence of the simple monoamine deficit hypotheses that has not been met: the implication that monoamine precursors are effective in the treatment of depression and amine-depleting agents are effective in the treatment of mania has not been sustained (Healy, 1987b; Zis and Goodwin 1982).

Furthermore, although the early antidepressants reversed the behavioral syndrome induced by reserpine in mice, not all of the more recently introduced effective agents do so (J. Maj et al., 1984). In addition, there is evidence that many classic antidepressants, far from increasing brain monoamine levels, may even decrease them through actions on monoamine turnover or through inhibition of monoamine biosynthesis (Bruinvels, 1972; Carlsson et al., 1969; Ogren et al., 1982).

There is also a notable delay in the onset of the therapeutic effects of antidepressants compared with the immediate onset of pharmacologic effects on monoamine systems. This led to other hypotheses. The first alternative proposal was put forward by Ashcroft et al. (1972). They suggested that the pathologic lesion in depression might lie postsynaptically in monoaminergic receptors rather than simply in amine levels. The delay in responsiveness could be accounted for by the length of time it takes receptors to adapt.

This subsequently led to hypotheses of β-adrenergic receptor supersensitivity and α_2 autoreceptor supersensitivity. The β and α receptor hypotheses are consistent with the earlier theories in that hypersensitive α_2 receptors, if presynaptic, might bring about a functional depletion of norepinephrine and β-adrenergic receptors are a postsynaptic target for norepinephrine.

β-Adrenergic Receptor Supersensitivity

Vetulani et al. (1976) reported that antidepressant agents of different pharmacologic types brought about a down-regulation of rat cortical β receptor density. This led to the inference that β receptors might be supersensitive in depression, with antidepressants acting to down-regulate them (Sulser, 1978). It has been reported that all current antidepressants bring about a reduction in β receptor number after long-term but not short-term administration (Sulser, 1984). These results have been replicated widely, except with administration of the tetracyclic antidepressants (Costa et al., 1986; Sugrue, 1980). However, it also appears that similar effects can be brought about by chlorpromazine (J. Blumberg et al., 1976), cocaine, and amphetamine (Banerjee et al., 1979).

Furthermore, the length of time taken to induce down-regulation can be as short as a few days (Asakura et al., 1982; Schultz et al., 1981; Sethy and Harris, 1981). Particularly rapid down-regulation has been induced with combinations of imipramine or desipramine and yohimbine (Jones and Olpe, 1983; Salama et al., 1983) and with various antidepressants combined with phenoxybenzamine (Crews et al., 1981), but none of these combinations have been reported to bring about comparably rapid clinical response (Charney et al., 1986). In addition, there have been problems in attempting to replicate the findings in species other than the rat (Hu et al., 1980) and even in all strains of rats (Kopanski et al., 1983). It appears that there are regional variations in antidepressant effects on β receptors and even variations within the population of limbic β receptors, with some down-regulating and others not (Biegon and Israeli, 1986).

A further point concerns the functional effects of altered postsynaptic β receptor density. Given the heterogeneity of the findings, it would be helpful to know what behavioral function was being modulated along with the postsynaptic receptor and by how much before deciding whether the changes are clinically relevant. Receptor down-regulation might occur but still leave net neurotransmission unchanged. Work on the postsynaptic β receptor hypothesis has largely ignored these questions.

Nevertheless, as β receptor down-regulation is one of the most consistently reported effects of antidepressants, occurring in response to antidepressants of a variety of pharmacologic classes, there has been considerable interest in investigating the β receptor hypothesis in clinical populations. Suitable models have been difficult to find. Lymphocyte β receptors have been used, but care must be taken in interpreting the results because lymphocyte populations are heterogeneous and both subsets of lymphocytes and their receptors show pronounced circadian changes (Healy et al., 1985).

Healy et al. (1985) reported an increase in lymphocyte β-adrenergic receptor density in depression, which normalized on recovery. However, Mann et al. (1985) found no differences between depressed and control groups, whereas Carstens et al. (1987) found reductions in β-adrenergic receptor density. Using a method potentially free from the above complications but also far removed from conditions that might exist in a depressive illness, the culture of lymphocytes in an artificial medium, Wright et al. (1984) found decreased β-adrenergic receptor density on cells in lymphoblastoid cell cultures from patients with manic-depressive disorder compared with unaffected relatives and other controls.

A further approach has been to examine pineal β receptors by assessing melatonin output after challenge with the β receptor antagonist clenbuterol (Thompson et al., 1985). Results of this study did not indicate that antidepressants induced a significant change in β receptor–mediated function. In a related study, Thompson et al. (1983) found that treatment with desipramine led to an increased output of melatonin in depressed subjects that was not found in normal persons, which indicated a net increase in functional noradrenergic neurotransmission rather than the decrease that is implied by the β receptor down-regulation hypothesis.

α₂-Adrenergic Receptor Supersensitivity

It has been postulated that noradrenergic neurons carry presynaptic α₂ autoreceptors, which act to reduce the synaptic release of norepinephrine (Starke, 1977). Crews and Smith (1978) reported that α₂ receptors adapt to long-term desipramine treatment and that this adaptation, which took 3 weeks to become established, involved effects on noradrenergic transmission that were substantially greater than those occurring acutely, in response to blockage of norepinephrine reuptake. These findings led to the proposal that the α₂ autoreceptor might be supersensitive in depression, leading to a functional depletion of norepinephrine, and that antidepres-

sants might act to desensitize it (R.M. Cohen et al., 1980).

There have been difficulties in replicating this finding with antidepressants other than desipramine (Schoffelmeer et al., 1984). In addition, it appears that there are regional variations in effects on α₂ receptor number after desipramine administration, with desensitization occurring in some brain areas but not in other areas (Johnson et al., 1980; Salama et al., 1983).

A number of possible tests of the hypothesis have generated considerable interest. One method has been to measure β₂ receptor density in binding studies of platelet α₂ receptors both in depression and after antidepressant treatment. The other method has been to assess function by challenge of pituitary α₂ receptor by neuroendocrine means.

Platelet Receptor Binding

Garcia-Sevilla and co-workers (1981a,b) reported that platelet α₂ receptor density was increased in depressed patients, returning to normal with effective antidepressant treatment. There has been some support for this finding from studies using either [³H]clonidine or [³H]dihydroergocriptine as radioligands. Both these agents are α₂ agonists. However, studies using radiolabeled antagonists, such as [³H]yohimbine, [³H]rauwolscine, or ³H-labeled UK-14,304, failed to find increased receptor density (Table 61–1).

Variations that are based on the radioligand used suggest caution in the interpretation of the findings (Kafka and Paul, 1986). It is possible that differences in the affinity of the α receptors affects the measurements. There are both low- and high-affinity α₂ receptors. The agonist ligands bind to the high-

Table 61–1. PLATELET α RECEPTOR BINDING IN DEPRESSION

B_{max} **Lower Than in Controls***
Wood and Coppen (1981)
Carstens et al. (1986a)

No Difference
Daiguji et al. (1981)
Lenox et al. (1983)
Pimoule et al. (1983)
Stahl et al. (1983)
Campbell et al. (1985)
Braddock et al. (1986)
Horton et al. (1986)
Theodorou et al. (1986, 1991)
Georgotas et al. (1987)

B_{max} **Higher Than in Controls***
Garcia-Sevilla et al. (1981a, 1987)
Kafka et al. (1981)
Healy et al. (1983, 1985)
Siever et al. (1984)
Doyle et al. (1985)
Takeda et al. (1989)

*B_{max} = receptor density.

affinity sites, whereas the antagonist ligands bind preferentially to the low-affinity sites. Accordingly, these findings would be consistent with a specific increase in the number of high-affinity sites in depression. In an attempt to test for this possibility, Theodorou et al. (1991) tested for binding using ^{3}H-labeled UK-14,304, an agonist for the high-affinity site, and used [^{3}H]yohimbine to displace binding to sites other than the high-affinity site. They were unable to demonstrate any specific increase in high-affinity binding sites, which leaves the position regarding platelet α_2 binding still uncertain.

It must also be kept in mind that changes in platelet receptors may be epiphenomena of the illness rather than indicators of some generalized adrenergic receptor defect. There have also been reports that platelet α receptor number is increased in anorexia nervosa (Heufelder et al., 1985; Luck et al., 1983), suggesting perhaps effects of undernourishment or hormonal influences, although Whitehouse et al. (1991) were unable to confirm this finding. Furthermore, Horton et al. (1986) reported effects of antidepressants on platelet α_2 receptor density, which were independent of changes in clinical state. These findings emphasize the necessity of studying only drug-free subjects or subjects who have been withdrawn from antidepressants for considerable lengths of time.

Finally, it must be asked what an alteration in receptor density, if demonstrated, would mean. The platelet lacks a nucleus and reflects the result of earlier formation in the bone marrow. Platelet populations vary in age and size, and alterations in receptor number could be determined by such factors. It is not clear if platelet receptors can adapt, and they may be influenced by the medium in which they correlate. Receptor number does not necessarily parallel function. Garcia-Sevilla et al. (1990) provided some evidence that increased platelet α_2 receptor density in depression is accompanied by an increased responsiveness to aggregating effects of epinephrine. However, the findings are not unambiguous, in that Healy et al. (1991c) noted that neither the density of high- or low-affinity α_2 receptors nor their various affinities correlate with circulating epinephrine or norepinephrine levels as one might expect if they were being functionally regulated by these hormones.

Neuroendocrine Testing

An alternative avenue for the investigation of α_2-adrenergic receptor function has been through neuroendocrine challenge testing. Infusions of clonidine, an α_2 agonist, produce increases in plasma growth hormone concentration (Checkley, 1980). In depressed patients, this increase has consistently been reported to be attenuated (Charney et al., 1982; Checkley et al., 1981; Katona et al., 1986). It has been argued that this blunting is indicative of an α_2-adrenergic receptor defect in depression (Checkley

et al., 1981). Such findings, however, do not directly support the original hypothesis of Crews and Smith (1978), which involved presynaptic autoreceptors, as the α_2 receptor involved in the release of growth hormone appears to lie postsynaptically (McWilliam and Meldrum, 1983).

In addition to causing the release growth hormone, clonidine also produces an inhibition of release of norepinephrine and dihydroxyphenylethyleneglycol from the peripheral nervous system. These peripheral effects probably reflect central noradrenergic tone (Healy et al., 1991c). Siever et al. (1984) found that clonidine-induced inhibition was attenuated in depressed subjects and argued that this supported a hypothesis of α_2 receptor dysfunction in depression. However, Charney et al. (1982) and Healy et al. (1991c) found no differences between depressed and control subjects in plasma amine response to challenge.

In addition, Siever and Uhde (1984) found that growth hormone responses were blunted in patients with unipolar but not bipolar disorder and were significantly lower in postmenopausal female controls than in other controls, a finding replicated by Horton et al. (1986). In separate studies, Siever and co-workers found blunted responsiveness in obsessive compulsive (Siever et al., 1983) and in panic disorders (Uhde et al., 1986). Finally, blunting of growth hormone responses to clonidine was also reported in hypertensive patients (Struthers et al., 1985).

There appears to be an increase in the basal output of growth hormone in depressed patients (Mendlewicz et al., 1985). This might have a negative feedback effect, inhibiting further release on challenge testing, thereby prohibiting inferences to an adrenergic receptor defect. In addition, Katona et al. (1986) reported an association between blunted response to clonidine and dexamethasone nonsuppression, which raised the possibility that abnormalities in growth hormone output may be secondary to hypercortisolemia. This finding is in line with a recognition that hormonal challenge responses reflect responses in complex systems rather than the functioning of single receptors (Gibbs, 1986).

SEROTONIN RECEPTORS

Ever since Brodie's initial findings that reserpine depleted 5-HT, there have been proponents of a 5-HT hypothesis of depression (see Carlsson, 1990). At present, there are more empirical findings overall in favor of a disturbance of 5-HT functioning than for a catecholaminergic dysfunction.

The development of antidepressants that specifically inhibit 5-HT reuptake has strengthened the case for an involvement of 5-HT in affective disorders. The original tertiary amine tricyclic antidepressants imipramine and amitriptyline were known to block both 5-HT and norepinephrine uptake (Axelrod et al., 1961, 1963). The demonstration that their metabolites, desipramine and nortriptyline, were also antidepressants and far more potent at blocking norepinephrine than 5-HT uptake, suggested that catecholamines were more important than indolamines in depression.

However, in the 1970s, Arvid Carlsson (Carlsson, 1990) designed and synthesized a specific 5-HT reuptake inhibitor, zimeldine. Clinical trials indicated that this and subsequently introduced 5-HT reuptake inhibitors, such as fluoxetine and fluvoxamine, are effective antidepressants.

Although these results redressed the balance and restored 5-HT to a position of importance, it remains unclear why some drugs acting predominantly on noradrenergic systems are antidepressants, whereas other drugs acting on 5-HT systems are also antidepressant. There are furthermore some indications that drugs acting on 5-HT systems have effects on anxiety in addition to being antidepressant (Healy, 1991b). The newly developed $5-HT_{1a}$ partial agonists buspirone, ipsapirone, gepirone, and flesinoxan appear to be broadly anxiolytic. The 5-HT reuptake–inhibiting antidepressants appear to be more anxiolytic than non–5-HT reuptake–inhibiting antidepressants. In addition, early clinical trials of $5-HT_3$ receptor antagonists suggested a role for these compounds in anxiety (Healy, 1991a).

The clinical finding that adding lithium to tricyclic antidepressants sometimes produces a dramatic response in treatment-resistant depression also provided some impetus to the 5-HT hypotheses (De Montigny et al., 1988). This finding resulted from studies aimed at determining whether lithium sensitized human postsynaptic 5-HT receptors as it did in animals. Lithium was shown to bring about an increased functional sensitivity of postsynaptic receptors, but in addition it produced dramatic clinical responses in some of the treatment-resistant subjects to whom it was given (De Montigny et al., 1988).

A novel strategy was used to support the role of 5-HT in antidepressant effects (Delgado et al., 1990). In patients showing remission of depression while receiving antidepressant alone or with lithium, dietary tryptophan depletion was found to produce a rapid return of symptoms.

Serotonin Receptor Sensitivity

Attempts to investigate 5-HT receptor function in depression were hampered compared with corresponding efforts in the case of catecholamine systems by gaps in the knowledge of these receptors and technical problems in studying them. An increasing number of 5-HT receptors have been identified, with the development of specific ligands. In the early 1980s, when ligand-binding evidence indicated two receptors, $5-HT_1$ and $5-HT_2$, Fozard (1984) proposed that there would probably be at least four distinct subtypes. His prediction has been remarkably prescient, with $5-HT_{1a}$, $5-HT_{1c}$, $5-HT_2$, and $5-HT_3$ receptors recognized in humans and $5-HT_{1d}$ and $5-HT_4$ receptors proposed but not yet generally accepted (Healy, 1991a).

Aprison et al. (1978) and Sherman (1979) postulated a supersensitivity of serotoninergic receptors in depression. Peroutka and Snyder (1980) reported that chronic antidepressant treatments down-regulated $5-HT_2$ receptor densities. Subsequent receptor-binding studies suggested that most, but probably not all, antidepressants bring about decreases in $5-HT_2$ receptor density after long-term administration (Costa et al., 1986).

In addition, electrophysiologic studies indicated a change in $5-HT_2$ receptor function after long-term treatment with antidepressants (De Montigny and Aghajanian, 1978), although these findings noted a sensitization of 5-HT function, rather than the desensitization that decreased receptor density might lead one to expect. Comparable findings were reported in platelet studies by Healy et al. (1985). Using 5-HT–stimulated platelet aggregation as a test of function, these authors found decreased responsiveness in depression, with an increased responsiveness developing in the course of treatment. Wood et al. (1985) replicated these effects of treatment but not the original decrease in sensitivity. Cowen et al. (1989) reported no differences between control and depressed subjects for platelet $5-HT_2$ receptor density, but they also found that antidepressant treatments increased $5-HT_2$ receptor density on platelets from depressed patients, a finding that contrasts with the effects of these drugs on rat cortical $5-HT_2$ receptor numbers. Such findings indicate the ambiguities associated with receptor research: the precise relations between changes in functional sensitivity and receptor number are as yet unknown.

Serotonin Neuroendocrine Challenge Tests

A number of studies have now been conducted in depression using a variety of serotoninergic challenge agents, such as the 5-HT precursors 5-hydroxytryptophan and L-tryptophan, the 5-HT agonist quipazine, the antagonist methysergide, and 5-HT uptake inhibitors such as clomipramine. It was initially claimed that these were unlikely to yield clear-cut results, as none of these agents are specific either to any one 5-HT receptor or to the 5-HT system as a whole—with most also having pronounced catecholaminergic effects (van Praag et al., 1987). However, using an L-tryptophan challenge, Glue et al. (1986) found that lithium treatment led to increases in prolactin output in response to L-tryptophan. Clomipramine was also shown to enhance prolactin responses (Anderson and Cowen, 1986). It was suggested that these effects are mediated through $5-HT_{1a}$ receptors (Glue et al., 1986).

Subsequent studies in depressed subjects yielded

somewhat more complicated findings. Patients without significant weight loss appear to have blunted growth hormone and prolactin responses to L-tryptophan, whereas those with weight loss have enhanced responses (Deakin et al., 1990; G.M. Goodwin et al., 1987). In a study of lithium enhancement of antidepressant treatment in resistant depression, Cowen et al. (1989) found that lithium enhanced prolactin release in response to L-tryptophan, although this enhancement bore little relation to subsequent therapeutic outcome. Kasper et al. (1990) reported that fenfluramine also increased prolactin release but that these increases were correlated neither with the severity of illness nor with treatment outcome, although changes in responsiveness were brought about by antidepressants, depending on whether they acted at 5-HT uptake sites or not.

Serotonin Transport and [³H]Imipramine Binding

In contrast to studies of 5-HT receptors, the measurement of a different system, the 5-HT uptake system in platelets and synaptosomes, is a sensitive and reproducible assay. The α_2 receptor studies on platelets or the lymphocyte β receptor studies have been hypothesis driven; in contrast, it was fortuitously discovered by Tuomisto and Tukiainen (1976) that platelet 5-HT uptake is reduced in subjects who are depressed.

This finding has since been replicated extensively (Table 61–2) and appears to be specific to depression, not being found in schizophrenia or other disorders (Healy and Leonard, 1987). The reduction in uptake rates appears to be restored to normal by effective treatment with antidepressants (Healy et al., 1986a, b; Meltzer et al., 1981) and appears to occur whether the patient is being treated with drugs active at the uptake sites, such as nortriptyline (Meltzer et al.,

Table 61–2. PLATELET SEROTONIN UPTAKE RATES IN DEPRESSION

V_{max} **Lower Than in Controls***
Tuomisto and Tukiainen (1976)
Coppen et al. (1978)
Scott et al. (1979)
Tuomisto et al. (1979)
Born et al. (1980)
Aberg-Wistedt et al. (1981)
Malmgren et al. (1981)
Meltzer et al. (1981, 1983)
Stahl et al. (1982)
Healy et al. (1983, 1986—9 [AM])
Wood et al. (1983)
Butler and Leonard (1986)
Faludi et al. (1988)

No Difference
Kaplan and Mann (1982)
Healy et al. (1986—noon)
A. Roy et al. (1987)

*V_{max} = maximal uptake rate.

Table 61–3. PLATELET [³H]IMIPRAMINE BINDING IN DEPRESSION

Lower Than in Controls
Asarch et al. (1980)
Briley et al. (1980)
Paul et al. (1981)
Raismann et al. (1981)
Suranyi-Cadotte et al. (1982, 1985)
Wood et al. (1983)
Lewis and McChesney (1985)
Schneider et al (1985, 1987)
Wagner et al. (1985)
Nankai et al. (1986)
Poirier et al. (1986)
Takeda et al. (1989)

No Change
Berrettini et al. (1982)
Gentsch et al. (1985)
Mellerup et al. (1982)
Baron et al. (1983, 1986)
Whittaker et al. (1984)
Hrdina et al. (1985)
Tang and Morris (1985)
Braddock et al. (1986)
Carstens et al. (1986b)
Horton et al. (1986)
Muscettola et al. (1986)
Desmedt et al. (1987)
Georgotas et al. (1987)
Kanof et al. (1987)
A. Roy et al. (1987)
Healy et al. (1990)

1981), dothiepin (Healy et al., 1986b), fluvoxamine (Wood et al., 1983); agents having no effect at this uptake site, such as mianserin and nomifensine; or electroconvulsive therapy (Butler and Leonard, 1986; Coppen et al., 1978; Healy et al., 1986b). It is not yet clear how such a normalization is brought about, as it is not a natural consequence of simple exposure of these transport proteins to antidepressants (Healy and Leonard, 1987).

Technical advances have revealed the existence of a high-affinity [³H]imipramine-binding site, found on serotoninergic nerve terminals and on platelets and apparently associated with the 5-HT transport site (Briley et al., 1980; Paul et al., 1980). A number of initial and subsequent reports suggested that there are also reductions in the number of these binding sites on platelets in depression, apparently consonant with findings of reductions in 5-HT uptake in depression (Table 61–3).

However, other studies failed to replicate the finding of reduced [³H]imipramine binding in depression (see Table 61–3). In addition, unlike diminished 5-HT uptake, which at present appears to be a state-dependent phenomenon normalizing with recovery, decreased [³H]imipramine binding has been reported long after the index depression has resolved (Raisman et al., 1981).

Although there is uncertainty as to whether [³H]imipramine binding is lowered in depression, there is a degree of consensus on the finding that antidepressant treatments increase it (Healy et al.,

1990, 1991a). However, it is not clear if this increase bears any relation to clinical response. It appears to occur in both responders and nonresponders (Healy et al., 1990), in normal subjects (Healy et al., 1991a), and within a week of commencing treatment (Healy et al., 1991a).

The precise relation between high-affinity [³H]imipramine-binding sites and 5-HT uptake is still obscure. Binding to this site occurs at concentrations of imipramine in the nanomolar (10^{-9} M) range, whereas uptake inhibition needs considerably higher concentrations (10^{-7} M) of the drug (Segonzac et al., 1985; Tuomisto, 1974). At the concentrations necessary to inhibit uptake, imipramine also binds to a low-affinity site (Ieni et al., 1984; Reith et al., 1983), and it is not yet clear what effects binding to this site might have on 5-HT uptake.

Furthermore, when first reported, high-affinity [³H]imipramine-binding sites were thought to be generic antidepressant-binding sites, but this appears not to be the case, as other antidepressants such as [³H]desipramine bind at high affinity to different sites (Biegon and Rainbow, 1983), as do [³H]mianserin (Costa et al., 1986) and [³H]nortriptyline (Biegon, 1984). It has also been reported that all antidepressants investigated bind at therapeutic concentrations to a low-affinity [³H]imipramine-binding site (Gross-Isseroff et al., 1989). However, neither the functional effects of binding to this low-affinity site nor the densities of these sites in depressed subjects have been elucidated.

A great deal of the confusion in [³H]imipramine-binding studies resulted because this impure radioligand binds to a number of different sites on platelets. The radiolabeling of specific 5-HT reuptake inhibitors, such as paroxetine, may help to settle this matter (Mellerup and Plenge, 1986).

The existence of [³H]imipramine-binding sites has also stimulated interest in the question of the nature of the endogenous ligand that modulates 5-HT transport. One candidate for this has been the acute phase protein α_1-acid glycoprotein (Abraham et al., 1987). This protein has been reported to inhibit phagocytosis, inhibit platelet aggregation, and reduce binding to the 5-HT transporter site (Kremer et al., 1988), all of which changes have been reported in depression (McAdam et al., 1991).

There have been a number of reports that levels of α_1-acid glycoprotein are elevated in depression, although hitherto no correlation has been demonstrated between this elevation and alterations in [³H]imipramine-binding variables (Brinkschulte et al., 1982; Calil et al., 1982; Healy et al., 1991b; Nemeroff et al., 1990). Future studies may need to correlate the more specific [³H]paroxetine binding with levels of α_1-acid glycoprotein or other acute-phase proteins.

OTHER NEUROTRANSMITTERS

Neurotransmitters other than norepinephrine or 5-HT have also been implicated in depression. There

has been a hypothesis related to dopamine (Downs et al., 1986; Randrup and Braestrup, 1977), and considerable evidence can be offered that antidepressants bring about changes in dopaminergic systems after long-term administration (Leonard, 1984; Willner, 1983). Dopamine, of all the catecholamines, seems most involved in motivation and in the reinforcement of behavior (Gallistel et al., 1981; Willner, 1983). However, if dopamine depletion were responsible for depression, one might expect a high incidence of neuroleptic-induced depression, which does not occur.

Hypotheses related to acetylcholine have also been put forward (Dilsaver, 1986; Janowsky et al., 1972). Cholinergic mechanisms have been implicated in the disturbances of sleep, particularly rapid eye movement sleep disturbances, and in the lack of drive found in depression, as well as the pathophysiology of cortisol hypersecretion (Dilsaver, 1986). However, although the most marked acute clinical effects of many antidepressants are their atropinic side effects, antidepressant efficacy generally does not correspond to potency on cholinergic receptor systems (Costa et al., 1986).

There are also some grounds for implicating opioid systems in depression (G.C. Davis, 1983). Opiates have long been known to give symptomatic relief in depression (Kuhn, 1970), and endogenous opioids appear to be mobilized in distressing circumstances and to modulate dysphoria (M.R. Cohen et al., 1984; G.C. Davis, 1983). M.R. Cohen et al. (1984) administered high-dose naloxone infusions to volunteer subjects with no ill effects other than a mild degree of loss of concentration and a mild dysthymia. The same challenge administered to a schizophrenic population appeared to produce beneficial effects (M.R. Cohen et al., 1985). However, when given to depressed persons, this challenge elicited pronounced dysphoria (M.R. Cohen et al., 1984). Allied with this are findings that patients with a major depressive disorder are less sensitive than controls or other psychiatric patients to painful stimuli (G.C. Davis et al., 1979). Antidepressants also interact with opiate and other receptors in the brain (Biegon and Samuel, 1979; Reichenberg et al., 1985).

It has been suggested that there may be a decrease in γ-aminobutyric acid (GABA)–ergic tone in depression (Costa et al., 1986). In support, there is some evidence that the GABA agonists progabide and fengabine have antidepressant effects (Leonard, 1986), although the only placebo-controlled study failed to confirm this (Paykel et al., 1991). There are also findings of lowered GABA levels in CSF of depressed subjects (Lloyd et al., 1986). Most antidepressants also up-regulate GABA$_B$-binding sites (Costa et al., 1986).

There is evidence (see earlier) that antidepressants down-regulate β-adrenergic receptors, up-regulate 5-HT$_2$ receptors and 5-HT transport sites, up-regulate GABA$_B$-binding sites, and increase opiate responsiveness (Reisine and Soubrie, 1982) and responsiveness to the opiate neuromodulator substance P (Jones and Olpe, 1983). They bind to muscarinic, histaminergic, serotoninergic, opiate, and adrenergic receptors (Ogren et al., 1982; Segonzac et al., 1985). It is possible, therefore, that antidepressant efficacy resides in multiple actions on a number of different neurotransmitter systems rather than a primary action on a specific neurotransmitter system.

NEUROENDOCRINE DISTURBANCES

There appear to be abnormalities in the output of most hormones in depression, including cortisol (Fullerton et al., 1968; Sachar et al., 1973), prolactin (Hallbreich et al., 1979; Mendlewicz et al., 1980), thyrotropin (Kjellmar et al., 1984; Weeke and Weeke, 1980), growth hormone (Mendlewicz et al., 1985), melatonin (Beck-Friis et al., 1985), and β-endorphin (Matthews et al., 1986). These studies all reported abnormalities in the 24-hour pattern of hormone secretion on serial sampling, where none had been apparent on single sample. Common to these reports is a consistent elevation or reduction in the hormone and a diminished range in the levels of the hormone found during a 24-hour period.

These basal abnormalites appear to accompany abnormalities in neuroendocrine challenge tests. Thus, there is a failure of suppression of cortisol in reponse to dexamethasone challenge (Carroll et al., 1976) along with the blunting of the thyrotropin response to thyrotropin-releasing hormone (Gold et al., 1980) and a blunting of growth hormone output in reponse to α-adrenergic agonists (see earlier [Checkley et al., 1981; Katona et al., 1986]).

The failure of suppression of cortisol in response to dexamethasone, first reported by Carroll et al. (1976), is the most widely cited biologic marker of major depressive disorders. Nonsuppression is also found in poststroke depressions (Starkstein and Robinson, 1989). It occurs in up to 50% of subjects with a major depressive disorder, but it has also been reported in eating disorders and dementia. The origins of the abnormality remain unclear.

A case can be made for hippocampus-related neuropeptide disturbances. Increased secretion of corticotropin-releasing factor leads to the secretion of adrenocorticotropin and thereby cortisol. This may be responsible for the hypercortisolemia found in depression and in part the anxiety that invariably accompanies depression (Britton et al., 1986). Some evidence that corticotropin-releasing factor may mediate both hypercortisolemia and anxiety comes from studies in which it has been found that dexamethasone nonsuppression is most likely to occur in depressed subjects who are also highly anxious (Kasper and Beckman, 1983; Whiteford et al., 1987).

With regard to the origins of the basal endocrine abnormalities in depression and also those found on neuroendocrine challenge tests, it has been suggested that this pattern of widespread abnormality in many hormones reflects a generalized dysregulation of neurotransmitter systems (Siever and Davis, 1985). As most of the hormones involved are regulated by dopaminergic, noradrenergic, serotoninergic, opioid, cholinergic, GABAergic, and peptide influences (Tuomisto and Mannisto, 1985) and as the pituitary system has considerable built-in redundancy (Gibbs, 1986), it is unlikely that the pattern of defects found in depression can be explained in terms of one common neurotransmitter abnormality.

However, a hypothesis that dysregulation is the disturbance in depression lacks explanatory power. It does not yield precise predictions, as any abnormal finding can be termed the consequence of a dysregulation. Nor does it permit inferences about the probable origin of such a disturbance. An alternative hypothesis is one of a circadian rhythm disturbance. Circadian hypotheses of desynchronized or phase-advanced rhythms do not appear to account satisfactorily for the abnormalities found. Healy and Waterhouse (1990, 1991) have suggested that some of the abnormalities may be due to a disturbance of circadian rhythms consequent on changes in social or environmental factors in much the way that jet lag or shift work produces changes.

POSTMORTEM STUDIES

Access to the central neurobiology of the affective disorders is achieved via postmortem studies. Patients who commit suicide have been seen as particularly likely to yield useful information in this way. Early studies focused on the concentrations of neurotransmitters, metabolites, and enzymes, but it now appears that these are too unstable after death for the results of such studies to be reliable (Hardy and Dodd, 1983; Rosser, 1984). In contrast, most neurotransmitter receptor sites appear stable for up to 96 hours post mortem (Hardy and Dodd, 1983). This led to a number of studies that examined receptor binding in postmortem brain tissue of suicides. The findings have not been consistent.

An increase in 5-HT$_2$ receptor numbers in the frontal cortex of patients who commit suicide was reported by Arora and Meltzer (1989), Mann et al. (1986), and Stanley and Mann (1983), but not by Cheetham et al. (1988), Cooper et al. (1985), Crow et al. (1984), or Owen et al. (1986). After reviewing the findings, Cheetham et al. (1991) suggested that common to the reports of an increase in 5-HT$_2$ receptor density have been histories of violent suicide. In the only postmortem study of 5-HT$_2$ receptors in depressed subjects after death by natural means, McKeith et al. (1987) found no increase in 5-HT$_2$ receptor density.

Increased muscarinic receptor binding in the frontal cortex of patients who commit suicide was reported by Meyerson et al. (1982) but not by Kaufman et al. (1983) or Stanley (1984).

An increase in β-adrenergic receptor binding was found in the frontal cortices of patients who commit suicide by Biegon and Israeli (1988), and Mann and Stanley (1984), but not by Crow et al. (1984), De Parmentier et al. (1990), or Meyerson et al. (1982). Ferrier et al. (1986) found no increases in β-adrenergic receptor binding in depressed subjects dying of natural causes.

Decreased imipramine-binding site densities were reported in the frontal cortex by Crow et al. (1984) and by Stanley et al. (1982) and in the hypothalamus by Paul et al. (1984), but Meyerson et al. (1982) found increased binding, Crow and colleagues were later unable to replicate their earlier findings (Owen et al., 1986), and Arora and Meltzer (1989) found no difference. An autoradiographic study by Gross-Isseroff et al. (1989) reported binding as being reduced in the postcentral gyrus, the insular cortex, and the claustrum; increased in the hippocampus; and unchanged in the frontal cortex. Arató et al. (1987) also reported that the right hemisphere has double the [³H]imipramine-binding site density found on the left but that this is reversed in persons who commit suicide. Using [³H]paroxetine, Lawrence et al. (1990) found no differences between control and suicide subjects and no regional or hemispheric differences.

Developments such as quantitative histochemistry and autoradiography, which permit more precise measurement of variation within brain areas (Biegon, 1986), may lead to greater consistency in future findings, as undoubtedly some of the apparent discrepancies result from sampling of different brain areas. These developments may also assist in the determination of the neurophysiologic significance of whatever findings emerge.

It must be noted that these studies do not necessarily bear on depression because persons who commit suicide comprise a heterogeneous group, including alcoholics, schizophrenics, and subjects with personality disorder. There are complexities consequent on the mode of death (e.g., anoxia because of respiratory distress and intercurrent physical illnesses); recent drug treatment may also cloud the issue. The findings of alterations in 5-HT systems in those who commit suicide, if confirmed, would complement the findings from CSF 5-HIAA studies indicative of abnormalities in 5-HT systems in suicidal states. The methodologic caveat regarding alcohol in the 5-HIAA studies should also be borne in mind here.

CONCLUSIONS

In spite of much work, therefore, results of studies of the neurobiology of affective disorders are at present inconclusive. The key problem has been the absence of good methods for examining localized neurotransmitter and functional changes. There is a reliance on the effects of antidepressant drugs, which consistently involve monoamine systems. Although these do not necessarily implicate causes of disorder,

they do at least suggest that these neurotransmitters are important in the systems regulating mood.

Better methods of functional study in humans, such as positron emission tomography, are likely to advance this field considerably. Most positron emission tomographic studies of affective disorders so far have been limited to measures of cerebral metabolic activity, and localization is somewhat crude. As specific ligands for monoamine receptors are developed, this technique and other methods of functional imaging that are likely to be developed offer considerable promise.

References

(Key references are designated with an asterisk.)
Aberg-Wistedt A., Jostell K.G., Ross S.B., et al. Effects of zimelidine and desipramine on serotonin and noradrenaline uptake mechanisms in relation to plasma concentrations and to therapeutic effects during treatment of depression. *Psychopharmacology (Berl.)* 74:297–305, 1981.
Abraham K.I., Ieni J.R., Meyerson L.R. Purification and properties of a human plasma endogenous modulator for the platelet tricyclic binding/serotonin and transport complex. *Biochim. Biophys. Acta* 923:8–21, 1987.
Agren H. Symptom pattern in unipolar and bipolar depressions correlating with monoamine metabolites in the cerebrospinal fluid. *Psychiatry Res.* 3:225–236, 1980.
Anderson I.M., Cowen P.J. Clomipramine enhances the prolactin response to L-tryptophan. *Br. J. Clin. Pharmacol.* 22:216, 1986.
Annitto W., Shopsin B. Neuropharmacology of mania. In Shopsin B., ed. *Manic Illness.* New York, Academic Press, pp. 105–164, 1979.
Aprison M.H., Takahashi R., Tachiki K. Hypersensitive serotonin receptors involved in clinical depression—a theory. In Naber B., Aprison M.H., eds. *Neuropharmacology and Behavior.* New York, Plenum Publishing, pp. 23–53, 1978.
Arató M., Tekes K., Tóthfalusi L., et al. Serotonergic split brain and suicide. *Psychiatry Res.* 21:355–356, 1987.
Arora R.C., Meltzer H.Y. Serotonergic measures in the brains of suicide victims: 5HT₂ binding sites in the frontal cortex of suicide subjects and controlled subjects. *Am. J. Psychiatry* 146:730–736, 1989.
Asakura M., Tsukumoto T., Kasegawa K. Modification of rat brain alpha₂ and beta adrenergic receptor sensitivity following long-term treatment with antidepressants. *Brain Res.* 235:192–197, 1982.
Asarch K.B., Shih J., Kulesar A. Decreased ³H-imipramine binding in depressed males and females. *Commun. Psychopharmacol.* 4:425–432, 1980.
Asberg M., Bertilsson L., Tuck D., et al. Indoleamine metabolism in the cerebrospinal fluid of depressed patients before and during treatment with nortriptyline. *Clin. Pharmacol. Ther.* 14:277–283, 1973.
*Asberg M., Thoren P., Traskman L., et al. Serotonin depression—a biochemical subgroup within the affective disorders? *Science* 191:478–479, 1976.
Ashcroft G., Crawford T., Eccleston E. 5-Hydroxyindole compounds in the cerebrospinal fluid of patients with psychiatric or neurological diseases. *Lancet* 2:1049–1052, 1966.
*Ashcroft G., Eccleston D., Murray I. Modified amine hypothesis for the aetiology of affective illness. *Lancet* 2:573–577, 1972.
*Axelrod J., Inscoe J.K. The uptake and binding of circulating serotonin and the effect of drugs. *J. Pharmacol. Exp. Ther.* 141:161–165, 1963.
Axelrod J., Whitby L., Hertting G. Effect of psychotropic drugs on the uptake of H³-norepinephrine by tissues. *Science* 133:383–384, 1961.
Banerjee S.P., Sharma V.K., Kung-Cheung L.S., et al. Cocaine and D-amphetamine induce changes in central beta-adrenergic

sensitivity: effects of acute and chronic drug treatment. *Brain Res.* 175:119–130, 1979.

Banki C.M., Arató M. Amine metabolites and neuroendocrine responses related to depression and suicide. *J. Affective Disord.* 5:223–232, 1983.

Baron M., Barkai A., Gruen R., et al. ³H-imipramine platelet binding sites in unipolar depression. *Biol. Psychiatry* 18:1403–1409, 1983.

Baron M., Borkai A., Gruen R., et al. Platelet [³H]imipramine binding in affective disorders: trait versus state characteristics. *Am. J. Psychiatry* 143:711–717, 1986.

Barrand M.A., Callingham B.A. The catecholamines; adrenaline, noradrenaline and dopamine. In Gray C.H., James V.H.T., eds. *Hormones in Blood.* 3rd ed. New York, Academic Press, pp. 55–121, 1985.

Beck-Friis J., Lyungren J-G., Thorén M., et al. Melatonin, cortisol, and ACTH in patients with major depressive disorder and healthy humans with special reference to the outcome of the dexamethasone supression test. *Psychoneuroendocrinology* 10:173–186, 1985.

Berrettini W.H., Nurnberger J.I. Jr., Post R.M., et al. Platelet ³H-imipramine binding in euthymic bipolar patients. *Psychiatry Res.* 7:215–219, 1982.

Biegon A. The complex binding of tricyclic antidepressants to rat brain: the case of nortriptyline. *Brain Res.* 32:347–351, 1984.

Biegon A. Effect of chronic desipramine treatment on dihydroalprenolol, imipramine and desipramine binding sites; a quantitative autoradiographic study in the rat brain. *J. Neurochem.* 47:77–80, 1986.

Biegon A., Israeli M. Localisation of the effects of electroconvulsive shock on beta adrenoceptors in the rat brain. *Eur. J. Pharmacol.* 123:329–334, 1986.

Biegon A., Israeli M. Regionally selective increases in beta-adrenergic receptor density in the brains of suicide victims. *Brain Res.* 442:199–203, 1988.

Biegon A., Rainbow T.C. Localisation and characterisation of [³H]desmethylimipramine binding in rat brain by quantitative autoradiography. *J. Neurosci.* 3:1069–1076, 1983.

Biegon A., Samuel D. Binding of a labelled antidepressant to rat brain tissue. *Biochem. Pharmacol.* 28:3361–3366, 1979.

Blumberg J., Vetulani J., Stawarz R., et al. The noradrenergic cyclic AMP generating system in the limbic forebrain: pharmacological characterisation and possible role of limbic noradrenergic mechanisms in the mode of action of antipsychotic drugs. *Eur. J. Pharmacol.* 37:357–366, 1976.

Blumberg P., Kopin I., Gordon E., et al. Conversion of MHPG to VMA: implications for the importance of urinary MHPG. *Arch. Gen. Psychiatry* 37:1095–1098, 1980.

Born G.V.R., Grignani G., Martin K. Long term effects of lithium on the uptake of 5-hydroxytryptamine by human platelets. *Br. J. Clin. Pharmacol.* 9:321–326, 1980.

Braddock L.E., Cowen P.J., Elliott J.M., et al. Binding of yohimbine and imipramine to platelets in depressive illness. *Psychol. Med.* 16:765–773, 1986.

*Briley M.S., Langer S.Z., Raisman R., et al. Tritiated imipramine binding sites are decreased in platelets of untreated depressed patients. *Science* 209:303–305, 1980.

Brinkschulte M., Gaertner H.J., Schied H.W., et al. Plasma protein binding of perazine and amitriptyline in psychiatric patients. *Eur. J. Clin. Pharmacol.* 22:367–373, 1982.

Britton K.T., Lee G., Dana R., et al. Activating and "anxiogenic" effects of corticotropin releasing factor are not inhibited by blockade of the pituitary-adrenal system with dexamethasone. *Life Sci.* 39:1281–1286, 1986.

Bruinvels J. Inhibition of the biosynthesis of 5-hydroxytryptamine in rat brain by imipramine. *Eur. J. Pharmacol.* 20:231–237, 1972.

Bulat M. Some criteria for the study of biochemical processes in CNS by analysis of cerebrospinal fluid. *Clin. Neuropharmacol.* 7(Suppl. 1):S153, 1984.

*Bunney W.E., Davis J.M. Norepinephrine in depressive reactions. *Arch. Gen. Psychiatry* 13:483–494, 1965.

Butler J., Leonard B.E. Post-partum depression and the effect of

nomifensine treatment. *Int. Clin. Psychopharmacol.* 1:244–252, 1986.

Calil H.N., Jostell K.G., Cowdry R.W., et al. Zimelidine and norzimeldine protein binding measured by equilibrium dialysis. *Clin. Pharmacol. Ther.* 31:522–527, 1982.

Campbell I.C., McKernan R., Checkley S., et al. Characterisation of platelet alpha₂ adrenoceptors and their measurement in control and depressed subjects. *Psychiatry Res.* 14:17–32, 1985.

Cannon W.B. *Bodily Changes in Pain, Hunger, Fear and Rage.* New York, Appleton-Century, 1929.

*Carlsson A. Early psychopharmacology and the rise in modern brain research. *J. Psychopharmacol.* 4:120–126, 1990.

Carlsson A., Rosengren E., Bertler A., et al. Effect of reserpine on metabolism of catecholamines. In Garattini S., Ghetti V., eds. *Psychotropic Drugs.* Amsterdam, Elsevier, 1957a.

Carlsson A., Shore P.A., Brodie B.B. Release of serotonin from blood platelets by reserpine in vitro. *J. Pharmacol. Exp. Ther.* 120:334–339, 1957b.

Carlsson A., Corrodi H., Fuxe K., et al. Effect of antidepressant drugs on the depletion of intraneuronal brain 5-hydroxytryptamine stores caused by 4-methyl-alpha-ethyl-meta-tyramine. *Eur. J. Pharmacol.* 5:357–366, 1969.

*Carroll B., Curtis G., Mendel J. Neuroendocrine regulation in depression. II. Discrimination of depressed from nondepressed patients. *Arch. Gen. Psychiatry* 33:1051–1057, 1976.

Carstens M.E., Engelbrecht A.H., Russell V.A., et al. Alpha₂ adrenoceptor levels on platelets of patients with major depressive disorder. *Psychiatry Res.* 18:321–331, 1986a.

Carstens M.E., Engelbrecht A.H., Russell V.A., et al. Imipramine binding sites on platelets of patients with major depressive disorder. *Psychiatry Res.* 18:333–342, 1986b.

Carstens M.E., Engelbrecht A.H., Russell V.A., et al. Beta-adrenoceptors on lymphocytes of patients with major depressive disorder. *Psychiatry Res.* 20:239–248, 1987.

Charney D.S., Heninger G.R., Sternberg D.E., et al. Adrenergic receptor sensitivity in depression. Effects of clonidine in depressed patients and healthy subjects. *Arch. Gen. Psychiatry* 39:290–294, 1982.

Charney D.S., Price L.H., Heninger G.R. Desipramine-yohimbine combination treatment of refractory depression. *Arch. Gen. Psychiatry* 43:1155–1161, 1986.

Checkley S.A. Neuroendocrine tests of monoamine function in man: a review of basic theory and its application to the study of depressive illness. *Psychol. Med.* 10:35–53, 1980.

Checkley S.A., Slade A.P., Shur E. Growth hormone and other responses to clonidine in patients with endogenous depression. *Br. J. Psychiatry* 138:51–55, 1981.

Cheetham S.C., Crompton M.R., Katona C.L.E., et al. Brain 5-HT2 receptor binding sites in depressed suicide victims. *Brain Res.* 443:272–280, 1988.

*Cheetham S.C., Katona C.L.E., Horton R.W. Post mortem studies of neurotransmitter biochemistry in depression and suicide. In Horton R.W., Katona C.L.E., eds. *Biological Aspects of Affective Disorders.* London, Academic Press, pp. 191–221, 1991.

Cohen M.R., Cohen R.M., Pickar D., et al. High dose naloxone in depression. *Biol. Psychiatry* 19:825–832, 1984.

Cohen M.R., Pickar D., Cohen R.M. High dose naloxone administration in schizophrenia. *Biol. Psychiatry* 20:573–575, 1985.

Cohen R.M., Campbell I.C., Cohen M.R., et al. Presynaptive noradrenergic regulation during depression and antidepressant drug treatment. *Psychiatry Res.* 3:93–105, 1980.

Cooper S.J., Kelly J.G., King D.J. Adrenergic receptors in depression: effects of electroconvulsive therapy. *Br. J. Psychiatry* 147:23–29, 1985.

Coppen A., Swade C., Wood K. Platelet 5HT accumulation in depressive illness. *Clin. Chim. Acta* 87:165–168, 1978.

Coppen A.J. The biochemistry of affective disorders. *Br. J. Psychiatry* 113:1237–1264, 1967.

Costa E., Ravizza L., Barbaccia M.L. Evaluation of current theories on the mode of action of antidepressant drugs. In Bartholini, G., Lloyd K.G., Morselli P.L., eds. *GABA and Mood Disorders: Experimental and Clinical Research.* New York, Raven Press, pp. 9–21, 1986.

Cowen P.J., McCance S.L., Cowen P.R., et al. Lithium increases 5HT mediated neuroendocrine responses in tricyclic resistant depression. *Psychopharmacology (Berl.)* 99:230–232, 1989.

Crews F.T., Smith C.B. Presynaptic alpha-receptor subsensitivity after long-term antidepressant treatment. *Science* 202:322–324, 1978.

Crews F.T., Paul S.M., Goodwin F.K. Acceleration of beta receptor desensitisation in combined administration of antidepressants and phenoxybenzamine. *Nature* 290:787–789, 1981.

Crow T.J., Cross A.J., Cooper S.J., et al. Neurotransmitter receptors and monoamine metabolites in the brain of patients with Alzheimer-type dementia and depression and suicides. *Neuropharmacology* 23:1561–1569, 1984.

Daiguji M., Meltzer H.Y., U'Prichard D.C. Human platelet alpha 2-adrenergic receptors: labelling with 3H-yohimbine, a selective antagonist ligand. *Life Sci.* 28:2705–2717, 1981.

Davis G.C. Endorphins and pain. *Psychiatr. Clin. North Am.* 6:473–487, 1983.

Davis G.C., Buchsbaum M.S., Bunney W.E. Analgesia to painful stimuli in affective illness. *Am. J. Psychiatry* 136:1148–1151, 1979.

Davis V.E., Cashaw J.L., Huff J.A., et al. Identification of 5-hydroxytryptophol as a serotonin metabolite in man. *Proc. Soc. Exp. Biol. Med.* 122:890–892, 1966.

Deakin J.F.W., Pennelli I., Upadhya A.J., et al. A neuroendocrine study of 5HT function in depression: evidence for biological mechanisms of endogenous and psychosocial causation. *Psychopharmacology (Berl.)* 101:85–92, 1990.

Delgado P.L., Charney D.S., Price L.H., et al. Serotonin function and the mechanism of antidepressant action. *Arch. Gen. Psychiatry* 47:411–415, 1990.

De Montigny C., Aghajanian G.K. Tricyclic antidepressants: long-term treatment increases responsivity of rat forebrain neurons to serotonin. *Science* 202:1303–1306, 1978.

*De Montigny C., Chaput Y., Blier P. Lithium augmentation of antidepressant treatments: evidence for an involvement of the 5HT system. In Briley M., Fillion G., eds. *New Concepts in Depression.* Basingstoke, Macmillan Publishing, pp. 144–160, 1988.

De Parmentier F., Cheetham S.C., Cromton M.R., et al. Brain beta-adrenoceptor binding sites in antidepressant free depressed suicide victims. *Brain Res.* 525:71–77, 1990.

Desmedt D.H., Egrise D., Mendlewicz J. Tritiated imipramine binding sites in affective disorders and schizophrenia. Influence of circannual variation. *J. Affective Disord.* 12:193–198, 1987.

Downs N.S., Britton K.T., Gibbs D.M., et al. Supersensitive endocrine responses to physostigmine in dopamine-depleted rats. A model of depression. *Biol. Psychiatry* 21:775–786, 1986.

Doyle M.C., George A.J., Ravindran A.V., et al. Platelet alpha adrenoceptor binding in elderly depressed patients. *Am. J. Psychiatry* 142:1489–1490, 1985.

Ebert M.H., Post R.M., Goodwin F.K. Effect of physical activity on urinary MHPG excretion in depressed patients. *Lancet* 2:766, 1972.

Faludi G., Magyar I., Tekes K., et al. Measurement of 3H-serotonin uptake in blood platelets in major depressive episodes. *Biol. Psychiatry* 23:833–836, 1988.

Feldstein A., Hoagland H., Freeman H., et al. The effect of ethanol ingestion on serotonin-C14 in man. *Life Sci.* 6:53–61, 1967.

Ferrier I.N., McKeith I.G., Cross A.J., et al. Post-mortem neurochemical studies in depression. *Ann. N. Y. Acad. Sci.* 487:128–142, 1986.

Fozard J.R. Neuronal 5HT receptors in the periphery. *Neuropharmacology* 23:1473–1486, 1984.

Frize E.D. Mental depression in hypertensive patients treated for long periods with high doses of reserpine. *N. Engl. J. Med.* 251:1006–1008, 1954.

Fullerton D., Wenzel F., Lohrenz F., et al. Circadian rhythm of adrenal cortical activity in depression. *Arch. Gen. Psychiatry* 19:674–681, 1968.

Gallistel C.R., Shizgal P., Yeomans J.S. A portrait of the substrate for self-stimulation. *Psychol. Rev.* 88:228–273, 1981.

Garcia-Sevilla J.A., Zis A.P., Hollingsworth P.J., et al. Platelet alpha₂ adrenergic receptors in major depressive disorder. Binding of tritiated clonidine before and after tricyclic antidepressant drug treatment. *Arch. Gen. Psychiatry* 38:1327–1333, 1981a.

Garcia-Sevilla J.A., Zis A.P., Zelnick T.C., et al. Tricyclic antidepressant drug treatment decreases alpha₂ adrenoreceptors on human platelet membranes. *Eur. J. Pharmacol.* 69:121–123, 1981b.

Garcia-Sevilla J.A., Udina C., Furster M.J., et al. Enhanced binding of 3H.(−)adrenaline to platelets of depressed patients with melancholia: effect of longterm clomipramine treatment. *Acta Psychiatr. Scand.* 75:150–157, 1987.

Garcia-Sevilla J.A., Padro D., Girart T., et al. Alpha-2-adrenoceptor–mediated inhibition of platelets adenylate cyclase and induction of aggregation in major depression. *Arch. Gen. Psychiatry* 47:125–132, 1990.

Gentsch C., Lichsteiner M., Gastpar M., et al. 3H-imipramine binding sites in platelets of hospitalized psychiatric patients. *Psychiatry Res.* 14:177–187, 1985.

Georgotas A., Schweitzer J., McCue R.E., et al. Clinical and treatment effects on 3H-clonidine and 3H-imipramine binding in elderly depressed patients. *Life Sci.* 40:2137–2143, 1987.

Gibbs D.M. Vasopressin and oxytocin: hypothalamic modulators of the stress response: a review. *Psychoneuroendocrinology* 11:131–140, 1986.

Glassman A. Indoleamines and affective disorders. *Psychosom. Med.* 31:107–144, 1969.

Glue P.W., Cowen P.J., Nutt D.J., et al. The effect of lithium on 5HT mediated neuroendocrine responses and platelet 5HT receptors. *Psychopharmacology (Berl.)* 90:398–402, 1986.

Gold M., Potash A., Ryan N., et al. TRF induced TSH response in unipolar, bipolar and secondary depressions: possible utility in clinical assessment and difficult diagnosis. *Psychoneuroendocrinology* 5:147–155, 1980.

Goodwin F.K., Post R.M. CSF amine metabolites in affective illness. *J. Psychiatr. Res.* 10:320, 1974.

Goodwin G.M., Fairburn C.G., Cowen P.J. Dieting changes serotonergic function in women, not men: implications for the aetiology of anorexia nervosa? *Psychol. Med.* 17:839–842, 1987.

Green A.R., Grahame-Smith D.G. 5-Hydroxy and other indoles in the C.N.S. In Iversen L.L., Iversen S.D., Snyder S.H., eds. *Handbook of Psychopharmacology.* Vol. 3. New York, Plenum Publishing, p. 169, 1975.

Gross-Isseroff R., Israeli M., Biegon A. Autoradiographic analysis of tritiated imipramine binding in the human brain post mortem: effects of suicide. *Arch. Gen. Psychiatry* 46:237–241, 1989.

Hallbreich J., Grunhaus L., Ben-David M. Twenty-four hour rhythm of prolactin in depressed patients. *Arch. Gen. Psychiatry* 36:1183–1186, 1979.

Hardy J.A., Dodd P.R. Metabolic and functional studies on post-mortem human brain. *Neurochem. Int.* 5:253–266, 1983.

Harris T.H. Depression induced by rauwolfia compounds. *Am. J. Psychiatry* 113:950, 1957.

Healy D. Rhythm and blues: neurochemical, neuropharmacological and neuropsychological implications of a hypothesis of circadian rhythm disturbance in the affective disorders. *Psychopharmacology (Berl.)* 93:271–285, 1987a.

*Healy D. The structure of psychopharmacological revolutions. *Psychiatr. Dev.* 4:349–376, 1987b.

Healy D. The marketing of 5HT: depression or anxiety. *Br. J. Psychiatry* 158:737–742, 1991a.

Healy D. What do 5HT re-uptake inhibitors do in obsessive compulsive disorders? *Hum. Psychopharmacol.* (in press b).

Healy D., Leonard B.E. Monoamine transport in depression; kinetics and dynamics. *J. Affective Disord.* 12:91–105, 1987.

Healy D., Waterhouse J.M. The circadian system and affective disorders: clocks or rhythms? *Chronobiol. Int.* 7:5–10, 1990.

*Healy D., Waterhouse J.M. Reactive rhythms and endogenous clocks. *Psychol. Med.* 21:557–564, 1991.

*Healy D., Williams J.M.G. Dysrhythmia, dysphoria and depression; the interaction of learned helplessness and circadian dysrhythmia in the pathogenesis of learned helplessness. *Psychol. Bull.* 103:163–178, 1988.

Healy D., Carney P.A., Leonard B.E. Monoamine related markers of depression: changes following treatment. *J. Psychiatr. Res.* 17:251–260, 1983.

Healy D., O'Halloran A., Carney P.A., et al. Peripheral adrenoceptors and serotonin receptors in depression: changes associated with treatment with trazodone and amitriptyline. *J. Affective Disord.* 9:285–296, 1985.

*Healy D., O'Halloran A., Carney P.A., et al. Variations in platelet 5HT uptake in control and depressed populations. *J. Psychiatr. Res.* 20:345–354, 1986a.

Healy D., O'Halloran A., Leonard B.E. Increases in platelet 5HT uptake rates following treatment with "uptake inhibiting" drugs. *Int. Clin. Psychopharmacol.* 1:332–339, 1986b.

Healy D., Theodorou A.E., Whitehouse A.M., et al. ^{3}H-imipramine binding to previously frozen platelet membranes from depressed patients, before and after treatment. *Br. J. Psychiatry* 157:208–215, 1990.

Healy D., Calvin J., Whitehouse J.M., et al. Alpha-1-acid glycoprotein in major depressive and eating disorders. *J. Affective Disord.* 22:13–20, 1991a.

Healy D., Paykel E.S., Whitehouse A.M., et al. Platelet ^{3}H-imipramine α_2-adrenoceptor binding in normal subjects during desipramine administration and withdrawal. *Neuropsychopharmacology* 4:117–124, 1991b.

Healy D., Paykel E.S., Whitehouse A.M., et al. Plasma noradrenaline, adrenaline and DHPG responses to clonidine in control and depressed subjects. *Psychopharmacology* (submitted c).

Heufelder A., Warnhoff M., Pirke K. Platelet alpha$_2$ adrenoceptors and adenylate cyclase in patients with anorexia and bulimia. *J. Clin. Endocrinol. Metab.* 61:1053–1060, 1985.

Hollister L.E., Davis K.L., Overall J.E., et al. Excretion of MHPG in normal subjects. *Arch. Gen. Psychiatry* 35:1410–1415, 1978.

*Horton R.W., Katona C.L.E., Theodorou A.E., et al. Platelet radioligand binding and neuroendocrine challenge tests in depression. *Ciba Found. Symp.* 123:84–105, 1986.

Hrdina P.D., Lapierre Y.D., Horn E.R., et al. Platelet ^{3}H-imipramine binding: a possible predictor of response to antidepressant treatment. *Prog. Neuropsychopharmacol. Biol. Psychiatry* 9:619–623, 1985.

Hu H.Y., Davis J.M., Heinze W.J., et al. Effect of chronic treatment with antidepressants on beta adrenergic receptor binding in guinea pig brain. *Biochem. Pharmacol.* 29:2895–2896, 1980.

Ieni J.R., Zukin S.R., van Praag H.M. Human platelets possess multiple [^{3}H]imipramine binding sites. *Eur. J. Pharmacol.* 106:669–672, 1984.

Janowsky D.S., El-Youssef M.K., Davis J.M., et al. A cholinergic-adrenergic hypothesis of mania and depression. *Lancet* 2:632–635, 1972.

Jeste D.V., Lorh J.B., Goodwin F.K. Neuro-anatomical studies of major affective disorders. A review and suggestions for further research. *Br. J. Psychiatry* 153:444–459, 1988.

Johnson R.W., Reisine T., Spotnitz S., et al. Effects of desipramine and yohimbine on alpha$_2$ and beta adrenergic sensitivity. *Eur. J. Pharmacol.* 67:123–127, 1980.

Jones R., Olpe H. Cortical neuronal responsiveness to substance P is enhanced following chronic but not acute administration of antidepressants. *Eur. J. Pharmacol.* 87:171–172, 1983.

Kafka M.S., Paul S.M. Platelet alpha adrenergic receptors in depression. *Arch. Gen. Psychiatry* 43:91–95, 1986.

Kafka M.S., Van Kammen D.P., Kleinman J.E., et al. Alpha-adrenergic receptor function in schizophrenia, affective disorders and some neurological diseases. *Commun. Psychopharmacol.* 4:477–486, 1981.

Kanof P.D., Coccaro E.F., Johns C.A., et al. Platelet [^{3}H]imipramine binding in psychiatric disorders. *Biol. Psychiatry* 22:278–286, 1987.

Kaplan R.D., Mann J.J. Altered platelet serotonin uptake kinetics in schizophrenia and depression. *Life Sci.* 31:583–588, 1982.

Kasper S., Beckman H. Dexamethasone suppression test in a pluridiagnostic approach: its relationship to psychopathological and clinical variables. *Acta Psychiatr. Scand.* 68:31–37, 1983.

Kasper S., Vieir A., Schmidt R., et al. Multiple hormone responses to stimulation with DL-fenfluramine in patients with major depression before and after antidepressant treatment. *Pharmacopsychiatry* 23:76–84, 1990.

Katona C.L.E., Theodorou A.E., Davies S.L., et al. Platelet binding and neuroendocrine responses in depression. In Deakin J.F.W., ed. *The Biology of Depression.* Oxford, Arlen Press, pp. 121–136, 1986.

Kaufman C.A., Gillin J.C., O'Laughlin T., et al. Muscarinic binding in suicides. In *New Research Abstracts. Proceedings 136th Annual Meeting of American Psychiatric Association.* Washington, DC, American Psychiatric Association, 1983.

Kjellmar B., Beck-Friis J., Harrygren J., et al. Twenty-four hour serum levels of TSH in affective disorders. *Acta Psychiatr. Scand.* 69:491–502, 1984.

Kopanski C., Turek M., Schultz J.E. Effects of longterm treatment of rats with antidepressants on adrenergic receptor sensitivity in cerebral cortex: structure-activity study. *Neurochem. Int.* 5:649–659, 1983.

Kremer J.M.H., Wilting J., Janssen L.H.M. Drug binding to human alpha-1-acid glycoprotein in health and disease. *Pharmacol. Rev.* 40:1–47, 1988.

Kuhn R. The treatment of depressive states with G22355 (imipramine HCl). *Am. J. Psychiatry* 115:459–464, 1958.

Kuhn R. The imipramine story. In Ayd F.J., Blackwell B., eds. *Discoveries in Biological Psychiatry.* Philadelphia, Lippincott, pp. 205–217, 1970.

Lake C.R., Pickar D., Ziegler M.G., et al. High plasma norepinephrine levels in patients with major affective disorder. *Am. J. Psychiatry* 139:1315–1318, 1982.

Lawrence K.M., De Parmentier F., Cheetham S.C., et al. Symmetrical hemispheric distribution of ^{3}H-paroxetine binding sites in post-mortem human brain from controls and suicides. *Biol. Psychiatry* 28:544–546, 1990.

Lenox R., Ellis J., Van-Riiper D., et al. Platelet alpha$_2$ adrenergic receptor activity in clinical studies of depression. In Usdin E., Goldstein M., Friedhoff A.J., et al., eds. *Frontiers of Neuropsychiatric Research.* New York, Macmillan Publishing, 1983.

Leonard B.E. Pharmacology of new antidepressants. *Prog. Neuropharmacol. Biol. Psychiatry* 8:97–108, 1984.

Leonard B.E. Neurotransmitter receptors, endocrine responses and the biological substrate of depression: a review. *Human Psychopharmacol.* 1:3–22, 1986.

Lewis D.A., McChesney C. Tritiated imipramine binding distinguishes among subtypes of depression. *Arch. Gen. Psychiatry* 42:485–488, 1985.

Lloyd K.G., Thoret F., Pilc A. GABA and the mechanism of action of antidepressant drugs. In Bartholini G., Lloyd K.G., Morselli P.L., eds. *GABA and Mood Disorders: Experimental and Clinical Research.* New York, Raven Press, pp. 32–42, 1986.

Loomer H.P., Saunders J.C., Kline N.S. A clinical and pharmacodynamic evaluation of iproniazid as a psychic energiser. *Psychiatr. Res. Rep.* 8:129–141, 1958.

Luck P., Mikhailidis D., Dashwood M., et al. Platelet hyperaggregability and increased alpha adrenoceptor density in anorexia nervosa. *J. Clin. Endocrinol. Metab.* 57:911–914, 1983.

Maas J.W. Biogenic amines and depression. *Arch. Gen. Psychiatry* 32:1357–1361, 1975.

Maas J.W., Fawcett J.A., Dekirmenjian K. Catecholamine metabolism, depressive illness and drug response. *Arch. Gen. Psychiatry* 26:252–262, 1972.

Maj J., Przegalinski E., Mogilnicka E. Hypotheses concerning the mode of action of antidepressant drugs. *Rev. Physiol. Biochem. Pharmacol.* 100:1–74, 1984.

Malmgren R., Asberg M., Olsson P., et al. Defective serotonin transport mechanism in platelets from endogenous depressive patients. *Life Sci.* 29:2649–2658, 1981.

Mann J.J., Stanley M. Postmortem monoamine oxidase enzyme kinetics in the frontal cortex of suicide victims and controls. *Acta Psychiatr. Scand.* 69:135–139, 1984.

Mann J., Brown R., Halper J., et al. Reduced sensitivity of lymphocyte beta-adrenergic receptors in patients with endogenous depression and psychomotor agitation. *N. Engl. J. Med.* 313:715–720, 1985.

Mann J.J., Stanley M., McBride P.A., et al. Increased serotonin$_2$ and beta adrenergic receptor binding in the frontal cortices of suicide victims. *Arch. Gen. Psychiatry* 43:954–959, 1986.

Matthews J., Akil H., Greden J., et al. Beta-endorphin/beta-lipotropin immunoreactivity in endogenous depression. *Arch. Gen. Psychiatry* 43:374–381, 1986.

McAdam C., Colahan F.S., Brophy J., et al. Alteration by a plasma factor of platelet aggregation and 5HT uptake in depression. *Biol. Psychiatry* (in press).

McKeith I.G., Marshall E.F., Ferrier I.N., et al. 5HT binding in post-mortem brain from patients with affective disorders. *J. Affective Disord.* 13:67–74, 1987.

McWilliam J.R., Meldrun B.S. Noradrenergic regulation of growth hormone secretion in the baboon. *Endocrinology* 112:234–239, 1983.

Meek J.L., Neff N.H. Is cerebrospinal fluid the major source for the removal of 5-hydroxyindoleacetic acid from the brain? *Neuropharmacology* 12:497–503, 1973.

Mellerup E.T., Plenge P. High affinity binding of ^{3}H-paroxetine and ^{3}H-imipramine to rat neuronal membranes. *Psychopharmacology* 89:436–439, 1986.

Mellerup E., Plenge P., Rosenberg R. ^{3}H-imipramine binding sites in platelets from psychiatric patients. *Psychiatry Res.* 7:221–227, 1982.

Meltzer H.Y., Arora R.C., Baber R., et al. Serotonin uptake by blood platelets of psychiatric patients. *Arch. Gen. Psychiatry* 38:1322–1326, 1981.

Meltzer H.Y., Arora R.C., Tricou B.J., et al. Serotonin uptake in blood platelets and the dexamethasone suppression test in depressed patients. *Psychiatry Res.* 8:41–47, 1983.

Mendlewicz J., VanCauten E., Linkowski P., et al. The 24 hour profile of prolactin in depression. *Life Sci.* 27:2015–2024, 1980.

Mendlewicz J., Linkowski P., Kerkhoffs M., et al. Diurnal hypersecretion of growth hormone in depression. *J. Clin. Endocrinol. Metab.* 60:505–512, 1985.

Meyerson L.R., Wenogle I.P., Abel M.S., et al. Human brain receptor alterations in suicide victims. *Pharmacol. Biochem. Behav.* 17:159–163, 1982.

Muscettola G., Wehr P., Goodwin F.K. Effect of diet on urinary MHPG. *Am. J. Psychiatry* 134:914–917, 1977.

Muscettola G., Di Lauro A., Giannini C.P. Platelet ^{3}H-imipramine binding in bipolar patients. *Psychiatry Res.* 18:343–353, 1986.

Nankai M., Yoshimoto S., Narita K., et al. Platelet ^{3}H-imipramine binding in depressed patients and its circadian variation in healthy controls. *J. Affective Disord.* 11:207–212, 1986.

Nemeroff C.B., Krishnan R.R., Blazer D.G., et al. Elevated plasma concentration of alpha-1-acid glycoprotein, a putative endogenous inhibitor of the tritiated imipramine binding site in depressed patients. *Arch. Gen. Psychiatry* 47:337–340, 1990.

Ogren S.O., Ross S.B., Hall H., et al. The pharmacology of zimelidine: a selective 5HT reuptake inhibitor. *Br. J. Clin. Pract. (Symp. Suppl.)* 19:27–41, 1982.

Oreland L., Widberg A., Asberg M., et al. Platelet monoamine oxidase activity and monoamine metabolites in cerebrospinal fluid in depressed and suicidal patients and in healthy controls. *Psychiatry Res.* 4:21–29, 1981.

Owen F., Chambers D.R., Cooper S.J., et al. Serotonergic mechanisms in brains of suicide victims. *Brain Res.* 362:185–188, 1986.

Paul S.M., Rehavi M., Skolnick P., et al. Demonstration of specific high affinity binding sites for [^{3}H] imipramine on human platelets. *Life Sci.* 26:953–959, 1980.

Paul S.M., Rehavi M., Skolnick P., et al. Depressed patients have decreased binding of tritiated imipramine to platelet serotonin transporter. *Arch. Gen. Psychiatry* 38:1315–1317, 1981.

Paul S.M., Rehavi M., Skolnick P., et al. High affinity binding of antidepressants to a biogenic amine transport site in human brain and platelets: studies in depression. In Post R.M., Ballenger J.C., eds. *Neurobiology of Mood Disorders.* Baltimore, Williams & Wilkins, pp. 845–853, 1984.

Paykel E.S., von Woeekom A.E., Walvers D.E., et al. Fengabine in depression: a placebo controlled study of a GABA-agonist. *Hum. Psychopharmacol.* 6:147–154, 1991.

Peroutka S.J., Snyder S.H. Longterm antidepressant treatment decreases spiroperidol-labelled serotonin receptor binding. *Science* 210:88–90, 1980.

Pimoule C., Briley M.S., Gay C., et al. ^{3}H-Rauwolscine binding in platelets from depressed patients and healthy volunteers. *Psychopharmacology (Berl.)* 79:308–312, 1983.

Poirier M.F., Benkelfat C., Loo H., et al. Reduced Bmax of ^{3}H-imipramine binding to platelets of depressed patients free of previous medication with 5HT uptake inhibitors. *Psychopharmacology (Berl.)* 89:456–461, 1986.

Post R.M., Goodwin F.K., Gordon E. Amine metabolites in the human cerebrospinal fluid: effects of cord transection and spinal fluid block. *Science* 179:897–898, 1973a.

Post R.M., Gordon E.K., Goodwin F.K. Central norepinephrine metabolites in affective illness: MHPG in the cerebrospinal fluid. *Science* 179:1002–1003, 1973b.

Post R.M., Kotin J., Goodwin F. Psychomotor activity and cerebrospinal fluid amine metabolites in affective illness. *Am. J. Psychiatry* 130:67–72, 1973c.

Raisman R., Sechter D., Briley M.S., et al. High affinity ^{3}H.imipramine binding in platelets from untreated and treated depressed patients compared to healthy volunteers. *Psychopharmacology (Berl.)* 75:368–371, 1981.

Randrup A., Braestrup C. Uptake inhibition of biogenic amines by newer antidepressant drugs; relevance to the dopamine hypothesis of depression. *Psychopharmacology (Berl.)* 53:309–314, 1977.

Reichenberg K., Gaillard-Plaza G., Montastrue J.L. Influence of naloxone on the antinociceptive effects of some antidepressant drugs. *Arch. Int. Pharmacodyn. Ther.* 275:78–85, 1985.

Reith M.E., Sershen H., Allen D., et al. High- and low-affinity binding of [^{3}H]imipramine in mouse cerebral cortex. *J. Neurochem.* 40:389–395, 1983.

Reisine T., Soubrie P. Loss of rat cerebral cortical opiate receptors following chronic desmethylimipramine treatment. *Eur. J. Pharmacol.* 77:39–44, 1982.

Ridges A.P. The amine hypothesis in relation to the present understanding of depressive illness. *Br. J. Clin. Pract. (Symp. Suppl.)* 7:12–21, 1980.

Rosser M. Biological markers in mental disorders: post-mortem studies. *J. Psychiatr. Res.* 18:457–465, 1984.

Roy A., Pickar D., Linnoila M., et al. Plasma norepinephrine levels in affective disorders. *Arch. Gen. Psychiatry* 42:1181–1185, 1985.

Roy A., Everett D., Pickar D., et al. Platelet tritiated imipramine binding and serotonin uptake in depressed patients and controls. *Arch. Gen. Psychiatry* 44:320–327, 1987.

Roy P., Post R.M., Rubinow D.R., et al. CSF 5HIAA and personal and family history of suicide in affectively ill patients: a negative study. *Psychiatry Res.* 10:263–274, 1984.

Sachar E., Hellman L., Roffwarg H., et al. Disrupted 24 hour pattern of cortisol secretion in psychotic depression. *Arch. Gen. Psychiatry* 28:19–24, 1973.

Salama A., Garcia A., Wang C.H., et al. Relationship between adaptive changes in brain alpha2 and beta adrenergic receptors following repeated imipramine, yohimbine and electro-convulsive shock treatment to rats. In Usdin E., Goldstein M., Friedhoff A.J., et al., eds. *Frontiers of Neuropsychiatric Research.* New York, Macmillan Publishing, 1983.

Scatton B., Loo H., Dennis T., et al. Decrease in plasma levels of 3,4-dihydroxyphenylethyleneglycol in major depression. *Psychopharmacology (Berl.)* 88:220–225, 1986.

*Schildkraut J.J. The catecholamine hypothesis of affective disorders: a review of supporting evidence. *Am. J. Psychiatry* 122:509–522, 1965.

Schildkraut J.J., Orsulak P., Schatzberg A., et al. Towards a biochemical classification of depressive disorders. *Arch. Gen. Psychiatry* 35:1427–1439, 1978.

Schneider L.S., Severson J.A., Sloane R.B. Platelet ^{3}H-imipramine binding in depressed elderly patients. *Biol. Psychiatry* 20:1232–1234, 1985.

Schneider L.S., Fredrickson E.R., Severson J.A., et al. ^{3}H-imipramine binding in depressed elderly: relationship to family history and clinical response. *Psychiatry Res.* 19:257–266, 1987.

Schoffelmeer A., Hoorneman E.R., Sminia P., et al. Presynaptic alpha 2- and postsynaptic beta-adrenoceptor sensitivity in slices of rat neocortex after chronic treatment with various antidepressant drugs. *Neuropharmacology* 23:115–119, 1984.

Schultz J.E., Siggins G.R., Schocker F.W., et al. Effects of prolonged treatment with lithium and tricyclic antidepressants on discharge frequency, norepinephrine responses and beta-receptor binding in rat cerebellum: a physiological and biochemical comparison. *J. Pharmacol. Exp. Ther.* 216:28–38, 1981.

Scott M., Reading H., Loudon J. Studies on human blood platelets in affective disorders. *Psychopharmacology (Berl.)* 60:131–135, 1979.

Segonzac A., Schoemaker H., Tateishi T., et al. 5-Methoxytryptoline, a competitive endocoid acting at [^{3}H]imipramine recognition sites in human platelets. *J. Neurochem.* 45:249–256, 1985.

Sethy V.H., Harris D.W. Effect of norepinephrine uptake blockade on beta adrenergic receptors of the rat cerebral cortex. *Eur. J. Pharmacol.* 75:53–56, 1981.

Sherman A. Time course of the effects of antidepressants on serotonin in rat neocortex. *Commun. Psychopharmacol.* 3:1–5, 1979.

Siever L.J., Davis K.L. Overview: toward a dysregulation hypothesis of depression. *Am. J. Psychiatry* 142:1017–1031, 1985.

Siever L.J., Uhde T. New studies and perspectives on the noradrenergic receptor system in depression: effects of the alpha₂ adrenergic agonist clonidine. *Biol. Psychiatry* 19:131–156, 1983.

Siever L.J., Uhde T.W. New studies and perspectives on the noradrenergic receptor system in depression: effects of the alpha 2-adrenergic agonist clonidine. *Biol. Psychiatry* 19:131–156, 1984.

Siever L.J., Insel T., Jimerson D., et al. Growth hormone response to clonidine in obsessive-compulsive patients. *Br. J. Psychiatry* 142:184–187, 1983.

Siever L.J., Kafka M.S., Targum S., et al. Platelet alpha adrenergic binding and biochemical responsiveness in depressed patients and controls. *Psychiatry Res.* 11:287–302, 1984.

Siever L.J., Uhde T.W., Jimerson D.C., et al. Indices of noradrenergic output in depression. *Psychiatry Res.* 19:59–73, 1986.

Sigg E., Soffer L., Gyermek L. Influence of imipramine and related psychoactive agents on the effect of 5HT and catecholamines on the rat's nictitating membrane. *J. Pharmacol. Exp. Ther.* 142:13–20, 1963.

Spector S., Shore P.A., Brodie B.B. Biochemical and pharmacological effects of the monoamine oxidase inhibitors, iproniazid, 1-phenyl-2-hydrazinopropane (JB 516) and 1-phenyl-3-hydrazinobutane (JB 835). *J. Pharmacol. Exp. Ther.* 128:15–21, 1960.

Spector S., Hirsch A.O., Brodie B.B. Association of behavioural effects of pargyline, a non-hydrazide monoamine oxidase inhibitor with increase in brain norepinephrine. *Int. J. Neuropharmacol.* 2:81–93, 1963.

Stahl S.M., Ciaranello R.D., Berger P.A. Platelet serotonin in schizophrenia and depression. In Ho B.T., ed. *Serotonin in Biological Psychiatry.* New York, Raven Press, 1982.

Stahl S.M., Woo D.J., Mefford I.N., et al. Hyperserotonemia and platelet serotonin uptake and release in schizophrenia and affective disorders. *Am. J. Psychiatry* 140:26–30, 1983.

Stanley M. Cholinergic binding in the frontal cortex of suicide victims. *Am. J. Psychiatry* 141:11–14, 1984.

Stanley M., Mann J.J. Increased serotonin₂ binding sites in frontal cortex of suicide victims. *Lancet* 1:214–216, 1983.

Stanley M., Virgilio J., Gershon S. Tritiated imipramine binding sites are decreased in the frontal cortex of suicides. *Science* 216:1337–1339, 1982.

Starke K. Regulation of noradrenergic release by presynaptic receptor systems. *Rev. Physiol. Biochem. Pharmacol.* 77:1–124, 1977.

Starkstein S.E., Robinson R.G. Affective disorders and cerebral vascular disease. *Br. J. Psychiatry* 154:170–182, 1989.

Struthers A.D., Brown M.J., Adams E.F., et al. The plasma noradrenaline and growth hormone response to alphamethyl-dopa and clonidine in hypertensive subjects. *Br. J. Clin. Pharmacol.* 19:311–317, 1985.

Sugrue M.F. Changes in rat brain monoaminergic transmission following chronic antidepressant administration. *Life Sci.* 26:423–429, 1980.

Sulser F. Functional aspects of the norepinephrine-coupled adenylate cyclase system in the limbic forebrain and its modification by drugs which precipitate and alleviate depression. *Pharmacopsychiatry* 11:43–52, 1978.

*Sulser F. Regulation and function of noradrenergic receptor systems in the brain. *Neuropharmacology* 23:255–261, 1984.

Sulser F., Bickel M.H. On the role of catecholamines in the antireserpinic action of desmethylimipramine. *Pharmacologist* 4:178, 1962.

Sulser F., Bickel M.H., Brodie B.B. The action of desmethylimipramine in counteracting sedation and cholinergic effects of reserpine like drugs. *J. Pharmacol. Exp. Ther.* 144:321, 1964.

Suranyi-Cadotte B.E., Wood P.L., Nair N.P.V., et al. Normalization of platelet [³H]imipramine binding in depressed patients during remission. *Eur. J. Pharmacol.* 85:357–358, 1982.

Suranyi-Cadotte B.E., Gauthier S., Lafaille F., et al. Platelet ³H-imipramine binding distinguishes depression from Alzheimer's dementia. *Life Sci.* 37:2305–2311, 1985.

Takeda T., Harada T., Otsaki S. Platelet ³H-clonidine and ³H-imipramine binding and plasma cortisol level in depression. *Biol. Psychiatry* 26:52–60, 1989.

Tang S.W., Morris J.M. Variation in human platelet ³H-imipramine binding. *Psychiatry Res.* 16:141–146, 1985.

Theodorou A.E., Hale A.S., Davies S.L., et al. Platelet high affinity adrenoceptor binding sites labelled with the agonist [³H] UK-14,304 in depressed patients and matched controls. *Eur. J. Pharmacol.* 126:329–332, 1986.

Theodorou A.E., Healy D., Paykel E.S., et al. High and low affinity binding to platelet alpha adenergic receptors in depression. *J. Affective Disord.* (in press).

Thompson C., Clearly S.A., Corn T., et al. Down-regulation at pineal beta-adrenoceptors in depressed patients treated with desipramine. *Lancet* 2:735, 1983.

Thompson C., Mezey G., Corn T., et al. The effect of desipramine upon melatonin and cortisol secretion in depressed and normal subjects. *Br. J. Psychiatry* 147:389–393, 1985.

Träskman L., Tybring G., Asberg M., et al. Monoamine metabolites in the CSF and suicidal behaviour. *Arch. Gen. Psychiatry* 38:631–636, 1981.

Träskman-Bendz L., Asberg M., Bertilsson L., et al. CSF monoamine metabolites of depressed patients during illness and after recovery. *Acta Psychiatr. Scand.* 69:333–342, 1984.

Tuomisto J. A new modification for studying 5HT uptake by blood platelets: a re-evaluation of tricyclic antidepressants as uptake inhibitors. *J. Pharm. Pharmacol.* 26:92–100, 1974.

Tuomisto J., Mannisto P. Neurotransmitter regulation of anterior pituitary hormones. *Pharmacol. Rev.* 37:249–332, 1985.

*Tuomisto J., Tukiainen E. Decreased uptake of 5-hydroxytryptamine in blood platelets from depressed patients. *Nature* 262:596–598, 1976.

Tuomisto J., Tukiainen E., Ahlfors U.G. Decreased uptake of 5-hydroxytryptamine in blood platelets from patients with endogenous depression. *Psychopharmacology (Berl.)* 65:141–147, 1979.

Uhde T.W., Vitone B.J., Siever L.J., et al. Blunted growth hormone response to clonidine in panic disorder patients. *Biol. Psychiatry* 21:1081–1084, 1986.

van Praag H.M. CSF 5HIAA and suicide in non-depressed schizophrenics. *Lancet* 1:977–978, 1983.

van Praag H.M. Biological suicide research: outcome and limitations. *Biol. Psychiatry* 21:1305–1323, 1986.

van Praag H.M., Korf J., Schut D. Cerebral monamines and depression; an investigation with the probenecid technique. *Arch. Gen. Psychiatry* 28:827–831, 1973.

van Praag H.M., Lemus C., Kahn R. Hormonal probes of the central serotonergic activity: do they really exist? *Biol. Psychiatry* 22:86–98, 1987.

Vestergaard P., Sorensen T., Hoppe E., et al. Biogenic amine metabolites in cerebrospinal fluid of patients with affective disorders. *Acta Psychiatr. Scand.* 58:88–96, 1978.

Vetulani J., Stawarz R.J., Dingell J.V., et al. A possible common mechanism of action of antidepressant treatments: reduction in the sensitivity of the noradrenergic cyclic AMP generating system in the rat limbic forebrain. *Naunyn Schmiedebergs Arch. Pharmacol.* 293:109–114, 1976.

Wägner A., Aberg-Wistedt A., Asberg M., et al. Lower ³H-imipramine binding in platelets from untreated depressed patients compared to healthy controls. *Psychiatry Res.* 16:131–139, 1985.

Weeke A., Weeke J. The 24 hour pattern of serum TSH in patients with endogenous depression. *Acta Psychiatr. Scand.* 62:69–74, 1980.

Whiteford H.A., Peabody C.A., Csernonsky J.G., et al. Elevated baseline and post dexamethasone cortisol levels—a reflection of severity or endogeneity? *J. Affective Disord.* 12:199–202, 1987.

Whitehouse A.M., Healy D., White W., et al. Platelet alpha to receptive binding and tritiated imipramine binding in subjects with anorexia nervosa and bulimia nervosa. *J. Affective Disord.* (submitted).

Whittaker P.M., Warsh J.J., Stancer H.C., et al. Seasonal variation in platelet ³H-imipramine binding: comparative values in control and depressed populations. *Psychiatry Res.* 11:127–131, 1984.

Willner P. Dopamine and depression: a review of recent evidence. *Brain Res.* 287:211–246, 1983.

Wood K., Coppen A.J. Platelet alpha-adrenoceptor sensitivity in depressive illness. *Adv. Biol. Psychiatry* 7:85–89, 1981.

Wood K., Swade C., Abou-Saleh M., et al. Drug plasma levels or lithium in patients with affective disorders. *Br. J. Clin. Pharmacol.* 15:365S–368S, 1983.

Wood K., Swade C., Abou-Saleh M., et al. Apparent supersensitivity of platelet 5HT receptors in lithium treated patients. *J. Affective Disord.* 8:69–72, 1985.

Wright A.F., Crichton D.N., Loufdon J.B., et al. Beta-adrenergic binding defects in cell lines from families with manic depressive disorder. *Ann. Hum. Genet.* 48:201–214, 1984.

Zis A.P., Goodwin F.K. The amine hypothesis. In Paykel E.S., ed. *Handbook of the Affective Disorders.* Edinburgh, Churchill Livingstone, pp. 175–190, 1982.

62

Neurologic Complications of Psychotropic Drugs

Larry E. Tune
J. Raymond DePaulo

This chapter considers neurologic and some neuropsychiatric complications of the following types of psychotropic drugs: lithium and neuroleptic, antiparkinsonian, and antidepressant drugs, all of which are regularly prescribed for patients with major psychiatric disorders. Because the adverse neuropsychiatric reactions to psychotropic drugs are so numerous, only those of great clinical importance are discussed: (1) disorders of consciousness, particularly delirium; (2) disorders of memory; (3) convulsive and myoclonic disorders; (4) disorders of movement and tone; and (5) the neuroleptic malignant syndrome. A brief discussion of the neural toxicity of lithium-neuroleptic combinations is included.

DELIRIUM

Delirium is a mental disorder characterized by a disturbance in consciousness (of varying severity) associated with global cognitive impairment and variable disturbances in mood, perception, and behavior (Folstein and McHugh, 1976). In establishing these criteria, the reliable assessment of consciousness has been most problematic; simple bedside tests of cognition such as the Mini-Mental State examination are the usual means of detecting and following the course of delirium (DePaulo et al., 1982; Folstein et al., 1975). In addition to the disordered mental functioning, certain physical symptoms may be present: tremor, asterixis, nystagmus, and incoordination. Diffuse slowing of electroencephalographic activity is also usually present.

Although no definitive pathophysiology has been established for delirium, acetylcholine dysfunction may be important in the development of most delir-

ious states (Blass and Plum, 1982). Several models of encephalopathy (including impairments in cardiovascular, pulmonary, hepatic, renal, endocrine, and brain function and toxic, hypoxic, and nutrition- and thiamine-deficient states) are associated with cholinergic abnormalities (Blass and Plum, 1982). In the clinical literature, the syndrome of anticholinergic intoxication has been known since antiquity (Lipowski, 1989). Cholinergic mechanisms may be involved in most cases of drug-induced delirium (Lipowski, 1989): anticholinergic drugs are frequently associated with delirium; delirium is reversed with physostigmine, even in cases not associated with typical anticholinergic agents (Nattel et al., 1979); and studies demonstrate elevated serum anticholinergic activity in many cases of postoperative delirium (Golinger et al., 1987; Tune et al., 1981). Drug-induced delirium may be the most common form of the disorder, particularly in the elderly. Psychotropic drugs of all varieties appear capable of inducing delirium, although those with obvious anticholinergic activity do so most frequently. Table 62–1 gives the relative anticholinergic activity of frequently used psychotropic medications.

Lithium Intoxication

Delirium resulting from lithium intoxication usually occurs at serum lithium levels greater than 1.5 mEq/L. Stupor, coma, and rarely death are more likely at serum levels exceeding 3.5 mEq/L.

The onset of the disorder is usually heralded by one or more premonitory symptoms. General lethargy is probably the most common of these. Stammering or other problems of speech articulation are

Table 62–1. PSYCHOTROPIC DRUGS AND
ANTICHOLINERGIC ACTIVITY

Drug*	IC_{50} (nmol/L) Rat Brain QNB†
Atropine sulfate	0.4
Trihexyphenidyl hydrochloride	0.6
Benztropine	1.5
Amitriptyline	10
Doxepin	44
Nortriptyline	57
Imipramine	78
Thioridazine	150
Chlorpromazine	1000
Perphenazine	10000
Fluphenazine	12000
Haloperidol	48000

*Twelve psychotropic drugs compared with atropine in their blocking of QNB binding to acetylcholine receptors. Lower concentrations (nanomolar) indicate greater anticholinergic activity.

†IC_{50} = 50% of inhibitory concentration; QNB = 3-quinuclidinyl benzilate.
Adapted from Snyder S.H., Yamamura H.I. Antidepressants and the muscarinic acetylcholine receptor. *Arch. Gen. Psychiatry* 34:236–239, 1977; and Snyder S.H., Banerjee S.P., Yamamura H.I., et al. Drugs, neurotransmitters, and schizophrenia. *Science* 184:1243–1253, 1974. Copyright 1974 by the AAAS.

quite frequent as well. Muscular jerks or fasciculations are often seen. Gastrointestinal upsets similar to those seen in the early phases of lithium treatment (nausea, vomiting, and diarrhea) occur in some cases but are notably absent in many patients (Hansen and Amdisen, 1978). When clouding of consciousness and delirium supervene, the mental state is not distinguishable from the delirium seen as the result of any other toxin.

The clinical course of the disorder (when it is recognized and lithium administration is discontinued) does not promptly respond to the descent of the serum lithium level; rather, the resolution of the delirium often lags 2 weeks behind the elimination of lithium from the serum (DePaulo et al., 1982). In addition, the course of severely affected patients may be punctuated by late-developing but usually self-limited complications such as temporary stupor or seizures, even after serum lithium levels are reduced to below usual therapeutic levels. Focal neurologic signs such as cranial nerve palsies and extrapyramidal signs may appear, suggesting a second pathologic process such as intracranial hemorrhage. The electroencephalogram, reflecting this clinical picture, is usually diffusely slow but may show focal changes in addition.

The principles of treatment are to stop lithium administration and give supportive care, to maintain fluid and electrolyte balance, and to encourage lithium excretion. Because nephrogenic diabetes insipidus is frequently associated with lithium therapy, hyperosmolar hypernatremic coma has resulted from attempts to promote lithium excretion via saline diuresis (Hansen and Amdisen, 1978). Because lithium is reabsorbed only in the proximal tubule and the descending loop of Henle in association with sodium, the use of distal-acting and loop diuretics does not enhance lithium excretion. Diuretic agents

with greater proximal activity such as aminophylline and acetazolamide promote lithium excretion to a much greater degree (Thomsen and Schou, 1968). However, no diuretic or fluid regimen can approximate hemodialysis as a rapid means of reducing the serum lithium level. Thus, prompt hemodialysis is the treatment of choice when the patient is clinically deteriorating (stuporous), when there is a problem with lithium excretion (recalling that lithium intoxication itself can induce a transient renal failure), and when the serum lithium level is high (>3.5 mEq/L).

Outcome in general seems related to the lithium level, the duration of the high lithium state, and premorbid susceptibility (e.g., cardiovascular condition) (Hansen and Amdisen, 1978). The outcome of intoxication with treatment is usually full recovery. A small number of patients have neurologic residua: parkinsonian signs, cerebellar signs, and dementia syndromes are the most frequent (Apte and Langston, 1983).

DISORDERS OF MEMORY AND ATTENTION NOT APPARENTLY RELATED TO CONSCIOUSNESS

Delirium is not the only cognitive side effect of psychotropic medications. Perhaps more common are subtle, significant, and disabling impairments of attention, memory deficiencies, and distractibility that may be the result of therapeutic doses of psychotropic medications. These side effects are usually seen with moderate-to-high doses (and blood levels) of medications. They are clinically relevant because they contribute significantly to morbidity. For example, Tune et al. (1982) showed, in outpatients with chronic schizophrenia whose condition was stabilized by medications, that impairments in recent memory and distractibility are significantly and positively associated with rising serum levels of anticholinergic medications.

The role of lithium in the pathogenesis of memory deficits is controversial. Some reports suggested that long-term lithium treatment leads to a decline in "intellectual efficiency" (Loo et al., 1981). However, most large studies (Smigan and Perris, 1983; Squire et al., 1980) showed that, in the long term, there are no significant impairments in memory function resulting from lithium therapy. Smigan and Perris (1983) studied 53 patients for 1 year; patients were maintained with lithium levels of approximately 0.6 mEq/L. At 1 year, there were no significant long-term memory deficits appreciated.

By contrast, Lund et al. (1982), in a study of 50 patients treated with long-term lithium administration, found that there was a relative lowering of "level of memory" and "perceptual processing" in lithium-treated patients when compared with level of attention, productivity, and emotional reactivity in this group when they were not receiving lithium. When these patients were compared with age-matched controls, there were no significant differences. These data tend to support the hypothesis that lithium induces a delay in the rate of information processing in clinically treated patients. This observation, that long-term lithium treatment produces a slowing of performance on certain tasks, particularly perceptual motor tasks, has been supported by other authors (Shaw et al., 1987; Squire et al., 1980).

CONVULSIVE AND MYOCLONIC DISORDERS

Most neuroleptic drugs, tricyclic antidepressants (especially imipramine), and lithium lower the seizure threshold. Generalized seizures have been reported to occur rarely at therapeutic dosages with these drugs. The risk is greatest after overdosage (Starkey and Lawson, 1980). However, the seizure risk may be somewhat higher than usual when dosages are being increased and when therapeutic dosages in high ranges are given. All neuroleptic agents (except thioridazine and mesoridazine) have been reported to cause grand mal or focal motor seizures. Pre-existing seizure disorder, abnormal electroencephalographic patterns, and central nervous system pathologic changes have been identified as predisposing factors (Sovner and DiMascio, 1978). Among novel antidepressants, amoxapine and maprotiline have been associated with seizures after overdosage (Bock et al., 1982).

Myoclonus (repetitive, brief nonrhythmic contractions of muscle groups) occurs frequently in lithium and tricyclic antidepressant intoxication. It has also been observed after treatment with monoamine oxidase inhibitors (R.M. Cohen et al., 1980). The pathophysiology is uncertain; however, Adams and Victor (1981) observed that "it seems logical to assume that myoclonus is caused by abnormal discharges of aggregates of motor neurons or interneurons, due either to directly enhanced excitability or to removal of some inhibitory mechanism." How psychotropic drugs would augment this process may be related to enhanced serotoninergic activity. Subthreshold doses of serotonin plus imipramine induced myoclonic seizures in guinea pigs apparently owing to imipramine's potentiation of serotonin via its blockade of 5-HT reuptake in the brain (Westheimer and Klawans, 1977). It is of some interest that myoclonus has also been seen in association with antidepressants that are apparently less potent at blocking serotonin reuptake, such as maprotiline (Kettl and DePaulo, 1983).

DISORDERS OF MOVEMENT AND TONE RESULTING FROM NEUROLEPTIC MEDICATIONS

Acute Dystonic Reactions

Acute dystonic reactions occur in 2–5% of patients taking neuroleptic agents. They typically occur within the first 7 days of treatment, often after the first dose (Marsden et al., 1975). Clinical examination reveals usually trismus, torticollis, occasionally arching of the back, jaw opening with tongue spasms, and occasionally forced eye deviation.

When Meldrum et al. (1977) administered haloperidol and other potent neuroleptic agents to Senegalese baboons, the baboons experienced dystonic reactions. By contrast, thioridazine, the most anticholinergic neuroleptic medication, did not produce acute dystonic reactions. Anticholinergic compounds (e.g., benztropine, 2 mg intravenously or intramuscularly) have proved highly effective in resolving acute dystonic reactions. The putative neurochemical mechanism can be understood by examining the relationship between nigrostriatal dopaminergic neurons and acetylcholine-producing interneurons within the corpus striatum. Because dopamine is an inhibitory neurotransmitter (Carlsson, 1970) in the corpus striatum, neuroleptic drugs have the effect of canceling this inhibitory effect on cholinergic interneurons. Acute dystonic reactions thus represent a state of relative acetylcholine excess within the striatum, a state that is corrected with the administration of anticholinergic compounds. Investigations involving positron emission tomograpy with ligands that selectively block dopamine D_2 receptors showed that extrapyramidal side effects typically occur when dopamine D_2 receptors are extensively blocked (>80% receptor occupancy) (L. Farde et al., unpublished observations).

Further support for this pathophysiologic model is provided by the finding that pretreatment of animals either with reserpine (which disrupts the granular storage of catecholamines) or with α-methyl-p-tyrosine (which prevents catecholamine synthesis) diminishes the frequency of dystonic reactions in animals (Marsden and Jenner, 1980). Patients with Parkinson's disease treated with levodopa (L-dopa) occasionally experience abnormal movements resembling the acute dystonic reactions seen with neuroleptic drug administration (Parkes et al., 1976).

Two mechanisms are important in understanding acute extrapyramidal side effects. The first is a compensatory mechanism within the dopaminergic neurotransmitter system as the use of neuroleptic medications continues. Changes in dopamine turnover are greatest with short-term treatment. With prolonged administration of neuroleptics, the effect of neuroleptic medications on dopamine turnover diminishes (Asper et al., 1973; Marsden and Jenner, 1980). Anticholinergic drugs also diminish the effects of neuroleptic drugs on dopamine turnover (Anden, 1972). The second mechanism is postsynaptic receptor supersensitivity. Of particular interest is the observation that when haloperidol or other neuroleptics are given as short-term treatment to rats, neuroleptic-induced stereotypy is enhanced. Short-term dosage of neuroleptic in animals may result in a supersensitive dopamine receptor. This acute dopamine receptor sensitivity may relate to the mechanism of such dystonic reactions.

Drug-Induced Movement Disorders: Parkinsonian Symptoms

Drug-induced parkinsonism resembles idiopathic Parkinson's disease. Both result from a relative deficiency of dopamine within the nigrostriatal dopaminergic pathway. Drug-induced parkinsonism is caused by postsynaptic dopamine receptor blockade by neuroleptic drugs. The result is a relative excess of acetylcholine within the striatum. Drug-induced parkinsonism has been caused by reserpine and tetrabenazine, both of which prevent dopamine storage presynaptically (Glowinski et al., 1966).

Under ordinary circumstances, extrapyramidal side effects occur in 20–40% of patients receiving neuroleptic agents. Marsden et al. (1975) stated that it is "probable that everyone would develop obvious clinical features of the disorder if given a big enough dose of neuroleptic drugs," suggesting that the incidence of extrapyramidal signs is dose dependent. However, several published studies involving megadose strategies with neuroleptic medications failed to show an increased incidence of extrapyramidal reactions (Dencker et al., 1981; McClelland et al., 1976). Most studies directly investigating the relationship between dose and incidence of extrapyramidal effects demonstrate a lack of correlation (Tune and Coyle, 1981).

Myrianthopoulos et al. (1962) observed that individuals who experience extrapyramidal side effects have a greater incidence of idiopathic parkinsonism in their families. Chase et al. (1970) studied the incidence of extrapyramidal reactions in a small population of schizophrenic patients. They found that patients who developed extrapyramidal sequelae showed an atypical cerebrospinal fluid response to neuroleptic medications (as measured by alterations in cerebrospinal fluid homovanillic acid levels). F. Ayd (1961) found that the age incidence of drug-induced parkinsonism parallels that of idiopathic parkinsonism. These scattered observations suggest that factors involving individual susceptibility are important in the pathophysiology of extrapyramidal side effects and have yet to be carefully elucidated.

Treatment of all acute extrapyramidal effects of neuroleptic drugs is use of anticholinergic medications to correct the state of relative cholinergic excess existing in the corpus striatum. In most instances, modest doses of benztropine mesylate (2–6 mg/day) or trihexyphenidyl (4–8 mg/day) are adequate to provide symptomatic relief. When standard doses fail to relieve extrapyramidal effects, it may be that patients do not achieve adequate serum blood levels of anticholinergic medications (Tune and Coyle, 1981). Most acute extrapyramidal symptoms abate if the dosage of anticholinergic drug is carefully increased while anticholinergic toxicity is diligently monitored.

Akathisia

Akathisia is characterized primarily by the subjective complaint of motor restlessness. Typically, the patient complains of an uncomfortable feeling of the "urge to move." In its most severe form, the patient paces about constantly. At some point, 10–20% of all patients receiving neuroleptic medications have this syndrome, typically in the first 2–4 weeks of treatment (although chronic akathisia has been described). It is of great clinical importance because, as Van Putten (1974) showed, this side effect is the most common reason given for failure to comply with the medication regimen.

Two hypotheses have been suggested to explain this syndrome. The first is supported by evidence in which blockade of mesocortical and mesolimbic dopaminergic pathways, alone or in addition to terminal projection areas in the frontal cingular areas, causes locomotor hyperactivity in rodents (Marsden and Jenner, 1980). If this hyperactivity is comparable with akathisia, the neuroanatomic basis of akathisia may be different from that of drug-induced parkinsonism; mesolimbic and mesocortical rather than nigrostriatal dopaminergic projections may be the affected neuroanatomic regions. Indeed, akathisia and drug-induced parkinsonism have been observed to coexist (Marsden and Jenner, 1980).

The second hypothesis implicates the blockade of the presynaptic dopamine autoreceptor, which results in increased dopamine release (Kebabian and Calne, 1979; Seeman, 1980). If this were the mechanism of akathisia (i.e., presynaptic rather than postsynaptic dopamine receptor blockade leading to a state of relative acetylcholine deficiency resulting from increased dopamine release), the variable response to anticholinergic compounds might be explained. This hypothesis is inconsistent with two observations. First, akathisia occurs in patients who receive large doses of neuroleptic medications. It would be difficult to explain akathisia as a result of presynaptic blockade when postsynaptic receptors were themselves presumably adequately blocked. Second, the administration of reserpine and tetrabenazine, compounds that diminish presynaptic release of dopamine, is associated with akathisia (Marsden and Jenner, 1980).

Tardive Dyskinesia

Tardive dyskinesia (TD) is usually a late manifestation of long-term neuroleptic treatment. Although it has been described after 1 month of treatment (American Psychiatric Association Task Force, 1979), it typically occurs after many years of neuroleptic administrations. Predisposing factors include (1) age: it is rare to develop TD before age 40 years, and the incidence steadily increases after age 55 years; (2) sex: women have repeatedly been shown to have TD significantly more often than men; and (3) previous brain damage (Gerlach, 1979; Waddingtan and Youssef, 1986). The typical clinical syndrome is oral-lingual-buccal dyskinesia: synchronous jaw movements accompanied by tongue protrusions, licking, or tongue rotating. Occasionally, the syndrome is more extensive and affects the arms, the trunk, and the legs. On rare occasions, the respiratory musculature is involved, leading to potentially life-threatening respiratory dyskinesias (Casey and Rabins, 1978).

The diagnosis of TD can be difficult to establish for several reasons. First, abnormal movements resembling those in TD have been described in individuals who have never received neuroleptic medications (American Psychiatric Association Task Force, 1979). Spontaneous dyskinesias occur in approximately 1% of the population; approximately 30% of patients receiving long-term neuroleptic medication experience similar dyskinesias. Second, according to numerous investigators (American Psychiatric Association Task Force, 1979; Rabins et al., 1981), the onset of symptoms typical of TD occurs when neuroleptic medication is either reduced or discontinued (withdrawal dyskinesia). These symptoms, unlike those of TD, may respond to anticholinergic medications.

The medical (and legal) concern is that TD is often permanent. Marsden et al. (1975) estimated that approximately 30% of patients who evidence symptoms of TD have them permanently. This observation is based largely on the results of point prevalence studies, which have been challenged by several groups (D. Casey, unpublished observations; Robinson and McCreadie, 1986). In the Nithsdale Schizophrenia Survey, for example, although the point prevalence of TD was approximately 30%, only 12% of patients showed persistent TD during a 3½-year period. In addition, the severity of TD fluctuated in 41% of patients, suggesting that dyskinesia is transient in some cases (Robinson and McCreadie, 1986).

The pathophysiology of TD is widely held to entail neuroleptic-induced supersensitivity of dopamine receptors (Carlsson, 1970; Klawans, 1973). This results in a state of relative acetylcholine deficiency within the corpus striatum. Treatment with neuroleptic drugs causes dopamine receptors to be sensitive to the effects of standard dopamine agonists (e.g., apomorphine). The development of pharmacologic supersensitivity has been shown in animals receiving reserpine, α-methyl-*p*-tyrosine, and chlorpromazine (Marsden and Jenner, 1980). Pharmacologic supersensitivity, even after the short-term use of neuroleptic medications, can result in increased numbers of dopamine receptors and possibly an increase in the sensitivity of adenylate cyclase to the stimulatory effects of dopamine. Marsden and Jenner (1980) demonstrated that dopamine receptor supersensitivity exists for 6 months after drug withdrawal.

Figure 62–1 provides a schematic approach to the management of TD. Few treatments have been shown to be effective. When the symptoms are observed, the first issue is to decide whether the patient can discontinue medications. More often than not, discontinuance of medications is not a viable option for patients receiving long-term neuroleptic treatment. It is possible to discontinue anticholinergic medications when symptoms of TD are first observed. Because anticholinergic agents increase the intensity and possibly the frequency of TD, this is of considerable clinical importance (Gerlach et al., 1974; Klawans, 1973; Klawans and Rubovits, 1974).

NEUROLEPTIC MALIGNANT SYNDROME

The neuroleptic malignant syndrome is an idiosyncratic reaction to the administration of neuroleptics (Delay and Deniker, 1968) or to withdrawal of amantadine (Simpson and Davis, 1984) (Table 62–2). It is characterized by fever, generalized rigidity, and obtundation. Table 62–3 lists the most common signs and symptoms associated with the disorder. Most patients recover completely after discontinuation of neuroleptic drug administration. Fatalities do occur, however. A significant number of patients are left with persisting neurologic signs and cognitive deficits

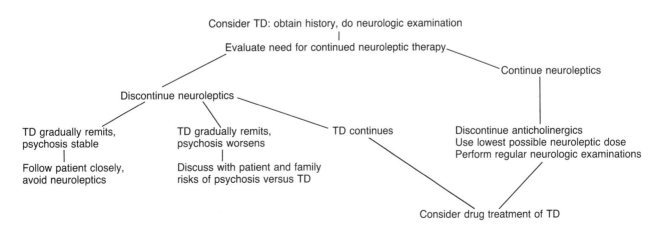

Figure 62–1. Management of tardive dyskinesia (TD). (Adapted from Rabins P., Tune L., McHugh P.R. Tardive dyskinesia. *Johns Hopkins Med. J.* 148:206–211, 1981.)

Table 62–2. MEDICATIONS TAKEN BY 53 PATIENTS WHO DEVELOPED NEUROLEPTIC MALIGNANT SYNDROME

Drug	Number of Patients
Neuroleptic(s) alone	20*
Neuroleptics plus anticholinergic†	15‡
Neuroleptic plus lithium	3§
Neuroleptics plus lithium plus anticholinergic†	6‖
Neuroleptics, other drugs not specified (13)	6
Lithium plus benzodiazepine	1
Tetrabenazine plus methyltyrosin	1
Withdrawal from levodopa/carbidopa and amantadine	1

*Two patients were also receiving anticonvulsants.
†Includes tricyclic antidepressants and/or antiparkinsonian drugs.
‡One patient had been abusing amphetamines for 10 years.
§One patient also received deanol.
‖One patient also received levodopa/carbidopa and amantadine.
Adapted from Levenson J.L. Neuroleptic malignant syndrome. *Am. J. Psychiatry* 142:1137–1145, 1985.

(e.g., dementias), especially when the neuroleptic malignant syndrome goes unrecognized for long periods. Its incidence is estimated to be 0.5–1.0% in patients given neuroleptic agents (Caroff, 1980). There is a suggestion that it may be a more likely result of high doses of high-potency neuroleptics, but it has been seen with single doses of low-potency preparations as well (Table 62–4).

Although the pathophysiology of neuroleptic malignant syndrome is not well understood, Kurlan et al. (1984) argued that dopamine receptor blockade may explain all the essential features of the disorder. The mechanism underlying the hyperthermia may be heat production attributable to striatal dopamine blockade–induced muscular rigidity and/or a direct hypothalamic thermoregulatory injury. In addition, a nonshivering autonomic thermogenic mechanism in which dopaminergic input is postulated may also play a significant role. The muscular rigidity is assumed to be a generalized and severe expression of the dopamine blockade–induced parkinsonian syn-

Table 62–3. CLINICAL AND LABORATORY SIGNS IN 53 PATIENTS WITH NEUROLEPTIC MALIGNANT SYNDROME

Clinical Sign	Percentage of Patients with Sign
Fever	98
Elevated serum creatine kinase level	91
Tachycardia	91
Rigidity	89
Altered consciousness	84
Leukocytosis	79
Abnormal blood pressure	74
Tachypnea	73
Profuse diaphoresis	67
Tremor	45
Incontinence	21

Adapted from Levenson J.L. Neuroleptic malignant syndrome. *Am. J. Psychiatry* 142:1137–1145, 1985.

Table 62–4. NEUROLEPTICS TAKEN BY 50 OF 53 PATIENTS WHO DEVELOPED NEUROLEPTIC MALIGNANT SYNDROME

Medication	Number of Patients*
Haloperidol	28
Fluphenazine	15
Chlorpromazine or derivatives	8
Trifluoperazine	6
Thioridazine	5
Thiothixene	2
Other	7

*The sum is greater than the total number of patients because many patients received more than one drug.
Adapted from Levenson J.L. Neuroleptic malignant syndrome. *Am. J. Psychiatry* 142:1137–1145, 1985.

drome. As noted earlier, the pathogenesis of the obtundation and/or delirium is unknown. It is of some interest that any one or two of the three central features may be seen in an occasional patient without the other feature or features (Greenblatt et al., 1978; Nakra and Hwu, 1982).

The treatments, aside from the discontinuation of neuroleptic administration, that have been reported to be a dramatic help in several cases include dantrolene sodium (to relieve rigidity and hyperpyrexia) and either levodopa or bromocriptine (Granato et al., 1983; May et al., 1983; Mueller et al., 1983). The comparison with anesthesia-induced malignant hyperpyrexia is useful in that both conditions involve the same muscular rigidity, pyrexia, elevation of creatine kinase level, and some response to dantrolene sodium. However, patients who have survived neuroleptic malignant syndrome have been shown not to have muscular sensitivity to halothane. In addition, a butyrophenone neuroleptic has been successfully used to treat the anesthesia-induced hyperpyrexia (Kurlan et al., 1984).

LITHIUM-NEUROLEPTIC COMBINATIONS

The suggestion in a case report (W.J. Cohen and Cohen, 1974) of permanent brain damage after the combined use of lithium and haloperidol merits some discussion. Cohen and Cohen reported four cases of older patients receiving substantial doses of lithium and haloperidol who developed a delirium, fever, and a variety of parkinsonian and cerebellar signs. Two of the four patients recovered fully after discontinuation of medications, whereas the other two patients were left with residual dementia and cerebellar syndromes. This picture resembles that after severe lithium intoxication, which as noted earlier, rarely produces similar residual findings. Depending on the extent of rigidity and fever, the symptom complex may be similar to that of neuroleptic malignant syndrome as well. Several neuroleptic-lithium combinations have been observed to induce reversible neurotoxic reaction. The neuroleptics associated with adverse effects include thioridazine, chlorpromazine, thiothixene, perphenazine, flupentixol, fluphenazine, and haloperidol (Prakash et al., 1983). It does not appear that haloperidol is associated with any unique risks in combination with lithium. Baastrup et al. (1976) reported 425 cases of lithium-haloperidol combination treatment without a single instance of neurotoxicity similar to that described by W.J. Cohen and Cohen (1974). It is clear that lithium and neuroleptics enhance each other's characteristic toxicities. However, the judicious use of these combinations in severe psychopathologic states (such as mania) is warranted and reasonably safe, assuming the use of modest dosages, short combined treatment intervals, and careful clinical monitoring (E.J. Ayd, 1975).

References

(Key references are designated with an asterisk.)

Adams R.D., Victor M. *Principles of Neurology.* 2nd ed. New York, McGraw-Hill, pp. 73–75, 1981.

Anden N.E. Dopamine turnover in the corpus striatum and the limbic system after treatment with neuroleptic and anti-acetylcholine drugs. *J. Pharm. Pharmacol.* 24:905–906, 1972.

*American Psychiatric Association Task Force. *Tardive Dyskinesia.* Washington, DC, American Psychiatric Press, Report No. 18. 1979.

Apte S.N., Langston J.W. Permanent neurological deficits due to lithium toxicity. *Ann. Neurol.* 13:453–455, 1983.

Asper H., Baggliolini M., Burki H.R., et al. Tolerance phenomena with neuroleptics: catalepsy, apomorphine stereotypies and striatal dopamine metabolism in the rat after single and repeated administration of loxapine and haloperidol. *Eur. J. Pharmacol.* 22:287–294, 1973.

Ayd E.J. Jr. Lithium-haloperidol for mania. Is it safe or hazardous? *Int. Drug Ther. Newslett.* 10:29–36, 1975.

Ayd F. A survey of drug induced extrapyramidal reactions. *J.A.M.A.* 175:1054–1060, 1961.

Baastrup P.C., Hollnagel P., Soprenson R., et al. Adverse reactions in treatment with lithium carbonate and haloperidol. *J.A.M.A.* 236:2645–2646, 1976.

*Blass J., Plum F. Metabolic encephalopathies in older adults. In Plum F., ed. *The Neurology of Aging.* New York, Davis, pp. 189–219, 1982.

Bock J.L., Cummings K.C., Jatlow P.I. Amoxapine overdose: a case report. *Am. J. Psychiatry* 139:1619–1620, 1982.

Carlsson A. Biochemical implications of dopa-induced actions on the central nervous system with particular reference to abnormal movements. In Barbeau A., McDowell F.H., eds. L-*Dopa and Parkinsonism.* Philadelphia, Davis, pp. 205–213, 1970.

Caroff S.N. The neuroleptic malignant syndrome. *J. Clin. Psychiatry* 41:79–83, 1980.

Casey D., Rabins P. Tardive dyskinesia as a life threatening illness. *Am. J. Psychiatry* 135:486–488, 1978.

Chase T.N., Schnur J.A., Gordon E.K. Cerebrospinal fluid monoamine catabolites in drug-induced extrapyramidal disorders. *Neuropharmacology* 9:265–268, 1970.

Cohen R.M., Pickar D., Murphy D.L. Myoclonus-associated hypomania during MAO-inhibitor treatment. *Am. J. Psychiatry* 136:105–106, 1980.

Cohen W.J., Cohen N.H. Lithium carbonate, haloperidol and irreversible brain damage. *J.A.M.A.* 230:1283–1287, 1974.

Delay J., Deniker P. Drug-induced extrapyramidal syndromes. In Viken P.J., Bruyn G.W., eds. *Handbook of Clinical Neurology.* Vol. 6. Amsterdam, North Holland, pp. 248–266, 1968.

Dencker S.J., Enoksson P., Johansson R., et al. Late (4–8 years) outcome of treatment with megadoses of fluphenazine enan-

thate in drug refractory schizophrenics. *Acta Psychiatr. Scand.* 63:1–12, 1981.

DePaulo J.R., Folstein M.F., Correa E.I. The course of delirium due to lithium intoxication. *J. Clin. Psychiatry* 43:447–449, 1982.

Folstein M.F., McHugh P.R. Phenomenological approach to the treatment of "organic" psychiatric syndromes. In Wolman B.B., ed. *The Therapist's Handbook: Treatment Methods of Mental Disorders.* New York, Van Nostrand Reinhold, pp. 279–286, 1976.

Folstein M.F., Folstein S.E., McHugh P.R. "Mini-Mental State," a practical method for grading the cognitive state of patients for the clinician. *J. Psychiatr. Res.* 12:189–198, 1975.

Gerlach J. Tardive dyskinesia. *Dan. Med. Bull.* 46:209–245, 1979.

Gerlach J., Reisby N., Randrup A. Dopaminergic hypersensitivity and cholinergic hypofunction in the pathophysiology of tardive dyskinesia. *Psychopharmacologia* 34:21–35, 1974.

Glowinski J., Iverson L.L., Axelrod J. Storage synthesis of norepinephine in the reserpine treated rat brain. *J. Pharmacol. Exp. Ther.* 151:385–399, 1966.

Golinger R.C., Peet T., Tune L. Association of elevated plasma anticholinergic activity with delirium in surgical patients. *Am. J. Psychiatry* 144:1218–1220, 1987.

Granato J.E., Stern B.J., Ringel A., et al. Neuroleptic malignant syndrome: successful treatment with dantrolene and bromocriptine. *Ann. Neurol.* 14:89–90, 1983.

Greenblatt D.J., Gross P.L., Harris J., et al. Fatal hyperthermia following haloperidol therapy of sedative hypnotic withdrawal. *J. Clin. Psychiatry* 39:57–59, 1978.

Hansen H.E., Amdisen A. Lithium intoxication. *Q. J. Med.* 47:123–144, 1978.

Kebabian J., Calne D.B. Multiple receptors for dopamine. *Nature* 277:92–96, 1979.

Kettl P., DePaulo J.R. Maprotiline-induced myoclonus. *J. Clin. Psychopharmacol.* 3:264–265, 1983.

Klawans H. The pharmacology of tardive dyskinesias. *Am. J. Psychiatry* 130:82–86, 1973.

Klawans H., Rubovits R. Effect of cholinergic and anticholinergic agents on tardive dyskinesia. *J. Neurol. Neurosurg. Psychiatry* 27:941–947, 1974.

Kurlan R., Hamill R., Shoulson I. Neuroleptic malignant syndrome. *Clin. Neuropharmacol.* 7:109–120, 1984.

Levenson J.L. Neuroleptic malignant syndrome. *Am. J. Psychiatry* 142:1137–1145, 1985.

Lipowski Z.J. *Delirium: Acute Brain Failure in Man.* Springfield, IL, Thomas, 1989.

Loo H., Bonnel J., Etevenon P., et al. Intellectual efficiency in manic-depressive patients treated with lithium. *Acta Psychiatr. Scand.* 64:423–430, 1981.

Lund Y., Nissen M., Rafaelsen O.J. Long-term lithium treatment and psychological functions. *Acta Psychiatr. Scand.* 65:233–244, 1982.

*Marsden C.D., Jenner P. The pathophysiology of extrapyramidal side effects of neuroleptic drugs. *Psychol. Med.* 10:55–72, 1980.

Marsden C.D., Tarsy D., Baldessarini R.J. Spontaneous and drug induced movement disorders in psychiatric patients. In Benson D.F., Blumer D., eds. *Psychiatric Aspects of Neurologic Disease.* New York, Grune & Stratton, pp. 219–266, 1975.

May D.C., Morris S.W., Steward R.M., et al. Neuroleptic malignant syndrome. Response to dantrolene sodium. *Ann. Intern. Med.* 98:183–184, 1983.

McClelland H., Farquharson R., Leybrun P., et al. Very high dose of fluphenazine. *Arch. Gen. Psychiatry* 33:1435–1439, 1976.

Meldrum B.S., Anlegark G.M., Marsden C.D. Acute dystonia as an idiosyncratic response to neuroleptic drugs in baboons. *Brain* 100:313–326, 1977.

Mueller P.S., Vester J.W., Fermaglich J.F. Neuroleptic malignant syndrome. Successful treatment with bromocriptine. *J.A.M.A.* 249:386–388, 1983.

Myriathopoulos W.C., Kurland A.A., Kurland L.T. Hereditary predisposition in drug induced parkinsonism. *Arch. Neurol.* 6:5–9, 1962.

Nakra B.R.S., Hwu H-G. Catatonic-like syndrome during neuroleptic therapy. *Psychosomatics* 23:769–770, 1982.

Nattel S., Bayne L., Ruedy J. Physostigmine in coma due to drug overdose. *Clin. Pharmacol. Ther.* 25:96–102, 1979.

Parkes J.D., Bedard P., Marsden C.D. Chorea and torsion in parkinsonism (letter). *Lancet* 2:155, 1976.

administration of lithium and a neuroleptic. *Compr. Psychiatry* 23:567–571, 1983.

Rabins P., Tune L., McHugh P.R. Tardive dyskinesia. *Johns Hopkins Med. J.* 148:206–211, 1981.

Robinson A.D.T., McCreadie R.G. The Nithesdale Schizophrenia Survey. V. Follow-up of tardive dyskinesia at 3½ years. *Br. J. Psychiatry* 149:621–623, 1986.

Seeman P. Brain dopamine receptors. *Pharmacol. Rev.* 32:229–313, 1980.

Shaw E.D., Stokes P.E., Mann J.J., et al. Effects of lithium carbonate on the memory of and motor speed of bipolar outpatients. *J. Abnorm. Psychol.* 96:64–69, 1987.

Simpson D.M., Davis G.C. Case report of neuroleptic malignant syndrome associated with withdrawal from amantadine. *Am. J. Psychiatry* 141:796–797, 1984.

Smigan L., Perris C. Memory functions and prophylactic treatment with lithium. *Psychol. Med.* 13:529–536, 1983.

Snyder S.H., Yamamura H.I. Antidepressants and the muscarinic acetylcholine receptor. *Arch. Gen. Psychiatry* 34:236–239, 1977.

Snyder S.H., Banerjee S.P., Yamamura H.I., et al. Drugs, neurotransmitters, and schizophrenia. *Science* 184:1243–1253, 1974.

Sovner R., DiMascio A. Extrapyramidal syndromes and other neurological side effects of psychotropic drugs. In Lipton M., DiMascio A., Killam K., eds. *Psychopharmacology: A Generation of Progress*. New York, Raven Press, pp. 1021–1032, 1978.

Squire L.R., Judd L.L., Janowski D., et al. Effects of lithium carbonate on memory and other cognitive functions. *Am. J. Psychiatry* 137:1042–1046, 1980.

Starkey I.R., Lawson A.A.H. Poisoning with tricyclic and related antidepressants—a ten-year review. *Q. J. Med.* 49:33–49, 1980.

Thomsen K., Schou M. Renal lithium excretion in man. *Am. J. Psychol.* 215:823–827, 1968.

Tune L.E., Coyle J.T. Acute extrapyramidal side effects: serum levels of neuroleptics and anticholinergic drugs. *Psychopharmacology (Berlin)* 75:9–15, 1981.

Tune L.E., Holland A., Folstein M.F., et al. Association of postoperative delirium with raised serum levels of anticholinergic drugs. *Lancet* 2:651–653, 1981.

Tune L.E., Strauss M.E., Lew M.F., et al. Serum levels of anticholinergic drugs and impaired recent memory in chronic schizophrenic patients. *Am. J. Psychiatry* 139:1460–1462, 1982.

Van Putten T. Why do schizophrenic patients refuse to take their drugs? *Arch. Gen. Psychiatry* 31:67–72, 1974.

Waddington J.L., Youssef H.A. An unusual cluster of tardive dyskinesia in schizophrenia: asociation with cognitive dysfunction and negative symptoms. *Am. J. Psychiatry* 143:1162–1165, 1986.

Westheimer R., Klawans H.L. The role of serotonin in the pathophysiology of myoclonic seizures associated with acute imipramine toxicity. *Neurology* 27:1175–1177, 1977.

63

Schizophrenia

Jack A. Grebb
Daniel R. Weinberger
Richard Jed Wyatt

Although many features of schizophrenia remain enigmatic, the conclusion that schizophrenia is a bona fide organic brain disorder is now incontrovertible. Residual doubts about this conclusion arise more from persistent philosophic questions about mental illness than from reasoned criticism of the clinical and research data. This chapter summarizes these data and presents a view of schizophrenia as a neuropsychiatric disorder.

During the past decade, psychiatric diagnosis has increasingly emphasized understandable, reliable, and valid descriptive terms. In the United States, the accepted diagnostic system is found in the *Diagnostic and Statistical Manual of Mental Disorders*, Third Edition, Revised (DSM-III-R) (American Psychiatric Association, 1987). DSM-III-R refers to schizophrenia as a disorder rather than a disease because there are no etiologic, pathophysiologic, or clinical data to warrant conceptualizing schizophrenia as a single disease entity. DSM-III-R defines schizophrenia using explicit inclusion and exclusion criteria, which attempt to be atheoretic regarding the cause of the disorder. The criteria are based only on information from the mental status examination and clinical history of the patient. The criteria, in brief, are as follows: (1) continuous signs of the disorder for at least 6 months, including severe psychotic symptoms (e.g., delusions, hallucinations, disordered verbal communication, and grossly bizarre behavior or affect) for at least 1 week; (2) deterioration in functioning in work, social relations, and self-care; (3) the absence of a full depressive or manic syndrome; (4) the absence of any other diagnosable organic mental disorder.

The application of criteria from DSM-III-R and its predecessors has remedied earlier problems with diagnostic reliability, which led, as in one study, to a twofold difference in the frequency of the diagnosis of schizophrenia between psychiatrists in London and psychiatrists in New York City (Cooper et al., 1972). The two most common misconceptions stemming from the previously vague psychiatric lexicon are that schizophrenia is somehow unique as a thought disorder and that it involves a split personality. Every sign or symptom of disordered thinking that is seen in schizophrenia can also be seen in mania and psychotic depression (Pope and Lipinski, 1981), as well as in diverse organic brain disorders (Maneros, 1988). Although patients with schizophrenia may seem to have fractured psyches, the term *split* inappropriately implies two parts and further confuses schizophrenia with a different disorder involving multiple personalities.

Many schemes have been proposed to subdivide or subtype patients with schizophrenia. These differentiations have resulted in limited clinical or research utility. On purely clinical grounds, DSM-III-R delimits five subtypes: disorganized (previously known as hebephrenic), catatonic, paranoid, undifferentiated, and residual. There is little evidence that genetic factors are specifically associated with these subtypes (Kendler et al., 1988). A newer approach has been to subtype schizophrenia as type I for those patients with predominantly productive, or positive, symptoms (e.g., hallucinations and delusions) and as type II for those patients with predominantly deficit, or negative, symptoms (e.g., affective flattening and anhedonia) (Crow et al., 1982; Walker and Levine, 1988). It is not clear that this approach offers any advantages over the previous subtyping schemes (Kay and Singh, 1989). Although not a formal subtype, late-onset schizophrenia (onset after 45 years old) may be associated more frequently with premorbid schizoid or paranoid traits; visual, tactile, and olfactory hallucinations; persecutory delusions; and perhaps, a more complete response to neuroleptic agents (Harris and Jeste, 1988; Pearlson et al., 1989).

DIFFERENTIAL DIAGNOSIS OF SCHIZOPHRENIA-LIKE SYMPTOMS

The differential diagnosis of schizophrenia-like symptoms includes neurologic and medical conditions that may be clinically indistinguishable from schizophrenia during some phase of their course (Table 63–1) (Davison, 1983; Davison and Bagley, 1969). Nonetheless, patients with neurologic illness associated with psychoses, in general, have more focal neurologic signs, more cognitive impairment, a greater fluctuation in their level of consciousness, and more insight into their illnesses than do patients with schizophrenia.

Table 63–1. DIFFERENTIAL DIAGNOSES OF SCHIZOPHRENIA-LIKE SYMPTOMS

Medical or Neurologic Disorders
Degenerative and/or metabolic illnesses
  Vitamin B$_{12}$ deficiency
  Cerebral lipoidoses
  Fahr's syndrome
  Hallervorden-Spatz disease
  Huntington's disease
  Metachromatic leukodystrophy
  Pellagra
  Wernicke-Korsakoff syndrome
  Wilson's disease
Disorders induced by drugs such as
  Amphetamine, belladonna, alkaloids, alcohol or barbiturate
    withdrawal, cocaine, disulfiram, lysergic acid diethylamide,
    mescaline, phenylpropylamine, tetrahydrocannabinol,
    phencyclidine
Endocrinopathies
  Thyroid
  Adrenal
Epilepsy
Infections
  Acquired immunodeficiency syndrome
  Creutzfeldt-Jakob disease
  Herpes encephalitis
  Neurosyphilis
Immunologic conditions
  Systemic lupus erythematosus
  Other vasculitides
Normal-pressure hydrocephalus
Stroke
Toxic
  Carbon monoxide poisoning
  Heavy metal exposure
Trauma (especially limbic frontal)
Tumor (especially limbic frontal)
Psychiatric (DSM-III-R) Disorders
Schizophrenia
Schizophreniform disorder
Brief reactive psychosis
Mood disorders
Schizoaffective disorder
Psychotic disorder not otherwise specified (atypical psychosis)
Delusional disorder
Personality disorders
  Schizotypal
  Schizoid
  Borderline
Factitious disorder with psychologic symptoms
Malingering
Autistic disorder
Pervasive developmental disorder (not otherwise specified)

Schizophrenia-like symptoms can also be present in a range of psychiatric disorders (see Table 63–1). Schizophreniform disorder is diagnosed when the symptoms of schizophrenia have been present for less than 6 months. The diagnosis of brief reactive psychosis is made when the symptoms are present for less than 1 month and there is a history of one or more psychosocial stressors of major proportions. Psychosis can be a symptom of mood disorders (previously called the affective disorders). The symptoms of mania can mimic the positive symptoms of schizophrenia, and the symptoms of depression can mimic the negative symptoms. A diagnosis of schizoaffective disorder is appropriate if a patient has symptoms of both a mood disorder and schizophrenia. Atypical psychosis is the diagnosis used when psychotic symptoms fit no other diagnostic category. In the delusional disorders (previously called the paranoid disorders), delusions—which can be persecutory, grandiose, somatic, jealous, or erotomanic—predominate over other symptoms. One of three personality disorders—schizotypal, schizoid, and borderline—may be an appropriate diagnosis if the patient has symptoms suggestive of schizophrenia but does not demonstrate these symptoms with enough severity to warrant a diagnosis of schizophrenia. To support a diagnosis of a personality disorder, the symptoms must be long-standing. A diagnosis of factitious disorder with psychologic symptoms necessitates that the symptoms be under the patient's voluntary control and that the motivation arise from psychodynamic issues, whereas malingering is identified when the goal of symptoms is more obviously self-serving. The differentiation between factitious disorder and malingering can be difficult.

In practice, if a child meets the diagnostic criteria for schizophrenia, she or he is considered to have schizophrenia occurring in childhood. There is no specific diagnosis of childhood schizophrenia. The symptoms of autistic disorder include a marked impairment of social interactions and communication, as well as a severely restricted range of interests. In infants and young children, autistic disorder is much more common than schizophrenia; however, if an infant or a young child evidences prominent delusions or hallucinations, schizophrenia is the appropriate diagnosis.

A number of insights into schizophrenia can be gained from the variety of neurologic diseases with schizophrenia-like symptoms. Disorders with unitary causes (e.g., tertiary syphilis and Huntington's disease) can have a wide range of psychopathologic symptoms (Caine and Shoulson, 1983), suggesting that the cause of one case of schizophrenia may, in another individual, produce a different psychiatric syndrome. Furthermore, a single neurologic syndrome (e.g., parkinsonism and dementia) can have many different causes, supporting the possibility that schizophrenia is a heterogeneous disorder.

It has also been observed that when psychotic symptoms are clinically evident in a neurologic disorder (e.g., Fahr's syndrome [Cummings et al., 1983], systemic lupus erythematosus [Feinglass et al., 1976], and metachromatic leukodystrophy [Haltia et al., 1980]), they tend to occur early in the course. As the disease progresses, and presumably as the pathologic alteration becomes more extensive, classic neurologic symptoms eclipse psychiatric ones. It is perhaps an important clue to the neuropathologic process of schizophrenia that what separates this psychiatric disorder from neurologic disorders is the failure of classic neurologic symptoms to develop. It is predictable, therefore, that the pathologic findings in schizophrenia would be more subtle than those of neurologic diseases and that the neuropathologic process would be relatively static.

It has been observed that younger adult patients are more likely than older adult patients to develop psychotic symptoms as part of the clinical picture of a neurologic disorder (Weinberger, 1987). An intrinsic property of the brain of young adults may make it more vulnerable to the development of psychotic symptoms as result of a variety of neuropathologic processes. Finally, there is clinical diversity in the medical and neurologic disorders listed in Table 63–1. For example, not all young adults who have cerebral lipoidosis have psychotic symptoms. This observation reflects the currently unanswerable question regarding what effects premorbid disposition and/or environment have on the development of psychiatric symptoms in either neurologic disorders or schizophrenia.

CLINICAL ASPECTS OF SCHIZOPHRENIA AND ITS TREATMENT

Epidemiology

Estimates of the incidence of schizophrenia in the United States and Europe range between 0.3 and 0.6 per 1000. The prevalence is between 0.25 and 1.0% (Hare, 1987). The prevalence of schizophrenia may vary geographically, but only to a small degree (Torrey, 1980). Onset is most common in the third decade of life and is rare before age 10 years or after age 40 years. Individuals of lower socioeconomic status in an urban environment may be at greater risk (Saugstad, 1989). There is excessive mortality among schizophrenic patients (Allebeck, 1989; Buda et al., 1989), probably related to an increased number of accidents, poor hygiene, and inadequate health care. Approximately 50% of schizophrenic patients have attempted suicide, with perhaps 10% succeeding during a 20-year follow-up (Tsuang, 1978). As is the case with all psychiatric patients, the best predictor of a future suicide attempt is a past suicide attempt. The abuse of a variety of stimulant drugs, but not sedatives, is more common among schizophrenic individuals than among other groups (Schneier and Siris, 1987).

Course and Prognosis

Historically, the course and prognosis of schizophrenia have been considered almost invariably to be characterized by deterioration. Since 1940, perhaps because of improved treatment or because of an evolution of the disorder itself, the course of schizophrenia seems to be less malignant. Bleuler (1972) summarized the findings of his longitudinal studies with schizophrenic patients identified between 1928 and 1943 by stating that "intensified therapeutic methods applied in recent decades [before the introduction of neuroleptics] have been able to combat with considerable success the catastrophe-schizophrenias" (i.e., schizophrenia with acute onset, severe and chronic symptoms, and no periods of remissions). Of the individuals studied in the era before effective antipsychotic drugs were available, 19 (10%) of 187 schizophrenic probands or their relatives experienced catastrophe-schizophrenia. Of the individuals whom Bleuler (1972) studied in the era after the introduction of effective antipsychotic drugs, only 3 (1%) of 262 schizophrenic probands or their relatives had catastrophe-schizophrenia. This difference in occurrence is statistically significant. Bleuler does not believe, however, that the therapeutic methods introduced in the 1930s affected the unfavorable outcomes of schizophrenic patients who had a more gradual onset.

Long-term follow-up studies using modern standardized diagnostic criteria and multiple measures of outcome (e.g., hospitalization and clinical and social state) found recovery rates of 20–50% in patients followed for 4–20 years (Ciompi, 1988). Nevertheless, 30–60% of schizophrenic patients are socially isolated, unemployed, and institutionalized for much of their lives (Scottish Schizophrenia Research Group, 1988). Several features predictive of more favorable outcome have been identified (Table 63–2) (Kay and Lindenmayer, 1987; McGlashan, 1986).

Genetic Considerations

Many research studies have demonstrated a clear genetic influence in the development of schizophrenia (McGuffin et al., 1987). The data from genetic studies indicate significantly higher rates of schizo-

Table 63–2. FEATURES PREDICTIVE OF MORE FAVORABLE OUTCOME IN SCHIZOPHRENIA

Later onset
Acute onset
Obvious precipitating factors
Good premorbid social, sexual, and work history
Affective symptoms (especially depression)
Absence of assaultiveness or violence
Married
Family history of mood disorders or alcoholism
Absence of a family history of schizophrenia
Female sex

phrenia in relatives of schizophrenic probands: 5% in parents, 10% in children. Monozygotic twins are approximately 30–50% concordant for schizophrenia, whereas dizygotic twins are 5–10% concordant, approximately the same rate as for nontwin siblings. Monozygotic twins reared apart have approximately the same concordance rate as those raised together, suggesting that a genetic factor influencing vulnerability, when present sufficiently, can overwhelm any nonspecific environmental differences.

The mode of genetic transmission is unknown. Although one group of investigators reported a linkage between markers on chromosome 5 and schizophrenia in a number of families (Sherrington et al., 1988), other investigators studying different pedigrees have not found a similar linkage (Detera-Wadleigh et al., 1989; Kennedy et al., 1988). Possible reasons for the lack of replicability include genetic heterogeneity, polygenic transmission, incomplete penetrance, and technical difficulties with the experimental methodologies (Owen and Mullan, 1990).

Given the current level of knowledge, it is possible to hypothesize that some schizophrenic patients have a disease that is purely genetic, some have a disease that is both genetic and environmental, and some have a disease representing primarily environmental impact on a normal brain. It is of note that 80–90% of schizophrenic patients do not have a first-degree relative with schizophrenia, and any model of this disorder must incorporate interaction between genetics and the environment.

Psychosocial Considerations

No carefully controlled studies identify a specific psychosocial factor in the development of schizophrenia (Liem, 1980). Proponents of the psychosocial cause of schizophrenia point to the discordance in monozygotic twins to support their position. It is important to remember, however, that few genetic illnesses of any type have 100% concordance in monozygotic twins. From the clinician's point of view, the absence of clear evidence supporting psychosocial etiologic factors makes the risks of inducing guilt in the family or resentment in the patient by implying such factors unacceptable. Furthermore, preconceived notions about psychosocial factors may augment the significant stigma experienced by schizophrenic individuals and their families (Wahl and Harman, 1989).

A role for psychosocial factors in affecting the course of schizophrenia has also been proposed. Perhaps analogous to the way that psychosocial stress affects the course of medical illnesses (e.g., diabetes, epilepsy, and multiple sclerosis), stressful life events (Dohrenwend and Egri, 1981) and family settings with high levels of expressed negative emotion (Koenigsberg and Handley, 1986) have been reported to increase the frequency and severity of schizophrenic relapses. When family therapy is spe-

cifically directed at the level of expressed emotion in affected families, it may reduce the number and severity of relapses (Falloon et al., 1985). Some researchers question a causal relationship between expressed negative emotion and relapse and suggest that families with higher expressed emotion are responding to more severely ill family members (Parker et al., 1988). It remains clear, however, that the combined use of pharmacotherapy and psychosocial support is more effective than either therapeutic modality alone (Wyatt et al., 1988). It also seems reasonable to provide support not only to the patient but also to the family to help them cope with this debilitating illness. There is no justifiable role, however, for long-term insight-oriented psychotherapy as the primary therapy for schizophrenia.

Biologic Treatments

Antipsychotic or neuroleptic medications are the single most effective treatment of schizophrenia, as measured by reducing acute psychotic symptoms, preventing relapse, and lowering the amount of time spent in the hospital (Davis et al., 1982). A common clinical error in the use of these drugs is the administration of doses that are higher than necessary (Cole, 1982). Unfortunately, research has not yet shown that measuring neuroleptic plasma concentrations is of clinical use, except perhaps as a gross measure of compliance and absorption.

The most serious neurologic adverse effects of antipsychotic drugs are tardive dyskinesia and neuroleptic malignant syndrome. The major medication-related correlate of the development of tardive dyskinesia is the total length of time that the patient receives neuroleptics. Neuroleptic malignant syndrome is a rare complication and is characterized by life-threatening autonomic instability, hyperthermia, and muscular rigidity. Its early symptoms can mimic catatonia, resulting in the incorrect clinical decision to increase the antipsychotic dosage rather than to discontinue the medication (Kaufmann and Wyatt, 1987).

A major pharmacologic advance in the treatment of schizophrenia has been the introduction of clozapine (Lieberman et al., 1989). Unlike other antipsychotic medications, clozapine is a weak dopamine D_2 receptor antagonist. Its antipsychotic mechanism of action remains uncertain. Clozapine has been reported to be significantly more effective in treating both the positive and negative symptoms of schizophrenia, especially in chronically ill patients. Clozapine has not been associated with the appearance of tardive dyskinesia. The administration of clozapine requires careful hematologic monitoring because the medicine is associated with agranulocytosis in 1–2% of patients in the first year of treatment. Unfortunately, this hematologic monitoring can cost as much as $9000/year.

Many other pharmacologic agents have been used

in treating schizophrenia. Most initial reports of positive results have not been replicated. Nonetheless, because of diagnostic difficulties in distinguishing schizophrenia from psychotic mood disorders, a trial of lithium carbonate and/or carbamazepine is warranted in some patients with a psychotic illness. Electroconvulsive therapy may be effective in patients with affective or catatonic symptoms and shorter durations of illness. Benzodiazepines may be useful in the treatment of catatonia and agitation. None of the myriad research clinical trials has yet produced data that would support the use of any other biologic treatments in routine clinical settings.

NEUROLOGIC FINDINGS IN SCHIZOPHRENIA

Whereas the preceding discussion emphasized what is reasonably well known about schizophrenia, the remainder of this chapter is about research findings and related hypothetic formulations. A general observation about many biologic measurements in schizophrenic populations is that this group usually has more interindividual variability than a control group. This is consistent with the clinical, and probable etiologic, heterogeneity of schizophrenia.

Physical Examination

Many studies indicate that patients with schizophrenia have more physical anomalies (Green et al., 1989) and abnormal neurologic findings than either affectively ill patients or normal controls. Minor, or soft, neurologic signs are found in 50–100% of schizophrenic patients (Heinrichs and Buchanan, 1988; Youssef and Waddington, 1988). The most consistently observed minor signs are motor stereotypies, tics, dystonic movements, poor coordination, and so-called frontal-release signs. Interruption of smooth ocular pursuit movements, paroxysmal saccadic eye movements, and episodic lateral deviation of the eyes are also frequently observed in patients with schizophrenia and their first-degree relatives (Holzman et al., 1988; Siever et al., 1989). Some studies correlated the presence of neurologic abnormalities with severity of illness, disordered thinking, abnormal behavior, asocial behavior, and violence, thus suggesting a parallelism between the evidence of brain disease and the severity of schizophrenia. Children at risk for schizophrenia, because of having an affected parent, show more abnormalities on neurologic examination, neuropsychologic testing, and electrophysiologic recordings (Erlenmeyer-Kimling et al., 1982).

Neuropsychologic Testing

Despite the long-standing definition of schizophrenia as a thought disorder in the presence of normal cognition, the conclusion is inescapable that the majority of schizophrenic patients have cognitive impairment (Seidman, 1983). The most consistent abnormalities are in attention as measured by the continuous performance test, in problem solving as assessed by the Wisconsin Card Sort Test, and in recall memory as assessed by the Wechsler Memory Scale. In a study of monozygotic twins discordant for schizophrenia, the affected twin in every pair performed more poorly than the unaffected twin on at least one of these tests (Goldberg et al., 1990). The deficits may be present at the onset of illness or early in its course (Goldberg and Weinberger, 1988; Goldberg et al., 1988). The patterns of cognitive deficits have been variously interpreted as suggesting left-sided (Robertson and Taylor, 1987), temporal (Gruzelier et al., 1988), or dorsolateral prefrontal dysfunction (Weinberger, 1988).

Electrophysiologic Testing

Abnormal electroencephalograms have been reported in 20–40% of patients with schizophrenia (Grebb et al., 1986). Nonspecific increases in theta and delta activity independent of drug treatment are the most frequently described findings. Computer-analyzed topographic electroencephalographic mapping has demonstrated generalized increases in slow activity (Karson et al., 1987). It has also been reported that a decrease in alpha activity may be associated with enlarged cerebral ventricles (Karson et al., 1988).

In Vivo Brain Metabolism Studies

The in vivo brain imaging techniques of regional cerebral blood flow and positron emission tomography (PET) have provided valuable insights into regional brain function in schizophrenia. The weight of data from regional cerebral blood flow studies indicates decreased frontal blood flow in schizophrenic individuals (Mathew et al., 1988), especially when the studies have been conducted with cognitive activation procedures specific for the dorsolateral prefrontal cortex (Fig. 63–1) (Weinberger et al., 1988). This inability to increase blood flow to the dorsolateral prefrontal cortex may be correlated with the presence of enlarged cerebral ventricles (Berman et al., 1987) and is specifically seen with cognitive tests of dorsolateral prefrontal cortex and not with cognitive tests of more posterior regions (Berman et al., 1988).

Unfortunately, PET studies have been less consistent in their conclusions, variously reporting left- or right-sided abnormalities, the presence or absence of hypofrontality, and hypoactivity or hyperactivity of deep brain nuclei. The inconsistent PET results probably reflect, in part, that most of the PET studies were performed with the subjects in the resting state, a physiologically variable condition that does not

PERCENT CHANGE MAPS OF WCS/NUMBERS

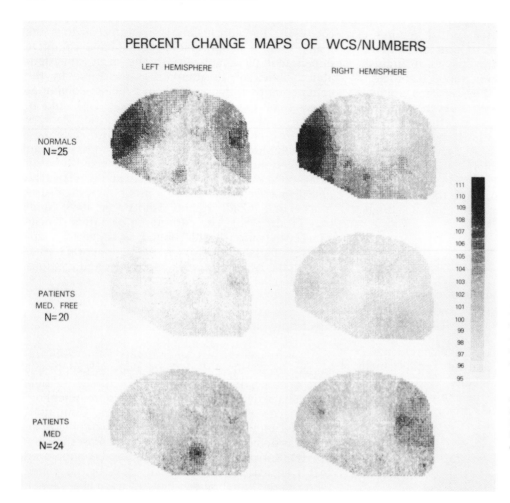

Figure 63–1. Regional cerebral blood flow study. Lateral view (anterior pole at left) of left and right hemisphere percent change in regional cerebral blood flow during the Wisconsin Card Sort (WCS) Test compared with regional cerebral blood flow during a number-matching control task. Data are for 25 normal control subjects *(top)*, 20 medication-free patients *(middle)*, and 24 antipsychotic drug–treated patients *(bottom)*. Note that the control subjects, unlike either patient group, show striking regional cerebral blood flow increases (i.e., darker shades) during the test, in an area corresponding to dorsolateral prefrontal cortex. (Adapted from Weinberger D.R., Berman K.F., Zec R.F. Physiological dysfunction of dorsolateral prefrontal cortex in schizophrenia: I. Regional cerebral blood flow [rCBF] evidence. *Arch. Gen. Psychiatry* 43:114–125, 1986; and Berman K.F., Zec R.F., Weinberger D.R. Physiological dysfunction of dorsolateral prefrontal cortex in schizophrenia: II. Role of neuroleptic treatment, attention, and mental effect. *Arch. Gen. Psychiatry* 43:126–130, 1986.)

control adequately for individual differences in the experience of the procedure (Weinberger and Berman, 1988). The question of whether there is an increase in the number of dopamine D_2 receptors in never-medicated patients with schizophrenia remains unresolved because one PET study found an increased number (Wong et al., 1986), whereas two other similar studies found no increase (Farde et al., 1990; Martinot et al., 1990).

In Vivo Anatomic Studies

The fundamental conclusion from computed tomographic (CT) and magnetic resonance imaging (MRI) studies is that there is incontrovertible evidence of brain pathologic change in schizophrenia. Well more than 50 controlled CT studies have reported lateral and third ventricular enlargement and dilated cortical sulci in schizophrenic individuals (Shelton and Weinberger, 1986). In the vast majority of studies, the degree of ventricular enlargement is not correlated with the length of illness, thereby suggesting that the pathologic alteration in most cases of schizophrenia is static and independent of drug treatment artifacts. Nevertheless, because occasional reports demonstrated a correlation between the duration of illness and the degree of ventricular

enlargement on CT scans, the possibility that the pathologic change may be progressive in some cases of schizophrenia cannot be ruled out. The lack of an association between these CT findings and identifiable treatment factors is supported by the demonstration of enlarged ventricles and dilated cortical sulci in first-episode patients; in addition, these same findings were reported in pneumoencephalographic studies before the introduction of neuroleptic drugs. Clinically, the patients with CT findings seem to have greater cognitive impairment, more deficit symptoms, poorer response to neuroleptic drugs, poorer premorbid social adjustment, and a more frequent history of perinatal complications and left-handedness. These associations suggest that patients with schizophrenia are a more neurologically impaired subgroup.

Several MRI studies suggested that medial temporal lobe structures (e.g., hippocampus and parahippocampal gyrus) may be up to 20% smaller in schizophrenic individuals (DeLisi et al., 1988; Suddath et al., 1989). More recent studies compared schizophrenic patients with well siblings, including discordant monozygotic twins (Suddath et al., 1989). These studies showed that the schizophrenic patients almost invariably have larger lateral and third ventricles and smaller hippocampi than their unaffected siblings (Fig. 63–2). These data suggest that a subtle

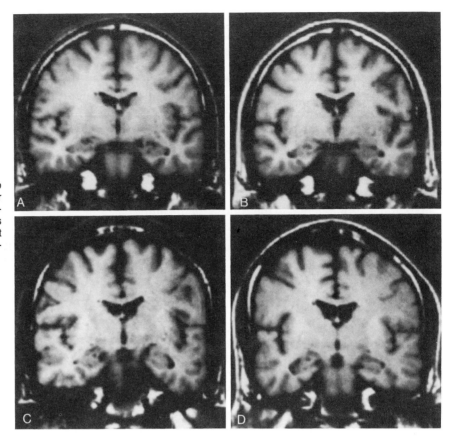

Figure 63–2. MRI coronal sections from two sets of monozygotic twins discordant for schizophrenia. Compared with the unaffected twins (*A* and *C*), the affected twins (*B* and *D*) demonstrate subtle enlargement of the lateral ventricles, even when the affected twin had small ventricles.

reduction of cerebral volume, especially in the anteromedial temporal lobe, may be present in most schizophrenic individuals.

Postmortem Brain Studies

The two main directions of postmortem brain studies have been neurochemical and morphometric. The most consistent neurotransmitter finding is an increased number of dopamine receptors, particularly in the nucleus accumbens (Kleinman et al., 1988). It remains unknown whether this increase is primary in schizophrenia or is related to treatment with antipsychotic drugs. Most postmortem studies have not reported the presence of pathologic gliosis, suggesting that schizophrenia is not associated with an active degenerative pathologic process. The most consistent postmortem finding, which was reported in at least six studies, is a relatively localized decrease in brain tissue volume in the anteromedial temporal lobe, including the hippocampus and the parahippocampal gyrus (Altshuler et al., 1990; Bogerts et al., 1985; Brown et al., 1986; Falkai et al., 1988; Jakob and Beckmann, 1986; Jeste and Lohr, 1989). Although most of these reports have been based on morphometric analyses, one study reported cytoarchitectural anomalies in entorhinal cortex that implicate a developmental disorder (Jakob and Beckmann, 1986). The postmortem data, combined with the results of MRI studies in young patients during life, represent compelling evidence for a temporal lobe lesion in schizophrenia.

NEUROPSYCHIATRIC INTEGRATION OF CLINICAL AND RESEARCH DATA

Anatomic Location

The most frequently implicated brain regions are the frontal cortex, the limbic system, and the diencephalon. The evidence implicating the frontal cortex, particularly the dorsolateral aspect, includes the similarity of neuropsychologic deficits in schizophrenia to symptoms associated with dorsolateral prefrontal lesions (Stuss and Benson, 1984). The neuropsychologic profile for lesions of the orbitomedial frontal cortex does not fit as well with schizophrenia as does the profile for lesions of the dorsolateral cortex. Evidence of cortical sulcal prominence on CT and MRI studies, eye tracking abnormalities (possibly representing a pathologic process in the frontal eye fields), regional cerebral blood flow abnormalities using cognitive activation procedures, and results of some of the PET studies also support physiologic dysfunction of the frontal cortex in schizophrenia.

A comprehensive review of neurologic conditions with schizophrenic-like symptoms suggested that the limbic system, particularly the temporal lobe and the diencephalon, is the region most frequently involved (Davison and Bagley, 1969). The postmortem studies demonstrating pathologic change in these regions and the CT and MRI data suggestive of diencephalic and temporal lobe pathologic processes support this observation.

It is not unreasonable that three different brain regions are implicated in schizophrenia. Much like the situation in the aphasias, lesions in different regions of a complex brain circuit may result in a set of syndromes involving the particular brain function. It is certainly reasonable to assume that a brain circuit involving the frontal cortex, the limbic system, and the diencephalon affects thinking and emotions. Indeed, this circuit constitutes much of the circuit of Papez and is fundamental to the concept of the limbic system (MacLean, 1990). The reciprocal innervations of the thalamus, the hippocampal region, and the frontal cortex are well established.

Pathophysiology

Some of the research data from CT, MRI, and postmortem studies suggest the presence of a relatively static lesion that is already present at the time symptoms first appear. It is not known whether this putative lesion is the result of degeneration and/or abnormal brain development. It is also not known whether the hypothesized degeneration or abnormal development results from a genetically determined defect, an environmental insult, or an interaction between the two. How this lesion remains clinically dormant for the first 2–3 decades of an individual's life and how it is then associated with functional decompensation are matters for speculation (Weinberger, 1987), but few leads exist to address these questions.

The dominant neurochemical hypothesis generating research during the past 3 decades has been that schizophrenia is caused by a hyperfunctional dopamine system. The major support for this is the close correlation between the clinical potencies of antipsychotic drugs and their abilities to block dopamine D_2 receptors (Wyatt, 1976). Other clinical research (e.g., cerebrospinal fluid studies of dopamine metabolites and postmortem brain studies) offers only limited evidence for this hypothesis, and it may be that blocking dopamine receptors is merely an effective way of controlling schizophrenic symptoms and does not relate to the primary functional pathophysiologic process in schizophrenia. The cloning and sequencing of the dopamine receptor family and the introduction of new antipsychotic drug treatments (e.g., clozapine) may help advance the neurochemical understanding of the treatment of schizophrenia.

SUMMARY

Schizophrenia is a disorder that involves the brain. Although the characteristics of the lesion and the pathophysiology of the disease process remain un-

certain, evidence is increasingly focusing on developmental abnormalities involving the anteromedial temporal lobe. There may well be multiple disease processes that result in the symptom pattern called schizophrenia. The further application of brain imaging techniques and molecular genetics and cellular neuroscience methods toward solving these mysteries will undoubtedly advance the understanding of schizophrenia.

References

(Key references are designated with an asterisk.)

Allebeck P. Schizophrenia: a life-shortening disease. *Schizophr. Bull.* 15:81–89, 1989.

Altshuler L.L., Casanova M.F., Goldberg T.E., et al. The hippocampus and parahippocampus in schizophrenic suicide and control brains. *Arch. Gen. Psychiatry* 47:1029–1034, 1990.

American Psychiatric Association. *Diagnostic and Statistical Manual of Mental Disorders, DSM-III-R.* 3rd ed. revised. Washington, DC, American Psychiatric Association, 1987.

Berman K.F., Zec R.F., Weinberger D.R. Physiological dysfunction of dorsolateral prefrontal cortex in schizophrenia: II. Role of neuroleptic treatment, attention, and mental effort. *Arch. Gen. Psychiatry* 43:126–130, 1986.

Berman K.F., Weinberger D.R., Shelton R.C., et al. A relationship between anatomical and physiological brain pathology in schizophrenia: lateral cerebral ventricular size predicts cortical blood flow. *Am. J. Psychiatry* 144:1277–1282, 1987.

Berman K.F., Illowsky B.P., Weinberger D.R. Physiological dysfunction of dorsolateral prefrontal cortex in schizophrenia. IV. Further evidence for regional and behavioral specificity. *Arch. Gen. Psychiatry* 45:616–622, 1988.

*Bleuler M. (1972) *The Schizophrenic Disorders: Long-Term Patient and Family Studies* (translated by S.M. Clemens). New Haven, CT, Yale University Press, p. 213, 1978.

Bogerts B., Meertz E., Schönfeldt-Bausch R. Basal ganglia and limbic system pathology in schizophrenia. *Arch. Gen. Psychiatry* 42:784–791, 1985.

Brown R., Colter N., Corsellis J.A.N., et al. Postmortem evidence of structural brain changes in schizophrenia. *Arch. Gen. Psychiatry* 43:36–42, 1986.

Buda M., Tsuang M.T., Fleming J.A. Causes of death in DSM-III schizophrenics and other psychotics (atypical group). *Arch. Gen. Psychiatry* 45:283–285, 1988.

Caine E.G., Shoulson I. Psychiatric syndromes in Huntington's disease. *Am. J. Psychiatry* 140:728–733, 1983.

Ciompi L. Learning from outcome studies. Toward a comprehensive biological-psychosocial understanding of schizophrenia. *Schizophr. Res.* 1:373–384, 1988.

Cole J.O. Psychopharmacology update—antipsychotic drugs: is more better? *McLean Hosp. J.* 7:61–87, 1982.

Cooper J.E., Kendell R.E., Gorland B.J., et al. *Psychiatric Diagnosis in New York and London.* New York, Oxford University Press, 1972.

Crow T.J., Cross A.J., Johnstone E.C., et al. Two syndromes in schizophrenia and their pathogenesis. In Henn F.A., Nasrallah H.A., eds. *Schizophrenia as a Brain Disease.* New York, Oxford University Press, pp. 196–234, 1982.

Cummings J.L., Gosenfeld L.F., Houlihan J.P., et al. Neuropsychiatric disturbance associated with idiopathic calcification of the basal ganglia. *Biol. Psychiatry* 18:591–601, 1983.

Davis J.M., Janicak P., Chang S., et al. Recent advances in the pharmacologic treatment of schizophrenic disorders. In Grinspoon L., ed. *Psychiatry 1982: The American Psychiatric Association Annual Review Psychiatry Updates.* Vol. I. Washington, DC, American Psychiatric Press, pp. 178–228, 1982.

Davison K. Schizophrenia-like psychoses associated with organic cerebral disorders: a review. *Psychiatr. Dev.* 1:1–31, 1983.

Davison K., Bagley C.R. Schizophrenia-like psychoses associated with

with organic disorders of the central nervous system: a review of the literature. *Br. J. Psychiatry* (special publication 4):113–184, 1969.

DeLisi L.E., Dauphinais I.D., Gershon E.S. Perinatal complications and reduced size of brain limbic structures in familial schizophrenia. *Schizophr. Bull.* 14:185–191, 1988.

Detera-Wadleigh S.D., Goldin L.R., Sherrington R., et al. Exclusion of linkage to 5q11–13 in families with schizophrenia and other psychiatric disorders. *Nature* 340:391–393, 1989.

Dohrenwend B.P., Egri G. Recent stressful life events and episodes of schizophrenia. *Schizophr. Bull.* 7:12–23, 1981.

Erlenmeyer-Kimling L., Cornblatt B., Friedman D., et al. Neurological, electrophysiological, and attentional deviations in children at risk for schizophrenia. In Henn F.A., Nasrallah H.A., eds. *Schizophrenia as a Brain Disease.* New York, Oxford University Press, pp. 61–98, 1982.

Falkai P., Bogerts B., Rozumek M. Limbic pathology in schizophrenia: the entorhinal region—a morphometric study. *Biol. Psychiatry* 24:515–521, 1988.

*Falloon I.R.H., Boyd J.L., McGill C.W., et al. Family management in the prevention of morbidity of schizophrenia. *Arch. Gen. Psychiatry* 42:887–896, 1985.

Farde L., Wisel F.-A., Stone-Elander S., et al. D$_2$ dopamine receptors in neuroleptic-naive schizophrenic patients. *Arch. Gen. Psychiatry* 47:213–219, 1990.

Feinglass E.J., Arnett F.C., Dorsch C.A., et al. Neuropsychiatric manifestations of systemic lupus erythematosus: diagnosis, clinical aspects, and relationship to other features of the disease. *Medicine* 55:323–339, 1976.

Goldberg T.E., Weinberger D.R. Probing prefrontal function in schizophrenia with neuropsychological paradigms. *Schizophr. Bull.* 14:179–183, 1988.

Goldberg T.E., Karson C.E., Leleszi J.P., et al. Intellectual impairment in adolescent psychosis. A controlled psychometric study. *Schizophr. Res.* 1:261–266, 1988.

Goldberg T.E., Ragland J.D., Gold J.M., et al. Neuropsychological assessment of monozygotic twins discordant for schizophrenia. *Arch. Gen. Psychiatry* 47:1066–1072, 1990.

Grebb J.A., Weinberger D.R., Morihisa J.M. Electroencephalogram and evoked potential studies of schizophrenia. In Nasrallah H.A., Weinberger D.R., ed. *Handbook of Schizophrenia.* Amsterdam, Elsevier, pp. 121–140, 1986.

Green M.F., Satz P., Gaier D.J., et al. Minor physical anomalies in schizophrenia. *Schizophr. Bull.* 15:91–99, 1989.

Gruzelier J., Seymour K., Wilson L., et al. Impairments on neuropsychologic tests of temporohippocampal and frontohippocampal functions and word fluency in remitting schizophrenia and affective disorders. *Arch. Gen. Psychiatry* 45:623–629, 1988.

Haltia T., Palo J., Haltia M., et al. Juvenile metachromatic leukodystrophy: clinical, biochemical, and neuropathologic studies in nine new cases. *Arch. Neurol.* 37:42–46, 1980.

Hare E.H. Epidemiology of schizophrenia and affective psychoses. *Br. Med. Bull.* 43:514–530, 1987.

Harris M.J., Jeste D.V. Late-onset schizophrenia: an overview. *Schizophr. Bull.* 14:39–55, 1988.

Heinrichs D.W., Buchanan R.W. Significance and meaning of neurological signs in schizophrenia. *Am. J. Psychiatry* 145:11–18, 1988.

Holzman P.S., Kringler E., Matthysse S., et al. A single dominant gene can account for eye tracking dysfunction and schizophrenia in offspring of discordant twins. *Arch. Gen. Psychiatry* 45:641–647, 1988.

Jakob H., Beckmann H. Prenatal developmental disturbances in the limbic allocortex in schizophrenics. *J. Neural Transm.* 65:303–326, 1986.

Jeste D.V., Lohr J.B. Hippocampal pathologic findings in schizophrenia. *Arch. Gen. Psychiatry* 46:1019–1024, 1989.

Karson C.N., Coppola R., Morihisa J.M., et al. Computed electroencephalographic activity mapping in schizophrenia. *Arch. Gen. Psychiatry* 44:514–517, 1987.

Karson C.N., Coppola R., Daniel D.G. Alpha frequency in schizophrenia: an association with enlarged cerebral ventricles. *Am. J. Psychiatry* 145:861–864, 1988.

Kaufmann C.A., Wyatt R.J. Neuroleptic malignant syndrome. In Meltzer, H.Y., ed. *Psychopharmacology: The Third Generation of Progress.* New York, Raven Press, pp. 1421–1430, 1987.

Kay S.R., Lindenmayer J.-P. Outcome predictors in acute schizophrenia. Prospective significance of background and clinical dimensions. *J. Nerv. Ment. Dis.* 175:152–160, 1987.

Kay S.R., Singh M.M. The positive-negative distinction in drug-free schizophrenic patients. Stability, response to neuroleptics, and prognostic significance. *Arch. Gen. Psychiatry* 46:711–718, 1989.

Kendler K.S., Gruenberg A.M., Tsuang M.T. A family study of the subtypes of schizophrenia. *Am. J. Psychiatry* 145:57–62, 1988.

Kennedy J.L., Giuffra L.A., Moises H.W., et al. Evidence against linkage of schizophrenia to markers on chromosome 5 in a northern Swedish pedigree. *Nature* 336:167–170, 1988.

Kleinman J.E., Casanova M.F., Jaskiw G.E. The neuropathology of schizophrenia. *Schizophr. Bull.* 14:209–216, 1988.

Koenigsberg H.W., Handley R. Expressed emotion: from predictive index to clinical construct. *Am. J. Psychiatry* 143:1361–1373, 1986.

*Lieberman J.A., Kane J.M., Johns C.A. Clozapine: guidelines for clinical management. *J. Clin. Psychiatry* 50:329–338, 1989.

Liem J.H. Family studies of schizophrenia: an update and commentary. *Schizophr. Bull.* 6:429–454, 1980.

*MacLean P.D. *The Triune Brain in Evolution.* New York, Plenum Publishing, pp. 269–313, 1990.

Marneros A. Schizophrenic first-rank symptoms in organic mental disorders. *Br. J. Psychiatry* 152:625–628, 1988.

Martinot J.-L., Peron Magnan P., Huret J.-D., et al. Striatal D$_2$ dopaminergic receptors assessed with positron emission tomography and [^{76}Br]bromospiperone in untreated schizophrenic patients. *Am. J. Psychiatry* 147:44–50, 1990.

Mathew R.J., Wilson W.H., Tant S.R., et al. Abnormal resting regional cerebral blood flow patterns and their correlates in schizophrenia. *Arch. Gen. Psychiatry* 45:542–549, 1988.

McGlashan T.H. The prediction of outcome in chronic schizophrenia. IV. The Chestnut Lodge follow-up study. *Arch. Gen. Psychiatry* 43:167–176, 1986.

McGuffin P., Murray R.M., Reveley A.M. Genetic influences on the psychoses. *Br. Med. Bull.* 43:531–556, 1987.

Owen M.J., Mullan M.J. Molecular genetic studies of manic-depression and schizophrenia. *Trends Neurosci.* 13:29–31, 1990.

Parker G., Johnston P., Hayward L. Parental "expressed emotion" as a predictor of schizophrenic relapse. *Arch. Gen. Psychiatry* 45:806–813, 1988.

Pearlson G.D., Kreger L., Rabins P.V., et al. A chart review study of late-onset and early-onset schizophrenia. *Am. J. Psychiatry* 146:1568–1574, 1989.

*Pope H.G., Lipinski J.F. Diagnosis in schizophrenia and manic-depressive illness. *Arch. Gen. Psychiatry* 35:811–828, 1978.

Robertson G., Taylor P.J. Laterality and psychosis: neuropsychological evidence. *Br. Med. Bull.* 43:634–650, 1987.

Saugstad L.F. Social class, marriage, and fertility in schizophrenia. *Schizophr. Bull.* 15:9–43, 1989.

Schneier F.R., Siris S.G. A review of psychoactive substance use and abuse in schizophrenia: patterns of drug choice. *J. Nerv. Ment. Dis.* 175:641–652, 1987.

Scottish Schizophrenia Research Group. The Scottish first episode schizophrenia study. V. One-year follow-up. *Br. J. Psychiatry* 152:470–476, 1988.

*Seidman L.J. Schizophrenia and brain dysfunction: an integration of recent neurodiagnostic findings. *Psychol. Bull.* 94:195–238, 1983.

Shelton R.C., Weinberger D.R. Computerized tomography in schizophrenia: a review and synthesis. In Nasrallah H.A., Weinberger D.R., eds. *Handbook of Schizophrenia.* Vol. I. *The Neurology of Schizophrenia.* Amsterdam, Elsevier, pp. 207–250, 1986.

Sherrington R., Brynjolfsson J., Petursson H., et al. Localization of a susceptibility locus for schizophrenia on chromosome 5. *Nature* 336:164–167, 1988.

Siever L.J., Coursey R.D., Alterman I.S., et al. Clinical, psychophysiological, and neurological characteristics of volunteers with impaired smooth pursuit eye movements. *Biol. Psychiatry* 26:35–51, 1989.

Stuss D.T., Benson D.F. Neuropsychological studies of the frontal lobes. *Psychol. Bull.* 95:3–28, 1984.

Suddath R.L., Casanova M.F., Goldberg T.E., et al. Temporal lobe pathology in schizophrenia: a quantitative magnetic resonance imaging study. *Am. J. Psychiatry* 146:464–472, 1989.

Suddath R.L., Chrisison G.W., Torrey E.F., et al. Anatomical abnormalities in the brains of monozygotic twins discordant for schizophrenia. *N. Engl. J. Med.* 322:789–794, 1990.

Torrey E.F. *Civilization and Schizophrenia.* New York, Aronson, 1980.

Tsuang M.T. Suicide in schizophrenics, manics, depressives, and surgical controls. A comparison with general population suicide mortality. *Arch. Gen. Psychiatry* 35:153–155, 1978.

Wahl O.F., Harman C.R. Family views of stigma. *Schizophr. Bull.* 15:131–139, 1989.

Walker E., Levine R.J. The positive/negative symptom distinction in schizophrenia. Validity and etiological relevance. *Schizophr. Res.* 1:315–328, 1988.

*Weinberger D.R. Implications of normal brain development for the pathogenesis of schizophrenia. *Arch. Gen. Psychiatry* 44:660–669, 1987.

Weinberger D.R. Schizophrenia and the frontal lobe. *Trends Neurosci.* 11:367–370, 1988.

Weinberger D.R., Berman K.F. Speculation on the meaning of cerebral metabolic hypofrontality in schizophrenia. *Schizophr. Bull.* 14:157–161, 1988.

Weinberger D.R., Berman K.F., Zec R.F. Physiological dysfunction of dorsolateral prefrontal cortex in schizophrenia: I. Regional cerebral blood flow (rCBF) evidence. *Arch. Gen. Psychiatry* 43:114–125, 1986.

Weinberger D.R., Berman K.F., Illowsky B.P. Physiological dysfunction of dorsolateral prefrontal cortex in schizophrenia. III. A new cohort and evidence for a monoaminergic mechanism. *Arch. Gen. Psychiatry* 45:609–615, 1988.

Wong D.F., Wagner H.N., Tune L.E., et al. Positron emission tomography reveals elevated D2 dopamine receptors in drug-naive schizophrenics. *Science* 234:1558–1563, 1986.

Wyatt R.J. Biochemistry and schizophrenia (part IV). Neuroleptics. Their mechanism of action: a review of the biochemical literature. *Psychopharmacol. Bull.* 12:5–50, 1976.

*Wyatt R.J., Alexander R.C., Egan M.F., et al. Schizophrenia, just the facts? *Schizophr. Res.* 1:3–18, 1988.

Youssef H.A., Waddington J.L. Primitive (developmental) reflexes and diffuse cerebral dysfunction in schizophrenia and bipolar affective disorder: overrepresentation in patients with tardive dyskinesia. *Biol. Psychiatry* 23:791–797, 1988.

Index

Note: Page numbers in *italics* refer to illustrations; page numbers followed by *t* refer to tables.

i

Mercury
neurotoxicity of, 1254–1255
Mescaline, 1281–1282
Mesencephalic or midbrain vesicle, 8
Mesencephalic reticular activating system
cortical processing of sensory stimuli and, 771
Mesencephalotomy, 868
Metabolic amblyopia, 427
Metabolic disorders
epilepsy and, 901
headaches of, 873–874
hereditary ataxias of, 1170–1171, 1171t
inherited types of
mental retardation of, 617–618
Metabolic disturbances
intellectual functions and, 67
Metabolic encephalopathies
human immunodeficiency virus type 1 and, 1326
Metabolic-genetic disorders
direct therapeutic approaches for, 675–679
indirect therapies for, 670, 671t–672t, 673–675
Metabolic myopathies. See also specific myopathies
contracture of, 143
cramps of, 143
exercise intolerance and, 138
metabolic abnormalities of, clinical manifestations and,138–139
muscle fatigue and, 135–136
muscle weakness and, 136–137, 137
of cytosolic and lysosomal deficiencies, 176t, 176–179,177–178
of uncertain pathogenesis, 186–188
overview of, 144
pain of, 142–143
symptomatic inconsistences of, 137
types of, 135, 136t
vs. chronic fatigue syndrome, 138
Metals. See also specific metals
neurotoxicity of, 1250–1257
Metastases
in spinal cord, 1099, 1099–1100
intracranial form of, 1093–1094, 1094t
of carcinoma, in thoracic spine, 1504
of leptomeninges, 1100–1102, 1101
of vertebral column
neurologic manifestations of, 1504
site of, 1094–1095
specific sites of, 1097–1103, 1099, 11101
to peripheral nerve, 1102–1103
Methotrexate
blood-brain barrier permeability and, 115
necrotizing leukoencephalopathy and, 1121, 1124t, 1124–1125
3-Methoxy-4-hydroxymandelic acid (vanillylmandelic acid), 50
3-Methoxy-4-hydroxyphenylglycol, 50
mood and, 816
Methsuximide
pharmacokinetics of, 940, 940t
Methyl bromide
neurotoxicity of, 1246
N-Methyl-D-aspartate
Huntington's disease and, 1164
in alcoholism and alcohol abuse, 1265
N-Methyl-D-aspartate receptors (NMDA receptors), 1162
1-Methyl-4-phenyl-4-propionoxypiperidine (MPPP), 1283

1-Methyl-4-phenyl–1,2,3,6-tetrahydropyridine (MPTP), 2, 1147, 1283
akinetic-rigid syndrome and, 313–314
α-Methylfentanyl (China White), 1283
Methylnitrosurea, 1074
Michel's defect, 443
Microencephaly, 619
β-Microglobulin
in leptomeningeal metastases, 1102
β₂-Microglobulin amyloidosis, 1461, 1461
Microlung metastases, 1095
Microneurography
of dorsal root injury, 862
Microneurography and intraneural microstimulation, 226
Microspikes or filopodia, 15
Microvasculitis of peripheral nerve, 1114–1115
Microvillar cell
for olfaction, 391, 391
Micturition
dyfunction of
abnormal electromyographic activity of, 523, 523
neural control of, 513–514, 514
physiology of, 514, 514
Micturition syncope, 957–958
Midbrain, 8
Migraine
associated features of, 875
cerebral blood flow and, 998
clinical studies of, 875–876
definition of, 873
frequency and duration of, 874
mechanisms of, present concepts of, 878–879
of basilar artery, 462
pathophysiology of, 876–878
precipitating and relieving factors of, 875
serotonin and, 877
serotonin receptors and, 877
site of, 874–875
time and mode of onset for, 874
Minerals
amyotrophic lateral sclerosis and, 1192
Miniature end-plate potentials (MEPP), 198
Minisatellites, 650
Minor's tremor, 359
Miosis
periodic form of, 498
Misery perfusion, 997
Mitochondria
functions of, 127
metabolic defects of, 182t, 182–186, 183–185, 185t
Mitochondrial disorders, 666–667
Mitochondrial myopathies
exercise intolerance of, 141–142
muscle weakness of, 141–142
Mitoxantrone
for multiple sclerosis, 1223
Mitral valve prolapse
cerebral thromboembolism and, 1421
Mitral valve stenosis
cerebral thromboembolism and, 1420–1421
Mixed connective tissue disease, 1482
Mixed expressive-receptive disorder, 632
Mixed transcortical motor aphasia, 738
M line, 127
Mnemonic strategies, 714–715

Mobius' syndrome, 381
Modality specificity
in short-term memory loss, 719
Modeling, computational
goal of, 1552
problems with, 1553
Molecular biology
principles of, 657–658
Mondini's defect, 443
Monoamine oxidase
catecholamine degradation and, 50, 50
serotonin metabolism and, 51, 51–52
Monoamines
metabolites of
studies of, 816–817
mood and, 815–816
pain modulation and, 886–887
studies of, 816–817
Monoclonus
of epilepsy, 903, 903t
Mononeuritis multiplex, 1114–1115
Mononeuropathies
characterization of, 259, 261
of human immunodeficiency virus type 1, 1321
uremic form of, 1460–1462, 1461–1462
Mononeuropathy multiplex, 261
Mood
catecholamine receptors and, 817–819, 818t
disorders of
postmortem studies of, 823–824
serotonin receptors and, 819–822, 821t
monoamines and
studies of, 816–817
original amine hypotheses and, 815–816
Morphemes, 627
Morphine
spinal administration of, 891
Morphologic differentiation
in neurogenesis, 8, 14–16, 15
Morphology, 627
Morquio's syndrome, 1501
Mossy fibers
neurotransmitters of, 326–327
of cerebellum, 321
rosettes of, 321
synaptic effects of, 324–325, 325
Motherese, 630
Motion sickness, 465, 466t
Motor control
cerebellum in, 300
cortical systems of, 304–305
subcortical systems of, 304–305
Motor cortex
functions of, 290
pyramidal tract neurons of, 290
Motor disorders. See also specific disorders
neuropharmacology of, 346–350
Motor dysfunction
damage of unimodal sensory association areas and, 755–756
Motor end plate, 124
Motor function
age-related changes of, 606
Motor loss
in peripheral nerve disorders, 244–246
in spinal root disorders, 244–246
Motor neglect
tests for, 770
Motor neuron diseases
acquired types of
amyotrophic lateral sclerosis. See Amyotrophic lateral sclerosis
primary lateral sclerosis, 1195–1196